Nutrition

Sixth Edition

Paul Insel
Stanford University

Don Ross
California Institute of Nutrition

Kimberley McMahon
Logan University

Melissa Bernstein
Rosalind Franklin University of Medicine and Science

JONES & BARTLETT
LEARNING

World Headquarters
Jones & Bartlett Learning
5 Wall Street
Burlington, MA 01803
978-443-5000
info@jblearning.com
www.jblearning.com

Jones & Bartlett Learning books and products are available through most bookstores and online booksellers. To contact Jones & Bartlett Learning directly, call 800-832-0034, fax 978-443-8000, or visit our website, www.jblearning.com.

Substantial discounts on bulk quantities of Jones & Bartlett Learning publications are available to corporations, professional associations, and other qualified organizations. For details and specific discount information, contact the special sales department at Jones & Bartlett Learning via the above contact information or send an email to specialsales@jblearning.com.

10022-8

Production Credits

VP, Executive Publisher: David D. Cella
Publisher: Cathy L. Esperti
Acquisitions Editor: Sean Fabery
Senior Development Editor: Nancy Hoffmann
Editorial Assistant: Carter McAllister
Director of Production: Jenny Corriveau
Production Manager: Dan Stone
Media Development Editor: Shannon Sheehan
Rights and Media Specialist: Merideth Tumasz
Production Services Manager: Colleen Lamy
VP, Manufacturing and Inventory Control: Therese Connell
Composition: Cenveo® Publisher Services
Cover and Headings Image: © Bertl123/Shutterstock
Printing and Binding: RR Donnelley
Cover Printing: RR Donnelley

Library of Congress Cataloging-in-Publication Data

Names: Insel, Paul M., author. | Ross, Don, 1952- author. | McMahon, Kimberley, author. | Bernstein, Melissa, author.
Title: Nutrition / Paul Insel, Don Ross, Kimberley McMahon, Melissa Bernstein.
Description: Sixth edition. | Burlington, Massachusetts : Jones & Bartlett Learning, [2017] | Preceded by Nutrition / Paul Insel...[et al.]. 5th ed. c2014. | Includes bibliographical references and index.
Identifiers: LCCN 2016018159 | ISBN 9781284100051
Subjects: | MESH: Nutritional Physiological Phenomena | Food | Nutritional Sciences
Classification: LCC QP141 | NLM QU 145 | DDC 612.3--dc23
LC record available at https://lccn.loc.gov/2016018159

6048

Printed in the United States of America
20 19 18 17 16 10 9 8 7 6 5 4 3 2 1

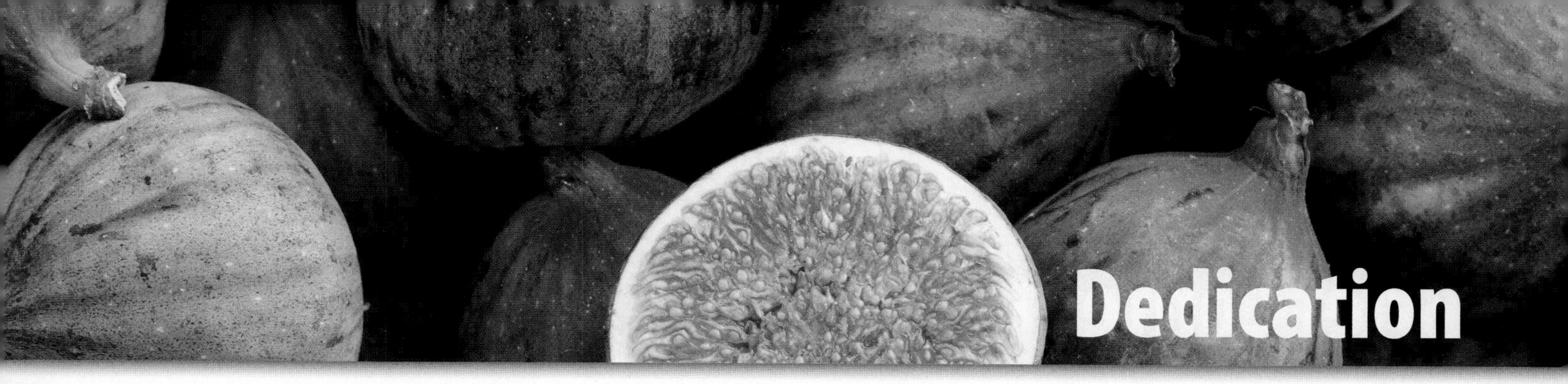

Dedication

To Michelle with love.
— Paul Insel

To Donna and Mackinnon for their sustenance of love, support, and patience.
— Don Ross

To my parents for their constant support and love.
— Kimberley McMahon

To my family with all my love.
— Melissa Bernstein

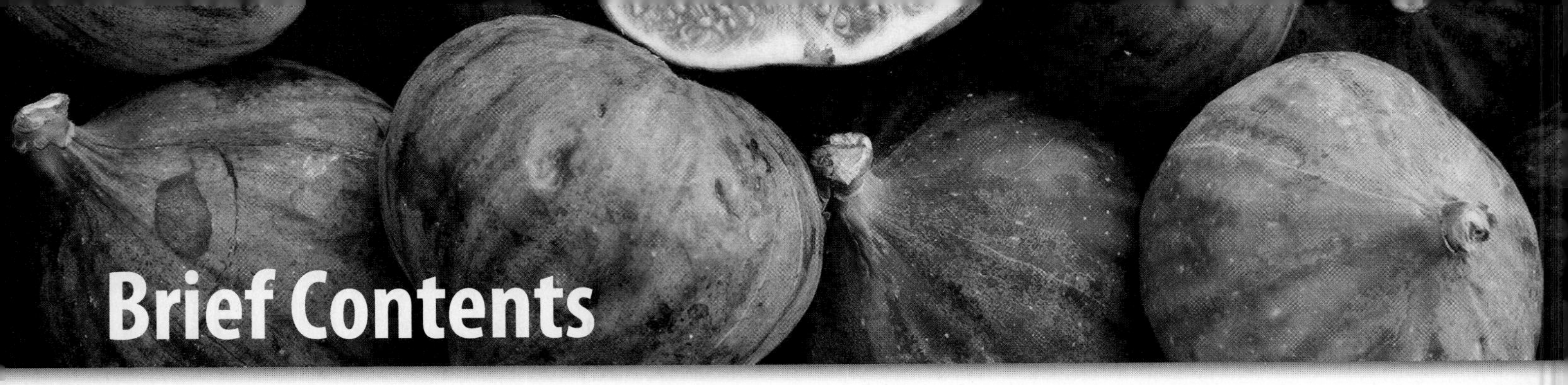

Brief Contents

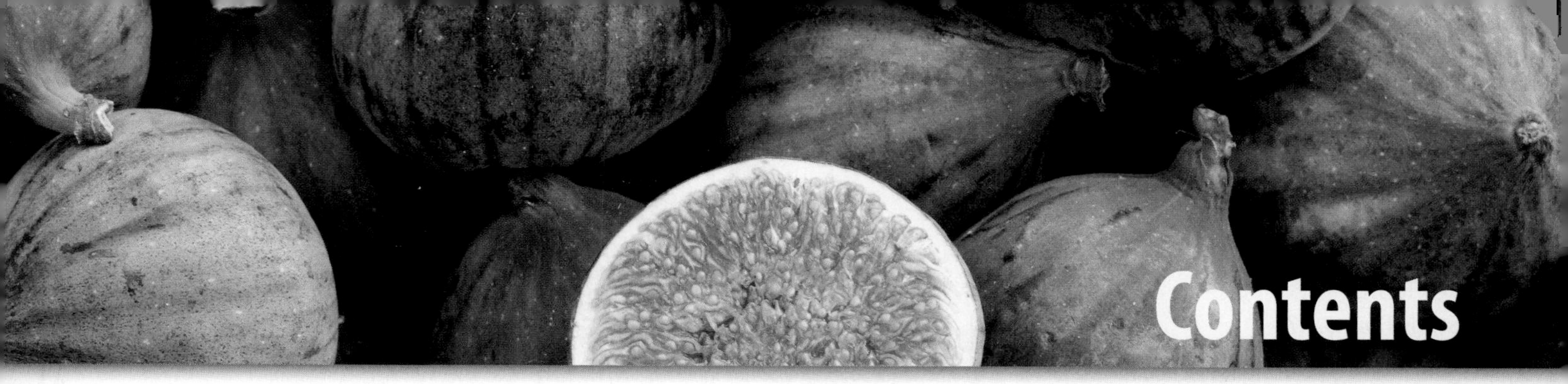

Contents

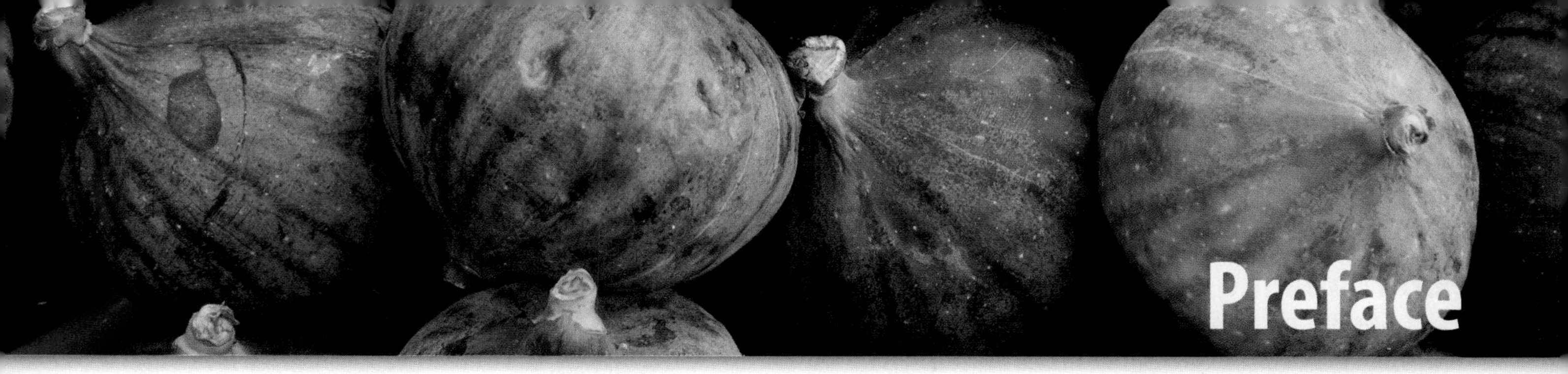

Preface

Welcome to the sixth edition of *Nutrition*. Changes in nutrition-related information have never been more exciting or important than they are today. *Nutrition* takes students on a fascinating journey beginning with curiosity and ending with a solid knowledge base and a healthy dose of skepticism for the endless ads and infomercials promoting "new" diets and food products. We want students to learn enough about their nutritional and health status to use this new knowledge in their everyday lives.

The new standards emerging in the science of nutrition inspire us to provide comprehensive, current, and accurate information on the most pressing issues. For example, you will find a focus on "the obesity epidemic" and the challenges the nutrition community is taking on to help resolve this chronic problem. You should find the overall content, organization, and features remain, but, within this framework, key topics and issues have been updated with new features and the most recent information available. Our goals in writing this book can be stated simply:

- To present science-based, accurate, up-to-date information in an accessible format
- To involve students in taking responsibility for their nutrition, health, and well-being
- To instill a sense of competence and personal power in students

The first of these goals means making expert knowledge about nutrition available to the individual. *Nutrition* presents current information to students about topics and issues that concern them—a balanced diet, nutritional supplements, weight management, exercise, and a multitude of others. Current, complete, and straightforward coverage is balanced with user-friendly features designed to make the text appealing.

Our second goal is to involve students in taking responsibility for their nutrition and health. To encourage students to think about the material they're reading and how it relates to their own lives, *Nutrition* uses innovative pedagogy and unique interactive features. We invite students to examine the issues and to analyze their nutrition-related behaviors.

Our third goal in writing *Nutrition* is the most important: to stimulate a sense of competence and personal power in the students who read this book. Everyone has the ability to monitor, understand, and affect his or her own nutritional behaviors.

Accessible Science

Nutrition makes use of the latest in learning theory and balances the behavioral aspects of nutrition with an accessible approach to scientific concepts. You will find this book to be a comprehensive resource that communicates nutrition both graphically and personally.

We present technical concepts in an engaging, nonintimidating way with an appealing parallel development of text and annotated illustrations. Illustrations in all chapters use consistent representations. For example, each type of nutrient has a distinct color and shape. Icons of an amino acid, a protein, a triglyceride, and a glucose molecule represent "characters" in the nutrition story and are instantly recognizable as they appear throughout the book.

This book is unique in the field of nutrition and leads the way in depicting important biological and physiological phenomena, such as emulsification, glucose regulation, digestion and absorption, and fetal development. Extensive graphic presentations make nutrition and physiological principles come alive.

Dietary Guidelines for Americans, 2015–2020

The *Dietary Guidelines for Americans, 2015–2020* reflects advances in the scientific understanding of the importance of improving diets and increasing physical activity, two of the most important factors reducing obesity and preventing chronic diseases in Americans. Eating a healthy balance of nutritious foods continues as a central point in the *Dietary Guidelines*, which serves to provide Americans with the information they need in order to make informed choices about their diet. Focused on science-based recommendations on food and nutrition, the *Dietary Guidelines for Americans, 2015–2020* empowers the American public to make shifts in what they eat and drink diet in favor of good health. As you read this text, look for key recommendations of the *Dietary Guidelines* highlighted in the margins.

Food Labeling

The Food and Drug Administration announced a new and redesigned Nutrition Facts label that will be required on most packaged food by July 2018. In an effort to encourage consumers to make more informed decisions, changes on the new label include such things as highlighting calories per serving and serving sizes more prominently, featuring a separate line showing how much sugar has been added to the food, and including updated Dietary Value information. The new label is discussed in Chapter 2, "Nutrition Guidelines and Assessment," and has been incorporated into all Label to Table features found throughout the text.

New to this Edition

For this edition, the latest scientific evidence, recommendations, and national standards have been incorporated throughout each chapter.

Key Highlights

- Updated content reflects the *Dietary Guidelines for Americans, 2015–2020* released in January 2016, as well as the redesigned Nutrition Facts label, released in May 2016.
- The new Getting Personal feature, found in most of the end-of-chapter Learning Portfolios, encourages students to apply their nutritional knowledge to understanding their own diets.
- Revised statistics and data incorporated throughout the text reflect the current state of nutrition in America and the world.
- Revised food source charts in the vitamins and minerals chapters more clearly convey common sources for vitamins and minerals.
- Updated Position Statements from the Academy of Nutrition and Dietetics, the American Heart Association, and other organizations appear throughout the text.
- Updated references utilize the latest science in the field.
- New and updated FYI, Going Green, and Quick Bite features provide in-depth discussions of controversial issues and topics for classroom discussion.

Chapter 1—Food Choices

- New section discusses the impact of eating away from home
- New FYI feature: "The Affordable Care Act and Nutrition"
- New Quick Bite features: "Try It Again, You Just Might Like It," "Does Being Overweight Spread from Person to Person?" and "High-Fructose Corn Syrup"
- Updated section on the impact of healthy food experiences early in life on forming healthy eating habits throughout the life cycle
- Updated discussion of the effect TV advertisements have on childhood nutrition

Chapter 2—Nutrition Guidelines and Assessment

- Revised description and discussion of the Nutrition Facts label, reflecting changes announced in May 2016
- New discussion of FDA regulations regarding the labeling of gluten-free foods
- New Going Green feature: "Is the American Diet Contributing to a Warmer Planet?"
- New Quick Bite feature: "Variety is Key"
- Revised FYI feature: "Portion Distortion"

Spotlight on Dietary Supplements and Functional Foods

- New table highlights groups for whom nutritional supplementation may be recommended
- Revised FYI feature: "Defining Complementary and Integrative Health"
- Updated Position Statement from the Academy of Nutrition and Dietetics: "Functional Foods"

Chapter 3—Digestion and Absorption

- New FYI feature: "Celiac Disease and Gluten Sensitivity"
- New Quick Bite feature: "Living Without a Gallbladder"
- Updated discussion regarding the link between red meat consumption and colorectal cancer
- Updated Nutrition Science in Action feature: "Screen Time and Diet Quality"
- Updated FYI feature: "Bugs in Your Gut? Health Effects of Intestinal Bacteria"
- Streamlined description of emulsification and its role in fat digestion
- In-depth discussion of the effect of medications on food absorption

Chapter 4—Carbohydrates

- New table summarizing the effects of fiber on digestion and absorption, and the health benefits of these effects
- New comparison of soluble and insoluble fibers
- New discussion of agave sweeteners
- Streamlined discussion of artificial sweeteners, with new table summarizing nonnutritive sweeteners and sweet substances
- Expanded discussion of resistant starches
- Expanded FYI features: "The Glycemic Index of Foods: Useful or Useless?" and "Unfounded Claims Against Sugars," with new sections on "Sugar and Type 2 Diabetes" and "High-Fructose Corn Syrup (HFCS), Obesity, and Disease"

Chapter 5—Lipids

- New sections providing recommendations for omega fatty acid intake and summarizing the health effects of omega-3 fatty acids
- New Position Statement from the Academy of Nutrition and Dietetics: "Fatty Acids for Healthy Adults"
- Streamlined section on fat replacers
- Revised Going Green feature: "Fish: Good For You and the Environment"
- Revised FYI feature: "Fats on the Health Store Shelf," which now delves into coconut oil and grapeseed oil
- Revised table incorporating American Heart Association Diet and Lifestyle Recommendations
- Updated American Heart Association Position Statement: "Omega-3 Fatty Acids"

Chapter 6—Proteins and Amino Acids

- New discussion regarding whether eating more protein helps build more muscle
- New table providing dietary suggestions for vegetarians
- New FYI feature: "High Protein Diets and Supplements"
- New Quick Bite feature: "Eating Lower on the Food Chain is Good for the Planet"
- New Position Statement from the Academy of Nutrition and Dietetics: "Vegetarian Diets"
- Revised Going Green feature: "Send in the Proteins"
- Revised FYI feature: "Do Athletes Need More Protein?" incorporating latest information from the Academy of Nutrition and Dietetics

Chapter 7—Alcohol

- New discussion of the prehistoric origins of alcohol
- Revised description of alcohol metabolism

Chapter 8—Metabolism

- Updated information on the role of carnitine in cardiovascular efficiency during exercise

Chapter 9—Energy Balance

- New discussion of digital private counseling programs
- New Quick Bite feature "The Raw Foods Diet"
- New description of metabolically healthy obesity
- Revised section on FDA-approved weight-loss medications
- Updated section on portion distortion phenomenon
- Updated Going Green feature: "Salad Days"
- Updated discussions regarding over-the-counter drugs, dietary supplements, and surgery for weight loss

Spotlight on Obesity

- New section on the link between gut microbiota and obesity
- New Quick Bite features: "Can You Pick Your Partners?" and "Your Microbiota and You"
- New statistics concerning obesity rates in Asia and the Middle East
- Revised FYI feature: "U.S. Obesity Trends: A Relentless Increase"

Chapter 10—Fat-Soluble Vitamins

- New table summarizes fat-soluble vitamins, their functions, and the results of deficiency and megadoses
- New table compares fat-soluble and water-soluble vitamins
- New table lists common carotenoids and their potential benefits

Chapter 11—Water-Soluble Vitamins

- New table summarizes water-soluble vitamins, their functions, and the results of deficiency and megadoses

Chapter 12—Water and Major Minerals

- New section discusses minerals in fluid balance

- Updated Going Green feature: "The Thirst for Water Resources"
- Updated FYI feature: "Tap, Filtered, or Bottled: Which Water is Best?"

Chapter 13—Trace Minerals

- New discussion of arsenic levels in rice-based products
- New reference to sea salts as sources of iodine

Chapter 14—Sports Nutrition

- New discussion of exercise intensity, muscle-strengthening exercises, and flexibility and neuromotor exercises
- New section on ephedrine
- Updated coverage of protein and hydration recommendations for athletes
- Updated discussion of nutrition supplements and ergogenic aids
- Updated section on caffeine
- Expanded discussion of the American Medical Association and American College of Sports Medicine's *Exercise is Medicine* initiative

Spotlight on Eating Disorders

- New introduction of the acronym OSFED (Other Specified Feeding or Eating Disorder)

Chapter 15—Diet and Health

- New section on nutrition informatics
- New Quick Bite features: "Adaptation Gone Awry, "Smartphones Advance Artificial Pancreas," and "What Smells in Blood Pressure?"
- Revised section delving into whether intakes of saturated and trans fat and cholesterol should be limited

Chapter 16—Life Cycle: Maternal and Infant Nutrition

- New Position Statement from the Academy of Nutrition and Dietetics: "Nutrition and Lifestyle for a Healthy Pregnancy Outcome"
- New table presenting a meal plan for a vegan pregnancy

Chapter 17—Life Cycle: From Childhood Through Adulthood

- New content discussing the increase in use of e-cigarettes among American high school students
- Updated information relating to lead toxicity
- Revised Quick Bite feature: "The Dangers of Teenage Smoking"

Chapter 18—Food Safety and Technology

- New FYI feature: "Are Nutrigenomics in Your Future?"
- New table listing food safety mistakes
- New information regarding the FDA's voluntary plan to phase out the use of certain antibiotics for enhanced food production in farm animals
- Revised section on genetically engineered foods
- Revised table providing USDA's labeling requirements for organic foods
- Updated Going Green feature: "Ocean Pollution and Mercury Poisoning"

Chapter 19—World View of Nutrition

- New Quick Bite features: "Urban Food Production" and "Tackling Food Insecurity"
- Expanded information on iodine deficiency disorders
- Revised table provides poverty guidelines based on household size
- Updated Position Statement from the Academy of Nutrition and Dietetics: "Addressing World Hunger, Malnutrition, and Food Insecurity"

The Pedagogy

Nutrition focuses on teaching behavioral change, personal decision making, and up-to-date scientific concepts in a number of novel ways. This interactive approach addresses different learning styles, making it the ideal text to ensure mastery of key concepts. Beginning with Chapter 1, the material engages students in considering their own behavior in light of the knowledge they are gaining. The pedagogical aids that appear in most chapters include the following:

The **Think About It** questions at the beginning of each chapter present realistic nutrition-related situations and ask students to consider how they would behave in such circumstances.

The **Chapter Menu** at the beginning of each chapter gives students a preview of topics that will be covered.

Learning Objectives focus students on the key concepts of each chapter and the material they will learn.

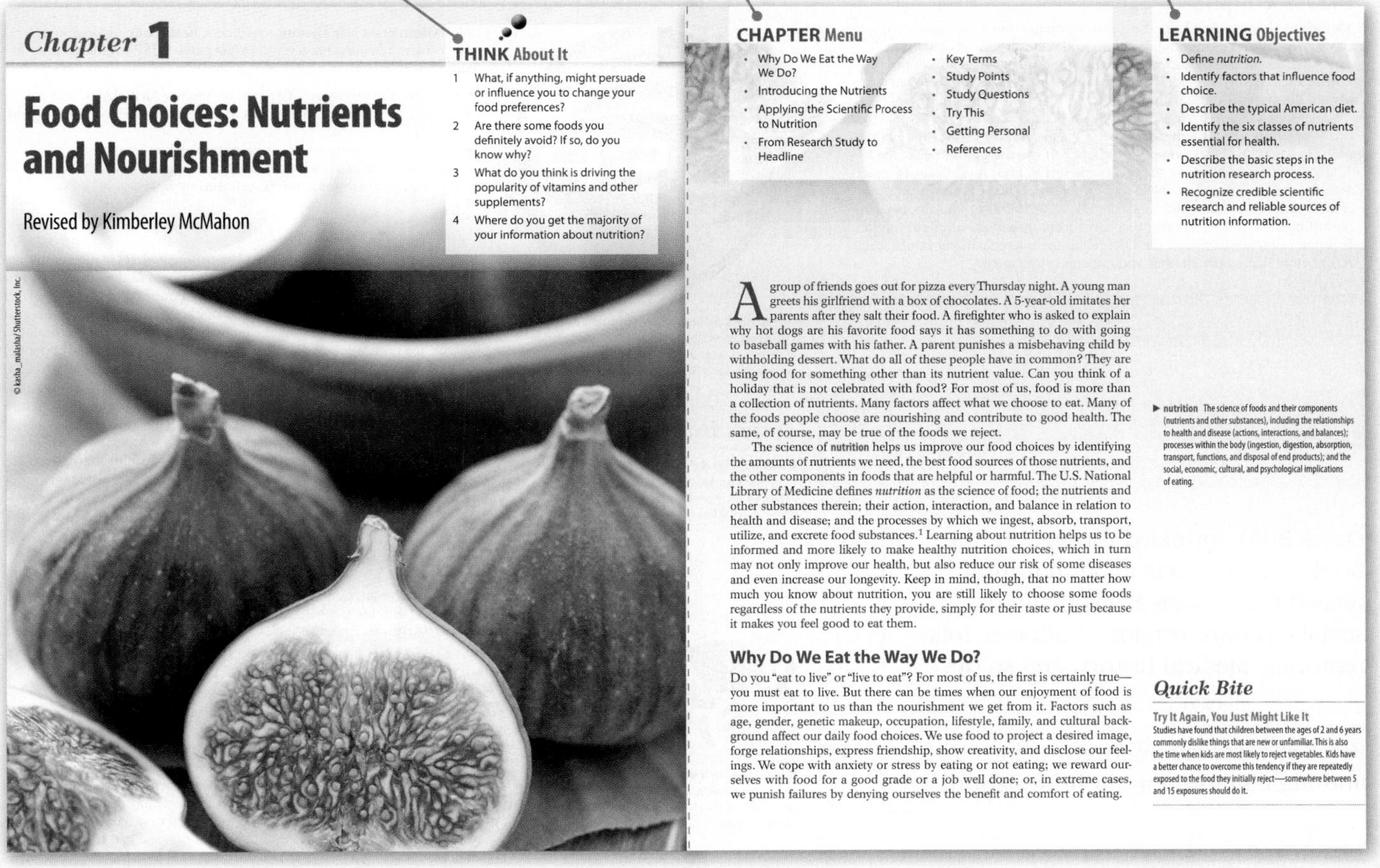
Chapter 1

Food Choices: Nutrients and Nourishment

Revised by Kimberley McMahon

THINK About It

1 What, if anything, might persuade or influence you to change your food preferences?
2 Are there some foods you definitely avoid? If so, do you know why?
3 What do you think is driving the popularity of vitamins and other supplements?
4 Where do you get the majority of your information about nutrition?

© kasha_malasha/ Shutterstock, Inc.

CHAPTER Menu

- Why Do We Eat the Way We Do?
- Introducing the Nutrients
- Applying the Scientific Process to Nutrition
- From Research Study to Headline
- Key Terms
- Study Points
- Study Questions
- Try This
- Getting Personal
- References

LEARNING Objectives

- Define *nutrition.*
- Identify factors that influence food choice.
- Describe the typical American diet.
- Identify the six classes of nutrients essential for health.
- Describe the basic steps in the nutrition research process.
- Recognize credible scientific research and reliable sources of nutrition information.

A group of friends goes out for pizza every Thursday night. A young man greets his girlfriend with a box of chocolates. A 5-year-old imitates her parents after they salt their food. A firefighter who is asked to explain why hot dogs are his favorite food says it has something to do with going to baseball games with his father. A parent punishes a misbehaving child by withholding dessert. What do all of these people have in common? They are using food for something other than its nutrient value. Can you think of a holiday that is not celebrated with food? For most of us, food is more than a collection of nutrients. Many factors affect what we choose to eat. Many of the foods people choose are nourishing and contribute to good health. The same, of course, may be true of the foods we reject.

The science of **nutrition** helps us improve our food choices by identifying the amounts of nutrients we need, the best food sources of those nutrients, and the other components in foods that are helpful or harmful. The U.S. National Library of Medicine defines *nutrition* as the science of food; the nutrients and other substances therein; their action, interaction, and balance in relation to health and disease; and the processes by which we ingest, absorb, transport, utilize, and excrete food substances.[1] Learning about nutrition helps us to be informed and more likely to make healthy nutrition choices, which in turn may not only improve our health, but also reduce our risk of some diseases and even increase our longevity. Keep in mind, though, that no matter how much you know about nutrition, you are still likely to choose some foods regardless of the nutrients they provide, simply for their taste or just because it makes you feel good to eat them.

▶ **nutrition** The science of foods and their components (nutrients and other substances), including the relationships to health and disease (actions, interactions, and balances); processes within the body (ingestion, digestion, absorption, transport, functions, and disposal of end products); and the social, economic, cultural, and psychological implications of eating.

Why Do We Eat the Way We Do?

Do you "eat to live" or "live to eat"? For most of us, the first is certainly true—you must eat to live. But there can be times when our enjoyment of food is more important to us than the nourishment we get from it. Factors such as age, gender, genetic makeup, occupation, lifestyle, family, and cultural background affect our daily food choices. We use food to project a desired image, forge relationships, express friendship, show creativity, and disclose our feelings. We cope with anxiety or stress by eating or not eating; we reward ourselves with food for a good grade or a job well done; or, in extreme cases, we punish failures by denying ourselves the benefit and comfort of eating.

Quick Bite

Try It Again, You Just Might Like It
Studies have found that children between the ages of 2 and 6 years commonly dislike things that are new or unfamiliar. This is also the time when kids are most likely to reject vegetables. Kids have a better chance to overcome this tendency if they are repeatedly exposed to the food they initially reject—somewhere between 5 and 15 exposures should do it.

- People with **malabsorption syndromes** such as cystic fibrosis often take large nutrient doses to compensate for nutritive losses and to override intestinal barriers to absorption.
- Megadoses of vitamin B_{12} can overcome the malabsorption seen in pernicious anemia, a condition in which a key substance needed for vitamin B_{12} absorption is lacking.

A vitamin at megadose levels can have *pharmacological activity*—that is, it acts as a drug. Nicotinic acid (niacin) is a good example. At usual levels (around 10 or 20 milligrams), it functions as a vitamin, but at levels 50 or 100 times higher it acts as a drug to lower blood lipid levels. Niacin has been used since the 1950s as a lipid-altering drug for low-density lipoprotein (LDL) cholesterol and is currently an effective agent available for raising high-density lipoprotein (HDL) cholesterol.[8] Like any drug, though, it can have serious side effects.[9]

▶ **malabsorption syndromes** Conditions that result in imperfect, inadequate, or otherwise disordered gastrointestinal absorption.

Position Statement: American Heart Association

Vitamin and Mineral Supplements

The American Heart Association recommends that healthy people get adequate nutrients by eating a variety of foods in moderation, rather than by taking supplements.

"The Dietary Recommended Intakes (DRIs) published by the Institute of Medicine are the best available estimates of safe and adequate dietary intakes," says the AHA. "There aren't sufficient data to suggest that healthy people benefit by taking certain vitamin or mineral supplements in excess of the DRIs." Moreover, "vitamin or mineral supplements aren't a substitute for a balanced, nutritious diet that limits excess calories, saturated fat, trans fat, sodium and dietary cholesterol. This dietary approach has been shown to reduce coronary heart disease risk in both healthy people and those with coronary disease."

Reprinted with permission, www.heart.org, © 2014 American Heart Association, Inc.

Position Statements from distinguished organizations such as the Academy of Nutrition and Dietetics, the American College of Sports Medicine, and the American Heart Association relate to the chapter topics and bolster the assertions made by the authors by showcasing concurrent opinions held by some of the leading organizations in nutrition and health.

Megadosing Beyond Conventional Medicine: Orthomolecular Nutrition

In 1968, Linus Pauling, the best-known advocate of megadosing, coined the term **orthomolecular medicine**. To him, *orthomolecular* meant achieving the optimal nutrient levels in the body.[10] Few nutritionists argue with the importance of optimum nutrition. In fact, some nutritionists share Pauling's concerns that the typical diet is too refined and processed to provide adequate nutrients and that intake equal to RDA values may not be high enough to achieve optimal body levels.

Most nutritionists would argue, however, with the high doses Pauling recommended to attain those optimal body levels and with the therapeutic value he and his followers attributed to those doses. Most notably, Pauling suggested in the early 1970s that an optimal daily intake of vitamin C was 2,000 milligrams—more than 30 times the current Daily Value. (See **FIGURE SF.2**.) Dr. Pauling claimed megadoses of vitamin C prevented or cured the common cold. Although many researchers have attempted to confirm this theory, studies do not support the idea that vitamin C prevents colds. A few studies found that colds were slightly less severe or less frequent in those who took high doses of vitamin C, but most studies found no beneficial effect.[11]

▶ **orthomolecular medicine** The preventive or therapeutic use of high-dose vitamins to treat disease.

Key Terms are in boldface type the first time they are mentioned. Their definitions also appear in the margins near the relevant textual discussion, making it easy for students to review material.

Drawbacks of Megadoses

Megadose vitamins and minerals remain popular, but when taken without recommendation or prescription from a qualified health professional, they can cause problems. Because high doses of a nutrient can act as a drug, with a drug's risk of adverse side effects, people who choose to take megadoses should always check first with their doctors.

THINK About 1

Excesses of some nutrients can create deficits of other nutrients. High doses of supplemental minerals, especially calcium, iron, zinc, and copper, can interfere with absorption of the others.[12] If you use high doses of the fat-soluble vitamin A, it is easy to reach toxic levels. Even megadoses of water-soluble vitamins can be problematic; for example, nerve damage can result from vitamin B_6 at 50 to 100 times the DV. **FIGURE SF.3** lists some more examples of medical side effects that can occur from megadose supplementation. It is good practice to review the DRI tables for tolerable upper intake levels (UL) before taking any vitamin and mineral supplement.

FIGURE SF.9 U.S. Pharmacopeia verification mark. Dietary supplements can earn the USP-Verified mark through a comprehensive testing and evaluation process.

Registered trademark of The United States Pharmacopeial Convetion. Used with permission.

verification mark helps assure consumers, health care professionals, and supplement retailers that a product has passed USP's rigorous program and does the following:

- Contains the ingredients declared on the product label
- Contains the amount or strength of ingredients declared on the product label
- Meets requirements for limits on potential contaminants
- Has been manufactured properly by complying with USP and FDA standards for current good manufacturing practices (cGMPs)

Fraudulent Products

Some health advocates consider the burgeoning market of dietary supplements an unwelcome return to the "snake oil" era of the late nineteenth and early twentieth centuries, when "magic" potions and cures were sold door-to-door and at county fairs and markets. The Internet and social media marketing are changing the industry because they are a prominent vehicle for promoting and selling products, reaching millions of people worldwide instantly at any time.

Most manufacturers work hard to ensure the quality of their products, yet some supplements on the market are nothing more than a mixture of ineffective ingredients. In recent years, the FDA has found hundreds of fraudulent products that contain hidden or deceptively labeled ingredients.[33] Most frequently recalled products with potentially harmful ingredients are those that are promoted for weight loss, sexual enhancement, and bodybuilding. When considering the use of dietary supplements, do your homework—make sure the product is safe and effective. It's always a good idea to ask your health care professional for help in distinguishing between reliable and questionable information.

Quick Bite

Jell-O and Your Nails

You may have heard that taking gelatin can make your nails stronger. Not true. Fingernails get their strength from sulfur in amino acids. Gelatin has no sulfur-containing amino acids.

Quick Bites sprinkled throughout the book offer fun facts about nutrition-related topics such as exotic foods, social customs, origins of phrases, folk remedies, medical history, and so on.

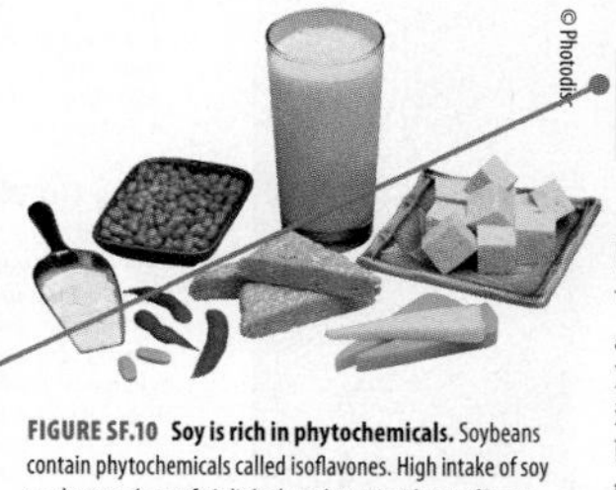

© Photodisc

FIGURE SF.10 Soy is rich in phytochemicals. Soybeans contain phytochemicals called isoflavones. High intake of soy products such as tofu is linked to a lower incidence of heart disease and cancer.

Key Concepts When **2017 Open Range Light 319RLS** considering a dietary supplement, it is important to consider the product and its claims carefully. Be aware that some products may promise more than they can deliver. A good indicator of quality is the USP verification mark, but this does not guarantee that a product will fulfill its claims.

Key Concepts summarize previous text and highlight important information.

Functional Foods

What do garlic, tomato sauce, tofu, and oatmeal all have in common? They aren't in the same food group, nor do they have the same nutrient composition. Instead, all of these foods could be considered "functional foods." Although there is not yet a legal definition for the term, a **functional food** is widely considered to be a food or food component that provides a health benefit beyond basic nutrition.[34] Garlic contains sulfur compounds that may reduce heart disease risk, and tomato sauce is rich in **lycopene**, a compound that may reduce prostate cancer risk. The soy protein in tofu and the fiber in oatmeal can help reduce the risk of heart disease. (See **FIGURE SF.10**.) The functional food industry has grown rapidly since its birth in Japan in the late 1980s and in 2014, reached almost $177 billion dollars of sales worldwide. In the U.S., functional food and beverage sales account for 5 percent of the overall food market.[35–37]

THINK About 3

▶ **functional food** A food that may provide a health benefit beyond basic nutrition.

▶ **lycopene** One of a family of plant chemicals, the carotenoids. Others in this big family include alpha-carotene and beta-carotene.

▶ **phytochemicals** Substances in plants that may possess health-protective effects, even though they are not essential for life.

Phytochemicals Make Foods Functional

Many functional foods get their health-promoting properties from naturally occurring compounds that are not considered nutrients but are called **phytochemicals**. Although the word *phytochemical* may sound intimidating, its

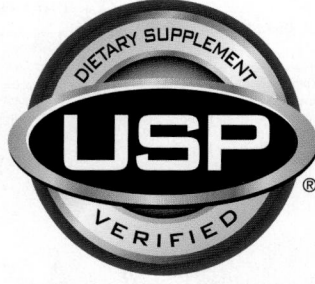

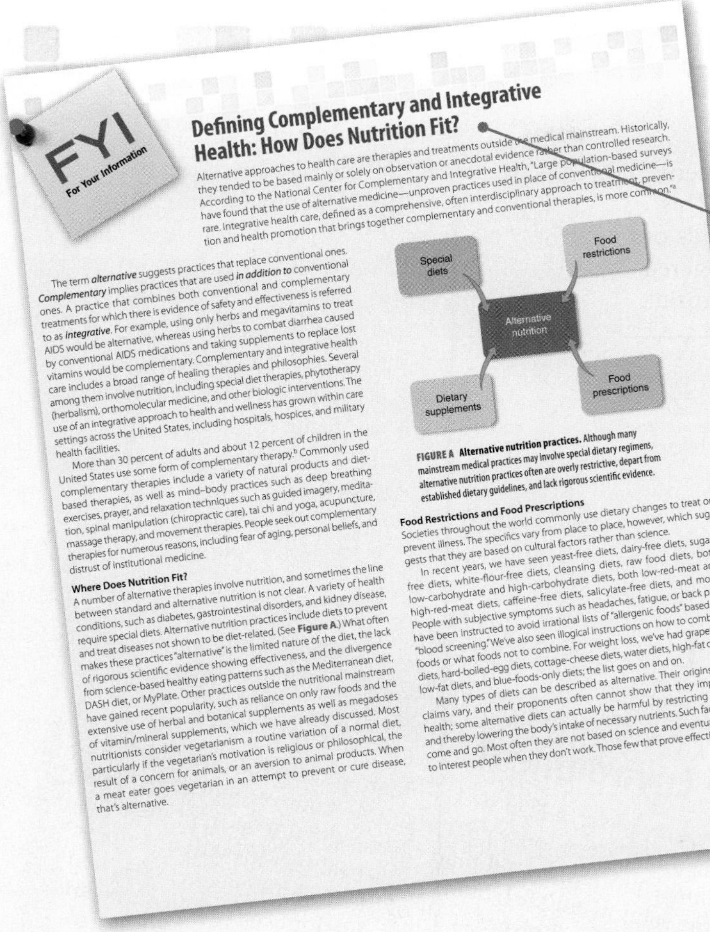

FYI For Your Information

Defining Complementary and Integrative Health: How Does Nutrition Fit?

Alternative approaches to health care are therapies and treatments outside the medical mainstream. Historically, they tended to be based mainly or solely on observation or anecdotal evidence rather than controlled research. According to the National Center for Complementary and Integrative Health, "Large population-based surveys have found that the use of alternative medicine—unproven practices used in place of conventional medicine—is rare. Integrative health care, defined as a comprehensive, often interdisciplinary approach to treatment, prevention and health promotion that brings together complementary and conventional therapies, is more common."[a]

The term ***alternative*** suggests practices that replace conventional ones. ***Complementary*** implies practices that are used ***in addition to*** conventional ones. A practice that combines both conventional and complementary treatments for which there is evidence of safety and effectiveness is referred to as ***integrative***. For example, using only herbs and megavitamins to treat AIDS would be alternative, whereas using herbs to combat diarrhea caused by conventional AIDS medications and taking supplements to replace lost vitamins would be complementary. Complementary and integrative health care includes a broad range of healing therapies and philosophies. Several among them involve nutrition, including special diet therapies, phytotherapy (herbalism), orthomolecular medicine, and other biologic interventions. The use of an integrative approach to health and wellness has grown within care settings across the United States, including hospitals, hospices, and military health facilities.

More than 30 percent of adults and about 12 percent of children in the United States use some form of complementary therapy.[b] Commonly used complementary therapies include a variety of natural products and diet-based therapies, as well as mind–body practices such as deep breathing exercises, prayer, and relaxation techniques such as guided imagery, meditation, spinal manipulation (chiropractic care), tai chi and yoga, acupuncture, massage therapy, and movement therapies. People seek out complementary therapies for numerous reasons, including fear of aging, personal beliefs, and distrust of institutional medicine.

Where Does Nutrition Fit?

A number of alternative therapies involve nutrition, and sometimes the line between standard and alternative nutrition is not clear. A variety of health conditions, such as diabetes, gastrointestinal disorders, and kidney disease, require special diets. Alternative nutrition practices include diets to prevent and treat diseases not shown to be diet-related. (See **Figure A**.) What often makes these practices "alternative" is the limited nature of the diet, the lack of rigorous scientific evidence showing effectiveness, and the divergence from science-based healthy eating patterns such as the Mediterranean diet, DASH diet, or MyPlate. Other practices outside the nutritional mainstream have gained recent popularity, such as reliance on only raw foods and the extensive use of herbal and botanical supplements as well as megadoses of vitamin/mineral supplements, which we have already discussed. Most nutritionists consider vegetarianism a routine variation of a normal diet, particularly if the vegetarian's motivation is religious or philosophical, the result of a concern for animals, or an aversion to animal products. When a meat eater goes vegetarian in an attempt to prevent or cure disease, that's alternative.

FIGURE A Alternative nutrition practices. Although many mainstream medical practices may involve special dietary regimens, alternative nutrition practices often are overly restrictive, depart from established dietary guidelines, and lack rigorous scientific evidence.

Food Restrictions and Food Prescriptions

Societies throughout the world commonly use dietary changes to treat or prevent illness. The specifics vary from place to place, however, which suggests that they are based on cultural factors rather than science.

In recent years, we have seen yeast-free diets, dairy-free diets, sugar-free diets, white-flour-free diets, cleansing diets, raw food diets, both low-carbohydrate and high-carbohydrate diets, both low-red-meat and high-red-meat diets, caffeine-free diets, salicylate-free diets, and more. People with subjective symptoms such as headaches, fatigue, or back pain have been instructed to avoid irrational lists of "allergenic foods" based on "blood screening." We've also seen illogical instructions on how to combine foods or what foods not to combine. For weight loss, we've had grapefruit diets, hard-boiled-egg diets, cottage-cheese diets, water diets, high-fat diets, low-fat diets, and blue-foods-only diets; the list goes on and on.

Many types of diets can be described as alternative. Their origins and claims vary, and their proponents often cannot show that they improve health; some alternative diets can actually be harmful by restricting foods and thereby lowering the body's intake of necessary nutrients. Such fad diets come and go. Most often they are not based on science and eventually fail to interest people when they don't work. Those few that prove effective and

FYI (For Your Information) offers more in-depth discussions of controversial and timely topics, such as unfounded claims about the effects of sugar, whether athletes need more protein, and the usefulness of the glycemic index.

Containing new and current scientific research, **Nutrition Science in Action** is an exciting feature that walks students through science experiments involving nutrition. Each *Nutrition Science in Action* presents observations and hypotheses or study questions, an experimental plan, and results, conclusions, and discussions that allow students to apply their knowledge of nutrition to real-life experiments outside of the classroom.

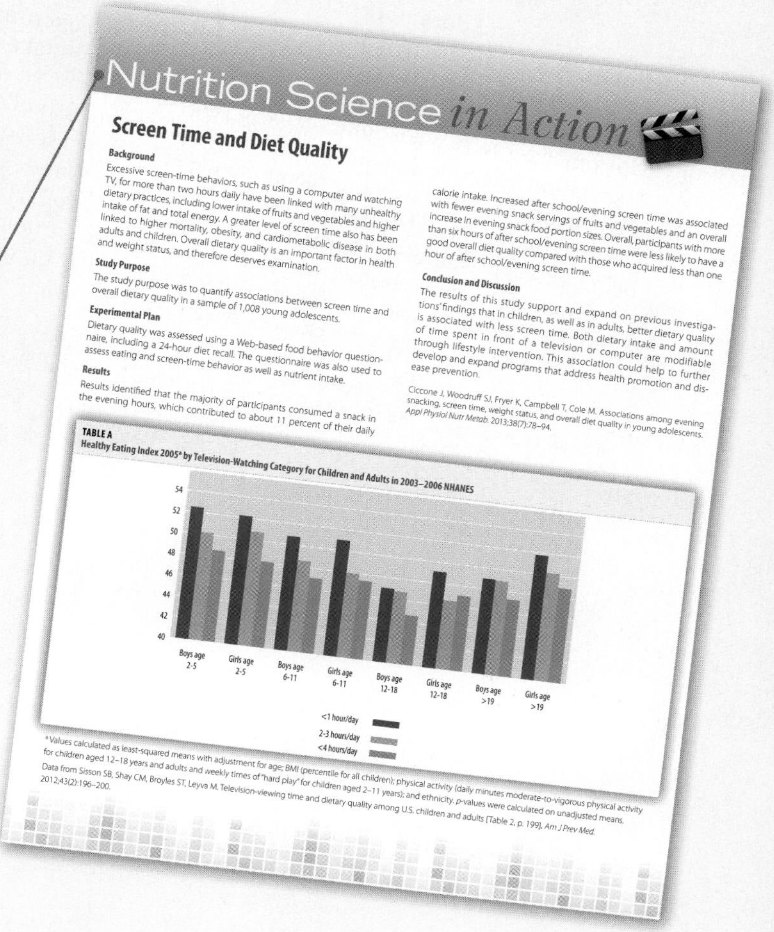

Nutrition Science *in Action*

Screen Time and Diet Quality

Background

Excessive screen-time behaviors, such as using a computer and watching TV, for more than two hours daily have been linked with many unhealthy dietary practices, including lower intake of fruits and vegetables and higher intake of fat and total energy. A greater level of screen time also has been linked to higher mortality, obesity, and cardiometabolic disease in both adults and children. Overall dietary quality is an important factor in health and weight status, and therefore deserves examination.

Study Purpose

The study purpose was to quantify associations between screen time and overall dietary quality in a sample of 1,008 young adolescents.

Experimental Plan

Dietary quality was assessed using a Web-based food behavior questionnaire, including a 24-hour diet recall. The questionnaire was also used to assess eating and screen-time behavior as well as nutrient intake.

Results

Results identified that the majority of participants consumed a snack in the evening hours, which contributed to about 11 percent of their daily calorie intake. Increased after school/evening screen time was associated with fewer evening snack servings of fruits and vegetables and an overall increase in evening snack food portion sizes. Overall, participants with more than six hours of after school/evening screen time were less likely to have a good overall diet quality compared with those who acquired less than one hour of after school/evening screen time.

Conclusion and Discussion

The results of this study support and expand on previous investigations' findings that in children, as well as in adults, better dietary quality is associated with less screen time. Both dietary intake and amount of time spent in front of a television or computer are modifiable through lifestyle intervention. This association could help to further develop and expand programs that address health promotion and disease prevention.

Ciccone J, Woodruff SJ, Fryer K, Campbell T, Cole M. Associations among evening snacking, screen time, weight status, and overall diet quality in young adolescents. *Appl Physiol Nutr Metab*. 2013;38(7):78–94.

TABLE A
Healthy Eating Index 2005[a] by Television-Watching Category for Children and Adults in 2003–2006 NHANES

[a] Values calculated as least-squared means with adjustment for age; BMI (percentile for all children); physical activity (daily minutes moderate-to-vigorous physical activity for children aged 12–18 years and adults and weekly times of "hard play" for children aged 2–11 years); and ethnicity. *p*-values were calculated on unadjusted means.

Data from Sisson SB, Shay CM, Broyles ST, Leyva M. Television-viewing time and dietary quality among U.S. children and adults [Table 2, p. 199]. *Am J Prev Med*. 2012;43(2):196–200.

Updated to reflect the most current environmental concerns, **Going Green** boxes address the nutrition community's concern about the importance of environmental issues in our time. This environmental theme runs through each chapter and expands our nutrition focus to show that we are all citizens of an endangered planet with opportunities to reduce our environmental footprint.

Going Green

Fish: Good for You and the Environment

Fatty fish or fatty meat? What is a "good" source of fat, a lean protein high in vitamins and minerals, and does not contribute to the production of methane greenhouse gas? Fish! Methane, produced by farm animals, is a powerful greenhouse gas and is considered 20 times more powerful than carbon dioxide at trapping solar energy. In comparison, no methane is produced from harvesting salmon, and fish offers you a healthier meal than a ribeye steak. Choosing to eat fish while decreasing your beef intake not only will give you all of the health benefits associated with omega-3 fatty acids, but also will potentially decrease dangerous greenhouse gas production. An American Heart Association scientific statement on fish consumption, fish oils, omega fatty acids, and cardiovascular disease emphasizes the benefits of eating fish and recommends at least two servings of fish per week. Eicosapentaenoic acid (EPA) and docosahexaenoic acid (DHA) are the omega-3 fatty acids found in oily fish, with mackerel, salmon, trout, sardines, and herring being excellent sources. Approximately 1 gram of EPA/DHA can be obtained from 100 grams (3.5 ounces) of oily fish.

There are many choices when it comes to incorporating healthful fats into your diet. Just remember, even though these fatty acids provide a "good" source of fat, don't go overboard. Fat is still fat, even if it is good for you and for the environment, so make your choices wisely.

Data from Rigby A. Omega-3 choices: fish or flax? *Today's Dietitian*. 2004;6(1):37; Hernandez E. Omega-3 oils as food ingredients [webcast]. 2007. Institute of Food Technologists; and Mantzioris E, Cleland LG, Gibson RA, et al. Biochemical effects of a diet containing foods enriched with n-3 fatty acids. *Am J Clin Nutr*. 2000;72:42–48.

Label to Table helps students apply their new decision-making skills at the supermarket. It walks students through the various types of information that appear on food labels, including government-mandated terminology, misleading advertising phrases, and amounts of ingredients. This feature has been updated for this edition to reflect the new labeling guidelines released by the FDA in May 2016.

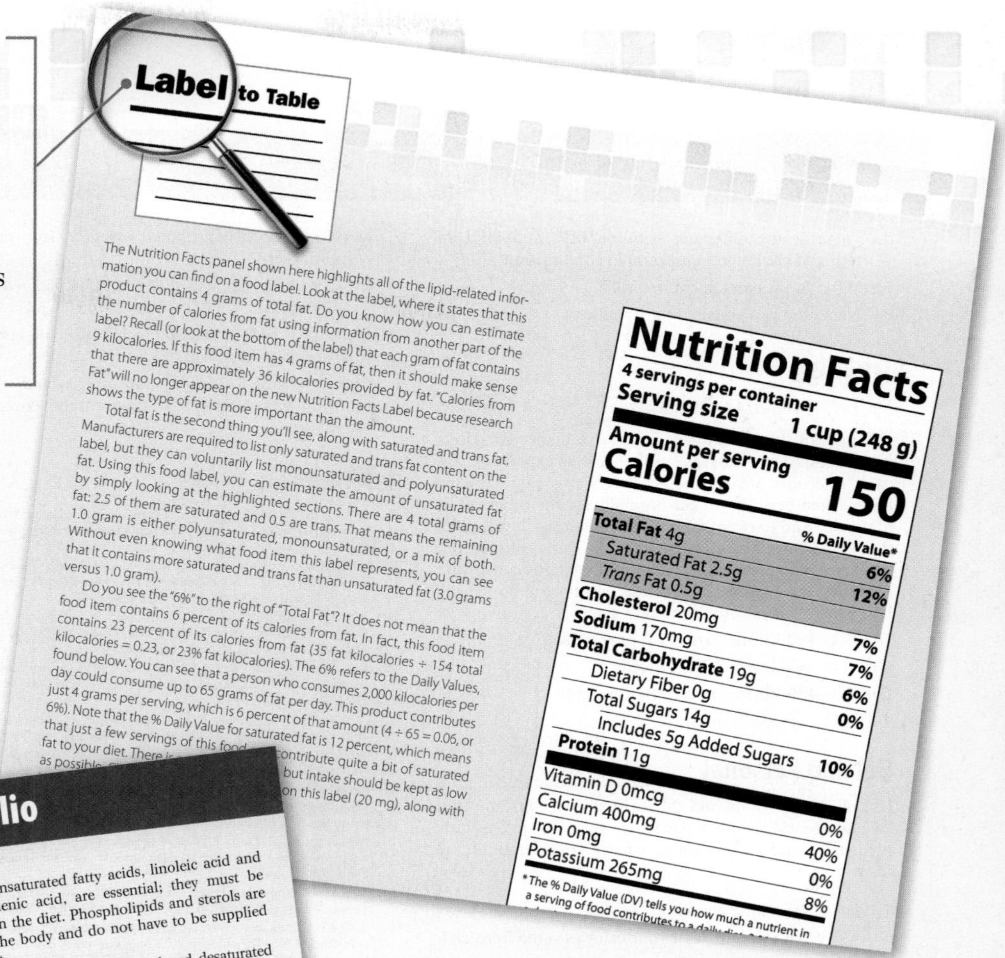

Label to Table

The Nutrition Facts panel shown here highlights all of the lipid-related information you can find on a food label. Look at the label, where it states that this
product contains 4 grams of total fat. Do you know how you can estimate
the number of calories from fat using information from another part of the
label? Recall (or look at the bottom of the label) that each gram of fat contains
9 kilocalories. If this food item has 4 grams of fat, then it should make sense
that there are approximately 36 kilocalories provided by fat. "Calories from
Fat" will no longer appear on the new Nutrition Facts Label because research
shows the type of fat is more important than the amount.
Total fat is the second thing you'll see, along with saturated and trans fat.
Manufacturers are required to list only saturated and trans fat content on the
label, but they can voluntarily list monounsaturated and polyunsaturated
fat. Using this food label, you can estimate the amount of unsaturated fat
by simply looking at the highlighted sections. There are 4 total grams of
fat: 2.5 of them are saturated and 0.5 are trans. That means the remaining
1.0 gram is either polyunsaturated, monounsaturated, or a mix of both.
Without even knowing what food item this label represents, you can see
that it contains more saturated and trans fat than unsaturated fat (3.0 grams
versus 1.0 gram).
Do you see the "6%" to the right of "Total Fat"? It does not mean that the
food item contains 6 percent of its calories from fat. In fact, this food item
contains 23 percent of its calories from fat (35 fat kilocalories ÷ 154 total
kilocalories = 0.23, or 23% fat kilocalories). The 6% refers to the Daily Values,
found below. You can see that a person who consumes 2,000 kilocalories per
day could consume up to 65 grams of fat per day. This product contributes
just 4 grams per serving, which is 6 percent of that amount (4 ÷ 65 = 0.06, or
6%). Note that the % Daily Value for saturated fat is 12 percent, which means
that just a few servings of this food ... contribute quite a bit of saturated
fat to your diet. There ... but intake should be kept as low
as possible ... on this label (20 mg), along with

Nutrition Facts
4 servings per container
Serving size 1 cup (248 g)
Amount per serving
Calories 150
% Daily Value*
Total Fat 4g
Saturated Fat 2.5g 6%
Trans Fat 0.5g 12%
Cholesterol 20mg
Sodium 170mg 7%
Total Carbohydrate 19g 7%
Dietary Fiber 0g 6%
Total Sugars 14g 0%
Includes 5g Added Sugars
Protein 11g 10%
Vitamin D 0mcg
Calcium 400mg 0%
Iron 0mg 40%
Potassium 265mg 0%
8%
*The % Daily Value (DV) tells you how much a nutrient in a serving of food contributes to a daily ...

The **Learning Portfolio** at the end of each chapter condenses all aspects of nutrition information that students need to solidify their understanding of the material. The various formats will appeal to students according to their individual learning and studying styles.

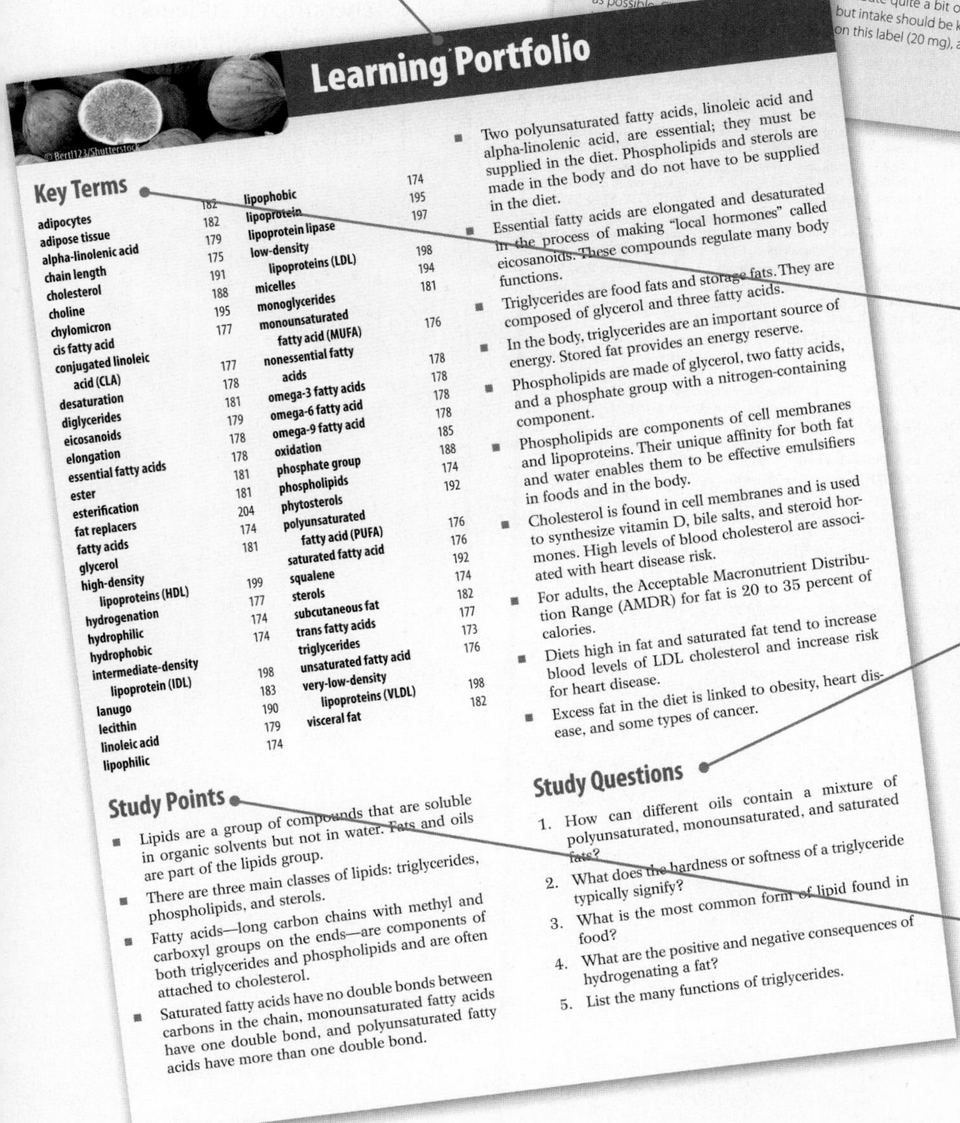

Learning Portfolio

© Bert1123/Shutterstock

Key Terms

adipocytes
adipose tissue
alpha-linolenic acid
chain length
cholesterol
choline
chylomicron
cis fatty acid
conjugated linoleic acid (CLA)
desaturation
diglycerides
eicosanoids
elongation
essential fatty acids
ester
esterification
fat replacers
fatty acids
glycerol
high-density lipoproteins (HDL)
hydrogenation
hydrophilic
hydrophobic
intermediate-density lipoprotein (IDL)
lanugo
lecithin
linoleic acid
lipophilic

182 182 179 175 191 188 195 177 177 178 181 179 178 178 181 181 204 174 181 199 177 174 174 198 183 190 179 174

lipophobic
lipoprotein
lipoprotein lipase
low-density lipoproteins (LDL)
micelles
monoglycerides
monounsaturated fatty acid (MUFA)
nonessential fatty acids
omega-3 fatty acids
omega-6 fatty acid
omega-9 fatty acid
oxidation
phosphate group
phospholipids
phytosterols
polyunsaturated fatty acid (PUFA)
saturated fatty acid
squalene
sterols
subcutaneous fat
trans fatty acids
triglycerides
unsaturated fatty acid
very-low-density lipoproteins (VLDL)
visceral fat

174 195 197 198 194 181 176 178 178 178 178 185 188 174 192 176 176 192 174 182 177 173 176 198 182

Study Points

- Lipids are a group of compounds that are soluble in organic solvents but not in water. Fats and oils are part of the lipids group.
- There are three main classes of lipids: triglycerides, phospholipids, and sterols.
- Fatty acids—long carbon chains with methyl and carboxyl groups on the ends—are components of both triglycerides and phospholipids and are often attached to cholesterol.
- Saturated fatty acids have no double bonds between carbons in the chain, monounsaturated fatty acids have one double bond, and polyunsaturated fatty acids have more than one double bond.
- Two polyunsaturated fatty acids, linoleic acid and alpha-linolenic acid, are essential; they must be supplied in the diet. Phospholipids and sterols are made in the body and do not have to be supplied in the diet.
- Essential fatty acids are elongated and desaturated in the process of making "local hormones" called eicosanoids. These compounds regulate many body functions.
- Triglycerides are food fats and storage fats. They are composed of glycerol and three fatty acids.
- In the body, triglycerides are an important source of energy. Stored fat provides an energy reserve.
- Phospholipids are made of glycerol, two fatty acids, and a phosphate group with a nitrogen-containing component.
- Phospholipids are components of cell membranes and lipoproteins. Their unique affinity for both fat and water enables them to be effective emulsifiers in foods and in the body.
- Cholesterol is found in cell membranes and is used to synthesize vitamin D, bile salts, and steroid hormones. High levels of blood cholesterol are associated with heart disease risk.
- For adults, the Acceptable Macronutrient Distribution Range (AMDR) for fat is 20 to 35 percent of calories.
- Diets high in fat and saturated fat tend to increase blood levels of LDL cholesterol and increase risk for heart disease.
- Excess fat in the diet is linked to obesity, heart disease, and some types of cancer.

Study Questions

1. How can different oils contain a mixture of polyunsaturated, monounsaturated, and saturated fats?
2. What does the hardness or softness of a triglyceride typically signify?
3. What is the most common form of lipid found in food?
4. What are the positive and negative consequences of hydrogenating a fat?
5. List the many functions of triglycerides.

Key Terms list all new vocabulary alphabetically with the page number of the first appearance. This arrangement allows students to review any term they do not recall and turn immediately to the definition and discussion of it in the chapter. This approach also promotes the acquisition of knowledge, not simply memorization.

Study Questions encourage students to probe deeper into the chapter content, making connections and gaining new insights. Although these questions can be used for pop quizzes, they will also help students to review, especially students who study by writing out material.

Study Points summarize the content of each chapter with a synopsis of each major topic. The points are in the order in which they appear in the chapter, so related concepts flow together.

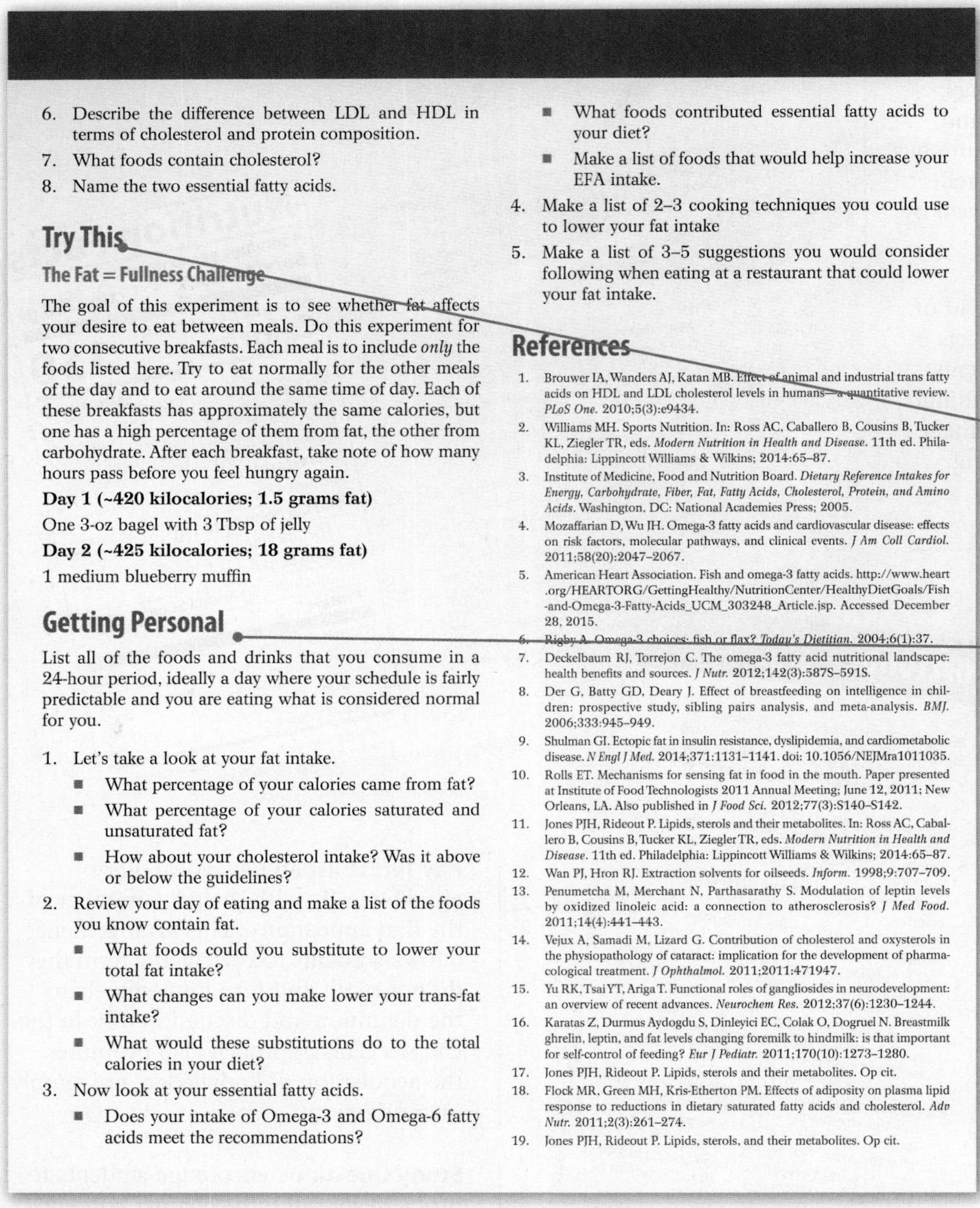

6. Describe the difference between LDL and HDL in terms of cholesterol and protein composition.
7. What foods contain cholesterol?
8. Name the two essential fatty acids.

Try This

The Fat = Fullness Challenge

The goal of this experiment is to see whether fat affects your desire to eat between meals. Do this experiment for two consecutive breakfasts. Each meal is to include *only* the foods listed here. Try to eat normally for the other meals of the day and to eat around the same time of day. Each of these breakfasts has approximately the same calories, but one has a high percentage of them from fat, the other from carbohydrate. After each breakfast, take note of how many hours pass before you feel hungry again.

Day 1 (~420 kilocalories; 1.5 grams fat)

One 3-oz bagel with 3 Tbsp of jelly

Day 2 (~425 kilocalories; 18 grams fat)

1 medium blueberry muffin

Getting Personal

List all of the foods and drinks that you consume in a 24-hour period, ideally a day where your schedule is fairly predictable and you are eating what is considered normal for you.

1. Let's take a look at your fat intake.
   - What percentage of your calories came from fat?
   - What percentage of your calories saturated and unsaturated fat?
   - How about your cholesterol intake? Was it above or below the guidelines?
2. Review your day of eating and make a list of the foods you know contain fat.
   - What foods could you substitute to lower your total fat intake?
   - What changes can you make lower your trans-fat intake?
   - What would these substitutions do to the total calories in your diet?
3. Now look at your essential fatty acids.
   - Does your intake of Omega-3 and Omega-6 fatty acids meet the recommendations?
   - What foods contributed essential fatty acids to your diet?
   - Make a list of foods that would help increase your EFA intake.
4. Make a list of 2–3 cooking techniques you could use to lower your fat intake
5. Make a list of 3–5 suggestions you would consider following when eating at a restaurant that could lower your fat intake.

References

1. Brouwer IA, Wanders AJ, Katan MB. Effect of animal and industrial trans fatty acids on HDL and LDL cholesterol levels in humans—a quantitative review. *PLoS One*. 2010;5(3):e9434.
2. Williams MH. Sports Nutrition. In: Ross AC, Caballero B, Cousins B, Tucker KL, Ziegler TR, eds. *Modern Nutrition in Health and Disease*. 11th ed. Philadelphia: Lippincott Williams & Wilkins; 2014:65–87.
3. Institute of Medicine, Food and Nutrition Board. *Dietary Reference Intakes for Energy, Carbohydrate, Fiber, Fat, Fatty Acids, Cholesterol, Protein, and Amino Acids*. Washington, DC: National Academies Press; 2005.
4. Mozaffarian D, Wu JH. Omega-3 fatty acids and cardiovascular disease: effects on risk factors, molecular pathways, and clinical events. *J Am Coll Cardiol*. 2011;58(20):2047–2067.
5. American Heart Association. Fish and omega-3 fatty acids. http://www.heart.org/HEARTORG/GettingHealthy/NutritionCenter/HealthyDietGoals/Fish-and-Omega-3-Fatty-Acids_UCM_303248_Article.jsp. Accessed December 28, 2015.
6. Rigby A. Omega-3 choices: fish or flax? *Today's Dietitian*. 2004;6(1):37.
7. Deckelbaum RJ, Torrejon C. The omega-3 fatty acid nutritional landscape: health benefits and sources. *J Nutr.* 2012;142(3):587S–591S.
8. Der G, Batty GD, Deary J. Effect of breastfeeding on intelligence in children: prospective study, sibling pairs analysis, and meta-analysis. *BMJ*. 2006;333:945–949.
9. Shulman GI. Ectopic fat in insulin resistance, dyslipidemia, and cardiometabolic disease. *N Engl J Med.* 2014;371:1131–1141. doi: 10.1056/NEJMra1011035.
10. Rolls ET. Mechanisms for sensing fat in food in the mouth. Paper presented at Institute of Food Technologists 2011 Annual Meeting; June 12, 2011; New Orleans, LA. Also published in *J Food Sci.* 2012;77(3):S140–S142.
11. Jones PJH, Rideout P. Lipids, sterols and their metabolites. In: Ross AC, Caballero B, Cousins B, Tucker KL, Ziegler TR, eds. *Modern Nutrition in Health and Disease*. 11th ed. Philadelphia: Lippincott Williams & Wilkins; 2014:65–87.
12. Wan PJ, Hron RJ. Extraction solvents for oilseeds. *Inform.* 1998;9:707–709.
13. Penumetcha M, Merchant N, Parthasarathy S. Modulation of leptin levels by oxidized linoleic acid: a connection to atherosclerosis? *J Med Food*. 2011;14(4):441–443.
14. Vejux A, Samadi M, Lizard G. Contribution of cholesterol and oxysterols in the physiopathology of cataract: implication for the development of pharmacological treatment. *J Ophthalmol.* 2011;2011:471947.
15. Yu RK, Tsai YT, Ariga T. Functional roles of gangliosides in neurodevelopment: an overview of recent advances. *Neurochem Res.* 2012;37(6):1230–1244.
16. Karatas Z, Durmus Aydogdu S, Dinleyici EC, Colak O, Dogruel N. Breastmilk ghrelin, leptin, and fat levels changing foremilk to hindmilk: is that important for self-control of feeding? *Eur J Pediatr.* 2011;170(10):1273–1280.
17. Jones PJH, Rideout P. Lipids, sterols and their metabolites. Op cit.
18. Flock MR, Green MH, Kris-Etherton PM. Effects of adiposity on plasma lipid response to reductions in dietary saturated fatty acids and cholesterol. *Adv Nutr.* 2011;2(3):261–274.
19. Jones PJH, Rideout P. Lipids, sterols, and their metabolites. Op cit.

Try This activities are provide suggestions for hands-on activities that encourage students to put theory into practice. It will especially help students whose major learning style is experimental.

Getting Personal encourages students to consider their newly gained knowledge in the context of their own diets.

The Integrated Learning and Teaching Package

Integrating the text with constructive instructor resources is crucial to deriving their full benefit. Based on feedback from instructors and students, Jones & Bartlett Learning has made the following resources available to qualified instructors:

- Test Bank, including more than 1,250 questions
- Slides in PowerPoint format, featuring more than 500 slides
- Instructor's Manual, containing lecture outlines, discussion questions, and answers to the in-text Study Questions
- Image Bank, supplying key figures from the text
- Sample Syllabus, showing how a course can be structured around this text
- Transition Guide, providing guidance in switching from the previous edition

An interactive eBook is available with study questions that reinforce key concepts as well as 36 scientifically based animations that give students an accurate, accessible explanation of the major scientific concepts and physiological principles presented in *Nutrition*.

Diet analysis software is an important component of the behavioral change and personal decision-making focus of a nutrition course. **EatRight Analysis**, developed by ESHA Research, provides software that enables students to analyze their diets by calculating their nutrient intake and comparing it to recommended intake levels. EatRight Analysis offers dietary software online at EatRight.jblearning.com. With this online tool, you and your students can access personal records from any computer with Internet access. Through a variety of reports, students learn to make better choices regarding their diet and activity habits.

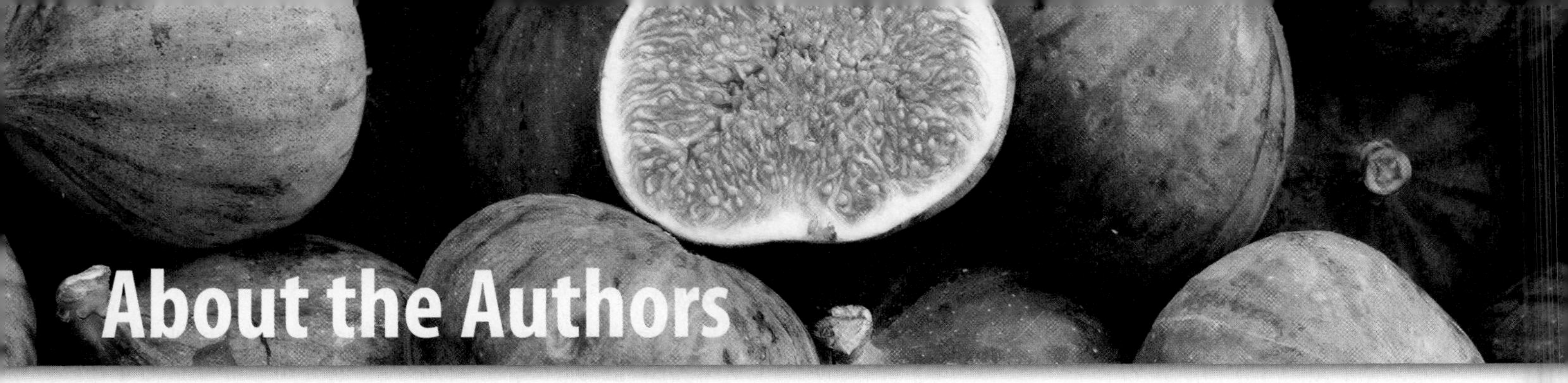

About the Authors

The *Nutrition* author team represents a culmination of years of teaching and research in nutrition science and psychology. The combined experience of the authors yields a balanced presentation of both the science of nutrition and the components of behavioral change.

Dr. Paul Insel is Consulting Associate Professor of Psychiatry at Stanford University (Stanford, California). In addition to being the principal investigator on several nutrition projects for the National Institutes of Health (NIH), he is the senior author of the seminal text in health education and has co-authored several best-selling nutrition books.

Don Ross is Director of the California Institute of Human Nutrition (Redwood City, California). For more than 20 years, he has co-authored multiple textbooks and created educational materials about health and nutrition for consumers, professionals, and college students. He has special expertise in communicating complicated physiological processes with easily understood graphical presentations. The National Institutes of Health selected his *Travels with Cholesterol* for distribution to consumers. His multidisciplinary focus brings together the fields of psychology, nutrition, biochemistry, biology, and medicine.

Kimberley McMahon is a Registered Dietitian, Licensed Dietitian, and University Instructor. She received her undergraduate degree from Montana State University and master's degree from Utah State University. She has taught nutrition courses for the past 20 years in both traditional and online settings. She currently teaches in the Master of Science in Nutrition and Human Performance program at Logan University (Chesterfield, Missouri). In addition to *Nutrition*, she is a co-author of *Discovering Nutrition* and of *Eat Right! Healthy Eating in College and Beyond* and has contributed to and authored textbook chapters on a variety of nutrition topics. Her interests and experience are in the areas of wellness, weight management, sports nutrition, lifecycle nutrition, and eating disorders.

Dr. Melissa Bernstein is a Registered Dietitian, Licensed Dietitian, and Fellow of the Academy of Nutrition and Dietetics. She received her doctoral degree from the Gerald J. and Dorothy R. Friedman School of Nutrition Science and Policy at Tufts University in Boston, MA. Dr. Bernstein has been a nutrition educator for almost 25 years. In her position as Assistant Professor in the Department of Nutrition at Rosalind Franklin University of Medicine and Science (North Chicago, Illinois), she is innovative in creating engaging and challenging online nutrition courses. Her interests include nutrition throughout the life stages, physical activity and wellness, and nutritional biochemistry. Dr. Bernstein is the coauthor of the *Position of the Academy of Nutrition and Dietetics: Food and Nutrition for Older Adults: Promoting Health and Wellness*. In addition to co-authoring *Discovering Nutrition* and *Nutrition for the Older Adult,* she has contributed, authored, and reviewed textbook chapters and peer-reviewed journal publications on nutrition and nutrition for older adults.

Contributors

The following contributors revised chapters for this edition:

Cynthia Blanton, PhD, RD
Idaho State University

Chapter 19 World View of Nutrition

Carolyn Dunn, PhD, RD
North Carolina State University

Chapter 7 Alcohol

Diane L. McKay, PhD, FACN
Tufts University

Chapter 4 Carbohydrates

Emily Mohn, PhD
Tufts University

Chapter 4 Carbohydrates

Veronica J. Oates, PhD
Tennessee State University

Chapter 12 Water and Major Minerals

Diane K. Tidwell, PhD, RD
Missisippi State University

Chapter 13 Trace Minerals

The following made contributions to previous editions of this text:

Janine T. Baer, PhD, RD
University of Dayton

Toni Bloom, MS, RD, CDE
San Jose State University

Boyce W. Burge, PhD
California Institute of Human Nutrition

Eileen G. Ford, MS, RD
Drexel University

Ellen B. Fung, PhD, RD
University of Pennsylvania

Michael I. Goran, PhD
University of Southern California

Nancy J. Gustafson, MS, RD, FADA
Director, Sawyer County Aging Unit, WI

Marc Hellerstein, MD, PhD
University of California, Berkeley

Rita H. Herskovitz, MS
University of Pennsylvania

Nancy I. Kemp, MD
University of California, San Francisco

Sarah Harding Laidlaw, MS, RD, MPA
Editor, Nutrition in Complementary Care, *DPG*

Rick D. Mattes, MPH, PhD, RD
Purdue University

Maye Musk, MS, RD
Past President of the Consulting Dietitians of Canada

Joyce D. Nash, PhD

C.J. Nieves
University of Florida

Elizabeth Peck, MS, RD, LD

Rachel Stern, MS, RD, CNS
North Jersey Community Research Initiative

Lisa Stollman, MA, RD, CDE, CDN
State University of New York, Stony Brook

Barbara Sutherland, PhD
University of California, Davis

R. Elaine Turner, PhD
University of Florida

Isabelle Vachon, RD

Debra M. Vinci, PhD, RD, CD
Appalachian State University

Stella L. Volpe, PhD, RD, FACSM
University of Massachusetts

Reviewers

Michelle D. Aldrich, PhD
Laramie County College College

Sandra D. Baker, EdD, PhD
University of Delaware

Gregory Bonikowske, DC, CNS, CFMP
Carroll University

Dale E. Brigham, PhD
University of Missouri

Wendy Buchan, PhD, RDN
California State University, Sacramento

Diane E. Carson, PhD
Chapman University

Janet Colson, PhD, RD
Middle Tennessee State University

Robert T. Davidson, PhD
Logan University

Lora N. Day, MA, RD/LD
University of Texas at Dallas

Cathy R. Deimeke, RDN
Paradise Valley Community College

Johanna H. Donnenfield, MS, RD
Scottsdale Community College

Kamal Dulai, PhD
University of California, Merced

Virginia B. Gray, PhD, RDN
California State University, Long Beach

Shelley Holden, EdD
University of South Alabama

Arlene Hoogewerf, PhD
Calvin College

Cindy Hudson, MS, RD, LD
Hinds Community College

Mary Ann Meesig Jondle, PhD
Notre Dame College of Ohio

Charlotte F. Kooima, RDN, LD, LN
Dordt College

Linda Y. Kosa-Postl, PhD
Cascadia College

Maureen Mason, MS, RD
Arizona State University

Kasuen Mauldin, PhD, RD
San Jose State University

Diane L. McKay, PhD, FACN
Tufts University

Lisa Moran, MSHS, RDMS, RVT, PhD
Jefferson Community and Technical College

Adam Pennell, MS
California State University, Bakersfield

Rizwana Rahim, PhD
East/West University

Amy Reuter, MS, RDN
City University of Seattle

Kristina von Castel-Roberts, PhD, RDN, LDN
University of Florida

Tony Ward, MS, ATC, CES
Shawnee State University

Lynne Zeman, MS
Kirkwood Community College

Reviewers of Previous Editions

Namanjeet Ahluwalia, PhD
Pennsylvania State University

Nancy K. Amy, PhD
University of California, Berkeley

R. James Barnard, PhD
University of California, Los Angeles

Susan I. Barr, PhD, RDN
University of British Columbia

Richard C. Baybutt, PhD
Kansas State University

Beverly A. Benes, PhD, RD
University of Nebraska, Lincoln

Marion Birdsall, PhD, RD
University of Pennsylvania

Cynthia Blanton, PhD, RD
Idaho State University

Shelley H. Bradford
University of South Alabama

Melanie Tracy Burns, PhD, RD
Eastern Illinois University

N. Joanne Caid, PhD
California State University, Fresno

Jau-Jiin Chen, PhD, RD
University of Nevada, Las Vegas

Jo Carol Chezem, PhD, RD
Ball State University

Beverly E. Conway, MS
Williston State College

Jane B. Dennis, PhD, RD
Tarleton State University

Holly A. Dieken, PhD, MS, BS, RD
University of Tennessee, Chattanooga

Betty J. Forbes, RD, LD
West Virginia University

Debra K. Goodwin, PhD, RD
Jacksonville State University

Margaret Gunther, PhD
Palomar Community College

Shelley R. Hancock, MS, RD, LD
University of Alabama

Donna V. Handley, MS, RD
University of Rhode Island

Jeffrey Harris, DrPH, MPH, CNS, RD
West Chester University

Nancy Gordon Harris, MS, RD, LDN
East Carolina University

Diana Himmel, RDH, MS
Tunxis Community College

Sharon Himmelstein, PhD, MNS, RD, LD
Central New Mexico University

Craig A. Horswill, PhD
University of Illinois, Chicago

Georgette Howell, MS, RD
Montgomery County Community College

Michael Jenkins
Kent State University

Simon Jenkins, DPhil
University of Bath

Mary Beth Kavanagh, MS, RD, LD
Case Western Reserve University

Zaheer Ali Kirmani, PhD, RD, LD
Sam Houston State University

Char Kooima, RD LD
Dordt College

Anda Lam, MS, RD
Pasadena City College

Samantha R. Logan, DrPH, RD
University of Massachusetts

Colleen Loveland, MS, RD, LD, CDE
Dallas County Community College

Mary-Pat Maciolek, MBA, RD
Middlesex County College

Patricia Z. Marincic, PhD, RD, LD, CLE
College of Saint Benedict/Saint John's University

Melissa J. Martilotta, MS, RD
Pennsylvania State University

Keith R. Martin, PhD
Pennsylvania State University

Glen F. McNeil, MS, RD/LD
Fort Hays State University

Liza Merly, MS
Florida International University, University Park

Mark S. Meskin, PhD, RD, FADA
California State Polytechnic University, Pomona

Kristin Moline, MSEd
Lourdes College

Katherine O. Musgrave, MS, RD, CAS
University of Maine, Orono

Deborah Myers, MS, RD, LD
Bluffton University

J. Dirk Nelson, PhD
Missouri Southern State College

Anne O'Donnell, MS, MPH, RD
Santa Rosa Junior College

Susan Okonkowski, MPH, RD
Washtenaw Community College

Martha Olson, RN, BSN, MS
Iowa Lakes Community College

Rebecca S. Pobocik, PhD, RD
Bowling Green State University

John A. Polagruto, PhD, MS
Sacramento City College

Alayne Ronnenberg, ScD
University of Massachusetts, Amherst

Susan T. Saylor, RD, EdD
Shelton State University

Brian Luke Seaward, PhD
Paramount Wellness Institute

Sanjay Singh, PhD
East-West University

Mohammad R. Shayesteh, PhD, RD, LD
Youngstown State University

LuAnn Soliah, PhD, RD
Baylor University

Bernice Gales Spurlock, PhD
Hinds Community College

Tammy J. Stephenson, PhD
University of Kentucky

James H. Swain, PhD, RD, LD
Case Western Reserve University

Joy E. Swanson, PhD
Cornell University

Jill K. Thein, M.S.
Notre Dame College

Margaret Kay Trigiano
South College

Priya Venkatesan, MS, RD, CLE
Pasadena City College

Sharonda Wallace, PhD, MPH, RD
California State Polytechnic University

Janelle Walter, PhD
Baylor University

Brenda E. Wingard-Haynes, MS, CNE
Milwaukee Area Technical College

Shahla M. Wunderlich, PhD
Montclair State University

Najat Yahia, PhD, RD, LD
Central Michigan University

Joseph J Zielinski, MPH, RD
State University of New York, Brockport

Jennifer Zimmerman, MS, RD
Tallahassee Community College

Nancy Zwick, MED, RD, LD
Northern Kentucky University

Acknowledgments

We would like to thank the following people for their hard work and dedication, as they have helped make this new edition a reality. A special thank you to Sean Fabery and our entire editorial staff from Jones & Bartlett Learning, including Nancy Hoffmann, Carter McAlister, and Cathy Esperti. We would also like to acknowledge and express our thanks to Dan Stone for his production help, Andrea DeFronzo for marketing our texts, Shannon Sheehan for her assistance with the artwork, and Merideth Tumasz for her photo research and permissions work. We thank you all for your efforts, dedication, and guidance.

Thanks to Diane L. McKay, Emily Mohn, Carolyn Dunn, Veronica J. Oates, Diane K. Tidwell, and Cynthia Blanton for their contributions to this edition, which have helped to further strengthen the scientific foundation of *Nutrition*. We would also like to thank Feon Cheng for her work in updating the instructor supplements, as well as Mackinnon Ross for her research assistance.

Finally, we would like to express the utmost gratitutde to the more than twenty-five instructors who provided feedback about the previous edition as well as draft chapters of this edition.

Nutrition

Sixth Edition

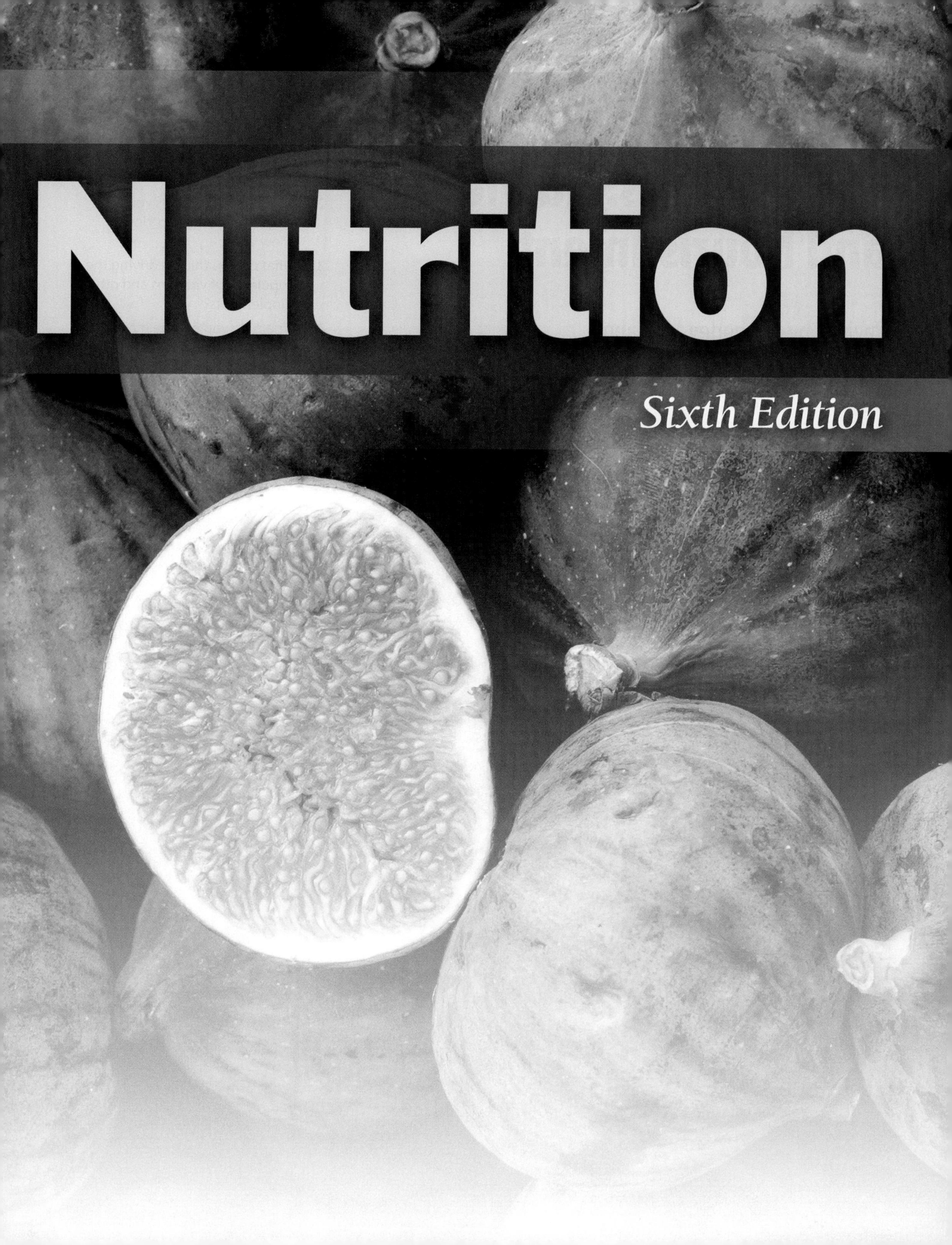

Chapter 1

Food Choices: Nutrients and Nourishment

Revised by Kimberley McMahon

THINK About It

1 What, if anything, might persuade or influence you to change your food preferences?
2 Are there some foods you definitely avoid? If so, do you know why?
3 What do you think is driving the popularity of vitamins and other supplements?
4 Where do you get the majority of your information about nutrition?

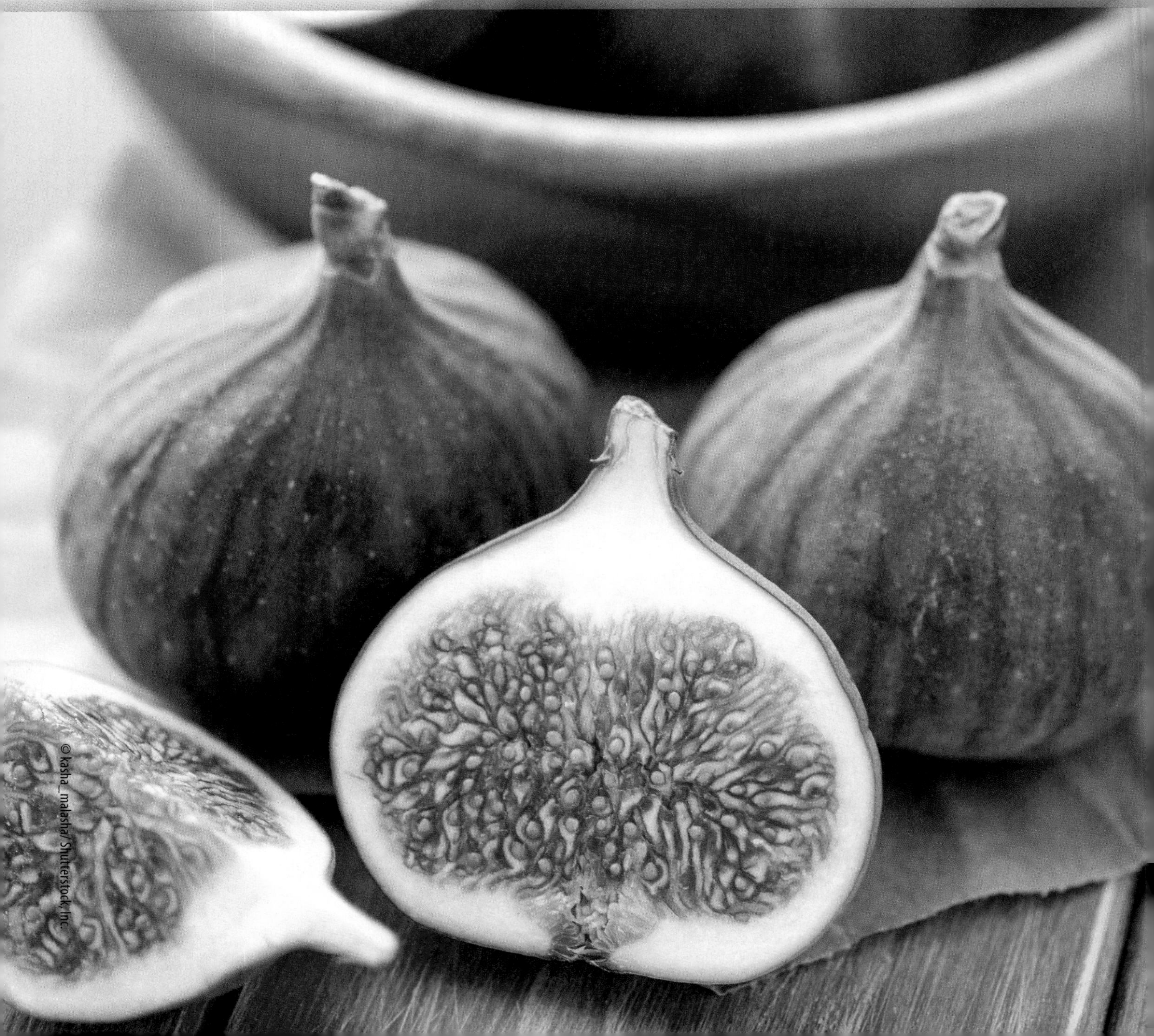

© Kasha_malasha/Shutterstock, Inc.

CHAPTER Menu

LEARNING Objectives

- Define *nutrition.*
- Identify factors that influence food choice.
- Describe the typical American diet.
- Identify the six classes of nutrients essential for health.
- Describe the basic steps in the nutrition research process.
- Recognize credible scientific research and reliable sources of nutrition information.

A group of friends goes out for pizza every Thursday night. A young man greets his girlfriend with a box of chocolates. A 5-year-old imitates her parents after they salt their food. A firefighter who is asked to explain why hot dogs are his favorite food says it has something to do with going to baseball games with his father. A parent punishes a misbehaving child by withholding dessert. What do all of these people have in common? They are using food for something other than its nutrient value. Can you think of a holiday that is not celebrated with food? For most of us, food is more than a collection of nutrients. Many factors affect what we choose to eat. Many of the foods people choose are nourishing and contribute to good health. The same, of course, may be true of the foods we reject.

The science of **nutrition** helps us improve our food choices by identifying the amounts of nutrients we need, the best food sources of those nutrients, and the other components in foods that are helpful or harmful. The U.S. National Library of Medicine defines *nutrition* as the science of food; the nutrients and other substances therein; their action, interaction, and balance in relation to health and disease; and the processes by which we ingest, absorb, transport, utilize, and excrete food substances.[1] Learning about nutrition helps us to be informed and more likely to make healthy nutrition choices, which in turn may not only improve our health, but also reduce our risk of some diseases and even increase our longevity. Keep in mind, though, that no matter how much you know about nutrition, you are still likely to choose some foods regardless of the nutrients they provide, simply for their taste or just because it makes you feel good to eat them.

▶ **nutrition** The science of foods and their components (nutrients and other substances), including the relationships to health and disease (actions, interactions, and balances); processes within the body (ingestion, digestion, absorption, transport, functions, and disposal of end products); and the social, economic, cultural, and psychological implications of eating.

Why Do We Eat the Way We Do?

Do you "eat to live" or "live to eat"? For most of us, the first is certainly true—you must eat to live. But there can be times when our enjoyment of food is more important to us than the nourishment we get from it. Factors such as age, gender, genetic makeup, occupation, lifestyle, family, and cultural background affect our daily food choices. We use food to project a desired image, forge relationships, express friendship, show creativity, and disclose our feelings. We cope with anxiety or stress by eating or not eating; we reward ourselves with food for a good grade or a job well done; or, in extreme cases, we punish failures by denying ourselves the benefit and comfort of eating.

Quick Bite

Try It Again, You Just Might Like It

Studies have found that children between the ages of 2 and 6 years commonly dislike things that are new or unfamiliar. This is also the time when kids are most likely to reject vegetables. Kids have a better chance to overcome this tendency if they are repeatedly exposed to the food they initially reject—somewhere between 5 and 15 exposures should do it.

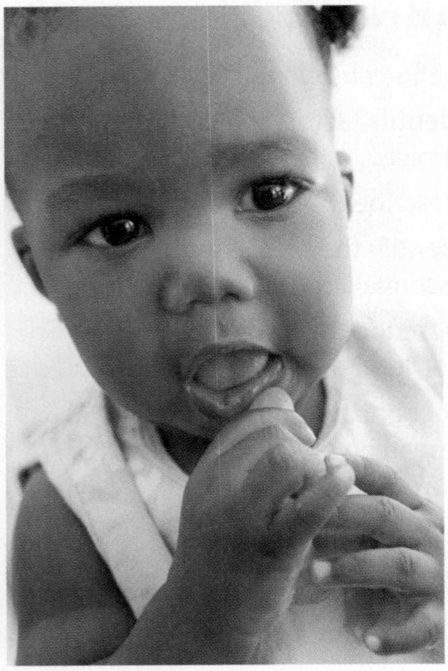

© Monkey Business Images/ShutterStock, Inc.

FIGURE 1.1 Adventures in eating. Babies and toddlers are willing to try new things, generally after repeated exposure.

► **neophobia** A dislike for anything new or unfamiliar.

Personal Preferences

THINK About It 1

What we eat reveals much about who we are. Food preferences begin early in life, and then change as we interact with parents, friends, and peers. Further experiences with different people, places, and situations often cause us to expand or change our preferences. Taste and other sensory factors such as texture are the most important things that influence our food choices; next are cost and convenience.[2]

Age is also a factor in food preferences. Consider taste preferences and how they might be influenced even before birth. Science shows that, when compared to adults, children naturally prefer higher levels of sweet and salty tastes and reject bitter tastes.[3] This might help explain why children are drawn to more unhealthy food choices within our current food environment—an environment composed of high-salt, high-refined-sugar foods. In support of this idea, studies have found that sensory experiences, beginning early in life, can shape preferences in both a positive and a negative way.[4] For example, expecting mothers who consume diets rich in healthy foods can help develop their child's taste preferences in a positive way because flavors from foods that the mother eats are transmitted to amniotic fluid and to mother's milk, creating an environment in which breastfed infants are more accepting of these flavors. In contrast, infants fed formula learn to prefer its unique flavor profile and may have more difficulty initially accepting flavors not found in formula, such as those of fruit and vegetables.[5] Having healthy food experiences early in life may go a long way toward promoting healthy eating throughout a person's life span.

Although young children prefer sweet or familiar foods, babies and toddlers are generally willing to try new things (see **FIGURE 1.1**). Experimental evidence suggests children repeatedly exposed to a variety of foods, particularly when the caregiver focuses on the child's willingness to eat a food, are more likely to accept these foods; as a result, the child will add more variety to their diet and, therefore, eat more healthfully.[6]

Preschoolers typically go through a period of food **neophobia**, a dislike for anything new or unfamiliar. School-age children tend to accept a wider array of foods, and teenagers are strongly influenced by the preferences and habits of their peers. If you track the kinds of foods you have eaten in the past year, you might be surprised to discover how few basic foods your diet includes. By the time we reach adulthood, we have formed a core group of foods we prefer. Of this group, only about 100 basic items account for 75 percent of our food intake.

Like many aspects of human behavior, food choices are influenced by many interrelated factors. Generally, hunger and satiety dictate when we eat, but what we choose to eat is not always determined by physiological or nutritional needs. When we consider that our food preferences are also dictated by factors such as sensory properties of foods (taste, smell, and texture), emotional and cognitive factors (habits, comfort/discomfort foods, food advertising and promotion, eating away from home, etc.), and environmental factors (economics, lifestyle, food availability, culture, religion, and socioeconomics), we can better understand why we choose to eat the foods that we do (see **FIGURE 1.2**).

Environmental Factors

Economic
Lifestyle
Availability
Cultural influences
Religion
Socio-ecological model

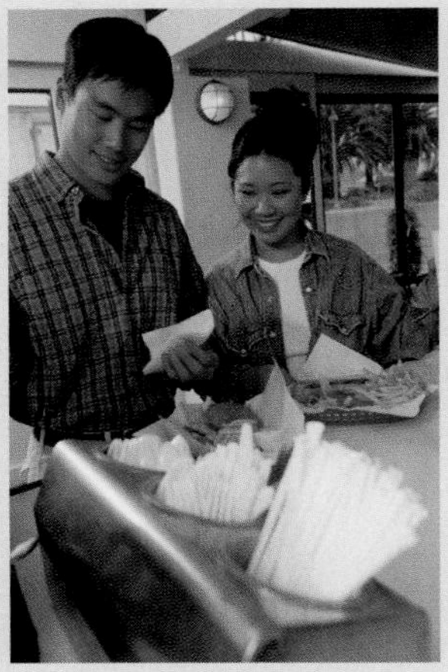

© Photodisc

Personal Preference

Sensory influences (taste, smell, texture) Habit
Comfort/discomfort foods
Food advertising and promotion
Eating away from home
Food and diet trends
Social factors
Nutrition and health belief

FIGURE 1.2 Factors that affect food choices. We often select a food to eat automatically without thought. But, in fact, our choices are complex events involving the interactions of a multitude of factors.

Sensory Influences: Taste, Smell, and Texture

In making food choices, what appeals to our senses contributes to our personal preferences. People often refer to **flavor** as a collective experience that describes both taste and smell. Texture also plays a part. You may prefer foods that have a crisp, chewy, or smooth texture. You may reject foods that feel grainy, slimy, or rubbery. Other sensory characteristics that affect food choice are color, moisture, and temperature.

▶ **flavor** The collective experience that describes both taste and smell.

We are familiar with the classic four tastes—sweet, sour, bitter, and salty—but studies show that there are more. One of these additional taste sensations is **umami**, which is a Japanese term for the taste produced by glutamate.[7] It is the brothy, meaty, savory flavor in foods such as meat, seafood, and vegetables. Monosodium glutamate (MSG) enhances this flavor when it is added to such foods.

▶ **umami [ooh-MA-mee]** A Japanese term that describes a delicious meaty or savory sensation. Chemically, this taste detects the presence of glutamate.

Emotional and Cognitive Influences

Habits

Your eating and cooking habits likely reflect what you learned from your parents. We typically learn to eat three meals a day, at about the same times each day. Quite often we eat the same foods, particularly for breakfast (e.g., cereal and milk) and lunch (e.g., sandwiches). This routine makes life convenient, and we don't have to think much about when or what to eat. But we don't have to follow this routine! How would you feel about eating mashed potatoes for breakfast and cereal for dinner? Some people might get a stomach ache just thinking about it, whereas others may enjoy the prospect of doing things differently. Look at your eating habits and see how often you make the same choices every single day.

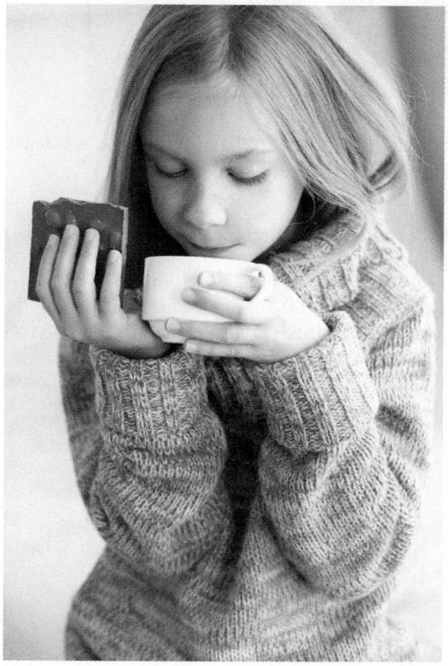
© Alena Ozerova/Shutterstock, Inc.

FIGURE 1.3 **Comfort foods.** Depending on your childhood food experiences, a bowl of traditional soup, a remembered sweet, or a mug of hot chocolate can provide comfort in times of stress.

Comfort/Discomfort Foods

Our desire for particular foods often is based on behavioral motives, even though we may not be aware of them. For some people, food becomes an emotional security blanket. Consuming our favorite foods can make us feel better, relieve stress, and allay anxiety (see **FIGURE 1.3**). Starting in the first days of life, food and affection are intertwined. Breastfed infants, for example, experience physical, emotional, and psychological satisfaction when nursing. As we grow older, this experience is continually reinforced. For example, chicken soup and hot tea with honey may be favorites when we feel under the weather because someone had prepared these foods for us when we were not feeling well. If we were rewarded for good behavior with a particular food (e.g., ice cream, candy, cookies), our positive feelings about that food can persist for a lifetime. In contrast, at some point, you may have gotten sick soon after eating a certain food and you still avoid that food.

THINK About It 2

Food Advertising and Promotion

Aggressive and sometimes deceptive advertising programs can influence a person's food-buying decision; therefore, it may not surprise you that some of the most popular food purchases are high-fat and high-sugar baked goods and alcoholic beverages. We are, however, seeing more innovative and aggressive advertising that promotes milk, meat, cranberries, and other more nutrient-dense products.

According to the Federal Trade Commission (FTC), businesses spend $9.6 billion annually marketing food and beverages. More than $1.79 billion specifically targets children and adolescents, promoting items such as sugared

Quick Bite

Sweetness and Salt

Salt can do more than just make your food taste salty. Researchers at the Monell Chemical Senses Center demonstrated that salt also suppresses the bitter flavors in foods. When combined with chocolate, for example, in a chocolate-covered pretzel, salt blocks some of the bitter flavor, making the chocolate taste sweeter. This may explain why people in many cultures salt their fruit.

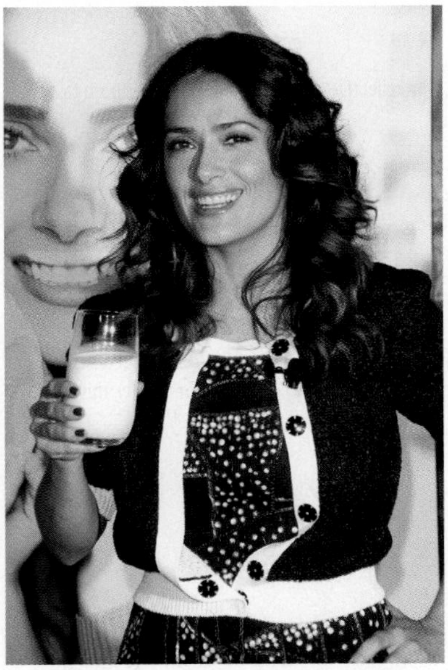
© s_bukley/Shutterstock, Inc.

FIGURE 1.4 Healthy advertising. Got milk? Is an example of a successful healthy advertising campaign.

▶ **calorie** The general term for energy in food; used synonymously with the term *energy*. Often used instead of *kilocalorie* on food labels, in diet books, and in other sources of nutrition information.

breakfast cereals, fast food, and soft drinks.[8] It is easy to see that from television to online marketing, a lot of money is being spent to promote certain products. Children and teens see about 12–16 TV advertisements per day for products generally high in saturated fat, sugar, or sodium.[9] Some researchers have linked the high prevalence of obesity among American children to their exposure to TV food advertisements. When compared to other countries, the contribution of TV food ads for children ages 6 to 11 years old to the occurrence of childhood obesity was greatest among the American population.[10]

Some advertising is positive. Ads like the one shown in **FIGURE 1.4**, for example, can be helpful, especially to consumers whose diets need improvement.

Eating Away from Home

Americans spend almost half of their food budget on foods prepared away from home.[11] Many people, however, underestimate the amount of **calories**, the general term for the amount of energy in food, and the amount of fat in foods prepared away from home, which is likely contributing to increasing weight and obesity.[12] This trend has promoted an increase in the interest for information on calories, fat, and sodium, as well as other nutrients on restaurant menus. When calories are present on menus, people order foods with fewer calories compared to menus without calories identified,[13] and parents order fewer calories for their children.[14] The Food and Drug Administration (FDA) has implemented guidelines in which nutrition labeling in chain restaurants and similar retail food establishments will provide consumers with clear and consistent nutrition information in a direct and accessible manner for the foods they eat and buy.

Food and Diet Trends

The popularity of different diets can influence changes in food product consumption. Beginning in the late 1980s, low-fat diets became popular and were accompanied by an explosion of reduced-fat, low-fat, and fat-free products. When the "low-carb" diet became popular, so did the rise in low-carb or no-carb products. Diet and health-related products also compete for consumer dollars. For example, sales of gluten-free products in the United States continue to rise due to the increased diagnosis of celiac disease and the belief that eliminating gluten, a protein found in wheat and related grains such as barley and rye, from the diet will treat other conditions as well.[15]

Social Factors

Social factors exert a powerful influence on food choice. Food is often at the center of family reunions, social gatherings, and office holiday parties. Perhaps even more influential, though, are the messages from peers about what to eat or how to eat.

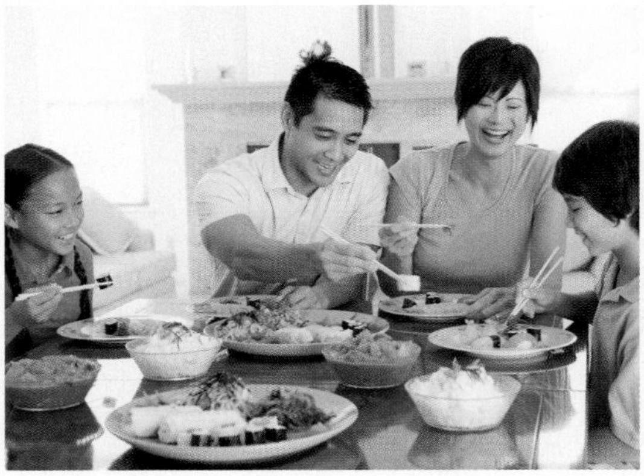
© iStockphoto/Thinkstock

FIGURE 1.5 Social facilitation. Interactions with others can affect your eating behaviors.

As **FIGURE 1.5** illustrates, eating is a social event that brings together people for a variety of purposes (e.g., religious or cultural celebrations, business meetings, family dinners). Social pressures, however, can restrict our food intake and selection. We might, for example, order nonmeat dishes when dining with a group of vegetarian friends.

Knowledge of Health and Nutrition

Many people select and emphasize certain foods they think are "good for them" (see **FIGURE 1.6**). Consumer health beliefs, perceptions of disease susceptibility, and desires to take action to prevent or delay disease onset can have powerful influences on diet and food choices. For example, people who feel vulnerable to disease and believe that dietary change might lead to positive results are more likely to pay attention to information about links among dietary choices, dietary fat, and health risks. A desire to lose weight or alter one's physical appearance also can be a powerful force shaping decisions to accept or reject particular foods. How nutrition information is delivered to consumers may also play a role in food choices. One study that compared the type of nutrition information provided, education levels, and obesity predominance in three different countries (France, Canada, and the United States) supported the idea that a "science" or nutrient approach to food might not result in appropriate food choices, indicating that in these instances consumers lose sight of the big picture and that a more practical approach to nutrition education may lead to better overall food choices.[16] Furthermore, consumers are placing higher priority on foods for health and seeking foods with more protein, less sugars, and minimal processing.[17]

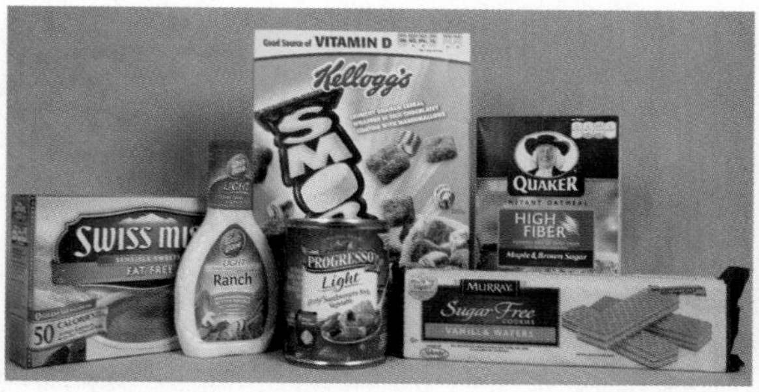

FIGURE 1.6 Where do you get your nutrition information? We are constantly bombarded by food messages. Which sources do you find most influential? Are they the most reliable?

Key Concepts Many factors influence our decisions about what to eat and when to eat. Some of the main factors include personal preferences such as taste, texture, and smell; our habits with eating; the emotional connections of comfort or discomfort that are linked to certain foods; advertisements and promotions; and whether we choose to eat our meals at home or away from home. The cultural environment in which people live also has a major influence on what foods they choose to eat.

Environment

Your environment—where you live, how you live, who you live with—has a lot to do with what you choose to eat. People around us influence our food choices, and we generally prefer the foods we grew up eating. Environmental factors that influence our food choices include economics, lifestyle, culture, and religion. Where you live and the surrounding climate also influence which foods are most accessible to you. Environmental factors such as location and climate affect food costs, a major determinant of food choice. In the United States, our environment and the choices we make play a large role in the current obesity epidemic. The **obesogenic environment** is used to describe how many Americans live: in an environment that promotes overconsumption of calories while at the same time discouraging physical activity. Other environmental factors that influence our food choices include economics, lifestyle, availability, cultural influences, religion, and the social-ecological model.

▶ **obesogenic environment** Circumstances in which a person lives, works, and plays that promote the overconsumption of calories and discourage physical activity and calorie expenditure.

Economics

Where you live and the surrounding climate not only influence which foods are most accessible to you, but also affect food costs, which are a major determinant of food choice. You may have "lobster taste" but a "hot dog budget." The types of foods purchased and the percentage of income used for food are affected by total income. Households spend more money on food when incomes rise. In 2012, middle-income families spent an average of $5,798 on food, representing about 12 percent of income. In contrast, the lowest-income households spent an average of $3,502 on food, representing 35 percent of income.[18] How much does it cost to follow dietary recommendations? For adults on a 2,000-calorie per day diet, the cost of meeting the *Dietary Guidelines for Americans* recommendations for fruit and vegetable consumption is $2.00 to $2.50 per day, according to an analysis by the U.S. Department of Agriculture (USDA).[19]

Lifestyle

Another influential factor is lifestyle. Our fast-paced society has little time or patience for food preparation. Convenience foods, from frozen entrées to

Going Green

Are you taking part in the green revolution? What are your environmental concerns?

Are you familiar with the terms *eco-friendly, carbon footprint, greenhouse gases, global climate,* and *global warming*? These phrases reflect new perspectives on our interrelated world, signaling our recent awareness of an environment in trouble. Our continuing abuse of our environment has resulted in a global climatic backlash: widespread disruptions threaten irreversible damage to our planet. The result could be a far less livable planet, inhospitable to a way of life we have taken for granted. Some green protesters are taking action. For example, to stop Brazilian rainforest destruction, some soya traders refuse to sell soy from deforested areas of the Amazon.

It is important to focus on our nutrition environment. Here are several examples of the new green technology. Only three kinds of plants supply 65 percent of the global food supply. You might be surprised to learn that they are rice, wheat, and corn. With amazing efficiency, farmers can turn plant products into animal protein with aquaculture, a fancy word for fish farming, which has realized the fastest growth of global food production and now accounts for more than 30 percent of fish consumption in the world. Again, although modern agricultural methods depend heavily on fertilizers, pesticides, and herbicides, we can also turn to newer, ecologically friendly farming technologies that increasingly lower costs and preserve the quality of soils. And although surrounded by controversy, genetically modified crops and foods are used to resist pests and increase yields and are finding a niche in our nutrition environment.

Quick Bite

Dietary Guidelines for Americans, 2015

"Positive changes in individual diet and physical activity behaviors, and in the environmental contexts and systems that affect them, could substantially improve health outcomes."

Reproduced from U.S. Department of Agriculture and U.S. Department of Health and Human Services. *Dietary Guidelines for Americans, 2015.* 8th ed. Washington, DC: U.S. Government Printing Office; February 2015.

complete meals "in a box," saturate supermarket shelves. Rising incomes and busier lifestyles have led consumers to spend less time cooking and more time taking advantage of the convenience of food prepared away from home.

Availability

Poor access to healthy, nutritious foods can negatively affect health and well-being. Approximately 23.5 million Americans, including 6.5 million children, live in nutritional wastelands commonly referred to as "food deserts." Food deserts are low-income areas where residents lack access to a supermarket or large grocery store to buy affordable fruits, vegetables, whole grains, low-fat milk, and other foods that make up the full range of a healthy diet.[20]

Not only do many people who live in food deserts lack the ability to get fresh, healthy, and affordable foods easily, but they often rely on "quick markets" that offer mostly highly processed, high-sugar, and high-fat foods. Their communities often lack healthy food providers, such as grocery stores and farmers' markets. In these neighborhoods, food needs typically are served by inexpensive restaurants and convenience stores, which offer few fresh foods. As part of its Let's Move! initiative, the Healthy Food Financing Initiative (HFFI) plans to help revitalize neighborhoods by eliminating food deserts that exist across urban and rural America.[21]

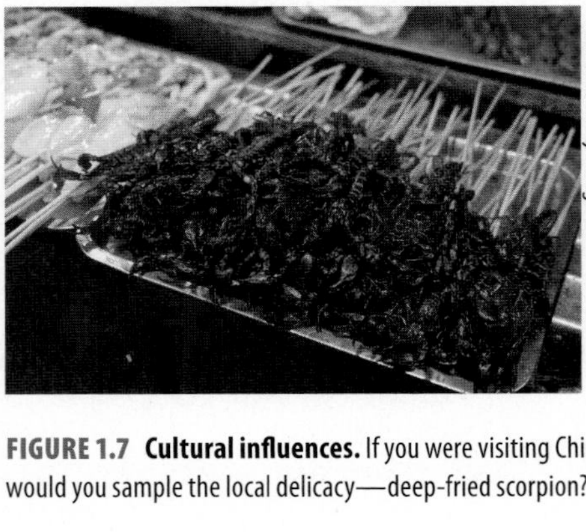

© ksbank/Getty Images

FIGURE 1.7 Cultural influences. If you were visiting China, would you sample the local delicacy—deep-fried scorpion?

Cultural Influences

One of the strongest influences on food preferences is tradition or cultural background. In all societies, no matter how simple or complex, eating is the primary way of initiating and maintaining human relationships.

To a large extent, culture defines our attitudes. "One man's food is another man's poison." Look at **FIGURE 1.7**. How does the photo make you feel? Insects, maggots, and entrails are delicacies to some, whereas just the thought of ingesting them is enough to make others cringe. Cultural forces are so powerful that if you were permitted only a single question to establish someone's

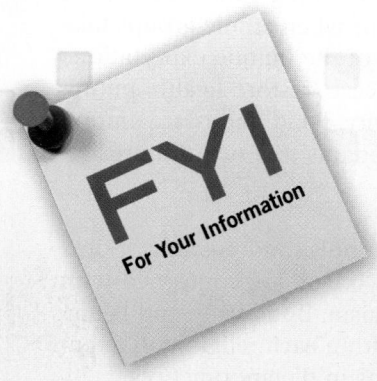

FYI For Your Information

Food and Culture

Do you ever wonder why people choose prickly pears over apples or pomegranates over blueberries? For the most part, food choices are a result of what people are accustomed to or what they have learned. Dietary habits are as diverse as individuals, and culture plays a key role in the food choices people make. Cultural influences often determine what roles various foods play in dietary habits, health beliefs, and everyday behaviors. As cultural diversity becomes more common among populations, regional food favorites become less foreign. Although beliefs and traditions can be modified through geography, economics, or experiences, core values and customs typically remain similar within a specific group.[a–c]

Food plays a major role in most religions and religious customs. Religious beliefs usually are learned early and can define certain dietary habits. For example, Jewish dietary laws specify that foods must be *kosher*. To be kosher, meat must come from animals that chew their cud, have split hooves, and are free from blemishes to their internal organs. Fish must have fins and scales. Pork, crustaceans and shellfish, and birds of prey are not kosher. Kosher laws prohibit eating meat and milk at the same meal or even preparing or serving them with the same plates and utensils. Islam identifies acceptable foods as Halal and has rules similar to those of Judaism for the slaughtering of animals. Islam prohibits the consumption of pork, the flesh of clawed animals, alcohol, and other intoxicating drugs. The Church of Jesus Christ of Latter Day Saints disapproves of coffee, tea, and alcoholic beverages. Most Hindus are vegetarians and do not eat eggs, and some avoid onions and garlic. The Orthodox Jain religion in India forbids eating meat or animal products (e.g., milk, eggs) and any root vegetables (e.g., potatoes, carrots, garlic). In Buddhism, mind-altering substances or intoxicating beverages are prohibited, but dietary habits vary considerably based on the sect and geographic location.[d] Some Buddhists follow strict forms of vegetarianism whereas others do not. In Christianity and many other religions, food plays a key role in religious ceremonies and various religious holidays, from what foods may or may not be eaten (e.g., no meat on Fridays during Lent) to when foods can be consumed (e.g., only from sundown to sunrise during Islam's Ramadan). Food plays an important role not only in physical survival, but also in many people's spiritualism.

Many cultures have traditional medical practices based on the belief that nature is composed of two opposing forces. In traditional Chinese medicine, for example, these forces, called *yin* and *yang*, must be in proper balance for good health.[e] It is believed that excesses in either direction cause illness. The illness must then be treated by giving foods of the opposite force. This idea of balance or harmony, accompanied by terms describing illness and foods as either cold (e.g., banana, fish, juices) or hot (e.g., beef, nuts, ginger) or yin or yang, also is found in other Asian cultures, including India and the Philippines, and in Latin American cultures and ethnicities.

Numerous cultures view a variety of foods as having medicinal properties. Treatments commonly use assorted herbs, herbal teas, and special foods. From generation to generation, knowledge of such remedies is passed on. Remarkably, various cultures all over the world use remedies based on similar common substances, such as chamomile, garlic, and honey. These familiar substances often are more trusted and are considered safer than modern medicines. In addition to traditions and culture, the complete array of herbs and foods used daily and also as medicines is based on the geographic region, growing conditions, and climate.

The interplay of diet and culture helps to define a person's values, preferences, and practices. As a result, even in the face of changing world events and populations, neither is abandoned easily or quickly. Just as there is diversity in individuals and families, there is also diversity within cultures. One must be alert to avoid the assumption that all people of a specific culture eat, believe, or follow traditions in the exact same manner. Even so, the question arises: What impact will our increasing mobility and globalization have on food choice? Undoubtedly, cultural interactions and exposure to various cuisines will increase. Will this expand our appreciation and preservation of cultural culinary practices and result in the formation of new hybrid cuisines?

[a] Welcome to food, culture and tradition. http://www.food-links.com. Accessed December 18, 2015.

[b] EthnoMed. Cultures. http://ethnomed.org/culture. Accessed December 18, 2015.

[c] PBS. The meaning of food: food and culture. http://www.pbs.org/opb/meaningoffood/ Accessed April 10, 2015.

[d] HerbMed. Top 20 herbs. http://www.herbmed.org/#param.wapp?sw_page=top20. Accessed December 18, 2015.

[e] China Highlights. Chinese medicinal cuisine/food therapy. http://www.chinahighlights.com/travelguide/chinese-food/medicinal-cuisine.htm. Accessed December 18, 2015.

food preferences, a good choice would be "What is your ethnic background?" (See the FYI feature "Food and Culture.")

Knowledge, beliefs, customs, and habits all are defining elements of human culture. Although genetic characteristics tie people of ethnic groups together, culture is a learned behavior and, consequently, can be modified through education, experience, and social and political trends.[22]

In many cultures, food has symbolic meanings related to family traditions, social status, and health. In fact, many folk remedies rely on food. Some of these have gained wide acceptance, such as the use of spices and herbal teas for purposes ranging from allaying anxiety to preventing cancer and heart disease. Just as cultural distinctions eventually blur when ethnic groups take part in the larger American culture, so do many of the unique expectations about the ability of certain foods to prevent disease, restore health among those with various afflictions, or enhance longevity. Food habits are among the last practices to change when an immigrant adapts to a new culture.[23]

Religion

Food is an important part of religious rites, symbols, and customs. Some religious rules apply to everyday eating whereas others are concerned with special celebrations. Christianity, Judaism, Hinduism, Buddhism, and Islam, for example, all have distinct dietary laws, but within each religion, different interpretations of these laws give rise to variations in dietary practices.

Social-Ecological Model

The social-ecological model included in the *Dietary Guidelines for Americans* (**FIGURE 1.8**) is designed to illustrate how individual factors, environmental settings, various sectors of influence, and social and cultural elements of society overlap to form the food and physical activity choices of an individual.[24] You can use the social-ecological model to think about how your current food and physical activity choices affect your calorie balance and risk for chronic diseases.

Quick Bite

Nerve Poison for Dinner?

The puffer fish is a delicacy in Japan. Danger is part of its appeal; eating a puffer fish can be life threatening! The puffer fish contains a poison called tetrodotoxin (TTX), which blocks the transmission of nerve signals and can be fatal. Chefs who prepare the puffer fish must have special training and licenses to prepare the fish properly so that diners feel nothing more than a slight numbing feeling.

Quick Bite

Does Being Overweight Spread from Person to Person?

The spread of obesity in social networks appears to be a factor in the obesity epidemic. Likewise, this also suggests that it may be possible for peers to have the same effect in the opposite direction, slowing the spread of obesity.

Key Concepts The cultural environments in which people grow up have a major influence on what foods they prefer, what foods they consider edible, and what foods they eat in combination and at what time of day. Many factors work to define a group's culture: environment, economics, access to food, lifestyle, traditions, and religious beliefs. As people from other cultures immigrate to new lands, they adopt new behaviors consistent with their new homes. However, food habits are among the last to change. The social-ecological model of food and physical activity behavior shows how individual factors, environmental settings, sectors of influence, and cultural social values influence our food and physical activity behavior.

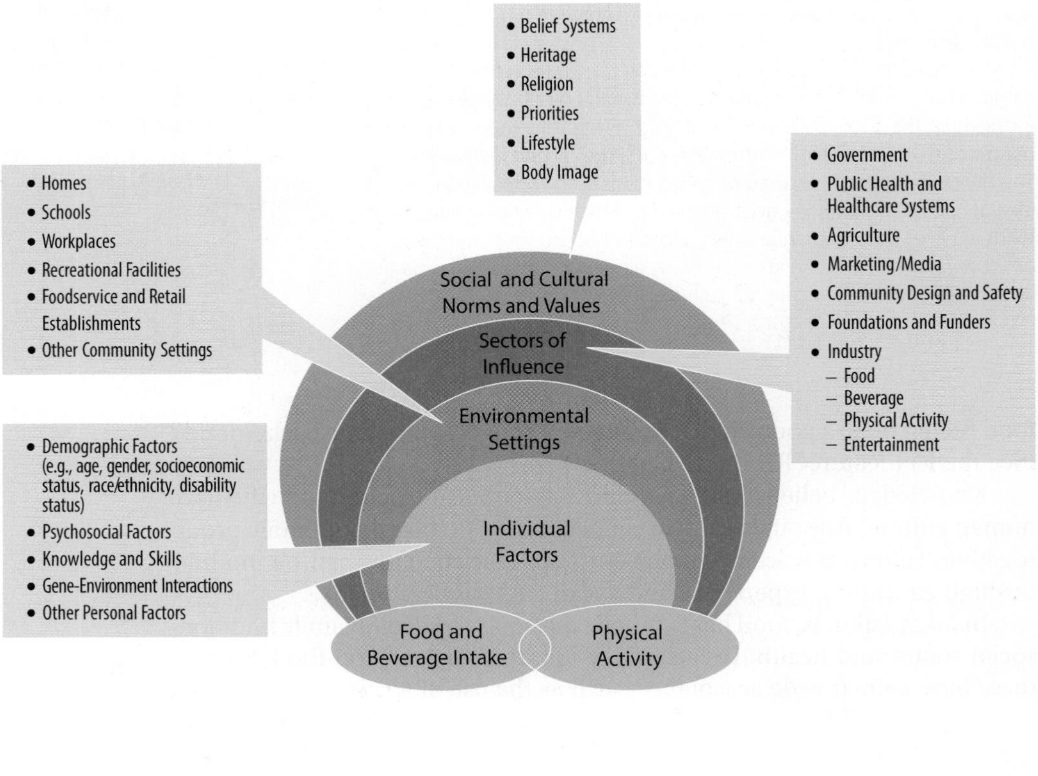

FIGURE 1.8 A social-ecological framework for nutrition and physical activity decisions.

Modifed from Centers for Disease Control and Prevention. Division of Nutrition, Physical Activity, and Obesity. State Nutrition, Physical Activity and Obesity (NPAO) Program: Technical Assistance Manual. January 2008, page 36. Accessed April 21, 2010. http://www.cdc.gov/obesity/ downloads/TA_Manual_1_31_08.pdf; Institute of Medicine. Preventing Childhood Obesity: Health in the Balance, Washington (DC): The National Academies Press; 2005, page 85; Story M, Kaphingst KM, Robinson-O'Brien R, Glanz K. Creating healthy food and eating environments: Policy and environmental approaches. Annu Rev Public Health 2008;29:253–272.

The American Diet

Surveys involving large amounts of people are conducted in the United States to determine what foods are consistently being eaten. The U.S. government uses data collected by the U.S. Department of Health and Human Services called the National Health and Nutrition Examination Survey (NHANES), which combines interviews and physical examinations for data collection. What, then, is a "typical American diet"? As a country influenced by the practices of so many cultures, religions, backgrounds, and lifestyles, there is no easy or single answer to this question. The U.S. diet is as diverse as Americans themselves, even though many people around the world imagine that the American diet consists mainly of hamburgers, french fries, and cola drinks. Our fondness for fast food and the marketability of such restaurants overseas make them seem like icons of American culture—and many of the stereotypes are true.

So, how healthful is the "American" diet? The average American falls short of the USDA's MyPlate recommendations for vegetables, dairy, and fruit. **TABLE 1.1** shows average U.S. consumption compared to the MyPlate recommendations (see **Table 1.1**).[25]

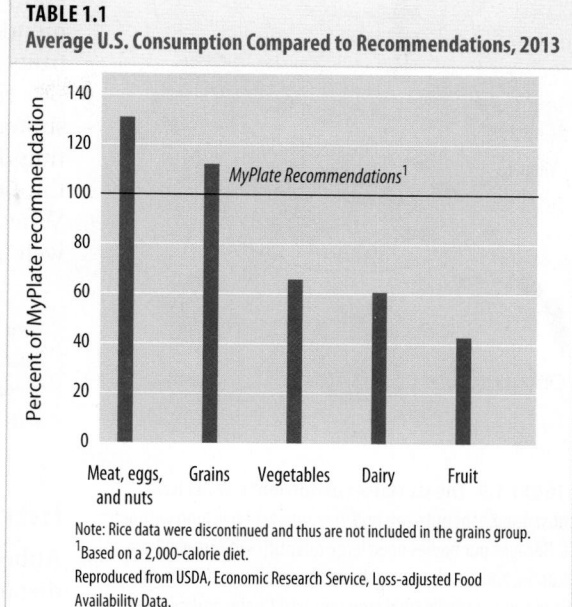

TABLE 1.1
Average U.S. Consumption Compared to Recommendations, 2013

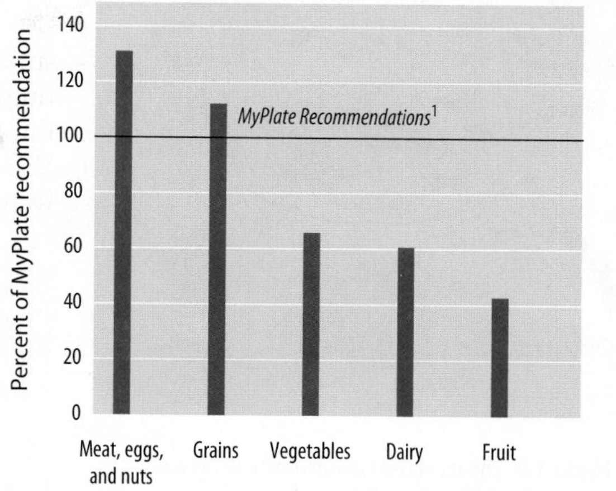

Note: Rice data were discontinued and thus are not included in the grains group.
[1]Based on a 2,000-calorie diet.
Reproduced from USDA, Economic Research Service, Loss-adjusted Food Availability Data.

For individuals age 2 years and older, the estimated average total intakes of the following foods all fall well below the Dietary Guidelines: fruit intake is 1.03 cups, with 33% consumed as fruit juice; vegetable intake is 1.47 cups, of which 22% was potatoes and 20% was tomatoes; whole grains consumption is less than 1 ounce, average dairy intake is 1.8 cups, of which 44% is cheese and 51% was fluid milk; average solid fat intake is 37 grams, oil is 25 grams, and sugar intake is estimated to be 18.4 teaspoon equivalents.[26] (See **TABLE 1.2**.)

Americans are not eating enough nutrient-dense foods and eating too much of the foods known to be harmful. Together, solid fats and added sugars alone contribute many empty calories. Soda, sugar-sweetened beverages, and grain-based desserts are the major sources of added sugars for many Americans. Regular cheese, grain-based desserts, and pizza are the top contributors of solid and saturated fat in the American diet. In addition, Americans of all age groups are eating more than the recommended amounts of sodium, mainly in the form of processed foods.[27]

Although good health and nutrition information can be found in multiple publications and at a variety of venues, this doesn't necessarily translate into better food choices. People are not natural nutritionists, and they generally don't know which foods to choose for good health. So, it is not surprising when national surveys indicate that although Americans know that nutrition

TABLE 1.2
Estimated Average Intake Compared to the *Dietary Guidelines or Americans*, 2015–2020

	Estimated Average Intake	Recommended Intake
Fruit	1.03 cups	2 cups per day
Vegetables	1.47 cups	2 ½ cups per day
Whole grains	< 1 ounce per day	> 3 ounces per day
Dairy	1.8 cups	3 cups per day
Solid fat intake	37 grams	Limit solid fat intake
Sugar	18.4 teaspoon equivalents	<10% of calories per day

Data from Bowman, S. Clemens J, Friday J, Moshfegh, A. Food Patterns Equivalents Intakes from Food: Mean Amounts Consumer per Individual, What We Eat In America, NHANES 2011-12; Tables 1-4. http://www.ars.usda.gov/research/publications/publications.htm?seq_no_115=312662

Quick Bite

High Fructose Corn Syrup (HFCS)

High fructose corn syrup (HFCS) is a desired ingredient for food manufacturers because it provides the sweet taste we get from table sugar, it works well in a number of different products helping maintain longer shelf life, and is inexpensive compared to other sweeteners. HFCS is a likely ingredient in foods such as soft drinks and other canned beverages, ice cream, cereal, baked goods, and snack foods. But, did you know that HFCS can also be found in products that do not taste sweet, such as sliced bread, processed meats, and condiments? Reading food labels is the easiest way to determine if a food has HFCS added.

and food choices are important factors in health, few have made recommended changes such as eating less fat, sugar, and salt, and eating more fruits and vegetables.

You are in a position to gather more information than the average consumer. By using this book to expand your study of nutrition, you will be getting the full story: the nutrients we need for good health, the science behind the health messages, and the food choices it will take to implement them. Whether you use this information is up to you, but at least you will be a well-informed consumer!

Key Concepts "American" cuisine is truly a melting pot of cultural contributions to foods and tastes. Although Americans receive and believe many messages about the role of diet in good health, these beliefs do not always translate into better food choices. The typical American diet contains too much sodium, solid fat, saturated fat, and sugar and not enough fruits, vegetables, low-fat dairy, and whole-grain foods.

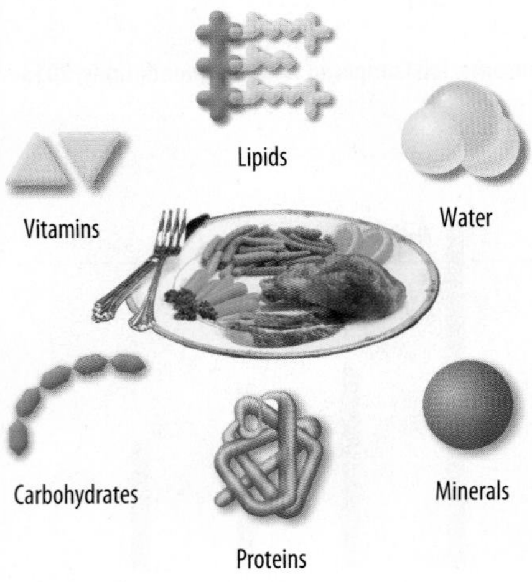

FIGURE 1.9 The six classes of nutrients. Water is the most important nutrient, and we cannot survive long without it. Because our bodies need large quantities of carbohydrate, protein, and fat, they are called macronutrients. Our bodies need comparatively small amounts of vitamins and minerals, so they are called micronutrients.

Introducing the Nutrients

Although we give food meaning through our culture and experience and make dietary decisions based on many factors, ultimately the reason for eating is to obtain nourishment—nutrition.

Just like your body, food is a mixture of chemicals, some of which are essential for normal body function. These essential chemicals are called **nutrients**. You need nutrients for normal growth and development, for maintaining cells and tissues, for fuel to do physical and metabolic work, and for regulating the hundreds of thousands of body processes that go on inside you every second of every day. Further, food must provide these nutrients; the body either cannot make these **essential nutrients** or cannot make enough of them. There are six classes of nutrients in food: carbohydrates, lipids (fats and oils), proteins, vitamins, minerals, and water (see **FIGURE 1.9**). For normal human growth, development, and maintenance, the diet must supply about 45 essential nutrients.

▶ **nutrients** Any substances in food that the body can use to obtain energy, synthesize tissues, or regulate functions.

▶ **essential nutrients** Substances that must be obtained in the diet because the body either cannot make them or cannot make adequate amounts of them.

Definition of Nutrients

In studying nutrition, we focus on the functions of nutrients in the body so that we can see why they are important in the diet. However, to define a nutrient in technical terms, we focus on what happens in its absence. A nutrient is a chemical the absence of which from the diet for a long enough time results in a specific change in health; we say that a person has a deficiency of that nutrient. A lack of vitamin C, for example, can eventually lead to scurvy. A diet with too little iron can result in iron-deficiency anemia. To complete the definition of a nutrient, it also must be true that putting the essential chemical back in the diet reverses the change in health, if done before permanent damage occurs. For example, if taken early enough, supplements of vitamin A can reverse the effects of deficiency on the eyes. If not, prolonged vitamin A deficiency can cause permanent blindness.

Nutrients are not the only chemicals in food. Other substances add flavor and color, some contribute to texture, and others such as caffeine have physiological effects on the body. **Phytochemicals** are compounds in plants that are believed to provide health benefits beyond the traditional nutrients. **Zoochemicals** are the animal equivalent of phytochemicals in plants. Although not nutrients, nor considered essential in the diet, these chemicals have important health benefits. For instance, research suggests that phytochemicals in fruits and vegetables provide **antioxidant** activity, which can reduce risk for heart disease or cancer.[28]

▶ **phytochemicals** Substances in plants that possess health-protective effects, even though they are not essential for life.

▶ **zoochemicals** The animal equivalent of phytochemicals in plants that are believed to provide health benefits beyond the traditional nutrients that foods contain.

▶ **antioxidant** A substance that combines with or otherwise neutralizes a free radical, thus preventing oxidative damage to cells and tissues.

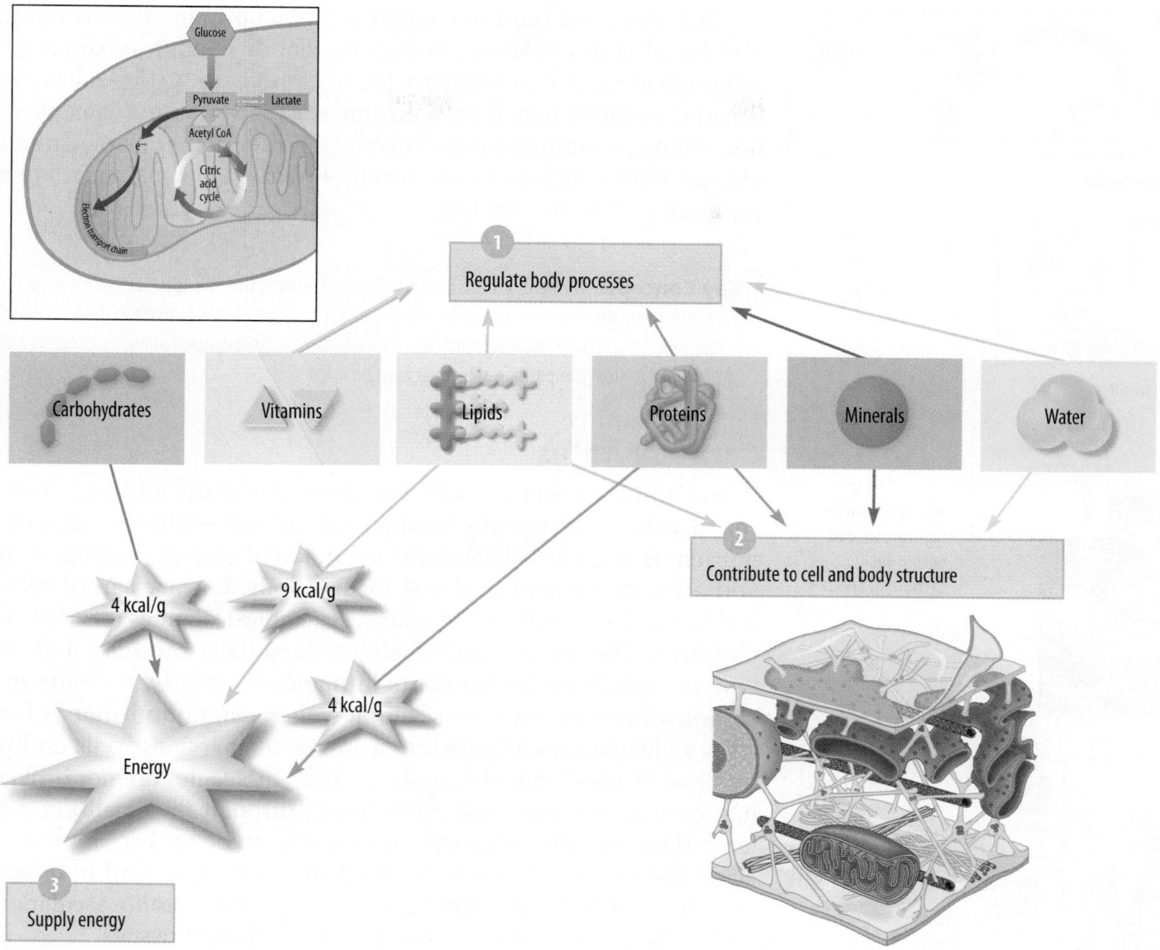

FIGURE 1.10 Nutrients have three general functions in your body. (1) Micronutrients, some lipids and proteins, and water help regulate body processes such as blood pressure, energy production, and temperature. (2) Lipids, proteins, minerals, and water help provide structure to bone, muscle, and other cells. (3) Macronutrients supply energy to power muscle contractions and cellular functions.

The six classes of nutrients serve three general functions: They provide energy, regulate body processes, and contribute to body structures (see **FIGURE 1.10**). Although virtually all nutrients can be said to influence body processes, and many contribute to body structures, only proteins, carbohydrates, and fats are sources of energy.

Because the body needs large quantities of carbohydrates, proteins, and fats, they are called **macronutrients**; vitamins and minerals are called **micronutrients** because the body needs comparatively small amounts of these nutrients.

In addition to their functions, there are several other key differences among the classes of nutrients. First, the chemical composition of nutrients varies widely. One way to divide the nutrient groups is based on whether the compounds contain the element carbon. Most substances that contain carbon are **organic** substances; most of those that do not are **inorganic**. Carbohydrates, lipids, proteins, and vitamins are all organic; minerals and water are not. Structurally, nutrients can be very simple—minerals such as sodium are single elements, although we often consume them as larger compounds (e.g., sodium chloride, which is table salt). Water also is very simple in structure. The organic nutrients have more complex structures—the carbohydrates, lipids, and proteins we eat are made of smaller building blocks, whereas the vitamins are elaborately structured compounds.

▶ **macronutrients** Nutrients, such as carbohydrate, fat, or protein, that are needed in relatively large amounts in the diet.

▶ **micronutrients** Nutrients, such as vitamins and minerals, that are needed in relatively small amounts in the diet.

▶ **organic** In chemistry, any compound that contains carbon, except carbon oxides (e.g., carbon dioxide) and sulfides and metal carbonates (e.g., potassium carbonate). The term *organic* also is used to denote crops that are grown without synthetic fertilizers or chemicals.

▶ **inorganic** Any substance that does not contain carbon, excepting certain simple carbon compounds such as carbon dioxide and carbon monoxide. Common examples include table salt (sodium chloride) and baking soda (sodium bicarbonate).

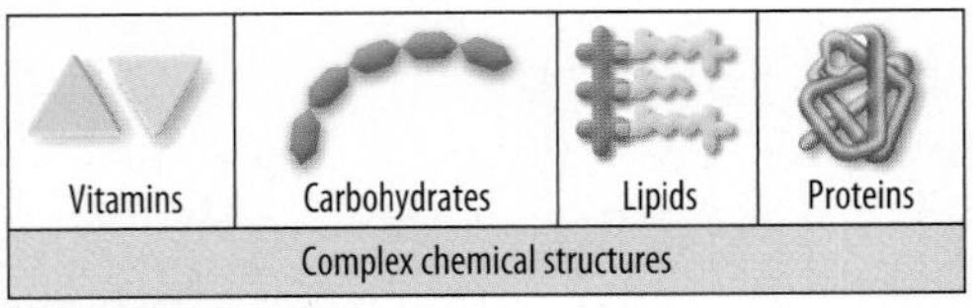

Organic – contains carbon

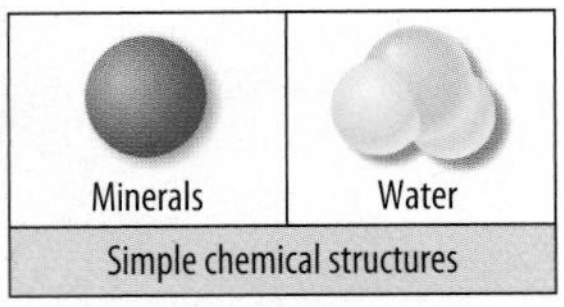

Inorganic – no carbon

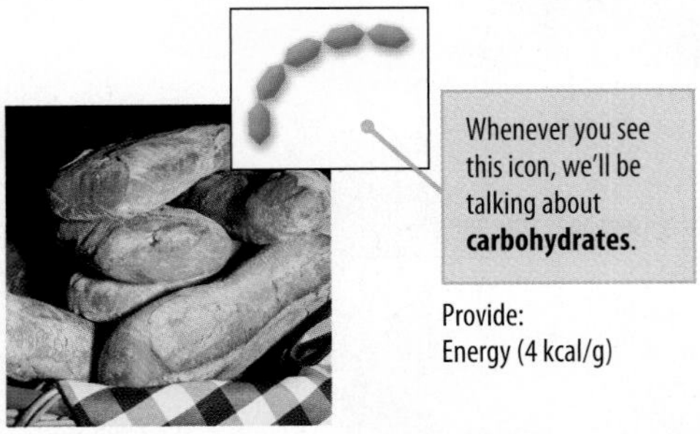

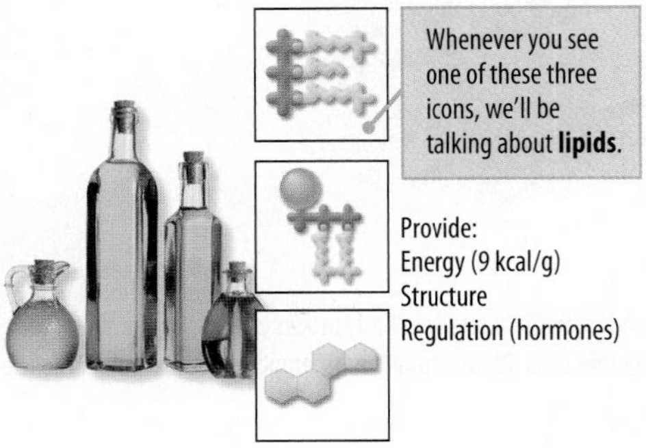

Whenever you see one of these three icons, we'll be talking about **lipids**.
Provide:
Energy (9 kcal/g)
Structure
Regulation (hormones)

It is rare for a food to contain just one nutrient. Meat is not just protein and bread is not solely carbohydrate. Foods contain mixtures of nutrients, although in many cases protein, fat, or carbohydrate dominates. So, although bread is certainly rich in carbohydrates, it also contains some protein, a little fat, and many vitamins and minerals. If you're eating whole-grain bread, you also get fiber, which is not technically a nutrient, but an important compound for good health nonetheless.

Key Concepts Nutrients are the essential chemicals in food that the body needs for normal functioning and good health and that must come from the diet because they either cannot be made in the body or cannot be made in sufficient quantities. Six classes of nutrients—carbohydrates, proteins, lipids, vitamins, minerals, and water—can be described by their composition or by their function in the body.

Carbohydrates

If you think of water when you hear the word *hydrate*, then the word *carbohydrate*—or literally "hydrate of carbon"—tells you exactly what this nutrient is made of. **Carbohydrates** are made of carbon, hydrogen, and oxygen and are a major source of fuel for the body. Dietary carbohydrates are the starches and sugars found in grains, vegetables, legumes (dry beans and peas), and fruits. We also get carbohydrates from dairy products and from fiber, a type of carbohydrate that exists in plants. Your body converts most dietary carbohydrates to glucose, a simple sugar compound that is found in the body's circulation and provides a source of energy for cells and tissues. The monosaccharide units that make up fiber molecules are not broken down by human digestive enzymes. Fiber passes through the small intestine into the large intestine, where bacteria metabolize some and some short-chain fatty acids and gas are also formed. It is glucose that we find in **circulation**, or the movement of substances through the vessels of the cardiovascular or lymphatic system, providing a source of energy for cells and tissues.

Lipids

The term **lipids** refers to substances we know as fats and oils but also to fatlike substances in foods, such as cholesterol and phospholipids. Lipids are organic compounds and, like carbohydrates, contain carbon, hydrogen, and oxygen. Fats and oils—or, more correctly, **triglycerides**—are another major fuel source for the body. In addition, triglycerides, cholesterol, and phospholipids have other important functions: providing structure for body cells, carrying the fat-soluble vitamins (A, D, E, and K), and providing the starting material (cholesterol) for making many **hormones**. Dietary sources of lipids include the fats and oils we cook with or add to foods, the naturally occurring fats in meats and dairy products, and some less obvious plant sources, such as coconut, olives, and avocado.

Proteins

Proteins are organic compounds made of smaller building blocks called **amino acids**. Unlike carbohydrates and lipids, amino acids contain nitrogen as well as carbon, hydrogen, and oxygen. Proteins are found in a variety of foods, but meats and dairy products are among the most concentrated sources. Grains, **legumes**, and vegetables all contribute protein to the diet, whereas fruits contribute negligible amounts. The amino acids that we get from dietary protein combine with the amino acids made in the body to make hundreds of different body proteins. Proteins are the main structural material in the body. They are also important components in blood, cell membranes, enzymes, and immune factors.[29] Proteins regulate body processes and can also be used for energy.

- ▶ **carbohydrates** Compounds, including sugars, starches, and dietary fibers, that usually have the general chemical formula $(CH_2O)n$, where *n* represents the number of CH_2O units in the molecule. Carbohydrates are a major source of energy for body functions.
- ▶ **circulation** Movement of substances through the vessels of the cardiovascular or lymphatic system.
- ▶ **lipids** A group of fat-soluble compounds that includes triglycerides, sterols, and phospholipids.
- ▶ **triglycerides** Fats composed of three fatty acid chains linked to a glycerol molecule.
- ▶ **hormones** Chemical messengers that are secreted into the blood by one tissue and act on cells in another part of the body.
- ▶ **proteins** Large, complex compounds consisting of many amino acids connected in varying sequences and forming unique shapes.
- ▶ **amino acids** Organic compounds that function as the building blocks of protein.
- ▶ **legumes** A family of plants with edible seed pods, such as peas, beans, lentils, and soybeans; also called pulses.

Vitamins

Vitamins are organic compounds that contain carbon and hydrogen and perhaps nitrogen, oxygen, phosphorus, sulfur, or other elements. The main function of vitamins is to help regulate many body processes such as energy production, blood clotting, and calcium balance. Vitamins help to keep organs and tissues functioning and healthy. Because vitamins have such diverse functions, a lack of a particular vitamin can have widespread effects. Although the body does not break down vitamins to yield energy, vitamins have vital roles in the extraction of energy from carbohydrate, fat, and protein.

THINK About It 3

Each of the 13 vitamins belongs in one of two groups: fat-soluble or water-soluble. The four fat-soluble vitamins—A, D, E, and K—have very diverse roles. What they have in common is the way they are absorbed and transported in the body and the fact that they are more likely to be stored in larger quantities than the water-soluble vitamins are. The water-soluble vitamins include vitamin C and eight B vitamins: thiamin (B_1), riboflavin (B_2), niacin (B_3), pyridoxine (B_6), cobalamin (B_{12}), folate, pantothenic acid, and biotin. Most of the B vitamins are involved in some way with the pathways for energy metabolism. Vitamins are found in a wide variety of foods, not just fruits and vegetables—although these are important sources—but also meats, grains, legumes, dairy products, and even fats. Choosing a well-balanced diet usually makes vitamin supplements unnecessary. In fact, when taken in large doses, vitamin supplements (especially those containing vitamins A, D, B_6, or niacin) can be harmful.

Minerals

Structurally, **minerals** are simple, inorganic substances. Minerals are important for keeping your body healthy because they are used for many different functions. There are two kinds of minerals: macrominerals and trace minerals. **Macrominerals** are minerals your body needs in relatively large amounts compared to other minerals and include calcium, phosphorus, magnesium, sodium, potassium, chloride, and sulfur.[30] The body needs the remaining minerals in only very small amounts. These **microminerals**, or **trace minerals**, include iron, zinc, copper, manganese, molybdenum, selenium, iodine, and fluoride. As with vitamins, the functions of minerals are diverse. Minerals can be found in structural roles (e.g., calcium, phosphorus, and fluoride in bones and teeth) as well as regulatory roles (e.g., control of fluid balance, regulation of muscle contraction).

Food sources of minerals are just as diverse. Although we often associate minerals with animal foods, such as meats and milk, plant foods are important sources as well. Deficiencies of minerals, except iron, calcium, iodine (in patients with cystic fibrosis and people who are pregnant), and selenium, are generally uncommon. A balanced diet provides enough minerals for most people. However, individuals with iron-deficiency anemia may need iron supplements, and others may need calcium supplements if they cannot or will not drink milk or eat dairy products. As is true for vitamins, excessive intake of some minerals as supplements can be toxic.

Water

Water is the most essential nutrient. We can survive far longer without any of the other nutrients in the diet, indeed without food at all, than we can without water. Like minerals, water is inorganic. Water has many roles in the body, including temperature control, lubrication of joints, and transportation of nutrients and wastes.

Because your body is nearly 60 percent water, regular fluid intake to maintain adequate hydration is important. Water is found not only in beverages,

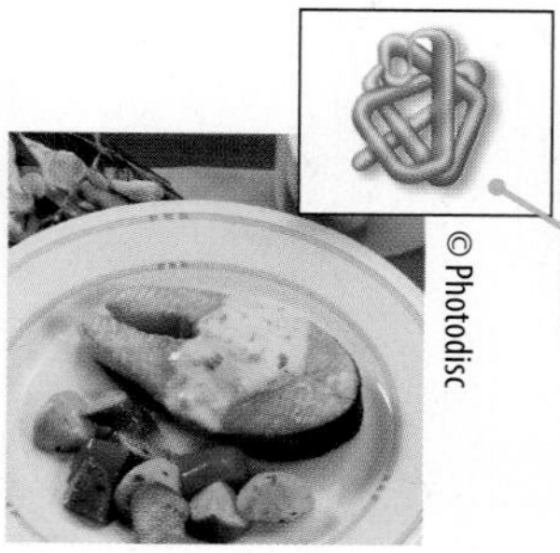

© Photodisc

Whenever you see this icon, we'll be talking about **proteins.**

Provide:
Energy (4 kcal/g)
Structure
Regulation

▶ **vitamins** Organic compounds necessary for reproduction, growth, and maintenance of the body. Vitamins are required in miniscule amounts.

▶ **minerals** Inorganic compounds needed for growth and for regulation of body processes.

▶ **macrominerals** Major minerals required in the diet and present in the body in large amounts compared with trace minerals.

▶ **microminerals** See *trace minerals*.

▶ **trace minerals** Minerals present in the body and required in the diet in relatively small amounts compared with major minerals; also known as *microminerals*.

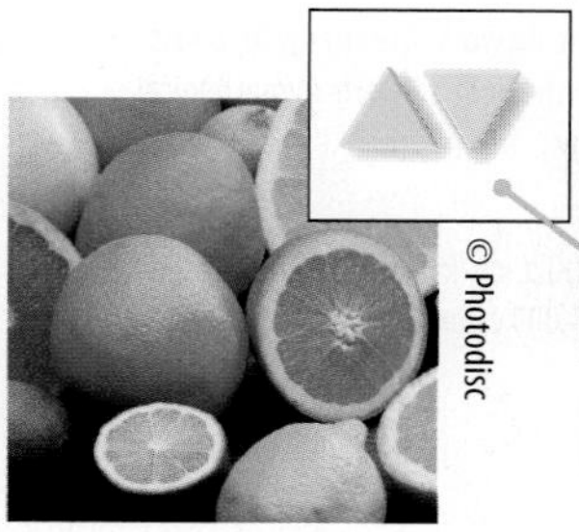

© Photodisc

Whenever you see these icons, we'll be talking about **vitamins.**

Provide:
Regulation

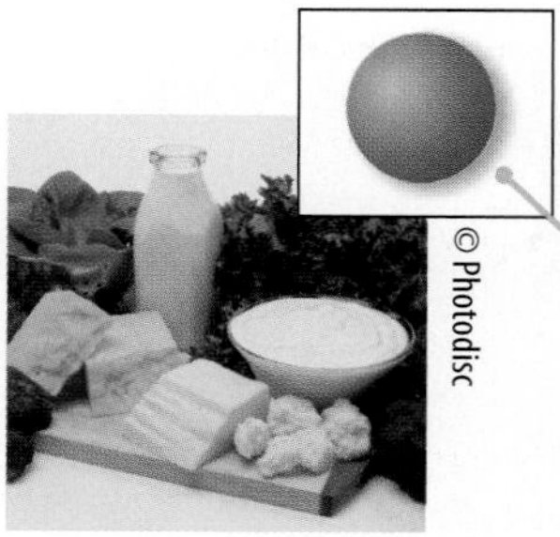

© Photodisc

Whenever you see this icon, we'll be talking about **minerals.**

Provide:
Regulation
Structure

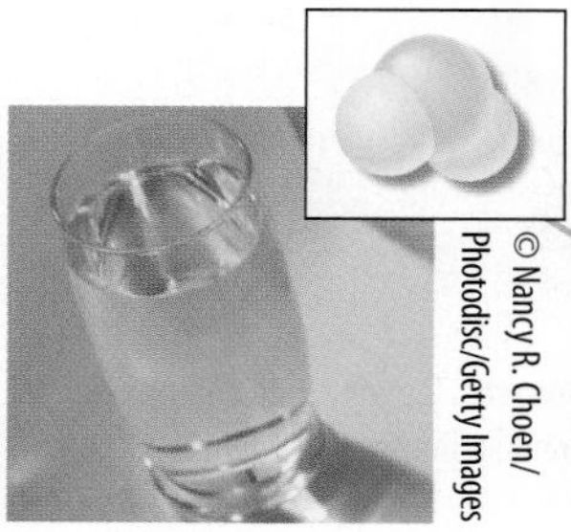

© Nancy R. Chen/Photodisc/Getty Images

Whenever you see this icon, we'll be talking about **water.**

Provides:
Regulation
Structure

but also in most food products. Fruits and vegetables in particular are high in water content. Through many chemical reactions, the body makes some of its own water, but this is only a fraction of the amount needed for normal function.

Key Concepts The body needs larger amounts of carbohydrates, lipids, and proteins (macronutrients) than vitamins and minerals (micronutrients). Carbohydrates, lipids, and proteins provide energy; proteins, vitamins, minerals, water, and some fatty acids regulate body processes; and proteins, lipids, minerals, and water contribute to body structure.

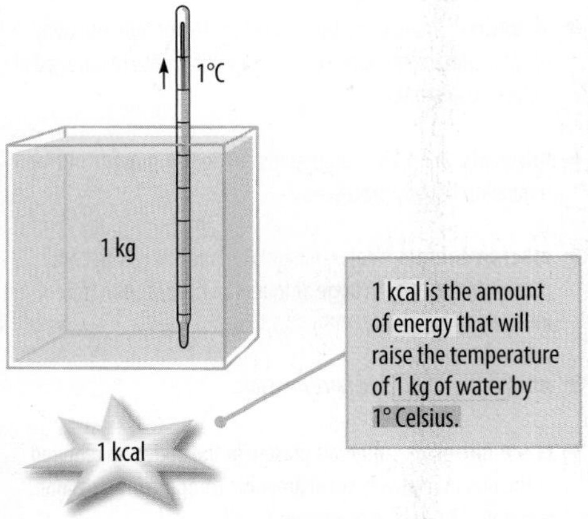

Nutrients and Energy

One major reason we eat food, and the nutrients it contains, is for **energy**. Every cellular reaction, every muscle movement, and every nerve impulse requires energy. Three of the nutrient classes—carbohydrates, lipids (triglycerides only), and proteins—are energy sources. Although not considered a nutrient, another energy source is alcohol. When we speak of the energy in foods, we are really talking about the *potential* energy that foods contain.

Different scientific disciplines use different measures of energy. In nutrition, we discuss the potential energy in food, or the body's use of energy, in units of heat called **kilocalories** (1,000 calories). One kilocalorie (or kcal) is the amount of energy (heat) it would take to raise the temperature of 1 kilogram (kg) of water by 1 degree Celsius. For now, this may be an abstract concept, but, as you learn more about nutrition, you will discover how much energy you likely need to fuel your daily activities. You also will learn about the amounts of potential energy in various foods. You'll find that food labels, diet books, and other sources of nutrition information generally use the term *calorie* rather than *kilocalorie*. Technically, the potential energy in foods is best measured in kilocalories; however, the term *calorie* has become familiar and commonplace. Throughout the text, we will use the terms *calorie* and *kilocalorie (kcal)* to mean generally the same thing.

▶ **energy** The capacity to do work. The energy in food is chemical energy, which the body converts to mechanical, electrical, or heat energy.

▶ **kilocalories (kcal)** [KILL-oh-kal-oh-rees] Units used to measure food energy (1,000 calories = 1 kilocalorie).

Energy in Foods

Energy is available from foods because foods contain carbohydrate, fat, and protein. These nutrients can be broken down completely (metabolized) to yield energy in a form that cells can use. When completely metabolized in the body, carbohydrate and protein yield 4 kilocalories of energy for every gram (g) consumed; fat yields 9 kilocalories per gram; and alcohol contributes 7 kilocalories per gram (see **FIGURE 1.11**). Therefore, the energy available from a given food or from a total diet is reflected by the amount of each of these substances consumed. Because fat is a concentrated source of energy, adding or removing fat from the diet can have a big effect on available energy.

How Can We Calculate the Energy Available from Foods?

To calculate the energy available from food, multiply the number of grams of fat, carbohydrate, and protein by 9, 4, and 4, respectively; then, add the results.

Here is an example:

One bagel with ½ ounce of cream cheese contains 39 grams of carbohydrate, 10 grams of protein, and 16 grams of fat, so:

Carbohydrate	39 grams × 4 calories per gram = 156 kcal
Protein	10 grams × 4 calories per gram = 40 kcal
Fat	16 grams × 9 calories per gram = 144 kcal
Total	**340 kcal**

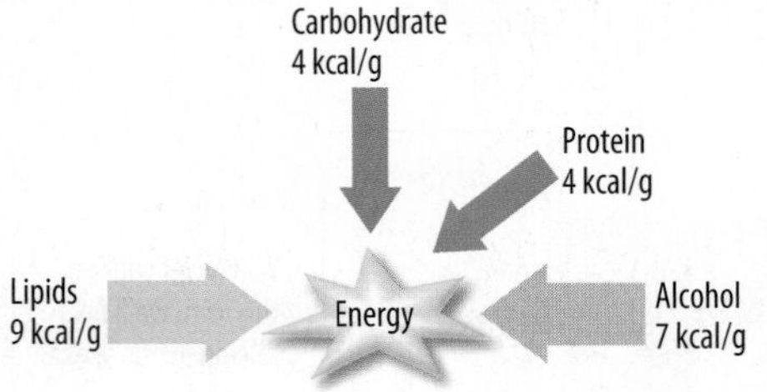

FIGURE 1.11 Energy sources. Carbohydrate, fat, protein, and alcohol provide different amounts of energy per gram.

Be Food Smart: Calculate the Percentages of Calories in Food

To calculate the *percentage* of calories that carbohydrate, protein, and fat each contribute to the total, divide the amount of kcal from each nutrient (carbohydrate, protein, fat) by the total amount of kcal and then multiply by 100.

For example, to determine the percentage of calories from fat in a bagel with cream cheese:

% of energy as carbohydrates = 156 kcal/340 kcal
= 0.459 × 100 = 46% kcal from carbohydrate

% of energy from protein = 40 kcal/340 kcal
= 0.118 × 100 = 12% kcal from protein

% of energy from fat = 144 kcal/340 kcal
= 0.423 × 100 = 42% kcal from fat

Current health recommendations suggest limiting fat intake to about 20 to 35 percent of *total* energy intake. You can monitor this for yourself in two ways. If you like counting fat grams, you can first determine your suggested maximum fat intake. For example, if you need to eat 2,000 kilocalories each day to maintain your current weight, at most 35 percent of those calories can come from fat:

2,000 kcal × 0.35 = 700 kcal from fat

700 kcal from fat ÷ 9 kcal/g = 77.8 g of fat

Therefore, your maximum fat intake should be about 78 grams/day. You can check food labels to see how many fat grams you typically eat.

Another way to monitor your fat intake is to know the percentage of calories that come from fat in various foods. If the proportion of fat in each food choice throughout the day exceeds 35 percent of calories, then the day's total of fat will be too high as well. Some foods contain virtually no fat calories (e.g., fruits, vegetables) whereas others are nearly 100 percent fat calories (e.g., margarine, salad dressing). Being aware that a snack like the bagel with cream cheese provides 42 percent of its calories from fat can help you select lower-fat foods at other times of the day.

Diet and Health

What does it mean to be healthy? The World Health Organization (WHO) defines health as "a state of complete physical, mental, and social well-being and not merely the absence of disease or infirmity."[31] Although we often focus on the last part of that definition, "the absence of disease or infirmity," the first part is equally important. As you have learned, nutrition is an important part of physical, mental, and social well-being. It also is important for preventing disease.

Disease can be defined as "an impairment of the normal state of the living animal or plant body or one of its parts that interrupts or modifies the performance of the vital functions" and can arise from environmental factors or specific infectious agents, such as bacteria or viruses.[32] Diseases can be *acute* (short-lived illnesses that arise and resolve quickly) or *chronic* (diseases with a slow onset and long duration). Although nutrition can affect our susceptibility to acute diseases—and contaminated food is certainly a source of acute disease—our food choices are more likely to affect our risk for developing chronic diseases such as heart disease or cancer. Other lifestyle factors, such as smoking and exercise, in addition to genetic factors, also determine who gets sick and who remains healthy. The 10 leading causes of death are listed in **TABLE 1.3**. Nutrition plays a role in the prevention or treatment of

Calculating the Energy Available from Foods and Percentage of Macronutrients in Your Diet

Example: If you know the amount of carbohydrates, protein, and fat that you eat each day, you can calculate the total amount of calories as well as the percentage of calories from each nutrient. In this example if you eat 275 g of carbohydrate, 75 g of protein and 67 g of fat you have eaten 2,000 kcal because:

275 g carbohydrate × 4 kcal/g = 1,100 kcal

75 g protein × 4 kcal/g = 300 kcal

67 g fat × 9 kcal/g = 600 kcal (rounded from 603 kcal)

Total = 2,000 kcal

Calculating the Percentage of Kilocalories from Carbohydrate, Protein, and Fat

Example:

275 g carbohydrate × 4 kcal/m = 1,100 kcal

1,100 kcal ÷ 2,000 kcal × 100 = 55% carbohydrate kcal

75 g protein × 4 kcal/g = 300 kcal

300 kcal ÷ 2,000 kcal × 100 = 15% protein kcal

67 g fat × 9 kcal/g = 600 kcal (rounded from 603 kcal)

600 kcal ÷ 2,000 kcal × 100 = 30% fat kcal

In this example, the 2,000 kcal have provided 55% of calories from carbohydrate, 15% of calories from protein, and 30% of calories from fat. As you will learn later, this macronutrient breakdown falls within the recommended intake ranges.

TABLE 1.3
Leading Causes of Death: United States

Rank	Cause of Death
1	Heart disease[a]
2	Cancer[a]
3	Chronic lower respiratory diseases
4	Stroke
5	Accidents (unintentional injuries)
6	Alzheimer's disease
7	Diabetes mellitus[a]
8	Influenza and pneumonia
9	Kidney disease[a]
10	Intentional self-harm (suicide)

[a] Causes for which nutrition is thought to be important in the prevention or treatment of the condition.

Reproduced from Kochanek KD, Xu J, Murphy SL, Miniño AM, Kung H-C. Deaths: preliminary data for 2009. *National Vital Statistics Reports.* 2011;59(4). http://www.cdc.gov/nchs/data/nvsr/nvsr59/nvsr59_04.pdf. Accessed December 18, 2015.

more than half of the conditions listed. Heart disease and cancer, together, account for almost half of all deaths.[33]

The foods we choose to eat do more than provide us with an adequate diet. The balance of energy sources can affect our risk of chronic disease. For example, high-fat diets have been linked to heart disease and cancer. Excess calories contribute to obesity, which also increases disease risk. Other nutrients, such as the minerals sodium, chloride, calcium, and magnesium, affect blood pressure, and a lack of the vitamin folate prior to conception and in early pregnancy can cause serious birth defects. Non-nutrient components in the diet (e.g., phytochemicals) may have antioxidant or immune-enhancing properties that also can keep us healthy. The choices we make can reduce our disease risk as well as provide energy and essential nutrients.

Physical Activity

A sedentary lifestyle is also a significant risk factor for chronic disease. Physically active people generally outlive those who are inactive, and, as a risk factor for heart disease, inactivity can be almost as significant as high blood pressure, smoking, or high blood cholesterol. Physical activity plays a significant role in long-term weight management. Current physical activity guidelines recommend that children and adolescents participate in 60 minutes or more of physical activity each day. Children should be encouraged to participate in activities that are age-appropriate, are enjoyable, and offer variety. Aerobic activity should make up most of a child's activity time, but muscle strengthening, such as gymnastics or doing push-ups, and bone strengthening, such as jumping rope or running, count as well. For adults, the Centers for Disease Control and Prevention set the recommendations to be measured as a weekly total, with the understanding that one can reach the suggested weekly time goals by breaking up exercise time into smaller chunks. Recommendations for adults include 150 minutes of moderate-intensity aerobic activity every week and muscle-strengthening activity on 2 or more days a week, or 75 minutes of vigorous-intensity aerobic activity every week and muscle-strengthening activities on 2 or more days a week.[34]

Key Concepts All cells and tissues need energy to keep the body functioning. Energy in foods and in the body is measured in kilocalories. The carbohydrates, lipids, and proteins in food are potential sources of energy, meaning that the body can extract energy from them. Excess energy intake is a contributing factor to obesity, a major public health issue. All individuals should aim to be physically active.

Applying the Scientific Process to Nutrition

Whether it's identifying essential nutrients, establishing recommended intake levels, or exploring the effects of vitamins on cancer risk, scientific studies are the cornerstone of nutrition. Although we may use creative, artistic talents to choose and serve a pleasing array of healthful foods, the fundamentals of nutrition are developed through the scientific process of observation and inquiry.

▶ **hypotheses** Scientists' educated guesses to explain phenomena.

The scientific process enables researchers to test the validity of **hypotheses** that arise from observations of natural phenomena. A hypothesis is a supposition or proposed explanation made on the basis of limited evidence as a starting point for further investigation. For example, it was common knowledge in the eighteenth century that sailors on long voyages would likely develop scurvy (which we now know results from a deficiency of vitamin C). Scurvy had been recognized since ancient times, and its common symptoms—pinpoint skin hemorrhages, swollen and bleeding gums, joint pain, fatigue and lethargy, and psychological changes such as depression and hysteria—were well known. Native populations discovered plant foods that would cure this illness; among Native Americans, these included cranberries in the Northeast and many tree extracts in other parts of the country. From observations such as these come questions that lead to hypotheses, or "educated guesses," about factors that might be responsible for the observed phenomenon. Scientists then test hypotheses using appropriate research designs. Poorly designed research can produce useless results or false conclusions. By following the steps of the scientific process (**FIGURE 1.12**), researchers can minimize influences that may arise during a research study (such as bias, prejudice, or coincidence). The scientific process (also referred to as the scientific method) follows these general steps: (1) Make observations, ask questions, or describe phenomena; (2) formulate a hypothesis to explain the observation, question, or phenomena; (3) test the hypothesis by conducting an experiment; (4) analyze data and draw conclusions; and (5) communicate results indicating whether or not the hypothesis is accepted.

Nutrition research is exciting and always changing. Scientists ask questions to be answered and define problems to be solved. Investigators choose a study design that will best answer their research question or hypothesis. Throughout the research process, researchers must follow rigorous ethical procedures in all areas of the study design. Common study designs used in nutrition research are defined in **TABLE 1.4**.

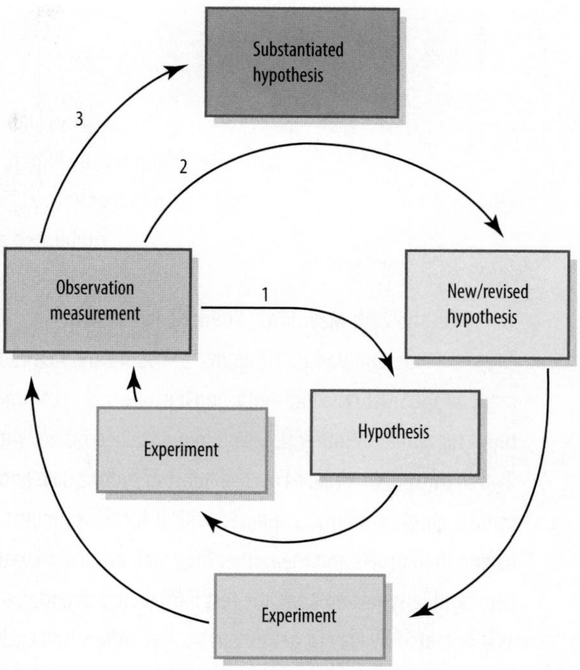

FIGURE 1.12 The scientific process. The scientific process (also referred to as the scientific method) follows these general steps: (1) make observations; (2) formulate a hypothesis; (3) test the hypothesis; (4) analyze the data and draw conclusions; and (5) communicate results.

TABLE 1.4
Common Study Designs Used in Nutrition Research

Study Type	Description
Human Studies	
Epidemiological studies	An epidemiological study compares disease rates among population groups and attempts to identify related conditions or behaviors such as diet and smoking habits. Epidemiological studies can provide useful information about relationships but often do not clarify cause and effect. The results of these studies show **correlations**—relationships between two or more factors; however, they do not establish or address cause and effect. Epidemiological studies can provide important clues and insights that lead to animal and human studies that can further clarify diet and disease relationships. The relationship between inadequate vitamin C intake and scurvy is one example of this.
Case control studies	**Case control studies** are small-scale epidemiological studies in which individuals who have a condition (e.g., breast cancer) are compared with similar individuals who do not have the condition. Researchers then identify factors other than the disease in question that differ between the two groups. These factors provide researchers with clues about the cause, progression, and prevention of the disease.
Clinical trials	**Clinical trials**, also called **intervention studies**, are controlled studies where some type of intervention (e.g., nutrient supplement, controlled diet, exercise program) is used to determine its impact on certain health parameters. These studies include an **experimental group** (the people experience the intervention) and a **control group** (similar people who are not treated). Scientists measure aspects of health or disease in each group and compare the results.
Animal Studies	Animal studies can provide preliminary data that often lead to human studies or can be used to study hypotheses that cannot be tested on humans. Although animal studies give scientists important information that furthers nutrition knowledge, the results of animal studies cannot be extrapolated directly to humans. Animal studies need to be followed with cell culture studies and ultimately human clinical studies to determine specific effects in humans.
Cell Culture Studies	Another way to study nutrition is to isolate specific types of cells and grow them in the laboratory. Scientists then can use these cells to study the effects of nutrients or other components on metabolic processes in the cell. An important area of nutrition research, called **nutrigenomics**, explores the effect of specific nutrients and other chemical compounds on gene expression. This area of molecular biology helps us explain individual differences in chronic disease risk factors and may lead to designing diets based on an individual's genetic profile.

▶ **correlations** Connections co-occurring more frequently than can be explained by chance or coincidence but without a proven cause.

▶ **case control studies** Investigations that use a group of people with a particular condition rather than a randomly selected population. These cases are compared with a control group of people who do not have the condition.

▶ **clinical trials** Studies that collect large amounts of data to evaluate the effectiveness of a treatment.

▶ **intervention studies** See *clinical trials*.

▶ **experimental group** A set of people being studied to evaluate the effect of an event, substance, or technique.

▶ **control group** A set of people used as a standard of comparison to the experimental group. The people in the control group have characteristics similar to those in the experimental group and are selected at random.

▶ **nutrigenomics** The study of how nutrition interacts with specific genes to influence a person's health.

James Lind: A Treatise of the Scurvy in Three Parts.
Containing an inquiry into the Nature, Causes and Cure of that Disease,
together with a Critical and Chronological View of what has been
published on the subject. A. Millar, London, 1753.

On the 20th May, 1747, I took twelve patients in the scurvy on board the Salisbury at sea. Their cases were as similar as I could have them. They all in general had putrid gums, the spots and lassitude, with weakness of their knees. They lay together in one place, being a proper apartment for the sick in the fore-hold; and had one diet in common to all, viz., water gruel sweetened with sugar in the morning; fresh mutton broth often times for dinner; at other times puddings, boiled biscuit with sugar ect.; and for supper barley, raisins, rice and currants, sago and wine, or the like. Two of these were ordered each, a quart of cyder a day. Two others took twenty five gutts of elixir vitriol three times a day upon an empty stomach, using a gargle strongly acidulated with it for their mouths. Two others took two spoonfuls of vinegar three times a day upon an empty stomach, having their gruels and their other food well acidulated with it, as also the gargle for the mouth. Two of the worst patients, with the tendons in the ham rigid (a symptom none the rest had) were put under, a course of sea water. Of this they drank half a pint every day and sometimes more or less as it operated by way of gentle physic. Two others had each, two oranges and one lemon given them every day. These they eat with greediness at different times upon an empty stomach. They continued but six days under, this course, having consumed the quantity that could be spared. The two remaining patients took the bigness of a nutmeg three times a day of an electuray recommended by an hospital surgeon made of garlic, mustard seed, rad. raphan., balsam of Peru and gum myrrh, using for common drink narley water well acidulated with tamarinds, by a decoction of wich, with the addition of cremor tartar, they were gently purged three or four times during the course.

The consequence was that the most sudden and visible good effects were perceived from the use of the oranges and lemons; one of those who had taken them being at the end of six days fit four duty. The spots were not indeed at that time quite off his body, nor his gums sound; but without any other medicine than a gargarism or, elixir of vitriol he became quite healthy before we came into Plymouth, which was on the 16th June. The other was the best recovered of any in his condition, and being now deemed pretty well was appointed nurse to the rest of the sick...

As I shall have occasion elsewhere to take notice of the effects of other medicines in this disease, I shall here only observe that the result of all my experiments was that oranges and lemons were the most effectual remedies for this distemper at sea. I am apt to think oranges preferable to lemons...

FIGURE 1.13 The first clinical trial. In 1753, physician James Lind reported the careful process of his clinical trial among British sailors afflicted with scurvy.

James Lind's experiments with sailors aboard the *Salisbury* in 1747 are considered to be the first dietary clinical trial (see **FIGURE 1.13**). His observation that oranges and lemons were the only dietary elements that seemed to cure scurvy was an important finding. However, it took more than 40 years before the British Navy began routinely giving all sailors citrus juice or fruit, such as lemons or limes—a practice that led to the nickname "limeys" when referring to British sailors. It took nearly 200 years (until the 1930s) for scientists to isolate the compound we call vitamin C and show that it had antiscurvy properties.[35] The chemical name for vitamin C, ascorbic acid, comes from its role as an antiscorbutic (antiscurvy) compound.

Modern clinical trials include several important elements: random assignment to groups, use of placebos, and the double-blind method. Subjects are assigned randomly—as by the flip of a coin—to the experimental group or the control group. Randomization potentially reduces, minimizes, or eliminates selection and volunteer bias. People in the experimental group receive the treatment or specific protocol (e.g., consuming a certain nutrient at a specific level). People in the control group do not receive the treatment but usually receive a **placebo**. A placebo is an imitation treatment (such as a sugar pill) that looks the same as the experimental treatment but has no effect. The placebo also is important for reducing bias because subjects do not know if they are receiving the intervention and are less inclined to alter their responses or reported symptoms based on what they think should happen. The *expectation* that a medication will be effective can be nearly as effective as the medication itself—a phenomenon called the **placebo effect**. Because the placebo effect can exert a powerful influence, research studies must take it into account.

When the members of neither the experimental nor the control group know what treatment they are receiving, we say the subjects are "blinded" to the treatment. If a clinical trial is designed so that neither the subjects nor the researchers collecting data are aware of the subjects' group assignments (experimental or control), the study is called a **double-blind study**. This reduces the possibility that researchers will see the results they want to see even if these results do not occur. In this case, another member of the research team holds the code for subject assignments and does not participate in the data collection. Double-blind, placebo-controlled clinical trials are considered the gold standard of nutrition studies. These studies can show clear cause-and-effect relationships but often require large numbers of subjects and are expensive and time consuming to conduct.

▶ **placebo** An inactive substance that is outwardly indistinguishable from the active substance whose effects are being studied.

▶ **placebo effect** A physical or emotional change that is not caused by properties of an administered substance. The change reflects participants' expectations.

▶ **double-blind study** A research study set up so that neither the subjects nor the investigators know which study group is receiving the placebo and which is receiving the active substance.

Key Concepts The scientific method is used to expand our nutrition knowledge. Hypotheses are formed from observations and are then tested by experiments. Epidemiological studies observe patterns in populations. Animal and cell culture studies can test the effects of various treatments. For human studies, randomized, double-blind, placebo-controlled clinical trials are the best research tools for determining cause-and-effect relationships.

From Research Study to Headline

What about the health headlines we see in the newspapers, hear on television, or read on the Internet daily? Consumers often are confused by what they see as the "wishy-washiness" of scientists—for example, coffee is good, then coffee is bad. Margarine is better than butter.... No wait, maybe butter is better after all. These contradictions, despite the confusion they cause, show us that nutrition is truly a science: dynamic, changing, and growing with each new finding.

Publishing Experimental Results

Once an experiment is complete, scientists publish the results in a scientific journal to communicate new information to other scientists. Generally, before articles are published in scientific journals, other scientists who have expert knowledge of the subject critically review them. This **peer review** greatly reduces the chance that low-quality research is published. Peer-reviewed journals such as the *American Journal of Clinical Nutrition* and the *Journal of the Academy of Nutrition and Dietetics* are not the main sources of information presented in the popular media. Often, a new article becomes a 30-second sound bite that often fails to reflect the original data. In some cases, the study may be distorted, with its results misstated or overstated (see **FIGURE 1.14**).

▶ **peer review** An appraisal of research against accepted standards by professionals in the field.

Quick Bite

Controlling the Pesky Placebo

When researchers tested the effectiveness of a medication in reducing binge eating among people with bulimia, they used a double-blind, placebo-controlled study to eliminate the placebo effect. After a baseline number of binge-eating episodes was determined, 22 women with bulimia were given the medication or a placebo. After a period of time, the number of binge-eating episodes was reassessed. The group taking the medication had a 78 percent reduction in binge-eating episodes. Sounds good, right? But, the placebo group had a similar reduction of 70 percent. The placebo effect was nearly as powerful as the medication.

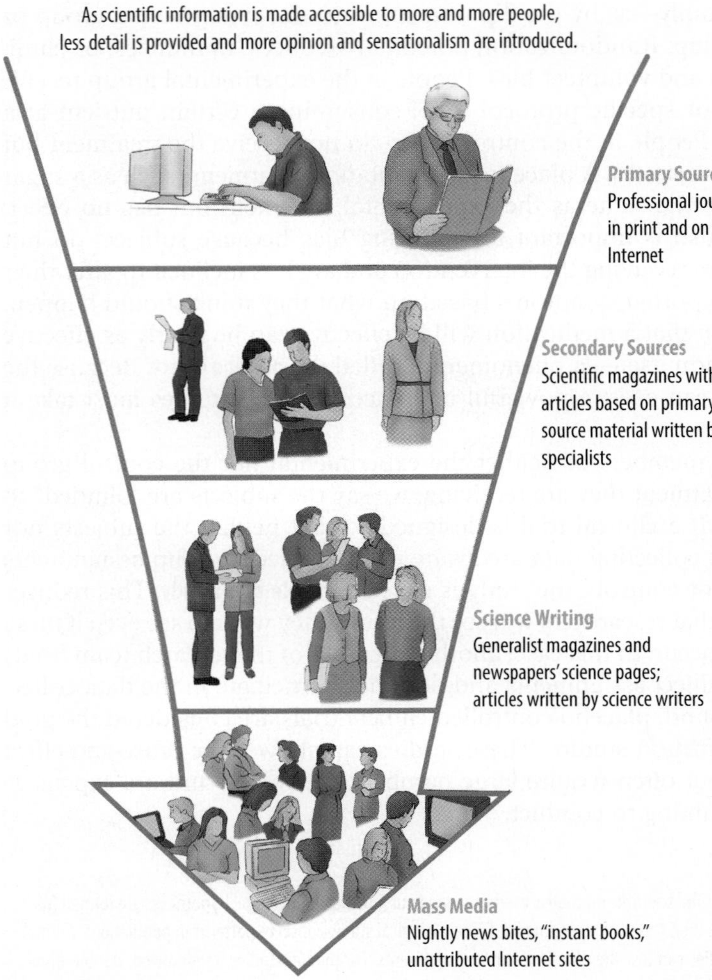

As scientific information is made accessible to more and more people, less detail is provided and more opinion and sensationalism are introduced.

Secondary Sources
Scientific magazines with articles based on primary source material written by specialists
Science Writing

Mass Media
Nightly news bites, "instant books," unattributed Internet sites

FIGURE 1.14 Sorting facts and fallacies. From original research to the evening news, each step along the way introduces biases as information is summarized and restated. Whether on television, radio, the Internet or in print, the best consumer information cites sources for reported facts.

Sorting Facts and Fallacies in the Media

THINK About It 4

People tend to believe what they hear repeatedly. Even when it has no basis in fact, a claim can seem credible if heard often enough. For example, do you believe that sugar makes kids hyperactive? There is little scientific evidence

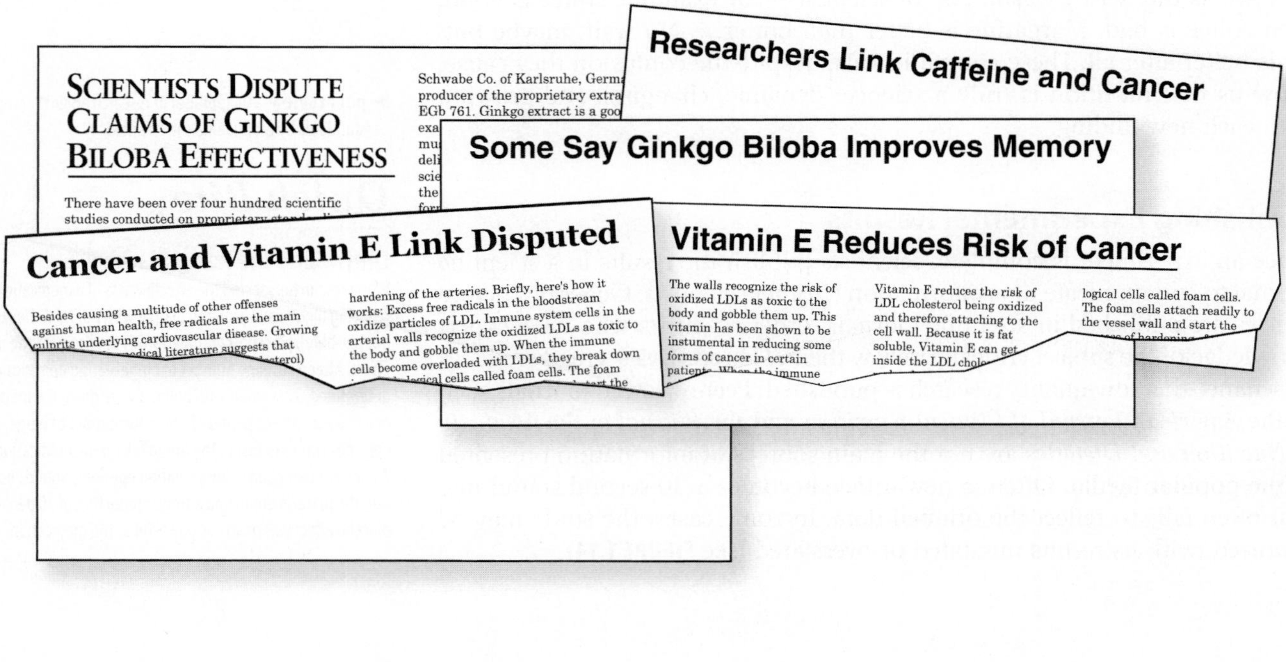
Scientists Dispute Claims of Ginkgo Biloba Effectiveness
There have been over four hundred scientific studies conducted on proprietary standardized
Schwabe Co. of Karlsruhe, Germany producer of the proprietary extract EGb 761. Ginkgo extract is a goo
Researchers Link Caffeine and Cancer
Some Say Ginkgo Biloba Improves Memory
Cancer and Vitamin E Link Disputed
Besides causing a multitude of other offenses against human health, free radicals are the main culprits underlying cardiovascular disease. Growing
hardening of the arteries. Briefly, here's how it works: Excess free radicals in the bloodstream oxidize particles of LDL. Immune system cells in the arterial walls recognize the oxidized LDLs as toxic to the body and gobble them up. When the immune cells become overloaded with LDLs, they break down
Vitamin E Reduces Risk of Cancer
The walls recognize the risk of oxidized LDLs as toxic to the body and gobble them up. This vitamin has been shown to be instumental in reducing some forms of cancer in certain
Vitamin E reduces the risk of LDL cholesterol being oxidized and therefore attaching to the cell wall. Because it is fat soluble, Vitamin E can get inside the LDL chole
logical cells called foam cells. The foam cells attach readily to the vessel wall and start the

to support this claim! Although news stories may be based on reports in the scientific literature, the media can distort the facts through omission of details.

Evaluating Information on the Internet

Surfing the Web has made life easier in many ways. You can buy a car, check stock prices, search out sources for a paper you're writing, chat with like-minded people, and stay up-to-date on news or sports scores. Hundreds of websites are devoted to nutrition and health topics, and you may be asked to visit such sites as part of your course requirements. So, how do you evaluate the quality of information on the Web? Can you trust what you see?

First, it's important to remember that there are no rules for posting on the Internet. Anyone who has the equipment can set up a website and post any content he or she likes. Although the Health on the Net Foundation has set up a Code of Conduct for medical and health websites, following its eight principles is completely voluntary.[36]

Second, consider the source, if you can tell what it is. Many websites do not specify where the content came from, who is responsible for it, or how often it is updated. If the site lists the authors, what are their credentials? Who sponsors the site itself? Educational institutions (.edu), government agencies (.gov), and organizations (.org) generally have more credibility than commercial (.com) sites, where selling rather than educating is the primary motive. Identifying the purpose for a site can give you more clues about the validity of its content.

Third, when you see claims for nutrients, dietary supplements, or other products and the results of studies or other information, keep in mind the scientific method and the basics of sound science. Who did the study? What type of study was it? How many subjects? Was it double-blind? Were the results published in a peer-reviewed journal? Think critically about the content, look at other sources, and ask questions of experts before you accept information as truth. What is true of books, magazines, and newspapers also applies to the Internet: Just because it is in print or online doesn't mean it's true.

Finally, be on the lookout for "junk science"—sloppy methods, interpretations, and claims that lead to public misinformation. The Food and Nutrition Science Alliance (FANSA) is a coalition of several health organizations, including the Academy of Nutrition and Dietetics. FANSA has developed the "10 Red Flags of Junk Science" to help consumers identify potential misinformation. Use these red flags to evaluate websites.

The 10 Red Flags of Junk Science[37]

1. Recommendations that promise a quick fix
2. Dire warnings of danger from a single product or regimen
3. Claims that sound too good to be true
4. Simplistic conclusions drawn from a complex study
5. Recommendations based on a single study
6. Statements refuted by reputable scientific organizations
7. Lists of "good" and "bad" foods
8. Recommendations made to help sell a product
9. Recommendations based on studies that were not peer reviewed
10. Recommendations from studies that ignore differences among individuals or groups

Use the Internet; it's fun and can be educational. Don't forget about the library, though, because many scientific journals are not available online. Treat claims as "guilty until proven innocent"—in other words, don't accept what you read at face value until you have evaluated the science behind it. If it sounds too good to be true, it probably is!

FYI For Your Information

The Affordable Care Act and Nutrition

The Affordable Care Act (ACA), also known as Obamacare, was signed into law on March 23, 2010. By 2014, much of the new policy had been implemented. Here is a brief summary of health coverage, costs, and care provided by the law.[a]

Coverage

- *Ends pre-existing condition exclusions:* Health plans can no longer deny or limit benefits due to a pre-existing condition.
- *Keeps young adults covered:* If you are under 26, you may be eligible to be covered under your parents' health plan.
- *Ends arbitrary withdrawals of insurance coverage:* Insurers can no longer cancel your coverage just because you made an honest mistake.
- *Guarantees the right to appeal:* You now have the right to ask that your plan reconsider its denial of payment.

Costs

- *Ends lifetime limits on coverage:* There are no longer limits on the amount paid out for most benefits over a lifetime.
- *Reviews premium increases:* Insurance companies must now publicly justify any unreasonable rate hikes.
- *Helps you get the most from your premium dollars:* The majority of your premium dollars (amount charged for your plan) must be spent primarily on health care—not administrative costs.

Care

- *Covers preventive care at no cost to you:* You may be eligible for recommended preventive health services with no copayment.
- *Protects your choice of doctors:* From your plan's network, you can choose the primary care doctor you want.
- *Removes insurance company barriers to emergency services:* You can seek emergency care at a hospital outside of your health plan's network.[b]

Benefits to College Students

Before the ACA, what was health insurance like for college students? Most colleges required students to either purchase health insurance or continue enrollment in their parents' plans. As previously mentioned, under the ACA students are now able to stay on their parents' health-insurance plans until age 26—even if they are married or have coverage through employers.

Since 2014, college students, like other sectors of the population, have had to abide by the "individual mandate" in the ACA, which requires most people to obtain insurance or pay tax penalties. That's where the *exchanges* come in for students who aren't on their parents' plans and don't want to purchase insurance through their schools: Each state provides health insurance exchanges for qualified Americans to purchase affordable coverage. Each state also has its own exchange that offers a variety of coverage options from private, state-regulated insurance companies—often cheaper than other options. However, the National Center for Public Policy calculated that a college student's penalty for nonenrollment ($325 or 2% of income in 2015) could be cheaper in the short-term (if you don't get sick) than paying for health insurance.

Alternatively, students who can't afford insurance may qualify for Medicaid if their income is below a certain threshold. To see whether you're eligible, check with your state department of health insurance.

Another option for those under 30 is to purchase a *catastrophic health plan*. These plans usually feature low monthly premiums, but the insured are required to pay all their medical costs up to a certain amount, usually several thousand dollars. The insurance company pays for essential health benefits over that amount, essentially providing participants with protection in the event of serious accidents or illnesses.

Finally, individuals with nonimmigrant status, including people on worker visas and student visas, can qualify for insurance coverage through the exchanges.[c]

Heath Care Reform, Preventive Care, and Nutrition

The ACA emphasizes prevention through wellness plans, outreach campaigns, and more opportunities to see registered dietitian nutritionists. The law supports counseling and behavioral interventions in the areas of obesity, breastfeeding, chronic diseases, blood pressure, and cholesterol. It requires most plans to cover calcium and vitamin D testing for women over 60 at risk for osteoporosis, anemia screening for most pregnant women, folic acid pills, and type 2 diabetes screening for adults with high blood pressure.

The ACA also requires proper nutrition labeling in chain restaurants and vending machines, which informs consumers about calories so that they will be aware of the recommended daily caloric intake and its effect on obesity. Should the consumer request it, the following information must be available on menus or display items: total calories, calories from fat, total fat, saturated fat, cholesterol, trans fat, sodium, total carbohydrates, sugars, dietary fiber, and protein.[d,e]

[a] U.S. Department of Health and Human Services, Health Resources and Services Administration, Maternal and Child Health. The Affordable Care Act (ACA) and the nutrition workforce: A summary report. http://www.mchb.hrsa.gov/training/pgm-hi-nutri.asp. Accessed December 18, 2015.

[b] HealthCare.gov. Accessed May 6, 2015.

[c] *Christian Science Monitor.* Obamacare 101: What to know if you opt out of buying health insurance. http://www.csmonitor.com/USA/DC-Decoder/2013/1001/Obamacare-101-What-to-know-if-you-opt-out-of-buying-health-insurance. Accessed December 18, 2015.

[d] Obamacare Facts. Summary of provisions in the Patient Protection and Affordable Care Act. http://obamacarefacts.com/summary-of-provisions-patient-protection-and-affordable-care-act. Accessed December 18, 2015.

[e] WebMD. Understanding the Affordable Care Act and women's health. http://www.webmd.com/health-insurance/covered-preventive-tests-screenings. Accessed January 15, 2015.

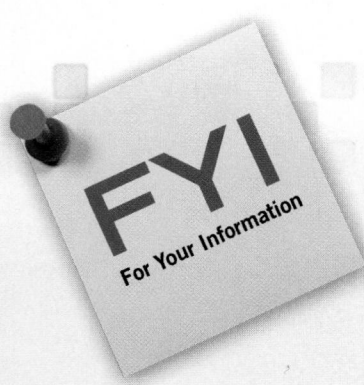

As you learn about nutrition, you will undoubtedly be more aware not only of your eating and shopping habits, but also of nutrition-related information in the media. As you see and hear reports, stop to think carefully about what you are hearing. Headlines and news reports often overstate the findings of a study. Two other things to keep in mind: One study does not provide all the answers to our nutrition questions; and if it sounds too good to be true, it probably is!

Your study of nutrition is just beginning. As you learn about the essential nutrients, their functions, and food sources, be alert to your food choices and the factors that influence them. When the discussion turns to the role of diet in health, think about your preconceived ideas and evaluate your beliefs in light of the current scientific evidence. Keep an open mind, but also think critically. Most of all, remember that food is more than the nutrients it provides; it is part of the way we enjoy and celebrate life!

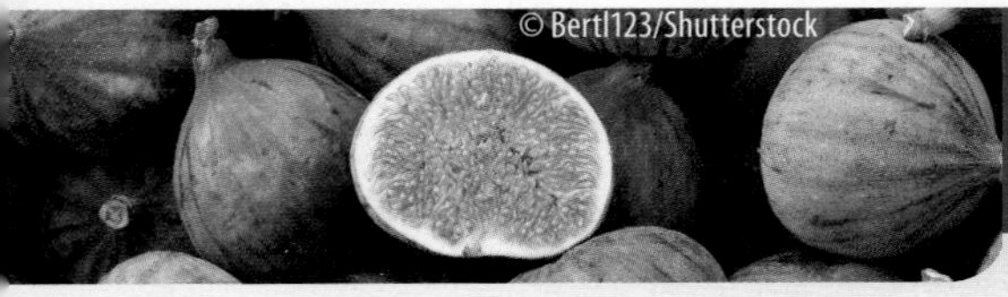
© Bertl123/Shutterstock

Learning Portfolio

Key Terms

Study Points

- Most people make food choices for reasons other than nutrient value.
- Taste and texture are the two most important factors that influence food choices.
- In all cultures, eating is the primary way of maintaining social relationships.
- Although most North Americans know about healthful food choices, their eating habits do not always reflect this knowledge.
- Food is a mixture of chemicals. Essential chemicals in food are called nutrients.
- Carbohydrates, lipids, proteins, vitamins, minerals, and water are the six classes of nutrients found in food.
- Nutrients have three general functions in the body: They serve as energy sources, structural components, and regulators of metabolic processes.
- Vitamins regulate body processes such as energy metabolism, blood clotting, and calcium balance.
- Minerals contribute to body structures and to regulating processes such as fluid balance.
- Water is the most important nutrient in the body. We can survive much longer without the other nutrients than we can without water.
- Energy in foods and the body is measured in kilocalories. Carbohydrates, fats, and proteins are sources of energy.
- Carbohydrate and protein have a potential energy value of 4 kilocalories per gram, and fat provides 9 kilocalories per gram.
- Scientific studies are the cornerstone of nutrition. The scientific method uses observation and inquiry to test hypotheses.
- Double-blind, placebo-controlled clinical trials are considered the gold standard of nutrition studies.
- Research designs used to test hypotheses include epidemiological, animal, cell culture, and human studies.
- Information in the public media is not always an accurate or complete representation of the current state of the science on a particular topic.

Study Questions

1. Name three sensory aspects of food that influence our food choices.
2. How do our health beliefs affect our food choices?
3. List the six classes of nutrients.
4. List the 13 vitamins.
5. What determines whether a mineral is a macromineral or a micromineral (trace mineral)?
6. How many kilocalories are in 1 gram of carbohydrate? One gram of protein? One gram of fat?

7. What is an epidemiological study?
8. What is the difference between an experimental and a control group?
9. What is a placebo?

Try This

Try a New Cuisine Challenge

Expand your culinary taste buds and try a new cuisine. Go to the grocery store or nearby restaurant and select a cuisine you are not very familiar with. If you go out to eat, take some friends along for dinner so that you can order and share more than one dish. While you're there, don't be afraid to ask questions about the menu so that you can gain a better understanding of the foods, preparation techniques, spices, and even the cultural meaning attached to some of the dishes. If you select food from the grocery store, choose food or dishes with minimal preparation—maybe something from the frozen section. As you try the new food(s), think about your eating experience in terms of sensory properties. Are the smells, flavors, and textures different from what you are used to eating? Do you like the new foods you are trying, and/or do you think that after multiple exposures to the food you would learn to like it?

Food Label Puzzle

The purpose of this exercise is to put the individual pieces of the food label together to determine how many kilocalories are in a serving. Pick six foods in your dorm room or home that have complete food labels. On a separate sheet of paper, write down the value for grams of total carbohydrate, protein, and fat in one serving. Now, using information from this chapter, calculate the amount of calories per serving, using the macronutrient amounts. Check your answer against the package information. Remember that the term *calories* on a food label is really referring to kilocalories. Your job is to determine how many kilocalories are in a serving of each of these foods. You can do this by putting together the individual pieces (carbohydrate, protein, and fat). If you need help, review this chapter and pay close attention to the section on the energy-yielding nutrients. How many kilocalories does each have per gram? You may find that the results of your calculations don't exactly match the numbers on the label. Within labeling guidelines, food manufacturers can round values.

Getting Personal

Why Are You Eating?

Choose one day this week to evaluate why you are eating. Using the table below, list all of the foods and drinks that you consume in a 24-hour period. Select a day where your schedule is fairly predictable and you are eating what is considered normal for you. Using factors that influence food choices as discussed in the section "Why Do We Eat the Way We Do?," identify why you consumed each food that you ate. Example reasons could be: you felt hungry; you wanted the flavor of a particular food that was available; it is a habit to eat at that particular time; or everyone else was eating right then. Keep in mind that there may be more than one reason for eating. Also, using the Hunger/Fullness scale below, rate how hungry you were before you started eating and rate how full you were after you finished eating.

Time	Food or Drink	Amount	Why I Ate	Hunger and Fullness Rating: Before	Hunger and Fullness Rating: After

Rating System to Determine How Hungry and How Full You Are Feeling

0 or 1: Empty feeling in your stomach; you feel grumpy and irritable.

2 or 3: Feeling very hungry; you want to eat just about any type of food.

4: Feeling some hunger pangs; particular foods are starting to sound good to you.

5: Neutral; you have no strong feelings of hunger or fullness.

6 or 7: Satisfied; you are content with your recent food choices and the amount of food that you have eaten.

8: Full; you feel like you may have overeaten just a bit.

9: Stuffed; you feel like you have overeaten.

10: Sick feeling in your stomach; you feel like you ate much more than you should have.

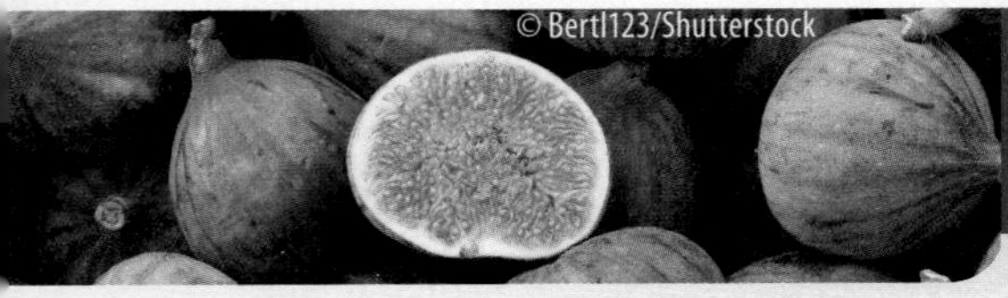

© Bertl123/Shutterstock

Learning Portfolio (continued)

Questions to ask yourself

- Was there one reason that you ate that appeared more often than any other? If so, what was that reason?
- Are health and nutrition concerns ever a reason for your eating? If not, how can you make eating for health and nutrition concerns a priority?
- Looking at your hunger and fullness ratings, are you eating when you are hungry and stopping when you are satisfied? What changes can you make to become a more mindful and healthy eater?

*Hunger and Fullness Scale adapted from: Tribole E, Resch E. *Intuitive Eating: A Revolutionary Program That Works*. New York: St. Martin's Griffin; 2003.

References

1. National Institutes of Health, U.S. National Library of Medicine. Joint collection development policy: human nutrition and food. February 27, 1998. http://www.nlm.nih.gov/pubs/cd_hum.nut.html. Accessed December 18, 2015.
2. Kittler PG, Sucher KP, Nelms M. *Food and Culture*. 6th ed. Belmont, CA: Wadsworth; 2011.
3. Mennella JA. Ontogeny of taste preferences: basic biology and implications for health. *Am J Clin Nutr*. 2014;99(3):704S–711S. Epub January 22, 2014.
4. Ibid.
5. Ibid.
6. Ibid.
7. Bachmanov AA, Bosak NP, Lin C, et al. Genetics of taste receptors. *Curr Pharm Des*. 2014;20(16):2669–83
8. Federal Trade Commission. FTC releases follow-up study detailing promotional activities, expenditures, and nutritional profiles of food marketed to children and adolescents. December 21, 2012. http://www.ftc.gov/news-events/press-releases/2012/12/ftc-releases-follow-study-detailing-promotional-activities. Accessed December 18, 2015.
9. Powell LM, Harris JL, Fox T. Food marketing expenditures aimed at youth: putting the numbers in context. *Am J Prev Med*. 2013;45(4):453–461.
10. Goris JM,, Petersen S, Stamatakis E, Veerman JL. Television food advertising and the prevalence of childhood overweight and obesity. A multicountry comparison. *Public Health*. 2010;13:1003.
11. Larson N, Story M. *Menu Labeling: Does Providing Nutrition Information at the Point of Purchase Affect Consumer Behavior? A Research Synthesis*. Healthy Eating Research. A National Program of the Robert Wood Johnson Foundation. June 2009. http://www.rwjf.org/en/research-publications/find-rwjf-research/2009/06/menu-labeling.html. Accessed December 18, 2015.
12. Burton S, Creyer E, Kees J, et al. Attacking the obesity epidemic: The 27 potential health benefits of providing nutrition information in restaurants. *Am J Public Health*. 2006;96(9):1669–1675.
13. Roberto CA, Larsen PD, Agnew H, Baik J, Browneli KD. Evaluating the impact of menu labeling on food choices and intake. *Am J Public Health*. 2010;100(2):312–318. Epub December 17, 2009.
14. Tandon PS, Wright J, Zhou C, Rogers CB, Christakis DA. Nutrition menu labeling may lead to lower-calorie restaurant meal choices for children. *Pediatrics*. 2010;125(2):244–248. Epub January 25, 2010.
15. National Foundation for Celiac Awareness. Spins: annual gluten-free sales reach $12.4 billion. September 18, 2012. http://www.celiaccentral.org/celiac-disease-in-the-news/gluten-free-sales-reach-12-billion-spins-8561/. Accessed December 18, 2015.
16. Laulais L, Doyon M, Ruffeux B, Kaiser H. Consumer knowledge about dietary fats: another French paradox? *Br Food J*. 2012;114(1):108–120.
17. Layman DK. Eating patterns, diet quality and energy balance: a perspective about applications and future directions for the food industry. *Physiol Behav*. 2014;134:126–130.
18. U.S. Department of Agriculture. Food prices and spending. February 2014. http://www.ers.usda.gov/data-products/ag-and-food-statistics-charting-the-essentials/food-prices-and-spending.aspx#.UznDOyjPCLE. Accessed December 18, 2015.
19. Hayden S, Hyman J, Buzby JC, Frazao E, Carlson A. *How Much Do Fruit and Vegetables Cost?* Economic Information Bulletin No. (EIB-71). USDA Economic Research Service. February 2011. http://www.ers.usda.gov/publications/eib-economic-information-bulletin/eib71.aspx#.UzxaZSjPCLE. Accessed December 18, 2015.
20. Economic Research Service. Food desert locator: documentation. http://www.ers.usda.gov/data-products/food-access-research-atlas.aspx. Accessed December 18, 2015.
21. Let's Move! Taking on "food deserts." http://www.letsmove.gov/blog/2010/02/24/taking-food-deserts. Accessed December 18, 2015.
22. Bryant CA, DeWalt KM, Courtney A, Schwartz J. *The Cultural Feast: An Introduction to Food and Society*. 2nd ed. Belmont, CA: Wadsworth; 2004.
23. Kittler, Sucher, Nelms. *Food and Culture*.
24. U.S. Department of Agriculture, U.S. Department of Health and Human Services. *Dietary Guidelines for Americans, 2015-2020*. 8th ed. Washington, DC: US Government Printing Office; January 2016.

25. USDA Ag and Food Statistics: Charting the Essentials. Food Availability and Consumption. http://www.ers.usda.gov/data-products/ag-and-food-statistics-charting-the-essentials/food-availability-and-consumption.aspx#.U44CfJRdVor)
26. Blisard N, Stewart H. *Food Spending in American Households 2003–2004.* Economic Information Bulletin (EIB-23). U.S. Department of Agriculture, Economic Research Service. March 2007. http://www.usda.gov/wps/portal/usda/usdahome?contentidonly=true&contentid=ERS_Agency_Splash.xml. Accessed 2/2/2016
27. Bowman, S. Clemens J, Friday J, Moshfegh, A. Food Patterns Equivalents Intakes from Food: Mean Amounts Consumer per Individual, What We Eat In America, NHANES 2011-12; Tables 1-4. http://www.ars.usda.gov/research/publications/publications.htm?seq_no_115=312662
28. U.S. Department of Agriculture, U.S. Department of Health and Human Services. *Dietary Guidelines for Americans, 2010.* 7th ed. Washington, DC: U.S. Government Printing Office; December 18, 2015.
29. Luo WP, Fang YJ, Lu MS, et al. High consumption of vegetable and fruit colour groups is inversely associated with the risk of colorectal cancer: a case-control study. *Br J Nutr*. 2015;16:1–10.
30. Food and Nutrition Board. *Dietary Reference Intakes for Energy, Carbohydrate, Fiber, Fat, Fatty Acids, Cholesterol, Protein, and Amino Acids.* Washington, DC: Food and Nutrition Board; 2002.
31. MedlinePlus. Minerals. http://www.nlm.nih.gov/medlineplus/minerals.html. Accessed December 18, 2015.
32. Centers for Disease Control and Prevention. Physical activity basics: how much physical activity do you need? http://www.cdc.gov/physicalactivity/everyone/guidelines/index.html. Accessed December 18, 2015.
33. Ross A, Caballero B, Cousins R, Tucker K, Ziegler T. *Modern Nutrition in Health and Disease*. 11th ed. Philadelphia: Lippincott Williams & Wilkins; 2014.
34. Kochanek KD, Xu J, Murphy SL, Miniño AM, Kung H-C. Deaths: preliminary data for 2009. *National Vital Statistics Reports*. 2011;59(4). http://www.cdc.gov/nchs/data/nvsr/nvsr59/nvsr59_04.pdf. Accessed December 18, 2015.
35. U.S. Department of Health and Human Services. 2008 physical activity guidelines: chapter 4: active adults. http://www.health.gov/paguidelines/guidelines/chapter4.aspx. Accessed December 18, 2015.
36. Levine M, Katz A, Padayatty SJ. Vitamin C. In: Shils ME, Shike M, Ross AC, et al., eds. *Modern Nutrition in Health and Disease*. 10th ed. Philadelphia: Lippincott Williams & Wilkins; 2006.
37. Health on the Net Foundation. The HON code of conduct for medical and health web sites (HONcode). http://www.hon.ch/HONcode/Conduct.html. Accessed December 18, 2015.
38. Academy of Nutrition and Dietetics. Practice Paper: Nutrition Informatics. Bolume 112, issue 11, page 1859 (November 2012) http://www.eatrightpro.org/resource/practice/position-and-practice-papers/practice-papers/practice-paper-nutrition-informatics. Accessed 2/2/2016.

Chapter 2

Nutrition Guidelines and Assessment

Revised by Kimberley McMahon

THINK About It

1. Do you think that the food choices you make today will effect your future health?
2. Have you ever taken a very large dose of a vitamin or mineral? If so, why? How did you determine whether it was safe?
3. Do you eat the same foods most days, or do you select a variety of foods from day to day?

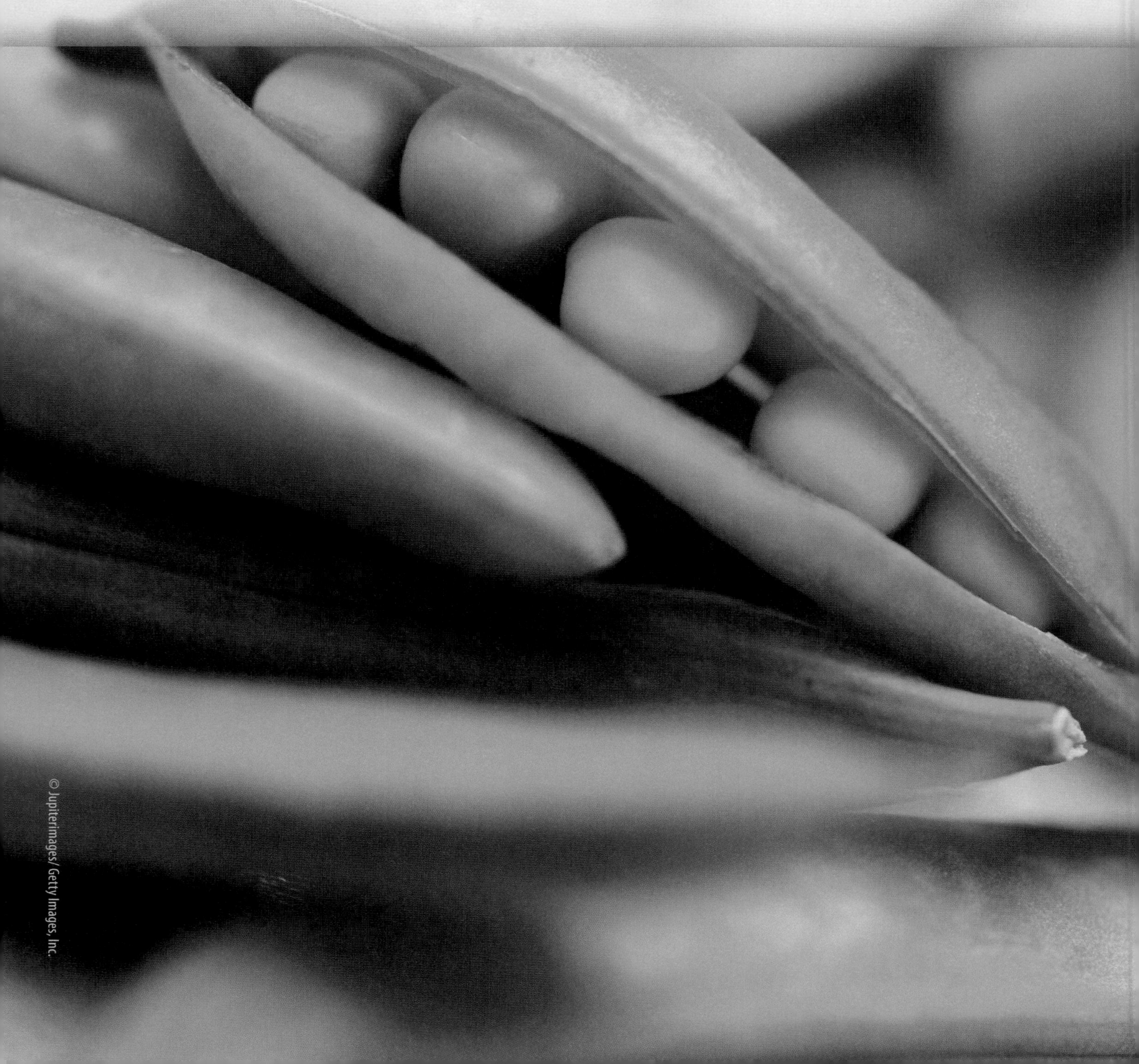

© Jupiterimages/Getty Images, Inc.

CHAPTER Menu

- Linking Nutrients, Foods, and Health
- Dietary Guidelines
- From Dietary Guidelines to Planning: What You Will Eat
- Exchange Lists
- Recommendations for Nutrient Intake: The DRIs
- Food Labels
- Nutrition Assessment: Determining Nutritional Health
- Nutrition Assessment Methods
- Key Terms
- Study Points
- Study Questions
- Try This
- Getting Personal
- References

LEARNING Objectives

- Describe and discuss the nutrition concepts of adequacy: balance, calorie control, nutrient density, moderation, and variety.
- List the key recommendations of the *Dietary Guidelines for Americans, 2015-2020.*
- Define the Dietary Reference Intake values: DRI, EAR, RDA, AI, and DV.
- Identify five mandatory components of a food label.
- List and describe four major factors in nutrition assessment of an individual.

So, you want to be healthier—maybe that's why you are taking this course! You probably already know that a well-planned diet is one important element of being healthy. Although most of us know that the foods we choose to eat have a major impact on our health, we aren't always certain about what choices to make. Choosing the right foods isn't made any easier when we are bombarded by headlines and advertisements: Eat less fat! Get more fiber in your diet! Moderation is the key! Build strong bones with calcium!

For many Americans, nutrition is simply a lot of hearsay, or maybe the latest slogan coined from last week's news headlines. Conversations about nutrition start with "*They* say you should…" or "Now *they* think that…". Have you ever wondered who "they" are and why "they" are telling you what to eat or what not to eat?

It's no secret that a healthy population is a more productive population, so many of our nutrition guidelines come from the federal government's efforts to improve our overall health. Thus, the government is one "they." Undernutrition and overnutrition are examples of two nutrition problems that government policy has addressed.

Many important elements of nutrition policy focus on relieving **undernutrition** in some population groups. Let's look at some examples. To prevent widespread deficiencies, the government requires food manufacturers to add nutrients to certain foods: iodine to salt, vitamin D to milk, and thiamin, riboflavin, niacin, iron, and folic acid to enriched grains. Another example is the creation of dietary standards, such as the Dietary Reference Intakes, which make it easier to define adequate diets for large groups of people.

▶ **undernutrition** Poor health resulting from depletion of nutrients caused by inadequate nutrient intake over time. It is now most often associated with poverty, alcoholism, and some types of eating disorders.

Overnutrition, or the excessive intake of food, especially in unbalanced proportions, has led to changes in public policy as well. Health researchers have discovered links between diet and obesity, high blood pressure, cancer, and heart disease. As a result, nutritionists suggest that we make informed food choices by reducing our intake of excess calories, sodium, saturated fats, added sugar, refined grains, and trans fats, and at the same time, be physically active. Another aspect of nutrition policy is shaped by the public's desire to know what is in the food they eat. This need has led to increased nutrition information on food labels. Public education efforts have resulted in the development of teaching tools such as MyPlate.

▶ **overnutrition** The long-term consumption of an excess of nutrients. The most common type of overnutrition in the United States results from the regular consumption of excess calories, fats, saturated fats, and cholesterol.

New information about diet and health will continue to drive public policy. This chapter explores diet-planning tools, dietary guidelines, and current dietary standards and discusses how to evaluate nutritional health. How does your diet compare with these current guidelines and standards?

Quick Bite

Early "Laws" of Health

Galen might be among the best-known physicians who ever lived. During the second century, Galen expounded his "laws of health"—eat proper foods, drink the right beverages, exercise, breathe fresh air, get enough sleep, have a daily bowel movement, and control your emotions. Isn't it interesting that these core concepts are still recommended today?

Linking Nutrients, Foods, and Health

We all know that what we eat affects our health. Nutrition science has made many advances in identifying essential nutrients and the foods in which they are found. Eating foods with all the essential nutrients prevents nutritional deficiencies such as scurvy (vitamin C deficiency) or pellagra (deficiency of the B vitamin niacin). In the United States, few people suffer nutritional deficiencies as a result of dietary inadequacies. More often, Americans suffer from chronic diseases such as heart disease, cancer, hypertension, and diabetes—all linked to overconsumption and lifestyle choices. Your future health depends on today's lifestyle choices, including your food choices.

THINK About It 1

Living in a high-tech world, we expect immediate solutions to long-term problems. Wouldn't it be interesting if we could avoid the consequences of overeating by taking a pill, drinking a beverage, or getting a shot? As you know, no magic food, nutrient, or drug exists. Instead, we have to rely on healthful foods, exercise, and lifestyle choices to reduce our risk of chronic disease—a task that challenges many Americans. Tools are available to help us select healthful foods to eat. The U.S. Department of Agriculture's MyPlate food guidance system and the Exchange Lists are two common and comprehensive tools. Although different, these tools rely on the same core nutrition concepts: adequacy, balance, calorie (energy) control, nutrient density, moderation, and variety. These underlying concepts help to keep the focus of healthy eating on a total diet approach.[1] Let's look at how each concept can shape our eating patterns.

Adequacy

Having an adequate diet means that the foods you choose to eat provide all the essential nutrients, fiber, and energy in amounts sufficient to support growth and maintain health.[2] Many Americans consume more calories than they need without getting 100 percent of the recommended intakes for a number of nutrients. Take, for example, a meal of soda pop, two hard-shell beef tacos, and cinnamon breadsticks. Although this meal provides foods from different food groups, it is high in sugar and fat and low in many of the vitamins and minerals found in fruits and vegetables. Occasionally skipping fruits and vegetables at a meal does not create a vitamin or mineral deficiency; however, dietary habits that skimp on fruits and vegetables most of the time provide an overall inadequate diet. Most people could improve the adequacy of their diet by choosing meals and snacks that are high in vitamins and minerals but low to moderate in energy (calorie) content. Doing so offers important benefits: normal growth and development of children, health promotion for people of all ages, and reduction of risk for a number of chronic diseases that are major public health problems.[3]

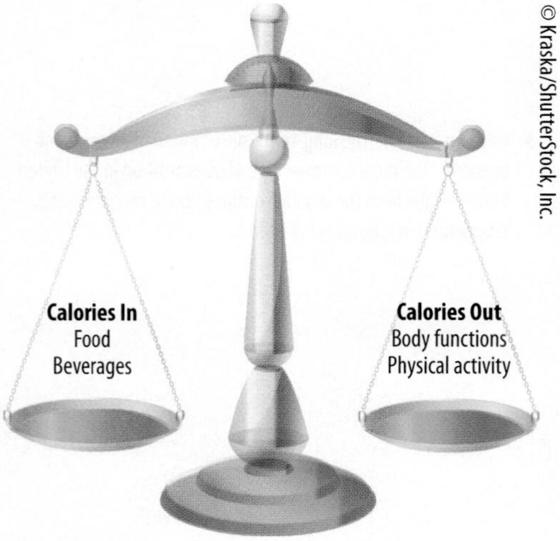

© Kraska/ShutterStock, Inc.

Energy Balance Equation

Data from Centers for Disease Control and Prevention.

Balance

A healthful diet requires a balance of a variety of foods (grains, vegetables, fruits, oil, milk, and meat and beans), energy sources (carbohydrate, protein, and fat), and other nutrients (vitamins and minerals). Your diet can also be balanced in a complementary way when the foods you choose to eat provide you with adequate nutrients. The trick is to consume enough, but not too much, from all the different food groups.

Calorie Control

It can be a challenge to identify the amount of calories you need to maintain or achieve a healthy weight. Although complicated by a number of factors, the formula for weight maintenance seems simple: If you eat the same amount of calories that you use each day, your weight will stay the same. If you eat more calories than you use, you will gain weight, and if you eat less than you use, you will lose weight. In this chapter, we focus on how to choose foods by learning how to get the most nutrients without wasting calories. This is a lesson on budgeting: you should demand value for your expenditures. Just as each of us has a monetary budget—a limited amount of money to spend on things such as food, rent, books, and transportation—in a sense we all have a calorie budget as well. Once you determine how many calories your body uses each day and how to manipulate your calorie expenditure to reach certain health goals, you will be making food choices to match your calorie needs. Every time you eat, you are choosing to spend some of your calorie budget for that day. Those who spend their budget wisely tend to be healthier than those who do not. Let's put the concept of calorie control together with nutrient density to see how it works.

Nutrient Density

The concern that Americans' diets are becoming increasingly energy-rich but nutrient-poor has focused attention on the nutrient content of individual foods relative to the energy they provide.[4] Understanding nutrient density can help explain how overeating can nevertheless result in undernutrition, and it also can help people make informed food choices.

The **nutrient density** of food provides a clue to how "healthy" a food is. It is a ratio of nutrient content to energy content. Nutrient-dense foods provide

▶ **nutrient density** A description of the healthfulness of foods. Foods high in nutrient density are those that provide substantial amounts of vitamins and minerals and relatively few calories; foods low in nutrient density are those that supply calories but relatively small amounts of vitamins and minerals (or none at all).

Going Green

Is the American Diet Contributing to a Warmer Planet?

Our food choices not only contribute to our state of health, both current and future, but also are a significant part of greenhouse gas emissions known as carbon footprint. The impact includes production, transport, processing, packaging, storage, and preparation of food that is delivered to our dinner plates. The food sector contributes 15–30 percent of all greenhouse gas emissions, the primary promoter of global warming. The average American diet creates 2.8 tons of carbon dioxide (CO_2) emissions per person per year, which far exceeds the 2.2 tons of CO_2 emissions generated by Americans driving cars and trucks.

Some foods can result in damage to both our health and the environment. For example, the highly processed foods that have become a big part of our diets are low sources of good nutrition and often require barrels of oil to create. How can we make eating healthier and also more environmentally friendly? Choose plant-based foods. Because they are healthy and protect natural resources, many nutritionists favor an emphasis on plant-based foods in our diets.

Although grains and sweets have less environmental impact, animal-derived foods such as meat and dairy with higher levels of greenhouse gas emissions have more nutritional value. Can we choose both and optimize the levels of nutrient density as well as lower greenhouse gas emissions? The answer is not as simple as reducing or excluding animal-based products and replacing them with plants or grains just because these food sources are more sustainable. When optimizing a diet with regard to sustainability, it is crucial to account for the nutritional value and not solely focus on impacts per kilogram of products, because any dietary recommendations to reduce greenhouse gas emissions must also meet dietary requirements. Current research has demonstrated that a sustainable diet that meets the dietary requirements for health combined with lower greenhouse gas emissions can be achieved without eliminating meat or dairy products, but rather through various food combinations that are associated with different environmental impacts.

Drewnowski A, Rehm CD, Martin, A, et al. Energy and nutrient density of foods in relation to their carbon footprint. *Am J Clin Nutr.* 2015;101(1):184–191; Werner LB, Flysjo A, Tholstrup T. Greenhouse gas emissions of realistic dietary choices in Denmark: the carbon footprint and nutritional value of dairy products. *Food Nutr Res.* 2014;58.

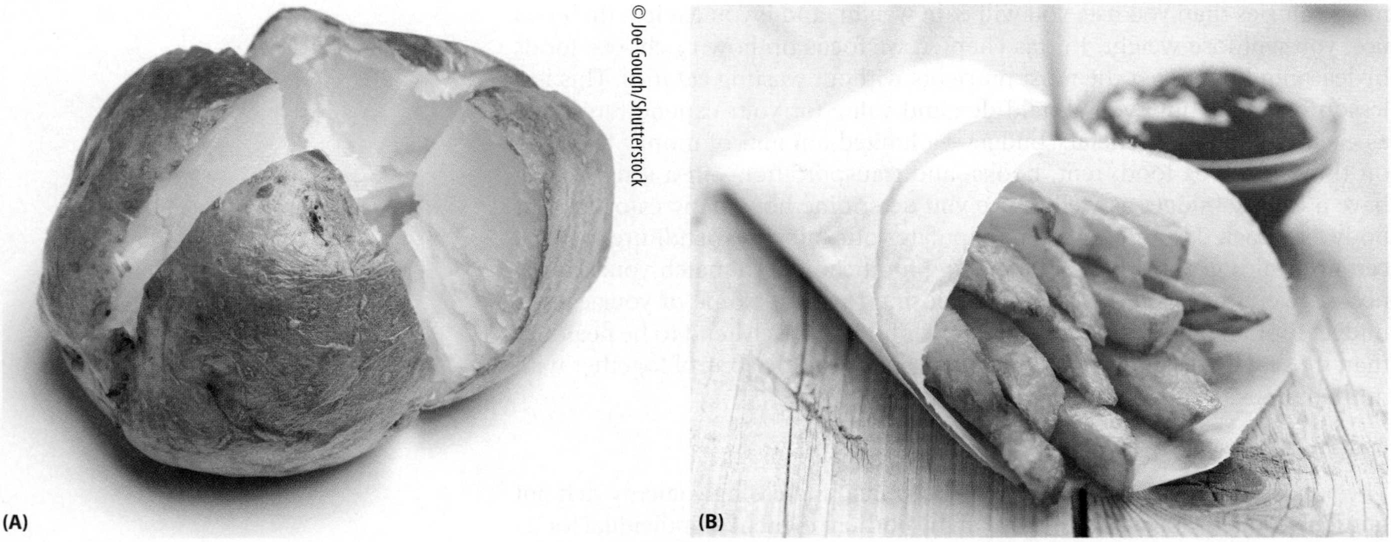

FIGURE 2.1 Nutrient density. Based on the amount of nutrients per total calories, the plain baked potato is more nutrient dense than the same amount of French fries.

substantial amounts of vitamins and minerals and relatively few calories.[5] Foods that are low in nutrient density supply calories but relatively small amounts of vitamins and minerals, sometimes none at all.[6] A food high in calories but low in vitamins and minerals is less nutrient dense than one that has a high vitamin and mineral content compared with its overall calories.

Consider a potato as an example. We can prepare a potato in many different ways. We can eat baked potatoes, mashed potatoes with toppings, or French fries. Depending on how it is cooked and what is added to it before we eat it, the nutrient density of a potato changes. The most nutrient-dense form of this potato would be a plain baked potato, which provides the most vitamins and minerals with relatively few calories. The least nutrient-dense version of this potato is French fries, because frying a food adds a lot more calories without adding more vitamins and minerals. In this case, the proportion of vitamins and minerals is low compared to the overall higher calorie content. French fries are not nutrient dense (See **FIGURE 2.1**).

Some foods with little or no added sugar or fat are high-nutrient-density food choices. For example, you might decide to eat a pear instead of a handful of caramel corn. Both provide about the same amount of calories. By choosing to eat the pear instead of the caramel corn, however, you are working toward meeting your daily nutrient needs while gaining more nutrients within the calories consumed, thereby selecting a more nutrient-dense and overall more healthy food choice.

Moderation

Not too much or too little—that's what moderation means. Moderation does not mean that you have to eliminate low-nutrient-density foods from your diet, such as soft drinks and candy, but rather that you can include them occasionally. Moderation entails not taking anything to extremes. You probably have heard that vitamin C has positive effects, but that doesn't mean huge doses of this essential nutrient are appropriate for you. It's also important to remember that substances that are healthful in small amounts can sometimes be dangerous in large quantities. For example, the body needs zinc for hundreds of chemical reactions, including those that support normal growth, development, and immune function. Too much zinc, however, can cause deficiency of copper, another essential mineral, which can lead to impaired immune function.

THINK About It 2

Being moderate in your diet means that you do not restrict or completely eliminate any one type of food, but rather that all types of food can fit into a healthful diet.

Food guides and their graphics convey the message of moderation by showing suggested amounts of different food groups. Appearing in diverse shapes, food guides from other countries reflect their cultural contexts. Japan, for example, uses the shape of a spinning top (see **FIGURE 2.2**).

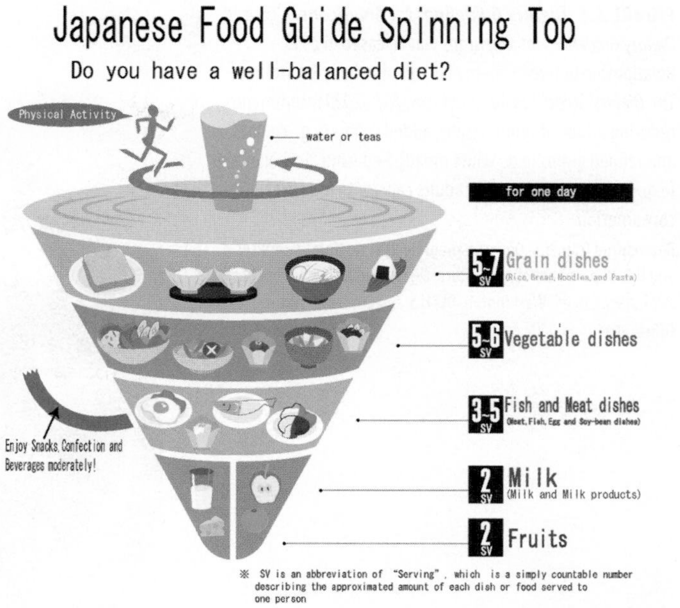

FIGURE 2.2 Dietary guidelines around the world. Global differences in environment, culture, socioeconomics, and behavior create significant differences in the foods that make up our diets. Despite this, dietary guidelines from one country to the next show surprising similarities. Whether a country has only 3 guidelines or as many as 23, all share similar basic recommendations. For example, the Japanese dietary guidelines use a spinning top. The United States uses a plate, and Canada uses a rainbow. Mexico and most European countries use a circular form.

Courtesy of the Japanese Ministry of Health, Labor and Welfare/USDA.

Variety

How many different foods do you eat on a daily basis? Ten? Fifteen? Would it surprise you that one of Japan's dietary guidelines suggests eating 30 different foods each day?[7] Now *that's* variety! Variety means including a lot of different foods in the diet: not just different food groups such as fruits, vegetables, and grains, but also different foods from each group. Eating two bananas and three carrots each and every day might give you the minimum number of recommended daily servings of fruits and vegetables, but it doesn't add much variety.

THINK About It 3

Variety is important for a number of reasons. Eating a variety of fruits, for example, provides a broader mix of vitamins, minerals, and phytochemicals than if you eat the same one or two fruits most of the time. Choosing a variety of protein sources gives you a different balance of fats and other nutrients. Variety can add interest and excitement to your meals while preventing boredom with your diet. Perhaps most important, variety in your diet helps ensure that you get all the nutrients you need. Studies have shown that people who have varied diets are more likely to meet their overall nutrient needs.[8]

There are no magic diets, foods, or supplements. Instead, your overall, long-term food choices can bring you the benefits of a nutritious diet. A healthful diet is something you create over time, not the way you eat on any given day. Using the principles of adequacy, balance, calorie (energy) control, nutrient density, moderation, and variety can help you attain and achieve healthy eating habits, which in turn will contribute to your overall healthy lifestyle. Let's take a look at some general guidance for making those food choices.

Key Concepts Food and nutrient intake play a major role in health and risk of disease. For most Americans, overnutrition is more of a problem than undernutrition. The diet-planning principles of adequacy, balance, calorie (energy) control, nutrient density, moderation, and variety are important concepts in choosing a healthful diet.

Quick Bite

Variety Is Key

Mothers often say, "Eat your vegetables." Studies show that adding variety in the vegetables you eat is a good indicator of overall increased vegetable consumption. It may cost a little more today, but eating different types of vegetables is related to better overall diet quality and a larger quantity of vegetables consumed. The small increase in cost at the grocery store now likely will save you more than money in the future. So experiment a little, and try something other than your usual carrots and green beans at dinner.

Dietary Guidelines

To help citizens improve their overall health, many countries have developed dietary guidelines—simple, easy-to-understand statements about food choices, food safety, and physical activity. This section examines dietary guidelines for the United States and Canada.

Dietary Guidelines for Americans

In 1980, the **U.S. Department of Agriculture (USDA)** and the **U.S. Department of Health and Human Services (DHHS)** jointly released the first edition of the *Dietary Guidelines for Americans.* Revised guidelines have been released every five years

- **U.S. Department of Agriculture (USDA)** The government agency that monitors the production of eggs, poultry, and meat for adherence to standards of quality and wholesomeness. The USDA also provides public nutrition education, performs nutrition research, and administers the WIC program.
- **U.S. Department of Health and Human Services (DHHS)** The principal federal agency responsible for protecting the health of all Americans and providing essential human services. The agency is especially concerned with those Americans who are least able to help themselves.

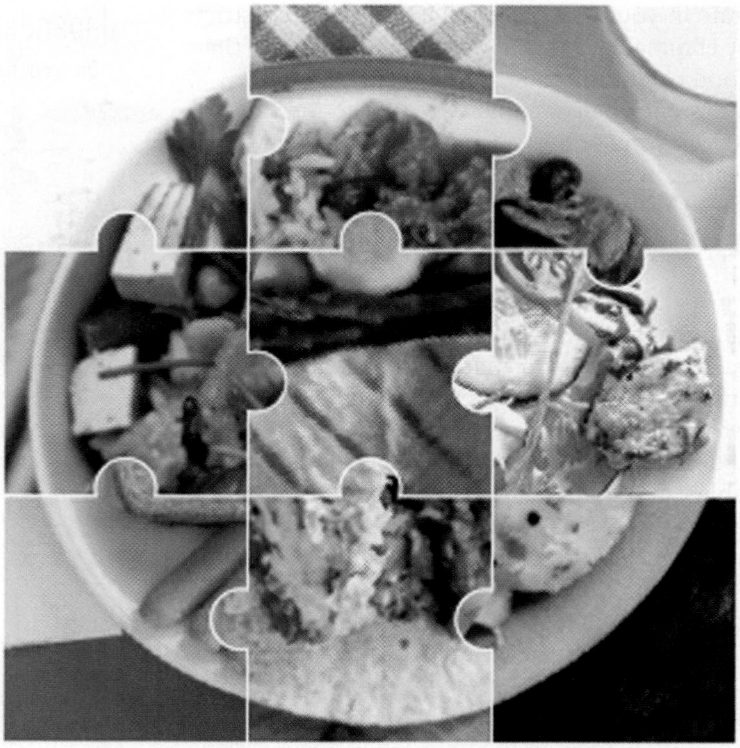

FIGURE 2.3 ***Dietary Guidelines for Americans.*** A revised *Dietary Guidelines for Americans* was released in 2015. Relationship between energy balance and body fat storage. The *Dietary Guidelines for Americans, 2015-2020* recommends reducing intake of sodium (salt), added sugars (e.g., cookies), and refined grains (e.g., white bread). Reducing alcohol intake (e.g., beer) is a strategy that adults can use to reduce calorie consumption.

Reproduced from U.S. Department of Health and Human Services and U.S. Department of Agriculture. *Dietary Guidelines for Americans, 2015-2020.* 8th ed. Washington, DC: U.S. Government Printing Office; 2015.

as scientific information about links between diet and chronic disease is updated. The *Dietary Guidelines for Americans* provides science-based advice that suggests how nutrition and physical activity can help promote health across the lifespan and reduce the risk for major chronic diseases in the U.S. population ages 2 years and older.[9] The food and physical activity choices you make every day affect your health—how you feel today, tomorrow, and in the future.

▶ ***Dietary Guidelines for Americans, 2015-2020*** The *Dietary Guidelines for Americans* are the foundation of federal nutrition policy and are developed by the U.S. Department of Agriculture (USDA) and the U.S. Department of Health and Human Services (DHHS). These science-based guidelines are intended to reduce the number of Americans who develop chronic diseases such as hypertension, diabetes, cardiovascular disease, obesity, and alcoholism.

The ***Dietary Guidelines for Americans, 2015-2020*** (see **FIGURE 2.3**) is designed as a tool for professionals to help individuals and their families consume a healthy, nutritionally adequate diet. The *Dietary Guidelines for Americans, 2015-2020* is based on research that looks at the relationship between overall eating patterns, health, and risk of chronic disease. Advances in research have provided a greater understanding of, and focus on, the importance of healthy eating patterns as a whole, and how foods and beverages act in combination to affect health. Recommendations within the *Guidelines* are what experts have determined to be the best advice for Americans to reduce the risk for chronic diseases such as heart disease, cancer, diabetes, stroke, osteoporosis, and obesity. These guidelines are the cornerstone of federal nutrition policy and education. They are used to develop educational materials and to aid in the design and implementation of nutrition-related programs, such as the National School Lunch Program and Meals on Wheels. The *Dietary Guidelines for Americans* serves as the basis for nutrition messages and consumer materials developed by nutrition educators and health professionals for the general public.[10]

Lifestyle choices, including a poor diet and lack of physical activity, are the most important factors that contribute to the overweight and obesity epidemic that is currently affecting men, women, and children throughout the United States. Even in individuals who are not overweight, a poor diet and physical inactivity are well known to be associated with the major causes of morbidity and mortality. Currently, the number of Americans who are overweight or obese is at an all-time high; as a consequence, the risk for various chronic diseases is also on the rise. Furthermore, among the population of overweight and obese individuals, many are undernourished in several key nutrients. In an effort to address this growing problem, the *Dietary Guidelines for Americans, 2015-2020* focuses on the integration of government, agriculture, health care, business, educators, and communities working together to encourage individuals to make healthy lifestyle changes.[11] The main objective of these guidelines is to encourage eating patterns and regular physical activity for the American people. These *Guidelines* emphasize a total diet approach by encouraging us to think holistically about what we eat and drink. They also emphasize meeting nutritional needs by including nutrient-dense foods that contain essential vitamins and minerals, dietary fiber, and other naturally occurring substances that have positive health effects. The *Guidelines* offer practical tips for how people can make changes within their own diet as a way to integrate healthier choices. Examples of these practical tips include: consuming more vegetables, fruits, whole grains, fat-free and low-fat dairy products, and seafood; consumption of foods with less sodium, saturated and trans fats, added sugars, and refined grains; and an increase in daily physical activity.

The Dietary Guidelines, 2015-2020 provide five overarching guidelines that encourage healthy eating patterns, recognizing that individuals will need to make shifts in their food and beverage choices to achieve a healthy pattern, and acknowledge that all segments of our society—food producers, grocery stores, restaurants, families, and policymakers—have a role to play in supporting healthy choices. These guidelines also emphasize that a healthy eating pattern is not a rigid prescription, but rather an adaptable framework in which individuals can enjoy foods that meet their personal, cultural, and traditional preferences and fit within their budget and lifestyle.

Overarching Guidelines

1. **Follow a healthy eating pattern across the lifespan.** All food and beverage choices matter. Choose a healthy eating pattern at an appropriate calorie level to help achieve and maintain a healthy body weight, support nutrient adequacy, and reduce the risk of chronic disease.
2. **Focus on variety, nutrient density, and amount.** To meet nutrient needs within calorie limits, choose a variety of nutrient-dense foods across and within all food groups in recommended amounts.
3. **Limit calories from added sugars and saturated fats and reduce sodium intake.** Consume foods low in added sugars, saturated fats, and sodium. Cut back on foods and beverages higher in these components to amounts that fit within healthy eating patterns.
4. **Shift to healthier food and beverage choices.** Choose nutrient-dense foods and beverages across and within all food groups in place of less healthy choices. Consider cultural and personal preferences to make these shifts easier to accomplish and maintain.
5. **Support healthy eating patterns for all.** Everyone has a role in helping to create and support healthy eating patterns in multiple settings nationwide, from home to school to work to communities.

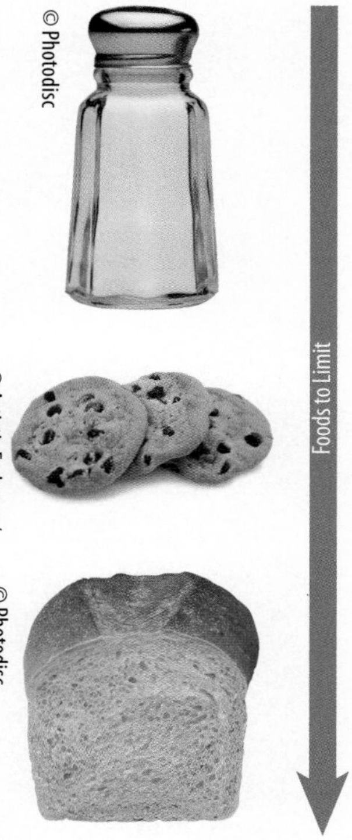

© Photodisc

© Artistic Endeavor/ ShutterStock, Inc.

© Photodisc

Key Recommendations from the *Dietary Guidelines for Americans 2015-2020*

Key recommendations provide further guidance on how individuals can follow the five guidelines. These should be applied in their entirety, given the interconnected relationship that each dietary component can have with others.

Dietary Guidelines for Americans, 2015-2020
Key Recommendations

- Follow a healthy eating pattern that accounts for all foods and beverages within an appropriate calorie level
- Consume less than 10 percent of calorie per day from added sugars
- Consume less than 10 percent of calories per day from saturated fats
- Consume less than 2,300 mg per day of sodium
- If alcohol is consumed, it should be consumed in moderation-up to one drink per day for women and up to two drinks per day for men-and only by adults of legal drinking age.
- Meet the Physical Activity Guidelines for Americans

Looking further into the *Dietary Guidelines* you can determine what foods to increase in our diets, as well as what foods to limit. For most Americans, foods to eat more of in our diet include:

- A variety of vegetables from all of the subgroups—dark green, red and orange, legumes (beans and peas), starchy, and other types
- Fruits, especially whole fruits
- Grains, at least half of which are whole grains
- Fat-free or low-fat dairy, including milk, yogurt, cheese, and/or fortified soy beverages
- A variety of protein foods, including seafood, lean meats and poultry, eggs, legumes, and nuts, seeds, and soy products
- Oils

In order to follow healthy eating patterns, individuals should limit the following foods:

- Saturated fats and *trans* fats
- Added sugars
- Sodium

In addition, individuals of all ages should meet *Physical Activity Guidelines for Americans* to help promote health and reduce the risk of chronic disease Americans should aim to achieve and maintain a healthy body weight. The relationship between diet and physical activity contributes to calorie balance and managing body weight. The *Physical Activity Guidelines for Americans* suggests that adults should do the equivalent of 150 minutes of moderate-intensity aerobic activity each week—that's an average of only 30 minutes a day, five days a week. For children and adolescents age 6 years and older, the recommendation is 60 minutes or more of physical activity per day.[12]

The environment in which many Americans live, work, learn, and play can be a roadblock for many people trying to achieve or maintain a healthy body weight. Having been described as an obesogenic environment, this way of life is a significant contributor to America's obesity epidemic because it affects both sides of the calorie balance equation.[13] In our modern lifestyle, the availability of high-calorie, palatable, inexpensive food is coupled with many mechanized labor-saving devices. The result is that we live in an environment that often promotes overeating while at the same time discourages physical activity.

A Roadmap to the 2015-2020 Edition of the Dietary Guidelines for Americans

Previous editions of the *Dietary Guidelines* have made suggestions that individuals follow particular dietary patterns. The current *Dietary Guidelines* are different in this way. In recognizing that people do not eat individual nutrients, but rather combinations of different foods that provide a variety of nutrients, which forms an overall eating pattern providing a cumulative effect on one's health. Because of this, eating patterns and their food and nutrient characteristics are a primary emphasis of recommendations in the 2015-2020 edition of the the *Dietary Guidelines*. As of such, three chapters make up this edition.

Although the primary focus of the *Dietary Guidelines* is on nutrition, because of its critical and complementary role in promoting health and in preventing disease, the importance of meeting the *Physical Activity Guidelines for Americans* is discussed throughout these *Guidelines*. Examples of health benefits as well as tips for helping you to adopt the Dietary Guidelines' key recommendations can be found in **TABLE 2.1**.

Chapter 1. Key Elements of Healthy Eating Patterns

This chapter focuses on the first three Guidelines as well as the Key Recommendations. The first three guidelines are: "*Follow a healthy eating pattern across the lifespan; Focus on variety, nutrient density, and amount; and limit calories from added sugars and saturated fats and reduce sodium intake.* This chapter discusses the relationship of diet and physical activity to health and

TABLE 2.1
2015–2020 Dietary Guidelines for Americans: Benefits, Behaviors, and Tips

	Dietary Guideline Recommendation Benefits to Your Health	Goals or Behaviors That could Make You Healthier	How-to-Tips
Follow a healthy eating pattern across the lifespan	• Individuals throughout all stages of the lifespan should have eating patterns that promote overall health and help prevent chronic disease • Choose a healthy eating pattern at an appropriate calorie level to help achieve and maintain a healthy body weight, support nutrient adequacy, and reduce the risk of chronic disease	• Consume foods and drinks to meet, not exceed, calorie needs. • Plan ahead to make healthy food choices • Track food and calorie intake • Reduce portion sizes, especially of high-calorie foods • Choose healthy food options when eating away from home	• Know your calorie needs • Prepare and pack healthy snacks at home to be eating at school or at work
Focus on variety, nutrient density, and amount	• Choose a variety of nutrient-dense foods across and within all food groups in recommended amounts	• Eat five or more servings of vegetables and fruit daily, make up of a variety of choices • Choose foods which contain nutrients and other beneficial substances that have not been "diluted" by the addition of calories from added solid fats, sugars, or refined starches, or by the solid fats naturally present in food	• Add dark-green, red, and orange vegetables to soups, stews, casseroles, and stir-fries and other main and side dishes • Add beans or peas to salad, soups, and side dishes, or serve as a mina dish • Have raw, cut-up vegetables and fruit handy for a quick side dish snacks, salad, for desserts • When eating out, choose a vegetable as a side dish
Limit calories from added sugars and saturated fats and reduce sodium intake	• Cut back on foods and beverages high in added sugars, saturated fats and sodium to amounts that fit within healthy eating patterns • Limit added sugars to less than 10 percent of calories per day • Limit saturated fat intake to less than 10 percent of calories per day • Limit sodium to less than 2,300 mg per day (adults) • Eating a diet that includes saturated fat, trans fat, and dietary cholesterol raises low-density lipoprotein (LDL), or "bad" cholesterol levels, which increases the risk of coronary heart disease (CHD)	• Replace saturated fats with polyunsaturated fats • Be aware of the most likely sources of trans fat in your diet, such as many pastry items and donuts, deep-fried foods, many types of snack chips, cookies, and crackers	• Eat less cake, cookies, ice cream, other desserts, and candy • Include foods which provide monounsaturated and polyunsaturated fats, such as olive oil and nuts in your diet • Limit intake of foods high in saturated and trans fats such as ground beef and full fat dairy products

(*continues*)

TABLE 2.1
2015–2020 Dietary Guidelines for Americans: Benefits, Behaviors, and Tips ***(Continued)***

	Dietary Guideline Recommendation Benefits to Your Health	Goals or Behaviors That could Make You Healthier	How-to-Tips
Shift to healthier food and beverage choices	• Choose nutrient-dense foods and beverages across and within all food groups • Excessive alcohol consumption has no benefits, and the health and social hazards of heavy alcohol intake are numerous and well known	• Drink an adequate amount of water each day • Choose foods and drinks with added sugars or caloric sweeteners (sugar-sweetened beverages) less frequently • If you are of legal drinking age and you if alcohol is consumed, do so in moderation • Mixing alcohol and caffeine is not recognized as safe by the FDA	• Drink few or no regular sodas, sports drinks, energy drinks, and fruit drinks • Choose water, fat-free milk, 100 percent fruit juice, or unsweetened tea or coffee as drinks • If alcohol is consumed limit to no more than one drink per day for women and two drinks per day for men • Avoid excessive (heavy or binge) drinking • Avoid alcohol if you are pregnant or may become pregnant
Support healthy eating patterns for all	• Everyone has a role in helping to create and support healthy eating patterns in multiple settings*	• Systems, organizations, and businesses and industries, all have important role in helping individuals make healthy choices • Professionals can work with individuals in a variety of settings to adapt their choices to develop a healthy eating pattern tailored to accommodate physical health, cultural, ethnic, traditional, and personal preferences, as well as personal food budgets and other issues of accessibility	• Make healthy food choices at home and away-from-home

Modified from U.S. Department of Health and Human Services and U.S. Department of Agriculture. 2015–2020 *Dietary Guidelines for Americans*. 8th Edition. December 2015. Available at http://health.gov/dietaryguidelines/2015/guidelines/.

TABLE 2.2
Healthy U.S.-Style Eating Pattern at the 2,000-Calorie Level

Food Group	Amount in the 2,000-Calorie-Level Pattern
Vegetables	2 ½ c-eq/day
• Dark green	1 ½ c-eq/wk
• Red and orange	5 ½ c-eq/wk
• Legumes (beans and peas)	1 ½ c-eq/wk
• Starchy	5 c-eq/wk
• Other	4 c-eq/wk
Fruits	2 c-eq/day
Grains	6 oz-eq/day
• Whole grains	≥ 3oz-eq/day
• Refined grains	≤ 3 oz-eq/day
Dairy	3 c-eq/day
Protein Foods	5 ½ oz-eq/day
• Seafood	8 oz-eq/wk
• Meats, poultry, eggs	26 oz-eq/wk
• Nuts, seeds, soy products	5 oz-eq/wk
Oils	27 g/day
Limit on Calories for Other Uses (% of calories)	270 kcal/day (14%)

Reproduced from U.S. Department of Health and Human Services and U.S. Department of Agriculture. 2015–2020 Dietary Guidelines for Americans. 8th Edition. December 2015. Available at http://health.gov/dietaryguidelines/2015/guidelines/

explains the principles of a healthy eating pattern. The dietary recommendation examples are based off of a 2,000-calorie level as shown in (**TABLE 2.2**).

To help determine if a 2,000-calorie diet is right for you, refer to the Estimated Daily Calorie Needs (**TABLE 2.3**).

Two additional USDA Food Patterns, the Healthy Mediterranean-Style Eating Pattern, and the Healthy Vegetarian Eating Pattern are found in the Appendix of the Guidelines. All of the eating plans emphasize fruits, vegetables, whole grains, beans and peas, fat-free and low-fat milk and milk products, and healthy oils as well as including less red meat and more seafood than the typical American diet. The Mediterranean diet, given its name as the eating pattern associated with those cultures bordering the Mediterranean Sea, has been associated with positive health outcomes such as lower rates of heart disease. The Mediterranean-Style eating pattern includes more fruits and seafood and less dairy compared to the Healthy U.S-Style Pattern. The Healthy Vegetarian Pattern modifies the Healthy U.S-Style Pattern by eliminating meat, poultry, and fish while adding more soy products, legumes, nuts, seeds, and whole grains. Dairy and eggs are included; however, the Vegetarian Pattern can be modified based on individual food restrictions.

The core elements of this chapter is the importance of consuming overall healthy eating patterns, including vegetables, fruits, grains, dairy, protein foods, and oils, eaten within an appropriate calorie level and in forms with limited amounts of saturated fats, added sugars, and sodium.

Chapter 2. Shifts Needed To Align with Healthy Eating Patterns

This chapter focuses on the fourth Dietary Guideline, "*Shift to healthier food and beverage choices.*" This chapter compares current food and nutrient intakes in the U.S. to recommendations and describes the shifts in dietary choices that are needed to align current intakes with current recommendations. Within this chapter, small shifts in food choices, both within and across food groups, encourage Americans that changes in food choices over the course of a week,

TABLE 2.3
Estimated Daily Calorie Needs

AGE (YEARS)	SEDENTARY[a]	MODERATELY ACTIVE[b]	ACTIVE[c]
Female			
2–3	1000	1000–1200	1000–1400
4–8	1200–1400	1400–1600	1400–1800
9–13	1400–1600	1600–2000	1800–2200
14–18	1800	2000	2400
19–30	1800–2000	2000–2200	2400
31–50	1800	2000	2200
51+	1600	1800	2000–2200
Male			
2–3	1000	1000–1400	1000–1400
4–8	1200–1400	1400–1600	1600–2000
9–13	1600–2000	1800–2200	2000–2600
14–18	2000–2400	2400–2800	2800–3200
19–30	2400–2600	2600–2800	3000
31–50	2200–2400	2400–2600	2800–3000
51+	2000–2200	2200–2400	2600–2800

[a]A lifestyle that includes only the light physical activity associated with typical day-to-day life

[b]A lifestyle that includes physical activity equivalent to walking about 1.5 to 3 miles per day at 3 to 4 miles per hour (30–60 minutes a day of moderate physical activity), in addition to the light physical activity associated with typical day-to-day life

[c]A lifestyle that includes physical activity equivalent to walking more than 3 miles per day at 3 to 4 miles per hour (60 or more minutes a day of moderate physical activity), in addition to the light physical activity associated with typical day-to-day life

U.S. Department of Health and Human Services and U.S. Department of Agriculture. 2015–2020 Dietary Guidelines for Americans. 8th Edition. December 2015. Available at http://health.gov/dietaryguidelines/2015/guidelines/.

a day, or even a meal can make a big difference (see **FIGURES 2.4**, **2.5**, and **2.6**). The following provides small shift examples:

Instead of	Choose
High calorie snacks	Nutrient-dense snacks
Fruit products with added sugars	Fresh fruit
Refined grains	Whole grains
Snacks with added sugars (candy bar)	Unsalted snacks (unsalted peanuts)
Solid fats	Unsaturated oils
Beverages with added sugars (soda pop)	No-sugar added beverages (water)

Most Americans would agree that they need to shift intakes in order to meet the suggested eating patterns of the *Dietary Guidelines*; however, young children and older Americans generally are closer to the recommendations than are adolescents and young adults.

In addition to shifting food choices, most individuals would benefit from making shifts to increase the amount of physical activity they engage in each week. This shift can come from limiting screen time and time spent on other sedentary activities.

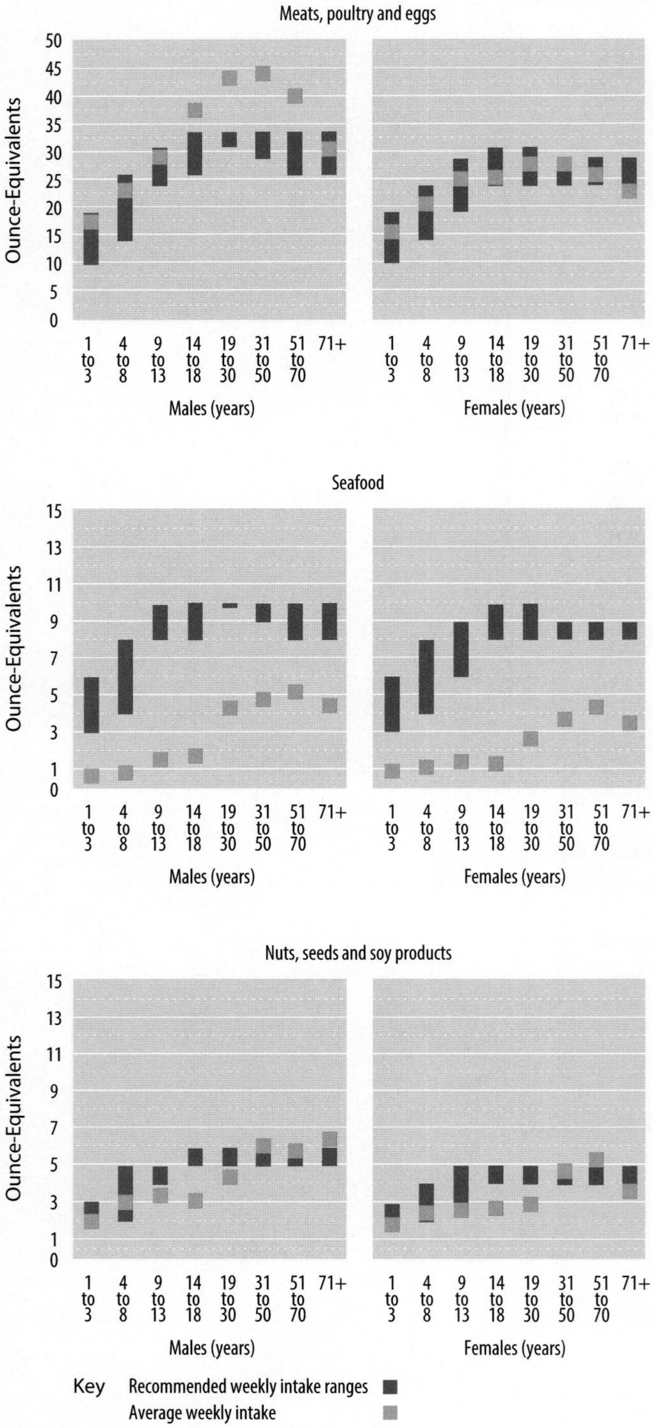

FIGURE 2.4 Average protein foods subgroup intake. Average Protein Foods Subgroup Intakes in ounce-Equivalents per Week by Age-Sex Groups, Compared to Ranges of Recommended Intake.

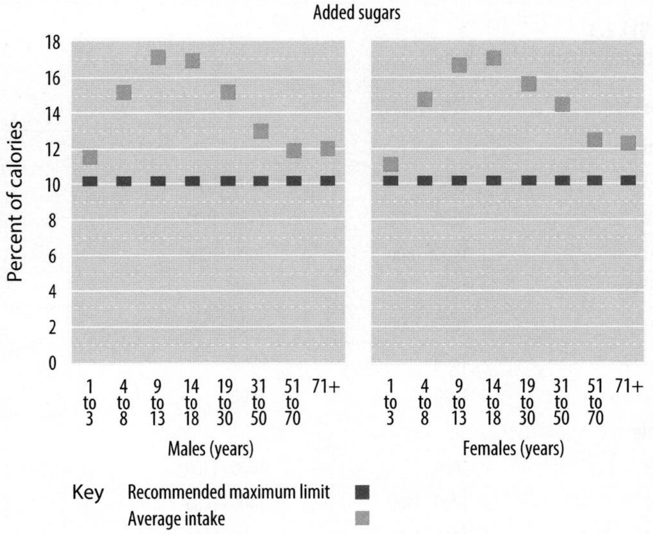

FIGURE 2.5 Intake of added sugars. Average intakes of added sugars as a percent of calories per day by age-sex group, in comparison to the *Dietary Guidelines'* maximum limit of less than 10 percent of calories.

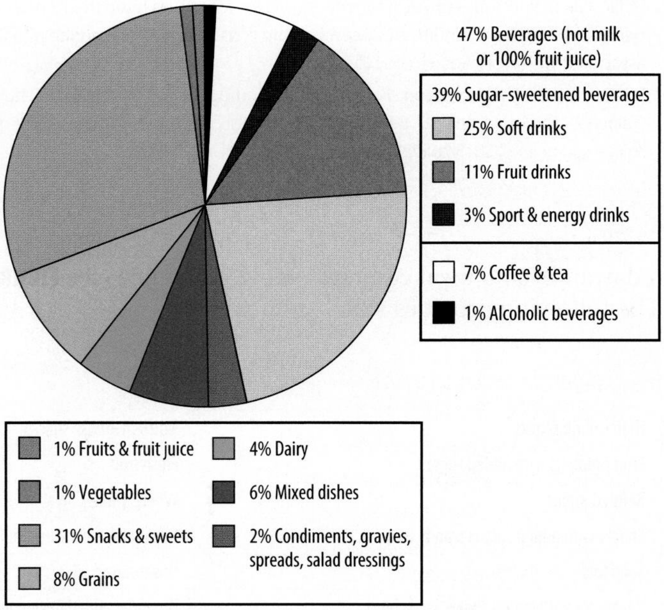

FIGURE 2.6 Sources of added sugars. Food category sources of added sugars in the U.S. population ages 2 years and older.

Chapter 3. Everyone Has a Role in Supporting Healthy Eating Patterns

This chapter focuses on the fifth guideline, "*Support healthy eating patterns for all.*" It explains how all individuals and segments of society have an important role to play in supporting healthy eating and physical activity choices. Coordination and collaboration between individuals and all aspects of society is needed to create a new model in which healthy lifestyle choices at home, school, work, and in the community are easy, accessible, affordable, and normative. As suggested in the Social-Ecological Model used in these *Dietary Guidelines* (see **FIGURE 2.7**), various factors have a role in helping individuals shift their everyday food, beverage, and physical activity choices to align with the suggestions that make up the *Dietary Guidelines*.

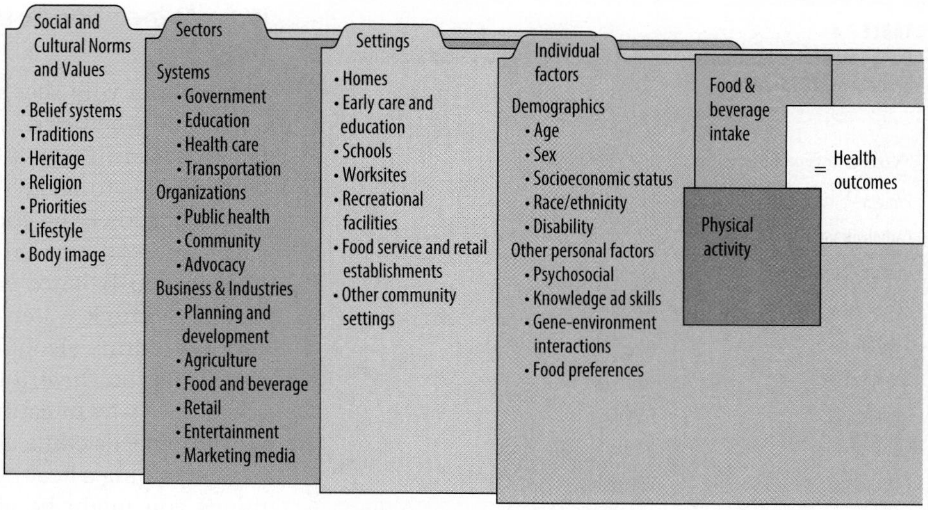

FIGURE 2.7 A social-ecological framework for nutrition and physical activity decisions.
Data from Health.gov. 2015. http://health.gov/dietaryguidelines/2015/guidelines/chapter-3/social-ecological-model/.

Components of this chapter also encourages use of **MyPlate**, the USDA's current icon and primary food group symbol, as a guide to support healthy eating patterns. As part of the government's healthy eating initiative, MyPlate is an easy-to-understand visual image intended to empower people with the information they need to make healthy food choices and create eating habits consistent with the *Dietary Guidelines for Americans, 2015-2020*. Because we eat from plates, the design of the MyPlate icon identifies visually how much room on a plate each food group should occupy. It is the objective of this tool to remind people to think about, create, and make better, more balanced food choices. MyPlate uses the image of a dinner plate divided into four sections: fruits, vegetables, grains, and proteins, with a smaller plate (or glass) representing a serving of dairy. MyPlate is accompanied by a supporting website, www.ChooseMyPlate.gov, which provides tools, resources, and practical information on dietary assessment, nutrition education, and other user-friendly nutrition information.

Unlike the USDA's former food guide systems, MyPlate does not suggest particular foods or specific serving sizes and does not even mention desserts or sweets. It is not intended to tell people what to eat, but to empower them to make their own healthy choices and to use this visual icon as a sensible guide.[16]

Quick Bite

Pass Up the Salt

We require only a few hundred milligrams of sodium each day, but this would be unpalatable. Given our current high-salt food environment, it would also be difficult to achieve. The average intake of sodium is about 3,400 mg per day, whereas the Dietary Guidelines recommend no more than 1,500 mg, or 3/4 teaspoon per day. The guideline is to eat less sodium, but not down to the level of actual requirements.

The Appendices

The appendices of the *Dietary Guidelines for Americans, 2015-2020* are made up of 14 additional resources to support the content of the chapters. Included in the appendices are recommendations for the *Physical Activity Guidelines for Americans*; calorie needs by age, sex, and level of physical activity; a basic Healthy U.S.-Style Eating Pattern; two additional examples of healthy eating patterns; a glossary of terms; and nutritional goals for various age-sex groups. A list of select government resources on diet and physical activity, additional information on alcohol, lists of food sources of nutrients of public health concern, and food safety principles and guidance are also provided.

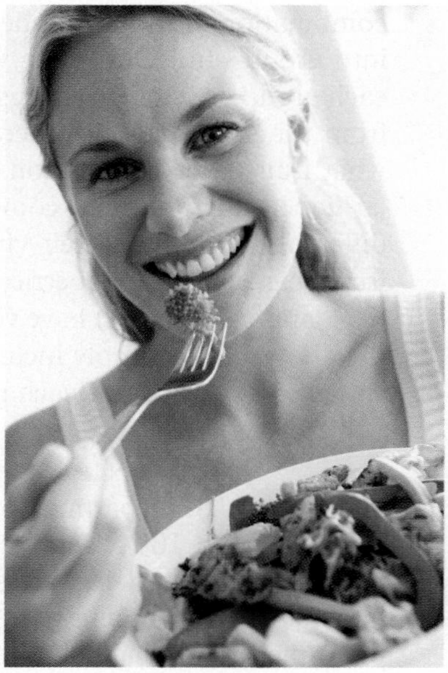
© Monkey Business Images/ShutterStock, Inc.

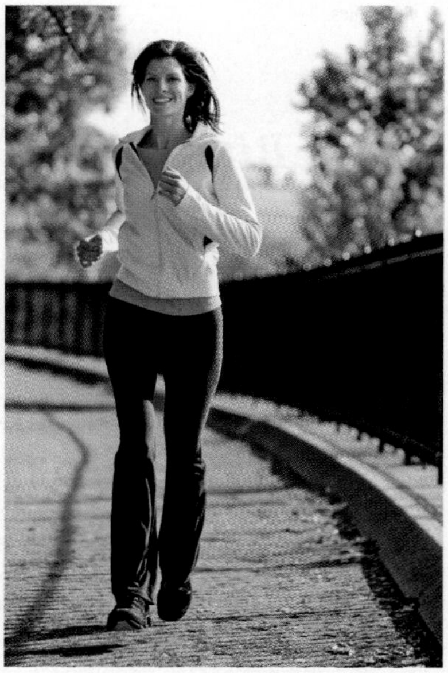
© iStockphoto/Thinkstock

TABLE 2.4
Daily Targets for Nutrients as Addressed in the *Dietary Guidelines for Americans, 2015-2020*

Nutrient or Food Group	Target Amount per Day for Adult Female Ages 19–30
Protein	46 gm (10-35% kcal)
Carbohydrate	130 gm (45-65% kcal)
Dietary fiber	28 gm
Added sugars	<10% kcal
Total fat	20-35% kcal
Saturated fat	<10% kcal
Linoleic acid	12 gm
Linolenic acid	1.1 gm
Calcium	1,000 mg
Iron	18 mg
Magnesium	310 mg
Phosphorus, mg	700 mg
Potassium	4,700 mg
Sodium	2,300 mg
Vitamin A	700 mg RAE
Vitamin E	15 mg AT
Vitamin D	600 IU
Vitamin C	75 mg

Data from U.S. Department of Agriculture and U.S. Department of Health and Human Services. *Dietary Guidelines for Americans, 2015-2020.* 8th ed. Washington, DC: U.S. Government Printing Office; 2015.

Ways to Incorporate the Dietary Guidelines into Your Daily Life

Think about your diet and consider your overall food intake to determine whether it is consistent with the *Dietary Guidelines for Americans, 2015-2020*. Choose more fruits, vegetables, and whole grains to make sure you are getting all the nutrients you need while lowering your intake of saturated fat, trans fat, added sugar, and sodium. Eat fewer high-fat toppings and fried foods to help you balance energy intake and expenditure. Exercise regularly. Drink water more often than soft drinks, and if you choose to drink alcohol at all, use caution.

Using the *Dietary Guidelines* as your road map for finding a healthier way of eating, you might find it easier to meet your nutrition needs while also protecting your health and achieving or maintaining a healthy weight along the way. Table 2.1 suggests things you might be able to change in your own diet or lifestyle. Pick one or two suggestions or come up with some simple changes of your own to try that incorporate the *Dietary Guidelines for Americans, 2015-2020* into your daily life. **TABLE 2.4** summarizes daily limits or targets for a number of nutrients addressed in the *Dietary Guidelines*.

Key Concepts Dietary guidelines are recommendations based on current science that guide people toward more healthful choices. The *Dietary Guidelines for Americans, 2015-2020* provide five overarching guidelines that encourage healthy eating patterns, recognize that individuals will need to make shifts in their food and beverage choices to achieve a healthy pattern, and acknowledge that all segments of our society have a role to play in supporting healthy choices.

From Dietary Guidelines to Planning: What You Will Eat

By understanding the *Dietary Guidelines for Americans*, you will be able to identify characteristics that can make your diet and your lifestyle healthy. The next step is to translate your knowledge into healthful food choices. For many years, nutritionists and teachers have used **food groups** to illustrate the proper combination of foods in a healthful diet. Even young children can sort food into groups and fill a plate with foods from each group. The foods within each group are similar because of their origins—fruits, for example, all come from the same part of different plants. But from a nutritional perspective, what fruits have in common is the balance of macronutrients and the similarities in micronutrient composition. Even so, the foods in one group can differ significantly in their vitamin and mineral profiles; for example, some fruits (e.g., citrus, strawberries, and kiwi) are rich in vitamin C, whereas others (e.g., apples, bananas) have very little. Here again, we can see the importance of variety, of not simply including different food groups but also choosing a variety of foods *within* each group.

▶ **food groups** Categories of similar foods, such as fruits or vegetables.

Quick Bite

How Well Do School Cafeterias Follow Nutrition Guidelines?

About one in three kids and teenagers is obese, and high-fat school lunches might be part of the problem. Until recently, the USDA's nutritional standards for school meals had not been updated in more than 15 years. With the majority of school-age kids and teens getting 30 to 50 percent of their total calories from cafeteria meals each day, it's important that these meals be as healthy as possible. The Healthy, Hunger-Free Kids Act, which was passed in 2010, (1) boosts the nutrition quality of school lunches by requiring fewer calories, less sodium, and more fresh fruits, vegetables, and whole grains; (2) expands the number of students enrolled in free- and reduced-cost meals; and (3) puts into place a plan to eliminate things like vending machines from school cafeterias.

A Brief History of Food Group Plans

When the U.S. Department of Agriculture published its first dietary recommendations in 1894, specific vitamins and minerals had not even been discovered.[15] The initial guide stressed the importance of consuming enough fat and sugar and energy-rich foods to support daily activity. Because people performed more manual labor in those days, many people were simply not

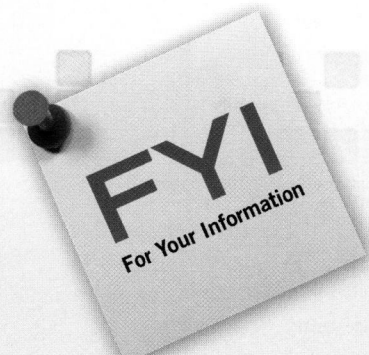

FYI
For Your Information

MyPlate: Foods, Serving Sizes, and Tips

Grains	Amount Equal to 1 Ounce	Common Portions and Ounce Equivalents
Bagels	1 "mini" bagel	1 large bagel = 4 ounce equivalents
Biscuits	1 small (2″ diameter)	1 large (3″) = 2 ounce equivalents
Breads	1 regular slice	2 regular slices = 2 ounce equivalents
Bulgur	½ cup cooked	
Cornbread	1 small piece (2½″ × 1¼″ × 1¼″)	1 medium piece = 2 ounce equivalents
English muffin	½ muffin	1 muffin = 2 ounce equivalents
Muffins	1 small (2½″ diameter)	1 large (3½″ diameter) = 3 ounce equivalents
Oatmeal	½ cup cooked	
Pancakes	1 pancake (4½″ diameter)	3 pancakes (4½″ diameter) = 3 ounce equivalents
Popcorn	3 cups, popped	1 microwave bag, popped = 4 ounce equivalents
Ready-to-eat cereals	1 cup flakes; 1¼ cups puffed	
Rice	½ cup cooked (1 ounce dry)	1 cup cooked = 2 ounce equivalents
Pasta	½ cup cooked (1 ounce dry)	1 cup cooked = 2 ounce equivalents
Tortillas	1 small (6″ diameter)	1 large (12″ diameter) = 4 ounce equivalents

Tips: Make at least half your grains whole grains. Choose foods that name one of the following first on the label's ingredient list: brown rice, bulgur, graham flour, oatmeal, whole oats, whole rye, whole wheat, wild rice. Go easy on high-fat or sugary toppings.

Vegetables	Amount Equal to 1 Cup of Vegetables
Dark-Green Vegetables	
Spinach, romaine, collards, mustard greens, kale, other leafy greens	2 cups raw or 1 cup cooked
Broccoli	1 cup chopped or florets
Orange Vegetables	
Carrots	1 cup raw or cooked 2 medium whole 1 cup baby chopped, sliced, or cooked
Pumpkin, sweet potato, winter squash	1 cup chopped, sliced, or cooked

Vegetables	Amount Equal to 1 Cup of Vegetables
Starchy Vegetables	
Corn	1 cup or 1 large ear (8″ to 9″ long)
Green peas	1 cup
White potatoes	1 cup diced or mashed 1 medium potato, boiled or baked
Other Vegetables	
Bean sprouts	1 cup cooked
Green beans	1 cup cooked
Tomatoes	1 large raw whole (3″)

Tips: Vary your veggies. Make half your plate fruits and vegetables. Eat more dark-green vegetables, more orange vegetables, and more dry beans. Buy fresh vegetables in season for best taste and lowest cost. Buy vegetables that are easy to prepare.

(*continues*)

Fruit	Amount Equal to 1 Cup of Fruit	Milk	Amount Equal to 1 Cup of Milk
Apple	1 small	Milk	1 cup
Applesauce	1 cup	Yogurt	1 regular container (8 ounces) or 1 cup yogurt
Banana	1 large (8″ to 9″ long)	Cheese	1½ ounces hard cheese
Melon	1 cup diced or melon balls		⅓ cup shredded cheese
Grapes	1 cup whole; 32 seedless grapes		2 ounces processed cheese
Canned fruit or diced raw fruit	1 cup		2 cups cottage cheese
Orange or peach	1 large	Milk-based desserts	1 cup pudding made with milk
Strawberries	About 8 large berries		1 cup frozen yogurt
100% fruit juice	1 cup	Soymilk	1 cup calcium-fortified soymilk

Tips: Focus on fruit. Make half your plate fruits and vegetables. Eat a variety of fruit. Choose fresh, frozen, canned, or dried fruit. Go easy on juices. When choosing a juice, look for "100% juice" on the label.
Tips: Get your calcium-rich foods. Switch to fat-free or low-fat milk. If you don't or can't consume milk, get your calcium-rich foods by choosing lactose-free or other calcium sources such as calcium-fortified juices, cereals, breads, soy beverages, or rice beverages.

Meat and Beans	Amount Equal to 1 Ounce	Common Portions and Ounce Equivalents
Cooked lean beef, pork, ham	1 ounce	1 small steak = 3½ to 4 ounce equivalents
Cooked chicken or turkey without skin	1 ounce	1 small lean hamburger = 2 to 3 ounce equivalents 1 small chicken breast half = 3 ounce equivalents
Cooked fish or shellfish	1 ounce	1 can tuna, drained = 3 to 4 ounce equivalents 1 salmon steak = 4 to 6 ounce equivalents 1 small trout = 3 ounce equivalents
Eggs	1 egg	
Nuts and seeds	½ ounce of nuts (12 almonds, 24 pistachios, 7 walnut halves) ½ ounce of seeds, roasted 1 tablespoon of peanut butter	
Dry beans and peas	¼ cup cooked beans or peas ¼ cup baked beans, refried beans ¼ cup tofu 1 ounce tempeh 2 tablespoons hummus	

Tips: Go lean with protein. Choose low-fat or lean meats and poultry. Bake it, broil it, or grill it. Vary your choices, with more fish, beans, peas, nuts, and seeds.
Oils
Common oils: Vegetable oils (canola, corn, cottonseed, olive, safflower, soybean, sunflower)
Foods naturally high in oils:
Nuts
Olives
Some fish
Avocados
Tips: Know your oils. Oils are not a food group, but they provide essential nutrients. Make most of your fat sources from fish, nuts, and vegetable oils. Limit solid fats such as butter, stick margarine, shortening, and lard.

Modified from U.S. Department of Agriculture Center for Nutrition Policy and Promotion. Food Groups, MyPlate. http://www.choosemyplate.gov/myplate/.

getting enough calories. Canada's Official Food Rules (1942) recommended a weekly serving of liver, heart, or kidney and regular doses of fish liver oils—good sources of vitamins A and D. Later food group plans, including the Basic Four that was popular from the 1950s through the 1970s, focused on fruits, vegetables, grains, dairy products, and meats and their substitutes. After the development of the *Dietary Guidelines for Americans* in 1980, the USDA developed a new food guide that would promote overall health and be consistent with the *Dietary Guidelines*; thus, the Food Guide Pyramid was developed. Updated again and renamed in 2005, the USDA MyPyramid food guidance system was intended to be a visual reminder for individuals to make healthy food choices and be physically active every day. By law, the *Dietary Guidelines for Americans* is reviewed, updated if necessary, and published every five years, bringing us to the most current version, the *Dietary Guidelines for Americans, 2015-2020* (see **FIGURE 2.8**).

Position Statement: Academy of Nutrition and Dietetics

Total Diet Approach to Communicating Food and Nutrition Information

It is the position of the Academy of Nutrition and Dietetics that the total diet or overall pattern of food eaten is the most important focus of a healthful eating style. All foods can fit within this pattern, if consumed in moderation with appropriate portion size and combined with regular physical activity. The Academy of Nutrition and Dietetics strives to communicate healthful eating messages to the public that emphasize a balance of food and beverages, rather than any one food or meal.

Reproduced from Position of the American Dietetic Association: total diet approach to healthy eating. *J Am Diet Assoc.* 2013;113(2):307–317. Reprinted with permission from the American Academy of Nutrition and Dietetics.

Canada's Guidelines for Healthy Eating

Promoting healthy eating habits among Canadians has been a priority of Health Canada for many years. Health Canada is the federal department responsible for helping the people of Canada maintain and improve their health. In the 1980s, a high priority was given to developing a single set of dietary guidelines. The result of this effort was the 1990 ***Nutrition Recommendations for Canadians*** and ***Canada's Guidelines for Healthy Eating***. This report updated the existing dietary standards and provided a scientific description of the characteristics of a healthy dietary pattern.

▶ ***Nutrition Recommendations for Canadians*** A set of scientific statements that provide guidance to Canadians for a dietary pattern that will supply recommended amounts of all essential nutrients while reducing the risk of chronic disease.

▶ ***Canada's Guidelines for Healthy Eating*** Key messages that are based on the 1990 *Nutrition Recommendations for Canadians* and that provide positive, action-oriented, scientifically accurate eating advice to Canadians.

Quick Bite

SuperTracker: My Foods, My Fitness, My Health

The MyPlate website includes an interactive diet and physical activity tool called SuperTracker. You can use it to get your own personalized nutrition and physical activity plan. Track your foods and physical activities to see how they stack up to recommendations. Get tips and support to help you make healthier choices and plan ahead. Visit www.supertracker.usda.gov.

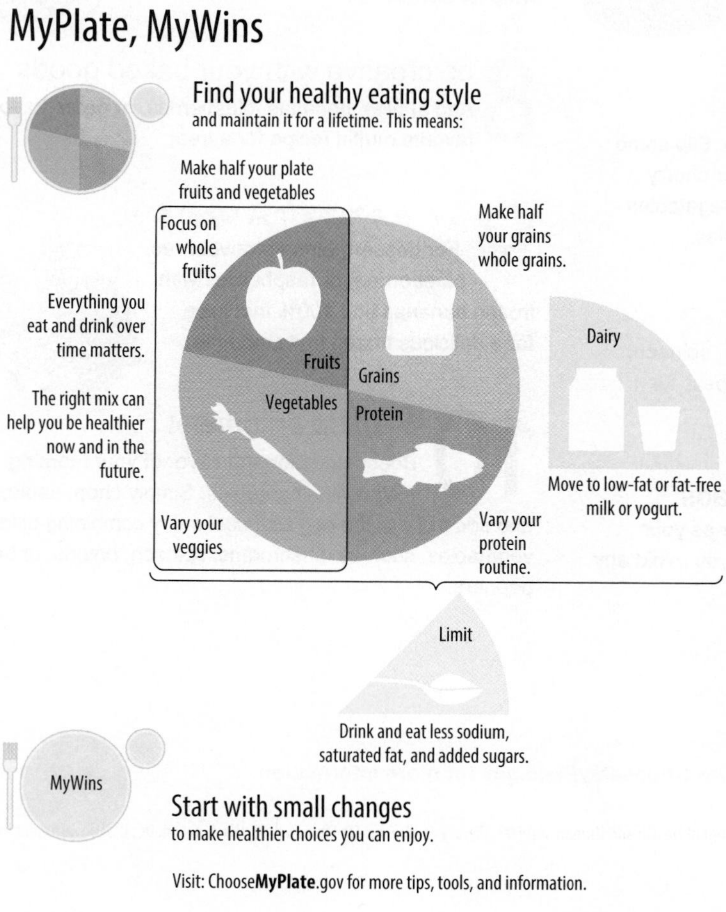

MyPlate, MyWins
Find your healthy eating style
and maintain it for a lifetime. This means:
Make half your plate fruits and vegetables
Focus on whole fruits
Make half your grains whole grains.
Everything you eat and drink over time matters.
The right mix can help you be healthier now and in the future.
Fruits
Grains
Vegetables
Protein
Dairy
Move to low-fat or fat-free milk or yogurt.
Vary your veggies
Vary your protein routine.
Limit
Drink and eat less sodium, saturated fat, and added sugars.
MyWins
Start with small changes
to make healthier choices you can enjoy.
Visit: ChooseMyPlate.gov for more tips, tools, and information.

FIGURE 2.8 MyPlate. Released in 2011, MyPlate is an Internet-based educational tool that helps consumers implement the principles of the *Dietary Guidelines for Americans 2015-2020* and other nutritional standards. Courtesy of the USDA.

10 tips
Nutrition Education Series

liven up your meals with vegetables and fruits

ChooseMyPlate.gov

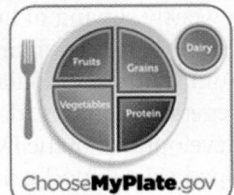

10 tips to improve your meals with vegetables and fruits

Discover the many benefits of adding vegetables and fruits to your meals. They are low in fat and calories, while providing fiber and other key nutrients. Most Americans should eat more than 3 cups—and for some, up to 6 cups—of vegetables and fruits each day. Vegetables and fruits don't just add nutrition to meals. They can also add color, flavor, and texture. Explore these creative ways to bring healthy foods to your table.

1 fire up the grill
Use the grill to cook vegetables and fruits. Try grilling mushrooms, carrots, peppers, or potatoes on a kabob skewer. Brush with oil to keep them from drying out. Grilled fruits like peaches, pineapple, or mangos add great flavor to a cookout.

2 expand the flavor of your casseroles
Mix vegetables such as sauteed onions, peas, pinto beans, or tomatoes into your favorite dish for that extra flavor.

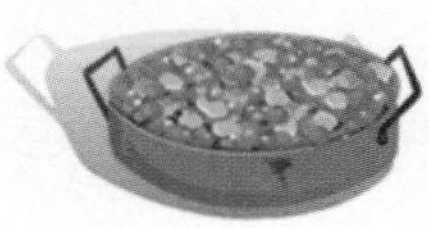

3 planning something Italian?
Add extra vegetables to your pasta dish. Slip some peppers, spinach, red beans, onions, or cherry tomatoes into your traditional tomato sauce. Vegetables provide texture and low-calorie bulk that satisfies.

4 get creative with your salad
Toss in shredded carrots, strawberries, spinach, watercress, orange segments, or sweet peas for a flavorful, fun salad.

5 salad bars aren't just for salads
Try eating sliced fruit from the salad bar as your dessert when dining out. This will help you avoid any baked desserts that are high in calories.

6 get in on the stir-frying fun
Try something new! Stir-fry your veggies—like broccoli, carrots, sugar snap peas, mushrooms, or green beans—for a quick-and-easy addition to any meal.

7 add them to your sandwiches
Whether it is a sandwich or wrap, vegetables make great additions to both. Try sliced tomatoes, romaine lettuce, or avocado on your everday sandwich or wrap for extra flavor.

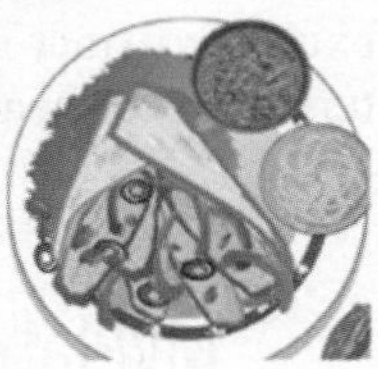

8 be creative with your baked goods
Add apples, bananas, blueberries, or pears to your favorite muffin recipe for a treat.

9 make a tasty fruit smoothie
For dessert, blend strawberries, blueberries, or raspberries with frozen bananas and 100% fruit juice for a delicious frozen fruit smoothie.

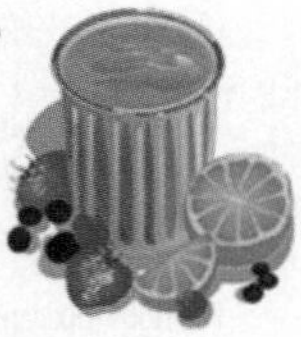

10 liven up an omelet
Boost the color and flavor of your morning omelet with vegetables. Simply chop, saute, and add them to the egg as it cooks. Try combining different vegetables, such as mushrooms, spinach, onions, or bell peppers.

Go to www.ChooseMyPlate.gov for more information.

Reproduced from U.S. Department of Agriculture and U.S. Department of Health and Human Services. *Dietary Guidelines.* Tip Sheet No. 10. Washington, DC: U.S. Government Printing Office; 2011.

As science advanced and nutritional concerns changed, Canada's official food rules evolved into ***Eating Well with Canada's Food Guide***. (See **FIGURE 2.9**.) The amounts and types of foods recommended in the *Food Guide* are based on the nutrient reference values of the Dietary Reference Intakes (DRIs). The foods pictured in the *Food Guide* reflect the diversity of foods available in Canada. The "rainbow" used by the *Food Guide* places foods into four groups: Vegetables and Fruit, Grain Products, Milk and Alternatives, and Meat and Alternatives. The *Food Guide* describes the kinds of foods to choose from each group. For example, under the Milk and Alternatives group, the *Food Guide* suggests, "Drink fortified soy beverages if you do not drink milk." *Eating Well with Canada's Food Guide* illustrates that vegetables, fruits, and grains should be the major part of the diet, with milk products and meats consumed in smaller amounts.

The *Food Guide* also provides a "bar" that shows how many daily servings are recommended for each age group and gives examples of serving sizes. The *Food Guide* provides specific advice for different ages and stages. Limiting foods and beverages high in calories, fat, sugar, or salt is recommended, as is label-reading.

The current edition of *Eating Well with Canada's Food Guide* recommends that Canadians do the following[14]:

- Eat at least one dark-green and one orange vegetable each day.
- Enjoy vegetables and fruit prepared with little or no added fat, sugar, or salt.
- Eat vegetables and fruits more often than juice.
- Select whole grains for at least half of one's grain products.
- Choose grain products that are low in fat, sugar, or salt.
- Drink skim, 1 percent, or 2 percent milk each day.
- Consume meat alternatives, such as beans, lentils, and tofu, often.
- Eat at least two *Food Guide* servings of fish each week.
- Select lean meat and alternatives prepared with little or no added fat or salt.
- Include a small amount of unsaturated fat each day.
- Satisfy thirst with water.
- Limit foods and beverages high in calories, fat, sugar, or salt.
- Be active every day.

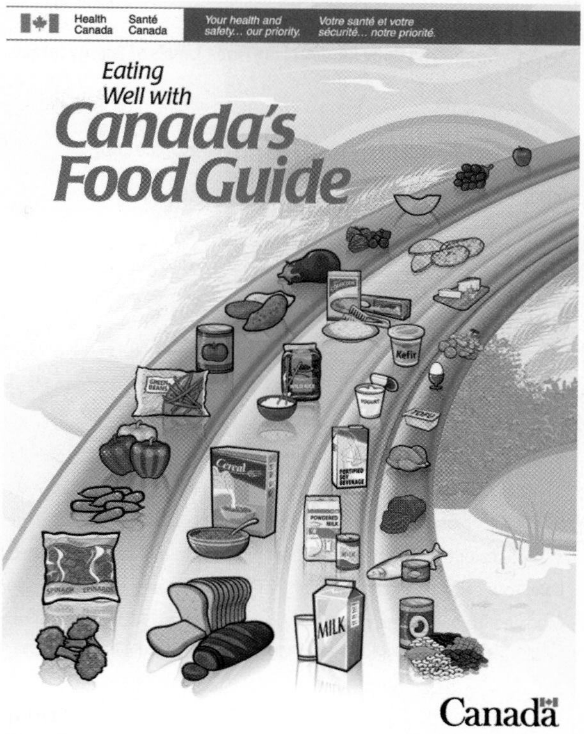

FIGURE 2.9 ***Eating Well with Canada's Food Guide.*** The rainbow portion of *Canada's Food Guide* sorts food into groups from which people can make wise food choices.

▶ ***Eating Well with Canada's Food Guide*** Recommendations to help Canadians select foods to meet energy and nutrient needs while reducing the risk of chronic disease. The *Food Guide* is based on the *Nutrition Recommendations for Canadians* and *Canada's Guidelines for Healthy Eating* and is a key nutrition education tool for Canadians aged 4 years and older.

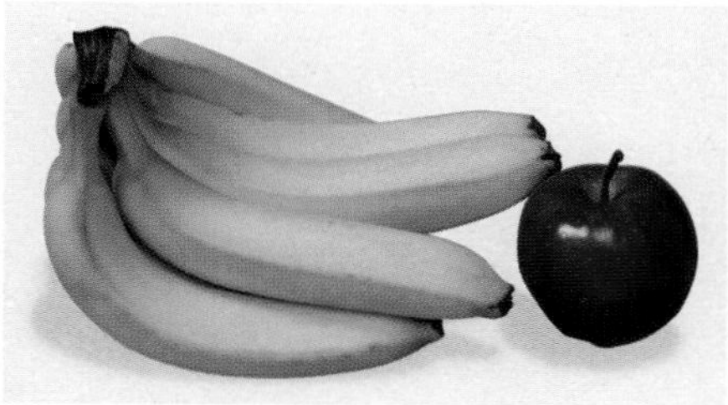

2–4 servings of fruit per day.

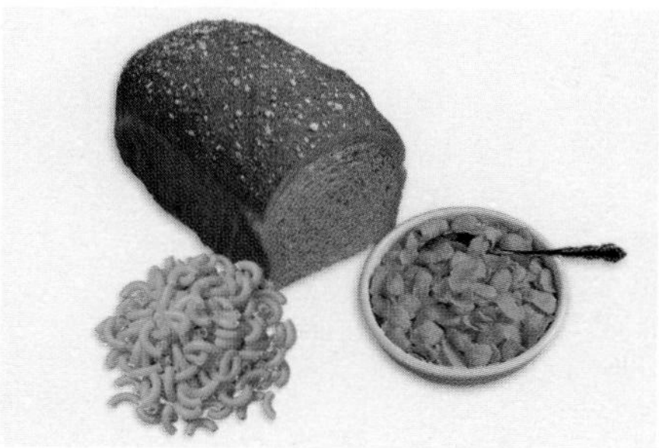

6–11 servings of bread, rice, and cereal per day.

Following the eating pattern of *Canada's Food Guide* will help people to get enough vitamins, minerals, and other nutrients; reduce the risk of obesity, type 2 diabetes, heart disease, certain types of cancer, and osteoporosis; and achieve overall health and vitality. The Health Canada website (www.healthcanada.gc.ca/foodguide) includes a link to My Food Guide, which is an interactive tool for personalizing the information in *Canada's Food Guide*.

Canada's Physical Activity Guide, released in January 2011 by the Canadian Society for Exercise Physiology, recommends that children ages 5 to 11 and youth ages 12 to 17 should get at least 60 minutes of moderate-to-vigorous-intensity physical activity daily. Adults ages 18 to 64 and older adults age 65 and older should get at least 150 minutes of moderate- to vigorous-intensity aerobic physical activity per week, in bouts of 10 minutes or more.

Using MyPlate or *Canada's Food Guide* in Diet Planning

The first step in using MyPlate or *Canada's Food Guide* for diet planning is to determine the amount of calories you should eat each day. **TABLE 2.5** shows the recommended amounts of food for three calorie-intake levels. It also gives

TABLE 2.5
MyPlate Suggested Daily Amounts for Three Levels of Energy Intake

	Energy Intake Level		
Food Group	**Low (1,400 kcal)[a]**	**Moderate (2,000 kcal)[b]**	**High (2,800 kcal)[c]**
Grains	5 oz eq	6 oz eq	10 oz eq
Vegetables	1½ cups	2½ cups	3½ cups
Fruits	1½ cups	2 cups	2½ cups
Milk	2 cups	3 cups	3 cups
Meat and beans	4 oz eq	5½ oz eq	7 oz eq
Oils	4 teaspoons	6 teaspoons	8 teaspoons
Empty calories allowed[d]	117 kilocalories	270 kilocalories	426 kilocalories

[a] 1,400 kilocalories is about right for many young children.

[b] 2,000 kilocalories is about right for teenage girls, active women, and many sedentary men.

[c] 2,800 kilocalories is about right for teenage boys and many active men.

[d] Empty calorie allowance is the remaining amount of calories needed for all food groups, assuming that those choices are fat-free or low-fat and with no added sugars.

Note: Your calorie needs may be higher or lower than those shown. Women may need more calories when they are pregnant or breastfeeding.

Modified from U.S. Department of Agriculture and U.S. Department of Health and Human Services. *Dietary Guidelines for Americans, 2010.* 7th ed. U.S. Government Printing Office; 2010. Courtesy of U.S. Department of Agriculture and U.S. Department of Health and Human Services.

you an idea of how MyPlate varies with different energy needs. Next, become familiar with the types of food in each group, the number of recommended servings, and the appropriate serving sizes. For an intuitive guide to serving sizes, see **TABLE 2.6**, and plan your meals and snacks using the suggested serving sizes for your appropriate calorie level.

Let's start to plan a 2,000-calorie diet. Beginning with breakfast, you could plan to have the following: 1 cup (1 oz) of ready-to-eat cereal, ½ cup of skim milk, 1 slice of whole wheat toast with 1 teaspoon of butter, and 1 cup of orange juice.

Continue to plan your meals and snacks for the rest of the day with the amount of servings you have remaining for each food group. In this case, it would be as shown in **TABLE 2.7**. Keep in mind that what you consider a serving might differ from the sizes defined in MyPlate. Research shows that Americans' serving sizes for common foods such as pasta, cookies, cereal, soft drinks, and French fries have increased significantly.[17] Do large portions promote overeating and obesity? See the FYI feature "Portion Distortion" for a scientific exploration related to this question.

Sometimes it's difficult to figure out how to account for foods that are mixtures of different groups—lasagna, casseroles, or pizza, for example. Try separating such foods into their ingredients (e.g., pizza contains crust, tomato sauce, cheese, and toppings, which might be meats or vegetables) to estimate the amounts. You should be able to come up with a reasonable approximation. All in all, MyPlate and *Canada's Food Guide* are easy-to-use guidelines that can help you select a variety of foods.

Be aware of foods that contain many calories but have little or no nutrients, such as cookies, pastries, and donuts. Note in Table 2.7 that for a 2,000-calorie food plan, 270 calories are remaining and allowed to be used even when all the other food groups are accounted for. However, this accounting with leftover calories assumes that all food choices are fat-free or low-fat and do not have added sugars. What does this mean? If you are already in the habit of choosing low-fat and low-sugar options, you have a few calories to play with each day. These calories can be used for a higher-fat choice or for some sugar in your iced tea. But watch out! Those calories get used up quickly.

TABLE 2.6
Playing with MyPlate Portions Your Favorite Sports and Games Can Help You Visualize MyPlate Portion Sizes

Grains	1 cup dry cereal 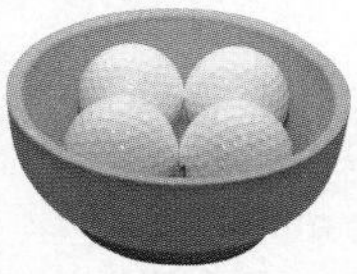 4 golf balls	2-ounce bagel 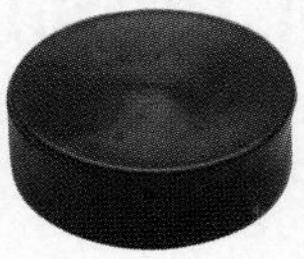 1 hockey puck	½ cup cooked cereal, rice, or pasta 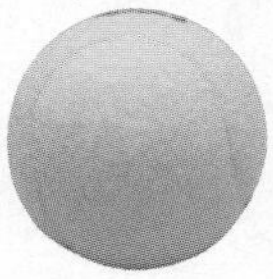 tennis ball
Vegetables	1 cup of vegetables 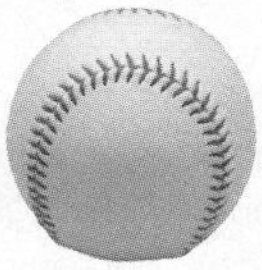		
Fruits	1 medium fruit (equivalent of 1 cup of fruit) 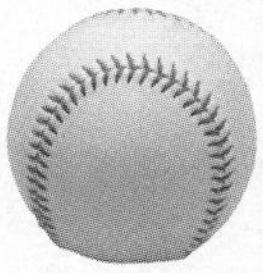		
Oils	1 teaspoon vegetable oil 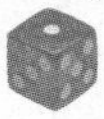 1 die (11/16″ size)	1 tablespoon salad dressing  1 jacks ball	
Milk	1 ½ ounces of hard cheese 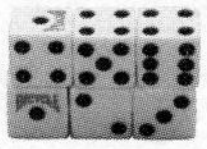 6 dice (11/16″ size)	1/3 cup of shredded cheese  1 billiard ball or raquetball	
Meat and beans	3 ounces cooked meat 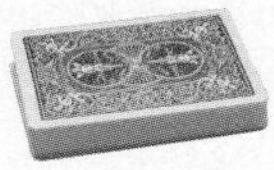 1 deck of playing cards	2 tablespoons hummus  1 ping pong ball	

One regular 12-ounce soft drink would take up 150 discretionary calories; an extra tablespoon of dressing on your salad is 100 calories.

Using the ChooseMyPlate.gov website is easy and informative. Getting a personalized plan, learning healthy eating tips, getting weight loss information, planning a healthy menu, and analyzing your diet are examples of what ChooseMyPlate.gov offers. The website is an excellent way to help guide you through the necessary steps of putting the *Dietary Guidelines* into practice, while at the same time teaching good nutrition and providing appropriate physical activity information.

Key Concepts MyPlate is a complete food guidance system based on the *Dietary Guidelines for Americans* and Dietary Reference Intakes to help Americans make healthy food choices and remind them to be active every day. The interactive tools on the ChooseMyPlate.gov website can help you monitor your food choices. *Eating Well with Canada's Food Guide* illustrates the dietary guidelines for Canadians and the Dietary Reference Intakes. These graphic tools show the appropriate balance of food groups in a healthful diet: more whole grains, low-fat dairy, vegetables, and fruits and less meat, and added fats and sugars.

TABLE 2.7
Sample 2,000 calorie diet showing *Empty Calories Allowed*

Food Group	Total Recommended for 2,000-Calorie Diet	Amount Used at Breakfast	Amount Left for Remainder of the Day
Grains	6 oz eq	2 oz eq	4 oz eq
Vegetables	2½ cups	0	2½ cups
Fruits	2 cups	1 cup	1 cup
Dairy	3 cups	½ cup	2½ cups
Protein	5½ oz eq	0	5½ oz
Oils	6 tsp	1 tsp	5 tsp
Empty calories allowed	267 calories	0	267 calories

Data from U.S. Department of Agriculture and U.S. Department of Health and Human Services. *Dietary Guidelines for Americans, 2010.* 7th ed. Washington, DC: U.S. Government Printing Office; December 2010.

FYI For Your Information

Portion Distortion

How do portions and serving sizes differ? According to the National Institutes of Health, a *portion* of food is defined as the amount of food that you choose to eat at one time, whereas a *serving* is a specific amount of food or drink.[a] Many foods that are packaged as a single portion actually contain multiple servings. Sometimes the portion size and serving size are the same, but not always. Check the food label to see how much of a portion of the foods you like to eat counts as one serving.

Over the past few years, portions have grown significantly in supermarkets, restaurants, and even in our own homes.[b] The prevalence of obesity continues to be of great concern to both adults and children in the United States, and increasing portion sizes can have a lot to do with this increasing weight.

Many factors contribute to Americans' growing waistlines, but one observation in particular cannot be overlooked: The incidence of obesity has increased in parallel with increasing portion sizes.[c] Consider this: Adults today consume an average of 300 more calories per day than they did in the year 1985.[d] Is this just a coincidence, or do larger portion sizes have something to do with it? In almost every eating situation, we are now confronted by huge portions, which are perceived as "normal" or "a great value." Americans have created the perception that large portion sizes are appropriate, creating an environment of *portion distortion*.[e] We find portion distortions in restaurants, where the jumbo-sized portions are consistently 250 percent larger than the regular portions.[f] We even find portion distortions in our homes, where the sizes of our bowls and glasses have steadily increased and where the surface area of the average dinner plate has increased 36 percent since 1960.[g] Research shows that people unintentionally consume more calories when offered larger portions.[h] Consuming larger portion sizes can contribute to positive energy balance, which, over time, leads to weight gain and ultimately can result in obesity.

The phenomenon of portion distortion has the potential to hinder weight loss, weight maintenance, and health improvement efforts. Consider right-sizing the portions of food that you choose to eat. This just might bring super-size benefits to your health.

To see whether you know how today's portions compare to the portions available 20 years ago, take the interactive portion distortion quizzes on the National Heart, Lung, and Blood Institute's Portion Distortion webpage (www.nhlbi.nih.gov/health/educational/wecan/eat-right/portion-distortion.htm). You can also learn about the amount of physical activity required to burn off the extra calories provided by today's portions.

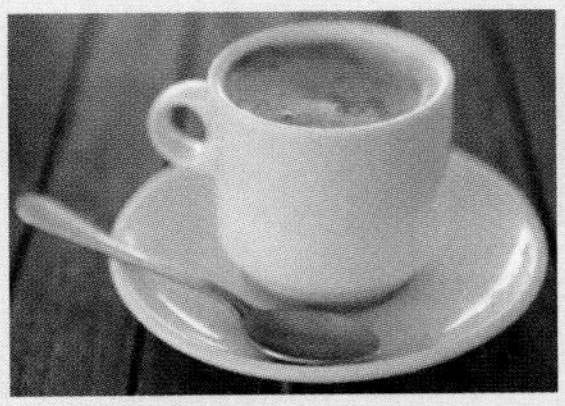

© holbox/ShutterStock, Inc.

8 oz with milk and sugar

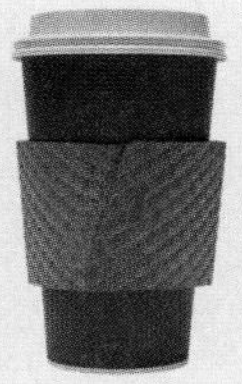

© iStockphoto/Thinkstock

16-oz mocha coffee

[a] American Heart Association, Robert Woods Johnson Foundation. A nation at risk: obesity in the United States. http://www.rwjf.org/en/library/research/2006/11/a-nation-at-risk--statistical-sourcebook--presents-facts-about-o.html

[b] Ibid.

[c] Schwartz J, Byrd-Bredbenner C. Portion distortion: typical portion sizes selected by young adults. *J Am Diet Assoc.* 2006;106(9):1412–1418.

[d] American Heart Association, Robert Woods Johnson Foundation. Op cit.

[e] Wansink B, van Ittersum K. Portion size me: downsizing our consumption norms. *J Am Diet Assoc.* 2007;7(7):1103–1106.

[f] Ibid.

[g] Ibid.

[h] Herman P, Polivy J, Pliner P, Vartanian L, Mechanisms underlying the portion-size effect. *Physiol Behav.* 2015 15;144:129–136. Epub March 20, 2015.

Exchange Lists

▶ **Exchange Lists** Lists of foods that in specified portions provide equivalent amounts of carbohydrate, fat, protein, and energy. Any food in an Exchange List can be substituted for any other without markedly affecting macronutrient intake.

Another food label tool for diet planning that uses food groups is called the **Exchange Lists**. Like MyPlate, the Exchange Lists divide foods into groups. Diets can be planned by choosing a certain number of servings, or exchanges, from each group each day. The original purpose of the Exchange Lists was to help people with diabetes plan diets that would provide consistent levels of energy and carbohydrates—both of which are essential for dietary management of diabetes. For this reason, foods are organized into groups or lists not only by the type of food (e.g., fruits or vegetables), but also by the amount of macronutrients (carbohydrate, protein, and fat) in each portion. The portions are defined so that each exchange has a similar composition. For example, 1 fruit exchange is ½ cup of orange juice or 17 small grapes or 1 medium apple or ½ cup of applesauce. All these exchanges have approximately 60 kilocalories,

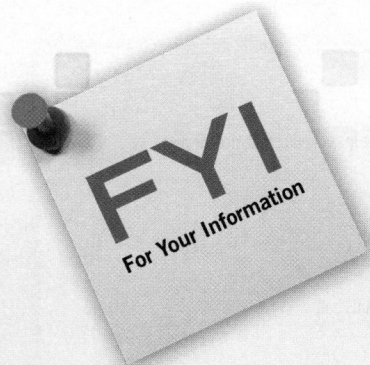

15 grams of carbohydrate, 0 grams of protein, and 0 grams of fat. In the Exchange Lists, starchy vegetables such as potatoes, corn, and peas are grouped with breads and cereals instead of with other vegetables because their balance of macronutrients is more like bread or pasta than carrots or tomatoes.

FIGURE 2.10 shows the amounts of carbohydrate, protein, fat, and kilocalories in one exchange from each group, along with a sample serving size. For a complete set of the Exchange Lists, go to NIH Food Exchange Lists (https://www.nhlbi.nih.gov/health/educational/lose_wt/eat/fd_exch.htm).

Using the Exchange Lists in Diet Planning

In addition to their use by people with diabetes, Exchange Lists are used in many weight-control programs. Planning a diet using the Exchange Lists is done in much the same manner as using MyPlate. The first step is to become very familiar with the components of each group, the variations in fat content for dairy and meat lists, and ways that other foods may be included. Then, an individual diet plan can be used to select meals and snacks throughout the day. An exchange-based diet plan specifies the number of exchanges to be consumed from each group at each meal. For example, a 1,500-kilocalorie weight reduction diet plan might have the following meal pattern:

Breakfast:	2 starch, 1 fruit, 1 milk, 1 fat
Lunch:	3 meat, 2 starch, 1 fruit, 1 vegetable, 1 fat
Snack:	1 milk, 1 starch, 1 fat
Dinner:	2 meat, 1 starch, 2 vegetable, 2 fat
Snack:	2 starch, 1 fruit

Using this pattern and a complete set of the Exchange Lists, you could then plan out a day or week of menus. Here's one sample:

Breakfast:	½ cup orange juice, ¾ cup corn flakes, 1 cup 2% milk, 1 slice toast, 1 tsp margarine
Lunch:	3 oz cooked hamburger on bun, 1 tsp mayonnaise, ½ cup baby carrots, 1 medium apple
Snack:	¾ cup low-fat yogurt, ½ bagel with 1 tbsp cream cheese
Dinner:	2 oz cooked pork chop, ½ cup rice with 1 tsp margarine, ½ cup yellow squash and ½ cup zucchini stir-fried in 1 tsp vegetable oil
Snack:	1 toasted English muffin, 1 medium pear

Key Concepts The Exchange Lists are a diet-planning tool that use the idea of food groups, but define groups specifically in terms of macronutrient (carbohydrate, fat, and protein) content. Individual diet plans can be developed for people who need to control energy or carbohydrate intake, such as for weight control or management of diabetes mellitus.

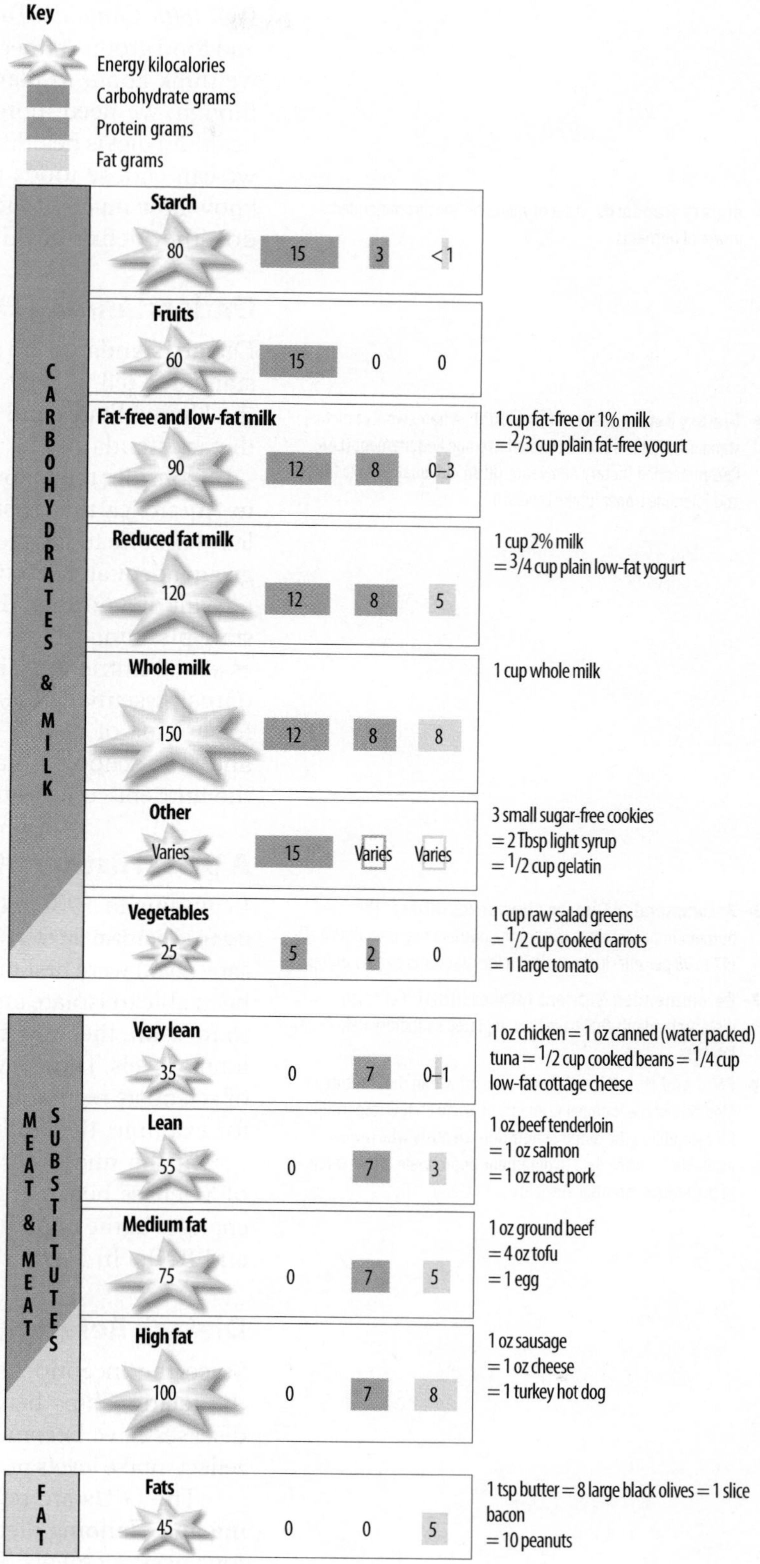

FIGURE 2.10 Exchange Lists. The Exchange Lists are a widely used system for meal planning for people with diabetes. They are also helpful for people interested in healthy eating and weight control.
Data from *Exchange Lists for Meal Planning*. Alexandria, VA: Academy of Nutrition and Dietetics; 2003.

Recommendations for Nutrient Intake: The DRIs

So far, the tools described (*Dietary Guidelines for Americans*, MyPlate, *Eating Well with Canada's Food Guide*, and Exchange Lists) deal with whole foods and food groups rather than individual nutrient values; after all, foods are what we think about in planning our daily meals and shopping lists. Sometimes, though, we need more specific information about our nutritional needs—a healthful diet is healthful because of the balance of *nutrients* it contains. Before we can choose foods that meet our needs for specific nutrients, we need to know how much of each nutrient we require daily. This is what **dietary standards** do—they define healthful diets in terms of specific amounts of the nutrients.

▶ **dietary standards** A set of values for the recommended intake of nutrients.

Understanding Dietary Standards

Dietary standards are sets of recommended intake values for nutrients. These standards tell us how much of each nutrient we should have in our diets. In the United States and Canada, the **Dietary Reference Intakes (DRIs)** are the current dietary standards.

▶ **Dietary Reference Intakes (DRIs)** A framework of dietary standards that includes Estimated Average Requirement (EAR), Recommended Dietary Allowance (RDA), Adequate Intake (AI), and Tolerable Upper Intake Level (UL).

Consider the following scenario. You are running a research center located in Antarctica that is staffed by 60 people. Because staff will not be able to leave the site to get meals, you must provide all their food. You must keep the group adequately nourished; you certainly don't want anyone to become ill as a result of a nutrient deficiency. How would you (or the nutritionist you hire) start planning? How can you be sure to provide adequate amounts of the essential nutrients? The most important tool would be a set of dietary standards! Essentially the same scenario faces those who plan and provide food for groups of people in more routine circumstances—the military, prisons, and even schools. To assess nutritional adequacy, diet planners can compare the nutrient composition of their food plans to recommended intake values.

A Brief History of Dietary Standards

Beginning in 1938, Health Canada published dietary standards called **Recommended Nutrient Intakes (RNIs)**. In the United States, the **Recommended Dietary Allowances (RDAs)** were first published in 1941. By the 1940s, nutrition scientists had been able to isolate and identify many of the nutrients in food. They were able to measure the amounts of these nutrients in foods and to recommend daily intake levels. These levels became the first RNI and RDA values. Committees of scientists regularly reviewed the standards and published revised editions; for example, the tenth (and final) edition of RDAs was published in 1989.

▶ **Recommended Dietary Allowances (RDAs)** The nutrient intake levels that meet the nutrient needs of almost all (97 to 98 percent) individuals in a life-stage and gender group.

▶ **Recommended Nutrient Intakes (RNIs)** Canadian dietary standards that have been replaced by Dietary Reference Intakes.

▶ **Food and Nutrition Board** A board within the Institute of Medicine of the National Academy of Sciences. It is responsible for assembling the group of nutrition scientists who review available scientific data to determine appropriate intake levels of the known essential nutrients.

In the mid-1990s, the **Food and Nutrition Board** of the National Academy of Sciences began a partnership with Health Canada to make fundamental changes in the approach to setting dietary standards and to replace the RDAs and RNIs. In 1997, the first set of DRIs was published.

Dietary Reference Intakes

Since the inception of the RDAs and RNIs, we have learned more about the relationships between diet and chronic disease, and nutrient-deficiency diseases have become rare in the United States and Canada. The new DRIs reflect intake levels not just for dietary adequacy, but also for optimal nutrition.

The DRIs are reference values for nutrient intakes to be used in assessing and planning diets for healthy people (see **FIGURE 2.11**). The DRIs include four basic elements: Estimated Average Requirement (EAR), Recommended Dietary Allowance (RDA), Adequate Intake (AI), and Tolerable Upper Intake Level (UL). Underlying each of these values is the definition of a **requirement** as the "lowest continuing intake level of a nutrient that, for a specific indicator of

▶ **requirement** The lowest continuing intake level of a nutrient that prevents deficiency in an individual.

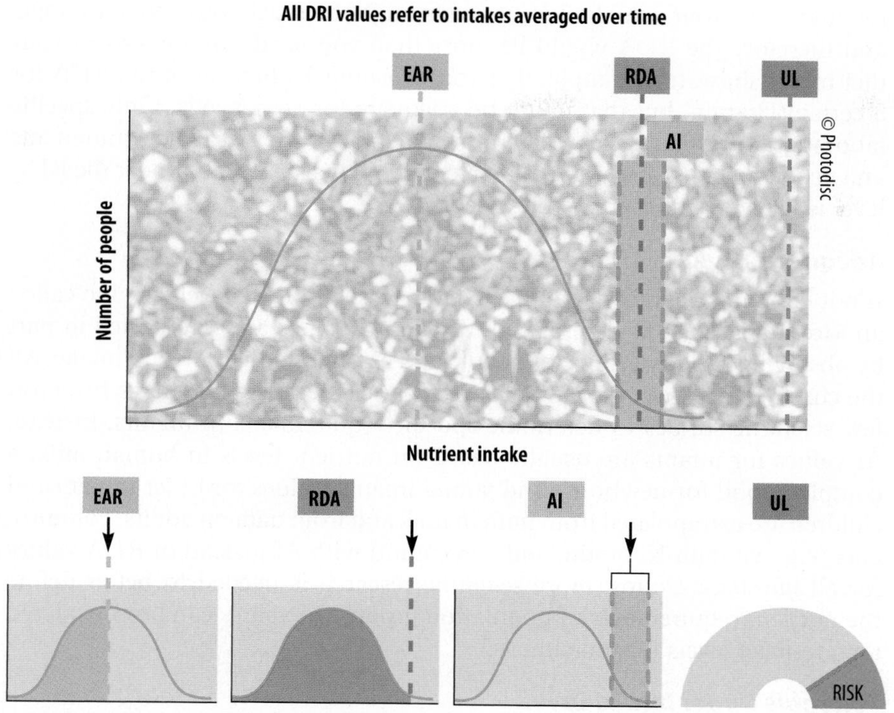

The **Estimated Average Requirement** is the nutrient intake level estimated to meet the needs of 50% of the individuals in a life-stage and gender group.

The **Recommended Dietary Allowance** is the nutrient intake level that is sufficient to meet the needs of 97–98% of the individuals in a life-stage and gender group. The RDA is calculated from the EAR.

Adequate Intake is based upon expert estimates of nutrient intake by a defined group of healthy people. These estimates are used when there is insufficient scientific evidence to establish an EAR. AI is not equivalent to RDA.

Tolerable Upper Intake Level is the maximum level of daily nutrient intake that poses little risk of adverse health effects to almost all of the individuals in a defined group. In most cases, supplements must be consumed to reach a UL.

FIGURE 2.11 Dietary Reference Intakes. The Dietary Reference Intakes are a set of dietary standards that include Estimated Average Requirement (EAR), Recommended Dietary Allowance (RDA), Adequate Intake (AI), and Tolerable Upper Intake Level (UL).

adequacy, will maintain a defined level of nutriture in an individual."[18-21] In other words, a requirement is the smallest amount of a nutrient you should take in on a regular basis to remain healthy. In the DRI report on macronutrients, two other concepts were introduced: the Estimated Energy Requirement (EER) and the Acceptable Macronutrient Distribution Ranges (AMDRs).[22]

Estimated Average Requirement

The **Estimated Average Requirement (EAR)** reflects the amount of a nutrient that would meet the needs of 50 percent of the people in a particular life-stage (age) and gender group. For each nutrient, this requirement is defined using a specific indicator of dietary adequacy. This indicator could be the level of the nutrient or one of its breakdown products in the blood, or the amount of an enzyme associated with that nutrient.[23] The EAR is used to set the RDA; EAR values also can be used to assess dietary adequacy or plan diets for groups of people.

▶ **Estimated Average Requirement (EAR)** The intake value that meets the estimated nutrient needs of 50 percent of individuals in a specific life-stage and gender group.

Recommended Dietary Allowance

The Recommended Dietary Allowance (RDA) is the daily intake level that meets the needs of most people (97 to 98 percent) in a life-stage and gender group. The RDA is set at two standard deviations above the EAR. A nutrient will not have an RDA value if there are not enough scientific data available to set an EAR value.

People can use the RDA value as a target or goal for dietary intake and make comparisons between actual intake and RDA values. It is important to remember, however, that the RDAs do not define an *individual's* nutrient requirements. Your actual nutrient needs might be much lower than average, and therefore the RDA would be more than you need. An analysis of your diet might show, for example, that you consume 45 percent of the RDA for a certain vitamin, but that might be adequate for your needs. Only specific laboratory or other tests can determine a person's true nutrient requirements and actual nutritional status. An intake that is consistently at or near the RDA level is likely to be meeting your needs.

Adequate Intake

▶ **Adequate Intake (AI)** The nutrient intake that appears to sustain a defined nutritional state or some other indicator of health (e.g., growth rate or normal circulating nutrient values) in a specific population or subgroup. AI is used when there is insufficient scientific evidence to establish an EAR.

If not enough scientific data are available to set an EAR level, a value called an **Adequate Intake (AI)** is determined instead. AI values are determined in part by observing healthy groups of people and estimating their dietary intake. All the current DRI values for infants are AI levels because there have been too few scientific studies to determine specific requirements in infants. Instead, AI values for infants are usually based on nutrient levels in human milk, a complete food for newborns and young infants. Values for older infants and children are extrapolated from human milk and from data on adults. For nutrients (e.g., vitamin K, biotin, and chromium) with AI instead of RDA values for all life-stage groups, more scientific research is needed to better define the nutrient requirements of population groups. AI values can be considered target intake levels for individuals.

Tolerable Upper Intake Level

▶ **Tolerable Upper Intake Levels (ULs)** The maximum levels of daily nutrient intakes that are unlikely to pose health risks to almost all of the individuals in the group for whom they are designed.

Tolerable Upper Intake Levels (ULs) have been defined for many nutrients. Consumption of a nutrient in amounts higher than the UL could be harmful. The ULs have been developed partly in response to the growing interest in dietary supplements that contain large amounts of essential nutrients. The UL is *not* to be used as a target for intake but rather should be a cautionary level for people who regularly take nutrient supplements.

Estimated Energy Requirement

▶ **Estimated Energy Requirement (EER)** Dietary energy intake that is predicted to maintain energy balance in a healthy adult of a defined age, gender, weight, height, and level of physical activity consistent with good health.

The **Estimated Energy Requirement (EER)** is defined as the energy intake that is estimated to maintain energy balance in healthy, normal-weight individuals. It is determined using an equation that considers weight, height, age, and physical activity. Different equations are used for males and females and for different age groups.

Acceptable Macronutrient Distribution Ranges

▶ **Acceptable Macronutrient Distribution Ranges (AMDRs)** Range of intakes for a particular energy source that are associated with reduced risk of chronic disease while providing adequate intakes of essential nutrients.

Acceptable Macronutrient Distribution Ranges (AMDRs) indicate the recommended balance of energy sources in a healthful diet. These values consider the amounts of macronutrients needed to provide adequate intake of essential nutrients while reducing the risk for chronic disease. The AMDRs are shown in **TABLE 2.8**.

TABLE 2.8
Acceptable Macronutrient Distribution Ranges for Adults

Fat	20–35%
Carbohydrate	45–65%
Protein	10–35%
Omega-6 polyunsaturated fatty acids	5–10%
Alpha-linolenic acid	0.6–1.2%

Note: All values are percentage of energy intake.

Reproduced from Institute of Medicine, Food and Nutrition Board. *Dietary Reference Intakes for Energy, Carbohydrate, Fiber, Fat, Fatty Acids, Cholesterol, Protein, and Amino Acids.* Copyright © 2005 by the National Academy of Sciences, courtesy of the National Academies Press, Washington, DC.

Use of Dietary Standards

The most appropriate use of DRIs is to plan and evaluate diets for large groups of people. Remember the Antarctica scenario at the beginning of this section? If you had planned menus and evaluated the nutrient composition of the foods that would be included and if the average nutrient levels of those daily menus met or exceeded the RDA/AI levels, you could be confident that your group would be adequately nourished. If you had a very large group—thousands of soldiers, for instance—the EAR would be a more appropriate guide.

Dietary standards are also used to make decisions about nutrition policy. The Special Supplemental Food Program for Women, Infants, and Children (WIC), for example, takes into account the DRIs as it provides food or vouchers for food. The goal of this federally funded supplemental feeding program is to improve the nutrient intake of low-income pregnant and breastfeeding women, their infants, and young children. The guidelines for school lunch and breakfast programs are also based on DRI values.

Often, we use dietary standards as comparison values for individual diets. It can be interesting to see how your daily intake of a nutrient compares with the RDA or AI. However, an intake that is less than the RDA/AI doesn't necessarily mean deficiency; your individual requirement for a nutrient can be less than the RDA/AI value. You can use the RDA/AI values as targets for dietary intake, while avoiding nutrient intake that exceeds the UL.

Key Concepts Dietary standards are levels of nutrient intake recommended for healthy people. These standards help the government set nutrition policy and also can be used to guide the planning and evaluation of diets for groups and individuals. The Dietary Reference Intakes are the dietary standards for the United States and Canada. These standards focus on maintaining optimal health and lowering the risks of chronic disease, rather than simply on dietary adequacy.

Food Labels

Now that you understand diet-planning tools and dietary standards, let's focus on your use of these tools—for example, when making decisions at the grocery store. One of the most useful tools in planning a healthful diet is the **food label**.

Specific federal regulations control what may and may not appear on a food label and what *must* appear on it. The **Food and Drug Administration (FDA)** is responsible for ensuring that foods sold in the United States are safe, wholesome, and properly labeled. The Health Products and Food Branch of Health Canada has similar responsibilities. Only a small category of foods, such as spices and flavorings, is not required by the FDA to have a particular food label. Such foods are exempted because they do not provide a significant amount of nutrients. Deli items and ready-to-eat foods that are prepared and sold in retail establishments also do not require a food label.[24] Raw fruits and vegetables and fresh fish generally do not carry food labels either; however, these foods fall under the FDA's voluntary, point-of-purchase nutrition information program, which establishes that the nutrition information for grocery stores' most commonly purchased items must be posted somewhere near where that food is sold.[25] The FDA's jurisdiction applies to packaged foods except for certain meat, poultry and processed egg products, because these foods are regulated by the U.S. Department of Agriculture Food Safety and Inspection Service.

In May of 2016 the FDA introduced updates to the Nutrition Facts Panel. Until then, and aside from adding trans fat to the list of required nutrients in 2006, the Nutrition Facts Label has not changed since 1994. Food manufacturers have until the year 2018 to implement the required label changes, therefore consumers can still see both the old and the new version of the Nutrition Facts Panel. Let's take a closer look at Food Lables.

▶ **food label** Labels required by law on virtually all packaged foods and having five requirements: (1) a statement of identity; (2) the net contents (by weight, volume, or measure) of the package; (3) the name and address of the manufacturer, packer, or distributor; (4) a list of ingredients; and (5) nutrition information.

▶ **Food and Drug Administration (FDA)** The federal agency responsible for ensuring that foods sold in the United States (except for eggs, poultry, and meat, which are monitored by the USDA) are safe, wholesome, and labeled properly. The FDA sets standards for the composition of some foods, inspects food plants, and monitors imported foods. The FDA is an agency of the U.S. Department of Health and Human Services (DHHS).

Ingredients and Other Basic Information

The label on a food you buy today has been shaped by many sets of regulations. As **FIGURE 2.12** shows, food labels have five mandatory components:

1. A statement of identity/name of the food
2. The net weight of the food contained inside of the package, not including the weight of the package
3. The name and address of the manufacturer, packer, or distributor
4. A list of ingredients in descending order by weight
5. Nutrition information

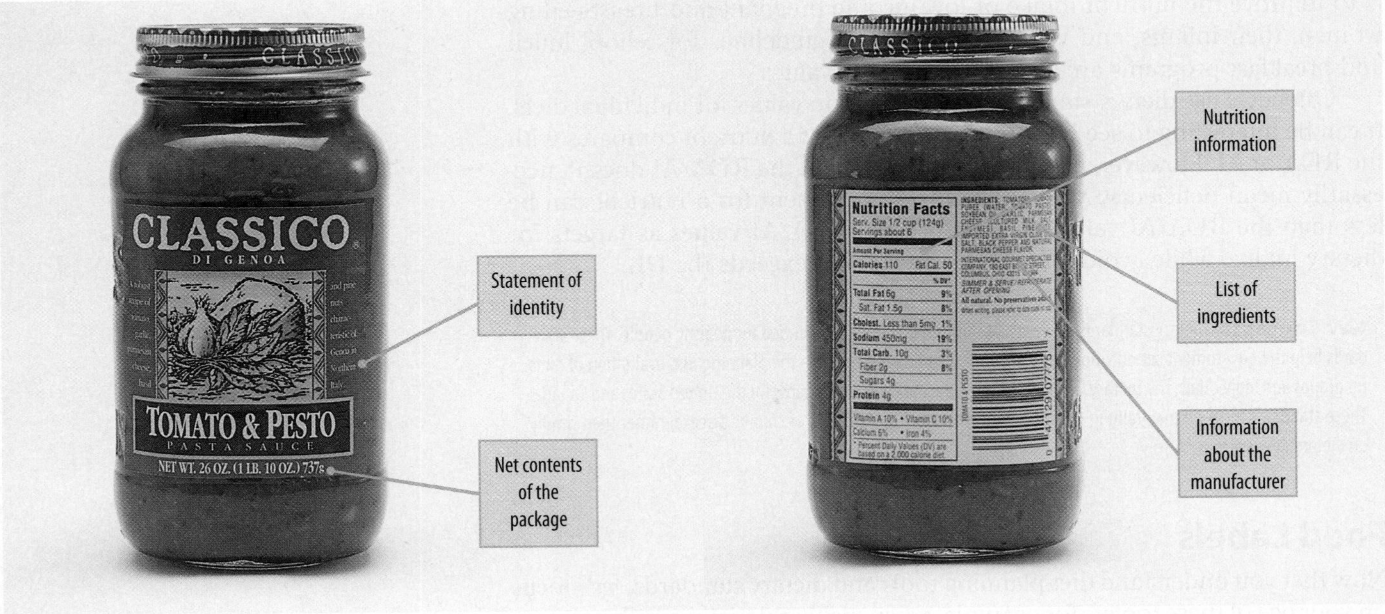

FIGURE 2.12 The five mandatory requirements for food labels. Federal regulations determine what may and may not appear on food labels.

▶ **statement of identity** A mandate that commercial food products prominently display the common or usual name of the product or identify the food with an "appropriately descriptive term."

The **statement of identity** requirement means that the product must prominently display the common or usual name of the product or identify the food with an "appropriately descriptive term." For example, it would be misleading to label a fruit beverage containing only 10 percent fruit juice as a "juice." The statement of net package contents must accurately reflect the quantity in terms of weight, volume, measure, or numerical count. Information about the manufacturer, packer, or distributor gives consumers a way to contact someone in case they have questions about the product.

Ingredients must be listed by common or usual name, in descending order by weight; thus, the first ingredient listed is the primary ingredient in that food product. Let's compare the ingredient list of two cereals:

> *Cereal A ingredients:* Milled corn, sugar, salt, malt flavoring, high-fructose corn syrup
>
> *Cereal B ingredients:* Sugar, yellow corn flour, rice flour, wheat flour, whole oat flour, partially hydrogenated vegetable oil (contains one or more of the following oils: canola, soybean, cottonseed), salt, cocoa, artificial favor, corn syrup

In Cereal B, the first ingredient listed is sugar, which means this cereal contains more sugar by weight than any other ingredient. Cereal A's primary ingredient is milled corn. That can make quite a difference in the amount (grams) of sugar a cereal contains!

As you probably have noticed, when the ingredient list includes the artificial sweetener aspartame, it also displays a warning statement. Also, preservatives and other additives in foods must be listed, along with an explanation of their function. Accurate and complete ingredient information is vital for people with food allergies who must avoid certain food components. The labels of foods that contain any of the eight major food allergens (egg, wheat, peanuts, milk, tree nuts, soy, fish, and crustaceans) are required to include common names when listing these ingredients.

Nutrition Facts Panel

The **Nutrition Facts Panel** informs the consumer about the nutritional value of a food product, enabling an informed shopper to compare similar products.

Using both the new and the older version of the Nutrition Facts Panel, (see **FIGURE 2.13**) let's take a closer look at it's elements. The heading "Nutrition Facts" stands out clearly. Just under the heading is information about the number of servings and serving size per container. It is important to note the serving size because all the nutrient information that follows is based on that amount of food, and the listed serving size might be different from what you usually eat. One change to the new Label is that the serving sizes described on the package are required to more closely reflect the amounts of that food in which people typically eat, something that has certainly changed since the last serving size requirements were published in 1993. People should recognize that the serving size does not necessarily reflect the recommended portion size, but rahter the amount of that food that is generally eaten in one sitting. In addition, calories and nutrition information must be declared for the entire package.

▶ **Nutrition Facts Panel** A portion of the food label that states the content of selected nutrients in a food in a standard way prescribed by the Food and Drug Administration. By law, Nutrition Facts must appear on nearly all processed food products in the United States and the new Nutrition Fact Label is intended to make it easier for consumers to make informed decisions about the foods that they are eating. For example, the new Label includes the addition of nutrients which better reflect people's adequate, over- or under-consumption of nutrients and vitamins such as added sugar, Vitamin D and potassium.

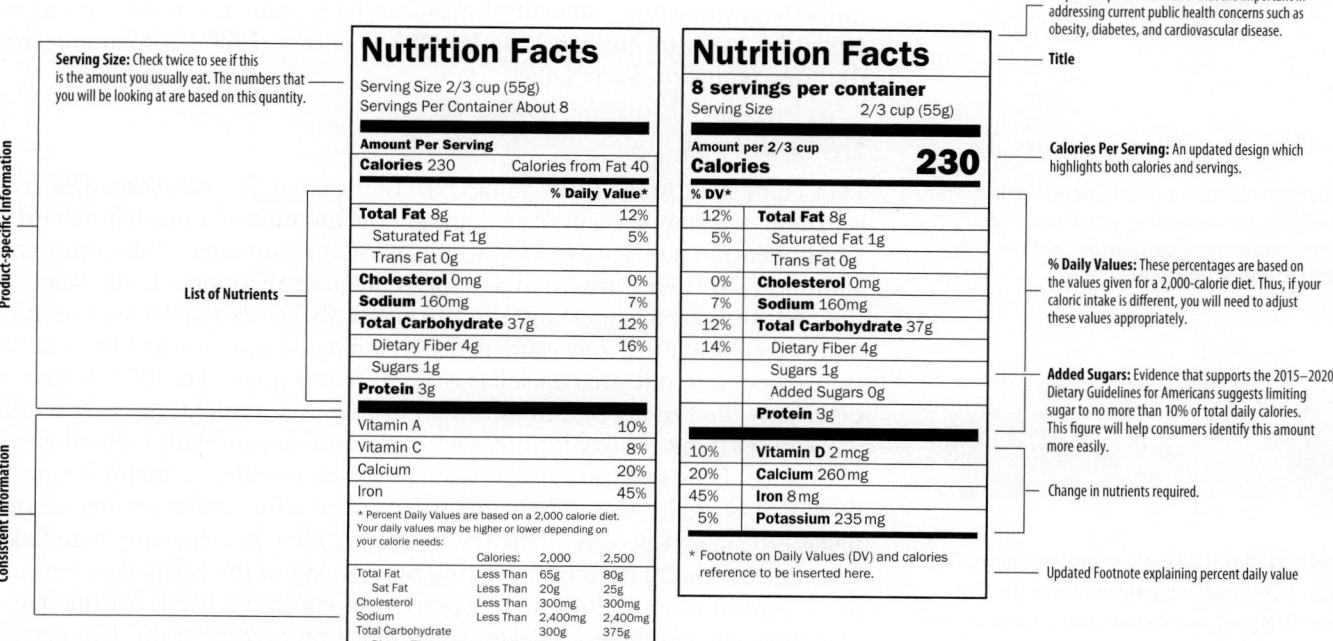

FIGURE 2.13 The Nutrition Facts panel. Comparison of the previous and new Nutrition Facts Panel.

The next part of the label shows a list of nutrients with % Daily Values. "Calories from Fat" will be removed from the old label because research shows that the type of fat is more important than the total amount. "Total Fat," "Saturated Fat," "Trans Fat" and "Cholesterol" will continue to be required on the label. In addition, Sodium, Total Carbohydrates, Dietary Fiber, Total Sugars, Added Sugars, and Protein are also included on this part of the Label. This information is given both in quantity (grams or milligrams per serving) and as a percentage of the Daily Value—a comparison standard specifically for food labels. (This standard is described in the following section.) Updated daily values for the nutrients sodium, dietary fiber, vitamin D, and potassium on the new label will now be consistent with the Institute of Medicine recommendations and the 2015-2020 Dietary Guidelines for Americans. Vitamin D and potassium tend to be nutrients that people are not getting enough of, therefore these nutrients wil be included on the Label. The % DV for calcium and iron will continue to be required, along with the actual gram amounts. Vitamin A and C will no longer be required because deficiencies of these vitamins are rare. These nutrients can be included on a voluntary basis. Listed next are percentages of Daily Values for vitamin D, Calcium, Iron and Potassium. which are the only micronutrients that must appear on all standard labels. Manufacturers can choose to include information about other nutrients, such as potassium, polyunsaturated fat, additional vitamins, or other minerals, in the Nutrition Facts panel. However, if they make a claim about an optional component (e.g., "good source of vitamin E") or **enrich** or **fortify** the food, the manufacturers must include specific nutrition information for these added nutrients. This information must be included even when government regulations require enrichment or fortification, such as the fortification of milk with vitamin D to prevent rickets (a bone disease in children that results from vitamin D deficiency) and the fortification of grain products with folic acid to reduce the risk of birth defects. Food products that come in small packages (e.g., gum, candy, tuna) or that have little nutritional value (e.g., diet soft drinks) can have abbreviated versions of the Nutrition Facts on the label, as **FIGURE 2.14** shows. **FIGURE 2.15** summarizes the New Nutrition Facts Label.

▶ **enrich** To add vitamins and minerals lost or diminished during food processing, particularly the addition of thiamin, riboflavin, niacin, folic acid, and iron to grain products.

▶ **fortify** Refers to the addition of vitamins or minerals that were not originally present in a food.

Daily Values

Let's come back to the Daily Values part of the label. The **Daily Values (DVs)** are a set of dietary standards used to compare the amount of a nutrient (or other component) in a serving of food to the amount recommended for daily consumption. Nutrients are listed as a percentage of the food's Daily Value on the Nutrition Facts panel, and the Percent Daily Values (%DV) are based on a 2,000-calorie diet. Your estimated needs may be more or less than 2,000 calories per day, but you can still use the %DV as a guide. The %DV helps you determine if a serving of a food is high or low in a nutrient. In other words, you can see if this food contributes a lot or a little to your daily recommended allowance. Let's say you rely on your breakfast cereal as a major source of dietary fiber intake. Comparing two packages, you find that a serving of cornflakes cereal has 4 percent of the DV for dietary fiber, but choosing bran-flakes cereal gives you 20 percent. By eating one serving of the cornflakes, you will get 4 percent of an estimated 100 percent of your fiber needs for the day. If you choose to eat the bran flakes, you will get 20 percent of the 100 percent estimated needs of fiber for the day. You don't have to know anything about grams to see which food is higher in fiber.

▶ **Daily Values (DVs)** A single set of nutrient intake standards developed by the Food and Drug Administration to represent the needs of the "typical" consumer; used as standards for expressing nutrient content on food labels.

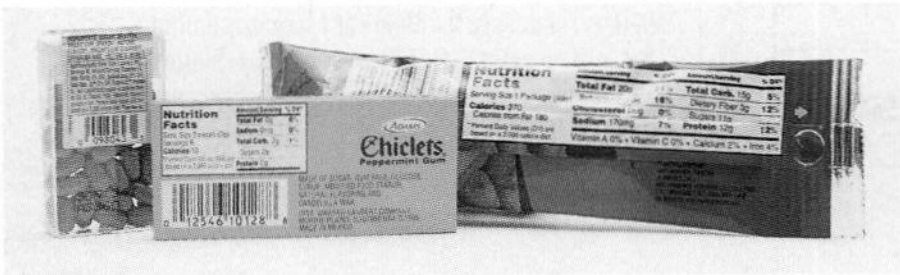

FIGURE 2.14 Nutrition Facts on small packages. When a product package has insufficient space to display a full Nutrition Facts panel, manufacturers may use an abbreviated version.

Nutrient Content Claims

The Nutrition Labeling and Education Act (NLEA) and the associated FDA regulations allow food manufacturers to make **nutrient content claims** using a variety of descriptive terms on labels, such as *low fat* and *high fiber*. The FYI feature "Definitions for Nutrient Content Claims on Food Labels" contains a list of terms that may be used. The FDA has made an effort to make the terms meaningful, and the regulations have reduced the number of potentially misleading label statements. It would be misleading, for example, to print "cholesterol free" on a can of vegetable shortening—a food that is 100 percent fat and high in saturated and trans-fatty acids (types of fat that raise blood cholesterol levels). Although true, this type of statement misleads consumers who associate "cholesterol free" with "heart healthy." Under the NLEA regulations, statements about low cholesterol content can be used only when the product is also low in saturated fat (less than 2 grams per serving).

▶ **nutrient content claims** These claims describe the level of a nutrient or dietary substance in the product, using terms such as *good source*, *high*, or *free*.

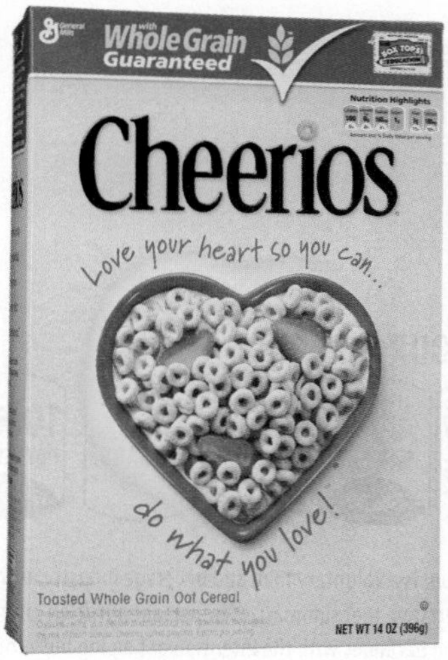

© smartstock/iStockphoto.com

The FDA recently made a ruling on food labels for the term *gluten-free*. The rule will be helpful for people who have celiac disease, a digestive and autoimmune disorder that results in damage to the lining of the small intestine when foods with gluten are eaten. Gluten is a protein that occurs naturally in wheat, rye, barley, and cross-bred hybrids of these grains. The rule requires that to be labeled 'gluten free' each kilogram of the product must contain less than 20 milligrams of the protein, and the food cannot contain any of the following: an ingredient that is any type of wheat, rye, barley, or crossbreeds of these grains; an ingredient derived from these grains that has not been processed to remove gluten; and an ingredient derived from these grains that has been processed to remove gluten, if it results in the food containing 20 or more parts per million of gluten.[27] Most people with a gluten allergy can tolerate gluten in small amounts, and this amount is consistent with the threshold established by other countries and international bodies that set food safety standards.[26]

In addition to the content claims defined in the regulations, companies may submit to the FDA a notification of a new nutrient content claim based on "an authoritative statement from an appropriate scientific body of the United States Government or the National Academy of Sciences."[29]

Health Claims

With the passage of the NLEA, manufacturers also were allowed to add health claims to food labels. A **health claim** is a statement that links one or more dietary components to reduced risk of disease—such as a claim that calcium helps reduce the risk of osteoporosis. Before the NLEA was passed, products making such claims were considered drugs, not foods.

▶ **health claim** Any statement that associates a food or a substance in a food with a disease or health-related condition. The FDA authorizes health claims.

A health claim must be supported by scientifically valid evidence for it to be approved for use on a food label. Regulations require a finding of "significant scientific agreement" before the FDA may authorize a new health claim. In addition, there are specific criteria for the use of claims. For example, a high-fiber food that is also high in fat is not eligible for a health claim. So far, the FDA has approved the following health claims:

- *Calcium, vitamin D, and osteoporosis:* Adequate calcium and vitamin D along with regular exercise may reduce the risk of osteoporosis.
- *Dietary fat and cancer:* Low-fat diets may reduce the risk for some types of cancer.

- *Dietary fiber, such as that found in whole oats, barley, and psyllium seed husk, and coronary heart disease (CHD):* Diets low in fat and rich in these types of fiber can help reduce the risk of heart disease.
- *Dietary noncarcinogenic carbohydrate sweeteners and dental caries (tooth decay):* Foods sweetened with sugar alcohols do not promote tooth decay.
- *Dietary saturated fat and cholesterol and coronary heart disease (CHD):* Diets high in saturated fat and cholesterol increase risk for heart disease.
- *Dietary saturated fat, cholesterol, and trans fat and heart disease:* Diets low in saturated fat and cholesterol and as low as possible in trans fat may reduce the risk of heart disease.
- *Fiber-containing grain products, fruits, and vegetables and cancer:* Diets low in fat and rich in high-fiber foods may reduce the risk of certain cancers.
- *Fluoridated water and dental caries:* Drinking fluoridated water may reduce the risk of dental caries.
- *Folate and neural tube defects:* Adequate folate intake prior to and early in pregnancy may reduce the risk of neural tube defects (a birth defect).
- *Fruits and vegetables and cancer:* Diets low in fat and rich in fruits and vegetables may reduce the risk of certain cancers.
- *Fruits, vegetables, and grain products that contain fiber, particularly pectins, gums, and mucilages, and CHD:* Diets low in fat and rich in these types of fiber may reduce the risk of heart disease.
- *Plant sterol/stanol esters and CHD:* Diets low in saturated fat and cholesterol that contain significant amounts of these additives may reduce the risk of heart disease.
- *Potassium and high blood pressure/stroke:* Diets that contain good sources of potassium may reduce the risk of high blood pressure and stroke.
- *Sodium and hypertension (high blood pressure):* Low-sodium diets may help lower blood pressure.
- *Soy protein and CHD:* Foods rich in soy protein as part of a low-fat diet may help reduce the risk of heart disease.
- *Substitution of saturated fat with unsaturated fat and heart disease:* Replacing saturated fat with similar amounts of unsaturated fats may reduce the risk of heart disease.
- *Whole-grain foods and CHD or cancer:* Diets high in whole-grain foods and other plant foods and low in total fat, saturated fat, and cholesterol may help reduce the risk of heart disease and certain cancers.

A new health claim may be proposed at any time, so this list might expand in the future. The most current information on label statements and claims can be found on the Food tab of the FDA website at www.fda.gov.[28]

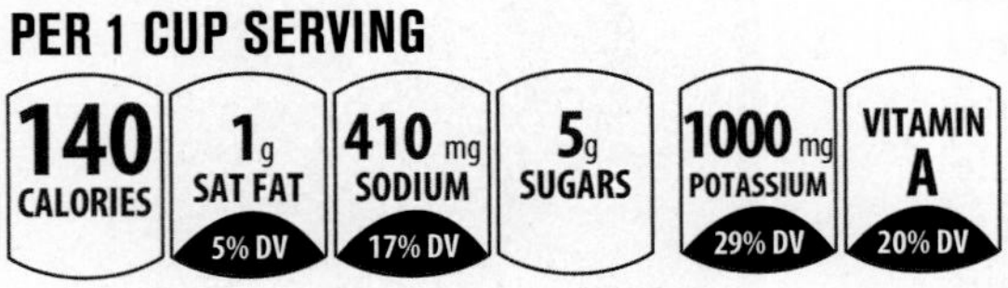

PER 1 CUP SERVING
140 CALORIES
1g SAT FAT 5% DV
410 mg SODIUM 17% DV
5g SUGARS
1000 mg POTASSIUM 29% DV
VITAMIN A 20% DV

Facts Up Front is a voluntary food and beverage industry nutrient-based labeling initiative that summarizes important nutrition information on the front of food packages with the intention of helping busy consumers make healthier food choices.

Courtesy of Grocery Manufacturers Association, available at http://www.factsupfront.org.

Structure/Function Claims

▶ **structure/function claims** These statements may claim a benefit related to a nutrient-deficiency disease (e.g., *vitamin C prevents scurvy*) or describe the role of a nutrient or dietary ingredient intended to affect a structure or function in humans (e.g., *calcium helps build strong bones*).

Food labels also may contain **structure/function claims** that describe potential effects of a food, food component, or dietary supplement component on body structures or functions, such as bone health, muscle strength, and digestion. As long as the label does not claim to diagnose, cure, mitigate, treat, or prevent a disease, a manufacturer can claim that a product "helps promote immune health" or is an "energizer" if *some* evidence can be provided to support the claim. Currently, structure/function claims on foods must be related to the food's nutritive value. Many scientists are concerned

FYI For Your Information

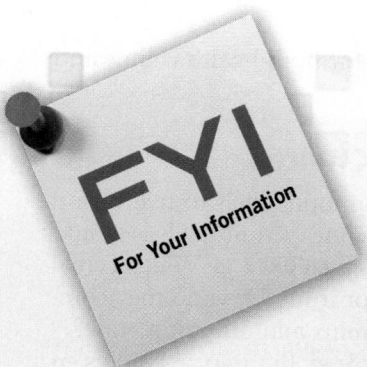

Definitions for Nutrient Content Claims on Food Labels

Free: Food contains no amount (or trivial or "physiologically inconsequential" amounts). May be used with one or more of the following: fat, saturated fat, cholesterol, sodium, sugar, and calories. Synonyms include *without, no, and zero.*

Fat-free: Less than 0.5 gram of fat per serving.

Saturated fat-free: Less than 0.5 gram of saturated fat per serving, and less than 0.5 gram of trans fatty acids per serving.

Cholesterol-free: Less than 2 milligrams of cholesterol and 2 grams or less of saturated fat per serving.

Sodium-free: Less than 5 milligrams of sodium per serving.

Sugar-free: Less than 0.5 gram of sugar per serving.

Calorie-free: Fewer than 5 calories per serving.

Low: Food can be eaten frequently without exceeding dietary guidelines for one or more of these components: fat, saturated fat, cholesterol, sodium, and calories. Synonyms include *little, few,* and *low source of.*

Low-fat: 3 grams or less per serving.

Low-saturated-fat: 1 gram or less of saturated fat per serving; no more than 15 percent of calories from saturated fat.

Low-cholesterol: 20 milligrams or less and 2 grams or less of saturated fat per serving.

Low-sodium: 140 milligrams or less per serving.

Very-low-sodium: 35 milligrams or less per serving.

Low-calorie: 40 calories or less per serving.

Lean and extra lean: Describe the fat content of meal and main dish products, seafood, and game meat products.

Lean: Less than 10 grams of fat, 4.5 grams or less saturated of fat, and less than 95 milligrams of cholesterol per serving and per 100 grams.

Extra lean: Less than 5 grams of fat, less than 2 grams of saturated fat, and less than 95 milligrams of cholesterol per serving and per 100 grams.

High: Food contains 20 percent or more of the Daily Value for a particular nutrient in a serving.

Good source: Food contains 10 to 19 percent of the Daily Value for a particular nutrient in one serving.

Reduced: Nutritionally altered product containing at least 25 percent less of a nutrient or of calories than the regular or reference product. *Note:* A "reduced" claim cannot be used if the reference product already meets the requirement for "low."

Less: Food, whether altered or not, contains 25 percent less of a nutrient or of calories than the reference food. *Fewer* is an acceptable synonym.

Light: This descriptor can have two meanings:

1. A nutritionally altered product contains one-third fewer calories or half the fat of the reference food. If the reference food derives 50 percent or more of its calories from fat, the "light" version must contain 25 percent or less calories (which is 50 percent of the reference food fat content) from fat.
2. The sodium content of a low-calorie, low-fat food has been reduced by 50 percent. Also, *light in sodium* may be used on a food in which the sodium content has been reduced by at least 50 percent.

Note: The term *light* can still be used to describe such properties as texture and color as long as the label clearly explains its meaning (e.g., *light brown sugar, light and fluffy*).

More: A serving of food, whether altered or not, contains more of a nutrient that is at least 10 percent of the Daily Value more than the reference food. This also applies to *fortified, enriched,* and *added* claims, but in those cases, the food must be altered.

Healthy: A *healthy* food must be low in fat and saturated fat and contain limited amounts of cholesterol (less than 60 milligrams) and sodium (less than 360 milligrams for individual foods and less than 480 milligrams for meal-type products). In addition, a single-item food must provide at least 10 percent or more of one of the following: vitamin A or C, iron, calcium, protein, or fiber. A meal-type product, such as a frozen entrée or dinner, must provide 10 percent of two or more of these vitamins or minerals, or protein or fiber, in addition to meeting the other criteria. Additional regulations allow the term *healthy* to be applied to raw, canned, or frozen fruits and vegetables and enriched grains even if the 10 percent nutrient content rule is not met. However, frozen or canned fruits or vegetables cannot contain ingredients that would change the nutrient profile.

Fresh: Food is raw, has never been frozen or heated, and contains no preservatives. *Fresh frozen, frozen fresh,* and *freshly frozen* can be used for foods that are quickly frozen while still fresh. Blanched foods also can be called fresh.

Percent fat-free: Food must be a low-fat or a fat-free product. In addition, the claim must reflect accurately the amount of nonfat ingredients in 100 grams of food.

Implied claims: These are prohibited when they wrongfully imply that a food contains or does not contain a meaningful level of a nutrient. For example, a product cannot claim to be made with an ingredient known to be a source of fiber (such as "made with oat bran") unless the product contains enough of that ingredient (e.g., oat bran) to meet the definition for "good source" of fiber. As another example, a claim that a product contains "no tropical oils" is allowed, but only on foods that are "low" in saturated fat, because consumers have come to equate tropical oils with high levels of saturated fat.

Data from Food and Drug Administration. Guidance for industry: a food labeling guide (9. Appendix A: definitions of nutrient content claims). October 2009. http://www.fda.gov/food/guidanceregulation/guidancedocumentsregulatoryinformation/labelingnutrition/ucm064911.htm. Accessed January 25, 2016.

Nutrition Facts

8 servings per container	
Serving size	**2/3 cup (55g)**
Amount per serving Calories	**230**
	% Daily Value*
Total Fat 8g	**10%**
Saturated Fat 1g	**5%**
Trans Fat 0g	
Cholesterol 0mg	**0%**
Sodium 160mg	**7%**
Total Carbohydrate 37g	**13%**
Dietary Fiber 4g	**14%**
Total Sugars 12g	
Includes 10g Added Sugars	**20%**
Protein 3g	
Vitamin D 2mcg	10%
Calcium 260mg	20%
Iron 8mg	45%
Potassium 235mg	6%

* The % Daily Value (DV) tells you how much a nutrient in a serving of food contributes to a daily diet. 2,000 calories a day is used for general nutrition advice.

Nutrition Facts

8 servings per container	
Serving size	**2/3 cup (55g)**
Amount per serving Calories	**250**
	% Daily Value*
Total Fat 10g	**13%**
Saturated Fat 3g	**15%**
Trans Fat 0g	
Cholesterol 0mg	**0%**
Sodium 220mg	**9%**
Total Carbohydrate 37g	**13%**
Dietary Fiber 4g	**14%**
Total Sugars 12g	
Includes 10g Added Sugars	**20%**
Protein 4g	
Vitamin D 2mcg	10%
Calcium 260mg	20%
Iron 8mg	45%
Potassium 235mg	6%

* The % Daily Value (DV) tells you how much a nutrient in a serving of food contributes to a daily diet. 2,000 calories a day is used for general nutrition advice.

FIGURE 2.15 Comparing product labels. Labels might looks similar, but appearances can be deceptive. Compare the amounts of saturated fat and sodium in these two products.

▶ **nutrition assessment** Measurement of the nutritional health of the body. It can include anthropometric measurements, biochemical tests, clinical observations, and dietary intake, as well as medical histories and socioeconomic factors.

about the lack of a consistent scientific standard for both health claims and structure/function claims.

Using Labels to Make Healthful Food Choices

What's the best way to start using information on food labels to make food choices? Let's look at a couple examples. Perhaps one of your goals is to add more iron to your diet. Compare the cereal labels in **FIGURE 2.15**. Which cereal contains a higher percentage of the Daily Value for iron? How do they compare in terms of sugar content? What about vitamins and other minerals?

Maybe it's a frozen entrée you're after. Look at the two examples in Figure 2.17. Which is the best choice nutritionally? Are you sure? Sometimes the answer is not clear-cut. Product A is higher in sodium, whereas Product B has more saturated and trans fat. It would be important to know about the rest of your dietary intake before deciding. Do you already have quite a bit of sodium in your diet, or are you likely to add salt at the table? Maybe you never salt your food, so a bit extra in your entrée is okay. If you know that your saturated fat intake is already a bit high, however, Product A might be a better choice. To make the best choice, you should know which substances are most important in terms of your own health risks. The label is there to help you make these types of food decisions.

Key Concepts Making food choices at the grocery store is your opportunity to implement the *Dietary Guidelines for Americans* and your MyPlate-planned diet. The Nutrition Facts panel on most packaged foods contains not only specific amounts of nutrients shown in grams or milligrams, but also comparisons between amounts of nutrients in a food and recommended intake values. These comparisons are reported as %DV (Daily Values). The %DV information can be used to compare two products or to see how individual foods contribute to the total diet.

Nutrition Assessment: Determining Nutritional Health

In a nutritional sense, what does it mean to be healthy? Nutritional health is quite simply obtaining all nutrients in amounts needed to support body processes. We can measure nutritional health in a number of ways. Taken together, such measurements can give you insight into your current and long-term well-being. The process of measuring nutritional health is usually termed **nutrition assessment**.

Nutrition assessment serves a variety of purposes. It can help evaluate nutrition-related risks that can jeopardize a person's current or future health. Generally, nutrition assessment is a routine part of the nutritional care of hospitalized patients because it includes anthropometric measurements, biochemical values, and clinical observations. In this setting, nutrition assessment not only identifies risks, but also measures the effectiveness of treatment. In public health, nutrition assessment helps to identify people in need of nutrition-related interventions and to monitor the effectiveness of intervention programs. Sometimes assessments determine the nutritional health of an entire population—identifying health risks common in a population group so that specific policy measures can be developed to combat them.

The Continuum of Nutritional Status

Your nutritional status can be seen as a point along a continuum, with undernutrition and overnutrition at the extremes. Chronic undernutrition results in the development of nutritional deficiency diseases, as well as conditions of energy and protein malnutrition, and can lead to death. Unlike starvation, undernutrition is a condition in which *some* food is being consumed, but the intake is not nutritionally adequate. Although chronic undernutrition and associated deficiency diseases were common in the United States in the 1800s and early 1900s, today they are rare. Undernutrition now is most often associated with extreme poverty, alcoholism, illness, or some types of eating disorders.

Overnutrition is the chronic consumption of more than is necessary for good health. Specifically, overnutrition is the regular consumption of excess calories, fats, saturated fats, or cholesterol—all of which increase risk for chronic disease. Today, nutrition-related chronic diseases such as heart disease, cancer, stroke, and diabetes are among the 10 leading causes of death in the United States. All these problems have been linked to dietary excess. (Remember that epidemiological [population] studies can show associations between various factors and diseases, but these correlations do not necessarily indicate cause and effect.) Between these two extremes lies a region of good health. Good food and lifestyle choices, a balanced diet, and regular exercise help to reduce the risk of chronic disease and delay its onset, keeping us in a region of good health for more of our lifetime.

Nutrition Assessment of Individuals

In health care settings, a registered dietitian or physician can do an individual nutrition assessment of a patient or client. Depending on the purpose of the nutrition assessment, the measures can be very comprehensive and detailed. A dietitian can then use this information to plan individualized nutrition counseling. Nutrition assessment measures are often repeated to assess the effectiveness of nutrition counseling.

Nutrition Assessment of Populations

Population-based nutrition assessment is done in conjunction with programs to monitor the status of nutrition in the United States or Canada or as part of large-scale epidemiological studies. Typically, nutrition assessment of populations is not as comprehensive as an assessment of an individual. One of the largest ongoing nationwide surveys of dietary intake and health status is the National Health and Nutrition Examination Survey (NHANES). The survey is unique in that it combines interviews and physical examinations. Data from NHANES have told us a great deal about the nutritional status and dietary intake of our population. This information is released periodically as the *What We Eat in America* report. Another tool for monitoring the dietary intake of Americans is the Continuing Survey of Food Intake by Individuals (CSFII).

Nutrition Assessment Methods

Just as there is not only one measure of physical fitness, there is not just one indicator of nutritional health. Nutrients play many roles in the body, so measures of nutritional status must look at many factors. Often these factors are called the **ABCDs of nutrition assessment**: anthropometric measurements, biochemical tests, clinical observations, and dietary intake. (See **TABLE 2.9**.)

▶ **ABCDs of nutrition assessment** Nutrition assessment components: anthropometric measurements, biochemical tests, clinical observations, and dietary intake.

Anthropometric Measurements

Anthropometric measurements are physical measurements of the body, such as height and weight, head circumference, girth measurement, or skin-fold measurements.

▶ **anthropometric measurements** Measurements of the physical characteristics of the body, such as height, weight, head circumference, girth, and skinfold measurements. Anthropometric measurements are particularly useful in evaluating the growth of infants, children, and adolescents and in determining body composition.

Height and Weight

To provide useful information, height and weight must be accurately measured. For infants and very young children, measurement of height is really

TABLE 2.9
The ABCDs of Nutrition Assessment

Assessment Method	Why It's Done
Anthropometric measures	Measure growth in children; show changes in weight that can reflect diseases (e.g., cancer, thyroid problems); monitor progress in fat loss
Biochemical tests	Measure blood, urine, and feces for nutrients or metabolites that indicate infection or disease
Clinical observations	Assess change in skin color and health, hair texture, fingernail shape, etc.
Dietary intake	Evaluate diet for nutrient (e.g., fat, calcium, protein) or food (e.g., number of fruits and vegetables) intake

measurement of recumbent length (that is, length when they are lying down). Careful measurement of length at each checkup gives a clear indication of a child's growth rate. Standard growth charts show how the child's growth compares with that of others of the same age and sex. For children 2 to 20 years old, charts illustrating growth are based on standing height, or stature.

The standing height of older children and adults can be determined with a tape measure fixed to a wall and a sliding right-angle headboard for reading the measurement. Aging adults lose some height as a result of bone loss and curvature, so it is important to *measure* height and not simply rely on remembered values.

To convert pounds to kilograms, divide the number of pounds by 2.2

pounds ÷ 2.2 = kilograms

Weight is a critical measure in nutrition assessment. It is used to assess children's growth, predict energy expenditure and protein needs, and determine body mass index. Weight should be measured using a calibrated scale. For assessments that need a high degree of accuracy, subtract the weight of the clothing. Because many calculations and standards use metric measures of height and weight, it's important to be familiar with standard conversion factors.

To convert inches to centimeters, multiply the number of inches by 2.54

inches × 2.54 = centimeters

For the anthropometric assessment of infants and young children, a third measurement is common: head circumference. This is measured using a flexible tape measure placed snugly around the head. Head circumference measures are compared with standard growth charts and are another useful indicator of normal growth and development, especially during rapid growth from birth to age 3 years.

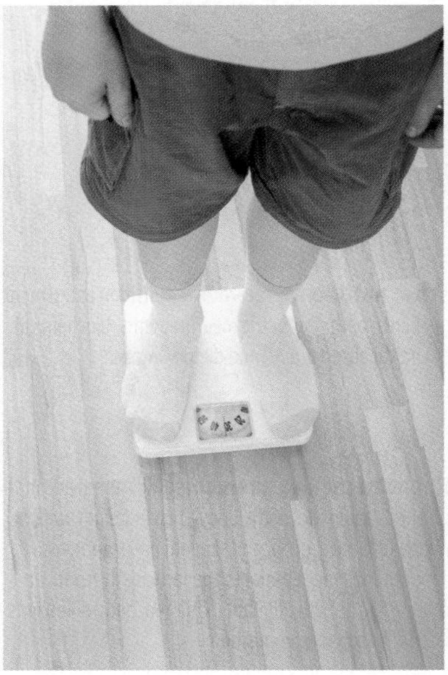
© iStockphoto/Thinkstock

Body Mass Index

Body mass index (BMI) is a useful tool to screen an individual for the weight categories of underweight, healthy weight, overweight, or obese. BMI is determined using a numerical formula of a person's weight in kilograms divided by the square of height in meters. BMI can be a reasonably accurate measure of the health risks associated with body weight. Although BMI is a useful measurement across populations, this measurement has limitations in the assessment of individuals because it does not take into account the distribution of body fat, or overall percent body fat of an individual.

Waist Circumference

One of the simplest means of determining body fat distribution uses waist circumference. Waist circumference can be accurately determined using a flexible tape measure placed just above the upper hip bone, snug to the body, and parallel to the floor. The total distance around the waist is the waist circumference measurement. Waist circumference is a good indicator of abdominal fat and risk for chronic diseases in adults.[29]

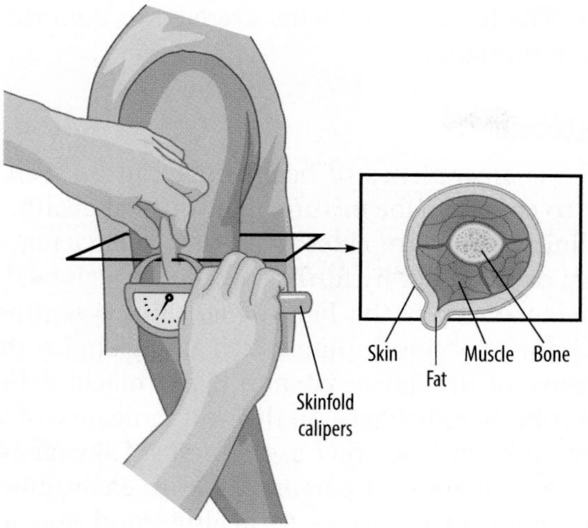

FIGURE 2.16 Skinfold measurements. A significant amount of the body's fat stores lies just beneath the skin, so when done correctly, skinfold measurements can provide an indication of body fatness. An inexperienced or careless measurer, however, can easily make large errors. Skinfold measurements can also be an effective tool for monitoring malnutrition.

Skinfolds

Skinfold measurements serve a variety of purposes. Because a significant amount of the body's fat stores is located right beneath the skin (subcutaneous fat), skinfold measurements at various sites around the body can give a good indication of body fatness. This information can be used to evaluate the physical fitness of an athlete or predict the risk of obesity-related disorders. Skinfold measurements also are useful in cases of illness; the maintenance of fat stores in a patient's body is a valuable indicator of dietary adequacy. Skinfold measurements are made with special calipers (see **FIGURE 2.16**). For reliable measurements, training in the use of calipers is essential. Skinfold measurements can be used to estimate the percentage of body fat or can be compared with percentile tables for specific sex and age categories.

▶ **skinfold measurements** A method to estimate body fat by measuring with calipers the thickness of a fold of skin and subcutaneous fat.

Biochemical Tests

Because of their relation to growth and body composition, anthropometric measurements give a broad picture of nutritional health—whether the diet contains enough calories and protein to maintain normal patterns of growth, normal body composition, and normal levels of lean body mass. However, anthropometric measures do not give specific information about *nutrients*. For that information, a variety of biochemical tests is useful.

Biochemical assessment measures a nutrient or metabolite (a related compound) in one or more body fluids, such as blood or urine, or in feces. For example, the concentration of albumin (an important transport protein) in the blood can be an indicator of the body's protein status. If little protein is eaten, the body produces smaller amounts of body proteins such as albumin.

▶ **biochemical assessment** Assessment by measuring a nutrient or its metabolite in one or more body fluids, such as blood and urine, or in feces. Also called laboratory assessment.

Biochemical assessments can include measurements of a nutrient metabolite, a storage or transport compound, an enzyme that depends on a vitamin or mineral, or another indicator of the body's functioning in relation to a particular nutrient. These measures usually are a better indicator of nutritional status than directly measuring blood levels of nutrients such as vitamin A or calcium. The levels of nutrients excreted in the urine or feces also provide valuable information.

Clinical Observations

▶ **clinical observations** Assessment by evaluating the characteristics of well-being that can be seen in a physical exam. Nonspecific, clinical observations can provide clues to nutrient deficiency or excess that can be confirmed or ruled out by biochemical testing.

Clinical observations—the characteristics of health that can be seen during a physical exam—help to complete the picture of nutritional health. Although often nonspecific, clinical signs are clues to nutrient deficiency or excess that can be confirmed or ruled out by further testing. In a clinical nutrition examination, a clinician observes the hair, nails, skin, eyes, lips, mouth, bones, muscles, and joints. Specific findings, such as cracking at the corners of the mouth (suggestive of riboflavin, vitamin B_6, or niacin deficiency) or petechiae (small, pinpoint hemorrhages on the skin indicative of vitamin C deficiency), need to be followed by other assessments. Clinical assessment should also include an evaluation of personal, social, environmental, and lifestyle factors that could impact access to healthy food and nutritional well-being.

Dietary Intake

A picture of nutritional health would not be complete without information about dietary intake. Dietary information can confirm the lack or excess of a dietary component suggested by anthropometric, biochemical, or clinical evaluations.

There are a number of ways to collect dietary intake data. Each has strengths and weaknesses. It is important to match the method to the type and quantity of data needed. Remember, too, that the quality of information obtained about people's diets often relies heavily on people's memories, as well as their honesty in sharing those recollections. How well do you remember *everything* you ate yesterday?

Quick Bite

Nutrition and Nails

Do your nails have white marks or ridges? Contrary to popular belief, that does not necessarily mean you have a vitamin deficiency. Usually a slight injury to the nail causes white marks or ridges.

Diet History

The most comprehensive form of dietary intake data collection is **diet history**. In this method, a skilled interviewer finds out not only what the client has been eating in the recent past, but also the client's long-term food consumption habits. The interviewer's questions also address other risk factors for nutrition-related problems, such as economic issues.

▶ **diet history** Record of food intake and eating behaviors that includes recent and long-term habits of food consumption. Conducted by a skilled interviewer, the diet history is the most comprehensive form of dietary intake data collection.

▶ **food records** Detailed information about day-to-day eating habits; typically includes all foods and beverages consumed for a defined period, usually three to seven consecutive days.

▶ **weighed food records** Detailed food records obtained by weighing foods before eating and then weighing leftovers to determine the exact amount consumed.

Food Record

Food records, or diaries, provide detailed information about day-to-day eating habits. Typically, a person records all foods and beverages consumed during a defined period, usually three to seven consecutive days. Because food records are recorded concurrently with intake, they are less prone to inaccuracy from lapses in memory. The data are completely self-reported; therefore, food records are not accurate if the person fails to record all items or changes their usual food intake while completing the record. To make food records more precise, the items in a meal can be weighed before consumption. Remaining portions are weighed at the end of the meal to determine exactly how much was eaten. **Weighed food records** are much more time consuming to complete.

▶ **food frequency questionnaire (FFQ)** A questionnaire for nutrition assessment that asks how often the subject consumes specific foods or groups of foods, rather than what specific foods the subject consumes daily. Also called food frequency checklist.

Food Frequency Questionnaire

A **food frequency questionnaire (FFQ)** asks how often the subject consumes specific foods or groups of foods, rather than what specific foods the subject consumes daily. A food frequency questionnaire might ask, for example, "How often do you drink a cup of milk?" with the response options of daily, weekly, monthly, and so on. This information is used to estimate that person's average daily intake.

Although food frequency questionnaires do not require a trained interviewer and can be relatively quick to complete, there are disadvantages to this method of data collection. One problem is that it is often difficult to translate people's response to how often they drink milk, or how many cups of milk they drink per week, into specific nutrient values without more detailed information. More important, food frequency questionnaires require a person to average, over a long period, foods consumed erratically in portions that are sometimes large and sometimes small.

24-Hour Dietary Recall

The **24-hour dietary recall** is the simplest form of dietary intake data collection. In a 24-hour recall, the interviewer takes the client through a recent 24-hour period (usually midnight to midnight) to determine what foods and beverages the client consumed. To get a complete, accurate picture of the subject's diet, the interviewer must ask probing questions such as "Did you put anything on your toast?" but not leading questions such as "Did you put butter and jelly on your toast?" Comprehensive population surveys frequently use 24-hour recalls as the main method of data collection. Although a single 24-hour recall is not very useful for describing the nutrient content of an individual's overall diet (there's too much day-to-day variation), in large-scale studies it gives a reasonably accurate picture of the average nutrient intake of a population. Multiple dietary recalls also are useful for estimating the nutrient intake of individuals.

▶ **24-hour dietary recall** A form of dietary intake data collection. The interviewer takes the client through a recent 24-hour period (usually midnight to midnight) to determine what foods and beverages the client consumed.

Methods of Evaluating Dietary Intake Data

Once the data are collected, the next step is to determine the nutrient content of the diet and evaluate that information in terms of dietary standards or other reference points. This is commonly done using nutrient analysis software. Computer programs remove the tedium of looking up foods in tables of nutrient composition; large databases allow for simple access to food composition, and the computer does the math automatically.

Comparison to Dietary Standards

It is possible to compare a person's nutrient intake to dietary standards such as the RDA or AI values. Although this will give a quantitative idea of dietary adequacy, it cannot be considered a definitive evaluation of a person's diet because we don't know that individual's specific nutrient requirements. The bottom line is that comparisons of individual diets to RDA or AI values should be interpreted with caution.

Comparison to MyPlate and the Dietary Guidelines for Americans

The MyPlate system has several online tools for assessment of dietary intake. Individuals (or evaluators) can use the SuperTracker feature on the ChooseMyPlate.com website to compare a typical day's intake to the MyPlate groups and *Dietary Guidelines*. Although these evaluations usually are not specific, they give a general idea of whether the subject's diet is high or low in saturated fat, or whether the subject is eating enough fruits, vegetables, and whole grains.

Outcomes of Nutrition Assessment

When taken together, anthropometric measures, biochemical tests, clinical exams, and dietary evaluation, along with the individual's family history, socioeconomic situation, and other factors, give a complete picture of nutritional health. A client's assessment can lead to a recommendation for a diet change to reduce weight or blood cholesterol, the addition of a vitamin or mineral supplement to treat a deficiency, the identification of abnormal growth resulting from inadequate infant feeding, or simply the affirmation that dietary intake is adequate for current nutrition needs.

Key Concepts Nutrition assessment involves the collection of various types of data—anthropometric measurements, biochemical tests, clinical observations, and dietary intake—for a complete picture of one's nutritional health. Such data are compared to established standards to diagnose nutritional deficiencies, identify dietary inadequacies, or evaluate progress as a result of dietary changes.

Learning Portfolio

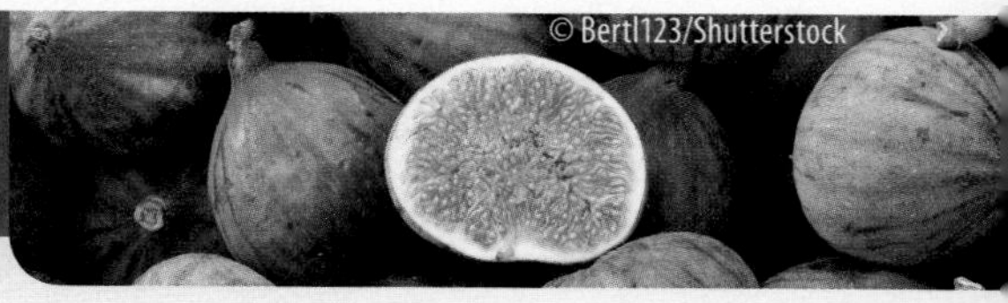

Key Terms

Study Points

- The diet-planning principles of adequacy, balance, calorie (energy) control, nutrient density, moderation, and variety are important concepts in choosing a healthful diet.
- The *Dietary Guidelines for Americans* gives consumers advice regarding general components of the diet.
- MyPlate is a graphic representation of a food guidance system that supports the principles of the *Dietary Guidelines for Americans.*
- Each food group in MyPlate has a recommended daily amount based on calorie needs. A variety of foods from each group can supply all the nutrients.
- The Exchange Lists are a diet-planning tool most often used for diabetic or weight-control diets.
- Servings for each food in the Exchange Lists are grouped so that equal amounts of carbohydrate, fat, and protein are provided by each choice.
- Dietary standards are values for individual nutrients that reflect recommended intake levels. These values are used for planning and evaluating diets for groups and individuals.
- The Dietary Reference Intakes are the current dietary standards in the United States and Canada. The DRIs consist of several types of values: EAR, RDA, AI, UL, EER, and AMDR.
- Nutrition information on food labels can be used to determine a more healthful diet.
- Label information not only provides the gram or milligram amounts of the nutrients present, but also gives a percentage of Daily Values so that the consumer can compare the amount in the food to the amount recommended for consumption each day.
- Nutrition assessment is a process of determining the overall health of a person as related to nutrition.
- Nutrition assessment involves four major evaluations: anthropometric measurements, biochemical tests, clinical observations, and dietary intake.

Study Questions

1. Define undernutrition and overnutrition.
2. What is the purpose of the *Dietary Guidelines for Americans*?
3. What are the recommended amounts for each food group of MyPlate for a 2,000-calorie diet?
4. Describe how the exchange system works and why people with diabetes might use it.
5. List and define four main Dietary Reference Intake categories.

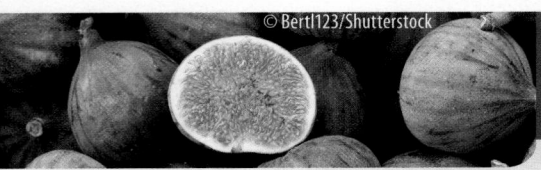

Learning Portfolio (continued)

6. List five mandatory components found on all food labels.
7. The standard Nutrition Facts panel shows information on which nutrients?
8. What is the purpose of the "% Daily Value" listed next to most nutrients on food labels?
9. Define three types of claims that might be found on food labels.

Try This

Are You a MyPlate Pleaser?

Keep a detailed food diary for three days. Make sure to include things you drink, along with the amounts (e.g., cups, ounces, tablespoons) of each food or beverage. How well do you think your intake matches the *Dietary Guidelines* and MyPlate recommendations? To find out, go to ChooseMyPlate.gov and click on SuperTracker, and then on Food Tracker. This feature allows you to do an online assessment of your food intake. Follow the instructions to Create Your Profile. Then, click on Proceed to Food Intake and enter each food you ate for one day. When you are done, you can click on Analyze Your Food Intake and see the comparisons to the *Dietary Guidelines* and MyPlate. How did you do? From which groups did you tend to eat more than is recommended? Were there any groups for which you did not meet the recommendations? Was there a day-to-day variation in the number of servings you ate of each group? Use the results of this activity to plan ways you can improve your diet. You might want to visit this site frequently to monitor changes you are making in your food intake.

Grocery Store Scavenger Hunt

On your next trip to the grocery store, find a food item that has any number other than a "0" listed for the two vitamins and minerals required to be listed on the food label %DV. It doesn't matter whether you choose a cereal, soup, cracker, or snack item, as long as it has numbers other than "0" for all four items. Once you're home, calculate the number of milligrams of calcium, iron, and vitamin C found in each serving of your food. Next, take a look at vitamin A: How many International Units (IUs) does each serving of your product have? If you can calculate these, you should have a better understanding of % Daily Values.

Getting Personal

How well are You Following the *Dietary Guidelines*?

Advice provided by the *Dietary Guidelines for Americans* can help you determine the healthfulness of your diet. Using these guidelines as an evaluation tool, they can also help identify shifts you can make on the road to a more healthy lifestyle. Using the checklist below, consider your own eating habits and evaluate them against the recommendations. An example 2,000 Calorie Level is provided. Table A3-1 of the *Dietary Guidelines 2015-2020* provide recommendations for a variety of calorie levels.

Food Group	Suggested Amount/Day Based on 2,000 Calorie Level	Other Calorie Level Suggestions	My Intake Each Day	Did I Meet the Recommendations?	
				Yes	No
Dark-green vegetables	2 ½ cup				
Red and orange vegetables	5 ½ cup				
Legumes (beans and peas)	1 ½ cup				
Starchy vegetables	5 cups				

Food Group	Suggested Amount/Day Based on 2,000 Calorie Level	Other Calorie Level Suggestions	My Intake Each Day	Did I Meet the Recommendations?	
				Yes	No
Other vegetables	4 cups				
Fruits	2 cup				
Grains	6 oz				
Dairy	3 cup				
Protein foods	5 ½ oz				
• Seafood	8 oz/wk				
• Meats, poultry, eggs	26 oz/wk				
• Nuts, seeds, soy products	5 oz/wk				
Oil	27 gm				
Limit on calories for other uses	270 Cal or 14% of calorie intake				
Physical Activity Guidelines	equivalent of 150 minutes of moderate-intensity aerobic activity each week				

Serving Sizes and Equivalents

Food Group	Serving Sizes and Equivalents
Grains	1 ounce-equivalent = 1 slice of bread; 1 small muffin; 1 cup ready-to-eat cereal flakes; or ½ cup cooked cereal, rice, grains, or pasta
Vegetables	1 cup or equivalent (1 serving) = 1 cup raw or cooked vegetables; 2 cup raw leafy salad greens; or 1 cup vegetable juice
Fruits	1 cup or equivalent (1 serving) = 1 cup fresh, canned, or frozen fruit; 1 cup fruit juice; 1 small whole fruit; or ½ cup dried fruit
Dairy	1 cup or equivalent = 1 cup milk or yogurt; 1½ oz natural cheese; or 2 oz processed cheese
Protein Foods	1 ounce-equivalent = 1 oz lean meat, poultry, or fish; ¼ cup cooked dry beans or tofu; 1 egg; 1 tablespoon peanut butter; or ½ oz nuts or seeds
Oils	1 teaspoon or equivalent = 1 teaspoon vegetable oil or 1 tablespoon mayonnaise-type salad dressing

For each of the food groups that you did not meet the recommended intake amounts each day consider shifts you can make in your eating habits that will improve your intake. List three measurable goals to help achieve these changes:

To make my diet and lifestyle more healthy, I can:

1) ______________________________

2) ______________________________

3) ______________________________

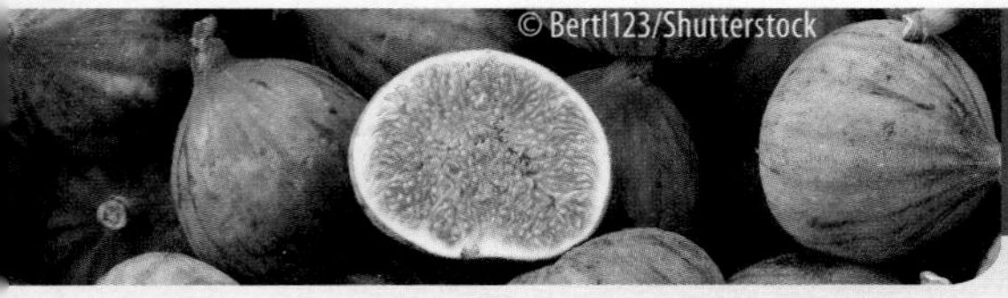

Learning Portfolio (continued)

References

1. Nitzke S, Freeland-Graves J. Position of the American Dietetic Association: total diet approach to communicating food and nutrition information. *J Am Diet Assoc*. 2007;107(7):1224–1232.
2. U.S. Department of Agriculture and U.S. Department of Health and Human Services. *Dietary Guidelines for Americans, 2015-2020*. 8th ed. Washington, DC: U.S. Government Printing Office; 2015.
3. Ibid.
4. Ibid.
5. Pennington J, Kandiah J, Nicklas T, et al. Practice paper of the American Dietetic Association: nutrient density: meeting nutrient goals within calorie needs. *J Am Diet Assoc*. 2007;107(5):860–869.
6. Ibid.
7. Uauy R, Hertrampf E, Dangour AD. Food-based dietary guidelines for healthier populations: international considerations. In: Shils ME, Shike M, Ross AC, et al., eds. *Modern Nutrition in Health and Disease*. 10th ed. Baltimore, MD: Lippincott Williams & Wilkins; 2006.
8. Foote JA, Murphy SP, Wilkens LR, et al. Dietary variety increases the probability of nutrient adequacy among adults. *J Nutr*. 2004;134:1779–1785.
9. U.S. Department of Agriculture and U.S. Department of Health and Human Services. Scientific report of the 2015 Dietary Guidelines Advisory Committee. http://www.health.gov/dietaryguidelines/2015-scientific-report/04-integration.asp. Accessed January 26, 2016.
10. Ibid.
11. Ibid.
12. U.S. Department of Health and Human Services. *Physical Activity Guidelines for Americans*. Washington, DC: Author; 2008. http://www.health.gov/paguidelines/guidelines. Accessed January 26, 2016.
13. U.S. Department of Agriculture and U.S. Department of Health and Human Services. *Dietary Guidelines for Americans, 2010*. Op cit.
14. Health Canada. *Eating Well with Canada's Food Guide*. http://www.hc-sc.gc.ca/fn-an/food-guide-aliment/index-eng.php. Accessed January 26, 2016.
15. Davis C, Saltos E. Chapter 2. Dietary recommendations and how they have changed over time. http://www.ers.usda.gov/media/91022/aib750b_1_.pdf. Accessed January 26, 2016.
16. U.S. Department of Agriculture. First lady, Agriculture Secretary Vilsack and Surgeon General Benjamin launch MyPlate icon as a new reminder to help consumers to make healthier food choices. Press release. June 2, 2011. http://www.usda.gov/wps/portal/usda/usdahome?contentid=2011/06/0225_xml&contentidonly=true. Accessed October 4, 2012.

17. Burger KS, Kern M, Coleman KJ. Characteristics of self-selected portion size in young adults. *J Am Diet Assoc*. 2007;3:611–618.

18. Institute of Medicine, Food and Nutrition Board. *Dietary Reference Intakes for Calcium, Phosphorus, Magnesium, Vitamin D, and Fluoride*. Washington, DC: National Academies Press; 1997.

19. Institute of Medicine, Food and Nutrition Board. *Dietary Reference Intakes for Thiamin, Riboflavin, Niacin, Vitamin B-6, Folate, Vitamin B-12, Pantothenic Acid, Biotin, and Choline*. Washington, DC: National Academies Press; 1998.

20. Institute of Medicine, Food and Nutrition Board. *Dietary Reference Intakes for Vitamin C, Vitamin E, Selenium, and Carotenoids*. Washington, DC: National Academies Press; 2000.

21. Institute of Medicine, Food and Nutrition Board. *Dietary Reference Intakes for Vitamin A, Vitamin K, Arsenic, Boron, Chromium, Copper, Iodine, Iron, Molybdenum, Nickel, Silicon, Vanadium, and Zinc*. Washington, DC: National Academies Press; 2001.

22. Institute of Medicine, Food and Nutrition Board. *Dietary Reference Intakes for Energy, Carbohydrate, Fiber, Fat, Fatty Acids, Cholesterol, Protein, and Amino Acids*. Washington, DC: National Academies Press; 2005.

23. American Dietetic Association. Practice paper of the American Dietetic Association: using the Dietary Reference Intakes. *J Am Diet Assoc*. 2011;111:762–770.

24. U.S. Food and Drug Administration. FDA proposed updates to Nutrition Facts label on food packages. FDA news release. February 27, 2014. http://www.fda.gov/NewsEvents/Newsroom/PressAnnouncements/ucm387418.htm. Accessed January 2016.

25. Ibid.

26. Ibid.

27. U.S. Food and Drug Administration. 'Gluten-free' now means what it says. http://www.fda.gov/ForConsumers/ConsumerUpdates/ucm363069.htm. Accessed January 26, 2016.

28. Taylor MR. A new era of "gluten-free" labeling. FDA Voice. August 5, 2014. http://blogs.fda.gov/fdavoice/index.php/2014/08/a-new-era-of-gluten-free-labeling. Accessed January 26, 2016.

29. Park HR, Shin SR, Han AL, Jeong YJ. The correlation between the triglyceride to high density lipoprotein cholesterol ratio and computed tomography-measured visceral fat and cardiovascular disease risk factors in local adult male subjects. *J Fam Med*. 2015 Nov;36(6):335-40

Spotlight on Dietary Supplements and Functional Foods

Revised by Melissa Bernstein

THINK About It

1. How much do you know about the safety of high doses of nutrient supplements?
2. Would you ask your physician before taking an herbal supplement?
3. When choosing food, what health benefits do you consider beyond basic nutrition?
4. If a friend told you about a new food product that is guaranteed to improve your memory, would you try it?

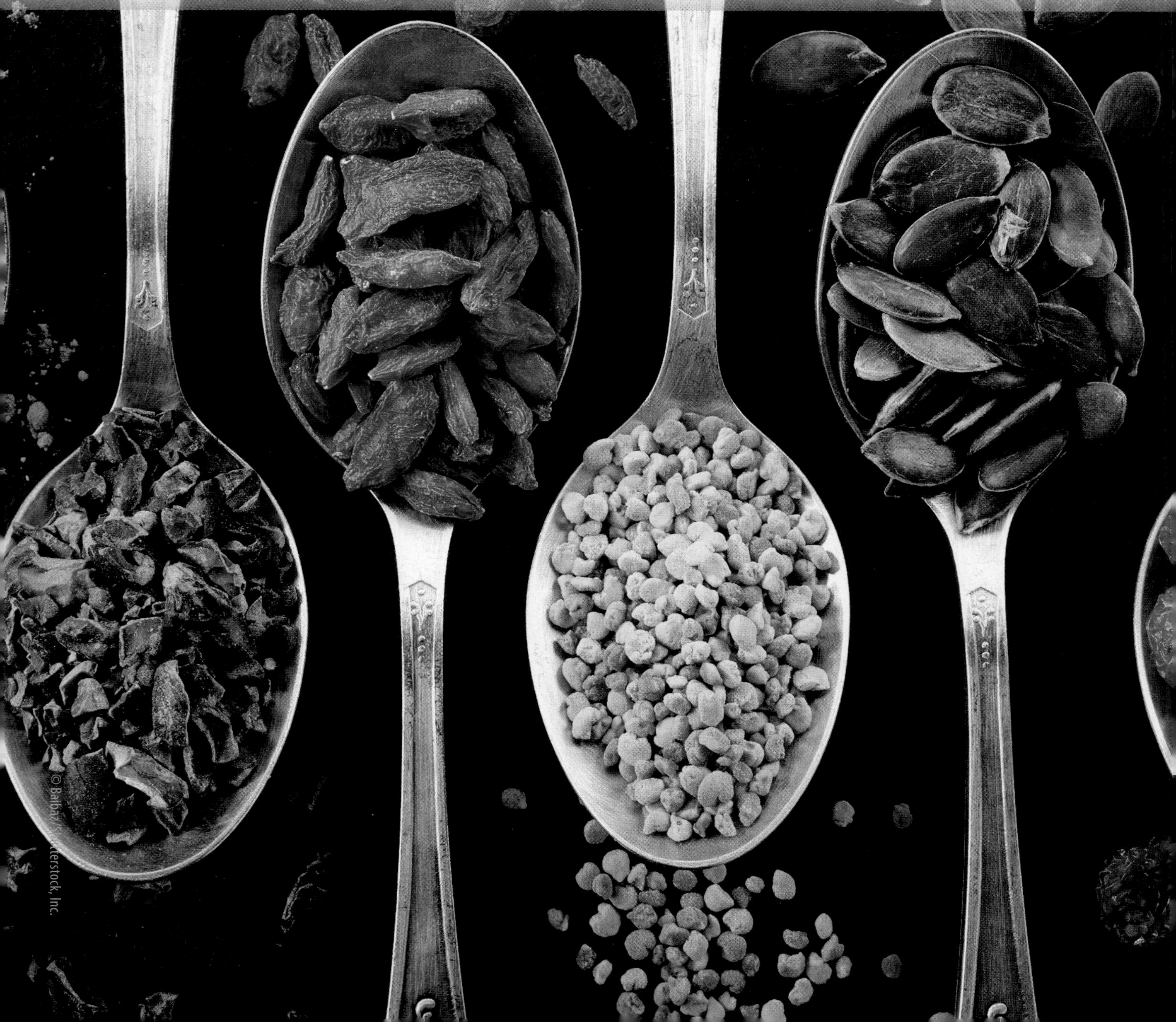

CHAPTER Menu

- Dietary Supplements: Vitamins and Minerals
- Dietary Supplements: Natural Health Products
- Dietary Supplements in the Marketplace
- Functional Foods
- Study Points
- Study Questions
- Try This
- Getting Personal
- References

LEARNING Objectives

- Describe how dietary supplements are regulated in the food supply.
- Discuss the potential benefits and harmful effects of dietary supplements and herbal supplements.
- List individuals for whom dietary supplements would be considered appropriate.
- Discuss functional foods and give three to five examples, including the food source and potential benefit.
- Define phytochemicals.

When she feels down, Jana takes the herb St. John's wort to give her a lift. Whenever she has the option, Sherina chooses calcium-fortified foods. Carlos swears by creatine in his muscle-building regimen. Jason tries a new energy bar with added ginkgo biloba, hoping it will improve his memory. Others in search of better health turn to massage therapy, meditation, organic diets, homeopathy, acupuncture, and many other practices.

Any trip to the grocery store will tell you that a new era in product development is here—one in which food products are more often touted for what they contain (e.g., soy **isoflavones**, vitamins and minerals, herbal ingredients) than for what they lack (e.g., sugar, fat, cholesterol). Beverages, energy bars, and teas marketed as functional foods sit side by side on the store shelves with traditional foods. The market for **dietary supplements**—which are much more than the simple vitamins and minerals our parents knew—continues to grow.

This spotlight looks at dietary supplements, functional foods, and the role of nutrition in complementary and **integrative health care**. We will discuss not only the claims made for products and therapies in terms of current scientific knowledge, but also the regulatory and safety issues. Making decisions about nutrition and health requires both consumers and professionals to stay informed and consult reliable sources before trying a new product or embarking on a new health regimen.

▶ **isoflavones** Plant chemicals that include genistein and daidzein and may have positive effects against cancer and heart disease. Also called *phytoestrogens*.

▶ **dietary supplements** Products taken by mouth in tablet, capsule, powder, gelcap, or other nonfood form that contain one or more of the following: vitamins, minerals, amino acids, herbs, enzymes, metabolites, or concentrates.

▶ **integrative health care** A comprehensive, often interdisciplinary approach to treatment, prevention, and health promotion that brings together complementary and conventional therapies.

Dietary Supplements: Vitamins and Minerals

Dietary supplements come in various forms—vitamins, minerals, amino acids, herbs, extracts, enzymes, and many others. The marketplace includes a wide variety of products claiming to do everything from enhancing immune function to improving memory and mood. Dietary supplement use is common in the United States among adults, with over half the population using at least one, the most common of which are multivitamin/mineral dietary supplements.[1,2] **TABLE SF.1** lists many popular supplements, claims, and important cautions. Despite the enticing claims made for many nonnutrient supplements, scientific evidence has confirmed health benefits for some dietary supplements but not others. It is always important to look for reliable sources of information on dietary supplements and evaluate the claims made about them.[3]

TABLE SF.1
Some Commonly Used Dietary Supplements and Their Claims

Supplement	Claimed Benefit	What Does the Science Say?
Beta-carotene	Prevents cancer and heart disease, boosts immunity, improves eye health	Diets rich in beta-carotene–containing fruits and vegetables reduce heart disease and cancer risk. Supplements have not been shown to be beneficial. Taking supplements may increase lung cancer risk in smokers. In combination with vitamin C, vitamin E, and zinc, may slow progression of age-related macular degeneration.
Chromium picolinate	Builds muscle, helps with blood glucose control in diabetes, promotes weight loss, reduces cholesterol	No solid evidence that chromium picolinate supplements perform as claimed or benefit healthy people. Some evidence that supplements may harm cells.
Coenzyme Q_{10}	Prevents heart disease, improves health of people with heart disease and hypertension, cure-all	May have value in preexisting heart disease, but benefits for healthy people are unproven.
Cranberry	Prevents and treats urinary tract infections (UTIs)	There is some evidence that cranberry can help to *prevent* urinary tract infections; however, the evidence is not definitive, and more research is needed. Cranberry has not been shown to be effective as a *treatment* for an existing urinary tract infection.
Creatine	Increases muscle strength and size, improves athletic performance	May enhance power and strength for some athletes, but is ineffective for casual exercisers and distance athletes.
Echinacea	Protects against and cures colds, boosts immunity	Study results are mixed on whether echinacea can prevent or effectively treat upper respiratory tract infections such as the common cold. Other studies have shown that echinacea may be beneficial in treating upper respiratory infections.
Ephedra	Weight control, herbal "high," decongestant	Ephedra raises heart rate and blood pressure, causes gastrointestinal problems, and is dangerous for people with diabetes, hypertension, or heart disease. According to the Food and Drug Administration (FDA) there is little evidence of ephedra's effectiveness, except for short-term weight loss—and the increased risk of heart problems and stroke outweighs any benefits. The FDA has prohibited sales of ephedra-containing supplements.
Feverfew	Prevents migraines	Some evidence of reduced severity and frequency of migraines, but high dropout rates in studies. Study results are mixed and there is not enough evidence available to assess whether feverfew is beneficial for other uses.
Flaxseed and flaxseed oil	Laxative, lowers cholesterol levels, prevents cancer	Studies of flaxseed preparations to lower cholesterol levels show mixed results. Some studies suggest that alpha-linolenic acid found in flaxseed and flaxseed oil may benefit people with heart disease. Flaxseed might reduce the risk of certain cancers; however, research does not yet support a recommendation for this use.
Garlic	Lowers blood pressure and blood cholesterol, reduces cancer risk	There is some evidence that garlic reduces cholesterol and blood pressure. Dietary garlic may reduce cancer risk; however, results are conflicting.
Ginkgo biloba	Improves blood flow and circulatory disorders, prevents or cures absentmindedness, memory loss, dementia	Studies on ginkgo biloba have found it to be ineffective in lowering the overall incidence of dementia and Alzheimer's disease in older adults, improving memory, slowing cognitive decline, lowering blood pressure, or reducing the incidence of hypertension; there is conflicting evidence on the efficacy of ginkgo for tinnitus.
Ginseng	Improves athletic performance, fights fatigue, helps control blood glucose in people with diabetes, reduces cancer risk	No evidence that ginseng has any beneficial effects. Many products on the market contain no ginseng.
Glucosamine and chondroitin sulfate	Relieve arthritis pain, slow progression of arthritis	Some evidence of reduced pain and improved symptoms, although more studies are needed. Do not reverse arthritis. Variable amounts in products.
Kava	Promotes relaxation and relieves anxiety	The FDA has issued a warning that using kava supplements has been linked to a risk of severe liver damage. Banned in Switzerland, Germany, and Canada.
Melatonin	Promotes sleep, counters jet lag, improves sex life, prevents migraine	May be effective for jet lag; studies are contradictory relative to sleep. No evidence for anti-aging or sex-drive claims. No data on long-term safety.
Milk thistle	Reduces liver damage in alcoholic liver disease, promotes general liver health	Previous studies suggested that milk thistle may benefit the liver by protecting and promoting the growth of liver cells, fighting oxidation, and inhibiting inflammation. However, results from small clinical trials of milk thistle for liver diseases have been mixed or found no benefit.
Saw palmetto	Shrinks prostate, reduces symptoms of benign prostatic hyperplasia, prevents prostate cancer	Several small studies suggest that saw palmetto may be effective for treating benign prostatic hyperplasia (BPH) symptoms. However, in a 2011 study saw palmetto did not reduce the urinary symptoms associated with BPH more than placebo; a review of the research concluded that saw palmetto has not been shown to be more effective than placebo for this use.
St. John's wort	Alleviates depression, promotes emotional well-being	Some studies of St. John's wort have reported benefits for depression; however, others have not. St. John's wort has not been found to be any more effective than placebo in treating depression.
Valerian	Enhances sleep, reduces stress and anxiety	Valerian may be helpful for insomnia. Results are inconclusive to date; much more research is needed.

Data from National Center for Complementary and Integrative Health (NCCIH). Herbs at a glance. http://nccih.nih.gov/health/herbsataglance.htm. Accessed December 20, 2015; National Institutes of Health, Office of Dietary Supplements. Dietary supplement fact sheets. http://ods.od.nih.gov/factsheets/list-all. Accessed December 20, 2015.

"Should I take a vitamin (or mineral) supplement?" Apparently many people already have answered that question for themselves: Multivitamin/mineral supplements and other single-vitamin or -mineral supplements are popular and are taken by a substantial percentage of Americans.[4] Dietary supplement use generally falls into two categories: (1) moderate doses that are in the range of the Daily Values (DVs) or levels you might eat in a nutrient-rich diet and (2) **megadoses**, or high levels that are typically multiples of the DVs and much greater amounts than diet alone could supply.

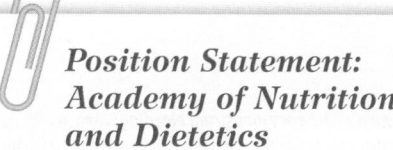

▶ **megadoses** Doses of a nutrient that are 10 or more times the recommended amount.

Moderate Supplementation

The most common reasons people use supplements are to improve or maintain health, yet less than a quarter of adults who take dietary supplements do so based on a recommendation from a health care provider.[4] Health care practitioners often recommend moderate nutrient supplementation for people with elevated nutrient needs and for people who may not always eat a well-balanced diet.[5] **TABLE SF.2** gives some examples of people for whom nutritional supplementation may be recommended.

In addition to those listed in Table SF.2, other groups may also be vulnerable to nutrient inadequacies, such as individuals who are food insecure, are alcohol/drug dependent, or have altered nutritional needs due to an illness or medication use. Many people take nutrient supplements to ensure they meet their nutritional needs. However, taking supplements to "fix" a poor diet is not a perfect solution. Experts advocate achieving healthy dietary patterns through healthy, nutrient-dense food and beverage choices rather than nutrient or dietary supplements except when needed.[6] According to the Academy of Nutrition and Dietetics, "focusing on variety, moderation, and proportionality in the context of a healthy lifestyle, rather than targeting specific nutrients or foods, can help reduce consumer confusion and prevent unnecessary reliance on supplements."[7] Foods provide not only nutrients, but also fiber and other health-promoting phytochemicals. For the most healthful benefits, whenever possible, meet your nutritional needs with food.

If you are one of those people who should take multivitamin/mineral supplements, look for brands that contain no more than 100 percent of the Daily Value unless otherwise instructed by your doctor. (See **FIGURE SF.1**.) Although many products have appropriate nutrient levels, some formulas are irrational and unbalanced, with less than 10 percent of the Daily Value of some nutrients and more than 1,000 percent of others.

Position Statement: Academy of Nutrition and Dietetics

Nutrient Supplementation

It is the position of the American Dietetic Association that the best nutrition-based strategy for promoting optimal health and reducing the risk of chronic disease is to wisely choose a wide variety of foods. Additional nutrients from supplements can help some people meet their nutrition needs as specified by science-based nutrition standards such as the Dietary Reference Intakes.

Reproduced from Marra MV, Boyar AP. Position of the American Dietetic Association: nutrient supplementation. *J Am Diet Assoc*. 2009;109(12):2073–2085.

Key Concepts Vitamin and mineral supplements are popular; however, it is better to obtain nutrients from food. Some conditions and circumstances make it difficult to meet nutritional needs through food alone or to consume enough food to accommodate increases in nutrient needs. Multivitamin/mineral supplements should be well balanced, with doses no greater than about 100 percent of the Daily Value of each nutrient.

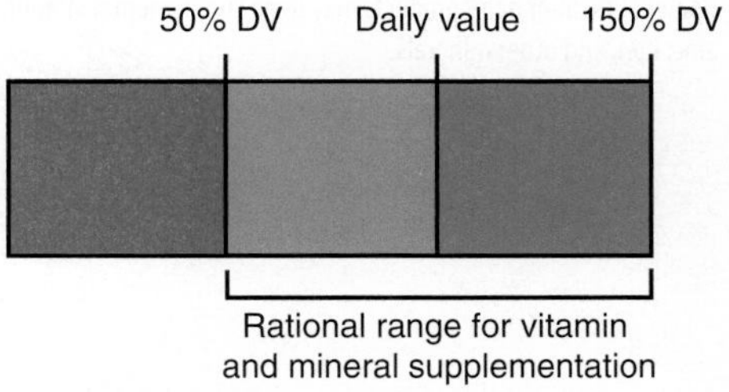

FIGURE SF.1 Moderate supplementation. Health care practitioners often recommend moderate nutrient supplementation for people with elevated nutrient needs and for people who have consistently poor diets.

Megadoses in Conventional Medical Management

High doses of vitamins and minerals have become so much a part of treating certain illnesses that when physicians prescribe these nutrients, many see themselves as following "standard medical practice" rather than as "practicing nutrition." Here are some situations in which physicians may prescribe a vitamin or mineral at megadose levels:

- When a medication dramatically depletes or destroys the stores or blocks the functions of vitamins or minerals, megadosing can overcome these effects. For example, folic acid and vitamin B_6 are used during long-term treatment with some tuberculosis drugs.

TABLE SF.2
People for Whom Nutrition Supplementation May Be Recommended

Women of childbearing age who may become pregnant as well as pregnant and breastfeeding women: Taking supplemental folic acid prior to and during pregnancy can reduce the incidence of birth defects. During pregnancy, it's hard to meet the increased needs for iron and other nutrients through diet alone. Morning sickness makes it even harder. When a woman breastfeeds, some of her nutrient needs are even higher than they were in pregnancy.	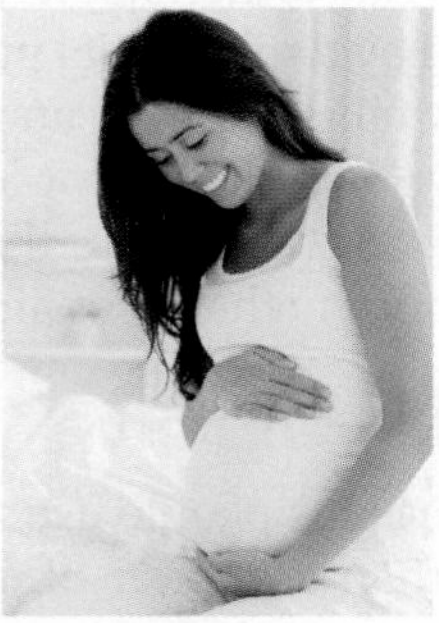 © wavebreakmedia ltd/ShutterStock
Women with heavy menstrual bleeding: Women with high iron losses may need a supplement, but they should not take high doses of iron without a doctor's recommendation. Lab tests can show whether a woman gets enough blood-building nutrients or whether she needs supplements.	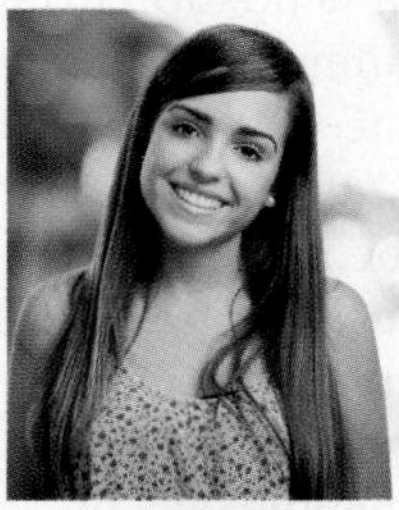 © Asier Romero/ShutterStock
Children: A supplement can help balance the diets of picky eaters or children on a food jag (eating only a few specific foods), and it can ease parental worries. Children who do not consume the recommended amounts of vitamin D–fortified milk may need supplemental vitamin D.	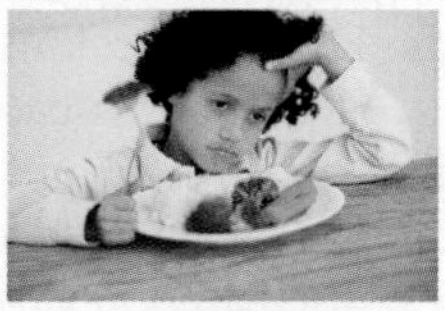 © PeopleImages/ iStockphoto
Infants: If their access to sunlight is restricted, infants may need supplemental vitamin D. Doctors also may prescribe fluoride in areas where water is not fluoridated.	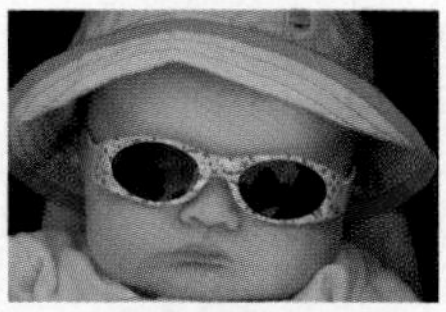 © elaine hudson/ Shutterstock
People with severe food restrictions: Supplements may help people with food restrictions, either self-imposed or medically prescribed such as those on a strict weight-loss diet, those who have eating disorders, those who have mental illnesses, and those who limit their eating because of social or emotional situations.	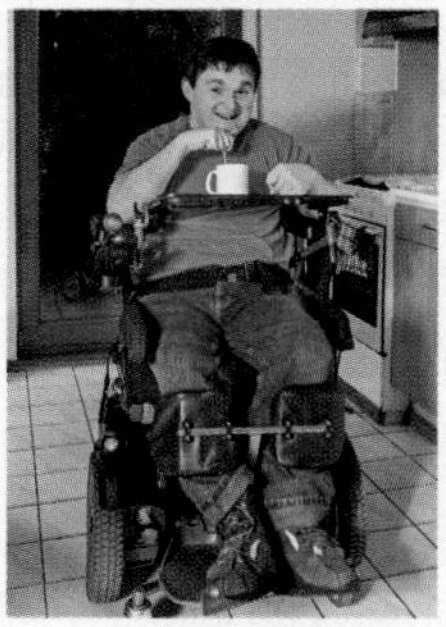 © Belushi/Shutterstock
Strict vegetarians and vegans who abstain from animal foods and dairy products: People who don't eat meat or dairy products may need supplemental vitamin B_{12}, vitamin D, and perhaps calcium, zinc, iron, and other minerals.	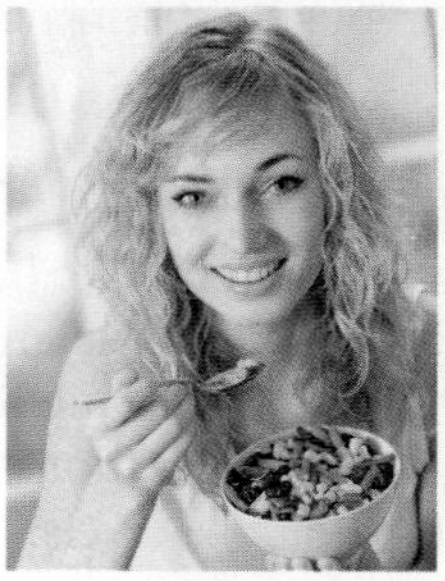 © Vitalii Gubin/Getty Images
Older adults: Because inadequate stomach acid (which is needed for normal absorption of vitamin B_{12}) is common among older people, older adults may need extra vitamin B_{12}. When older adults have limited exposure to the sun and their diets lack dairy products, they should take supplements of vitamin D, calcium, and possibly other nutrients to help maintain bone health.	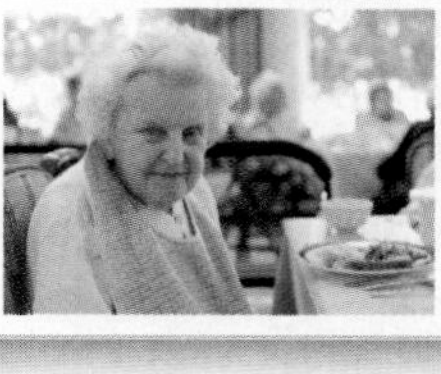 © Pell Studio/ ShutterStock

- People with **malabsorption syndromes** such as cystic fibrosis often take large nutrient doses to compensate for nutritive losses and to override intestinal barriers to absorption.
- Megadoses of vitamin B_{12} can overcome the malabsorption seen in pernicious anemia, a condition in which a key substance needed for vitamin B_{12} absorption is lacking.

A vitamin at megadose levels can have *pharmacological activity*—that is, it acts as a drug. Nicotinic acid (niacin) is a good example. At usual levels (around 10 or 20 milligrams), it functions as a vitamin, but at levels 50 or 100 times higher it acts as a drug to lower blood lipid levels. Niacin has been used since the 1950s as a lipid-altering drug for low-density lipoprotein (LDL) cholesterol and is currently an effective agent available for raising high-density lipoprotein (HDL) cholesterol.[8] Like any drug, though, it can have serious side effects.[9]

▶ **malabsorption syndromes** Conditions that result in imperfect, inadequate, or otherwise disordered gastrointestinal absorption.

> ***Position Statement: American Heart Association***
>
> **Vitamin and Mineral Supplements**
>
> The American Heart Association recommends that healthy people get adequate nutrients by eating a variety of foods in moderation, rather than by taking supplements.
>
> "The Dietary Recommended Intakes (DRIs) published by the Institute of Medicine are the best available estimates of safe and adequate dietary intakes," says the AHA. "There aren't sufficient data to suggest that healthy people benefit by taking certain vitamin or mineral supplements in excess of the DRIs." Moreover, "vitamin or mineral supplements aren't a substitute for a balanced, nutritious diet that limits excess calories, saturated fat, trans fat, sodium and dietary cholesterol. This dietary approach has been shown to reduce coronary heart disease risk in both healthy people and those with coronary disease."
>
> Reprinted with permission, www.heart.org, © 2014 American Heart Association, Inc.

Megadosing Beyond Conventional Medicine: Orthomolecular Nutrition

In 1968, Linus Pauling, the best-known advocate of megadosing, coined the term **orthomolecular medicine**. To him, *orthomolecular* meant achieving the optimal nutrient levels in the body.[10] Few nutritionists argue with the importance of optimum nutrition. In fact, some nutritionists share Pauling's concerns that the typical diet is too refined and processed to provide adequate nutrients and that intake equal to RDA values may not be high enough to achieve optimal body levels.

Most nutritionists would argue, however, with the high doses Pauling recommended to attain those optimal body levels and with the therapeutic value he and his followers attributed to those doses. Most notably, Pauling suggested in the early 1970s that an optimal daily intake of vitamin C was 2,000 milligrams—more than 30 times the current Daily Value. (See **FIGURE SF.2**.) Dr. Pauling claimed megadoses of vitamin C prevented or cured the common cold. Although many researchers have attempted to confirm this theory, studies do not support the idea that vitamin C prevents colds. A few studies found that colds were slightly less severe or less frequent in those who took high doses of vitamin C, but most studies found no beneficial effect.[11]

▶ **orthomolecular medicine** The preventive or therapeutic use of high-dose vitamins to treat disease.

Drawbacks of Megadoses

Megadose vitamins and minerals remain popular, but when taken without recommendation or prescription from a qualified health professional, they can cause problems. Because high doses of a nutrient can act as a drug, with a drug's risk of adverse side effects, people who choose to take megadoses should always check first with their doctors.

THINK About It 1

Excesses of some nutrients can create deficits of other nutrients. High doses of supplemental minerals, especially calcium, iron, zinc, and copper, can interfere with absorption of the others.[12] If you use high doses of the fat-soluble vitamin A, it is easy to reach toxic levels. Even megadoses of water-soluble vitamins can be problematic; for example, nerve damage can result from vitamin B_6 at 50 to 100 times the DV. **FIGURE SF.3** lists some more examples of medical side effects that can occur from megadose supplementation. It is good practice to review the DRI tables for tolerable upper intake levels (UL) before taking any vitamin and mineral supplement.

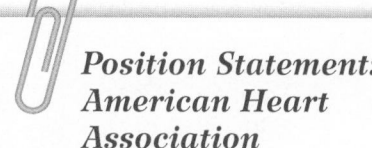

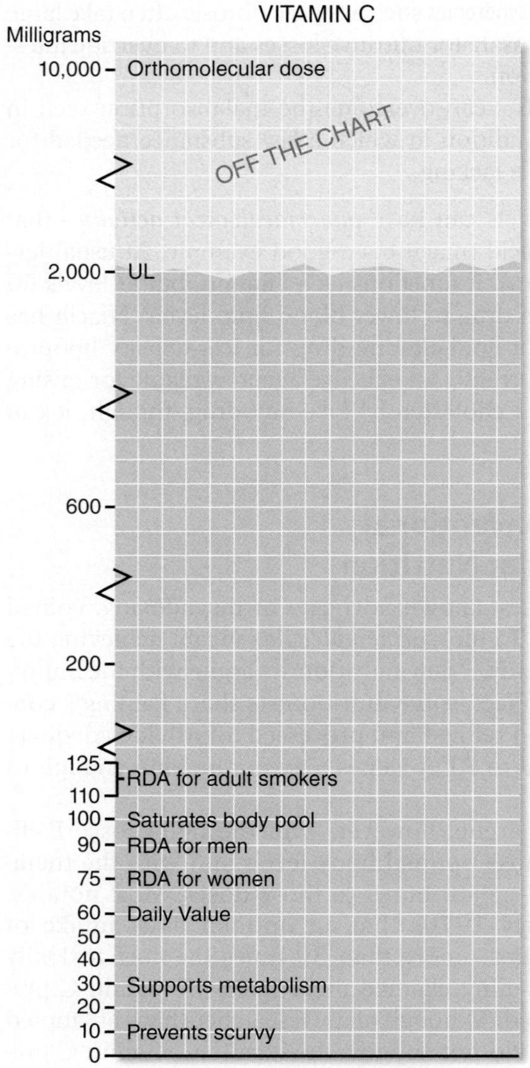

FIGURE SF.2 Vitamin C megadoses. Megadoses of vitamin C are much higher intakes than currently recommended.

Key Concepts High doses (megadoses) of vitamins or minerals turn nutrients into drugs—chemicals with pharmacological activity. Although there may be medical reasons for prescribing high-dose supplements, they should be taken under a physician's supervision. Many claims for high-dose supplements are not supported by clinical studies.

Supplement	Common Side Effect of Megadoses
Iron	Constipation
Vitamin C	Diarrhea
Folic acid	Breakthrough seizures for those on antiseizure medication
Vitamin K	Disrupts balance of blood-clotting medication
Vitamin E	Bleeding problems during surgery
Antioxidant formulas	Counteract some chemotherapy and radiation treatments

FIGURE SF.3 Side effects. Some common side effects of megadose dietary supplements.

▶ **herbal therapy (phytotherapy)** The therapeutic use of herbs and other plants to promote health and treat disease.

Dietary Supplements: Natural Health Products

Supplementation with herbal and other "natural" products is a popular form of integrative medicine. (See **FIGURE SF.4**.) The 1990s saw a dramatic rise in the popularity of dietary supplements—a trend that continues into the 2000s. Currently in the United States, more than 150 million people use dietary supplements, accounting for $32 billion in annual sales.[13] Health Canada estimates that 71 percent of Canadians have consumed natural health products: herbs, vitamins and minerals, and homeopathic products.[14] **Herbal therapy (phytotherapy)** is nothing new, however. Most cultures have long traditions of using plants (and some animal products) to treat illness or sustain health. For centuries, there were no other medicines. Even now, most of the world's people depend primarily on plants for medications; in some remote areas, modern medicines are just not obtainable.

Traditional herbalists know their patients and individualize their herbal remedies accordingly. Those who turn to the mass market for herbal supplements rarely receive such attention and are likely to be confused by nutrition and health-related claims that surround foods and supplements.

In the Western world, the assumption that "natural" is better than "chemical" or "synthetic" has launched the market for "natural" foods to a $12.9-billion industry, with "all natural" becoming the second most common claim to be found on new food labels in recent years.[15] Consumers naively interpret claims such as "100% natural" to mean the product is more wholesome, nutritious, and healthy.

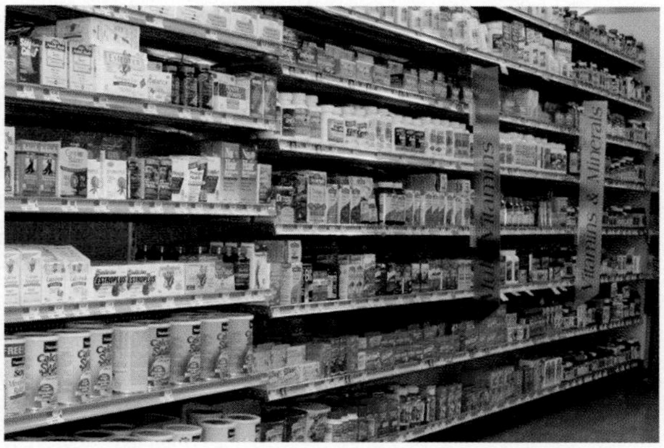

FIGURE SF.4 Use of herbal supplements has grown significantly in recent years.

Helpful Herbs, Harmful Herbs

Until recently, most research on herbs was published in obscure or foreign-language journals that were hard to locate or read. Traditional herbal medical practices are difficult to study in a controlled manner because they use plants to make teas or soups, a far cry from the purified extracts and herbal blends sold in a supermarket. Nevertheless, for some herbs, researchers have enough data to plan carefully controlled studies.

In 1998, Congress established the National Center for Complementary and Alternative Medicine (NCCAM) at the **National Institutes of Health (NIH)** to stimulate, develop, and support research on complementary and alternative medicine (CAM) for the benefit of the public. The NIH agency with primary responsibility for research on promising health approaches that already are in use by the American public was renamed at the end of 2014 to the **National Center for Complementary and Integrative Health (NCCIH)**.[16] The NCCIH is an advocate for quality science, rigorous and relevant research, and encouraging objective inquiry into which CAM practices work, which do not, and why. The mission of the NCCIH "is to define, through rigorous scientific investigation, the usefulness and safety of complementary and integrative health approaches and their roles in improving health and health care."[17] (For more information about how to define complementary and integrative medicine, see the FYI feature "Where Does Nutrition Fit?".) According to the NCCIH, natural products are the most common type used in a complementary approach, as shown in **FIGURE SF.5**. Approximately one-third of American adults and almost 12 percent of children ages 4–17 used complementary health approaches in 2012.[18] Almost 18 percent of American adults used a nonvitamin/nonmineral natural product in recent years; fish oil/omega-3s were the most commonly used natural product among adults.[19] Some natural products have been

Quick Bite

Culinary Herbs Are Not Medicinal Herbs—Or Are They?

Herbs used in cooking are called *culinary herbs* to distinguish them from medicinal herbs. But culinary herbs are also rich in phytochemicals. Some examples are beta-carotene in paprika, the antioxidants in rosemary, the mild antibiotic allicin in garlic, and the mild antiviral curcumin in turmeric.

▶ **National Institutes of Health (NIH)** A U.S. Department of Health and Human Services agency composed of 27 separate institutes and centers with a mission to advance knowledge and improve human health.

▶ **National Center for Complementary and Integrative Health (NCCIH)** A National Institutes of Health organization established to stimulate, develop, and support objective scientific research on complementary and alternative medicine for the benefit of the public.

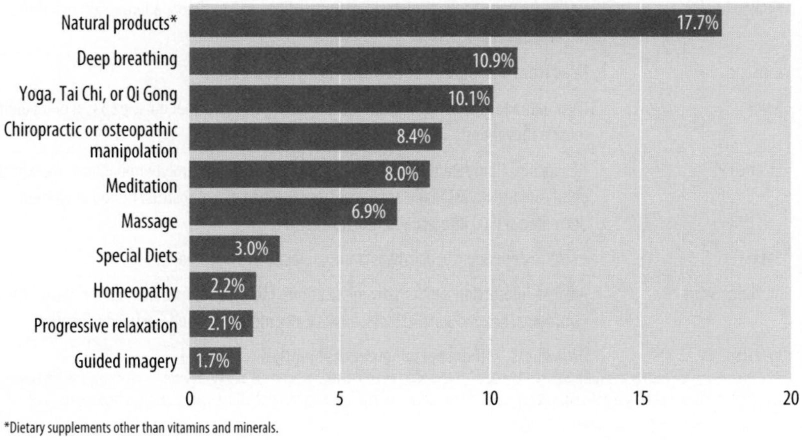

FIGURE SF.5 Ten most common complementary health approaches among adults.

Reproduced from Clark, TC, Black LI, Stussman BJ, Barnes PM, Nahin RL. Trends in the use of complementary health approaches among adults: United States, 2002-2012. National Health Statistics reports; no 79. Hyattsville, MD.: National Center for Health Statistics, 2015.

studied in large, scientific trials, and although there are indications that some may be helpful, many have failed to show anticipated effects (Table SF.1). The suggested benefits of other herbs are based not on scientific study but on years of informal observation: Mint helps indigestion; ginger helps nausea and motion sickness; lemon perks appetite; chamomile helps insomnia. More research is still needed about the effects of these products in the human body and about their safety and potential interactions with medicines and with other natural products.

If you're considering using an herb, remember this important rule of thumb: Any herb that is strong enough to help you can be strong enough to hurt you. Like any medicine, herbs can have side effects, and herbs can be contraindicated. Herbs can interfere with standard medicines. They can affect the way the body processes both over-the-counter and prescription medications, causing the medications to not work the way they should, and therefore can make people with underlying health problems quite sick.[20] Herbal products and supplements may not be safe if you have certain health problems or take certain medications.

THINK About It 2

Some herbs and herbalist treatments are downright dangerous. (See **TABLE SF.3**.) Some hazardous therapies even use lead or arsenic, known poisons. St. John's wort, ginseng, ginkgo biloba, garlic, grapefruit juice, hawthorn, saw palmetto, danshen, echinacea, yohimbe, licorice, and black cohosh are examples of common herbal remedies known to be potentially dangerous for people taking medications for cardiovascular disease.[21] Other herbs, such as ephedra (ma huang), chaparral, and comfrey, have also been shown to be dangerous.

Quality control is a big issue in herbal medicines. In 2007, the FDA issued final regulations requiring current good manufacturing practices (cGMPs) for the manufacturing, packaging, labeling, and storage of dietary supplements. Under the regulations, manufacturers are required to evaluate the identity, purity, strength, and composition of their products and ensure proper labeling.[22]

Quick Bite

Office of Dietary Supplements

The Office of Dietary Supplements (ODS) is a Congressionally mandated office in the National Institutes of Health (NIH). The mission of the ODS is to strengthen knowledge and understanding of dietary supplements by evaluating scientific information, stimulating and supporting research, disseminating research results, and educating the public to foster an enhanced quality of life and health for the U.S. population.

TABLE SF.3
Potential Adverse Effects of Selected Herbs

Herb	Adverse Effects
Chamomile (tea)	Allergic reaction
Echinacea	Allergic reaction, gastrointestinal side effects
Ephedra	Stroke, heart attack, sudden death, seizures
Ginkgo biloba	Headache, nausea, gastrointestinal upset, diarrhea, dizziness, allergic skin reactions, increased bleeding risk
Ginseng	Headaches, insomnia, diarrhea, itching, nervousness
Kava	Liver damage, including hepatitis and liver failure; abnormal muscle spasm or involuntary muscle movements
Licorice	Headaches; fluid retention; increased blood pressure; electrolyte imbalance; weakness, paralysis, and occasionally brain damage; absence of a menstrual period in women, decreased sexual interest and function in men
Senna	Laxative dependency, diarrhea, cramps, electrolyte disturbances
St. John's wort	Adverse interactions with many medications, increased sensitivity to light, gastrointestinal symptoms, headaches, dizziness, anxiety, dry mouth, fatigue, sexual dysfunction
Valerian	Drowsiness; withdrawal symptoms if abruptly discontinued

Medline Plus. Herbs and supplements. http://www.nlm.nih.gov/medlineplus/druginfo/herb_All.html. Accessed December 20, 2015.

Other Dietary Supplements

The supplement market used to include only vitamins, minerals, and a handful of other products, such as brewer's yeast and sea salt. Today there are thousands more products, with new ones continuously popping up.

Supplement categories, for example, now include protein powders, amino acids, carotenoids, **bioflavonoids**, digestive aids, fatty acid formulas and special fats, lecithin and phospholipids, probiotics, products from sharks and other sea animals, algae, metabolites such as coenzyme Q_{10} and **nucleic acids**, glandular extracts, garlic products, and fibers such as guar gum. Supplement producers also blend these products with herbs and nutrients, resulting in the countless array of individual and combination supplements sold today. In many cases, labeling and advertising claims extend beyond current knowledge about these products. Although some are useful, many are of dubious benefit, and wise consumers look for scientific evidence and reliable medical guidance before wasting their money or, worse, risking their health.

▶ **bioflavonoids** Naturally occurring plant chemicals, especially from citrus fruits, that reduce the permeability and fragility of capillaries.

▶ **nucleic acids** A family of more than 25,000 molecules found in chromosomes, nucleoli, mitochondria, and the cytoplasm of cells.

Key Concepts Herbal products are among the many dietary supplements available today. Herbal medicine has a long history in many cultures. Although there is anecdotal support for the use of many herbal products, there is little scientific evidence to back it up. The FDA has set standards for production and sale of herbal supplements. It is important to remember that any herb that is strong enough to help you can also be strong enough to hurt you. Before taking any supplements, it's a good idea to consult your health care practitioner.

Dietary Supplements in the Marketplace

Although some dietary supplements have drug-like actions (e.g., niacin reducing cholesterol levels), government agencies regulate supplements differently from drugs. Manufacturers often make a wide variety of claims for product effects without having to provide scientific evidence to support those claims. The freedoms of speech and press prevail; in practical terms, almost anything goes. Promotional books, infomercials, magazine articles, CDs and DVDs, lectures, staged interviews, podcasts, and web pages—all are protected by the First Amendment, and their authors have the freedom to inform or to deceive. It's up to the listener or reader to distinguish fact from fiction. (See **FIGURE SF.6**.)

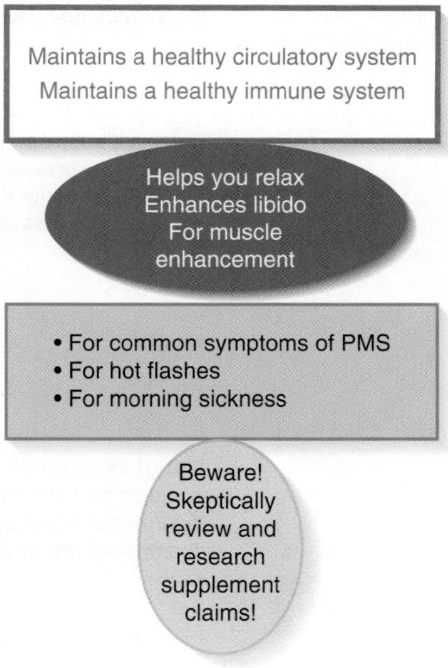

FIGURE SF.6 Dietary supplement label claims. Although claims such as these appear on dietary supplement labels, they do not have to be approved by the FDA. All should be viewed with skepticism.

The FTC and Supplement Advertising

The Federal Trade Commission (FTC) in the U.S. Department of Commerce is responsible for ensuring that advertisements and commercials are truthful and do not mislead. The agency depends on and encourages voluntary self-monitoring by the supplement industry. This industry is creative in its advertising campaigns, fabricating the benefits of many supplements, and is resourceful in finding loopholes in federal regulations to continue selling products. In pursuing deceptive companies, the FTC gives priority to cases that put people's health and safety at serious risk or that affect sick and vulnerable consumers, allowing many products to be falsely marketed without repercussions.

The FDA and Supplement Regulation

The Food and Drug Administration has primary responsibility for regulating labeling and content of dietary supplements under the Federal Food, Drug, and Cosmetic Act, as amended by the 1994 **Dietary Supplement Health and Education Act (DSHEA)**.[23] How do you know a product is a "dietary supplement"? Simple. The law defines *dietary supplements*, in part, as products that are taken by mouth

▶ **Dietary Supplement Health and Education Act (DSHEA) [da-shay]** Legislation that regulates dietary supplements.

that contain a "dietary ingredient."[24] Dietary supplements include vitamins, minerals, herbs or botanicals, and amino acids as well as other substances such as enzymes, organ tissues, metabolites, extracts, or concentrates used to supplement the diet.

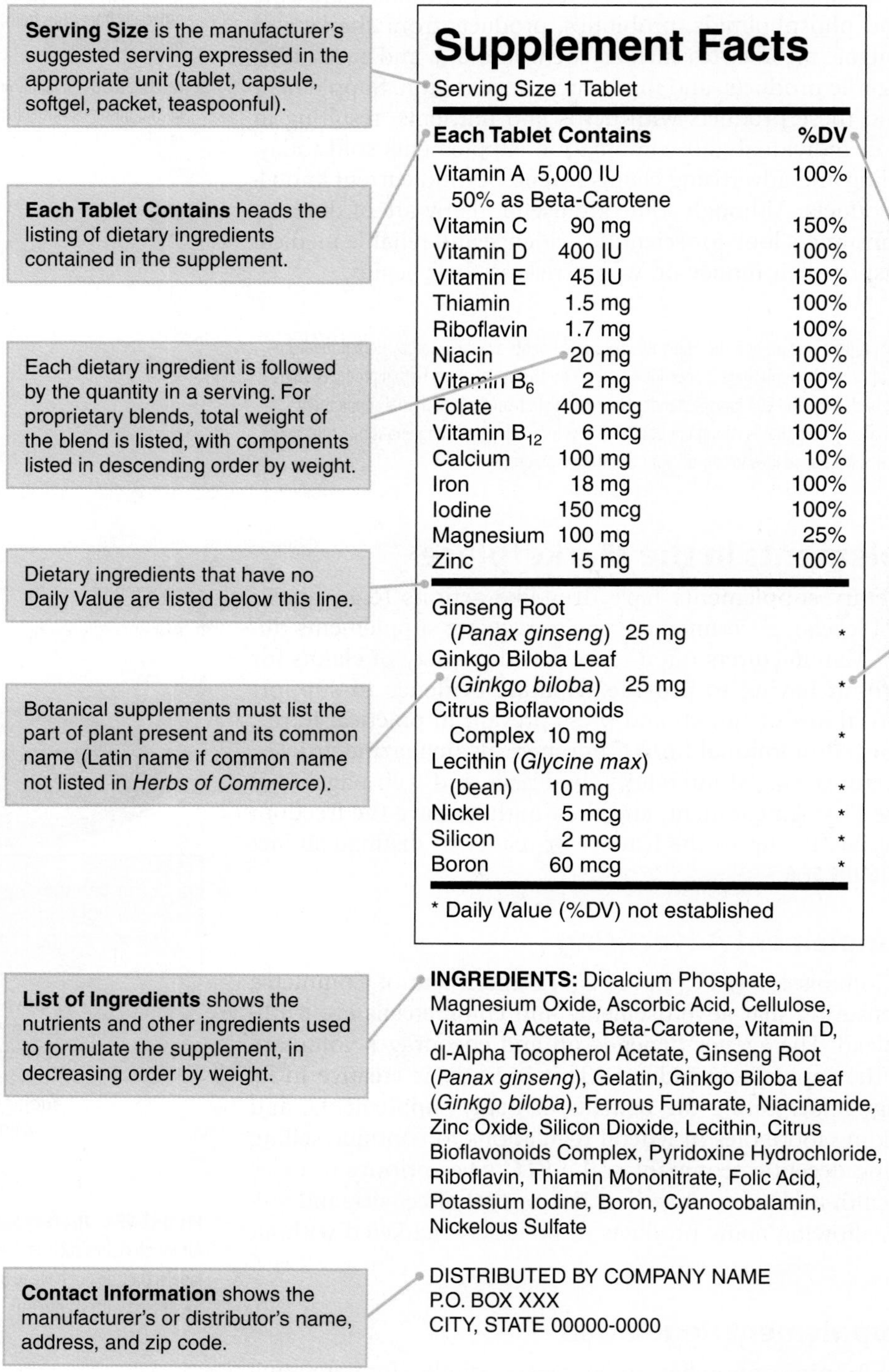
Serving Size is the manufacturer's suggested serving expressed in the appropriate unit (tablet, capsule, softgel, packet, teaspoonful).
Each Tablet Contains heads the listing of dietary ingredients contained in the supplement.
Each dietary ingredient is followed by the quantity in a serving. For proprietary blends, total weight of the blend is listed, with components listed in descending order by weight.
Dietary ingredients that have no Daily Value are listed below this line.
Botanical supplements must list the part of plant present and its common name (Latin name if common name not listed in Herbs of Commerce).
List of Ingredients shows the nutrients and other ingredients used to formulate the supplement, in decreasing order by weight.
Contact Information shows the manufacturer's or distributor's name, address, and zip code.
%DV indicates the percentage of the Daily Value of each nutrient that a serving provides.
An asterisk under %DV indicates that a Daily Value is not established for that ingredient.
Supplement Facts
Serving Size 1 Tablet
Each Tablet Contains %DV
Vitamin A 5,000 IU 100%
50% as Beta-Carotene
Vitamin C 90 mg 150%
Vitamin D 400 IU 100%
Vitamin E 45 IU 150%
Thiamin 1.5 mg 100%
Riboflavin 1.7 mg 100%
Niacin 20 mg 100%
Vitamin B6 2 mg 100%
Folate 400 mcg 100%
Vitamin B12 6 mcg 100%
Calcium 100 mg 10%
Iron 18 mg 100%
Iodine 150 mcg 100%
Magnesium 100 mg 25%
Zinc 15 mg 100%
Ginseng Root (Panax ginseng) 25 mg *
Ginkgo Biloba Leaf (Ginkgo biloba) 25 mg *
Citrus Bioflavonoids Complex 10 mg *
Lecithin (Glycine max) (bean) 10 mg *
Nickel 5 mcg *
Silicon 2 mcg *
Boron 60 mcg *
* Daily Value (%DV) not established
INGREDIENTS: Dicalcium Phosphate, Magnesium Oxide, Ascorbic Acid, Cellulose, Vitamin A Acetate, Beta-Carotene, Vitamin D, dl-Alpha Tocopherol Acetate, Ginseng Root (Panax ginseng), Gelatin, Ginkgo Biloba Leaf (Ginkgo biloba), Ferrous Fumarate, Niacinamide, Zinc Oxide, Silicon Dioxide, Lecithin, Citrus Bioflavonoids Complex, Pyridoxine Hydrochloride, Riboflavin, Thiamin Mononitrate, Folic Acid, Potassium Iodine, Boron, Cyanocobalamin, Nickelous Sulfate
DISTRIBUTED BY COMPANY NAME
P.O. BOX XXX
CITY, STATE 00000-0000

FIGURE SF.7 Supplement Facts panel. Similar to the Nutrition Facts panel on food labels, the Supplement Facts panel required on dietary supplement labels shows the product composition.

Dietary supplements are *not* drugs. A drug is intended to diagnose, cure, mitigate, treat, or prevent disease. Before marketing, drugs must undergo extensive studies of effectiveness, safety, interactions with other substances, and dosing. The FDA gives formal premarket approval to a drug and monitors its safety after the drug is on the market. If a drug is subsequently shown to be dangerous, the FDA can act quickly to have it removed from the market. None of this is true for dietary supplements. The current law gives the FDA only limited authority over supplements, making it difficult for the government to remove unsafe supplements from the marketplace. The FDA does not evaluate the safety and effectiveness of supplements before they hit the marketplace. There are some legislators in Congress who want to improve the law by requiring supplement makers to put safer products on the shelves and label products more clearly.[25] The objective is to ensure that consumers can tell the difference between dietary supplements that are safe and those that have potentially serious side effects or drug interactions.

Quick Bite

Pronouncing the Acronym

The Dietary Supplement Health and Education Act of 1994 is better known by its acronym DSHEA, pronounced "da-shay."

Supplement Labels

Like food labels, supplement labels have mandatory and optional information. All labels on dietary supplements must include ingredient information and a **Supplement Facts panel**.[26] You'll notice in **FIGURE SF.7** that the format is similar to the Nutrition Facts panel on food labels. Supplements that contain *proprietary blends*—products or techniques exclusive to the manufacturer—are not required to list specific amounts of each ingredient.[27]

▶ **Supplement Facts panel** Content label that must appear on all dietary supplements.

Supplement labels, like food labels, may contain health claims, structure/function claims, and nutrient content claims. (See **FIGURE SF.8**.) Qualified health claims may also apply to dietary supplements.

Manufacturers can use structure/function claims without FDA authorization and can base their claims on their own review and interpretation of the scientific literature. Structure/function claims are easy to spot because they are accompanied by the following disclaimer: "This statement has not been evaluated by the Food and Drug Administration. This product is not intended to diagnose, treat, cure, or prevent any disease."[28] A dietary supplement with a label claiming to cure or treat a specific condition is considered an unapproved drug.[29]

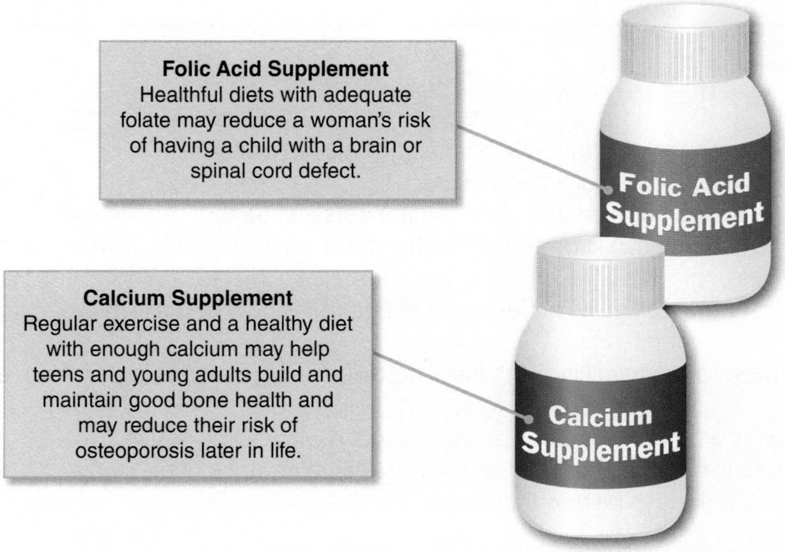

Folic Acid Supplement
Healthful diets with adequate folate may reduce a woman's risk of having a child with a brain or spinal cord defect.
Calcium Supplement
Regular exercise and a healthy diet with enough calcium may help teens and young adults build and maintain good bone health and may reduce their risk of osteoporosis later in life.
Folic Acid Supplement
Calcium Supplement

FIGURE SF.8 Health claims for supplements. Calcium and folic acid supplements may carry health claims similar to these model statements.

Data from U.S. Food and Drug Administration.

FYI For Your Information

Shopping for Supplements

Thinking about buying a dietary supplement? Before you do, ask yourself, "Why do I need this supplement?" and "Is it suitable for me?" Think about your typical diet and what it may be lacking. Remember, the word *supplement* means just that—a product meant to supplement your food. A well-chosen supplement can be beneficial under some circumstances, especially if your diet is limited. However, if you're healthy and eat a good balance of healthful foods, supplements probably won't help you much.

It's a good idea to let your doctor know your supplement plans. Some supplements are contraindicated during pregnancy or lactation; others should not be used with certain chronic illnesses. Supplements sometimes interfere with the action of medicines. Some slow blood clotting, which is a concern if surgery is planned.

To a great extent, you will need to rely on your own understanding of diet and nutrition to make your selection. And, you must rely on the supplement manufacturer for the product's safety, its purity, potency, and cleanliness, and the label's accuracy. If you are concerned about potential side effects or contraindications, you will probably need to contact the manufacturer or distributor.

Choose Quality

In 2010, the FDA finalized guidelines for current good manufacturing practices by supplement manufacturers.[a] Additionally, you should also use tip-offs to judge a quality company—the kind you would expect to have good quality control procedures and to manufacture, store, and transport products safely and carefully.

A quality company will not promise miracles on its website, in catalogues, in commercials or advertisements, or in in-store promotions. A quality company will not manipulate statistics or distort research findings in an attempt to mislead you. And a quality company will take care with its labels, print materials, and Web information.

Confirm Supplement Ingredients

Use resources that analyze and confirm supplement content, dose, and purity. ConsumerLab.com is one such service. Pharmaceutical researchers also report findings on supplement label accuracy; a search on PubMed can lead you to this information.

Look for the U.S. Pharmacopeia (USP) logo (USP verification mark) on supplement labels. The mark certifies that the USP has found the ingredients consistent with those stated on the label; that the supplement has been manufactured in a safe, sanitary, controlled facility; and that the product dissolves or disintegrates to release nutrients in the body. However, the USP does not test the supplement's efficacy.

Choose Freshness

Finding the freshest supplement is often easier if you shop in a retail store. Choose a store where turnover is likely to be quick, and check expiration dates. Supplements should be displayed away from direct sunlight, bright lights, or nearby heat sources, because heat ages many supplements.

Expect Accountability

How easily can you obtain information about the product? Look for a phone number on the label so you can call with questions or to report side effects. On websites, look for a domestic address and phone number, in addition to an email contact. Does a knowledgeable company representative respond to your questions, or is the only person available one who reads a scripted response?

If you're shopping online but are uncertain whether the supplement is right for you, check the Web retailer's return policy. A Web retailer that also has a brick-and-mortar outlet near your locale may be preferable.

[a]Food and Drug Administration. Guidance for industry: Current good manufacturing practice in manufacturing, packaging, labeling, or holding operations for dietary supplements; small entity compliance guide. December 2010. http://www.fda.gov/Food/GuidanceRegulation/GuidanceDocumentsRegulatoryInformation/DietarySupplements/ucm238182.htm. Accessed December 20, 2015.

Be a Safe and Informed Consumer

When buying supplements, follow this advice from the Food and Drug Administration:

- Let your health care professional advise you on sorting reliable information from questionable information.
- Contact the manufacturer for information about the product you intend to use.
- Be aware that some supplement ingredients, including nutrients and plant components, can be toxic. Also, some ingredients and products can be harmful when consumed in large amounts, when taken for a long time, or when used in combination with certain other drugs, substances, or foods.
- Do not self-diagnose any health condition. Work with health care professionals to determine how best to achieve optimal health.
- Do not substitute a dietary supplement for a prescription medicine or therapy, or for the variety of foods important to a healthful diet.
- Do not assume that the term *natural* in relation to a product ensures that the product is wholesome or safe.
- Be wary of hype and headlines. Sound health advice is generally based on research over time, not a single study.
- Learn to spot false claims. If something sounds too good to be true, it probably is.

Food and Drug Administration. FDA 101: dietary supplements. http://www.fda.gov/ForConsumers/ConsumerUpdates/ucm050803.htm. Accessed December 20, 2015.

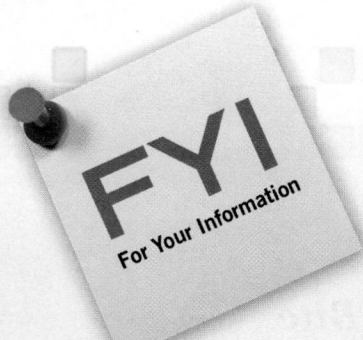

Canadian Regulations

Beginning January 1, 2004, all natural health products sold in Canada have been subject to Health Canada's Natural Health Products Regulations.[30] By definition, natural health products include vitamins, minerals, herbal remedies, and homeopathic medicines. Health Canada has developed a product approval system whereby each product must meet the requirements of the Natural Health Products Regulations to acquire a license and be legally sold in Canada. Authorization requires evidence of safety and efficacy. The regulations also include provisions for on-site licensing, good manufacturing practices, labeling and packaging requirements, and adverse reaction reporting. The Canadian regulations go further than DSHEA in terms of assuring the safety and efficacy of supplements.

Key Concepts Dietary supplements are neither foods nor drugs, and the government regulates their manufacture and sale differently than it does for foods, additives, and drugs. The FTC and FDA monitor advertising and labeling of dietary supplements. A Supplement Facts panel is now required on labels. Canada's regulations for natural health products require premarket approval and product licensing.

Choosing Dietary Supplements

Knowledge of nutrition science is your most valuable tool for evaluating a supplement. Read each label and judge each implied claim in light of what you know. For tips on choosing supplements, see the FYI feature "Shopping for Supplements." Ask the following questions:

- *Is the quantity enough to have an effect, or is it trivial?* What will happen if you take more than you need?
- *Is the product new to you?* Learn about it from the many reliable resources available. Evaluate the product in light of scientific research.
- *Can the supplement cross the intestine and travel to its presumed site of action in the body?* There are little data on the absorption and **bioavailability** of herbal preparations and other types of non-nutrient supplements.
- *Can this supplement interact with any prescription or over-the-counter medications?* Some combinations of supplements or using some supplements together with either prescription or OTC medications could produce potentially harmful adverse effects.
- *Does the product promise too much?* A product touted to control high blood cholesterol, hangnails, psoriasis, and insomnia is unlikely to do much of anything.
- *Who is selling the product?* Alternative practitioners, dietitians, and even physicians sometimes sell the supplements they recommend—which is a possible conflict of interest that could compromise their objectivity. The Academy of Nutrition and Dietetics has issued guidelines for practitioners' recommendations and sales of supplements.[31]
- *What is the evidence?* Carefully evaluate the reliable scientific evidence to support the use of the dietary supplement for the intended purpose. A good place to start your research for current and accurate information are the NIH websites for the NCCIH (http://nccih.nih.gov) and the Office of Dietary Supplements (http://ods.od.nih.gov).

Even the best-intentioned, most carefully considered supplement can prove ineffective or even risky. A good indicator of quality is the voluntary **U.S. Pharmacopeia (USP)** verification mark (see **FIGURE SF.9**), which verifies that the product meets the U.S. Pharmacopeia's standards for product purity, accuracy of ingredient labeling, and proper manufacturing practices.[32] The USP

▶ **bioavailability** A measure of the extent to which a nutrient becomes available to the body after ingestion and thus is available to the tissues.

▶ **U.S. Pharmacopeia (USP)** Established in 1820, the USP is a nonprofit health care organization that sets quality standards for a range of health care products.

verification mark helps assure consumers, health care professionals, and supplement retailers that a product has passed USP's rigorous program and does the following:

- Contains the ingredients declared on the product label
- Contains the amount or strength of ingredients declared on the product label
- Meets requirements for limits on potential contaminants
- Has been manufactured properly by complying with USP and FDA standards for current good manufacturing practices (cGMPs)

FIGURE SF.9 U.S. Pharmacopeia verification mark. Dietary supplements can earn the USP-Verified mark through a comprehensive testing and evaluation process.

Fraudulent Products

Some health advocates consider the burgeoning market of dietary supplements an unwelcome return to the "snake oil" era of the late nineteenth and early twentieth centuries, when "magic" potions and cures were sold door-to-door and at county fairs and markets. The Internet and social media marketing are changing the industry because they are a prominent vehicle for promoting and selling products, reaching millions of people worldwide instantly at any time.

Most manufacturers work hard to ensure the quality of their products, yet some supplements on the market are nothing more than a mixture of ineffective ingredients. In recent years, the FDA has found hundreds of fraudulent products that contain hidden or deceptively labeled ingredients.[33] Most frequently recalled products with potentially harmful ingredients are those that are promoted for weight loss, sexual enhancement, and bodybuilding. When considering the use of dietary supplements, do your homework—make sure the product is safe and effective. It's always a good idea to ask your health care professional for help in distinguishing between reliable and questionable information.

Quick Bite

Jell-O and Your Nails

You may have heard that taking gelatin can make your nails stronger. Not true. Fingernails get their strength from sulfur in amino acids. Gelatin has no sulfur-containing amino acids.

Key Concepts When considering a dietary supplement, it is important to consider the product and its claims carefully. Be aware that some products may promise more than they can deliver. A good indicator of quality is the USP verification mark, but this does not guarantee that a product will fulfill its claims.

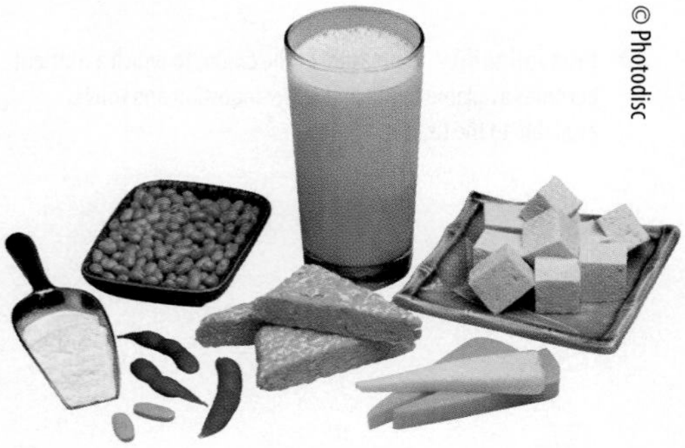

FIGURE SF.10 Soy is rich in phytochemicals. Soybeans contain phytochemicals called isoflavones. High intake of soy products such as tofu is linked to a lower incidence of heart disease and cancer.

Functional Foods

What do garlic, tomato sauce, tofu, and oatmeal all have in common? They aren't in the same food group, nor do they have the same nutrient composition. Instead, all of these foods could be considered "functional foods." Although there is not yet a legal definition for the term, a **functional food** is widely considered to be a food or food component that provides a health benefit beyond basic nutrition.[34] Garlic contains sulfur compounds that may reduce heart disease risk, and tomato sauce is rich in **lycopene**, a compound that may reduce prostate cancer risk. The soy protein in tofu and the fiber in oatmeal can help reduce the risk of heart disease. (See **FIGURE SF.10**.) The functional food industry has grown rapidly since its birth in Japan in the late 1980s and in 2014, reached almost $177 billion dollars of sales worldwide. In the U.S., functional food and beverage sales account for 5 percent of the overall food market.[35–37]

THINK About It 3

- **functional food** A food that may provide a health benefit beyond basic nutrition.
- **lycopene** One of a family of plant chemicals, the carotenoids. Others in this big family include alpha-carotene and beta-carotene.
- **phytochemicals** Substances in plants that may possess health-protective effects, even though they are not essential for life.

Phytochemicals Make Foods Functional

Many functional foods get their health-promoting properties from naturally occurring compounds that are not considered nutrients but are called **phytochemicals**. Although the word *phytochemical* may sound intimidating, its

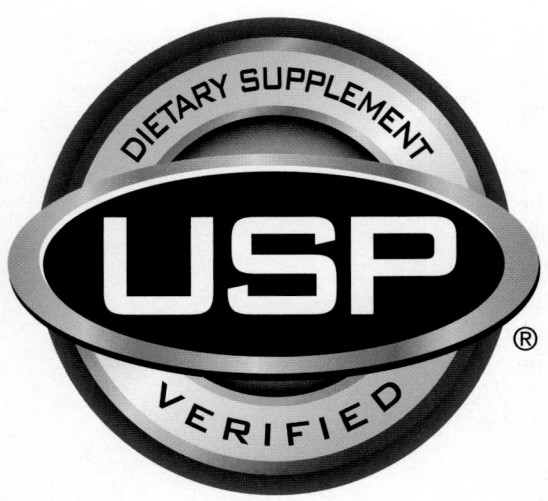

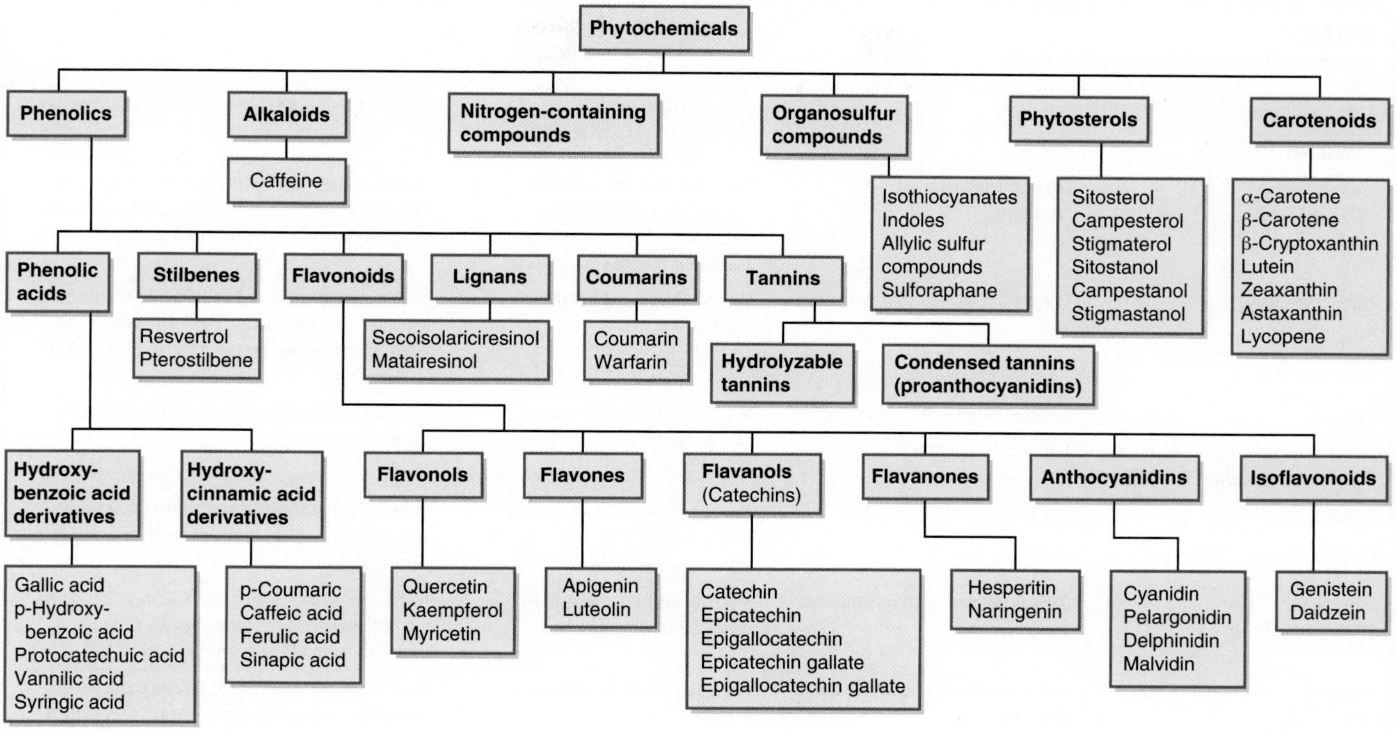

FIGURE SF.11 Classification of well-known dietary phytochemicals. Dietary phytochemicals from plant foods including fruits, vegetables, and whole grains have complementary and overlapping mechanisms of action for health and disease prevention. Dietary phytochemicals can be divided into six general categories. The most related to human health and well-being are the phenolics and carotenoids.

Reproduced from *Adv Nutr.* 2013;4(3):384S–392S. Published online May 6, 2013. Copyright © 2013 American Society for Nutrition.

meaning is simple: "plant chemical." A vitamin is a food substance essential for life. Phytochemicals, in contrast, are substances in plants that may affect health, even though they are not essential for life. Phytochemicals are complex chemicals that vary from plant to plant. They include pigments, antioxidants, and thousands of other compounds, many of which have been associated with protection from heart disease, vision loss, hypertension, cancer, and diabetes. The flow chart in **FIGURE SF.11** shows the classifications of the most well-known dietary phytochemicals that affect human health. **TABLE SF.4** lists many examples of phytochemicals and their potential benefits.

Plants contain phytochemicals in abundance because these substances are of benefit to the plant itself. For example, an orange has at least 170 distinct phytochemicals. Individually and together, these compounds help plants resist the attacks of bacteria and fungi, the ravages of free radicals, and high levels of ultraviolet light from the sun. When we eat these plants, the phytochemicals end up in our tissues and provide many of the same protections that benefit plants.

Phytochemicals are part of the reason why the *Dietary Guidelines for Americans* recommends that we eat a variety of fruits and vegetables each day, especially dark-green, red, and orange vegetables and beans and peas.[38] The emphasis also can literally be seen in the MyPlate food plan, which encourages you to make half your plate fruits and vegetables.[39] Fruits and vegetables are naturally low in fat and calories and tend to be rich in fiber, potassium, and vitamins. In addition, studies consistently show that people who consume more fruits and vegetables tend to have lower rates of common chronic diseases.

Quick Bite

Functional Food Decisions

Are you a health-conscious consumer who seeks out functional foods? More than half of consumers "strongly" agree that functional foods offer health benefits. The top functional foods named by consumers included fruits and vegetables, fish and seafood, dairy, meat and poultry, herbs/spices, fiber, tea/green tea, nuts, whole grains, water, cereal, and oat products. The top three food components people look for when choosing foods and beverages for themselves and their children are fiber, whole grains, and protein.

TABLE SF.4
Examples of Functional Components in Foods

Class/Components	Sources[a]	Potential Benefits	Tips for Including Healthful Components in the Diet
Carotenoids			
Beta-carotene	Carrots, pumpkin, sweet potato, cantaloupe	Neutralizes free radicals that may damage cells; bolsters cellular antioxidant defenses; can be made into vitamin A in the body	For beta-carotene–rich french fries, try sweet potatoes coated lightly with olive oil or fat-free cooking spray, and add spices to taste (e.g., pepper, rosemary, thyme).
Lutein, zeaxanthin	Kale, collards, spinach, corn, eggs, citrus	May contribute to maintenance of healthy vision	For a simple way to enjoy kale, purchase a prewashed and destemmed ready-to-eat bag. Toss lightly with olive or peanut oil and salt, and then roast for 10–12 minutes at 425 degrees.
Lycopene	Tomatoes and processed tomato products, watermelon, red/pink grapefruit	May contribute to maintenance of prostate health	Try adding 1 cup tomato sauce to sautéed zucchini for a colorful side dish.
Dietary (Functional and Total) Fiber			
Insoluble fiber	Wheat bran, corn bran, fruit skins	May contribute to maintenance of a healthy digestive tract; may reduce the risk of some types of cancer	Try adding a little dry wheat bran when making smoothies or muffins to bulk up the fiber content; this may help keep you full longer.
Beta-glucan[b]	Oat bran, oatmeal, oat flour, barley, rye	May reduce risk of coronary heart disease (CHD)	Instant oatmeal packets are easily stored in your backpack or desk drawer to have on hand when you missed breakfast or need a hearty afternoon snack.
Soluble fiber[b]	Psyllium seed husk, peas, beans, apples, citrus fruit	May reduce risk of CHD and some types of cancer	Try adding canned beans (black, pinto, or garbanzo) to a quesadilla or an omelet, or enjoy them cold in a mixed green salad.
Whole grains[b]	Cereal grains, whole wheat bread, oatmeal, brown rice	May reduce risk of CHD and some types of cancer; may contribute to maintenance of healthy blood glucose levels	Did you know that air-popped popcorn is a great low-fat source of whole grains? Try spicing up your popcorn with garlic powder and cinnamon or rosemary and parmesan cheese.
Fatty Acids			
Monounsaturated fatty acids (MUFAs)[b]	Tree nuts, olive oil, canola oil	May reduce risk of CHD	For a quick and healthy on-the-go snack with heart-healthy fats make snack bags of mixed nuts (e.g., almonds, pecans). Throw in some dried fruit for an antioxidant boost.
Polyunsaturated fatty acids (PUFAs): omega-3 fatty acids, alpha-linolenic acid (ALA)	Walnuts, flax	May contribute to maintenance of heart health; may contribute to maintenance of mental and visual function	When cooking, try substituting a tablespoon of flaxseed oil in a recipe that calls for canola or olive oil, once or twice a week. Add ground flax to baked products, smoothies, yogurt, and hot cereal.
PUFAs: omega-3 fatty acids, docosahexaenoic acid (DHA) / eicosapentaenoic acid (EPA)[b]	Salmon, tuna, and other fish oils	May reduce risk of CHD; may contribute to maintenance of mental and visual function	Salmon or tuna that is canned in water or in a shelf-stable pouch can make easy and affordable meals.
Conjugated linoleic acid (CLA)	Beef and lamb; some cheese	May contribute to maintenance of desirable body composition and healthy immune function	Try something fun at your next cookout by preparing kebabs for the grill by alternating beef and vegetables.
Flavonoids			
Anthocyanins: cyanidin, delphinidin, malvidin	Berries, cherries, red grapes	Bolster cellular antioxidant defenses; may contribute to maintenance of brain function	For a cold treat, try frozen berries. They are also tasty additions to any yogurt and can help to cool and flavor your oatmeal in the morning.
Flavanols: catechins, epicatechins, epigallocatechin, procyanidins	Tea, cocoa, chocolate, apples, grapes	May contribute to maintenance of heart health	Go ahead and indulge in an occasional piece of chocolate.
Flavanones: hesperetin, naringenin	Citrus fruits	Neutralize free radicals, which may damage cells; bolster cellular antioxidant defenses	Squeeze half an orange and half a lemon into a small dish; add olive or flax oil and dashes of salt, pepper, and basil for a perfectly refreshing salad dressing.
Flavonols: quercetin, kaempferol, isorhamnetin, myricetin	Onions, apples, tea, broccoli	Neutralize free radicals, which may damage cells; bolster cellular antioxidant defenses	Caramelized onions make a sweet and tasty garnish to many main dishes. Sautee onions over low heat in oil until a deep gold color; add on top of prepared steak, chicken, fish, or whole grain.
Proanthocyanidins	Cranberries, cocoa, apples, strawberries, grapes, wine, peanuts, cinnamon	May contribute to maintenance of urinary tract health and heart health	Grab an apple or a bunch of grapes for a snack—what could be easier than that?

TABLE SF.4
Examples of Functional Components in Foods (*Continued*)

Class/Components	Sources[a]	Potential Benefits	Tips for Including Healthful Components in the Diet
Isothiocyanates			
Sulforaphane	Cauliflower, broccoli, broccoli sprouts, cabbage, kale, horseradish	May enhance detoxification of undesirable compounds; bolsters cellular antioxidant defenses	Keep frozen broccoli and cauliflower on hand for an easy dinner side dish.
Phenolic Acids			
Caffeic acid, ferulic acid	Apples, pears, citrus fruits, some vegetables, coffee	May bolster cellular antioxidant defenses; may contribute to maintenance of healthy vision and heart health	Love your morning coffee? Good news—coffee is a powerful source of antioxidants.
Plant Stanols/Sterols			
Free stanols/sterols[b]	Corn, soy, wheat, wood oils, fortified foods and beverages	May reduce risk of CHD	Get your free stanols/sterols from fortified foods such as bread containing whole-wheat flour, low-fat yogurt, and some cereals.
Stanol/sterol esters[b]	Stanol ester dietary supplements, fortified foods and beverages, including table spreads	May reduce risk of CHD	Many table spreads (butter or margarine alternatives) are now fortified with stanol and/or sterol esters. Check labels for other commercial products now commonly fortified with stanols and sterols, including orange juices, yogurt beverages, chocolate, and granola bars.
Polyols			
Sugar alcohols[b]: xylitol, sorbitol, mannitol, lactitol	Some chewing gums and diet candies	May reduce risk of dental caries	Reduce your risk for dental caries and curb your appetite by chewing gum containing xylitol after eating.
Prebiotics			
Inulin, fructo-oligosaccharides (FOS), polydextrose	Whole grains, onions, some fruits, garlic, honey, leeks, fortified foods and beverages	May improve gastrointestinal health; may improve calcium absorption	You can get prebiotics by simply adding honey to some of your routine meals. Try honey in your oatmeal or yogurt, or use in place of sugar as a sweetener.
Probiotics			
Yeast, *Lactobacilli*, *Bifidobacteria*, and other specific strains of beneficial bacteria	Certain yogurts and other cultured dairy and nondairy products	May improve gastrointestinal health and systemic immunity; benefits are strain-specific	For an easy way to add probiotics into your diet, choose from a variety of flavored yogurts with probiotics.
Phytoestrogens			
Isoflavones: daidzein, genistein	Soybeans and soy-based foods	May contribute to maintenance of bone health, healthy brain, and immune function; for women, may contribute to maintenance of menopausal health	Get your isoflavones by getting soft, silken tofu and adding it to the cheese mixture used to make lasagna.
Lignans	Flax, rye, some vegetables	May contribute to maintenance of heart health and healthy immune function	Add ground flaxseeds to a smoothie or a recipe for baked goods to pack a lignan punch!
Soy Protein			
Soy protein	Soybeans and soy-based foods	May reduce risk of CHD	Soybeans are also called edamame. Look for edamame in the frozen section to easily prepare as a healthy snack or party sampler. Edamame that has been cooked and removed from the pod adds great flavor and extra protein to any salad.
Sulfides/Thiols			
Diallyl disulfide, allyl methyl trisulfide	Garlic, onions, leeks, scallions	May enhance detoxification of undesirable compounds; may contribute to maintenance of heart health and healthy immune function	Scallions, or green onions, are milder than traditional onions and are commonly added at the last minute to salads or cooked sauces as a garnish. Leeks can also be an easy substitute, but are more commonly used in soups.
Dithiolethiones	Cruciferous vegetables, varieties of cabbage, bok choy, Brussels sprouts, kale	May enhance detoxification of undesirable compounds; may contribute to maintenance of healthy immune function	Use cabbage to make a variety of slaws and add to fresh salads. Bok choy is great in any stir-fry or raw in a salad with Asian dressing.

[a] Examples are not an all-inclusive list.

[b] FDA-approved health claim established for component.

Modified from the International Food Information Council Foundation. Functional foods. July 2011. http://www.foodinsight.org/Content/3842/Final%20Functional%20Foods%20Backgrounder.pdf. Accessed December 20, 2015.

▶ **phytoestrogens** Compounds that have weak estrogen activity in the body.

▶ **free radicals** Short-lived, highly reactive chemicals often derived from oxygen-containing compounds, which can have detrimental effects on cells, especially DNA and cell membranes.

Benefits of Phytochemicals

What are some of the specific benefits of phytochemicals? People who eat tomatoes and processed tomato products take in lycopene, which is associated with a decreased risk of chronic diseases, such as cancer and cardiovascular diseases.[40] Scientists believe that the large consumption of soy products in Asian countries contributes to lower rates of colon, prostate, uterus, and breast cancers.[41] Depending on the source of the isoflavones, the kind of cancer, and the study population, the outcomes of these studies are occasionally conflicting.[42] The foods and herbs with the highest anticancer activity include garlic, soybeans, cabbage, ginger, and licorice as well as the family of vegetables that includes celery, carrots, and parsley. The benefits of phytochemicals seem to be as varied as the phytochemicals themselves, with ongoing and exciting health-promoting perks being elucidated by nutrition scientists even today.

How do phytochemicals work to prevent chronic disease? A number of phytochemicals, including those from soybeans and from the cabbage family, are able to modify estrogen metabolism or block the effect of estrogen on cell growth. Such compounds are known as **phytoestrogens**. Other phytochemicals neutralize **free radicals**. Free radicals (active oxidants) are continually produced in our cells and over time can result in damage to DNA and important cell structures. Eventually, this damage can promote both cancer and cell aging. Many different plant chemicals, such as the pigments in grapes and red wine (see **FIGURE SF.12**), are able to neutralize or reduce concentrations of free radicals, thus protecting us against the development of both cancer and heart disease. Phytochemicals in fruits and vegetables have a number of other potential benefits. Lutein and zeaxanthin are carotenoids (plant pigments) found in dark-green leafy vegetables, corn, and egg yolks. Increased consumption of these compounds is associated with a lower incidence and slower progression of age-related macular degeneration, the leading cause of blindness in older people.[43,44]

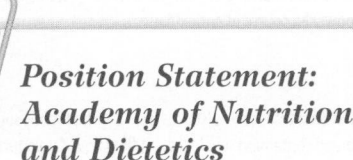

Position Statement: Academy of Nutrition and Dietetics

Functional Foods

It is the position of the Academy of Nutrition and Dietetics to recognize that although all foods provide some level of physiological function, the term *functional foods* is defined as whole foods along with fortified, enriched, or enhanced foods that have a potentially beneficial effect on health when consumed as part of a varied diet on a regular basis at effective levels based on significant standards of evidence. The Academy supports Food and Drug Administration–approved health claims on food labels when based on rigorous scientific substantiation.

Position of the Academy of Nutrition and Dietetics: functional foods. *J Acad Nutr Diet*. 2013;113:1096–1103.

Adding Phytochemicals to Your Diet

After learning about all the powerful health-protecting effects of phytochemicals, you are likely wondering how you can simply and quickly change your own food choices to include more. Before you reach for your next slice of bread, it is worth remembering that refined wheat, the source of white flour, has lost more than 99 percent of its phytochemical content. Because phytochemicals are so beneficial, why can't we just purify the important ones and add them to our diet as supplements, the way we put vitamins back into white flour after processing? The short answer is that we don't know enough about how phytochemicals function. There are still unidentified bioactive compounds in foods, such as phytochemicals, that have potential health benefits; however, the precise role, requirement, interactions, and toxicity levels of many of these substances remain unclear. Furthermore, whole foods might contain additional nutritional substances that have not yet been elucidated, and their health benefits might not be maintained when components are isolated and consumed as supplements or fortification ingredients.[45] Thus, appropriate food choices, rather than supplements, should be the foundation for achieving nutritional adequacy. Table SF.4 has some practical suggestions that require minimal effort.

Many phytochemicals appear to act synergistically, both fighting free radicals and blocking the negative effects of hormones. Yet there is no doubt that consumption of plant foods containing multiple antioxidants is strongly associated with health benefits. The weight of evidence and experience strongly favors finding a place for more fruits and vegetables in the diet. (See **FIGURE SF.13**.)

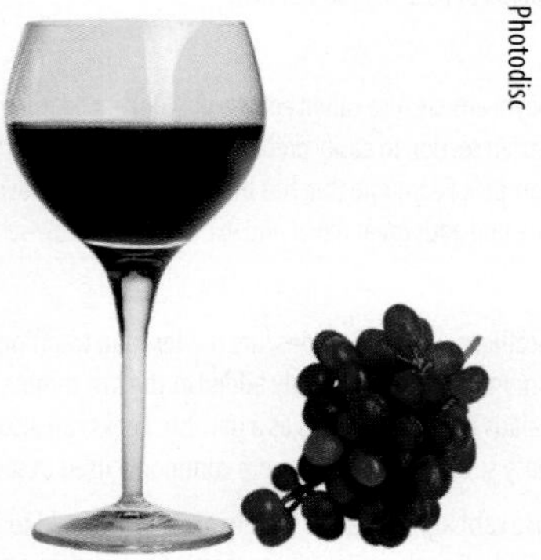

© Photodisc

FIGURE SF.12 Grapes, red wine, and heart disease. Grapes and red wine contain phytochemicals that appear to reduce the risk of heart disease. Studies show that moderate consumption of alcohol independently reduces heart disease risk.

The MyPlate graphic and the Fruits & Veggies—More Matters logo both encourage fruit and vegetable consumption. In addition, MyPlate's advice to "Make at least half your grains whole grains" helps promote intake of disease-fighting phytochemicals naturally found in whole grains. Changing your diet to include more functional foods and fewer empty calories needn't be painful. Sometimes you can have your pizza and eat it too. Next time, ask for your pizza loaded with vegetables. Whole-wheat crust would be a plus. The combination of lycopene from tomato sauce, quercetin from onions, and carotenoids and glucarates from colored peppers can turn your pizza into a phytochemical cornucopia.

fruits & veggies more matters®

Courtesy of FruitsandVeggiesMatter.org

FIGURE SF.13 The National Fruit and Vegetable Program. This program encourages Americans to increase their consumption of fruits and vegetables for better health. It is a public–private partnership, consisting of government agencies, nonprofit groups, and industry. For more information, visit www.fruitsandveggiesmorematters.org.

Foods Enhanced with Functional Ingredients and Additives

Phytochemicals are not the only substances that make foods functional. Another type of functional food is one that gets its health-promoting properties from what has been added during processing. Calcium-fortified orange juice, breakfast cereals fortified with folic acid, yogurt with live active cultures, and margarines with added plant sterol and plant stanol esters are examples. (See **FIGURE SF.14**.) Health properties come from added nutrients, bacteria, fiber, or other substances. Some are foods and beverages that contain added herbal compounds, such as those sold in pill form as dietary supplements. The result is a wide variety of products making an often confusing array of label statements and health claims. There are instances where functional foods do not deliver the health benefit they claim; consumers should be skeptical of products that sound too good to be true.

Using additives to create functional foods raises questions of how much should be used and how much is safe. In addition, although there are guidelines for the use of vitamins and minerals in the fortification of food and for the use of approved food additives, not much is known about what happens to many novel ingredients, such as botanical extracts, when they are put into a food. Tea beverages with enhanced antioxidant content and yogurt with

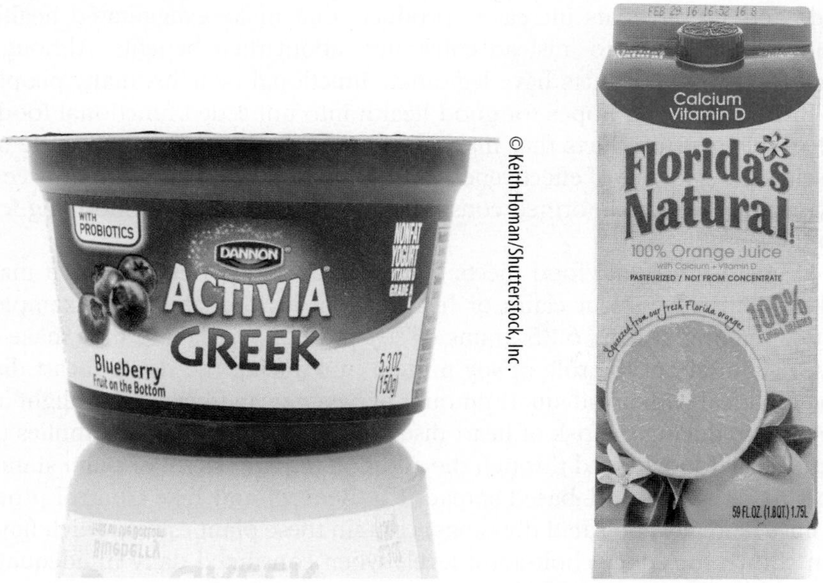

© Keith Homan/Shutterstock, Inc.

© Keith Homan/Shutterstock, Inc.

FIGURE SF.14 Examples of foods with functional ingredients.

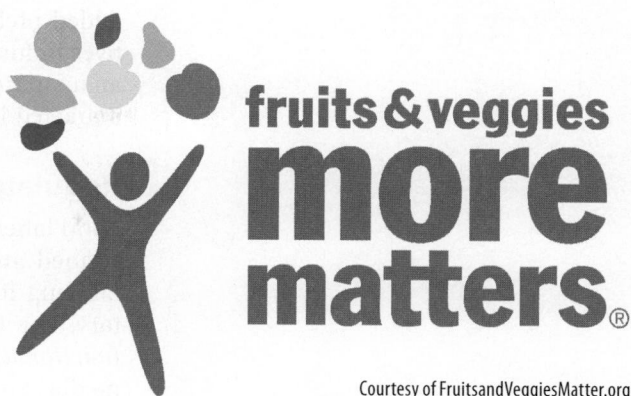

added prebiotic or probiotics, for example, are common examples of additives in functional foods with intended health benefits. Any food containing an unapproved food additive is considered adulterated and cannot legally be marketed in the United States.

Regulatory Issues for Functional Foods

Food labeling is required for most prepared foods, such as breads, cereals, canned and frozen foods, snacks, desserts, drinks, and so on. Nutrition labeling for raw produce such as fruits and vegetables and fish is voluntary. The FDA refers to these products as *conventional* foods. The terms *functional foods* and *nutraceuticals* are widely used in the marketplace and media. Such foods are regulated by the FDA under the authority of the Federal Food, Drug, and Cosmetic Act, even though they are not specifically defined by law.[46] Although this may sound a little confusing, a *food* is a product that we eat or drink as well as all the components of that product. This definition distinguishes a food from a *drug*, which is a substance intended to diagnose, cure, mitigate, treat, or prevent disease. Foods also are distinct from *dietary supplements*, which are products intended to supplement the diet but that do not represent themselves as a conventional food, meal, or diet.

Although some manufacturers have tried to market functional products as dietary supplements rather than foods to take advantage of broader allowances for label claims, the FDA's position is that products that are conventional foods and beverages are subject to the regulations for food and not for dietary supplements. A substance added to a food for health benefits must still conform to FDA regulations for food.

Quick Bite

Early Food Laws
In 1202, King John of England proclaimed the first English food law, the Assize of Bread, which prohibited adulteration of bread with such ingredients as ground peas or beans.

Quick Bite

Old Concept, New Frontier
Functional foods are a new frontier of nutrition and food science, but the idea has been around for centuries. Hippocrates, the father of modern medicine, proclaimed, "Let food be your medicine, and medicine be your food."

Key Concepts Functional foods provide health benefits beyond basic nutrition. Phytochemicals are "plant chemicals" that include thousands of compounds, pigments, and natural antioxidants, many of which are associated with protection from heart disease, hypertension, cancer, and diabetes. Just like conventional foods, functional foods are subject to FDA regulations for claims and safety.

Health Claims for Functional Foods

As consumer choices continue to expand and the abundance of functional foods and supplements increases, products that make exaggerated health claims will continue to mislead consumers about their benefits. Although many foods and products have legitimate functional benefits, many people put their money and hopes for good health into unneeded functional foods and supplement products that make misleading health claims with little or no scientific evidence of effectiveness.[47] To avoid wasting money on unnecessary products, be an informed consumer (see the FYI feature "Shopping for Supplements").

When a functional food meets the appropriate FDA guidelines, it may make a nutrient content claim or health claim on the label. For example, tofu containing at least 6.25 grams of soy protein per serving may make a health claim about the role of soy protein in reducing the risk of heart disease. Oatmeal with an adequate amount of beta-glucan fiber can highlight its benefit in reducing the risk of heart disease. Another health claim applies to a functional food created through the addition of plant sterol or plant stanol esters to a vegetable-oil–based spread. The Benecol and Take Control product lines (spreads and salad dressings) contain these plant esters, which have been shown to reduce cholesterol levels when consumed daily in adequate amounts.[48] (See **FIGURE SF.15**.)

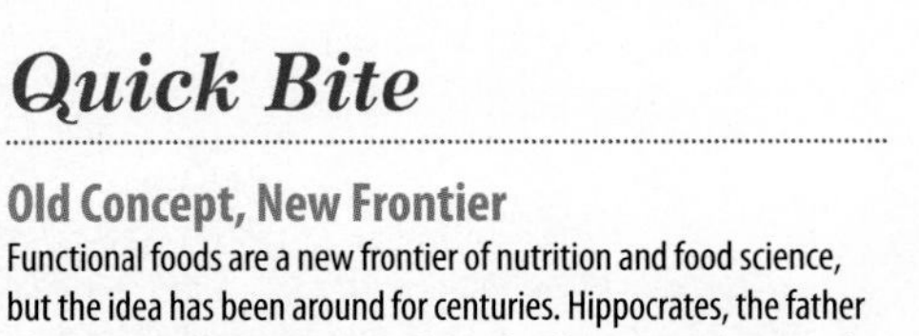

FIGURE SF.15 Some functional foods can make health claims. Manufacturers have obtained approval from the FDA to make health claims for these margarine products.

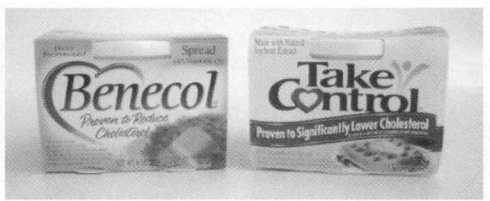

Structure/Function Claims for Functional Foods

Structure/function claims on conventional or functional foods must be based on the food's nutritive value. An example is orange juice with added vitamin C, vitamin E, and zinc to "support your natural defenses." However, structure/function claims are not as stringently regulated by the FDA as health claims. So, at present, many manufacturers are making claims about non-nutrients in foods and their effects on body structure or function. For example, a cereal with added St. John's wort and kava extract is "accented with herbs to support emotional and mental balance," and a bottled tea is "infused with memory-enhancing ginkgo biloba and Panax ginseng." Consumers should beware; many companies continue to deliberately confuse consumers by exaggerating the health effects or ingredients of their products, despite the FDA sending warning letters to food manufacturers about misleading labeling.[49]

THINK About It 4

Key Concepts Under FDA guidelines, a functional food's label may have a nutrient content claim, health claim, or structure/function claim. A structure/function claim promotes a substance's effect on the structure or function of the body. For foods, the claimed effect must be based on the food's "nutritive value." Currently, many manufacturers make structure/function claims about non-nutrients in foods.

Quick Bite

Mayonnaise Protects Against Strokes

Is this claim science or snake oil? Studies show that foods rich in vitamin E help protect against heart disease and stroke. In one study of stroke reduction in postmenopausal women, mayonnaise was the most concentrated food source of vitamin E. But to claim that mayonnaise prevents strokes is unwarranted and overstates the evidence.

Strategies for Functional Food Use

So, should you run out and fill your shopping cart with functional foods? Which ones would you buy? The best course of action is to stick with what scientists have agreed upon so far. First, fruits and vegetables promote health and reduce disease risk through a whole host of natural phytochemicals. Use the list of foods and phytochemicals in Table SF.4 to enhance your shopping list with nature's functional foods. Second, consider nutrient-fortified products when a particular nutrient is lacking in your diet and you either don't like or can't eat good food sources of that nutrient. For example, if you are allergic to milk and dairy products, consider calcium-fortified orange juice as a nutritious way to get the calcium you need. Third, *read, read, read* about functional foods, and be skeptical when you evaluate what's on the Internet. Table SF.5 lists some questions to ask when assessing the credibility of websites. For more tips on how to evaluate health information on the Internet, visit the Office of Dietary Supplements website.[50] Do your homework by looking at scientific articles—your instructor can help you find and interpret studies of functional food components. Finally, be critical of advertising and hype—if it sounds too good to be true, it probably is!

Quick Bite

The Yin and Yang of Food

The early theory of yin and yang had its genesis during the Yin and Zhou dynasties in China (1766 B.C.E.–256 B.C.E.). The yin force is passive, downward flowing, and cold. Conversely, the yang force is aggressive, upward rising, and hot. The concept of balance and harmony between these life forces is the basis upon which food and herbs are used as medicine. In traditional Chinese healing methods, disease is viewed as the result of an imbalance of these energies in the body. To balance these energies, according to this view, your diet should balance yin foods and yang foods. Yin (cold) foods include milk, honey, fruit, and vegetables; yang (hot) foods include beef, poultry, seafood, eggs, and cheese. Foods are also classified as sweet (earth), bitter (fire), sour (wood), pungent (metal), and salty (water). Each class supposedly has specific effects on different parts of the body.

Questions to Ask to Assess the Credibility of Websites

Checking Out a Health Website: Five Quick Questions

Many online health resources are useful, but others may present information that is inaccurate or misleading, so it's important to find sources you can trust and to know how to evaluate their content.

If you're visiting a health website for the first time, these five quick questions can help you decide whether the site is a helpful resource.

Who? Who runs the website? Can you trust them?

What? What does the site say? Do its claims seem too good to be true?

When? When was the information posted or reviewed? Is it up-to-date?

Where? Where did the information come from? Is it based on scientific research?

Why? Why does the site exist? Is it selling something?

National Institutes of Health, National Center for Complementary and Alternative Medicine. Finding and evaluating online resources on complementary health approaches. http://nccih.nih.gov/health/webresources#ask. Accessed December 21, 2015.

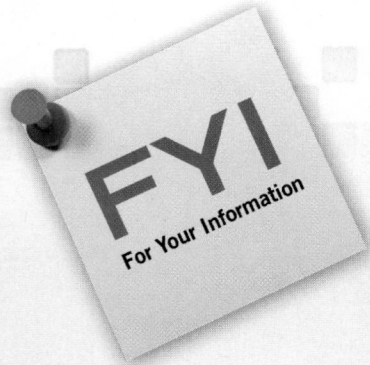

FYI
For Your Information

Defining Complementary and Integrative Health: How Does Nutrition Fit?

Alternative approaches to health care are therapies and treatments outside the medical mainstream. Historically, they tended to be based mainly or solely on observation or anecdotal evidence rather than controlled research. According to the National Center for Complementary and Integrative Health, "Large population-based surveys have found that the use of alternative medicine—unproven practices used in place of conventional medicine—is rare. Integrative health care, defined as a comprehensive, often interdisciplinary approach to treatment, prevention and health promotion that brings together complementary and conventional therapies, is more common."[a]

The term *alternative* suggests practices that replace conventional ones. *Complementary* implies practices that are used *in addition to* conventional ones. A practice that combines both conventional and complementary treatments for which there is evidence of safety and effectiveness is referred to as *integrative*. For example, using only herbs and megavitamins to treat AIDS would be alternative, whereas using herbs to combat diarrhea caused by conventional AIDS medications and taking supplements to replace lost vitamins would be complementary. Complementary and integrative health care includes a broad range of healing therapies and philosophies. Several among them involve nutrition, including special diet therapies, phytotherapy (herbalism), orthomolecular medicine, and other biologic interventions. The use of an integrative approach to health and wellness has grown within care settings across the United States, including hospitals, hospices, and military health facilities.

More than 30 percent of adults and about 12 percent of children in the United States use some form of complementary therapy.[b] Commonly used complementary therapies include a variety of natural products and diet-based therapies, as well as mind–body practices such as deep breathing exercises, prayer, and relaxation techniques such as guided imagery, meditation, spinal manipulation (chiropractic care), tai chi and yoga, acupuncture, massage therapy, and movement therapies. People seek out complementary therapies for numerous reasons, including fear of aging, personal beliefs, and distrust of institutional medicine.

Where Does Nutrition Fit?

A number of alternative therapies involve nutrition, and sometimes the line between standard and alternative nutrition is not clear. A variety of health conditions, such as diabetes, gastrointestinal disorders, and kidney disease, require special diets. Alternative nutrition practices include diets to prevent and treat diseases not shown to be diet-related. (See **Figure A**.) What often makes these practices "alternative" is the limited nature of the diet, the lack of rigorous scientific evidence showing effectiveness, and the divergence from science-based healthy eating patterns such as the Mediterranean diet, DASH diet, or MyPlate. Other practices outside the nutritional mainstream have gained recent popularity, such as reliance on only raw foods and the extensive use of herbal and botanical supplements as well as megadoses of vitamin/mineral supplements, which we have already discussed. Most nutritionists consider vegetarianism a routine variation of a normal diet, particularly if the vegetarian's motivation is religious or philosophical, the result of a concern for animals, or an aversion to animal products. When a meat eater goes vegetarian in an attempt to prevent or cure disease, that's alternative.

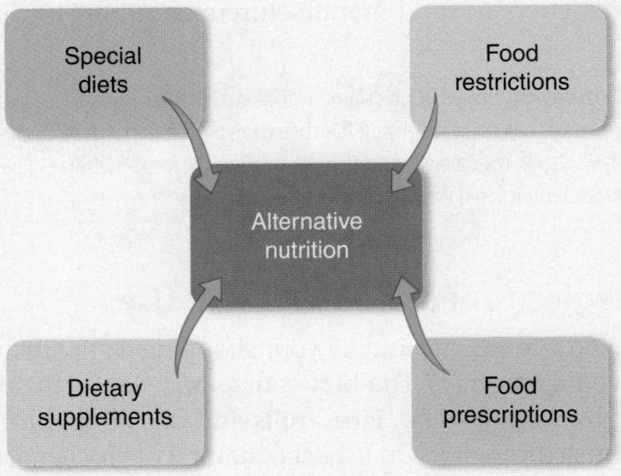

FIGURE A Alternative nutrition practices. Although many mainstream medical practices may involve special dietary regimens, alternative nutrition practices often are overly restrictive, depart from established dietary guidelines, and lack rigorous scientific evidence.

Food Restrictions and Food Prescriptions

Societies throughout the world commonly use dietary changes to treat or prevent illness. The specifics vary from place to place, however, which suggests that they are based on cultural factors rather than science.

In recent years, we have seen yeast-free diets, dairy-free diets, sugar-free diets, white-flour-free diets, cleansing diets, raw food diets, both low-carbohydrate and high-carbohydrate diets, both low-red-meat and high-red-meat diets, caffeine-free diets, salicylate-free diets, and more. People with subjective symptoms such as headaches, fatigue, or back pain have been instructed to avoid irrational lists of "allergenic foods" based on "blood screening." We've also seen illogical instructions on how to combine foods or what foods not to combine. For weight loss, we've had grapefruit diets, hard-boiled-egg diets, cottage-cheese diets, water diets, high-fat diets, low-fat diets, and blue-foods-only diets; the list goes on and on.

Many types of diets can be described as alternative. Their origins and claims vary, and their proponents often cannot show that they improve health; some alternative diets can actually be harmful by restricting foods and thereby lowering the body's intake of necessary nutrients. Such fad diets come and go. Most often they are not based on science and eventually fail to interest people when they don't work. Those few that prove effective and

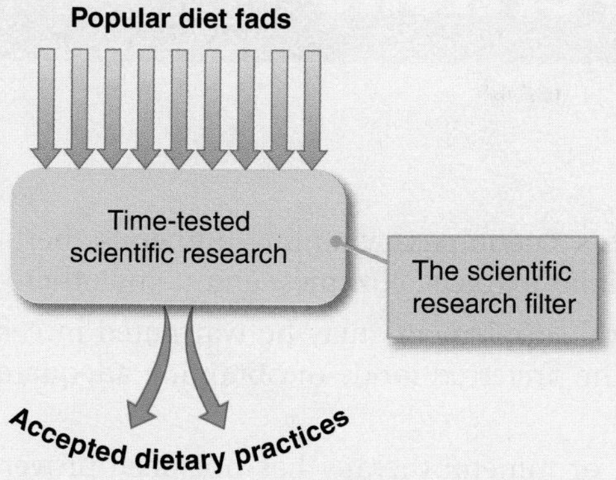

FIGURE B Many apply but few are chosen. Dietary practices with a scientific basis and proven efficacy are incorporated into conventional nutrition and diet therapy.

have a scientific basis become *integrated* into conventional nutrition and diet therapy. (See **Figure B**.)

[a] National Institutes of Health, National Center for Complementary and Integrative Health. NIH complementary and integrative health agency gets new name. https://nccih.nih.gov/news/press/12172014. Accessed December 21, 2015.

[b] National Institutes of Health, National Center for Complementary and Integrative Health. Complementary, alternative, or integrative health: what's in a name? https://nccih.nih.gov/health/integrative-health. Accessed December 21, 2015.

Label to Table

If you picked up a multivitamin/mineral container from your drugstore shelf, would you know how to read the label? Look at this Supplement Facts panel from a basic multivitamin/mineral supplement. Here are some questions that you might have:

1. If you were a 20-year-old woman who knew she wasn't consuming enough calcium, would this supplement allow you to get your recommended intake?
2. If 25 percent of the vitamin A in this supplement comes from beta-carotene, where does the rest come from?
3. What trend do you see in the amounts of B vitamins?
4. What trend do you see in the amounts of bone minerals?
5. What trend do you see in the amounts of antioxidant vitamins?

Supplement Facts

Daily Multivitamin/Mineral Dietary Supplement

USP USP has tested and verified ingredients, potency, and manufacturing process. USP sets official standards for Dietary Supplements. For more information, go to www.uspverified.org.

Serving Size 1 tablet

Each Tablet Contains	%DV	Each Tablet Contains	
Vitamin A 10,000 I.U.	200%	Iodine 150 mcg	100%
25% as beta-carotene			
Vitamin C 120 mg	200%	Magnesium 100 mg	25%
Vitamin D 400 IU	100%	Zinc 22.5 mg	150%
Vitamin E 60 IU	200%	Selenium 45 mcg	64%
Vitamin K 25 mcg	31%	Copper 3 mg	150%
Thiamin (vit. B_1) 1.5 mg	100%	Manganese 2.5 mg	125%
Riboflavin (vit. B_2) 1.7 mg	100%	Chromium 100 mcg	83%
Niacin 20 mg	100%	Molybdenum 25 mcg	33%
Vitamin B_6 2 mg	100%	Chloride 36.3 mg	1%
Folate (folic acid) 400 mcg	100%	Sodium less than 5 mg	less than 1%
Vitamin B_{12} 6 mcg	100%	Potassium 40 mg	1%
Biotin 30 mcg	10%	Nickel 5 mcg	*
Pantothenic acid 10 mg	100%	Tin 10 mcg	*
Calcium 162 mg	16%	Silicon 2 mg	*
Iron 9 mg	50%	Vanadium 10 mcg	*
Phosphorus 109 mg	11%	Boron 150 mcg	*

* Daily Value (%DV) not established

Reprinted with permission from The United States Pharmacopeial Convention, 12601 Twinbrook Parkway, Rockville, Maryland 20852.

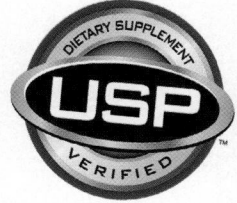

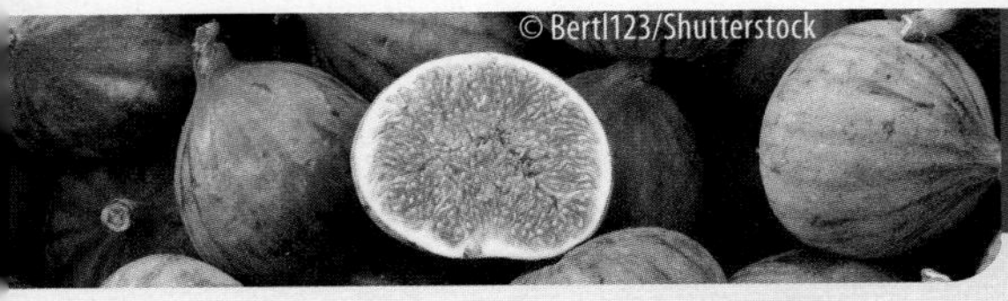

© Bertl123/Shutterstock

Learning Portfolio

Key Terms

bioavailability	89
bioflavonoids	85
Dietary Supplement Health and Education Act (DSHEA)	85
dietary supplements	77
free radicals	94
functional food	90
herbal therapy (phytotherapy)	82
integrative health care	77
isoflavones	77
lycopene	90
malabsorption syndromes	81
megadoses	79
National Center for Complementary and Integrative Health (NCCIH)	83
National Institutes of Health (NIH)	83
nucleic acids	85
orthomolecular medicine	81
phytochemicals	90
phytoestrogens	94
Supplement Facts panel	87
U.S. Pharmacopeia (USP)	89

Study Points

- Dietary supplements encompass vitamins, minerals, herbal products, amino acids, glandular extracts, enzymes, and many other products.
- Vitamin and mineral supplements may be warranted in certain circumstances, although the preferred mode of obtaining adequate nutrition is through foods.
- Megadose vitamin or mineral therapy has not been proven effective in the treatment of cancer, colds, or heart disease. Moreover, such megadoses act more like drugs than nutrients in the body and should be approached with caution.
- Herbal medicine is a traditional form of healing in many cultures. Some herbal medicines have shown enough promise to warrant large-scale clinical studies involving supplements. However, herbal products can have side effects and can interfere with prescription medications.
- Dietary supplements are regulated according to the provisions of the Dietary Supplement Health and Education Act of 1994 (DSHEA). Unlike drugs and additives, dietary supplements do not need premarket approval.
- Claims for dietary supplements can include health claims, structure/function claims, and nutrient content claims.
- Dietary supplements must have a Supplement Facts panel on the label.
- Consumers should carefully evaluate claims and evidence for dietary supplements and consult their physician before taking a supplement.
- A functional food is considered to be a food that may provide a health benefit beyond basic nutrition.
- Phytochemicals are plant chemicals responsible for the health-promoting properties of many functional foods.
- Consumption of plant foods containing multiple antioxidants is strongly associated with health benefits. Scientific evidence strongly supports eating at least five servings of fruits and vegetables daily and emphasizing whole grains.
- Complementary and integrative health care comprises practices developed outside the medical mainstream that are being practiced together with conventional medicine. Integrative approaches include a broad range of therapies, many of which include nutrition. People seek them for a variety of reasons, including environmental concerns and a fear of aging.

Study Questions

1. How do you know a product is a dietary supplement?
2. If a dietary supplement product label contains the words, "High in vitamin E," what type of claim is it making? What other claims can a supplement make?
3. What things should someone do before purchasing supplements?
4. What are phytochemicals, and how do they benefit plants and humans?
5. Name three chronic diseases that consuming functional foods may help prevent or treat.
6. What are some of the possible complications involved in using herbal medicines?
7. What role does nutrition have in complementary and integrative health?

Try This

Finding Functional Beverages

This exercise will familiarize you with the many beverages that contain functional ingredients now available to consumers. Take a trip to your grocery store and spend some time in the beverage aisles. You may want to check out the chilled juice section in addition to the bottled teas and juice beverages. Pick out about 10 different products that have either a nutrient or herbal compound added and try to identify how many have nutrient content claims, health claims, and structure/function claims. Note the prices of these products. How does their nutritional content compare to a 100-percent fruit juice like orange juice? How does it compare to soda?

Take a Walk on the "Web Side"

This exercise will familiarize you with various websites that promote and sell supplements. Do an Internet search with keywords affiliated with supplements. Try *vitamins*, *minerals*, *supplements*, *herbs*, and even some specific terms like *chromium picolinate* and *ginseng*. On the websites you visit, how is the nutrition information presented? Do the supplement's benefits sound too good to be true? See if you can spot a fraud. Use the information in the "Fraudulent Products" section of this chapter to identify the accuracy of the product information you find.

References

1. Gahche J, Bailey R, Burt V, et al. Dietary supplement use among U.S. adults has increased since NHANES III (1988–1994). NCHS Data Brief No. 61. April 2011. http://www.cdc.gov/nchs/data/databriefs/db61.pdf. Accessed December 21, 2015.
2. Bailey RL, Gahche JJ, Miller PE, Thomas PR, Dwyer JT. Why US adults use dietary supplements. *JAMA Intern Med.* 2013;173(5):355–361. doi: 10.1001/jamainternmed.2013.2299.
3. National Center for Complementary and Integrative Health. Using dietary supplements wisely. https://nccih.nih.gov/health/supplements/wiseuse.htm. Accessed December 21, 2015.
4. Position of the Academy of Nutrition and Dietetics: nutrient supplementation. *J Am Diet Assoc.* 2009;109:2073–2085.
5. Bailey, Gahche, Miller, Thomas, Dwyer. Why US adults use dietary supplements. Op cit.
6. Position of the Academy of Nutrition and Dietetics: Nutrient supplementation. Op cit.
7. National Institutes of Health, Office of Dietary Supplements. A compilation of dietary supplement statements from the scientific report of the 2015 Dietary Guidelines Advisory Committee. February 2015. http://ods.od.nih.gov/pubs/2015_DGAC_Scientific_Report_ODS_Compiled_DS_Statements.pdf. Accessed December 21, 2015.
8. Position of the Academy of Nutrition and Dietetics: functional foods. *J Acad Nutr Diet.* 2013;113:1096–1103.
9. Hochholzer W, Berg DD, Giugliano RP. The facts behind niacin. *Ther Adv Cardiovasc Dis.* 2011;5(5):227–240. doi: 10.1177/1753944711419197. Epub September 5, 2011.
10. *Physicians' Desk Reference 2011*. 65th ed. Montvale, NJ: Thompson Healthcare; 2010.
11. Pauling L. Orthomolecular psychiatry. Varying the concentrations of substances normally present in the human body may control mental disease. *Science.* 1968;160(3825):265–271.
12. Institute of Medicine, Food and Nutrition Board. *Dietary Reference Intakes for Vitamin C, Vitamin E, Selenium, and Carotenoids*. Washington, DC: National Academies Press; 2000.
13. Institute of Medicine, Food and Nutrition Board. *Dietary Reference Intakes for Vitamin A, Vitamin K, Arsenic, Boron, Chromium, Copper, Iron, Manganese, Molybdenum, Nickel, Silicon, Vanadium, and Zinc*. Washington, DC: National Academies Press; 2001.

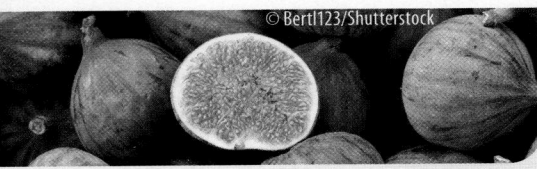
© Bertl123/Shutterstock

Learning Portfolio (continued)

14. Council for Responsible Nutrition. Dietary supplements: safe, beneficial and regulated. http://www.crnusa.org/CRNRegQandA.html. Accessed December 21, 2015.
15. Health Canada. About natural health products. http://www.hc-sc.gc.ca/dhp-mps/prodnatur/about-apropos/cons-eng.php. Accessed December 21, 2015.
16. Silverglade B, Ringel Heller I. Food labeling chaos. The case for reform. 2010. Center for Science in the Public Interest. http://cspinet.org/new/pdf/food_labeling_chaos_report.pdf. Accessed December 21, 2015.
17. National Institutes of Health, National Center for Complementary and Integrative Health. NIH complementary and integrative health agency gets new name. https://nccih.nih.gov/news/press/12172014. Accessed December 21, 2015.
18. Ibid.
19. National Institutes of Health, National Center for Complementary and Integrative Health. Use of complementary health approaches in the U.S. What complementary and integrative approaches do Americans use? Key findings from the 2012 National Health Interview Survey. https://nccih.nih.gov/research/statistics/NHIS/2012/key-findings. Accessed December 21, 2015.
20. Ibid.
21. Kennedy DA, Seely D. Clinically based evidence of drug–herb interactions: A systematic review. *Expert Opin Drug Saf.* 2010;9(1):79–124.
22. Tachjian A, Maria V, Jahangir A. Use of herbal products and potential interactions in patients with cardiovascular diseases. *J Am Coll Cardiol.* 2010; 55(6):515–525.
23. U.S. Food and Drug Administration. FDA issues dietary supplements final rule. FDA press release. June 22, 2007. http://www.fda.gov/newsevents/newsroom/pressannouncements/2007/ucm108938.htm. Accessed December 21, 2015.
24. U.S. Food and Drug Administration. Regulatory information. Dietary Supplement Health and Education Act of 1994. http://www.fda.gov/regulatoryinformation/legislation/significantamendmentstothefdcact/ucm148003.htm. Accessed February 3, 2016.
25. U.S. Food and Drug Administration. FDA 101: dietary supplements. http://www.fda.gov/ForConsumers/ConsumerUpdates/ucm050803.htm. Accessed December 21, 2015.
26. S.1425 (113th): Dietary Supplement Labeling Act of 2013. https://www.govtrack.us/congress/bills/113/s1425. Accessed December 21, 2015.
27. U.S. Food and Drug Administration. Guidance for industry. Dietary supplement labeling guide. http://www.fda.gov/food/guidanceregulation/guidancedocumentsregulatoryinformation/dietarysupplements/ucm2006823.htm. Accessed December 21, 2015.
28. National Institutes of Health, Office of Dietary Supplements. Dietary supplements. Background information. http://ods.od.nih.gov/factsheets/DietarySupplements-HealthProfessional/. Accessed December 21, 2015.
29. U.S. Food and Drug Administration. Structure/function claims. http://www.fda.gov/Food/IngredientsPackagingLabeling/LabelingNutrition/ucm2006881.htm. Accessed December 21, 2015.
30. U.S. Food and Drug Administration. Dietary supplements. http://www.fda.gov/Food/Dietarysupplements/default.htm. Accessed December 21, 2015.
31. Health Canada. Drugs and health products. About natural health product regulation in Canada. http://www.hc-sc.gc.ca/dhp-mps/prodnatur/about-apropos/index-eng.php. Accessed December 21, 2015.
32. Academy of Nutrition and Dietetics. Guidelines regarding the recommendation and sale of dietary supplements: Full text. http://www.eatrightpro.org/resource/career/code-of-ethics/ethics-education-resources/guidelines

-regarding-the-recommendation-and-sale-of-dietary-supplements-full-text. Accessed December 21, 2015.
33. U.S. Pharmacopeial Convention. Home page. http://www.usp.org. Accessed December 21, 2015.
34. U.S. Food and Drug Administration. Beware of fraudulent dietary supplements. http://www.fda.gov/forconsumers/consumerupdates/ucm246744.htm. Accessed December 21, 2015.
35. Position of the Academy of Nutrition and Dietetics: Functional foods. Op cit.
36. Daniells S. What's driving functional food and beverage growth? Snacking, convenience, and customer behavior. November 20, 2014. http://www.nutraingredients-usa.com/Markets/What-s-driving-functional-food-and-beverage-growth-Snacking-convenience-and-consumer-behavior. Accessed February 3, 2016.
37. Pearson L. Global functional food analysis. http://reportlinker.com/ci02036/Functional-Food.html. Accessed December 21, 2015.
38. U.S. Department of Agriculture and U.S. Department of Health and Human Services. *Dietary Guidelines for Americans, 2015-2020*. 8th ed. Washington, DC: U.S. http://health.gov/dietaryguidelines/2015/guidelines/ Accessed February 3, 2016.
39. U.S. Department of Agriculture. MyPlate. http://www.choosemyplate.gov. Accessed December 21, 2015.
40. Mordente A, Guantario B, Meucci E, et al. Lycopene and cardiovascular diseases: An update. *Curr Med Chem*. 2011;18(8):1146–1163.
41. Andres S, Abraham K, Appel KE, Lampen A. Risks and benefits of dietary isoflavones for cancer. *Crit Rev Toxicol*. 2011;41(6):463–506.
42. Ibid.
43. Wong IY, Koo SC, Chan CW. Prevention of age-related macular degeneration. *Int Ophthalmol*. 2011;31(1):73–82.
44. Olson JH, Erie JC, Bakri SJ. Nutritional supplementation and age-related macular degeneration. *Semin Ophthalmol*. 2011;26(3):131–136.
45. Position of the Academy of Nutrition and Dietetics: Functional Foods. *J Acad Nutr Diet*. 2013;113:1096–1103.
46. U.S. Food and Drug Administration. Labeling and nutrition. http://www.fda.gov/food/ingredientspackaginglabeling/labelingnutrition/default.htm. Accessed May 13, 2015.
47. Position of the Academy of Nutrition and Dietetics: functional foods. *J Acad Nutr Diet*. 2013;113:1096–1103.
48. U.S. Food and Drug Administration. Guidance for industry: a food labeling guide. 11. Appendix C: health claims. http://www.fda.gov/food/guidanceregulation/guidancedocumentsregulatoryinformation/labelingnutrition/ucm064919.htm. Accessed December 21, 2015.
49. Silverglade, Ringel Heller. Food labeling chaos. The case for reform. Op cit.
50. National Institutes of Health, Office on Dietary Supplements. Health information. How to evaluate health information on the Internet: questions and answers. http://ods.od.nih.gov/Health_Information/How_To_Evaluate_Health_Information_on_the_Internet_Questions_and_Answers.aspx. Accessed December 21, 2015.

Chapter 3

Digestion and Absorption

Revised by Kimberley McMahon

THINK About It

1. Your friend warns you that eating some foods together is not healthful. Is this likely to change your eating behavior?
2. How good are you at identifying tastes?
3. Have you ever noticed that food sometimes tastes sweeter after chewing it for a while?
4. You feel particularly happy and you find that a meal prepared by your friend tastes especially good. Any connection?

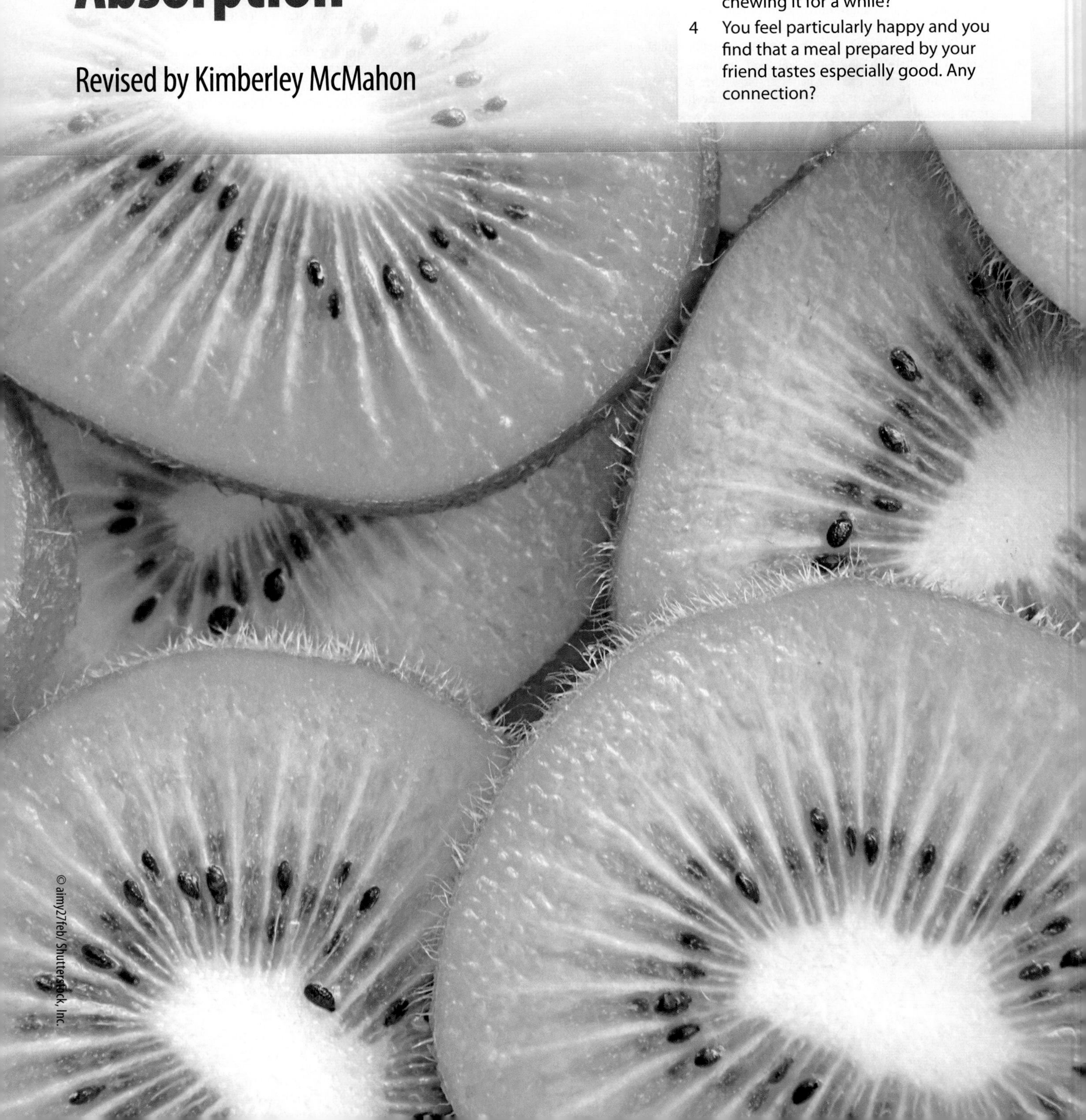

© aimy27feb/ Shutterstock, Inc.

CHAPTER Menu

- Taste and Smell: The Beginnings of Our Food Experience
- The Gastrointestinal Tract
- Overview of Digestion: Physical and Chemical Processes
- Overview of Absorption
- Assisting Organs
- Putting It All Together: Digestion and Absorption
- Circulation of Nutrients
- Signaling Systems: Command, Control, and Defense
- Influences on Digestion and Absorption
- Nutrition and GI Disorders
- Key Terms
- Study Points
- Study Questions
- Getting Personal
- References

LEARNING Objectives

- Describe the basic components and functions of digestive system organs.
- Sequence the steps for digestion of food and absorption of nutrients through the digestive system.
- Explain the role of enzymes and hormones required for digestion and absorption of nutrients.
- Explain how nutrients are absorbed by, circulated through, and eliminated from the body.
- Identify factors that influence digestion, absorption, and nutrient transport in the body.
- Examine common nutritional and digestive system disorders, common approaches to prevention, and likely treatments.

The aroma of food that we like to eat fills the air—roasted garlic, pasta sauce, chocolate chip cookies. You start to anticipate a delicious food experience; after all, you haven't eaten for six or seven hours and all of a sudden your mouth waters and your digestive juices are working. Even before you eat, thoughts from your brain signal your body to prepare for food. Before we begin digesting and absorbing, our senses of taste and smell first attract us to foods we are likely to consume. In this way, the process of digestion begins even before we eat, and it continues until all of the food we have eaten has moved from our mouth through the gastrointestinal tract.

The body's machinery to process food and turn it into nutrients is not only efficient, but also elegant. The action unfolds in the digestive tract in two stages: **digestion**—the breaking apart of foods into smaller and smaller units—and **absorption**—the movement of those small units from the gut into the bloodstream or lymphatic system for circulation. Your digestive system is designed to digest carbohydrates, proteins, and fats simultaneously, while preparing other substances—vitamins, minerals, and cholesterol, for example—for absorption. Despite promotions for enzyme supplements and diet books that recommend consuming food or nutrient groups separately, scientific research does not support these claims. Unless you have a specific medical condition, your digestive system is ready, willing, and able to digest and absorb the foods you eat, in whatever combination you eat them.

THINK About It 1

▶ **digestion** The process of transforming the foods we eat into units for absorption.

▶ **absorption** The movement of substances into or across tissues; in particular, the passage of nutrients and other substances into the walls of the gastrointestinal tract and then into the bloodstream.

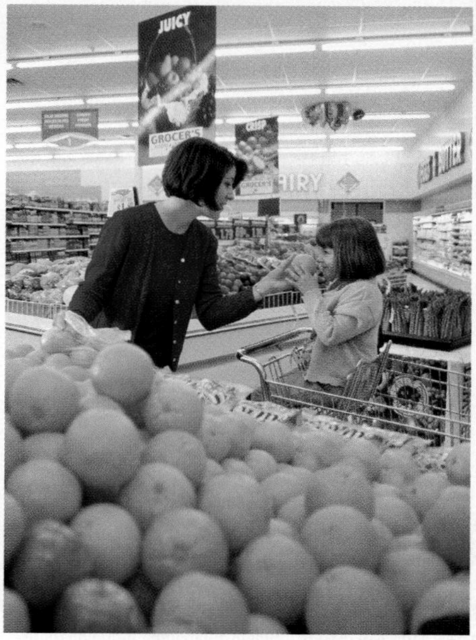

© Photodisc/ Getty Images

Taste and Smell: The Beginnings of Our Food Experience

THINK About It 2

You probably wouldn't eat a food if it didn't appeal in some way to your senses. Odors around us, such as the smell of bread baking, stimulate nerve cells inside of the nose. In the mouth, taste, as well as texture and temperature, combine with odors to produce a perception of flavor. You recognize flavors mainly through the sense of smell. If you hold your nose while eating chocolate, for example, you will have trouble identifying it—even though you can distinguish the food's sweetness or bitterness. That's because the familiar flavor of chocolate is sensed largely by odor, as is the well-known flavor of coffee.

The sight, smell, thought, taste, and in some cases even the sound of food can trigger a set of physiologic responses known as the **cephalic phase responses**. These responses (see **FIGURE 3.1**) are innate and learned physiological responses to sensory signals (such as sight, smell, thought, and taste) that prepare the gastrointestinal (GI) tract for processing the foods we eat.

▶ **cephalic phase responses** The responses of the parasympathetic nervous system to the sight, smell, thought, and sound of food. Also called preabsorptive phase responses.

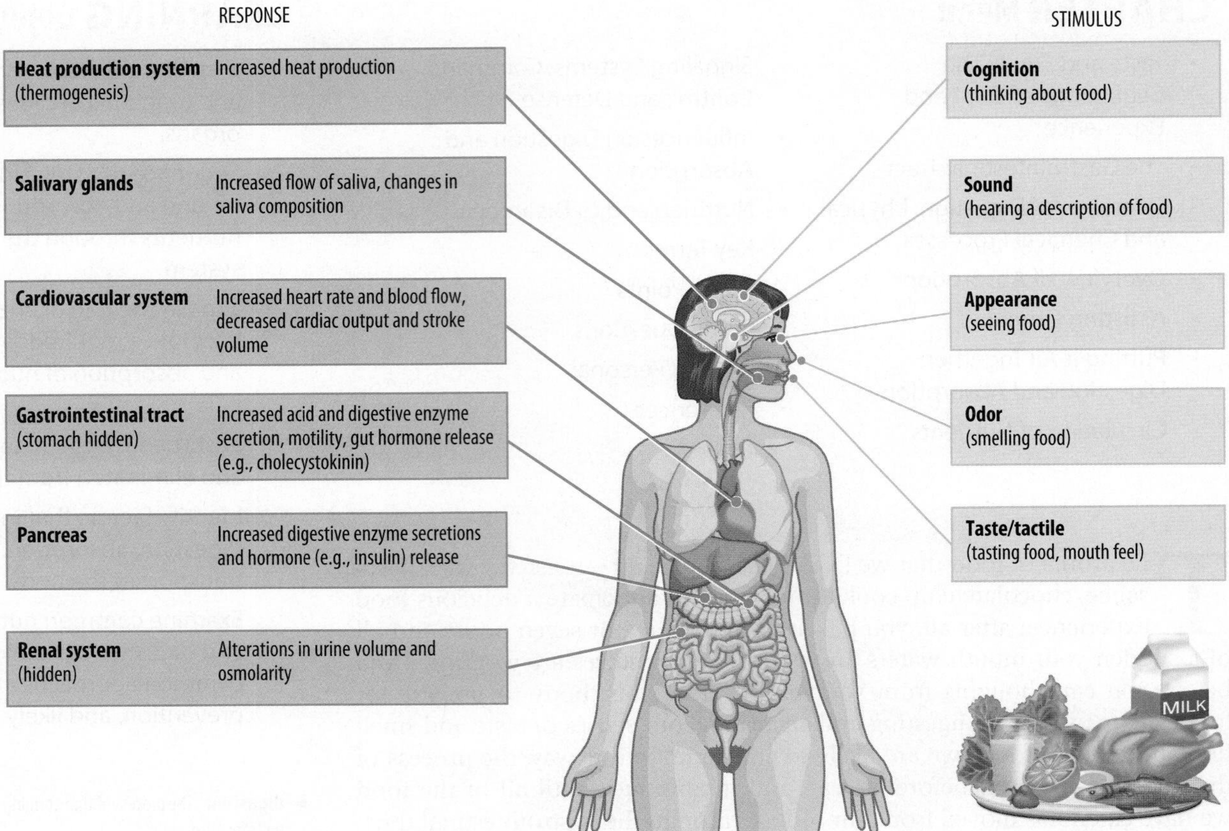

FIGURE 3.1 The cephalic (preabsorptive) phase responses. In response to sensory stimulation, your body primes its resources to better absorb and use anticipated nutrients.

For example, thinking of food can stimulate the cerebral cortex, sending a message to the hypothalamus, then on to the vagus nerve, and then to the stomach, to secrete gastric juices—all of which help prepare the stomach for the consumption of food. If no food is consumed, the response diminishes. Eating prolongs the stimulation of the salivary and gastric cells.

Key Concepts Taste and smell are the first interactions we have with food. The flavor of a particular food is really a combination of olfactory, gustatory, and other stimuli. Smell (olfactory) receptors receive stimuli through odor compounds. Taste (gustatory) receptors in the mouth sense flavors. Other nerve cells (the common chemical senses) are stimulated by other chemical factors. If one of these stimuli is missing, our sense of flavor is incomplete.

The Gastrointestinal Tract

If, instead of teasing the body with mere sights and smells, we actually sit down to a meal and experience the full flavor and texture of foods, the real work of the digestive tract begins. For the food we eat to nourish our bodies, we need to digest it (break it down into smaller units), absorb it (move it from the gut into circulation), and finally transport it to the tissues and cells of the body. The digestive process starts in the mouth and continues as food journeys down the GI tract. Nutrients are absorbed at various points along the GI tract, meaning they move from the GI tract into circulatory systems so they can be transported throughout the body. If there are problems along the way, with either incomplete digestion or inadequate absorption, the cells

Quick Bite

How Many Taste Buds Do You Have?

We have almost 10,000 taste buds in our mouths, including those on the roofs of our mouths. In general, females have more taste buds than males.

will not receive the nutrients they need to grow, perform daily activities, fight infection, and maintain health. A closer look at the gastrointestinal tract can help you see just how amazing this organ system is.

Organization of the GI Tract

The **gastrointestinal (GI) tract**, also known as the alimentary canal, is a long, hollow tube that begins at the mouth and ends at the anus. The specific parts include the mouth, esophagus, stomach, small intestine, large intestine, and rectum (see **FIGURE 3.2**). With the help of the assisting organs—the salivary

▶ **gastrointestinal (GI) tract [GAS-troh-in-TES-tin-al]** The connected series of organs and structures used for digestion of food and absorption of nutrients; also called the alimentary canal or the digestive tract. The GI tract contains the mouth, esophagus, stomach, small intestine, large intestine (colon), rectum, and anus.

Functional Organization	Anatomical Organization	Organs Role in Digestion
Ingestion	Mouth	Breakdown of food. Along with the enzyme amylase, startch digestion begins here.
	Esophagus	Moves food from the mouth to the stomach.
Digestion and Absorption	Stomach	Secretes gastric juices and acid, which aid in digestion. Mixes food and converts it into liquid chyme. Kills pathogenic (disease-causing) bacteria that might have been ingested. Starts the digestion of protein. Starts the digestion of fat Secretes intrinsic factor which is necessary for Vitamin B12 absorption. Slowly releases chyme into the small intestine.
	Small intestine	Where the digestion of protein, fat and carbohydrates is completed. Where the majority of nutrients are absorbed.
	Large intestine	Absorbs water and electrolytes. Forms and stores feces. Where most gut microbiota exist.
Assisting Organs	Salivary glands	Secrete saliva which moistens food, allowing for more easy swallowing.
	Liver	Produces bile, which aids in the digestion and absorption of fat.
	Gallbladder	Stores and concentrates bile from the liver.
	Pancreas	Secretes enzymes that affect digestion and absorption. Releases hormones which help to regulate metabolism and how nutrients are used in the body.
Elimination	Rectum	Holds and releases feces via the anus.

FIGURE 3.2 Anatomic and functional organization of the GI tract.
Although digestion begins in the mouth, most digestion occurs in the stomach and small intestine. Absorption primarily takes place in the small intestine.

glands, liver, gallbladder, and pancreas—the GI tract turns food into small molecules that the body can absorb and use. The GI tract has an amazing variety of functions, including the following:

1. Ingestion—the receipt and softening of food
2. Transport of ingested food
3. Secretion of digestive enzymes, acid, mucus, and bile
4. Absorption of end products of digestion
5. Movement of undigested material
6. Elimination—the excretion of waste products

A Closer Look at Gastrointestinal Structure

Often described as a hollow tube, the structure of the GI tract is much more complex. As you can see in **FIGURE 3.3**, there are several layers to this tube:

- The innermost layer, called the **mucosa**, is a layer of epithelial (lining) cells and glands.
- Next is the **submucosa**, which is made up of loose, fibrous connective tissue, glands, blood vessels, and nerves. Here, substances, including nutrients, are carried both to and from the GI tract.
- Continuing outward are two layers of muscle fibers that help to move food through the GI tract:
  - First is a layer of **circular muscle**, where muscle fibers go around the tube.
  - Next is a layer of **longitudinal muscle**, where fibers lie lengthwise along the tube.
- Finally, the outer surface, or **serosa**, provides a covering and protection for the entire GI tract. The serosa secretes fluids that help to protect the GI tract and reduce friction as it and other organs move.

▶ **mucosa [myu-KO-sa]** The innermost layer of a cavity. The inner layer of the gastrointestinal tract, also called the intestinal wall. It is composed of epithelial cells and glands.

▶ **submucosa** The layer of loose, fibrous connective tissue under the mucous membrane.

▶ **circular muscle** Layers of smooth muscle that surround organs, including the stomach and the small intestine.

▶ **longitudinal muscle** Muscle fibers aligned lengthwise.

▶ **serosa** A smooth membrane composed of a mesothelial layer and connective tissue. The intestines are covered in serosa.

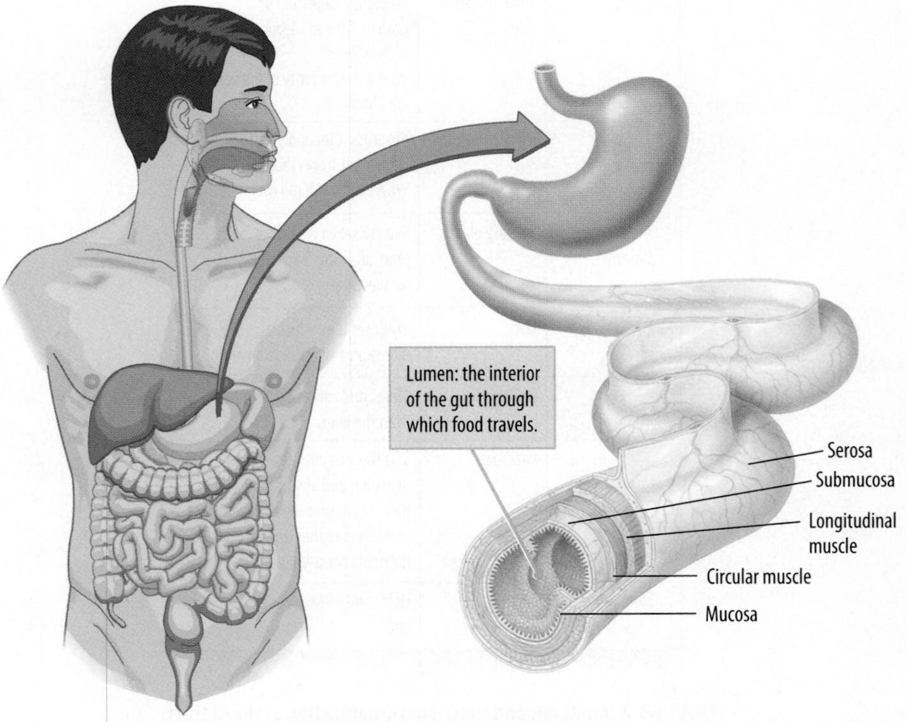

FIGURE 3.3 Structural organization of the GI tract wall. Your intestinal tract is a long, hollow tube lined with mucosal cells and surrounded by layers of muscle cells.

At points along the tract, where one organ connects with another (e.g., where the esophagus meets the stomach), the muscles are thicker and form **sphincters** (see **FIGURE 3.4**). By alternately contracting and relaxing, these muscular rings act like one-way doors, allowing the mixture of food and digestive juices to flow into an organ but not back out.

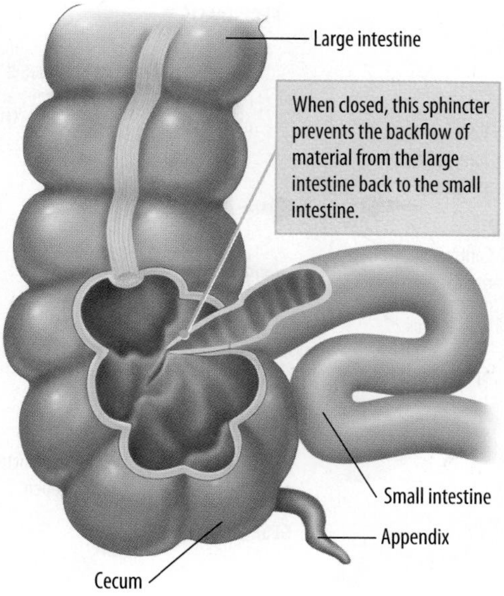
Large intestine
When closed, this sphincter prevents the backflow of material from the large intestine back to the small intestine.
Small intestine
Appendix
Cecum

FIGURE 3.4 Sphincters in action. Movement from one section of the GI tract to the next is controlled by muscular valves called sphincters. When closed, this sphincter (the ileocecal valve) prevents the backflow of material from the large intestine back to the small intestine.

Key Concepts The gastrointestinal tract consists of the mouth, esophagus, stomach, small intestine, large intestine, and rectum. The function of the GI tract is to ingest, digest, and absorb nutrients and eliminate waste. The general structure of the GI tract consists of many layers, including an inner mucosal lining, a layer of connective tissue, layers of muscle fibers, and an outer covering layer. Sphincters are muscular valves along the GI tract that control movement from one part to the next.

Overview of Digestion: Physical and Chemical Processes

The breakdown of food into smaller units and finally into absorbable nutrients involves both chemical and physical processes. The physical process comes first, as food is broken up into smaller pieces. Chewing starts this breakup, and muscular contractions of the GI tract continue it. As the GI tract breaks up food, it mixes the food with various secretions and moves the mixture (called **chyme**) along the GI tract. Enzymes, along with other chemicals, help complete the breakdown process and promote absorption of nutrients.

The Physical Movement and Breakdown of Food

Distinct muscular actions of the GI tract take the food on its journey. From mouth to anus, wavelike muscular contractions called **peristalsis** transport food and nutrients along the length of the GI tract. Peristaltic waves from the stomach muscles occur about three times per minute. In the small intestine, circular and longitudinal bands of muscle contract approximately every four to five seconds. Peristaltic contractions of the small intestine often are continuations of contractions that began in the stomach. The large intestine uses slow peristalsis to move the waste products of digestion (feces).

Segmentation, a series of muscular contractions that occurs in the small intestine, divides and mixes the chyme. Every few centimeters along the gut wall, alternating constrictions "chop" the contents into smaller portions. Segmentation also increases absorption by bringing chyme into contact with the intestinal wall. **FIGURE 3.5** shows peristalsis and segmentation.

The Chemical Breakdown of Food

During the chemical process of digestion, enzymes divide nutrients into compounds small enough for absorption.

Enzymes are proteins that **catalyze**, or speed up, chemical reactions but are not altered in the process. In digestion, these chemical reactions divide substances into smaller compounds by a process called **hydrolysis** (breaking apart by water), as **FIGURE 3.6** shows. Most of the digestive enzymes can be identified by name; they commonly end in *–ase* (amylase, lipase, and so on). For example, the enzyme needed to digest sucr*ose* is sucr*ase*.

In addition to enzymes, other chemicals support the digestive process. These include acid in the stomach, a neutralizing base in the small intestine, bile that prepares fat for digestion, and mucus secreted along the GI tract. This mucus does not break down food but lubricates it and protects the cells that line the GI tract from the strong digestive chemicals. Along the GI tract, fluids containing various enzymes and other substances are added to the consumed food. In fact, the volume of fluid secreted into the GI tract is about 7,000 milliliters (about 7½ quarts) per day.[1] **TABLE 3.1** shows the average input and output of fluids in the GI tract each day.

▶ **sphincters** [SFINGK-ters] Circular bands of muscle fibers that surround the entrance or exit of a hollow body structure (e.g., the stomach) and act as valves to control the flow of material.

▶ **chyme [KIME]** A mass of partially digested food and digestive juices moving from the stomach into the duodenum.

▶ **peristalsis [per-ih-STAHL-sis]** The wavelike, rhythmic muscular contractions of the GI tract that propel its contents down the tract.

▶ **segmentation** Periodic muscle contractions at intervals along the GI tract that alternate forward and backward movement of the contents, thereby breaking apart chunks of the food mass and mixing in digestive juices.

▶ **enzymes [EN-zimes]** Large proteins in the body that accelerate the rate of chemical reactions but are not altered in the process.

▶ **catalyze** To speed up a chemical reaction.

▶ **hydrolysis** A reaction that breaks apart a compound through the addition of water.

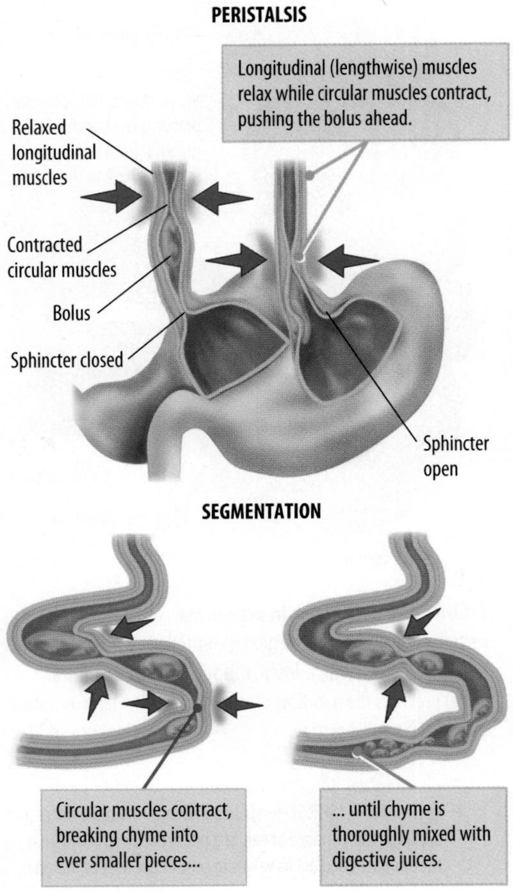
PERISTALSIS
Longitudinal (lengthwise) muscles relax while circular muscles contract, pushing the bolus ahead.
Relaxed longitudinal muscles
Contracted circular muscles
Bolus
Sphincter closed
Sphincter open
SEGMENTATION
Circular muscles contract, breaking chyme into ever smaller pieces...
... until chyme is thoroughly mixed with digestive juices.

FIGURE 3.5 Peristalsis and segmentation. Peristalsis and segmentation help break up, mix, and move food through the GI tract.

TABLE 3.1
Average Daily Fluid Input and Output

Source	Amount (mL)
Fluid Input	
Food and beverages	2,000
Saliva	1,500
Gastric secretions	2,500
Pancreatic secretions	1,500
Bile	500
Small intestine secretions	1,000
Total input	**9,000**
Fluid Output	
Small intestine absorption	7,500
Large intestine absorption	1,400
Feces	100
Total output	**9,000**

Data from Klein S, Cohn SM, Alpers DH. Alimentary tract in nutrition. In: Shils ME, Shike M, Ross AC, et al., eds. *Modern Nutrition in Health and Disease*. 11th ed. Philadelphia: Lippincott Williams & Wilkins; 2014:102–109.

Key Concepts Digestion involves both physical and chemical activity. Physical activity includes chewing and the movement of muscles along the GI tract that divide food into smaller pieces and mix it with digestive secretions. Chemical digestion is the breaking of bonds in nutrients, such as carbohydrates or proteins, to produce smaller units. Enzymes—proteins that encourage chemical processes—catalyze these hydrolytic reactions.

▶ **lumen** Cavity or hollow channel in any organ or structure of the body.

Overview of Absorption

Food is broken apart during digestion, and it is then moved from the GI tract into circulation and on to the cells. Many of the nutrients—vitamins, minerals, and water—do not need to be digested before they are absorbed. But the energy-yielding nutrients—carbohydrate, fat, and protein—are too large to be absorbed intact and must be digested first. When ready for absorption, how are nutrients moved from the interior, or **lumen**, of the gut through the lining cells (mucosa) and into circulation?

The Four Roads to Nutrient Absorption

One of four different processes allows nutrients to be absorbed from the GI tract into circulation: passive diffusion, facilitated diffusion, active transport, and endocytosis (see **FIGURE 3.7**).

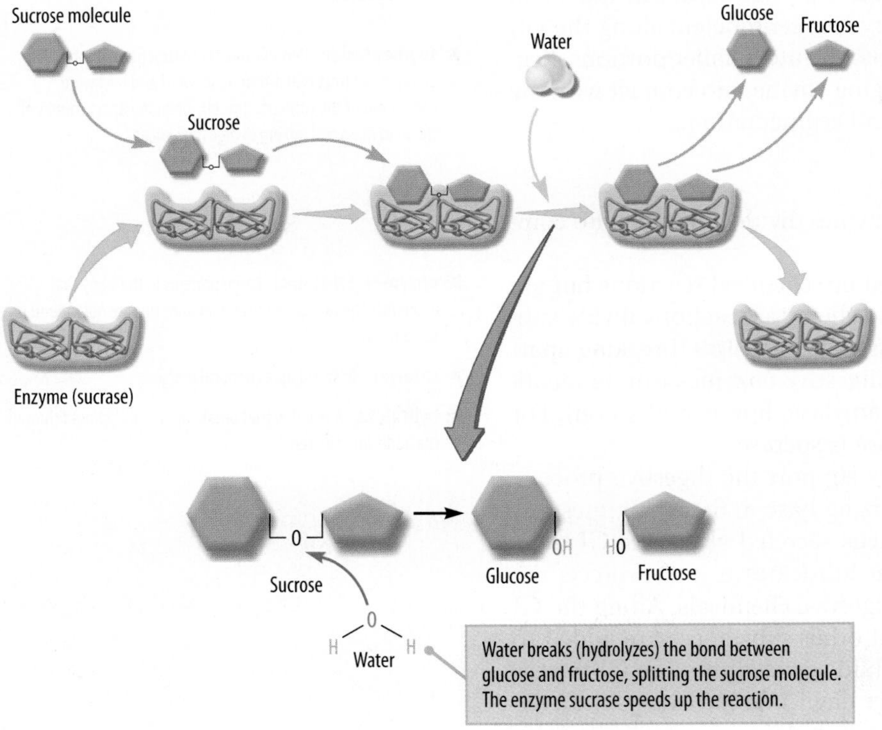
Sucrose molecule
Sucrose
Water
Glucose
Fructose
Enzyme (sucrase)
O
OH
HO
Sucrose
Glucose
Fructose
H
Water
H
Water breaks (hydrolyzes) the bond between glucose and fructose, splitting the sucrose molecule. The enzyme sucrase speeds up the reaction.

FIGURE 3.6 Water and enzymes in chemical reactions. Enzymes speed up (catalyze) chemical reactions. When water breaks a chemical bond, the action is called hydrolysis.

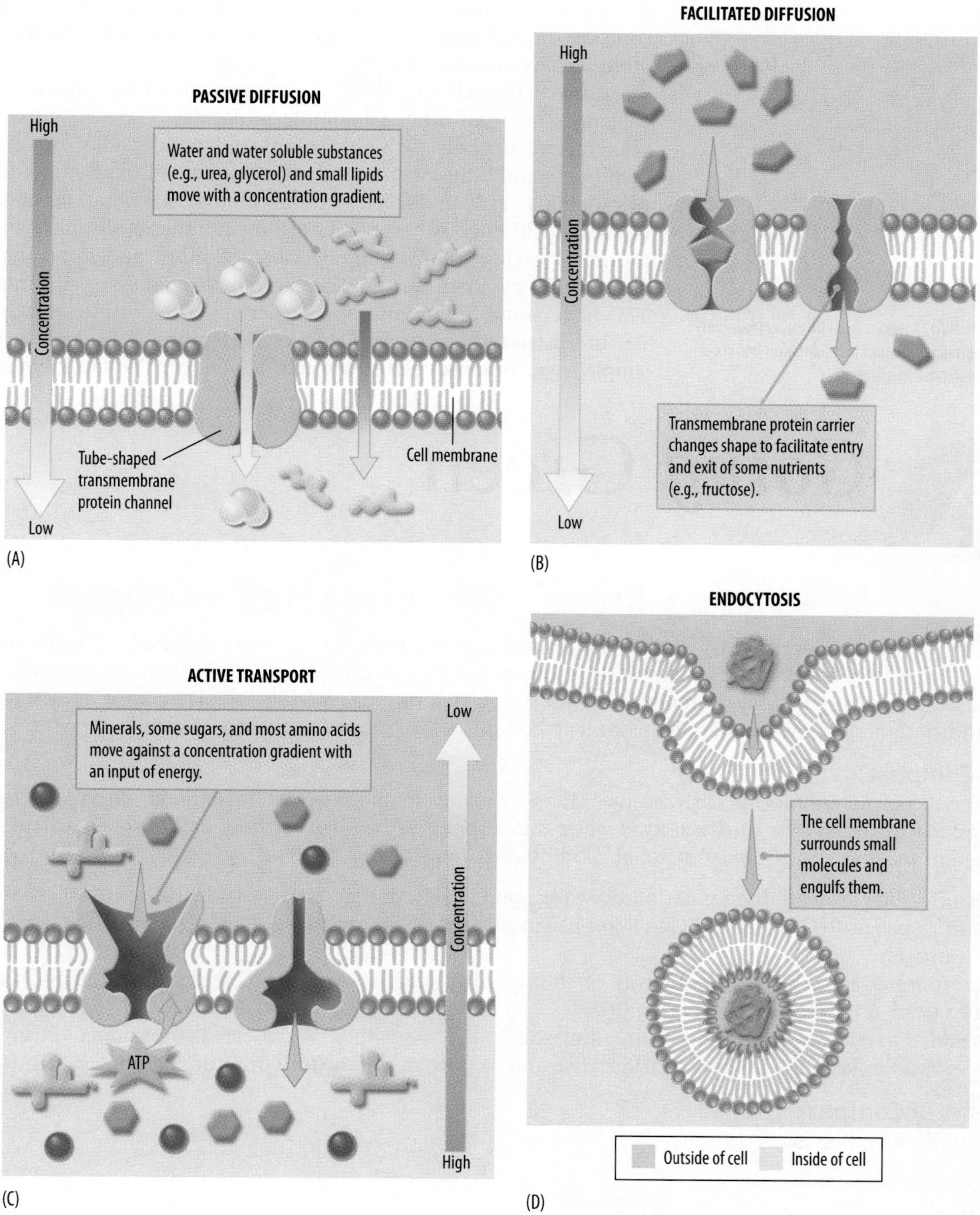
PASSIVE DIFFUSION
High
Water and water soluble substances (e.g., urea, glycerol) and small lipids move with a concentration gradient.
Concentration
Tube-shaped transmembrane protein channel
Cell membrane
Low
(A)
FACILITATED DIFFUSION
High
Concentration
Transmembrane protein carrier changes shape to facilitate entry and exit of some nutrients (e.g., fructose).
Low
(B)
ACTIVE TRANSPORT
Minerals, some sugars, and most amino acids move against a concentration gradient with an input of energy.
Low
Concentration
ATP
High
(C)
ENDOCYTOSIS
The cell membrane surrounds small molecules and engulfs them.
Outside of cell
Inside of cell
(D)

FIGURE 3.7 (a) **Passive diffusion.** Using passive diffusion, some substances easily move into and out of cells, either through protein channels or directly through the cell membrane. (b) **Facilitated diffusion.** Some substances need a little assistance to enter and exit cells. A transmembrane protein helps out by changing shape. (c) **Active transport.** Some substances need a lot of assistance to enter cells. Similar to swimming upstream, energy is needed for the substance to penetrate despite an unfavorable concentration gradient. (d) **Endocytosis.** Cells can use their cell membranes to engulf a particle and bring it inside the cell. The engulfing portion of the membrane separates from the cell wall and encases the particle in a vesicle.

Passive diffusion is the movement of molecules without the expenditure of energy through the cell membrane, through either special protein channels or intermolecular gaps in the cell membrane. **Concentration gradients** (e.g., meaning that one side of the cell wall has a higher concentration of molecules than the other side of the cell wall) drive passive diffusion. Molecules cross permeable cell membranes as a result of random movements that tend to equalize

▶ **passive diffusion** The movement of substances into or out of cells without the expenditure of energy or the involvement of transport proteins in the cell membrane. Also called simple diffusion.

▶ **Concentration gradients** A driver of passive diffusion in which one side of the cell wall has a higher concentration of molecules than the other side of the cell wall.

the concentration of substances on both sides of a membrane. The larger the concentration of molecules on one side of the cell membrane, the faster those molecules move across the membrane to the area of lower concentration.

Because the cell membrane mainly consists of fat-soluble substances, it welcomes fats and other fat-soluble molecules. Oxygen, nitrogen, carbon dioxide, and alcohols are highly soluble in fat and readily dissolve in the cell membrane and diffuse across it. Large amounts of oxygen are delivered this way, passing easily into a cell's interior almost as if it had no membrane barrier at all. Although water crosses cell membranes easily, most water-soluble nutrients (carbohydrates, amino acids, vitamins, and minerals) cannot be absorbed by passive diffusion. They need help to cross into the intestinal cells. This help comes in the form of a carrier and also requires energy.

▶ **facilitated diffusion** A process by which carrier (transport) proteins in the cell membrane transport substances into or out of cells down a concentration gradient.

In **facilitated diffusion**, special carriers help transport a substance (such as the simple sugar fructose) across the cell membrane. The facilitating carriers are

Going Green

Air + Water + Brown Stuff + Green Stuff = Compost!

Planned decomposition of plants and once-living materials to create enriched soil is the way to recycle your yard and kitchen wastes. It also is a critical step in disposing of garbage needlessly sent to landfills. Compost makes an earthy-smelling, dark, crumbly substance rich in nutrients for house plants or garden soil. Finished compost can be applied to lawns and gardens to help condition the soil and replenish nutrients.

What's in Compost?

The recipe for successful compost is fairly simple. Microorganisms (some too small to see, and others such as millipedes, sowbugs, and earthworms) turn yard and food waste into compost. Air, water, carbon, and nitrogen are the other ingredients needed to make useful compost material. Compost is made in the following way:

- "Brown stuff," such as dead dried plant parts (leaves, pine needles), newspaper, or sawdust, provides carbon.
- "Green stuff," such as fresh, recently living items like freshly cut grass, kitchen vegetable scraps, weeds, and other plants, provides nitrogen.
- Air is incorporated into the mixture by way of churning (by the microorganisms at work as well as by mixing with a shovel or using a rotating movement).
- Water is added to each layer of compost mixture as the pile is assembled. Water can also be added during the decomposition process to keep the microorganisms alive and to prevent the mixture from drying out.

The Benefits of Compost

Compost can do the following:

- Suppress plant diseases and pests
- Reduce or eliminate the need for chemical fertilizers
- Promote higher yields of agricultural crops
- Facilitate reforestation, wetlands restoration, and habitat revitalization efforts by amending contaminated, compacted, and marginal soils
- Cost-effectively remediate soils contaminated by hazardous waste
- Remove solids, oil, grease, and heavy metals from stormwater runoff
- Capture and destroy 99.6 percent of industrial volatile organic chemicals (VOCs) in contaminated air
- Provide cost savings of at least 50 percent over conventional soil, water, and air pollution remediation technologies, where applicable

What to Compost

Not all items can be composted. Those items in the "In" list can be included in a compost pile, whereas those in the "Out" list should be excluded.

The In List

- Some types of animal manure
- Clean paper, shredded newspaper, cardboard rolls
- Coffee grounds, filters, tea bags
- Cotton rags, wool rags
- Dryer and vacuum cleaner lint
- Eggshells, nut shells
- Fireplace ashes
- Fruits and vegetables
- Grass clippings, yard trimmings, leaves, houseplants, hay, and straw
- Hair and fur
- Sawdust, wood chips

The Out List

- Black walnut tree leaves or twigs (might release substances harmful to plants)
- Coal or charcoal ash (might contain substances harmful to plants).
- Dairy products (create odor problems and attract pests such as rodents and flies)
- Diseased or insect-ridden plants (infect other plants)
- Fats, grease, lard, or oils (create odor problems; attract pests such as rodents and flies)
- Meat or fish bones and scraps (create odor problems; attract pests such as rodents and flies)
- Pet wastes, such as dog or cat feces or soiled cat litter (might contain parasites, bacteria, germs, pathogens, and viruses harmful to humans)
- Yard trimmings treated with chemical pesticides (might kill beneficial composting organisms)

Modified from U.S. Environmental Protection Agency. Basic information: composting. http://www3.epa.gov/region5/waste/solidwaste/compost/index.htm. Accessed 2/4/2016

proteins that reside in the cell membrane. The diffusing molecule becomes lightly bound to the carrier protein, which changes its shape to open a pathway for the diffusing molecules to move into or out of the cell. Concentration gradients also help to drive facilitated diffusion, which is passive and can move substances only from a region of higher concentration to one of lower concentration.

Some substances need energy to move across a cell membrane, a process called **active transport**. Substances that usually require active transport across some cell membranes include many minerals (sodium, potassium, calcium, iron, chloride, and iodide), several sugars (glucose and galactose), and most amino acids (simple components of protein). These substances can move from the intestine even though their concentration in the intestinal lumen is lower than their concentration in the absorptive cell.

▶ **active transport** The movement of substances into or out of cells against a concentration gradient. Active transport requires energy (ATP) and involves carrier (transport) proteins in the cell membrane.

Most substances either diffuse or are actively transported across cell membranes, but some are engulfed and ingested in a process known as **endocytosis**. In endocytosis, a portion of the cell membrane forms a sac around the substance to be absorbed, pulling it into the interior of the cell. When cells ingest small molecules and fluids, the process is known as **pinocytosis**. A similar ingestion process, **phagocytosis**, is used by specialized cells to absorb large particles.

▶ **endocytosis** The uptake of material by a cell by the indentation and pinching off of its membrane to form a vesicle that carries material into the cell.

▶ **pinocytosis** The process by which cells internalize fluids and macromolecules. To do so, the cell membrane invaginates and forms a pocket around the substance. From *pino*, "drinking," and *cyto*, "cell."

▶ **phagocytosis** The process by which cells engulf large particles and small microorganisms. Receptors on the surface of cells bind these particles and organisms to bring them into large vesicles in the cytoplasm. From *phago*, "eating," and *cyto*, "cell."

Key Concepts Absorption through the GI cell membranes occurs by one of four basic processes. Passive diffusion occurs when nutrients (e.g., water) permeate the intestinal wall without a carrier or energy expenditure. Facilitated diffusion occurs when a carrier brings substances (e.g., fructose) into the absorptive intestinal cell without expending energy. Active transport requires energy (ATP) to transport a substance (e.g., glucose, galactose) across a cell membrane in an unfavorable direction. Endocytosis (phagocytosis or pinocytosis) occurs when the absorptive cell's membrane engulfs particles or fluids (e.g., absorption of antibodies from breast milk).

Assisting Organs

Although food does not travel through these organs, the salivary glands, liver, gallbladder, and pancreas all have critical roles in the digestive process. The

GI tract works together with these organs, which assist digestion by providing fluid, acid neutralizers, enzymes, and **emulsifiers**.

▶ **emulsifiers** Agents that blend fatty and watery liquids by promoting the breakdown of fat into small particles and stabilizing their suspension in aqueous solution.

Salivary Glands

▶ **salivary glands** Glands in the mouth that release saliva.

We have three pairs of **salivary glands** (parotid, sublingual, and submandibular) located in or near the mouth, which secrete saliva into the oral cavity (see **FIGURE 3.8**). Saliva moistens food, lubricating it for easy swallowing. Saliva also contains enzymes that begin the process of chemical digestion. We secrete approximately 1,500 milliliters (about 1.5 quarts) of saliva each day. The mere sight, smell, or thought of food can start the flow of saliva.

Liver

▶ **liver** The largest glandular organ in the body, it produces and secretes bile, detoxifies harmful substances, and helps metabolize carbohydrates, lipids, proteins, and micronutrients.

▶ **bile** An alkaline, yellow-green fluid that is produced in the liver and stored in the gallbladder. The primary constituents of bile are bile salts, bile acids, phospholipids, cholesterol, and bicarbonate. Bile emulsifies dietary fats, aiding fat digestion and absorption.

The **liver** produces and secretes 600 to 1,000 milliliters of **bile** daily. Bile is a yellow-green, pasty material that helps digest fat. It contains water, bile salts and acids, pigments, cholesterol, phospholipids (a type of fat molecule), and electrolytes (electrically charged minerals). Bile tastes bitter, which is why the word *bile* has come to denote bitterness. Bile acts as an emulsifier by reducing large globs of fat to smaller globs, similar to how dish soap separates a layer of fat into smaller particles. This process of emulsification does not break bonds in fat molecules, but rather increases the surface area of fat, allowing more contact between fat molecules and enzymes in the small intestine. Emulsification makes fat digestion more efficient.

Bile is stored and concentrated in your gallbladder and released to the small intestine on demand. After it has done its work, most bile salts are reabsorbed and returned to the liver for recycling. This recirculation is known as the **enterohepatic** (*entero* meaning "intestines," and *hepatic* referring to the liver) **circulation** of bile salts (see **FIGURE 3.9**).

▶ **enterohepatic circulation [EN-ter-oh-heh-PAT-ik]** Recycling of certain compounds between the small intestine and the liver. For example, bile acids move from the liver to the gallbladder, and then into the small intestine, where they are absorbed into the portal vein and transported back to the liver.

The liver also is a detoxification center that filters toxic substances from the blood and alters their chemical forms. These altered substances might be sent to the kidney for excretion or carried by bile to the small intestine and removed from the body in feces. The liver is a chemical factory, performing more than 500 chemical functions that include the production of blood proteins, cholesterol, and sugars. The liver is also a dynamic warehouse that stores vitamins, hormones, cholesterol, minerals, and sugars, releasing them to the bloodstream as needed.

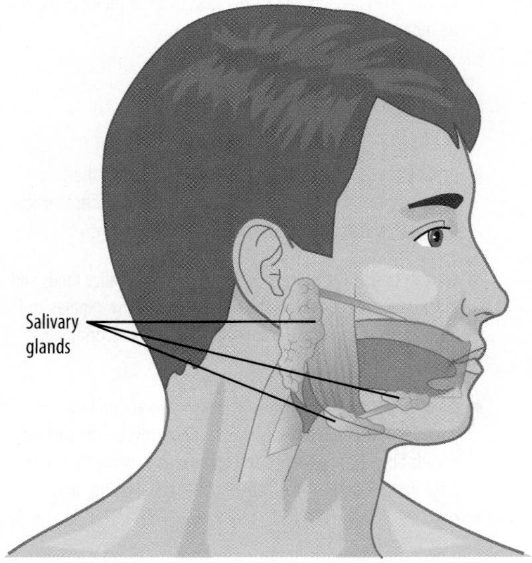

Salivary glands

FIGURE 3.8 The salivary glands. The three pairs of salivary glands supply saliva, which moistens and lubricates food. Saliva also contains salivary enzymes that begin the digestion of starch.

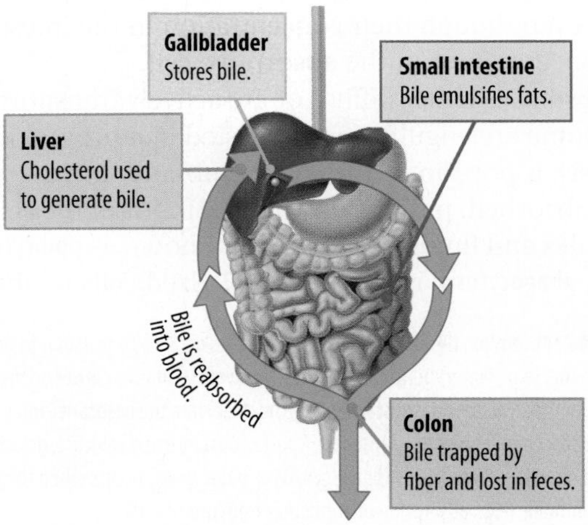

Gallbladder
Stores bile.
Small intestine
Bile emulsifies fats.
Liver
Cholesterol used to generate bile.
Bile is reabsorbed into blood.
Colon
Bile trapped by fiber and lost in feces.

FIGURE 3.9 Enterohepatic circulation. During this recycling process, bile travels from the liver to the gallbladder and then to the small intestine, where it assists digestion. In the small intestine, most of the bile is reabsorbed and sent back to the liver for reuse.

Gallbladder

The primary function of the **gallbladder** is to store and concentrate bile from the liver. The gallbladder is a small, muscular, pear-shaped sac nestled in a depression on the right underside of the liver. This organ holds about a quarter of a cup of bile and is the storage stop for bile between the liver and the small intestine. The gallbladder fills with bile and thickens it until a hormone released after eating signals the gallbladder to squirt out its colorful contents.

The gallbladder is normally relaxed and full between meals. When dietary fats enter the small intestine, they stimulate the production of **cholecystokinin (CCK)**, a hormone, in the intestinal wall. Cholecystokinin causes the gallbladder to contract and the sphincter of Oddi, which is at the end of the common bile duct, to relax. Like a squeeze bulb, the gallbladder squirts bile into the duodenum (the upper part of the small intestine)—about 500 milliliters each day. The common bile duct also carries digestive enzymes from the pancreas.

▶ **gallbladder** A pear-shaped sac that stores and concentrates bile from the liver.

▶ **cholecystokinin (CCK) [ko-la-sis-toe-KY-nin]** A hormone produced by cells in the small intestine that stimulates the release of digestive enzymes from the pancreas and bile from the gallbladder.

Quick Bite

Living Without a Gallbladder

When the gallbladder is removed, bile is delivered into the intestine rather than being stored in the gallbladder. For the first few weeks after surgery, a low-fat diet is recommended. This gives the body time to adjust to having no stored bile. After that, most people go back to eating the way they did before the surgery.

Pancreas

The **pancreas** secretes enzymes that affect the digestion and absorption of nutrients in the small intestine. During the course of a day, the pancreas secretes about 1,500 milliliters of fluid, which contains mostly water, bicarbonate, and digestive enzymes. The pancreas also releases hormones that are involved in other aspects of nutrient use by the body. For example, the pancreatic hormones insulin and glucagon regulate blood glucose levels. The combination of these two functions makes the pancreas one of the most important organs in the digestion and use of food.

▶ **pancreas** An organ that secretes enzymes that affect the digestion and absorption of nutrients and that releases hormones, such as insulin, that regulate metabolism as well as the disposition of the end products of food in the body.

Key Concepts The salivary glands, liver, gallbladder, and pancreas all make important contributions to the digestive process. The salivary glands release saliva, which contains mucus and enzymes, into the mouth. The liver produces bile, which is stored in the gallbladder and released into the small intestine, where bile helps to prepare fats for digestion. The pancreas also secretes liquid that contains bicarbonate and several types of enzymes into the small intestine.

Putting It All Together: Digestion and Absorption

Up to this point, we have focused on structures, mechanisms, and processes, providing a general idea of the workings of the GI tract. Now let's look at the whole process—a journey along the GI tract—to see what happens and how digestion and absorption are accomplished.

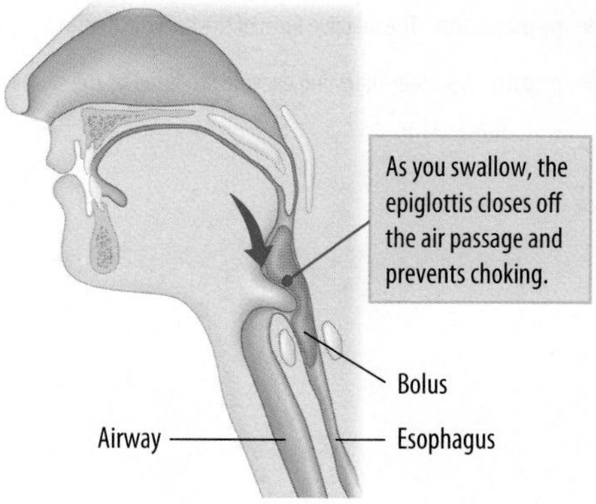

As you swallow, the epiglottis closes off the air passage and prevents choking.
Bolus
Airway
Esophagus

FIGURE 3.10 Swallowing. Your epiglottis didn't completely do its job if you have ever had a drink go "down the wrong pipe" and choked.

Mouth

As soon as you put food in your mouth, the digestive process begins. As you chew, you break down food into smaller pieces, increasing the surface area available to enzymes. Saliva contains the enzyme salivary **amylase** (ptyalin), which breaks down starch into small sugar molecules. Food remains in the mouth for only a short time, so only about 5 percent of the starch is completely broken down. The next time you eat a cracker or piece of bread, chew slowly and notice the change in the way it tastes. It gets sweeter. That's the salivary amylase breaking down the starch into sugar. Salivary amylase continues to work until the strong acid content of the stomach deactivates it. To start the process of fat digestion, the cells at the base of the tongue secrete another enzyme, **lingual lipase**. The overall impact of lingual lipase on fat digestion, though, is small.

THINK About It 3

Saliva and other fluids, including mucus, blend with the food to form a **bolus**, a chewed, moistened lump of food that is soft and easy to swallow. When you swallow, the bolus slides past the epiglottis, a valve-like flap of tissue that closes off your air passages so that you don't choke. The bolus then moves rapidly through the **esophagus** to the stomach, where it is digested further. **FIGURE 3.10** shows the process of swallowing.

▶ **amylase** [AM-ih-lace] A salivary enzyme that catalyzes the hydrolysis of amylose, a starch. Also called *ptyalin*.

▶ **lingual lipase** A fat-splitting enzyme secreted by cells at the base of the tongue.

▶ **bolus [BOH-lus]** A chewed, moistened lump of food that is ready to be swallowed.

▶ **esophagus [ih-sof-uh-gus]** The food pipe that extends from the pharynx to the stomach, about 25 centimeters long.

▶ **stomach** The enlarged, muscular, saclike portion of the digestive tract between the esophagus and the small intestine, with a capacity of about 1 quart.

▶ **esophageal sphincter** The opening between the esophagus and the stomach that relaxes and opens to allow the bolus to travel into the stomach, and then closes behind it. Also acts as a barrier to prevent the reflux of gastric contents. Commonly called the cardiac sphincter.

▶ **hydrochloric acid** An acid of chloride and hydrogen atoms made by the gastric glands and secreted into the stomach. Also called gastric acid.

▶ **pH** A measurement of the hydrogen ion concentration, or acidity, of a solution. It is equal to the negative logarithm of the hydrogen ion (H^+) concentration expressed in moles per liter.

▶ **mucus** A slippery substance secreted in the GI tract (and other body linings) that protects cells from irritants such as digestive juices.

▶ **pepsinogen** The inactive form of the enzyme pepsin.

▶ **pepsin** A protein-digesting enzyme produced by the stomach.

Stomach

The bolus enters the **stomach** through the **esophageal sphincter**, also called the cardiac sphincter, which immediately closes to keep the bolus from sliding back into the esophagus. Quick and complete closure by the esophageal sphincter is essential to prevent the acidic stomach contents from backing up into the esophagus, causing the pain and tissue damage called heartburn.

Nutrient Digestion in the Stomach

The stomach cells produce secretions that are collectively called gastric juice. Included in this mixture are water, hydrochloric acid, mucus, pepsinogen (the inactive form of the enzyme pepsin), the enzyme gastric lipase, the hormone gastrin, and intrinsic factor.

- **Hydrochloric acid** makes the stomach contents extremely acidic, dropping the **pH** to 2, compared with a neutral pH of 7. (See **FIGURE 3.11**.) This acidic environment kills many pathogenic (disease-causing) bacteria that might have been ingested and also aids in the digestion of protein. **Mucus** secreted by the stomach cells coats the stomach lining, protecting these cells from damage by the strong gastric juice. Hydrochloric acid works in protein digestion in two ways. First, it demolishes the functional, three-dimensional shape of proteins, unfolding them into linear chains; this increases their vulnerability to attacking enzymes. Second, it promotes the breakdown of proteins by converting the enzyme precursor **pepsinogen** to its active form, **pepsin**.

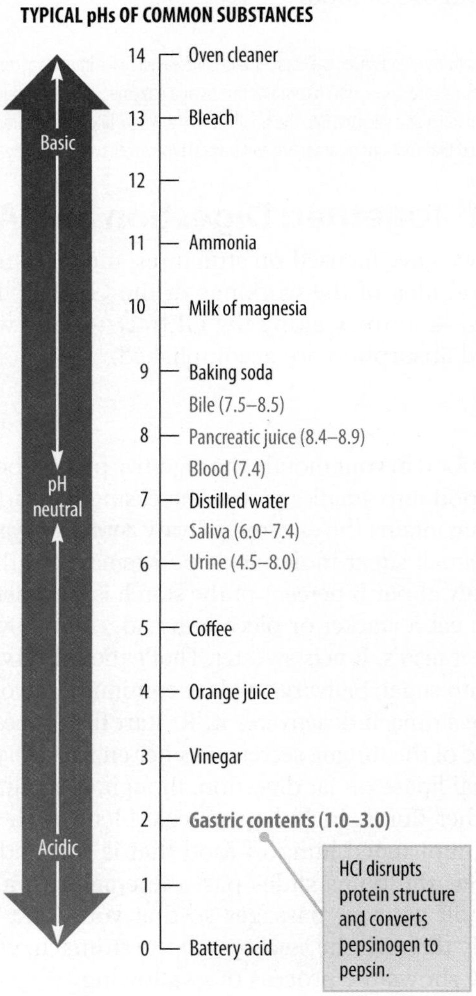

FIGURE 3.11 The pH scale. Because pancreatic juice has a pH around 8, it can neutralize the acidic chyme, which leaves the stomach with a pH around 2.

- Pepsin then begins breaking the links in protein chains, cutting dietary proteins into smaller and smaller pieces.
- Stomach cells also produce an enzyme called **gastric lipase**. It has a minor role in the digestion of lipids, specifically triglycerides with an abundance of short-chain fatty acids.
- **Gastrin**, another component of gastric juice, is a hormone that stimulates gastric secretion and motility.
- **Intrinsic factor** is a substance necessary for the absorption of vitamin B_{12} that occurs farther down the GI tract, near the end of the small intestine. In the absence of intrinsic factor, only about one-fiftieth of ingested vitamin B_{12} is absorbed.

▶ **gastric lipase** An enzyme in the stomach that hydrolyzes certain triglycerides into fatty acids and glycerol.

▶ **gastrin [GAS-trin]** A polypeptide hormone released from the walls of the stomach mucosa and duodenum that stimulates gastric secretions and motility.

▶ **intrinsic factor** A glycoprotein released from parietal cells in the stomach wall that binds to and aids in absorption of vitamin B_{12}.

After swallowing, salivary amylase continues to digest carbohydrates. After about an hour, acidic stomach secretions become well mixed with the food. This increases the acidity of the food and effectively blocks further salivary amylase activity.

Do you sometimes feel your stomach churning? An important action of the stomach is to continue mixing food with GI secretions to produce the semi-liquid chyme. To accomplish this, the stomach has an extra layer of diagonal muscles. These, along with the circular and longitudinal muscles, contract and relax to mix food completely. When the chyme is ready to leave the stomach, about 30 to 40 percent of carbohydrate, 10 to 20 percent of protein, and less than 10 percent of fat have been digested.[2] The stomach slowly releases the chyme through the **pyloric sphincter** into the small intestine. The pyloric sphincter then closes to prevent the chyme from returning to the stomach (see **FIGURE 3.12**).

▶ **pyloric sphincter [pie-LORE-ic SFINGK-ter]** A circular muscle that forms the opening between the stomach and the duodenum. It regulates the passage of food into the small intestine.

▶ **small intestine** The tube (approximately 10 feet long) where the digestion of protein, fat, and carbohydrate is completed, and where the majority of nutrients are absorbed. The small intestine is divided into three parts: the duodenum, the jejunum, and the ileum.

The stomach normally empties in one to four hours, depending on the types and amounts of food eaten. Carbohydrates speed through the stomach in the shortest time, followed by protein and fat. Thus, the higher the fat content of a meal, the longer it will take to leave the stomach.

Nutrient Absorption in the Stomach

Although much digestion has been accomplished by the time chyme leaves the stomach, very little absorption has occurred. The stomach absorbs weak acids, such as alcohol and aspirin, and a few fat-soluble compounds. Chyme moves on to the small intestine—the digestive and absorptive workhorse of the gut.

Small Intestine

The **small intestine** completes the digestion of protein, fat, and nearly all carbohydrates, and it absorbs most nutrients. As you can see in

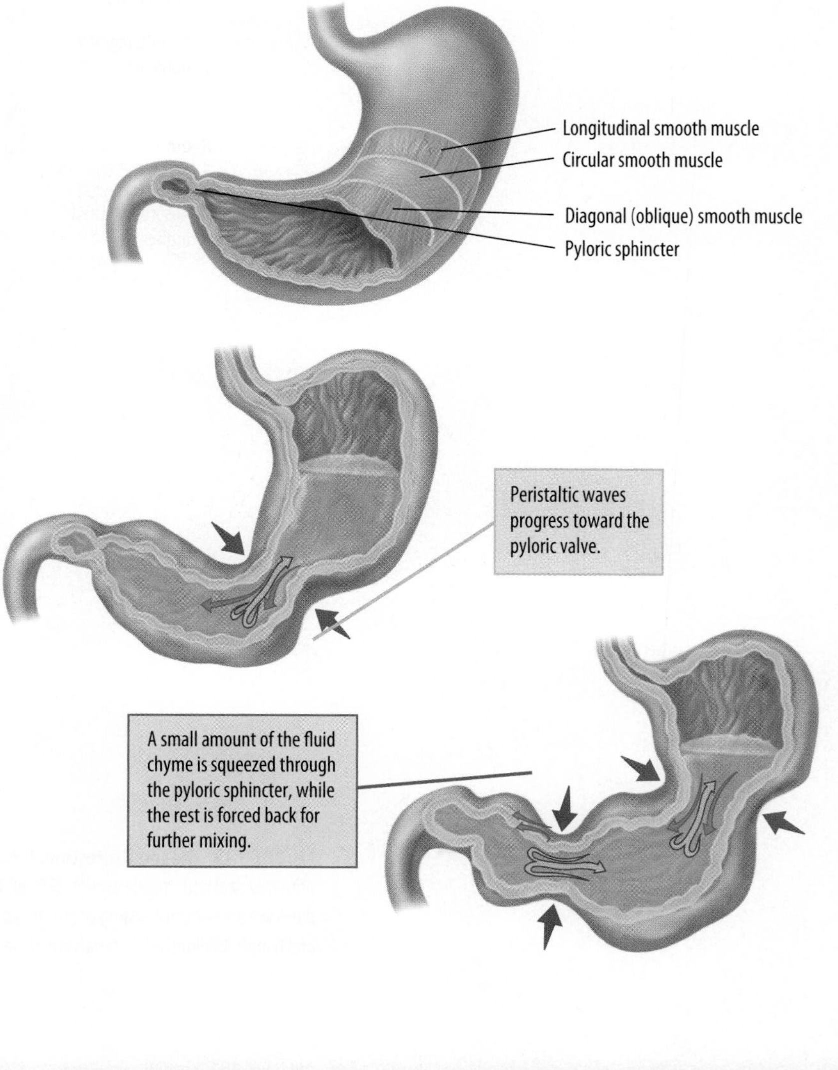

FIGURE 3.12 The stomach. The stomach churns and mixes food with stomach secretions. Hydrochloric acid unfolds proteins and stops salivary amylase action, while pepsin begins protein digestion. The pyloric sphincter controls movement of chyme from the stomach to the small intestine.

▶ **duodenum [doo-oh-DEE-num or doo-AH-den-um]** The portion of the small intestine closest to the stomach. The duodenum is 10 to 12 inches long and wider than the remainder of the small intestine.

▶ **jejunum [je-JOON-um]** The middle section (about 4 feet) of the small intestine, lying between the duodenum and ileum.

▶ **ileum [ILL-ee-um]** The terminal segment (about 5 feet) of the small intestine, which opens into the large intestine.

▶ **digestive secretions** Substances released at different places in the GI tract to speed the breakdown of ingested carbohydrates, fats, and proteins into smaller compounds that can be absorbed by the body.

FIGURE 3.13, the small intestine is a tube about 3 meters long (about 10 feet), divided into three parts:

- **Duodenum** (the first 25 to 30 centimeters—10 to 12 inches)
- **Jejunum** (about 120 centimeters—about 4 feet)
- **Ileum** (about 150 centimeters—about 5 feet)

Most digestion occurs in the duodenum, where the small intestine receives **digestive secretions** from the pancreas, gallbladder, and its own glands. The remainder of the small intestine primarily absorbs previously digested nutrients.

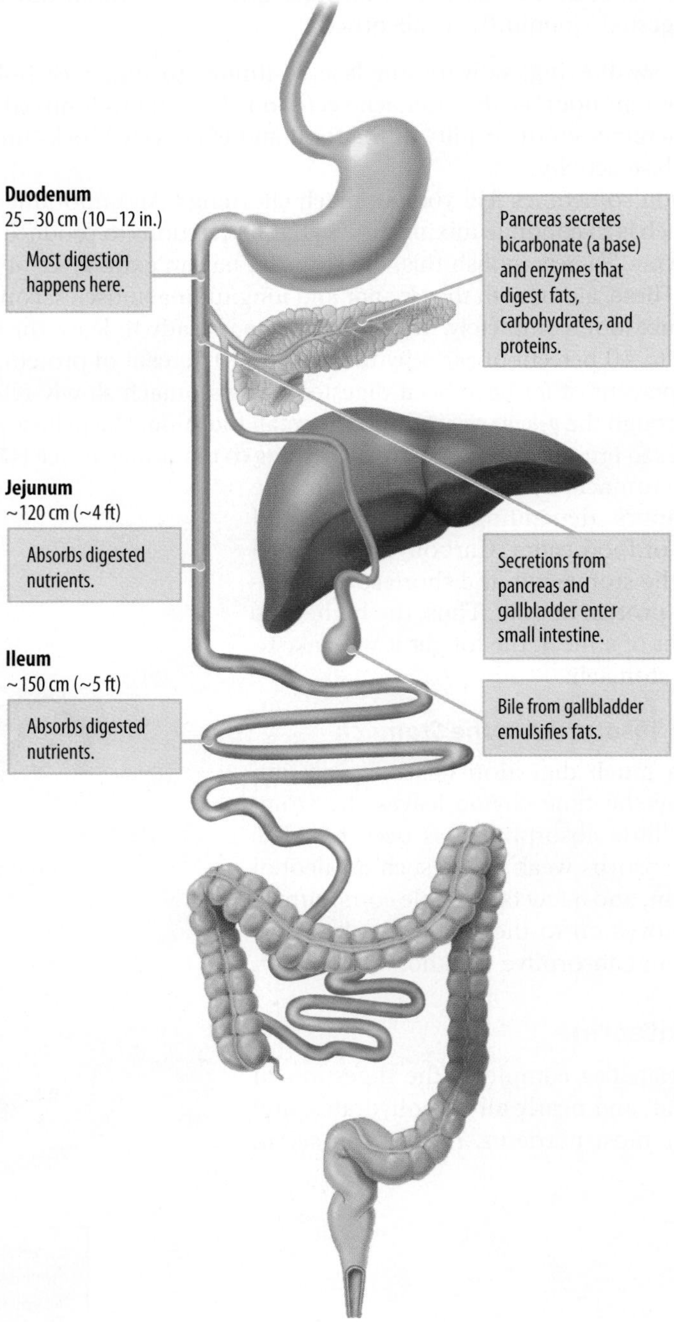
Duodenum
25–30 cm (10–12 in.)
Most digestion happens here.
Pancreas secretes bicarbonate (a base) and enzymes that digest fats, carbohydrates, and proteins.
Jejunum
~120 cm (~4 ft)
Absorbs digested nutrients.
Secretions from pancreas and gallbladder enter small intestine.
Ileum
~150 cm (~5 ft)
Absorbs digested nutrients.
Bile from gallbladder emulsifies fats.

FIGURE 3.13 The small intestine. The duodenum is mainly responsible for digesting food; the jejunum and ileum primarily deal with the absorption of food. The duodenum secretes mucus, enzymes, and hormones along with other digestive juices from assisting organs to aid digestion. All along the intestinal walls, nutrients are absorbed into blood and lymph. Undigested materials are passed on to the large intestine.

Nutrient Digestion in the Small Intestine

In the duodenum, bicarbonate from the pancreas neutralizes the acidic chyme from the stomach. The slow delivery of chyme through the pyloric sphincter (about 2 milliliters per minute) allows chyme to be adequately neutralized. This is important because the enzymes of the small intestine need a more neutral environment to work effectively. The stimulus for release of bicarbonate from the pancreas is the hormone **secretin**. This hormone is released from intestinal cells in response to the appearance of chyme. Pancreatic juice contains a variety of digestive enzymes that help to digest fats, carbohydrates, and proteins. Secretions from the intestinal wall cells add enzymes to complete carbohydrate digestion.

The presence of fat in the duodenum stimulates the release of stored bile by the gallbladder. The specific signal comes from the intestinal hormone cholecystokinin. Lipids ordinarily do not mix with water, but bile acts as an emulsifier, keeping lipid molecules mixed with the watery chyme and digestive secretions. Without the action of bile, lipids might not come into contact with pancreatic lipase, and digestion would be incomplete.

With the pancreatic and intestinal enzymes working together, digestion progresses nicely, leaving smaller protein, carbohydrate, and lipid compounds ready for absorption. Other nutrients, such as vitamins, minerals, and cholesterol, are not digested and generally are absorbed unchanged.

Just as the small intestine accomplishes much of the nutrient digestion, it is also responsible for most nutrient absorption. Its structure makes the process of absorption efficient and complete. In most cases, more than 90 percent of ingested carbohydrate, fat, and protein is absorbed. To see how this is possible, we need to examine the structure of the small intestine.

▶ **secretin [see-CREET-in]** An intestinal hormone released during digestion that stimulates the pancreas to release water and bicarbonate.

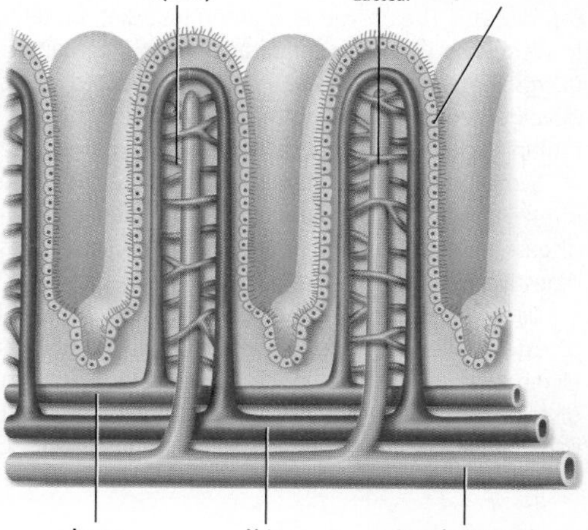

FIGURE 3.14 The absorptive surface of the small intestine. To maximize the absorptive surface area, the small intestine is folded and lined with finger-like villi. You have a surface area the size of a tennis court packed into your gut.

Absorptive Structures of the Small Intestine

The small intestine packs a gigantic surface area into a small space. As you can see in **FIGURE 3.14**, the interior surface of the small intestine is wrinkled into folds, tripling the absorptive surface area. These folds are carpeted with fingerlike projections called **villi** that expand the absorptive area another 10-fold. Each cell lining the surface of each villus is covered with a "brush border" containing as many as 1,000 hair-like projections called **microvilli**. The microvilli increase the surface area another 20 times. Taken together, the folds plus the villi and microvilli yield a 600-fold increase in surface area. In fact, your 10-foot (3-meter) long small intestine has an absorptive surface area of more than 300 square yards (250 or more square meters)—equivalent to the surface of a tennis court!

▶ **villi** Small, finger-like projections that blanket the folds in the lining of the small intestine. Singular is villus.

▶ **microvilli** Minute, hairlike projections that extend from the surface of absorptive cells facing the intestinal lumen. Singular is microvillus.

Nutrient Absorption in the Small Intestine

As nutrients journey through the small intestine, they are trapped in the folds and projections of the intestinal wall and absorbed through the microvilli into the lining cells. Depending on your diet, each day your small intestine absorbs several hundred grams of carbohydrate, 60 or more grams of fat, 50 to 100 grams of amino acids, and 7 to 8 liters of water. But the total absorptive capacity of the healthy small intestine is far greater. It actually has the capacity to absorb as much as several kilograms of carbohydrate, 500 grams of fat, 500 to 700 grams of amino acids, and 20 or more liters of water per day.[3] Approximately 85 percent of the water absorption by the gut occurs in the jejunum.[4]

Nutrients absorbed through the intestinal lining pass into the interior of the villi. Each villus contains blood vessels (veins, arteries, and capillaries) and a **lymph** vessel (known as a **lacteal**) that transport nutrients to other parts of your body. Water-soluble nutrients are absorbed directly into the bloodstream.

▶ **lacteal** A small lymphatic vessel in the interior of each intestinal villus that picks up chylomicrons and fat-soluble vitamins from intestinal cells.

▶ **lymph** Fluid that travels through the lymphatic system, made up of fluid drained from between cells and large fat particles.

FYI For Your Information

Celiac Disease and Gluten Sensitivity

Unexplained iron-deficiency anemia, fatigue, bone or joint pain, bone fractures, seizures or migraines, canker sores inside the mouth, and an itchy skin rash are some of the symptoms that adults can experience if they have celiac disease. For children, common symptoms include such things as abdominal bloating and pain, chronic diarrhea, constipation, weight loss, fatigue, and dental enamel defects of the permanent teeth.

Celiac disease is an autoimmune disorder of the small intestine that is triggered by eating gluten. Susceptibility to celiac disease is hereditary, and the disorder affects about 1 in 100 people worldwide. Is there any treatment for this disease? The answer is a gluten-free diet. Gluten is a protein found in foods such as wheat, rye, and barley, as well as malt, soy sauce, and triticale (a cross between wheat and rye). Left untreated, celiac disease can lead to development of other autoimmune disorders such as type 1 diabetes and multiple sclerosis, anemia, osteoporosis, and others.

Symptoms of celiac disease may not be the same for everyone, making the condition sometimes difficult to diagnose. Some people with this disease have no symptoms at all, whereas others experience a variety of digestive symptoms.

Gluten sensitivity is a condition with symptoms similar to those of celiac disease; however, in these individuals, symptoms improve when gluten is eliminated from the diet. One difference between gluten sensitivity and celiac disease is that those with gluten sensitivity do not experience small intestine damage or develop the antibodies found in celiac disease. Similar to celiac disease, the body reacts negatively to eating foods that contain gluten. Symptoms of gluten sensitivity include, but are not limited to, abdominal pain, bloating, diarrhea, constipation, headaches, bone or joint pain, and chronic fatigue.

It is important not to self-diagnose gluten sensitivity or celiac disease. Foods that contain gluten can also be good sources of other nutrients, and eliminating them unnecessarily may compromise your diet. If you think you have celiac disease or gluten sensitivity, talk to your health care provider about testing before you start a gluten-free diet. Pharmaceutical companies are racing to develop drugs that will cure or treat celiac disease.

Celiac Disease Foundation. Celiac disease. http://celiac.org/celiac-disease/. Accessed December 21, 2015; National Institutes of Health. Welcome to the National Institutes of Health (NIH) celiac disease awareness campaign. http://celiac.nih.gov. Accessed December 21, 2015.

- **ileocecal valve** The sphincter at the junction of the small and large intestines.
- **large intestine** The tube (about 5 feet long) extending from the ileum of the small intestine to the anus. The large intestine includes the appendix, cecum, colon, rectum, and anal canal.
- **cecum** The blind pouch at the beginning of the large intestine into which the ileum opens from one side and which is continuous with the colon.
- **colon** The portion of the large intestine extending from the cecum to the rectum. It is made up of four parts—the ascending, transverse, descending, and sigmoid colons. Although often used interchangeably with the term *large intestine*, these terms are not synonymous.
- **rectum** The muscular final segment of the intestine, extending from the sigmoid colon to the anus.

Fat-soluble lipid compounds are absorbed into the lymph rather than directly into the blood.

Absorption takes place along the entire length of the small intestine. Most minerals, with the exception of the electrolytes sodium, chloride, and potassium, are absorbed in the duodenum and upper part of the jejunum. Carbohydrates, amino acids, and water-soluble vitamins are absorbed along the jejunum and upper ileum, whereas lipids and fat-soluble vitamins are absorbed primarily in the ileum. At the very end of the small intestine, the terminal ileum is the site of vitamin B_{12} absorption. If there is damage to the lower small intestine, or surgical removal of this section in the treatment of cancer and other diseases, malabsorption of fat-soluble vitamins and vitamin B_{12} is likely.

The small intestine suffers constant wear and tear as it propels and digests the chyme. The intestinal lining is renewed continually as the mucosal cells are replaced every two to five days. When the chyme has completed its 3- to 10-hour journey through the small intestine, it passes through the **ileocecal valve**, the connection to the large intestine.

The Large Intestine

The chyme's next stop is the **large intestine**. As **FIGURE 3.15** shows, this tube is about 5 feet (1.5 meters) long and includes the **cecum**, **colon**, **rectum**, and anal canal. As chyme fills the cecum, a local reflex signals the ileocecal valve to close, preventing material from reentering the ileum of the small intestine.

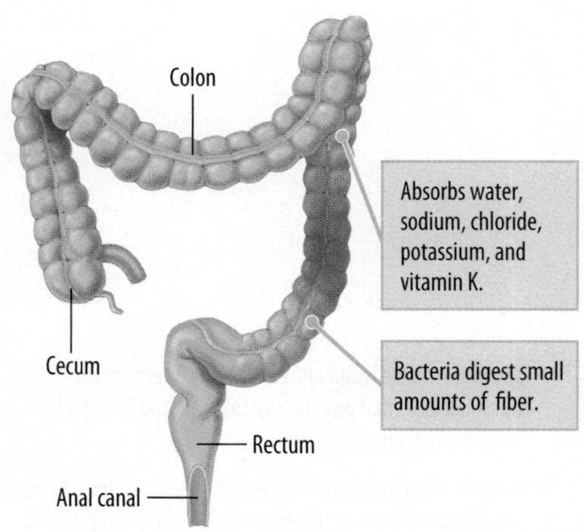
Colon
Absorbs water, sodium, chloride, potassium, and vitamin K.
Bacteria digest small amounts of fiber.
Cecum
Rectum
Anal canal

FIGURE 3.15 The large intestine. In the large intestine, bacteria break down dietary fiber and other undigested carbohydrates, releasing acids and gas. The large intestine absorbs water and minerals and forms feces for excretion.

Digestion in the Large Intestine

The peristaltic movements of the large intestine are sluggish compared with those of the small intestine. Normally, 18 to 24 hours are required for material to traverse its length. During that time, the colon's large population of bacteria digests small amounts of fiber, providing a negligible number of calories daily.[5] Of more significance are the other substances formed by this bacterial activity, including vitamin K, vitamin B_{12}, thiamin, riboflavin, biotin, and various gases that contribute to flatulence.[6] Other than bacterial action, no further digestion occurs in the large intestine.

Nutrient Absorption in the Large Intestine

Minimal nutrient absorption takes place in the large intestine, limited to water, sodium, chloride, potassium, and some of the vitamin K produced by bacteria. Although vitamin B_{12} is also produced by colonic bacteria, it is not absorbed. The colon dehydrates the watery chyme, removing and absorbing most of the remaining fluid. Of the approximately 1,000 milliliters of material that enter the large intestine, only about 150 milliliters remain for excretion as feces. The semisolid feces, consisting of roughly 60 percent solid matter (food residues, which include dietary fiber, bacteria, and digestive secretions) and 40 percent water, then passes into the rectum. In the rectum, strong muscles hold back the waste until it is time to defecate. The rectal muscles then relax, and the anal sphincter opens to allow passage of the stool out the anal canal.[7] **FIGURE 3.16** summarizes nutrient absorption along the GI tract.

▶ **vascular system** A network of veins and arteries through which the blood carries nutrients. Also called the circulatory system.

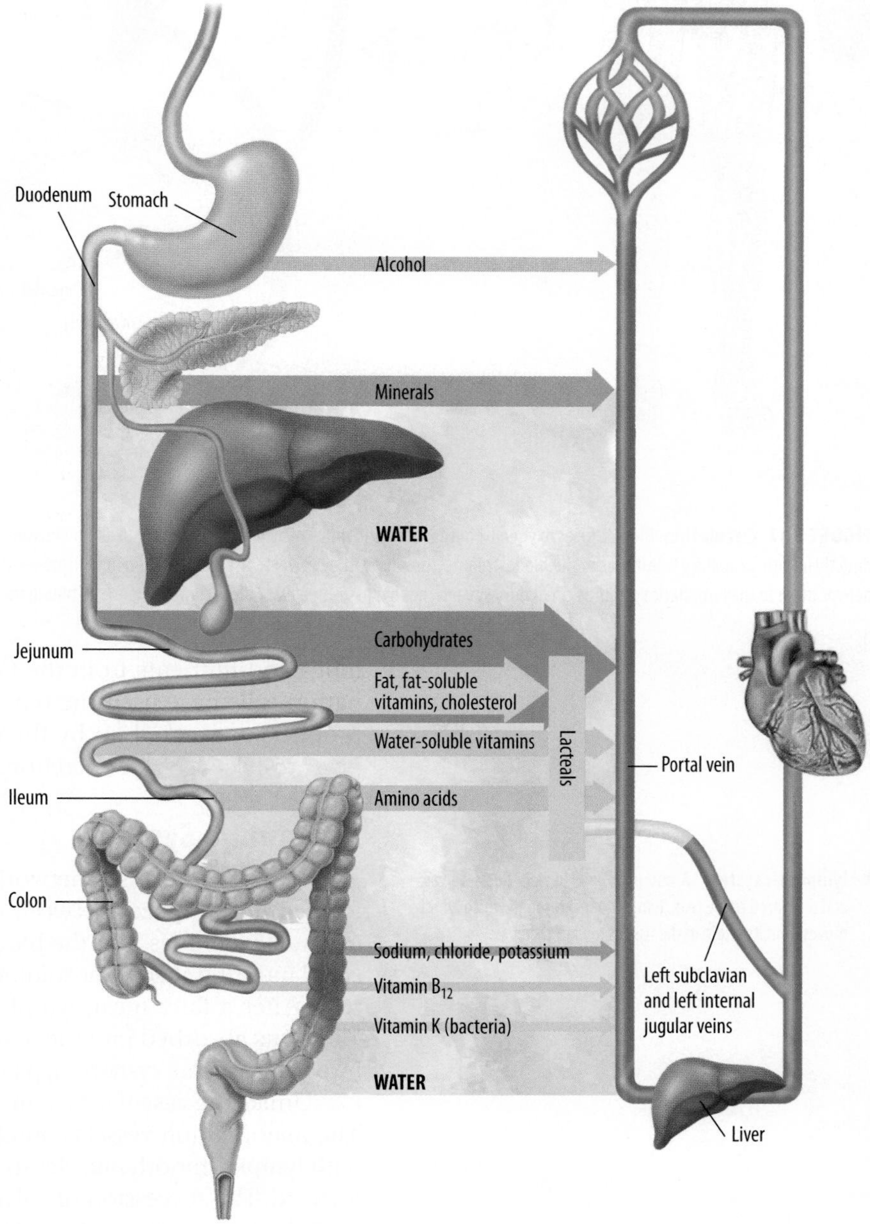

FIGURE 3.16 Absorption of nutrients.

Circulation of Nutrients

After foods are digested and nutrients are absorbed, the nutrients are transported by the vascular and lymphatic systems to specific destinations throughout the body. Let's take a closer look at how each of these circulatory systems delivers nutrients to the places they are needed.

Vascular System

The **vascular system** is a network of veins and arteries through which the blood carries nutrients (see **FIGURE 3.17**). The heart is the pump that keeps the blood circulating through the body. From intestinal cells, water-soluble nutrients are absorbed directly into tiny capillary tributaries of the bloodstream, where they travel to the liver before being dispersed throughout the body. Blood carries oxygen from the

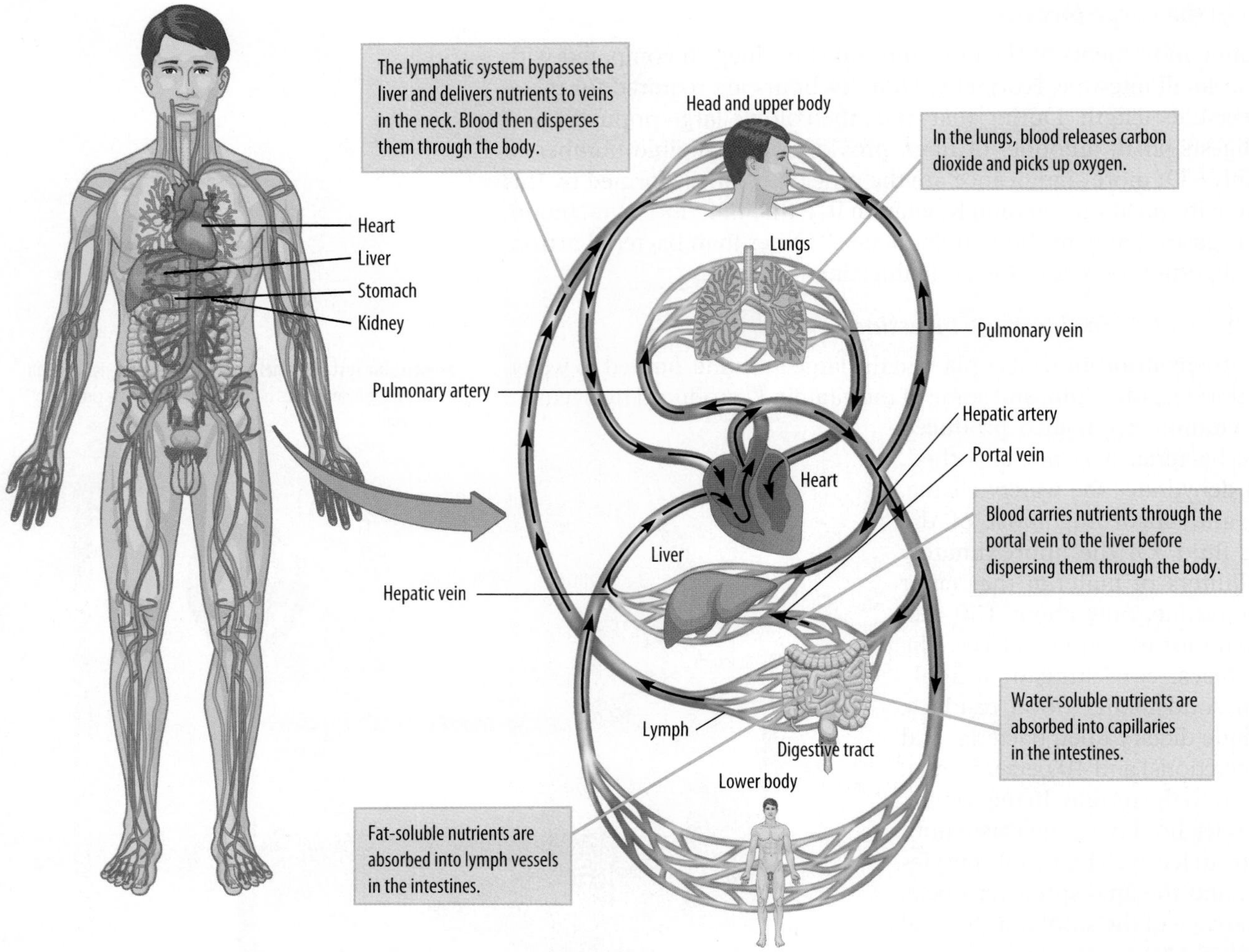
The lymphatic system bypasses the liver and delivers nutrients to veins in the neck. Blood then disperses them through the body.
Head and upper body
In the lungs, blood releases carbon dioxide and picks up oxygen.
Heart
Liver
Stomach
Kidney
Lungs
Pulmonary vein
Pulmonary artery
Hepatic artery
Portal vein
Heart
Blood carries nutrients through the portal vein to the liver before dispersing them through the body.
Liver
Hepatic vein
Water-soluble nutrients are absorbed into capillaries in the intestines.
Lymph
Digestive tract
Lower body
Fat-soluble nutrients are absorbed into lymph vessels in the intestines.

FIGURE 3.17 Circulation. Blood carries oxygen from the lungs and nutrients from the GI system to all body tissues. Intestinal cells absorb water-soluble nutrients and deliver them directly into tiny capillary tributaries of the bloodstream. From there, they travel to the liver before being dispersed throughout the body. Intestinal cells absorb fat-soluble nutrients and deliver them to the lymphatic system, a circulatory system that bypasses the liver before connecting to the bloodstream.

lungs and nutrients from the GI system to all body tissues. Once the destination cells have used the oxygen and nutrients, carbon dioxide and waste products are picked up by the blood and transported to the lungs and kidneys, respectively, for excretion.

Lymphatic System

▶ **lymphatic system** A system of small vessels, ducts, valves, and organized tissue (e.g., lymph nodes) through which lymph moves from its origin in the tissues toward the heart.

The **lymphatic system** is a network of vessels that drain lymph, the clear fluid formed in the spaces between cells. Lymph moves through this system and eventually empties into the bloodstream near the neck. Lymph vessels in the small intestine absorb fat-soluble nutrients and most end products of fat digestion. After a fatty meal, lymph can become as much as 1 to 2 percent fat. Nutrients absorbed into the lymphatic system, unlike those absorbed directly into the vascular system, bypass the liver before entering the bloodstream.

Unlike the vascular system, the lymphatic system has no pumping organ. The major lymph vessels contain one-way valves; when the vessels are filled with lymph, smooth muscles in the vessel walls contract and pump the lymph forward. The succession of valves allows each segment of the vessel to act as an independent pump. Lymph also is moved along by skeletal muscle contractions that squeeze the vessels.

The lymphatic system also performs an important cleanup function. Proteins and large particulate matter in tissue spaces cannot be absorbed directly into the blood capillaries, but they easily enter the lymphatic system, where they are carried away for removal. This removal process is essential—without it a person would die within 24 hours from buildup of fluid and materials around the cells.[8]

Excretion and Elimination

Excretion regulates the concentrations of minerals and other substances in the body and removes the waste products of metabolism. Do not confuse the metabolic waste removed by excretion with digestive waste removed by elimination. Metabolic waste arises from all of the chemical reactions that take place in cells throughout the body. Digestive waste never passes into cells—it is the unabsorbed "leftovers" that pass along and out of the GI tract.

The primary organs of excretion are the lungs and kidneys. The lungs excrete water and carbon dioxide. The kidneys filter the blood and excrete substances to remove waste and maintain the body's water and ion balance. The kidneys excrete salts; nitrogen-containing wastes, such as urea; small amounts of other substances; and water. This watery mix is called urine. The kidneys vary the amount and concentration of urine to help maintain constant physiological conditions within the body.

Key Concepts Digestion begins in the mouth with the action of salivary amylase. Food material next moves down the esophagus to the stomach, where it mixes with gastric secretions. Protein digestion is begun through the action of pepsin, while salivary amylase action ceases because of the low pH level of the stomach. Some substances, such as alcohol, are absorbed directly from the stomach. The liquid material (chyme) next moves to the small intestine. Here, secretions from the gallbladder, pancreas, and intestinal lining cells complete the digestion of carbohydrates, proteins, and fats. The end products of digestion, along with vitamins, minerals, water, and other compounds, are absorbed through the intestinal wall and into circulation. Undigested material and some liquid move on to the large intestine, where water and electrolytes are absorbed, leaving waste material to be excreted as feces.

Signaling Systems: Command, Control, and Defense

How does your body keep the complex processes of digestion, absorption, and nutrient transport running smoothly? The nervous system, your body's communication network, carries commands and feedback to and from tissues throughout the body. Signals delivered by the nervous system can trigger the release of hormones—chemical messengers that control and coordinate biological activities. The gastrointestinal tract also is a major player in your immune system, a coordinated system of cells and tissues that defends against invading microorganisms.

Nervous System

Nerves carry information back and forth between tissues and the brain. Chemicals called neurotransmitters send signals to either excite or suppress nerves, thereby stimulating or inhibiting activity in various parts of the body.

The **central nervous system (CNS)** regulates GI activity in two ways. The **enteric nervous system** is a local system of nerves in the gut wall that is stimulated both by the chemical composition of chyme and by the stretching of the GI lumen that results from food in the GI tract. This stimulation leads to nerve impulses that enhance the muscle and secretory activity along the tract. The enteric nervous system plays an essential role in the control of motility, blood flow, water and electrolyte transport, and acid secretion in the GI tract. A branch of the

Quick Bite

The Clever Colon

Although it has been presumed that the colon has no digestive function, research shows that the human colon can be an important digestive site in patients who are missing significant sections of their intestines. These patients can actually absorb energy from starch and nonstarch polysaccharides in the colon.

▶ **central nervous system (CNS)** The brain and the spinal cord. The central nervous system transmits signals that control muscular actions and glandular secretions along the entire GI tract.

▶ **enteric nervous system** A network of nerves located in the gastrointestinal wall.

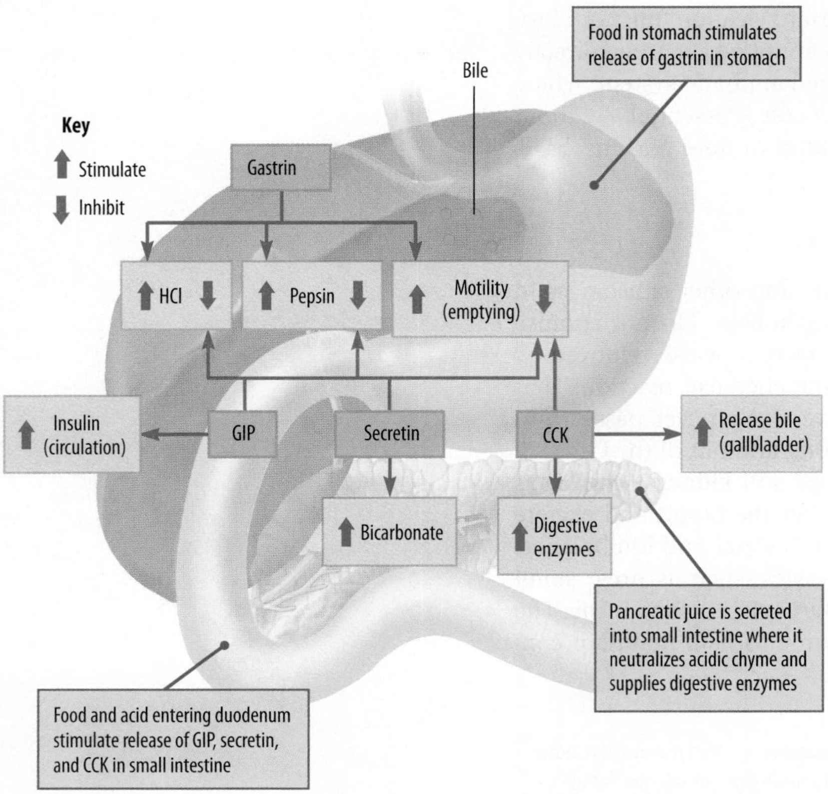

FIGURE 3.18 Hormonal regulation of digestion. In response to food moving through the digestive tract, hormones control the increase and decrease of digestive activities.

autonomic nervous system (the portion of the CNS that controls organ function) responds to the sight, smell, and thought of food. This branch of the CNS carries signals to and from the GI tract through the vagus nerve and enhances GI motility and secretion. In the past, treatments for some ulcers and other GI ailments included severing the vagus nerve, a measure that brought temporary, but not long-term, relief from pain.

Hormonal System

Hormones also are involved in GI regulation (see **FIGURE 3.18**). As defined earlier, hormones are chemical messengers that are produced at one location and travel in the bloodstream to affect another location in the body. Some GI hormones, however, are secreted by and active in the same tissue.

Gastrointestinal hormonal signals increase or decrease GI motility and secretions and influence your appetite by sending signals to the central nervous system. Some GI hormones function as growth factors for the gastrointestinal mucosa and pancreas.

The four major hormones that regulate the GI function are gastrin, secretin, cholecystokinin, and gastric inhibitory peptide.

- Gastrin is released by cells in the stomach in response to distention of the stomach, nerve impulses from the vagus nerve, and the presence of chemicals such as alcohol and caffeine. Gastrin increases muscle movement in the stomach and enhances release of hydrochloric acid and pepsinogen to encourage digestion.
- Secretin is released by cells along the duodenal wall when acidic chyme begins to move into the duodenum. Secretin opposes the action of gastrin; it reduces gastric secretion and motility, and stimulates the pancreas to release bicarbonate to neutralize chyme.
- Cholecystokinin (CCK) is released by cells along the small intestine as the amino acids and fatty acids from digestion begin to enter the small intestine. CCK stimulates the pancreas to secrete enzymes, stimulates the gallbladder to contract and release bile, and slows gastric emptying.
- **Gastric inhibitory peptide (GIP)** is also released from the intestinal mucosal cells in response to fat and glucose in the small intestine. As its name implies, GIP inhibits gastric secretion, motility, and emptying. In addition, GIP stimulates the release of insulin, which is necessary for glucose utilization.

Taken together, nerve cells and hormones coordinate the movement and secretions of the GI tract so that enzymes are released when and where they are needed and chyme moves at a rate that optimizes digestion and absorption. Side effects from abdominal surgery can slow or halt movement through the GI tract for hours or days. Researchers are investigating strategies for stimulating the release of hormones to improve postoperative GI movement and speed recovery.

Key Concepts Both hormonal and nervous system signals regulate gastrointestinal activity. Nerve cells in both the enteric and autonomic nervous systems control muscle movement and secretory activity. Key hormones involved in regulation are gastrin, secretin, cholecystokinin, and gastric inhibitory peptide. The net effect of these regulators is to coordinate GI movement and secretion for optimal digestion and absorption of nutrients.

▶ **autonomic nervous system** The part of the central nervous system that regulates the automatic responses of the body; consists of the sympathetic and parasympathetic systems.

▶ **gastric inhibitory peptide (GIP) [GAS-trik in-HIB-ih-tor-ee PEP-tide]** A hormone released from the walls of the duodenum that slows the release of the stomach contents into the small intestine and stimulates release of insulin from the pancreas.

Screen Time and Diet Quality

Background

Excessive screen-time behaviors, such as using a computer and watching TV, for more than two hours daily have been linked with many unhealthy dietary practices, including lower intake of fruits and vegetables and higher intake of fat and total energy. A greater level of screen time also has been linked to higher mortality, obesity, and cardiometabolic disease in both adults and children. Overall dietary quality is an important factor in health and weight status, and therefore deserves examination.

Study Purpose

The study purpose was to quantify associations between screen time and overall dietary quality in a sample of 1,008 young adolescents.

Experimental Plan

Dietary quality was assessed using a Web-based food behavior questionnaire, including a 24-hour diet recall. The questionnaire was also used to assess eating and screen-time behavior as well as nutrient intake.

Results

Results identified that the majority of participants consumed a snack in the evening hours, which contributed to about 11 percent of their daily calorie intake. Increased after school/evening screen time was associated with fewer evening snack servings of fruits and vegetables and an overall increase in evening snack food portion sizes. Overall, participants with more than six hours of after school/evening screen time were less likely to have a good overall diet quality compared with those who acquired less than one hour of after school/evening screen time.

Conclusion and Discussion

The results of this study support and expand on previous investigations' findings that in children, as well as in adults, better dietary quality is associated with less screen time. Both dietary intake and amount of time spent in front of a television or computer are modifiable through lifestyle intervention. This association could help to further develop and expand programs that address health promotion and disease prevention.

Ciccone J, Woodruff SJ, Fryer K, Campbell T, Cole M. Associations among evening snacking, screen time, weight status, and overall diet quality in young adolescents. *Appl Physiol Nutr Metab*. 2013;38(7):78–94.

TABLE A
Healthy Eating Index 2005[a] by Television-Watching Category for Children and Adults in 2003–2006 NHANES

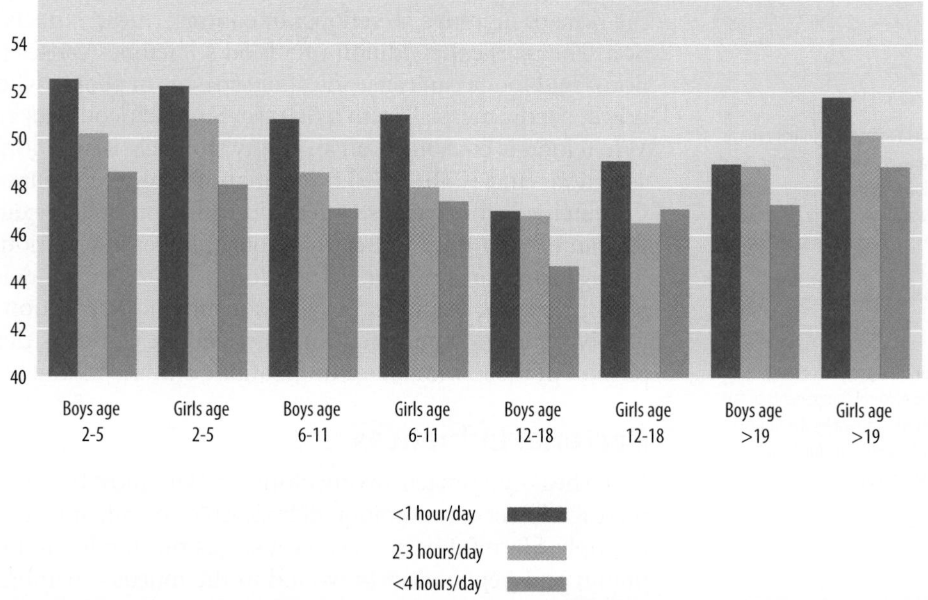

[a] Values calculated as least-squared means with adjustment for age; BMI (percentile for all children); physical activity (daily minutes moderate-to-vigorous physical activity for children aged 12–18 years and adults and weekly times of "hard play" for children aged 2–11 years); and ethnicity. *p*-values were calculated on unadjusted means.

Data from Sisson SB, Shay CM, Broyles ST, Leyva M. Television-viewing time and dietary quality among U.S. children and adults [Table 2, p. 199]. *Am J Prev Med.* 2012;43(2):196–200.

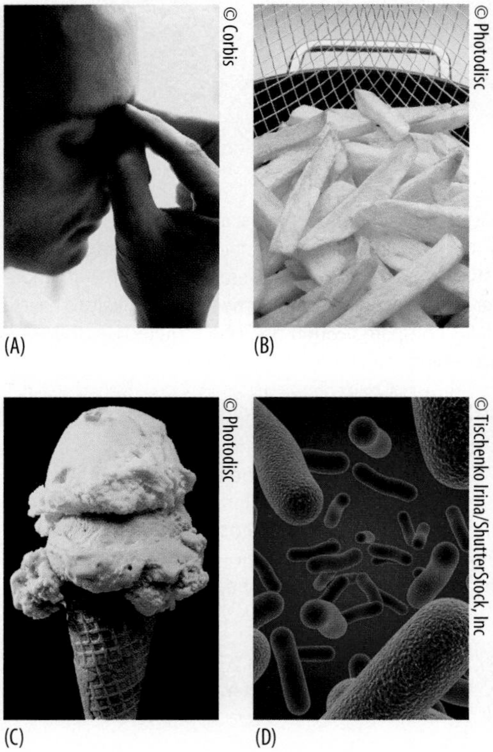

FIGURE 3.19 Negative factors for digestion. (a) Stress. (b) High-temperature fat frying. (c) Cold foods. (d) Bacteria.

Key Concepts Absorbed nutrients are carried by either the vascular or lymphatic system. Water-soluble nutrients are absorbed directly into the bloodstream, carried to the liver, and then distributed around the body. Fat-soluble vitamins and large lipid molecules are absorbed into the lymphatic vessels and are carried by this system before entering the vascular system.

Influences on Digestion and Absorption

Psychological Influences

The taste, smell, and presentation of foods can have a positive effect on digestion. Just the thought of food can trigger saliva production and peristalsis. Stressful emotions such as depression and fear can have the reverse effect (see **FIGURE 3.19**); they stimulate the brain to activate the autonomic nervous system. This results in decreased gastric acid secretion, reduced blood flow to the stomach, inhibition of peristalsis, and reduced propulsion of food.[9] The next time you sit down to a holiday meal, notice how you feel at the sight of your family's traditional foods as well as smells from your childhood. Happiness and positive memories add to the enjoyment of food, whereas sadness can bring on a poor appetite or stomach upset. THINK About It 4

Chemical Influences

The type of protein you eat and the way it is prepared affect digestion. Plant proteins tend to be less digestible than animal proteins. Cooking food usually denatures protein (uncoils its three-dimensional structure), which increases digestibility. Cooking meat softens its connective tissue, making chewing easier and increasing the meat's accessibility to digestive enzymes. Food processing produces chemicals that can influence digestive secretions. For example, frying foods in fat at very high temperatures produces small amounts of **acrolein**,[10] which decreases the flow of digestive secretions; in contrast, meat extracts can stimulate digestion. The physical condition of a food sometimes causes problems with digestion. Cold foods can cause intestinal spasms in people who suffer from irritable bowel syndrome or Crohn's disease. Stomach contents can affect absorption. When food is consumed on an empty stomach, it has more contact with gastric secretions and is absorbed faster than if it were consumed on a full stomach. Certain medicines can also affect food absorption. For example, the medication Reglan (a drug used to treat heartburn) increases GI motility, which decreases food absorption. In turn, certain foods can enhance, delay, or decrease drug absorption. For example, certain foods impair absorption of many antibiotics, and tyramine, a component in cheese and a vasoconstrictor, can cause hypertension in those who take a monoamine oxidase inhibitor (MAOI) medication.

Bacterial Influences

In the healthy stomach, hydrochloric acid kills most bacteria. In conditions where there is a lower concentration of hydrochloric acid, more bacteria can survive and multiply. Harmful bacteria can cause gastritis (an inflammation of the stomach lining) and peptic ulcer (a wound in the mucous membranes lining the stomach or duodenum). Bacteria that cause foodborne illness resist the germicidal effects of hydrochloric acid, causing trouble or damage to the digestive process.

The large intestine maintains a large population of bacteria. These bacteria can form several vitamins and digest small amounts of fiber, producing a small amount of energy. These bacteria also synthesize gases, such as hydrogen, ammonia, and methane, as well as acids and various substances that contribute to the odor of feces. If the digestion and absorption of food in the small intestine are incomplete, the undigested material enters the large intestine, where bacterial action produces excessive gas, and possibly bloating and pain.

Quick Bite

Short Bowel Syndrome

Patients who suffer from short bowel syndrome commonly have difficulty absorbing fat-soluble vitamins. To enhance absorption, treatment includes taking a fat-soluble vitamin supplement that easily mingles with water. These patients also might need to take intramuscular shots of B_{12} because they are unable to absorb this water-soluble vitamin.

▶ **acrolein** A pungent decomposition product of fats, generated from dehydrating the glycerol components of fats; responsible for the coughing attacks caused by the fumes released by burning fat. This toxic, water-soluble liquid vaporizes easily and is highly flammable.

Key Concepts Psychological, chemical, and bacterial factors can influence the processes of digestion and absorption. Emotions can influence GI motility and secretion. The temperature and form of food also can affect digestive secretions. Although stomach acid kills many types of bacteria, some are resistant to acid and cause foodborne illness. Helpful bacteria in the large intestine can cause bloating and gas if they receive and begin to digest food components that are normally digested in the small intestine.

Nutrition and GI Disorders

"I have butterflies in my stomach." "It was a gut-wrenching experience." Our language contains many references to the connection between emotional distress and the GI tract. Most of us have experienced a queasy stomach or intestinal pain right before an important event, such as a special date, big exam, or job interview. Through its many neurochemical connections with the gut, the brain exerts a profound influence on GI function. Nearly all GI disorders are influenced to some degree by emotional state. However, a number of illnesses that were once attributed largely to emotional stress, such as peptic ulcer disease, have been shown to be caused primarily by infection and other physical causes. **FIGURE 3.20** shows some common ailments that affect the GI tract.

Although stress management can help and medical intervention might be required, we can prevent and manage most GI disorders with diet. For instance, adding fiber-rich foods (see **TABLE 3.2**) and water to the diet reduces intestinal pressure, decreases the time food byproducts remain in the colon, and promotes bowel regularity. Eating a healthful diet, exercising, and maintaining a healthy weight are all good ways to help prevent and/or manage most GI disorders.

Quick Bite

Gastrointestinal Flora Abound

Your entire body has about 100 trillion cells, but this is only one-tenth the number of protective microorganisms normally living in your body. More than 500 bacterial species live in your GI tract.

TABLE 3.2
Fiber Content of Foods

Food Group	Serving Size	Fiber (g)
Legumes		
Kidney beans	1 cup, cooked	13.1
Lentils	1 cup, cooked	15.6
Split peas	1 cup, cooked	16.3
Fruit		
Dried plums	½ cup	6.2
Apple with skin	1 small	3.6
Peach with skin	1 large	2.6
Vegetables		
Broccoli	1 cup, raw	2.4
Carrot	2 medium, raw	3.4
Tomato	1 large, raw	2.2
Grains		
Wheat bran-flake cereal	1 ounce	5.3
Bulgur wheat	½ cup, cooked	4.1
Whole-wheat bread	1 slice	1.9
Brown rice	½ cup, cooked	1.8
Spaghetti, enriched white	½ cup, cooked	1.3
White bread	1 slice	0.7
White rice	½ cup, cooked	0.3

Data from U.S. Department of Agriculture, Agricultural Research Service. USDA National Nutrient Database for Standard Reference, Release 28. 2015. http://www.ars.usda.gov/ba/bhnrc/ndl. Accessed December 21, 2015.

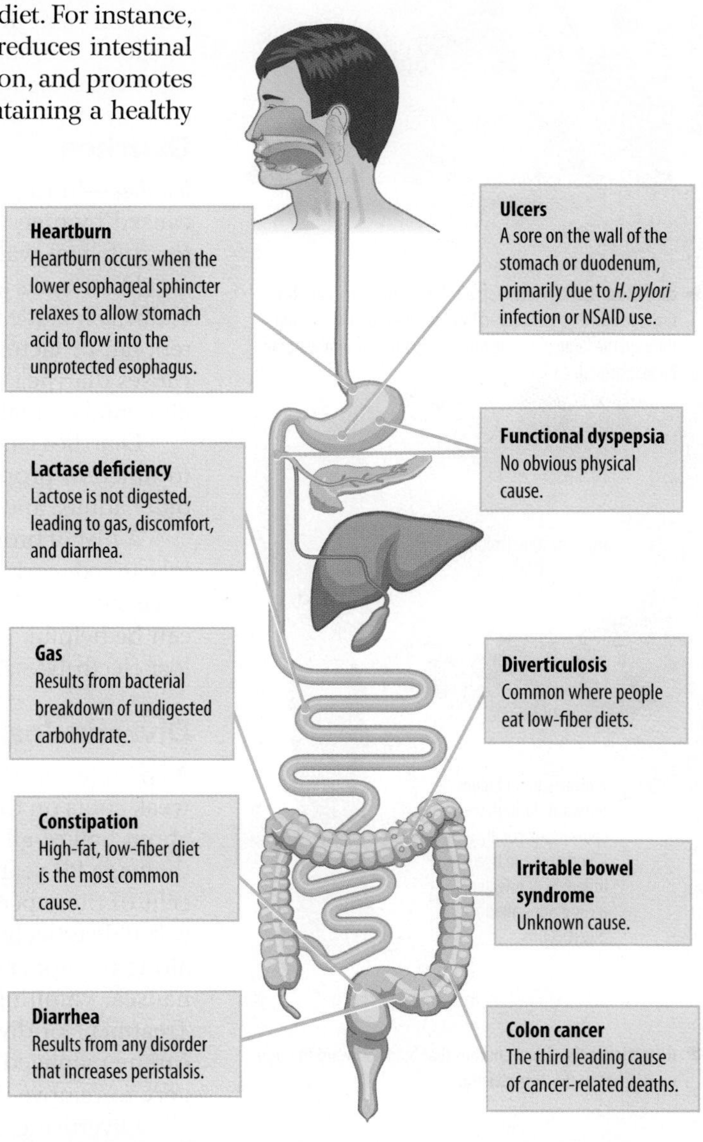

Heartburn
Heartburn occurs when the lower esophageal sphincter relaxes to allow stomach acid to flow into the unprotected esophagus.
Ulcers
A sore on the wall of the stomach or duodenum, primarily due to *H. pylori* infection or NSAID use.
Functional dyspepsia
No obvious physical cause.
Lactase deficiency
Lactose is not digested, leading to gas, discomfort, and diarrhea.
Gas
Results from bacterial breakdown of undigested carbohydrate.
Diverticulosis
Common where people eat low-fiber diets.
Constipation
High-fat, low-fiber diet is the most common cause.
Irritable bowel syndrome
Unknown cause.
Diarrhea
Results from any disorder that increases peristalsis.
Colon cancer
The third leading cause of cancer-related deaths.

FIGURE 3.20 Gastrointestinal symptoms and disorders can occur all along the GI tract.

Constipation

▶ **constipation** Infrequent and difficult bowel movements, followed by a sensation of incomplete evacuation.

Constipation is defined as having a bowel movement fewer than three times per week.[11] With constipation, stools are usually hard, dry, small in size, and difficult to eliminate. People who are constipated might find it painful to have a bowel movement and often experience straining, bloating, and the sensation of a full bowel.

Constipation is a symptom, not a disease. Almost everyone experiences constipation at some point. Although stress, inactivity, cessation of smoking, or various illnesses can lead to constipation, a diet low in fiber and water and high in fats is a common cause. Some fibers, such as the pectins in fruits and gums in beans, dissolve easily in water and take on a soft, gel-like texture in the intestines. Other fibers, such as the cellulose in wheat bran, pass almost unchanged through the intestines. The bulk and soft texture of fiber help prevent hard, dry stools that are difficult to pass. People who eat plenty of high-fiber foods are not likely to become constipated. When eating a high-fiber diet, one should also include plenty of liquids to prevent dehydration. Liquids such as water and juice add fluid to the colon and bulk to stools, making bowel movements softer and easier to pass. The caffeine in many liquids (e.g., coffee, tea, many soft drinks) is a mild diuretic (a substance that increases urine production). Although treatment depends on the cause, severity, and duration, in most cases dietary changes help relieve symptoms and prevent constipation.

Quick Bite

Halt! Who Goes There?

Be they friend or foe, antibiotics kill microorganisms in your GI tract, frequently causing diarrhea. Some pharmaceutical drugs have gastrointestinal side effects.

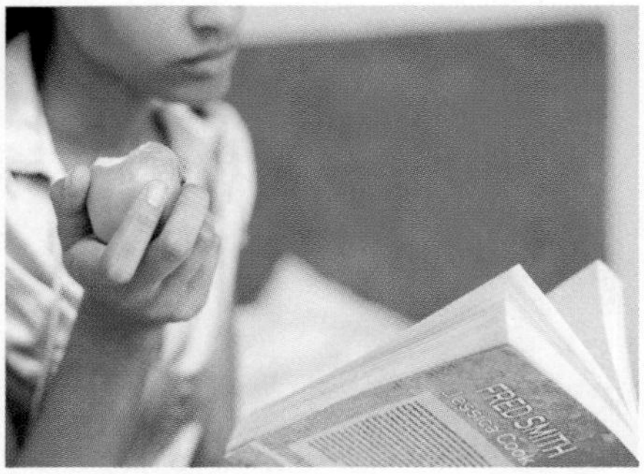

© Jupiterimages/Polka Dot/Thinkstock

Diarrhea

▶ **diarrhea** Loose, watery stools that occur more than three times in one day; it is caused by digestive products moving through the large intestine too rapidly for sufficient water to be reabsorbed.

Diarrhea—loose, watery stools that occur more than three times in one day—is caused by digestive products moving though the large intestine too rapidly for sufficient water to be reabsorbed.

Diarrhea is a symptom of many disorders that cause increased peristalsis. Culprits include stress, intestinal irritation or damage, and intolerance to gluten, fat, or lactose. Eating food contaminated with bacteria or viruses often causes diarrhea when the digestive tract speeds the offending food along the alimentary canal and out of the body.

Diarrhea can cause dehydration, which means the body lacks enough fluid to function properly. Dehydration is particularly dangerous in children and older adults, and it must be treated promptly to avoid serious health problems.

A diet of broth, tea, and toast and avoidance of lactose, caffeine, and sorbitol can reduce diarrhea until it subsides. As stools form, you can gradually introduce more foods. Pectin, a form of dietary fiber found in apples and citrus peel, can be helpful. Also, include foods high in potassium, if tolerated, to replace lost electrolytes. Fluid replacement is also important to avoid dehydration.

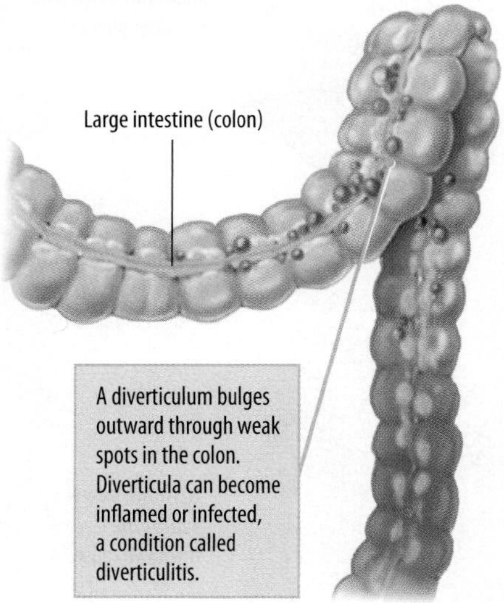

Large intestine (colon)
A diverticulum bulges outward through weak spots in the colon. Diverticula can become inflamed or infected, a condition called diverticulitis.

Diverticulosis

▶ **diverticulosis** Small pouches that bulge outward through weak spots on the digestive tract.

As people age, the colon develops small pouches that bulge outward through weak spots on the digestive tract. Known as **diverticulosis**, this condition afflicts about half of all Americans aged 60 to 80 years, and almost everyone older than age 80 years. Although it usually causes few problems, in 10 to 25 percent of these people the pouches become infected or inflamed—a condition called diverticulitis. Symptoms of diverticulitis include abdominal pain, usually along the upper left side of the lower abdomen. If the area is infected, fever, nausea, vomiting, chills, cramping, constipation, or bleeding may develop. Treatment of diverticulitis depends on its severity. Generally, this condition can be managed with diet, but serious cases of diverticulitis may require surgery to remove the affected part of the colon.

Diverticulosis and diverticulitis are common in developed or industrialized countries—particularly the United States, England, and Australia—where

FYI For Your Information

Bugs in Your Gut? Health Effects of Intestinal Bacteria

Unseen and unnoticed, millions and millions of bacteria call your GI tract home. Although we often associate bacteria with illness, the right kinds of bacteria in the gut actually protect us from disease. The human microbiome is the population of more than 100 trillion microorganisms in our gut, mouth, skin, and elsewhere in our bodies and has been linked to improved digestion, intestinal regularity, enhanced GI immune function, improved lactose tolerance, reduced risk of developing allergies, and even reduced risk of colorectal cancer. So, how can we be good hosts to our intestinal guests, keeping them well fed and happy? The answer might be in food products and dietary supplements known as probiotics and prebiotics.

Probiotics are foods (or supplements) that contain live microorganisms. Many types of bacteria are categorized as probiotics, and most fall into one of two groups: *Lactobacillus* and *Bifidobacterium*, both found in dairy products. *Lactobacillus* is thought to help alleviate diarrhea and also can help lactose-intolerant individuals digest lactose. *Bifidobacterium* is believed to ease the symptoms of irritable bowel syndrome. Research suggests that probiotics work by replacing "good" bacteria in your body, can lower the amount of "bad" bacteria in your system, and can help balance your "good" and "bad" bacteria to keep your body working well.

The term *prebiotic* describes a specialized plant fiber that nourishes the "good" bacteria that already exist in your GI tract. This nondigestible food product can be fermented by gastrointestinal bacteria and stimulates the growth or activity of "good" gut bacteria.

So, how does feeding the bacteria in your gut improve your health? Successful colonization of helpful bacteria allows them to outnumber (and outeat) disease-causing bacteria, thus reducing the likelihood of foodborne illness and other infections. Studies in young children show that supplementation with *Lactobacillus* reduced the severity and duration of diarrhea caused by rotavirus, a common infectious agent in daycare centers. Some probiotics enhance the ability of the gut to act as a barrier to infectious agents and might also adjust the activity of the immune system.

In addition to promoting the growth and function of beneficial bacteria, prebiotics might have other health effects. Some prebiotics have been shown to enhance absorption of calcium and magnesium. Others inhibit growth of lesions in the gut, which in turn reduces colorectal cancer risk. Although lipid-lowering effects have been attributed to prebiotics, the limited data available show inconsistent effects on cholesterol and triglycerides.

Fermented milk products such as yogurt and kefir are one way to keep your gut happy. Look for a seal adopted by the National Yogurt Association to identify products that contain a minimum of 100 million live lactic acid bacteria per gram of yogurt. Not all brands of yogurt contain live, active cultures. Supplemental probiotics must have sufficient numbers of live bacteria to be useful; currently, identification and standardization procedures are lacking. Prebiotics are found in whole grains, onions, bananas, garlic, artichokes, and a variety of fortified foods, beverages, and dietary supplements. Although results are preliminary, food and supplement sources of probiotics and prebiotics might be another useful way to improve gut microflora and overall health.

See the "Bacterial Influences" section for more information.

low-fiber diets are common. Diverticular disease is rare in Asian and African countries, where people eat high-fiber, vegetable-based diets.

A low-fiber diet can make stools hard and difficult to pass. If the stool is too hard, muscles must strain to move it. This is the main cause of increased pressure in the colon, which causes weak spots to bulge outward.

Increasing the amount of fiber in the diet, along with adequate fluid intake, may reduce symptoms of diverticulosis and prevent complications such as diverticulitis. Fiber keeps stools soft and lowers pressure inside the colon so that bowel contents can move through easily. During acute attacks of diverticulitis, following a low-fiber diet and avoiding foods that may contribute to nausea or pain, such as caffeine, spicy foods, chocolate, and milk products, is recommended. Once symptoms of diverticulitis have resided, gradual transition to a high-fiber diet (25–35 grams per day) is recommended. Additional benefits of fiber are listed in **TABLE 3.3**.

TABLE 3.3
Benefits of Fiber

- Helps control weight by delaying gastric emptying and providing a feeling of fullness
- Improves glucose tolerance by delaying the movement of carbohydrate into the small intestine
- Reduces risk for heart disease by binding with bile (which contains cholesterol) in the intestine and causing it to be excreted, which in turn helps to lower blood cholesterol levels
- Promotes regularity and reduces constipation by pulling water from the colon, which increases stool weight and decreases transit time
- Guards against diarrhea by absorbing excess fluid in the bowel and acting to firm up loose stool
- Reduces the risk of diverticulosis by decreasing pressure within the colon, decreasing transit time, and increasing stool weight

Modified from Institute of Medicine, Food and Nutrition Board. *Dietary Reference Intakes for Energy, Carbohydrate, Fiber, Fat, Fatty Acids, Cholesterol, Protein, and Amino Acids.* Washington, DC: National Academies Press; 2005.

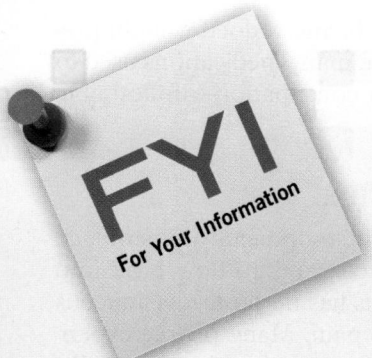

If cramps, bloating, and constipation are problems, a doctor might prescribe a short course of pain medication. However, many medications used to treat such symptoms can cause either diarrhea or constipation—undesirable side effects for people with diverticulosis.

Heartburn and Gastroesophageal Reflux

Heartburn occurs when the sphincter between the esophagus and stomach relaxes inappropriately, allowing the stomach's contents to flow back into the esophagus. Unlike the stomach, the esophagus has no protective mucous lining, so acid can damage it quickly and cause pain. Many people experience occasional heartburn, but for some, heartburn is a chronic, often daily, event and a symptom of a more serious disorder called **gastroesophageal reflux disease (GERD)**. GERD, along with obesity, is a key risk factor for esophageal cancer.[12] GERD has a variety of causes, and many treatment strategies involve lifestyle and nutrition.

▶ **gastroesophageal reflux disease (GERD)** A condition in which gastric contents move backward (reflux) into the esophagus, causing pain and tissue damage.

Diet recommendations include avoiding foods and beverages that can weaken the esophageal sphincter, including chocolate, peppermint, fatty foods, coffee, and alcoholic beverages. Foods and beverages that can irritate a damaged esophageal lining, such as citrus fruits and juices, tomato products, and pepper, also should be avoided. Individual response to food varies, so many people with GERD use trial and error to determine what foods cause discomfort.

Decreasing both the portion size and the fat content of meals can help. High-fat meals remain in the stomach longer than low-fat meals. This creates back pressure on the lower esophageal sphincter. Eating meals at least two to three hours before bedtime can lessen reflux by allowing partial emptying and a decrease in stomach acidity. Elevating the head of the bed 4 to 8 inches or sleeping on a specially designed wedge reduces heartburn by allowing gravity to minimize reflux of stomach contents into the esophagus.

In addition, cigarette smoking weakens the lower esophageal sphincter (LES), and being overweight often worsens symptoms. Stopping smoking is important, and many overweight people find relief when they lose weight.

Irritable Bowel Syndrome

Irritable bowel syndrome (IBS) is a common, functional gastrointestinal disorder with estimated worldwide prevalence of 10–15 percent[13] and significantly higher prevalence in women than in men.[14] This poorly understood condition causes abdominal pain, altered bowel habits (such as diarrhea or constipation), and cramps.[15] Often, IBS is just a mild annoyance, but for some people it can be disabling.

▶ **irritable bowel syndrome (IBS)** A disruptive state of intestinal motility with no known cause. Symptoms include constipation, abdominal pain, and episodic diarrhea.

The cause of IBS remains a mystery, but emotional stress and specific foods clearly aggravate the symptoms in most sufferers.[16] Beans, chocolate, milk products, and large amounts of alcohol are frequent offenders. Fat in any form (animal or vegetable) is a strong stimulus of colonic contractions after a meal. Caffeine causes loose stools in many people, but it is more likely to affect those with IBS. Women with IBS might have more symptoms during their menstrual periods, suggesting that reproductive hormones can increase IBS symptoms.

The good news about IBS is that although its symptoms can be uncomfortable, it does not shorten life span or progress to more serious illness. IBS can usually be controlled with diet and lifestyle modifications and judicious use of medication. A diet strategy referred to as FODMAP (low fermentable oligosaccharides, disaccharides, monosaccharides, and polyol diet) has been shown to decrease symptoms caused by IBS. The short-chain carbohydrates (oligo-, di-, and monosaccharides) are incompletely absorbed in the GI tract and can be easily fermented by gut bacteria. The fermentation and osmosis created by these undigested sugars are a cause of major IBS symptoms such as gas, pain, and diarrhea,[17] and eliminating these foods from the diet can help prevent such undesirable symptoms. Stress management is an important part of treatment for IBS as well. This includes stress reduction (relaxation) training and relaxation therapies such as meditation, counseling and support, regular exercise, changes to stressful situations in your life, and adequate sleep.[18]

IBS sufferers may have abnormal patterns of intestinal motility or might be hypersensitive to GI stimuli, but research results are inconclusive. Although the exact causes of IBS are not well understood, it is likely that a number of physical and psychosocial factors combine to trigger this disorder.

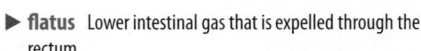

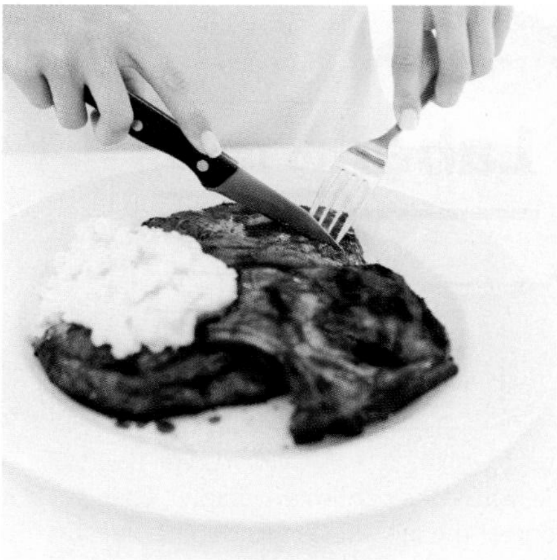

Colorectal Cancer

After lung cancer, colorectal cancer—cancer of the colon or rectum—is the second leading cause of cancer-related deaths in the United States.[19] Many studies suggest that consumption of large amounts of red and processed meats, along with low intake of fiber and the protective phytochemicals found in fruits, vegetables, and whole grains, might be responsible for the high incidence of colorectal cancer.[20] It is important to recognize, however, that other dietary factors (i.e., Western lifestyle; high intake of refined sugars and alcohol; and low intake of fruits, vegetables, and fiber) and behavioral factors (i.e., low physical activity, high smoking prevalence, high body mass index) limit the ability to isolate the effects of red meat consumption as an independent variable.[21,22]

The link between colorectal cancer and the consumption of cooked and processed red meat is attributed to chemical carcinogens that arise during the cooking process.[23] Observational and case control studies support the idea that fiber-rich diets reduce colorectal cancer risk, and scientists have hypothesized a number of possible ways that fiber might be protective.[24] These include dilution of carcinogens in a bulkier stool, more rapid transit of carcinogens through the GI tract, and lower colon pH resulting from bacterial fermentation of fiber.

Gas

Everyone has gas and eliminates it by burping or passing it through the rectum. Gas is made primarily of odorless vapors. The unpleasant odor of flatulence comes from bacteria in the large intestine that release small amounts of gases that contain sulfur. Although having gas is common, it can be uncomfortable and embarrassing.

Gas in the stomach is commonly caused by swallowing air. Everyone swallows small amounts of air when they eat and drink. However, eating or drinking rapidly, chewing gum, smoking, or wearing loose dentures can cause some people to take in more air. Burping is the way most swallowed air leaves the stomach. The remaining gas moves into the small intestine, where it is partially absorbed. A small amount travels into the large intestine for release through the rectum. (The stomach also releases carbon dioxide when stomach acid and bicarbonate mix, but most of this gas is absorbed into the bloodstream and does not enter the large intestine.)

Frequent passage of rectal gas can be annoying, but it's seldom a symptom of serious disease. **Flatus** (lower intestinal gas) composition depends largely on dietary carbohydrate intake and the activity of the colon's bacterial population.

▶ **flatus** Lower intestinal gas that is expelled through the rectum.

Most foods that contain carbohydrates can cause gas. By contrast, fats and proteins cause little gas. In the large intestine, bacteria partially break

Label to Table

As you've learned in this chapter, fiber is one of the few things you do not digest fully. Instead, fiber moves through the GI tract and most of it leaves the body in feces. If it's not digested, then why all the fuss about eating more fiber? A healthy intake of fiber can lower your risk of cancer and heart disease and help with bowel regularity. So, how do you know which foods have fiber? You have to check out the food label!

This Nutrition Facts panel is from the label on a loaf of whole-wheat bread. The highlighted sections show you that every slice of bread contains 3 grams of fiber. The 12% listed to the right of that refers to the Daily Values below. Look at the Daily Values at the far right of the label, and note that there are two numbers listed for fiber. One (25 g) is for a person who consumes about 2,000 kilocalories per day, and the other (30 g) is for a 2,500-kilocalorie level. It should be no surprise that if you are consuming more calories, you should also be consuming more fiber. The 12% Daily Value is calculated using the 2,000-kilocalorie fiber guideline as follows:

$$\frac{\text{3 grams fiber per slice}}{\text{25 grams Daily Value}} = 0.12\text{, or } 12\%$$

This means if you make a sandwich with two slices of whole-wheat bread, you're getting 6 grams of fiber and almost one-quarter (24% Daily Value) of your fiber needs per day. Not bad! Be careful, though; many people inadvertently buy wheat bread thinking that it's as high in fiber as ***whole-wheat*** bread, but it's not. Whole-wheat bread contains the whole (complete) grain, but wheat bread often is stripped of its fiber. Check the label before you buy your next loaf.

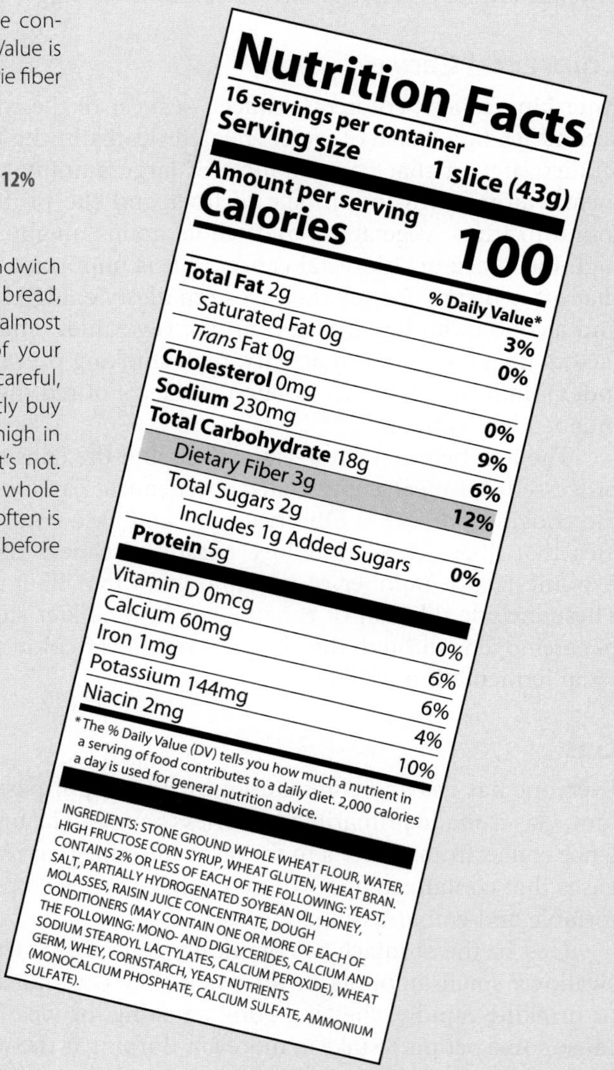
Nutrition Facts
16 servings per container
Serving size 1 slice (43g)
Amount per serving
Calories 100
% Daily Value*
Total Fat 2g 3%
Saturated Fat 0g 0%
Trans Fat 0g
Cholesterol 0mg 0%
Sodium 230mg 9%
Total Carbohydrate 18g 6%
Dietary Fiber 3g 12%
Total Sugars 2g
Includes 1g Added Sugars 0%
Protein 5g
Vitamin D 0mcg 0%
Calcium 60mg 6%
Iron 1mg 6%
Potassium 144mg 4%
Niacin 2mg 10%
* The % Daily Value (DV) tells you how much a nutrient in a serving of food contributes to a daily diet. 2,000 calories a day is used for general nutrition advice.
INGREDIENTS: STONE GROUND WHOLE WHEAT FLOUR, WATER, HIGH FRUCTOSE CORN SYRUP, WHEAT GLUTEN, WHEAT BRAN. CONTAINS 2% OR LESS OF EACH OF THE FOLLOWING: YEAST, SALT, PARTIALLY HYDROGENATED SOYBEAN OIL, HONEY, MOLASSES, RAISIN JUICE CONCENTRATE, DOUGH CONDITIONERS (MAY CONTAIN ONE OR MORE OF EACH OF THE FOLLOWING: MONO- AND DIGLYCERIDES, CALCIUM AND SODIUM STEAROYL LACTYLATES, CALCIUM PEROXIDE), WHEAT GERM, WHEY, CORNSTARCH, YEAST NUTRIENTS (MONOCALCIUM PHOSPHATE, CALCIUM SULFATE, AMMONIUM SULFATE).

down undigested carbohydrate, producing hydrogen, carbon dioxide, and, in about one-third of people, methane. Eventually these gases exit through the rectum.

Foods that produce gas in one person might not cause gas in another. Some common bacteria in the large intestine can destroy the hydrogen that other bacteria produce. The balance of the two types of bacteria explains why some people have more gas than others do.

Carbohydrates that commonly cause gas are raffinose and stachyose, found in large quantities in beans; lactose, the natural sugar in milk; fructose, a common sweetener in soft drinks and fruit drinks; and sorbitol, found naturally in fruits and used as an artificial sweetener. Most starches, including potatoes, corn, noodles, and wheat, produce gas as they are broken down in the large intestine. Rice is the only starch that does not cause gas. The fiber in oat bran, beans, peas, and most fruits is not broken down until it reaches the large intestine, where digestion causes gas. In contrast, the fiber in wheat bran and some vegetables, such as green beans, cauliflower, zucchini, and celery, passes essentially unchanged through the intestines and produces little gas.

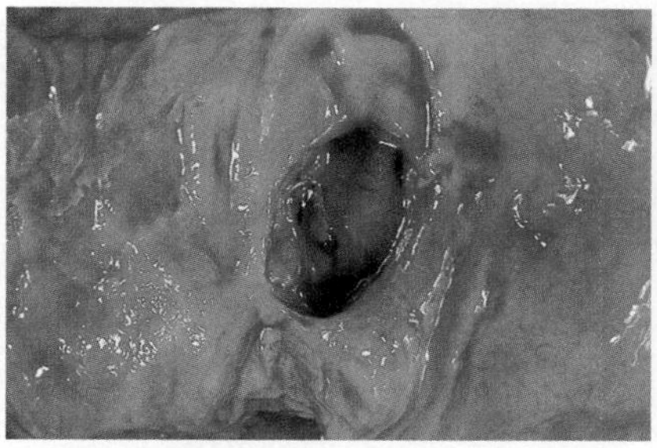

FIGURE 3.21 Stomach ulcer.

Ulcers

A gnawing, burning pain in the upper abdomen is the classic sign of a peptic **ulcer**, which also can cause nausea, vomiting, loss of appetite, and weight loss. A peptic ulcer is a sore that forms in the duodenum (duodenal ulcer) or the lining of the stomach (gastric ulcer) (see **FIGURE 3.21**).

▶ **ulcer** A craterlike lesion that occurs in the lining of the stomach or duodenum; also called a peptic ulcer to distinguish it from a skin ulcer.

It was once assumed that stress was a major factor in the development of peptic ulcer disease, particularly in people with "intense" personalities. Diet also was thought to be important, with spicy foods often cast as a major villain. But much to the amazement of most of the medical community, research in the 1980s and 1990s confirmed that infection with a bacterium, *Helicobacter pylori* (see **FIGURE 3.22**), actually causes most ulcers. *H. pylori* are spiral-shaped bacteria found in the stomach that can cause ulcers by damaging the mucous coating that protects the lining of the stomach and duodenum. Once *H. pylori* have damaged the mucous coating, powerful stomach acid can penetrate into the stomach and duodenum, irritating the lining of the stomach or duodenum, causing an ulcer.[25]

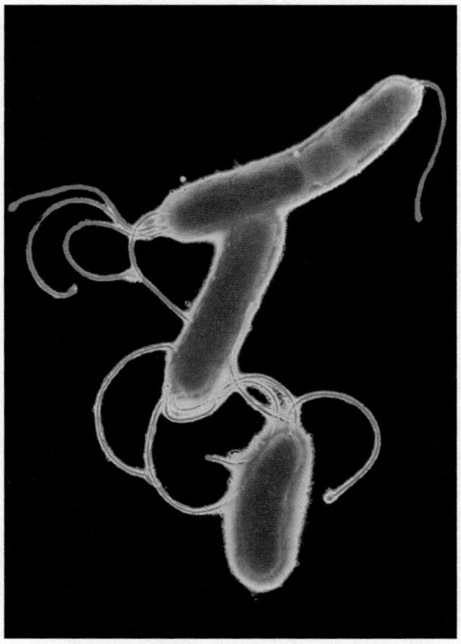

FIGURE 3.22 Helicobacter pylori.

Excessive use of nonsteroidal anti-inflammatory drugs (NSAIDs), such as aspirin, ibuprofen, and naproxen sodium, also is a common cause of ulcers. NSAIDs cause ulcers by interfering with the GI tract's ability to protect itself from acidic stomach juices. Normally, the stomach and duodenum employ three defenses against digestive juices: mucus that coats the lining and shields it from stomach acid; the chemical bicarbonate, which neutralizes acid; and blood circulation, which aids in cell renewal and repair. NSAIDs hinder all these protective mechanisms. With the defenses down, digestive juices can cause ulcers by damaging the sensitive lining of the stomach and duodenum. Fortunately, NSAID-induced ulcers usually heal once the person stops taking the medication.

If you had ulcers in the 1950s, you would have been told to quit your high-stress job and switch to a bland diet. Today, ulcer sufferers are usually treated with an antimicrobial regimen aimed at eradicating *H. pylori*. However, resistance to available antibiotics is mounting and treatment remains a daunting task for the practicing physician.[26] Although personality and life stress are no longer considered significant factors in the development of most ulcers, relapse after treatment is more common in people who are emotionally stressed or suffering from depression.

Quick Bite

Flatulence Facts

Researchers studying pilots and astronauts during the 1960s made some interesting discoveries. The average person inadvertently swallows air with food and drink and subsequently expels approximately 1 pint of gas per day, composed of 50 percent nitrogen. Another 40 percent is composed of carbon dioxide and the products of aerobic bacteria in the intestine.

Functional Dyspepsia

▶ **dyspepsia** A condition also known as upset stomach or indigestion; refers to difficulty with digestion.

Chronic pain in the upper abdomen that has no obvious physical cause (such as inflammation of the esophagus, peptic ulcer, or gallstones) is referred to as **functional dyspepsia**. As with IBS, the cause of functional dyspepsia is unknown, although hypersensitivity to GI stimuli, abnormal GI motility, and psychosocial problems have all been suggested as possible causes.[27] *H. pylori* may also be a factor in some cases of functional dyspepsia.

The treatment of functional dyspepsia includes drugs that speed up the transit of food through the upper part of the intestinal tract, agents that decrease stomach acid production, and antibiotics. Just as with IBS, stress reduction techniques such as meditation and biofeedback can often improve the symptoms of functional dyspepsia.

Key Concepts GI disorders generally produce uncomfortable symptoms such as abdominal pain, gas, bloating, and change in elimination patterns. Some GI disorders, such as diarrhea, are generally symptoms of some other illness. Although medications are useful in reducing symptoms, many GI disorders are treatable with changes in diet, especially getting adequate fiber and fluids in the diet.

As you have seen, the gastrointestinal tract is the key to turning food and its nutrients into nourishment for our bodies. **FIGURE 3.23** shows the sites for digestion and absorption of the macronutrients using a piece of pizza as an example of a food that contains substantial amounts of carbohydrate, fat, and protein. A healthy GI tract is an important factor in our overall health and well-being.

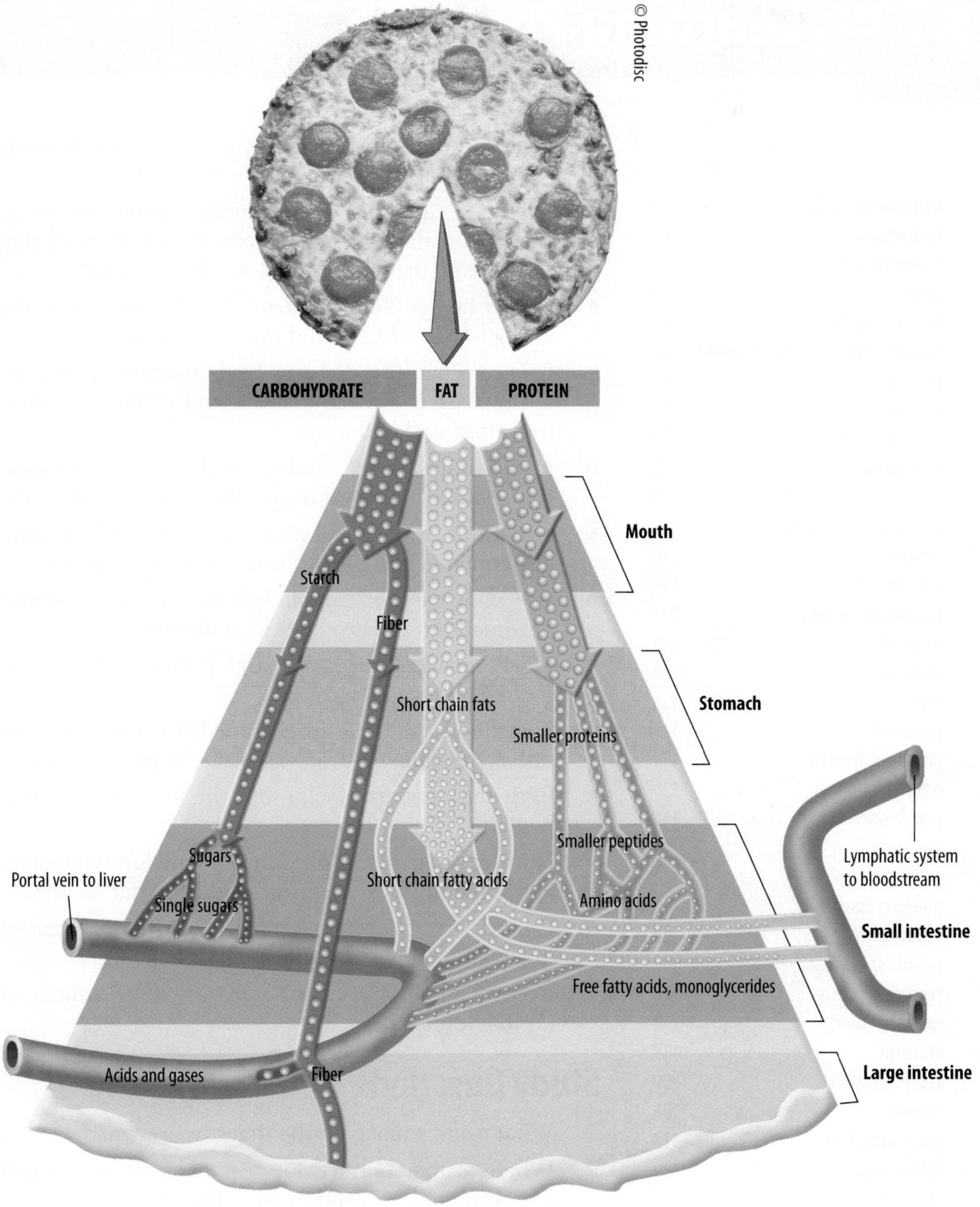

FIGURE 3.23 Fate of a piece of pizza. When you eat a piece of pizza, what happens to the carbohydrate, fat, and protein?

- *Carbohydrate:* Enzymes in the mouth begin the breakdown of starch. Stomach acid halts carbohydrate digestion. In the small intestine, enzymes break down carbohydrate, which is absorbed into the blood. In the large intestine, bacteria digest small amounts of fiber. The remainder is eliminated in feces.
- *Fat:* The stomach absorbs a few short-chain fatty acids into the blood, but most fat is broken down and absorbed in the small intestine, where it enters the lymphatic system.
- *Protein:* Stomach acid unfolds proteins, and enzymes begin protein breakdown. The small intestine completes the breakdown to amino acids, which enter the blood.

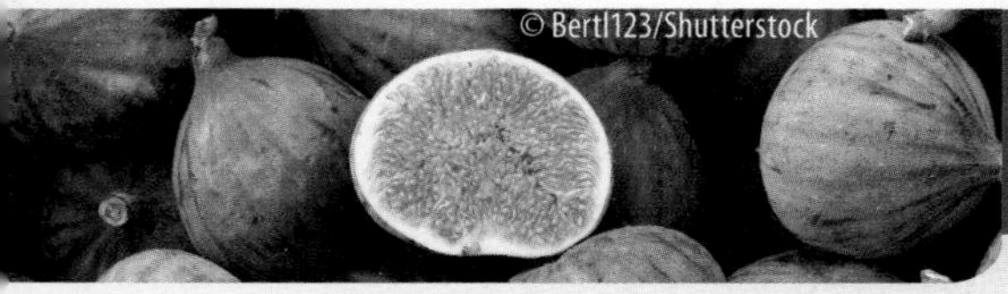
© Bertl123/Shutterstock

Learning Portfolio

Key Terms

absorption	105
acrolein	126
active transport	113
amylase	115
autonomic nervous system	124
bile	114
bolus	115
catalyze	109
cecum	120
central nervous system (CNS)	123
cephalic phase responses	105
cholecystokinin (CCK)	115
chyme	109
circular muscle	108
colon	120
concentration gradients	111
constipation	128
diarrhea	128
digestion	105
digestive secretions	118
diverticulosis	128
duodenum	118
dyspepsia	134
emulsifiers	114
endocytosis	113
enteric nervous system	123
enterohepatic circulation	114
enzymes	109
esophageal sphincter	116
esophagus	115
facilitated diffusion	112
flatus	131
gallbladder	115
gastric inhibitory peptide (GIP)	124
gastric lipase	117
gastrin	117
gastroesophageal reflux disease (GERD)	130
gastrointestinal (GI) tract	107
hydrochloric acid	116
hydrolysis	109
ileocecal valve	120
ileum	118
intrinsic factor	117
irritable bowel syndrome (IBS)	130
jejunum	118
lacteal	119
large intestine	120
lingual lipase	115
liver	114
longitudinal muscle	108
lumen	110
lymph	119
lymphatic system	122
microvilli	119
mucosa	108
mucus	116
pancreas	115
passive diffusion	111
pepsin	116
pepsinogen	116
peristalsis	109
pH	116
phagocytosis	113
pinocytosis	113
pyloric sphincter	117
rectum	120
salivary glands	114
secretin	119
segmentation	109
serosa	108
small intestine	117
sphincters	109
stomach	116
submucosa	108
ulcer	133
vascular system	121
villi	119

Study Points

- The GI tract is a tube that can be divided into regions: the mouth, esophagus, stomach, small intestine, large intestine, and rectum.
- Digestion and absorption of the nutrients in foods occur at various sites along the GI tract.
- Digestion involves both physical processes (e.g., chewing, peristalsis, segmentation) and chemical processes (e.g., the hydrolytic action of enzymes).
- Absorption is the movement of molecules across the lining of the GI tract and into circulation.
- Four mechanisms are involved in nutrient absorption: passive diffusion, facilitated diffusion, active transport, and endocytosis.
- In the mouth, food is mixed with saliva for lubrication. Salivary amylase begins the digestion of starch.
- Secretions from the stomach lower the pH of stomach contents and begin the digestion of proteins.
- The pancreas and gallbladder secrete material into the small intestine to help with digestion.
- Most chemical digestion and nutrient absorption occur in the small intestine.
- Electrolytes and water are absorbed from the large intestine. Remaining material, waste, is excreted as feces.
- Both the nervous system and the hormonal system regulate GI tract processes.
- Numerous factors affect GI tract functioning, including psychological, chemical, and bacterial factors.
- Problems that occur along the GI tract can affect digestion and absorption of nutrients.
- Dietary changes are important in the treatment of GI disorders.

Study Questions

1. What organs make up the digestive system?
2. Where in the GI tract does the majority of nutrient digestion and absorption take place?
3. Describe the path food follows as it travels through the digestive system. Summarize the muscular actions that take place along the way.
4. Name three "assisting" organs that are not part of the GI tract but that are needed for proper digestion. What are their roles in digestion?
5. List three nutrients that are transported by the cardiovascular system and three nutrients that are transported first through the lymphatic system before being transported to body tissues in the cardiovascular system.
6. What is gastroesophageal reflux disease?

Getting Personal

Are you following a diet that helps to keep your gut healthy? What we usually eat can either help maintain a healthy GI tract or cause GI trouble.

For each of the following questions, determine if this is a dietary habit you "usually do," you "sometimes do," or you "never do." To ensure that you are eating a diet that keeps your GI tract healthy, consider improving those things that you sometimes or never do by turning them into eating habits that you usually do.

Eating Habits	Usually Do	Sometimes Do	Never Do
I eat at least seven servings of fruits and vegetables every day.			
For breakfast I choose whole grains, nuts, and berries instead of foods like low-fiber, refined cereal.			
For lunch I select sandwiches or wraps on a whole-grain tortilla or whole-grain bread and add veggies.			
For a snack I choose fresh veggies, fruit, whole-grain crackers, almonds, avocado, or air-popped popcorn.			
I drink 8–10 cups of water each day.			
I limit foods that are high in fat, and if I eat meat, I choose lean cuts.			
I include probiotics (such as low-fat yogurt) in my diet.			
I exercise regularly, getting at least 30 minutes of exercise each day.			

References

1. Klein S, Cohn SM, Alpers DH. Alimentary tract in nutrition. In: Shils ME, Shike M, Ross AC, et al., eds. *Modern Nutrition in Health and Disease*. 10th ed. Philadelphia: Lippincott Williams & Wilkins; 2006:1115–1142.
2. Guyton AC, Hall JE. *Textbook of Medical Physiology*. 12th ed. Philadelphia: WB Saunders; 2010.
3. Ibid.
4. Klein, Cohn, Alpers. Alimentary tract in nutrition. Op cit.
5. El Kaoutari A, Armougom F, Raoult D, Henrissat B. Gut microbiota and digestion of polysaccharides. *Med Sci* (Paris). 2014;30(3):259–265.
6. Guyton, Hall. *Textbook of Medical Physiology*. Op cit.
7. Ibid.
8. Ibid.
9. Mahan LK, Escott-Stump S. *Krause's Food Nutrition and Diet Therapy*. 12th ed. Philadelphia: WB Saunders; 2008.
10. U.S. Department of Health and Human Services, Agency for Toxic Substances and Disease Registry. Toxicological profile for acrolein. http://www.atsdr.cdc.gov/ToxProfiles/tp.asp?id=557&tid=102. Accessed December 22, 2015.
11. National Digestive Diseases Information Clearinghouse. Constipation. February 2006. NIH Pub. no. 06-2754. http://digestive.niddk.nih.gov/ddiseases/pubs/constipation/index.htm. Accessed December 22, 2015.
12. Cheung, WY, Zhai R, Bradbury P, et al. Single nucleotide polymorphisms in the matrix metalloproteinase gene family and the frequency and duration of gastroesophageal reflux disease influence the risk of esophageal adenocarcinoma. *Int J Cancer*. 2012;131(11):2478–2486.
13. National Institute of Diabetes and Digestive and Kidney Diseases. Definition and facts for irritable bowel syndrome. http://www.niddk.nih.gov/health-information/health-topics/digestive-diseases/irritable-bowel-syndrome/Pages/definition-facts.aspx. Accessed December 22, 2015.
14. Anbardan SJ, Daryani NE, Fereshtehnejad SM, et al. Gender role in irritable bowel syndrome: a comparison of Irritable Bowel Syndrome Module (ROME III) between male and female patients. *J Neurogastroenterol Motil*. 2012;18(1):70–77.
15. National Institute of Diabetes and Digestive and Kidney Diseases. Definition and facts for irritable bowel syndrome.
16. Konturek PC, Brzozowski T, Konturek SJ. Stress and the gut: pathophysiology, clinical consequences, diagnostic approach and treatment options. *J Physiol Pharmacol*. 2011;62(6):591–599.
17. Shepherd SJ, Halmos E, Glance S. The role of FODMAPS in irritable bowel syndrome. *Curr Opin Clin Nutr Metab Care*. 2014;17(6):605–609.
18. Konturek, Brzozowski, Konturek. Stress and the gut: pathophysiology, clinical consequences, diagnostic approach and treatment options. Op cit.
19. Centers for Disease Control and Prevention. Colorectal (colon) cancer. http://www.cdc.gov/cancer/colorectal. Accessed December 22, 2015.
20. Zur Hausen H. Red meat consumption and cancer: reasons to suspect involvement of bovine infectious factors in colorectal cancer. *Int J Cancer*. 2011;130(11):2475–2483.
21. World Health Organization. *Diet, Nutrition and the Prevention of Chronic Diseases: Report of the Joint WHO/FAO Expert Consultation*. Geneva, Switzerland: World Health Organization; 2003. WHO Technical Report Series 916. http://www.who.int/dietphysicalactivity/publications/trs916/en. Accessed December 22, 2015.
22. Gingras D, Belliveau R. Colorectal cancer prevention through dietary and lifestyle modifications. *Cancer Microenviron*. 2011;4(2):133–139.
23. Zur Hausen H. Red meat consumption and cancer: reasons to suspect involvement of bovine infectious factors in colorectal cancer. Op cit.
24. Cao Y, Gao X, Zhang W, et al. Dietary fiber enhances TGF-β signaling and growth inhibition in the gut. *Am J Physiol Gastrointest Liver Physiol*. 2011;301(1):G156–G164.
25. Shahid SK. Novel anti-*Helicobacter pylori* therapies. *Pharm Pat Anal*. 2014;3(4):411–427.
26. National Institute of Diabetes and Digestive and Kidney Diseases. Symptoms and causes of peptic ulcer disease. How do *H. pylori* cause a peptic ulcer and peptic ulcer disease? http://www.niddk.nih.gov/health-information/health-topics/digestive-diseases/peptic-ulcer/Pages/symptoms-causes.aspx. Accessed December 22, 2015.
27. Ates F, Francis DO, Vaezi MF. Refractory gastroesophageal reflux disease: Advances and treatment. *Expert Rev Gastroenterol Hepatol*. 2014;8(6):657–667.

Chapter 4

Carbohydrates

Revised by Diane McKay and Emily Mohn

THINK About It

1 When you think of the word *carbohydrate*, what foods come to mind?

2 How does your dietary fiber intake stack up?

3 Many people choose honey or agave instead of white sugar because they think they are more "natural." What do you think?

4 Do you prefer artificial or nonnutritive sweeteners to sugar? Explain why or why not.

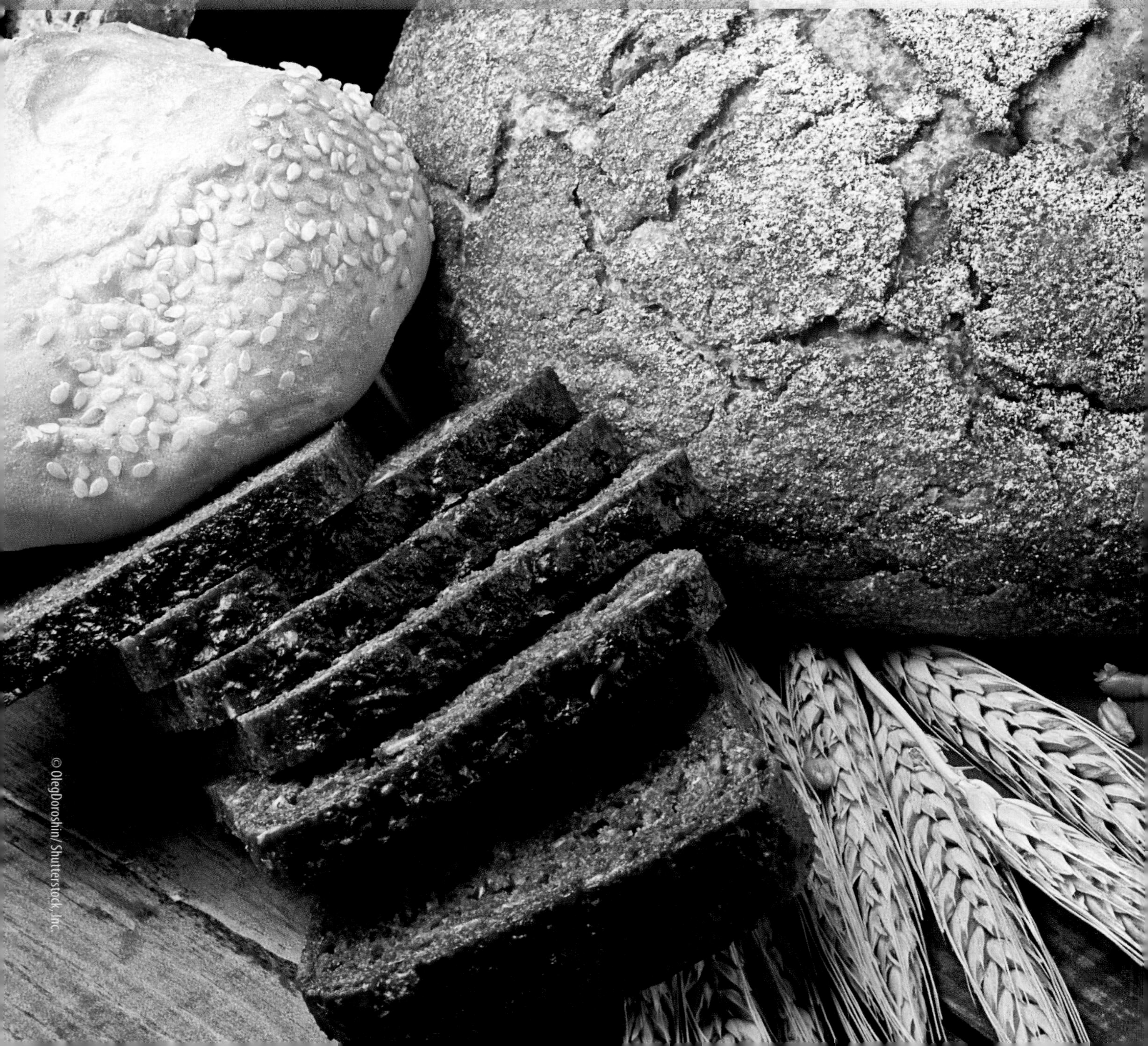

CHAPTER Menu

LEARNING Objectives

- Differentiate between disaccharides, oligosaccharides, and polysaccharides.
- Explain how carbohydrates are digested and absorbed in the body.
- Explain the effects of fiber in the gastrointestinal tract.
- Explain the functions of carbohydrates in the body.
- Discuss diabetes, including etiology, types, risk factors, and management.
- Make healthy carbohydrate selections for an optimal diet.
- Analyze the contributions of carbohydrates to health.

Does sugar causes diabetes? Will too much sugar make a child hyperactive? Does excess sugar contribute to criminal behavior? What about starch? Does it really make you fat? These and other questions have been asked about sugar and starch—dietary carbohydrates—over the years. But where do these ideas come from? What is myth and what is fact? Are carbohydrates important in the diet? Or, as some diets suggest, should we eat only small amounts of carbohydrates? What links, if any, are there between carbohydrates in your diet and your health?

Most of the world depends on carbohydrate-rich plant foods for daily sustenance. In some countries, 80 percent or more of daily calorie intake is carbohydrates. Rice provides the bulk of the diet in Southeast Asia, as does corn in South America, cassava in certain parts of Africa, and wheat in Europe and North America (see **FIGURE 4.1**). Besides providing energy, foods rich in carbohydrates, such as whole grains, legumes, fruits, and vegetables, are also good sources of vitamins, minerals, dietary fiber, and phytochemicals that can help lower the risk of chronic diseases.

THINK About It 1

Generous carbohydrate intake should provide the foundation for any healthful diet. Carbohydrates contain only 4 kilocalories per gram, compared with 9 kilocalories per gram for fat. Thus, a diet rich in carbohydrates provides fewer calories and a greater volume of food than the typical fat-laden American diet. As you explore the topic of carbohydrates, think about some claims you have heard for and against eating lots of carbohydrates.

What Are Carbohydrates?

Plants use carbon dioxide from the air, water from the soil, and energy from the sun to produce carbohydrates and oxygen through a process called photosynthesis (see **FIGURE 4.2**). Carbohydrates are organic compounds that contain carbon (C), hydrogen (H), and oxygen (O) in the ratio of two hydrogen atoms and one oxygen atom for every one carbon atom (CH_2O). The sugar glucose, for example, contains 6 carbon atoms, 12 hydrogen atoms, and 6 oxygen atoms, giving this vital carbohydrate the chemical formula $C_6H_{12}O_6$. Two or more sugar molecules can be assembled to form increasingly complex carbohydrates. The two main types of carbohydrates in food are simple carbohydrates (sugars) and complex carbohydrates (starches and fiber).

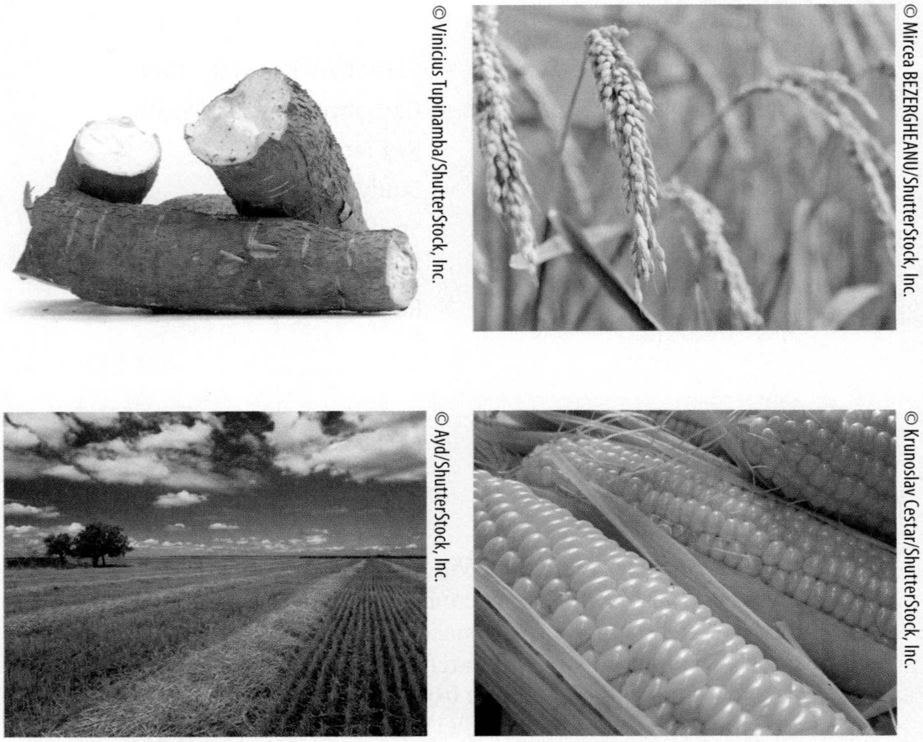

FIGURE 4.1 Cassava, rice, wheat, and corn. These carbohydrate-rich foods are dietary staples in many parts of the world.

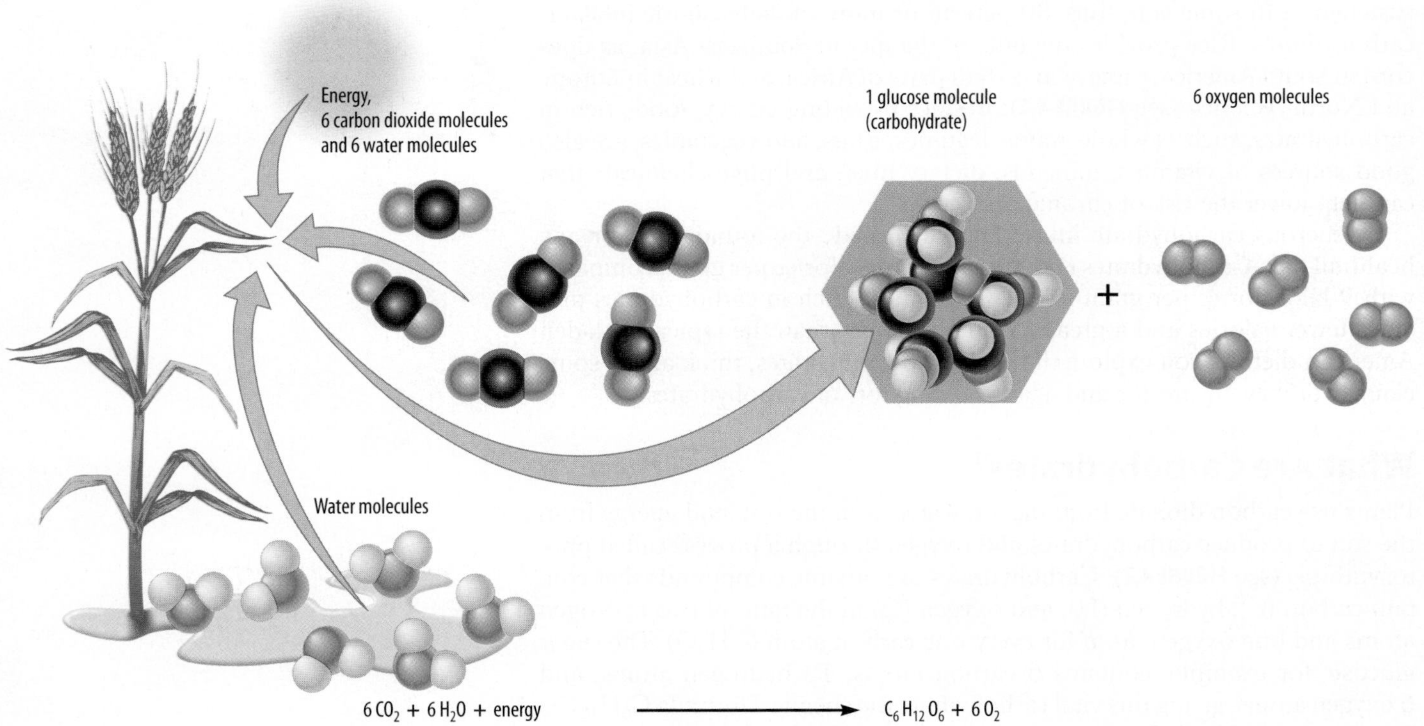

$$6\,CO_2 + 6\,H_2O + \text{energy} \longrightarrow C_6H_{12}O_6 + 6\,O_2$$

FIGURE 4.2 Plants make carbohydrates. Plants release oxygen as they use water, carbon dioxide, and energy from the sun to make carbohydrate (glucose) molecules.

Simple Carbohydrates: Monosaccharides and Disaccharides

Simple carbohydrates occur naturally as simple sugars in fruits, milk, and other foods. Plant carbohydrates also can be refined to produce sugar products such as table sugar or corn syrup. The two main types of sugars are monosaccharides and disaccharides. **Monosaccharides** consist of a single sugar molecule (*mono* meaning "one" and *saccharide* meaning "sugar"). **Disaccharides** consist of two sugar molecules chemically joined together (*di* meaning "two"). Monosaccharides and disaccharides give various degrees of sweetness to foods.

▶ **simple carbohydrates** Sugars composed of a single sugar molecule (a monosaccharide) or two joined sugar molecules (a disaccharide).

▶ **monosaccharides** Any sugars that are not broken down further during digestion and have the general formula $C_nH_{2n}O_n$, where $n = 3$ to 7. The common monosaccharides glucose, fructose, and galactose all have six carbon atoms ($n = 6$).

▶ **disaccharides** [dye-SACK-uh-rides] Carbohydrates composed of two monosaccharide units linked by a glycosidic bond. They include sucrose (common table sugar), lactose (milk sugar), and maltose.

Quick Bite

Is Pasta a Chinese Food?

Noodles were used in China as early as the first century; Marco Polo did not bring them to Italy until the 1300s.

Monosaccharides: The Single Sugars

The most common monosaccharides in the human diet are the following:

- Glucose
- Fructose
- Galactose

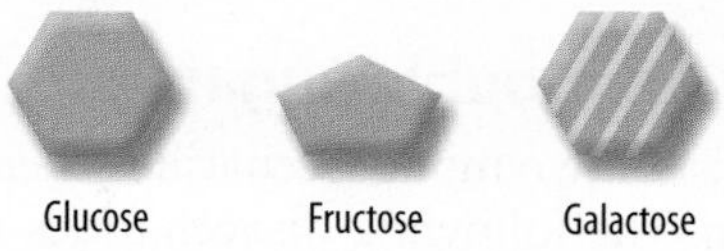

All three monosaccharides have six carbons, and all have the chemical formula $C_6H_{12}O_6$, but each has a different arrangement of these atoms. The carbon and oxygen atoms of glucose and galactose form a six-sided ring. The structures of glucose and galactose look almost identical except for the reversal of the OH and H groups on one carbon atom. The carbons and oxygen of fructose form a five-sided ring. Look carefully at **FIGURE 4.3** to find all six carbons.

Glucose

The monosaccharide **glucose** is the most abundant simple carbohydrate unit in nature. Also referred to as dextrose, glucose plays a key role in both foods and the body. Glucose imparts a mildly sweet flavor to food. It seldom exists as a monosaccharide in food but is usually joined to other sugars to form disaccharides, starch, or dietary fiber. Glucose makes up at least one of the two sugar molecules in every disaccharide.

In the body, glucose supplies energy to cells. The body closely regulates blood glucose (blood sugar) levels to ensure a constant fuel source for vital body functions. Glucose is virtually the only fuel used by the brain, except during prolonged starvation, when the glucose supply is low.

▶ **glucose** [GLOO-kose] A common monosaccharide containing six carbons that is present in the blood; also known as dextrose or blood sugar. It is a component of the disaccharides sucrose, lactose, and maltose and various complex carbohydrates.

Fructose

Also called levulose or fruit sugar, **fructose** tastes the sweetest of all sugars and occurs naturally in fruits and vegetables. Although the sugar in honey is about half fructose and half glucose, fructose is the primary source of the sweet taste. Food manufacturers use high-fructose corn syrup as an additive to sweeten many foods, including soft drinks, fruit beverages such as lemonade, desserts, candies, jellies, and jams. The term *high-fructose* is a little misleading—the fructose content of this sweetener is approximately 55%.

▶ **fructose** [FROOK-tose] A common monosaccharide containing six carbons that is naturally present in honey and many fruits; often added to foods in the form of high-fructose corn syrup. Also called levulose or fruit sugar.

Galactose

Galactose rarely occurs as a monosaccharide in food. It usually is chemically bonded to glucose to form lactose, the primary sugar in milk.

▶ **galactose** [gah-LAK-tose] A monosaccharide containing six carbons that can be converted into glucose in the body. In foods and living systems, galactose usually is joined with other monosaccharides.

Other Monosaccharides and Derivative Sweeteners

Pentoses are single sugar molecules that contain five carbons. Although they are present in foods in only small quantities, they are essential components

▶ **pentoses** Sugar molecules containing five carbon atoms.

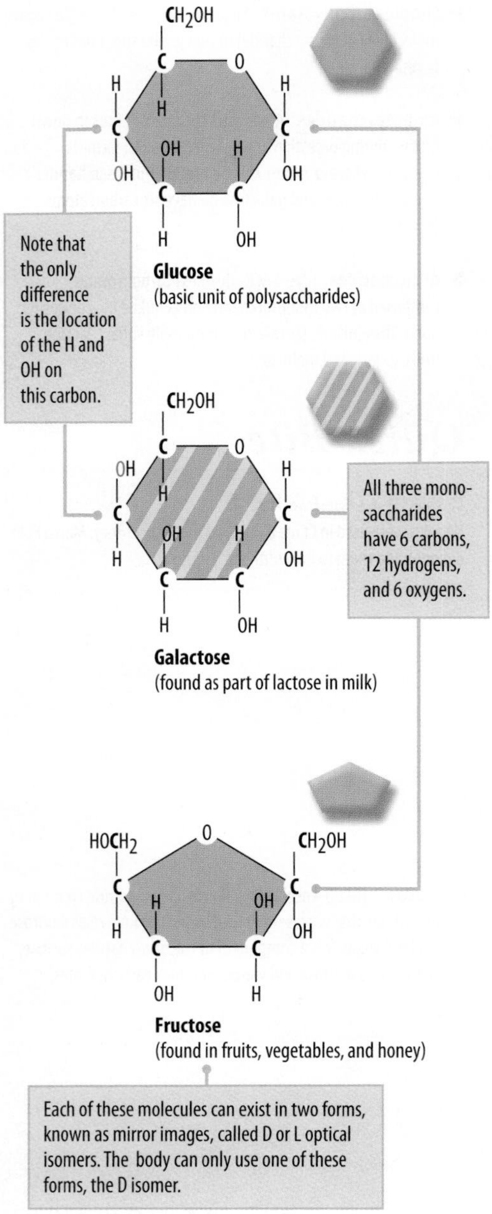

Note that the only difference is the location of the H and OH on this carbon.
Glucose
(basic unit of polysaccharides)
All three monosaccharides have 6 carbons, 12 hydrogens, and 6 oxygens.
Galactose
(found as part of lactose in milk)
Fructose
(found in fruits, vegetables, and honey)
Each of these molecules can exist in two forms, known as mirror images, called D or L optical isomers. The body can only use one of these forms, the D isomer.

FIGURE 4.3 The monosaccharides: glucose, galactose, and fructose. Because glucose and galactose share similar six-sided hexagonal structures, they can be difficult to tell apart. Fructose's five-sided pentagon stands out.

▶ **sugar alcohols** Compounds formed from monosaccharides by replacing a hydrogen atom with a hydroxyl group (–OH); commonly used as nutritive sweeteners. Also called polyols.

of nucleic acids, the genetic material of life (see **FIGURE 4.4**). The five-carbon sugar ribose is part of ribonucleic acid, or RNA. Another five-carbon sugar, deoxyribose, is a part of deoxyribonucleic acid, or DNA. Some pentoses also are components of indigestible gums and mucilages, which are classified as part of the dietary fiber component of foods.[1] Pentoses are synthesized in the body and therefore are not needed in the diet.

Sugar alcohols are derivatives of monosaccharides. Like other sugars, they taste sweet and supply energy to the body. However, they are absorbed more slowly than sugars, and the body processes them differently. Some fruits naturally contain minute amounts of sugar alcohols. Sugar alcohols such as sorbitol, mannitol, lactitol, and xylitol also are used as nutritive sweeteners in foods. For example, sorbitol, which is derived from glucose, sweetens sugarless gum, breath mints, and candy. For more information on sugar alcohols, see the "Nutritive Sweeteners" section later in this chapter.

Disaccharides: The Double Sugars

Disaccharides consist of two monosaccharides chemically joined by a process called condensation. The following disaccharides (see **FIGURE 4.5**) are important in human nutrition:

- Sucrose (common table sugar)
- Lactose (major sugar in milk)
- Maltose (product of starch digestion)

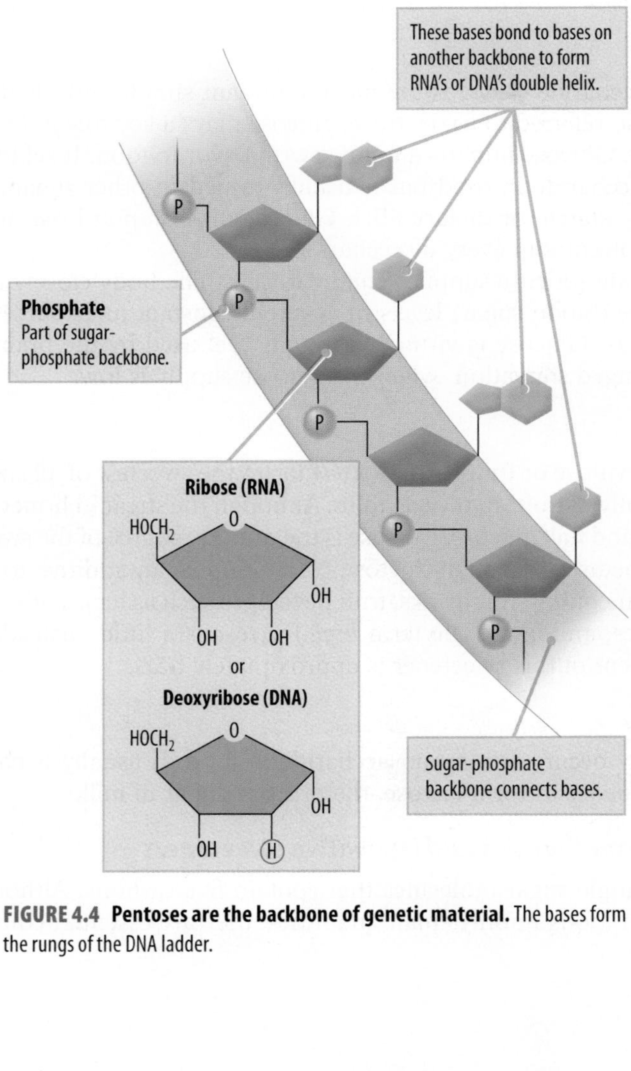

These bases bond to bases on another backbone to form RNA's or DNA's double helix.

Part of sugar-phosphate backbone.
Ribose (RNA)

Sugar-phosphate backbone connects bases.

FIGURE 4.4 Pentoses are the backbone of genetic material. The bases form the rungs of the DNA ladder.

Joining and Cleaving Sugar Molecules

Sugar molecules are joined or separated (cleaved) by the removal or addition of a molecule of water. A **condensation** reaction chemically joins two monosaccharides while removing an H from one sugar molecule and an OH from the other to form water (H_2O) (see **FIGURE 4.6**). A hydrolysis reaction separates disaccharides into monosaccharides (see **FIGURE 4.7**). During hydrolysis, the addition of a molecule of water splits the bond between the two sugar molecules, providing the H and OH groups necessary for the sugars to exist as monosaccharides. The digestion of carbohydrates involves hydrolysis reactions.

Sucrose

Sucrose, most familiar to us as table sugar, is composed of one molecule of glucose and one molecule of fructose. Sucrose provides some of the natural sweetness of honey, maple syrup, fruits, and vegetables. Manufacturers use a refining process to extract sucrose from the juices of sugar cane or sugar beets. Full refining removes impurities; white sugar and powdered sugar are so highly refined they are virtually 100 percent sucrose. When a food label lists *sugar* as an ingredient, the term refers to sucrose.

Lactose

Lactose, or milk sugar, is composed of one molecule of glucose and one molecule of galactose. Lactose gives milk and other dairy products a slightly sweet taste. Human milk has a higher concentration (approximately 7 grams per 100 milliliters) of lactose than cow's milk (approximately 4.5 grams per 100 milliliters), so human milk tastes sweeter than cow's milk.

Maltose

Maltose is composed of two glucose molecules. Maltose seldom occurs naturally in foods but is formed whenever long molecules of starch break down. Human digestive enzymes in the mouth and small intestine break down starch into maltose. When you chew a slice of fresh bread, you might detect a slightly sweet taste as starch breaks down into maltose. Starch also breaks down into maltose in germinating seeds. Maltose is fermented in the production of beer.

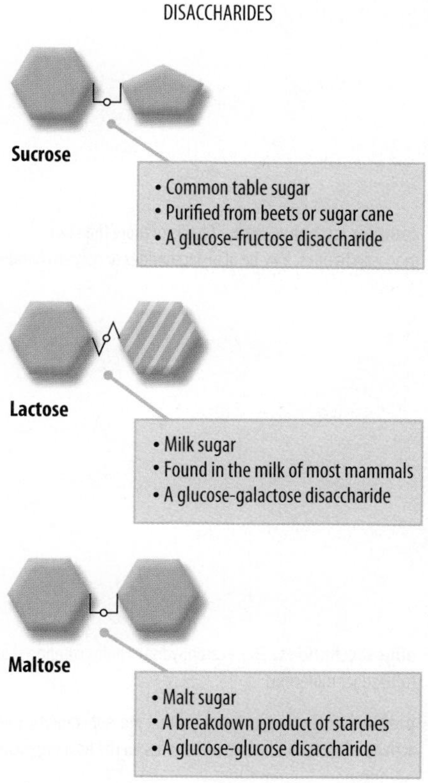
DISACCHARIDES
Sucrose
• Common table sugar
• Purified from beets or sugar cane
• A glucose-fructose disaccharide
Lactose
• Milk sugar
• Found in the milk of most mammals
• A glucose-galactose disaccharide
Maltose
• Malt sugar
• A breakdown product of starches
• A glucose-glucose disaccharide

FIGURE 4.5 The disaccharides: sucrose, lactose, and maltose. The three monosaccharides pair up in different combinations to form the three disaccharides.

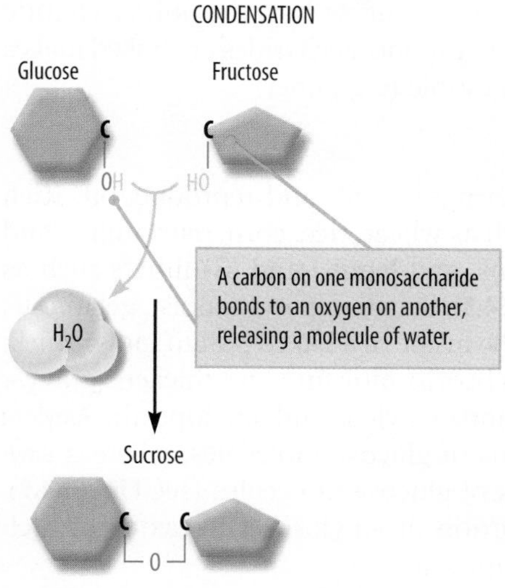
CONDENSATION
Glucose
Fructose
C
C
OH
HO
A carbon on one monosaccharide bonds to an oxygen on another, releasing a molecule of water.
H2O
Sucrose
C
C
O

FIGURE 4.6 Condensation reactions form disaccharides.

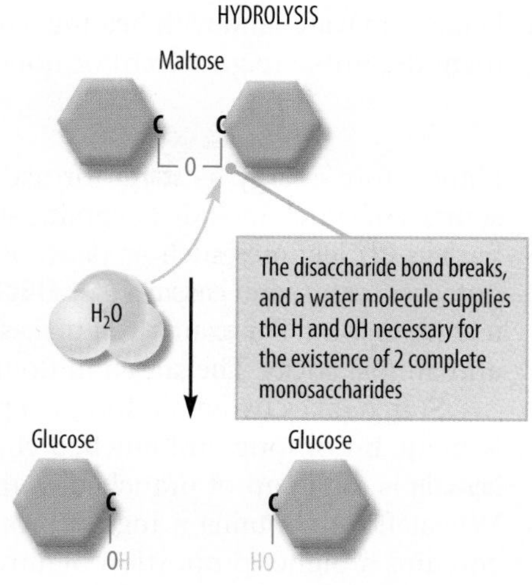
HYDROLYSIS
Maltose
C
C
O
The disaccharide bond breaks, and a water molecule supplies the H and OH necessary for the existence of 2 complete monosaccharides
H2O
Glucose
Glucose
C
C
OH
HO

FIGURE 4.7 Hydrolysis reactions split disaccharides into monosaccharides.

▶ **condensation** In chemistry, a reaction in which a covalent bond is formed between two molecules by removal of a water molecule.

▶ **sucrose** [SOO-crose] A disaccharide composed of one molecule of glucose and one molecule of fructose joined together. Also known as table sugar.

▶ **lactose** [LAK-tose] A disaccharide composed of glucose and galactose; also called milk sugar because it is the major sugar in milk and dairy products.

▶ **maltose** [MALL-tose] A disaccharide composed of two glucose molecules; sometimes called malt sugar. Maltose seldom occurs naturally in foods but is formed whenever long molecules of starch break down.

Key Concepts Carbohydrates are composed of carbon, hydrogen, and oxygen and can be categorized as simple or complex. Simple carbohydrates include monosaccharides and disaccharides. The monosaccharides glucose, fructose, and galactose are single sugar molecules. The disaccharides sucrose, lactose, and maltose are double sugar molecules. A condensation reaction joins two monosaccharides to form a disaccharide.

Complex Carbohydrates

▶ **complex carbohydrates** Chains of more than two monosaccharides. May be oligosaccharides or polysaccharides.

Complex carbohydrates are chains of more than two sugar molecules. Short carbohydrate chains can have as few as three monosaccharide molecules, but long chains, the polysaccharides, can contain hundreds or even thousands.

Oligosaccharides

▶ **oligosaccharides** Short carbohydrate chains composed of 3 to 10 sugar molecules.

▶ **prebiotics** Group of compounds that promote growth and activity of bacteria that impart benefits on the host organism.

▶ **microbiota** Community of beneficial and pathogenic microorganisms that inhabit the body.

Oligosaccharides (*oligo* meaning "scant") are short carbohydrate chains of 3 to 10 sugar molecules. They are found naturally, at least in small amounts, in many plant foods, such as onions, legumes, wheat, asparagus, and jicama. Dried beans, peas, and lentils contain the two most common oligosaccharides—raffinose and stachyose.[2] Raffinose is formed from three monosaccharide molecules—one galactose, one glucose, and one fructose. Stachyose is formed from four monosaccharide molecules—two galactose, one glucose, and one fructose. The body cannot break down raffinose or stachyose, but they are readily broken down by intestinal bacteria and are responsible for the familiar gaseous effects of foods such as beans.

Human milk contains large amounts of complex oligosaccharides,[3] which, for breastfed infants, serve a function similar to dietary fiber in adults—making stools easier to pass. Certain human milk oligosaccharides can also act as **prebiotics**, resisting digestion in the small intestine and reaching the colon to modulate the **microbiota** of infants by increasing good bacteria in their gut.[4] Some of these oligosaccharides can also protect infants from disease-causing agents by binding to them in the intestine. Oligosaccharides in human milk also provide sialic acid, a compound essential for normal brain development.[5]

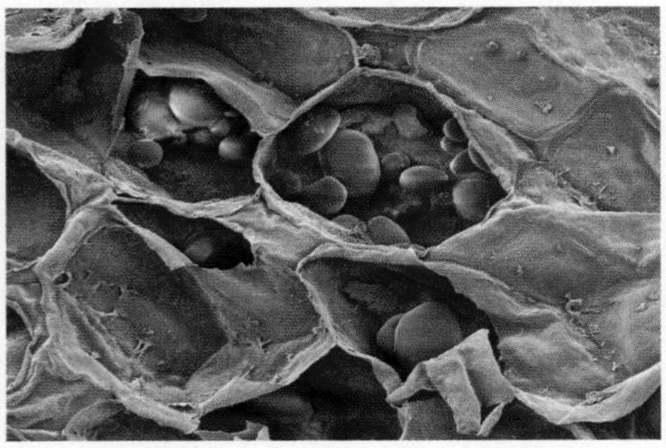

FIGURE 4.8 A scanning electron micrograph of a potato tuber cell shows the starch granules where energy is stored.

Polysaccharides

▶ **polysaccharides** Long carbohydrate chains composed of more than 10 sugar molecules. Polysaccharides can be straight or branched.

▶ **starch** The major storage form of carbohydrate in plants; starch is composed of long chains of glucose molecules in a straight (amylose) or branching (amylopectin) arrangement.

▶ **amylose** [AM-ih-los] A straight-chain polysaccharide composed of glucose units.

▶ **amylopectin** [am-ih-low-PEK-tin] A branched-chain polysaccharide composed of glucose units.

Polysaccharides (*poly* meaning "many") are long carbohydrate chains of monosaccharides. Some polysaccharides form straight chains, whereas others branch off in all directions. Such structural differences affect how the polysaccharide behaves in water and with heating. The way monosaccharides are linked makes them digestible (e.g., starch) or nondigestible (e.g., fiber).

Starch

Plants store energy as **starch** for use during growth and reproduction. Rich sources of starch include (1) grains such as wheat, rice, corn, oats, millet, and barley; (2) legumes such as peas, beans, and lentils; and (3) tubers such as potatoes, yams, and cassava (see **FIGURE 4.8**). Starch imparts a moist, gelatinous texture to food. For example, it makes the inside of a baked potato moist, thick, and almost sticky. The starch in flour absorbs moisture and thickens gravy.

Starch takes two main forms in plants: amylose and amylopectin. **Amylose** is made up of long, unbranched chains of glucose molecules, whereas **amylopectin** is made up of branched chains of glucose molecules (see **FIGURE 4.9**). Wheat flour contains a higher proportion of amylose, whereas cornstarch contains a higher proportion of amylopectin.

The proportion of amylose to amylopectin in a food affects its functional properties. For example, food manufacturers often thicken gravies for frozen foods with cornstarch (rich in branched amylopectin) because it forms thicker, more stable gels than gravies thickened with wheat flour (rich in unbranched amylose).

In the body, amylopectin is digested more rapidly than amylose.[6] Although the body easily digests most starches, there is a subgroup of starches known as **resistant starches (RSs)**, which are not digested in the small intestine. There are several different types of RSs. Some are found in whole-grain foods and are resistant to digestion because they are physically inaccessible to amylase. Raw potatoes, unripened bananas, and some legumes, such as white beans, contain a type of RS that resists digestion due to the nature of the starch granule. The process of heating and cooling certain foods produces RS as well. An example of this would be cooked-and-cooled potatoes or bread. Finally, RS can also be manufactured from starch through chemical modification. It is estimated that Americans, on average, consume between 3 and 8 grams of RS per day.[7] Because RS passes through the small intestine intact, it can be classified as a form of fiber. RS shares many of the same health benefits as dietary fiber, which will be described in greater detail later in the chapter. Briefly, RS can slow rates of glucose absorption into the blood, lower cholesterol absorption and reabsorption, add bulk to feces, promote growth of healthy gut bacteria, and produce beneficial short-chain fatty acids for use in the colon.[8]

Glycogen

Glycogen, also called animal starch, is the storage form of carbohydrate in living animals (see **FIGURE 4.9**). After slaughter, tissue enzymes break down most glycogen within 24 hours. Although some organ meats, such as kidney, heart, and liver, contain small amounts of carbohydrate, meat from muscle contains none.[9] Because plant foods also contain no glycogen, it is a negligible carbohydrate source in our diets. Glycogen does, however, play an important role in our bodies as a readily mobilized store of glucose.

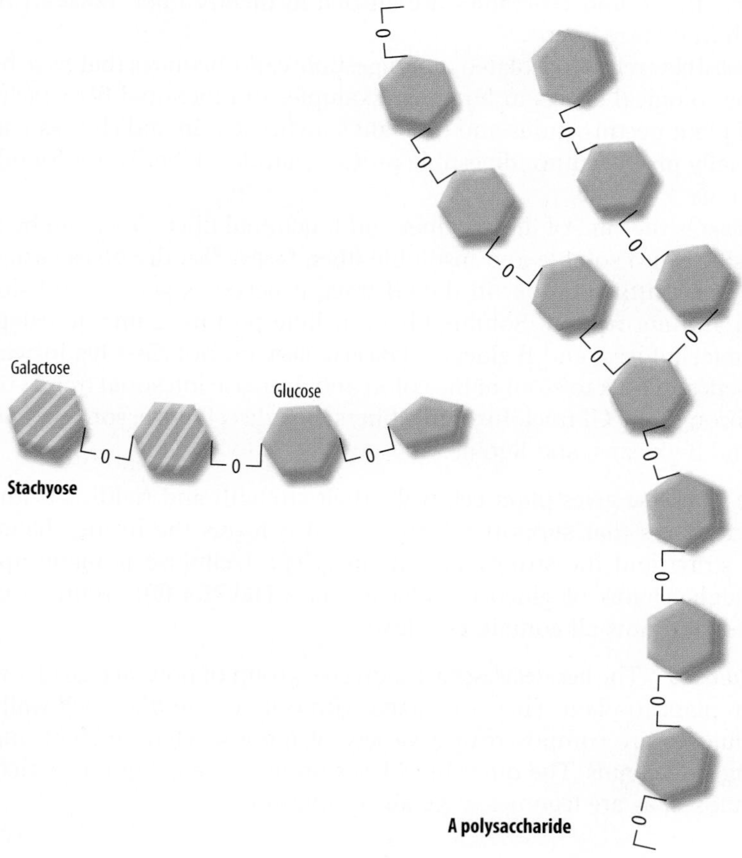

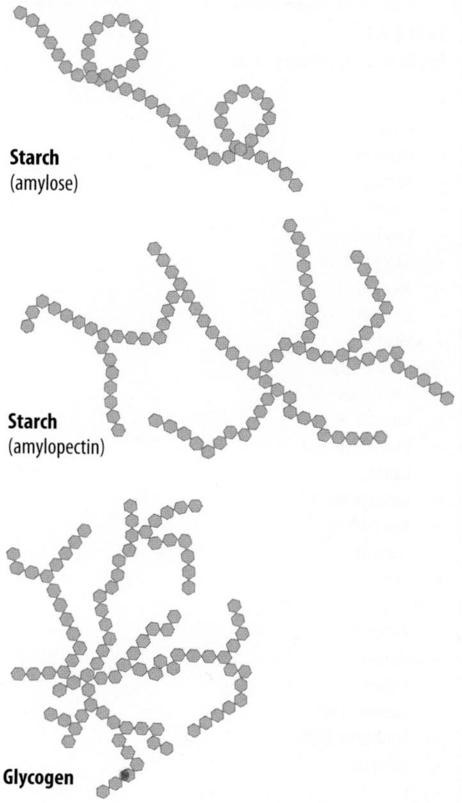

FIGURE 4.9 Starch and glycogen. Plants have two main types of starch—amylose, which has long unbranched chains of glucose, and amylopectin, which has branched chains. Animals store glucose in highly branched chains called glycogen.

▶ **resistant starch** A starch that is not digested.

▶ **glycogen** [GLY-ko-jen] A very large, highly branched polysaccharide composed of multiple glucose units. Sometimes called animal starch, glycogen is the primary storage form of glucose in animals.

TABLE 4.1
Foods Rich in Dietary Fiber

Fruits
- Apples
- Bananas
- Berries
- Cherries
- Cranberries
- Grapefruit
- Mangos
- Oranges
- Pears

Vegetables
- Asparagus
- Broccoli
- Brussels sprouts
- Carrots
- Green peppers
- Red cabbage
- Spinach
- Sprouts

Nuts and Seeds
- Almonds
- Peanuts
- Pecans
- Sesame seeds
- Sunflower seeds
- Walnuts

Legumes
- Most legumes

Grains
- Brown rice
- Oat bran
- Oatmeal
- Wheat-bran cereals
- Whole-wheat breads

Data from Shils ME, Olson JA, Shike M, Ross AC, eds. Modern Nutrition in Health and Disease. 10th ed. Philadelphia: Lippincott Williams & Wilkins, 2006.

Glycogen is composed of long, highly branched chains of glucose molecules. Its structure is similar to amylopectin, but glycogen is much more highly branched. When we need extra glucose, glycogen in our cells can be broken down rapidly into single glucose molecules. Because enzymes can attack only the ends of glycogen chains, the highly branched structure of glycogen multiplies the number of sites available for enzyme activity.

Skeletal muscle and the liver are the two major sites of glycogen storage. In muscle cells, glycogen provides a reservoir of glucose for strenuous muscular activity. Liver cells also use glycogen to regulate blood glucose levels. If necessary, liver glycogen can provide as much as 100 to 150 milligrams of glucose per minute to the blood at a sustained rate for up to 12 hours.[10]

Normally, the body can store only about 200 to 500 grams of glycogen at a time.[11] Some athletes practice a carbohydrate-loading regimen by gradually tapering off rigorous training and emphasizing high-carbohydrate meals a few days to one week before competition. This can increase the amount of stored glycogen by 20 to 40 percent above normal, providing a competitive edge for marathon running and other endurance events.[12]

Fiber

All types of plant foods—including fruits, vegetables, legumes, and whole grains—contain **dietary fiber**. Dietary fiber consists of nondigestible carbohydrates and lignins that are intact and intrinsic in plants. Many types of dietary fiber resemble starches—they are polysaccharides, but are not digested in the human gastrointestinal (GI) tract. Examples of these nonstarch polysaccharides include cellulose, hemicellulose, pectins, gums, and beta-glucans (β-glucans). Oligosaccharides also are considered to be dietary fiber. Whole-grain foods such as brown rice, rolled oats, and whole-wheat breads and cereals; legumes such as kidney beans, garbanzo beans (chickpeas), peas, and lentils; fruits; and vegetables are all rich in dietary fiber. **TABLE 4.1** lists foods rich in dietary fiber.

Functional fiber refers to isolated, nondigestible carbohydrates that have beneficial physiological effects in humans. Examples of functional fiber include extracted plant pectins, gums and resistant starches, chitin and chitosan, and commercially produced nondigestible polysaccharides. Fiber is not found in animal foods.

Total fiber is the sum of dietary fiber and functional fiber. Fiber can be further classified into soluble and insoluble fiber. **Soluble fiber** dissolves easily in water. When it attracts water in the GI tract, it becomes gel-like and slows digestion and absorption. Soluble fibers include pectins, gums, mucilages, some hemicelluloses, and β-glucans. **Insoluble fibers** do not dissolve in water. These fibers add bulk to stool in the colon and decrease intestinal transit time of food through the GI tract. Insoluble fibers include cellulose, some hemicelluloses and β-glucans, and lignins.

Cellulose **Cellulose** gives plant cell walls their strength and rigidity. It forms the woody fibers that support tall trees. It also forms the brittle shafts of hay and straw and the stringy threads in celery. Cellulose is made up of long, straight chains of glucose molecules (see **FIGURE 4.10**). Grains, fruits, vegetables, and nuts all contain cellulose.

Hemicelluloses The **hemicelluloses** are a diverse group of polysaccharides that vary from plant to plant. They are mixed with cellulose in plant cell walls.[13] Hemicelluloses are composed of a variety of monosaccharides with many branching side chains. The outer bran layer on many cereal grains is rich in hemicelluloses, as are legumes, vegetables, and nuts.

- ▶ **dietary fiber** Carbohydrates and lignins that are naturally in plants and are nondigestible; that is, they are not digested and absorbed in the human small intestine.
- ▶ **functional fiber** Isolated nondigestible carbohydrates, including some manufactured carbohydrates, that have beneficial effects in humans.
- ▶ **total fiber** The sum of dietary fiber and functional fiber.
- ▶ **soluble fiber** Nondigestible carbohydrates that dissolve in water.
- ▶ **insoluble fiber** Nondigestible carbohydrates that do not dissolve in water.
- ▶ **cellulose** [SELL-you-los] A straight-chain polysaccharide composed of hundreds of glucose units linked by beta bonds. It is nondigestible by humans and a component of dietary fiber.
- ▶ **hemicelluloses** [hem-ih-SELL-you-los-es] A group of large polysaccharides in dietary fiber that are fermented more easily than cellulose.

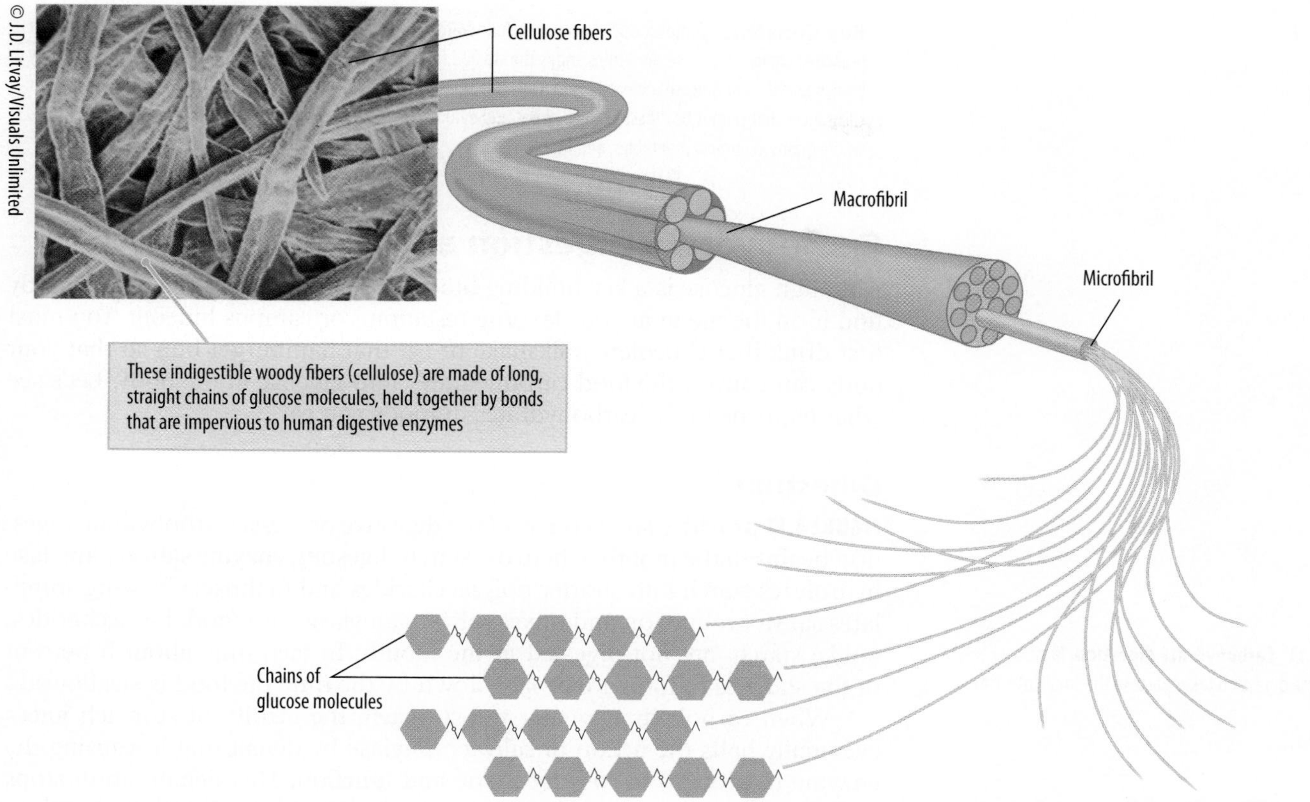
© J.D. Litvay/Visuals Unlimited
Cellulose fibers
Macrofibril
Microfibril
These indigestible woody fibers (cellulose) are made of long, straight chains of glucose molecules, held together by bonds that are impervious to human digestive enzymes
Chains of glucose molecules

FIGURE 4.10 The structure of cellulose. Cellulose forms the nondigestible, fibrous component of plants and is part of grasses, trees, fruits, and vegetables.

Pectins **Pectins** are gel-forming polysaccharides found in all plants, especially fruits. The pectin in fruits acts like a cement that gives body to fruits and helps them keep their shape. When fruit becomes overripe, pectin breaks down into monosaccharides and the fruit becomes mushy. When mixed with sugar and acid, pectin forms a gel that the food industry uses to add firmness to jellies, jams, sauces, and salad dressings.

Gums and Mucilages Like pectin, **gums** and **mucilages** are thick, gel-forming fibers that help hold plant cells together. The food industry uses plant gums such as gum arabic, guar gum, locust bean gum, and xanthan gum, and mucilages such as carrageenan to thicken, stabilize, or add texture to foods such as salad dressings, puddings, pie fillings, candies, sauces, and even drinks. **Psyllium** (the husk of psyllium seeds) is a mucilage that becomes very viscous when mixed with water. It is the main component in the laxative Metamucil and is being added to some breakfast cereals.

Lignins **Lignins** are not actually carbohydrates. Rather, these nondigestible substances make up the woody parts of vegetables such as carrots and broccoli and the seeds of fruits such as strawberries.

β-Glucans **β-glucans** are polysaccharides of branched glucose units. These fibers are found in large amounts in barley and oats. β-glucan fiber is especially effective in lowering blood cholesterol levels (see the section "Carbohydrates and Health" later in this chapter).

Chitin and Chitosan **Chitin** and **chitosan** are polysaccharides found in the exoskeletons of crabs and lobsters and in the cell walls of most fungi. Chitin and chitosan are primarily consumed in supplement form. Although they are marketed as useful for weight control, published research does not support this claim.

Quick Bite

"An Apple a Day Keeps the Doctor Away"

Most likely this adage persisted over time because of the actual health benefits from apples. Apples have a high pectin content, a soluble fiber known to be an effective GI regulator.

- **pectins** A type of dietary fiber found in fruits.
- **gums** Dietary fibers, which contain galactose and other monosaccharides, found between plant cell walls.
- **mucilages** Gelatinous soluble fibers containing galactose, mannose, and other monosaccharides; found in seaweed.
- **psyllium** The dried husk of the psyllium seed.
- **lignins** [LIG-nins] Insoluble fibers composed of multi-ring alcohol units that constitute the only noncarbohydrate component of dietary fiber.
- **β-glucans** Functional fiber, consisting of branched polysaccharide chains of glucose, that helps lower blood cholesterol levels. Found in barley and oats.
- **chitosan** Polysaccharide derived from chitin.
- **chitin** A long-chain structural polysaccharide of slightly modified glucose. Found in the hard exterior skeletons of insects, crustaceans, and other invertebrates; also occurs in the cell walls of fungi.

Key Concepts Complex carbohydrates include starch, glycogen, and fiber. Starch is composed of straight or branched chains of glucose molecules and is the storage form of energy in plants. Glycogen is composed of highly branched chains of glucose molecules and is the storage form of energy in animals. Fibers include many different substances that cannot be digested by enzymes in the human intestinal tract and are found in plant foods, such as whole grains, legumes, vegetables, and fruits.

Carbohydrate Digestion and Absorption

Although glucose is a key building block of carbohydrates, you can't exactly find it on the menu at your favorite restaurant or campus hideout. You must first drink that chocolate milkshake or eat that hamburger bun so that your body can convert the food carbohydrates into glucose in the body. Let's see what happens to the carbohydrates in foods you eat.

Digestion

FIGURE 4.11 provides an overview of the digestive process. Carbohydrate digestion begins in the mouth, where the starch-digesting enzyme salivary amylase hydrolyzes starch into shorter polysaccharides and maltose. Chewing stimulates saliva production and mixes salivary amylase with food. Disaccharides, unlike starch, are not digested in the mouth. In fact, only about 5 percent of the starches in food are broken down by the time the food is swallowed.

When carbohydrates enter the stomach, the acidity of stomach juices eventually halts the action of salivary amylase by denaturing it, causing the enzyme (a protein) to lose its shape and function. This denaturation stops carbohydrate digestion, which restarts in the small intestine. Soluble fibers, such as pectins and gums, tend to delay digestive activity by slowing stomach emptying, thus providing a feeling of fullness after a meal.

Most carbohydrate digestion takes place in the small intestine. As the stomach contents enter the small intestine, the pancreas secretes pancreatic

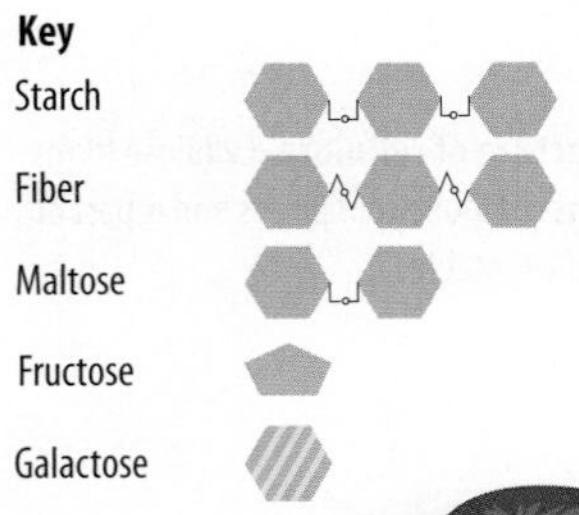

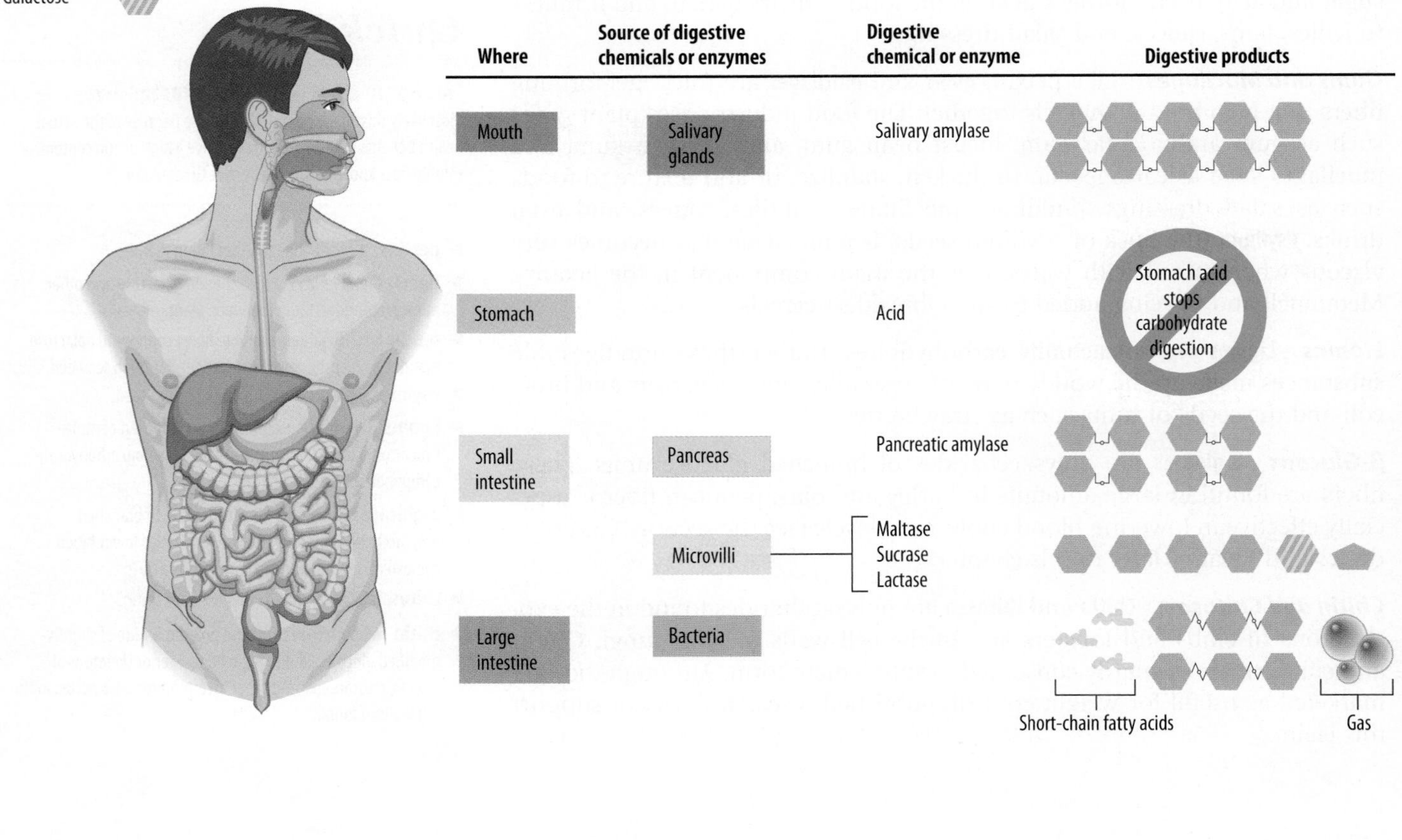

FIGURE 4.11 Carbohydrate digestion. Most carbohydrate digestion takes place in the small intestine.

amylase into the small intestine. **Pancreatic amylase** continues the digestion of starch, breaking it into many units of the disaccharide maltose.

Meanwhile, enzymes attached to the brush border (microvilli) of the mucosal cells lining the intestinal tract go to work. These digestive enzymes, called brush border disaccharidases, break disaccharides into monosaccharides to be absorbed. The enzyme maltase splits maltose into two glucose molecules. The enzyme sucrase splits sucrose into glucose and fructose. The enzyme lactase splits lactose into glucose and galactose.

The bonds that link glucose molecules in complex carbohydrates are called glycosidic bonds. The two forms of these bonds, **alpha (α) bonds** and **beta (β) bonds**, have important differences (see **FIGURE 4.12**). Human enzymes easily break alpha bonds, making glucose available from the polysaccharides starch and glycogen. Our bodies don't have enzymes to break most beta bonds found in fiber. With fiber remaining intact in the small intestine, it can act as a bulky barrier between other nutrients (e.g., glucose) and the brush border, delaying their digestion and absorption. Furthermore, soluble fiber can bind cholesterol and bile acids in the GI tract, inhibiting their absorption and enhancing their excretion in the stool. This can lead to lower blood cholesterol levels and, subsequently, decrease the risk for heart disease.

Beta bonds also link the galactose and glucose molecules in the disaccharide lactose, but the enzyme lactase is specifically tailored to attack this small molecule. People with a sufficient supply of the enzyme lactase can break these bonds. When lactase is lacking, however, the beta bonds remain unbroken and lactose remains undigested until bacteria in the colon can attack it.

Enzymes are highly specific; they speed up only certain reactions and work on only certain molecules. Humans lack the digestive enzymes needed to break down the oligosaccharides raffinose and stachyose, for example. The commercial product Beano is an enzyme preparation. When taken immediately before eating beans or other gas-forming vegetables, Beano helps break oligosaccharides into monosaccharides so the body can absorb them.

Indigestible carbohydrates remain intact as they enter the large intestine. These carbohydrates can be fiber or resistant starch, or the small intestine might have lacked the necessary enzymes to break them down. In the large intestine, bacteria partially ferment (break down) undigested carbohydrates and produce gas and short-chain fatty acids. These fatty acids are absorbed into the colon and are used for energy by the colon cells. In addition, these fatty acids might reduce the risk of developing gastrointestinal disorders, cancers, and cardiovascular disease.[14]

Some fibers, particularly cellulose (insoluble) and psyllium (soluble), pass through the large intestine unchanged and therefore produce little gas. Instead, these fibers add to the stool weight and water content, making it easier to pass. By making stools easier to pass, insoluble fibers reduce the risk of constipation, diverticular disease (formation of bulging pouches in the colon that can become infected), and colon cancer.

Absorption

Monosaccharides are absorbed into the mucosal cells lining the small intestine by two different mechanisms. Fructose is absorbed by facilitated diffusion, whereas glucose and galactose depend on an active transport mechanism. A sodium-dependent glucose transport protein helps move glucose and galactose across the intestinal cell's membrane. The carrier protein in the cell membrane is first loaded with sodium, and then either glucose or galactose can attach to it.[15] Energy for this process is provided by the hydrolysis of adenosine triphosphate (ATP). Fructose absorption is slower than that of glucose or galactose. In the villi, absorbed monosaccharides pass through the intestinal mucosal

- **pancreatic amylase** Starch-digesting enzyme secreted by the pancreas.
- **alpha (α) bonds** Chemical bonds linking two monosaccharides (glycosidic bonds) that can be broken by human intestinal enzymes, releasing the individual monosaccharides. Maltose and sucrose contain alpha bonds.
- **beta (β) bonds** Chemical bonds linking two monosaccharides (glycosidic bonds) that cannot be broken by human intestinal enzymes. Cellulose contains beta bonds.

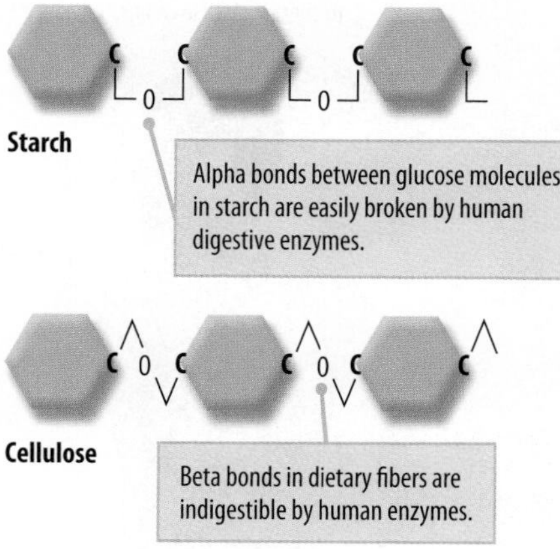

FIGURE 4.12 Alpha bonds and beta bonds. Human digestive enzymes can easily break the alpha bonds in starch, but they cannot break the beta bonds in cellulose.

cells and enter the bloodstream. Glucose, galactose, and fructose molecules travel to the liver by the portal vein, where galactose and fructose are converted into glucose or used for energy. The liver stores and releases glucose as needed to maintain constant blood glucose levels. **FIGURE 4.13** illustrates the digestion and absorption of carbohydrates. **TABLE 4.2** summarizes the effects of fiber on digestion and absorption and the health benefits of these effects.

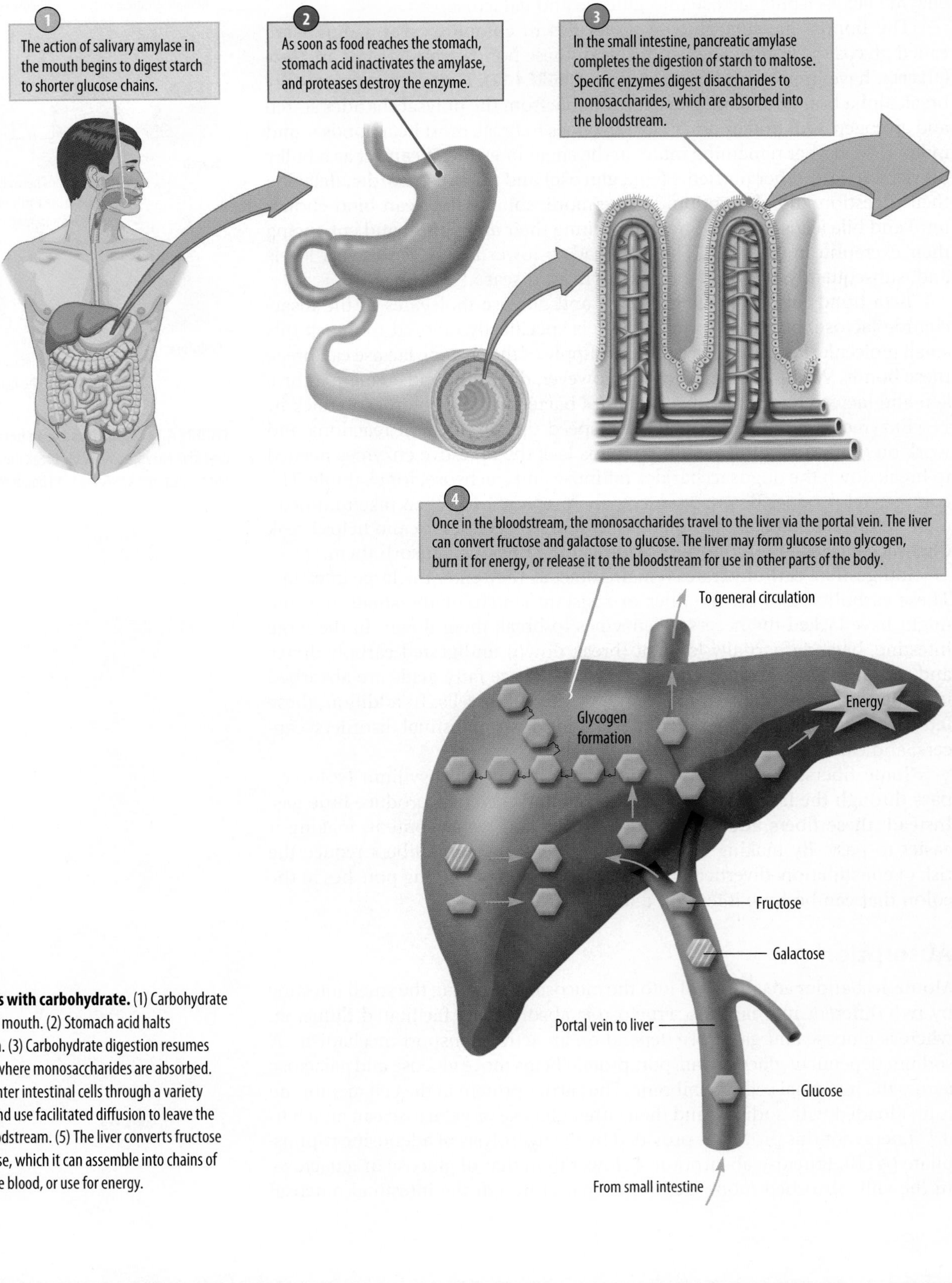

1
The action of salivary amylase in the mouth begins to digest starch to shorter glucose chains.
2
As soon as food reaches the stomach, stomach acid inactivates the amylase, and proteases destroy the enzyme.
3
In the small intestine, pancreatic amylase completes the digestion of starch to maltose. Specific enzymes digest disaccharides to monosaccharides, which are absorbed into the bloodstream.
4
Once in the bloodstream, the monosaccharides travel to the liver via the portal vein. The liver can convert fructose and galactose to glucose. The liver may form glucose into glycogen, burn it for energy, or release it to the bloodstream for use in other parts of the body.
To general circulation
Energy
Glycogen formation
Fructose
Galactose
Portal vein to liver
Glucose
From small intestine

FIGURE 4.13 Travels with carbohydrate. (1) Carbohydrate digestion begins in the mouth. (2) Stomach acid halts carbohydrate digestion. (3) Carbohydrate digestion resumes in the small intestine, where monosaccharides are absorbed. (4) Monosaccharides enter intestinal cells through a variety of transport proteins and use facilitated diffusion to leave the cells and enter the bloodstream. (5) The liver converts fructose and galactose to glucose, which it can assemble into chains of glycogen, release to the blood, or use for energy.

TABLE 4.2
Summary of the Effects and Health Benefits of Fiber in the GI Tract

Digestive System	Effect on Digestion/Absorption	Health Benefit
Mouth	• Increased chewing	Eating less at a meal promotes calorie control. Reduces risk for *obesity*.
Stomach	• Increased feeling of fullness/satiety • Increased stomach distention • Delayed gastric emptying	Eating less between meals promotes calorie control. Reduces risk for *obesity*.
Small intestine	• Delays absorption of nutrients by physically blocking from brush border and digestive enzymes • Decreases glycemic and insulin response • Binds cholesterol/bile acids and prevents absorption	Reduces risk for *type 2 diabetes* and *heart disease*.
Large intestine	• Promotes growth of healthy bacteria • Fermentation produces beneficial short-chain fatty acids • Adds bulk to feces; decreases intestinal transit time	Reduces risk of *colon cancer* and *diverticular disease*. Reduces *constipation*.

Key Concepts Carbohydrate digestion takes place primarily in the small intestine, where digestible carbohydrates are broken down and absorbed as monosaccharides. Bacteria in the large intestine partially ferment resistant starch and some types of fiber, producing gas and a few short-chain fatty acids that can be absorbed through the large intestine and used for energy. The liver converts absorbed monosaccharides into glucose.

Carbohydrates in the Body

Through the processes of digestion and absorption, the carbohydrates from our varied diet of vegetables, fruits, grains, and milk ultimately become glucose. Glucose has one major role—to supply energy for the body.

Normal Use of Glucose

Cells throughout the body depend on glucose for energy to drive chemical processes. Although most—but not all—cells can also burn fat for energy, the body needs some glucose to burn fat efficiently.

When we eat food, our bodies immediately use some glucose to maintain normal blood glucose levels. We store excess glucose as glycogen in liver and muscle tissue. Insulin and glucagon, two hormones produced by the pancreas, closely regulate blood glucose levels.

Using Glucose for Energy

Glucose is the primary fuel for most cells in the body and the preferred fuel for the brain, red blood cells, nervous system, fetus, and placenta. Even when fat is burned for energy, a small amount of glucose is needed to break down fat completely. To obtain energy from glucose, cells must first take up glucose from the blood. Once glucose enters cells, a series of metabolic reactions break it down into carbon dioxide and water, releasing energy in a form that the body can use.[16]

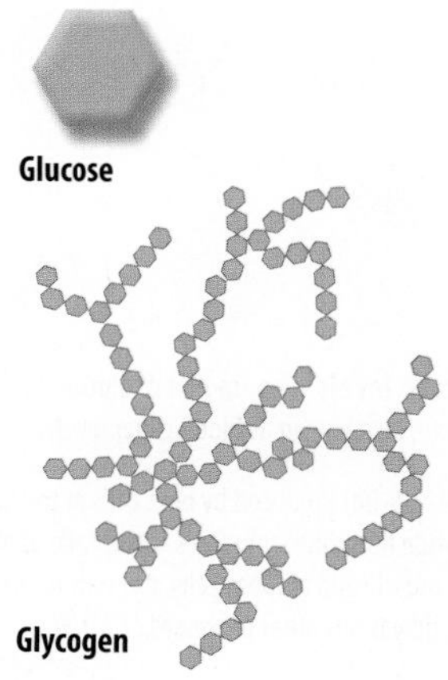

Storing Glucose as Glycogen

To store excess glucose, the body assembles it into the long, branched chains of glycogen. Glycogen can be broken down quickly, releasing glucose for energy as needed. Liver glycogen stores are used to maintain normal blood glucose levels and account for about one-third of the body's total glycogen stores. Muscle glycogen stores are used to fuel muscle activity and account for about two-thirds of the body's total glycogen stores.[17] The body can store only limited amounts of glycogen—usually enough to last from a few hours to one day, depending on activity level.[18]

Sparing Body Protein

In the absence of carbohydrate, both proteins and fats can be used for energy. Although most cells can break down fat for energy, brain cells and developing red blood cells require a constant supply of glucose.[19] (After an extended period of starvation, the brain adapts and is able to use ketone bodies from fat breakdown for part of its energy needs.) If glycogen stores are depleted and glucose is not provided in the diet, the body must make its own glucose from protein to maintain blood levels and supply glucose to the brain. Adequate consumption of dietary carbohydrate spares body proteins from being broken down and used to make glucose.

Preventing Ketosis

▶ **ketone bodies** Molecules formed when insufficient carbohydrate is available to completely metabolize fat. Formation of ketone bodies is promoted by a low glucose level and high acetyl CoA level within cells.

▶ **ketosis** [kee-TOE-sis] Abnormally high concentration of ketone bodies in body tissues and fluids.

Even when fat provides the fuel for cells, cells require a small amount of carbohydrate to completely break down fat to release energy. When no carbohydrate is available, the liver cannot break down fat completely. Instead, it produces small compounds called **ketone bodies**.[20] Most cells can use ketone bodies for energy.

When ketone bodies are produced more quickly than the body can use them, ketone levels build up in the blood and can cause a condition known as **ketosis**. People vulnerable to ketosis include those who consume only small amounts of carbohydrate or who cannot metabolize blood glucose normally. Ketosis is most commonly caused by very low carbohydrate diets, starvation, uncontrolled diabetes mellitus, and chronic alcoholism. Ketosis also can develop when fluid intake is too low to allow the kidneys to excrete excess ketone bodies. As the concentration of ketone bodies increases, the blood becomes too acidic. The body loses water as it excretes excess ketones in urine, and dehydration is a common consequence of ketosis. To prevent ketosis, the body needs a minimum of 50 to 100 grams of carbohydrate daily.[21]

Key Concepts Glucose circulates in the blood to provide immediate energy to cells. The body stores excess glucose in the liver and muscle as glycogen. The body needs adequate carbohydrate intake to prevent the breakdown of body proteins to fulfill glucose or energy needs. The body needs some carbohydrate to completely break down fat and prevent the buildup of ketone bodies in the blood.

Regulating Blood Glucose Levels

The body closely regulates **blood glucose levels** (also known as blood sugar levels) to maintain an adequate supply of glucose for cells. If blood glucose levels drop too low, a person becomes shaky and weak. If blood glucose levels rise too high, a person becomes sluggish and confused and can have difficulty breathing.

Two hormones produced by the pancreas tightly control blood glucose levels.[22] When blood glucose levels rise after a meal, special pancreatic cells called beta cells release the hormone insulin into the blood. **Insulin** acts like a key, "unlocking" the cells of the body and allowing glucose to enter and fuel them. Insulin works on receptors on the surface of cells, increasing their affinity for glucose and increasing glucose uptake by cells. It also stimulates liver and muscle cells to store glucose as glycogen. As glucose enters cells to deliver energy or be stored as glycogen, blood glucose levels return to normal. (See **FIGURE 4.14a**.)

▶ **blood glucose levels** The amount of glucose in the blood at any given time. Also known as blood sugar levels.

▶ **insulin** [IN-suh-lin] Produced by beta cells in the pancreas, this polypeptide hormone stimulates the uptake of blood glucose into muscle and adipose cells, the synthesis of glycogen in the liver, and various other processes.

▶ **glucagon** [GLOO-kuh-gon] Produced by alpha cells in the pancreas, this polypeptide hormone promotes the breakdown of liver glycogen to glucose, thereby increasing blood glucose. Glucagon secretion is stimulated by low blood glucose levels and by growth hormone.

When an individual has not eaten in a while and blood glucose levels begin to fall, alpha cells in the pancreas release another hormone, **glucagon**. Glucagon stimulates the breakdown of glycogen stores to release glucose into the bloodstream. (See **FIGURE 4.14b**.) It also stimulates gluconeogenesis, or the

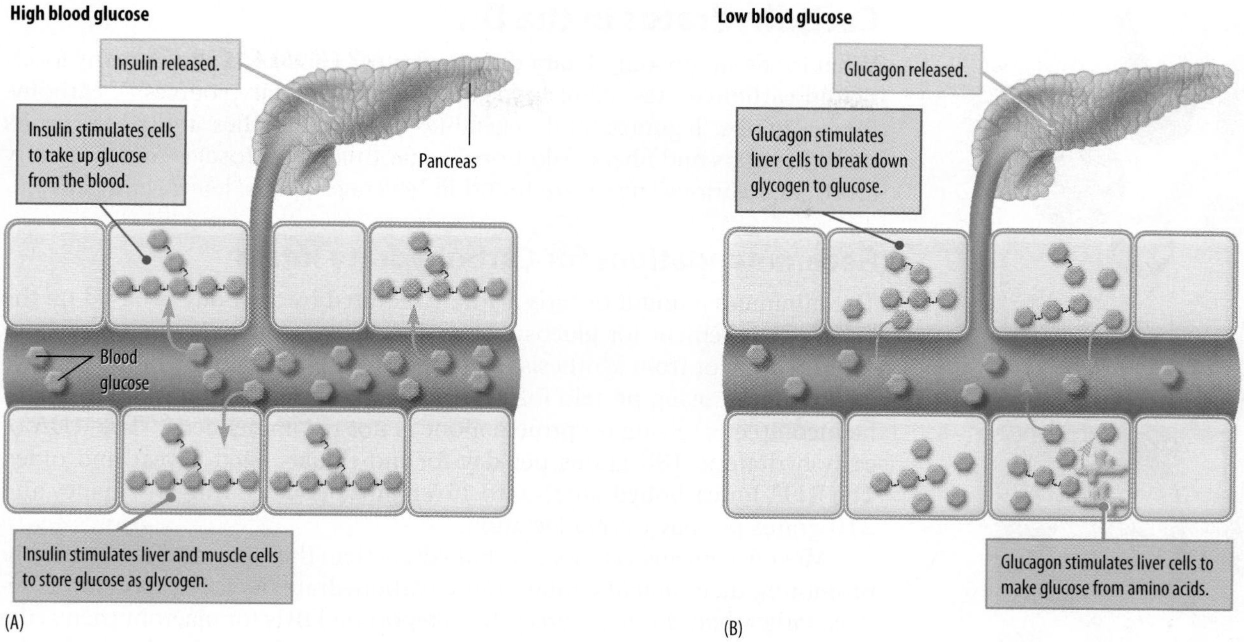
High blood glucose
Insulin released.
Insulin stimulates cells to take up glucose from the blood.
Pancreas
Blood glucose
Insulin stimulates liver and muscle cells to store glucose as glycogen.
(A)
Low blood glucose
Glucagon released.
Glucagon stimulates liver cells to break down glycogen to glucose.
Glucagon stimulates liver cells to make glucose from amino acids.
(B)

FIGURE 4.14 Regulating blood glucose levels. Insulin and glucagon have opposing actions. (a) Insulin acts to lower blood glucose levels, and (b) glucagon acts to raise them.

synthesis of glucose from protein. Another hormone, **epinephrine** (also called adrenaline), exerts effects similar to glucagon to ensure that all body cells have adequate energy for emergencies. Released by the adrenal glands in response to sudden stress or danger, epinephrine is called the fight-or-flight hormone.

Different foods vary in their effect on blood glucose levels. Foods rich in simple carbohydrates or starch but low in fat or fiber tend to be digested and absorbed rapidly. This rapid absorption causes a corresponding large and rapid rise in blood glucose levels.[23] The body reacts to this rise by pumping out extra insulin, which in turn lowers blood sugar levels. Other foods—especially those rich in dietary fiber, resistant starch, or fat—cause a less dramatic blood glucose response accompanied by smaller swings in blood glucose levels.

The **glycemic index** measures the effect of a food on blood glucose levels. The **glycemic load** is similar to the glycemic index except that it accounts for the amount of carbohydrates in a serving of a given food. Foods with a high glycemic index and/or glycemic load cause a faster and higher rise in blood glucose, whereas foods with a low glycemic index/glycemic load cause a slower rise in blood glucose.[24,25] See the FYI feature "The Glycemic Index of Foods: Useful or Useless?" to learn more about using glycemic index and glycemic load as a guide for a healthy diet.

▶ **epinephrine** A hormone released in response to stress or sudden danger, epinephrine raises blood glucose levels to ready the body for "fight or flight." Also called adrenaline.

▶ **glycemic index** A measure of the effect of food on blood glucose levels. It is the ratio of the blood glucose value after eating a particular food to the value after eating the same amount of white bread or glucose.

▶ **glycemic load** The glycemic index of a food adjusted for the amount of carbohydrate in one serving: (glycemic index × g carbohydrate per serving)/100.

▶ **diabetes mellitus** A chronic disease in which uptake of blood glucose by body cells is impaired, resulting in high glucose levels in the blood and urine. Type 1 is caused by decreased pancreatic release of insulin. In type 2, target cells (e.g., fat and muscle cells) lose the ability to respond normally to insulin.

Inadequate Regulation of Blood Glucose Levels: Diabetes Mellitus

When people have **diabetes mellitus**, their bodies either do not produce enough insulin (most common in type 1 diabetes) or do not use insulin properly (most common in type 2 diabetes). If diabetes is not treated and controlled, blood glucose levels are chronically elevated, causing serious complications and premature death.[26] Although scientists don't completely understand the causes of diabetes, both genetics and environmental factors (obesity and lack of exercise, for example) appear to be involved. A high-sugar diet alone does not directly cause diabetes.

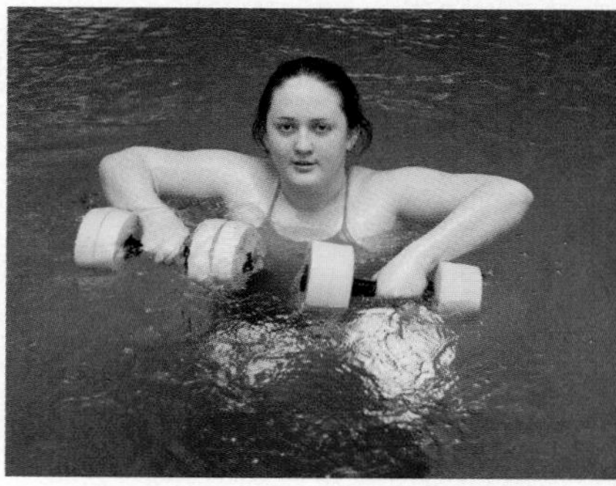

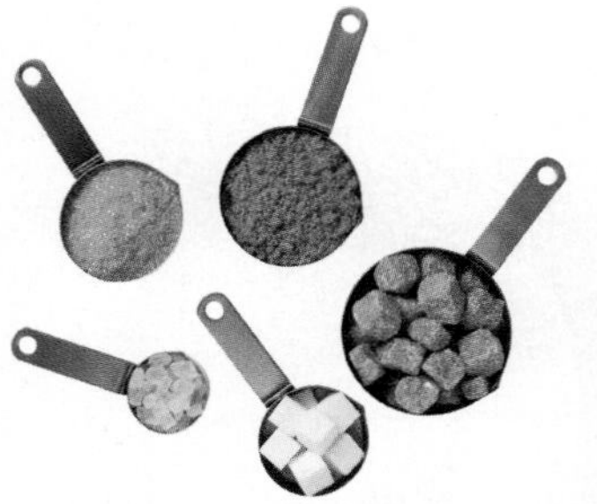

© Photodisc

Table and brown sugar and corn syrup are rich in sucrose, a simple carbohydrate.

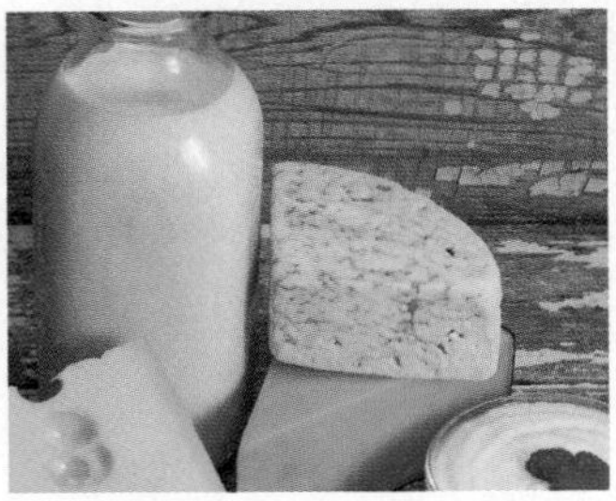

© Comstock/Thinkstock

Milk and milk products are rich in lactose, a simple carbohydrate.

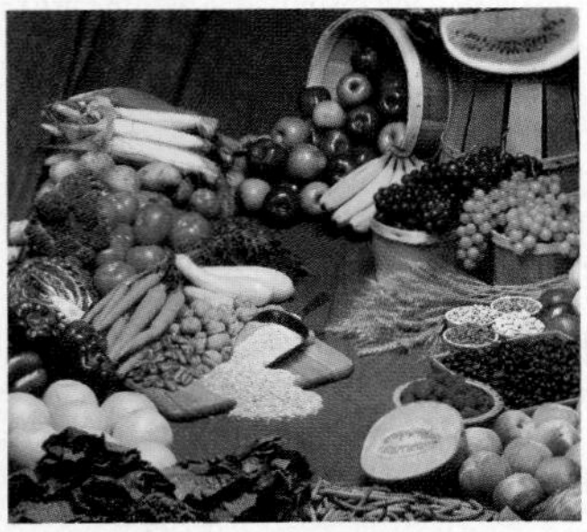

Photo by Keith Weller. Courtesy of USDA.

Fruits and vegetables provide simple sugars, starch, and fiber.

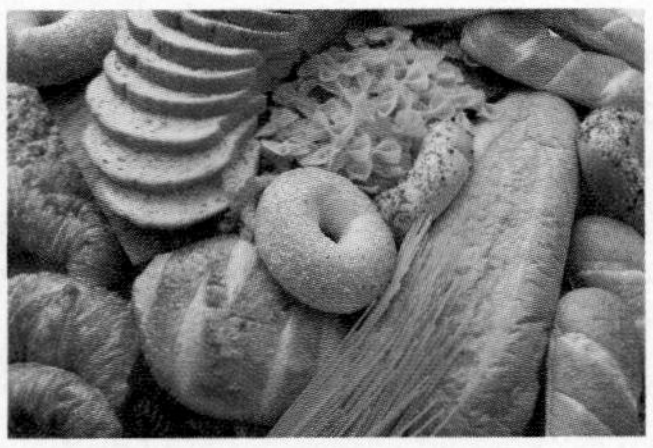

© Morgan Lane Photography/ShutterStock, Inc.

Bread, cornmeal, rice, and pasta are rich in starch and, sometimes, dietary fiber.

FIGURE 4.15 Carbohydrate sources.

Carbohydrates in the Diet

What foods supply our dietary carbohydrates? **FIGURE 4.15** shows many foods rich in carbohydrates. Plant foods are our main dietary sources of carbohydrates: grains, legumes, and vegetables provide starches and fibers; fruits provide sugars and fibers. Additional sugar (mainly lactose) is found in dairy foods, and various sugars are found in beverages, jams, jellies, and candy.

Recommendations for Carbohydrate Intake

The minimum amount of carbohydrate required by the body is based on the brain's requirement for glucose. This glucose can come either from dietary carbohydrate or from synthesis of glucose from protein in the body. Because adaptation to using protein for glucose and ketone bodies for energy might be incomplete, relying on protein alone is not recommended.[27] The RDA of carbohydrate is 130 grams per day for individuals aged 1 year and older. The RDA for carbohydrate rises to 175 grams per day during pregnancy and 210 grams per day during lactation.

Most Americans eat more carbohydrate than this amount. In fact, health-promoting diets *should* contain more carbohydrate, focusing more on complex, rather than simple, sources. In its report on DRIs for macronutrients, the Food and Nutrition Board developed recommended ranges of intake for the energy-yielding nutrients. The Acceptable Macronutrient Distribution Range (AMDR) for carbohydrate is 45 to 65 percent of kilocalories. For an adult who eats about 2,000 kilocalories daily, this represents 225 to 325 grams of carbohydrate. The Daily Value for carbohydrates is 300 grams per day, representing 60 percent of the calories in a 2,000-kilocalorie diet.

The *Dietary Guidelines for Americans, 2015–2020* suggest that we limit intake of added sugars in an effort to build healthy eating patterns."[28] One key recommendation is to choose and prepare nutrient dense foods and beverages with little added sugar.[28A] Although the AMDR for added sugars is no more than 25 percent of daily energy intake, a point at which the micronutrient quality of the diet declines, many sources suggest that added sugar intake should be even lower. For example, the *Dietary Guidelines* and World Health Organization recommend limiting added sugar to less than 10 percent of total energy intake.

The *Dietary Guidelines for Americans, 2015–2020* also recommend that we consume a healthy eating pattern that includes a variety of vegetables from all the subgroups, including dark-green, red, and orange, legumes (beans and peas), starchy and other vegetables; fruits, especially whole fruits; and grains, at least half of which are whole grains.[29] In doing so, individuals can meet the recommendations for fiber. It is important to choose a variety of fruits, vegetables, and whole grains, along with legumes, in order to consume a healthy balance of both soluble and insoluble fiber. In general, fruits, oat bran, barley, and legumes contain soluble fiber, whereas most other whole grains and vegetables contain insoluble fiber. However, most high-fiber foods contain some combination of both. For example, fruits, like apples, contain insoluble fiber in their skin, and some vegetables, like carrots and broccoli, contain a fair amount of soluble fiber. The Adequate Intake (AI) value for total fiber is 38 grams per day for men aged 19 to 50 years, and 25 grams per day for women in the same age group. For men and women over 50 years, fiber recommendations are set at 30 grams per day and 21 grams per day, respectively, due to decreased calorie needs. The AI for fiber is based on a level of intake (14 grams per 1,000 kilocalories) that provides the greatest risk reduction for heart disease.[30] The Daily Value for fiber used on food labels is 25 grams.

Quick Bite

Carbohydrate Companions

The word *companion* comes from the Latin *companio*, meaning "one who shares bread."

Current Consumption

American adults currently consume about 49 to 50 percent of their energy intake as carbohydrate, which falls within the AMDR; however, this does not account for the quality of the carbohydrates consumed. According to the National Health and Nutrition Examination Survey (NHANES) data, 13 percent of the population has an added sugar intake of more than 25 percent of calories, with a mean equivalent of added sugar intake of about 83 grams per day.[31] About one-third of the added sugar intake for Americans comes from nondiet soft drinks in the form of white sugar and high-fructose corn syrup. This is of concern because as soft drink consumption rises, energy intake increases, but milk consumption and the vitamin and mineral quality of the diet decline.[32] Many studies suggest that rising soft drink and sugar-sweetened beverage consumption is a factor in overweight and obesity, even among very young children.[33] Regular soft drinks, sugary sweets, sweetened grains, and regular fruitades/drinks comprise 72 percent of the intake of added sugar.[34]

Most Americans do not consume enough dietary fiber, with usual intakes averaging only 15 grams per day.[35] This is due to the fact that Americans do not meet the recommended intakes of fruits, vegetables, and whole grains. With the exception of older women (51 years and older), fewer than 5 percent of individuals in all other life-stage groups have fiber intakes meeting or exceeding the AI.[36] The major sources of dietary fiber in the American diet are white flour and potatoes, not because they are concentrated fiber sources, but because they are widely consumed.[37]

THINK About It 2

Choosing Carbohydrates Wisely

The 2015-2020 *Dietary Guidelines for Americans* encourages us to consume a healthy eating pattern that contains fruits, vegetables, legumes. whole grains, and fat-free or low-fat milk while keeping calorie intake under control. These foods are all good sources of carbohydrates and many other nutrients. Choosing a variety of whole fruits and vegetables, and in particular including choices from all vegetable subgroups (dark-green vegetables, orange vegetables, legumes, starchy vegetables, and other vegetables), provides fiber as well as vitamin A, vitamin C, folate, and potassium.

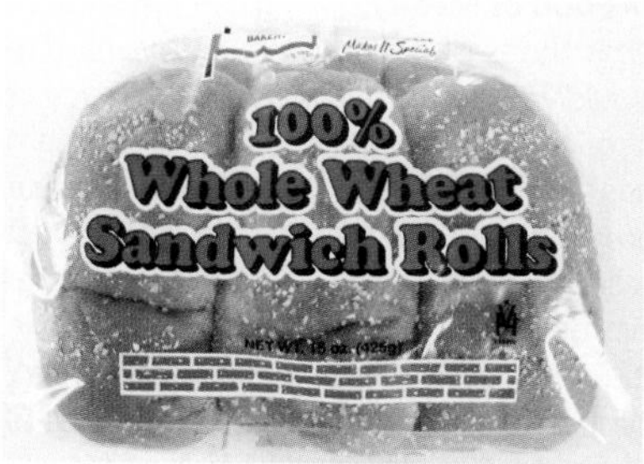

Strategies for Increasing Fiber Intake

Along with fruits and vegetables, whole grains are important sources of fiber. Whole kernels of grains consist of four parts: germ, endosperm, bran, and husk (see **FIGURE 4.16**). The **germ**, the innermost part at the base of the kernel,

▶ **germ** The innermost part of a grain, located at the base of the kernel, that can grow into a new plant. The germ is rich in protein, oils, vitamins, and minerals.

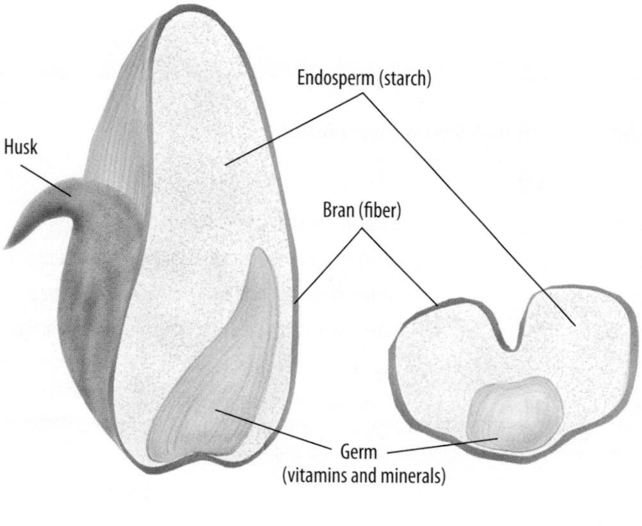

FIGURE 4.16 Anatomy of a kernel of grain. Whole kernels of grains consist of four parts: germ, endosperm, bran, and husk.

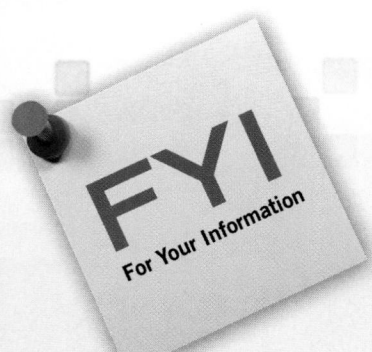

FYI For Your Information

The Glycemic Index of Foods: Useful or Useless?

Although controversial, the glycemic index is a valuable and easy-to-use concept.[a] Some contend that although it is promising, more definitive data are needed before this concept should be promoted for widespread public use.[b] Several popular weight-loss diets use the glycemic index to guide food choices.

How Is the Glycemic Index Measured?

The glycemic index classifies foods or meals based on their potential to raise blood glucose levels. It compares the change in blood glucose after eating a sample food to the change expected from eating an equal amount of available carbohydrate from a standard food such as white bread or pure glucose.[c] Thus, the glycemic index is expressed as a percentage, ranging from 1 to 100, with 100 being the standard food.

Foods with a high glycemic index trigger a sharp rise in blood glucose, followed by a dramatic fall, often to levels that are transiently below normal. In contrast, low-glycemic-index foods trigger slower and more modest changes in blood glucose levels.

What Factors Affect the Glycemic Index of a Food or Meal?

The glycemic index of a food is not always easy to predict. Would you expect a high-sugar food such as ice cream to have a high glycemic index? Ice cream actually has a low index because its fat slows sugar absorption. On the other hand, wouldn't you expect complex carbohydrate foods such as bread or potatoes to have a low glycemic index? In fact, the starch in white bread and cooked potatoes is readily absorbed, so each has a high value.[d] The glycemic indices of some common foods are listed in **Table A**, and lower-glycemic-index substitutions are given in **Table B**.

The type of carbohydrate, the cooking process, and the presence of fat and dietary fiber all affect a food's glycemic index.[e,f] Because fiber can delay gastric emptying and create a physical barrier between nutrients and digestive enzymes, fiber slows the absorption of glucose, thus lowering the glycemic index of foods.[g] In a person's diet, it is the glycemic index of mixed meals, referred to as the glycemic load of a meal, rather than the individual foods, that counts.[h] That is, the glycemic load takes the glycemic index and accounts for the amount of carbohydrate consumed. Glycemic load is calculated by multiplying the glycemic index of a food by carbohydrate content in one serving. Because the glycemic index is expressed as a percentage, the resulting value must then be divided by 100. It is important to note that a high glycemic index food may not necessarily have a high glycemic load if there is only a small amount of carbohydrate in a serving. Watermelon is a good example of this. It has a high glycemic index of 72, but a lower glycemic load because it is mostly water, and the carbohydrate content in a serving is relatively low.[i]

TABLE A
Glycemic Index of Some Foods Compared to Pure Glucose[a]

Food	Glycemic Index	Food	Glycemic Index
Bakery Products		Skim milk	36
Cake	67	**Fruits**	
Waffles	76	Apples	38
Bread		Bananas	52
White bread	73	Pineapple	59
Whole-wheat bread, whole-meal flour	71	**Legumes**	
		Black-eyed peas	42
Breakfast Cereals		Lentils	29
Bran	42	**Pasta**	
Corn flakes	81	Spaghetti	42
Oatmeal	58	Macaroni	47
Cereal Grains		**Vegetables**	
Barley	25	Carrots	47
Sweet corn	53	Baked potatoes	85
White rice, long grain	56	Green peas	48
Bulger	45	**Candy**	
Dairy Foods		Jelly beans	78
Ice cream	61	Life Savers	70

[a] Glycemic response to pure glucose is 100.

Data from Foster-Powell K, Holt SHA, Brand-Miller JC. International table of glycemic index and glycemic load values: 2002. *Am J Clin Nutr.* 2002;76:5–56.

TABLE B
Sample Substitutions for High-Glycemic-Index Foods[a]

High-Glycemic-Index Food	Low-Glycemic-Index Alternative
Bread, wheat or white	Oat bran, rye, or pumpernickel bread
Processed breakfast cereal	Unrefined cereal such as oats (either muesli or oatmeal) or bran cereal
Plain cookies and crackers	Cookies made with nuts and whole grains such as oats
Cakes and muffins	Cakes and muffins made with fruit, oats, or whole grains
Bananas	Apples
White potatoes	Sweet potatoes, pastas, or legumes

[a] Low glycemic index = 56 or less; medium = 56–69; and high = 70 or more.

Why Do Some Researchers Believe the Glycemic Index Is Useful?

Foods with a high glycemic load will cause dramatic increases in blood glucose, which can lead to large spikes in insulin and a subsequent drop in blood glucose, often temporarily falling below baseline glucose levels. Dips in blood glucose can increase hunger after a meal, and increased insulin can have negative effects on fat metabolism and storage. Therefore, the health benefits of following a low-glycemic-load diet can be significant. Diets that emphasize low-glycemic-index foods decrease the risk of developing type 2 diabetes and improve blood sugar control in people who are already afflicted.[j] Epidemiological studies suggest that such diets, which tend to be higher in fiber, reduce the risk of colon and other cancers[k] and might help reduce the risk of heart disease as well. Diets with a low glycemic load are associated with higher high-density lipoprotein (HDL) cholesterol levels and with reduced incidence of heart attack.[l] Also, studies indicate that the effectiveness of low-fat, high-carbohydrate diets for weight loss can be improved by reducing their glycemic load.[m,n]

Why Do Some Researchers Believe the Glycemic Index Is Useless?

Some researchers question the usefulness of conclusions drawn primarily from epidemiological studies.[o,p] Epidemiological studies can show association but cannot prove causation. Also, researchers worry about the inconsistencies in the use of glucose or white bread as the standard and the wide variations in measured glycemic responses to individual foods.

Many believe that the glycemic index is too complex for most people to use effectively. The position of the American Diabetes Association is that the glycemic index and load can provide additional benefit in the management of diabetes over that observed when total carbohydrate is considered alone.[q]

What's the Bottom Line?

Like many other nutrition issues, the glycemic index needs further study. We need to continue to identify the influence of processing techniques on the glycemic index and agree on methodologies and standards for measuring it. Most researchers also call for prospective, long-term clinical trials to evaluate the effects of low-glycemic-index and low-glycemic-load diets in chronic disease risk reduction and treatment.[r] Until then, encouraging the consumption of whole-grain, minimally refined cereal products and other low-glycemic-index foods won't hurt, and it might help to improve health!

a. Mondazzi L, Arcelli, E. Glycemic index in sport nutrition. *J Am Coll Nutr.* 2009; 28(suppl):455S–463S.
b. Thomas DE, Elliott EJ. The use of low-glycaemic index diets in diabetes control. *Br J Nutr.* 2010;104(6):797–802.
c. Udani J, Singh B, Barrett M, Preuss H. Lowering the glycemic index of white bread using a white bean extract. *Nutr J.* 2009;8:52.
d. Williams SM, Venn BJ, Perry T, Brown R, Wallace A, Mann JI, Green TJ. Another approach to estimating the reliability of glycaemic index. *Br J Nutr.* 2008;100(2):354–372.
e. Bohado-Singh PS, Riles CK, Wheatley AO, Lowe HI. Relationship between processing method and the glycemic indices of ten sweet potato cultivars commonly consumed in Jamaica. *J Nutr Metab.* 2011;584832: http://www.hindawi.com/journals/jnme/2011/584832/cta/.
f. Wolever TM, Bhaskaran K. Use of glycemic index to estimate mixed-meal glycemic response. *Am J Clin Nutr.* 2012;95(1):256–257.
g. Scazzina F, Siebenhandl-Ehn S, Pellegrini N. The effect of dietary fibre on reducing glycemic index of bread. *Br J Nutr.* 2013;109:1163–1174.
h. Fabricatore AN, Ebbeling CB, Wadden TA, Ludwig DS. Continuous glucose monitoring to assess the ecologic validity of dietary glycemic index and glycemic load. *Am J Clin Nutr.* 2011;94(6):1519–1524.
i. Foster-Powell K, Holt SHA, Brand-Miller JC. International table of glycemic index and glycemic load values: 2002. *Am J Clin Nutr.* 2002;76:5–56.
j. Finley C, Barlow C, Halton T, Haskell W. Glycemic index, glycemic load, and prevalence of the metabolic syndrome in the Cooper Center Longitudinal Study. *J Am Diet Assoc.* 2010;110(12):1820–1829.
k. Cari K. Low-glycemic load diets: how does the evidence for prevention of disease measure up? *J Am Diet Assoc.* 2010;110(12):1818–1819.
l. Ibid.
m. Ibid.
n. Collinson A, Lindley R, Campbell A, Waters I, Lindley T, Wallace A. An evaluation of an Internet-based approach to weight loss with low glycaemic load principles. *J Hum Nutr Diet.* 2011;24(2):192–195.
o. Raben A. Should obese patients be counseled to follow a low-glycaemic index diet? No. *Obes Rev.* 2002;3(4):245–256.
p. Pi-Sunyer FX. Glycemic index and disease. *Am J Clin Nutr.* 2002;76(suppl):290S–298S.
q. American Diabetes Association. Nutrition recommendations and interventions for diabetes: a position statement of the American Diabetes Association. *Diabetes Care.* 2007;30(suppl 1):S48–65.
r. Esfahani A, Wong JM, Mirrahimi A, Villa CR, Kendall CW. The application of the glycemic index and glycemic load in weight loss: a review of the clinical evidence. *IUBMB Life.* 2011;63(1):7–13.

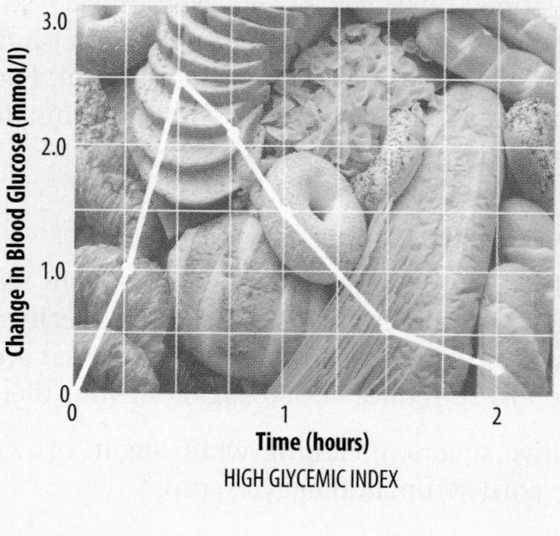

HIGH GLYCEMIC INDEX

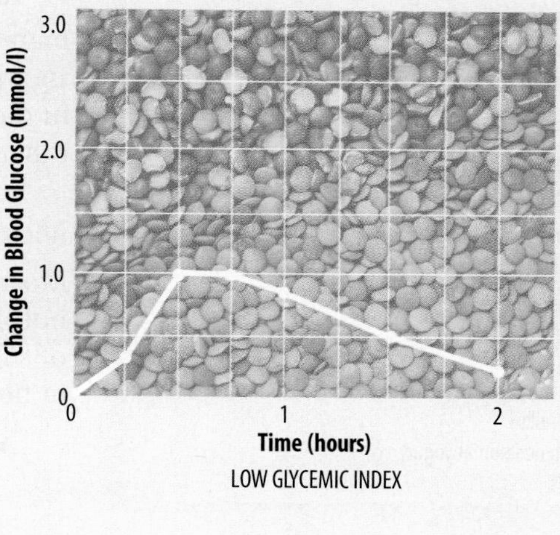

LOW GLYCEMIC INDEX

▶ **endosperm** The largest, middle portion of a grain kernel. The endosperm is high in starch to provide food for the growing plant embryo.

▶ **bran** The layers of protective coating around the grain kernel that are rich in dietary fiber and nutrients.

▶ **husk** The inedible covering of a grain kernel. Also known as the chaff.

is the portion that grows into a new plant. It is rich in protein, oils, vitamins, and minerals. The **endosperm** is the largest, middle portion of the grain kernel. It is high in starch and provides food for the growing plant embryo. The **bran** is composed of layers of protective coating around the grain kernel and is rich in dietary fiber. The **husk** is an inedible covering.

When grains are refined—making white flour from wheat, for example, or making white rice from brown rice—the process removes the outer husk and bran layers and sometimes the inner germ of the grain kernel. Because the bran and germ portions of the grain contain much of the dietary fiber, vitamins, and minerals, the nutrient content of whole grains is far superior to that of refined grains. Although food manufacturers add iron, thiamin, riboflavin, and niacin back to white flour to enrich it, they usually do not add back dietary fiber and nutrients such as vitamin B_6, calcium, phosphorus, potassium, magnesium, and zinc, which are also lost in processing.

Read food labels carefully to choose foods that contain whole grains. Terms such as *whole-wheat*, *whole-grain*, *rolled oats*, and *brown rice* indicate that the entire grain kernel is included in the food. Even better, look for the words *100 percent whole grain* or *100 percent whole wheat*. To increase your fiber intake:

- Eat more whole-grain breads, cereals, pasta, and rice, as well as more fruits, vegetables, and legumes.
- Eat fruits and vegetables with the peel, if possible. The peel is high in fiber.
- Add fruits to muffins and pancakes.
- Add legumes—such as lentils and pinto, navy, kidney, and black beans—to casseroles and mixed dishes as a meat substitute.
- Substitute whole-grain flour for all-purpose flour in recipes whenever possible.
- Use brown rice instead of white rice.
- Substitute oats for flour in crumb toppings.
- Choose high-fiber cereals.
- Choose whole fruits rather than fruit juices.
- Choose whole vegetables rather than vegetable juice.

When increasing your fiber intake, do so gradually and drink plenty of fluids to allow your body to adjust. Add just a few grams a day; otherwise, abdominal cramps, gas, bloating, and diarrhea or constipation can result. Parents and caregivers should also emphasize foods rich in fiber for children older than 2 years but must take care that these foods do not fill a child up before energy and nutrient needs are met. **TABLE 4.3** lists various foods that are high in simple and complex carbohydrates.

TABLE 4.3
High-Carbohydrate Foods

High in Complex Carbohydrates
- Bagels
- Cereals
- Corn
- Crackers
- Legumes
- Peas
- Popcorn
- Potatoes
- Rice Cakes
- Squash
- Tortillas

High in Simple Carbohydrates

Naturally Present
- Fruits
- Fruit juices
- Plain nonfat yogurt
- Skim milk

Added
- Cake
- Candy
- Cookies
- Frosting
- Gelatin
- High-sugar breakfast cereals
- Jams
- Jellies
- Sherbet
- Soft drinks
- Sweetened nonfat yogurt
- Syrups

Although health food stores, pharmacies, and even grocery stores sell many types of fiber supplements, most experts agree that you should first try to get fiber from whole foods rather than from a supplement. Foods rich in dietary fiber contain a variety of fibers as well as vitamins, minerals, and other phytochemicals that offer important health benefits.

Moderating Added Sugar Intake

Most of us enjoy the taste of sweet foods, and there's no reason why we should not. But for some individuals, habitually high sugar intake, specifically that of sugar added during processing of foods, crowds out foods that are higher in fiber, vitamins, and minerals. To reduce added sugars in your diet:

- Use less of all nutritive sugars, including white sugar, brown sugar, honey, high-fructose corn syrup, and agave syrup.

- Limit consumption of soft drinks, high-sugar breakfast cereals, candy, ice cream, and sweet desserts.
- Use fresh or frozen fruits and fruits canned in natural juices or light syrup for dessert and to sweeten waffles, pancakes, muffins, and breads.

Read ingredient lists carefully. Food labels list the total grams of sugar in a food, which includes both sugars naturally present in foods and sugars added to foods. Many terms for added sweeteners appear on food labels. Foods likely to be high in sugar list some form of sweetener as the first, second, or third ingredient on labels. **TABLE 4.4** lists various forms of sugar used in foods.

Sugar substitutes can help many people lower sugar intake, but foods with these substitutes might not provide less energy than similar products containing nutritive sweeteners. Rather than sugar, other energy-yielding nutrients, such as fat, are the primary source of the calories in these foods. Also, as sugar substitute use in the United States has increased, so has sugar consumption—an interesting paradox!

TABLE 4.4
Forms of Sugar Used in Foods

- Agave syrup
- Brown rice syrup
- Brown sugar
- Concentrated fruit juice sweetener
- Confectioner's sugar
- Corn syrup
- Dextrose
- Fructose
- Galactose
- Glucose
- Granulated sugar
- High-fructose corn syrup
- Invert sugar
- Lactose
- Levulose
- Maltose
- Mannitol
- Maple sugar
- Molasses
- Natural sweeteners
- Raw sugar
- Sorbitol
- Turbinado sugar
- White sugar
- Xylitol

Key Concepts Current recommendations suggest that Americans consume at least 130 grams of carbohydrate per day. An intake of total carbohydrates representing between 45 and 65 percent of total energy intake and a fiber intake of 14 grams per 1,000 kilocalories are associated with reduced heart disease risk. Added sugar should account for no more than 10 percent of daily energy. Americans generally eat too little fiber, far less than the Adequate Intake (AI) of 38 grams per day for men and 25 grams per day for women age 19 to 50 years. An emphasis on consuming whole grains, legumes, fruits, and vegetables would help to increase fiber intake.

Nutritive Sweeteners

Nutritive sweeteners are digestible carbohydrates and therefore provide energy. They include monosaccharides, disaccharides, and sugar alcohols from either natural or refined sources. White sugar, brown sugar, honey, maple syrup, glucose, fructose, xylitol, sorbitol, and mannitol are just some of the many nutritive sweeteners used in foods. One slice of angel food cake, for example,

▶ **nutritive sweeteners** Substances that impart sweetness to foods and that can be absorbed and yield energy in the body. Simple sugars, sugar alcohols, and high-fructose corn syrup are the most common nutritive sweeteners used in food products.

Going Green

Whole Grains: Delicious, Easy to Prepare, Affordable, Good for Your Health, and Good for the Environment

Whole-grain products are the perfect fit for a healthy body and a healthy environment. Remember that, by definition, whole grains are not processed. These "whole" foods require ingestion and digestion in the way that they come in nature—together. Whole grains possess an array of health benefits that other foods do not. Studies show that people who eat whole grains have a lower body mass index, lower total cholesterol, and lower waist-to-hip ratio. In addition, as a less processed food, whole grains save on CO_2 production and lighten your carbon footprint.

Whole grains are convenient, easy to prepare, generally inexpensive, and found in a number of delicious foods. Many options are available for adding whole grains to your diet. A simple way to include more grains is to substitute them for the more processed version, such as using whole-grain bread instead of white bread, or brown rice instead of white rice. Foods rich in whole grains also make great snack foods. Whole-grain ready-to-eat cereal, snack crackers, and popcorn are all great choices. So, the next time you are tempted to choose a highly processed snack, such as potato chips, a doughnut, or chocolate chip cookies, consider a whole-grain option instead. Such a change just might add years to your life, and life to the planet!

contains about 5 teaspoons of sugar. Fruit-flavored yogurt contains about 7 teaspoons of sugar. Even two sticks of chewing gum contain about 1 teaspoon of sugar. Whether sweeteners come from natural sources or are refined, all are broken down in the small intestine and absorbed as monosaccharides and provide energy. Because all these absorbed monosaccharides end up as glucose, the body cannot tell whether the monosaccharides came from honey or table sugar.

THINK About It 3

The sugar alcohols in sugarless chewing gums and candies are also nutritive sweeteners, but the body does not digest and absorb them fully, so they provide only about 2 kilocalories per gram, compared with the 4 kilocalories per gram that other sugars provide.

Natural Sweeteners Natural sweeteners such as honey and maple syrup contain monosaccharides and disaccharides that make them taste sweet. Honey contains a mix of fructose and glucose—the same two monosaccharides that make up sucrose. Bees make honey from the sucrose-containing nectar of flowering plants. Real maple syrup contains primarily sucrose and is made by boiling and concentrating the sap from sugar maple trees. Most maple-flavored syrups sold in grocery stores, however, are made from corn syrup with maple flavoring added.

Many fruits also contain sugars that impart a sweet taste. Usually the riper the fruit, the higher its sugar content—a ripe pear tastes sweeter than an unripe one.

▶ **refined sweeteners** Composed of monosaccharides and disaccharides that have been extracted and processed from other foods.

Refined Sweeteners **Refined sweeteners** are monosaccharides and disaccharides that have been extracted from plant foods. White table sugar is sucrose extracted from either sugar beets or sugar cane. Molasses is a by-product of the sugar-refining process. Most brown sugar is really white table sugar with molasses added for coloring and flavor.

Manufacturers make high-fructose corn syrup by treating cornstarch with acid and enzymes to break down the starch into glucose. Then, different enzymes convert about half the glucose to fructose. High-fructose corn syrup has about the same sweetness as table sugar but costs less to produce. An increase in high-fructose corn syrup in soft drinks and other processed foods accounts for much of the increased use of sweeteners in the United States since the 1970s.[38,39] High fructose consumption can contribute to obesity and high triglyceride levels.[40]

Another sweetener increasing in popularity is agave syrup. Agave sweeteners are generally derived from the blue agave plant, which is also used to make tequila. Similar to high-fructose corn syrup, these sweeteners are highly processed and contain more fructose than glucose. Agave contains more calories per tablespoon than table sugar; however, it is 1.5 times sweeter. Therefore, you may lower calorie intake, but only by using smaller amounts of agave than you would table sugar. Research on potential health benefits of using agave sweeteners is limited; the American Diabetes Association states that agave consumption should be limited, just like sugar, honey, high-fructose corn syrup, and maple syrup.[41]

▶ **polyols** See *sugar alcohols*.

Sugar Alcohols The sugar alcohols sorbitol, xylitol, and mannitol occur naturally in a wide variety of fruits and vegetables and are commercially produced from other carbohydrates such as sucrose, glucose, and starch. Also known as **polyols**, these sweeteners are not as sweet as sucrose, but they do have the advantage of being less likely to cause tooth decay. Manufacturers use sugar alcohols to sweeten sugar-free products, such as gum and mints, and to add bulk and texture, provide a cooling sensation in the mouth, and retain moisture in foods. When sugar alcohols are used as the sweetener, the product might be sugar- (sucrose-) free, but it is not calorie-free. Check the label to be sure. An excessive intake of sugar alcohols can cause diarrhea.[42]

Nonnutritive Sweeteners

THINK About It 4

Gram for gram, most **nonnutritive sweeteners** (also called artificial sweeteners) are many times sweeter than nutritive sweeteners are. As a consequence, food manufacturers can use much less artificial sweetener to sweeten foods. Although some nonnutritive sweeteners do provide energy, their energy contribution is minimal, given the small amounts used.

The most common nonnutritive sweeteners in the United States are saccharin, aspartame, and acesulfame K. Cyclamates, which were banned in the United States in 1969 because of cancer concerns, are still used in Canada and many other countries. For people who want to decrease their intake of sugar and energy while still enjoying sweet foods, artificial sweeteners offer an alternative. Also, artificial sweeteners do not contribute to tooth decay. **TABLE 4.5** summarizes current nonnutritive sweeteners and sweet substances typically used in the United States.

TABLE 4.5
Summary of Nonnutritive Sweeteners and Sweet Substances

Nonnutritive Sweetener	Relative Sweetness to Sucrose	FDA Approval?	Typical Foods Where Sweetener Is Added	Acceptable Daily Intake (mg/kg body weight)
Saccharin	300×	Yes	Tabletop sweetener, beverages, fruit juices, drink mix	15
Aspartame	200–250×	Yes	Beverages, gelatin desserts, gums, fruit spreads	50[a]
Acesulfame K	200×	Yes	Gum, powdered drink mixes, nondairy creamers, gelatins, pudding	15
Sucralose	600×	Yes	Baked goods, beverages, gelatin desserts, frozen dairy desserts, tabletop sweetener	5
d-Tagatose	75–90%	Generally recognized as safe	Derived from lactose	—
Trehalose[b]	50%	Generally recognized as safe	Found naturally in mushrooms, lobster, shrimp, baker's/brewer's yeast	—
Neotame	7,000–13,000×	Yes	Tabletop sweetener	0.3
Stevioside	300×	No[c]	Sold as dietary supplement in U.S.	—

[a] Set for general population. Individuals with **phenylketonuria (PKU)** should control phenylalanine intake from all sources, including aspartame.

[b] Generally used more for textural properties than sweetness. Provides 4 kcal/g but produces lower glycemic response than glucose.

[c] Rebaudioside A (a specific steviol glycoside) has been approved by the FDA as a food additive.

Data from U.S. Department of Health and Human Services, U.S. Food and Drug Administration. Additional information about high-intensity sweeteners permitted for use in food in the United States. http://www.fda.gov/food/ingredientspackaginglabeling/foodadditivesingredients/ucm397725.htm#Advantame. Accessed December 23, 2015.

Quick Bite

Why Is Honey Dangerous for Babies?

Because honey and Karo syrup (corn syrup) can contain spores of the bacterium *Clostridium botulinum*, they should never be fed to infants younger than 1 year. Infants do not produce as much stomach acid as older children and adults, so these spores can germinate in an infant's GI tract and cause botulism, a deadly foodborne illness.

▶ **nonnutritive sweeteners** Substances that impart sweetness to foods but supply little or no energy to the body; also called artificial sweeteners or alternative sweeteners. They include acesulfame, aspartame, saccharin, and sucralose.

▶ **saccharin** [SAK-ah-ren] An artificial sweetener that tastes about 300 to 700 times sweeter than sucrose.

▶ **aspartame** [AH-spar-tame] An artificial sweetener composed of two amino acids and methanol. It is 200 times sweeter than sucrose. Its trade name is NutraSweet.

▶ **acesulfame K** [ay-SUL-fame kay] An artificial sweetener that is 200 times sweeter than common table sugar (sucrose). Because it is not digested and absorbed by the body, acesulfame contributes no calories to the diet and yields no energy when consumed.

▶ **sucralose** An artificial sweetener made from sucrose; it was approved for use in the United States in 1998 and has been used in Canada since 1992. Sucralose is nonnutritive and about 600 times sweeter than sugar.

▶ **d-tagatose** An artificial sweetener derived from lactose that has the same sweetness as sucrose with only half the calories.

▶ **trehalose** A disaccharide of two glucose molecules, but with a linkage different from maltose. Used as a food additive and sweetener.

▶ **neotame** An artificial sweetener similar to aspartame, but that is sweeter and does not require a warning label for phenylketonurics.

▶ **stevioside** A dietary supplement, not approved for use as a sweetener, that is extracted and refined from *Stevia rebaudiana* leaves.

▶ **phenylketonuria (PKU)** An inherited disorder caused by a lack or deficiency of the enzyme that converts phenylalanine to tyrosine.

Nutrition Science *in Action*

Sugar-Sweetened and Artificially Sweetened Beverages and Type 2 Diabetes Mellitus

Background

In the United States, the prevalence of obesity and type 2 diabetes has risen dramatically in recent years. Some studies have revealed that sugar-sweetened beverage (SSB) consumption is a risk factor for weight gain and type 2 diabetes mellitus (T2DM). It is unclear if artificially sweetened beverages (ASBs) such as diet colas and other diet drinks should be recommended as a replacement for SSBs because some studies suggest that ASB consumption is also associated with an increased risk for T2DM.

Study Purpose

To examine the associations of SSBs and ASBs with T2DM in a well-characterized cohort of men (Health Professionals Follow-Up Study) and to determine alternative beverages that should be considered in populations at risk for T2DM.

Experimental Plan

In 1986, 51,529 men aged 40–75 years were recruited to form the Health Professionals Follow-Up Study (HPFS). Questionnaires were mailed to participants every other year to assess lifestyle factors and health status, including the consumption of SSBs, ASBs, and new diagnosis of type 2 diabetes. All participants in the HPFS with baseline type 2 diabetes, cardiovascular disease, cancer (except nonmelanoma skin cancer), or an implausible energy intake (< 800 or > 4,200 kcal/day) were excluded, leaving 40,389 participants for this analysis. Participants were followed over 20 years.

Results

SSB consumption was associated with a significant increase in risk for type 2 diabetes after adjustment for both age and confounding variables (family history, health status, pre-enrollment weight change, dieting, total energy intake, and BMI). The consumption of ASBs was significantly associated with risk for type 2 diabetes in the age-adjusted model; however, after statistical adjustment for confounding variables, ASBs were no longer associated with risk for type 2 diabetes.

Conclusion and Discussion

In the all-male HPFS cohort the consumption of SSBs significantly increased the risk of type 2 diabetes, independent of age and lifestyle factors. The association between ASBs and diabetes risk was largely explained by health status, pre-enrollment weight change, dieting, and BMI. After adjustment for these factors, there was no longer any association between ASB and diabetes risk. Substituting sugar-sweetened beverages with ASBs, low-fat milk, fruit juice, coffee, and tea are supported by the study findings.

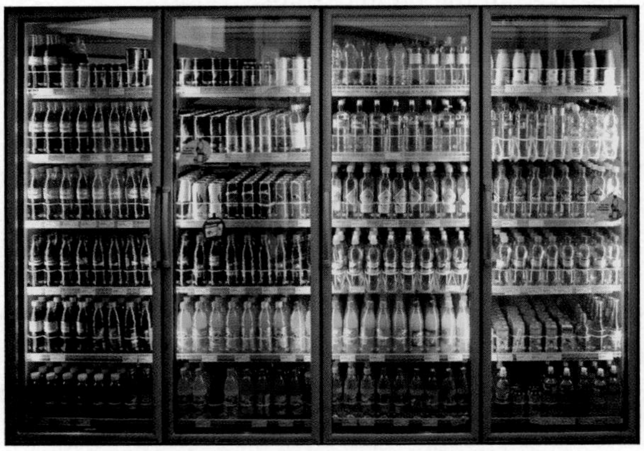

Data from de Koning L, Malik VS, Rimm EB, Willett WC, Hu FB. Sugar-sweetened and artificially sweetened beverage consumption and risk of type 2 diabetes in men. *Am J Clin Nutr.* 2011;93:1321–1327.

Key Concepts Sweeteners add flavor to foods. Nutritive sweeteners provide energy, whereas nonnutritive sweeteners provide little or no energy. The body cannot tell the difference between sugars derived from natural and refined sources.

Carbohydrates and Health

Carbohydrates contribute both positively and negatively to health. On the up side, foods rich in fiber help keep the gastrointestinal tract healthy and can reduce the risk of heart disease and cancer. On the down side, excess sugar can contribute to weight gain, poor nutrient intake, and tooth decay.

Sugar and Dental Caries

High sugar intake contributes to **dental caries**, or cavities. (See **FIGURE 4.17**.) When bacteria in the mouth feed on sugars, they produce acids that eat away tooth enamel and dental structure, causing dental caries. Although these bacteria quickly metabolize sugars, they feed on any carbohydrate, including starch.

The longer a carbohydrate remains in the mouth or the more frequently it is consumed, the more likely it will promote dental caries. Foods that stick to the teeth, such as caramel, licorice, crackers, sugary cereals, and cookies, are more likely to cause dental caries than foods that are quickly washed out of the mouth. High-sugar beverages such as soft drinks are more likely to cause dental caries when they are sipped slowly over an extended period of time. A baby should never be put to bed with a bottle because the warm milk or juice might remain in the mouth all night, providing a ready source of carbohydrate for bacteria to break down.

Snacking on high-sugar foods throughout the day provides a continuous intake of carbohydrate that nourishes the bacteria in your mouth, promoting the formation of dental caries. Good dental hygiene, adequate fluoride, and a well-balanced diet for strong tooth formation can help prevent cavities.[43]

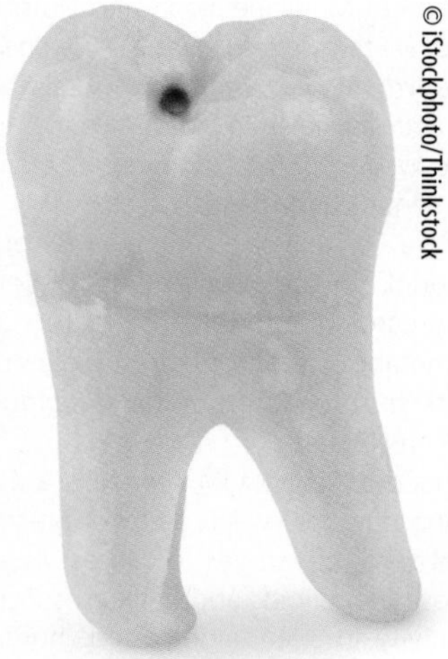

© iStockphoto/Thinkstock

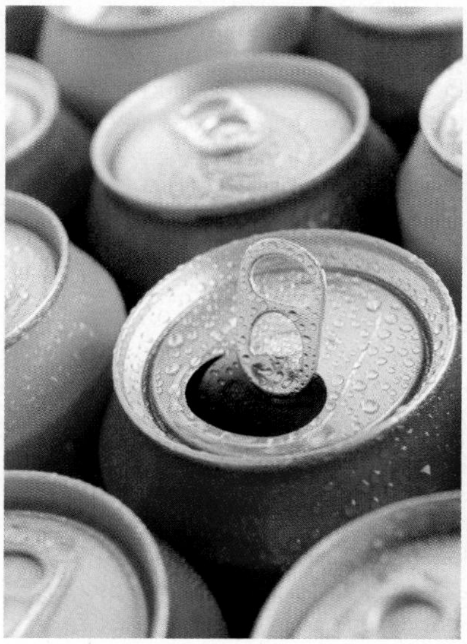

© Monkey Business Images/Shutterstock, Inc.

Position Statement: Academy of Nutrition and Dietetics

Use of Nutritive and Nonnutritive Sweeteners

It is the position of the Academy of Nutrition and Dietetics that consumers can safely enjoy a range of nutritive and nonnutritive sweeteners when consumed within an eating plan that is guided by current federal nutrition recommendations, such as the *Dietary Guidelines for Americans* and the Dietary References Intakes, as well as individual health goals and personal preference.

Reproduced from Position of the American Dietetic Association: use of nutritive and nonnutritive sweeteners. *J Acad Nutr Diet.* 2012;112:739-758. Copyright © 2012. Reprinted with permission from Elsevier.

▶ **dental caries** [KARE-ees] Destruction of the enamel surface of teeth caused by acids resulting from bacterial breakdown of sugars in the mouth.

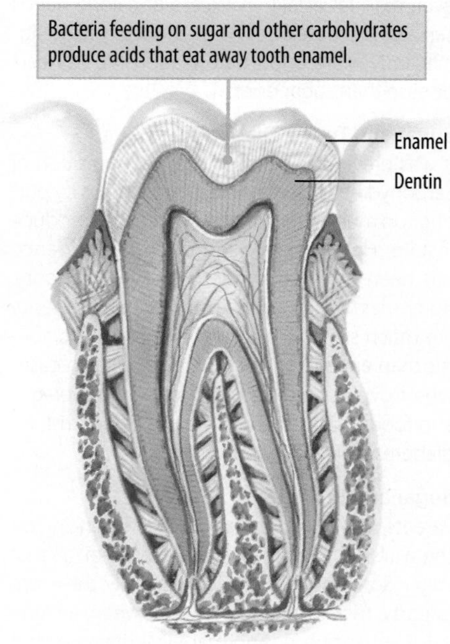
Bacteria feeding on sugar and other carbohydrates produce acids that eat away tooth enamel.
Enamel
Dentin

FIGURE 4.17 Dental health. Good dental hygiene, adequate fluoride, and proper nutrition help maintain healthy teeth. A well-balanced diet contains vitamins and minerals crucial for healthy bones and teeth. To help prevent dental caries, avoid continuous snacking on high-sugar foods, especially those that stick to the teeth.

FYI For Your Information

Unfounded Claims Against Sugars

Sugar has become the vehicle for diet zealots to create a new crusade. Cut sugar to trim fat! Bust sugar! Break the sugar habit! These battle cries falsely demonize sugar as a dietary villain. But what are the facts?

Sugar and Obesity

Many people believe that sugar is fattening and causes obesity. Sugar is a carbohydrate, and all carbohydrates provide 4 kilocalories per gram. Excess energy intake from any source (sugar, fat, or protein) will cause obesity, but sugar by itself is no more likely to cause obesity than the other macronutrients. The increased availability of low-fat and fat-free foods has not reduced obesity rates in the United States, with rates remaining constant over the past 10 years.[a] Some speculate that consumers equate fat-free with calorie-free and eat more of these foods, not realizing that fat-free foods often have a higher sugar content, which makes any calorie savings negligible. Also, foods high in added sugars often have low nutrient value and become "extras" in the diet. High intake of added sugar is associated with increased total energy intake.[b]

Sugar and Heart Disease

Risk factors for heart disease include a genetic predisposition, smoking, high blood pressure, high blood cholesterol levels, diabetes, and obesity. Sugar by itself does not cause heart disease.[c] However, if intake of high-sugar foods contributes to obesity, then risk for heart disease increases. In addition, excessive intake of refined sugar can alter blood lipids in carbohydrate-sensitive people, increasing their risk for heart disease. However, high fat intake in excess of calorie needs can also promote obesity. Thus, obesity has a significantly more important relationship to heart disease than sugar does.

Sugar and Type 2 Diabetes

It was previously believed that consumption of carbohydrate-rich meals caused diabetes by putting too much strain on the pancreas to produce insulin. However, enough scientific evidence has been produced now to dispel this theory. Body mass index (BMI) and abdominal obesity are much stronger risk factors for type 2 diabetes than any single nutrient.[d] However, in cases where overconsumption of sugar-rich beverages and foods leads to an excess of calories, risk for diabetes increases.

Sugar and Behavior

Parents continue to talk about kids "bouncing off the walls" at birthday parties because of "all that sugar." So, what's going on? Most likely, the event (a party, trick-or-treating for Halloween, a carnival) is enhancing kids' normal levels of excitement and enthusiasm. From a brain chemistry perspective, carbohydrates actually have a calming effect by increasing production of the sleep-inducing chemical serotonin! Well-controlled research studies have found no consistent link between sugar and hyperactivity, so blame the excitement of the party, but not the sugar, for kids' "wild" behavior.[e–g]

In 1978, Dan White blamed his gunning down the mayor of San Francisco on an emotional state created by his change in diet from healthy foods to Twinkies and other sugary foods, a legal strategy that became known as the Twinkie defense. Claims that sugar causes criminal behavior in adults are unfounded. Studies show no association between high sugar intake and adult behavior.[h]

High-Fructose Corn Syrup (HFCS), Obesity, and Disease

In the early 2000s, sucrose began to be replaced with high-fructose corn syrup in the U.S. diet. Since this time, scientists have observed concurrent increases in weight gain/body fatness and consumption of HFCS. As a result, HFCS quickly became villainized as the source of the obesity epidemic. When investigated further, researchers determined that people who consume the most HFCS weigh more than those who consume less. These individuals also take in more calories than their leaner counterparts.[i] Therefore, it appears that HFCS consumption is correlated to obesity risk; however, it remains unclear whether HFCS actually *causes* obesity and its related comorbidities. Studies in both animals and humans indicate that consumption of fructose may cause abdominal weight gain and increase blood triglycerides more than glucose does.[j] Furthermore, fructose absorption does not promote insulin secretion, which plays a role in suppressing appetite. Therefore, consuming more fructose may lead to increased calorie consumption. However, HFCS is a combination of fructose *and* glucose; thus, it remains unclear whether the negative effects of HFCS would be as dramatic as those of pure fructose. Consuming an HFCS beverage at every meal for 10 weeks, however, has been shown to increase blood triglycerides in overweight and obese women.[k]

Although consuming HFCS-sweetened beverages in excess of calorie needs will lead to weight gain and increased risk for diseases related to obesity, there is no concrete evidence indicating that the consumption of HFCS within a calorie-controlled diet will cause significant health problems. Therefore, similar to recommendations for added sugars and other sweeteners, individuals should aim to limit their consumption of HFCS, but can enjoy it in moderation as a part of a healthy, balanced diet.

a. Fryar DC, Carroll MD, Ogden CL. Prevalence of overweight, obesity, and extreme obesity among adults: United States, 1960–1962 through 2011–2012. CDC/National Center for Health Statistics. 2014. http://www.cdc.gov/nchs/data/hestat/obesity_adult_11_12/obesity_adult_11_12.htm. Accessed December 23, 2015.

b. Dietary Guidelines Advisory Committee. *Report of the Dietary Guidelines Advisory Committee on the Dietary Guidelines for Americans, 2005*. January 31, 2005. http://www.health.gov/dietaryguidelines/dga2005/report. Accessed December 23, 2015.

c. Institute of Medicine, Food and Nutrition Board. *Dietary Reference Intakes for Energy, Carbohydrate, Fiber, Fat, Fatty Acids, Cholesterol, Protein, and Amino Acids*. Washington, DC: National Academies Press; 2005.

d. Bray GA, Jablonski KA, Fujimoto WY et al. Relation of central adiposity and body mass index to the development of diabetes in the Diabetes Prevention program. *Am J Clin Nutr*. 2008;87:1212–1218.

e. White JW, Wolraich M. Effect of sugar on behavior and mental performance. *Am J Clin Nutr*. 1995;62:S242–S249.

f. Wolraich ML, Lindgren SD, Stumbo PJ, et al. Effects of diets high in sucrose or aspartame on the behavior and cognitive performance of children. *N Engl J Med*. 1994;330:301–307.

g. Institute of Medicine, Food and Nutrition Board. *Dietary Reference Intakes for Energy, Carbohydrate, Fiber, Fat, Fatty Acids, Cholesterol, Protein, and Amino Acids*. Op cit.

h. White, Wolraich. Effect of sugar on behavior and mental performance. Op cit.

i. Dhingra R, Sullivan L, Jacques PF et al. Soft drink consumption and risk of developing cardiometabnolic risk factors and the metabolic syndrome in middle-aged adults in the community. *Circulation*. 2007;116:480–488.

j. Stanhope KL, Schwarz JM, Keim NL et al. Consuming fructose-sweetened, not glucose-sweetened, beverages increases visceral adiposity and lipids and decreases insulin sensitivity in overweight/obese humans *J Clin Invest*. 2009;119:1322–1334.

k. Swarbrick MM, Stanhope KL, Elliott SS et al. Consumption of fructose-sweetened beverages for 10 weeks increases postprandial triacylglycerol and apolipoprotein-B concentrations in overweight and obese women. *Br J Nutr*. 2008;100:947–952.

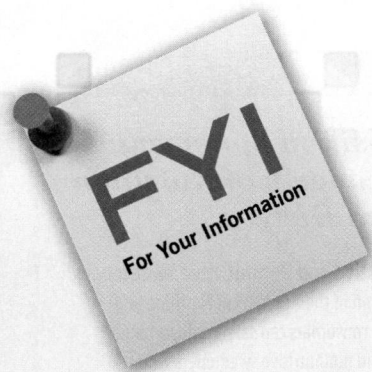

Fiber and Obesity

Foods rich in fiber are usually low in fat and energy. They also are more filling, offer a greater volume of food for fewer calories, and take longer to eat. Once eaten, foods high in soluble fiber take longer to leave the stomach and they attract water, giving a feeling of fullness. Consider the following three apple products, which have the same energy content but different fiber content: a large apple containing 5 grams of dietary fiber, ½ cup of applesauce containing 2 grams of fiber, and ¾ cup of apple juice containing 0.2 grams of fiber. For most of us, the whole apple would be more filling and satisfying than the applesauce or apple juice.

Studies show that people who consume more fiber weigh less than those who consume less fiber, suggesting that fiber intake has a role in weight control. Although research supports a role for dietary fiber in reducing hunger and promoting satiety, studies on specific types of fiber have produced inconsistent results.[44]

Fiber and Type 2 Diabetes

Populations with a high intake of dietary fiber have a low incidence of type 2 diabetes. Epidemiological evidence suggests that intake of soluble fibers can delay glucose uptake and smooth out the blood glucose response, thus providing a protective effect against diabetes.[45] Current dietary recommendations for people with type 2 diabetes advise a high intake of foods rich in dietary fiber.[46]

Fiber and Cardiovascular Disease

High blood cholesterol levels increase risk for heart disease. Dietary trials using high doses of oat bran, which is high in soluble fiber, show blood cholesterol reductions of 2 percent per gram of intake.[47] Because every 1 percent decrease in blood cholesterol levels decreases the risk of heart disease by 2 percent, high fiber intake can decrease the risk of heart disease substantially. Studies show a 20 to 40 percent difference in heart disease risk between the highest and lowest fiber intake groups.[48]

Soluble fiber from oat bran, legumes, and psyllium might lower serum cholesterol levels by binding bile acids in the gastrointestinal tract and preventing their reabsorption into the body. Bile acids are made from cholesterol in the liver and are secreted into the intestinal tract to aid with fat absorption. When dietary fiber prevents their reabsorption, new bile acids must be made in the liver from cholesterol, reducing blood cholesterol levels. The short-chain fatty acids produced from bacterial fermentation of insoluble fiber in the large intestine can also inhibit cholesterol synthesis.[49]

Studies also show an association between high intake of whole grains and low risk of heart disease.[50] Whole grains contain not only fiber, but also antioxidants, which protect against cellular damage that promotes heart disease. It is likely that the combination of compounds found in grains, rather than any one component, explains the protective effects against heart disease.[51,52] Consuming at least three 1-ounce servings of whole grains each day can reduce heart disease risk.[53]

Fiber and Gastrointestinal Disorders

Insoluble fiber, particularly cellulose from cereal grains, helps promote healthy gastrointestinal functioning. High fiber intake also helps in treating certain gastrointestinal disorders.[54]

Quick Bite

Sugar Overload

In many affluent countries, sugar consumption is nearly 100 pounds per capita per year. The United States averages 103 pounds of sugar per person per year—roughly half as refined sugar and half as corn sweeteners (especially high-fructose corn syrup). Boys aged 12 to 19 years consume nearly 160 pounds per year, and girls the same ages consume 114 pounds annually.

Quick Bite

Liquid Candy

In the United States, corn sweeteners are primarily consumed in carbonated soft drinks (25.4 pounds per year), fruitades and drinks (8.2 pounds), and syrup and sweet toppings (4.1 pounds). In all, 36.3 percent of sugar and corn sweeteners is consumed in carbonated soft drinks, fruitades, and other nonalcoholic drinks.

Dietary Guidelines for Americans, 2015-2020

Key Recommendations

The *Dietary Guidelines'* Key Recommendations for healthy eating patterns should be applied in their entirety, given the interconnected relationship that each dietary component can have with others.

Consume a healthy eating pattern that accounts for all foods and beverages within an appropriate calorie level.

A healthy eating pattern includes:

- A variety of vegetables from all of the subgroups—dark-green, red and orange, legumes (beans and peas), starchy, and other
- Fruits, especially whole fruits
- Grains, at least half of which are whole grains
- Fat-free or low-fat dairy, including milk, yogurt, cheese, and/or fortified soy beverages
- A variety of protein foods, including seafood, lean meats and poultry, eggs, legumes (beans and peas), and nuts, seeds, and soy products
- Oils

A healthy eating pattern limits:

- Saturated fats and *trans* fats, added sugars, and sodium
    - Consume less than 10 percent of calories per day from added sugars
    - Consume less than 10 percent of calories per day from saturated fats

(*continued*)

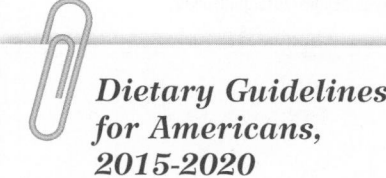

- Consume less than 2,300 milligrams (mg) per day of sodium
- If alcohol is consumed, it should be consumed in moderation—up to one drink per day for women and up to two drinks per day for men—and only by adults of legal drinking age.

In tandem with the recommendations above, Americans of all ages—children, adolescents, adults, and older adults—should meet the *Physical Activity Guidelines for Americans* to help promote health and reduce the risk of chronic disease. Americans should aim to achieve and maintain a healthy body weight. The relationship between diet and physical activity contributes to calorie balance and managing body weight.

Reproduced from Department of Health and Human Services and U.S. Department of Agriculture. *2015–2020 Dietary Guidelines for Americans*. 8th Edition. December 2015. Available at http://health.gov/dietaryguidelines/2015/guidelines/.

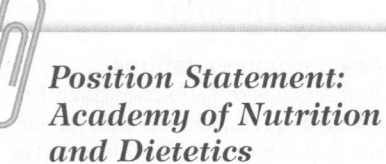

Position Statement: Academy of Nutrition and Dietetics

Health Implications of Dietary Fiber

It is the position of the Academy of Nutrition and Dietetics that the public should consume adequate amounts of dietary fiber from a variety of plant foods.

Reproduced from Position of the American Dietetic Association: health implications of dietary fiber. *J Am Diet Assoc.* 2008;108:1716–1731. Copyright © 2008.

Quick Bite

Fierce Fiber and Flatulence

The Jerusalem artichoke surpasses even dry beans in its capacity for promoting flatulence. This artichoke contains large amounts of nondigestible carbohydrate. After passing through the small intestine undigested, the fiber is attacked by gas-generating bacteria in the colon.

Diets rich in fiber add bulk and increase water in the stool, softening the stool and making it easier to pass. Insoluble fiber also accelerates passage of food through the intestinal tract, promoting regularity. If fluid intake is also ample, high fiber intake helps prevent and treat constipation, hemorrhoids (swelling of rectal veins), and diverticular disease (development of pouches on the intestinal wall).

Negative Health Effects of Excess Fiber

Despite its health advantages, high fiber intake can cause problems, especially for people who drastically increase their fiber intake in a short period of time. If you increase your fiber intake, you also should increase your water intake to prevent the stool from becoming hard and impacted. A sudden increase in fiber intake also can cause increased intestinal gas and bloating. These problems can be prevented both by increasing fiber intake gradually over several weeks and by drinking plenty of fluids.

High fiber intake can also bind small amounts of minerals in the GI tract and prevent them from being absorbed. In particular, fiber binds the minerals zinc, calcium, and iron. For people who get enough of these minerals, the recommended amounts of dietary fiber do not significantly affect mineral status.[55]

If the diet contains high amounts of fiber, some people, such as young children and older adults, can become full before meeting their energy and nutrient needs. Because of limited stomach capacity, they must be careful that their fiber intake does not interfere with their ability to consume adequate energy and nutrients.

Because of the bulky nature of fibers, excess consumption is likely to be self-limiting. Although a high fiber intake might cause occasional adverse gastrointestinal symptoms, serious chronic adverse effects have not been observed. As part of an overall healthful diet, a high intake of fiber does not produce significant deleterious effects in healthy people. Therefore, a Tolerable Upper Intake Level (UL) is not set for fiber.

Key Concepts High sugar intake promotes dental caries and can contribute to nutrient deficiencies by replacing more nutritious foods in the diet. High intake of foods rich in dietary fiber offers many health benefits, including reduced risk of obesity, type 2 diabetes, cardiovascular disease, and gastrointestinal disorders. Increase fiber intake gradually while drinking plenty of fluids; children and older adults with small appetites should take care that their energy needs are still met. The DRIs do not contain a UL for fiber.

Label to Table

This label highlights all the carbohydrate-related information you can find on a food label. Look at the center of the Nutrition Facts label, and you'll see the Total Carbohydrates along with the carbohydrate "subgroups": Dietary Fiber, Total Sugars and Added Sugars. Recall that carbohydrates are classified into simple carbohydrates and the two complex carbohydrates starch and fiber.

Using this food label, you can determine all three of these components. There are 19 total grams of carbohydrate, with 14 grams coming from sugars of which 11 grams are added to the food and 0 grams from fiber. This means the remaining 5 grams must be from starch, which is not required to be listed separately on the label.

"Added sugars," in grams and as percent Daily Value, will now be included on the label. Scientific data shows that it is difficult to meet nutrient needs while staying within calorie limits if you consume more than 10 percent of your total daily calories from added sugar, and this is consistent with the 2015–2020 Dietary Guidelines for Americans. Because the Daily Values are based on a caloric intake of 2,000 calories that means you should limit your intake of added sugar to less than 200 calories or 50g each day.

Without even knowing what food this label represents, you can decipher that it contains a high proportion of added sugar (11 of the 19 grams) and is probably sweet. If this is a fruit juice, that level of sugar would be expected; but if this is cereal, you'd be getting a lot more sugar than complex carbohydrates, and probably not be making the best choice! You can use the information from the 'Added Sugars' to help make informed food decisions.

Do you see the 6% listed to the right of "Total Carbohydrates"? This doesn't mean that the food item contains 6 percent of its calories from carbohydrate. Instead, it refers to the daily allotment (or Daily Value) of carbohydrates listed at the bottom of the label. There you can see that a person consuming 2,000 kilocalories per day should consume 300 grams of carbohydrates each day. This product contributes 19 grams per serving, which is just 6 percent of the Daily Value of 300 grams per day. Note that the % Daily Value for fiber is 0% because this food item lacks fiber.

Recall that carbohydrates contain 4 kilocalories per gram. Armed with this information and the product's calorie information, can you calculate the percentage of calories that come from carbohydrate?

Here's how:

19 g carbohydrate × 4 kcal per g
= 76 carbohydrate kcal

76 carbohydrate kcal ÷ 154 total kcal
= 0.49 or 49% carbohydrate kcal

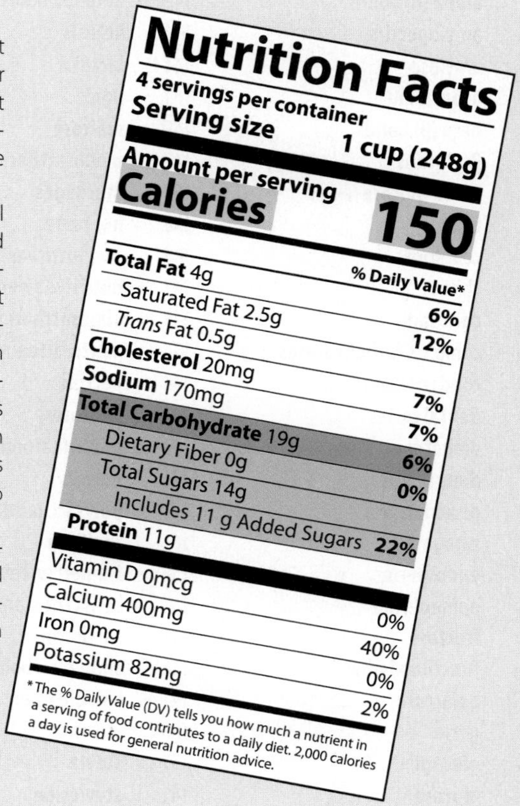

Nutrition Facts
4 servings per container
Serving size 1 cup (248g)
Amount per serving
Calories 150
% Daily Value*
Total Fat 4g
Saturated Fat 2.5g 6%
Trans Fat 0.5g 12%
Cholesterol 20mg
Sodium 170mg 7%
Total Carbohydrate 19g 7%
Dietary Fiber 0g 6%
Total Sugars 14g 0%
Includes 11 g Added Sugars 22%
Protein 11g
Vitamin D 0mcg
Calcium 400mg 0%
Iron 0mg 40%
Potassium 82mg 0%
2%
* The % Daily Value (DV) tells you how much a nutrient in a serving of food contributes to a daily diet. 2,000 calories a day is used for general nutrition advice.

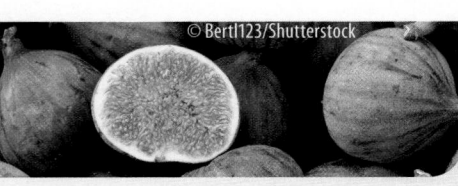

Learning Portfolio

Key Terms

acesulfame K	161	**insulin**	152
alpha (α) bonds	149	**ketone bodies**	152
amylopectin	144	**ketosis**	152
amylose	144	**lactose**	143
aspartame	161	**lignins**	147
beta (β) bonds	149	**maltose**	143
β-glucans	147	**monosaccharides**	141
blood glucose levels	152	**mucilages**	147
bran	158	**neotame**	161
cellulose	146	**nonnutritive sweeteners**	161
chitin	147	**nutritive sweeteners**	159
chitosan	147	**oligosaccharides**	144
complex carbohydrates	144	**pancreatic amylase**	149
condensation	143	**pectins**	147
dental caries	163	**pentoses**	141
diabetes mellitus	153	**phenylketonuria (PKU)**	161
dietary fiber	146	**polyols**	160
disaccharides	141	**polysaccharides**	144
d-tagatose	161	**psyllium**	147
endosperm	158	**refined sweeteners**	160
epinephrine	153	**resistant starch**	145
fructose	141	**saccharin**	161
functional fiber	146	**simple carbohydrates**	141
galactose	141	**soluble fiber**	146
germ	155	**starch**	144
glucagon	152	**stevia**	
glucose	141	**stevioside**	161
glycemic index	153	**sucralose**	161
glycogen	145	**sucrose**	143
gums	147	**sugar alcohols**	142
hemicelluloses	146	**total fiber**	146
husk	158	**trehalose**	161
insoluble fiber	146		

Study Points

- Carbohydrates include simple sugars and complex carbohydrates.
- Monosaccharides are the building blocks of carbohydrates.
- Three monosaccharides are important in human nutrition: glucose, fructose, and galactose.
- The monosaccharides combine to make disaccharides: sucrose, lactose, and maltose.
- Starch, glycogen, and fiber are long chains (polysaccharides) of glucose units.
- Fibers are indigestible polysaccharides that can be classified as soluble or insoluble.
- Carbohydrates are digested by enzymes from the mouth, pancreas, and small intestine and absorbed as monosaccharides.
- The liver converts the monosaccharides fructose and galactose to glucose.
- Blood glucose levels rise after eating and fall between meals. Two pancreatic hormones, insulin and glucagon, regulate blood glucose levels, preventing extremely high or low levels.
- The main function of carbohydrates in the body is to supply energy. In this role, carbohydrates spare protein for use in making body proteins and allow for the complete breakdown of fat as an additional energy source.
- Carbohydrates are found mainly in plant foods as starch, fiber, and sugar.
- In general, Americans consume more sugar and less whole grains and fiber than is recommended.
- Carbohydrate intake can affect health. Excess sugar can contribute to low nutrient intake, excess energy intake, and dental caries.
- Diets high in complex carbohydrates, including fiber, have been linked to reduced risk for GI disorders, heart disease, and cancer.

Study Questions

1. Describe the difference between starch and fiber.
2. What type of fiber is pectin? What beneficial effects does it have in the stomach and small intestine during digestion?
3. How will eating excessive amounts of carbohydrate affect health?
4. What are the negative consequences of eating too little carbohydrate?

5. What are the negative consequences of eating too little fiber? Too much fiber?
6. Which foods contain carbohydrates?
7. What advantage does the branched-chain structure of glycogen provide compared with a straight chain of glucose?
8. Which blood glucose regulation hormone is secreted in the recently fed state? The fasting state?
9. Describe the structure of a monosaccharide, disaccharide, and polysaccharide.
10. In an effort to lose weight, you decide to follow a diet of 1,200 calories with 225 grams of carbohydrate. Calculate the percentage of carbohydrate in this diet and compare this amount to the Daily Value recommendations. Daily Value recommendations for carbohydrate are 300 grams per day. Compare this amount to the recommendation for the overall percentage of carbohydrate, which is 45 to 65 percent of total calories.

Try This

The Fiber-Type Experiment

This experiment is to help you understand the difference between sources of dietary fiber. Go to the store and buy a small amount of raw bran. It is usually sold in a bin at a health food store or near the hot cereals in a grocery store. Also purchase some pectin (near the baking items) or some Metamucil (in the pharmacy section). Once you're home, fill two glasses with water and put the raw bran in one glass and the pectin or Metamucil in the other. Stir each glass for a minute or two and watch what happens. Describe the differences. What would happen in your GI tract? What type of fiber is pectin? What type of fiber is in bran?

The Sweetness of Soda

This experiment is to help you understand the amount of sugar found in a can of soda. Take a glass and fill it with 12 ounces (1½ cups) of water. Using a measuring spoon, add 10 to 12 teaspoons of sugar to the water. Stir the sugar water until all the sucrose has dissolved. Now sip the water. Does it taste sweet? It shouldn't taste any sweeter than a can of regular soda. This is the amount of sugar found in one 12-ounce can!

References

1. Eastwood M. *Principles of Human Nutrition*. New York: Chapman & Hall; 1997.
2. Institute of Medicine, Food and Nutrition Board. *Dietary Reference Intakes for Energy, Carbohydrate, Fiber, Fat, Fatty Acids, Cholesterol, Protein, and Amino Acids (Macronutrients)*. Washington, DC: National Academies Press; 2005. http://www.nap.edu/read/10490/chapter/1.
3. Marcobal A, Borboza M, Froehlich JW, et al. Consumption of human milk oligosaccharides by gut-related microbes. *J Agric Food Chem*. 2010;58(9): 5334–5340.
4. Musilova S, Rada V, Vikova E, Bunesova V. Beneficial effects of human milk oligosaccharides on gut microbiota. *Benef Microbes*. 2014;5:273–283.
5. Fong B, Ma K, McJarrow P. Quantification of bovine milk oligosaccharides using liquid chromatography-selected reaction monitoring—mass spectrometry. *J Agric Food Chem*. 2011;59(18):9788–9795.
6. Institute of Medicine, Food and Nutrition Board. *Dietary Reference Intakes for Energy, Carbohydrate, Fiber, Fat, Fatty Acids, Cholesterol, Protein, and Amino Acids (Macronutrients)*. Op cit.
7. Murphy MM, Douglass JS, Birkett A. Resistant starch intakes in the United States. *J Am Diet Assoc*. 2008;108:67–78.
8. Sajilata MG, Singhal RS, Kulkarni PR. Resistant starch—a review. *Comp Rev Food Sci Food Safety*. 2006;5:1–17.
9. Cross HR. Meat processing. *Encyclopaedia Britannica*. http://www.britannica.com/EBchecked/topic/371756/meat-processing. Accessed December 23, 2015.
10. Rapoport B. Metabolic factors limiting performance in marathon runners. *PLoS Comput Biol*. 2010;6(10).
11. Ibid.
12. Sedlock DA. The latest on carbohydrate loading: a practical approach. *Curr Sports Med Rep*. 2008;7(4):209–213.
13. Schisti C, Richter A, Blandr A, Richt A. Hemicellulose concentration and composition in plant cell walls under extreme carbon source-sink imbalances. *Physiologia Plantarum*. 2010;139(3):241–255.
14. Grabitske H, Slavin J. Low-digestible carbohydrates in practice. *J Am Diet Assoc*. 2008;108(10):1677–1681.
15. Hall JE. *Guyton and Hall Textbook of Medical Physiology*. 12th ed. Philadelphia: Elsevier Saunders; 2012.
16. Berg JM, Tymoczko JL, Stryer L. *Biochemistry*. 6th ed. New York: WH Freeman; 2007.
17. Martini FH. *Fundamentals of Anatomy and Physiology*. 9th ed. San Francisco, CA: Benjamin Cummings; 2011.
18. Ibid.
19. Ibid.
20. Position of the Academy of Nutrition and Dietetics: weight management. *J Am Diet Assoc*. 2009;109(2):330–346.
21. Institute of Medicine, Food and Nutrition Board. *Dietary Reference Intakes for Energy, Carbohydrate, Fiber, Fat, Fatty Acids, Cholesterol, Protein, and Amino Acids*. Washington, DC: National Academies Press; 2005.
22. Franz MJ, Powers MA, Leontos C, et al. The evidence for medical nutrition therapy for type 1 and type 2 diabetes in adults. *J Am Diet Assoc*. 2010;110(12):1852–1889.
23. Institute of Medicine, Food and Nutrition Board. *Dietary Reference Intakes for Energy, Carbohydrate, Fiber, Fat, Fatty Acids, Cholesterol, Protein, and Amino Acids (Macronutrients)*. Op cit.

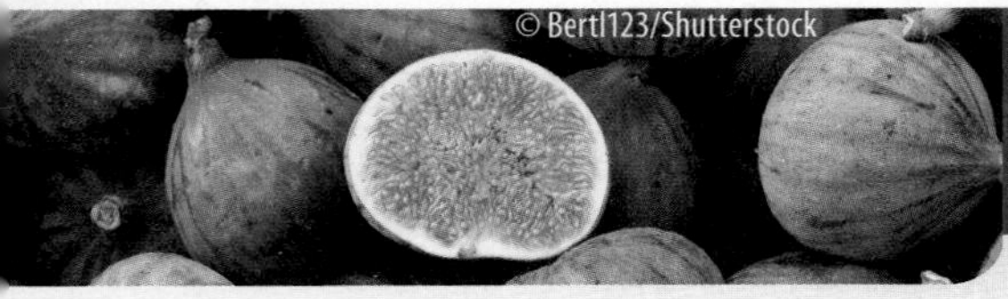
© Bertl123/Shutterstock

Learning Portfolio (continued)

24. Nansel TR, Gellar L, McGill A. Effect of varying glycemic index meals on blood glucose control assessed with continuous glucose monitoring in youth with type 1 diabetes on basal-bolus insulin regimens. *Diabetes Care.* 2008;31(4):695–697.
25. Rovner AJ, Nansel TR, Gellar L. The effect of a low-glycemic diet vs a standard diet on blood glucose levels and macronutrient intake in children with type 1 diabetes. *J Am Diet Assoc.* 2009;109(2):303–307.
26. Centers for Disease Control and Prevention. National Diabetes Statistics Report: Estimates of Diabetes and Its Burden in the United States, 2014. Atlanta, GA: U.S. Department of Health and Human Services; 2014.
27. Institute of Medicine, Food and Nutrition Board. *Dietary Reference Intakes for Energy, Carbohydrate, Fiber, Fat, Fatty Acids, Cholesterol, Protein, and Amino Acids (Macronutrients)*. Op cit.
28. U.S. Department of Agriculture and U.S. Department of Health and Human Services. *Dietary Guidelines for Americans, 2010.* 7th ed. Washington, DC: U.S. Government Printing Office; December 2010.
29. U.S. Department of Health and Human Services and U.S. Department of Agriculture. *2015–2020 Dietary Guidelines for Americans*. 8th Edition. December 2015. Available at http://health.gov/dietaryguidelines/2015/guidelines/.
30. Ibid.
31. Institute of Medicine, Food and Nutrition Board. *Dietary Reference Intakes for Energy, Carbohydrate, Fiber, Fat, Fatty Acids, Cholesterol, Protein, and Amino Acids (Macronutrients)*. Op cit.
32. Dietary Guidelines Advisory Committee. *Report of the Dietary Guidelines Advisory Committee on the Dietary Guidelines for Americans, 2010.* Washington, DC: U.S. Department of Agriculture and U.S. Department of Health and Human Services; May 2010. http://www.cnpp.usda.gov/Publications/DietaryGuidelines/2010/DGAC/Report/2010DGACReport-camera-ready-Jan11-11.pdf.
33. U.S. Department of Health and Human Services and U.S. Department of Agriculture. *2015–2020 Dietary Guidelines for Americans*. 8th Edition. December 2015. Available at http://health.gov/dietaryguidelines/2015/guidelines/.
34. Navga RM. Childhood obesity and unhappiness. The influence of soft drinks and fast food consumption. *J Happiness Studies*. 2010;11(3):261–275.
35. Marriott BP, Olsho L, Hadden L, Connor P. Intake of added sugars and selected nutrients in the United States, National Health and Nutrition Examination Survey (NHANES) 2003–2006. *Cr Rev Food Sci Nutr*. 2010;50:228–258.
36. U.S. Department of Health and Human Services and U.S. Department of Agriculture. *2015–2020 Dietary Guidelines for Americans*. 8th Edition. December 2015. Available at http://health.gov/dietaryguidelines/2015/guidelines/.
37. Marriott BP, Olsho L, Hadden L, Connor P. Intake of added sugars and selected nutrients.
38. U.S. Department of Health and Human Services and U.S. Department of Agriculture. *2015–2020 Dietary Guidelines for Americans*. 8th Edition. December 2015. Available at http://health.gov/dietaryguidelines/2015/guidelines/.
39. Giboney M, Sigman-Grant M, Stanton JL, Keast DR. Consumption of sugars. *Am J Clin Nutr*. 1995;62(suppl):178S–194S
40. Coulston AM, Johnson RK. Sugar and sugars: myth and realities. *J Am Diet Assoc*. 2002;102:351–353.
41. White J, Foreyt J, Elanson K, Angelopoulos T. High-fructose corn syrup; controversies and common sense. *Am J Lifestyle Med*. 2010;4(6):515–520.
42. Horton J. The Truth About Agave. WebMD Feature. External Link on USDA Food and Nutrition Center *Nutritive and Nonnutritive Sweetener Resources*. Accessed 22 July 2015 http://www.webmd.com/diet/the-truth-about-agave?page=1
43. Position of the American Dietetic Association: use of nutritive and nonnutritive sweeteners. *J Am Diet Assoc*. 2004;104:255–275.
44. American Dental Association. *Fluoridation Facts*. Chicago: American Dental Association; 2005. http://www.ada.org/~/media/ADA/Member%20Center/FIles/fluoridation_facts.ashx.
45. Slavin JL. Position of the American Dietetic Association: health implications of dietary fiber. *J Am Diet Assoc*. 2008;108(10):1716–1731.
46. Institute of Medicine, Food and Nutrition Board. *Dietary Reference Intakes for Energy, Carbohydrate, Fiber, Fat, Fatty Acids, Cholesterol, Protein, and Amino Acids (Macronutrients)*. Op cit.

47. Slavin. Position of the American Dietetic Association: health implications of dietary fiber. Op cit.

48. Institute of Medicine, Food and Nutrition Board. *Dietary Reference Intakes for Energy, Carbohydrate, Fiber, Fat, Fatty Acids, Cholesterol, Protein, and Amino Acids (Macronutrients)*. Op cit.

49. Ibid.

50. Hosseini E, Grootaert C, Verstraete W, Van de Wiele T. Propionate as a health-promoting microbial metabolite in the human gut. *Nutr Rev*. 2011;69(5):245–258.

51. Finks SW, Airee A, Chow SL, Macaulay TE, Moranville MP, Rogers KC, Trujillo TC. Key articles of dietary interventions that influence cardiovascular mortality. *Pharmacotherapy*. 2012;32(4): e54-87.

52. Slavin JL, Jacobs D, Marquart L, Wiemer K. The role of whole grains in disease prevention. *J Am Diet Assoc*. 2001;101:780–785.

53. Johnston C. Functional foods as modifiers of cardiovascular disease. *Am J Lifestyle Med*. 2009;3(1 suppl):39S–43S.

54. Slavin. Position of the American Dietetic Association: health implications of dietary fiber. Op cit.

55. Brownawell AM, Caers W, Gibson GR, Kendall CW, Lewis KD, Ringel Y, Slavin JL. Prebiotics and the health benefits of fiber: current regulatory status, future research, and goals. *J Nutr*. 2012;142(5):962–974.

56. Institute of Medicine, Food and Nutrition Board. *Dietary Reference Intakes for Energy, Carbohydrate, Fiber, Fat, Fatty Acids, Cholesterol, Protein, and Amino Acids (Macronutrients)*. Op cit.

Chapter 5

Lipids

Revised by Melissa Bernstein

THINK About It

1 How important is fat to the foods you think of as tasty?
2 What is your view about the value of body fat?
3 What's your take on the differences between fat and cholesterol?
4 What's your understanding of "good" versus "bad" cholesterol?

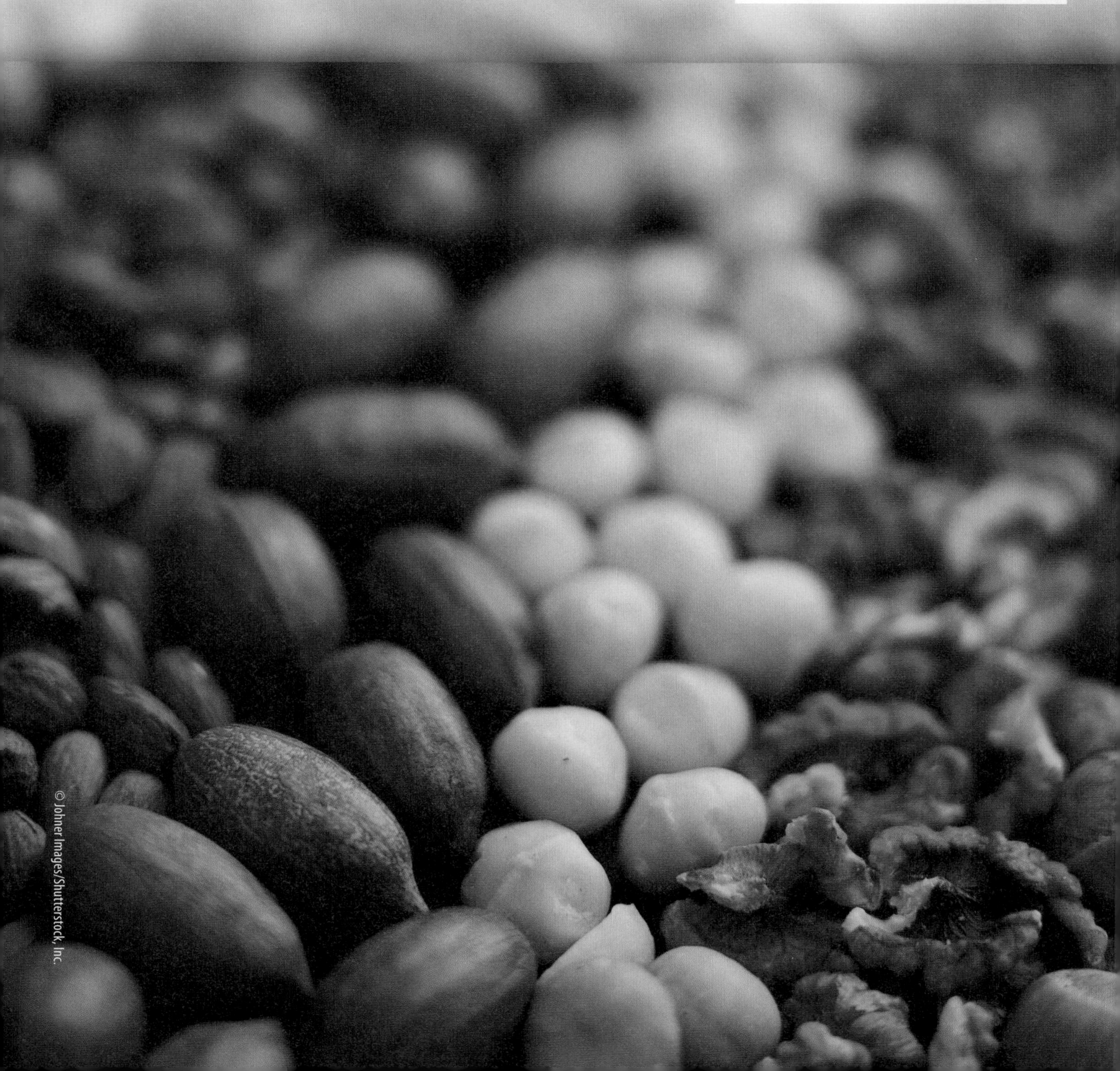

CHAPTER Menu

- What Are Lipids?
- Fatty Acids Are Key Building Blocks
- Triglycerides
- Phospholipids
- Sterols
- Lipids in the Body
- Transportation of Lipids in the Body
- Lipids in the Diet
- Lipids and Health
- Key Terms
- Study Points
- Study Questions
- Try This
- Getting Personal
- References

LEARNING Objectives

- Differentiate between types of fatty acids according to chain length, saturation, location of double bond, and whether they are essential or nonessential.
- Explain how lipids are digested, absorbed, and transported in the body.
- Differentiate between VLDL, LDL, and HDL cholesterol using their key components and their role in the development of atherosclerosis.
- Suggest healthy fat selections for an optimal diet.
- Describe possible health problems associated with a high-fat diet.

Maria and Rachel are trying to lose weight. Maria swears by a new diet program that allows you to eat all the fat you want but no high-carbohydrate, "starchy" foods. Her diet is working—she's already lost 10 pounds! Then there's Rachel, whose goal is to eat zero grams of fat. She's fat-obsessed—always insisting on "fat-free" everything and constantly annoying her friends with information about the number of fat grams in whatever they eat. As you listen to Maria and Rachel compare dieting stories, you wonder which one has the right approach to fat consumption, or even whether there *is* a right approach. On the one hand, it seems that you hear a lot about American high-fat diets and high rates of obesity and heart disease. On the other hand, can a "no-fat" diet be healthy? Are all low-fat and no-fat products really more nutritious? Is there a way to include dietary fat in a healthy diet?

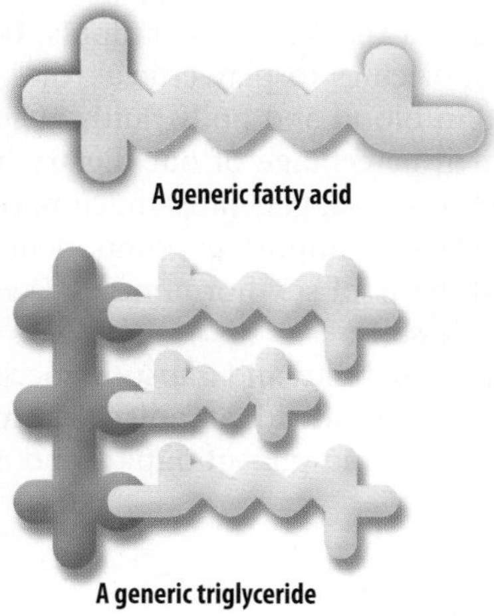

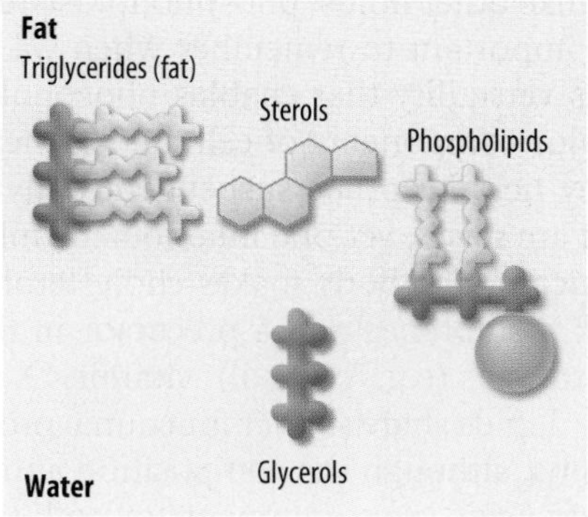

Fat is an essential nutrient. Although our bodies are very good at making and storing fat in the form of triglycerides, they cannot make some types of fatty acids (a component of triglycerides), so these compounds must come from the diet. Dietary **triglycerides**—the fats we eat in fried foods, cream cheese, vegetable oil, or salad dressing—are one type of a larger group of compounds called lipids. Cholesterol, another lipid, is familiar to most Americans, but you may not realize that your body makes cholesterol and that your dietary cholesterol makes only a small contribution to the total amount in your body. All lipids have important roles, but, at the same time, too much triglyceride or too much cholesterol can increase the risk for chronic disease.

▶ **triglycerides** The major form of lipids in food and in the body. They are composed of three fatty acids attached to a glyceride backbone. Triglycerides are the body's main storage form of energy and source of fuel for the body cells, with the exception of nervous system and red blood cells, which prefer glucose.

Fats contribute greatly to the flavor and texture of foods. When you take out the fat, sometimes you have to boost the flavor with sugar, sodium, or other additives to have a tasty product. This means that fat-free foods sometimes aren't any lower in calories or sugar than regular food—so Rachel can't eat the whole box of fat-free cookies and still expect to lose weight! Overeating calories, whether they come from fat, carbohydrate, or protein, will lead to energy storage as fat and, ultimately, increases in body weight. Once you have an idea of the role of lipids in the body and in foods, you'll be able to apply the principles of balance, variety, and moderation in selecting a healthful, enjoyable diet with neither too much nor too little fat.

THINK About It 1

What Are Lipids?

The term *lipids* applies to a broad range of organic molecules that dissolve easily in organic solvents such as alcohol, ether, or acetone, but are much less soluble in water. Lipids generally are **hydrophobic** (averse to water; literally "water-fearing") and **lipophilic** (soluble in fat and fat solvents; literally "fat-loving"). In contrast, water-soluble substances are, not surprisingly, **hydrophilic** (attracted to water, "water loving") and **lipophobic** (averse to fat solvents, "fat fearing"). Lipids vary in their solubility, with some being very hydrophobic and others less so. The main classes of lipids found in foods and in the body are triglycerides, phospholipids, and sterols.

Triglycerides are the largest category of lipids. In the body, fat cells store triglycerides in adipose tissue. In foods, we call triglycerides "fats and oils," with fats usually being solid and oils being liquid at room temperature. Overall, however, the choice of terminology—*fat, triglyceride, oil*—is somewhat arbitrary, and the terms are often used interchangeably. In this chapter, when we use the word *fat* or *oil*, we are referring to triglycerides.

About 2 percent of dietary lipids are **phospholipids.** They are found in foods of both plant and animal origin, and the body also makes those that it needs. Unlike other lipids, phospholipids are soluble in both fat and water. This will be important to remember when we talk about the functions of lipids. It is this versatility that enables phospholipid molecules to play crucial roles as major components of cell membranes and in blood and body fluids, where they help keep fats suspended. Only a small percentage of our dietary lipids are **sterols**, yet one infamous member, cholesterol, generates much public concern. The body makes cholesterol, which is an important component of cell membranes and a precursor in the synthesis of sex hormones, adrenal hormones (e.g., cortisol), vitamin D, and bile salts.

Lipids share similar functional properties, solubility, and transport mechanisms, although the composition and structure of individual molecules vary. Fatty acids are components of both triglycerides and phospholipids and are often attached to cholesterol.

Fatty Acids Are Key Building Blocks

Fatty acids determine the characteristics of a fat, such as whether it is solid or liquid at room temperature. Fatty acids that are not joined to another compound, such as the glycerol of a triglyceride, are sometimes called "free" fatty acids to emphasize that they are unattached. Some free fatty acids have their own distinct flavor. Butyric acid, for example, is the fatty acid that gives butter its flavor (see **FIGURE 5.1**).

Although there are many kinds of fatty acids, they are basically chains of carbon atoms with an organic acid (carboxyl) group (–COOH) at one end and a methyl group ($-CH_3$) at the other end.

- **hydrophobic** Insoluble in water.
- **lipophilic** Attracted to fat and fat solvents; fat-soluble.
- **hydrophilic** [high-dro-FILL-ik] Can mix with or dissolve in water ("water-loving"). Hydrophilic compounds are polar and soluble in water.
- **lipophobic** Adverse to fat solvents; insoluble in fat and fat solvents.
- **phospholipids** Compounds that consist of a glycerol molecule bonded to two fatty acid molecules and to a phosphate group with a nitrogen-containing component. Phospholipids have both hydrophilic and hydrophobic regions that make them good emulsifiers.
- **sterols** A category of lipids that includes cholesterol. Sterols are hydrocarbons with several rings in their structures.
- **fatty acids** Compounds containing a long hydrocarbon chain with a carboxyl group (–COOH) at one end and a methyl group ($-CH_3$) at the other end.

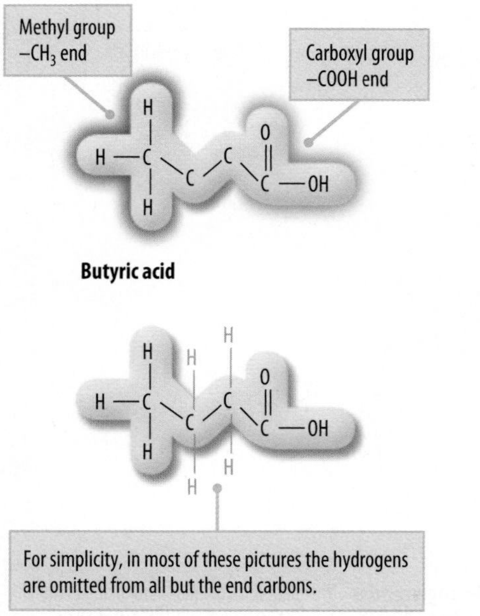
Methyl group
$-CH_3$ end
Carboxyl group
–COOH end
Butyric acid
For simplicity, in most of these pictures the hydrogens are omitted from all but the end carbons.

FIGURE 5.1 Fatty acid structure. The basic structure of a fatty acid is a carbon chain with a methyl end ($-CH_3$) and an acid (carboxyl) end (–COOH). Butyric acid (shown here) is a fatty acid found in butter fat.

Chain Length

Fatty acids differ in **chain length** (the number of carbons in the chain). Foods contain fatty acids with chain lengths of 4 to 24 carbons, and most have an even number of carbons. They are grouped as short-chain (fewer than 6 carbons), medium-chain (6 to 10 carbons), and long-chain (12 or more carbons) fatty acids (see **FIGURE 5.2**). The shorter the carbon chain, the more liquid the fatty acid (the lower its melting point) (see **FIGURE 5.3**). Shorter fatty acids also are more water-soluble, a property that affects their absorption in the digestive tract.

Each carbon in these chains can be numbered for identification, but it's important to know from which end the counting begins. In organic chemistry, the scientific naming of fatty acids counts from the carbon at the acid (COOH) end. This carbon is the alpha carbon, and the carbon at the methyl (CH_3) end is the omega carbon. They are named after the first and last letters of the Greek alphabet, respectively (see **FIGURE 5.4**). As you'll see later, nutritionists identify double bonds by their location relative to the omega carbon.

Saturation

Within a fatty acid chain, each carbon atom has four bonds. When a carbon is joined to adjacent carbons with single bonds (–C–C–C–), it still has two bonds available

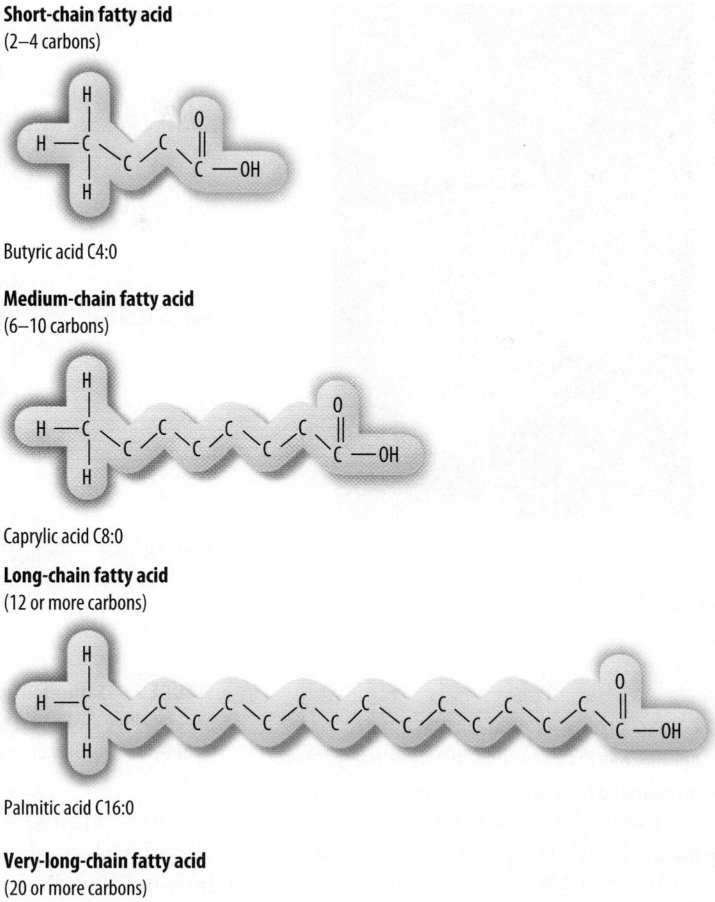

FIGURE 5.2 Fatty acid chain lengths. Fatty acids can be classified by their chain length as short-, medium-, or long-chain fatty acids.

▶ **chain length** The number of carbons that a fatty acid contains. Foods contain fatty acids with chain lengths of 4 to 24 carbons, and most have an even number of carbons.

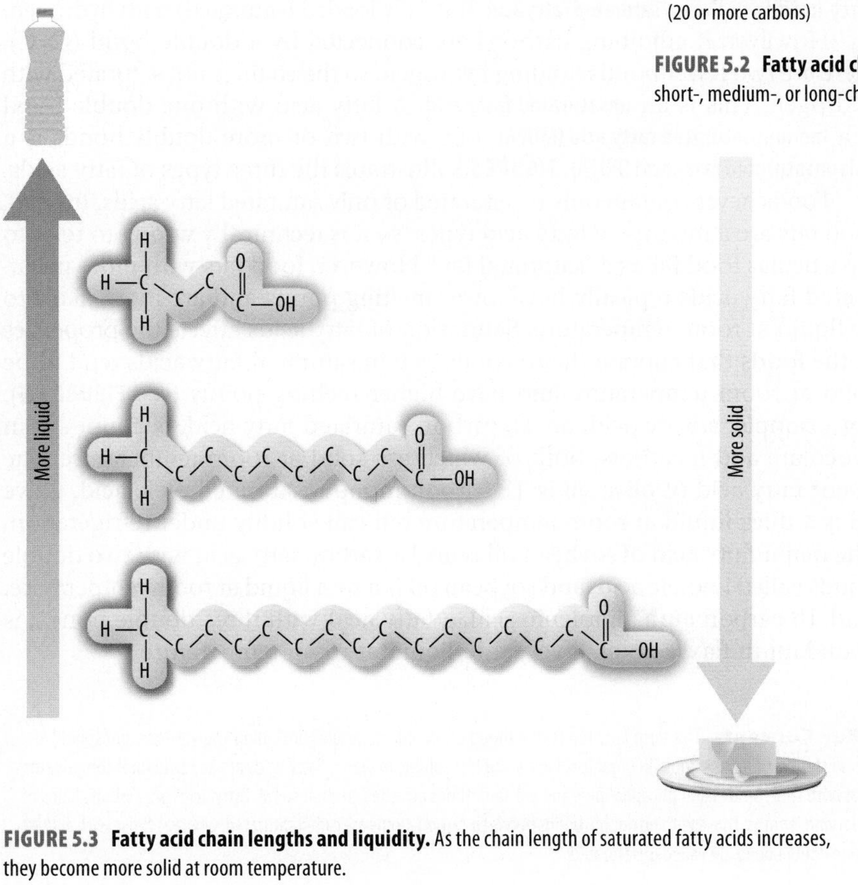

FIGURE 5.3 Fatty acid chain lengths and liquidity. As the chain length of saturated fatty acids increases, they become more solid at room temperature.

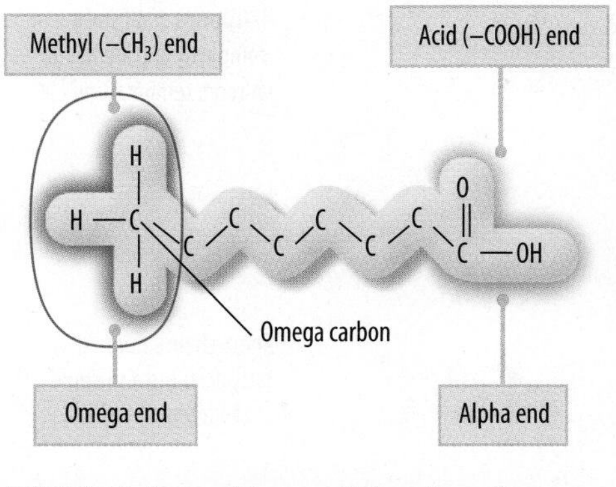

FIGURE 5.4 Fatty acid nomenclature. The carbons are identified by their locations in the chain. Although some disciplines count from the alpha carbon, nutritionists count from the omega carbon.

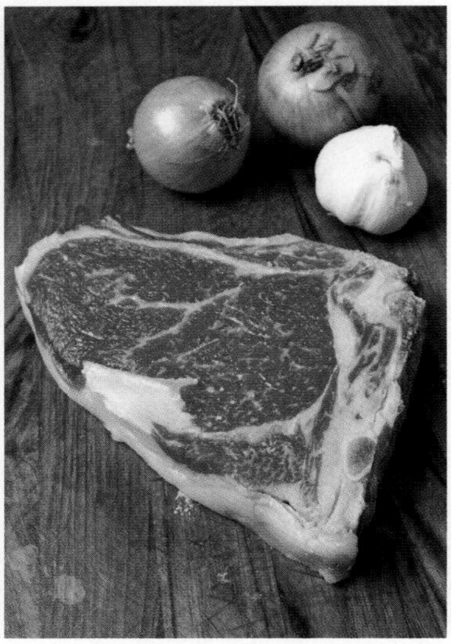

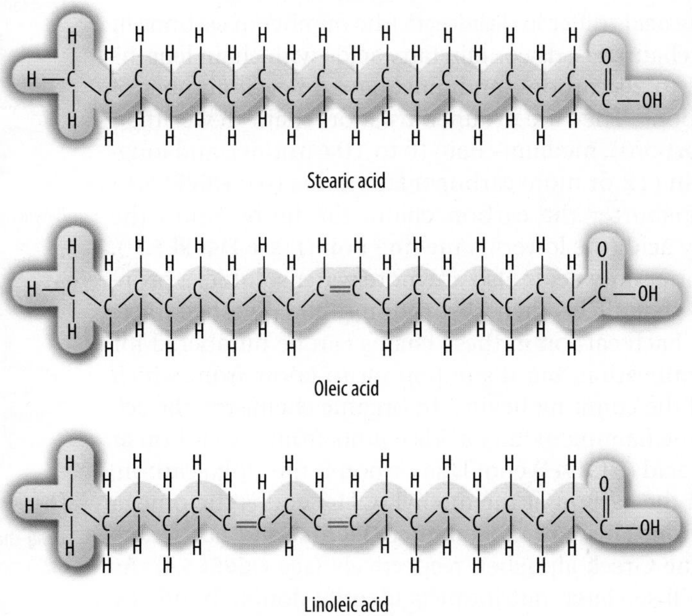
Type of Fatty Acid
Name and Chemical Structure
Saturated
Stearic acid
Monounsaturated
Oleic acid
Polyunsaturated
Linoleic acid

FIGURE 5.5 Saturated, monosaturated, and polyunsaturated fatty acids. All fatty acids have the same basic structure. Hydrogens saturate the carbon chain of a saturated fatty acid. Unsaturated fatty acids are missing some hydrogens and have one (mono) or more (poly) carbon–carbon double bonds.

- **saturated fatty acid** A fatty acid completely filled by hydrogen with all carbons in the chain linked by single bonds.
- **unsaturated fatty acid** A fatty acid in which the carbon chain contains one or more double bonds.
- **monounsaturated fatty acid (MUFA)** A fatty acid in which the carbon chain contains one double bond.
- **polyunsaturated fatty acid (PUFA)** A fatty acid in which the carbon chain contains two or more double bonds.

for other atoms, such as hydrogen atoms. If all the carbons in the chain are joined with single bonds and the remaining bonds are filled with hydrogen, the fatty acid is called a **saturated fatty acid**. It is fully loaded (saturated) with hydrogen.

However, if adjoining carbons are connected by a double bond (C=C), there are two fewer bonds holding hydrogen, so the chain is not saturated with hydrogen. This is an **unsaturated fatty acid**. A fatty acid with one double bond is a **monounsaturated fatty acid (MUFA)**; one with two or more double bonds is a **polyunsaturated fatty acid (PUFA)**. **FIGURE 5.5** illustrates the three types of fatty acids.

Foods never contain only unsaturated or only saturated fatty acids. Instead, food fats are a mixture of fatty acid types, so it is technically wrong to refer to a particular food fat as a "saturated fat." However, food fats with more unsaturated fatty acids typically have lower melting points and are more likely to be liquid at room temperature. Saturation of fatty acids affects the properties of the foods that contain them. Foods rich in saturated fatty acids tend to be solid at room temperature and have higher melting points (see **FIGURE 5.6**). For example, stearic acid, an 18-carbon saturated fatty acid, is abundant in chocolate and meat fats, both of which are solid at room temperature. The major fatty acid of olive oil is 18-carbon monounsaturated oleic acid. Olive oil is a thick liquid at room temperature but can solidify under refrigeration. The major fatty acid of soybean oil is an 18-carbon fatty acid with two double bonds called linoleic acid, and soybean oil is a thin liquid at room temperature. And 18-carbon alpha-linolenic acid, a fatty acid with three double bonds, is abundant in flaxseed oil, a very thin liquid at room temperature.

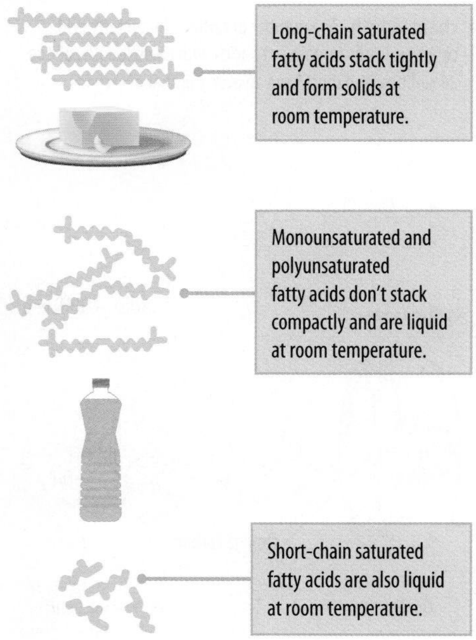
Long-chain saturated fatty acids stack tightly and form solids at room temperature.
Monounsaturated and polyunsaturated fatty acids don't stack compactly and are liquid at room temperature.
Short-chain saturated fatty acids are also liquid at room temperature.

FIGURE 5.6 Liquid or solid at room temperature? Short-chain and unsaturated fatty acids cannot pack tightly together and tend to be more liquid than long-chain saturated fatty acids are.

Key Concepts The term *lipid* refers to a group of organic molecules, including triglycerides, phospholipids, and sterols, that are soluble in organic solvents and less soluble in water. Fatty acids are key structural components of both triglycerides and phospholipids and are sometimes attached to cholesterol. Fatty acids are carbon chains of varying lengths. Those with no double bonds between carbon atoms are called saturated, whereas those with at least one double bond are called unsaturated.

Geometric and Positional Isomers

Otherwise identical unsaturated fatty acids can exist in different geometric forms, or isomers. In most naturally occurring unsaturated fatty acids, the hydrogens next to double bonds are on the same side of the carbon chain. This is called a *cis* formation. The carbon chain of a ***cis* fatty acid** is bent. If the double bond is altered, moving the hydrogens across from each other, the formation is called *trans* and the carbon chain is more straight (see **FIGURE 5.7**). Most of the naturally occurring unsaturated fatty acids are *cis* fatty acids. Although there are small amounts of ***trans* fatty acids** in meats and dairy products from cows and sheep, a commercial process of **hydrogenation** creates most of the *trans* fatty acids in our diets. The process of hydrogenation adds hydrogen to an unsaturated fatty acid, thereby making it more saturated. This process also straightens the fatty acid to a *trans* configuration. Most *trans* fatty acids are monounsaturated, but a small number are fatty acids with two double bonds. You probably have heard about the health concerns surrounding *trans* fatty acids. *Trans* fatty acids have been shown to raise low-density lipoprotein (LDL) cholesterol levels and are also associated with reducing plasma high-density lipoprotein (HDL), and therefore increase one's risk for heart disease.[1] Dietary *trans* fatty acids are discussed in more detail later in this chapter.

Conjugated linoleic acid (CLA) is a collective term for a group of geometric and positional isomers of linoleic acid in which the double bonds (*trans* or *cis*) are conjugated; that is, the double bonds occur without an intervening carbon atom that is not part of a double bond. CLA supplementation is purported to have several health benefits and has been studied for its potential to reduce lipid uptake by adipose cells, decrease body fat, and produce favorable changes in body composition; however, additional research is needed to establish CLA's antiobesity effects.[2]

Small amounts of *trans* fatty acids and conjugated linoleic acid are present in all diets. They can serve as a source of fuel energy for the body. However, there are no known requirements for *trans* fatty acids and conjugated linoleic acid for specific body functions.[3]

▶ ***cis* fatty acid** Unsaturated fatty acid in which the hydrogens surrounding a double bond are both on the same side of the carbon chain, causing a bend in the chain. Most naturally occurring unsaturated fatty acids are *cis* fatty acids.

▶ ***trans* fatty acids** Unsaturated fatty acids in which the hydrogens surrounding a double bond are on opposite sides of the carbon chain. This straightens the chain, and the fatty acid becomes more solid.

▶ **hydrogenation** [high-dro-jen-AY-shun] A chemical reaction in which hydrogen atoms are added to carbon–carbon double bonds, converting them to single bonds. Hydrogenation of monounsaturated and polyunsaturated fatty acids reduces the number of double bonds they contain, thereby making them more saturated.

▶ **conjugated linoleic acid (CLA)** A polyunsaturated fatty acid in which the position of the double bonds has moved so that a single bond alternates with two double bonds.

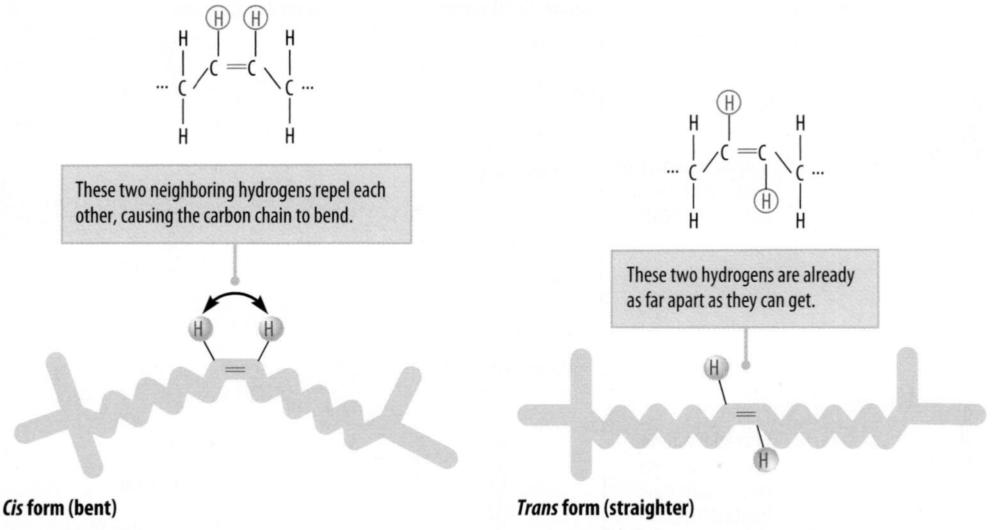
These two neighboring hydrogens repel each other, causing the carbon chain to bend.
These two hydrogens are already as far apart as they can get.
Cis form (bent)
Trans form (straighter)

FIGURE 5.7 *Cis* and *trans* fatty acids. Fatty acids with the bent *cis* form are more common in food than the *trans* form. *Trans* fatty acids are most commonly found in hydrogenated fats, such as those in stick margarine, shortening, and deep-fat-fried foods.

Essential and Nonessential Fatty Acids

The body is a good chemist, synthesizing most fatty acids as it needs them. The liver adds carbons in a process called **elongation** to build storage and structural fats, to manufacture the fat in breast milk, or to make fatty acids for use in other compounds. The body also synthesizes oleic acid, an omega-9 fatty acid, by removing hydrogens from carbons 9 and 10 of saturated stearic acid, thus creating a double bond at carbon 9. This process is called **desaturation**. Oleic acid can be elongated further and desaturated to create other necessary fatty acids.

- **elongation** Addition of carbon atoms to fatty acids to lengthen them into new fatty acids.
- **desaturation** Insertion of double bonds into fatty acids to change them into new fatty acids.
- **omega-9 fatty acid** Any polyunsaturated fatty acid in which the first double bond starting from the methyl ($-CH_3$) end of the molecule lies between the ninth and tenth carbon atoms.
- **omega-3 fatty acids** Any polyunsaturated fatty acid in which the first double bond starting from the methyl ($-CH_3$) end of the molecule lies between the third and fourth carbon atoms.
- **omega-6 fatty acid** Any polyunsaturated fatty acid in which the first double bond starting from the methyl ($-CH_3$) end of the molecule lies between the sixth and seventh carbon atoms.
- **nonessential fatty acids** The fatty acids that your body can make when they are needed. It is not necessary to consume them in the diet.
- **essential fatty acids** The fatty acids that the body needs but cannot synthesize, and which must be obtained from diet.

Omega-3, Omega-6, and Omega-9 Fatty Acids

The location of the double bond closest to the omega (methyl) end of the fatty acid chain identifies a fatty acid's family. Oleic acid has one double bond, at carbon 9 (counting from the omega end of the chain) and is classified as an **omega-9 fatty acid**. Linoleic acid has double bonds at both carbon 6 and carbon 9. Because the first double bond occurs at carbon 6, it is an **omega-6 fatty acid**. **Omega-3 fatty acids** such as alpha-linolenic acid have a double bond at carbon 3, plus two or more additional double bonds (see **FIGURE 5.8**). All of these fatty acids can be burned for energy. When the body uses them to synthesize new compounds, however, the omega-3, omega-6, and omega-9 classes behave quite differently.

Because your body can make saturated and omega-9 fatty acids, it is not essential to get them in your diet. We therefore call them **nonessential fatty acids**. Do not confuse "nonessential" with "unimportant." Your body ensures that there is an adequate supply of nonessential fatty acids by making them when they are needed.

Our bodies cannot produce carbon–carbon double bonds before the ninth carbon from the methyl end, so we cannot manufacture certain fatty acids such as omega-6 linoleic or omega-3 alpha-linolenic acids. They must come from food, so they're called **essential fatty acids** (EFAs) (see **FIGURE 5.9**). Deficiency of essential fatty acids is extremely rare. It typically occurs only with severe fat malabsorption or prolonged intravenous feeding without supplemental fat. A lack of linoleic acid leads to a scaly skin rash and dermatitis, poor growth in children, and a lowered immune response.

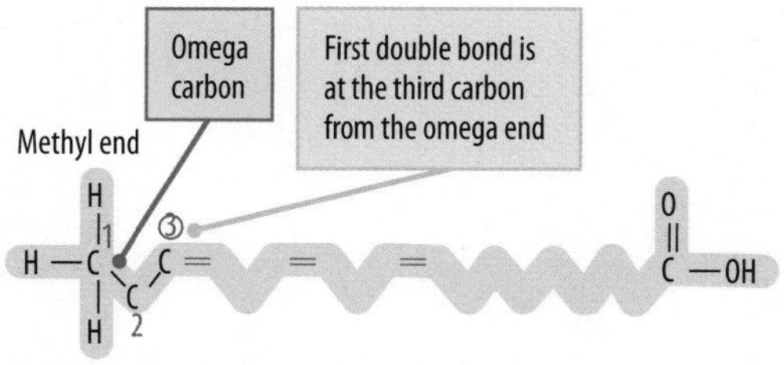

Alpha-linolenic, an omega-3 fatty acid

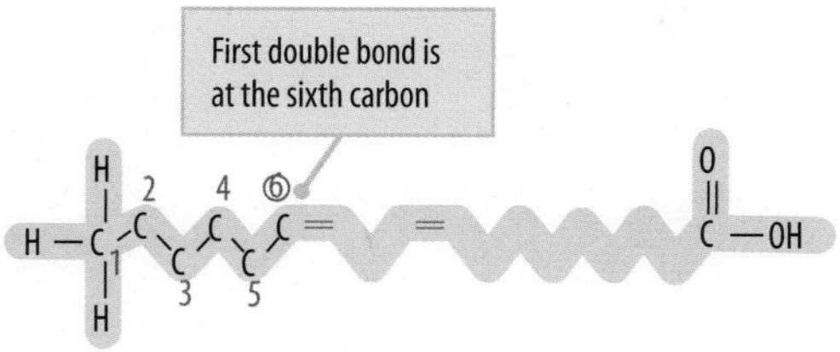

Linoleic, an omega-6 fatty acid

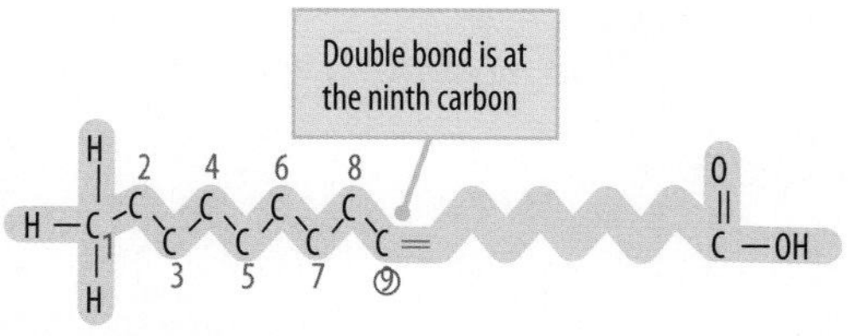

Oleic, an omega-9 fatty acid

FIGURE 5.8 Omega-3, omega-6, and omega-9 fatty acids. Unsaturated fatty acids can be classified by counting from the omega carbon to the location of the first double bond.

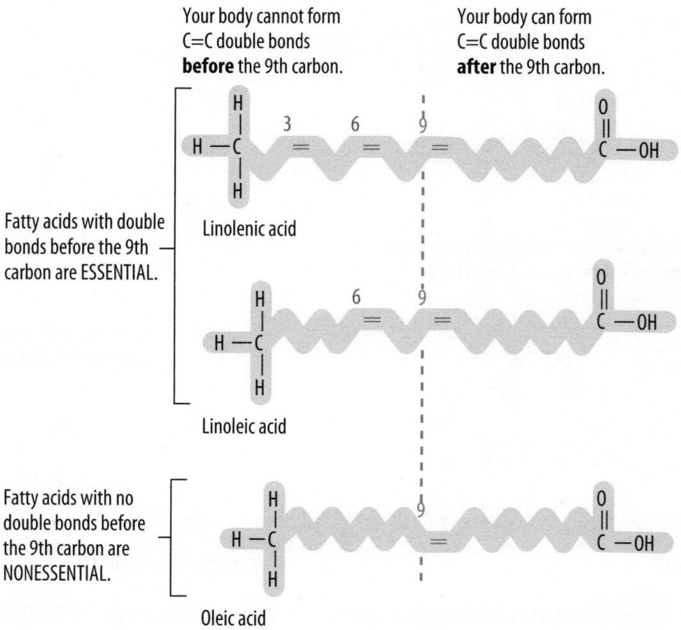

FIGURE 5.9 Essential and nonessential fatty acids. Your body makes some types of fatty acids, but others are essential to obtain from your diet.

Building Eicosanoids and Omega-3 and Omega-6 Fatty Acids

You metabolize most of the fatty acids you eat to supply your energy needs, but a small proportion become crucial chemical regulators. The **eicosanoids** (also called prostanoids) are one such group of regulators. These signaling molecules contain 20 or more carbons (*eikosi* is the Greek word for "twenty"). They have profound localized effects through their influence on inflammatory processes, blood vessel dilation and constriction, blood clotting, and more. Because they don't circulate throughout the body as hormones do, scientists sometimes call eicosanoids "local" hormones.

▶ **eicosanoids** A class of hormonelike substances formed in the body from long-chain fatty acids.

▶ **linoleic acid [lin-oh-LAY-ik ah-sid]** An essential omega-6 fatty acid that contains 18 carbon atoms and 2 carbon–carbon double bonds (18:2).

Eicosanoids are made from unsaturated long-chain fatty acids from membrane phospholipids or circulating free fatty acids. The liver elongates these fatty acids 2 carbons at a time until the carbon chains have 20 or 22 carbons. Elongation alternates with desaturation. Once the fatty acid reaches 20 carbons, the body can convert it to one or more of the eicosanoids, such as thromboxanes, prostaglandins, prostacyclins, lipoxins, and leukotrienes. Eicosanoids can have opposing physiologic effects depending on whether they are derived from omega-3, omega-6, or omega-9 fatty acids. Here, we concentrate on eicosanoids derived from the essential fatty acids—that is, from the omega-3s and omega-6s, over which we probably have the most dietary control and where most interest currently lies.

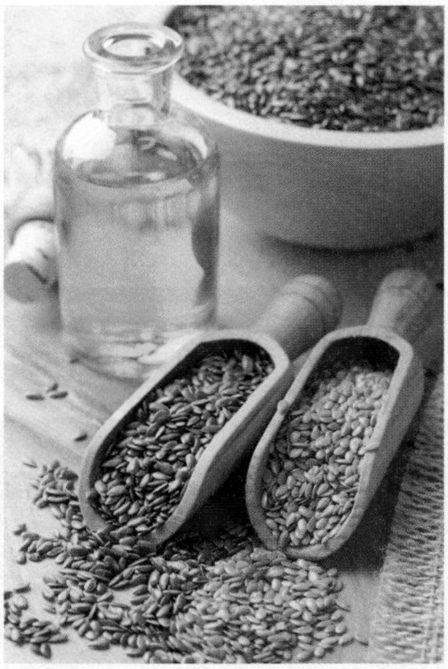

© iStockphoto/Thinkstock

The Omega-6 Fatty Acids

Linoleic acid, an 18-carbon essential fatty acid with two double bonds (18:2), is our main dietary omega-6 fatty acid. In a sequence of elongation and desaturation steps, our bodies convert linoleic acid to arachidonic acid, a 20-carbon fatty acid with four double bonds (20:4). To simplify a very complex picture, a series of eicosanoids is then formed from arachidonic acid (see **TABLE 5.1**), and these eicosanoids have the overall effect of constricting blood vessels, promoting blood clotting, and promoting inflammation.

Good sources of the 18-carbon omega-6 fatty acid linoleic acid include seeds, nuts, and the richest sources, common vegetable oils such as corn oil. Small amounts of arachidonic acid, a 20-carbon omega-6 fatty acid, are found in meat, poultry, and eggs but not in plant foods.

▶ **alpha-linolenic acid [al-fah lin-oh-LEN-ik ah-sid]** An essential omega-3 fatty acid that contains 18 carbon atoms and 3 carbon–carbon double bonds (18:3).

The Omega-3 Fatty Acids

Alpha-linolenic acid is an 18-carbon essential fatty acid with three double bonds (18:3). It can ultimately be elongated and desaturated to EPA (eicosapentaenoic acid), with 20 carbons and five double bonds (20:5), and DHA (docosahexaenoic acid), with 22 carbons and six double bonds (22:6). (See **TABLE 5.2**.) However, for these reactions to take place, it must compete with the omega-6s (and even with polyunsaturated trans fatty acids) for the same enzymes, so only a portion of alpha-linolenic acid is converted to EPA and DHA. Eicosanoids formed from the omega-3 fatty acid alpha-linolenic acid have opposing "heart-healthy" effects of dilating blood vessels, discouraging blood clotting, and reducing inflammation. The role of omega-3 fatty acids in decreasing the risk of abnormal heartbeat, lowering triglyceride levels, and slowing atherosclerotic plaque growth have attracted interest for reducing risk for vascular disease.[4,5] Additional health benefits that have been associated with omega-3 fatty acids include the secondary prevention of chronic diseases and an association with the following[6,7]:

- *Inflammatory conditions:* Improves rheumatoid arthritis, psoriasis, asthma, and some skin conditions.
- *Ulcerative colitis and Crohn's disease:* Reduces the severity of symptoms.

TABLE 5.1
Omega-6 to Eicosanoids

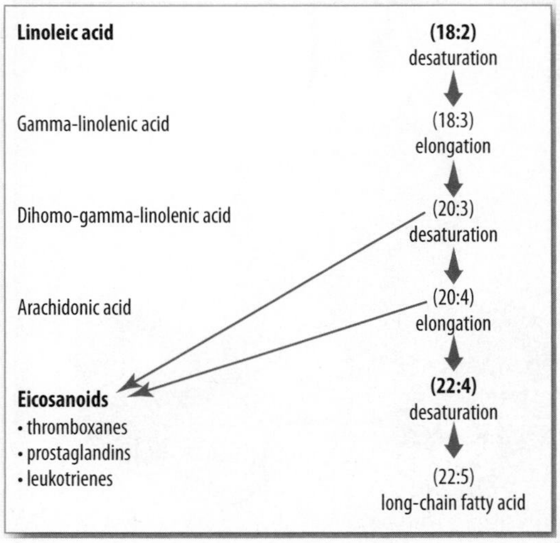

TABLE 5.2
Omega-3 to Eicosanoids

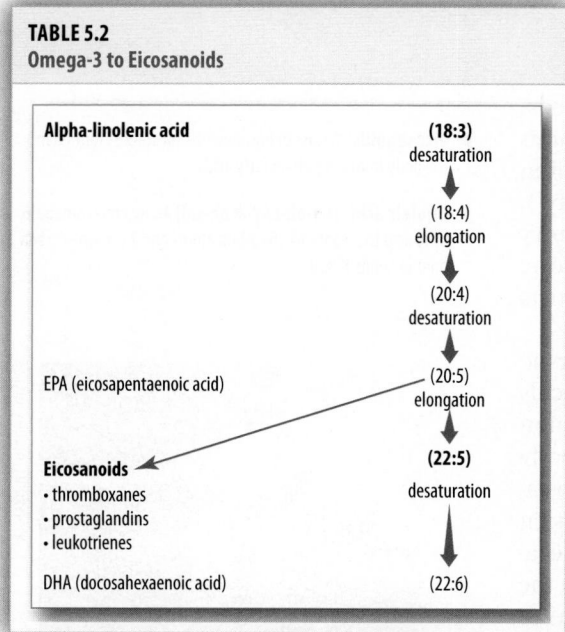

Alpha-linolenic acid	**(18:3)**
	desaturation ↓
	(18:4)
	elongation ↓
	(20:4)
	desaturation ↓
EPA (eicosapentaenoic acid)	(20:5)
	elongation ↓
Eicosanoids ← (from 20:5) • thromboxanes • prostaglandins • leukotrienes	**(22:5)**
	desaturation ↓
DHA (docosahexaenoic acid)	(22:6)

- *Cardiovascular disease:* Lowers triglycerides and raises high-density lipoprotein cholesterol levels, improves blood circulation, reduces clotting, improves vascular function, and lowers blood pressure.
- *Type 2 diabetes mellitus (T2DM):* Reduces hyperinsulinemia and insulin resistance.
- *Renal disease:* Preserves renal function in IgA nephropathy; potentially reduces vascular access thrombosis in hemodialysis patients and is cardioprotective.
- *Mental function:* Reduces severity of several mental conditions such as Alzheimer's disease, depression, and bipolar disorder; improvement in children with attention deficit hyperactivity disorder and dyslexia has also been noted.
- *Growth and development:* Neurodevelopment and function of the brain and also the retina of the eye where visual function is affected.

As a result of the findings regarding growth and development, DHA (along with omega-6 arachidonic acid) is now being added to selected infant formulas.

Plant foods are generally rich in polyunsaturated fatty acids. Soybean oil, canola oil, and walnuts contain alpha-linolenic acid, the essential omega-3 fatty acid. However, the most generous source is flaxseed (or linseed) oil, which is more than 50 percent alpha-linolenic acid. Longer-chain omega-3s—EPA and DHA—are found in fatty fish and in fish oil supplements. See the FYI feature "Fats on the Health Store Shelf." **TABLE 5.3** lists the omega-3 fatty acids in some foods.

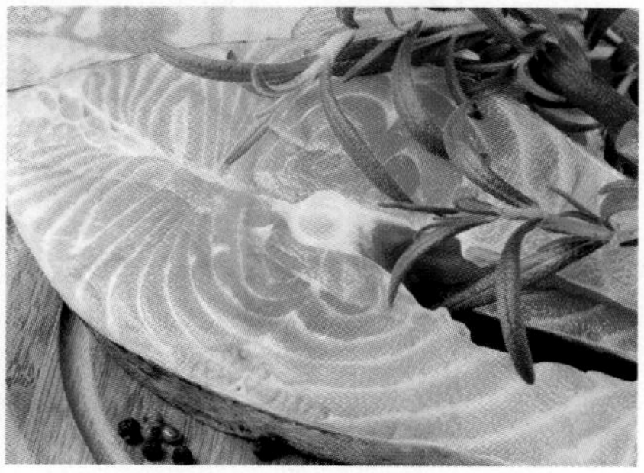
© iStockphoto/Thinkstock

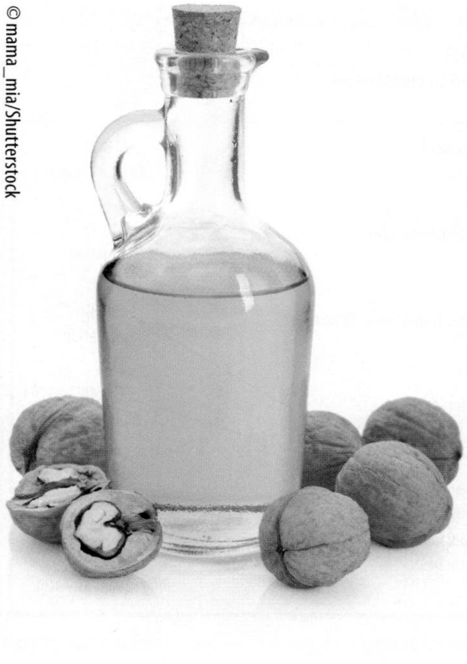
© mama_mia/Shutterstock

Key Concepts Unsaturated fatty acids can have *cis* or *trans* double bonds. The body can make many of the fatty acids it needs, but it cannot make linoleic or alpha-linolenic acids, so these are dietary essentials. The body can elongate and desaturate essential fatty acids to form other important compounds, such as eicosanoids.

TABLE 5.3
Omega-3 Fatty Acids in Selected Foods

	18:3 (mg)	20:5 (EPA) (mg)	22:6 (DHA) (mg)
1 Tbsp canola oil	1,279		
1 Tbsp soybean oil	923		
1 Tbsp walnut oil	1,414		
1 Tbsp flaxseed oil	7,258		
3 oz canned sockeye salmon (fatty fish)		440	637
3 oz cooked mackerel (fatty fish)		428	594
3 oz flounder (lean fish)		143	112
3 oz cooked shrimp		115	120
1 Tbsp cod liver oil		938	1,492
1 Tbsp salmon oil		1,771	2,480

Fish and seafood also contain small amounts of 18:3, which are not included on this table.

It sounds like a lot of omega-3. But remember, these are milligrams! Dietary fat is usually measured in grams. The 267 milligrams (0.267 g) of EPA and DHA in a serving of shrimp is not much in relation to a diet that has 50+ grams of fat and is a bit less than half the recommendation for daily intake.

Data from U.S. Department of Agriculture, Agricultural Research Service. USDA Nutrient Database for Standard Reference, Release 25. 2012. www.ars.usda.gov/ba/bhnrc/ndl. Accessed 1/20/13.

Triglycerides

Triglycerides are the major lipids in both the diet and the body. Triglycerides add flavor and texture (and calories!) to foods and are an important source of the body's energy.

Triglyceride Structure

A triglyceride consists of three fatty acids attached to a molecule of glycerol. Both in food and in the body, most fatty acids exist as part of a triglyceride molecule. Alone, **glycerol** is a thick, smooth liquid often used in the food industry. Chemically it is an alcohol, a simple three-carbon molecule with an alcohol (hydroxyl) group (–OH) at each carbon. Glycerol is the backbone of a triglyceride. It is always the same, whereas the fatty acids attached to it can vary considerably. Chemically speaking, a triglyceride is an **ester**, a combination of an alcohol and a fatty acid. An ester forms when a hydrogen and an oxygen from the fatty acid's carboxyl (acid) group combine with a hydrogen from the alcohol's hydroxyl (alcohol) group. Because the reaction produces a molecule of water, it is called a condensation reaction. An ester linkage now chemically joins the altered fatty acid and alcohol, a process called **esterification**.

Esterification produces triglycerides, **diglycerides** (two fatty acids attached to a glycerol), and **monoglycerides** (one fatty acid attached to a glycerol). **FIGURE 5.10** illustrates the formation of a triglyceride. Our foods contain relatively small amounts of mono- and diglycerides, mostly as food additives used for their emulsifying or blending qualities.

Triglyceride Functions

Although some of us, like Rachel at the beginning of this chapter, think of fat as something to avoid, fat is a key nutrient with important body functions. Fat serves many essential functions in the body. In addition to providing a valuable source of stored energy, lipids are essential to normal cellular structure and function. **FIGURE 5.11** shows the functions of triglycerides.

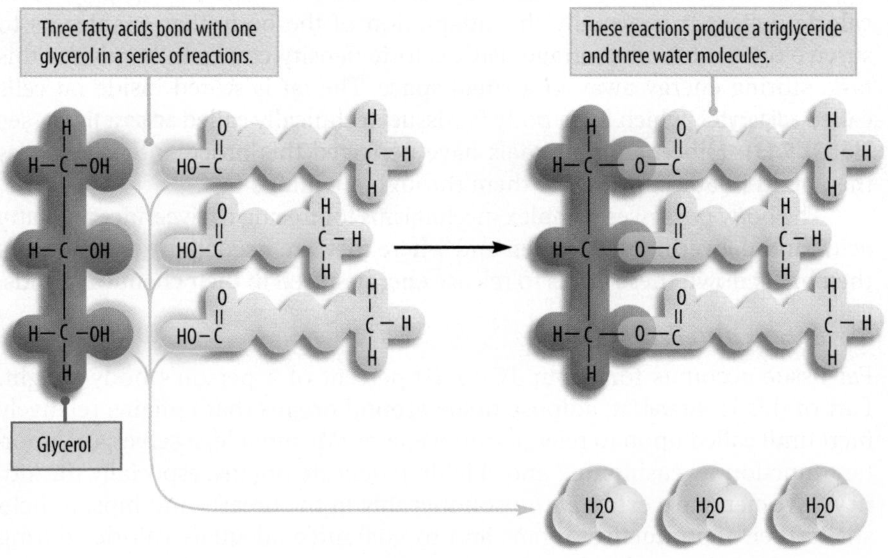

FIGURE 5.10 Forming a triglyceride. Condensation reactions attach three fatty acids to a glycerol backbone to form a triglyceride. These reactions release water.

Position Statement: American Heart Association

Omega-3 Fatty Acids

The American Heart Association recommends eating fish (particularly fatty fish) at least two times (two servings) a week. Each serving is 3.5 ounces cooked, or about ¾ cup of flaked fish. Fatty fish like salmon, mackerel, herring, lake trout, sardines, and albacore tuna are high in omega-3 fatty acids.

Increasing omega-3 fatty acid consumption through foods is preferable. However, those with coronary artery disease may not get enough omega-3 by diet alone. These people may want to talk to their doctor about supplements. And for those with high triglycerides, even larger doses could help.

Reproduced from American Heart Association. Fish and omega-3 fatty acids. 2015. http://www.heart.org/HEARTORG/GettingHealthy/NutritionCenter/HealthyDietGoals/Fish-and-Omega-3-Fatty-Acids_UCM_303248_Article.jsp. Accessed December 23, 2015.

- ▶ **glycerol** [GLISS-er-ol] An alcohol that contains three carbon atoms, each of which has an attached hydroxyl group (–OH). It forms the backbone of mono-, di-, and triglycerides.
- ▶ **ester** A chemical combination of an organic acid (e.g., fatty acid) and an alcohol. When hydrogen from the alcohol combines with the acid's hydrogen and oxygen, water is released and an ester linkage is formed. A triglyceride is an ester of three fatty acids and glycerol.
- ▶ **esterification** [e-ster-ih-fih-KAY-shun] A condensation reaction in which an organic acid (e.g., fatty acid) combines with an alcohol with the loss of water, creating an ester.
- ▶ **diglycerides** Molecules composed of glycerol combined with two fatty acids.
- ▶ **monoglycerides** Molecules composed of glycerol combined with one fatty acid.

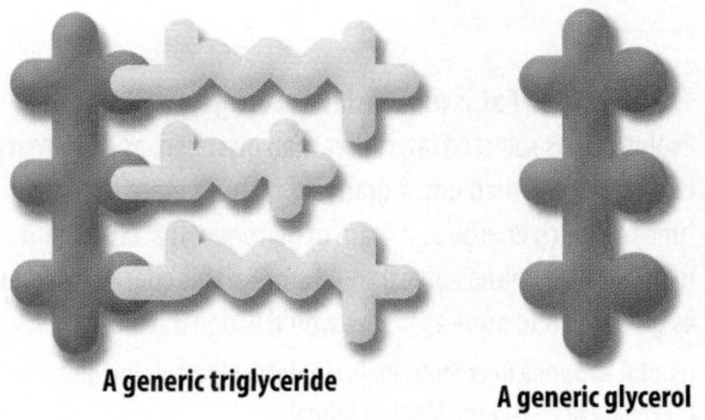

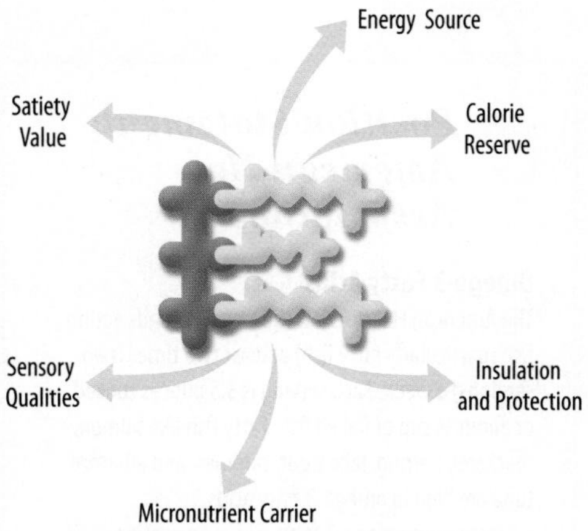

FIGURE 5.11 Functions of triglycerides. Fat performs a number of essential functions in the body.

© Photodisc

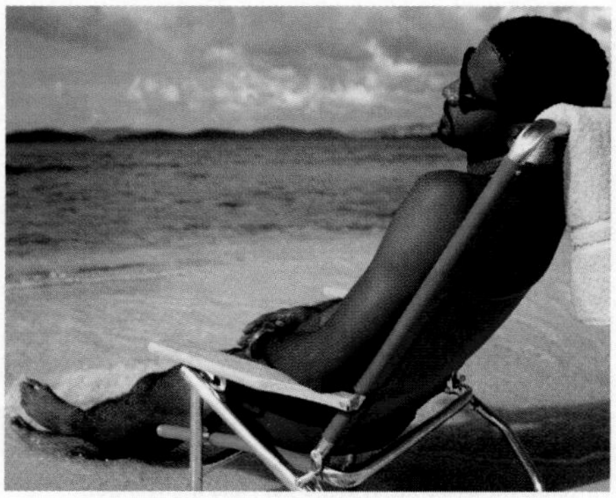

FIGURE 5.12 Fat is a major energy source. When at rest, muscles prefer to use fat for fuel.

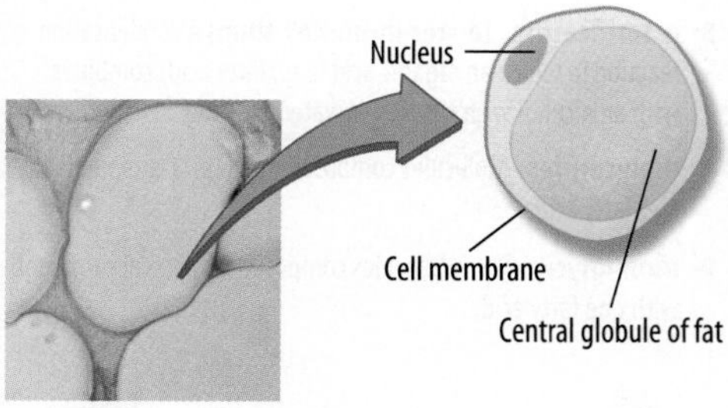

FIGURE 5.13 Fat is an efficient storage medium. Evolution has selected fat, rather than glycogen, as its primary energy storage medium. A gram of fat stores more than six times as much energy as a gram of glycogen. If a 155-pound man (with 20 pounds of fat) could store all his energy reserves as glycogen and none as fat, he would weigh 255 pounds!

(Photo) © Donna Beer Stolz, Ph.D., Center for Biologic Imaging, University of Pittsburgh Medical School.

- **adipocytes** Fat cells.
- **adipose tissue** Body fat tissue.
- **visceral fat** Fat stores that cushion body organs.
- **subcutaneous fat** Fat stores under the skin.

Energy Source

Fat is a rich and efficient source of calories. Under normal circumstances, dietary and stored fat supply about 60 percent of the body's resting energy needs. Like carbohydrate, fat is *protein-sparing*; that is, fat is burned for energy, sparing valuable proteins for their important roles as muscle tissue, enzymes, antibodies, and other functions. Different body tissues preferentially use different sources of calories. Glucose is virtually the sole fuel for the brain except during prolonged starvation, and fat is the preferred fuel of muscle tissue at rest (see **FIGURE 5.12**). During physical activity, glucose and glycogen join fat in supplying energy.

High-fat foods are higher in calories than either high-protein or high-carbohydrate foods. One gram of fat contains 9 kilocalories, compared with only 4 kilocalories in a gram of carbohydrate or protein, or 7 kilocalories per gram of alcohol. For example, a tablespoon of corn oil (pure fat) has 120 kilocalories, whereas a tablespoon of sugar (pure carbohydrate) has only 50 kilocalories.

The high concentration of calories in fat can be advantageous to good health in some circumstances. Fat's caloric density is especially important when energy needs are high. An infant, for example, who needs ample energy for fast growth but whose stomach can hold only a limited amount of food, needs the high fat content of breast milk or infant formula to get enough calories. When inappropriately put on a low-fat diet, infants and young children do not grow and develop properly. Other people with high energy needs include athletes, individuals who are physically active in their jobs, and people who are trying to regain weight lost as a result of illness.

Of course, fat's caloric density has a negative side. In practical terms, 9 kilocalories per gram translates to about 115 to 120 kilocalories per tablespoon of pure fat (e.g., vegetable oil). That makes it very easy to get too many fat calories, and dietary fat in excess of a person's energy needs is a major contributor to obesity.

Energy Reserve

We store excess dietary fat as body fat to hold us over during periods of calorie deficit. It is actually this adaptation of the body that enables us to survive times of food shortage. Fat's caloric density comes in handy for this task, storing energy away in a small space. The fat is stored inside fat cells called **adipocytes**, which form body fat tissue, technically called **adipose tissue** (see **FIGURE 5.13**). Hibernating animals have perfected this process; the fat stores they build in autumn can see them through a winter's fast.

The body possesses complex mechanisms for freeing triglycerides and fatty acids and delivering them when and where they are needed for energy. Cells then break down these lipids to release energy stored in their chemical bonds.

Insulation and Protection

Fat tissue accounts for about 15 to 30 percent of a person's body weight. Part of this is **visceral fat**, adipose tissue around organs that remains relatively inert until called upon to release stored energy. Meanwhile, it serves an important function by cushioning and shielding delicate organs, especially the kidneys. Women have extra fat, most noticeably in the breasts and hips, to help shield their reproductive organs and to guarantee adequate calories during pregnancy. Lying under the skin, where it protects and insulates the body, is other fat tissue called **subcutaneous fat**. Perhaps nowhere is fat's structural role more dramatic than in the brain, which is 60 percent fat.[8] Ectopic fat, the excess storage of triglycerides in non-adipose tissue locations, leads to an accumulation of fat in vital organs and blood vessels, which appears to impair their function and disrupt metabolic processes contributing to insulin resistance and increased risk of T2DM, unfavorable blood lipid levels, and cardiometabolic disease.[9] **FIGURE 5.14** shows the primary areas of fat storage in women and men.

THINK About It 2

Can a person have too little body fat? Just ask someone whose body fat has been depleted by illness. It hurts to sit and it hurts to lie down. For people without enough body fat, cool temperatures are intolerable and even room temperature can be uncomfortably cool. Women stop menstruating and become infertile. Children stop growing. Skin deteriorates from pressure sores or from fatty acid deficiency and can become covered with fine hair called **lanugo**. Illness, involuntary starvation, and famine can deplete fat to this extent, as can excessive dieting and exercise.

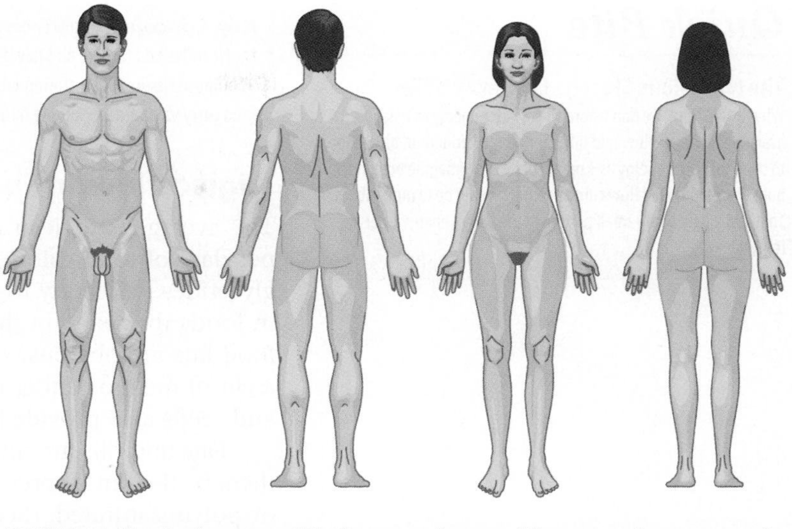

FIGURE 5.14 Sites for fat storage differ for men and women. Whereas men often store excess fat in their abdomens, women tend to store it in their hips.

▶ **lanugo [lah-NEW-go]** Soft, downy hair that covers a normal fetus from the fifth month but is shed almost entirely by the time of birth. It also appears on semistarved individuals who have lost much of their body fat, serving as insulation normally provided by body fat.

Carrier of Fat-Soluble Compounds

As you can see in **FIGURE 5.15**, dietary fats dissolve and transport micronutrients such as fat-soluble vitamins and fat-soluble phytochemicals such as carotenoids. Phytochemicals, although not essential (their lack does not cause a deficiency disease), have emerged as contributors to optimal health.

Dietary fats carry other fat-soluble substances through the digestive process, improving intestinal absorption and bioavailability. For example, the body absorbs more lycopene, the healthful red-colored phytochemical in tomatoes, if the tomatoes are served with a little oil or salad dressing. People who suffer from fat malabsorption disorders risk deficiency of fat-soluble micronutrients, so many must use supplements.

Removing a food's lipid portion—for example, removing butterfat from milk—also removes fat-soluble vitamins. In the case of most dairy products, vitamin A and sometimes vitamin D is replaced. Refining wheat grain to white flour extends shelf life, but removes the lipid-rich germ portion. Vitamin E is lost with the germ and is not replaced, which is another good reason to eat more whole-grain bread products. Fat-soluble vitamins also can be destroyed in fat processing; for example, some vitamin E is lost in processing vegetable oils.

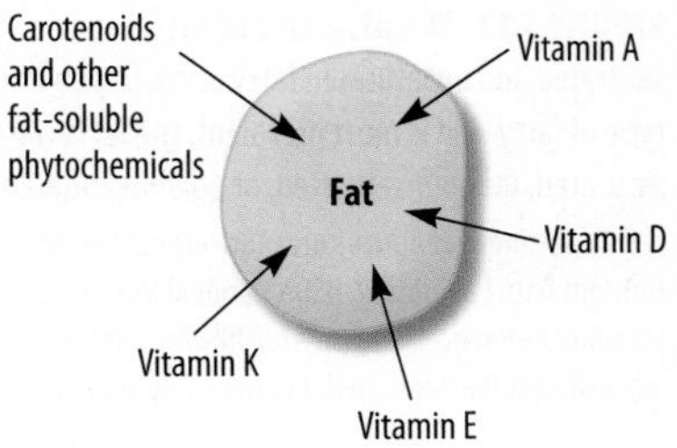

FIGURE 5.15 Fat is a micronutrient carrier. Fat holds more than just energy. It also carries important nutrients such as fat-soluble vitamins and carotenoids.

Sensory Qualities

As a food component or as an ingredient, fat contributes greatly to the flavor, odor, and texture of food (see **FIGURE 5.16**). Simply put, it makes food taste good. Flavorful volatile chemicals are dissolved in the fat of a food; heat sends them into the air, producing mouth-watering odors that perk up appetites. Fats have a rich, satisfying feeling in the mouth. Fats make baked goods tender and moist. And fats can be heated to high temperatures for frying, which seals in flavors and cooks food quickly. These are all good qualities—but too good for many people who find high-fat foods irresistible and eat too much of them. Alas, fat's most appealing attributes are also serious drawbacks to maintaining a healthful diet. Current research findings have implications for the design of foods that mimic the pleasant texture of fat in the mouth but have low energy content.[10] Such fat alternatives may prove to be useful in the prevention and treatment of overweight and obesity.

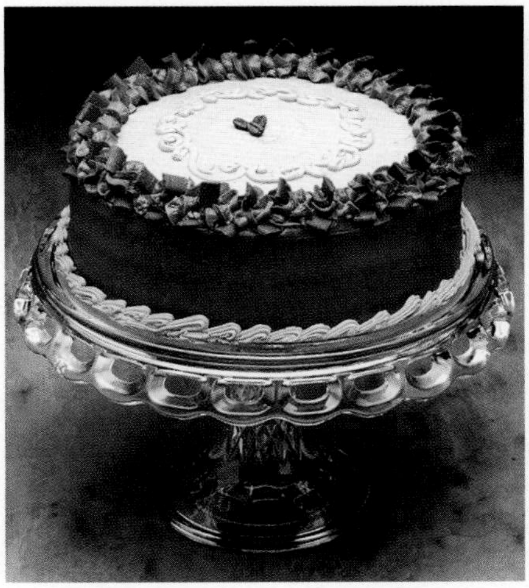

FIGURE 5.16 Fat imparts a rich sensory quality to food.

Quick Bite

The Marvelous Storage Efficiency of Fat

Why do you think we don't store all our extra energy as readily available glycogen? It would take more than 6 pounds of glycogen to store the same energy as 1 pound of fat. Just imagine how much bulkier we would be! How cumbersome it would be to move about. That's why only a very small portion of the body's energy reserve is glycogen.

Key Concepts Triglycerides are formed when a glycerol molecule combines with three fatty acids. Dietary triglycerides add texture and flavor to food and are a concentrated source of calories. The body stores excess calories as adipose tissue. While storing energy, adipose tissue also insulates the body and cushions its organs. The fats in food carry valuable fat-soluble nutrients into the body and help with their absorption.

Triglycerides in Food

The average American diet contains about 35–40 percent (80–130 grams per day) of total calories from fat; of that, more than 90% comes from triglycerides.[11] Dietary triglycerides are found in a variety of fats and oils and in foods that contain them, such as salad dressing and baked goods. Some food fats are obvious, such as butter, margarine, cooking oil, and fat along a cut of meat or under the skin of chicken. Baked goods, snack foods, nuts, and seeds also provide fat, but less noticeably.

Fats and oils are mixtures of many triglycerides, but we often categorize them by their most prevalent type of fatty acid—saturated, monounsaturated, or polyunsaturated. (See **FIGURE 5.17**.) Canola oil, for example, often is classified as a monounsaturated fat because most of the fatty acids in canola oil are the monounsaturated fatty acid oleic acid. Coconut oil, on the other hand, is considered a saturated fat because the most prevalent fatty acids are saturated. Although these classifications are useful, they do not always tell

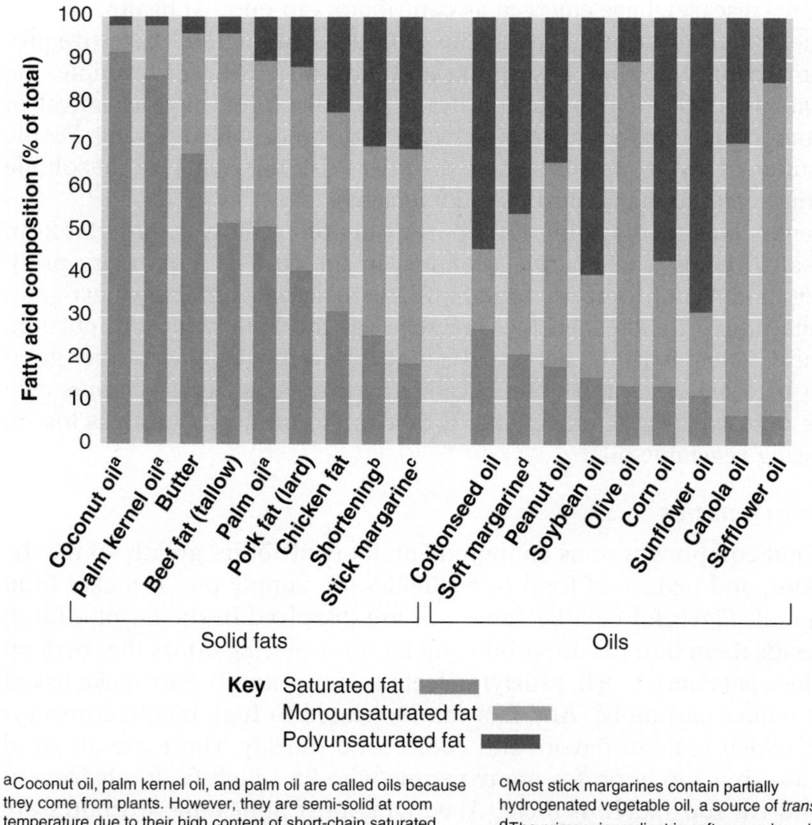

[a]Coconut oil, palm kernel oil, and palm oil are called oils because they come from plants. However, they are semi-solid at room temperature due to their high content of short-chain saturated fatty acids. They are considered solid fats for nutritional purposes.

[b]Partially hydrogenated vegetable oil shortening, which contains *trans* fats.

[c]Most stick margarines contain partially hydrogenated vegetable oil, a source of *trans* fats.

[d]The primary ingredient in soft margarine with no *trans* fats is liquid vegetable oil.

FIGURE 5.17 The diversity of fats. Fats are mixtures of saturated and unsaturated fatty acids. Depending on which type of fatty acid is most prevalent, the fat is classified as saturated, monounsaturated, or polyunsaturated.

U.S. Department of Agriculture, Agricultural Research Service, Nutrient Data Laboratory. USDA National Nutrient Database for Standard Reference, Release 22, 2009. Available at http://www.ars.usda.gov/ba/bhnrc/ndl. Accessed July 19, 2010.

the whole story. For example, saturated stearic acid appears to affect blood cholesterol differently than saturated palmitic acid does.

Commercial Processing of Fats

In nature, almost all fats exist in combination with other macronutrients: They generally occur along with starches in plant foods and with proteins in animal foods. In earlier times, the only concentrated fats and oils available to people were obtained by very simple processing: rendering fats from meats and poultry; skimming or churning the butterfat from milk; skimming the oil from ground nuts; or pressing a few oil-rich plant parts such as coconuts or olives.

Technology that came into use in the 1920s allowed production of pure vegetable oils.[12] By efficiently removing edible oil from its source, processing has increased the availability of calories worldwide. Processing reduces waste and prevents spoilage during normal use and storage. It does so by inhibiting the destructive processes of hydrolysis and oxidation.

Hydrolysis is the process that occurs in products containing unrefined fats and oils that also contain enzymes that hydrolyze oil by splitting fatty acids from triglycerides. Free fatty acids then perpetuate the damaging hydrolysis. Refining destroys the hydrolytic enzymes and removes most free fatty acids.

The more unsaturated an oil (the more double bonds it has), the more vulnerable it is to **oxidation**. Oxidation occurs when an unsaturated fat comes in contact with air, and oxygen atoms attach at double-bond sites on the fatty acid chain. Oxidation rapidly turns fats rancid, and oxidized fats damage body tissues, particularly blood vessels.[13] Fortunately, people avoid bad-tasting rancid fats. Exposure to light increases the rate of oxidation and shortens shelf life. The presence of small amounts of metals, which typically are removed by refining, also promotes oxidation. Naturally occurring vitamin E inhibits oxidation, which explains why it and other antioxidants are often added to oils.

▶ **oxidation** Oxygen attaches to the double bonds of unsaturated fatty acids. Rancid fats are oxidized fats.

Unfortunately, processing also has a negative side. To achieve stability and uniform taste, potentially healthful phospholipids, plant sterols, and other phytochemicals are removed, and a significant portion of the natural vitamin E is lost. Oils have become so familiar that we often forget they are highly processed, highly refined foods. Further processing of oils into solid fats such as margarine or shortening also produces some undesirable changes.

To get a liquid vegetable oil to act like a solid fat, it must be at least partially hydrogenated. Hydrogenation involves breaking some of the double bonds in unsaturated fatty acids and adding hydrogen. This process produces a harder, more saturated fat—one that is more effective for making baked goods and snack foods, and one that spreads like butter. Although hydrogenation protects the fat from oxidation and rancidity, it also changes some of the double bonds in the fat's structure to the trans configuration, leading many to wonder whether margarine is a better alternative to butter (see the FYI feature "Which Spread for Your Bread?").

Key Concepts Triglycerides are found mainly in foods we think of as fats and oils, but also in nuts, seeds, meats, and dairy products. Saturated fatty acids are found mainly in animal foods and tropical oils, whereas polyunsaturated fatty acids are found in vegetable oils and other plant foods. Unsaturated fatty acids are susceptible to spoilage by oxidation. Hydrogenation of oils protects fats from oxidation but creates trans fatty acids, which increases risk for heart disease.

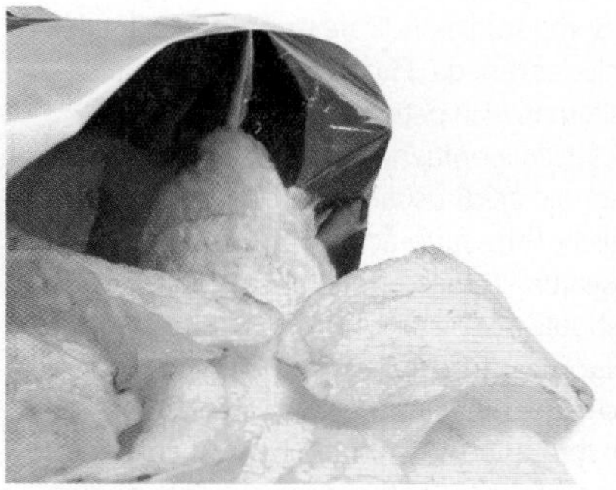

©Bragin Alexey/ShutterStock, Inc.

Going Green

Fish: Good for You and the Environment

Fatty fish or fatty meat? What is a "good" source of fat, a lean protein high in vitamins and minerals, and does not contribute to the production of methane greenhouse gas? Fish! Methane, produced by farm animals, is a powerful greenhouse gas and is considered 20 times more powerful than carbon dioxide at trapping solar energy. In comparison, no methane is produced from harvesting salmon, and fish offers you a healthier meal than a ribeye steak. Choosing to eat fish while decreasing your beef intake not only will give you all of the health benefits associated with omega-3 fatty acids, but also will potentially decrease dangerous greenhouse gas production. An American Heart Association scientific statement on fish consumption, fish oils, omega fatty acids, and cardiovascular disease emphasizes the benefits of eating fish and recommends at least two servings of fish per week. Eicosapentaenoic acid (EPA) and docosahexaenoic acid (DHA) are the omega-3 fatty acids found in oily fish, with mackerel, salmon, trout, sardines, and herring being excellent sources. Approximately 1 gram of EPA/DHA can be obtained from 100 grams (3.5 ounces) of oily fish.

There are many choices when it comes to incorporating healthful fats into your diet. Just remember, even though these fatty acids provide a "good" source of fat, don't go overboard. Fat is still fat, even if it is good for you and for the environment, so make your choices wisely.

FYI For Your Information

Fats on the Health Store Shelf

Many claims made for lipid products sold as supplements may not hold up under scientific scrutiny. You may not even recognize these products as lipids, especially because their long, complicated names are often abbreviated. The amount of lipids and calories in most of these products is quite small.

EPA and DHA in Fish Oil Capsules

These omega-3 fatty acids are thought to help lower blood pressure, reduce inflammation, reduce blood clotting, and lower high serum triglyceride levels.[a] Some studies indicate that nutrition intake that includes omega-3 fatty acids is a viable treatment alternative in patients with psoriasis.[b]

EPA (eicosapentaenoic acid) and DHA (docosahexaenoic acid) usually make up only about one-third of the fatty acids in fish oil capsules, and research studies often use multiple doses. These should not be taken without close medical supervision because their blood-thinning properties can cause bleeding. Because fish oil is highly unsaturated, antioxidant vitamins are included to prevent oxidation. Another problem, though not health related, is that fish oil capsules often leave a fishy aftertaste. The aftertaste can be avoided by taking the fish oil capsules with meals or at bedtime. A concentrated, purified, FDA-approved prescription form of omega-3 fatty acids has been developed that has a minimal aftertaste.[c] Findings from an analysis of randomized trials, however, do not suggest that fish oil supplements provide any cardiovascular benefits.[d]

Flaxseed Oil Capsules

Flaxseed oil is an unusually good source of omega-3 alpha-linolenic acid, which accounts for about 55 percent of its fatty acids. Like fish oil, flaxseed oil is highly unsaturated, and thus very susceptible to rancidity. Capsules protect the oil from oxygen, but limit the dose. A half-tablespoon of canola oil has about as much omega-3 as a capsule of flaxseed oil but adds more calories. DHA and EPA are considered more potent omega-3 fatty acids than alpha-linolenic is.

GLA in Borage, Evening Primrose, or Black Currant Seed Oil Capsules

These oils contain 9 to 24 percent GLA (gamma linolenic acid), the omega-6 desaturation product of linoleic acid. Studies of GLA's effects on skin diseases and heart conditions have been disappointing, and research on potential benefits of GLA supplements in rheumatoid arthritis has been conflicting.[e]

Medium-Chain Triglycerides

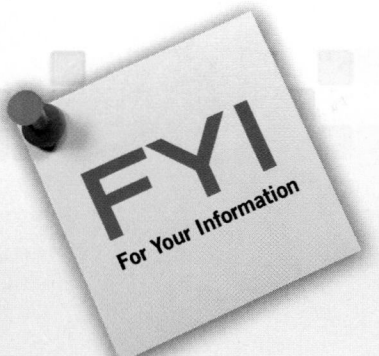

Medium-chain triglycerides (MCTs) can be purchased as such or found as ingredients in "sports" drinks and foods. Because MCTs are absorbed easily, they are marketed to athletes as a noncarbohydrate source of quick, concentrated energy. However, they have no specific performance benefits. A tablespoon of MCT contains about 100 kilocalories.

Lecithin Oil or Granules

Lecithin supplements are derived from soybeans and are a mixture of phospholipids. They are often promoted as emulsifiers that lower cholesterol, but because dietary phospholipids are broken down by the enzyme lecithinase in the intestine, they cannot have this effect. They may be useful as a source of choline. Because choline is the precursor of acetylcholine (a neurotransmitter), lecithin is promoted for treating Parkinson's and Alzheimer's diseases, which are associated with low levels of acetylcholine in the brain. Unfortunately, these claims have little scientific support.[f]

Conjugated Linoleic Acid

Conjugated linoleic acid (CLA) is linoleic acid with only one saturated bond between its two double bonds. It is promoted as an aid for reducing body fat and has been suggested to have anticancer properties. Studies show that CLA supplementation or consumption of foods enriched with CLA has favorable effects on LDL cholesterol levels.[g]

Dehydroepiandrosterone

Dehydroepiandrosterone (DHEA) is a testosterone precursor formed from cholesterol. It is present in the body in large quantities during adolescence, peaks in the 20s, and gradually declines with age. Many elderly people have low levels, and levels also dip during serious illnesses. With only a few exceptions, attempts to use DHEA for illnesses or to slow aging have been disappointing. Researchers generally use doses many times greater than those in over-the-counter supplements, levels that may cause hairiness in women and, more seriously, a risk of liver problems.[h]

Shark Liver Oil and Squalene Capsules

Squalene, an intermediary compound in the synthesis of cholesterol in the body, and shark liver oil, which contains squalene, are said to help liver, skin, and immune function. The basis for these claims is unclear.

Coconut Oil

The health claims regarding coconut oil tout the benefits of this dietary "superfood" for everything from promoting weight loss to protecting against cancer, dissolving kidney stones, promoting oral health, curing thyroid disease, boosting immune function, and warding off Alzheimer's disease. In addition to being called a dietary superfood, coconut oil has been used as a natural moisturizer and personal hair care product.

There are three common types of dietary coconut oil.

- *Virgin or cold pressed:* This is considered unrefined because the oil is extracted from the fruit of fresh, mature coconuts without using high temperatures or chemicals. The extra-virgin type has some antioxidant properties from phenolic compounds.
- *Refined:* Also called conventional, this coconut oil is made from dried coconut meat that is often chemically bleached and deodorized.
- *Partially hydrogenated coconut oil:* Some food manufacturers may use this form of coconut oil that's further processed, transforming some of the unsaturated fats into trans fats found in foods such as commercial baked goods.

One tablespoon of coconut oil provides 117 calories, 14 grams total fat (12 grams saturated fat, 0.8 gram monounsaturated fat, and 0.2 gram polyunsaturated fat), no protein or carbohydrate, and only trace amounts of iron and vitamins E and K. Coconut oil is 92 percent saturated fat, the highest amount of saturated fat of any fat, but like all other plant-based fats it has the benefits from phytochemicals and does not contain cholesterol or trans fat unless it has been commercially hydrogenated.

The unfortunate truth is that there isn't yet enough scientific evidence to support any of the claims about coconut oil's potential health benefits.[i,j] And despite the public hype, the American Heart Association recommends consumers stay away from tropical oils such as coconut oil.[k]

Grapeseed Oil

A relative newcomer in the specialty oil market, grapeseed oil is made from extracting oil from the seeds of grapes that are left over in wine production. Grapeseed oils and extracts contain antioxidants and omega fatty acids and therefore claim to be good for your health. Although the benefits of consuming grapes and moderate amounts of wine have been proven, evidence of the health effects of grapeseed oil and grapeseed extract requires further investigation.[l]

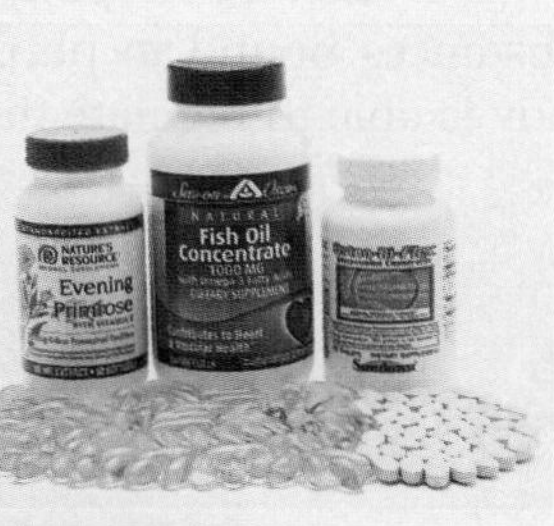

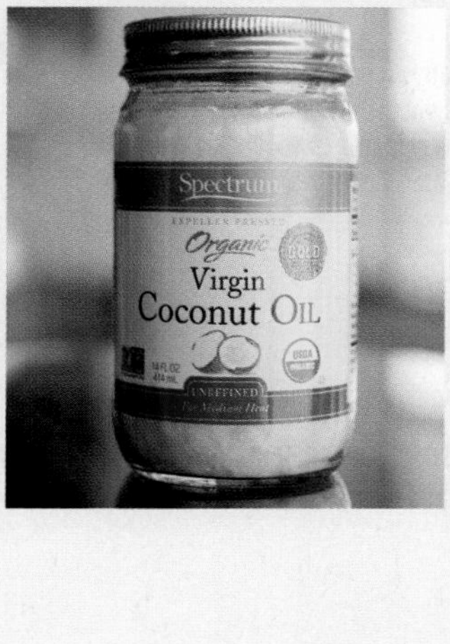

a. Meyer BJ. Are we consuming enough long chain omega-3 polyunsaturated fatty acids for optimal health? *Prostaglandins Leukot Essent Fatty Acids*. 2011;85(5):275–280.

b. Ricketts JR, Rothe MJ, Grant-Kels JM. Nutrition and psoriasis. *Clin Dermatol*. 2010;28(6);615–626.

c. Abete P, Testa G, Galizia G, et al. PUFA for human health: diet or supplementation? *Curr Pharm Des*. 2009;15(36):4186–4190.

d. Chowdhury R, Warnakula S, Kunutsor S, et al. Association of dietary, circulating, and supplement fatty acids with coronary risk: a systematic review and meta-analysis. *Ann Intern Med*. 2014;160(6):398–406. doi: 10.7326/M13-1788.

e. Cameron M, Gagnier JJ, Crubaskk S. Herbal therapy for treating rheumatoid arthritis. *Cochrane Database Syst Rev*. 2011;(2):CD002948.

f. Sarubin Fragakis A, Tomson CA. *The Health Professional's Guide to Popular Dietary Supplements*. 3rd ed. Chicago: Academy of Nutrition and Dietetics; 2006.

g. Derakhshande-Rishehri SM, Mansourian M, Kelishadi R, Heidari-Beni M. Association of foods enriched with conjugated linoleic acid (CLA) and CLS supplements with lipid profile in human studies: a systematic review and meta-analysis. *Public Health Nutr*. 2015;18(11):2041–2054.

h. Christensen JJ, Rruum JM, Christiansen JS, et al. Long-term dehydroepiandrosterone substitution in female adrenocortical failure, body composition, muscle function, and bone metabolism—a randomized trial. *Eur J Endocrinol*. 2011;165(2):293–300.

i. Newgent J. Coconut oil—what is it all about? Academy of Nutrition and Dietetics. http://jackienewgent.com/wp-content/uploads/2013/07/Coconut-Oil-What-is-it-All-About_eatright.org_07_2013.pdf. Accessed May 1, 2014.

j. Schardt D. Coconut oil. June 2012. *Nutrition Action Health Letter*. http://www.cspinet.org/nah/articles/coconut-oil.html. Accessed December 24, 2015.

k. American Heart Association. Fats and oils: AHA recommendation. http://www.heart.org/HEARTORG/GettingHealthy/FatsAndOils/Fats101/Fats-and-Oils-AHA-Recommendation_UCM_316375_Article.jsp. Accessed December 24, 2015.

l. University of Maryland Medical Center. Grape seed. http://umm.edu/health/medical/altmed/herb/grape-seed. Accessed December 24, 2015.

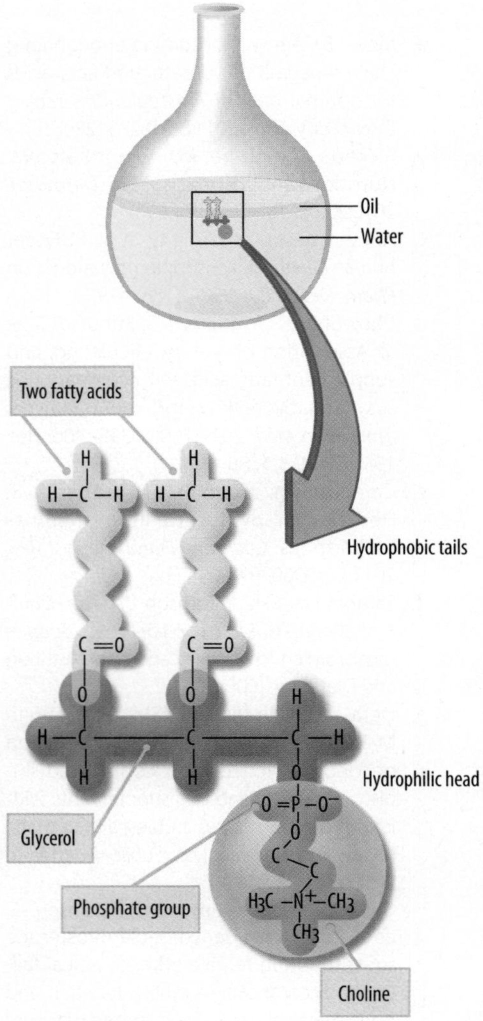

FIGURE 5.18 Phospholipid. Phospholipids are molecules of two fatty acids attached to a glycerol molecule with a phosphate group and a nitrogen-containing component. A phospholipid is soluble in both oil and water. This is a useful property for transporting fatty substances in the body's watery fluids.

▶ **phosphate group** A chemical group ($-PO_4$) on a larger molecule, where the phosphorus is single-bonded to each of the four oxygens and the other bond of one of the oxygens is attached to the rest of the molecule. Often hydrogen atoms are attached to the oxygens. Sometimes there are double bonds between the phosphorus and an oxygen.

▶ **choline** A nitrogen-containing compound that is part of phosphatidylcholine, a phospholipid. Choline is also part of the neurotransmitter acetylcholine. The body synthesizes choline from the amino acid methionine.

Phospholipids

Phospholipids are similar to triglycerides in that they contain both glycerol and fatty acids. However, important differences in their structure make phospholipids entirely different in terms of function. Phospholipids are synthesized by the body and not needed in the diet.

Phospholipid Structure

Phospholipids have a chemical structure similar to that of triglycerides, except that one of the fatty acids is replaced by another compound. Phospholipids are diglycerides—two fatty acids attached to a glycerol backbone. A **phosphate group** with a nitrogen-containing component, such as choline, occupies the third attachment site. **FIGURE 5.18** shows the structure of a phospholipid.

The phosphate–nitrogen component of phospholipids is hydrophilic, so a phospholipid is compatible with both fat and water: Fatty acids in their diglyceride area attract fats while their phosphate–nitrogen component attracts water-soluble substances.

Phospholipid Functions

Because phospholipids have both hydrophobic and hydrophilic regions, they are ideal emulsifiers (compounds that help keep fats suspended in a watery environment) and are often used in foods to keep oil and water mixed. This same property makes phospholipids a perfect structural element for cell membranes—able to communicate with the watery environments of blood and cell fluids, yet with a lipid portion that allows other lipids to enter and exit cells.

Cell Membranes

Phospholipids are major components of cell membranes. Cell membranes are a double layer of phospholipids that selectively allow both fatty and water-soluble substances into the cell (see **FIGURE 5.19**). They also provide a temporary store of fatty acids, donating them for short-term energy needs or for synthesis into regulatory chemicals (e.g., eicosanoids). One phospholipid, phosphatidylcholine, whose **choline** component eventually becomes part of the major neurotransmitter acetylcholine, plays an especially important role in nerve cells. By keeping fatty acids, choline, and other biologically active substances bound in phospholipids and freeing them only as needed, the body is able to regulate them closely.

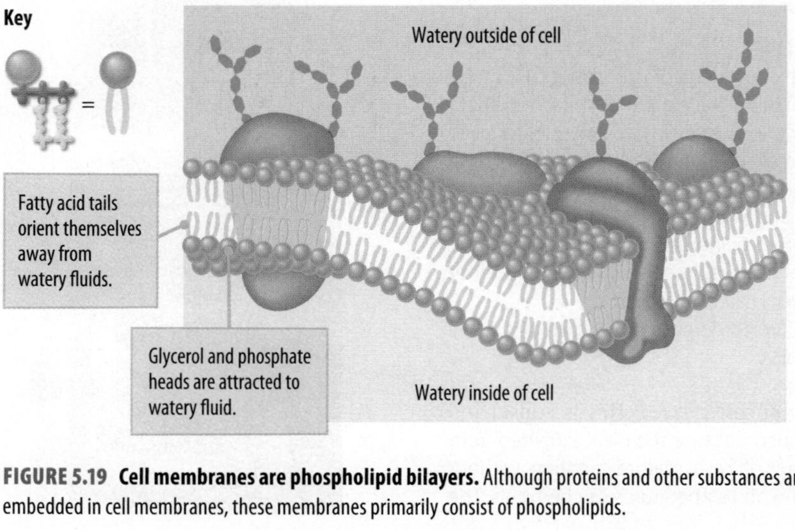

FIGURE 5.19 Cell membranes are phospholipid bilayers. Although proteins and other substances are embedded in cell membranes, these membranes primarily consist of phospholipids.

FYI For Your Information

Which Spread for Your Bread?

Okay, it's time to see if you can put some of your new knowledge about lipids to work. You're standing in front of the dairy case ready to pick out the best spread. But, wow! So many choices. Of course, there's butter, which has been around for thousands of years —wholesome, natural, and creamy; sometimes there's just no substitute for the real thing. Margarine is the more recent choice of many and has come to be more familiar than butter to some consumers. Then, what's this "vegetable oil spread"? The one that says it "helps promote healthy cholesterol levels"?

Butter

When it comes to heart health, butter is the most traditional choice; however, it has some serious disadvantages: (1) it's high in saturated fat; (2) it contains cholesterol; and (3) like other fats, it's high in calories.

Here are the facts: 1 tablespoon of butter provides:

- 100 kcal
- 11 g fat
- 7 g saturated fat
- 0 g trans fat
- 30 mg cholesterol
- 85 mg sodium
- 8% Daily Value for vitamin A

The ingredients are simple: "cream, salt, annatto (added seasonally)." Annatto is a natural coloring (a carotenoid) that is used to keep the color of butter consistent, despite what dairy cows might have been grazing on.

If you like the taste of butter but want a bit less saturated fat and cholesterol, you can buy "whipped butter." The ingredients are the same, but the incorporation of air reduces calories, fat, saturated fat, cholesterol, and sodium by 30 to 40 percent.

Margarine

Margarine was developed to be a substitute for butter. Made from vegetable oils, it appears to be more healthful; as a plant-derived food, it's certainly cholesterol-free, and vegetable oils contain more unsaturated fatty acids than butter. Inconveniently, though, unsaturated oils are liquid, and without extra processing, margarine would run right off any slice of bread. Hydrogenated oils are needed to produce a spreadable consistency. But, as you know, hydrogenation increases the number of saturated and trans fatty acids in a fat, and both of these are associated with higher blood cholesterol levels.

Looking at the label of a standard stick of margarine, you'll find the following per tablespoon:

- 100 kcal
- 11 g fat
- 2 g saturated fat
- 2 g trans fat
- 3.5 g polyunsaturated fat
- 3.5 g monounsaturated fat
- 0 mg cholesterol
- 115 mg sodium
- 10% Daily Value for vitamin A

Compared with butter, margarine has the same amount of calories and fat (a fact unknown to many consumers!), less saturated fat and cholesterol, and a bit more sodium and vitamin A. The PUFA and MUFA content of butter is not listed because these are not required elements of the Nutrition Facts label.

Turning to the list of ingredients, we find "liquid soybean oil, partially hydrogenated soybean oil, water, whey, salt, soy lecithin, and vegetable mono- and diglycerides (emulsifiers), sodium benzoate (a preservative), vitamin A palmitate, beta carotene (color)." Nothing unusual, especially now that you know what lecithin and mono- and diglycerides are.

Spreads and Other Butter Imitators

Beyond the traditional stick margarine, there are numerous "light," "soft," "whipped," "squeeze," and "spread" products. These items do not fit the legal definition of "margarine," so the term ***vegetable oil spread*** is generally used. In terms of ingredients, these products have more liquid oil and water and less partially hydrogenated oils than margarine. More emulsifiers might be needed, along with flavors (including salt) and colors. The result typically is fewer calories, saturated fat, and still no cholesterol.

Some products tout the inclusion of canola or olive oil for more healthful MUFA. Others indicate "no trans fatty acids" and have no hydrogenated oils on the list. Several spreads contain plant sterols or stanols that reduce intestinal absorption of cholesterol.[a]

Cholesterol-Lowering Margarines

Stanols are plant sterols similar in structure to cholesterol. Ingested plant sterols compete with and inhibit cholesterol absorption. Studies show that consumption of stanols produces favorable lipoprotein lipid changes in men and women with hypercholesterolemia.[b]

The "cholesterol-lowering" margarines Benecol and Take Control contain plant esters and plant sterols. Research on the extent of the ability for products such as Benecol and Take Control to improve cholesterol levels is split. Although some studies show a benefit secondary to their use, others have found that the agents have a modest ability to lower LDL cholesterol and are not effective in all conditions, nor do they have an effect on

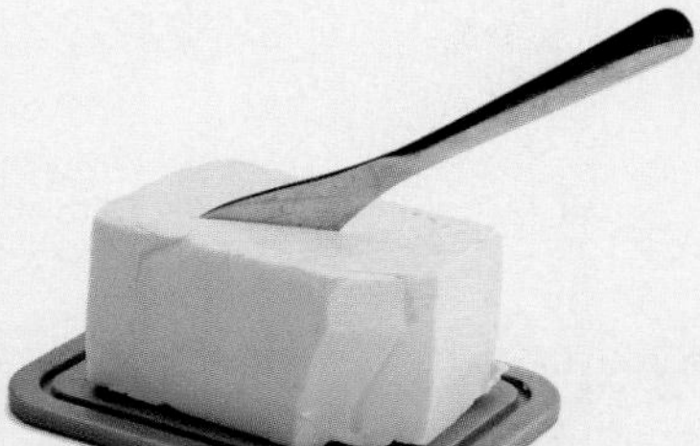

© Multiart/ShutterStock, Inc.

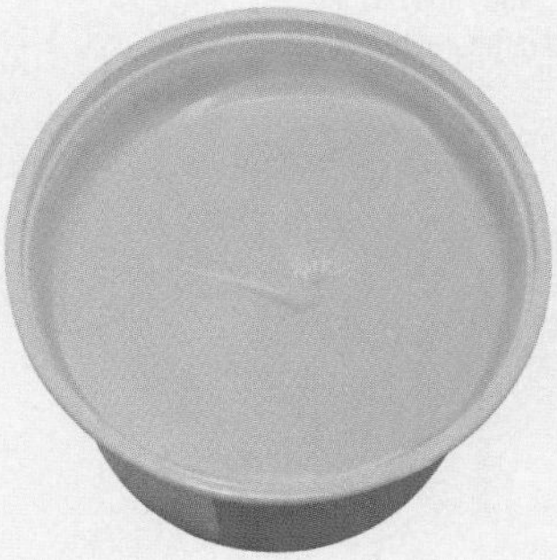

© Denise Campione/ShutterStock, Inc.

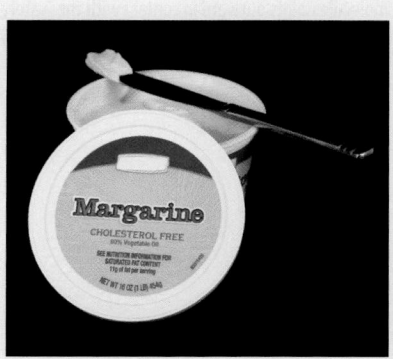

HDL cholesterol or triglyceride levels.[c] You should communicate with a physician if you choose to use stanol- or sterol-ester-containing margarines in an effort to improve cholesterol levels.

Making Choices

The spread you choose can depend on your purpose. There are times, and foods, where nothing but real butter will do. If you've ever tried baking cookies with a soft, reduced-fat spread, you know the outcome ... and probably will use butter, margarine, or vegetable shortening next time. Remember, your overall goal is to limit total fats as well as saturated and trans fatty acids. Using less butter or margarine on the whole will do that. Choosing a margarine or spread with liquid vegetable oil as the first ingredient (meaning that the amount of hydrogenated oil is less) will reduce not only saturated fat, but also trans fat. Although the latest scientific research on the topic found no evidence of dangers from saturated fat, it did confirm the link between trans fats and heart disease; and these findings should not be used as a green light to eat more butter and other foods rich in saturated fat.[d] Most importantly, you should not lose sight of the bigger picture, which is the part all fats play in your total diet. Moderation is the key—making choices that consider your whole diet helps you stay in line with heart-healthy recommendations.

a. Clifton P. Lowering cholesterol—a review on the role of plant *sterols. Aust Fam Physician.* 2009;38(4):218–221.
b. Maki KC, Lawless AL, Reeves MS, et al. Lipid-altering effects of a dietary supplement tablet containing free plant sterols and stanols in men and women with primary hypercholesterolemia: a randomized, placebo-controlled crossover trial. *Int J Food Sci Nutr.* 2011;63(4):476–482.
c. Doggrell SA. Lowering LDL cholesterol with margarine containing plant stanol/sterol esters: is it still relevant in 2011? *Complement Ther Med.* 2011;19(1):37–46.
d. Chowdhury R, Warnakula S, Kunutsor S, et al. Association of dietary, circulating, and supplement fatty acids with coronary risk: a systematic review and meta-analysis. *Ann Intern Med.* 2014;160(6):398–406. doi: 10.7326/M13-1788.

Lipid Transport

The ability of phospholipids to combine both fatty and watery substances comes in handy throughout the body. In the stomach, dietary phospholipids help break fats into tiny particles for easier digestion. In the intestine, phospholipids from bile continue emulsifying. And in the watery environment of blood, phospholipids coat the surface of the lipoproteins that carry lipid particles to their destinations in the body.

Emulsifiers (Lecithins)

► **lecithin** In the body, a phospholipid with the nitrogenous component choline. In foods, lecithin is a blend of phospholipids with different nitrogenous components.

In the body and in foods of animal origin, phosphatidylcholine is also called **lecithin**. However, for food additives or supplements, the term *lecithin* is used for a mix of phospholipids derived from plants (usually soybeans). Understandably, this inconsistent terminology has caused confusion.

Lecithins are used by the food industry as emulsifiers to combine two ingredients that don't ordinarily mix, such as oil and water (see **FIGURE 5.20**). In high-fat powdered products (e.g., dry milk, milk replacers, coffee creamers),

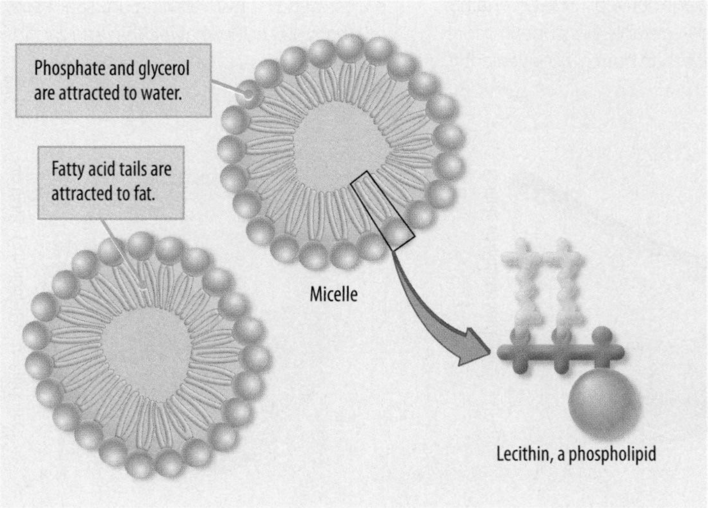

Phosphate and glycerol are attracted to water.
Fatty acid tails are attracted to fat.
Micelle
Lecithin, a phospholipid

FIGURE 5.20 Phospholipids and emulsification. Phospholipids form water-soluble packages called micelles that suspend fat-soluble compounds in watery media. In a micelle, the phospholipids form into a water-soluble ball with a fatty core. The hydrophilic head of each phospholipid molecule points outward in contact with the watery medium, whereas the hydrophobic tails point inward in contact with the fatty core.

lecithins help to mix hydrophobic compounds with water. Lecithins in salad dressing, for example, increase dispersion and reduce fat separation. Lecithin is even added to chewing gum to increase its shelf life, prolong flavor release, and prevent the gum from sticking to teeth and dental work.

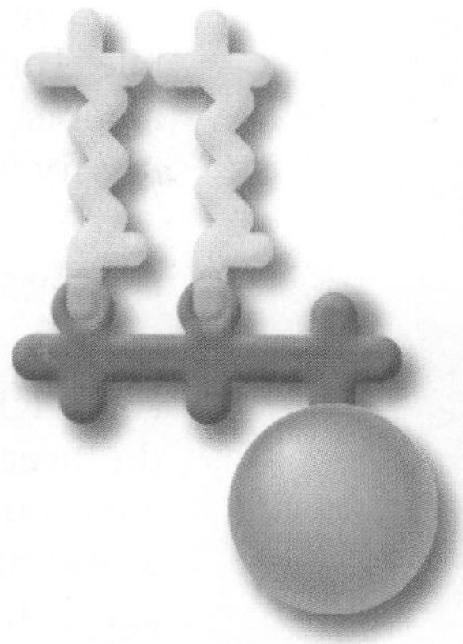

A generic phospholipid

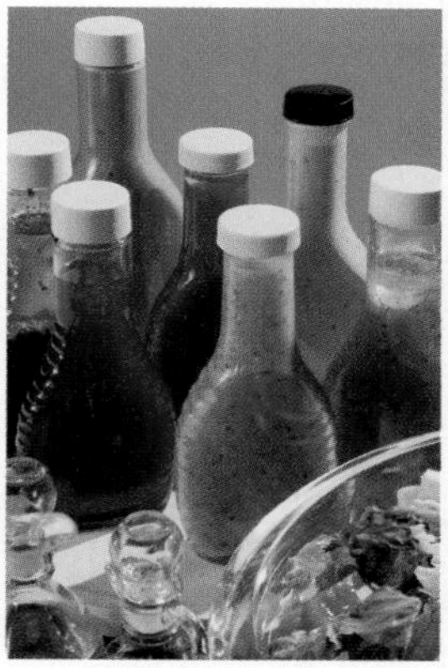

©Comstock/Thinkstock

Phospholipids in Food

Phospholipids occur naturally throughout the plant and animal world, albeit in small amounts compared with triglycerides. They are most abundant in egg yolks, liver, soybeans, and peanuts. Naturally occurring phospholipids are often lost when foods are processed, but other phospholipids are frequently used as food additives. Overall, a typical diet contains only about 2 grams per day. However, phospholipids are not a dietary essential because your body can readily synthesize them from available raw materials.

Key Concepts Phospholipids are diglycerides (glycerol plus two fatty acids) with a molecule containing a phosphate–nitrogen group attached at the third attachment point of glycerol. This structure gives the phospholipid both hydrophobic and hydrophilic regions, contributing to its functional properties. Phospholipids are major components of cell membranes and act as emulsifiers. They also store fatty acids for release into the cell and serve as a source of choline. Phospholipids are not needed in the diet because the body can synthesize them.

Quick Bite

The Power of Yolk

A single raw egg yolk is capable of emulsifying many cups of oil. Cooks take advantage of the natural emulsifying ability of egg yolk phospholipids to emulsify and stabilize preparations such as mayonnaise (oil and vinegar emulsion) and hollandaise sauce (butter and lemon juice emulsion). Food producers use phospholipid emulsifiers in processed foods, which today provide much of our intake.

Sterols

Although classified as lipids, sterols are quite different from triglycerides and phospholipids, both in structure and function.

Sterol Structure

THINK About It 3

Whereas triglycerides and phospholipids have fingerlike structures, sterols are hydrocarbons with a multiple-ring structure (see **FIGURE 5.21**). Like triglycerides, sterols are lipophilic and hydrophobic. Unlike triglycerides and phospholipids, most sterols contain no fatty acids.

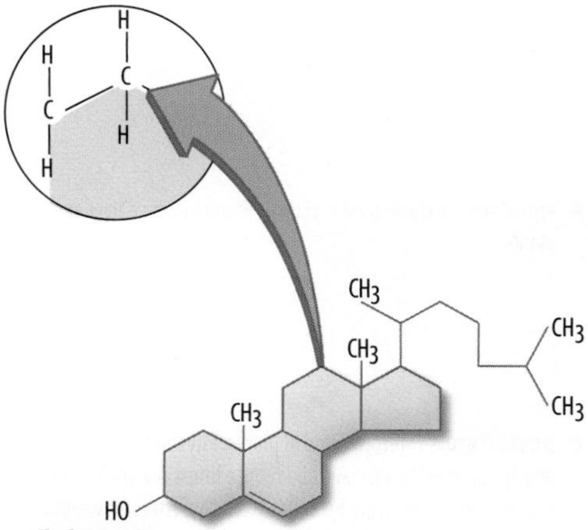

Cholesterol

FIGURE 5.21 Sterols. Sterols are a group of lipids that are multiple ring structures. Because of its role in heart disease, cholesterol has become the best-known sterol.

▶ **cholesterol [ko-LES-te-rol]** A waxy lipid (sterol), the chemical structure of which contains multiple hydrocarbon rings.

Cholesterol Functions

Because of the publicity generated by its role in atherosclerosis (heart disease), **cholesterol** is the best-known sterol. But cholesterol is a necessary, important substance in the body; it becomes a problem only when excessive amounts accumulate in the blood. Like phospholipids, it is a major structural component of all cell membranes and is especially abundant in nerve and brain tissue. In fact, most cholesterol resides in body tissue, not in the blood serum or plasma that is routinely tested for cholesterol levels.

Cholesterol is important not only in cell membranes, but also as a precursor molecule. For example, vitamin D is synthesized from cholesterol. Cholesterol is the precursor of five major classes of sterol hormones: progesterones, glucocorticoids, mineralocorticoids, androgens, and estrogens (see **FIGURE 5.22**). Progesterone is essential for maintaining a healthy pregnancy. Glucocorticoids (such as cortisol) increase the formation of liver glycogen and the breakdown of fat and protein. Mineralocorticoids (primarily aldosterone) help control blood pressure. Androgens (such as testosterone) promote the development of male sex characteristics, and estrogens promote the development of female sex characteristics. When testosterone is synthesized from cholesterol, an intermediate called DHEA (dehydroepiandrosterone) is formed. DHEA has become a popular nutritional supplement, marketed with the largely unfulfilled promise that it will boost potency and restore youth.

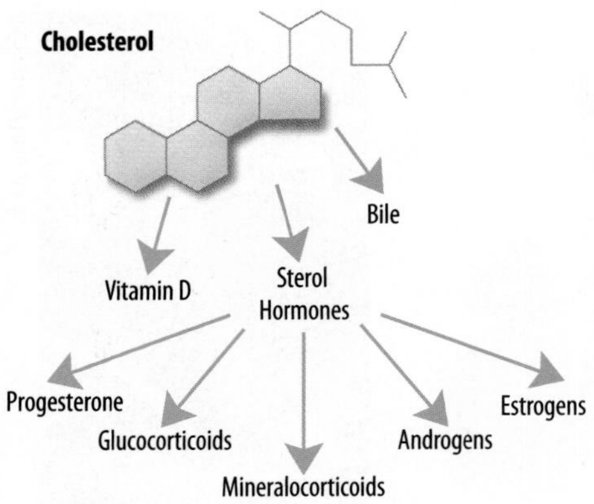

FIGURE 5.22 Cholesterol is a precursor of vitamin D and sterol hormones.

The liver uses cholesterol to manufacture bile salts, which are secreted in bile. The gallbladder stores and concentrates the bile. On demand, the gallbladder releases the bile into the small intestine, where bile salts emulsify dietary fats.

Cholesterol Synthesis

Because the body can synthesize cholesterol, it is not needed in the diet. Although researchers believe all cells synthesize at least some cholesterol, the liver is the primary cholesterol-manufacturing site, and the intestines contribute appreciable amounts. In fact, your body produces approximately 1,000 milligrams of cholesterol per day, far more than is found in the average diet. This production level attests to cholesterol's biological importance. In the lens of the eye, which has a high concentration of cholesterol, on-site cholesterol synthesis may be essential for preventing cataracts.[14] Animal studies suggest that the brain makes almost all the cholesterol incorporated into it during development.[15]

Sterols in Food

Cholesterol occurs only in foods of animal origin. It is distributed based on its biological roles: It is highest in the brain, high in the liver and other organ meats, and moderate in muscle tissue. Because it is fat-soluble, cholesterol is found in the butterfat portion of dairy products. Egg yolks are high in cholesterol, with about 212 milligrams per large egg. (The egg white contains no cholesterol.) Breast milk is moderately high, suggesting the importance of cholesterol during early growth and development, including its importance for an infant's self-control of feeding.[16] The typical American consumes between 250 and 700 milligrams of cholesterol and 250 milligrams of plant sterols each day.[17]

TABLE 5.4 lists the amounts of cholesterol in some common foods.

Aside from cholesterol and vitamin D, few dietary sterols have nutritional significance. Whale liver and plants contain the cholesterol precursor **squalene**, an intermediary compound in the synthesis of cholesterol. Although whale liver is not a common item in U.S. grocery stores, squalene capsules are sold as dietary supplements with the unproven claim that squalene speeds healing and helps liver, skin, and immune function. The basis for these claims is unclear. Plants contain a number of other sterols (phytosterols) that are poorly absorbed. **Phytosterols** are of current interest because they reduce intestinal absorption of cholesterol and are used as a cholesterol-lowering food ingredient in certain vegetable oil spreads.

▶ **squalene** A cholesterol precursor found in whale liver and plants.

▶ **phytosterols** Sterols found in plants. Phytosterols are poorly absorbed by humans and reduce intestinal absorption of cholesterol. They have been used as a cholesterol-lowering food ingredient.

Along with saturated fatty acids (SFAs), dietary cholesterol is a target for reducing plasma total and LDL cholesterol; however, many studies show that diets low in SFAs and cholesterol are less effective in improving the lipid profile in obese individuals and in patients with metabolic syndrome. In contrast, lean persons are more responsive to reductions in dietary SFA and cholesterol.[18]

Key Concepts Sterols are hydrocarbons with a distinctive ring structure. Cholesterol is the best-known sterol; other sterols are hormones or hormone precursors. Cholesterol is an important precursor compound and a key component of cell membranes. High levels of blood cholesterol increase the risk of heart disease. Cholesterol is found only in foods of animal origin. Because the body can make all it needs, cholesterol is not a dietary essential.

Lipids in the Body

Like the other macronutrients (carbohydrates and proteins), most lipids are broken into smaller compounds for absorption in the gastrointestinal tract.

TABLE 5.4
Cholesterol in Selected Foods

Food	Approximate Cholesterol (mg)	
1 oz cheddar cheese	28	As the fat content of dairy foods drops, so do cholesterol levels.
1 cup cottage cheese (1 percent fat)	9	
1 cup cottage cheese (4 percent fat)	36	
1 cup skim milk	5	
1 cup whole milk	24	
1 tablespoon half & half	6	
1 tablespoon whipping cream	21	
1 tablespoon butter	31	
1 tablespoon lard	12	
1 tablespoon margarine or vegetable oil	0	
3 oz lean meat	74	
3 oz lean pork	73	Notice that skeletal muscle from all kinds of animals has similar levels of cholesterol regardless of its differing fat content
3 oz ground beef	76	
3 oz chicken breast	73	
3 oz flounder	48	
3 oz salmon	54	
3 oz crabmeat	45	
3 oz lobster meat	60	
1 large egg	186	
3 oz beef kidney	609	Cholesterol is especially high in organ meats.
3 oz beef liver	324	
3 oz beef brain	1,696	

Note: The values provided offer a general idea of the amount of cholesterol in various foods. Cholesterol values are quite variable, differing by time of year; the animals' origin, species, or breed; processing; and more. One thing is always true, though: Cholesterol is never found in plant foods.

Data from U.S. Department of Agriculture, Agricultural Research Service, Nutrient Data Laboratory. USDA National Nutrient Database for Standard Reference, Release 28. Version Current: September 2015. Internet: http://www.ars.usda.gov/nea/bhnrc/ndl. Accessed February 3, 2016.

However, because lipids generally are not water-soluble and digestive secretions are all water-based, the body must treat lipids a bit differently to digest and transport them.

Lipid Digestion

Because triglycerides are not water-soluble and the enzymes needed to digest them are found in a watery environment, preparing triglycerides for digestion is a more elaborate process than for either carbohydrates or proteins. But don't worry! Your digestive system is up to the task. Physical actions (chewing, peristalsis, and segmentation) combined with various emulsifiers allow digestive enzymes to do their work and change dietary fat into molecules that can be digested and absorbed.

Quick Bite

Would You Pay More for Cholesterol-Free Mushrooms?

Several years ago, some plant foods were promoted with labels claiming they were "cholesterol free." As you might expect, the FDA found this misleading because plant foods never contain cholesterol unless an animal product such as butter or egg has been added. Regulations no longer allow the implication that cholesterol has been removed from a naturally cholesterol-free food. Rather than saying "cholesterol-free mushrooms," labels must now say "mushrooms, a cholesterol-free food."

Beginning in the mouth, a combination of chewing and the work of lingual lipase gets the digestive process rolling, with the small amount of dietary phospholipid providing emulsification. In the stomach, gastric lipase joins in, and the stomach's churning and contractions keep the fat dispersed. Diglycerides that form in the breakdown process become emulsifiers, too. After two to four hours in the stomach, about 30 percent of dietary triglycerides have been broken down into diglycerides and free fatty acids.[19]

Fat in the small intestine stimulates the release of the hormones cholecystokinin (CCK) and secretin from duodenal cells. CCK signals the gallbladder to contract, sending bile down the bile duct to the duodenum. Secretin signals the pancreas to release pancreatic juice rich in pancreatic lipase, which joins bile just before it reaches the duodenum, where the two substances mix with the watery chyme.

Bile contains a large quantity of bile salts and the phospholipid lecithin. These components are the key elements that emulsify fat, breaking globules into smaller pieces so water-soluble pancreatic lipase can attack the surface. This emulsification process increases the total surface area of fats by as much as 1,000-fold.[20] Many common household detergents remove grease with this same action of emulsification.

As bile breaks up clumps of triglycerides into small pieces and keeps them suspended in solution, pancreatic lipase breaks off one fatty acid at a time. Pancreatic juice contains enormous amounts of pancreatic lipase—enough to digest all accessible triglycerides within minutes. When the lipase has completed its work, most of the dietary triglycerides have been split into monoglycerides and free fatty acids (see **FIGURE 5.23**).

▶ **micelles** Tiny emulsified fat packets that can enter enterocytes. The complexes are composed of emulsifier molecules oriented with their hydrophobic part facing inward and their hydrophilic part facing outward toward the surrounding aqueous environment.

Bile salts surround the products of fat digestion, forming **micelles**—water-soluble globules with a fatty core. The micelles transport the monoglycerides and free fatty acids through the watery intestinal environment to the brush border of the intestinal mucosal cells for absorption.

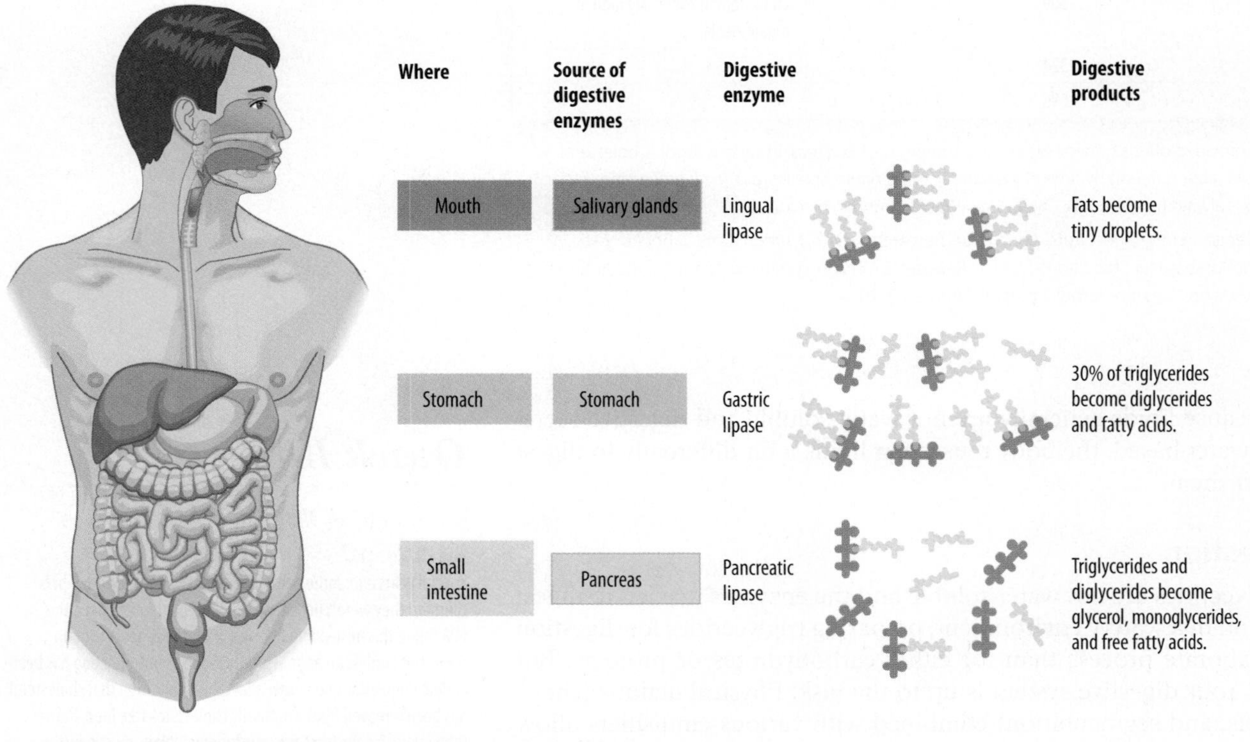

Where
Source of digestive enzymes
Digestive enzyme
Digestive products
Mouth
Salivary glands
Lingual lipase
Fats become tiny droplets.
Stomach
Stomach
Gastric lipase
30% of triglycerides become diglycerides and fatty acids.
Small intestine
Pancreas
Pancreatic lipase
Triglycerides and diglycerides become glycerol, monoglycerides, and free fatty acids.

FIGURE 5.23 Triglyceride digestion. Most triglyceride digestion takes place in the small intestine.

Phospholipid digestion follows a similar pathway, with phospholipases as well as other lipases participating in the process and with the added release of the phospholipid's phosphate and nitrogen components.

Lipid Absorption

Normally, triglyceride digestion and absorption are very efficient, and it is abnormal to find more than 6 or 7 percent of ingested lipids still intact in fecal matter. Most fat absorption takes place in the duodenum or jejunum of the small intestine. Micelles carry the monoglycerides and long-chain fatty acids to the surfaces of the microvilli in the brush border, even penetrating the recesses between individual microvilli. Here, the monoglycerides and long-chain fatty acids immediately diffuse into the intestinal cells (enterocytes). The unabsorbed bile salts return to the interior of the small intestine to ferry another load of monoglycerides and fatty acids. In the last section of the small intestine (the ileum), bile salts are absorbed. They return through the portal vein to the liver, where they are once again secreted as part of bile. This bile recycling pathway—the liver to the intestine, and the intestine to the liver—is called *enterohepatic circulation.*

As monoglycerides and fatty acids pass into the intestinal cells, they re-form into triglycerides. Most of the triglycerides, cholesterol, and phospholipids join protein carriers to form a **lipoprotein**. When this assemblage leaves the intestinal cell, it is called a **chylomicron**. The chylomicrons make their way to the central lacteal of the villi, where they enter the lymph system, to be propelled through the thoracic duct and emptied into veins in the neck.

Absorption of glycerol and of short-chain and medium-chain fatty acids is more direct. They are absorbed directly into the bloodstream rather than forming triglycerides and entering the lymph system. These fatty acids can diffuse directly into the capillaries of the villi because they are more water-soluble than longer-chain fatty acids. **FIGURE 5.24** illustrates the digestion and absorption of triglycerides.

One or two hours after you eat, dietary fat begins to appear in the bloodstream. Fat levels peak after 3 to 5 hours, and fats are generally cleared by 10 hours. That's why health professionals instruct people to fast for 12 hours before having blood drawn for lipid testing.

▶ **lipoprotein** Complexes that transport lipids in the lymph and blood. They consist of a central core of triglycerides and cholesterol surrounded by a shell composed of proteins and phospholipids. The various types of lipoproteins differ in size, composition, and density.

▶ **chylomicron** **[kye-lo-MY-kron]** A large lipoprotein particle formed in intestinal cells following the absorption of dietary fats. A chylomicron has a central core of triglycerides and cholesterol surrounded by phospholipids and proteins.

Digestion and Absorption of Sterols

Digestion does little to change cholesterol and other sterols, which are poorly absorbed compared with triglycerides. Cholesterol can be esterified (attached to a fatty acid) prior to absorption. When there is dietary fat in the intestine, cholesterol absorption increases. When there are plenty of plant sterols and dietary fiber in the intestine, especially fiber from fruits, vegetables, oats, peas, and beans, cholesterol absorption decreases. Overall, only about 50 percent of dietary cholesterol is absorbed, and that proportion decreases as cholesterol intake increases. Because certain fibers bind bile salts and cholesterol and carry them out of the colon, health professionals often recommend eating foods rich in soluble fiber to lower blood cholesterol.

Key Concepts Digestion breaks down most lipids into glycerol, free fatty acids, monoglycerides, and, in the case of phospholipids, a nitrogenous compound. In the small intestine, long-chain fatty acids and monoglycerides are absorbed primarily into the lymphatic system. Glycerol, short-chain fatty acids, and medium-chain fatty acids are absorbed directly into the blood. Sterols are mostly unchanged by digestion, and their absorption is relatively poor.

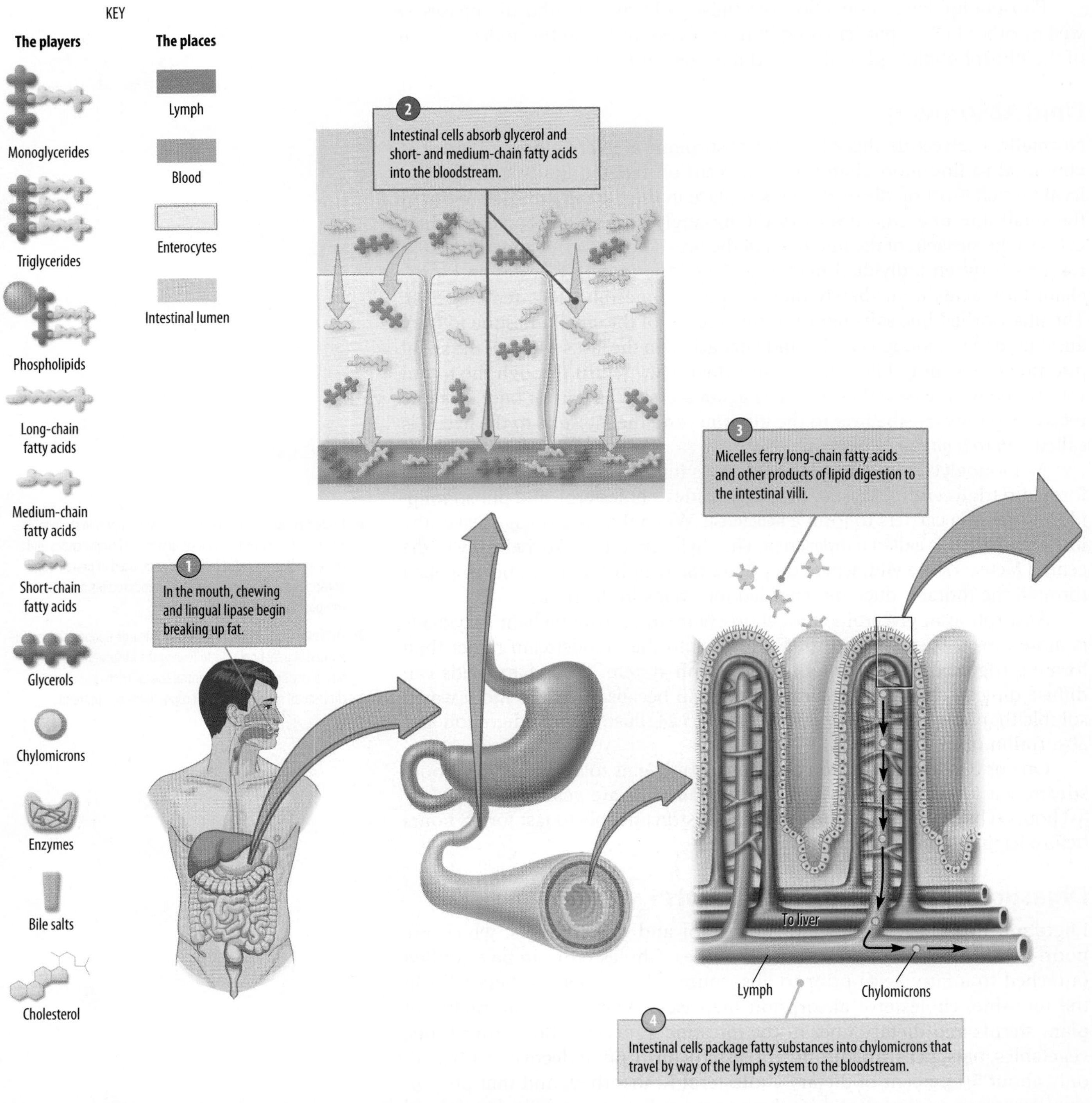
KEY
The players
The places
Monoglycerides
Triglycerides
Phospholipids
Long-chain fatty acids
Medium-chain fatty acids
Short-chain fatty acids
Glycerols
Chylomicrons
Enzymes
Bile salts
Cholesterol
Lymph
Blood
Enterocytes
Intestinal lumen
1 In the mouth, chewing and lingual lipase begin breaking up fat.
2 Intestinal cells absorb glycerol and short- and medium-chain fatty acids into the bloodstream.
3 Micelles ferry long-chain fatty acids and other products of lipid digestion to the intestinal villi.
To liver
Lymph
Chylomicrons
4 Intestinal cells package fatty substances into chylomicrons that travel by way of the lymph system to the bloodstream.

FIGURE 5.24A Digestion and absorption of triglycerides. Minimal fat digestion takes place in the mouth and stomach. In the small intestine, bile salts and lecithin break up and disperse fatty lipids in tiny globules. Enzymes attack these globules, breaking down triglycerides and phospholipids into fatty acids and other component parts. Glycerol and short- and medium-chain fatty acids are absorbed directly into the bloodstream.

Transportation of Lipids in the Body

The digestive tract is not the only place where lipids need special handling to move in a water-based environment. To be transported around the body in the bloodstream, lipids must be specially packaged into lipoprotein carriers.

Lipoproteins have a lipid core of triglycerides and cholesterol esters (cholesterol linked to fatty acids) surrounded by a shell of phospholipids with embedded

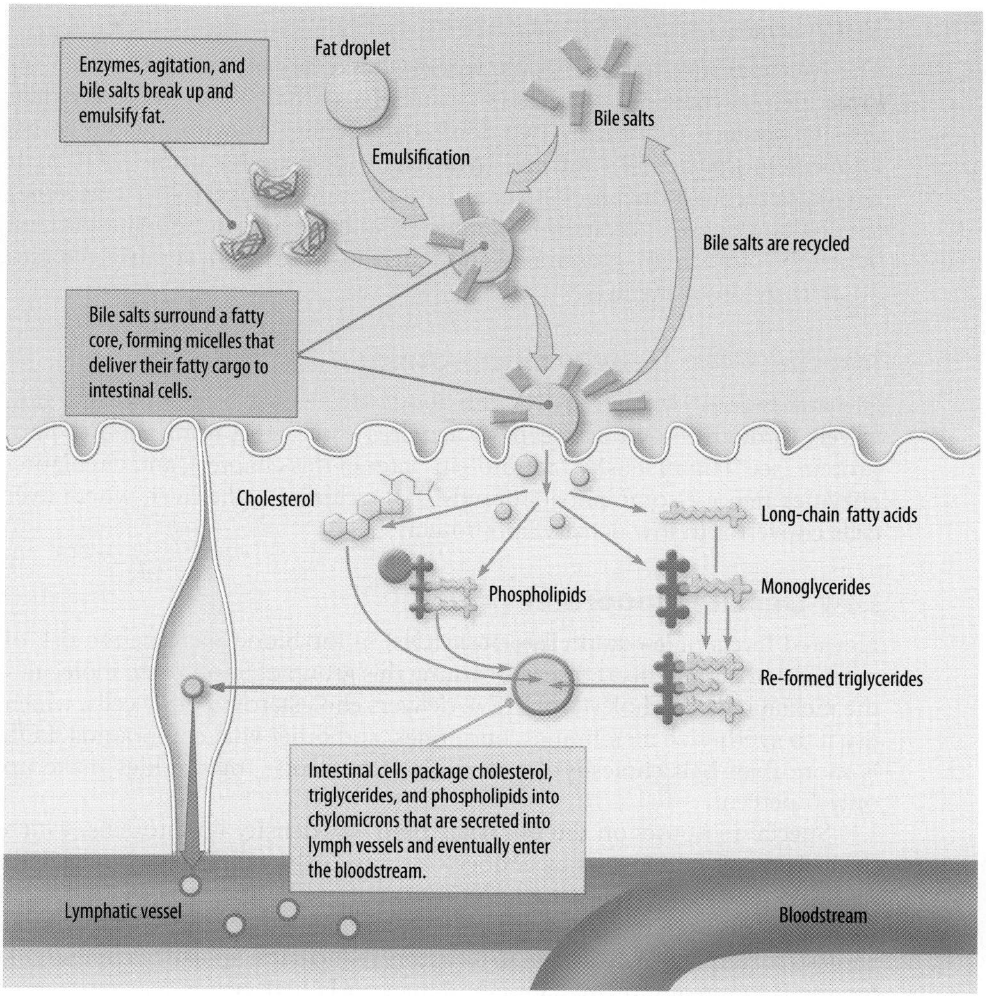

Enzymes, agitation, and bile salts break up and emulsify fat.
Fat droplet

FIGURE 5.24B Digestion and absorption of triglycerides. Bile salts surround the remaining products of fat digestion, forming water-soluble micelles that carry fat to intestinal cells, where it is absorbed and repackaged for transport by the lymphatic system.

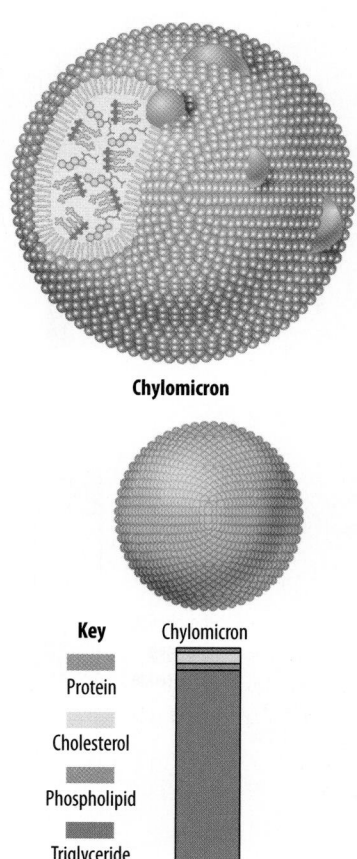

proteins and cholesterol. They can transport water-insoluble (hydrophobic) lipids through the watery environment of the bloodstream. Lipoproteins differ mainly by size, density, and the composition of their lipid cores. In general, as the percentage of triglyceride drops, the density increases. A lipoprotein with a small core that contains little triglyceride is much denser than a lipoprotein with a large core composed mostly of triglycerides. The protein shell portion of the lipoproteins contains apolipoproteins that assist the lipoprotein in its function.

Chylomicron

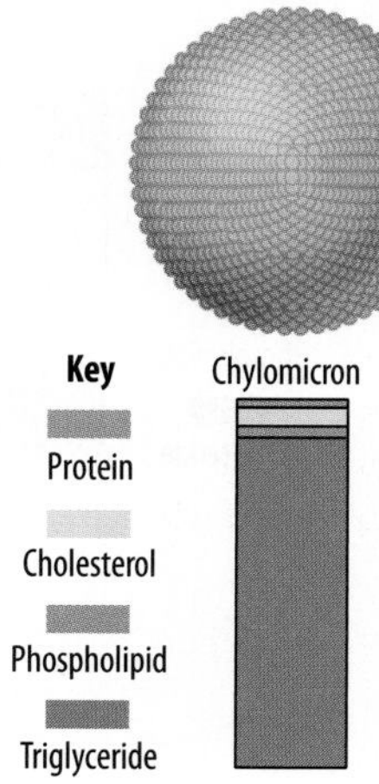

Chylomicrons

Chylomicrons formed in the intestinal tract enter the lymphatic system, travel through the thoracic duct, and flow into the bloodstream at the jugular veins of the neck. As they enter the bloodstream, chylomicrons are large, fatty lipoproteins. Chylomicrons are about 90 percent fat, but as they circulate through the capillaries they gradually give up their triglycerides.

An enzyme located on the capillary walls, called **lipoprotein lipase**, breaks apart the chylomicrons and removes a triglyceride, breaking it into free fatty acids and glycerol. These components enter adipose cells as needed, where they are reassembled into triglycerides. Alternatively, fatty acids can be taken up by muscle and oxidized for energy or remain in circulation and return to the liver.[21] After about 10 hours, little is left of a circulating chylomicron except cholesterol-rich remnants. The liver picks up these chylomicron remnants and uses them as raw material to build very-low-density lipoproteins.

▶ **lipoprotein lipase** The major enzyme responsible for the hydrolysis of plasma triglycerides.

▶ **very-low-density lipoproteins (VLDLs)** The triglyceride-rich lipoproteins formed in the liver. VLDL enters the bloodstream and is gradually acted upon by lipoprotein lipase, releasing triglyceride to body cells.

▶ **intermediate-density lipoproteins (IDLs)** The lipoproteins formed when lipoprotein lipase strips some of the triglycerides from VLDL. Containing about 40 percent triglycerides, this type of lipoprotein is more dense than VLDL and less dense than LDL. Also called a VLDL remnant.

▶ **low-density lipoproteins (LDLs)** The cholesterol-rich lipoproteins that result from the breakdown and removal of triglycerides from intermediate-density lipoprotein in the blood.

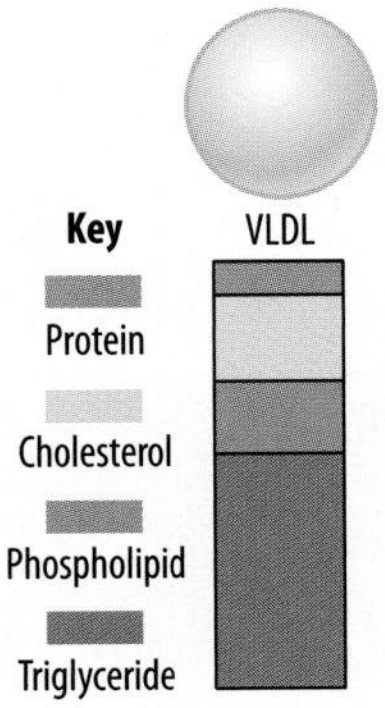

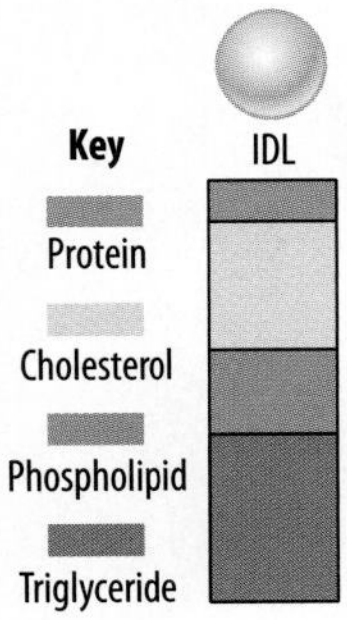

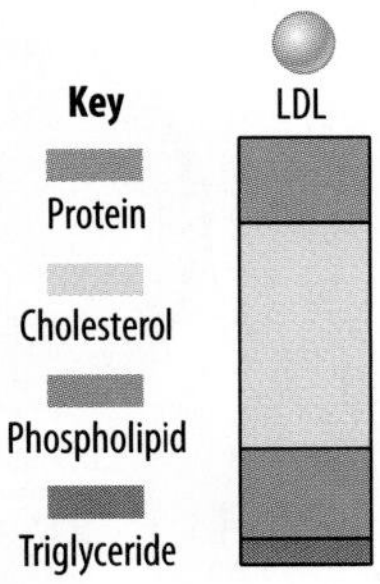

Very-Low-Density Lipoprotein

The liver and intestines assemble **very-low-density lipoproteins (VLDLs)** with a triglyceride-rich core—for relative size, think of a softball. VLDL has a very low density because it is nearly two-thirds triglyceride. As with chylomicrons, lipoprotein lipase splits off and hydrolyzes triglycerides from VLDL as it circulates through the bloodstream. As VLDL loses triglycerides, it becomes smaller and denser, gradually becoming an intermediate-density lipoprotein. When the diet is high in saturated and trans fat, more VLDL and triglycerides are released from the liver.[22]

Intermediate-Density Lipoprotein

Intermediate-density lipoproteins (IDLs) are about 40 percent triglyceride. As IDL travels through the bloodstream, it acquires cholesterol from another lipoprotein (see "High-Density Lipoprotein" later in this chapter), and circulating enzymes remove some phospholipids. IDL returns to the liver, where liver cells convert it to low-density lipoprotein.

Low-Density Lipoprotein

Elevated levels of **low-density lipoproteins (LDLs)** in the blood increase the risk of atherosclerosis and heart disease, earning this group of lipoprotein molecules the nickname "bad cholesterol." LDL delivers cholesterol to body cells, which use it to synthesize membranes, hormones, and other vital compounds. LDL is more than half cholesterol and cholesterol esters; triglycerides make up only 6 percent.

THINK About It 4

Special receptors on the cell walls bind low-density lipoproteins, which the cell engulfs and ingests by endocytosis. Inside the cell, LDL is broken into its component parts, releasing its load of cholesterol.

When the LDL receptors on liver cells bind LDL, they help control blood cholesterol levels.[23] A lack of LDL receptors reduces the uptake of cholesterol, forcing it to remain in circulation at dangerously high levels.

Low-density lipoprotein also is picked up by scavenger receptors. These are a different type of receptor that has a particular affinity for altered (oxidized) LDL. When smoking, diabetes, high blood pressure, or infections injure blood vessel walls, the body's emergency repair team swings into action. It mobilizes white blood cells, which travel to the site of the injury and bury themselves in the blood vessel wall. Certain white blood cells with scavenger receptors bind and ingest LDL. As LDL degrades, it releases its cholesterol. Over time, this process leads to an accumulation of cholesterol and the development of plaque that thickens and narrows the artery, a condition known as atherosclerosis (see **FIGURE 5.25**).

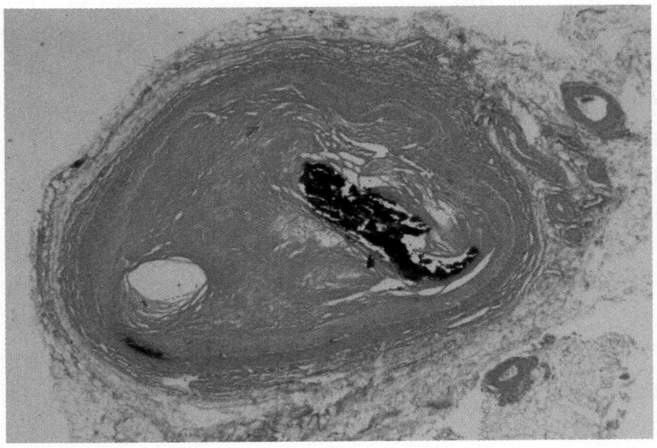

FIGURE 5.25 Plaque buildup in a coronary artery.

High-Density Lipoprotein

High-density lipoproteins (HDLs) are a group of lipoproteins that appear to protect against atherosclerosis, earning HDL cholesterol the nickname "good cholesterol." The liver and intestines make HDL, which is about 5 percent triglyceride, a fat content similar to LDL. On the other hand, HDL is only about 20 percent cholesterol, much less than LDL, which is more than 50 percent cholesterol. HDL has a higher protein content than any other lipoprotein.

In the bloodstream, HDL picks up cholesterol released by dying cells and from cell membranes as they are renewed. HDL also picks up cholesterol from arterial plaques, reducing their accumulation. HDL hands off cholesterol to other lipoproteins, especially IDL, which return the cholesterol to the liver for recycling. Low HDL levels increase risk for atherosclerotic heart disease, whereas high HDL levels have a protective effect.[24]

THINK About It 4

▶ **high-density lipoproteins (HDLs)** The blood lipoproteins that contain high levels of protein and low levels of triglycerides. Synthesized primarily in the liver and small intestine, HDL picks up cholesterol released from dying cells and other sources and transfers it to other lipoproteins.

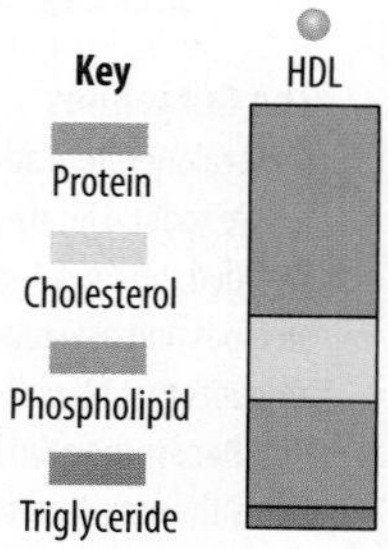

Key Concepts Lipoprotein carriers transport lipids in the blood. Chylomicrons, formed in the intestinal mucosal cells, transport lipids from the digestive tract into circulation. VLDL carries lipids from the liver to the other body tissues, delivering triglycerides and gradually becoming IDL. The liver takes up IDL and assembles LDL, the main carrier of cholesterol. High blood levels of LDL cholesterol, the "bad cholesterol," have been shown to be a risk factor for heart disease. Circulating HDL picks up cholesterol and sends it back to the liver for recycling or excretion. A relatively high level of HDL cholesterol, the "good cholesterol," reduces risk for heart disease.

Lipids in the Diet

Now that you know something about lipids and their importance in the body, you can see that Rachel's no-fat approach to life has serious flaws. A very low fat intake can make it difficult to get adequate amounts of vitamin E and essential fatty acids, which may also increase risk of heart disease.[25] At the other extreme, consumption of too much dietary fat can contribute unwanted calories and lead to obesity. A high-fat, low-carbohydrate diet tends to contribute extra calories that lead to weight gain. When high-fat diets are high in saturated and trans fat, increased LDL cholesterol levels and higher heart disease risk result.[26] A total diet approach, such as balancing calories from fat and carbohydrate rather than just targeting a reduction in fat alone, has become the focus of healthy eating and heart-protective dietary research.[27] Let's discuss the recommended amounts and balance of lipids in a healthful diet.

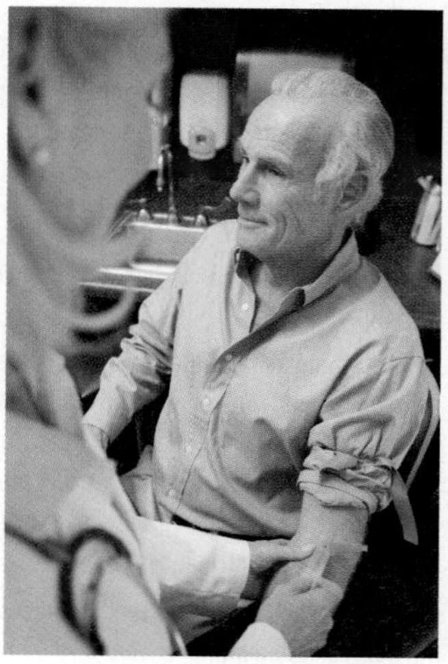

© Photodisc

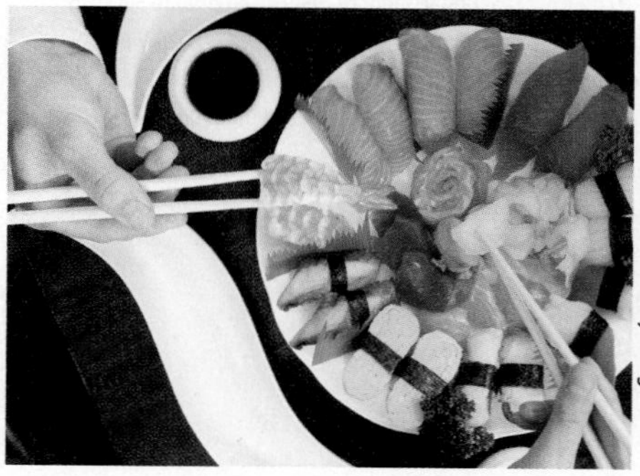

© John A. Rizzo/Photodisc/Getty Images

Recommendations for Fat Intake

In the 1990s, the American Heart Association (AHA), the National Cholesterol Education Program (NCEP) of the National Institutes of Health, and the *Dietary Guidelines for Americans* established specific target levels for intake of lipids. These guidelines limit total fat, trans fat and saturated fat intake and the total amount of cholesterol in the diet.

In 2006, the AHA released revised diet and lifestyle recommendations (see **TABLE 5.5**). One of the most significant changes from prior guidelines was a recommendation to consume at least two weekly servings of oily fish, such as tuna or salmon. These recommendations support the AHA's Diet and Lifestyle Goals for Cardiovascular Disease Risk Reduction.[28] Consuming an overall healthy diet and aiming for a healthy body weight are two of the AHA's goals. Recently, researchers also have focused on the balance of calories from fat and carbohydrate rather than just targeting a reduction in fat.

In 2002, the National Academy of Sciences published its report on Dietary Reference Intakes (DRIs) for the macronutrients.[31] This report recommends an Acceptable Macronutrient Distribution Range (AMDR) for fat of 20 to

Quick Bite

Doctors, Name Your Fat Syndrome

There are several conditions of high blood fats:

- *Hypercholesterolemia:* High total cholesterol.
- *Hypertriglyceridemia:* High triglycerides.
- *Hyperlipidemia:* Can be high triglycerides, high cholesterol, or both. The term is often used along with a more detailed classification, such as "hyperlipidemia type II." It is sometimes shortened to "lipidemia."
- *Dyslipidemia:* Abnormal lipid levels, usually too high.

Position Statement: Dietary Guidelines for Americans, 2015–2020

The Guidelines

Limit calories from added sugars and saturated fats and reduce sodium intake. Consume an eating pattern low in added sugars, saturated fats, and sodium. Cut back on foods and beverages higher in these components to amounts that fit within healthy eating patterns.

Key Recommendations

A healthy eating pattern includes:

- Fat-free or low-fat dairy, including milk, yogurt, cheese, and/or fortified soy beverages
- A variety of protein foods, including seafood, lean meats and poultry, eggs, legumes (beans and peas), and nuts, seeds, and soy products
- Oils

A healthy eating pattern limits:

- Saturated fats and trans fats, added sugars, and sodium

Key Recommendations that are quantitative are provided for several components of the diet that should be limited. These components are of particular public health concern in the United States, and the specified limits can help individuals achieve healthy eating patterns within calorie limits:

- Consume less than 10 percent of calories per day from saturated fats

Data from U.S. Department of Health and Human Services and U.S. Department of Agriculture. *2015 – 2020 Dietary Guidelines for Americans*. 8th Edition. December 2015. Available at http://health.gov/dietaryguidelines/2015/guidelines/.

TABLE 5.5
American Heart Association Diet and Lifestyle Recommendations

The 2014 American Heart Association Diet and Lifestyle Recommendations are designed to assist individuals in reducing cardiovascular disease risk.
Use up as many calories as you take in.
• Start by knowing how many calories you should be eating and drinking to maintain your weight. • Don't eat more calories than you know you can burn up every day. • Increase the amount and intensity of your physical activity to match the number of calories you take in. • Aim for at least 30 minutes of moderate physical activity on most days of the week or—best of all—at least 30 minutes every day.
Eat a variety of nutritious foods from all the food groups.

• Eating a variety of fruits and vegetables may help you control your weight, cholesterol, and blood pressure.
• To get the nutrients you need, eat a dietary pattern that emphasizes
  • Fruits and vegetables
  • Whole grains
  • Low-fat dairy products
  • Poultry, fish, and nuts while limiting red meat and sugary foods and beverages
• Many diets fit this pattern, including the DASH (Dietary Approaches to Stop Hypertension) eating plan.

Eat less of the nutrient-poor foods.
• You could use your daily allotment of calories on a few high-calorie foods and beverages, but you probably wouldn't get the nutrients your body needs to be healthy. • Limit foods and beverages high in calories but low in nutrients. Also limit the amount of saturated fat, trans fat, and sodium you eat.
As you make daily food choices, base your eating patterns on these recommendations:
• Choose lean meats and poultry without skin and prepare them without added saturated and trans fat. • Eat fish at least twice a week. Research shows that eating oily fish containing omega-3 fatty acids may help lower your risk of death from coronary artery disease. • Select fat-free, 1-percent-fat, and low-fat dairy products. • Cut back on foods containing partially hydrogenated vegetable oils to reduce trans fat in your diet. • To lower cholesterol, reduce saturated fat to no more than 5 to 6 percent of total calories. For someone eating 2,000 calories a day, that's about 13 grams of saturated fat. • Cut back on beverages and foods with added sugars. • Choose and prepare foods with little or no salt. To lower blood pressure, aim to eat no more than 2,400 milligrams of sodium per day. Reducing daily intake to 1,500 mg is desirable because it can lower blood pressure even further. • If you drink alcohol, drink in moderation. That means one drink per day if you're a woman and two drinks per day if you're a man. • Follow the American Heart Association recommendations when you eat out, and keep an eye on your portion sizes.
Also, don't smoke tobacco—and avoid secondhand smoke.

Reprinted with permission, www.heart.org ©2014 American Heart Association, Inc.

35 percent of calories for adults. This is balanced with 45 to 65 percent of calories from carbohydrates and 10 to 35 percent of calories from protein. Because children have higher energy needs, the AMDR for younger ages is more liberal: 30 to 40 percent of calories for children aged 1 to 3 years, and 25 to 35 percent of calories for those aged 4 to 18 years. For infants, the Adequate Intake (AI) for fat is 31 grams per day from birth to 6 months of age, and 30 grams per day for ages 7 to 12 months. AIs or RDAs were not set for older children and adults because there is no defined fat intake level that promotes optimal growth, maintains fat balance, or reduces chronic disease risk. In short, scientists suggest that humans can adapt to a wide range of fat intakes. By keeping total fat intake within the AMDR and getting most of our fat from vegetable oils, fish, and nuts, we can move closer to meeting recommendations.

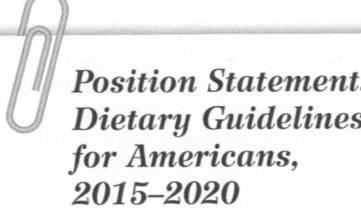

Many nutritionists were surprised to find that the DRI committee did not set a Tolerable Upper Intake Level (UL) for fat or cholesterol. The committee concluded that there were no defined levels of intake that separated "healthful" from "harmful" and that any increase in saturated fat, trans fat, or cholesterol in the diet increased LDL cholesterol levels and heart disease risk. Because it would be virtually impossible to completely exclude these lipids from the diet, the committee recommended that saturated fat, trans fat, and cholesterol intake be minimized. Substituting monounsaturated and polyunsaturated sources improves blood lipid values, with the most favorable results produced by replacing saturated fat with monounsaturated fat.[32]

The *Dietary Guidelines for Americans, 2015-2020* aligns with the recommendations from the DRI committee those of the American Heart Association (see **FIGURE 5.26**). The recommendation for total fat intake is the AMDR: 20 to 35 percent of calories for adults. Saturated fat and trans fat should be limited and replaced with better fats, such as monounsaturated and polyunsaturated fats. For those who need to lower their blood cholesterol, saturated fat should be reduced to no more than 5 or 6% of total calories.[33] *Dietary Guidelines* and American Heart Association Recommendations also suggests that we keep trans fat intake as low as possible. The Daily Values on food labels are 65 grams of total fat (29 percent of the calories in a 2,000-kilocalorie diet), 20 grams of saturated fat (9 percent of calories), and 300 milligrams of cholesterol. Additionally, partially hydrogenated oils, the major source of dietary trans fat in processed foods, are no longer Generally Recognized as Safe (GRAS), and trans fat information is now required on food labels. No Daily Value has been set, but consumers can use this information to choose foods to minimize trans fat intake. In 2015, the FDA began taking steps to remove artificial trans fat from the food supply in an effort to reduce coronary heart disease.[34]

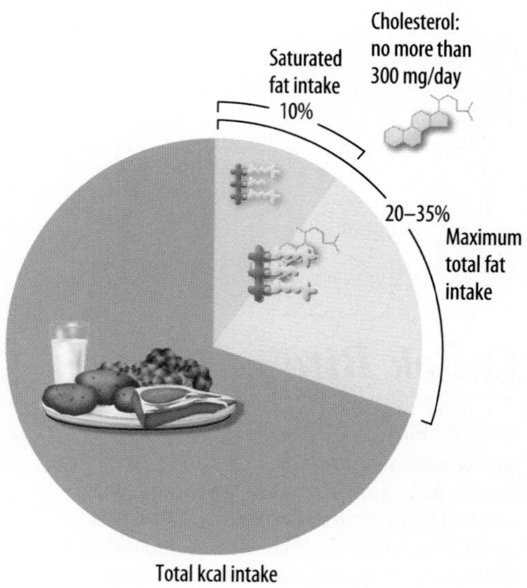

FIGURE 5.26 Recommended fat intake.
Recommendations for dietary fat intake are 20 to 35 percent of total calories. Saturated fat should supply no more than 10 percent of our total calories, or about one-third of our fat calories. Dietary trans fatty acids should be limited as much as possible.

U.S. Department of Agriculture, Agricultural Research Service. 2013. USDA National Nutrient Database for Standard Reference, Release 26. Nutrient Data Laboratory Home Page, http://www.ars.usda.gov/ba/bhnrc/ndl.

Recommendations for Omega Fatty Acid Intake

Fat is a critical nutrient, and although too much fat in the diet is not healthful, certain types of fat, such as omega-3s and omega-6s, are essential for good health.[35] On average, Americans consume approximately 1.6 grams of omega-3 fatty acids and almost 10 times more omega-6 fatty acids on a daily basis.[36] It is important to have the right balance of omega-3 and omega-6 fatty acids in your diet. Omega-6 fatty acid intake is often adequate when eating a typical American diet; however, recommendations for omega-3 fatty acids are not as easy to meet. Omega-3 fatty acids help reduce inflammation, whereas omega-6 fatty acids tend to promote inflammation. A proper balance between these two essential fatty acids helps to maintain, and even improve, health; an improper balance may contribute to the development of disease.

Because essential fatty acid deficiency is virtually nonexistent in the United States and Canada, the DRI committee relied on median intake levels of essential fatty acids to set AI levels. For adults aged 19 to 50, the AI for linoleic acid is 17 grams per day for men and 12 grams per day for women. The AI for alpha-linolenic acid is 1.6 grams per day for men and 1.1 grams per day for women. To fulfill our need for omega-6 fatty acids, linoleic acid should provide about 2 percent of our calories. Average U.S. consumption is much more than that. Two teaspoons of corn oil, which is a little more than half linoleic acid, would supply more than 2 percent of the calories in a 2,000-kilocalorie diet.

To meet these recommendations, most people need to eat more fish than meat.[37] The *Dietary Guidelines for Americans, 2015-2020* encourages a diet rich in omega-3 fatty acids as provided by seafood, which is a good source of polyunsaturated omega-3 fatty acids, eicosapentaenoic acid (EPA), and docosahexaenoic acid (DHA). A specific recommendation to consume 8 or more ounces of seafood per week is intended to supply dietary EPA and DHA at levels which are associated with reduced cardiac deaths among individuals with and without pre-existing cardiovascular disease.[38] Because shark, swordfish, king mackerel, and tilefish contain high levels of mercury, in the past the FDA and EPA recommended that women who may become pregnant, pregnant women, nursing mothers, and young children avoid eating these fish.[39] In June 2014, the FDA and EPA revised their advice on fish consumption for pregnant and breastfeeding women, those who might become pregnant, and young children. The two agencies currently advise that these populations eat more fish that is lower in mercury, such as salmon, anchovies, sardines, and trout for example, in order to gain desirable developmental and health benefits.[40]

It is important to try to get both enough and the right balance of essential fatty acids in our diets. Remember that consuming too much of the omega-3 fatty acids can have undesirable effects, such as suppressing immune function and prolonging bleeding time, so we should be cautious about the high levels of these fatty acids found in some supplements. The DRI committee set an AMDR for omega-6 fatty acids of 5 to 10 percent of energy and an AMDR for alpha-linolenic acid of 0.6 to 1.2 percent of energy.

Quick Bite

Just the Flax

Flax is nature's richest plant source of omega-3 fatty acids. Ounce for ounce, flaxseed oil has more alpha-linolenic acid than any other food. The oils in flaxseed are over 50% alpha-linolenic acid (ALA). Two tablespoons of ground flax has 2,800 milligrams of ALA (omega-3), 850 milligrams of linoleic acid (omega-6), 120 milligrams of lignans (phytoestrogens), and 4 grams of dietary fiber.

Health Effects of Omega Fatty Acids

Omega-3 fatty acids have attracted interest as potential factors in reducing risk for vascular disease. Additional health benefits that have been associated with omega-3 fatty acids include the secondary prevention of chronic diseases such as inflammatory conditions, GI disorders, and type 2 diabetes, as discussed in **TABLE 5.6**.

The American Heart Association recommends eating fish (particularly fatty fish) at least two times a week to reduce the risk of cardiovascular disease.[41] Fish is a good source of protein and doesn't have the high saturated fat that fatty meat products do. Fatty fish like mackerel, lake trout, herring, sardines,

TABLE 5.6
Potential Health Effects of Omega-3 Fatty Acids

Condition	Health Benefits
Inflammatory conditions	Improves rheumatoid arthritis, psoriasis, asthma, and some skin conditions.
Ulcerative colitis and Crohn's disease	Reduces the severity of symptoms.
Cardiovascular disease	Lowers triglycerides and raises HDL cholesterol levels, improves blood circulation, reduces clotting, improves vascular function, and lowers blood pressure.
Type 2 diabetes mellitus	Reduces hyperinsulinemia and insulin resistance.
Renal disease	Preserves renal function in IgA nephropathy; potentially reduces vascular access thrombosis in hemodialysis patients and is cardioprotective.
Mental function	Reduces severity of several mental conditions such as Alzheimer's disease, depression, and bipolar disorder; improvement in children with attention deficit hyperactivity disorder and dyslexia has also been noted.
Growth and development	Neurodevelopment and function of the brain and also the retina of the eye, where visual function is affected.

Data from Rigby A. Omega-3 choices: fish or flax? *Today's Dietitian*. 2004;6(1):37; Deckbaum RJ, Torrejon C. The omega-3 fatty acid nutritional landscape: health benefits and sources. *J Nutr*. 2012;142(3):587S-591S; Position of the Academy of Nutrition and Dietetics: dietary fatty acids for healthy adults. *J Acad Nutr Diet*. 2014;114:136–153.

albacore tuna, and salmon are high in two kinds of omega-3 fatty acids: eicosapentaenoic acid (EPA) and docosahexaenoic acid (DHA). Some people with high triglycerides and patients with cardiovascular disease may benefit from more omega-3 fatty acids than they can easily get from diet alone. These people should talk to their doctor about taking supplements to reduce heart disease risk. Because fish oil supplements can have potent effects, children, pregnant women, and nursing mothers should not take them without medical supervision.[42] EPA and DHA in fish oil capsules are thought to help lower blood pressure, reduce inflammation, reduce blood clotting, and lower high serum triglyceride levels.[43] Some studies indicate that nutrition intake that includes omega-3 fatty acids is a viable treatment alternative in patients with psoriasis.[44]

Conjugated linoleic acid (CLA) is linoleic acid with only one saturated bond between its two double bonds. It is promoted as an aid for reducing body fat and has been suggested to have anticancer properties. Studies show promising results, but more work is needed to identify specific functions of CLA and evaluate its long-term safety.[45] A systematic review of the scientific studies found only fair evidence that short-term supplementation with CLA can result in decreased body fat and increased fat-free mass; however, the evidence suggests no effect on body weight.[46]

Current Dietary Intakes

Dietary surveys report that mean fat intake in the U.S. population is about 33 percent of calories.[47] Although this value is within the recommended AMDR, about 25 percent of the population has a fat intake greater than 35 percent of calories. Fat intake as a percentage of calories is down from 36 percent in the early 1970s.[48]

Although the percentage of calories from fat dropped, average calorie intake increased, which means Americans actually are consuming more total grams of fat. Americans are consuming more sugar-sweetened beverages, food mixtures (e.g., prepared and convenience foods), processed grain snacks, and pastries.[49] Although intake of whole milk and fats and oils has declined, intake of fat from food mixtures is higher.[50] Snacks contribute a significant percentage of daily calories. Frequently reported snacks are cookies, candies, crackers, popcorn, and potato chips, all generally high in fat.

Current intake of saturated fat is about 11 percent of calories, a little higher than recommended.[51] Major sources of saturated fatty acids in the American diet include regular cheese; pizza; grain-based desserts; chicken and chicken mixed dishes; and sausage, hot dogs, bacon, and ribs. The typical American diet contains 14 to 25 times more omega-6 fatty acids than omega-3 fatty acids.[52] Intake of linoleic acid is estimated to be 6 percent of calories, with alpha-linolenic acid providing 0.75 of calories, and EPA plus DHA another 0.1 percent of calories. The amount of trans fat in the American diet has been declining over the past decades; however, it still appears to be in the range of 2 percent to 7 percent of total energy intake, significantly higher than the AHA recommendations to limit trans fat to less than 1 percent of energy.[53] **FIGURE 5.27** provides an overview of the dietary sources of fatty acids. By keeping total fat intake within the AMDR and getting most of our fat from vegetable oils, fish, and nuts, we can move closer to meeting recommendations.

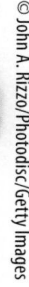

Fat Replacers: What Are They? Are They Safe? Do They Save Calories?

The food industry responded to the public health challenge of the 1990s to lower fat intake by making low-fat, low-calorie goodies that still taste good.

BASIC FATTY ACIDS

Saturated
Animal products (including dairy products), palm and coconut oils, and cocoa butter.

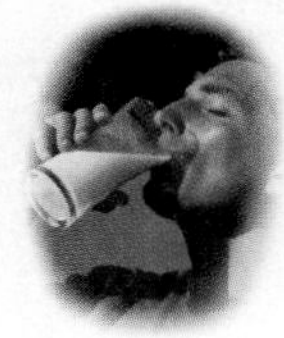
© Photodisc

Polyunsaturated
Sunflower, corn, soybean, and cottonseed oils.

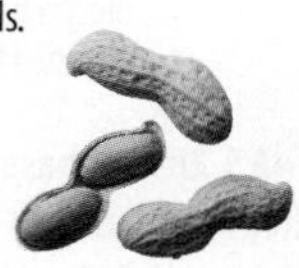
© Photodisc

Monounsaturated
Most nuts and olive, canola, peanut, and safflower oils.

TRANS FATTY ACIDS

Stick margarine (not soft or liquid margarine) and many fast foods and baked goods.

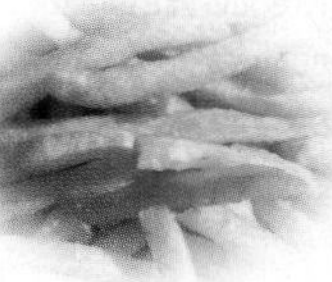
© Kirsta Mackey/ShutterStock, Inc.

ESSENTIAL FATTY ACIDS

Omega-3 fatty acids

Alpha-linolenic acid
Canola oil, soybeans, olive oil, many nuts (e.g., walnuts, peanuts, filberts, pistachios, pecans, almonds), seeds, and purslane (a green, leafy vegetable).

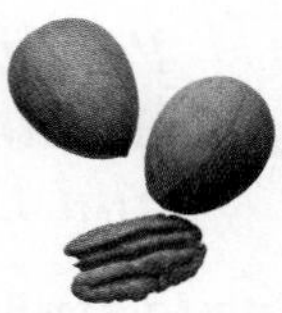
© Photodisc

DHA and EPA
Fish such as mackerel, tuna, salmon, herring, trout, and cod liver oil. The fish with the lowest amount of total fat include Atlantic cod, haddock, and pink salmon. Other fish high in omega-3 but also high in total fat are sardines and bluefish. Human milk.

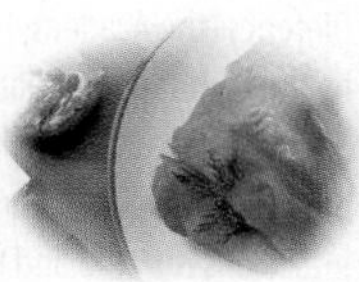
© John A. Rizzo/Photodisc/Getty Images

Omega-6 fatty acids

Linoleic acid
Plants (flax) and some vegetable oils (soybean and canola oil).

FIGURE 5.27 Overview of dietary sources of fatty acids.
Adapted from Cancer smart. Scientific American. 1998;4(3):9.

▶ **fat replacers** Compounds that imitate the functional and sensory properties of fats, but contain less available energy than fats.

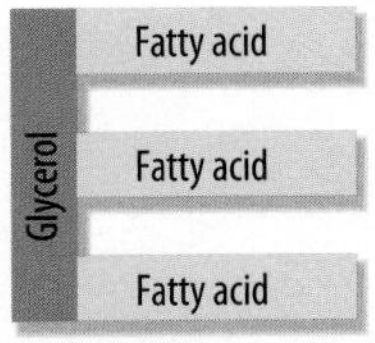

A triglyceride has three fatty acids attached to a glycerol backbone.

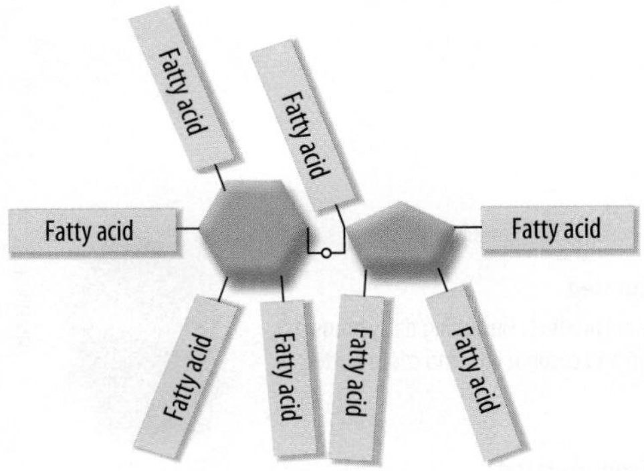

Olestra has six to eight fatty acids attached to a sucrose backbone.

FIGURE 5.28 Fat-based fat replacers' structure. The structure of fat-based fat replacers are unlike the structure of a triglyceride. Although fat-based fat replacers impart triglyceride-like qualities to food, your digestive enzymes cannot break them down.

Many different types of **fat replacers** have been developed, and over the years, thousands of fat-free, low-fat, and reduced-fat foods have hit grocery shelves.

Some fat replacers are carbohydrates: generally starches and fibers such as vegetable gums, cellulose, maltodextrins, and Oatrim (a fat replacer made from oats). Some are more digestible than others, but all provide far fewer than the 9 kilocalories per gram of fat. With their moist, thick textures, they mimic fat's richness and smooth "mouth feel."

Proteins provide the raw ingredients of other fat replacers. Food manufacturers can modify egg whites and whey from milk so that they are thick and smooth and hold water. Because this protein and water combination has fewer calories per gram than fat, it cuts calories.

The most high-tech fat replacers—and the most controversial—are the "fat-based" replacers, also called artificial fats. Manufacturers can alter the characteristics of the fatty acids—their number, length, arrangement, and saturation, for example—to vary properties such as melting point and consistency. Digestive enzymes do not recognize the fatty acid arrangement, so the fat replacement is not broken down and absorbed; therefore, fat-based fat replacers provide about half the calories of fat. (See **FIGURE 5.28**.) One advantage of fat-based fat replacers is their ability to withstand heat. However, a disadvantage is that the GI tract does not absorb fat-based fat replacers, leading to fat malabsorption symptoms in some people—diarrhea, gas, and cramps.

American fat and calorie intake has not declined with the growth in the fat-replacer market. It is clear that fat replacers won't help if people treat them simply as an excuse to eat more. Nor should "low-fat foods," which can have added sugar, be confused with "low-calorie foods." In general, eating less "fake" processed foods and instead eating more "real" foods—ones that have stood the test of time, those that are farmed or grown and harvested, not made in a factory—is good practice.

Lipids and Health

Elevated triglyceride levels are associated with cardiovascular disease. During 2009–2012, about one-quarter of the U.S. adult population aged 20 and over had elevated triglyceride levels. Factors that increase triglyceride levels include sedentary lifestyle, overweight and obesity, cigarette smoking, dietary simple sugars, trans fatty acids, and alcohol.[54]

When diets are consistently high in fat, several problems emerge. High-fat diets are typically high in calories and contribute to weight gain and obesity. For decades, health officials have warned that high intakes of saturated fat and trans fat increase risk for heart disease, and high-fat diets have been linked to several types of cancer. The recent results from a large study, however, found no evidence that people who ate higher levels of saturated fat had more heart disease than those who ate less saturated fat or that those who ate higher amounts of unsaturated fat or polyunsaturated fats benefitted.[55] These findings must be interpreted cautiously, however, because looking at individual nutrient groups such as dietary fats in isolation could be misleading; for example, people who change their diet to eat less saturated fat may replace it with other foods that are detrimental to cardiovascular health such as refined carbohydrates. So, where does that leave you? If you follow the dietary recommendations discussed earlier, you should reduce your risk for cardiovascular disease. Rather than strategies that emphasize exclusively one nutrient, such as dietary fat to reduce cardiovascular risk, focus instead on a "whole diet approach" such as increasing intake of fruits, vegetables, nuts, and fish.[56,57] There is more evidence that this type of diet not only reduces cardiovascular risk, but also other degenerative conditions.

Position Statement: Academy of Nutrition and Dietetics

Fatty Acids for Healthy Adults

It is the position of the Academy of Nutrition and Dietetics (the Academy) that dietary fat for the healthy adult population should provide 20 percent to 35 percent of energy, with an increased consumption of omega-3 polyunsaturated fatty acids and limited intake of saturated and trans fats. The Academy recommends a food-based approach through a diet that includes regular consumption of fatty fish, nuts and seeds, lean meats and poultry, low-fat dairy products, vegetables, fruits, whole grains, and legumes.

Position of the Academy of Nutrition and Dietetics: dietary fatty acids for healthy adults. *J Acad Nutr Diet.* 2014;114:136–153.

FYI For Your Information

Does "Reduced Fat" Reduce Calories? Don't Count on It!

Reducing fat intake is a common dietary recommendation, one that can help reduce risk for heart disease, cancer, and obesity. Given that fat is our most concentrated source of calories, we expect that a reduced-fat or low-fat food would have fewer calories than its unmodified counterpart. But is this always true?

Many reduced-fat products contain added sugar. Although sugar has fewer calories per gram than fat, the amount added can negate any difference in calories. If fat is your concern, low-fat or fat-free makes sense. But if you're trying to reduce fat *and* calories, modified products might not be a big help. So, be a smart shopper—check the label before you check out with a cartload of reduced-fat foods.

Sometimes low-fat and fat-free foods make a big difference in calories.

Food	Kilocalories
1 slice American cheese	50
1 slice nonfat American cheese	24
1 slice bologna	90
1 slice fat-free bologna	22
1 tablespoon mayonnaise	103
1 tablespoon fat-free mayonnaise/dressing	11

But sometimes they make almost no difference at all.

Food	Kilocalories
1 cup canned chicken vegetable soup	84
1 cup reduced-fat chicken vegetable soup	96
3 chocolate chip cookies (30 g)	144
3 reduced-fat chocolate chip cookies (30 g)	153
2 tablespoon peanut butter	188
2 tablespoon reduced-fat peanut butter	187
1 oz potato chips	154
1 oz reduced-fat potato chips	134

And don't forget to check the labels and ingredient list for added sugars. Many reduced-fat products contain added sugar. Although sugar has fewer calories per gram than fat, the amount added may negate any difference in calories. Many nutrition experts now believe that the highly refined carbohydrate and sugary foods in our diet are the primary culprits for adversely affecting risk of chronic conditions such as heart disease, obesity, type-2 diabetes, and cancer. Processed foods such as baked goods, sugar-sweetened beverages, and savory snacks, which in general supply our diets with little more than added sugar and trans fatty acids, should be the focus of dietary reform. You can start improving your diet by choosing these foods less often.

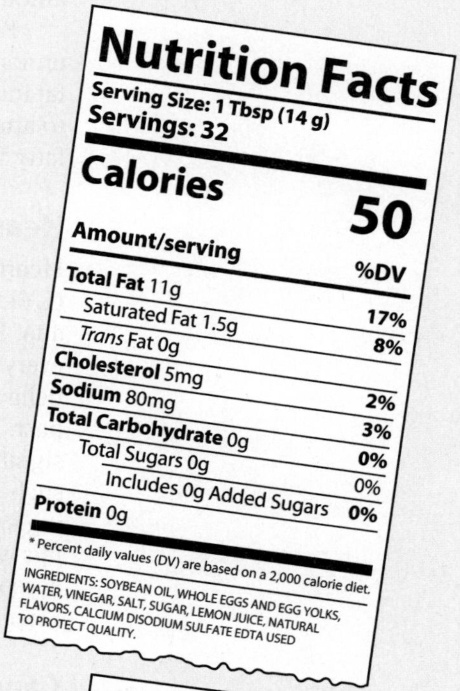
Nutrition Facts
Serving Size: 1 Tbsp (14 g)
Servings: 32
Calories
50
Amount/serving
%DV
Total Fat 11g
Saturated Fat 1.5g
17%
Trans Fat 0g
8%
Cholesterol 5mg
Sodium 80mg
2%
Total Carbohydrate 0g
3%
Total Sugars 0g
0%
Includes 0g Added Sugars
0%
Protein 0g
0%
* Percent daily values (DV) are based on a 2,000 calorie diet.
INGREDIENTS: SOYBEAN OIL, WHOLE EGGS AND EGG YOLKS, WATER, VINEGAR, SALT, SUGAR, LEMON JUICE, NATURAL FLAVORS, CALCIUM DISODIUM SULFATE EDTA USED TO PROTECT QUALITY.

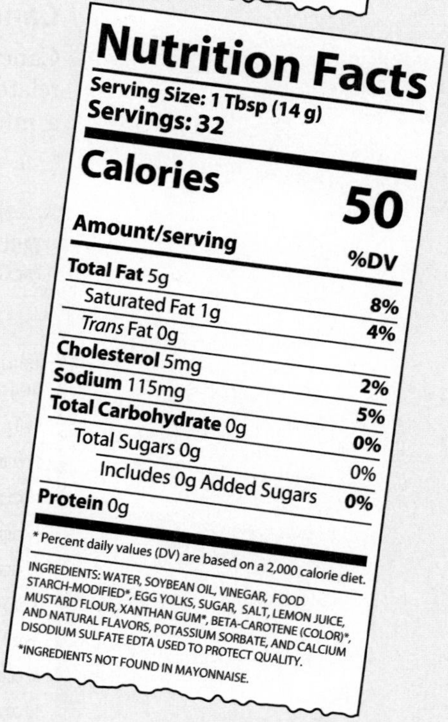
Nutrition Facts
Serving Size: 1 Tbsp (14 g)
Servings: 32
Calories
50
Amount/serving
%DV
Total Fat 5g
Saturated Fat 1g
8%
Trans Fat 0g
4%
Cholesterol 5mg
Sodium 115mg
2%
Total Carbohydrate 0g
5%
Total Sugars 0g
0%
Includes 0g Added Sugars
0%
Protein 0g
0%
* Percent daily values (DV) are based on a 2,000 calorie diet.
INGREDIENTS: WATER, SOYBEAN OIL, VINEGAR, FOOD STARCH-MODIFIED*, EGG YOLKS, SUGAR, SALT, LEMON JUICE, MUSTARD FLOUR, XANTHAN GUM*, BETA-CAROTENE (COLOR)*, AND NATURAL FLAVORS, POTASSIUM SORBATE, AND CALCIUM DISODIUM SULFATE EDTA USED TO PROTECT QUALITY.
*INGREDIENTS NOT FOUND IN MAYONNAISE.

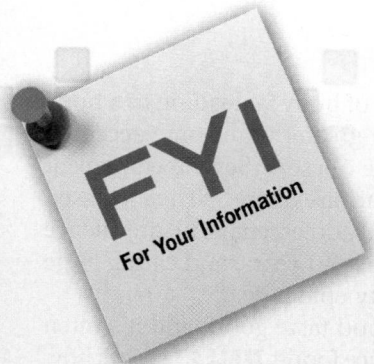

Data from U.S. Department of Agriculture, Agricultural Research Service, Nutrient Data Laboratory. USDA National Nutrient Database for Standard Reference, Release 28. Version Current: September 2015. Internet: http://www.ars.usda.gov/nea/bhnrc/ndl. Accessed February 4, 2016

Obesity

Obesity is defined as the excessive accumulation of body fat leading to a body weight in relation to height that is substantially greater than some accepted standard. More than one-third of U.S. adults are obese.[58] Seventeen percent of U.S. children and adolescents aged 2 to 19 years are obese.[59] The increased prevalence of obesity is a concern for children and adolescents. The prevalence of obesity has significantly increased over the past 30 years, and eating large amounts of dietary fat contributes to this obesity epidemic.[60]

Fat is a dense source of calories, it makes food taste good, and it's often unnoticed or "hidden" in restaurant and convenience foods. **TABLE 5.7** shows how fat increases the calorie content of foods. Standard advice to Americans trying to attain or maintain normal weight usually includes cutting back on fats and fatty foods, along with increasing physical activity and eating fewer calories.

Heart Disease

Heart disease and stroke are the principal types of cardiovascular disease (CVD), which is the leading cause of death in the United States and Canada. Heart disease claims one life every 90 seconds, accounting for 1 out of every 6 deaths in the United States alone.[61] Given the current state of diet behavior, nearly half of all Americans alive today will die from CVD. In the past 50 years, however, lifestyle changes and medical advances have led to significant progress in the fight against CVD. Eating more wholesome foods such as antioxidant-rich fresh fruits, vegetables, and whole grains; consuming smaller amounts of meat and poultry; and replacing trans and saturated fats with monounsaturated or omega-3 polyunsaturated fatty acids are widely accepted as important dietary patterns for heart protection. See the Nutrition Science in Action feature "Green Tea and Blood Lipids."

Cancer

Cancer usually develops over time. It results from a complex mix of factors related to lifestyle, heredity, and environment. Researchers have identified a number of factors that increase a person's chance of developing cancer.

TABLE 5.7
Fat Can Markedly Increase Calories in Food

	Approximate Calories	Approximate Fat (g)
1 small/medium serving (100 g) French-fried potatoes	312	15
100 g boiled potatoes	87	0.1
½ cup creamed cottage cheese	103	4.5
½ cup 1-percent low-fat cottage cheese	82	1.2
½ cup green beans with 1 teaspoon butter	56	4.0
½ cup green beans without butter	22	0.2
3 oz T-bone steak, untrimmed	225	14.9
3 oz T-bone steak, trimmed	161	7.4
½ cup vanilla ice cream	137	7.23
½ cup fat-free vanilla ice cream	92	0

Based on data from US Department of Agriculture, Agricultural Research Service, Nutrient Data Laboratory. USDA National Nutrient Database for Standard Reference, Release 28. Version Current: September 2015. Internet: http://www.ars.usda.gov/nea/bhnrc/ndl.

Although evidence suggests that between 30 and 40 percent of cancers are due to poor food choices and physical inactivity, the role of nutrition and diet in cancer development is complex. Some dietary factors may act as promoters; many others may have protective roles, blocking the cellular changes in one of the developmental stages.

The evidence linking dietary fat to cancer is inconclusive. The case looks strong when we compare cancer rates among countries: Overall cancer rates are generally higher in countries with high fat intake and lower in countries where people eat less fat. But in population studies within those countries, the evidence linking fat to cancer is weaker.

Healthy People 2020 objectives target reducing deaths from heart disease, stroke, cancer, and obesity-related comorbidities.[62] To accomplish these goals, dietitians and health professionals recommend lowering total fat intake, lowering saturated and trans fat intake, maintaining a healthy body weight, and exercising on a regular basis. Eating fruits, vegetables, legumes, and grains that contain fiber helps lower cholesterol levels, too. These foods contain antioxidants and B vitamins, such as B_6 and folate, that may also reduce the risk of heart disease. Substituting fish or soy foods for high-fat meats and cheeses can be beneficial as well.

Key Concepts Current recommendations suggest eating 20 to 35 percent of calories from fat, while keeping saturated fat, trans fat, and cholesterol intake as low as possible. Over the years, Americans have reduced their percentage of calories from fat but are eating more total calories and, as a result, more grams of fat. This is in spite of the increased availability of a wide variety of fat substitutes and lower-fat foods. Excessive fat intake has been linked to obesity, heart disease, and cancer.

Green Tea and Blood Lipids

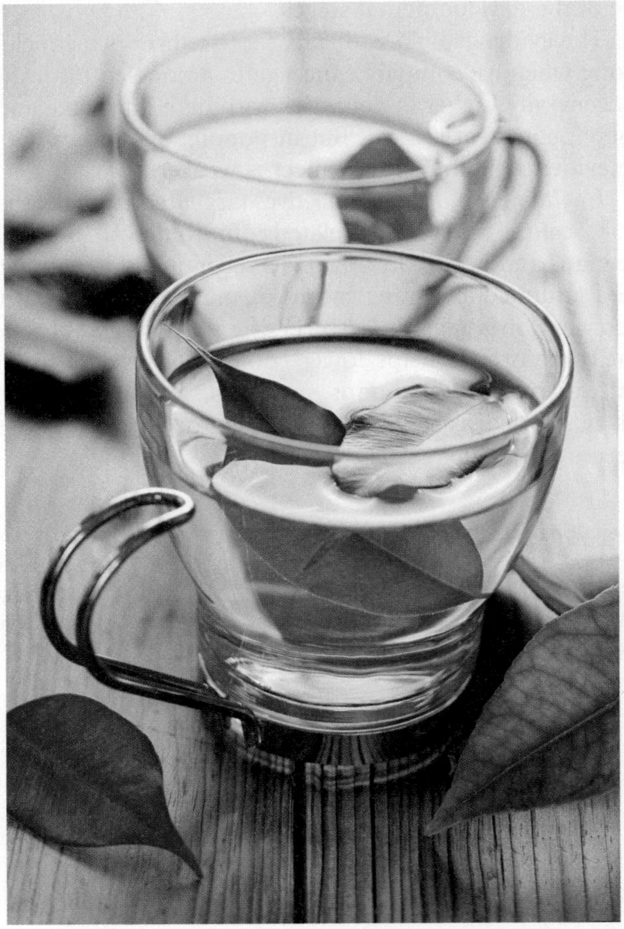

© Liv friis-larsen/Shutterstock

Background

The health benefits of green tea have been attributed to a group of antioxidants called polyphenols. Catechins comprise 80 to 90 percent of the polyphenols found in green tea. Results from animal studies suggest that green tea catechins (GTCs) can improve serum lipids by reducing lipid absorption in the intestines, promoting fecal excretion of cholesterol, and inhibiting enzymes involved in hepatic cholesterol synthesis. In humans, GTCs have been studied in randomized controlled trials for their potential lipid-lowing effects. However, the studies completed to date have had small sample sizes and conflicting results.

Study Purpose

To perform a systematic review and meta-analysis of randomized controlled trials evaluating the relationship between GTCs and serum lipid levels, including total, low-density lipoprotein (LDL) cholesterol, high-density lipoprotein (HDL) cholesterol, and triglycerides.

Experimental Plan

A literature search using scientific databases was conducted to identify randomized trials evaluating the use of GTCs and their effect on serum lipid levels. In addition, a manual search of references from primary or review articles was performed to identify additional suitable trials. Relevant data were abstracted and assessed for validity prior to being included in analysis. Ultimately, 20 trials were included in the meta-analysis.

Results

GTCs were associated with a significant reduction in total cholesterol and LDL cholesterol compared to the control. There was no significant effect of GTCs on HDL cholesterol or triglycerides. (See **Figure A**.)

Conclusion and Discussion

GTCs might have a beneficial effect on total and LDL cholesterol levels in human beings, but based on existing scientific literature they have not demonstrated an effect on HDL cholesterol or triglycerides. The ideal GTC dose, method of administration, and required length of supplementation still remain to be determined. In addition, future research should concentrate on the effect of specific catechin components on lipid values and aim to identify whether certain target populations can benefit from GTC supplementation.

Data from Kim A, Chiu A, Barone MK, et al. Green tea catechins decrease total and low-density lipoprotein cholesterol: a systematic review and meta-analysis. *J Am Diet Assoc.* 2011;111:1720–1729.

Label to Table

The Nutrition Facts panel shown here highlights all of the lipid-related information you can find on a food label. Look at the label, where it states that this product contains 4 grams of total fat. Do you know how you can estimate the number of calories from fat using information from another part of the label? Recall (or look at the bottom of the label) that each gram of fat contains 9 kilocalories. If this food item has 4 grams of fat, then it should make sense that there are approximately 36 kilocalories provided by fat. "Calories from Fat" will no longer appear on the new Nutrition Facts Label because research shows the type of fat is more important than the amount.

Total fat is the second thing you'll see, along with saturated and trans fat. Manufacturers are required to list only saturated and trans fat content on the label, but they can voluntarily list monounsaturated and polyunsaturated fat. Using this food label, you can estimate the amount of unsaturated fat by simply looking at the highlighted sections. There are 4 total grams of fat: 2.5 of them are saturated and 0.5 are trans. That means the remaining 1.0 gram is either polyunsaturated, monounsaturated, or a mix of both. Without even knowing what food item this label represents, you can see that it contains more saturated and trans fat than unsaturated fat (3.0 grams versus 1.0 gram).

Do you see the "6%" to the right of "Total Fat"? It does not mean that the food item contains 6 percent of its calories from fat. In fact, this food item contains 23 percent of its calories from fat (35 fat kilocalories ÷ 154 total kilocalories = 0.23, or 23% fat kilocalories). The 6% refers to the Daily Values, found below. You can see that a person who consumes 2,000 kilocalories per day could consume up to 65 grams of fat per day. This product contributes just 4 grams per serving, which is 6 percent of that amount (4 ÷ 65 = 0.06, or 6%). Note that the % Daily Value for saturated fat is 12 percent, which means that just a few servings of this food can contribute quite a bit of saturated fat to your diet. There is no DV for trans fat, but intake should be kept as low as possible. Cholesterol also is highlighted on this label (20 mg), along with its Daily Value contribution (7%).

Nutrition Facts

4 servings per container	
Serving size	**1 cup (248 g)**
Amount per serving	
Calories	**150**
	% Daily Value*
Total Fat 4g	**6%**
Saturated Fat 2.5g	**12%**
Trans Fat 0.5g	
Cholesterol 20mg	**7%**
Sodium 170mg	**7%**
Total Carbohydrate 19g	**6%**
Dietary Fiber 0g	**0%**
Total Sugars 14g	
Includes 5g Added Sugars	**10%**
Protein 11g	
Vitamin D 0mcg	0%
Calcium 400mg	40%
Iron 0mg	0%
Potassium 265mg	8%

*The % Daily Value (DV) tells you how much a nutrient in a serving of food contributes to a daily diet. 2,000 calories a day is used for general nutrition advice.

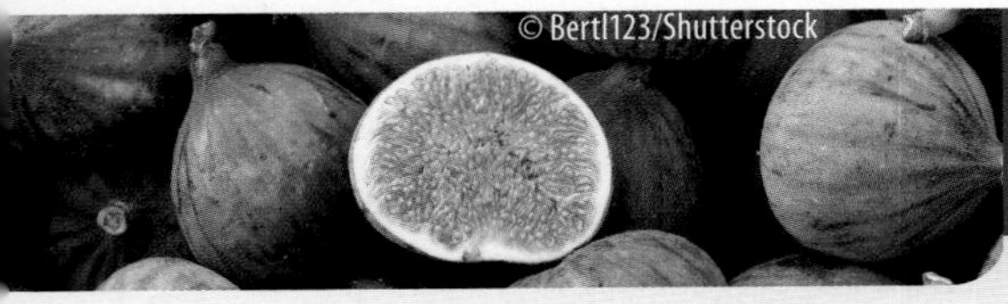

Learning Portfolio

Key Terms

adipocytes	182
adipose tissue	182
alpha-linolenic acid	179
chain length	175
cholesterol	191
choline	188
chylomicron	195
cis fatty acid	177
conjugated linoleic acid (CLA)	177
desaturation	178
diglycerides	181
eicosanoids	179
elongation	178
essential fatty acids	178
ester	181
esterification	181
fat replacers	204
fatty acids	174
glycerol	181
high-density lipoproteins (HDL)	199
hydrogenation	177
hydrophilic	174
hydrophobic	174
intermediate-density lipoprotein (IDL)	198
lanugo	183
lecithin	190
linoleic acid	179
lipophilic	174
lipophobic	174
lipoprotein	195
lipoprotein lipase	197
low-density lipoproteins (LDL)	198
micelles	194
monoglycerides	181
monounsaturated fatty acid (MUFA)	176
nonessential fatty acids	178
omega-3 fatty acids	178
omega-6 fatty acid	178
omega-9 fatty acid	178
oxidation	185
phosphate group	188
phospholipids	174
phytosterols	192
polyunsaturated fatty acid (PUFA)	176
saturated fatty acid	176
squalene	192
sterols	174
subcutaneous fat	182
trans fatty acids	177
triglycerides	173
unsaturated fatty acid	176
very-low-density lipoproteins (VLDL)	198
visceral fat	182

Study Points

- Lipids are a group of compounds that are soluble in organic solvents but not in water. Fats and oils are part of the lipids group.
- There are three main classes of lipids: triglycerides, phospholipids, and sterols.
- Fatty acids—long carbon chains with methyl and carboxyl groups on the ends—are components of both triglycerides and phospholipids and are often attached to cholesterol.
- Saturated fatty acids have no double bonds between carbons in the chain, monounsaturated fatty acids have one double bond, and polyunsaturated fatty acids have more than one double bond.
- Two polyunsaturated fatty acids, linoleic acid and alpha-linolenic acid, are essential; they must be supplied in the diet. Phospholipids and sterols are made in the body and do not have to be supplied in the diet.
- Essential fatty acids are elongated and desaturated in the process of making "local hormones" called eicosanoids. These compounds regulate many body functions.
- Triglycerides are food fats and storage fats. They are composed of glycerol and three fatty acids.
- In the body, triglycerides are an important source of energy. Stored fat provides an energy reserve.
- Phospholipids are made of glycerol, two fatty acids, and a phosphate group with a nitrogen-containing component.
- Phospholipids are components of cell membranes and lipoproteins. Their unique affinity for both fat and water enables them to be effective emulsifiers in foods and in the body.
- Cholesterol is found in cell membranes and is used to synthesize vitamin D, bile salts, and steroid hormones. High levels of blood cholesterol are associated with heart disease risk.
- For adults, the Acceptable Macronutrient Distribution Range (AMDR) for fat is 20 to 35 percent of calories.
- Diets high in fat and saturated fat tend to increase blood levels of LDL cholesterol and increase risk for heart disease.
- Excess fat in the diet is linked to obesity, heart disease, and some types of cancer.

Study Questions

1. How can different oils contain a mixture of polyunsaturated, monounsaturated, and saturated fats?
2. What does the hardness or softness of a triglyceride typically signify?
3. What is the most common form of lipid found in food?
4. What are the positive and negative consequences of hydrogenating a fat?
5. List the many functions of triglycerides.

6. Describe the difference between LDL and HDL in terms of cholesterol and protein composition.
7. What foods contain cholesterol?
8. Name the two essential fatty acids.

Try This

The Fat = Fullness Challenge

The goal of this experiment is to see whether fat affects your desire to eat between meals. Do this experiment for two consecutive breakfasts. Each meal is to include *only* the foods listed here. Try to eat normally for the other meals of the day and to eat around the same time of day. Each of these breakfasts has approximately the same calories, but one has a high percentage of them from fat, the other from carbohydrate. After each breakfast, take note of how many hours pass before you feel hungry again.

Day 1 (~420 kilocalories; 1.5 grams fat)

One 3-oz bagel with 3 Tbsp of jelly

Day 2 (~425 kilocalories; 18 grams fat)

1 medium blueberry muffin

Getting Personal

List all of the foods and drinks that you consume in a 24-hour period, ideally a day where your schedule is fairly predictable and you are eating what is considered normal for you.

1. Let's take a look at your fat intake.
   - What percentage of your calories came from fat?
   - What percentage of your calories saturated and unsaturated fat?
   - How about your cholesterol intake? Was it above or below the guidelines?
2. Review your day of eating and make a list of the foods you know contain fat.
   - What foods could you substitute to lower your total fat intake?
   - What changes can you make lower your trans-fat intake?
   - What would these substitutions do to the total calories in your diet?
3. Now look at your essential fatty acids.
   - Does your intake of Omega-3 and Omega-6 fatty acids meet the recommendations?
   - What foods contributed essential fatty acids to your diet?
   - Make a list of foods that would help increase your EFA intake.
4. Make a list of 2–3 cooking techniques you could use to lower your fat intake
5. Make a list of 3–5 suggestions you would consider following when eating at a restaurant that could lower your fat intake.

References

1. Brouwer IA, Wanders AJ, Katan MB. Effect of animal and industrial trans fatty acids on HDL and LDL cholesterol levels in humans—a quantitative review. *PLoS One.* 2010;5(3):e9434.
2. Williams MH. Sports Nutrition. In: Ross AC, Caballero B, Cousins B, Tucker KL, Ziegler TR, eds. *Modern Nutrition in Health and Disease.* 11th ed. Philadelphia: Lippincott Williams & Wilkins; 2014:65–87.
3. Institute of Medicine, Food and Nutrition Board. *Dietary Reference Intakes for Energy, Carbohydrate, Fiber, Fat, Fatty Acids, Cholesterol, Protein, and Amino Acids.* Washington, DC: National Academies Press; 2005.
4. Mozaffarian D, Wu JH. Omega-3 fatty acids and cardiovascular disease: effects on risk factors, molecular pathways, and clinical events. *J Am Coll Cardiol.* 2011;58(20):2047–2067.
5. American Heart Association. Fish and omega-3 fatty acids. http://www.heart.org/HEARTORG/GettingHealthy/NutritionCenter/HealthyDietGoals/Fish-and-Omega-3-Fatty-Acids_UCM_303248_Article.jsp. Accessed December 28, 2015.
6. Rigby A. Omega-3 choices: fish or flax? *Today's Dietitian.* 2004;6(1):37.
7. Deckelbaum RJ, Torrejon C. The omega-3 fatty acid nutritional landscape: health benefits and sources. *J Nutr.* 2012;142(3):587S–591S.
8. Der G, Batty GD, Deary J. Effect of breastfeeding on intelligence in children: prospective study, sibling pairs analysis, and meta-analysis. *BMJ.* 2006;333:945–949.
9. Shulman GI. Ectopic fat in insulin resistance, dyslipidemia, and cardiometabolic disease. *N Engl J Med.* 2014;371:1131–1141. doi: 10.1056/NEJMra1011035.
10. Rolls ET. Mechanisms for sensing fat in food in the mouth. Paper presented at Institute of Food Technologists 2011 Annual Meeting; June 12, 2011; New Orleans, LA. Also published in *J Food Sci.* 2012;77(3):S140–S142.
11. Jones PJH, Rideout P. Lipids, sterols and their metabolites. In: Ross AC, Caballero B, Cousins B, Tucker KL, Ziegler TR, eds. *Modern Nutrition in Health and Disease.* 11th ed. Philadelphia: Lippincott Williams & Wilkins; 2014:65–87.
12. Wan PJ, Hron RJ. Extraction solvents for oilseeds. *Inform.* 1998;9:707–709.
13. Penumetcha M, Merchant N, Parthasarathy S. Modulation of leptin levels by oxidized linoleic acid: a connection to atherosclerosis? *J Med Food.* 2011;14(4):441–443.
14. Vejux A, Samadi M, Lizard G. Contribution of cholesterol and oxysterols in the physiopathology of cataract: implication for the development of pharmacological treatment. *J Ophthalmol.* 2011;2011:471947.
15. Yu RK, Tsai YT, Ariga T. Functional roles of gangliosides in neurodevelopment: an overview of recent advances. *Neurochem Res.* 2012;37(6):1230–1244.
16. Karatas Z, Durmus Aydogdu S, Dinleyici EC, Colak O, Dogruel N. Breastmilk ghrelin, leptin, and fat levels changing foremilk to hindmilk: is that important for self-control of feeding? *Eur J Pediatr.* 2011;170(10):1273–1280.
17. Jones PJH, Rideout P. Lipids, sterols and their metabolites. Op cit.
18. Flock MR, Green MH, Kris-Etherton PM. Effects of adiposity on plasma lipid response to reductions in dietary saturated fatty acids and cholesterol. *Adv Nutr.* 2011;2(3):261–274.
19. Jones PJH, Rideout P. Lipids, sterols, and their metabolites. Op cit.

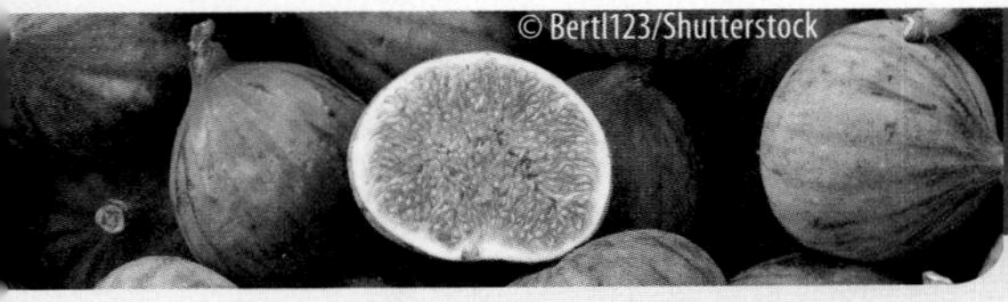

Learning Portfolio (continued)

20. Guyton AC, Hall JE. *Textbook of Medical Physiology.* 12th ed. Philadelphia: WB Saunders; 2012.
21. Dean JT, Rizk ML, Tan Y, et al. Ensemble modeling of hepatic fatty acid metabolism with a synthetic glyoxylate shunt. *Biophys J.* 2010;98(8):1385–1395.
22. Wood AC, Kabagambe EK, Borecki IB, Tiwari HK, Ordovas JM, Arnett DK. Dietary carbohydrate modifies the inverse association between saturated fat intake and cholesterol on very low-density lipoproteins. *Lipid Insights.* 2011;2011(4):7–15.
23. Zhao Z, Michaely P. Role of an intramolecular contact on lipoprotein uptake by the LDL receptor. *Biochem Biophys Acta.* 2011;1811(6):397–408.
24. Kleber ME, Grammer TB, Marz W. High-density lipoprotein (HDL) and cholesterol ester transfer protein (CETP): role in lipid metabolism and clinical meaning. *MMW Fortschr Med.* 2010:152(suppl 2):47–55.
25. U.S. Department of Health and Human Services and U.S. Department of Agriculture. *2015 – 2020 Dietary Guidelines for Americans.* 8th Edition. December 2015. Available at http://health.gov/dietaryguidelines/2015/guidelines/.
26. Ibid.
27. Position of the Academy of Nutrition and Dietetics: total diet approach to healthy eating. *J Acad Nutr Diet.* 2013;113:307–317.
28. American Heart Association Nutrition Committee, Lichtenstein AH, Appel LJ, Brands M, et al. Diet and lifestyle recommendations revision 2006: a scientific statement from the American Heart Association Nutrition Committee. *Circulation.* 2006;114(1):82–96.
29. U.S. Department of Agriculture and U.S. Department of Health and Human Services. *Dietary Guidelines for Americans.* Op cit.
30. Ibid.
31. Institute of Medicine, Food and Nutrition Board. *Dietary Reference Intakes for Energy, Carbohydrate, Fiber, Fat, Fatty Acids, Cholesterol, Protein, and Amino Acids.* Op cit.
32. Ibid.
33. American Heart Association. The American Heart Association's Diet and Lifestyle Recommendations. Updated Jan 20, 2016. http://www.heart.org/HEARTORG/HealthyLiving/HealthyEating/Nutrition/The-American-Heart-Associations-Diet-and-Lifestyle-Recommendations_UCM_305855_Article.jsp#.VrNsH7IrIdV.
34. U.S. Food and Drug Administration. FDA cuts trans fat in processed foods. June 16, 2015. http://www.fda.gov/ForConsumers/ConsumerUpdates/ucm372915.htm. Accessed December 28, 2015.
35. Position of the Academy of Nutrition and Dietetics: dietary fatty acids for healthy adults. *J Acad Nutr Diet.* 2014;114:136–153.
36. Mayo Clinic. Omega-3 fatty acids, fish oil, alpha-linolenic acid. http://www.mayoclinic.com/health/fish-oil/NS_patient-fishoil/DSECTION=dosing. Accessed May 18, 2015.
37. American Heart Association. Nutrition center. http://www.heart.org/HEARTORG/GettingHealthy/NutritionCenter/Nutrition-Center_UCM_001188_SubHomePage.jsp. Accessed December 28, 2015.
38. U.S. Department of Agriculture and U.S. Department of Health and Human Services. *Dietary Guidelines for Americans, 2010.* 7th ed. Washington, DC: U.S. Government Printing Office; 2010.
39. U.S. Department of Health and Human Services and Environmental Protection Agency. What you need to know about mercury in fish and shellfish. March 2004. http://www.fda.gov/food/resourcesforyou/consumers/ucm110591.htm. Accessed December 28, 2015.
40. Environmental Protection Agency. FDA and EPA issue updated draft advice for fish consumption/advice encourages pregnant women and breastfeeding mothers to eat more fish that are lower in mercury. June 9, 2014. http://yosemite.epa.gov/opa/admpress.nsf/596e17d7cac720848525781f0043629e/b8edc480d8cfe29b85257cf20065f826!OpenDocument. Accessed December 28, 2015.
41. American Heart Association. Fish and omega-3 fatty acids. Op cit.
42. Ibid.
43. Meyer BJ. Are we consuming enough long chain omega-3 polyunsaturated fatty acids for optimal health? *Prostaglandins Leukot Essent Fatty Acids.* 2011;85(5):275–280.

44. Ricketts JR, Rothe MJ, Grant-Kels JM. Nutrition and psoriasis. *Clin Dermatol.* 2010;28(6);615–626.
45. Racin NM, Watras AC, Carrel AL, et al. Effect of conjugated linoleic acid on body fat accretion in overweight or obese children. *Am J Clin Nutr.* 2010;91(5):1157–1164.
46. Academy of Nutrition and Dietetics. Evidence analysis library. http://andevidenceanalysislibrary.com. Accessed December 28, 2015.
47. Wright JD, Wang C-Y. Trends in intake of energy and macronutrients in adults from 1999–2000 through 2007–2008. U.S. Department of Health and Human Services, Centers for Disease Control and Prevention. http://www.cdc.gov/nchs/data/databriefs/db49.pdf. Accessed December 28, 2015.
48. Austin GL, Ogden LG, Hill JO. Trends in carbohydrate, fat, and protein intakes and association with energy intake in normal-weight, overweight, and obese individuals: 1971–2006. *Am J Clin Nutr.* 2011;93(4):836–843.
49. Office of Disease Prevention and Health Promotion. Scientific Report of the 2015 Dietary Guidelines Advisory Committee. Part A. Executive summary. http://www.health.gov/dietaryguidelines/2015-scientific-report/02-executive-summary.asp. Accessed December 28, 2015.
50. Position of the Academy of Nutrition and Dietetics: dietary fatty acids for healthy adults. Op cit.
51. Ibid.
52. de Batle J, Sauleda J, Balcells E, et al. Association between omega-3 and omega-6 fatty acid intakes and serum inflammatory markers in COPD. *J Nutr Biochem.* 2012;23(7):817–821.
53. Jones PJH, Rideout P. Lipids, sterols and their metabolites. Op cit.
54. Centers for Disease Control and Prevention. Trends in elevated triglyceride in adults: United States, 2001–2012. NCHS Data Brief No. 198. May 2015. http://www.cdc.gov/nchs/data/databriefs/db198.htm. Accessed December 28, 2015.
55. Chowdhury R, Warnakula S, Kunutsor S, et al. Association of dietary, circulating, and supplement fatty acids with coronary risk: a systematic review and meta-analysis. *Ann Intern Med.* 2014;160(6):398–406. doi: 10.7326/M13-1788.
56. Dalen JE, Devries S. Diets to prevent coronary heart disease 1957– 2013: what have we learned? *Am J Med.* May 2014 Volume 127, Issue 5, Pages 364–369. doi: 10.1016/j.amjmed.2013.12.014.
57. Position of the Academy of Nutrition and Dietetics: dietary fatty acids for healthy adults. Op cit.
58. Centers for Disease Control and Prevention. Adult obesity facts. http://www.cdc.gov/obesity/data/adult.html. Accessed December 28, 2015.
59. Centers for Disease Control and Prevention. Data and statistics. http://www.cdc.gov/obesity/data/index.html. Accessed December 28, 2015.
60. Ogden CL, Carroll MD, Kit BK, Flegal KM. Prevalence of obesity in the United States, 2009–2010. NCHS Data Brief No. 82. January 2012. http://www.cdc.gov/nchs/data/databriefs/db82.pdf. Accessed December 28, 2015.
61. American Heart Association. Heart disease and stroke continue to threaten U.S. health. American Heart Association annual statistical update. December 18, 2013. http://newsroom.heart.org/news/heart-disease-and-stroke-continue-to-threaten-u-s-healthdate. Accessed December 28, 2015.
62. Office of Disease Prevention and Health Promotion. Healthy people 2020. http://www.healthypeople.gov/2020/default.aspx. Accessed December 28, 2015.

Chapter 6

Proteins and Amino Acids

Revised by Melissa Bernstein

THINK About It

1 What's your understanding of the term *protein-sparing*?
2 What percentage of your energy intake do you think should come from protein?
3 Do you take amino acid or protein supplements? If so, why?
4 Do you follow a vegetarian-type diet, or have you ever considered it? Do you know of any environmental or health benefits of eating a more plant-based diet?

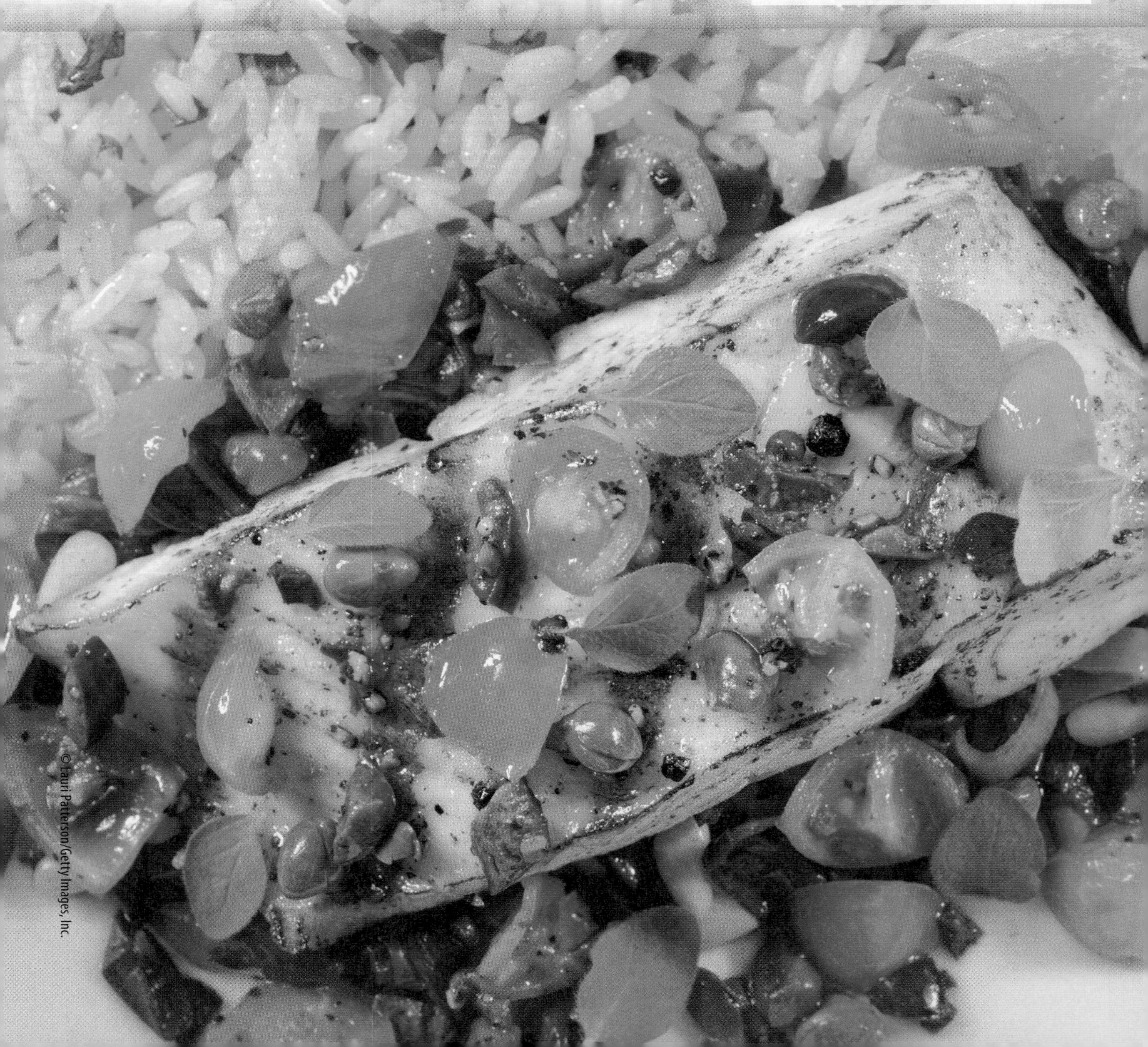

CHAPTER Menu

LEARNING Objectives

- Describe the structure, functions, and denaturation of proteins and amino acids.
- List the functions of proteins in the body.
- Describe the processes of digesting and absorbing proteins, amino acids, and peptides.
- Differentiate between essential amino acids and nonessential amino acids; and complete and incomplete proteins, and discuss their effect on protein quality.
- Interpret nitrogen balance in terms of protein status and nitrogen excretion.
- Make appropriate protein intake recommendations using AMDR guidelines and the AI or RDA for different age groups.
- Discuss the consequences of over- and underconsumption of protein in relation to health and disease.
- List the health benefits and risks of vegetarian diets.

Think of your favorite meal—perhaps a holiday feast, the foods you always ask for on your birthday, or something from a special restaurant. Was the meal you conjured up something along the lines of steak and baked potato; a lobster feast with corn on the cob; turkey with dressing, mashed potatoes, and all the trimmings; or maybe something simpler—a juicy hamburger and fries? What do all these meals have in common? In each case did you imagine a meat item as the focus of the plate, surrounded by various grains or vegetables? Maybe instead your thoughts were about a tofu stir fry surrounded with crisp vegetables; or perhaps a platter of red beans and rice, with melting cheddar cheese, fresh tomato salsa, avocado, corn, and cilantro; or even a steaming platter of chana pallak, a chickpea and spinach stew served with tomatoes, onions, and a hot fresh tandoori naan. In these vegetarian meals, protein also is a critical component; however, the plant products have the spotlight, providing protein along with other essential nutrients.

From a young age, you may have been taught that meat is an important source of protein and that protein helps us grow big and strong, which is true. However, overemphasizing meat can lead to neglecting other important plant-based proteins and nutrient-rich foods. Many food practices in the United States emphasize meat as the most important ingredient of the meal, and protein as the most important nutrient. But do such meals conform to your body's needs? Could other styles of eating be more healthful? For example, what about adding just a small amount of meat to a stir-fry of vegetables over rice? Or what about eliminating meat entirely from the diet? What makes the most sense nutritionally for long-term health?

From the body's perspective, protein is critically important. Protein is part of every cell, it is needed in thousands of chemical reactions, and it keeps us "together" structurally. But, as you are about to learn, the human body is so good at using the protein we feed it that our actual needs for dietary protein are relatively small. All foods made from meat, poultry, seafood, beans and peas, eggs, processed soy products, nuts, and seeds are considered "protein foods"—as you will learn, meat itself (including beef, pork, or chicken) doesn't need to be at the center of the plate to keep you healthy!

Why Is Protein Important?

The word *protein* was coined by the Dutch chemist Gerardus Mulder in 1838 and comes from the Greek word *protos*, meaning "of prime importance." Mulder discovered that proteins are a major component of all plant and animal

TABLE 6.1
Essential and Nonessential Amino Acids

Essential	Nonessential
Histidine	Alanine
Isoleucine	Arginine*
Leucine	Asparagine
Lysine	Aspartic acid
Methionine	Cysteine*
Phenylalanine	Glutamic acid
Threonine	Glutamine*
Tryptophan	Glycine*
Valine	Proline*
	Serine
	Tyrosine*

***Conditionally Essential Amino Acid**

▶ **wasting** The breakdown of body tissue such as muscle and organs for use as a protein source when the diet lacks protein.

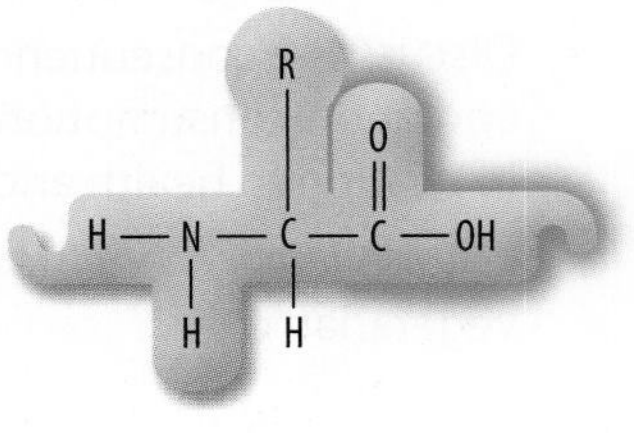

▶ **essential (indispensable) amino acids** Amino acids that the body cannot make at all or cannot make enough of to meet physiological needs. Essential amino acids must be supplied in the diet.

▶ **nonessential (dispensable) amino acids** Amino acids that the body can make if supplied with adequate nitrogen. Nonessential amino acids do not need to be supplied in the diet.

▶ **conditionally essential amino acids** Amino acids that are normally made in the body (nonessential) but become essential under certain circumstances, such as during critical illness.

Quick Bite

Bugburger, Anyone?

Did you know that bugs provide 10 percent of the protein consumed worldwide? What creepy crawler would you choose for your dinner plate? A grasshopper is 15 to 60 percent protein. Pound for pound, spiders have more protein than any other bug.

tissues, second only to water. Today we know that these intricately constructed molecules are vital to many aspects of health and play an integral role in every living cell. Our bodies use protein for functions such as replacing skin cells that slough off over time, producing antibodies to fight infections, and assisting in the essential body processes of water balance, nutrition transport, and muscle contractions.[1] Proteins are a source of energy and help keep skin, hair, and nails healthy.[2] Protein is absolutely critical for overall good health. Our bodies constantly assemble, break down, and use proteins, so we count on our diet to provide enough protein each day to replace what we use. When we eat more protein than we need, the excess either is used to make energy or is stored as fat.

Most people associate protein with animal foods such as beef, chicken, fish, or milk. However, plant foods such as dried beans and peas, grains, nuts, seeds, and vegetables also provide protein. Many protein-rich plant foods are also rich in vitamins and minerals. These plant foods usually are low in fat and calories.

People living in poverty can suffer from a shortage of both protein and energy in the diet. When the diet lacks protein, the body breaks down tissue such as muscle and uses it as a protein source. This causes loss, or **wasting**, of muscles, organs, and other tissues. Protein deficiency also increases susceptibility to infection and impairs digestion and absorption of nutrients. In the United States and other industrialized countries, most people are able to get more than enough protein to meet their physiological needs. In fact, a more common problem in these areas is excess intake of protein.

Amino Acids Are the Building Blocks of Proteins

Just as glucose is the basic building block of carbohydrates, amino acids are the basic building blocks of proteins. Proteins are sequences of amino acids. When building these sequences, your body chooses from the 20 different amino acids available. Nine of these amino acids are called **essential (indispensable) amino acids** because your body cannot make them and must get them in the diet. Your body can manufacture the remaining 11, called **nonessential (dispensable) amino acids**, when enough nitrogen, carbon, hydrogen, and oxygen are available. Nonessential amino acids do not need to be provided by your diet.

Some nonessential amino acids can become conditionally essential amino acids if the body cannot make them because of illness or the body lacks the necessary precursors or enzymes to make them. Tyrosine and cysteine are both considered **conditionally essential amino acids**. Under normal circumstances, your body makes tyrosine from the essential amino acid phenylalanine, and cysteine from either methionine or serine. However, if a disease or condition interferes with your ability to synthesize tyrosine or cysteine from its amino acid precursors, then your body will need tyrosine or cysteine from the diet. **TABLE 6.1** lists the essential and nonessential amino acids.

Tyrosine becomes an essential amino acid for people with phenylketonuria (PKU), a rare genetic disorder that impairs phenylalanine metabolism. Because people with PKU lack sufficient amounts of an enzyme needed to convert phenylalanine to tyrosine, tyrosine must be supplied in the diet. Phenylalanine intake must be carefully controlled because excess phenylalanine and its metabolic by-products (phenylketones) can build up and contribute to irreversible brain damage.[3] Because foods that have aspartame contain phenylalanine, they can be dangerous for people with PKU. When babies with PKU receive treatment starting at birth, their IQ development is unaffected.

Without treatment, they suffer severe mental retardation. Other amino acids also can become essential under certain circumstances. The amino acid glutamine is the main fuel for rapidly dividing cells and plays a key role in transporting nitrogen between organs.[4] Although normally considered nonessential, glutamine can become essential after trauma or during periods of critical illness that increase the body's need for it.[5] The amino acid arginine can also become essential in conditions of intestinal metabolic dysfunction or severe physiological stress.[6]

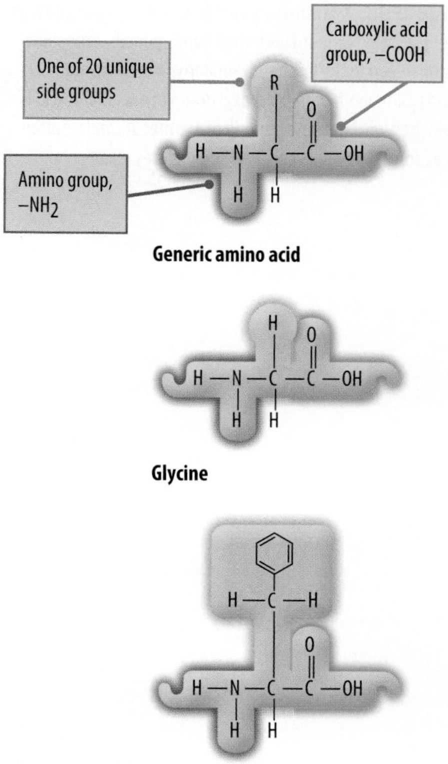

FIGURE 6.1 Structure of an amino acid. All amino acids have a similar structure. Attached to a carbon atom is a hydrogen (H), shown here but not in later illustrations of amino acids; an amino group ($-NH_2$); an acid group (–COOH); and a side group (R). The side group gives each amino acid its unique identity.

Amino Acids Are Identified by Their Side Groups

Amino acids (with the exception of proline) uniformly consist of a central carbon atom chemically bonded to one hydrogen atom (H), one carboxylic acid group (–COOH), one amino (nitrogen-containing) group ($-NH_2$), and one side group unique to each amino acid (R). The side group gives each amino acid its identity. It can vary from a simple hydrogen atom, as in glycine, to a complex ring of carbon and hydrogen atoms, as in phenylalanine. The side groups mean that amino acids differ in shape, size, composition, electrical charge, and pH. When amino acids are linked to form a protein, these characteristics work together to determine that protein's specific function. **FIGURE 6.1** shows the structure of an amino acid.

Key Concepts Amino acids, which consist of a central carbon atom bonded to a hydrogen atom, a carboxyl group, an amino group, and a side group, are the building blocks of proteins. Essential amino acids cannot be made by the body and must be supplied in the diet. Nonessential amino acids can be made in the body if there is an adequate supply of nitrogen, carbon, hydrogen, and oxygen.

Protein Structure: Unique Three-Dimensional Shapes and Functions

Proteins are very large molecules. Their chains of linked amino acids twist, fold, or coil into unique shapes. Just as we combine letters of the alphabet in different sequences to form an infinite variety of words, the body combines amino acids in different sequences to form a nearly infinite variety of proteins (see FYI feature "Scrabble Anyone?"). For this reason, protein molecules are more diverse than either carbohydrates or lipids are.

Amino Acid Sequence

Amino acids link in specific sequences to form strands of protein (often called peptides) up to hundreds of amino acids long. One amino acid is joined to the next by a **peptide bond**. To form a peptide bond, the carboxyl (–COOH) group of one amino acid bonds to the amino ($-NH_2$) group of another amino acid, releasing water (H_2O) in the process (see **FIGURE 6.2**). A **dipeptide** is two amino acids joined by a peptide bond, and a **tripeptide** is three amino acids joined by peptide bonds. The term **oligopeptide** refers to a chain of 4 to 10 amino acids, whereas a **polypeptide** contains more than 10 amino acids.[7] Proteins in the body and in the diet are long polypeptides, most with hundreds of linked amino acids.

Protein Shape

As its amino acids are assembled in the cell's cytoplasm, each protein chain assumes a unique three-dimensional shape that derives from the sequence and properties of its amino acids. The three-dimensional shape of a protein determines its function and its interaction with other molecules. As an example,

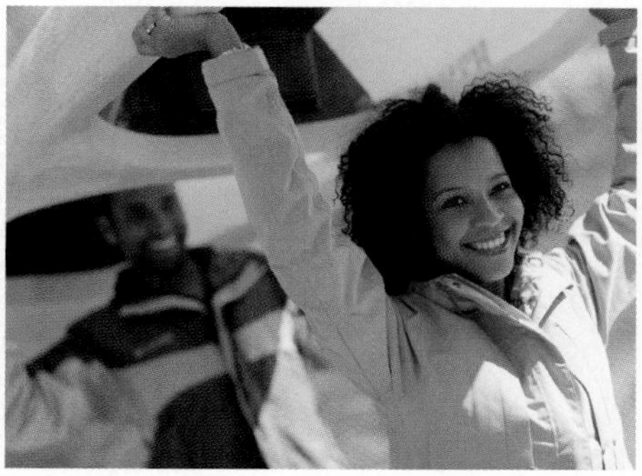

© Randy Faris/Corbis/age fotostock

- **peptide bond** The bond between two amino acids formed when a carboxyl (–COOH) group of one amino acid joins an amino ($-NH_2$) group of another amino acid, releasing water in the process.
- **dipeptide** Two amino acids joined by a peptide bond.
- **tripeptide** Three amino acids joined by peptide bonds.
- **oligopeptide** Four to 10 amino acids joined by peptide bonds.
- **polypeptide** More than 10 amino acids joined by peptide bonds.

FIGURE 6.2 Forming a peptide bond. Imagine a row of people facing forward with their hands joined—the right hand joined to the left hand. Similarly, when two amino acids join together, the carboxyl group of one amino acid is matched with the amino group of another. A condensation reaction forms a peptide bond and releases water.

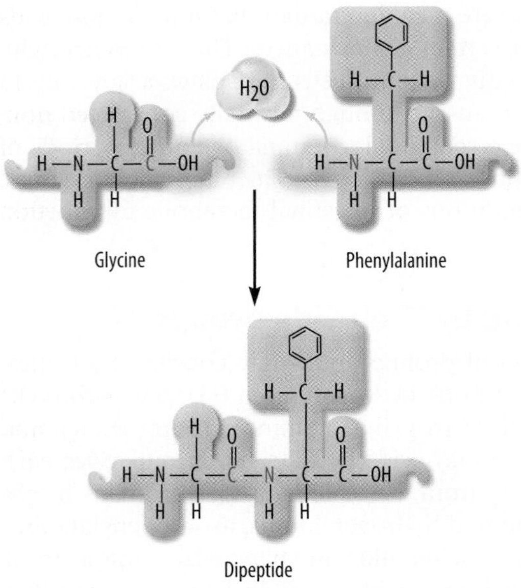

H₂O
Glycine
Phenylalanine
Dipeptide

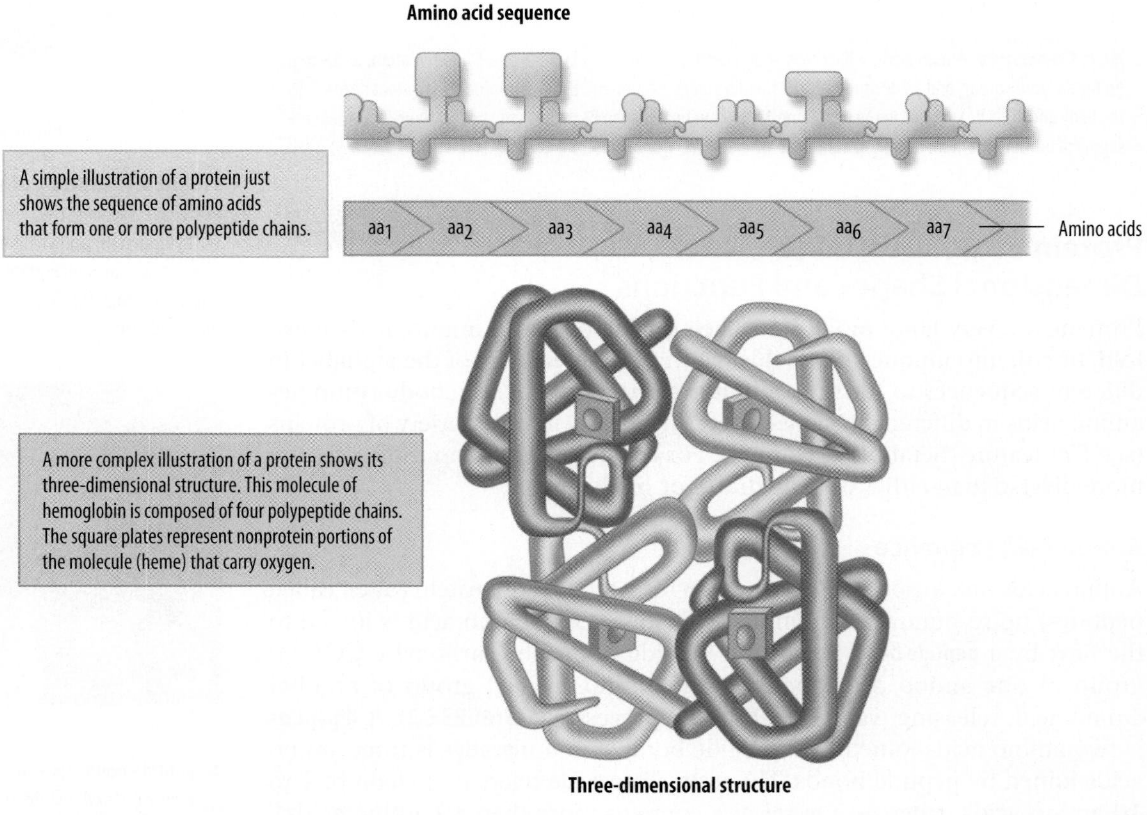

Amino acid sequence
A simple illustration of a protein just shows the sequence of amino acids that form one or more polypeptide chains.
aa1
aa2
aa3
aa4
aa5
aa6
aa7
Amino acids
A more complex illustration of a protein shows its three-dimensional structure. This molecule of hemoglobin is composed of four polypeptide chains. The square plates represent nonprotein portions of the molecule (heme) that carry oxygen.
Three-dimensional structure

FIGURE 6.3 Hemoglobin. Each protein becomes folded, twisted, and coiled into a shape all its own. This shape defines how a protein functions in your body. The simplest depiction of a protein reveals its unique sequence of amino acids.

▶ **hemoglobin** [HEEM-oh-glow-bin] The oxygen-carrying protein in red blood cells that consists of four heme groups and four globin polypeptide chains. The presence of hemoglobin gives blood its red color.

FIGURE 6.3 illustrates the unique folded and twisted shape of **hemoglobin**, the iron-carrying protein in red blood cells. In the lungs, hemoglobin binds oxygen and releases carbon dioxide. It then travels throughout the body, delivering oxygen to other tissues and picking up carbon dioxide for the return trip to the lungs.

Some amino acids carry electrical charges and therefore are attracted to the charged ends of water molecules (**hydrophilic amino acids**). In a watery environment, hydrophilic amino acids orient themselves on the outside of the folded protein chain in close contact with water molecules. Other amino acids are electrically neutral and do not interact with water (**hydrophobic amino acids**). In a watery environment, hydrophobic amino acids fold to the inside of the protein molecule. The amino acid cysteine, which has sulfur atoms in its side group, sometimes chemically bonds to another cysteine in the chain, creating a **disulfide bridge**, which helps stabilize the protein's structure.

▶ **hydrophilic amino acids** Amino acids that are attracted to water (water-loving).

▶ **hydrophobic amino acids** Amino acids that are repelled by water (water-fearing).

▶ **disulfide bridge** A bond between the sulfur components of two sulfur-containing amino acids that helps stabilize the structure of protein.

▶ **denaturation** An alteration in the three-dimensional structure of a protein resulting in an unfolded polypeptide chain that usually lacks biological activity.

Protein Denaturation: Destabilizing a Protein's Shape

Acidity, alkalinity, heat, alcohol, oxidation, and agitation can all disrupt the chemical forces that stabilize a protein's three-dimensional shape, causing it to unfold and lose its shape (denature), as shown in **FIGURE 6.4**. Because a protein's shape determines its function, denatured proteins lose their ability to function properly.

If you've ever cooked an egg, you've witnessed protein **denaturation**. As the egg cooks, some of its protein bonds break. As these proteins unfold, they bump into and bind to each other. Eventually, as these interconnections increase, the liquid egg coagulates to form a solid. Raw egg white proteins denature and stiffen as they are whipped, and milk proteins denature and curdle when acid is added.

In addition to risking a potentially serious bout of food poisoning, if an egg is eaten raw, its avidin protein can bind to the B vitamin biotin in the digestive tract, making the vitamin unavailable for absorption. Biotin deficiency is rare in the United States, and although not a safe dietary practice, it was once a trendy food fad to eat raw eggs. Thoroughly cooking the egg kills harmful bacteria and also denatures the avidin, destroying its ability to bind to biotin. Denaturation is the first step in breaking down protein for digestion. Stomach acids denature protein, uncoiling the structure into a simple amino acid chain that digestive enzymes can start breaking apart.

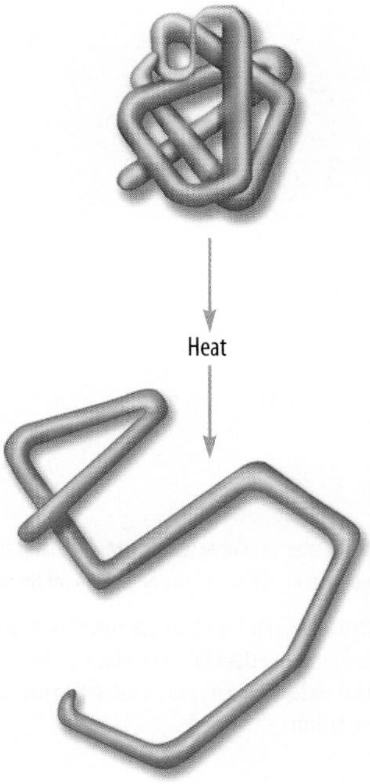

FIGURE 6.4 Denaturation. Heat, pH, oxidation, and mechanical agitation are some of the forces that can denature a protein, causing it to unfold and lose its functional shape.

Key Concepts Proteins are large molecules made up of amino acids joined in various sequences. Amino acids are joined by peptide bonds. Each protein assumes a unique three-dimensional shape depending on the sequence of its amino acids and the properties of their side groups. Acid, alkaline, heat, alcohol, and agitation can disrupt chemical forces that stabilize proteins, causing the proteins to denature, or lose their shape.

Functions of Body Proteins

The human body contains thousands of different proteins, each with a specific function determined by its unique shape. Some act as enzymes, speeding up chemical reactions. Others act as hormones, which are a kind of chemical messenger. Antibodies made of protein protect us from foreign substances. Proteins maintain fluid balance by pumping molecules across cell membranes and attracting water. They maintain the acid and base balance of body fluids by taking up or giving off hydrogen ions as needed. Finally, proteins transport many key substances such as oxygen, vitamins, and minerals to target cells throughout the body. **FIGURE 6.5** illustrates the functions of proteins in the human body.

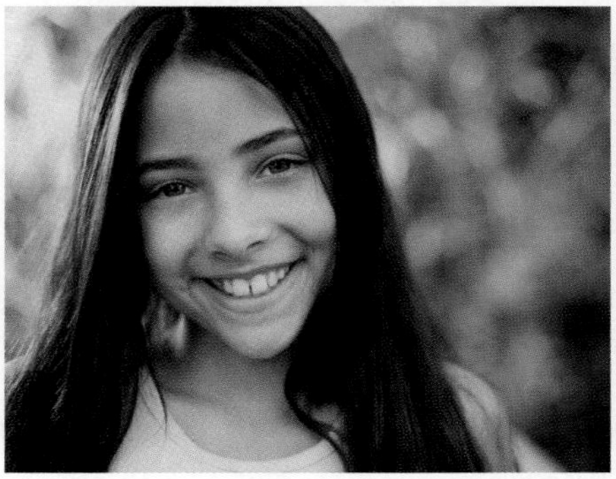

Structural and Mechanical Functions

Structures such as bone, skin, and hair owe their physical properties to unique proteins. **Collagen**, which appears microscopically as a densely packed long rod,

▶ **collagen** The most abundant fibrous protein in the body. Collagen is the major constituent of connective tissue, forms the foundation for bones and teeth, and helps maintain the structure of blood vessels and other tissues.

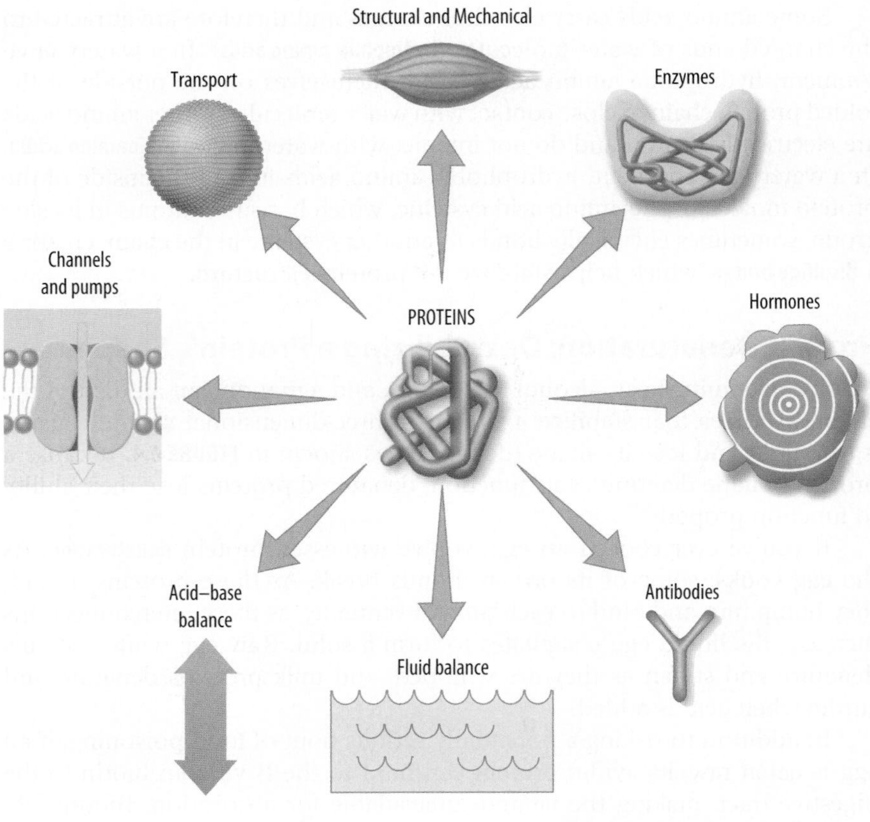

FIGURE 6.5 Functions of proteins. There are many different types of proteins, each with its particular role in the body.

▶ **keratin** A water-insoluble fibrous protein that is the primary constituent of hair, nails, and the outer layer of the skin.

▶ **motor proteins** Proteins that use energy and convert it into some form of mechanical work. Motor proteins are active in processes such as dividing cells, contracting muscle, and swimming sperm.

is the most abundant protein in mammals and gives skin and bones their elastic strength. Hair and nails are made of **keratin**, which is another dense protein made of coiled helices. Protein is essential for building these anatomical structures; therefore, protein deficiencies during a child's development can be disastrous. **FIGURE 6.6** shows structural proteins.

Motor proteins are exactly what their name implies: proteins that turn energy into mechanical work. In fact, these proteins perform the final step in converting our food into physical work. When you bike down a road or up a mountain, you are using your stored food energy to power minuscule molecular motors in your muscles. These molecular motors slide muscle proteins past each other, causing muscles to contract. As you pump the pedals, proteins turn that energy bar you ate into work. Similarly, specialized motor proteins are involved in a variety of processes, including cell division, muscle contraction, and sperm swimming.

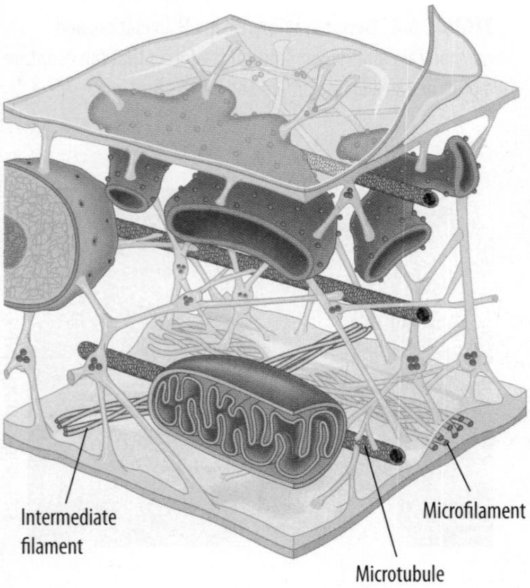

FIGURE 6.6 Structural proteins. Proteins provide structure to all cells, including hair, skin, nails, and bone. As part of muscle, they transform energy into mechanical movement.

Enzymes

Enzymes are proteins that catalyze chemical reactions without being destroyed in the process (see **FIGURES 6.7A** and **6.7B**). Every cell contains thousands of types of enzymes, each with its own purpose. During digestion, for example, enzymes help break down carbohydrates, proteins, and fats into monosaccharides, amino acids, and fatty acids for absorption into the body. Cellular enzymes release energy from these nutrients to fuel thousands of body processes. Enzymes also trigger the reactions that build muscle and tissue.

Our foods also contain enzymes, but these are inactivated (denatured) by cooking. Stomach acid denatures the enzymes in raw foods. You might

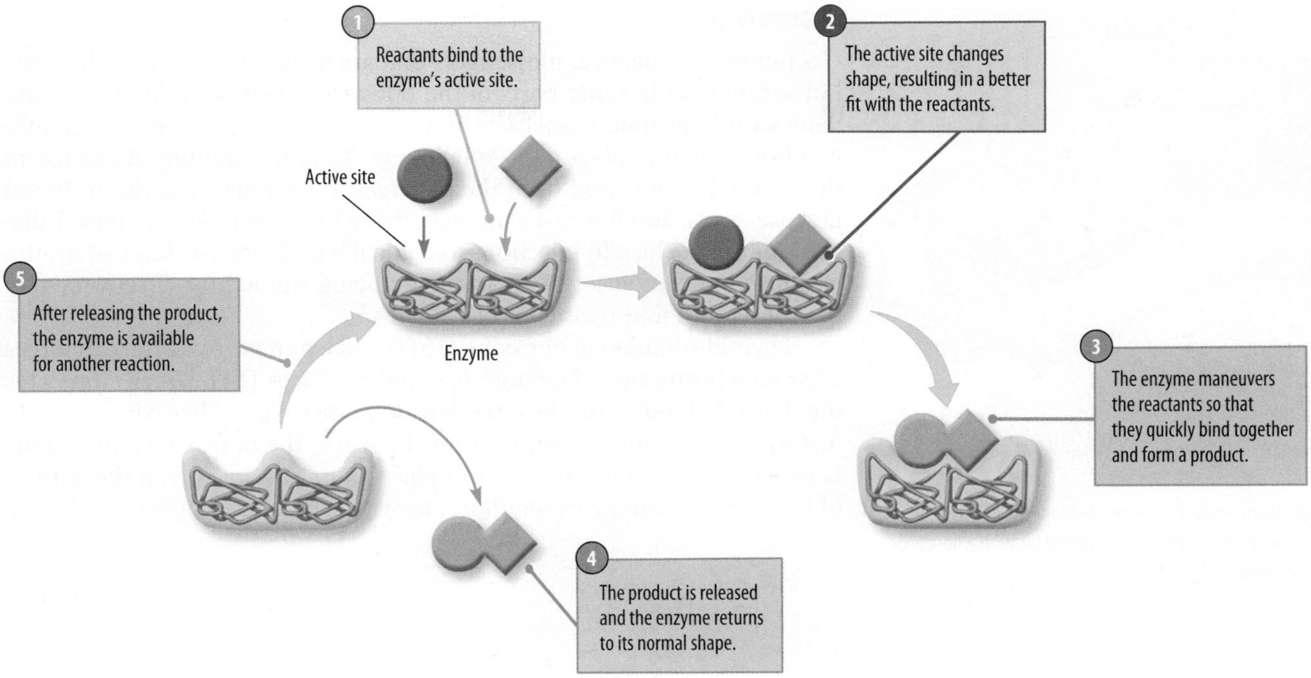

FIGURE 6.7A Enzymes. Enzymes catalyze (speed up) reactions that make or change substances.

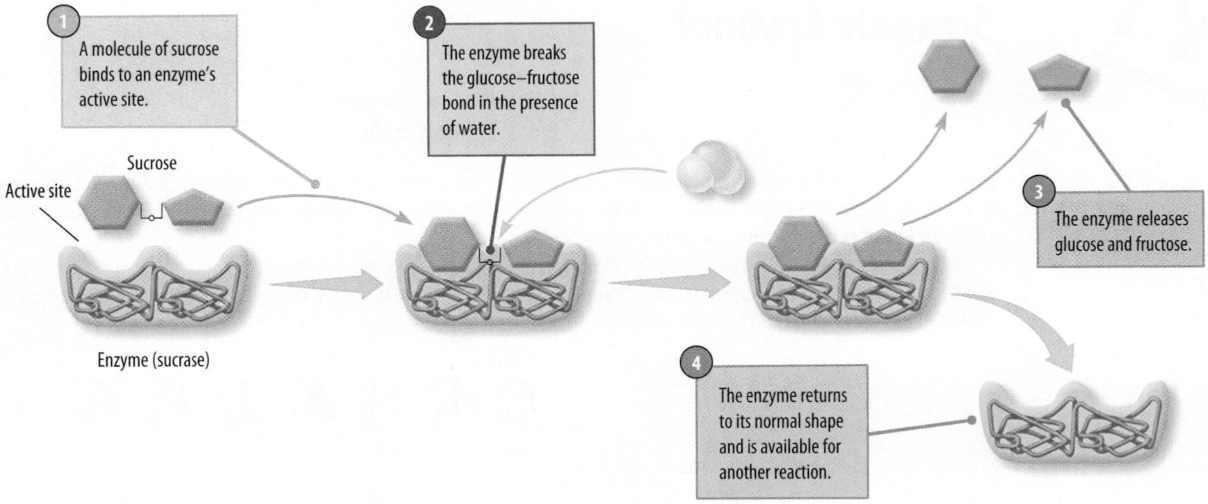

FIGURE 6.7B Enzymes catalyze reactions that break down molecules.

notice special purified enzymes being sold as supplements to enhance digestion. Most of the time, stomach acid denatures these enzymes so that they are unable to function in the intestinal tract. However, some enzyme supplements are coated with a special substance to protect them from stomach acid. For example, a specially coated tablet form of the enzyme lactase can help people with lactose intolerance. Coated enzymes temporarily help break down foods in the small intestine but eventually are digested themselves.

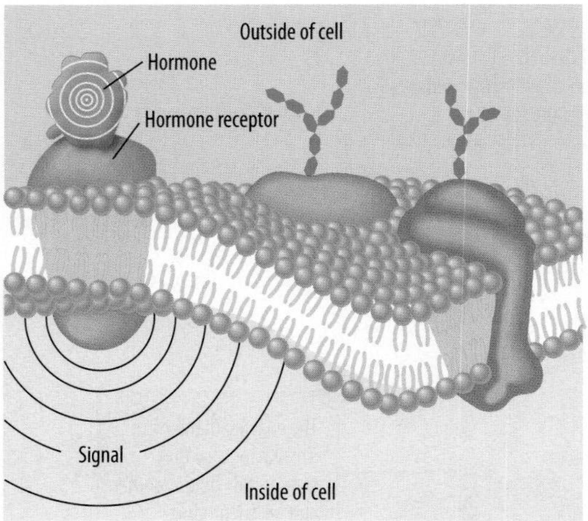

FIGURE 6.8 Hormones. Hormones are formed in one part of the body and are carried in the blood to a different location where they signal cells to alter activities.

Hormones

Hormones are chemical messengers that are made in one part of the body but act on cells in other parts of the body (see **FIGURE 6.8**). Many are proteins with important regulatory functions. Insulin, for example, is a protein hormone that plays a key role in regulating the amount of glucose in the blood. It is released from the pancreas in response to a rise in blood glucose levels, and functions to lower those levels. People with type 1 diabetes must take insulin injections to control blood glucose. Inhaled insulin and insulin taken as a pill are currently being studied for effectiveness in the prevention and treatment of diabetes.[8]

Thyroid-stimulating hormone (TSH) and leptin are two other examples of protein hormones. The pituitary gland produces TSH, which stimulates the thyroid gland to produce the hormone thyroxine. Thyroxine, a modified form of the amino acid tyrosine, increases the body's metabolic rate. Leptin is produced by fat cells and plays an important role in the control of food intake, energy expenditure, metabolism, and body weight.[9]

FYI For Your Information

Scrabble Anyone?

Scrabble tile = amino acid
word = protein chain

Making a meaningful word from available Scrabble tiles is a good analogy for the making of a functional protein chain from available amino acids. Just as we can make many different words from the same tiles, cells can make many different proteins from the same amino acids.

If your cells have all 20 amino acids at their disposal, these can be arranged in a bewildering number of combinations to create tens of thousands of different protein chains, just as all the letters of the alphabet can be used to make an almost unlimited number of words.

Key

Amino Acid		Scrabble Tile
Glutamic Acid	Glu	E
Isoleucine	Ile	I
Asparagine	Asn	N
Serine	Ser	S
Threonine	Thr	T
Lysine	Lys	K
Arginine	Arg	R

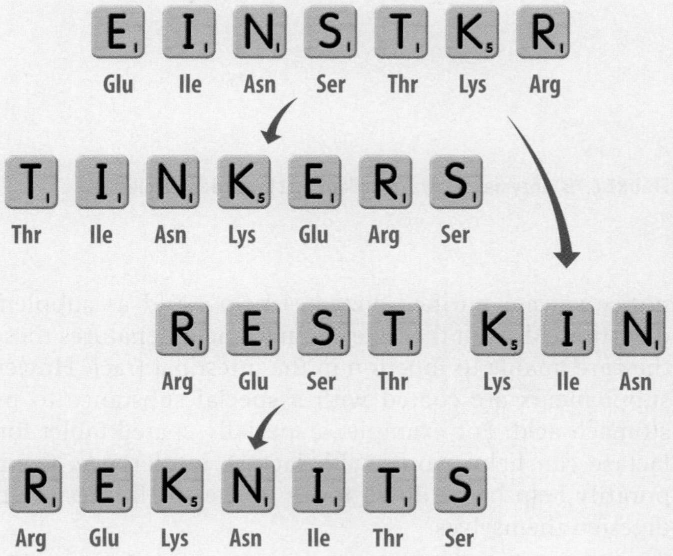

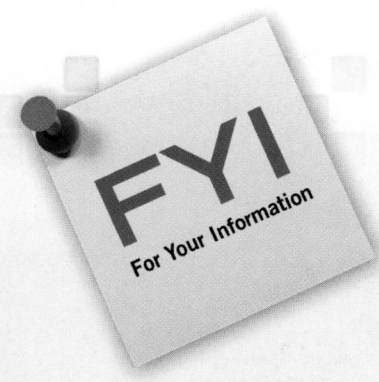

Immune Function

Proteins play an important role in the immune system, which is responsible for fighting invasion and infection by foreign substances (see **FIGURE 6.9**). **Antibodies** are blood proteins that attack and inactivate bacteria and viruses that cause infection. When your diet does not contain enough protein, your body cannot make as many antibodies as it needs. Your immune response is weakened, and your risk of infection and illness increases. Each protein antibody has a specific shape that allows it to attack and destroy a specific foreign invader. Once your immune system learns how to make a certain kind of antibody, your body can protect itself by quickly making that antibody the next time the same germ invades.

Viruses, such as those that cause the common cold, take over cells to replicate themselves. In a series of steps known as the **immune response**, your body mobilizes its defenses against the viral invaders. As part of the defense strategy, you produce protein antibodies that bind to the viruses, marking them for destruction. Even when the viruses are gone, special cells retain a memory of the particular virus so that a faster immune response can be mounted against future invasions. When people are immunized for a disease such as measles or mumps, they are actually getting a small amount of dead or inactivated virus in the injection. The dead virus cannot cause infection, but it does cue the body to make antibodies to the disease.

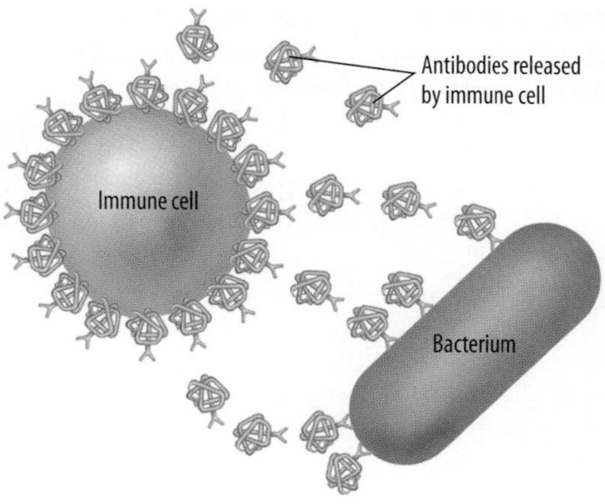

FIGURE 6.9 Proteins and the immune system. Protein antibodies are a crucial line of defense against invading bacteria and viruses.

- **antibodies** [AN-tih-bod-ees] Large blood proteins produced by B lymphocytes in response to exposure to particular antigens (e.g., a protein on the surface of a virus or bacterium). Each type of antibody specifically binds to and helps eliminate its matching antigen from the body. Once formed, antibodies circulate in the blood and help protect the body against subsequent infection.
- **immune response** A coordinated set of steps, including production of antibodies, that the immune system takes in response to an antigen.

Going Green

Send in the Proteins

In April 2010, in the Gulf of Mexico, the British Petroleum–owned *Deepwater Horizon* oil rig exploded and sank, killing 11 people. This explosion triggered a spill at the underwater oil well on which it was operating at the time, which gushed oil for 87 days, discharging an estimated 4.9 million barrels that had a devastating impact on precious marine life and wildlife habitats. Years later, dolphins and other marine life continued to die in record numbers, and other wildlife exposed to the spill developed deformities expected to be fatal. Scientists and researchers are still trying to understand the spill and its impact on marine life, the Gulf Coast, and human communities. The spill impacted over 1,000 miles of shoreline in Mississippi, Louisiana, Florida, Alabama, and Texas.

How can proteins help remedy this kind of catastrophe? In a method known as bioremediation, microorganisms naturally present in the soils help clean up groundwater contaminated with gasoline, solvents, and other contaminants. The superagents in this process are the enzymes—catalytic proteins—which consume toxic compounds and degrade them, transforming them into harmless carbon dioxide and water. These enzymes work just like those large proteins—also enzymes—that help us break down nutrients in digesting our food. This process is just one step in nature's biogeochemical recycling of organic compounds through the carbon cycle: Reservoirs of carbon are moved from plants to freshwater systems and soil to oceans, and eventually to the fossil fuels in sediments.

Nature's antidote, of course, takes many years to restore the environment to its former pristine state. To accelerate the process, scientists can stimulate the natural microbial community by pumping air, proteins, and other nutrients (fertilizers or molasses) underground, and then use the microorganisms to produce a sustained chemical reaction that breaks down the oil into molecules and base elements.

Similarly, wastewater treatment using bioremediation relies on the nutritional abilities of microbes to maintain clean water for us. Scientists continue to study and improve bioremediation technology and techniques, not only to clean up after oil spills, but also to restore many other environments that have been degraded.

FIGURE 6.10 Proteins in the blood. Blood proteins attract fluid into capillaries. This counteracts the force of the heart beating, which pushes fluid out of capillaries.

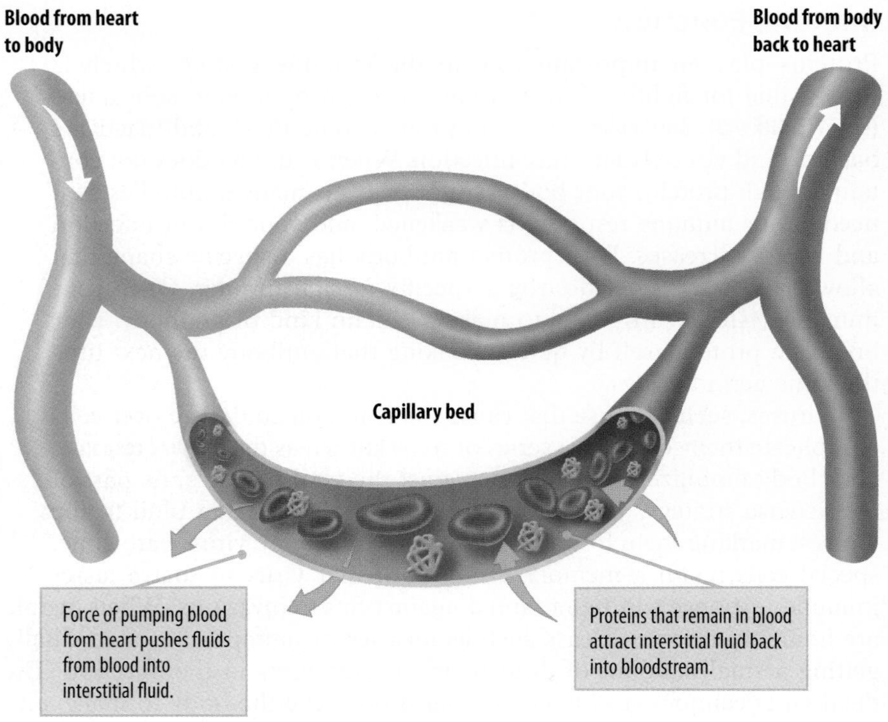
Blood from heart to body
Blood from body back to heart
Capillary bed
Force of pumping blood from heart pushes fluids from blood into interstitial fluid.
Proteins that remain in blood attract interstitial fluid back into bloodstream.

▶ **intracellular fluid** The fluid in the body's cells. It usually is high in potassium and phosphate and low in sodium and chloride. It constitutes about two-thirds of total body water.

▶ **extracellular fluid** The fluid located outside of cells. It is composed largely of the liquid portion of the blood (plasma) and the fluid between cells in tissues (interstitial fluid), with fluid in the GI tract, eyes, joints, and spinal cord contributing a small amount. It constitutes about one-third of body water.

▶ **interstitial fluid** [in-ter-STISH-ul] The fluid between cells in tissues. Also called intercellular fluid.

▶ **intravascular fluid** The fluid portion of the blood (plasma) contained in arteries, veins, and capillaries. It accounts for about 15 percent of the extracellular fluid.

▶ **edema** Swelling caused by the buildup of fluid between cells.

Fluid Balance

Fluids in the body are found inside cells (**intracellular fluid**) or outside cells (**extracellular fluid**). There are two types of extracellular fluid: fluid between cells (called intercellular fluid, or **interstitial fluid**) and fluid in the blood (**intravascular fluid**). These interior and exterior fluid levels must stay in balance for body processes to work properly.

Proteins in the blood help to maintain appropriate fluid levels in the vascular system (see **FIGURE 6.10**). The force of the heart's beating pushes fluid and nutrients from the capillaries out into the fluid surrounding the cells. But blood proteins such as albumin and globulin are too large to leave the capillary beds. These proteins remain in the capillaries, where they attract fluid. This provides a balancing and partially counteracting force that keeps fluid in the circulatory system.

If the diet lacks enough protein to maintain normal levels of blood proteins, fluid will leak into the surrounding tissue and cause swelling, also called **edema**. Children with protein malnutrition often suffer from severe edema. Reestablishing a diet adequate in protein and energy will allow the edema to subside.

Acid–Base Balance

The pH scale (which goes from 0 to 14) is a measure of the concentration of hydrogen ions in a substance. The higher the concentration of hydrogen ions, the lower the pH. Acids, with a high concentration of hydrogen ions, have a pH lower than 7; bases, with a low concentration of hydrogen ions, have a pH higher than 7. The lower the pH, the stronger the acid. The higher the pH, the stronger the base. The body works hard to keep the pH of the blood near 7.4, or nearly neutral. We can tolerate only small blood pH fluctuations without disastrous physiological consequences. Only a few hours with a blood pH above 8.0 or below 6.8 will cause death.

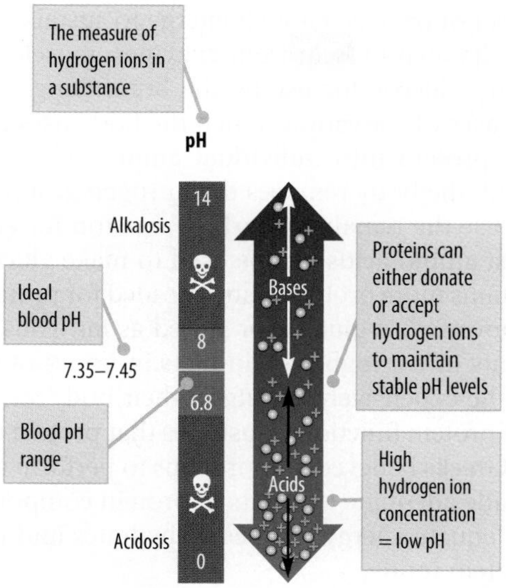

FIGURE 6.11 Proteins help maintain stable pH levels. Proteins act as buffers. When conditions are acidic, they pick up extra hydrogen ions. When conditions are alkaline, they donate hydrogen ions.

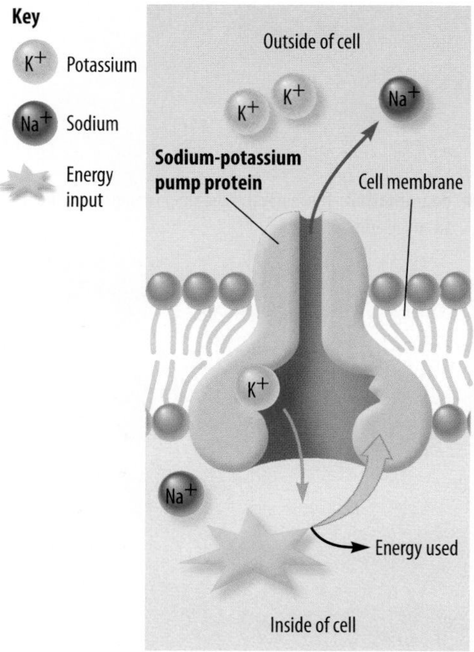

FIGURE 6.12 A transmembrane protein. Proteins form channels and pumps that help move substances into and out of cells.

Proteins help maintain stable pH levels in body fluids by serving as **buffers**; they pick up extra hydrogen ions when conditions are acidic, and they donate hydrogen ions when conditions are alkaline (see **FIGURE 6.11**). If proteins are not available to buffer acidic or alkaline substances, the blood can become too acidic or too alkaline, resulting in either **acidosis** or **alkalosis**. Both conditions can be serious; either can cause proteins to denature, which can lead to coma or death.

▶ **buffers** Compounds or mixtures of compounds that can take up and release hydrogen ions to keep the pH of a solution constant. The buffering action of proteins and bicarbonate in the bloodstream plays a major role in maintaining the blood pH at 7.35 to 7.45.

▶ **acidosis** An abnormally low blood pH (below about 7.35) resulting from increased acidity.

▶ **alkalosis** An abnormally high blood pH (above about 7.45) resulting from increased alkalinity.

Transport Functions

Many substances pass into and out of cells via proteins that cross cell membranes and act as channels and pumps. Channels allow substances to flow rapidly through the membranes by passive diffusion and require no input of energy. Pumps (active transporters), in contrast, must use energy to drive the transport of substances across membranes. In fact, sodium–potassium pumps, proteins that control cell volume and nerve impulses and drive the active transport of monosaccharides and amino acids, use more than one-third of the energy your body consumes at rest.[10] **FIGURE 6.12** shows a transmembrane protein.

Proteins also act as carriers, transporting many important substances in the bloodstream for delivery throughout the body. Lipoproteins, for example, package proteins with lipids so that lipid particles can be carried in the blood (see **FIGURE 6.13**). Other proteins carry fat-soluble vitamins, such as vitamin A, and certain other vitamins and minerals. Because protein carries vitamin A in the blood, protein deficiency contributes to vitamin A deficiency. The protein transferrin carries iron in the blood. In the liver, iron is stored as part of ferritin, a different protein.

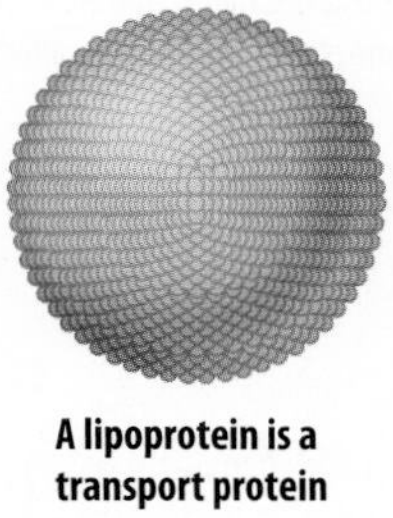

FIGURE 6.13 Proteins act as carriers. Lipoproteins have embedded proteins that help them transport fat and cholesterol in the blood.

Source of Energy and Glucose

THINK About It 1

Protein, like carbohydrates, when completely metabolized in the body yields 4 kilocalories of energy for every gram consumed. Although your body preferentially burns carbohydrate and fat for energy, if necessary it can use protein for energy or to make glucose. Thus, carbohydrate and fat are protein-sparing: They spare amino acids from being burned for energy and allow them to be used for protein synthesis.

If the diet does not provide enough energy to sustain vital functions, the body will sacrifice its own protein from enzymes, muscle, and other tissues to make energy and glucose for use by the brain, lungs, and heart. This is what happens in cases of starvation. When the body uses protein for energy, it first breaks the protein into individual amino acids. To release energy from an amino acid, the body removes the nitrogen group—a process called **deamination**. It can use the remaining carbon skeleton for energy. The carbon skeleton from most amino acids can be used to make glucose.

▶ **deamination** The removal of the amino group ($-NH_2$) from an amino acid.

If the diet contains more protein than is needed for protein synthesis, most of the excess is converted to glucose or stored as fat. Thus, people who take protein supplements or eat high-protein diets in hopes of increasing muscle mass may instead be expensively adding to their body fat.

This review of protein functions illustrates that protein is of "prime importance," just as the Greeks believed. For proteins to perform all these functions, the diet must provide adequate amounts of protein components. In addition, the body needs adequate energy from carbohydrates and fats, and adequate digestibility of protein foods.

Key Concepts In the body, proteins perform numerous vital functions that are determined by each protein's shape. As enzymes, they speed up chemical reactions; as hormones, they are chemical messengers. Protein antibodies protect the body from infection and illness; proteins also maintain fluid balance and acid–base balance and transport substances throughout the body. If needed, protein can also be used as a source of energy or glucose.

Protein Digestion and Absorption

Before your body can make a body protein from food protein, it must digest and absorb the protein you eat. **FIGURE 6.14** shows the process of protein digestion and absorption.

Protein Digestion

The first step in using dietary protein is digesting its long polypeptide chains into amino acids. As with the other energy-yielding nutrients, digestion requires enzymes from a number of sources. Digestion of protein begins in the stomach.

In the Stomach

In the stomach, hydrochloric acid (HCl) denatures a protein, unfolding it and making the amino acid chain more accessible to the action of enzymes. Glands in the stomach lining produce the proenzyme pepsinogen, an inactive **precursor** of the enzyme pepsin. When pepsinogen comes in contact with hydrochloric acid, it is converted to the active enzyme pepsin. The acidity of gastric juices is necessary for this enzyme to be active. It is most active at a (very acidic) pH of 2.5 and is inactive at a pH above 5.0. Gastric glands secrete hydrochloric acid at a pH of approximately 0.8. Once the hydrochloric acid is mixed with the gastric contents, the pH of the gastric juices falls to 2.5—the ideal medium for pepsin activity. By the time dietary protein leaves the stomach, pepsin has broken it down into individual amino acids and peptides of various lengths. Pepsin is responsible for about 10 to 20 percent of protein digestion.[11]

▶ **precursor** A substance that is converted into another active substance. Enzyme precursors also are called *proenzymes*.

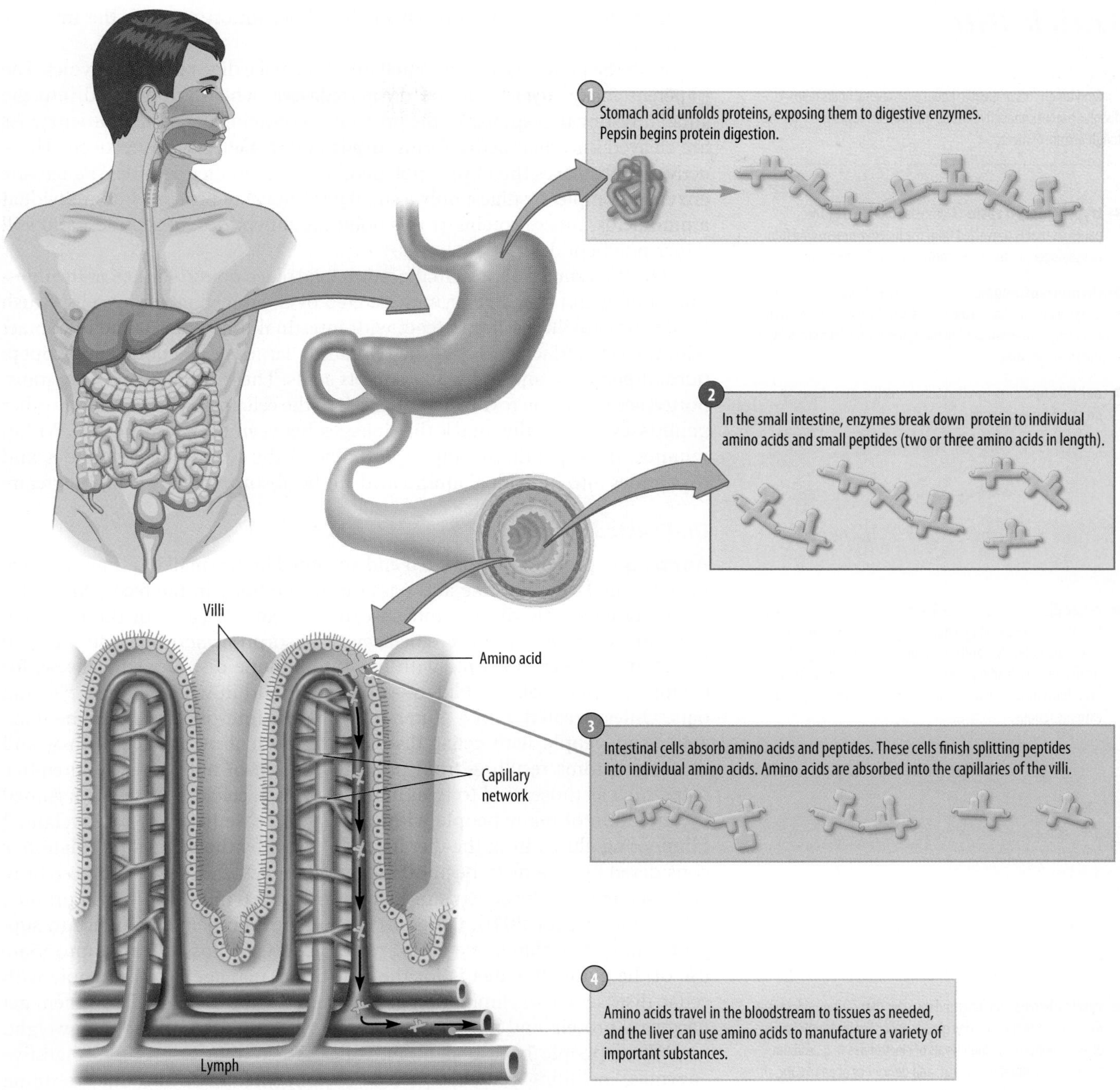
Stomach acid unfolds proteins, exposing them to digestive enzymes.
Pepsin begins protein digestion.
In the small intestine, enzymes break down protein to individual amino acids and small peptides (two or three amino acids in length).
Villi
Amino acid
Intestinal cells absorb amino acids and peptides. These cells finish splitting peptides into individual amino acids. Amino acids are absorbed into the capillaries of the villi.
Capillary network
Amino acids travel in the bloodstream to tissues as needed, and the liver can use amino acids to manufacture a variety of important substances.
Lymph

FIGURE 6.14 The breakdown of protein in the body. Digestion breaks down protein to amino acids that can be absorbed into the bloodstream.

In the Small Intestine

From the stomach, amino acids and polypeptides pass into the small intestine, where most protein digestion takes place. In the small intestine, **proteases** (protein-digesting enzymes) break down large peptides into smaller peptides. If a cell produces active forms of proteases, it will digest itself and break down its own cellular protein. However, cells employ a protective strategy. They produce and secrete most proteases as **proenzymes**, inactive forms of the

▶ **proteases** [PRO-tea-ace-ez] Enzymes that break down protein into peptides and amino acids.

▶ **proenzymes** Inactive precursors of enzymes.

Quick Bite

Softening Tough Meat

Cooking tough cuts of meat in liquid over several hours helps dissolve fibrous connective tissue, the proteins responsible for the tough texture of meat.

- **trypsinogen/trypsin** A protease produced by the pancreas that is converted from the inactive proenzyme form (trypsinogen) to the active form (trypsin) in the small intestine.
- **chymotrypsinogen/chymotrypsin** A protease produced by the pancreas that is converted from the inactive proenzyme form (chymotrypsinogen) to the active form (chymotrypsin) in the small intestine.
- **peptidases** Enzymes that act on small peptide units by breaking peptide bonds.
- **celiac disease** [SEA-lee-ak] A chronic autoimmune disorder that involves an inability to tolerate gluten, a protein found in wheat, barley, rye, and oats. If untreated, it damages the small intestine, leading to severe malabsorption of nutrients. Symptoms include diarrhea, fatty stools, swollen belly, and extreme fatigue.
- **cystic fibrosis** An inherited disorder that causes widespread dysfunction of the exocrine glands, resulting in chronic lung disease, abnormally high levels of electrolytes (e.g., sodium, potassium, chloride) in sweat, and deficiency of pancreatic enzymes needed for digestion.

enzymes, for later activation. This delayed activation protects the integrity of the cell.

Both the pancreas and the small intestine make digestive proenzymes. The pancreas makes **trypsinogen** and **chymotrypsinogen**, which are secreted into the small intestine in response to the presence of protein. Here, these proenzymes are cleaved into their active forms: **trypsin** and **chymotrypsin**, respectively. These activated proteases then break polypeptides into smaller peptides. Pancreatic enzymes completely digest only a small percentage of proteins into individual amino acids; most proteins at this point are dipeptides, tripeptides, and still larger polypeptides.

The final stages of protein digestion take place on the surface of the intestine's lining and require enzymes secreted by the intestinal lining cells. Brush border (microvilli) **peptidases** react with intestinal fluids that come in contact with the cell surface and split the remaining larger polypeptides into tripeptides, dipeptides, and individual amino acids. These smaller units are transported across the microvilli membranes into the cell. Inside the cell, many other peptidases specifically attack the linkages between the amino acids. Within minutes, these peptidases digest virtually all the remaining dipeptides and tripeptides into individual amino acids to be absorbed into the bloodstream.

Undigested Protein

Any parts of proteins not digested and absorbed in the small intestine continue through the large intestine and pass out of the body in the feces. Normally, the body efficiently digests and absorbs protein. Diseases of the intestinal tract, however, decrease the efficiency of absorption and increase nitrogen losses in the feces.[12] People with the autoimmune disorder **celiac disease**, for example, cannot tolerate gluten—a protein found in wheat, barley, rye, and oats. Unless treated with a gluten-free diet, the intestinal villi become damaged, and people with celiac disease have poor growth, weight loss, and other symptoms resulting from poor absorption of nutrients.[13] Gluten-free diets, such as those used to treat individuals with celiac disease, have gained the attention of many people without celiac disease trying to lose weight.[14] Eliminating gluten from the diet for weight loss by the general population is considered by experts to be another 'get-thin quick' fad. Aside from celebrity endorsements, flashy advertising claims, and $15.6 billion dollars in product sales estimated for 2016, there has yet to be experimental evidence to support claims that gluten-free eating promotes weight loss.[15] The appropriate use of the gluten-free diet is for the nutritional management of people with celiac disease where eliminating gluten from the diet actually helps them get necessary protein and nutrients so they can maintain a healthy body weight.

When people have **cystic fibrosis**, thick, sticky mucus prevents digestive enzymes, including proteases, from reaching the small intestine, resulting in poor digestion and absorption of protein and other nutrients.[15] Special enzyme preparations that contain protease, lipase, and amylase are needed to prevent malnutrition.

Amino Acid and Peptide Absorption

End products of protein digestion are absorbed as both amino acids and small peptides. Approximately 11 different transport mechanisms for amino acids have been identified within the absorptive cells of the small intestine.[16] Absorption of some amino acids requires active transport, whereas other amino acids are absorbed by facilitated diffusion (see **FIGURE 6.15**). Although the active transport process is the same for amino acids as it is for glucose and galactose, amino acids and monosaccharides use different transport proteins.

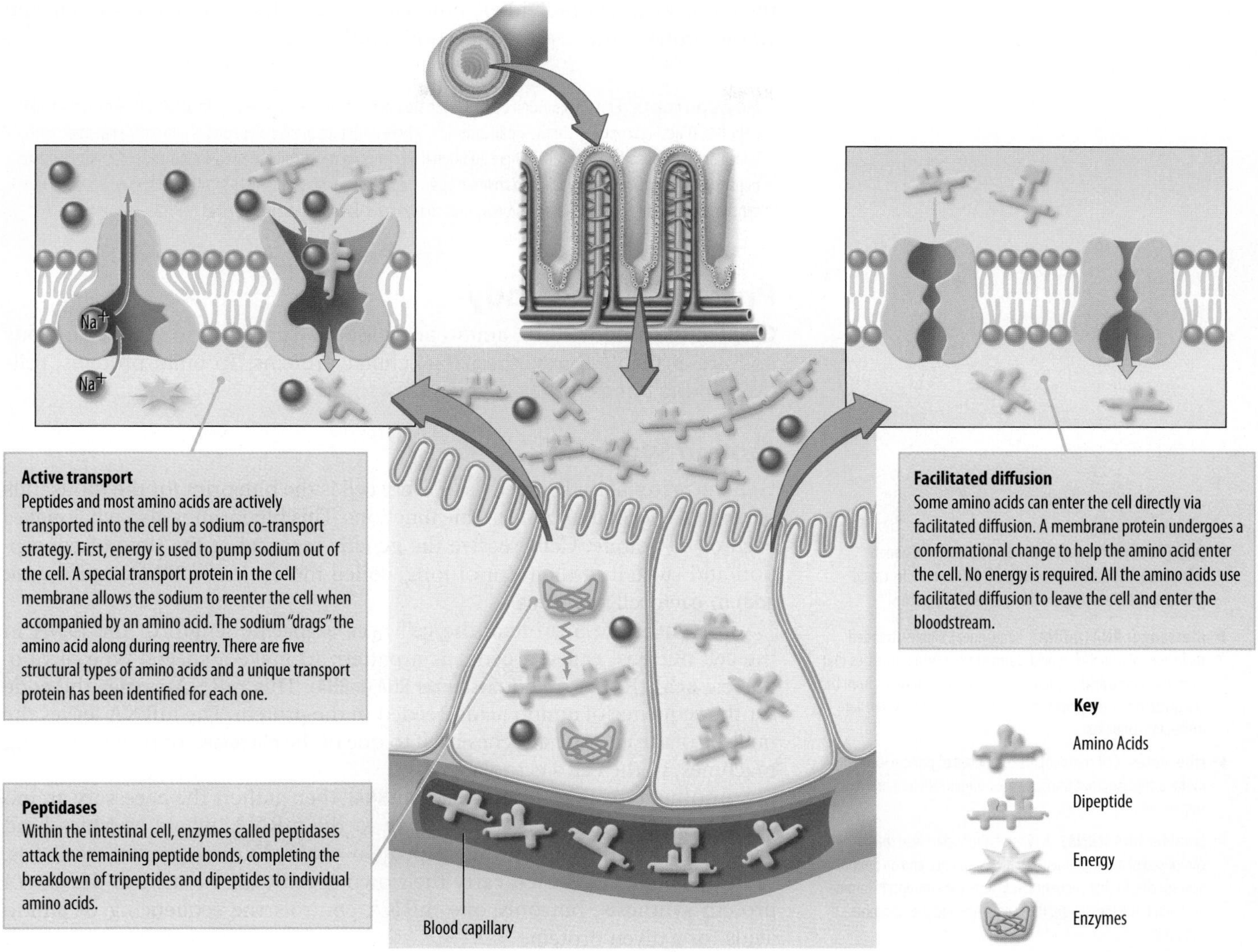

Na+
Na+
Active transport
Peptides and most amino acids are actively transported into the cell by a sodium co-transport strategy. First, energy is used to pump sodium out of the cell. A special transport protein in the cell membrane allows the sodium to reenter the cell when accompanied by an amino acid. The sodium "drags" the amino acid along during reentry. There are five structural types of amino acids and a unique transport protein has been identified for each one.
Peptidases
Within the intestinal cell, enzymes called peptidases attack the remaining peptide bonds, completing the breakdown of tripeptides and dipeptides to individual amino acids.
Blood capillary
Facilitated diffusion
Some amino acids can enter the cell directly via facilitated diffusion. A membrane protein undergoes a conformational change to help the amino acid enter the cell. No energy is required. All the amino acids use facilitated diffusion to leave the cell and enter the bloodstream.
Key
Amino Acids
Dipeptide
Energy
Enzymes

FIGURE 6.15 Protein absorption into an intestinal cell. Intestinal cells use active transport and facilitated diffusion to absorb amino acids.

Although there are several active transport mechanisms, similar amino acids share the same active transport system. The amino acids leucine, isoleucine, and valine, for example, all depend on the same carrier molecule for absorption. Normally, proteins in foods supply a mix of many amino acids, so amino acids that share the same transport system are absorbed fairly equally. If a person consumes a large amount of one particular amino acid, however, absorption of other amino acids that share the same transport system will be deficient. Thus, if you take a supplement of one amino acid, you might be interfering with the absorption of another amino acid from your diet.

Most protein absorption takes place in the cells that line the duodenum and jejunum. After they are absorbed, most amino acids and the few absorbed peptides are transported by the portal vein to the liver to be used for protein synthesis, energy needs, or conversion to carbohydrate or fat, or they are released into the bloodstream for transport to other cells.[17]

Some amino acids remain in the intestinal cells and are used to synthesize intestinal enzymes and new cells. More than 99 percent of protein enters the bloodstream as individual amino acids. Peptides are rarely absorbed, and whole proteins that escape digestion hardly ever are.

Key Concepts Protein digestion begins in the stomach, where the enzyme pepsin breaks proteins into smaller peptides. Digestion continues in the small intestine, where proteases break polypeptides into smaller peptide units, which are then absorbed into cells, where additional enzymes complete digestion to amino acids. Key enzymes are pepsin in the stomach and trypsin and chymotrypsin from the pancreas. Proteases (protein-digesting enzymes) are synthesized and secreted as inactive proenzymes so that cells do not digest themselves.

Proteins in the Body

Once in the bloodstream, amino acids are transported throughout the body and are available for synthesizing cellular proteins. To build proteins, cells use peptide bonds to link amino acids.

Protein Synthesis

Genetic material in the nucleus of every cell is the blueprint for the thousands of proteins needed to perform life functions. This blueprint is also what makes each of us unique. Cells receive the genetic material at the time of conception and store it in the form of long, coiled molecules of **DNA (deoxyribonucleic acid)** in each cell's nucleus.

To synthesize a protein, the cell uses a specific length of the DNA in the cell nucleus, called a gene, as a pattern to make a special type of ribonucleic acid (RNA) called **messenger RNA (mRNA)**. This mRNA carries the code for the sequence of amino acids needed in the protein. The mRNA leaves the nucleus of the cell and attaches itself to one of the **ribosomes**, or protein-making machines, in the cell's cytoplasm.

Another type of RNA, **transfer RNA (tRNA)**, then gathers the necessary amino acids from cell fluid and carries them to the mRNA, where enzymes bind each amino acid to the growing protein chain. During protein synthesis, thousands of tRNAs each carry their own specific amino acid to the site of protein synthesis, but only one mRNA controls the sequencing of amino acids for a given protein.

A third type of RNA, **ribosomal RNA (rRNA)**, is the major component of ribosomes. For many years, scientists assumed that rRNA primarily served as a structural framework for protein synthesis and had little catalytic function. With the discovery that RNA in general can play many catalytic roles, scientists now believe that rRNA has a major role in directing protein synthesis. **FIGURE 6.16** illustrates protein synthesis.

Just as one missing car part can stop an entire auto assembly line, one missing amino acid can stop synthesis of an entire protein in the cell. If a nonessential amino acid is missing during protein synthesis, the cell will either make that amino acid or obtain it from the liver through the bloodstream, and protein synthesis will continue. If an essential amino acid is missing, the body might break down its own protein to supply the missing amino acid. If a missing essential amino acid is unavailable, protein synthesis halts, and the partially completed protein is broken down into individual amino acids to be used elsewhere in the body.

Genetic defects in DNA also can cause problems in protein synthesis. People who have sickle cell anemia, for example, have a defect in the amino acid sequencing of their hemoglobin. A genetic error causes the substitution of the amino acid valine for glutamic acid in two locations in the protein chain. This simple error causes the shape of hemoglobin to change so much that the red blood cell becomes stiff and sickle-shaped instead of soft and

- **DNA (deoxyribonucleic acid)** The carrier of genetic information. Specific regions of each DNA molecule, called genes, act as blueprints for the synthesis of proteins.
- **messenger RNA (mRNA)** Long, linear, single-stranded molecules of ribonucleic acids formed from DNA templates that carry the amino acid sequence of one or more proteins from the cell nucleus to the cytoplasm, where the ribosomes translate mRNA into proteins.
- **ribosomes** Cell components composed of protein located in the cytoplasm that translate messenger RNA into protein sequences.
- **transfer RNA (tRNA)** A type of ribonucleic acid that is composed of a complementary RNA sequence and an amino acid specific to that sequence. It inserts the appropriate amino acid when the messenger RNA sequence and the ribosome call for it.
- **ribosomal RNA (rRNA)** A type of ribonucleic acid that is a major component of ribosomes. It provides a structural framework for protein synthesis and orchestrates the process.

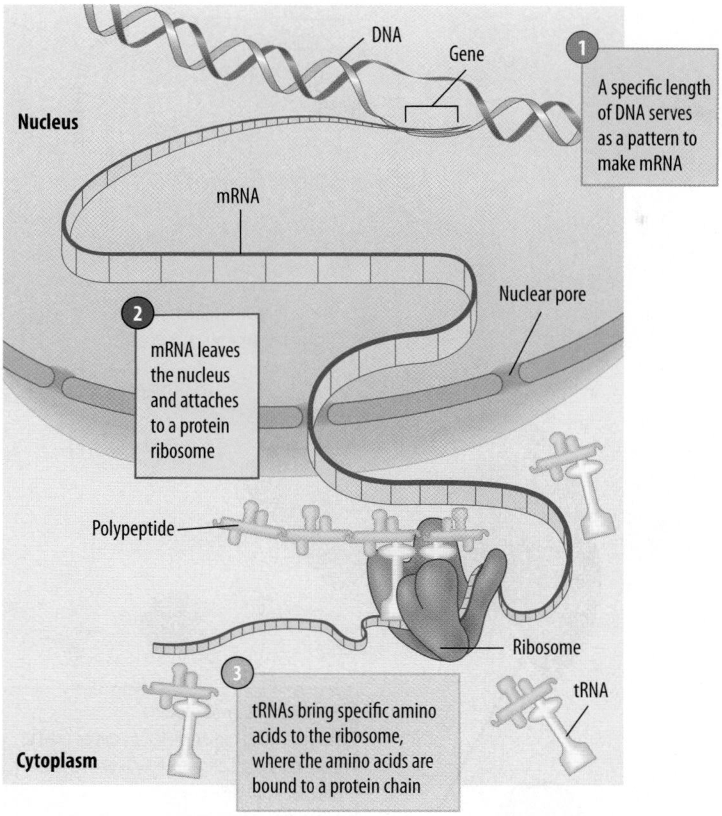
DNA
Gene
1
A specific length of DNA serves as a pattern to make mRNA
Nucleus
mRNA
Nuclear pore
2
mRNA leaves the nucleus and attaches to a protein ribosome
Polypeptide
Ribosome
3
tRNAs bring specific amino acids to the ribosome, where the amino acids are bound to a protein chain
tRNA
Cytoplasm

FIGURE 6.16 Protein synthesis. Ribosomes are our protein synthesis factories. mRNA carries manufacturing instructions from DNA in the cell nucleus to the ribosomes. tRNA collects amino acids in the correct sequence, and rRNA in the ribosome directs protein synthesis.

disk-shaped. Because this faulty protein cannot carry oxygen efficiently, it causes serious medical problems.

The Amino Acid Pool and Protein Turnover

Cells throughout the body constantly and simultaneously synthesize and break down protein. When cells break down protein, the protein's amino acids return to circulation (see **FIGURE 6.17**). These available amino acids, found throughout body tissues and fluids, are collectively referred to as the **amino acid pool**. Some of these amino acids can be used for protein synthesis; others might have their amino group removed and be used to produce energy or nonprotein substances such as glucose.

▶ **amino acid pool** The amino acids in body tissues and fluids that are available for new protein synthesis.

The constant recycling of proteins in the body is known as **protein turnover**. Each day, more amino acids in your body are recycled than are supplied in your diet. Of the approximately 300 grams of protein synthesized by the body each day, 200 grams are made from recycled amino acids.[20] This remarkable recycling capacity is the reason we need so little protein in our diet. Although our requirements are small, dietary protein is extremely important. When dietary protein is inadequate, increased breakdown of body protein replenishes the amino acid pool. This can lead to the breakdown of essential body tissue.

▶ **protein turnover** The constant synthesis and breakdown of proteins in the body.

Synthesis of Nonprotein Molecules

Amino acids serve other roles in addition to performing as components of peptides and proteins; they are precursors of many molecules with important biological roles. Your body makes nonprotein molecules from amino acids and the nitrogen they contain. The vitamin niacin, for example, is made from the amino acid tryptophan. Precursors of DNA, RNA, and many coenzymes

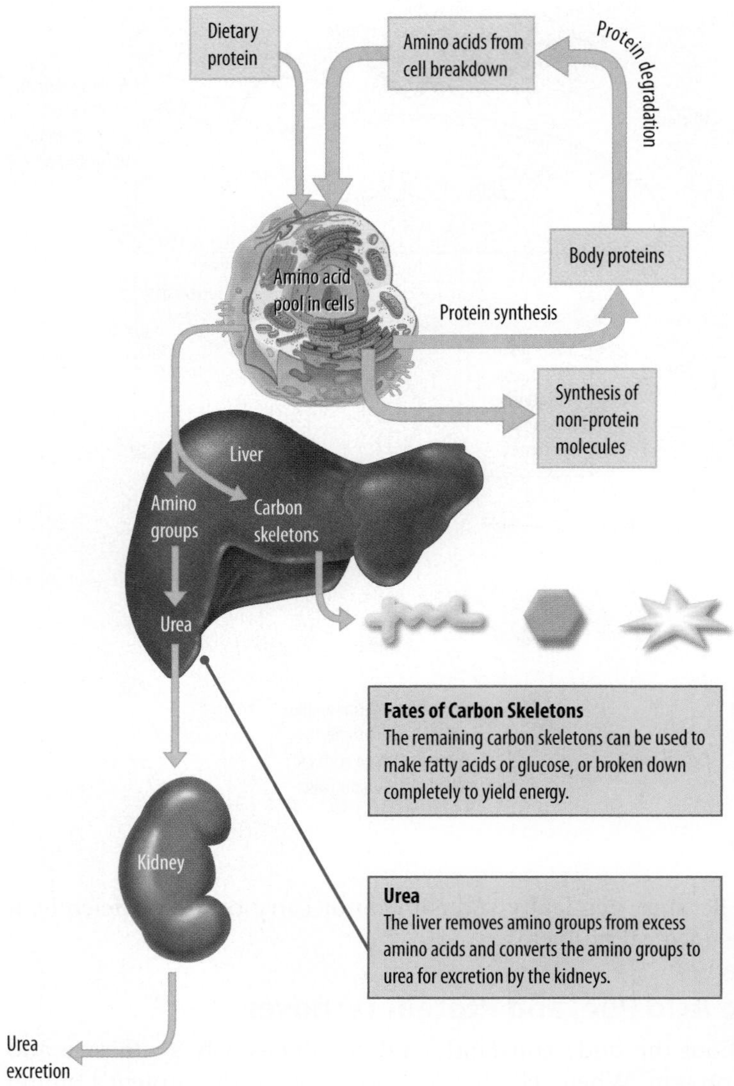
Dietary protein
Amino acids from cell breakdown
Protein degradation
Amino acid pool in cells
Body proteins
Protein synthesis
Synthesis of non-protein molecules
Liver
Amino groups
Carbon skeletons
Urea
Fates of Carbon Skeletons
The remaining carbon skeletons can be used to make fatty acids or glucose, or broken down completely to yield energy.
Kidney
Urea
The liver removes amino groups from excess amino acids and converts the amino groups to urea for excretion by the kidneys.
Urea excretion

FIGURE 6.17 Protein turnover. Cells draw upon their amino acid pools to synthesize new proteins. These small pools turn over quickly and must be replenished by amino acids from dietary protein and degradation of body protein. Dietary protein supplies about one-third and the breakdown of body protein supplies about two-thirds of the amino acids needed to synthesize roughly 300 grams of body protein daily.

▶ **neurotransmitters** Substances released at the end of a stimulated nerve cell that diffuse across a small gap and bind to another nerve cell or muscle cell, stimulating or inhibiting it.

derive in part from amino acids. Your body also uses amino acids to make **neurotransmitters**, chemicals that send signals from nerve cells to other parts of the body. The neurotransmitter serotonin, which helps regulate mood, is made from tryptophan. Norepinephrine and epinephrine (also called noradrenaline and adrenaline, respectively), which ready the body for action, are neurotransmitters made from tyrosine. Your body also uses tyrosine to make the skin pigment melanin and a hormone called thyroxine. The simple amino acid glycine combines with many toxic substances to make less harmful substances that the body can excrete. Your body uses the amino acid histidine to make histamine, a potent vasodilator (dilator of blood vessels) and a culprit in allergic reactions.

Protein and Nitrogen Excretion

Cells are constantly breaking down and recycling amino acids. Breakdown of an amino acid yields an amino group ($-NH_2$). This NH_2 molecule is unstable and is quickly converted to ammonia (NH_3). However, ammonia is toxic to cells, so it is expelled into the bloodstream as a waste product and carried to the liver. In the liver, an amino group and an ammonia group react with carbon dioxide through a series of reactions (known collectively as the urea cycle) to generate **urea** and water. The nitrogen-rich urea is transported from the liver by way of the bloodstream to the kidneys, where it is filtered from the blood and sent to the bladder for excretion in the urine. Small amounts of other nitrogen-containing compounds, such as ammonia, uric acid, and creatinine, are excreted in the urine as well. Some nitrogen also is lost through skin, sloughed-off gastrointestinal (GI) cells, mucus, hair and nail cuttings, and body fluids.

▶ **urea** The main nitrogen-containing waste product in mammals. Formed in liver cells from ammonia and carbon dioxide, urea is carried by the bloodstream to the kidneys, where it is excreted in the urine.

Nitrogen Balance

Because nitrogen is excreted as proteins are recycled or used, we can use the balance of nitrogen in the body to evaluate whether the body is getting enough protein (see **FIGURE 6.18**). To estimate the balance of nitrogen, and therefore

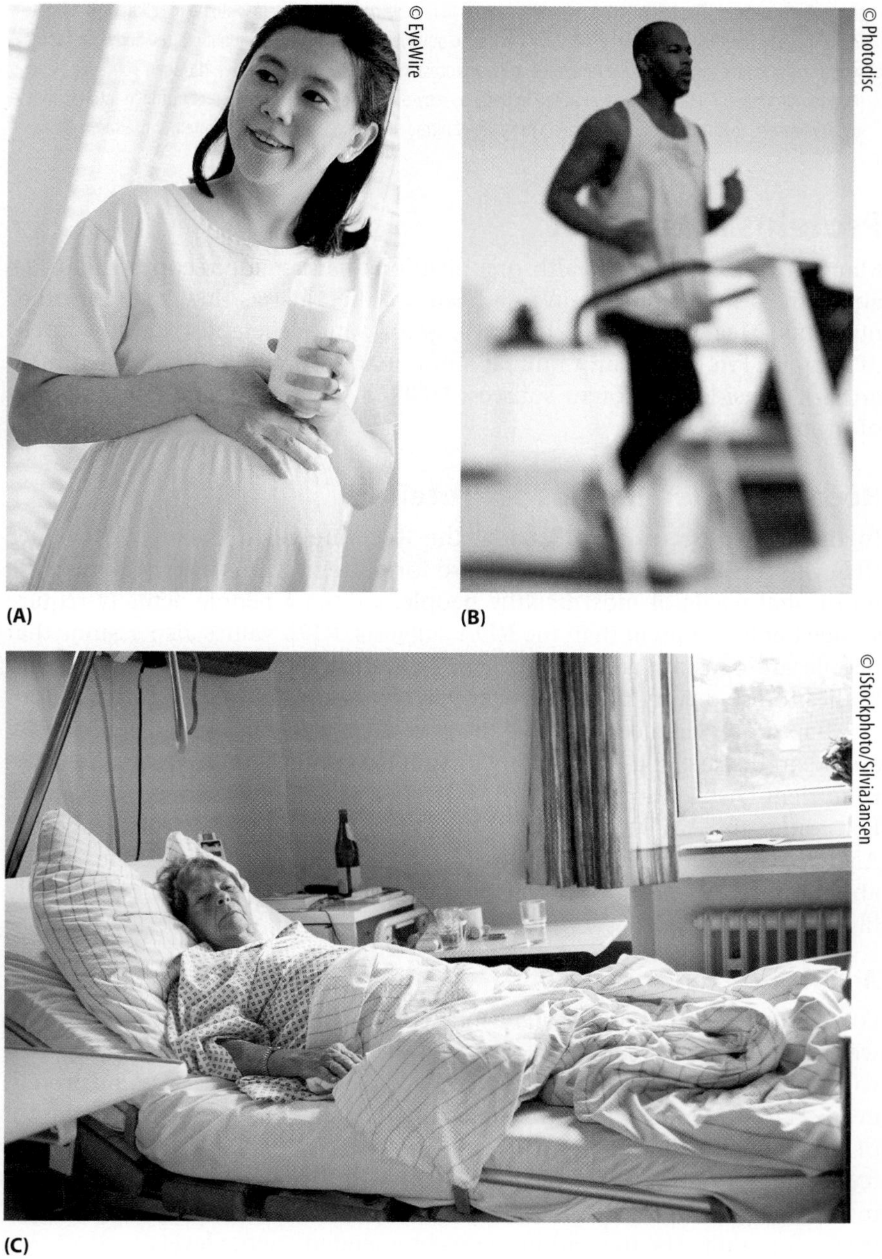

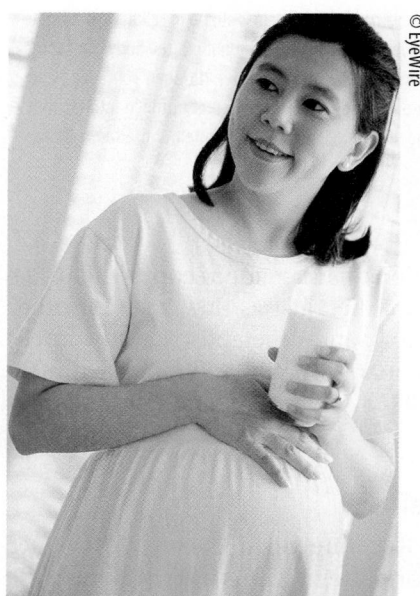

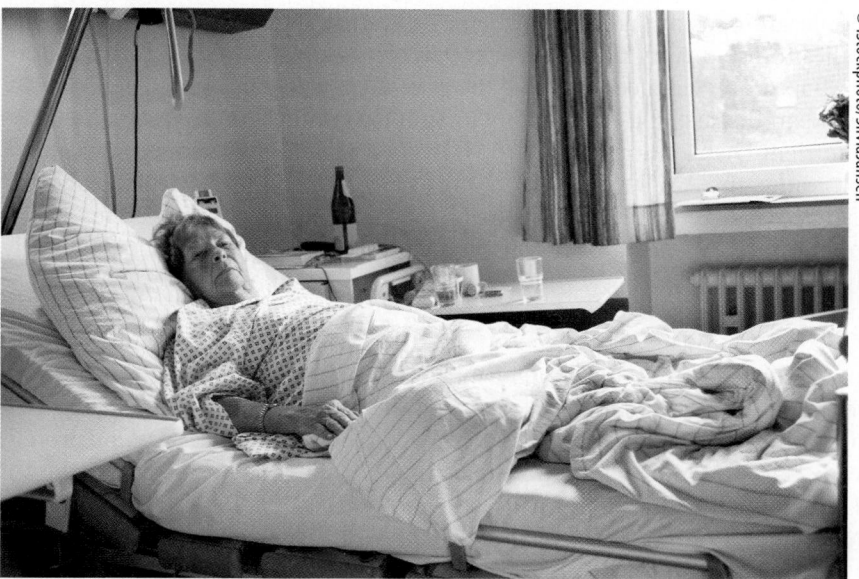

FIGURE 6.18 Protein (nitrogen) balance. Nitrogen balance reflects whether a person is gaining or losing protein. (A) A pregnant woman is adding protein, so she has a positive nitrogen balance. (B) A healthy person who is neither gaining nor losing protein is in nitrogen equilibrium. (C) A person who is severely ill and losing protein has a negative nitrogen balance.

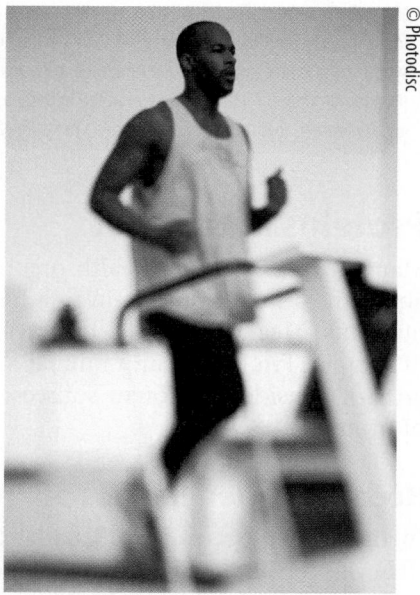

nitrogen balance = grams of nitrogen intake − grams of nitrogen output

protein in the body, nitrogen intake is compared to the sum of all sources of nitrogen excretion (urine, feces, skin, hair, and body fluids).[21]

If nitrogen intake exceeds nitrogen excretion, the body is said to be in **positive nitrogen balance**. Positive nitrogen balance means that the body is adding protein, as is the case for growing children, pregnant women, or people recovering from protein deficiency or illnesses. If nitrogen excretion exceeds nitrogen intake, the body is in **negative nitrogen balance**. This means that the body is losing protein. People who are starving or on extreme weight-loss diets or who suffer from fever, severe illnesses, or infections are in a state of negative nitrogen balance. If nitrogen intake equals nitrogen excretion, **nitrogen balance** is zero, and the body is in **nitrogen equilibrium**. Healthy adults are in nitrogen equilibrium, which means that their dietary protein intake is adequate to maintain and repair tissue. They have no net gain or loss of body protein, and they simply excrete excess dietary nitrogen.

- **positive nitrogen balance** Nitrogen intake exceeds the sum of all sources of nitrogen excretion.
- **negative nitrogen balance** Nitrogen intake is less than the sum of all sources of nitrogen excretion.
- **nitrogen balance** Nitrogen intake minus the sum of all sources of nitrogen excretion.
- **nitrogen equilibrium** Nitrogen intake equals the sum of all sources of nitrogen excretion; nitrogen balance equals zero.

Key Concepts The information that directs a cell to make a particular protein is stored in cellular DNA. Three forms of RNA—mRNA, tRNA, and rRNA—are needed to build body proteins. Cells throughout the body constantly synthesize and break down protein simultaneously, a process known as protein turnover. Nitrogen-containing end products of protein metabolism are excreted in urine by way of the kidneys. Comparison of nitrogen intake (from dietary protein) to nitrogen excretion gives a measure of nitrogen balance and indicates protein status in the body.

Proteins in the Diet

Many government and health organizations have made recommendations about the amount of protein in a healthful diet, just as they have for other nutrients. Meat, eggs, milk, legumes, grains, and vegetables are all sources of protein. Fruits contain minimal amounts of protein, and along with fats are not considered protein sources. **FIGURE 6.19** shows some good sources of protein.

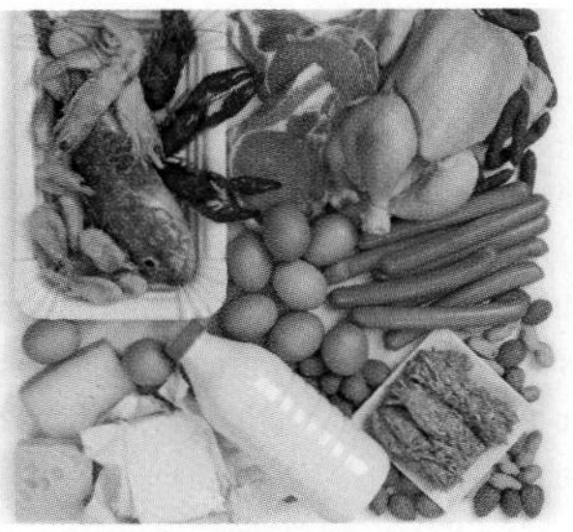

© iStockphoto/Thinkstock

Rich sources of protein include meats, fish, poultry, eggs, dairy products, legumes, and nuts.

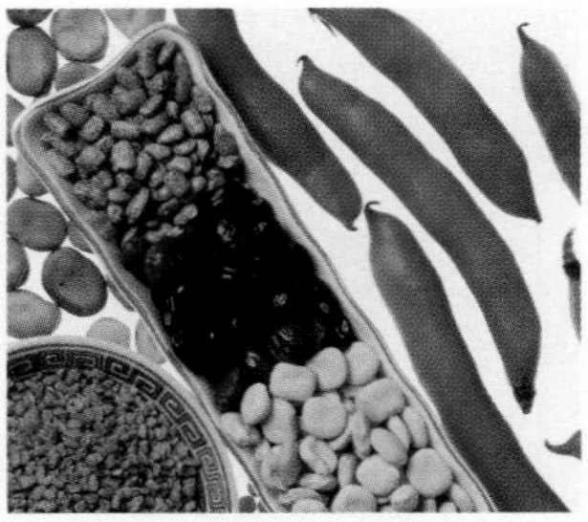

Photo by Keith Weller, Courtesy of USDA.

Legumes and nuts are important sources of protein for vegetarians.

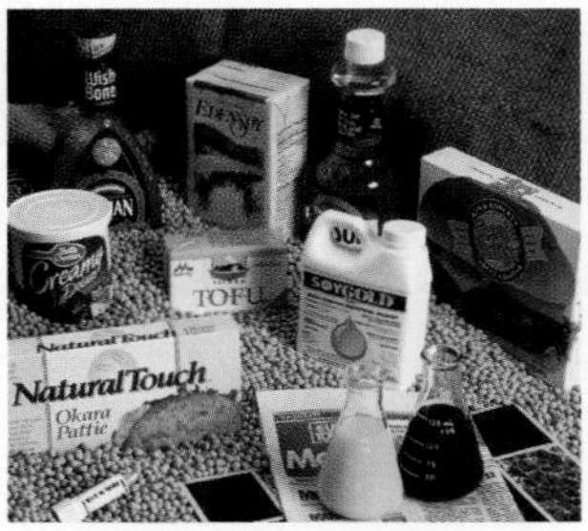

Photo by Scott Bauer, Courtesy of USDA.

Soybeans and soy products are plant sources of complete protein.

FIGURE 6.19 Protein sources. Meat, fish, eggs, dairy products, and soy are excellent protein sources. Legumes, grain products, starchy vegetables, nuts, and seeds also are good sources.

Recommended Intakes of Protein

In the United States and Canada, the Recommended Dietary Allowance (RDA) is the accepted dietary standard for protein. RDAs are set to meet the nutritional needs of most healthy people, so many people actually require somewhat less protein than the RDA suggests. RDA values also assume that people are consuming adequate energy and other nutrients to allow their bodies to use dietary protein for protein synthesis, rather than for energy.

Based on evidence to reduce the risk of chronic diseases such as obesity and heart disease, the Food and Nutrition Board developed Acceptable Macronutrient Distribution Ranges (AMDRs) for the energy-yielding nutrients.[22] For adults, the AMDR for fat is 20 to 35 percent of energy intake, and the AMDR for carbohydrate is 45 to 65 percent of energy intake. This leaves about 10 to 35 percent of energy intake from protein, a level that is typically higher than the RDA. THINK About It 2

Adults

For adults, the RDA for protein intake is 0.8 gram per kilogram of body weight.[23] In clinical situations that require precise assessments, ideal body weight (rather than actual body weight) is typically used to determine protein needs. The RDA for adults translates into a daily protein recommendation of 56 grams for the average adult male and 46 grams for the average adult female aged 19 to 24 years. When calculated as a percentage of average energy intake, the protein RDA for adults provides about 8 to 11 percent of energy intake for adults staying within the recommended energy levels.

Other Life Stages

Infants have the highest protein needs relative to body weight of any time of life (see **TABLE 6.2**). Protein is needed to support rapid growth during infancy. The Adequate Intake (AI) value for infants 0 to 6 months of age is based on the protein content of human milk and the average milk consumption of breastfed babies. Protein requirements per kilogram body weight gradually fall throughout childhood and adolescence until a person reaches adulthood.

Both pregnancy and lactation (production of breast milk) increase a woman's need for protein. The RDA for pregnant and lactating women is 1.1 grams of protein per kilogram body weight. This is an increase of about 25 grams per day over the female RDA for protein. Most American women already consume more than enough protein to support pregnancy and lactation.

The RDA for protein for all adults, regardless of age, is set at 0.8 gram protein per kilogram body weight. Although elderly people on average have less lean body mass to maintain than younger people, some experts believe that the daily protein requirement for people over the age of 50 should be higher than 0.8 gram per kilogram.[24] Evidence indicates that protein intake greater than the RDA can improve muscle mass, strength, and function in this population.[25] Immune status, wound healing, blood pressure, and bone health can also be improved by meeting protein needs in this group. Because energy needs decline with age, protein should provide a larger percentage of energy intake. An intake of 1.0–1.6 grams of protein per kilogram per day is a reasonable target for individuals older than 50 years.[26] To maximize protein efficiency, older adults should try to eat 25–30 grams of high-quality protein at each meal throughout the day.[27]

TABLE 6.2
Protein AI or RDA for Infants, Children, and Teens

Age	Protein AI or RDA (grams)
0 to 6 months	1.52
7 to 12 months	1.5
1 to 3 years	1.1
4 to 8 years	0.95
9 to 13 years	0.95
14 to 18 years	0.85

Data from Institute of Medicine, Food and Nutrition Board. *Dietary Reference Intakes for Energy, Carbohydrates, Fiber, Fat, Fatty Acids, Cholesterol, Protein, and Amino Acids (Macronutrients)*. Washington, DC: National Academies Press; 2005.

Physical Stress

Severe physical stress can increase the body's need for protein. Infections, burns, fevers, and surgery all increase protein losses, and the diet must replace that lost protein. A severe infection can increase protein requirements by one-third. Severe burns can increase requirements two to four times. Less severe physical stressors, such as a viral illness with a mild fever lasting only a few days, rarely increase protein requirements. Muscle-building activities, such as intense weight training, increase protein need much less than most people think. In fact, the typical American diet supplies an ample amount of protein for most people, even for bodybuilders. (See the FYI feature, "Do Athletes Need More Protein?")

Convert weight to kg
(pounds ÷ 2.2)
Multiply kg by 0.8 = Protein RDA in g

Male, 19–24 years old, 70 kg (154 lb)
70 kg × 0.8 g/kg = 56 g protein

Female, 19–24 years old, 57 kg (125 lb)
57 kg × 0.8 g/kg = 46 g protein

Protein Consumption

According to national survey data, the median daily intake of protein for women age 20 and older is about 68 grams of protein daily and men consume about 99 grams per day.[28] Individual intake of protein has a large range, but, based on average intake data, Americans are generally eating within the recommended range of 10 to 35 percent of calories from protein. Does eating more protein help you to build more muscle? No. If dietary intake of protein is greater than the body's protein requirements, the excess amino acids can be converted to glucose for energy or converted to fatty acids and stored as adipose tissue.[29] On the other hand, if your protein intake is insufficient, the body may break down stored protein in the muscles and transport the amino acids to more vital organs.[30] If energy intake falls dangerously low, protein amino acids can be taken from the muscles and sent to the liver to be converted into glucose.

Key Concepts Infants, who are growing rapidly, have the highest protein needs relative to body weight. The recommended intakes (AIs or RDAs) decline from 1.52 grams per kilogram for infants 0 to 6 months old to 0.8 gram per kilogram for adults. Pregnancy, lactation, and severe physical stress all can alter protein requirements. Adults currently consume about 15 percent of their energy as protein, a level that provides ample protein for most people.

Quick Bite

Mother's Milk

Because it contains less protein than cow's milk and, in particular, less casein protein, infants digest human milk more readily than they can digest cow's milk. Milks high in casein protein tend to form curds (clumps) in the stomach upon exposure to stomach acid. These tough curds are hard for digestive enzymes to break apart.

FYI For Your Information

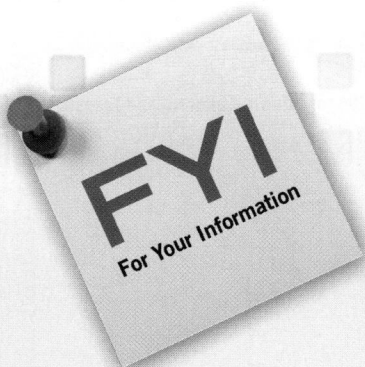

Do Athletes Need More Protein?

Athletes are not just pumping iron these days; they're also pumping protein supplements in hopes of building muscle and improving performance. Look inside many sports magazines and you'll see ads for protein or amino acid supplements targeted to athletes. You cannot force your body to build muscle by pumping in more protein than you need, any more than you can make your car run faster by adding more gas to a full tank. Extra protein does not build muscles; only regular workouts fueled by a mix of nutrients can achieve this goal.

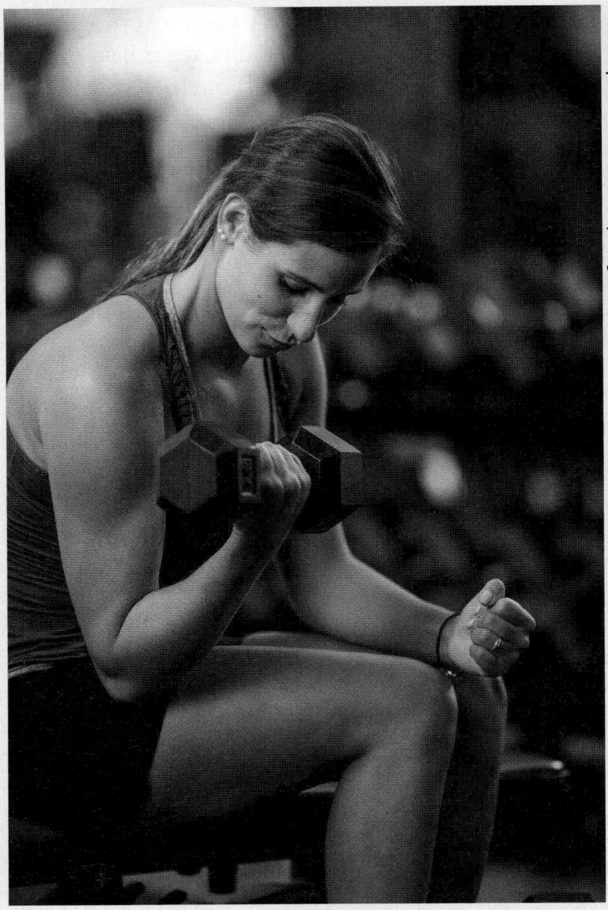

© Christopher Futcher/E+/Getty Images

Protein Requirements for Athletes

Many people assume that because muscle fibers are protein, building muscle must require protein. This is only partially true. The heavy resistance–type exercise that is needed to stimulate muscle growth must first be fueled by glucose and fatty acids (glucose is the predominant fuel). Little protein is used as a fuel source in resistance-type exercise. Some studies have shown that men who consume the RDA for protein (0.8 gram per kilogram body weight) and engage in heavy resistance exercise go into negative nitrogen balance. However, other studies have shown positive nitrogen balance and muscle hypertrophy during resistance training with intake at the RDA of 0.8 gram per kilogram per day.[a] The DRI committee reviewing evidence on macronutrients concluded that a higher RDA was not warranted for healthy adults doing resistance or endurance exercise.[b] Protein, however, is often recommended in amounts higher than the RDA to optimize athletic performance.[c] According to the Academy of Nutrition and Dietetics, endurance and strength athletes may need protein intakes in excess of the RDA[d] (see Position Statement figure/margin box). And according to the Position Stand by the International Society of Sports Nutrition, intakes of 1.4–2.0 grams per kilogram per day are needed for physically active individuals.[e]

Because Americans, on average, consume much more protein than they actually need, any increased need for athletes is most likely already being met. A male athlete in training (let's make his weight 70 kilograms [154 pounds]) might consume as many as 5,000 kilocalories per day. Even if his diet contained only 10 percent of calories as protein (the low side of the AMDR for protein, and lower than average), he would be getting about 126 grams of protein daily, about 1.8 grams per kilogram. It is unlikely that an athlete would not be able to meet his or her protein needs from a normal, mixed diet. Adequate intake and appropriate timing of protein ingestion have been shown to be beneficial in multiple exercise modes, including endurance, anaerobic, and strength exercise.[c]

Risks of Supplements

Maybe there's no benefit to taking protein or amino acid supplements, but there's no harm either, right? Not necessarily. If excess protein means excess calories, it could mean added weight as fat, not muscle, which can slow down your performance. Purified protein supplements can contribute to calcium losses, thereby harming bone health. Excess protein means excess nitrogen that must be excreted, which poses a risk for dehydration if fluid intake is inadequate. Supplements of single amino acids can interfere with absorption of other amino acids and can alter neurotransmitter activity. The bottom line is that protein or amino acid supplementation has not been shown to positively influence athletic performance and therefore should not be universally recommended.[f]

If you are a weekend athlete, there's no need to increase the protein in your diet and no reason to expect that doing so will help your performance. If you are a competitive athlete, choosing adequate calories from a wide variety of foods can ensure that you have an adequate protein intake. Supplements are unnecessary and expensive, and they can disrupt normal protein balance in the body. Play it safe; choose a healthful diet to fuel your exercise.

[a] Vieillevoye S, Poortmans JR, Duchateau J, Carpentie A. Effects of a combined essential amino acid/carbohydrate supplementation on muscle mass, architecture and maximal strength following heavy-load training. *Eur J Appl Physiol* 2010;110(3):479–488.

[b] Institute of Medicine, Food and Nutrition Board. *Dietary Reference Intakes for Energy, Carbohydrate, Fiber, Fat, Fatty Acids, Cholesterol, Protein, and Amino Acids (Macronutrients).* Washington, DC: National Academies Press; 2005. http://www.iom.edu/Global/News%20Announcements/~/media/C5CD2DD7840544979A549EC47E56A02B.ashx. Accessed December 29, 2015.

[c] Phillips SM. Dietary protein requirements and adaptive advantages in athletes. *Br J Nutr.* 2012;108(suppl 2):S158–S167.

[d] Position of the American Dietetic Association, Dietitians of Canada, and the American College of Sports Medicine: nutrition and athletic performance. *J Am Diet Assoc.* 2009;109:509–527.

[e] Campbell B, Kreider RB, Ziegenfuss T, et al. International Society of Sports Nutrition position stand: protein and exercise. *J Int Soc Sports Nutr.* 2007;4:8.

[f] Kreider RB, Campbell B. Protein for exercise and recovery. *Phys Sports Med.* 2009;37(2):12–21.

Protein Quality

Although both animal and plant foods contain protein, the quality of protein in these foods differs. Foods that supply all the essential amino acids in the proportions needed by the body are called **complete, or high-quality, proteins.** Foods that lack adequate amounts of one or more essential amino acids are called **incomplete, or low-quality, proteins**.

When a variety of foods provides ample dietary protein, the protein quality of foods is not a primary dietary concern. But whenever protein or energy intake is marginal, or when only one or a few plant foods are the main protein sources in the diet, protein quality is a critical issue.

▶ **complete (high-quality) proteins** Proteins that supply all the essential amino acids in the proportions the body needs.

▶ **incomplete (low-quality) proteins** Proteins that lack one or more amino acids.

Complete Proteins

Animal foods generally provide complete protein; that is, they provide all the essential amino acids in approximately the right proportions. One exception is gelatin, a protein derived from animal collagen that lacks the essential amino acid tryptophan.

Red meats, poultry, fish, eggs, milk, and milk products (all animal foods) contain complete protein. More than 20 percent of these foods' energy content is protein. For example, protein provides about 80 percent of the energy in water-packed tuna. There is also good news for vegetarians (discussed later in this chapter): The protein in soybeans is a notable exception to the rule that most plant proteins are incomplete. Protein isolated from soybeans provides a complete, high-quality protein equal to that of animal protein.[31] Although soy protein contains a lower proportion of the amino acid cysteine than does animal protein, the amount of soy typically consumed provides all the amino acids in sufficient amounts to meet the body's needs. Moreover, soybeans contain no cholesterol or saturated fat and are rich in isoflavonoids—phytochemicals that help reduce the risk of heart disease and cancer and improve bone health.

Americans, on average, obtain about 63 percent of their protein intake from animal foods.[32] (See **TABLE 6.3**.) In other parts of the world, animal proteins play a smaller role. In Africa and East Asia, for example, animal foods provide only 20 percent of protein intake.[33]

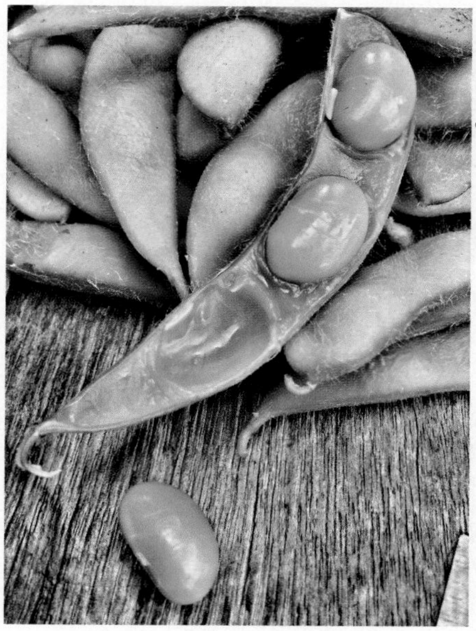

© successo images/Shutterstock

TABLE 6.3
Top 10 Sources of Protein for Children and Adolescents (ages 2–18) in the United States

Rank	Food	Grams of Protein Consumed[a]
1	Chicken and chicken mixed dishes	9.1
2	Pizza	5.6
3	Reduced-fat milk	5.5
4	Beef and beef mixed dishes	3.9
5	Burgers	3.8
6	Yeast breads	3.8
7	Pasta and pasta dishes	3.7
8	Whole milk	2.9
9	Mexican mixed dishes	2.7
10	Regular cheese	2.6

[a] Mean intake of protein 70 grams.

Modified from National Cancer Institute. Sources of protein among US children & adolescents, 2005–06. http://appliedresearch.cancer.gov/diet/foodsources/protein/. Accessed December 29, 2015.

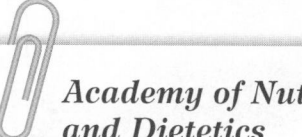

Academy of Nutrition and Dietetics

Excerpt from the Position of the American Dietetic Association, Dietitians of Canada, and the American College of Sports Medicine: Nutrition and Athletic Performance:

"Energy and macronutrient needs, especially carbohydrate and protein, must be met during times of high physical activity to maintain body weight, replenish glycogen stores, and provide adequate protein to build and repair tissue. . . . Protein recommendations for endurance and strength-trained athletes range from 1.2 to 1.7 g/kg (0.5 to 0.8 g/lb) body weight per day. These recommended protein intakes can generally be met through diet alone, without the use of protein or amino acid supplements. Energy intake sufficient to maintain body weight is necessary for optimal protein use and performance."

Position of the American Dietetic Association, Dietitians of Canada, and the American College of Sports Medicine: nutrition and athletic performance. *J Am Diet Assoc.* 2009;109:509–527.

TABLE 6.4
Examples of Complementary Food Combinations

- Beans and rice
- Beans and corn or wheat tortillas
- Rice and lentils
- Rice and black-eyed peas
- Pea soup with bread or crackers
- Chickpeas with sesame paste (hummus)
- Pasta with beans
- Peanut butter on bread

▶ **complementary protein** An incomplete food protein whose assortment of amino acids makes up for, or complements, another food protein's lack of specific essential amino acids so that the combination of the two proteins provides sufficient amounts of all the essential amino acids.

Quick Bite

Paleolithic Protein

Didn't our ancestors eat a lot of meat, too? Researchers estimate that hunter–gatherer populations' diets were about one-third meat and two-thirds vegetable. The meat from wild game, however, averages only one-seventh the fat of domesticated beef (about 4 grams of fat per 100 grams of wild meat, compared with 29 grams of fat per 100 grams of domestic meat). In addition, compared with the meat at your local supermarket, the fat contained in game animals that graze on the free range has five times as much polyunsaturated fat.

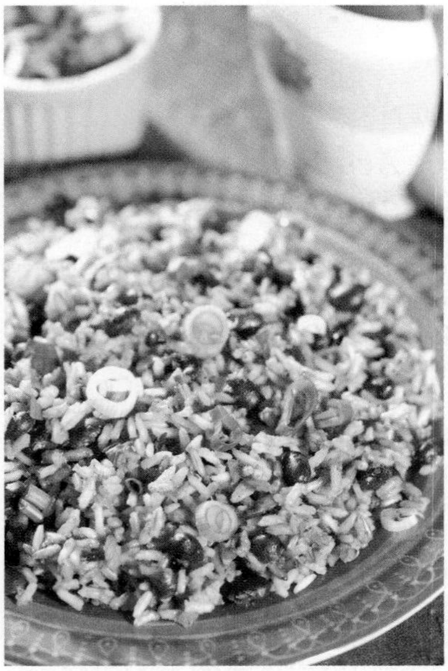

▶ **chemical scoring** A method to determine the protein quality of a food by comparing its amino acid composition with that of a reference protein. Also called *amino acid scoring*.

▶ **amino acid scoring** A method to determine the protein quality of a food by comparing its amino acid composition with that of a reference protein. Also called *chemical scoring*.

Incomplete and Complementary Proteins

With the exception of soy protein, the protein in plant foods is incomplete; that is, it lacks one or more essential amino acids and does not match the body's amino acid needs as closely as animal foods do. Although the protein in one plant food might lack certain amino acids, the protein in another plant food might be a **complementary protein** that completes the amino acid pattern. So, the protein of one plant food can provide the essential amino acid(s) that the other plant food is missing. **TABLE 6.4** lists some examples of complementary food combinations. Generally, when you combine grains with legumes, or legumes with nuts or seeds, you will get complete, high-quality protein.

For example, grain products such as pasta are low in the essential amino acid lysine but high in the essential amino acids methionine and cysteine. Legumes such as kidney beans are low in methionine and cysteine but high in lysine. In a dish that combines these foods, such as a pasta–kidney bean salad, the protein from pasta complements the protein from kidney beans so that together they provide a complete protein.

Small amounts of animal foods can also complement the protein in plant foods. For example, Asians often flavor rice with small amounts of beef, chicken, or fish, complementing the protein in the rice. Americans eat breakfast cereal with milk, which complements the protein in the cereal.

Protein complementation is important only for people who consume little to no animal proteins. For these people, eating a wide variety of plant protein sources is the key to obtaining adequate amounts of all the essential amino acids. When protein and energy intake are adequate, there is no need to plan complementary proteins at each meal.[34] In the past, it was mistakenly believed that complementary proteins needed to be eaten at the same meal for your body to use them together. Now studies show that your body can combine complementary proteins that are eaten within the same day, but not necessarily during the same meal.[35]

Boosting your intake of plant protein foods can provide additional excellent health benefits. High-protein plant foods are usually rich in vitamins, minerals, and dietary fiber. Plant foods contain no cholesterol and little fat, and they usually cost less than animal foods high in protein.

Evaluating Protein Quality and Digestibility

A high-quality protein (1) provides all the essential amino acids in the amounts the body needs, (2) provides enough other amino acids to serve as nitrogen sources for synthesis of nonessential amino acids, and (3) is easy to digest. If a food protein contains the right proportion of amino acids but cannot be digested and absorbed, it is useless to the body. We can measure protein quality in many ways, but any assessment of protein quality requires, at the least, information about the amino acid composition of the food protein. Protein quality might be assessed to plan a special diet or develop a new product such as infant formula.

Chemical, or Amino Acid, Scoring

A simple way to determine a food's protein quality is to compare its amino acid composition to that of a reference pattern of amino acids. This method is referred to as **chemical scoring** or **amino acid scoring**. The amino acid composition of the reference pattern closely reflects the amounts and proportions of amino acids that humans need. The Food and Nutrition Board has proposed an amino acid scoring pattern that uses the pattern of amino acids required by children aged 1 to 3 years.[36] If a protein meets the amino acid needs of growing preschool-aged children, then it also should meet the needs of almost all other segments of the population.

For each of the nine essential amino acids, researchers take the number of milligrams of the amino acid in one gram of food and divide it by the number of milligrams of that amino acid in the reference pattern. The result is multiplied by 100 to convert the figure to a percentage. For example, if a food contains only 65 percent of the lysine in the reference, the chemical score for the amino acid lysine is 65. The amino acid with the lowest score is the **limiting amino acid** (the amino acid present in the smallest amount relative to biological need). The chemical score of the food protein is the score of its limiting amino acid.

▶ **limiting amino acid** The amino acid in shortest supply during protein synthesis. Also the amino acid in the lowest quantity when evaluating protein quality.

> Chemical score* = mg of the essential amino acid in 1 g of test protein / mg of the essential amino acid in 1 g of reference protein
>
> * For a percentage value, multiply this result by 100.

Protein Efficiency Ratio

The **protein efficiency ratio (PER)** measures amino acid composition *and* accounts for digestibility. Researchers compare the weight gain of growing animals fed a test protein with the weight gain of growing animals fed a high-quality reference protein (e.g., casein, the main protein in cow's milk). Thus, this method measures how well the body can use the test protein, which reflects amino acid composition, digestibility, and availability. The PER is used to determine the protein quality of infant formulas.

▶ **protein efficiency ratio (PER)** Protein quality calculated by comparing the weight gain of growing animals fed a test protein with growing animals fed a high-quality reference protein. It depends on both the digestibility and the amino acid composition of a protein.

> protein efficiency ratio (PER) = weight gain in grams / protein intake in grams

Net Protein Utilization

Net protein utilization (NPU) measures how much dietary protein the body actually uses. Scientists carefully measure the nitrogen content of a test food, and then give the food to laboratory animals as their sole protein source. They then measure the animals' nitrogen excretion to determine how much of the food's nitrogen content is retained. The more nitrogen the animal retains from a food, the higher the protein quality of that food—that is, the more efficiently the animal is able to use the food protein to make body proteins.

▶ **net protein utilization (NPU)** Percentage of ingested protein nitrogen retained by the body. It measures the amount of dietary protein the body uses.

> net protein utilization (NPU) = (nitrogen retained / nitrogen intake) × 100

Biological Value

The **biological value (BV)** method determines how much of the nitrogen absorbed from a particular food protein is retained by the body for growth and/or maintenance. In general, if a protein has an essential amino acid composition similar to our needs, it will be more efficiently retained by the body.

Determining biological value is a tedious process because the key measures of urinary and fecal nitrogen output must be measured while subjects (human or animal) are consuming the test protein and again while they are on a nitrogen-free diet. The final value expresses nitrogen retention as a percentage of nitrogen absorption. Egg protein has a biological value of 100. This means that all the absorbed egg protein is retained by growing laboratory animals (100 percent). The biological value of the protein in corn is 60, meaning only 60 percent of the absorbed corn protein (and not all of it is absorbed) is retained for use by the body.

▶ **biological value (BV)** The extent to which protein in a food can be incorporated into body proteins. BV is expressed as the percentage of the absorbed dietary nitrogen retained by the body.

> biological value (BV) = (nitrogen retained / nitrogen absorbed) × 100

Protein Digestibility Corrected Amino Acid Score

The **protein digestibility corrected amino acid score (PDCAAS)** accounts for both the amino acid composition of a food and the digestibility of the protein. Egg protein provides all the amino acids that preschool children need (the reference standard) and is fully digested, so it has a PDCAAS of 1.0.

The U.S. Food and Drug Administration (FDA) recognizes the PDCAAS as the official method for determining the protein quality of most foods.[37] If the %DV for protein is listed on a food label, it must be based on the food's PDCAAS. It would be misleading to say that, for example, 8 grams of protein from tuna and 8 grams of protein from kidney beans would contribute equally to amino acid needs. Consequently, even though the number of grams of protein per serving might be the same, the %DV would be different for these two foods.

▶ **protein digestibility corrected amino acid score (PDCAAS)** A measure of protein quality that takes into account the amino acid composition of the food and the digestibility of the protein. It is calculated by multiplying the amino acid score by the percentage of the digestible food protein.

PDCAAS = chemical score × % digestibility of the protein

Key Concepts In general, animal foods provide complete protein that contains the right mix of all the essential amino acids. With the exception of soybean protein, plant foods contain incomplete protein—that is, proteins lacking one or more amino acids. Plant foods can be combined to complement each other's amino acid patterns. Researchers use many methods to determine protein quality, including chemical analysis of amino acid content and biological measures of the protein's digestibility, its retention in the body, or its ability to support growth.

Estimating Your Protein Intake

By this time, you might be wondering how much protein you consume in a typical day. To be accurate, you would need an inconvenient and expensive chemical analysis of your food intake. Instead, you can estimate your protein intake using more readily available information. First, food labels list the quantity of protein (in grams) in a serving of food. If you have a label for every food you consume, just add up the grams.

Another way to estimate your protein intake is to use the Exchange Lists. In the Exchange Lists, one starch exchange provides an average of 3 grams of protein, one milk exchange provides 8 grams, one vegetable exchange provides 2 grams, and one meat exchange provides 7 grams. Fruit and fat exchanges contribute 0 grams of protein. You also can use food composition tables or computer software to calculate your protein intake. As a reference point, if you consume the minimum number of servings recommended in MyPlate, you will get an ample amount of protein—more than enough to meet most people's protein needs.

Proteins and Amino Acids as Additives and Supplements

Proteins contribute to the structure, texture, and taste of food. They often are added to foods to enhance these properties. The milk protein casein is added to frozen dessert toppings. Gelatin is added to yogurt and fillings. **Protein hydrolysates**—proteins that have been broken down into amino acids and polypeptides—are added to many foods as thickeners, stabilizers, or flavor enhancers.

▶ **protein hydrolysates** Proteins that have been treated with acid or enzymes to break them down into amino acids and polypeptides.

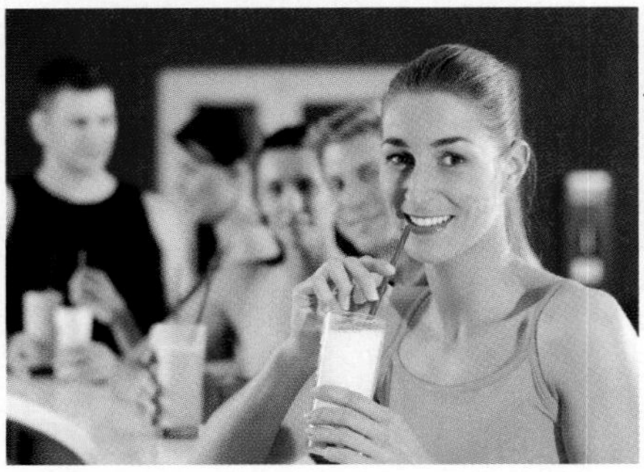

© iStockphoto/Thinkstock

Amino acids are also used as additives. Monosodium glutamate (sodium bound to the amino acid glutamic acid) is a flavor enhancer added to many foods. The artificial sweetener aspartame is a dipeptide composed of aspartic acid and phenylalanine.

Protein and amino acid supplements are sold to dieters, athletes, and people who suffer from certain diseases. An excess of a single amino acid in the digestive tract can impair absorption of other amino acids that use the same carrier for absorption, which could cause a deficiency of one or more amino acids and an unhealthy excess of the supplemented amino acid. A number of protein powders and amino acid cocktails are marketed with the claims that they enhance muscle building and exercise performance. Although anecdotal evidence for these products (from friends, website advertisements, and health food store clerks) can be convincing, only a handful of reliable scientific studies back up these claims. Remember, muscle work builds muscle strength and size, and muscles prefer carbohydrates to fuel this type of work.

THINK About It 3

Key Concepts You can use food labels to estimate your protein intake. Eating a diet that follows MyPlate will supply adequate amounts of protein. Supplements of protein or amino acids are rarely necessary and might be harmful.

Vegetarian Diets

What did Socrates, Plato, Albert Einstein, Leonardo da Vinci, William Shakespeare, Charles Darwin, and Mahatma Gandhi have in common? They all advocated a vegetarian lifestyle.[38,39] George Bernard Shaw, vegetarian, famous

TABLE 6.5
Religious Groups with Vegetarian Dietary Practices

Religious Group	Dietary Practices
Buddhism	Some sects lactovegetarian, other sects vegan
Hinduism	Generally lactovegetarian, but mutton or pork eaten occasionally
Jainism	Majority lactovegetarian, some vegan. Strict Jains will avoid root vegetables, honey, and some fruits and green vegetables.
Seventh-Day Adventists	Lacto-ovo-vegetarian emphasizing whole-grain foods; also avoid alcohol, tobacco, and caffeine

writer, and political analyst of the early 1900s, wrote, "A man fed on whiskey and dead bodies cannot do the finest work of which he is capable."[40] Meat-eaters often contend that vegetarian diets do not provide enough protein and other essential nutrients, but this is not necessarily the case. With careful planning, a diet that contains no animal products can be nutritionally complete and offer many health benefits. Just like a diet that contains animal products, a poorly planned vegetarian diet, however, can be nutritionally inadequate and pose health risks.

Why People Become Vegetarians

In some parts of the world where food is scarce, vegetarianism is not a choice but a necessity. Where food is abundant, people choose vegetarianism for various reasons. People might choose a vegetarian diet because of religious beliefs, concern for the environment, a desire to reduce world hunger and make better use of scarce resources, an aversion to eating another living creature, or concerns about cruelty to animals. Still others become vegetarians because they believe it is healthier for them. **TABLE 6.5** shows four religious groups and their vegetarian practices. Today, about 5 percent of Americans consistently follow a vegetarian diet, and between one-half to three-fourths of vegetarians are vegan, that is, they eat no animal products at all.[41] A quarter of Americans make dietary choices to limit their meat intake, and 47 percent eat at least one vegetarian meal weekly.[42]

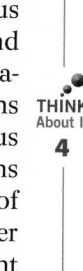

THINK About It 4

Types of Vegetarians

Although all vegetarians share the common practice of not eating meat and meat products, they differ greatly in specific dietary practices. Lacto-ovo-vegetarians use animal products such as milk, cheese, and eggs, but abstain from eating the flesh of animals. Vegans eat no animal-based foods, including food additives derived from animals or insects, and sweeteners such as honey, and may also avoid products such as cosmetics and medications made with animal-based ingredients. Fruitarians eat only raw fruit, nuts, and green foliage. Zen macrobiotic diets are mostly vegan and stress whole grains, locally grown vegetables, beans, sea vegetables, and soups. Extreme Zen macrobiotic diets can be very limited, such as a diet of primarily brown rice.

Some people eat a semi-vegetarian diet, avoiding red meats but eating small amounts of chicken or fish. The Mediterranean diet, known for reducing the risk of heart disease, is a semi-vegetarian diet rich in grains, pasta, vegetables, cheeses, and olive oil supplemented with small amounts of chicken and fish. **TABLE 6.6** lists common types of vegetarian diets and the foods typically included and excluded.

Quick Bite

Eating Lower on the Food Chain Is Good for the Planet

Eating less meat and more plant-based foods is one way to reduce your carbon footprint. Efforts to align diet with global sustainability point to vegetarian diets as an environmentally friendly way to eat. Diets that contain animal proteins require almost 3 times more water, 2.5 times more energy, 13 times more fertilizer, and almost 1.5 times more pesticides than vegetarian diets.

TABLE 6.6
Types of Vegetarian Diets

Type	Animal Foods Included	Foods Excluded
Semi-vegetarian	Dairy products, eggs, chicken, fish	Meats (beef, pork)
Pesco-vegetarian	Dairy products, eggs, and fish	Beef, pork, poultry
Lacto-ovo-vegetarian	Dairy products, eggs	Any animal flesh
Lactovegetarian	Dairy products	Any animal flesh, eggs
Fruitarian	None	All foods except raw fruits, nuts, and green foliage

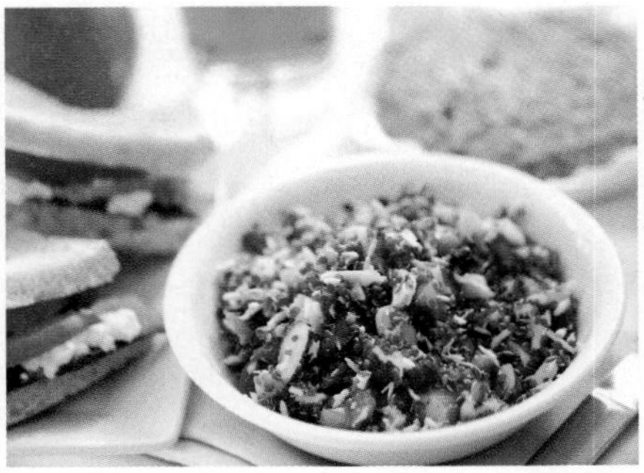
© kirin_photo/iStockphoto.com

Health Benefits of Vegetarian Diets

A carefully planned vegetarian eating pattern can be an important lifestyle behavior for good health. A vegetarian diet that is high in fiber and phytochemicals from fruits, vegetables, whole grains, legumes, nuts and seeds, and soy products, while at the same time low in processed foods and foods containing saturated fat and cholesterol, has been shown to provide tremendous benefits for prevention and treatment of chronic health conditions.[43] Vegetarian diets may contain less fat, saturated fat, and cholesterol and more magnesium and folate than nonvegetarian diets. Vegetarian diets that emphasize fresh fruits and vegetables can contain higher amounts of antioxidants such as beta-carotene and vitamins C and E, which protect the body from cell and tissue damage. Fruits and vegetables also contain dietary fiber and phytochemicals—substances that are not essential in the diet but can have important health effects.[44] Children and adolescents with vegetarian diets are more likely to be consistent with the dietary guidelines in Healthy People 2020.[45]

Vegetarians usually weigh less for their height than do nonvegetarians, partly because their diets provide less energy and partly because of other healthful lifestyle factors such as regular exercise.[46] Some studies have shown that hypertension occurs less frequently among vegetarians than among nonvegetarians, regardless of body weight or sodium intake. Intake of red meat has been linked to a higher risk of colorectal cancer. Vegetarians, including lacto-ovo and vegan, have reduced incidences of diabetes and lower rates of cancer than nonvegetarians, particularly for gastrointestinal cancer.[47,48]

Vegetarian-style diet patterns are associated with lower all-cause mortality.[49] Vegetarian-style eating patterns are being used for the prevention and therapeutic dietary treatment of numerous chronic conditions, including overweight and obesity, cardiovascular disease (hyperlipidemia, ischemic heart disease, and hypertension), diabetes, cancer, and osteoporosis.[50]

Health Risks of Vegetarian Diets

Simply eliminating animal products does not automatically lead to all the health perks of a vegetarian diet. Omitting foods from the diet actually comes with its own health risks. Although vegetarian diets offer many health benefits, certain types of vegetarian diets pose some unique nutritional risks. A vegetarian who simply avoids animal foods or includes lots of processed meat-free products while not eating a variety of whole foods, fruits, vegetables, and whole grains may miss out on essential nutrients and therefore may actually compromise their health. The more limited the vegetarian diet, the more likely are nutritional problems. Some individuals who adopt a vegetarian diet may have unhealthy or disordered eating patterns and eliminate animal foods as a method of weight management that can precede an eating disorder.

Poorly planned vegetarian diets can be low in many nutrients, particularly iron, zinc, calcium, vitamin D, vitamin B_{12}, and omega-3 fatty acids. The best sources of these nutrients are animal foods—red meat for iron and zinc, milk for calcium and vitamin D, and any animal foods for B_{12}. Because plant foods contain a form of iron called nonheme iron that is not as well absorbed as the heme iron in animal foods, vegetarians need to include more iron in their diets. Vitamin C and other compounds in fruits and vegetables aid iron absorption in the body. Protein consumed from a variety of plant foods can supply enough essential amino acids to meet the needs of vegetarians and vegans. Supplemental and fortified foods are useful to supply missing nutrients and help ensure nutritional adequacy.

Although vegetarian diets can be adequate for most people, they must be planned carefully for periods of rapid growth, such as for infants and young children, and for women who are pregnant or breastfeeding and the elderly.

Dietary Recommendations for Vegetarians

The *Dietary Guidelines for Americans, 2015–2020* and MyPlate dietary guidance include recommendations and a food guide for use in planning vegetarian diets.[51] Vegetarians who include milk, milk products, and eggs in their diet can easily meet their nutritional needs for protein and other essential nutrients, but like meat eaters, must take care to choose low-fat milk products and limit eggs to avoid excess saturated fat and cholesterol. **TABLE 6.7** lists some suggestions for vegetarians.

Because grains, vegetables, and legumes (soybeans, dried beans, and peas) all provide protein, vegans who eat a variety of foods also can meet their protein needs easily. Although most plant foods do not contain complete protein, eating complementary plant protein sources during the same day adequately meets the body's needs for protein production.

Vegans who avoid all animal products must supplement their diets with a reliable source of vitamin B_{12}, such as fortified soy milk. Although bacteria in some fermented foods and in the knobby growths of some seaweeds produce vitamin B_{12}, most vegans do not eat enough seaweeds and fermented foods to meet their vitamin B_{12} needs. Vegans also need a dietary source of vitamin D when sun exposure is limited. Additional suggestions for following a vegetarian diet, including healthy eating tips for vegetarians, can be found on the ChooseMyPlate.gov website.

Key Concepts Vegetarian diets eliminate animal products to various degrees. Vegetarian diets tend to be low in fat and high in fiber and phytochemicals, which might help reduce chronic disease risks. Careful diet planning is necessary for vegans and growing children to ensure that all nutrient needs are met.

TABLE 6.7
Nutritional Guidelines for Vegetarians

1. Choose a variety of foods, including whole grains, vegetables, fruits, legumes, nuts, seeds, and, if desired, dairy products and eggs.
2. Choose whole, unrefined foods often and minimize intake of processed, highly sweetened, fatty, and heavily refined foods.
3. Choose a variety of fruits and vegetables.
4. If animal foods such as dairy products and eggs are used, choose lower-fat dairy products and use both eggs and dairy products in moderation.
5. Include a regular source of vitamin B_{12} and, if sun exposure is limited, of vitamin D.

Position of the Academy of Nutrition and Dietetics: Vegetarian Diets, *J Am Diet Assoc.* 2009;109(7):1266–1282.

Position Statement: Academy of Nutrition and Dietetics

Vegetarian Diets

It is the position of the American Dietetic Association that appropriately planned vegetarian diets, including total vegetarian or vegan diets, are healthful, nutritionally adequate, and may provide health benefits in the prevention and treatment of certain diseases. Well-planned vegetarian diets are appropriate for individuals during all stages of the life cycle, including pregnancy, lactation, infancy, childhood, and adolescence, and for athletes. A vegetarian diet is defined as one that does not include meat (including fowl) or seafood, or products containing those foods. This article reviews the current data related to key nutrients for vegetarians including protein, n_3 fatty acids, iron, zinc, iodine, calcium, and vitamins D and B_{12}. A vegetarian diet can meet current recommendations for all of these nutrients. In some cases, supplements or fortified foods can provide useful amounts of important nutrients. An evidence-based review showed that vegetarian diets can be nutritionally adequate in pregnancy and result in positive maternal and infant health outcomes. The results of an evidence-based review showed that a vegetarian diet is associated with a lower risk of death from ischemic heart disease. Vegetarians also appear to have lower low-density lipoprotein cholesterol levels, lower blood pressure, and lower rates of hypertension and type 2 diabetes than nonvegetarians. Furthermore, vegetarians tend to have a lower body mass index and lower overall cancer rates. Features of a vegetarian diet that may reduce risk of chronic disease include lower intakes of saturated fat and cholesterol and higher intakes of fruits, vegetables, whole grains, nuts, soy products, fiber, and phytochemicals. The variability of dietary practices among vegetarians makes individual assessment of dietary adequacy essential. In addition to assessing dietary adequacy, food and nutrition professionals can also play key roles in educating vegetarians about sources of specific nutrients, food purchase and preparation, and dietary modifications to meet their needs.

Reproduced from Position of the Academy of Nutrition and Dietetics: vegetarian diets. *J Acad Nutr Diet.* 2015;115:801–810.

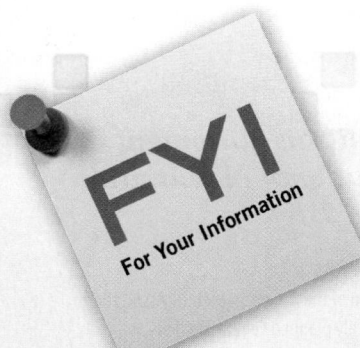

FYI For Your Information

High-Protein Plant Foods

Of the top 10 sources of protein in the American diet, only two sources—yeast breads and pasta—are plant-based (see Table 6.3). Lentils, a dense source of plant protein, don't even make the list. Yet look at the comparison between the nutritional profile of lentils and the profile of beef in **Table A**.

When we consider these two foods in light of the recommendations to reduce fat, saturated fat, and cholesterol while increasing fiber, it's no contest, the lentils win hands down! With all that lentils have going for them, you'd think more Americans would be eating them. Yet dried beans, peas, and lentils combined contribute less than 1 percent of the daily protein intake of Americans, whereas beef contributes 17.7 percent.

TABLE A
How Do Lentils Stack Up Against Beef?

	Cooked Lentils	Lean, Broiled Sirloin
Amount	1 cup	3 ounces
Energy	230 kcal	145 kcal
Protein	18 grams	24 grams
Fat	< 1 gram	5 grams
Cholesterol	0	73 milligrams
Carbohydrate	40 grams	0
Dietary Fiber	16 grams	0
Percent Calories from Fat	3%	31%

Data from U.S. Department of Agriculture, Agricultural Research Service, Nutrient Data Laboratory. USDA National Nutrient Database for Standard Reference, Release 28. September 2015. http://www.ars.usda.gov/nea/bhnrc/ndl. Accessed December 30, 2015.

High-protein plant foods also contribute complex carbohydrates, dietary fiber, and vitamins and minerals to the diet. Because these plant foods contain little fat, they are nutrient dense; that is, they provide a high amount of protein and nutrients relative to their energy contribution.

Sources of Plant Protein

Grains and grain products, legumes (lentils and dried beans and peas such as kidney beans or chickpeas), starchy vegetables, and nuts and seeds all provide protein (see **Table B**). A serving of a grain product or starchy vegetable provides an average of about 5 grams of protein, a serving of legumes provides 10 to 20 grams of protein, and a serving of vegetables provides about 3 grams of protein. Although a serving of these foods contains less protein than a serving of meat, you can eat more plant protein foods for fewer calories.

Complementing Plant Proteins

It's important to remember that plant proteins lack one or more of the essential amino acids needed to build body proteins, so individual plant proteins need to complement each other. A simple rule to remember in complementing plant proteins is that combining grains and legumes or combining legumes and nuts or seeds provides complete, high-quality protein.

Soy Protein

The protein in soybeans is a notable exception to the rule that most plant proteins are incomplete. Soy provides complete, high-quality protein comparable to that in animal foods. In addition, soybeans provide no saturated fat or cholesterol, and are rich in isoflavonoids—phytochemicals that help reduce risk of heart disease and cancer and improve bone health.

TABLE B
Plant Sources of Protein

Plant Protein Source	Grams of Protein	Kilocalories
Grain Products		
1 oat bran bagel (3-inch)	7	176
1 whole English muffin, whole-wheat	6	134
1 large flour tortilla (8-inch)	4	146
1 cup cooked spaghetti	8	221
1 cup cooked brown rice	5	216
1 cup cooked oatmeal	6	166
2 slices whole wheat bread	7	138
½ cup low-fat granola	4	191
Starchy Vegetables		
1 cup cooked corn	5	152
1 cup baked winter squash	2	76
1 medium baked potato with skin	4	161
Legumes		
½ cup tofu	8	92
1 cup cooked lentils	18	230
1 cup cooked kidney beans	15	225
Vegetables		
1 cup cooked broccoli	4	55
1 cup cooked cauliflower	2	29
1 cup cooked Brussels sprouts	4	56
Nuts and Seeds		
2 tablespoons peanut butter	8	188
¼ cup peanuts	9	207
¼ cup sunflower seeds	7	204

Data from U.S. Department of Agriculture, Agricultural Research Service, Nutrient Data Laboratory. USDA National Nutrient Database for Standard Reference, Release 28. September 2015. http://www.ars.usda.gov/nea/bhnrc/ndl. Accessed December 30, 2015.

Isoflavonoids act as antioxidants, protecting cells and tissues from damage. One specific isoflavonoid, genistein, inhibits growth of both breast and prostate cancer cells in the laboratory. Isoflavonoids protect LDL cholesterol (the kind of cholesterol associated with greater risk of heart disease) from oxidation. Oxidized LDL cholesterol contributes to the plaque buildup in

TABLE C
Soy Food Products and Uses

Food	Description
Tofu	Solid cake of curdled soy milk similar to soft cheese. Tofu comes in hard and soft varieties. It absorbs the flavors of the foods it is mixed with. Soft tofu can be substituted for cheese in pasta dishes, stuffed in large shell pasta, blended with fruit, or used to make pie filling. Hard tofu can be used in salads and shish-kabobs, and in place of meat in stir-fry or mixed dishes.
Tempeh	A flat cake made from fermented soybeans. It has a mild flavor and chewy texture. Tempeh can be grilled, included in sandwiches, or combined in casseroles.
Meat analogues	Meat alternatives made primarily of soy protein. Flavored and textured to resemble chicken, beef, and pork, they can be substituted for meat in mixed dishes, pizza, tacos, or sloppy joes.
Soy milk	The liquid of the soybean. It comes in regular and low-fat versions and in different flavors. Soy milk can be used plain or substituted for regular milk on cereals or in hot cocoa, puddings, or desserts.
Soy flour	Made from roasted soybeans ground into flour. Soy flour can replace up to one-quarter of the regular flour in a recipe.

arteries. The isoflavones in soybeans also act as phytoestrogens, helping to protect older women from cardiovascular disease and osteoporosis. Soy foods that contain most or all of the bean, such as soy milk, sprouts, flour, and tofu, are the best sources of these phytochemicals.

It is easy to incorporate a variety of soy foods into your diet. Tofu, tempeh, ground soy, soy milk, soy flour, and textured soy protein are soy-based products that can be included in many meals and snacks (see **Table C**).

The nutritional benefits of plant protein sources such as soy foods and other legumes, grains, and vegetables deserve a closer look. Most Americans would benefit from emphasizing plant protein foods in their diet. The next time you plan to make meatloaf, try making a lentil loaf instead.

The Health Effects of Too Little or Too Much Protein

Because protein plays such a vital role in so many body processes, protein deficiency can wreak havoc in numerous body systems. A lack of available protein means insufficient amounts of essential amino acids, which stops the synthesis of body proteins.

Protein deficiency occurs when energy and/or protein intake is inadequate. Adequate energy intake spares dietary and body proteins so they can be used for protein synthesis. Without adequate energy intake, the body burns dietary protein for energy rather than using it to make body proteins. Protein deficiency can occur even in people who eat seemingly adequate amounts of protein if the protein they eat is of poor quality or cannot be absorbed.

Although protein deficiency is widespread in poverty-stricken communities and in some nonindustrialized countries, most people in industrialized countries face the opposite problem—protein excess. The RDA for a 70-kilogram (154-pound) person is 56 grams; however, the average American man consumes approximately 100 grams of protein daily, and the average woman about 70 grams. Many meat-loving Americans eat far more protein.

Some research suggests that high protein intake contributes to risk for heart disease, cancer, and osteoporosis. However, because high protein intake often goes hand-in-hand with high intakes of saturated fat and cholesterol, the independent effects of high protein intake are difficult to determine.

Protein-Energy Malnutrition

Hunger and malnutrition are problems worldwide. In the United States, millions of families and individuals with food insecurity worry about where their food will come from and struggle to meet their basic nutritional needs. Worldwide, malnutrition is a debilitating and widespread problem that leaves individuals vulnerable to disease and death. A deficiency of protein, energy, or both in the diet is called **protein-energy malnutrition (PEM)**. Protein and energy intake are difficult to separate because diets adequate in energy usually are adequate in protein, and diets inadequate in energy inhibit the body's use of dietary protein for protein synthesis.

▶ **protein-energy malnutrition (PEM)** A condition resulting from long-term inadequate intakes of energy and protein that can lead to wasting of body tissues and increased susceptibility to infection.

FYI For Your Information

High-Protein Diets and Supplements

One trend commonly found in sports nutrition is the use of protein and amino acid supplements to build muscle. The theory is straightforward: because muscle mass is predominantly protein, eating more dietary protein must lead to building bigger muscles. In the 1990s, high-protein diets also became popular, not just for athletes, but also for those wanting to lose weight. Diets that contained very little fat and carbohydrate, with large percentages of calories coming from unscientifically recommended high amounts of dietary protein, were seen as the key to weight loss and peak athletic performance. Do you need more protein to lose weight or gain a competitive edge? Let's take a look at the evidence.

Browse through the weight-loss section of any major bookstore, and you will find books such as *Dr. Atkins' New Diet Revolution*, *The South Beach Diet*, *Sugar Busters*, and *Enter the Zone*. All of these books promote various high-protein diets for weight loss. These diets revisit the idea, popular in the 1970s (and with historical roots dating back nearly 200 years), that carbohydrates (starches and sugars) make us fat. Proponents of high-protein diets point to the fact that throughout the high-carb, low-fat 1980s and early 1990s and with the explosion of fat-free foods, Americans got fatter. They fail to note that although the percentage of calories from fat in U.S. diets has decreased, Americans are eating more total fat and total calories (and therefore more total grams of fat) and exercising less—a recipe for weight gain.

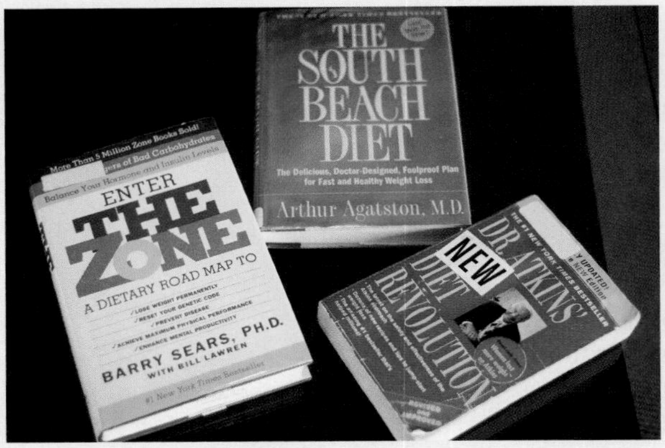

Do High-Protein, Low-Carbohydrate Diets Work?

The Atkins diet made headlines in November 2002 when researchers from Duke University presented results of a study comparing the Atkins diet to the American Heart Association's (AHA) low-fat diet at the AHA's annual scientific meeting. However, skeptics argued that the study, funded by the Atkins Center for Complementary Medicine, included too few people and failed to monitor participants' actual food intake and exercise levels. Since this report, several studies of low-carbohydrate diets have been published, some of which were funded by government sources. An early review of published studies concluded that participant weight loss on low-carbohydrate diets was mainly associated with decreased calorie intake rather than reduced carbohydrate content.[a] A study that compared four different types of popular weight-loss diets also confirmed that overall weight loss at one year was similar, regardless of diet.[b] More recently, a systematic review of high-protein versus low-protein diets on health outcomes found that higher-protein diets may improve risk factors for heart disease and diabetes, but the effects were minimal and potential for harm should be considered.[c] So, what explains reports of dramatic weight loss and no hunger while eating pork rinds, bacon, sausage, and steak? In the short term, removing carbohydrates from the diet causes the body to deplete glycogen stores, which results in a rapid loss of water. The ketosis that results from low carbohydrate intake can also enhance fluid loss. High protein intake tends to be satiating, and the monotony of the diet also blunts the appetite. However, findings seem to all point to one key feature: reducing calories for weight loss.

Are High-Protein, Low-Carbohydrate Diets Safe?

In a review of research on low-carbohydrate diets, insufficient evidence was found to recommend for or against this approach to weight loss.[d] Health concerns include accumulation of ketone bodies, abnormal insulin metabolism, impaired liver and kidney function, salt and water depletion, impaired renal function, and hyperlipidemia resulting from high fat intake. It is likely, though, that people who start a low-carbohydrate diet do not stay on it long enough to develop serious complications, although constipation, nausea, weakness, dehydration, and fatigue are common side effects.

If there were one best diet, we wouldn't have so many diet plans vying for our attention and money! What we know about our nutrient needs still points to the *Dietary Guidelines for Americans* for guidance: The best diet emphasizes fruits, vegetables, and whole grains with moderate amounts of lean protein. It can be difficult for individuals to follow a particular diet, especially those diets that are most restrictive. The most successful diet is the one a person can stick with.[e] For a diet to produce meaningful weight loss, the priority should be on reducing calories, not proportions of protein, carbohydrate, or fat.[f] Successful weight management requires permanent changes to eating habits and, more importantly, increased physical activity.

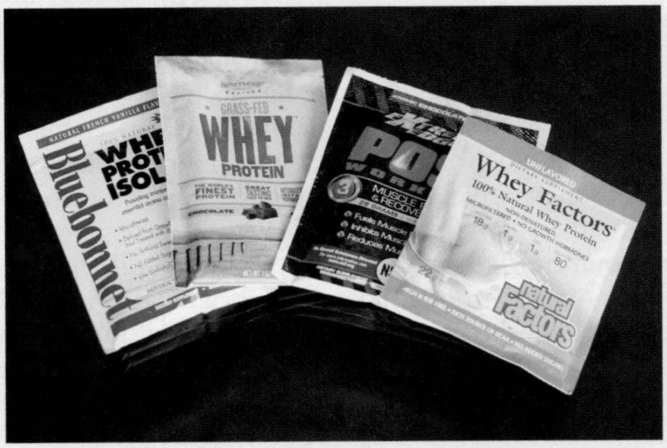

[a] Bravata DM, Sanders L, Huang J, et al. Efficacy and safety of low-carbohydrate diets: a systematic review. *JAMA*. 2003;289(14):1837–1850.

[b] Dansinger ML, Gleason JA, Griffith JL, et al. Comparison of the Atkins, Ornish, Weight Watchers, and Zone diets for weight loss and heart disease risk reduction: a randomized trial. *JAMA*. 2005;293:43–53.

[c] Santesso N, Akl EA, Bianchi M, et al. Effects of higher- versus lower-protein diets on health outcomes: a systematic review and meta-analysis. *Eur J Clin Nutr*. 2012;66(7):780–788.

[d] Levine MJ, Jones JM, Lineback DR. Low-carbohydrate diets: assessing the science and knowledge gaps, summary of an ILSI North America workshop. *J Am Diet Assoc*. 2006;106:2086–2094.

[e] Makris A, Foster GD. Dietary approaches to the treatment of obesity. *Psychiatr Clin North Am*. 2011;34(4):813–827.

[f] Sacks FM, Bray GA, Carey VJ, et al. Comparison of weight-loss diets with different compositions of fat, protein, and carbohydrates. *N Engl J Med*. 2009;360(9):859–873.

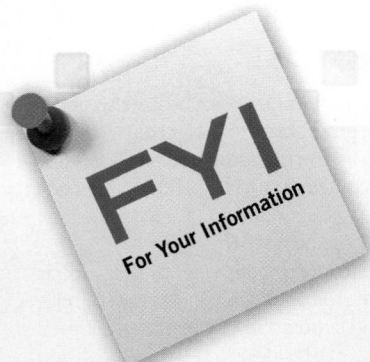

Although it can occur at all stages of life, PEM is most common during childhood, when protein is needed to support rapid growth. Childhood malnutrition is prevalent around the world and contributes to one-third of all deaths worldwide.[52] PEM symptoms can be mild or severe and exist in either acute or chronic forms.

Protein-energy malnutrition occurs in all parts of the world but is most common in Africa, South and Central America, East and Southeast Asia, and the Middle East. In industrialized countries, PEM occurs most often in populations living in poverty, in older adults, and in hospitalized patients with other conditions such as anorexia nervosa, AIDS, cancer, or malabsorption syndromes.[53]

There are two forms of severe PEM: **kwashiorkor** and **marasmus**. Severe protein deficiency is called kwashiorkor, whereas severe calorie and protein deficiency is called marasmus. In general, marasmus is an insufficient energy intake that does not meet the body's requirements. As a result, the body draws on its own stores, resulting in emaciation. In kwashiorkor, adequate carbohydrate consumption and decreased protein intake lead to decreased synthesis of visceral proteins, resulting in fluid accumulation and the appearance of a bloated or enlarged abdomen. See **FIGURE 6.20** for the signs and symptoms of kwashiorkor and marasmus.

▶ **kwashiorkor** A type of malnutrition that occurs primarily in young children who have an infectious disease and whose diets supply marginal amounts of energy and very little protein. Common symptoms include poor growth, edema, apathy, weakness, and susceptibility to infections.

▶ **marasmus** A type of malnutrition resulting from chronic inadequate consumption of protein and energy that is characterized by wasting of muscle, fat, and other body tissue.

Kwashiorkor

The term *kwashiorkor* is a Ghanaian word that describes the "illness of the first child when the second child is born." In many cultures, babies are breastfed until the next baby comes along. When the new baby arrives, the first baby is weaned from nutritious breast milk and placed on a watered-down version of the family's diet. In areas of poverty, this diet often is low in protein, or the consumed protein is not digested and absorbed easily.

One symptom of kwashiorkor that sets it apart from marasmus is edema, or swelling of body tissue, usually in the feet and legs. Lack of blood proteins reduces the force that keeps fluid in the bloodstream, allowing fluid to leak out into the tissues. Because proteins are unavailable to transport fat, it accumulates in the liver. Combined with edema, this accumulation produces a bloated belly. Other features of kwashiorkor include stunted weight and height; increased susceptibility to infection; dry, flaky skin, and sometimes skin sores; dry, brittle, and unnaturally blond hair; and changes in skin color. Because the energy deficit is usually not as severe (or as longstanding) in kwashiorkor as in marasmus, people with kwashiorkor may still have some body fat stores left.

Quick Bite

The Source of Salisbury Steak

Dr. James Salisbury, a London physician who lived in the late 1800s, believed humans to be two-thirds carnivorous and one-third herbivorous. He recommended a diet low in starch and high in lean meat, with lots of hot water to rinse out the products of fermentation. His diet regimen included broiled, lean, minced beef three times a day. Although we call it Salisbury steak as a courtesy to Dr. Salisbury's heritage, minced beef patties are really more like hamburgers.

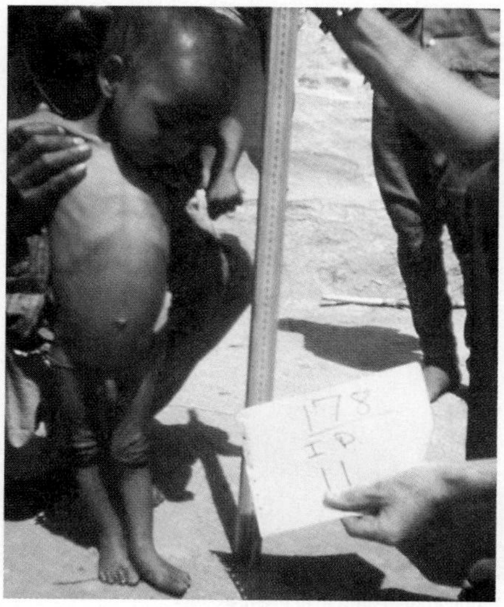

Courtesy of CDC/Dr. Lyle Conrad.

(A)

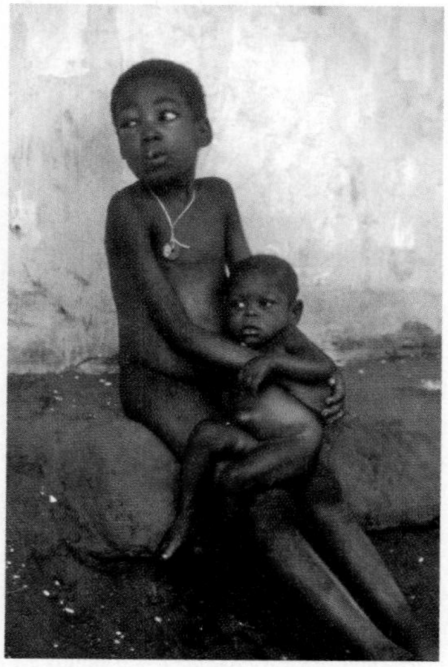

Courtesy of CDC/Dr. Edward Brink.

(B)

FIGURE 6.20 Kwashiorkor and marasmus. (A) Edema in the feet and legs and a bloated belly are symptoms of kwashiorkor. (B) Children with marasmus are short and thin for their age and can appear frail and wrinkled.

Kwashiorkor usually develops in children between 18 and 24 months of age, about the time weaning occurs. Its onset can be rapid and is often triggered by an infection or illness that increases the child's protein needs. In hospital settings, kwashiorkor can develop in situations where protein needs are extremely high (e.g., trauma, infection, burns), but dietary intake is poor. Kwashiorkor is associated with extreme poverty in developing countries and except for people with chronic illness, is rarely seen in affluent countries.

Marasmus

Marasmus is derived from the Greek word *marasmos*, which means "withering" or "to waste away." The condition develops more slowly than kwashiorkor and results from chronic PEM. Protein, energy, and nutrient intake are all grossly inadequate, depleting body fat reserves and severely wasting muscle tissue, including vital organs such as the heart. Growth slows or stops, and children are both short and very thin for their age. Metabolism slows and body temperature drops as the body tries to conserve energy. Children with marasmus are apathetic, often not even crying in an effort to conserve energy. Their hair is sparse and falls out easily. Because muscle and fat are used up, a child with marasmus often looks like a frail, wrinkled, elderly person.

Marasmus occurs most often in infants and children aged 6 to 18 months who are fed diluted or improperly mixed formulas. Because this is a time of rapid brain growth, marasmus can permanently stunt brain development and lead to learning disabilities. Marasmus also occurs in adults during cancer and starvation, including the self-imposed starvation of the eating disorder known as anorexia nervosa.

Excess Dietary Protein

In industrialized countries, an excess of protein and energy is more common than a deficiency. Generally, self-selected diets do not contain more than 40 percent of calories from protein.[54] Although high protein intake has been suggested to contribute to kidney problems, osteoporosis, heart disease, and cancer (see **FIGURE 6.21**), the Food and Nutrition Board did

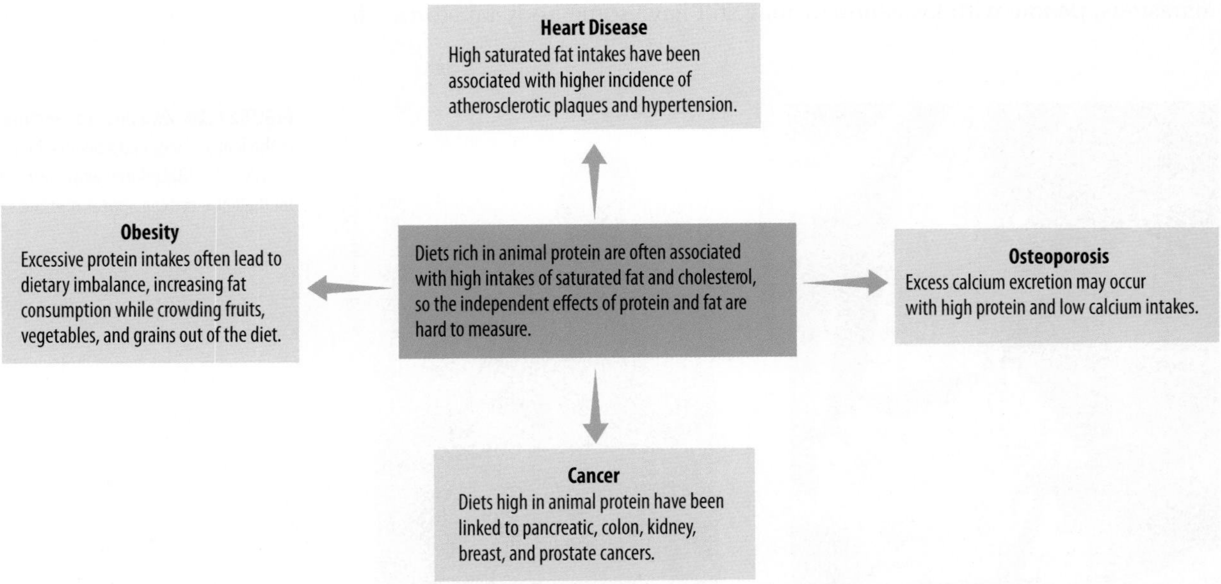

Heart Disease
High saturated fat intakes have been associated with higher incidence of atherosclerotic plaques and hypertension.
Obesity
Excessive protein intakes often lead to dietary imbalance, increasing fat consumption while crowding fruits, vegetables, and grains out of the diet.
Diets rich in animal protein are often associated with high intakes of saturated fat and cholesterol, so the independent effects of protein and fat are hard to measure.
Osteoporosis
Excess calcium excretion may occur with high protein and low calcium intakes.
Cancer
Diets high in animal protein have been linked to pancreatic, colon, kidney, breast, and prostate cancers.

FIGURE 6.21 Excess animal protein. In developed countries, excess protein and energy are a greater problem than protein deficiency.

not find the evidence supporting these links to be strong enough to set a UL for protein.[55]

Kidney Function

Because the kidneys must excrete the products of protein breakdown, there is concern that a high protein intake can strain kidney function and is especially harmful for people with kidney disease or diabetes. A diet with a higher proportion of calories coming from protein increases kidney filtration rate in healthy adults, suggesting that a high-protein diet may have long-term adverse consequence on kidney function.[56]

To prevent dehydration, it is important to drink plenty of fluids to dilute the by-products of protein breakdown for excretion. Human infants should not be fed unmodified cow's milk until they are at least 1 year old because the high protein concentration in cow's milk combined with an immature kidney system can cause excessive fluid losses and dehydration. (See the Nutrition Science in Action "High-Protein Diets and Kidney Function.")

Mineral Losses

The link between high-protein diets and osteoporosis is based on studies showing that a high protein intake increases calcium excretion, which could then contribute to bone mineral losses. However, these studies generally used purified proteins rather than food proteins. Studies of healthy postmenopausal women with an increase in dietary protein from 10 to 20 percent of energy slightly improved calcium absorption compared to a low-calcium diet, nearly compensating for the slight increase in urinary calcium excretion.[57] Other studies have found favorable effects on bone mineral density from increasing intake of protein in the presence of adequate dietary calcium and acid-neutralizing fruits and vegetables.[58]

Obesity

Some epidemiologic studies have shown a correlation between high protein intake and body fatness.[59] High-protein foods often are high in fat. A diet high in fat and protein can provide too much energy, contributing to obesity. Large amounts of high-protein foods displace fruits, vegetables, and grains—foods that contain fewer calories. Researchers have suggested that high dietary protein intake alters hormones and the body's response to hormones, including leptin, which regulates feeding centers in the brain to reduce food intake.[60] Some studies suggest that because of this effect on hormones, a high protein intake early in life increases the risk of obesity later in life.[61]

Heart Disease

Research has linked high intake of animal protein, especially processed meats, to high blood cholesterol levels and increased risk of heart disease, stroke, cancer, and diabetes.[62–65] Foods high in animal protein are also high in saturated fat and cholesterol. Whether protein alone—independent of fat—plays a role in the development of heart disease is less clear. Soy protein foods contain no saturated fat or cholesterol, and the FDA approved a health claim saying that soy protein is beneficial in reducing the risk of heart disease. Some epidemiologic studies, however, found that consuming soy protein has little or no effect on the risk factors for heart disease.[66] The researchers suggest that consuming soy protein products, such as tofu, soy butter, soy nuts, and some soy burgers, should be beneficial because of their low saturated fat content and high content of polyunsaturated fats, fiber, vitamins, and minerals. Using these and other soy foods to replace foods high in animal protein can reduce intake of saturated fat and cholesterol.[67] Choosing less red meat and

American Heart Association

High-Protein Diets

The American Heart Association doesn't recommend high-protein diets for weight loss. Some of these diets restrict healthful foods that provide essential nutrients and don't provide the variety of foods needed to adequately meet nutritional needs. People who stay on these diets very long might not get enough vitamins and minerals and face other potential health risks.

Quick Bite

Protein Makes for Springy Bugs

Resilin is an elastic rubberlike protein in insects, scorpions, and crustaceans. The springiness in the wing hinges of some insects, such as locusts and dragonflies, comes from the unique mechanical properties of resilin. The protein also is found in the stingers of bees and ants, the eardrums and sound organs of cicadas, and the little rubber balls in the hips of jumping fleas. The structural properties of resilin are similar to those of true rubber, which makes it very unusual among structural proteins.

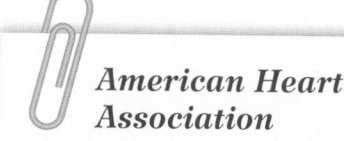

processed meat, in particular, could have beneficial effects towards reducing risk of type 2 diabetes and cardiovascular disease.[68]

Cancer

Some studies suggest a link between a diet high in animal protein foods and an increased risk for certain types of cancers, with a strong link between animal protein and colon cancer.[69] Prolonged high intake of both red meat (beef, pork) and processed meat (ham, smoked meats, sausage, bacon) has been associated with increased colon cancer risk and cancer mortality.[70,71]

Gout

▶ **gout** An intensely painful form of inflammatory arthritis that results from deposits of needlelike crystals of uric acid in connective tissue and/or the joint space between bones.

Gout is an immensely painful inflammatory arthritis caused by the accumulation of uric acid crystals in joints. Uric acid forms from the breakdown of nitrogen-containing compounds called purines. Uric acid normally dissolves in the blood and passes through the kidneys into the urine. In people with gout, uric acid builds up and forms sharp crystals that can collect around the joints, causing swelling and intense pain. Diets high in meats (especially red meats) and seafood and low in dairy products significantly increase the risk of gout—the most common form of inflammatory arthritis in men.[72] Total protein intake, however, is not correlated with an increased risk of gout.

Key Concepts Protein-energy malnutrition (PEM) is a common form of malnutrition in the developing world, with potentially devastating effects for children. PEM can manifest in two forms: kwashiorkor and marasmus. Among other symptoms, kwashiorkor is distinguished by edema, or swelling of the tissues. Marasmus results from chronic PEM and is distinguished by severe wasting of body fat and muscles. Excess dietary protein can contribute to obesity, heart disease, and certain forms of cancer. These links, however, might be attributable to the high fat intake that often accompanies high protein intake.

Nutrition Science *in Action*

High-Protein Diets and Kidney Function

Background

Little is known about the effect of low-carbohydrate, high-protein diets (such as the Atkins diet) on kidney function, especially in obese adults. Potential adverse effects of following such diets on kidney function include prolonged elevation in glomerular filtration rate (GFR), increased proteinuria, and derangements in electrolyte, acid–base, and bone mineral status. This is of particular concern in the obese population because obese persons are at risk for kidney failure and kidney-related abnormalities.

Hypothesis

In obese adults, following a low-carbohydrate, high-protein diet will be associated with greater adverse renal effects than following a low-fat weight-loss diet.

Experimental Plan

Three hundred and seven obese adults (BMI of 30–40 kg/m^2) ages 18–65 years and who weighed less than 136 kilograms (299 pounds) were recruited. Participants did not have serious medical illness, take lipid-lowering medications, have a blood pressure of greater than or equal to 140/90 mm Hg, were not pregnant or lactating, or were not taking medications that affect body weight. Participants were randomly assigned to either a low-carbohydrate, high-protein diet or a low-fat weight-loss diet for 24 months. Participants were provided with behavioral treatment weekly for 20 weeks, every other week for 20 weeks, and then every month for the remainder of the 2-year study period. Body weight and indicators of kidney function were measured throughout the study.

Results

The low-carbohydrate, high-protein diet was associated with small changes in measures of kidney function throughout the study as compared with the low-fat weight-loss diet. There was a minor reduction in serum creatinine and cystatin at 3 months and relative increases in creatinine clearance at 3 and 12 months; serum urea at 3, 12, and 24 months; and 24-hour urinary volume at 12 and 24 months. Urinary calcium excretion increased at 3 and 12 months without changes in bone mineral density or clinical diagnosis of new kidney stones.

Conclusion and Discussion

In obese individuals without preexisting kidney disease, following a low-carbohydrate, high-protein diet over a 2-year period is not associated with renal harm or significant changes in fluid and electrolyte balance as compared to a low-fat diet. Additional studies are needed to examine the longer-term effect of this diet on obese individuals with underlying chronic kidney disease, diabetes, and hypertension as well as those at risk for kidney stones.

Data from Friedman AN, Ogden LG, Foster GD, et al. Comparative effects of low-carbohydrate high-protein versus low-fat diets on the kidney. *Clin J Am Soc Nephrol.* 2012;7:1103–1111.

Label to Table

Have you ever visited a health food store and noticed all the protein powders, amino acid supplements, and high-protein bars? Do you believe claims like "protein boosts your energy level" or "amino acid *X* helps you build muscle" or "protein shakes are the best preworkout fuel"? You know from this chapter that protein is an important nutrient and that it's used to build and repair tissue. But do you need one of these supplements? Before reaching into your wallet, check out the Nutrition Facts of this protein powder and determine whether it's a good buy.

Take a look at this label and note how far down protein is on the list of nutrients. This deemphasized placement of protein was intentional to try to get consumers to deemphasize protein in their diets. You might recall that most Americans eat more protein than they need, and because much of that protein comes from animal foods, they are often getting excess saturated fat. Although there is a DV for protein (50 grams), manufacturers must first determine a food protein's quality before they can determine %DV. Manufacturers are not required to give the %DV for protein on food labels.

Do protein and amino acid supplements do what they claim to do? In terms of building muscle, exercise physiologists agree that it takes consistent muscle work (i.e., weight lifting) and a healthy diet that meets the body's calorie needs. Muscle building does not depend on extra protein. In fact, muscles use carbohydrate and fat for fuel, not protein, so these other nutrients are more important for effective workouts.

In terms of protein's ability to boost your energy level, recall that anything with calories (carbohydrates, proteins, and fats) provides the body with "energy." In fact, unlike carbohydrates and fats, only a small amount of protein is used for energy expenditure. Research shows that the best thing to eat prior to a workout is carbohydrate, not protein, because carbohydrate provides glucose for the muscle cells. Review this label again. What percentage of this protein powder's calories is from protein?

kcal 154

Protein = 11 grams × 4 kcal per gram

= 44 protein kcal

44 ÷ 154 = 0.28 or 28% protein kcal

Surprise, surprise! Only one-quarter of the powder's calories are protein anyway, so it's okay as a preworkout fuel not because of its protein content but because of its ample carbohydrate!

Nutrition Facts

18 servings per container

Serving size	**2 scoops**
Amount per serving	
Calories	**150**
	% Daily Value*
Total Fat 4g	**6%**
Saturated Fat 2.5g	**12%**
Trans Fat 0g	
Cholesterol 20mg	**7%**
Sodium 170mg	**7%**
Total Carbohydrate 17g	**6%**
Dietary Fiber 0g	**0%**
Total Sugars 14g	
Includes 10g Added Sugars	**20%**
Protein 11g	
Vitamin D 0mg	0%
Calcium 400mg	40%
Iron 0mg	0%
Potassium 185mg	5%

* The % Daily Value (DV) tells you how much a nutrient in a serving of food contributes to a daily diet. 2,000 calories a day is used for general nutrition advice.

Learning Portfolio

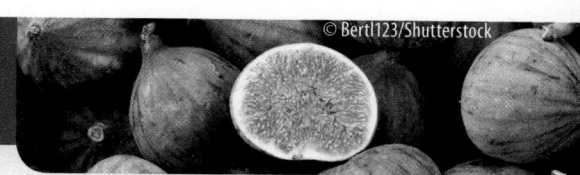
© Bertl123/Shutterstock

Key Terms

acidosis	225
alkalosis	225
amino acid pool	231
amino acid scoring	238
antibodies	223
biological value (BV)	239
buffers	225
celiac disease	228
chemical scoring	238
chymotrypsinogen/chymotrypsin	228
collagen	219
complementary protein	238
complete (high-quality) proteins	237
conditionally essential amino acids	216
cystic fibrosis	228
deamination	226
denaturation	219
dipeptide	217
disulfide bridge	219
DNA (deoxyribonucleic acid)	230
edema	224
essential amino acids	216
extracellular fluid	224
gout	250
hemoglobin	218
hydrophilic amino acids	219
hydrophobic amino acids	219
immune response	223
incomplete (low-quality) proteins	237
interstitial fluid	224
intracellular fluid	224
intravascular fluid	224
keratin	220
kwashiorkor	247
limiting amino acid	239
marasmus	247
messenger RNA (mRNA)	230
motor proteins	220
negative nitrogen balance	234
net protein utilization (NPU)	239
neurotransmitters	232
nitrogen balance	234
nitrogen equilibrium	234
nonessential amino acids	216
oligopeptide	217
peptidases	228
peptide bond	217
polypeptide	217
positive nitrogen balance	234
precursor	226
proenzymes	227
proteases	227
protein digestibility corrected amino acid score (PDCAAS)	239
protein efficiency ratio (PER)	239
protein hydrolysates	240
protein turnover	231
protein-energy malnutrition (PEM)	245
ribosomal RNA (rRNA)	230
ribosomes	230
transfer RNA (tRNA)	230
tripeptide	217
trypsinogen/trypsin	228
urea	233
wasting	216

Study Points

- Many vital compounds are proteins, including enzymes, hormones, transport proteins, and regulators of both acid–base and fluid balance.
- Proteins are long chains of amino acids.
- Amino acids are composed of a central carbon atom bonded to hydrogen, carboxyl, amino, and side groups.
- At least 20 amino acids are important in human nutrition; 9 of these amino acids are considered essential (must come from the diet), whereas the body can make the other 11 (nonessential) amino acids.
- The amino acid sequence of a protein determines its shape and function.
- Denaturing of proteins changes their shape and therefore their functional properties.
- Protein digestion begins in the stomach through the action of hydrochloric acid and the enzyme pepsin.
- Proteins are digested completely in the small intestine and absorbed by facilitated diffusion and active transport.
- Dietary protein is found in meats, dairy products, legumes, nuts, seeds, grains, and vegetables.
- In general, animal foods contain higher-quality protein than is found in plant foods.
- Protein needs are highest when growth is rapid, such as during infancy, childhood, and adolescence.
- The protein intake of most Americans exceeds their RDA.
- Protein deficiency is most common in developing countries and results in the conditions known as marasmus and kwashiorkor.
- Protein excess is harmful and can affect risk for osteoporosis, heart disease, cancer, and gout.

Study Questions

1. List the functions of body proteins.
2. Describe the differences among essential, nonessential, and conditionally essential amino acids.
3. Among the nutrient molecules, which element is unique to protein and how does it fit into the basic structure of an amino acid?
4. Why are most plant proteins considered incomplete?
5. What are complementary proteins? List three examples of food combinations that contain complementary proteins.
6. What health effects occur if you are protein deficient?
7. How is protein related to immune function?
8. Describe a vegan diet.
9. List the potential health benefits of a vegetarian diet.

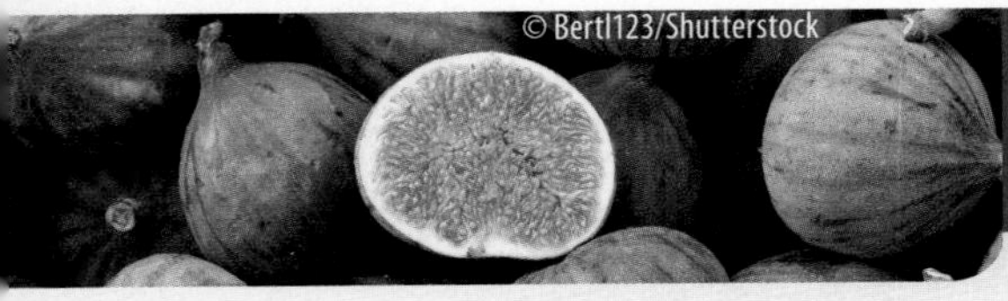

Learning Portfolio (continued)

Try This

The Sweetness of NutraSweet

The purpose of this experiment is to see the effect of high temperatures on the dipeptide known as NutraSweet (aspartame). Make a cup of hot tea (or coffee) and add one packet of Equal (one brand of aspartame). Stir and taste the tea; note its sweetness. Reheat the tea (in a microwave or on the stovetop) so that it boils for 30 to 60 seconds. After the tea cools, taste it. Does it still taste sweet? Why or why not?

The Vegetarian Challenge

The purpose of this activity is to eat a completely vegan diet for one day. Begin by making a list of your typical meals and snacks. Once the list is complete, review each food item and determine whether it contains animal products. Cross off items that contain animal products and circle the remaining vegan-friendly options. Double-check the circled list with a friend or roommate. You might have missed something! Create a full day's worth of meals and snacks using your circled foods as well as additional vegan options. Make sure your menu looks complete and nutritionally balanced. Try to stick to this menu for at least one day. Pay attention to deviations you make and whether these are vegan food choices.

Getting Personal

General instructions: List all of the foods and drinks that you consume in a 24-hour period, ideally a day where your schedule is fairly predictable and you are eating what is considered normal for you.

Take a minute to review your food intake with a special focus on protein.

Part A: Comparing your intake to the recommendations:

1. How do you think you did? Do you think you're lower or higher than the RDA?
2. Let's calculate your **RDA**. Your protein RDA is calculated as follows:

   ___ (your weight in pounds) ÷ 2.2 pounds = ___ kilograms × 0.8 g/kg/day = ___ g protein daily
3. Compare your protein RDA with your protein intake. Are you surprised by the results? Are you eating too much protein or just the right amount? How much more/less (grams) should you consume?
4. Another way to evaluate your protein intake is in terms of calories. What was your total kilocalorie intake ___? If your total protein intake is ___ grams, (×4 kcal/gram) =____kilocalories come from protein.

   a. We can include an example here: 96 g protein × 4 kcal/g = 384 kcal from protein. Assuming a 2,300 kcal diet, this amount is 17% of calories from protein and then compare to the recommended AMDR 10–35% calories from protein
5. What percentage of your total calories comes from protein? How does this compare to the **AMDR** for your caloric intake? General guidelines recommend that 10 to 35 percent of energy come from protein. (see sample calculation above). Does the percentage of protein in your diet fall in the recommended range?
6. Compare the two numbers (your RDA calculation vs your AMDR) numbers for recommended protein intake—do you meet the guidelines for protein intake using both recommendations? What could be the reason?

Part B: Now let's look at the protein containing foods in your diet:

7. What are the foods that contribute most to the protein in your diet?

8. **Activity:** Meatless Monday planning. Try to increased your plant based choices: For each animal product on your list, suggest a plant-based substitute for that food and compare the amount protein in the plant-based food to the animal product.
   a. Questions
      i. What happens to your protein intake when you go meatless? What effect does this have on your total calorie and fat intake?
      ii. What other nutrients could these changes affect?
      iii. What would be some challenges to eat a diet that is more plant-based?
      iv. List 3 foods plant-based foods that would be a good source of protein that you are willing to try.

References

1. Matthews DE. Proteins and amino acids. In: Ross AC, Caballero B, Cousins RJ, Tucker KL, Ziegler TR, eds. *Modern Nutrition in Health and Disease*. 11th ed. Baltimore, MD: Lippincott Williams and Wilkins; 2014.
2. Ibid.
3. Ribas GS, Sitta A, Wajner M, Vargas CR. Oxidative stress in phenylketonuria: what is the evidence? *Cell Mol Neurobiol.* 2011;31(5):653–662.
4. Ziegler TR. Glutamine. In: Ross AC, Caballero B, Cousins RJ, Tucker KL, Ziegler TR, eds. *Modern Nutrition in Health and Disease*. 11th ed. Baltimore, MD: Lippincott Williams and Wilkins; 2014.
5. Ibid.
6. Luiking YC, Castillo L, Deutz NEP. Arginine, citrulline and nitric oxide. In: Ross AC, Caballero B, Cousins RJ, Tucker KL, Ziegler TR, eds. *Modern Nutrition in Health and Disease*. 11th ed. Baltimore, MD: Lippincott Williams and Wilkins; 2014.
7. Gropper SG, Smith JL. *Advanced Nutrition and Human Metabolism*. 6th ed. Belmont CA. Wadsworth Cengage Learning; 2013.
8. Nathan DM. Diabetes: advances in diagnosis and treatment. *JAMA*. 2015;314(10):1052–1062. doi:10.1001/jama.2015.9536.
9. Marroqui L, Gonzalez A, Neco P, et al. Role of leptin in the pancreatic beta-cell: effects and signaling pathways. *J Mol Endocrinol.* 2012;49(1):R9–R17.
10. Berg JM, Tymoczko JL, Stryer L. *Biochemistry: A Short Course*. New York: Macmillan; 2009.
11. Hall J. *Guyton and Hall Textbook of Medical Physiology*. 13th ed. Philadelphia: Saunders; 2015.
12. Gropper, Smith. *Advanced Nutrition and Human Metabolism*. Op cit.
13. Pietzak M. Celiac disease, wheat allergy, and gluten sensitivity: when gluten free is not a fad. *J Parenter Enteral Nutr*. 2012;36(suppl 1):68S–75S. doi: 10.1177/0148607111426276.
14. Ibid.
15. Gaesser GA1, Angadi SS. Navigating the gluten-free boom. *JAAPA*. 2015 Aug;28(8). doi: 10.1097/01.JAA.0000469434.67572.a4 and Hartman LR. Gluten-Free Products Are Going Gangbusters. Food Processing Jul 29, 2015 http://www.foodprocessing.com/articles/2015/gluten-free-products-are-going-gangbusters/?show=all. Accessed February 4, 2016
16. Matthews. Proteins and amino acids. Op cit.
17. Ibid.
18. Gropper, Smith. *Advanced Nutrition and Human Metabolism*. Op cit.
19. Ibid.
20. Medeiros D, Wildman R. *Advanced Human Nutrition*. 3rd ed. Burlington, MA: Jones & Bartlett Learning; 2013.
21. Gropper, Smith. *Advanced Nutrition and Human Metabolism*. Op cit.
22. Institute of Medicine, Food and Nutrition Board. *Dietary Reference Intakes for Energy, Carbohydrate, Fiber, Fat, Fatty Acids, Cholesterol, Protein, and Amino Acids (Macronutrients)*. Washington, DC: National Academies Press; 2005. http://www.iom.edu/Global/News%20Announcements/~/media/C5CD2DD7840544979A549EC47E56A02B.ashx. Accessed December 30, 2015.
23. Ibid.
24. Position of the Academy of Nutrition and Dietetics: food and nutrition for older adults: promoting health and wellness. *J Acad Nutr Diet*. 2012;112:1255–1277.
25. Bernstein MA, Munoz N. *Nutrition for the Older Adult*. 2nd ed. Burlington, MA: Jones and Bartlett Learning; 2016.
26. Ibid.
27. Paddon-Jones D, Rasmussen B. Dietary protein recommendations and the prevention of sarcopenia. *Curr Opin Clin Nutr Metab Care*. 2009;12(1):86–90.
28. USDA What We Eat in America. NHANES 2011-2012 http://www.ars.usda.gov/Services/docs.htm?docid=18349 accessed January 25, 2016
29. Hall J. *Guton and Hall Textbook of Medical Physiology*. 12th ed. Philadelphia: Saunders/Elsevier; 2011.
30. Mahan LK, Escott-Stump S. *Krause's Food and Nutrition Therapy*. 13th ed. St. Louis, MO: Saunders Elsevier; 2008.
31. Michelfelder AJ. Soy: a complete source of protein. *Am Fam Physician*. 2009;79(1):43–47.
32. U.S. Department of Agriculture. Nutrient content of the U.S. food supply. http://www.cnpp.usda.gov/USfoodsupply Accessed June 5, 2015.
33. Ibid.

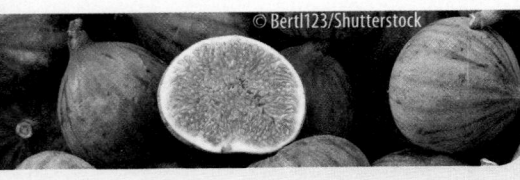

Learning Portfolio (continued)

34. Position of the Academy of Nutrition and Dietetics: vegetarian diets. *J Acad Nutr Diet*. 2015;115:801–810.
35. USDA ChooseMyPlate.gov Tips for Vegetarians http://www.choosemyplate.gov/tips-vegetarians accessed Jan 26, 2016
36. Institute of Medicine, Food and Nutrition Board. *Dietary Reference Intakes for Energy, Carbohydrate*. Op cit.
37. U.S. Food and Drug Administration. Guidance for industry: a food labeling guide. January 2013. http://www.fda.gov/Food/GuidanceRegulation/GuidanceDocumentsRegulatoryInformation/LabelingNutrition/ucm2006828.htm. Accessed December 30, 2015.
38. Ballenntine R. *Transition to Vegetarianism: An Evolutionary Step*. Honesdale, PA: Himalayan International Institute of Yoga Science and Philosophy; 1987.
39. Null G. *The Vegetarian Handbook: Eating Right for Total Health*. New York: St. Martin's Press; 1987.
40. Ibid.
41. Position of the American Dietetic Association: vegetarian diets. Op cit.
42. Ibid.
43. Ibid.
44. McEvoy CT, Temple N, Woodside JV. Vegetarian diets, low-meat diets and health: a review. *Public Health Nutr*. 2012;15(12):2287–2294. doi: 10.1017/S1368980012000936. Epub April 3, 2012.
45. Position of the American Dietetic Association: vegetarian diets. Op cit.
46. Orlich MJ, Singh PN, Sabaté J, et al. Vegetarian dietary patterns and mortality in Adventist Health Study 2. *JAMA Intern Med*. 2013;173(13):1230–1238. doi: 10.1001/jamainternmed.2013.6473.
47. Tonstad S, Stewart K, Oda K, Batech M, Herring RP, Fraser GE. Vegetarian diets and incidence of diabetes in the Adventist Health Study 2. *Nutr Metab Cardiovasc Dis*. 2013;23(4):292–299. doi:10.1016/j.numecd.2011.07.004. Epub October 7, 2011.
48. Tantamango-Bartley Y, Jaceldo-Siegl K, Fan J, Fraser G. Vegetarian diets and the incidence of cancer in a low-risk population. *Cancer Epidemiol Biomarkers Prev*. 2013;22(2):286–294. doi: 10.1158/1055-9965.EPI-12-1060. Epub November 20, 2012.
49. Orlich et al. Vegetarian dietary patterns and mortality in Adventist Health Study 2. Op cit.
50. Position of the American Dietetic Association: vegetarian diets. Op cit.
51. U.S. Department of Health and Human Services and U.S. Department of Agriculture. *2015–2020 Dietary Guidelines for Americans*. 8th Edition. December 2015. Available at http://health.gov/dietaryguidelines/2015/guidelines/. and U.S. Department of Agriculture. Healthy eating tips: tips for vegetarians. http://www.choosemyplate.gov/tips-vegetarians. Accessed Jan 26, 2016
52. Imdad A, Sadig K, Bhutta ZA, et al. Impaired glucose absorption in children with severe malnutrition. *J Pediatr*. 2011;158(2):282–287.
53. World Health Organization. WHO global database on child growth and malnutrition. 2014. http://www.who.int/nutgrowthdb/en. Accessed December 30, 2015.
54. Institute of Medicine, Food and Nutrition Board. *Dietary Reference Intakes for Energy, Carbohydrate*. Op cit.
55. Ibid.
56. Juraschek SP, Appel LJ, Anderson CA, Miller ER 3rd. Effect of a high-protein diet on kidney function in healthy adults: results from the OmniHeart trial.

Am J Kidney Dis. 2013;61(4):547–554. doi: 10.1053/j.ajkd.2012.10.017. Epub December 4, 2012.

57. Hunt JR, Johnson LK, Fariba Roughead ZK. Dietary protein and calcium interact to influence calcium retention: a controlled feeding study. *Am J Clin Nutr.* 2009;89(5):1357–1365.
58. Thrope MP, Evans EM. Dietary protein and bone health: harmonizing conflicting theories. *Nutr Rev.* 2011;69(4):215–230.
59. Hall KD. Predicting metabolic adaptation, body weight change, and energy intake in humans. *Am J Physiol Endocrin Metab.* 2010;298(3):E449–E466.
60. Gautron L, Elmquist JK. Sixteen years and counting: an update on leptin in energy balance. *J Clin Invest.* 2011;121(6):2087–2093.
61. Gunther AL, Remer T, Kroke A, Buyken AE. Early protein intake and later obesity risk: which protein sources at which time points throughout infancy and childhood are important for body mass index and body fat percentage at 7 y of age? *Am J Clin Nutr.* 2007;86(6):1765–1772.
62. Bernstein AM, Pan A, Rexrode KM, Stampfer M, Hu FB, Mozaffarian D, Willett WC. Dietary protein sources and the risk of stroke in men and women. *Stroke*. 2012;43(3):637–644. doi: 10.1161/STROKEAHA.111.633404. Epub December 29, 2011.
63. Pan A, Sun Q, Bernstein AM, et al. Red meat consumption and mortality: results from 2 prospective cohort studies. *Arch Intern Med.* 2012;172(7):555–563. doi: 10.1001/archinternmed.2011.2287. Epub March 12, 2012.
64. Micha R, Michas G, Mozaffarian D. Unprocessed red and processed meats and risk of coronary artery disease and type 2 diabetes—an updated review of the evidence. *Curr Atheroscler Rep.* 2012;14(6):515–524. doi: 10.1007/s11883-012-0282-8.
65. Feskens EJ, Sluik D, van Woudenbergh GJ. Meat consumption, diabetes, and its complications. *Curr Diab Rep.* 2013;13(2):298–306. doi: 10.1007/s11892-013-0365-0.
66. Messina M. Insights gained from 20 years of soy research. *J Nutr.* 2010;140(12):2289S–2295S.
67. Patisaul HB, Jefferson W. The pros and cons of phytoestrogens. *Neuroendocrinology.* 2010;31(4):400–419.
68. Micha, Michas, Mozaffarian. Unprocessed red and processed meats and risk of coronary artery disease and type 2 diabetes. Op cit.
69. Satia JA, Tseng M, Galanko JA, Sandler RS. Dietary patterns and colon cancer risk in Whites and African Americans in the North Carolina Colon Cancer Study. *Nutr Cancer.* 2009;61(2):179–193.
70. Corpet DE. Red meat and colon cancer: should we become vegetarians, or can we make meat safer? *Meat Sci.* 2011;89(3):310–316.
71. Hu J, La Vechia C, Morrison H, et al. Salt, processed meat and the risk of cancer. *Eur J Cancer Prev.* 2011;20(2):132–139.
72. Gout: epitome of painful arthritis. *Metabolism.* 2010;59(suppl 1):S32–S36.

Chapter 7

Alcohol

Revised by Carolyn Dunn

THINK About It

1. In a word or two, how would you describe alcohol? Is it a nutrient?
2. Compared with beer, what's your impression of the alcohol content of wine? How about compared with vodka?
3. Have you ever thought of alcohol as a poison?
4. After a night of drinking, your friend awakens with a splitting headache and asks you for a pain reliever. What would you recommend?

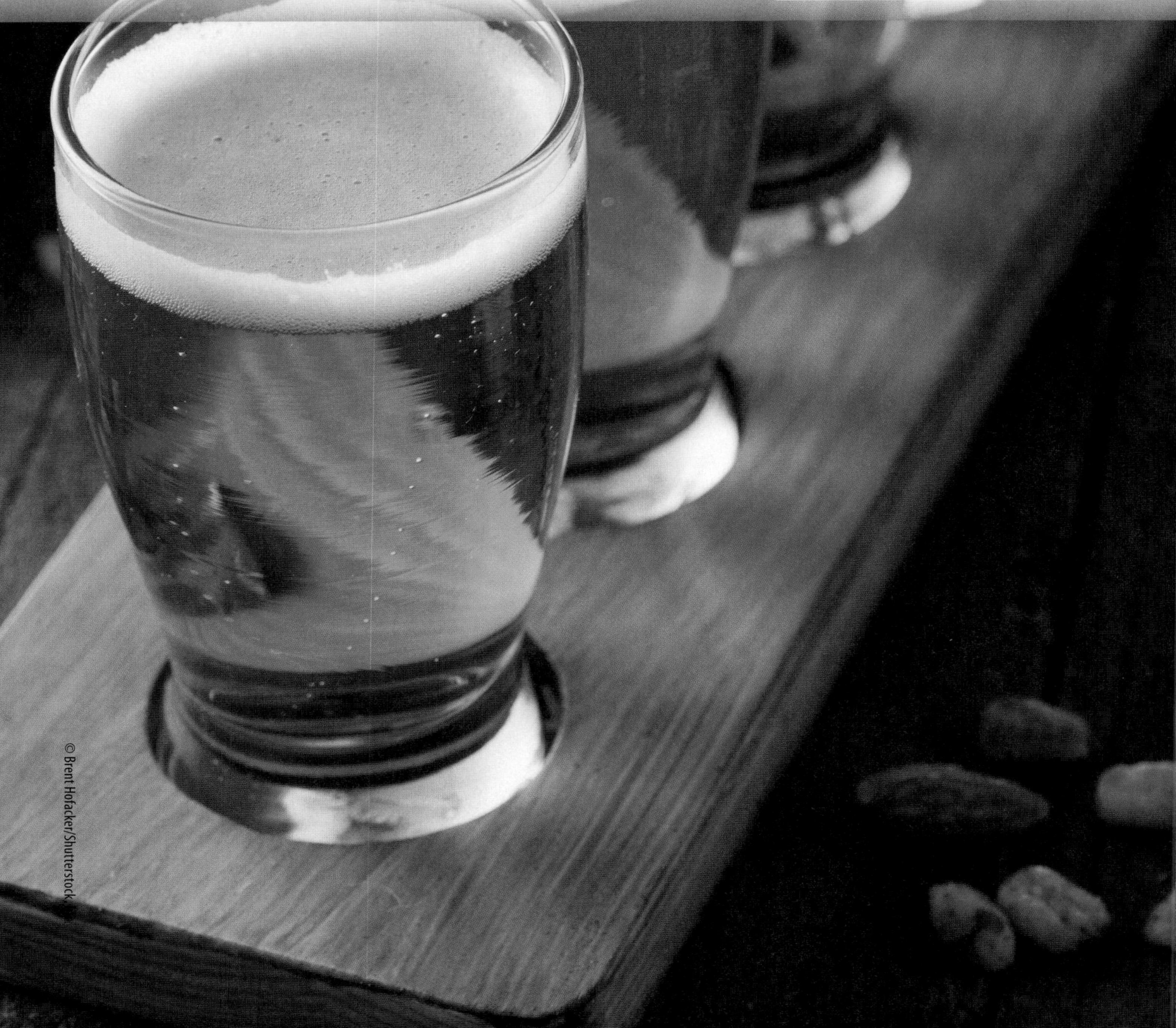

CHAPTER Menu

- History of Alcohol Use
- The Character of Alcohol
- Alcohol: Is It a Nutrient?
- Alcohol and Its Sources
- Alcohol Absorption and Metabolism
- When Alcohol Becomes a Problem
- Alcoholics and Malnutrition
- Does Alcohol Have Benefits?
- Key Terms
- Study Points
- Study Questions
- Try This
- References

LEARNING Objectives

- Describe the chemical characteristics of alcohol.
- Describe the process of alcohol metabolism and absorption.
- Explain ethnic, age, and gender differences in responses to alcohol consumption.
- Describe the effects of alcohol on the nervous system.
- Discuss the use and abuse of alcohol by college students and devise strategies to change the culture.
- Explain the effects of alcohol on the gastrointestinal system.
- Contrast the health benefits of moderate alcohol consumption with the harmful effects of inappropriate intake.

Think about alcohol. What image comes to mind: Grabbing a beer with a friend? A glass of wine with dinner? Or do you think of wild parties? Or out-of-control drinking? Violence? Car accidents? No other food or beverage has the power to elicit such strong, disparate images—images that reflect both the healthfulness of alcohol in moderation, the devastation of excess, and the political, social, and moral issues surrounding alcohol.

Alcohol has a long and checkered history. More drug than food, alcoholic beverages produce druglike effects in the body while providing little, if any, nutrient value other than calories. Yet, it still is important to consider alcohol in the study of nutrition. Alcohol is common to the diets of many people. In moderation, it can have health benefits; yet even small quantities can increase risks for birth defects and breast cancer. In large amounts, it interferes with our intake of nutrients as well as the body's ability to use them, and it causes significant damage to every organ system in the body. The *Dietary Guidelines for Americans, 2015* advises, "For people who drink, alcohol should be consumed in moderation defined as up to one drink per day for women and up to two drinks per day for men."[1]

For most people, alcohol consumption is a pleasant social activity. Moderate alcohol use does not harm most adults. Nonetheless, many people have serious trouble with drinking. Episodes of heavy drinking are common among adult populations and are on the rise.[2] In the United States, nearly 51 percent of adults 18 years of age and older are regular drinkers, whereas only 14 percent of adults 18 years of age and older drink infrequently.[3] More than half of the alcohol consumed by U.S. adults is consumed in binges. In the 18- to 20-year-old group, more than half (51 percent) binge drink.[4]

Heavy drinking can increase the risk for certain cancers. It can also cause liver cirrhosis, brain damage, and harm to the fetus during pregnancy. In addition, drinking increases the number of deaths from automobile crashes, recreational accidents, on-the-job accidents, homicide, and suicide. Excessive alcohol use is the third leading lifestyle-related cause of death for the nation.[5]

Drinking too much, at too young an age, is affecting young adults. Approximately 11 percent of alcohol consumed in the United States is by people under age (under 21 years of age). Underage alcohol use is more likely to kill young people than all illegal drugs combined.[6] For teenagers, the leading causes of death are accidents (unintentional injuries), homicide, and suicide.[7] Alcohol is the leading contributor to accidents and injury deaths for adolescents.[8]

Dietary Guidelines for Americans, 2015–2020

Key Recommendations

If alcohol is consumed, it should be consumed in moderation—up to one drink per day for women and two drinks per day for men—and only by adults of legal drinking age. For those who choose to drink, moderate alcohol consumption can be incorporated into the calorie limits of most healthy eating patterns.

Reproduced from U.S. Department of Agriculture and U.S. Department of Health and Human Services. *Dietary Guidelines for Americans, 2015*. 8th ed. Washington, DC: U.S. http://health.gov/dietaryguidelines/2015/guidelines/. Accessed March 24, 2015.

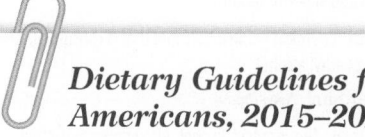

Quick Bite

Preferred Beverages
Beer is the national beverage of Germany and Great Britain. Wine is the national beverage of Greece and Italy.

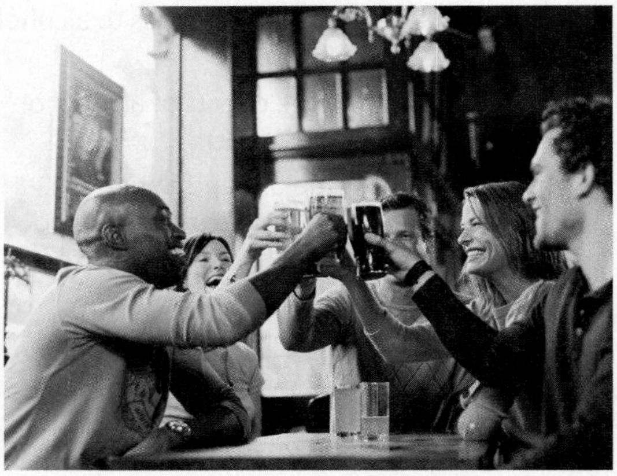
© Digital Vision/Thinkstock

History of Alcohol Use

Prehistoric humans were likely the first to consume alcohol, probably by accident, most likely in the form of fermented fruit. The fermented fruit would have had a taste that was unexpected and unlike what they were used to, but food was scarce so they ate it anyway. The alcohol that the fruit had produced as it fermented entered the bloodstream and produced the pleasing feelings associated with alcohol consumption. Evolution ultimately allowed humans to metabolize alcohol to make the calories available to the body.

Alcohol has had a prominent role throughout history. Old religious and medical writings frequently recommend its use, although with warnings for moderation. Thanks to alcohol's antiseptic properties, fermented drinks were safer than water during the centuries before modern sanitation, especially as people moved to towns and villages where water supplies were contaminated. Even mixing alcohol with dirty water afforded some protection from bacteria.[9]

At a time when life was filled with physical and emotional hardships, people valued alcohol for its analgesic and euphoric qualities. People relied on it to lift spirits, ease boredom, numb hunger, and dull the discomfort, even pain, of daily routine. Before the twentieth century, it was one of the few painkillers available in the Western world.

In sharp contrast to what is allowed today, drinking was often encouraged at the work site. Workers might be given alcohol as an inducement to do boring, painful, or dangerous jobs. Distilled spirits, beer, and wine accompanied sailors and passengers on all long voyages, supplying relatively pathogen-free fluid and calories. The British navy famously provided sailors on Royal Navy ships a ration of rum called a tot. The ration of two ounces of straight rum was given to officers; a watered-down version was given to junior sailors. This was a practice that was only discontinued in 1970. Legend has it that even the Puritans, a group known for rigid morality, disembarked at Plymouth Rock because their beer supply was depleted.[10]

The Character of Alcohol

Although there are many types of alcohol, the term **alcohol** commonly refers to the specific alcohol compound in beer, wine, and spirits (see **FIGURE 7.1**). Its technical name is **ethanol**, or **ethyl alcohol**. Ethanol is commonly abbreviated to EtOH, shorthand often preferred by health professionals. In this chapter, when we use the term *alcohol*, we are referring to ethanol.

Other types of alcohol are unsafe to drink. The simplest alcohol is **methanol**, also called **methyl alcohol** or **wood alcohol**, a solvent used in paints and for woodworking. Decades ago, some heavy drinkers thought they had discovered a way to save money—wood alcohol, used at that time to heat chafing dishes, was intoxicating but considerably cheaper than beer or wine. Unfortunately, methanol caused blindness and death. Methanol is no longer used in these products, but methanol poisoning from other sources still occurs.[11] Today, methanol is used in a number of consumer products, including paint strippers, duplicator fluid, model airplane fuel, and dry gas. Most windshield washer fluids are 50 percent methanol.

- **alcohol** Common name for ethanol or ethyl alcohol. As a general term, it refers to any organic compound with one or more hydroxyl (–OH) groups.
- **ethanol** Chemical name for alcohol that is consumed. Also known as ethyl alcohol.
- **ethyl alcohol** See *ethanol.*
- **methanol** The simplest alcohol. Also known as methyl alcohol and wood alcohol.
- **methyl alcohol** See *methanol.*
- **wood alcohol** Common name for methanol.

Alcohol: Is It a Nutrient?

Alcohol eludes easy classification. Like fat, protein, and carbohydrate, it provides energy. Laboratory experiments in the nineteenth century demonstrated that upon oxidation pure alcohol releases 7 kilocalories per gram, but many people doubted it actually produced energy in the body. These doubts were

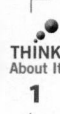

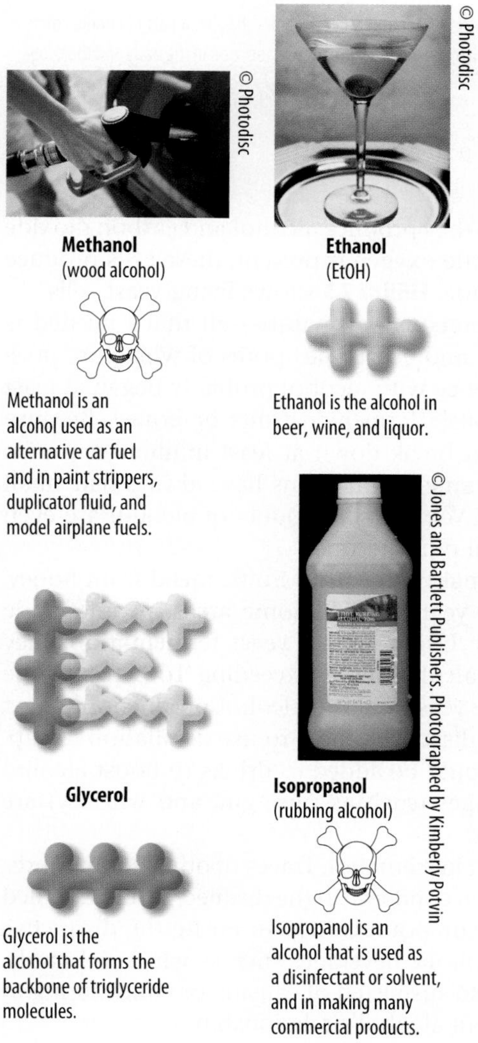
© Photodisc
© Photodisc
Methanol
(wood alcohol)
Ethanol
(EtOH)
Methanol is an alcohol used as an alternative car fuel and in paint strippers, duplicator fluid, and model airplane fuels.
Ethanol is the alcohol in beer, wine, and liquor.
© Jones and Bartlett Publishers. Photographed by Kimberly Potvin
Glycerol
Isopropanol
(rubbing alcohol)
Glycerol is the alcohol that forms the backbone of triglyceride molecules.
Isopropanol is an alcohol that is used as a disinfectant or solvent, and in making many commercial products.

FIGURE 7.1 Alcohols. Ethanol is not the only alcohol people consume. When people eat fat, they consume the alcohol glycerol. Consuming the alcohol methanol or isopropanol can be deadly.

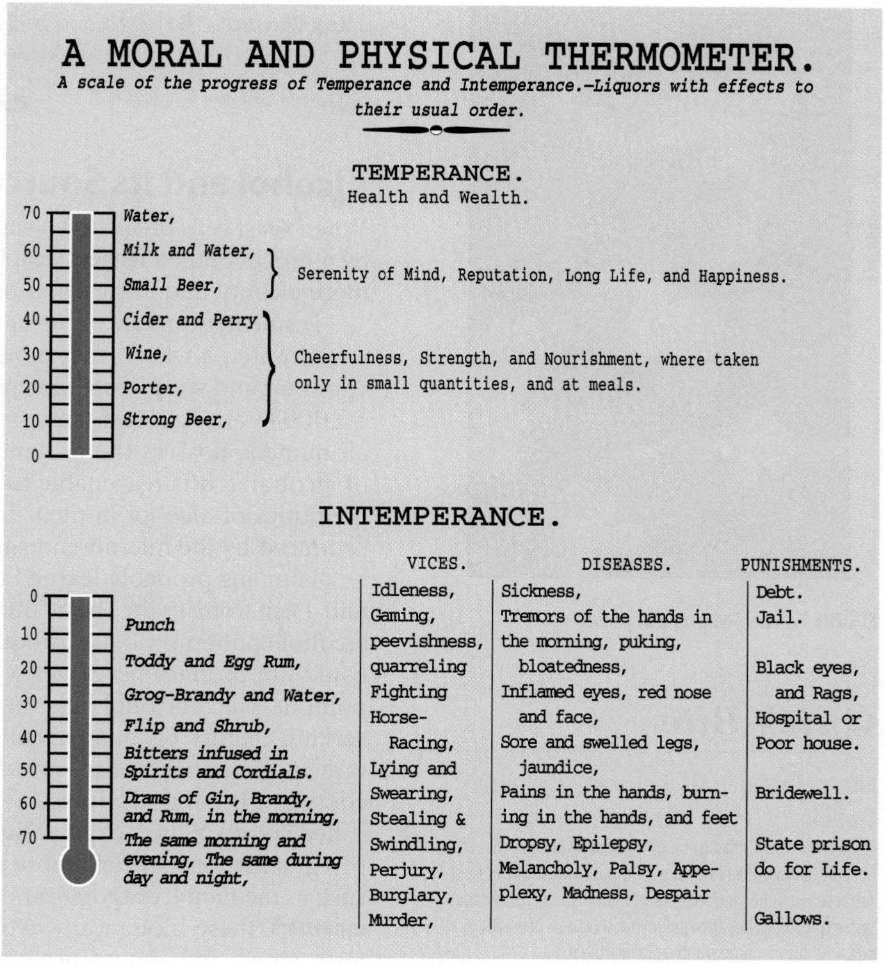

A MORAL AND PHYSICAL THERMOMETER.

A scale of the progress of Temperance and Intemperance.–Liquors with effects to their usual order.

TEMPERANCE.

Health and Wealth.

70	*Water,*	
60	*Milk and Water,*	Serenity of Mind, Reputation, Long Life, and Happiness.
50	*Small Beer,*	
40	*Cider and Perry*	Cheerfulness, Strength, and Nourishment, where taken only in small quantities, and at meals.
30	*Wine,*	
20	*Porter,*	
10	*Strong Beer,*	
0		

INTEMPERANCE.

		VICES.	DISEASES.	PUNISHMENTS.
0		Idleness,	Sickness,	Debt.
10	*Punch*	Gaming, peevishness,	Tremors of the hands in the morning, puking,	Jail.
20	*Toddy and Egg Rum,*	quarreling	bloatedness,	Black eyes,
30	*Grog-Brandy and Water,*	Fighting	Inflamed eyes, red nose and face,	and Rags,
40	*Flip and Shrub,*	Horse-Racing,	Sore and swelled legs,	Hospital or Poor house.
50	*Bitters infused in Spirits and Cordials.*	Lying and Swearing,	jaundice,	
60	*Drams of Gin, Brandy, and Rum, in the morning,*	Stealing &	Pains in the hands, burning in the hands, and feet	Bridewell.
70	*The same morning and evening, The same during day and night,*	Swindling, Perjury,	Dropsy, Epilepsy, Melancholy, Palsy, Appeplexy, Madness, Despair	State prison do for Life.
		Burglary, Murder,		Gallows.

FIGURE 7.2 A moral and physical thermometer of temperance and intemperance. As part of a late eighteenth-century temperance movement, Philadelphian Dr. Benjamin Rush (1745–1813) created the Moral and Physical Thermometer and distributed it to the clergy in a campaign against heavy drinking.

Reproduced from Rush B, 1823, An Inquiry into the Effects of Ardent Spirits upon the Human Body and Mind, 8th ed. (James Loring: Boston), 2-3.

the basis of the controversial conclusion that alcohol was not food—a conclusion used by early Prohibitionists in their fight against alcohol (see **FIGURE 7.2**). However, a classic series of experiments by energy researchers Francis Atwater and Wilbur Benedict showed that alcohol did indeed produce 7 kilocalories per gram in the body—findings that were a great disappointment to the Temperance Movement because they showed that alcohol was a food.[12]

But alcohol's status as a nutrient is more questionable. It is certainly different from any other substance in the diet. It provides energy but is not essential, performing no necessary function in the body. Unlike the nutrients, alcohol is not stored in the body. And for no nutrient are the dangers of overconsumption so dramatic and the window of safety so narrow. In the small amounts most people usually consume, alcohol acts as a drug, producing a pleasant euphoria. For some people it is addictive, with the characteristics of tolerance, dependence, and withdrawal symptoms. Certainly, alcohol is a substance available in the diet, but it does not meet the technical definition of a nutrient.

THINK About It 1

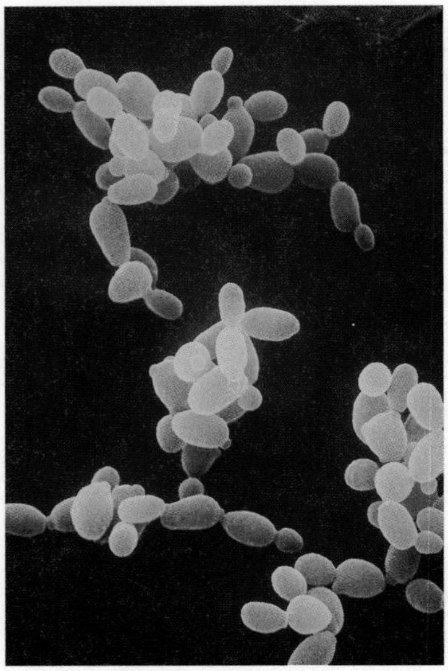
© David M. Phillips/Visuals Unlimited

FIGURE 7.3 A micrograph of yeast.

Key Concepts Alcohol—or, more specifically, the compound ethyl alcohol—has been part of people's diets for thousands of years. Although it provides calories, alcohol performs no essential function in the body and therefore is not a nutrient.

Alcohol and Its Sources

When yeast cells break down sugar, they produce alcohol and carbon dioxide by a process called **fermentation**. If little oxygen is present, these cells produce more alcohol and less carbon dioxide. **FIGURE 7.3** shows living yeast cells.

Fermentation can occur spontaneously in nature—all that's needed is sugar, water, a warm environment, and yeast (the spores of which are present in air and soil). Human experience with alcohol probably began at least 10,000 years ago with spontaneously fermented fruits or honey. Because all humans possess the enzymes to break down at least minimal amounts of alcohol,[13] it is reasonable to assume that humans have always had small quantities of alcohol in their diets. Very small amounts of alcohol are even produced by the microorganisms in our intestines.

Humans probably learned to make wine from fruits, mead from honey, and beer from grain about 5,000 years ago. In some areas, people made alcohol-containing dairy products. Using simple yeast fermentation, they could not produce beverages with alcohol levels exceeding 16 percent—the point at which alcohol kills off the yeast, halting alcohol production. Later, seventh-century Egyptian chemists discovered how to use distillation to capture concentrated alcohol, which could be added to drinks to boost alcohol content. Distilled alcoholic beverages (such as rum, gin, and whiskey) are called spirits, liquor, or hard liquor.

Distillation can yield more than just ethanol. Traces of other compounds, such as methanol, evaporate and then condense in the distilled product. Called **congeners**, these biologically active compounds help to create the distinctive taste, smell, and appearance of alcoholic beverages such as whiskey, brandy, and red wine. But congeners are also suspected of causing or contributing to hangovers[14] and might play a role in alcohol's relationship to cancer.

Beer, wine, and liquor have different alcohol levels: Most beer is up to 5 percent alcohol, although some beers exceed 6 percent. Many craft beers now on the market boast higher-than-average alcohol content, with some having 8–10 percent. Wine is usually 8–14 percent alcohol; however, some wine producers may add alcohol to soften the wine's taste (alcohol masks the harsh tannins that can be in some wine), increasing the alcohol content to 14.5–15.5 percent. Hard liquor is typically 35–45 percent alcohol. Beer and wine are labeled with the percentage of alcohol, but hard liquor is labeled by "proof," which is twice the alcohol percentage (an 80-proof whiskey is 40 percent alcohol).

THINK About It 2

Alcohol is a clear, colorless liquid used in chemistry labs. The purity is noted by the percent value; for example, 95 percent (close to the purest form of alcohol) still contains some water. The most unadulterated form of alcohol is vodka, which is alcohol, water, and almost nothing else; gin is similar, but flavored with juniper berries or other botanicals. Scotch, rum, rye, whiskey, and other liquors have residual flavor traces of the grain from which they were fermented or flavors introduced during storage. All liquors, however, offer little nutritional value besides energy. Beer and wine do contain unfermented carbohydrates and a trace of protein but, like liquor, have negligible minerals. With the exception of niacin in beer (a 12-ounce beer contains 1.8 milligrams of niacin, nearly 10 percent of the Daily Value), alcoholic beverages have negligible vitamins as well. **TABLE 7.1** shows the number of calories in various alcoholic beverages.

One serving of alcohol, or a **standard drink**, is defined as 12 ounces of regular beer, 5 ounces of wine (12 percent alcohol), or 1.5 ounces (a "jigger")

Quick Bite

Energy Drinks + Alcohol = A Recipe for Trouble

Think twice before mixing energy drinks with alcohol. These drinks not only increase the risk of alcohol toxicity, but also increase the risk of serious injury including heart rhythm problems, nervous system problems, impaired judgment, shortness of breath, dizziness, disorientation, and rapid heartbeat.[17]

▶ **fermentation** The anaerobic conversion of various carbohydrates to carbon dioxide and an alcohol or organic acid.

▶ **congeners** Biologically active compounds in alcoholic beverages that include nonalcoholic ingredients as well as other alcohols such as methanol. Congeners contribute to the distinctive taste and smell of the beverage and can increase intoxicating effects and subsequent hangover.

▶ **standard drink** One serving of alcohol (about 15 grams), defined as 12 ounces of beer, 4 to 5 ounces of wine, or 1.5 ounces of liquor.

TABLE 7.1
Calories in Selected Alcoholic Beverages

Beverage	Serving Size	Approximate Kilocalories
Beer (regular, 4.9% alcohol)	12 fl oz	153
Beer (craft, 6.9% alcohol)	12 fl oz	200
Beer (light)	12 fl oz	103
White wine	5 fl oz	121
Red wine	5 fl oz	125
Sweet dessert wine	3.5 fl oz	165
80-proof distilled spirits (gin, rum, vodka, whiskey)	1.5 fl oz	97

This table is a guide to estimate the caloric intake from various alcoholic beverages. Higher alcohol content and mixing alcohol with other beverages, such as calorically sweetened soft drinks, tonic water, fruit juice, or cream, increases the amount of calories in the beverage. Alcoholic beverages supply calories but provide few essential nutrients.

Data from U.S. Department of Agriculture, Agricultural Research Service. USDA National Nutrient Database for Standard Reference, Release 28. 2015. http://www.ars.usda.gov/ba/bhnrc/ndl. Accessed January 26, 2016.

of 80-proof liquor.[15] All contain roughly 15 grams (1 tablespoon) of pure alcohol. Most health professionals who speak of "moderate alcohol intake" usually mean no more than one (for women) or two (for men) servings in a day[16] (see **FIGURE 7.4**). Moderate intake is not an average of seven drinks per week, when there are six days of abstinence followed by seven drinks in one night! That's **binge drinking**, and it's dangerous.

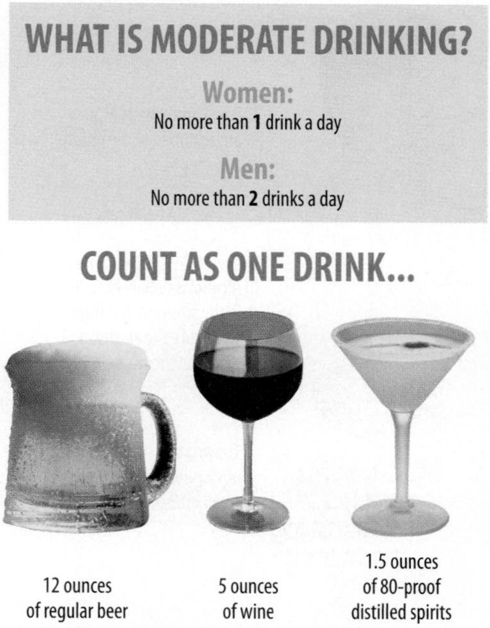
WHAT IS MODERATE DRINKING?
Women:
No more than 1 drink a day
Men:
No more than 2 drinks a day
COUNT AS ONE DRINK...
12 ounces of regular beer
5 ounces of wine
1.5 ounces of 80-proof distilled spirits

FIGURE 7.4 Moderate drinking.
Reproduced from USDA Center for Nutrition Policy and Promotion.

▶ **binge drinking** Consuming excessive amounts of alcohol in short periods of time.

Key Concepts Alcohol is formed when yeast ferments sugars to yield energy. Distillation methods produce concentrated solutions containing up to 95 percent alcohol. A typical serving of beer, wine, or distilled spirits contains about 15 grams of alcohol.

Alcohol Absorption and Metabolism

Alcohol absorption begins in the mouth and esophagus. Although alcohol absorption continues in the stomach, the small intestine efficiently absorbs most of the alcohol a person consumes.[19] (See **FIGURE 7.5**.)

You've heard it before: "Don't drink on an empty stomach." Eating before or with a drink slows down the rush of alcohol into the bloodstream in several ways. Food, especially if it contains fat, delays emptying of the stomach into the small intestine. The delay also provides a longer opportunity for oxidizing stomach enzymes to work. Food also dilutes the stomach contents, lowering the concentration of alcohol and its rate of absorption.

About 80 to 95 percent of alcohol is absorbed unchanged. However, some oxidation does take place in the digestive tract, mainly in the stomach, and the breakdown products join any remaining alcohol as it diffuses into the gut cells.[20] These products travel by way of the portal vein directly to the liver.

The body cannot store potentially harmful alcohol, so it works extra hard to get rid of it. To prevent alcohol from accumulating and destroying cells and organs, the body quickly breaks down alcohol and removes it from the blood. Alcohol breakdown always takes priority over the breakdown of carbohydrates, proteins, and fats.

Alcohol is metabolized in the liver primarily by the enzyme alcohol dehydrogenase (ADH). ADH metabolizes alcohol to **acetaldehyde**. It is then used for energy or converted to fat. One of the reasons why men can consume more

Quick Bite

How to Shock Your Surgeon

If a person who formerly misused alcohol neglects to disclose past alcohol use before undergoing surgery, the surgeon could be in for a big surprise. Even if the patient is now abstinent from alcohol use, his or her microsomal ethanol oxidizing system (MEOS) could still act like that of someone who currently misuses alcohol—operating at the faster speed it once needed to process alcohol quickly. The overactive MEOS would deplete anesthesia much quicker than expected. Theoretically, the patient could wake up in the middle of surgery, much to the shock of the surgeon. That's why anesthesiologists and surgeons ask their patients about alcohol use, past and present.

Quick Bite

Is the Alcoholic Beverage Industry Addicted to Alcohol Abuse?

The combined value of illegal and underage drinking and adult alcohol abuse to the alcoholic beverage industry is estimated to be at least $48.3 billion, or 37.5 percent of consumer expenditures for alcohol in 2001. Other estimates suggest the value might be closer to $62.9 billion (48.8 percent of expenditures).[18]

▶ **acetaldehyde** A toxic intermediate compound formed by the action of the alcohol dehydrogenase enzyme during the metabolism of alcohol.

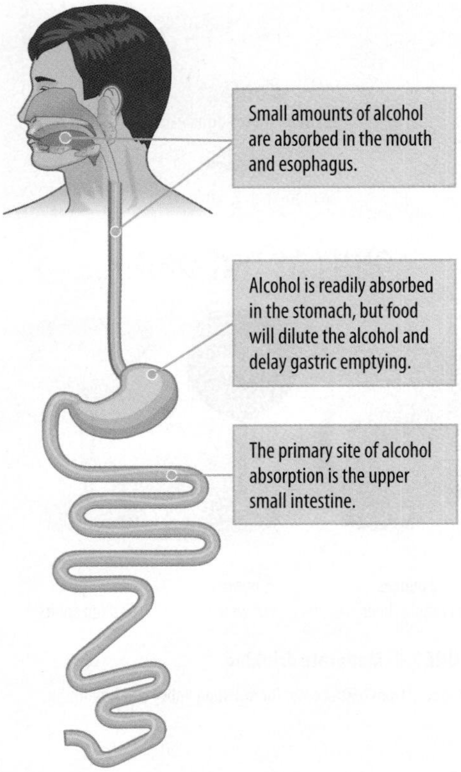

FIGURE 7.5 Alcohol absorption. Alcohol easily diffuses into and out of cells, so most alcohol is absorbed unchanged.

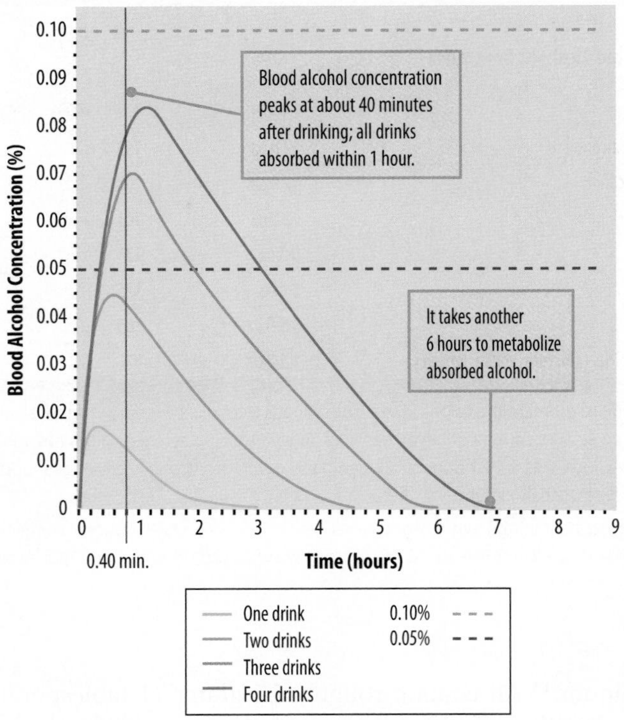

FIGURE 7.6 Blood alcohol concentration over time. Because the body breaks down alcohol at a relatively constant rate, it clears small amounts faster than large amounts.

Reproduced from Wilkinson PK, et al. Pharmacokinetics of ethanol after oral administration in the fasting state. J Pharmacokinet Biopharm. 1977;5(3):207-224. Reprinted with kind permission from Springer Science + Business Media B.V.

alcohol than women and not feel the effects is they have more of the enzyme alcohol dehydrogenase.

Clearing Alcohol from the Blood

The liver can break down only a certain amount of alcohol per hour, regardless of the amount in the bloodstream. In general, the amount of alcohol in the blood (blood alcohol concentration, or BAC) peaks 30 to 45 minutes after consuming one standard drink (see **FIGURE 7.6**). When absorption exceeds the liver's capacity, a bottleneck develops, and alcohol enters the general circulation. Alcohol diffuses rapidly, dispersing equally into all body fluids, including cerebrospinal fluid and the brain and, during pregnancy, into the placenta and fetus. About 10 percent of circulating alcohol is lost in urine, through the lungs, and through skin. Consequently, urine tests and breathalyzer tests both reflect concentrations of blood alcohol as well as alcohol levels in the brain and can indicate how much a person's mental and motor functions might be impaired.

Even after a person stops drinking, alcohol in the stomach and small intestine continues to enter the bloodstream and circulate throughout the body. Blood alcohol concentration continues to rise, and it is dangerous to assume the person will be fine by sleeping it off. Rapid binge drinking is especially dangerous because the victim can ingest a fatal dose of alcohol before becoming unconscious. Even if the victim lives, an alcohol overdose can lead to irreversible brain damage.

Excessive alcohol consumption deprives the brain of oxygen. The struggle to deal with an overdose of alcohol and lack of oxygen eventually causes the brain to shut down functions that regulate breathing and heart rate. This shutdown leads to a loss of consciousness and, in some cases, coma and death.

THINK About It 3

When a drinker passes out, the body is actually protecting itself: When you lose consciousness, you can't add more alcohol to your system. When you hear of an **alcohol poisoning** death, it usually is the result of consuming such a large quantity of alcohol in such a short period of time that the brain of the victim is overwhelmed. Heart and lung functions shut down, and the person dies.

▶ **alcohol poisoning** An overdose of alcohol. The body is overwhelmed by the amount of alcohol in the system and cannot break it down fast enough.

The Morning After

After a night of heavy alcohol consumption, the drinker might suffer from a pounding headache, fatigue, muscle aches, nausea, and stomach pain as well as a heightened sensitivity to light and noise—a **hangover** in full force. The sufferer might be dizzy, have a sense that the room is spinning, and be depressed, anxious, and irritable. Usually a hangover begins within several hours after the last drink, when the blood alcohol level is dropping. Symptoms normally peak about the time the alcohol level reaches zero, and they can continue for an entire day.[21]

▶ **hangover** The collection of symptoms experienced by someone who has consumed a large quantity of alcohol. Symptoms can include pounding headache, fatigue, muscle aches, nausea, stomach pain, heightened sensitivity to light and sound, dizziness, and possibly depression, anxiety, and irritability.

What causes a hangover? Scientists have identified several causes of the painful symptoms of a hangover (see **FIGURE 7.7**). Alcohol causes dehydration, which leads to headache and dry mouth. Alcohol directly irritates the stomach and intestines, contributing to stomach pain and vomiting. The sweating, vomiting, and diarrhea that can accompany a hangover cause additional fluid loss and electrolyte imbalance. Alcohol diverts liver activity away from glucose production, which can lead to low blood glucose (hypoglycemia), causing light-headedness and lack of energy. Alcohol also disrupts sleep patterns, interfering with the dream state and contributing to fatigue. The symptoms of a hangover are largely caused by an inflammatory response from your immune system similar to what is seen in an infection. In general, the greater the amount of alcohol consumed, the more likely a hangover will strike. However, some people experience a hangover after only one drink, whereas some heavy drinkers do not have hangovers.[22]

In addition, factors other than alcohol can contribute to the hangover. A person with a family history of alcoholism has increased vulnerability to hangovers. Mixing alcohol and drugs also is suspected of increasing the likelihood of a hangover. The congeners in most alcoholic beverages can contribute to more vicious hangovers.

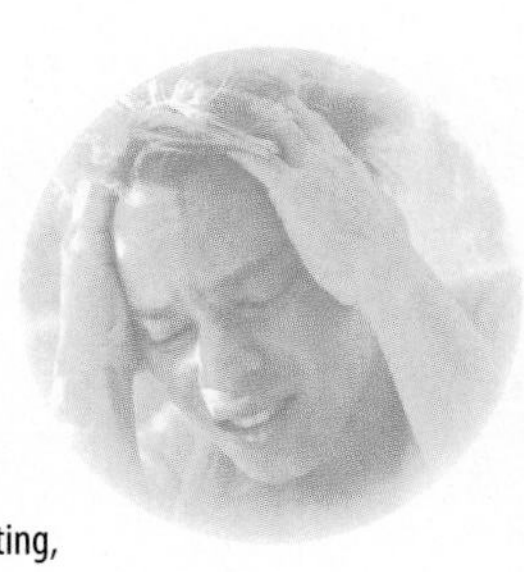

© Scott T. Baxter/Photodisc/Getty Images

Hangover Symptoms

Constitutional—fatigue, weakness, and thirst
Pain—headache and muscle aches
Gastrointestinal—nausea, vomiting, and stomach pains
Sleep and biological rhythms—decreased sleep, decreased dreaming when asleep
Sensory—vertigo and sensitivity to light and sound
Cognitive—decreased attention and concentration
Mood—depression, anxiety, and irritability
Sympathetic hyperactivity—tremor, sweating, increased pulse, and blood pressure

Possible Contributing Factors

Direct effects of alcohol
- Dehydration
- Electrolyte imbalance
- Gastrointestinal disturbances
- Low blood sugar
- Sleep and biological rhythm disturbances

Alcohol withdrawal
Alcohol metabolism (i.e., acetaldehyde toxicity)
Nonalcohol factors
- Compounds other than alcohol in beverages, especially the congener methanol
- Use of other drugs, especially nicotine
- Personality traits such as neuroticism,anger, and defensiveness
- Negative life events and feelings of guilt about drinking
- Family history for alcoholism

FIGURE 7.7 Hangovers. Factors other than just alcohol contribute to the misery of a hangover.

Treating a Hangover

How can you plan to minimize the symptoms of a hangover? You may want to consider these ways to help minimize the symptoms of a hangover[23]:

- Be sure to eat before you consume alcohol. Having a full stomach helps slow down the absorption of alcohol and gives the body more time to process the toxins.
- Drink in moderation. Limiting yourself to one drink per hour will give your body more time to process the alcohol.

So, what can you do about a hangover? Few treatments have undergone rigorous, scientific investigation. Time works best, however. Hangover symptoms usually disappear in 8 to 24 hours. No matter what you do to help get over your hangover, your body still has to clean up all the toxic by-products left over from the alcohol.[24] Eating bland foods that contain complex carbohydrates, such as toast or crackers, can combat low blood glucose and possibly nausea. Sleep can ease fatigue, and drinking nonalcoholic beverages can alleviate dehydration. Limited research suggests that taking vitamin B_6 or an extract from *Opuntia ficus indica* (a type of prickly pear cactus) before drinking can reduce the severity of hangover symptoms.[25] The prickly pear cactus extract might reduce three symptoms of hangover—nausea, dry mouth, and loss of appetite.[26] The best way to prevent a hangover, of course, is to abstain from alcohol use.

Certain medications also can relieve some symptoms. Antacids, for example, might relieve nausea and stomach pains. Aspirin can reduce headache and muscle aches, but could increase stomach irritation. Avoid acetaminophen because alcohol enhances its toxicity to the liver.[27] In fact, people who drink three or more alcoholic beverages per day should avoid all over-the-counter pain relievers and fever reducers. These heavy drinkers have an increased risk of liver damage and stomach bleeding from medicines that contain aspirin, acetaminophen (Tylenol), ibuprofen (Advil), naproxen sodium (Aleve), or ketoprofen (Orudis KT and Actron).[28]

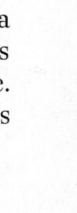

THINK About It 4

People with hangovers should avoid "the hair of the dog that bit you," a remedy that calls for drinking more alcohol. Additional drinking only enhances the toxicity of the alcohol previously consumed and extends the recovery time. The "hair of the dog" does little to relieve the hangover and only prolongs the pain and nausea.

Individual Differences in Responses to Alcohol

Individuals vary in their ability to break down alcohol and its products. As a consequence, they differ in their susceptibility to intoxication, hangover, and, in the long term, addiction and organ damage.

The result of individual differences is easiest to see in acute responses to alcohol. For example, when people of Asian descent drink alcohol, about half experience flushing around the face and neck, probably as a result of high blood levels of acetaldehyde—a toxic breakdown product.[29] The enzyme that catalyzes alcohol breakdown is lacking in the stomach. In the liver, the enzyme that breaks down acetaldehyde is present but in an inefficient form. These ethnic characteristics can explain why Asian ancestors depended on boiled water (for teas) as a source of safe fluid. In contrast, Europeans typically have the necessary enzymes to break down larger quantities of alcohol and their ancestors relied on fermentation to produce fluids that were safer to drink.[30]

Older people often find their tolerance for alcohol is less than it used to be. Because of decreased tolerance, the effects of alcohol, such as impaired coordination, occur at lower intakes in older adults than in younger people, whose tolerance increases with increased consumption. This reduced tolerance is compounded by an age-related decrease in body water, so blood alcohol concentrations in older people are likely to rise higher after drinking.[31]

Women and Alcohol

Men and women respond differently to alcohol (see **FIGURE 7.8**). Blood alcohol rises faster in women, so they become more intoxicated than do men with an equivalent dose of alcohol.[32] Accordingly, moderate drinking is usually defined as "two standard drinks for men and one for women."[33] Women also break down alcohol more slowly than men do. Several factors are responsible for alcohol's greater effect on women:

- *Body size and composition:* Women, on average, are smaller than men are and have smaller livers; thus, they have less capacity for processing alcohol. Women also have lower total body water and higher body fat than do men of comparable size. After alcohol is consumed, it diffuses uniformly into all body water, both inside and outside cells. Because of their smaller quantity of body water, women have higher concentrations of alcohol in their blood than men do after drinking equivalent amounts of alcohol.[34]
- *Less enzyme activity:* Compared to men, women also have less of the primary enzyme involved in the metabolism of alcohol (alcohol dehydrogenase)—about 40 percent less.[35] This contributes to higher blood alcohol concentrations and lengthens the time needed to break down and eliminate alcohol.[36]

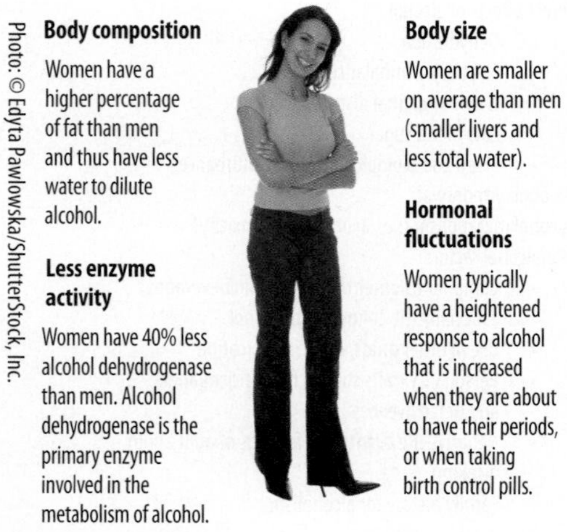

Photo: © Edyta Pawlowska/ShutterStock, Inc.
Body composition
Women have a higher percentage of fat than men and thus have less water to dilute alcohol.
Less enzyme activity
Women have 40% less alcohol dehydrogenase than men. Alcohol dehydrogenase is the primary enzyme involved in the metabolism of alcohol.
Body size
Women are smaller on average than men (smaller livers and less total water).
Hormonal fluctuations
Women typically have a heightened response to alcohol that is increased when they are about to have their periods, or when taking birth control pills.

FIGURE 7.8 Women and men respond differently to alcohol. Women tend to have a lower capacity for alcohol than men.

- *Chronic alcohol abuse:* Alcoholism and other abuses exact a greater physical toll on women than they do on men. Women who misuse alcohol have death rates 50 to 100 percent higher than those of men who do. Furthermore, a higher percentage of women who chronically misuse alcohol die from suicides, alcohol-related accidents, circulatory disorders, and cirrhosis of the liver.

Key Concepts Alcohol does not need to be digested prior to absorption and moves easily across the GI tract lining into the bloodstream. Once alcohol is absorbed, the liver breaks it down. Genetic and gender differences in the amount and activity levels of alcohol-related enzymes influence a person's response to consuming alcohol.

When Alcohol Becomes a Problem

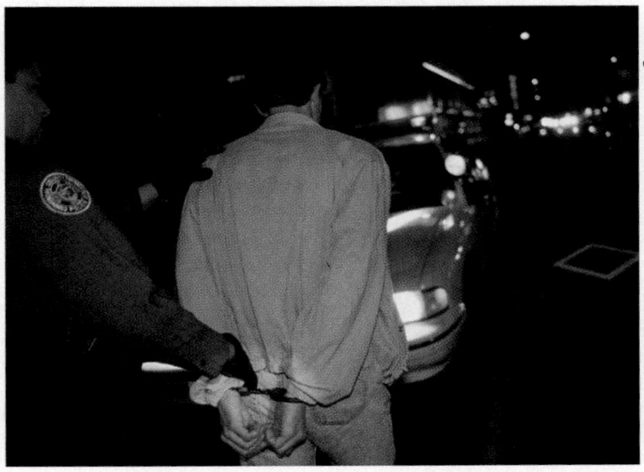

Alcohol affects every organ system in the body. In the short term, small amounts of alcohol change the levels of neurotransmitters in the brain, reducing inhibitions and physical coordination. In the long term, chronic intake of large amounts of alcohol damages the heart, liver, GI tract, and brain. When a pregnant woman drinks, alcohol can have a devastating effect on the development of her baby.

Alcohol in the Brain and the Nervous System

Alcohol diffuses readily into the brain, and because a small amount is absorbed from the mouth directly into circulating blood, its effects can be almost immediate, reaching the brain in as little as one minute after consumption. Alcohol can produce detectable impairments in memory after only a few drinks and, as the amount of alcohol increases, so does the degree of impairment. Large quantities of alcohol, especially when consumed quickly and on an empty stomach, can produce a blackout—that is, an interval of time for which the intoxicated person cannot recall key details of events, or even entire events. **FIGURE 7.9** shows the effects alcohol has on the brain.

Because alcohol is soluble in fat, it can easily cross the protective fatty membrane of nerve cells. There, it disrupts the brain's complex system for communicating between nerve cells. Neurotransmitters that excite nerve cells and those that inhibit nerve cells are thrown out of balance. Excess of some neurotransmitters produces sleepiness; high levels of others cause a loss of coordination; an imbalance of others impairs judgment and mental ability; and still other neurotransmitters perpetuate the desire to keep drinking, even when it's clearly time to stop. Changes in these messengers are suspected of leading to addiction and symptoms of alcohol withdrawal.[37] In the short run, they probably contribute to a hangover.

Alcohol's short-term effects are related to how much a person drinks. One or two drinks typically bring alcohol blood levels to 0.04 percent and usually cause only mild, pleasant changes in mood and release of inhibitions. With more drinks and rising blood alcohol levels, coordination, judgment, reaction time, and vision are increasingly impaired. In the United States and Canada, it is illegal for a person whose blood level of alcohol has reached or exceeds 0.08 percent to drive a motor vehicle. Studies show that certain skills required to drive a motor vehicle can become significantly impaired at a blood alcohol concentration as low as 0.05 percent.[38] A BAC of 0.04 percent is illegal nationwide for commercial drivers to operate a moving vehicle. **TABLE 7.2** shows the effects various amounts of alcohol have on mood and behavior. The acute effect

Quick Bite

Ancient Hangover Helpers

According to the ancient Persians, eating five almonds could prevent a hangover. The Romans and Greeks had a different solution: celery.

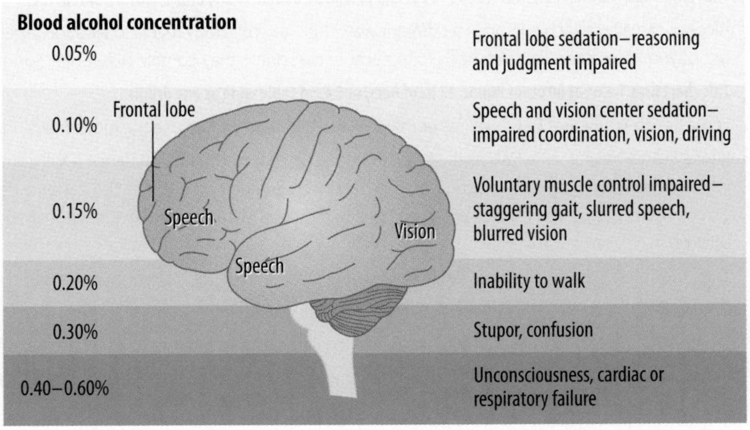

FIGURE 7.9 **Effects of alcohol on the brain.** As blood alcohol concentration rises, different parts of the brain are affected.

TABLE 7.2
Alcohol Impairment Chart

Men									
	Body Weight in Pounds								
	140	160	180	200	220	240	260	280	
Drinks	Approximate Blood Alcohol Percentage								
0	.00	.00	.00	.00	.00	.00	.00	.00	Only Safe Driving Limit
1	.03	.02	.02	.02	.02	.02	.01	.01	Impairment Begins
2	.05	.05	.04	.04	.03	.03	.02	.02	Driving Skills Affected
3	.08	.07	.06	.06	.05	.05	.04	.04	
4	.11	.09	.08	.08	.07	.06	.06	.05	Possible Criminal Penalties
5	.13	.12	.11	.09	.09	.08	.08	.07	
6	.16	.14	.13	.11	.10	.09	.09	.09	
7	.19	.16	.15	.13	.12	.11	.11	.10	Legally Intoxicated
8	.21	.19	.18	.17	.15	.13	.13	.12	
9	.24	.21	.20	.19	.17	.16	.15	.14	Criminal Penalties
10	.27	.23	.21	.19	.17	.16	.16	.15	

Women									
	Body Weight in Pounds								
	100	120	140	160	180	200	220	240	
Drinks	Approximate Blood Alcohol Percentage								
0	.00	.00	.00	.00	.00	.00	.00	.00	Only Safe Driving Limit
1	.05	.04	.03	.03	.03	.02	.02	.02	Impairment Begins
2	.09	.08	.07	.06	.05	.05	.04	.04	Driving Skills Affected
3	.14	.11	.10	.09	.08	.07	.06	.06	Possible Criminal Penalties
4	.18	.15	.13	.11	.10	.09	.08	.08	
5	.23	.19	.16	.14	.13	.11	.10	.09	
6	.27	.23	.19	.17	.15	.14	.12	.11	
7	.32	.27	.23	.20	.18	.16	.14	.13	Legally Intoxicated
8	.36	.30	.26	.23	.20	.18	.17	.15	
9	.41	.34	.29	.26	.23	.20	.19	.17	Criminal Penalties
10	.45	.38	.32	.28	.25	.23	.21	.19	

Note: Your body can get rid of one drink per hour. One drink is 1.25 oz of 80-proof liquor, 12 oz of beer, or 5 oz of table wine.

Reproduced with permission of the Pennsylvania Liquor Control Board's Bureau of Alcohol Education using data from the National Clearinghouse for Alcohol and Drug Information, Substance Abuse and Mental Health Services Administration.

THIS CHART IS INTENDED FOR INDIVIDUALS 21 YEARS OF AGE OR OLDER. IT IS A GUIDE, NOT A GUARANTEE.

Alcohol can affect each person in a different way. The way your body reacts to alcohol depends on your gender, how much you weigh, how quickly you drink, and whether or not you have eaten. You also need to remember that drinks may contain different amounts of alcohol.

This chart uses 1.5 oz of 80 proof liquor, 12 oz of beer, or 5 oz of table wine as one drink.

Females reach a higher BAC level faster than males. A woman should use the female version on the chart.

Pennsylvania has set .08% BAC as the legal limit for a Driving Under the Infl uence (DUI) conviction. You may be convicted of DUI at .05 % and above if there is supporting evidence of driving impairment. Commercial drivers can be convicted of DUI nationwide with a BAC level of .04%. A BAC reading is not necessary for an individual to be convicted of DUI. You may be convicted of DUI if there is circumstantial evidence that you imbibed a suffi cient amount of alcohol such that you are incapable of safe driving.

The Zero Tolerance Law (Section 3802(e) of the PA Vehicle Code, Title 75) lowered the Blood Alcohol Content (BAC) for minors (persons under 21) to .02%.

REMEMBER:

- A person must be 21 years of age or older to legally purchase, attempt to purchase, possess, consume, or transport any alcohol, liquor, malt or brewed beverages.
- Impairment begins with the fi rst drink - the only safe driving limit is .00%. • For safety's sake, never drive after drinking!

[Source: Refer to www.lcb.state.pa.us]

REFERENCES:

http://www.wikihow.com/Calculate-Blood-Alcohol-Content-(Widmark-Formula) http://www.alcohol.vt.edu/Students/alcoholEffects/estimatingBAC/index.htm http://www.ehow.com/how_7315381_calculate-estimated-blood-alcohol-content.html http://www.ctduiattorney.com/dui_information/calculating_bac.html

of a large alcohol intake—swallowed accidentally by children, for example—is hypoglycemia (low blood glucose) severe enough to kill.[39] Binge drinking, especially following several days of little food, also can be harmful or even deadly. The lack of food depletes glycogen stores, and heavy drinking suppresses gluconeogenesis. The resulting severe hypoglycemia is a medical emergency with the potential for coma and death.

A person who drinks heavily over a long period of time can have brain deficits that persist well after he or she achieves sobriety. This brain damage can range from memory loss to permanent debilitation that requires lifelong care. Exactly how alcohol affects the brain and the likelihood of reversing the impact of heavy drinking on the brain remain hot topics in alcohol research today.[40] Chronic misuse of alcohol produces many different mental disorders. Malnutrition is a probable factor in most of these, even when diet appears adequate. After years of drinking, brain cells become permanently damaged and unable to utilize nutrients properly.

Alcohol's Effect on the Gastrointestinal System

Years of heavy drinking and ongoing contact with alcohol and acetaldehyde eventually damage the gastrointestinal system, which in turn discourages eating, affects absorption of protective nutrients, and leaves the digestive lining even more vulnerable to damage as the vicious cycle continues.

Chronic irritation from alcohol and acetaldehyde erodes protective mucosal linings, causing inflammation and release of destructive free radicals. **Esophagitis** (inflammation of the esophagus), esophageal stricture (closing), and swallowing difficulties are common among alcoholics. When the stomach is exposed repeatedly to alcohol at high concentrations, **gastritis** (inflammation of the stomach) often develops. Alcoholics frequently have diarrhea and

▶ **esophagitis** Inflammation of the esophagus.

▶ **gastritis** Inflammation of the stomach.

FYI For Your Information

Myths About Alcohol

Myths and misunderstandings just keep circulating about alcohol. Some of these statements are partly true, but most are completely false. You might have heard some of the following:

- *Drinking isn't all that dangerous.* Wrong! One in three 18- to 24-year-olds admitted to emergency rooms for serious injuries is intoxicated. Alcohol use is also associated with homicides, suicides, and drowning.
- *I can manage to drive well enough after a few drinks.* No, it only takes a few drinks to raise your BAC level to 0.08 percent, too high to drive safely. Buzzed driving is drunk driving.
- *I can sober up quickly if needed.* No. It takes about three hours to eliminate the alcohol content of two drinks, depending on your weight and other factors. Nothing can speed up this process—not even coffee or cold showers.
- *Alcohol is a stimulant.* No. It's actually a depressant, but its initial depressing effect on inhibitions and judgment can make it seem stimulating.
- *Alcohol keeps you warm.* Partly true. It dilates blood vessels near the body's surface, giving a feeling of warmth. But as body heat escapes, alcohol cools the inner body.
- *Alcohol is an aphrodisiac.* Partly true. By suppressing inhibitions, it can loosen behavior. However, sexual function often is compromised by alcohol.
- *Most alcoholics don't live a productive life.* No. A high percentage of those with alcohol addiction lead productive lives, hold jobs, and have families.
- *Beer is a source of vitamins.* Partly true. Beer does contain a fair amount of niacin. But you'd need about 1 liter to fulfill daily niacin requirements. Levels of other vitamins are much lower.
- *Alcohol helps you sleep.* No. Alcohol disrupts sleep patterns, leading to a restless, unsatisfying sleep.
- *Laboratory animals love to drink.* No. Alcohol is usually given by tube feeding because most animals refuse to drink it willingly.
- *It's good to have a beer before breastfeeding.* No. Alcohol might be relaxing and allow milk to flow more readily, but alcohol concentrations in breast milk are similar to those in the mother's blood. Alcohol in breast milk reduces milk production by reducing the intensity of the infant's suckling.

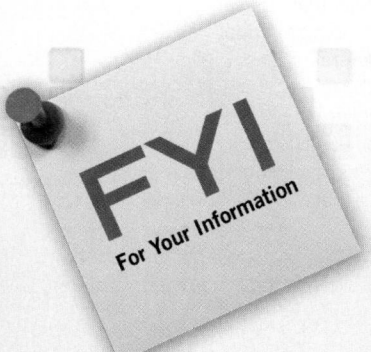

FYI For Your Information

Changing the Culture of Campus Drinking

From car crashes to alcohol poisoning, the culture of drinking on many college campuses puts students at grave risk. Alcohol use is pervasive among college students, many of whom are younger than the legal drinking age. Alcohol use is associated with 56 percent of motor-vehicle–related fatalities among persons aged 21 to 24 years.[a] Annually, at least 1,800 student deaths and nearly 600,000 unintentional injuries involve alcohol.[b] College students who drink are more likely to drink and drive, have failing grades, and have medical and legal problems. Increased rates of crime, traffic crashes, rapes and assaults, property damage, and other alcohol-related consequences affect both drinking and nondrinking students as well as members of the surrounding community. Each year, for example, students who have been drinking assault more than 696,000 of their classmates.[c,d]

The Culture of College Drinking

On many campuses, alcohol consumption is a rite of passage, and the influence of peers is an especially powerful force driving college problem drinking.[e] Traditions and beliefs handed down through generations of college drinkers reinforce the perception that alcohol is a necessary component of social success.[f,g] Many students arrive at college with a history of alcohol consumption and positive expectations about alcohol's effects. An ongoing study of the behaviors, attitudes, and values of American secondary school students, college students, and young adults finds that 37 percent of eighth graders and 72 percent of twelfth graders report having tried alcohol, with 24 percent of youth aged 12 to 20 years reporting binge drinking. Ten percent drove after drinking alcohol, and 28 percent rode with a driver who had been drinking alcohol.[h]

Rates of excessive alcohol use are highest at colleges and universities where fraternities and sororities are popular, where sports teams have a prominent role, and at schools located in the Northeast.[i] In the local community, tolerance of student drinking can permit alcoholic beverage outlets and advertising to be located near campus. Because of lax enforcement, selling alcohol to students younger than the legal drinking age often has few consequences. Also, underage students who are caught using fake IDs to obtain alcohol are seldom penalized.[j] Just look at the advertising and sale of alcoholic beverages on or near campuses, and the role of alcohol in college life is evident.

Alcohol Use and Abuse by College Students

In one 2010 study, approximately 70 percent of college students consumed some alcohol within 30 days of being surveyed.[k] Although some of these students are problem drinkers (e.g., frequent, heavy, episodic drinkers or those who display symptoms of dependence), others might drink moderately or misuse alcohol only occasionally (e.g., drink and drive infrequently). Surveys of drinking patterns show that college students are more likely than nonstudents of similar age to consume any alcohol, to drink heavily, and to engage in heavy episodic drinking. Young people who are not in college, however, are more likely to consume alcohol every day.[l] Even though college students tend to drink more, they are not at greater risk of alcohol-related problems.[m]

Results from the Fall 2010 American College Health Association National College Health Assessment revealed that 60 percent of college students reported using alcohol within the past 30 days.[n] Another survey questioned students about patterns and consequences of their alcohol use.[o] Thirty-two percent reported symptoms associated with alcohol abuse (e.g., drinking in hazardous situations and alcohol-related school problems), and 6 percent reported three or more symptoms of alcohol dependence (e.g., drinking more or longer than initially planned and experiencing increased tolerance to alcohol's effects). Students report that 91 percent of their alcohol consumption occurs in binges (68 percent occurs in frequent binges). What happens when these student binge-drinkers leave college? Surprisingly, most high-risk student drinkers reduce their consumption of alcohol. Nevertheless, some continue frequent, excessive drinking, leading to alcoholism or medical problems associated with chronic alcohol abuse.[p]

Binge Drinking

Binge drinking is especially worrisome, and it is widespread on college campuses. What is binge drinking? Binge drinking is defined as the consumption of at least five drinks in a row for men or four drinks in a row for women. Just over two in five students (44 percent) report binge drinking behaviors, and about one in four (23 percent) report bingeing frequently, defined as three or more times in a two-week period. Frequent binge drinkers average more than 14 drinks per week and account for more than 90 percent of the alcohol consumed by college students.[q] Most college binge drinkers drink not for sociability, but solely and purposefully to get drunk. Binge drinkers often do something they later regret—argue with friends, make fools of themselves, get sick, engage in unplanned (and often unprotected) sexual activity, or drive drunk. Afterward, they might forget where they were or what they did, but the consequences of the binge remain. These consequences can include alienated friends, a hangover, and embarrassment. Or the consequences could be much more serious—sexually transmitted disease, hospitalization, permanent injury, rape, pregnancy, or death.

Abstaining

There is a polarizing trend in college drinking, with binge drinkers at one extreme and abstainers at the other. One large study looked at characteristics of undergraduate U.S. college students and found that, overall, 20.5 percent of the students abstained from drinking alcohol, with predictors of abstention including the following[r]:

- The student's own negative attitude toward alcohol use
- Perception of friends' alcohol attitudes
- Male gender
- Age younger than 21 years
- Abstaining in high school
- Not a Greek member or pledge
- Not an athlete
- Not a smoker
- Not a marijuana user
- Participant in a religious group
- Working either 0 or 10+ hours per week for salary
- Having a mother who does not drink alcohol
- Having a close friend who does not drink alcohol

Prevention Strategies and Changing the Culture of Drinking

Changing the culture of college drinking represents the first step toward an effective prevention strategy, according to a task force of college presidents, alcohol researchers, and students established by the National Institute on Alcohol Abuse and Alcoholism. Their report emphasizes the need for collaboration among academic institutions, researchers, and the community to effect lasting change.[s]

The task force strongly supports the use of a "3-in-1 Framework" to target three primary audiences simultaneously: (1) individual students, including high-risk drinkers; (2) the student body as a whole; and (3) the surrounding community.[t,u]

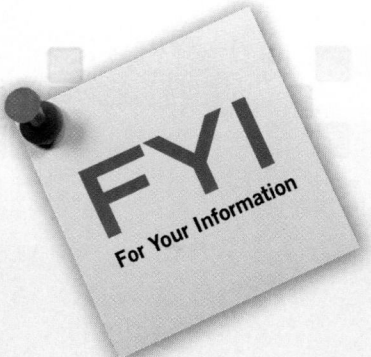

The task force reviewed potentially useful preventive interventions, grouping them into tiers according to evidence for their effectiveness. Other researchers support these steps to begin to change the culture of drinking on campus.[v,w]

Tier 1: Strategies Effective Among College Students

Strong evidence supports the following strategies:

- Simultaneously address alcohol-related attitudes and behaviors (e.g., refuting false beliefs about alcohol's effects while teaching students how to cope with stress without resorting to alcohol).
- Use survey data to counter students' misperceptions about their fellow students' drinking practices and attitudes toward excessive drinking.
- Increase student motivation to change drinking habits by providing nonjudgmental advice and progress evaluations.

Programs that combine these three strategies have proved effective in reducing alcohol consumption.[x]

Tier 2: Strategies Effective Among the General Population that Could Be Applied to College Environments

These strategies have proved successful in populations similar to those found on college campuses. Measures include the following:

- Increase enforcement of minimum legal drinking age laws.[y]
- Implement, enforce, and publicize other laws to reduce alcohol-impaired driving, such as zero-tolerance laws that reduce the legal blood alcohol concentration for underage drivers to near zero.[z]
- Increase the prices or taxes on alcoholic beverages.[aa]
- Institute policies and training for servers of alcoholic beverages to prevent sales to underage or intoxicated patrons.[ab]

Tier 3: Promising Strategies that Require Research

These strategies make sense intuitively or show theoretical promise, but their usefulness requires further testing. They include more consistent enforcement of campus alcohol regulations and increasing the severity of penalties for violating them, regulating happy hours, enhancing awareness of personal liability for alcohol-related harm to others, establishing alcohol-free dormitories, restricting or eliminating alcohol-industry sponsorship of student events while promoting alcohol-free student activities, and conducting social norms campaigns to correct exaggerated estimates of the overall level of drinking among the student body.

How Can I Say No to Drinking Alcohol and Still Fit in with My Friends?

Drinking alcohol is a personal decision. It is best to make your decision to drink or not to drink based on your own feelings, knowledge, and experiences. You might want to consider the following things before you are put in a position where alcohol is available[ac]:

- If you choose to abstain, make up your mind to say no before you are ever in the situation.
- Tell people that you feel better when you drink less.
- Stay away from people who give you a hard time about not drinking.
- Learn to hold a glass or beer bottle for a long time, and refill it with whatever you want (such as water or club soda).

[a] Centers for Disease Control and Prevention. Vital signs: binge drinking among high school students and adults—United States, 2009. *MMWR*. 2010;59(39):1274–1279.

[b] Hingson RW, Heeren T, Winter M, et al. Magnitude of alcohol-related mortality and morbidity among U.S. college students ages 18–24: changes from 1998 to 2001. *Ann Rev Pub Health*. 2005;26:259–279.

[c] College Drinking—Changing the Culture. A snapshot of annual high-risk college drinking consequences. July 2010. http://www.collegedrinkingprevention.gov/StatsSummaries/snapshot.aspx. Accessed May 1, 2012.

[d] Ibid.

[e] Ham LS, Hope DA. Incorporating social anxiety into a model of college student problematic drinking. *Addict Behav*. 2005;30(1):127–150.

[f] National Institute on Alcohol Abuse and Alcoholism. *A Call to Action: Changing the Culture of Drinking at U.S. Colleges*. Bethesda, MD: Author; 2002. NIH publication 02-5010.

[g] National Institute on Alcohol Abuse and Alcoholism. *Young Adult Drinking*. Bethesda, MD: Author; 2006. Alcohol Alert No. 68.

[h] Centers for Disease Control and Prevention. Alcohol and public health: fact sheets—underage drinking. October 2014. http://www.cdc.gov/alcohol/fact-sheets/underage-drinking.htm. Accessed January 27, 2016.

[i] Carter AC, Brandon KO, Goldman MS. The college and noncollege experience: a review of the factors that influence drinking behavior in young adulthood. *J Stud Alcohol Drugs*. 2010;71(5):472–475.

[j] Toomey TL, Lenk KM, Wagenaar AC. Environmental policies to reduce college drinking: an update of research findings. *J Stud Alcohol Drugs*. 2007;68(2):208–209.

[k] Wagoner K, Rhodes S, Lentz A, Wolfson M. Community organizing goes college: a practice-based model to implement environmental strategies to reduce high-risk drinking on college campuses. *Health Promot Pract*. 2010;11(6):817–827.

[l] Slutske WS. Alcohol use disorders among US college students and their non-college-attending peers. *Arch Gen Psychiatry*. 2005;62:321–327.

[m] Ibid.

[n] American College Health Association. National College Health Assessment II. Reference group executive summary. Fall 2010. http://www.achancha.org/docs/ACHA-NCHA-II_ReferenceGroup_ExecutiveSummary_Fall2010.pdf. Accessed October 16, 2015.

[o] Wechsler H, Nelson TF. What we have learned from the Harvard School of Public Health College Alcohol Study: focusing attention on college student alcohol consumption and the environmental conditions that promote it. *J Stud Alcohol Drugs*. 2008;69(4):481–490.

[p] McMambridge J, McAlaney J, Rowe R. Adult consequences of late adolescent alcohol consumption: a systematic review of cohort studies. *PLoS Med*. 2011;8(2):e1000413.

[q] Wechsler H, Nelson TF. What we have learned from the Harvard School of Public Health College Alcohol Study. Op cit.

[r] Huang JH, DeJong W, Towvim LG, Schneider SK. Sociodemographic and psychobehavioral characteristics of US college students who abstain from alcohol. *J Am Coll Health*. 2009;57(4):395–410.

[s] National Institute on Alcohol Abuse and Alcoholism. *A Call to Action*. Op cit.

[t] Hingson RW, Howland J. Comprehensive community interventions to promote health: implications for college-age drinking problems. *J Studies Alcohol*. 2002;(suppl 14):226–240.

[u] Holder HD, Gruenewald PJ, Ponicki WR, et al. Effect of community-based interventions on high-risk drinking and alcohol-related injuries. *JAMA*. 2000;284:2341–2347.

[v] Kingsbury JH, Gibbons FX, Gerrard M. The effects of social and health consequence framing on heavy drinking interventions among college students. *Brit Psychol Soc*. 2015;20:212–220.

[w] Scott-Sheldon LAJ, Carey KB, Elliott JC, Garey L, Carey MP. Efficacy of alcohol interventions for first-year college students: a meta-analysis review of randomized controlled trials. *J Consult Clin Psychol*. 2014;82(2):177–188.

[x] Larimer ME, Cronce JM. Identification, prevention, and treatment: a review of individual-focused strategies to reduce problematic alcohol consumption by college students. *J Studies Alcohol*. 2002;(suppl 14):148–163.

[y] Wagenaar AC, Toomey TL. Effects of minimum drinking age laws: review and analyses of the literature from 1960 to 2000. *J Studies Alcohol*. 2002;(suppl 14): 206–225.

[z] Wagenaar A, O'Malley P, LaFond L. Lowered legal blood alcohol limits for young drivers: effects on drinking, driving, and driving-after-drinking behaviors in 30 states. *Am J Pub Health*. 2001;91(5):801–804.

[aa] Cook PJ, Moore MJ. The economics of alcohol abuse and alcohol-control policies. *Health Aff*. 2002;21(2):120–133.

[ab] Toomey TL, Lenk KM, Wagenaar AC. Environmental policies to reduce college drinking. Op cit.

[ac] Anderson J, Vitale T, et al. *Eat Right! Healthy Eating in College and Beyond*. San Francisco: Pearson Benjamin Cummings; 2007:87.

malabsorption, evidence of intestinal damage. The mouth, throat, esophagus, stomach, and small and large intestines are all at greatly increased risk of cancer.[41] Smoking dramatically multiplies this risk.

Alcohol and the Liver

Breaking down and detoxifying alcohol is almost entirely the responsibility of the liver. So, it's not surprising that too much drinking hurts the liver more than any other site in the body. In the United States, heavy alcohol use is considered the most important risk factor for chronic liver disease. More than 29,000 people die annually in the United States as a result of chronic liver diseases and cirrhosis (nearly 10 deaths per 100,000 persons), according to the Centers for Disease Control and Prevention.[42]

The earliest evidence of liver damage is fat accumulation, which can appear after only a few days of heavy drinking. **Fatty liver** recedes with abstinence but persists with continued drinking (see **FIGURE 7.10**). Is fatty liver in and of itself harmful? The answer is controversial among liver researchers, with some experts suggesting it's a benign condition. However, studies show that 5 to 15 percent of people with alcoholic fatty liver who continue to drink develop liver fibrosis (excessive fibrous tissue) or cirrhosis (scarring) in only 5 to 10 years.[43]

▶ **fatty liver** Accumulation of fat in the liver, a sign of increased fatty acid synthesis.

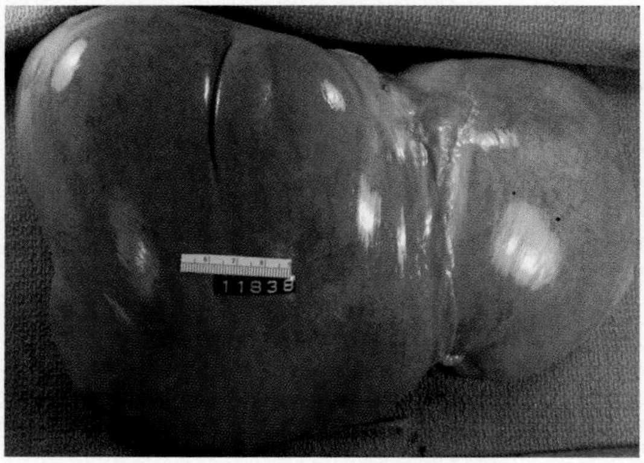

FIGURE 7.10 Fatty liver.

Fat accumulation is one of several factors resulting in alcoholic liver disease. With regular high intakes of alcohol, alcohol and acetaldehyde continually irritate and inflame the liver, producing alcoholic hepatitis (persistent inflammation of the liver) in 10 to 35 percent of heavy drinkers. The inflammatory process also generates free radicals that batter away at liver cells.[44] The destruction of liver cells becomes self-perpetuating, especially if antioxidant nutrients are unavailable to help break the cycle. If the intestines also have been damaged, toxins, including those produced by the gut's microorganisms, can cross the intestinal barrier into circulation, worsening inflammation.[45]

Alcoholic hepatitis is treatable, but it's often fatal. Alcoholic hepatitis also predisposes a person to liver cancer and cirrhosis, conditions that are usually fatal. With continued inflammation, the liver makes excessive collagen and becomes fibrous (fibrotic liver disease) and scarred (cirrhosis). This ultimately kills liver cells by choking off tiny blood vessels that nourish them. About 10 to 20 percent of heavy drinkers develop cirrhosis.[46]

Dietary changes can be helpful in treating liver disease, but abstinence from alcohol is essential. Reducing dietary fats somewhat reduces fat accumulation in the liver. Consuming adequate micronutrients and a healthful balance of macronutrients probably speeds recuperation from liver diseases in their earlier stages.[47] In late-stage liver disease, dietary restrictions, often of proteins, can slow disease progression or improve symptoms.

Fetal Alcohol Syndrome

▶ **fetal alcohol syndrome** A set of physical and mental abnormalities observed in infants born to women who abuse alcohol during pregnancy. Affected infants exhibit poor growth, characteristic abnormal facial features, limited hand–eye coordination, and mental retardation.

Fetal alcohol syndrome is perhaps the saddest result of alcohol consumption during pregnancy. Victims of this syndrome suffer a variety of congenital defects: mental retardation, coordination problems, and heart, eye, and genitourinary malformations, as well as low birth weight and slowed growth rate. Most apparent are characteristic facial abnormalities. Severe cases of fetal alcohol syndrome are rare, but subtle damage with one or two abnormalities, sometimes called "fetal alcohol effects," is probably much more widespread. This disorder, a major cause of mental retardation in the United States, is preventable.

Alcohol is especially damaging in the early weeks of pregnancy, before a woman might know she's pregnant. It crosses the placenta into the tiny body of the fetus, where its effects are grossly magnified. Both congeners and alcohol in alcoholic beverages can interfere with embryonic development by disrupting the body's use of vitamin A and folic acid, nutrients clearly required for fetal growth and development.[48]

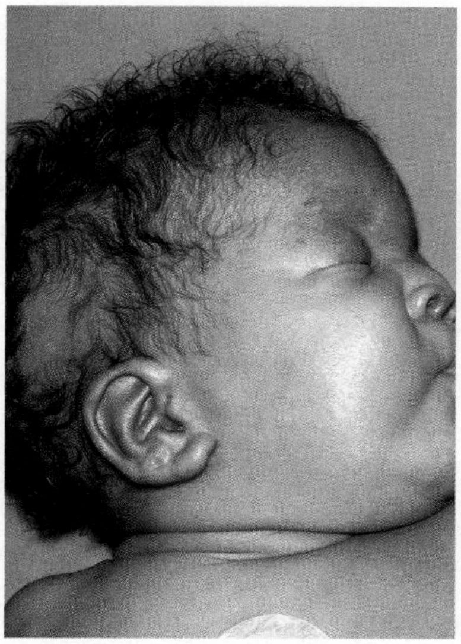

Relatively small amounts of alcohol can cause fetal alcohol syndrome. A safe level during pregnancy is not known; therefore, pregnant women should abstain from alcohol consumption. Unlike most other alcohol-related diseases, fetal alcohol damage does not require chronic intake. A binge—even having several drinks at a party—at the wrong moment of pregnancy can cause serious problems. However, population studies show that babies with neurodevelopmental problems are more common among women who drink more frequently during pregnancy.[49]

Official health advisories warn women against drinking alcohol if they are pregnant or considering becoming pregnant. Labels on alcoholic beverages must carry a warning for pregnant women. **FIGURE 7.11** shows the prevalence of binge drinking by women of childbearing age.[50]

Key Concepts Alcohol affects every organ system of the body. In the brain and nervous system, alcohol impairs coordination, judgment, reaction time, and vision. In the GI tract, alcohol damages cells of the esophagus and stomach and increases the risk for GI cancers. The liver is most affected by alcohol consumption, culminating in alcoholic hepatitis and cirrhosis after years of alcohol abuse. Alcohol intake during pregnancy can have devastating effects on fetal development.

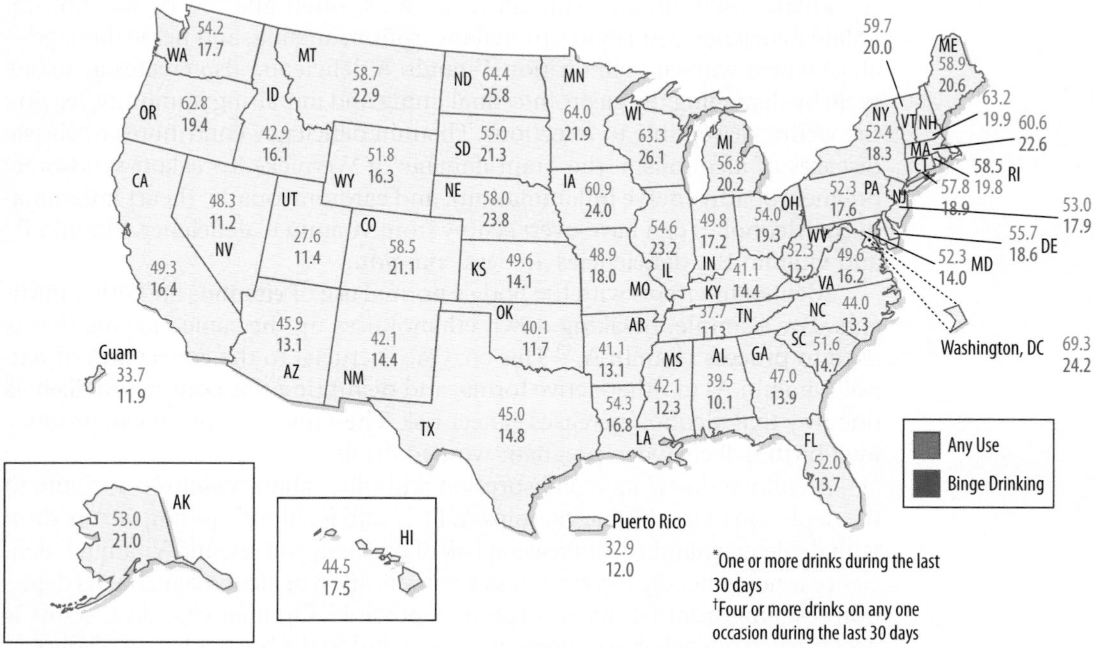

FIGURE 7.11 Prevalence of binge drinking among childbearing-aged women (18–44 years), by state: United States, 2010.

* Any Use = One or more drinks during the last 30 days. ** Binge = Four or more drinks on any one occasion during the last 30 days.

Courtesy of the Centers for Disease Control and Prevention.

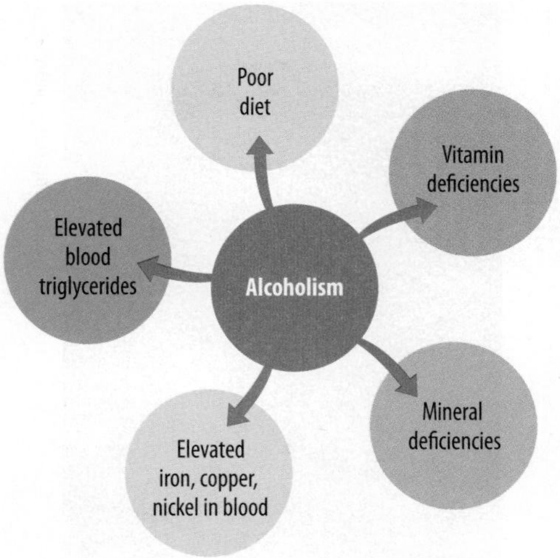

FIGURE 7.12 Alcoholism and malnutrition. Alcoholics' poor diets interact with alcohol's toxicity to worsen their malnutrition.

Alcoholics and Malnutrition

In the United States and Canada, where food is plentiful and fortification of foods with vitamins and minerals is common, overt nutrient deficiencies are rare—except among alcoholics. The results of their poor diet interact with the results of alcohol's toxicity—which include diarrhea, malabsorption, liver malfunction, bleeding, bone marrow changes, and hormonal changes—to worsen malnutrition (see **FIGURE 7.12**). In general, the more a person drinks, the worse the malnutrition.

Poor Diet

A nationally representative study found that as alcohol quantity increased, diet quality worsened, but as alcohol frequency increased, diet quality improved. Diet quality was poorest among the highest-quantity, lowest-frequency drinkers and best among the lowest-quantity, highest-frequency drinkers.[51]

Disordered eating is common among heavy drinkers, especially among women who chronically misuse alcohol.[52] Anxiety, depression, loneliness, and isolation are characteristics of some people who abuse alcohol, and all contribute to loss of appetite. So can physical pain. Lack of interest in food is common. There may be an aversion to many specific foods or to eating in general, especially after the experience of diarrhea, painful indigestion, or difficulty swallowing.

Heavy drinkers who get about half their calories from alcohol cannot eat enough to obtain adequate vitamins and minerals. Severely malnourished alcoholics often have multiple deficiencies.

Vitamin Deficiencies

Inadequate intake, poor absorption, increased vitamin destruction in the body, and urinary losses all contribute to vitamin deficiencies in the alcoholic. Alcohol also interferes with the conversion of vitamin precursors to active forms.

Folate, thiamin, and vitamin A are most often affected by alcoholism. Folate deficiency contributes to malabsorption, anemia, and nerve damage—all of which worsen malnutrition. Vitamin A deficiency also creates a vicious cycle by damaging the gastrointestinal lining and impairing immunity, leaving the victim susceptible to infections. Thiamin deficiency contributes to classic diseases of alcoholism: the brain damage of Wernicke-Korsakoff syndrome, polyneuropathy (nerve inflammation), and cardiomyopathy (heart inflammation). Alcoholics can have overt scurvy from vitamin C deficiency. Vitamin B_6 and vitamin B_{12} deficiencies are less common.

Alcohol interferes with the body's normal use of vitamins and other nutrients. For example, breaking down ethanol uses up the same enzyme that is used to process vitamin A.[53] This enzyme is crucial to the conversion of retinol (vitamin A) to other active forms, and disrupting this conversion likely is one way that alcohol increases cancer risk. The same disruption can produce fetal birth defects when pregnant women drink.

Alcohol-induced fat malabsorption and other abnormalities contribute to the depletion of fat-soluble vitamins A, D, E, and K. Blood-clotting factors drop with depleted vitamin K, increasing risk of bleeding and anemia. Vitamin E deficiency is not generally recognized as a complication of alcoholism, but its depletion resulting from fat malabsorption is possible. Optimal vitamin E status is necessary to quench free radicals generated during the breakdown of alcohol.[54]

Mineral Deficiencies

Alcoholics are commonly deficient in minerals such as calcium, magnesium, iron, and zinc. Alcohol itself does not seem to affect their absorption; rather, fluid losses and an inadequate diet are the primary culprits. Magnesium deficiency causes "shakes" similar to that seen in alcohol withdrawal. Chronic diarrhea and loss of epithelial tissue (caused by skin rashes or sloughing off of the digestive lining) can seriously deplete zinc, a mineral needed for immune function. In cases of bleeding, especially gastrointestinal blood loss, iron levels fall.

Not all minerals are lower in heavy drinkers than in nondrinkers. If there is no bleeding, a heavy drinker's iron levels tend to be higher than normal in the blood and liver, potentially contributing to harmful oxidation. Copper and nickel levels also might be elevated in advancing disease, but the reason and the effects are unclear.[55]

Macronutrients

Animal experiments can demonstrate a number of ways that alcohol alters digestion and breakdown of carbohydrate, fat, and protein, but the relevance to humans at usual levels of intake is not certain. Alcohol interferes with amino acid absorption, but its overall effect on protein balance appears minimal. It inhibits gluconeogenesis and lowers blood glucose levels, probably contributing to hangovers and, at the most extreme, causing acute, potentially lethal hypoglycemia if a person who drinks heavily neglects to eat.[56]

Alcohol's most dramatic effect is on fats. You have seen that alcohol causes fatty liver. On the one hand, excess alcohol has the undesirable effect of raising blood triglyceride levels, often significantly. Hyperlipidemia (high blood fats) is common among heavy drinkers. Abstinence and a balanced diet can usually return blood lipids to normal.[57] On the other hand, moderate alcohol use increases protective high-density lipoproteins (HDLs, or "good cholesterol"), an important factor in alcohol's relationship to the reduced risk for coronary artery disease.

Body Weight

Although alcoholic beverages provide minimal nutrient value, they do provide calories; alcohol contains 7 kilocalories per gram. Does alcohol consumption contribute to obesity? It appears likely. One reason for weight gain associated with alcohol intake is that the calories in alcohol can easily add up. Some cocktail-type drinks, such as margaritas or piña coladas, can contain more than 500 calories per drink! In addition, food choices that accompany drinking are generally low in nutrient density and high in calories, adding to an overall excess calorie intake. The excess calories promote body fat accumulation and weight gain.

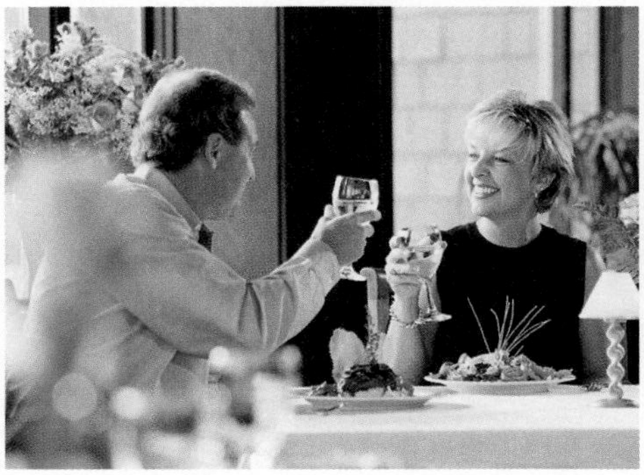
© Jupiterimages/liquidlibrary/Thinkstock

Key Concepts Alcohol interferes with normal nutrition by reducing the intake of nutrient-dense foods and by affecting the absorption, processing, and excretion of many vitamins and minerals. Alcohol contains a significant number of calories (7 kilocalories per gram), and heavy episodic drinkers tend to weigh more than light drinkers.

Does Alcohol Have Benefits?

Can a potentially harmful drink like alcohol play a role in a healthful diet? The consensus of health experts is that it can—but not for everyone. The question continues to arouse much debate, however, and even those supporting alcohol's usefulness often have reservations. Public health statements on alcohol are typically accompanied by plenty of "ifs" and "buts."

Consistent epidemiological evidence suggests that low to moderate drinking reduces mortality among some groups.[58] (**TABLE 7.3** gives definitions of different levels of drinking.) Compared with nondrinkers or heavy drinkers,

TABLE 7.3
How Much is Too Much?

Term	Definition
Moderate alcohol consumption	Moderate alcohol consumption, according to the 2015–2020 Dietary Guidelines for Americans, is up to 1 drink per day for women and up to 2 drinks per day for me
Low-risk Drinking	For women, low-risk drinking is defined as no more than 3 drinks on any single day and no more than 7 drinks per week. For men, it is defined as no more than 4 drinks on any single day and no more than 14 drinks per week. NIAAA research shows that only about 2 in 100 people who drink within these limits have an AUD.
Binge Drinking	NIAAA defines binge drinking as a pattern of drinking that brings blood alcohol concentration (BAC) levels to 0.08 g/dL. This typically occurs after 4 drinks for women and 5 drinks for men—in about 2 hours.
	The Substance Abuse and Mental Health Services Administration (SAMHSA), which conducts the annual National Survey on Drug Use and Health (NSDUH), defines binge drinking as drinking 5 or more alcoholic drinks on the same occasion on at least 1 day in the past 30 days.
Heavy Drinking	SAMHSA defines heavy drinking as drinking 5 or more drinks on the same occasion on each of 5 or more days in the past 30 days.
Alcohol Use Disorder (AUD)	AUDs are medical conditions that doctors diagnose when a patient's drinking causes distress or harm. The fourth edition of the Diagnostic and Statistical Manual (DSM–IV), published by the American Psychiatric Association, described two distinct disorders—alcohol abuse and alcohol dependence—with specific criteria for each. The fifth edition, DSM–5, integrates the two DSM–IV disorders, alcohol abuse and alcohol dependence, into a single disorder called alcohol use disorder, or AUD, with mild, moderate, and severe subclassifications.

NIAAA, National Institute on Alcohol Abuse and Alcoholism; SAMHSA, Substance Abuse and Mental Health Services Administration; WHO, World Health Organization; SAMHSA, Substance Abuse and Mental Health Services Administration.

Modified from http://www.niaaa.nih.gov/alcohol-health/overview-alcohol-consumption/alcohol-facts-and-statistics.

middle-aged and older adults who drink moderate amounts of alcohol have a lower risk of mortality from all causes.[59,60] This includes people with heart disease,[61] diabetes,[62] high blood pressure,[63] or a prior heart attack.[64] Consistent and growing evidence shows that alcohol reduces insulin resistance and might protect against heart disease by improving "good" cholesterol levels and reducing blood clotting.[65]

No evidence suggests that moderate drinking harmed the people in the studies. In fact, analysis of data from the Nurses' Health Study, which involves more than 12,000 participants, suggests that in women, up to one drink per day does not impair mental functioning and might actually decrease the risk of mental decline with age.[66]

Tracked against alcohol intake, death rates typically follow what statisticians describe as a U-shaped curve. Compared with people who rarely or never drink, people who drink slightly or moderately have lower total mortality rates. The lowest rate is seen in people who consume one drink per week. Increasing the number of drinks confers no additional benefit. In fact, as the number of drinks increases, the mortality rate rises. People who consume two drinks per day have about the same mortality rate as nondrinkers.[67] Beyond three drinks per day, the death rate rises dramatically.[68] Heavy alcohol consumption increases the risk of stroke, for example, whereas light or moderate drinking appears to reduce that risk.[69] Alcohol's primary benefit is to raise protective HDL cholesterol levels. It might also inhibit formation of blood clots, but this connection is less clear.[70] In addition, alcohol can have subjective benefits such as stress relief and relaxation.

In most studies, wine, beer, and spirits appear equal in offering protection against heart disease. Findings of reduced rates of nonfatal heart attacks among moderate drinkers support the view that protective benefits are due to the result of alcohol itself rather than other substances in alcoholic beverages.[71,72] However, international comparisons that highlight unexpectedly low rates of heart disease in France, despite a high-fat diet (the **French paradox**), suggest that red wine might have a unique protective effect. The apparent benefits of red wine could result from the overall healthier behavior of people who drink red wine. As yet, a direct connection between red wine and health benefits remains unproved.[73] Nevertheless, recognizing that alcohol generally confers moderate protection and noting the possibility that wine has a particular benefit, the Bureau of Alcohol, Tobacco, and Firearms, and Explosives granted permission for wine labels to include one of the following statements[74]:

> "The proud people who made this wine encourage you to consult your family doctor about the health effects of wine consumption."
>
> "To learn the health effects of wine consumption, send for the Federal Government's Dietary Guidelines for Americans."

Because of the many harmful effects of alcohol (see **FIGURE 7.13**), public health agencies and organizations caution against inappropriate drinking. Although low to moderate alcohol use might offer some benefit, these groups advise people to discuss their alcohol intake with their doctors, and they urge moderation. The U.S. Preventive Services Task Force recommends that primary care doctors routinely screen patients for unhealthy alcohol use and, when appropriate, intervene with a brief counseling session to reduce alcohol misuse.[75] Public health officials also point out that numerous groups should not drink any alcohol[76,77]:

- People who cannot restrict their alcohol intake to moderate levels
- Children and adolescents
- People taking medications that can interact with alcohol
- People who have an alcohol-related illness or another illness that will be worsened by alcohol
- People who plan to drive, operate machinery, or take part in other activities that require attention, skill, or coordination
- Women who are pregnant or who may become pregnant
- Women who are breastfeeding
- People with a personal or strong family history of alcoholism

Key Concepts Although alcohol has the potential to reduce risk for heart disease, most health organizations recommend moderate to no drinking. It is too early in the scientific investigation of alcohol's benefits to recommend alcohol intake for all adults. Some people, such as pregnant women, should not drink any alcohol.

▶ **French paradox** A phenomenon observed in the French, who have a lower incidence of heart disease than people whose diets contain comparable amounts of fat. Part of the difference has been attributed to the regular and moderate drinking of red wine.

American Heart Association

Alcohol

If you drink alcohol, do so in moderation. This means an average of one to two drinks per day for men and one drink per day for women. Drinking more alcohol increases such dangers as alcoholism, high blood pressure, obesity, stroke, breast cancer, suicide, and accidents. Also, it's not possible to predict in which people alcoholism will become a problem. Given these and other risks, the American Heart Association cautions people *not* to start drinking . . . if they do not already drink alcohol. Consult your doctor on the benefits and risks of consuming alcohol in moderation.

Quick Bite

A What?

An oenologist is an expert in the science of wine and wine making.

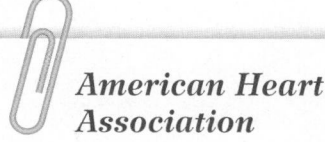

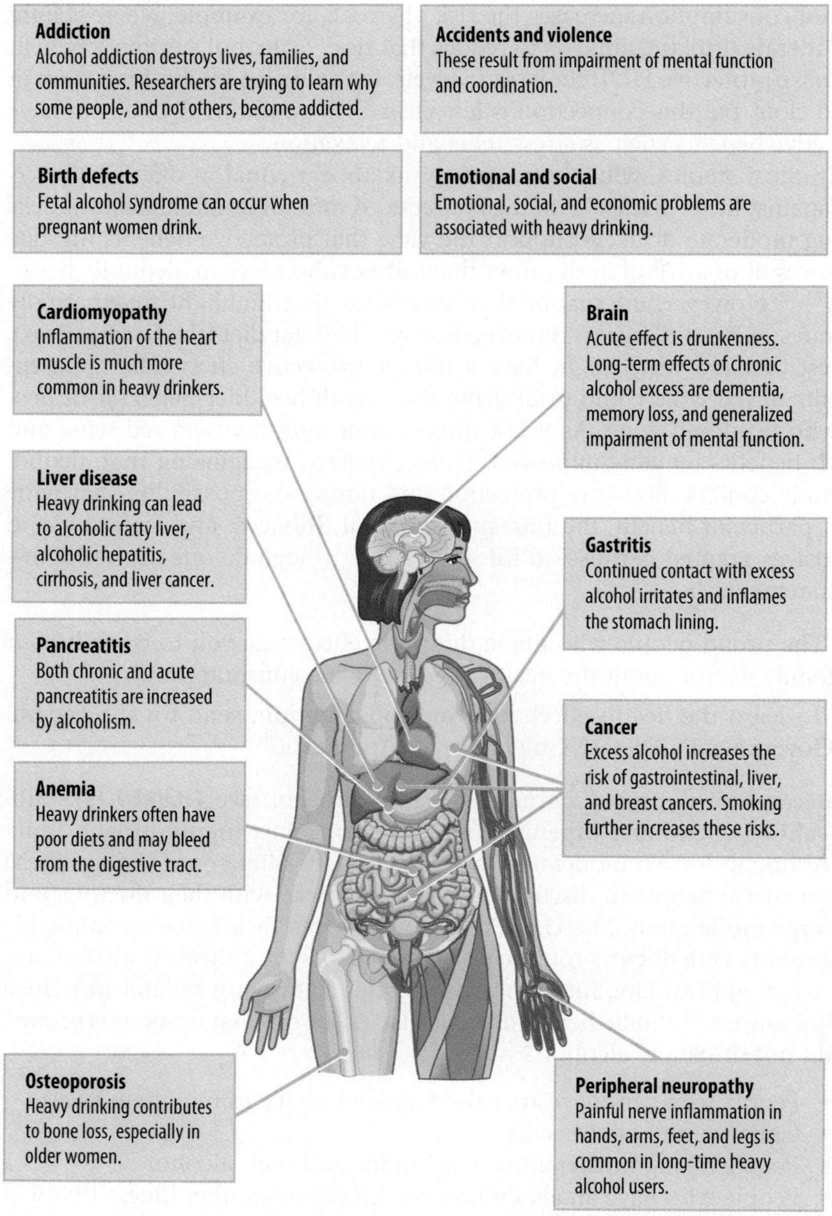

Addiction
Alcohol addiction destroys lives, families, and communities. Researchers are trying to learn why some people, and not others, become addicted.
Accidents and violence
These result from impairment of mental function and coordination.
Birth defects
Fetal alcohol syndrome can occur when pregnant women drink.
Emotional and social
Emotional, social, and economic problems are associated with heavy drinking.
Cardiomyopathy
Inflammation of the heart muscle is much more common in heavy drinkers.
Brain
Acute effect is drunkenness. Long-term effects of chronic alcohol excess are dementia, memory loss, and generalized impairment of mental function.
Liver disease
Heavy drinking can lead to alcoholic fatty liver, alcoholic hepatitis, cirrhosis, and liver cancer.
Gastritis
Continued contact with excess alcohol irritates and inflames the stomach lining.
Pancreatitis
Both chronic and acute pancreatitis are increased by alcoholism.
Cancer
Excess alcohol increases the risk of gastrointestinal, liver, and breast cancers. Smoking further increases these risks.
Anemia
Heavy drinkers often have poor diets and may bleed from the digestive tract.
Osteoporosis
Heavy drinking contributes to bone loss, especially in older women.
Peripheral neuropathy
Painful nerve inflammation in hands, arms, feet, and legs is common in long-time heavy alcohol users.

FIGURE 7.13 Harmful effects of alcohol. Because excess alcohol reaches all parts of the body, it causes a wide array of physical problems. Here are some of the ways alcohol can cause harm.

Label to Table

Have you ever wondered how much protein, carbohydrate, and fat are in a can of beer? If you've ever looked at a beer label, you know it's quite different from a food label. Look at the following information from a can of light beer and see if you can calculate the calories from carbohydrate, fat, and protein.

Serving size = 12 fl oz
Calories = 103 (kcal)
Carbohydrate = 5 g
Protein = 1 g
Fat = 0 g

First, to figure out how many calories come from the three macronutrients, multiply the number of grams by their respective calorie contribution per gram:

5 g carbohydrate × 4 kcal/g = 20 kcal from carbohydrate

1 g protein ×4 kcal/g = 4 kcal from protein

0 g fat × 9 kcal/g = 0 kcal from fat

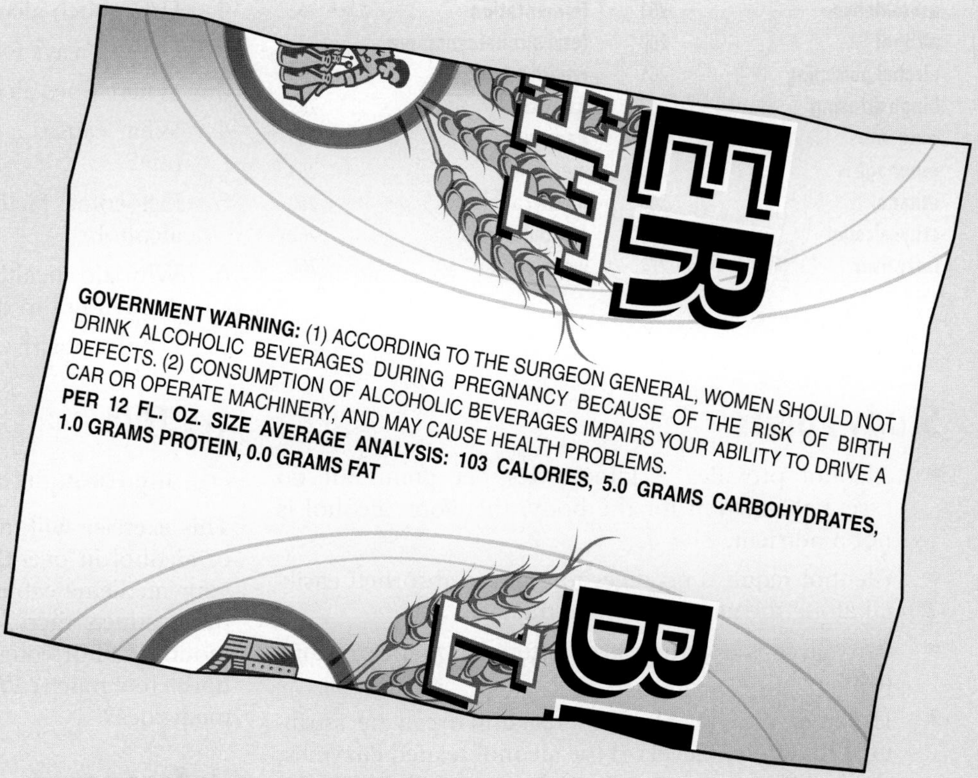
GOVERNMENT WARNING: (1) ACCORDING TO THE SURGEON GENERAL, WOMEN SHOULD NOT DRINK ALCOHOLIC BEVERAGES DURING PREGNANCY BECAUSE OF THE RISK OF BIRTH DEFECTS. (2) CONSUMPTION OF ALCOHOLIC BEVERAGES IMPAIRS YOUR ABILITY TO DRIVE A CAR OR OPERATE MACHINERY, AND MAY CAUSE HEALTH PROBLEMS.
PER 12 FL. OZ. SIZE AVERAGE ANALYSIS: 103 CALORIES, 5.0 GRAMS CARBOHYDRATES, 1.0 GRAMS PROTEIN, 0.0 GRAMS FAT

Uh-oh. Is this adding up correctly? So far, we have accounted for only 24 of the 103 kilocalories in this beer. Where are the other 79 kilocalories? Don't forget that many of the calories in beer come from alcohol, and it's easy to calculate just how many grams are in this can of light beer. Remember, alcohol has 7 kilocalories per gram, so the remaining 79 kilocalories come from 11 grams of alcohol (79 ÷ 7 = 11.3).

So, for the 103 kilocalories this beer provides, you get very little (if any) protein, carbohydrate, or fat. Instead, a majority of the calories come from alcohol. This holds true for the micronutrients as well: Beer contains negligible amounts of vitamins or minerals.

This is why people say alcoholic beverages have only "empty calories." They provide calories, but almost no nutrient value!

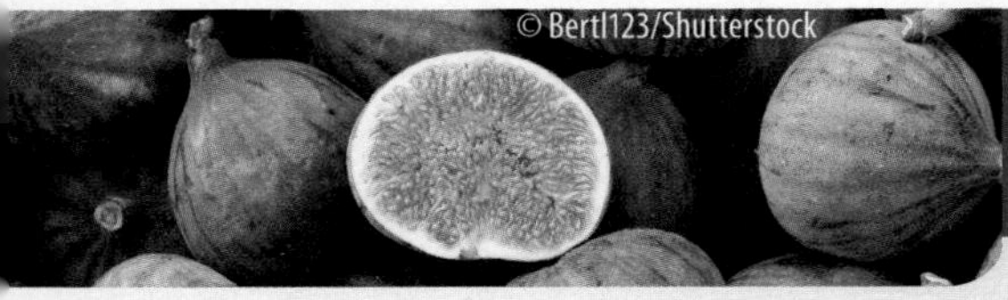

Learning Portfolio

Key Terms

acetaldehyde	263	fermentation	262
alcohol	260	fetal alcohol syndrome	272
alcohol poisoning	265	French paradox	277
binge drinking	263	gastritis	269
congeners	262	hangover	265
esophagitis	269	methanol	260
ethanol	260	methyl alcohol	260
ethyl alcohol	260	standard drink	262
fatty liver	272	wood alcohol	260

Study Points

- Alcohol provides 7 kilocalories per gram but no essential function for the body; therefore, alcohol is not a nutrient.
- Alcohol requires no digestion and is absorbed easily all along the gastrointestinal tract.
- Fatty liver is apparent even after one night of binge drinking.
- Different rates of alcohol breakdown can be attributed to different levels of the alcohol-related enzymes; these differences are caused by genetic and gender variations.
- Alcohol affects all organs in the body, but the most obvious effects are in the brain and nervous system, the GI system, and the liver.
- Malnutrition among alcoholics is common as a result of poor food choices and alcohol's interference with the absorption, breakdown, and excretion of nutrients.
- Fetal alcohol syndrome is one of the most devastating consequences of alcohol consumption, and it is preventable.
- Moderate alcohol consumption has been linked to reduced risk of heart disease.
- The potential benefits of moderate alcohol consumption might be related to effects on lipoprotein levels and the antioxidant components of beverages such as wine.
- Health organizations recommend moderate to no alcohol consumption.

Study Questions

1. How much alcohol is in beer, wine, and liquor?
2. List the ways food helps to delay or avoid inebriation.
3. Where does alcohol breakdown take place?
4. What causes a hangover? Is there any way to relieve one?
5. List some factors that affect our ability to process alcohol.
6. Why do health care professionals advise pregnant women not to drink alcohol?
7. List the positive and negative effects of alcohol.

Try This

Cruising Through the Medicine Cabinet

This exercise will increase your awareness of the amounts of alcohol in over-the-counter medications. Look through your medicine cabinet and check the ingredient lists of all the products there. In particular, take a close look at any mouthwash or cough syrup. Which products contain alcohol? How much? What do you think its purpose is in these medicines?

References

1. U.S. Department of Agriculture and U.S. Department of Health and Human Services. *Dietary Guidelines for Americans, 2015*. 8th ed. Washington, DC: U.S. http://health.gov/dietaryguidelines/2015/guidelines/. Accessed March 24, 2015.
2. Courtney KE, Polich J. Binge drinking in young adults: data, definitions, and determinants. *Psychol Bull*. 2009;135(1):142–156.
3. Centers for Disease Control and Prevention. Alcohol and public health: fact sheets—binge drinking. http://www.cdc.gov/alcohol/fact-sheets/binge-drinking.htm. Accessed January 27, 2016.
4. Ibid.
5. Centers for Disease Control and Prevention. Alcohol and public health: facts sheets—alcohol use and your health. http://www.cdc.gov/alcohol/fact-sheets/alcohol-use.htm. Accessed January 27, 2016.
6. National Institute on Alcohol Abuse and Alcoholism. *Underage Drinking: A Major Public Health Problem*. Bethesda, MD: Author; 2003. Alcohol Alert No. 59.
7. Minino AM. *Mortality Among Teenagers Aged 12–19 Years: United States, 1999–2006*. Hyattsville, MD: National Centers for Health Statistics; 2010. Data Brief No 37.
8. National Institute on Alcohol Abuse and Alcoholism. *Underage Drinking*. Op cit.
9. Roe DA. *Alcohol and the Diet*. Westport, CT: AVI Publishing; 1979.
10. Ibid.

11. Paasa R, Hovda KE, Jacobsen D. Methanol poisoning and long-term sequelae—a six year follow-up after a large methanol outbreak. *BMC Clin Pharmacol*. 2009;9:5.
12. Roe DA. *Alcohol and the Diet*. Op cit.
13. Haseba T, Ohno Y. A new view of alcohol metabolism and alcoholism—role of the high K_m class III alcohol dehydrogenase (ADH3). *Int J Environ Res Pub Health*. 2010;7(3):1076–1092.
14. Mitchinson A. Hangovers: uncongenial congeners. *Nature*. 2009;462(7276):992.
15. U.S. Department of Agriculture and U.S. Department of Health and Human Services. *Dietary Guidelines for Americans, 2015*. 8th ed. Washington, DC: U.S. http://health.gov/dietaryguidelines/2015/guidelines/. Accessed March 24, 2015. Op cit.
16. Doll R, Peto R, Boreham J, et al. Mortality in relation to alcohol consumption: a prospective study among male British doctors. *Int J Epidemiol*. 2005;34:199–204.
17. Marczinski CA, Fillmore MT, Bardgett ME, Howard MA. Effects of energy drinks mixed with alcohol on behavioral control: risks for college students consuming trendy cocktails. *Alcohol Clin Exp Res*. 2011;35:1282–1292.
18. Foster SE, Vaughan RD, Foster WH, Califano JA. Estimate of the commercial value of underage drinking and adult abusive and dependent drinking to the alcohol industry. *Arch Pediatr Adolesc Med*. 2006;160(5):473–478.
19. Zakhari S. Overview: how is alcohol metabolized by the body? *Alcohol Res Health*. 2006;29(4):245–254.
20. Ibid.
21. Verster JC, Penning R. Treatment and prevention of alcohol hangover. *Curr Drug Abuse Rev*. 2010;3(2):103–109.
22. Piasecki RM, Robertson BM, Epler AJ. Hangover and risk for alcohol use disorder: existing evidence and potential mechanisms. *Curr Drug Abuse Rev*. 2010;3(2):92–102.
23. Anderson J, Vitale T, et al. *Eat Right! Healthy Eating in College and Beyond*. San Francisco: Pearson Benjamin Cummings; 2007:85.
24. Ibid.
25. Tomczyk M, Zocko-Koncic M, Chrostek L. Phytotherapy of alcoholism. *Nat Prod Commun*. 2012;7(2):273–280.
26. Ibid.
27. Fruchter LL, Alexopoulou I, Lau KK. Acute interstitial nephritis with acetaminophen and alcohol intoxication. *Ital J Pediatr*. 2011;15(37):17.
28. Ibid.
29. Chen YC, Peng GS, Tsao TP, Wang MF, Lu RB, Yin SJ. Pharmacokinetic and pharmacodynamic basis for overcoming acetaldehyde-induced adverse reaction in Asian alcoholics, heterozygous for the variant *ALDH2*2* gene allele. *Pharmacogenet Genomics*. 2009;19(8):588–599.
30. Vallee BL. Alcohol in the Western world. *Sci Am*. June 1998:80–85.
31. Buffa R, Floris GU, Putzu PF, Marini E. Body composition variations in ageing. *Coll Antropol*. 2011;35(1):259–265.
32. Dufour MC. What is moderate drinking? *Alcohol Res Health*. 1999;23(1):1–14.
33. U.S. Department of Agriculture, Center for Nutrition Policy and Promotion. *Does Alcohol Have a Place in a Healthy Diet?* Washington, DC: Center for Nutrition Policy and Promotion; 1997. Nutrition Insights No. 4.
34. National Institute on Alcohol Abuse and Alcoholism. *Alcohol: An Important Women's Health Issue*. Bethesda, MD: Author; 2004. Alcohol Alert No. 62.
35. Swift R, Davidson D. Alcohol hangover: mechanisms and mediators. *Alcohol Health Res World*. 1998;22:54–60.
36. Baraona E, Abbittan CS, Dohmen K, et al. Gender differences in pharmacokinetics of alcohol. *Alcohol Clin Exp Res*. 2001;25:502–507.
37. Pinel JP. *Biopsychology*. Boston: Allyn & Bacon; 2006.
38. Friedman TW, Robinson SR, Yelland GW. Impaired perceptual judgment at low blood alcohol concentrations. *Alcohol*. 2011;45(7):711–718.
39. U.S. Department of Health and Human Services. *Hypoglycemia*. Washington, DC: National Institutes of Health; 2006. NIH publication 03-3926.
40. Parada M, Corral M, Caamano-Isorna F, et al. Binge drinking and declarative memory in university students. *Alcohol Clin Exp Res*. 2011;35(8):1475–1484.
41. Guha N, Boffetta P, et. al. Oral health and risk of squamous cell carcinoma of the head and neck and esophagus: results of two multicentric case-control studies. *Am J Epidemiol*. 2007;166(10):1159–1173.
42. Centers for Disease Control and Prevention. FastStats: chronic liver disease and cirrhosis. http://www.cdc.gov/nchs/fastats/liver-disease.htm. Accessed January 27, 2016.
43. Lieber CS. Alcoholic fatty liver: its pathogenesis and mechanism of progression to inflammation and fibrosis. *Alcohol*. 2004;34(1):9–19.
44. Dey A, Cederbaum AI. Alcohol and oxidative liver damage. *Hepatology*. 2006;43(2 suppl):S63–S74.
45. University of Maryland Medical Center. Liver disease: alcohol-induced liver disease. http://umm.edu/health/medical/ency/articles/alcoholic-liver-disease. Accessed April 30, 2012.
46. Ibid.
47. Bruha R, Dvorak K, Petrtyl J. Alcoholic liver disease. *World J Hepatol*. 2012;4(3):81–90.
48. Thompson BL, Levitt P, Stanwood GD. Prenatal exposure to drugs: effects on brain development and implications for policy and education. *Neuroscience*. 2009;10(4):303–312.
49. Centers for Disease Control and Prevention. Alcohol consumption among pregnant and childbearing-aged women—United States, 2002. *MMWR*. 2004;53:1178–1181.
50. Centers for Disease Control and Prevention. Fetal alcohol spectrum disorders (FASDs): data and statistics. http://www.cdc.gov/ncbddd/fasd/data.html. Accessed January 27, 2016.
51. Breslow RA, Guenther PM, Juan W, Graubard B. Alcoholic beverage consumption, nutrient intakes, and diet quality in the US adult population, 1999–2006. *J Am Diet Assoc*. 2010;110(4):551–562.
52. Harrop E, Marlatt GA. The comorbidity of substance use disorders and eating disorders in women: prevalence, etiology, and treatment. *Addict Behav*. 2010;35(5):392–398.
53. Chase JR, Poolman MG, Fell DA. Contribution of NADH increases to ethanol's inhibition of retinol oxidation by human ADH isoforms. *Alcohol Clin Exp Res*. 2009;33(4):571–580.
54. Lieber CS. Nutrition and diet in alcoholism. In: Shils ME, Olson JA, Shike M, eds. *Modern Nutrition in Health and Disease*. 9th ed. Philadelphia: Lippincott Williams & Wilkins; 2004.
55. Ibid.
56. Ibid.
57. Ibid.
58. MacArthur GJ, Smth MC, Meloti R, Heron J, et al. Patterns of alcohol use and multiple risk behavior by gender during early and late adolescence: the ALSPAC cohort. *J Public Health (Oxf)*. 2012;34(suppl 1):i20–i30.
59. National Institute on Alcohol Abuse and Alcoholism. *State of the Science Report on the Effects of Moderate Drinking*. Bethesda, MD. 2003.
60. U.S. Department of Agriculture and U.S. Department of Health and Human Services. *Dietary Guidelines for Americans, 2015*. 8th ed. Washington, DC: U.S. http://health.gov/dietaryguidelines/2015/guidelines/. Accessed March 24, 2015. Op cit.
61. Shuval K, Barlow CE, Chartier KG, Gabriel KP. Cardiorespiratory fitness, alcohol, and mortality in men: the Copper Center Longitudinal Study. *Am J Prev Med*. 2010;42(5):460–467.

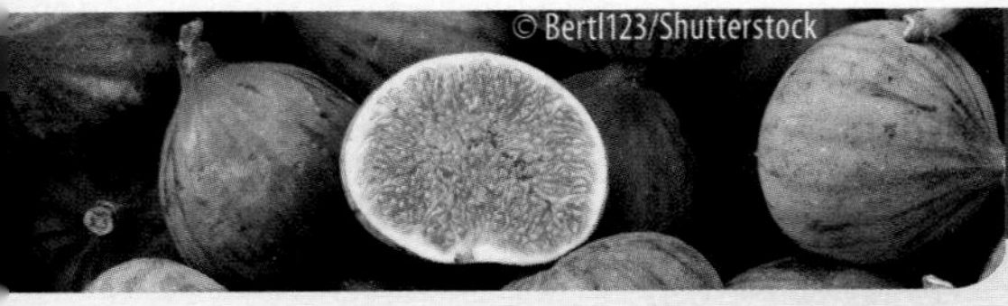

Learning Portfolio (continued)

62. Kim SJ, Kim DJ. Alcoholism and diabetes mellitus. *Diabetes Metab J.* 2012;36(2):108–115.
63. Malinski MK, Sesso HD, Lopez-Jimenez F, et al. *Alcohol consumption and cardiovascular mortality in hypertensive patients*. Paper presented at 41st Annual Conference on Cardiovascular Disease Epidemiology and Prevention; March 2, 2001; San Antonio, TX.
64. Shuval K, Barlow CE, Chartier KG, Gabriel KP. Cardiorespiratory fitness, alcohol, and mortality in men. Op cit.
65. Estruch R, Sacanella E, Mota F, et al. Moderate consumption of red wine, but not gin, decreases erythrocyte superoxide dismutase activity: a randomized cross-over trial. *Nutr Metab Cardiovasc Dis*. 2011;21(1):46–53.
66. Sun Q, Townsend MK, Okereke OI, et al. Alcohol consumption at midlife and successful ageing in women: a prospective cohort analysis in the Nurses' Health Study. *PLOS Med*. 2011;8(9):e1001090. http://www.plosmedicine.org/article/info%3Adoi%2F10.1371%2Fjournal.pmed.1001090. Accessed January 27, 2016.
67. Gaziano JM, Gaziano TA, Glynn RJ, et al. Light-to-moderate alcohol consumption and mortality in the Physicians' Health Study enrollment cohort. *J Am Coll Cardiol*. 2000;35:96–105.
68. Kloner RA, Rezkalla SH. To drink or not to drink? That is the question. *Circulation*. 2007;116:1306-1317.
69. Stockley CS. Is it merely a myth that alcoholic beverages such as red wine can be cardioprotective? *J Sci Food Agric*. 2012;92(9):1815–1821.
70. Ibid.
71. Bobak M, Skodova Z, Marmot M. Effect of beer drinking on risk of myocardial infarction: population based case-control study. *BMJ*. 2000;320:1378–1379.

72. Mukamal KJ, Conigrave KM, Mittleman MA, et al. Roles of drinking pattern and type of alcohol consumed in coronary heart disease in men. *N Engl J Med.* 2003;348:109–118.
73. Tjonneland A, Gronbaek M, Stripp C, Overvad K. Wine intake and diet in a random sample of 48,763 Danish men and women. *Am J Clin Nutr.* 1999;69:49–54.
74. U.S. Treasury Department, Bureau of Alcohol, Tobacco and Firearms. Treasury announces actions concerning labeling of alcoholic beverages. Press release. February 5, 1999.
75. Saitz R. Unhealthy alcohol use. *N Engl J Med.* 2005;352:596–607.
76. Pearson TA. Alcohol and heart disease. *Circulation.* 1996;94:3023–3025.
77. U.S. Department of Agriculture and U.S. Department of Health and Human Services. *Dietary Guidelines for Americans, 2015.* 8th ed. Washington, DC: U.S. http://health.gov/dietaryguidelines/2015/guidelines/. Accessed March 24, 2015. Op cit.

Chapter **8**

Metabolism

Revised by Don Ross

THINK About It

1 You are driving on "the energy highway." You stop at the tollbooth. What kind of currency do you need to pay the toll?

2 When you think of "cell power," what comes to mind?

3 What is meant by the saying "Fat burns in a flame of carbohydrate"?

4 When it comes to fasting, what's your body's first priority?

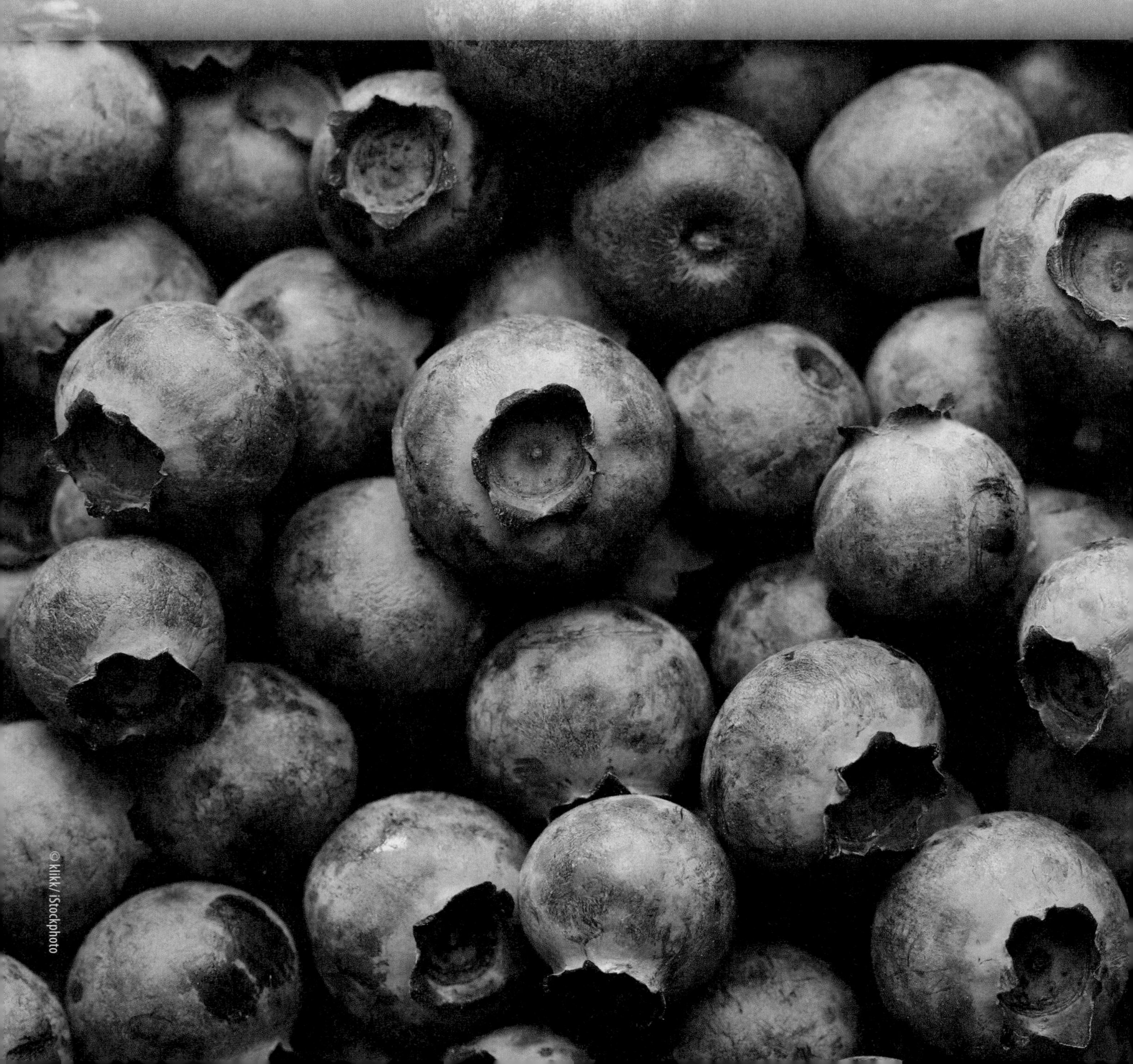

CHAPTER Menu

- Energy: Fuel for Work
- Who Are the Key Energy Players?
- Breakdown and Release of Energy
- Alcohol Metabolism
- Biosynthesis and Storage
- Regulation of Metabolism
- Special States
- Key Terms
- Study Points
- Study Questions
- Try This
- References

LEARNING Objectives

- Differentiate between anabolic and catabolic reactions.
- Describe ATP, NADH, $FADH_2$, and NADPH.
- Describe the process of extracting ATP from carbohydrates, fat, and protein.
- Trace the route of biosynthesis and the storage of glucose, fatty acids, and amino acids.
- Discuss the role of insulin in energy storage and glucose regulation.
- Discuss the roles of glucagon, cortisol, and epinephrine in the breakdown of glycogen and amino acids to make glucose by way of gluconeogenesis.
- Describe how the body achieves homeostasis in the feasting and fasting states.
- Explain how energy use differs in the states of psychological stress, diabetes, obesity, and exercise.

Your body is a wonderfully efficient factory. It accepts raw materials (food), burns some to generate power, uses some to produce finished goods, routes the rest to storage, and discards waste and by-products. Constant turnover of your stored inventory keeps it fresh. Your body draws on these stored raw materials to produce compounds, and nutrient intake replenishes the supply.

Do you ever wonder how your biological factory responds to changing supply and demand? Under normal circumstances, it hums along nicely with all processes in balance. When supply exceeds demand, your body stores the excess raw materials in inventory. When supply fails to meet demand, your body draws on these stored materials to meet its needs. Your biological factory never stops; even though a storage or energy-production process might dominate, all your factory operations are active at all times.

Collectively, these processes are known as **metabolism** (see **FIGURE 8.1**). Whereas some metabolic reactions break down molecules to extract energy, others synthesize building blocks to produce new molecules. To carry out metabolic processes, thousands of chemical reactions occur every moment in cells throughout your body. The most active metabolic sites include your liver, muscle, and brain cells.

▶ **metabolism** All chemical reactions within organisms that enable them to maintain life. The two main categories of metabolism are catabolism and anabolism.

Energy: Fuel for Work

To operate, machines need energy. Cars use gasoline for fuel, factory machinery uses electricity, and windmills rely on wind power. So, what about you? All cells require energy to sustain life. Even during sleep, your body uses energy for breathing, pumping blood, maintaining body temperature, delivering oxygen to tissues, removing waste products, synthesizing new tissue for growth, and repairing damaged or worn-out tissues. When awake, you need additional energy for physical movement (such as standing, walking, and talking) and for the digestion and absorption of foods.

Where does the energy come from to power your body's "machinery"? Biological systems use heat, mechanical, electrical, and chemical forms of energy. Our cells get their energy from **chemical energy** held in the molecular bonds of carbohydrates, fats, and protein—the energy macronutrients—as well as alcohol.[1] The chemical energy in foods and beverages originates as light energy from the sun. Green plants use light energy to make carbohydrate in a process called **photosynthesis**. In photosynthesis, carbon dioxide (CO_2) from the air combines with water (H_2O) from the earth to form a carbohydrate, usually glucose ($C_6H_{12}O_6$), and oxygen (O_2). Plants store glucose as starch and release oxygen into the atmosphere. Plants such as corn, peas, squash, turnips, potatoes, and rice store especially high amounts of starch in their edible parts. In the glucose molecule, the chemical bonds between the carbon

▶ **chemical energy** Energy contained in the bonds between atoms of a molecule.

▶ **photosynthesis** The process by which green plants use radiant energy from the sun to produce carbohydrates (hexoses) from carbon dioxide and water.

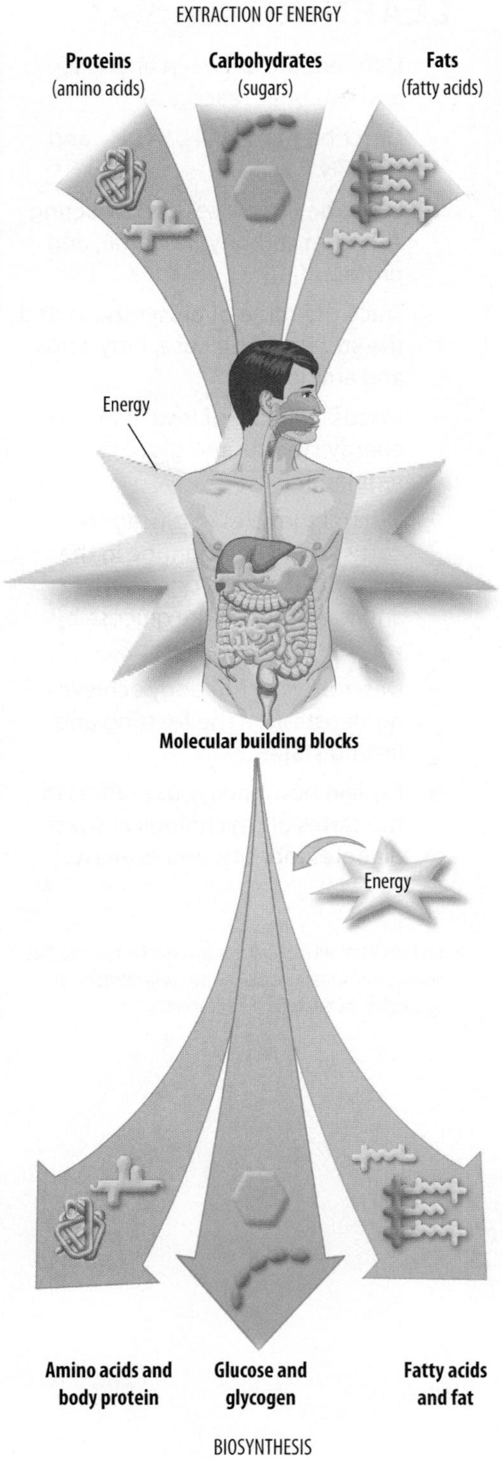

FIGURE 8.1 Metabolism. Cells use metabolic reactions to extract energy from food and to form building blocks for biosynthesis.

(C) and hydrogen (H) atoms hold energy from the sun. When our bodies extract energy from food and convert it to a form that our cells can use, we lose more than half of the total food energy as heat.[2]

Within any system (including the universe), the total amount of energy is constant. Although energy can change from one form to another and can move from one location to another, the system never gains or loses energy. This principle, called the first law of thermodynamics, is known as conservation of energy.

Transferring Food Energy to Cellular Energy

Although burning food releases energy as heat, we cannot use heat to power the many cellular functions that maintain life. Rather than using combustion, we transfer energy from food to a form that our cells can use (see **FIGURE 8.2**). This transfer is not completely efficient; we lose roughly

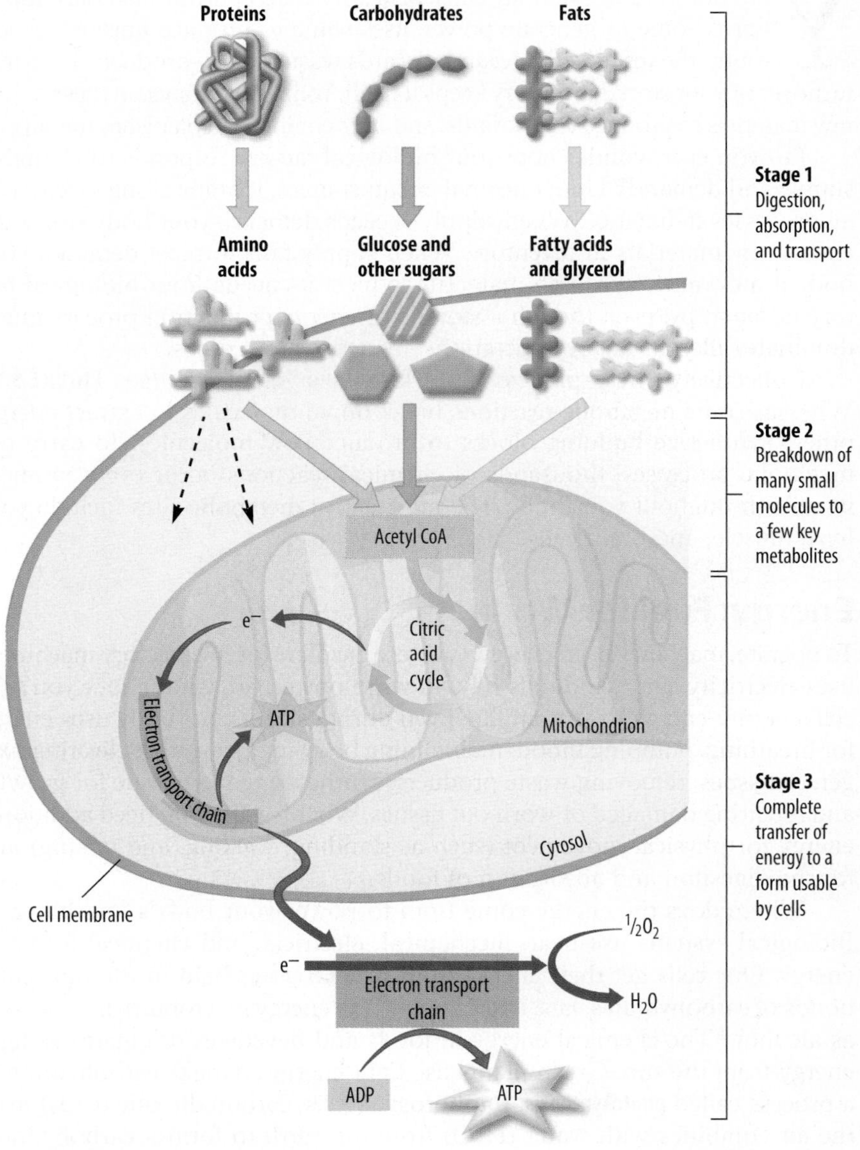

FIGURE 8.2 Energy extraction from food. In the first stage, the body breaks down food into amino acids, monosaccharides, and fatty acids. In the second stage, cells degrade these molecules to a few simple units, such as acetyl CoA, that are pervasive in metabolism. In the third stage, the oxygen-dependent reactions of the citric acid cycle and electron transport chain liberate large amounts of energy in the form of ATP.

half of the total food energy as heat as our bodies extract energy from food in three stages[3]:

- *Stage 1: Digestion, absorption, and transportation:* Digestion breaks food down into small subunits—simple sugars, fatty acids, monoglycerides, glycerol, and amino acids—that the small intestine can absorb. The circulatory system then transports these nutrients to tissues throughout the body.
- *Stage 2: Breakdown of many small molecules to a few key metabolites:* Inside individual cells, chemical reactions convert simple sugars, fatty acids, glycerol, and amino acids into a few key **metabolites** (products of metabolic reactions). This process liberates a small amount of usable energy.
- *Stage 3: Transfer of energy to a form that cells can use:* The complete breakdown of metabolites to carbon dioxide and water liberates large amounts of energy. The reactions during this stage are responsible for converting more than 90 percent of the available food energy to a form that our bodies can use.

▶ **metabolites** Any substances produced during metabolism.

What Is Metabolism?

Metabolism is a general term that encompasses all chemical changes occurring in living organisms. The term **metabolic pathway** describes a series of chemical reactions that either break down a large compound into smaller units (**catabolism**) or build more complex molecules from smaller ones (**anabolism**).[4] For example, when you eat bread or rice, the GI tract breaks down the starch into glucose units. Cells can further catabolize these glucose units to release energy for activities such as muscle contractions. Conversely, anabolic reactions take available glucose molecules and assemble them into glycogen for storage. **FIGURE 8.3** illustrates catabolism and anabolism.

Metabolic pathways are never completely inactive. Their activity continually ebbs and flows in response to internal and external events. Imagine, for example, that your instructor keeps you late and you have only five minutes

▶ **metabolic pathway** A series of chemical reactions that either break down a large compound into smaller units (catabolism) or synthesize more complex molecules from smaller ones (anabolism).

▶ **catabolism** [ca-TA-bol-iz-um] Any metabolic process whereby cells break down complex substances into simpler, smaller ones.

▶ **anabolism** [an-AH-bol-iz-um] Any metabolic process whereby cells convert simple substances into more complex ones.

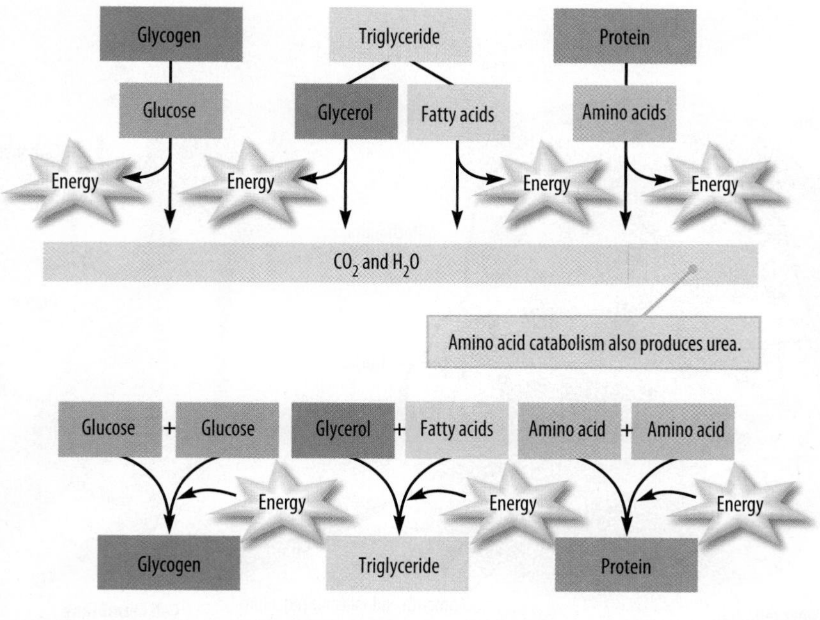

FIGURE 8.3 Catabolism and anabolism. Catabolic reactions break down molecules and release energy and other products. Anabolic reactions consume energy as they assemble complex molecules.

▶ **cells** The basic structural units of all living tissues, which have two major parts: the nucleus and the cytoplasm.

▶ **nucleus** The primary site of genetic information in the cell, enclosed in a double-layered membrane. The nucleus contains the chromosomes and is the site of messenger RNA (mRNA) and ribosomal RNA (rRNA) synthesis, the "machinery" for protein synthesis in the cytosol.

▶ **cytosol** The semifluid inside the cell membrane, excluding organelles. The cytosol is the site of glycolysis and fatty acid synthesis.

▶ **cytoplasm** The material of the cell, excluding the cell nucleus and cell membranes. The cytoplasm includes the semifluid cytosol, the organelles, and other particles.

▶ **organelles** Various membrane-bound structures that form part of the cytoplasm. Organelles, including mitochondria and lysosomes, perform specialized metabolic functions.

to get to your next class. As you hustle across campus, your body ramps up energy production to fuel the demand created by your rapidly contracting muscles. As you sit in your next class, your body continues to break down and extract glucose from the banana you recently ate. Your body reassembles the glucose into branched chains of glycogen to replenish the stores you depleted while running across campus.

The Cell Is the Metabolic Processing Center

Cells are the "work centers" of metabolism (see **FIGURE 8.4**). Although our bodies are made up of different types of cells (e.g., liver cells, brain cells, kidney cells, muscle cells), most have a similar structure. The basic animal cell has two major parts: the cell **nucleus** and a membrane-enclosed space called the **cytoplasm**. As we zoom in for a closer look, we see that the semifluid **cytosol** fills the cytoplasm. Floating in the cytosol are many **organelles**, small units that

Organelles

Endoplasmic reticulum (ER)
- An extensive membrane system extending from the nuclear membrane.
- Rough ER: The outer membrane surface contains ribosomes.
- Smooth ER: Devoid of ribosomes, the site of lipid synthesis.

Golgi apparatus
- A system of stacked membrane-encased discs.
- The site of extensive modification, sorting, and packaging of compounds for transport.

Lysosome
- Vesicle containing enzymes that digest intracellular materials and recycle the components.

Mitochondrion
- Contains two highly specialized membranes, an outer membrane and a highly folded inner membrane. Membranes are separated by narrow intermembrane space. Inner membrane encloses space called mitochondrial matrix.
- Often called the power plant of the cell. Site where most of the energy from carbohydrate, protein, and fat is captured in ATP (adenosine triphosphate).
- About 2,000 mitochondria in a cell.

Ribosome
- Site of protein synthesis.

Nucleus
- Contains genetic information in the DNA of chromosomes.
- Site of RNA synthesis—RNA needed for protein synthesis.
- Enclosed in a double-layered membrane.

Cytoplasm
- Enclosed in the cell membrane and separated from the nucleus by the nuclear membrane.
- Filled with particles and organelles which are dispersed in a clear semiliquid fluid called cytosol.

Cytosol
- The semifluid inside the cell membrane.
- Site of glycolysis and fatty acid synthesis.

Cell Membrane
- A double-layered sheet, made up of lipid and protein, that encases the cell.
- Controls the passage of substances in and out of the cell.
- Contains receptors for hormones and other regulatory compounds.

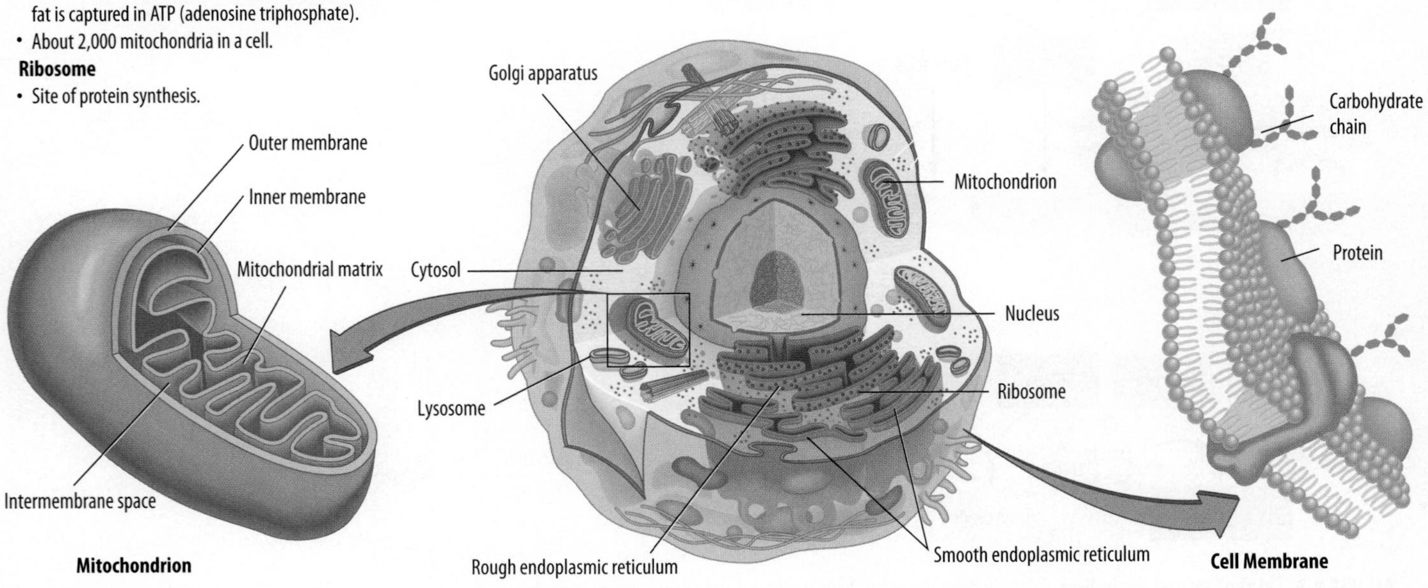

FIGURE 8.4 Cell structure. Liver cells, brain cells, kidney cells, muscle cells, and so forth all have a similar structure.

perform specialized metabolic functions. A large number of these organelles—the capsule-like **mitochondria**—are power generators that contain many important energy-producing pathways.

Enzymes, which are catalytic proteins, speed up chemical reactions in metabolic pathways. Many enzymes are inactive unless they are combined with certain smaller molecules called **cofactors**, which usually are derived from a vitamin or mineral. Vitamin-derived cofactors also are called **coenzymes**. All the B vitamins form coenzymes used in metabolic reactions.

Key Concepts Metabolism encompasses the many reactions that take place in cells to build tissue, produce energy, break down compounds, and do other cellular work. Anabolism refers to reactions that build compounds, such as protein or glycogen. Catabolism is the breakdown of compounds to yield energy. Mitochondria, the power plants within cells, contain many of the breakdown pathways that produce energy.

Who Are the Key Energy Players?

THINK About It 1

Certain compounds have recurring roles in metabolic activities. **Adenosine triphosphate (ATP)** is the fundamental energy molecule used to power cellular functions, so it is known as the universal energy currency. Two other molecules, **NADH** and **$FADH_2$**, are important couriers that carry energy for the synthesis of ATP. A similar energy carrier, **NADPH**, delivers energy for **biosynthesis**.

ATP: The Body's Energy Currency

To power its needs, your body must convert the energy in food to a readily usable form—ATP. This universal energy currency kick-starts many energy-releasing processes, such as the breakdown of glucose and fatty acids, and powers energy-consuming processes, such as building glucose from other compounds. Remember that making large molecules from smaller ones, like constructing a building from bricks, requires energy.

Production of ATP is the fundamental goal of metabolism's energy-producing pathways. Just as the ancient Romans could claim that all roads lead to Rome, you can say that, with a few exceptions, your body's energy-producing pathways lead to ATP production.

The ATP molecule has three phosphate groups attached to adenosine, which is an organic compound. Because breaking the bonds between the phosphate groups releases a tremendous amount of energy, ATP is an energy-rich molecule (see **FIGURE 8.5**). Cells can use this energy to power biological work. When a metabolic reaction breaks the first phosphate bond, it breaks down ATP to **adenosine diphosphate (ADP)** and **pyrophosphate (P_i)**. Breaking the remaining phosphate bond releases an equal amount of energy and breaks down ADP to **adenosine monophosphate (AMP)** and P_i.

Because the reaction can proceed in either direction, ATP and ADP are interconvertible, as **FIGURE 8.6** shows. When extracting energy from carbohydrate, protein, and fat, ADP binds P_i, forming a phosphate bond and capturing energy in a new ATP molecule. When the reaction flows in the opposite direction, ATP releases P_i, breaking a phosphate bond and liberating energy while re-forming ADP. This liberated energy can power biological activities such as motion, active transport across cell membranes, biosynthesis, and signal amplification.

The body's pool of ATP is a small, immediately accessible energy reservoir rather than a long-term energy reserve. The typical lifetime of an ATP molecule is less than one minute, and ATP production increases or decreases in direct relation to energy needs. At rest, you use about 40 kilograms of ATP in 24 hours (an average rate of about 28 grams per minute). In contrast, if you

▶ **mitochondria (mitochondrion)** The sites of aerobic production of ATP, where most of the energy from carbohydrate, protein, and fat is captured. Called the "power plants" of the cell, the mitochondria contain two highly specialized membranes, an outer membrane and a highly folded inner membrane, that separate two compartments, the internal matrix space and the narrow intermembrane space. A human cell contains about 2,000 mitochondria.

▶ **cofactors** Compounds required for an enzyme to be active. Cofactors include coenzymes and metal ions such as iron (Fe^{2+}), copper (Cu^{2+}), and magnesium (Mg^{2+}).

▶ **coenzymes** Organic compounds, often B-vitamin derivatives, that combine with an inactive enzyme to form an active enzyme. Coenzymes associate closely with these enzymes, allowing them to catalyze certain metabolic reactions in a cell.

▶ **adenosine triphosphate (ATP)** [ah-DEN-oh-seen try-FOS-fate] A high-energy compound that is the main direct fuel that cells use to synthesize molecules, contract muscles, transport substances, and perform other tasks.

▶ **NADH** The reduced form of nicotinamide adenine dinucleotide (NAD^+). This coenzyme, derived from the B vitamin niacin, acts as an electron carrier in cells and undergoes reversible oxidation and reduction.

▶ **$FADH_2$** The reduced form of flavin adenine dinucleotide (FAD). This coenzyme, which is derived from the B vitamin riboflavin, acts as an electron carrier in cells and undergoes reversible oxidation and reduction.

▶ **NADPH** The reduced form of nicotinamide adenine dinucleotide phosphate. This coenzyme, which is derived from the B vitamin niacin, acts as an electron carrier in cells, undergoing reversible oxidation and reduction. The oxidized form is $NADP^+$.

▶ **biosynthesis** Chemical reactions that form simple molecules into complex biomolecules, especially carbohydrate, lipids, protein, nucleotides, and nucleic acids.

▶ **adenosine diphosphate (ADP)** The compound produced upon hydrolysis of ATP and used to synthesize ATP. Composed of adenosine and two phosphate groups.

▶ **pyrophosphate (P_i)** Inorganic phosphate. This high-energy phosphate group is an important component of ATP, ADP, and AMP.

▶ **adenosine monophosphate (AMP)** Hydrolysis product of ADP and of nucleic acids. Composed of adenosine and one phosphate group.

Quick Bite

Key Players in the Energy Game

Each of the "key players" in the energy game has a common acronym by which it is usually called:

- *ATP:* Adenosine triphosphate
- *NAD^+:* Nicotinamide adenine dinucleotide (oxidized)
- *NADH:* Nicotinamide adenine dinucleotide (reduced)
- *$NADP^+$:* Nicotinamide adenine dinucleotide phosphate (oxidized)
- *NADPH:* Nicotinamide adenine dinucleotide phosphate (reduced)
- *FAD^+:* Flavin adenine dinucleotide (oxidized)
- *$FADH_2$:* Flavin adenine dinucleotide (reduced)

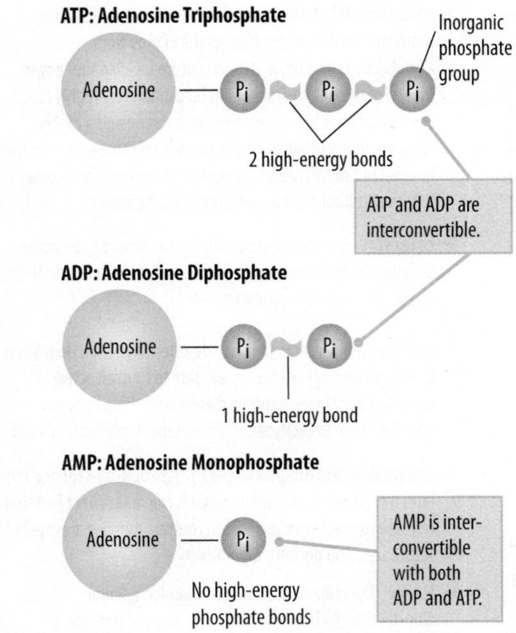

FIGURE 8.5 ATP, ADP, and AMP. Your body can readily use the energy in high-energy phosphate bonds. During metabolic reactions, phosphate bonds form or break to capture or release energy.

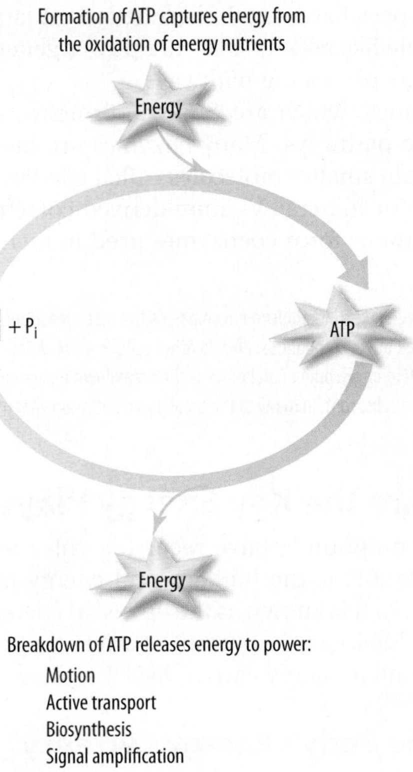

FIGURE 8.6 The ADP-ATP cycle. When extracting energy from nutrients, the formation of ATP from ADP + P_i captures energy. Breaking a phosphate bond in ATP to form DP + P_i releases energy for biosynthesis and work.

- **guanosine triphosphate (GTP)** A high-energy compound, similar to ATP but with three phosphate groups linked to guanosine.
- **nicotinamide adenine dinucleotide (NAD^+)** The oxidized form of nicotinamide adenine dinucleotide. This coenzyme, which is derived from the B vitamin niacin, acts as an electron carrier in cells, undergoing reversible oxidation and reduction. The reduced form is NADH. When a phosphate is present, the energy-carrying molecule is NADPH.
- **hydrogen ions** Also called a proton. This lone hydrogen has a positive charge (H^+). It does not have its own electron, but it can share one with another atom.

are exercising strenuously, you can use as much as 500 grams per minute! On average, you turn over your body weight in ATP every day.[5]

The molecule **guanosine triphosphate (GTP)** is similar to ATP and holds the same amount of available energy. Like ATP, GTP has high-energy phosphate bonds and three phosphate groups, but they are linked to guanosine rather than to adenosine. Energy-rich GTP molecules are crucial for vision and supply part of the power needed to synthesize protein and glucose. GTP readily converts to ATP.

NADH and $FADH_2$: The Body's Energy Shuttles

When breaking down nutrients, metabolic reactions release high-energy electrons. Further reactions transfer energy from these electrons to ATP (see **FIGURE 8.7**). To reach the site of ATP production, high-energy electrons hitch a ride on special molecular carriers. One major electron acceptor is **nicotinamide adenine dinucleotide (NAD^+)**, a derivative of the B vitamin niacin. The metabolic pathways have several energy-transfer points where an NAD^+ accepts two high-energy electrons and two **hydrogen ions** (two protons [$2H^+$]) to form NADH + H^+. For simplicity, the "+ H^+" often is dropped when talking about NADH.

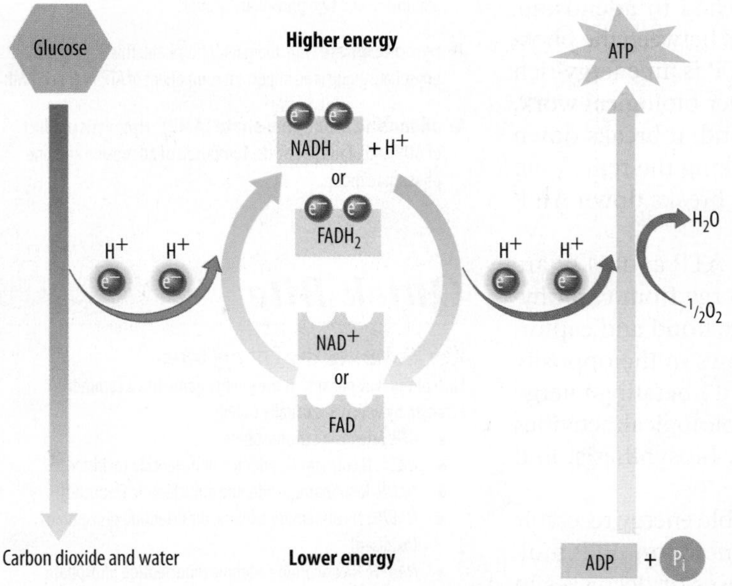

FIGURE 8.7 Energy transfer. As energy moves from glucose to ATP, molecules become high-energy or low-energy as they collect and transfer high-energy electrons and hydrogen ions (protons).

The other major electron acceptor is **flavin adenine dinucleotide (FAD)**, a derivative of the B vitamin riboflavin. When FAD accepts two high-energy electrons, it picks up two protons ($2H^+$) and forms $FADH_2$.

▶ **flavin adenine dinucleotide (FAD)** A coenzyme synthesized in the body from riboflavin. It undergoes reversible oxidation and reduction and thus acts as an electron carrier in cells. FAD is the oxidized form; $FADH_2$ is the reduced form.

NADPH: An Energy Shuttle for Biosynthesis

Energy powers the assembly of building blocks into complex molecules of carbohydrate, fat, and protein. NADPH, an energy-carrying molecule similar to NADH, delivers much of the energy these biosynthetic reactions require. The only structural difference between NADPH and NADH is the presence or absence of a phosphate group. Although both molecules are energy carriers, their metabolic roles are vastly different. Whereas the energy carried by NADH primarily produces ATP, nearly all the energy carried by NADPH drives biosynthesis. When a reaction transforms NADPH into $NADP^+$ (nicotinamide adenine dinucleotide phosphate), NADPH releases its cargo of two energetic electrons.

$NAD^+ + 2H^+ \leftrightarrow NADH + H^+$

NADH carries two high-energy electrons

$FAD + 2H^+ \leftrightarrow FADH_2$

$FADH_2$ carries two high-energy electrons

$NADPH + H^+ \leftrightarrow NADP^+ + 2H^+$

NADPH releases energy for biosynthesis when converted to $NADP^+$

Key Concepts ATP is the energy currency of the body. Your body extracts energy from food to produce ATP. NADH and $FADH_2$ are hydrogen and electron carriers that shuttle energy to ATP production sites. NADPH is also a hydrogen and electron carrier, but it shuttles energy for anabolic processes.

Breakdown and Release of Energy

The complete catabolism of carbohydrate, protein, and fat for energy occurs by way of several pathways. Although different pathways initiate the breakdown of these nutrients, complete breakdown eventually proceeds along two shared catabolic pathways—the citric acid cycle and the electron transport chain. This section first describes the pathways that catabolize glucose. It then discusses the steps that start the breakdown of fat and protein.

▶ **glycolysis** [gligh-COLL-ih-sis] The anaerobic metabolic pathway that breaks a glucose molecule into two molecules of pyruvate and yields two molecules of ATP and two molecules of NADH. Glycolysis occurs in the cytosol of a cell.

▶ **anaerobic** [AN-ah-ROW-bic] Referring to the absence of oxygen or the ability of a process to occur in the absence of oxygen.

▶ **pyruvate** The three-carbon compound that results from glycolytic breakdown of glucose. Pyruvate, the salt form of pyruvic acid, also can be derived from glycerol and some amino acids.

Extracting Energy from Carbohydrate

Cells extract usable energy from carbohydrate by four main pathways: glycolysis, conversion of pyruvate to acetyl CoA, the citric acid cycle, and the electron transport chain (see **FIGURE 8.8**). Although glycolysis and the citric acid cycle produce small amounts of energy, the electron transport chain is the major ATP production site.

Glycolysis

Glycolysis ("glucose splitting") is an **anaerobic** process; that is, it does not require oxygen. In the cytosol, this sequence of reactions splits each 6-carbon glucose molecule into two 3-carbon **pyruvate** molecules while producing a relatively small amount of energy.

Just as a pump requires priming, glycolysis requires the input of two ATP molecules to get started. In the later stages, various reactions produce energy-rich molecules of NADH and release four ATP molecules. Although glycolysis both consumes and releases energy, it produces more than it uses. Glycolysis is rapid, but it produces a comparatively small amount of ATP. The glycolysis of one glucose

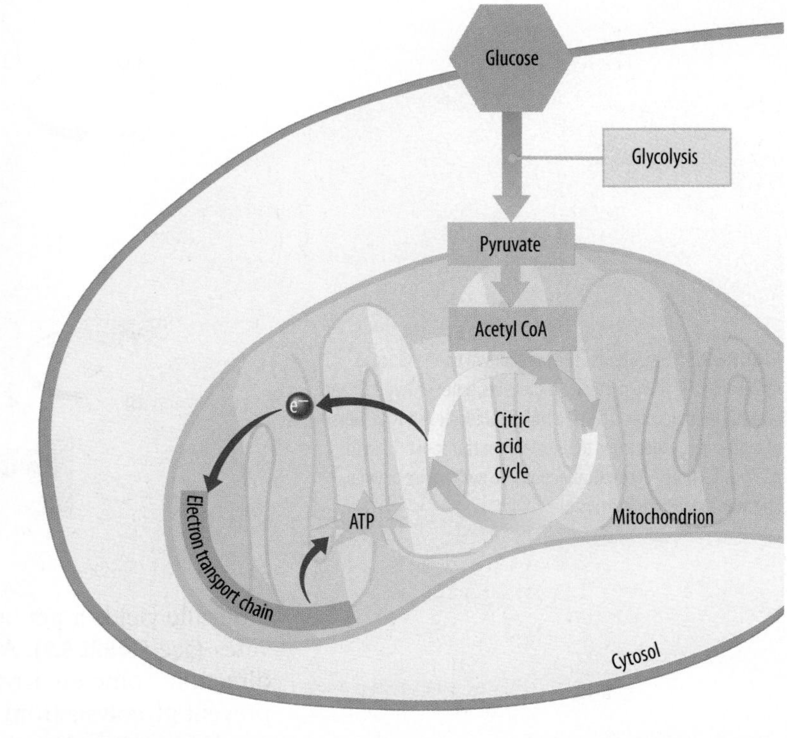

FIGURE 8.8 Obtaining energy from carbohydrate. The complete oxidation of glucose uses four major metabolic pathways: glycolysis, conversion of pyruvate to acetyl CoA, the citric acid cycle, and the electron transport chain. Glycolysis takes place in the cytosol. The remaining reactions take place in the mitochondria.

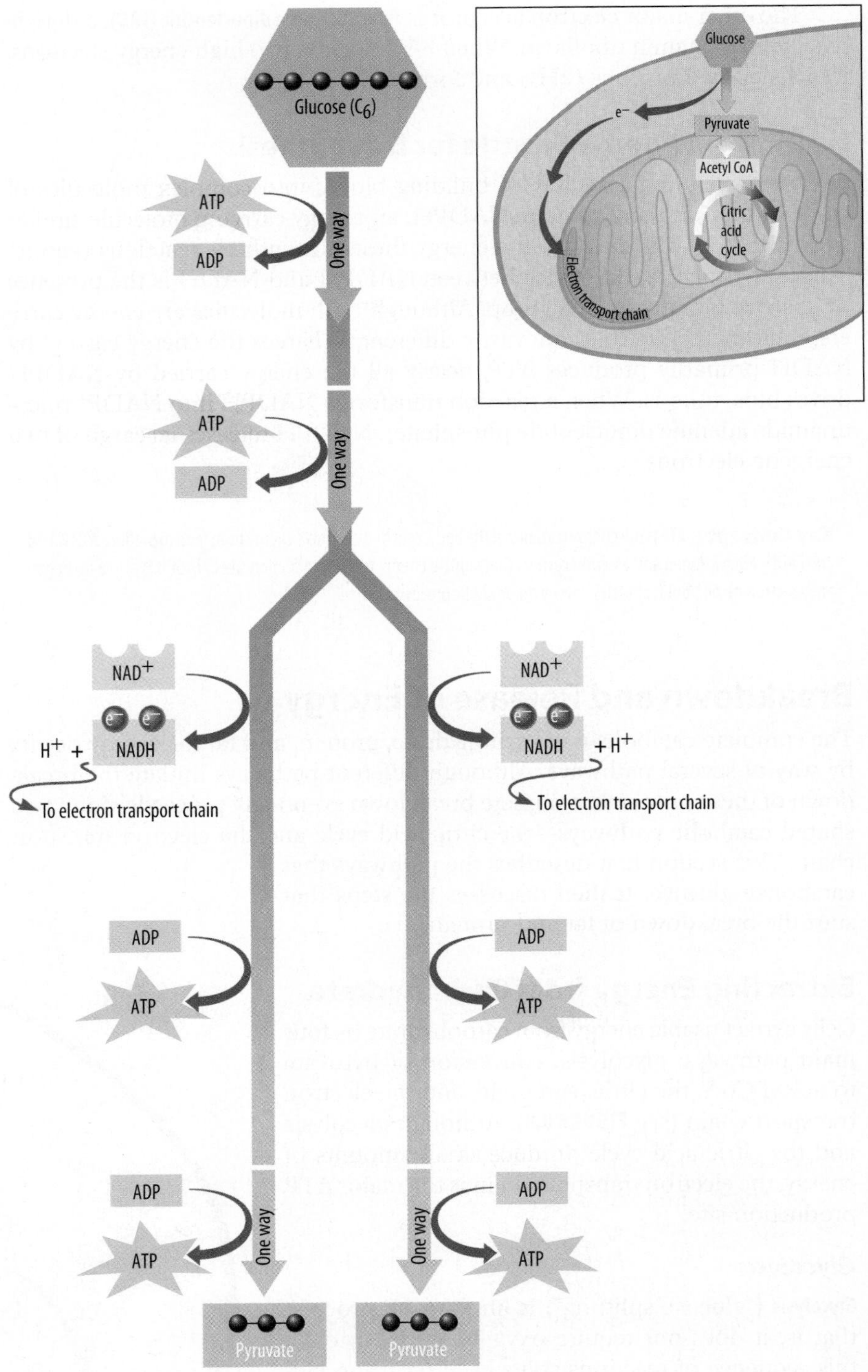

FIGURE 8.9 Glycolysis. The breakdown of one glucose molecule yields two pyruvate molecules, a net of two ATP and two NADH molecules. The two NADH molecules shuttle pairs of high-energy electrons to the electron transport chain for ATP production. Glycolytic reactions do not require oxygen, and some steps are irreversible.

molecule yields a net of two NADH and two ATP, along with the two pyruvates (see **FIGURE 8.9**). Although most glycolytic reactions can flow in either direction, some are irreversible, one-way reactions. These one-way reactions prevent glycolysis from running backward.

What about the other simple sugars, fructose and galactose? In liver cells, glycolysis usually breaks them down, and normally they are not available to other tissues.[6] Although fructose and galactose enter glycolysis at intermediate points, the end result is the same as for glucose. One molecule of glucose,

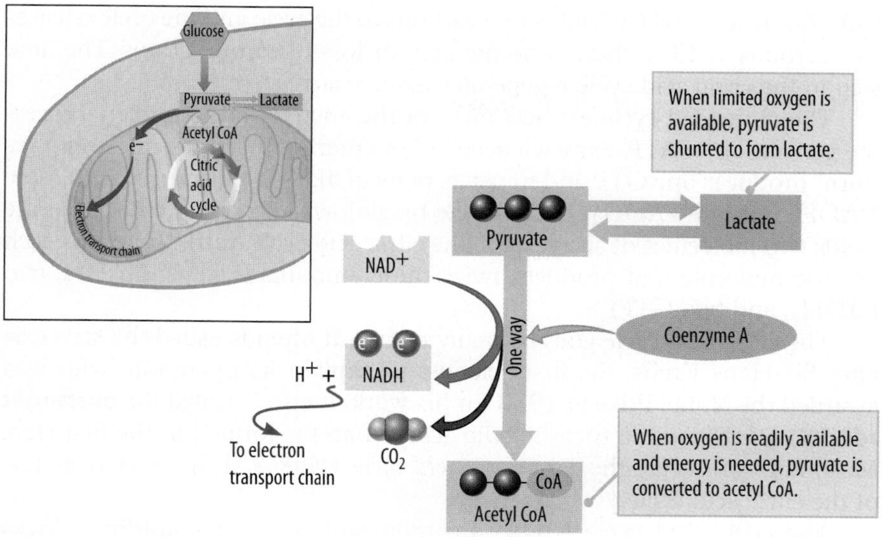

FIGURE 8.10 Conversion of pyruvate to acetyl CoA. When oxygen is readily available, each pyruvate formed from glucose yields one acetyl CoA, one CO_2, and one NADH. The NADH shuttles high-energy electrons to the electron transport chain for ATP production.

fructose, or galactose produces two NADH, a net of two ATP, and two pyruvates. Once glycolysis is complete, the pyruvate molecules easily pass from the cytosol to the interior of mitochondria, the cell's power generators, for further processing.

Conversion of Pyruvate to Acetyl CoA

When a cell requires energy, and oxygen is readily available, **aerobic** reactions in the mitochondria convert each pyruvate molecule to an **acetyl CoA** molecule. These reactions produce CO_2 and transfer a pair of high-energy electrons to form NADH (see **FIGURE 8.10**). The NADH shuttle carries the electrons to the electron transport chain.

Although many metabolic pathways can proceed either forward or backward, the formation of acetyl CoA from pyruvate is a one-way (irreversible) process. To form acetyl CoA, reactions remove one carbon from the three-carbon pyruvate and add **coenzyme A**, a molecule derived from the B vitamin pantothenic acid. After combining with oxygen, the carbon is released as part of carbon dioxide. Recall that glycolysis splits glucose into two pyruvate molecules, so we now have two NADH and two acetyl CoA molecules.

In rapidly contracting muscle, oxygen is in short supply, and pyruvate cannot form acetyl CoA. Instead, pyruvate is rerouted to form **lactate**, another three-carbon compound. Lactate is an alternative fuel that muscle cells can use or that liver cells can convert to glucose. When oxygen again becomes readily available, lactate is converted back to pyruvate, which irreversibly forms acetyl CoA.

Although pyruvate passes easily between the cytosol and the mitochondria, the mitochondrial membrane is impervious to acetyl CoA. The acetyl CoA produced from pyruvate is trapped inside the mitochondria, ready to enter the citric acid cycle.

Citric Acid Cycle

The **citric acid cycle** is an elegant set of reactions that proceed along a circular pathway in the mitochondria. To begin the cycle, acetyl CoA combines with **oxaloacetate**, freeing coenzyme A and yielding a six-carbon compound called citrate (citric acid). The coenzyme A leaves the cycle, becoming available to react with another pyruvate and form a new acetyl CoA. Subsequent reactions in the citric acid cycle transform citrate into a sequence of intermediate compounds as they remove two carbons and release them in two molecules of

▶ **aerobic** [air-ROW-bic] Referring to the presence of or need for oxygen. The complete breakdown of glucose, fatty acids, and amino acids to carbon dioxide and water occurs only through aerobic metabolism. The citric acid cycle and electron transport chain are aerobic pathways.

▶ **acetyl CoA** A key intermediate in the metabolic breakdown of carbohydrates, fatty acids, and amino acids. It consists of a two-carbon acetate group linked to coenzyme A, which is derived from pantothenic acid.

▶ **coenzyme A** Coenzyme A is a cofactor derived from the vitamin pantothenic acid.

▶ **lactate** The ionized form of lactic acid, a three-carbon acid. It is produced when insufficient oxygen is present in cells to oxidize pyruvate.

Quick Bite

When Glycolysis Goes Awry

Red blood cells do not have mitochondria, so they rely on glycolysis as their only source of ATP. They use ATP to maintain the integrity and shape of their cell membranes. A defect in red blood cell glycolysis can cause a shortage of ATP, which leads to deformed red blood cells. Destruction of these cells by the spleen leads to a type of anemia called hemolytic anemia.

▶ **citric acid cycle** The metabolic pathway occurring in mitochondria in which the acetyl portion (CH_3COO-) of acetyl CoA is oxidized to yield two molecules of carbon dioxide and one molecule each of NADH, $FADH_2$, and GTP. Also known as the *Krebs cycle* and the *tricarboxylic acid (TCA) cycle*.

▶ **oxaloacetate** A four-carbon intermediate compound in the citric acid cycle. Acetyl CoA combines with free oxaloacetate in the mitochondria, forming citrate and beginning the cycle.

CO_2. Because acetyl CoA adds two carbons to the cycle and the cycle releases two carbons as CO_2, there is no net gain or loss of carbon atoms. The final step in the citric acid cycle regenerates oxaloacetate.

The citric acid cycle extracts most of the energy that ultimately powers the generation of ATP. For each acetyl CoA entering the cycle, one complete "turn" produces one GTP and transfers pairs of high-energy electrons to three NADH and one $FADH_2$. Because the breakdown of one glucose molecule yields two molecules of acetyl CoA, the citric acid cycle "turns" twice for each glucose molecule and produces twice these amounts (i.e., six NADH, two $FADH_2$, and two GTP).

▶ **Krebs cycle** See *citric acid cycle.*

▶ **tricarboxylic acid (TCA) cycle** See *citric acid cycle.*

The citric acid cycle goes by many names. It often is called the **Krebs cycle** after Sir Hans Krebs, the first scientist to explain its operation, who was awarded the Nobel Prize in 1953 for his work. It also is called the **tricarboxylic acid (TCA) cycle** because a tricarboxylic acid (citrate) is formed in the first step. Most nutritionists use the term *citric acid cycle*. **FIGURE 8.11** shows an overview of the citric acid cycle.

The citric acid cycle is also an important source of building blocks for the biosynthesis of amino acids and fatty acids. Rather than using the cycle's intermediate molecules to complete the cycle, the cell might siphon them off for biosynthesis. Cells can use oxaloacetate, for example, to make glucose or certain amino acids. If alternate uses deplete the supply of oxaloacetate, the citric acid cycle can slow or even stop. Fortunately, cells can make oxaloacetate directly from pyruvate, easily replenishing the citric acid cycle's supply.

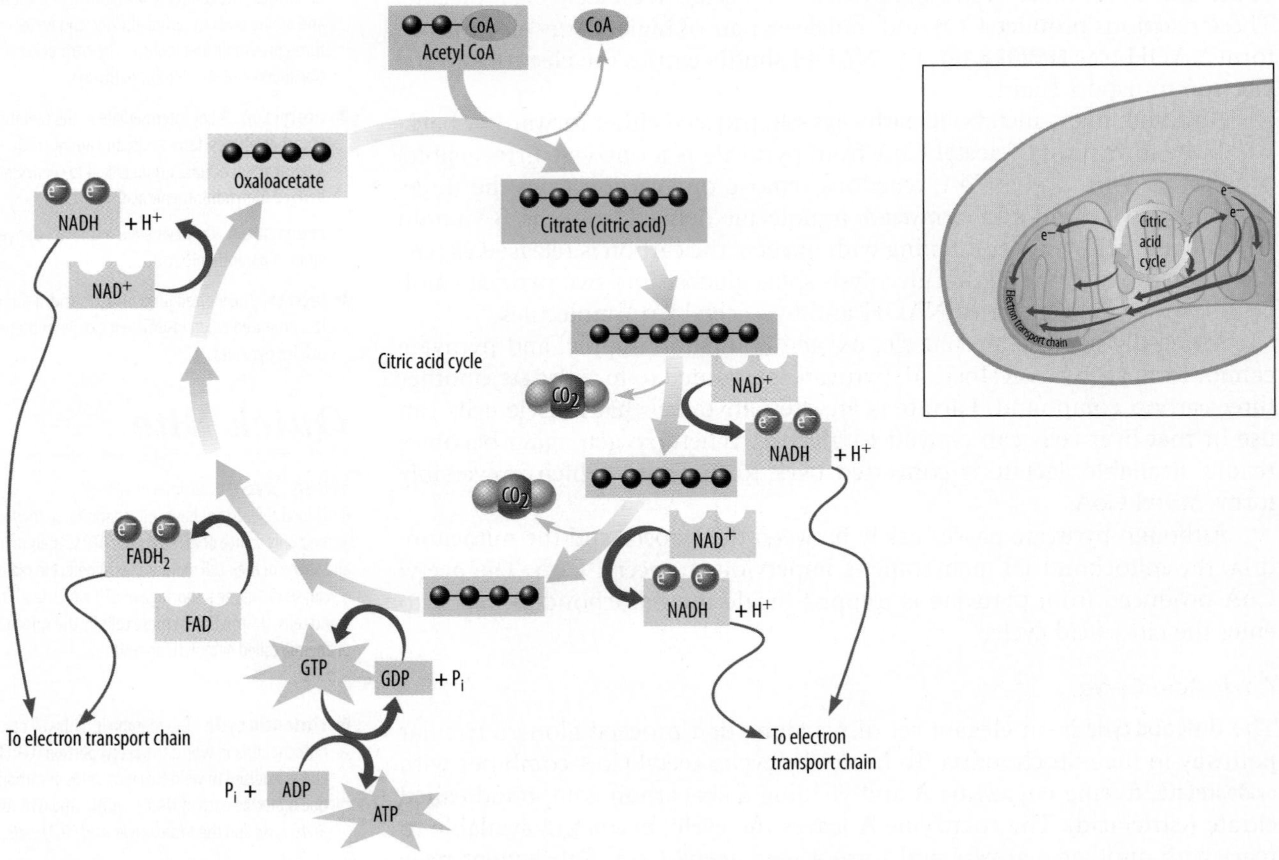

FIGURE 8.11 The citric acid cycle. This circular pathway accepts one acetyl CoA and yields two CO_2, three NADH, one $FADH_2$, and one GTP (readily converted to ATP). The electron shuttles NADH and $FADH_2$ carry high-energy electrons to the electron transport chain for ATP production.

Electron Transport Chain

The final step in glucose breakdown is a sequence of linked reactions that take place in the **electron transport chain**, which is located in the inner **mitochondrial membrane**. Most ATP is produced here, and as long as oxygen is available, it can dispense ATP and maintain exercise for hours. Because the mitochondrion is the site of both the citric acid cycle and the electron transport chain, it truly is the energy power plant of the cell.

THINK About It 2

NADH and $FADH_2$ now deliver their cargo of high-energy electrons. NADH produced in the mitochondria by the citric acid cycle delivers its pair of high-energy electrons to the beginning of the chain. In the inner mitochondrial membrane, these electrons are passed along a chain of linked reactions, giving up energy along the way to power the final production of ATP. At the end of the electron transport chain, oxygen accepts the energy-depleted electrons and reacts with hydrogen to form water. This formation of ATP coupled to the flow of electrons along the electron transport chain is called **oxidative phosphorylation** because it requires oxygen and it phosphorylates ADP (joins it to P_i) to form ATP (see **FIGURE 8.12**).

▶ **electron transport chain** An organized series of carrier molecules—including flavin mononucleotide (FMN), coenzyme Q, and several cytochromes—that are located in mitochondrial membranes and shuttle electrons from NADH and $FADH_2$ to oxygen, yielding water and ATP.

▶ **mitochondrial membrane** The mitochondria are enclosed by a double shell separated by an intermembrane space. The outer membrane acts as a barrier and gatekeeper, selectively allowing some molecules to pass through while blocking others. The inner membrane is where the electron transport chains are located.

▶ **oxidative phosphorylation** Formation of ATP from ADP and P_i coupled to the flow of electrons along the electron transport chain.

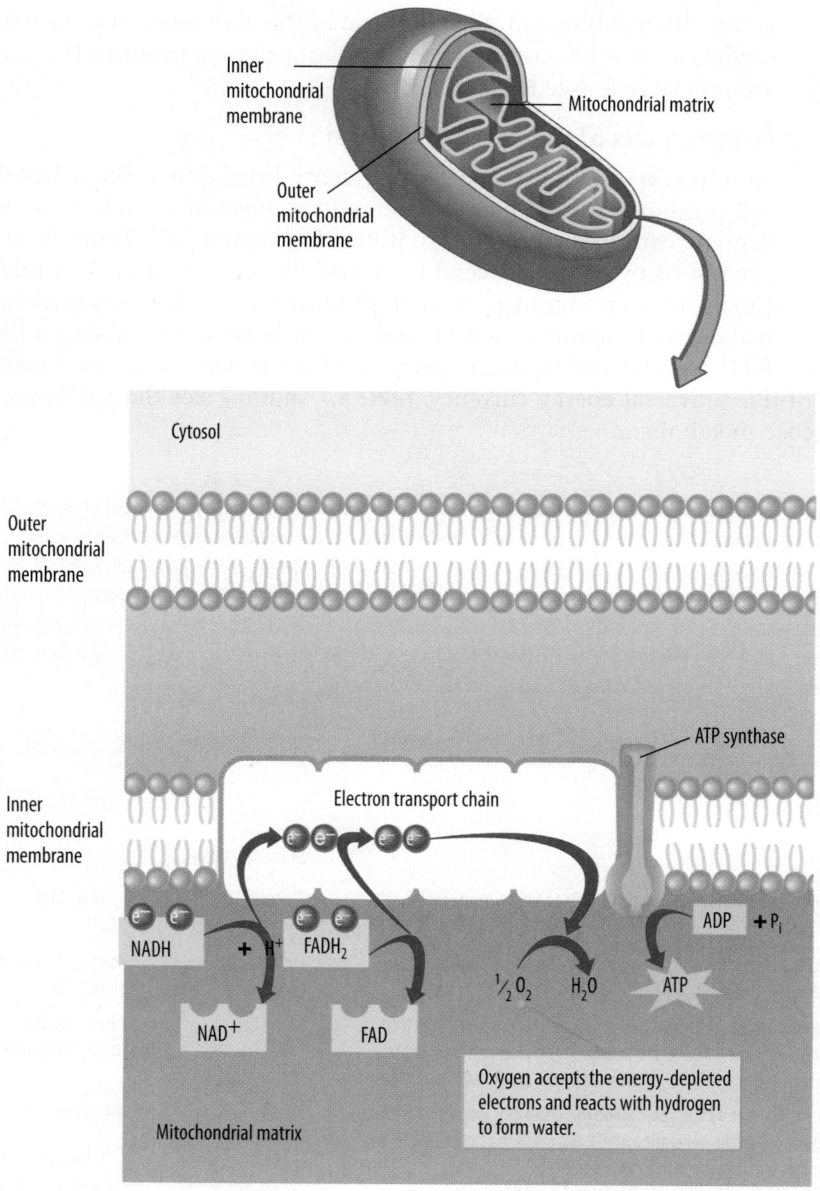

FIGURE 8.12 Electron transport chain. This pathway produces most of the ATP available from glucose. NADH molecules deliver pairs of high-energy electrons to the beginning of the chain. The pairs of high-energy electrons carried by $FADH_2$ enter this pathway farther along and produce fewer ATP than electron pairs carried by NADH. Whereas the electron pairs carried by NADH produce 2.5 ATP, those carried by $FADH_2$ produce 1.5 ATP. Water is the final product of the electron transport chain.

COMPLETE OXIDATION OF GLUCOSE

Pathway	ATP formed by pathway	ATP formed in electron transport chain
Glycolysis (1 Glucose)		
Net 2 ATP (4 produced – 2 used)	2	
2 NADH*		3 to 5
2 Pyruvate to 2 Acetyl CoA		
First pyruvate → Acetyl CoA		
1 NADH		2.5
Second pyruvate → Acetyl CoA		
1 NADH		2.5
Citric Acid Cycle (twice)		
First acetyl CoA → Citric acid cycle		
1 GTP (ATP)	1	
1 $FADH_2$		1.5
3 NADH		7.5
Second acetyl CoA → Citric acid cycle		
1 GTP (ATP)	1	
1 $FADH_2$		1.5
3 NADH		7.5
Subtotal	4	26 to 28
		Total = 30 to 32

* Each NADH formed in the cytosol by glycolysis will produce either 2.5 or 1.5 ATP in the electron transport chain.

FIGURE 8.13 Complete oxidation of glucose. These metabolic pathways and molecules move energy from glucose to ATP. Complete oxidation of one glucose molecule yields 30 to 32 ATP.

Without an oxygen "basket" at the end to accept the energy-depleted electrons, the transport of electrons down the chain would halt, stopping ATP production. Without ATP, there would be no power for our body's essential functions. If our oxygen supply were not rapidly restored, we would die.

Biochemists have revised their estimates of the amount of ATP produced by the electron transport chain. Historically, they believed that the complete breakdown of glucose produced 36 to 38 ATP, but the current estimate is 30 to 32 ATP.[7]

What about the electron pairs carried by NADH from glycolysis? Recall that glycolysis takes place in the cytosol, whereas the citric acid cycle and electron transport chain are located in the mitochondria. NADH in the cytosol cannot penetrate the outer mitochondrial membrane. Instead, cytosolic NADH transfers its high-energy electrons to special molecules that shuttle them across the outer mitochondrial membrane. Once inside the mitochondrion, the electron pair might be picked up by the formation of either NADH or $FADH_2$. Depending on which shuttle is formed, an electron pair from glycolytic NADH generates either 2.5 or 1.5 ATP. Because of this difference, the complete oxidation of a glucose molecule does not always produce the same amount of ATP (see **FIGURE 8.13**).

End Products of Glucose Catabolism

Now you've seen all the steps in glucose breakdown. What has the cell produced from glucose? The end products of complete catabolism are carbon dioxide (CO_2), water (H_2O), and ATP. Both the conversion of pyruvate to acetyl CoA and the citric acid cycle produce CO_2. The electron transport chain produces water. Whereas glycolysis makes small amounts of ATP and the citric acid cycle makes a little ATP as GTP, the electron transport chain generates the vast majority of this universal energy currency. **TABLE 8.1** summarizes the pathways of glucose metabolism.

Key Concepts The metabolism of glucose to yield energy occurs in several steps. Glycolysis breaks the six-carbon glucose molecule into two pyruvate molecules. Each pyruvate loses a carbon and combines with coenzyme A to form acetyl CoA, which then enters the citric acid cycle. Two carbons enter the cycle as part of acetyl CoA, and two carbons leave as part of two carbon dioxide molecules. Because two acetyl CoA molecules are formed from a single glucose molecule, the citric acid cycle operates twice. Finally, the NADH and $FADH_2$ formed in these pathways carry pairs of high-energy electrons to the electron transport chain, where ATP and water are produced. When completely oxidized, each glucose molecule yields carbon dioxide, water, and ATP.

TABLE 8.1
Summary of the Major Metabolic Pathways in Glucose Metabolism

Pathways	Location	Type	Summary	Starting Materials	End Products
Glycolysis	Cytosol	Anaerobic	A series of reactions that convert one glucose molecule to two pyruvate molecules.	Glucose, ATP	Pyruvate, ATP, NADH
Pyruvate to acetyl CoA	Mitochondria	Aerobic	Pyruvate from glycolysis combines with coenzyme A to form acetyl CoA while releasing carbon dioxide.	Pyruvate, coenzyme A	Acetyl CoA, carbon dioxide, NADH
Citric acid cycle	Mitochondria	Aerobic	This cycle of reactions degrades the acetyl portion of acetyl CoA and releases the coenzyme A portion. This cycle releases carbon dioxide and produces most of the energy-rich molecules, NADH and $FADH_2$, generated by the breakdown of glucose.	Acetyl CoA	Carbon dioxide, NADH, $FADH_2$, GTP
Electron transport chain	Mitochondria (membrane)	Aerobic	As the electrons from NADH and $FADH_2$ pass along this chain of transport proteins, they release energy to power the generation of ATP. Oxygen is the final electron acceptor and combines with hydrogen to form water.	NADH, $FADH_2$	ATP, water

Extracting Energy from Fat

To extract energy from fat, the body first breaks down triglycerides into their component parts, glycerol and fatty acids. Glycerol, a small three-carbon molecule, carries a relatively small amount of energy and can be converted by the liver to pyruvate or glucose. Fatty acids store nearly all the energy found in triglycerides.

The breakdown of fatty acids takes place inside the mitochondria. Before a fatty acid can cross into a mitochondrion, it must be linked to coenzyme A, which activates the fatty acid. Just as the input of ATP launched glycolysis, the input of ATP powers fatty acid activation. The breakdown of one ATP molecule to one AMP and two P_i provides the energy to drive this reaction. Although this activation reaction requires only one molecule of ATP, it breaks both of ATP's high-energy phosphate bonds and consumes the energetic equivalent of two ATP molecules (double the amount of energy released from the reaction $ATP \rightarrow ADP + P_i$).

Carnitine Shuttle

Without assistance, the activated fatty acid cannot get inside the mitochondria where fatty acid oxidation and the citric acid cycle operate. This entry problem is solved by **carnitine**, a compound formed from the amino acid lysine. Carnitine has the unique task of ferrying activated fatty acids across the mitochondrial membrane, from the cytosol to the interior of the mitochondrion. When carnitine is in short supply, the production of ATP slows. Based on its role in fatty acid oxidation, some people claim that carnitine supplements act as "fat burners." Although numerous studies have mixed results, some indicate that carnitine may increase fat oxidation and improve cardiovascular efficiency during exercise. Caution is warranted. The C-carnitine form can cause muscular weakness.[8]

▶ **carnitine** [CAR-nih-teen] A compound that transports fatty acids from the cytosol into the mitochondria, where they undergo beta-oxidation.

Beta-Oxidation

Once in the mitochondria, a process called **beta-oxidation** disassembles the fatty acid and converts it into several molecules of acetyl CoA (see **FIGURE 8.14**). Starting at the beta carbon of the fatty acid (the second carbon from the acid end), enzymes clip a two-carbon "link" off the end of the chain. Reactions convert this two-carbon link to one acetyl CoA while also transferring one pair of electrons to $FADH_2$ and another pair to NADH. This process repeats in stepwise fashion, shortening the chain by two carbons at a time until only a single two-carbon segment remains. This final two-carbon link simply becomes one acetyl CoA without producing $FADH_2$ and NADH.

▶ **beta-oxidation** The breakdown of a fatty acid into numerous molecules of the two-carbon compound acetyl coenzyme A (acetyl CoA).

In nature, almost all fatty acids have an even number of carbons. Although they can vary in length from 4 to 26 carbons, they often are 16 or 18 carbons long. If your body encounters an odd-numbered fatty acid, it breaks down this chain in the same way until it reaches a final three-carbon link. Rather than try to clip this link into smaller segments, a reaction joins it with coenzyme A. This three-carbon compound enters the citric acid cycle at a point farther along than acetyl CoA's entry point. Because it skips some of the early citric acid cycle reactions, it has a shorter journey than acetyl CoA and produces two fewer NADH molecules.

The Citric Acid Cycle and Electron Transport Chain Complete Fatty Acid Breakdown

Beta-oxidation of a fatty acid produces a flood of acetyl CoA that can enter the citric acid cycle. The citric acid cycle and electron transport chain complete the extraction of energy from fatty acids. Just as they processed acetyl

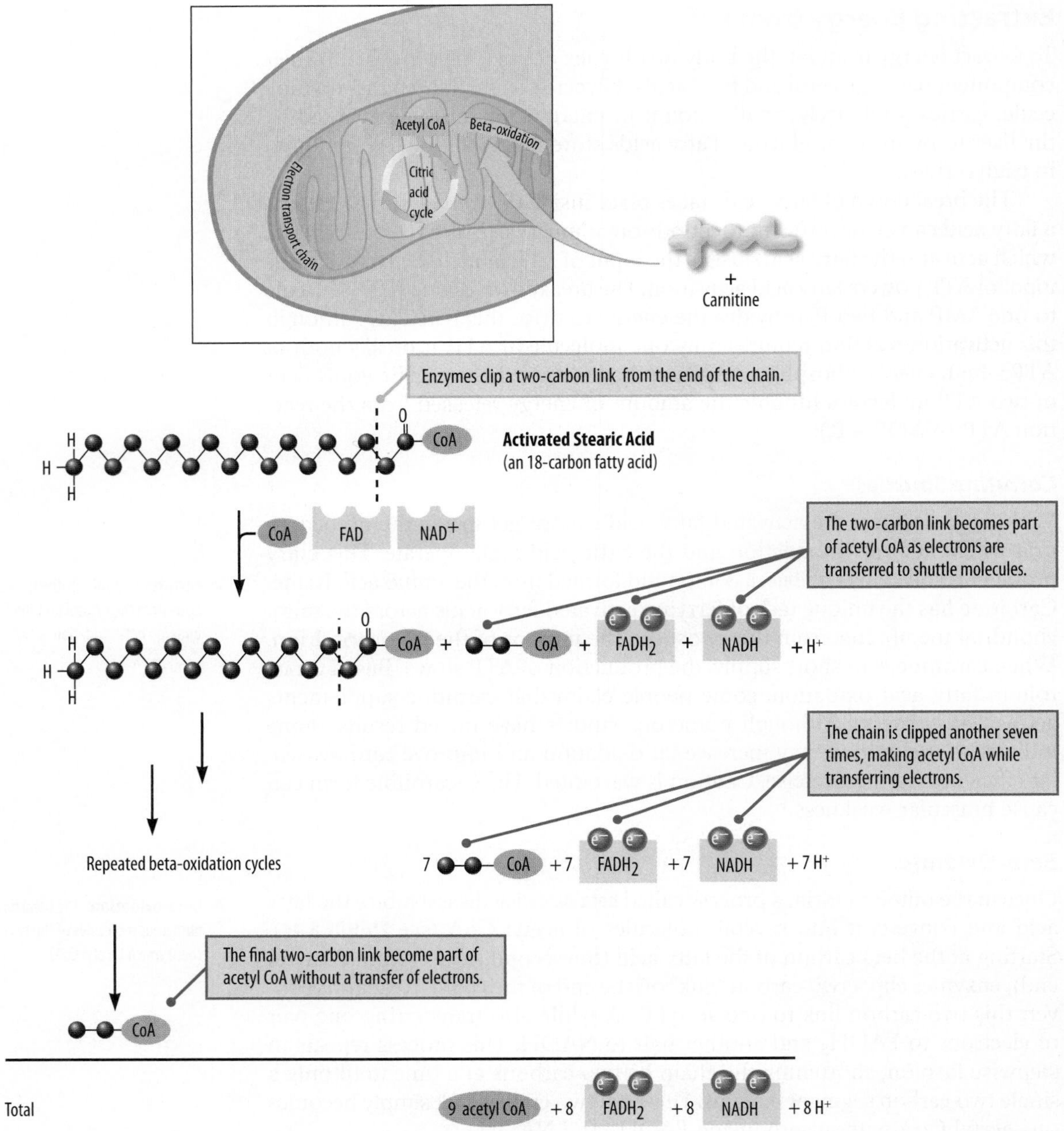

FIGURE 8.14 Beta-oxidation. Beta-oxidation reactions repeatedly clip the two-carbon end off a fatty acid until it is degraded entirely. Beta-oxidation of 18-carbon stearic acid produces nine acetyl CoA, eight $FADH_2$, and eight NADH.

CoA, NADH, and $FADH_2$ from glucose, these same pathways use acetyl CoA, NADH, and $FADH_2$ from fatty acids to produce ATP.

The end products of fatty acid breakdown are the same as those of glucose breakdown: carbon dioxide, water, and ATP. The exact amount of ATP depends on the length of the fatty acid chain. Because longer chains have more carbon bonds, beta-oxidation of longer chains produces more acetyl CoA and thus more ATP. The complete breakdown of an 18-carbon fatty acid, for example, produces 120 ATP (see **FIGURE 8.15**), whereas a 10-carbon fatty acid produces only 66 ATP. Because a fatty acid chain typically contains many more carbon atoms than a molecule of glucose, a single fatty acid produces substantially more ATP. For a single triglyceride with three 18-carbon fatty acids, complete breakdown of the fatty acids produces 360 ATP, more than 10 times the 32 ATP produced from the complete oxidation of glucose.

Fat Burns in a Flame of Carbohydrate

Acetyl CoA from beta-oxidation can enter the citric acid cycle only when fat and carbohydrate breakdown are synchronized. Without available oxaloacetate, acetyl CoA cannot start the citric acid cycle. Conditions such as starvation and consumption of high-fat, low-carbohydrate diets can deplete oxaloacetate, blocking acetyl CoA from entry. This reroutes the acetyl CoA to form a family of compounds called ketone bodies. (See the section "Making Ketone Bodies" later in this chapter.) Production of ketone bodies can occur with popular high-protein diets that are low in carbohydrate but also high in fat.

THINK About It 3

For fatty acid oxidation to continue efficiently and unchecked, reactions in the mitochondria must ensure a reliable supply of oxaloacetate. These reactions convert some pyruvate directly to oxaloacetate rather than to acetyl CoA. Because carbohydrate (glucose) is the original source of the pyruvate, and hence this oxaloacetate, scientists coined the adage "Fat burns in a flame of carbohydrate."

Pathway	ATP Yield
Beta-oxidation – stearic acid (C18:0)	
8 NADH	20
$8\ FADH_2$	12
Citric acid cycle – 9 acetyl CoA	
$1\ GTP \times 9 = 9\ GTP$	9
$3\ NADH \times 9 = 27\ NADH$	67.5
$1\ FADH_2 \times 9 = 9\ FADH_2$	13.5
Subtotal	122
ATP needed to start beta-oxidation	−2
Net yield	**120**

The grand total: 120 ATP from one molecule of stearic acid

FIGURE 8.15 The complete breakdown of stearic acid. The complete oxidation of one 18-carbon fatty acid yields about four times as much ATP as the complete oxidation of one glucose molecule.

Key Concepts Extracting energy from fat involves several steps. First, triglycerides are separated into glycerol and three fatty acids. Glycerol forms pyruvate and can be broken down to yield a small amount of energy. Beta-oxidation breaks down fatty acid chains to two-carbon links that form acetyl CoA, which enters the citric acid cycle. Beta-oxidation and the citric acid cycle form NADH and $FADH_2$, which carry pairs of high-energy electrons to the electron transport chain, where ATP and water are made. The complete breakdown of one triglyceride molecule yields water, carbon dioxide, and substantially more ATP than the complete breakdown of one glucose molecule.

Going Green

Biofuel Versus Fossil Fuel

Just as calories provide energy for our bodies, machine fuel supplies the energy for our lifestyles. We obtain calories from varied sources, and we obtain fuel from different sources. The two main fuel sources for machines are biofuel and fossil fuel. Both types of fuels present unique challenges in their impact on the environment, as well as on our carbon footprints.

Fossil fuels come from organisms that died millions of years ago. Coal is an example of a fossil fuel created from dead plant material that settled in swamps and underwent changes over millions of years. Fossil fuels are a nonrenewable resource because their replenishment rate is extremely low relative to their consumption rate. How do fossil fuels affect the environment? The prospecting and extracting, transporting, refining, and distribution of fossil fuel all contribute to greenhouse gas emissions and thus to climate change.

Biofuels can be produced from a number of different food crops that are derived directly or indirectly from photosynthesis. Although considered a renewable resource, this process raises environmental concerns and issues as well. The United States is the world's biggest producer of biofuels, derived mostly from corn. The environmental impacts of corn ethanol are significant. Soil erosion, in addition to the heavy use of nitrogen fertilizer and pesticides, leads to water and soil pollution. These factors, in turn, contribute to climate change. In addition, producing each gallon of ethanol requires 1,700 gallons of water (mostly to grow the corn) and generates 6 to 12 gallons of noxious organic effluent.[a]

Are biofuels a better alternative to fossil fuels? Some scientific research has established that some kinds of biofuel generate as much carbon dioxide as the fossil fuels they replace. Additionally, many people are focusing on how best to proceed globally with biofuel production in light of its potential impact on the world's food supply and hunger.[b]

One issue of increasing concern regards the quantity of arable land needed to produce biofuel rather than to produce food crops. Supporters of biofuel contend that biofuels are the only renewable alternative to fossil fuels and do generally result in greenhouse gas emission savings. Although there is great concern about the ultimate impact of biofuel production on hunger among the world's poorest people, the major increase in biofuels does have the potential to benefit the world's population living in poverty.[c]

So, what type of fuel is best for the environment? We do not have a definitive answer yet. Alternatives that have proven to be efficient for biofuel production are cellulose-containing materials, such as trees; grasses; woodchips; and field crop residues from wheat, rice straw, and cornstalks.[d] Until we have more definitive answers, we need to use every technique and strategy available. These will involve, in addition to experimenting with fuel sources, conservation of electricity and other resources. Small steps in energy conservation today can have a significant impact on your carbon footprint of tomorrow!

[a] Bournay E. *Atlas Environment du Monde Diplomatique 2007,* as cited in UNEP/GRID-Arendal. Biofuel versus fossil fuel. http://www.andjrnl.org/article/S0002-8223(07)01805-6/abstract. Accessed April 2, 2012.

[b] Stein K. Food vs biofuel. *J Am Diet Assoc.* 2007;107(11):1870.

[c] Ibid.

[d] Runge CF, Senauer B. How biofuels could starve the poor. *Foreign Affairs.* May/June 2007. https://www.foreignaffairs.com/articles/2007-05-01/how-biofuels-could-starve-poor. Accessed April 2, 2012.

Extracting Energy from Protein

Because protein has vital structural and functional roles, proteins and amino acids are not considered primary sources of energy. The primary and unique role of amino acids is to serve as building blocks for the synthesis of body protein and nitrogen-containing compounds. However, if energy production falters as a result of a lack of available carbohydrate and fat, protein comes to the rescue. During starvation, for example, energy needs take priority, so the body breaks down protein and extracts energy from the amino acid building blocks.

To use amino acids as an energy source, a process called deamination first strips off the amino group (–NH_2), leaving a "carbon skeleton" (see **FIGURE 8.16**). The liver quickly converts the amino group first to ammonia and then to urea, which the kidneys excrete in urine. When you eat more protein than you need, your kidneys excrete the excess nitrogen and your liver uses the carbon skeletons to produce energy, glucose, or fat. Much to the dismay of bodybuilders, when they attempt to build muscle by drinking pricey protein drinks, they can end up gaining fat instead!

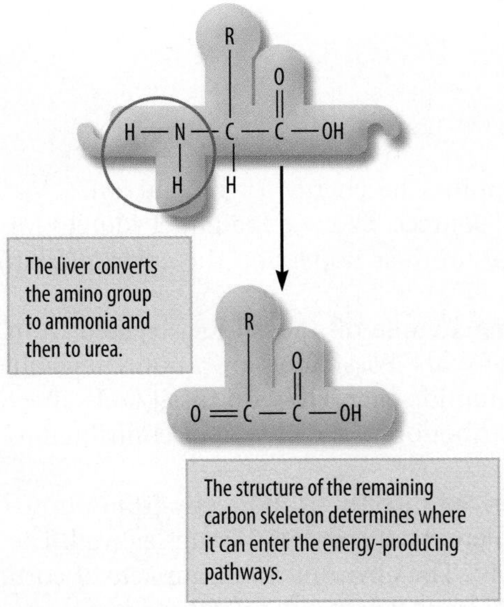
R
O
H—N—C—C—OH
H
H
The liver converts the amino group to ammonia and then to urea.
R
O
O=C—C—OH
The structure of the remaining carbon skeleton determines where it can enter the energy-producing pathways.

FIGURE 8.16 Deamination. A deamination reaction strips the amino group from an amino acid.

Carbon Skeletons Enter Pathways at Different Points

Like a crowd of people streaming into a concert through five different doors rather than one main entrance, carbon skeletons—unlike glucose—can enter the breakdown pathways at several different points. The carbon skeleton from each type of amino acid has a unique structure and number of carbon atoms. These characteristics determine the carbon skeleton's fate, be it pyruvate, acetyl CoA, ketone bodies, or one of the intermediates of the citric acid cycle.

End Products of Amino Acid Catabolism

The complete breakdown of an amino acid yields urea, carbon dioxide, water, and ATP. The carbon skeleton's point of entry into the breakdown pathways

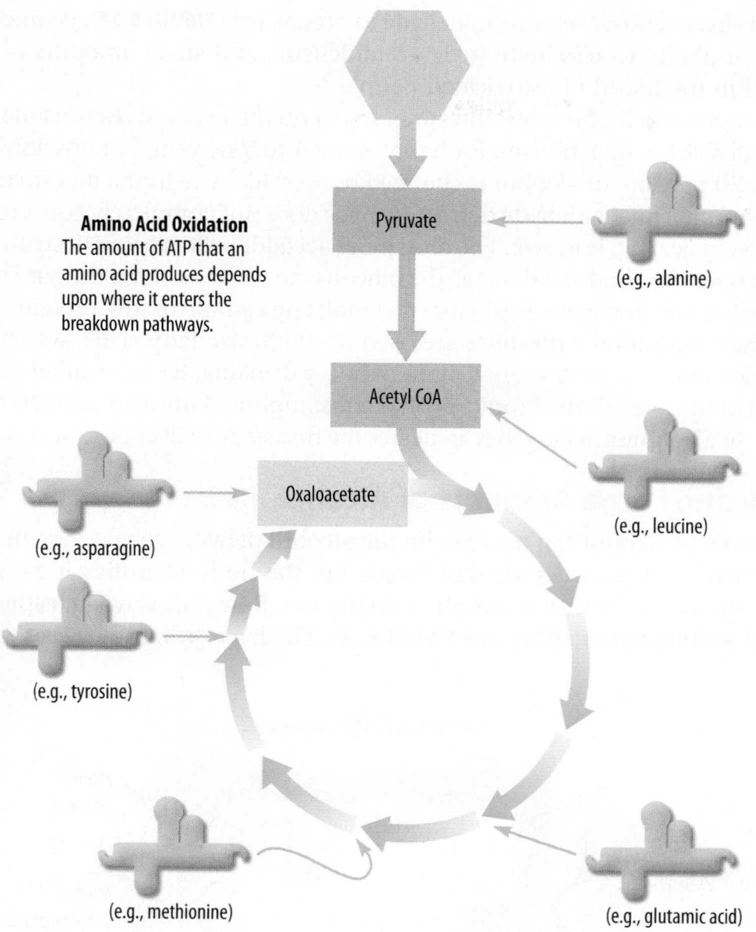

FIGURE 8.17 Extracting energy from amino acids. The carbon skeletons of amino acids have several different entrances to the breakdown pathways. Compared with glucose and fatty acids, amino acids yield much smaller amounts of energy (ATP).

determines the amount of ATP it produces. Whereas the complete breakdown of alanine, for example, produces 12.5 ATP, methionine produces only 5 ATP. Compared with glucose and fatty acids, no amino acid produces much ATP (see **FIGURE 8.17**).

Key Concepts To extract energy from amino acids, first deamination removes the amino groups, leaving behind carbon skeletons. The liver quickly converts these amino groups to urea and sends them to the kidneys for excretion. The carbon skeleton structure determines where it enters the catabolic pathways. Some carbon skeletons become pyruvate, others become acetyl CoA, and still others become intermediate compounds of the citric acid cycle. Complete breakdown of amino acids yields water, carbon dioxide, urea, and ATP.

Alcohol Metabolism

Alcohol metabolism takes priority over the breakdown of macronutrients. Because alcohol can accumulate and destroy cells and organs, the body metabolizes and removes it quickly. When the amount of alcohol consumed overwhelms the normal alcohol-metabolizing pathways, an alternate set of pathways helps handle the excess.

Metabolizing Small Amounts of Alcohol

Alcohol dehydrogenase (ADH) is a zinc-containing enzyme that catalyzes the conversion of small to moderate amounts of alcohol to acetaldehyde, a toxic substance. To avoid toxic buildup, another enzyme, **aldehyde dehydrogenase (ALDH)**,

▶ **alcohol dehydrogenase (ADH)** The enzyme that catalyzes the oxidation of ethanol and other alcohols.

▶ **aldehyde dehydrogenase (ALDH)** The enzyme that catalyzes the conversion of acetaldehyde to acetate, which forms acetyl CoA.

quickly and effectively converts acetaldehyde to acetate (see **FIGURE 8.18**). People differ in their ability to eliminate toxic acetaldehyde, and small amounts of it are found in the blood of intoxicated people.[9]

Dehydrogenases in the gastrointestinal tract and the liver are responsible for almost all alcohol metabolism. Probably about 4 to 9 percent, but possibly as much as 20 percent, of alcohol is changed to acetaldehyde in the digestive tract.[10] Gastrointestinal aldehyde dehydrogenase does not completely convert acetaldehyde to acetate, however. The remaining acetaldehyde is more destructive than alcohol itself and can damage the mucous membranes lining the gut.[11]

Liver cells break down alcohol before metabolizing carbohydrates, proteins, and fats. These breakdown products are used to synthesize fatty acids, which are assembled into fats. After a single bout of heavy drinking, fat accumulation can be seen in the liver. With chronic alcohol consumption, fatty acid synthesis accelerates. In alcoholics, a fatty liver indicates the first stage of liver destruction.

▶ **microsomal ethanol-oxidizing system (MEOS)** An energy-requiring enzyme system in the liver that normally metabolizes drugs and other foreign substances. When the blood alcohol level is high, alcohol dehydrogenase cannot metabolize it fast enough, and the excess alcohol is metabolized by MEOS.

Metabolizing Large Amounts of Alcohol

Large amounts of alcohol can overwhelm the alcohol dehydrogenase system, the usual metabolic path. As alcohol builds up, the body identifies it as a foreign substance and routes it into the primary overflow pathway, the **microsomal ethanol-oxidizing system (MEOS)** (see **FIGURE 8.19**). The liver ordinarily uses the

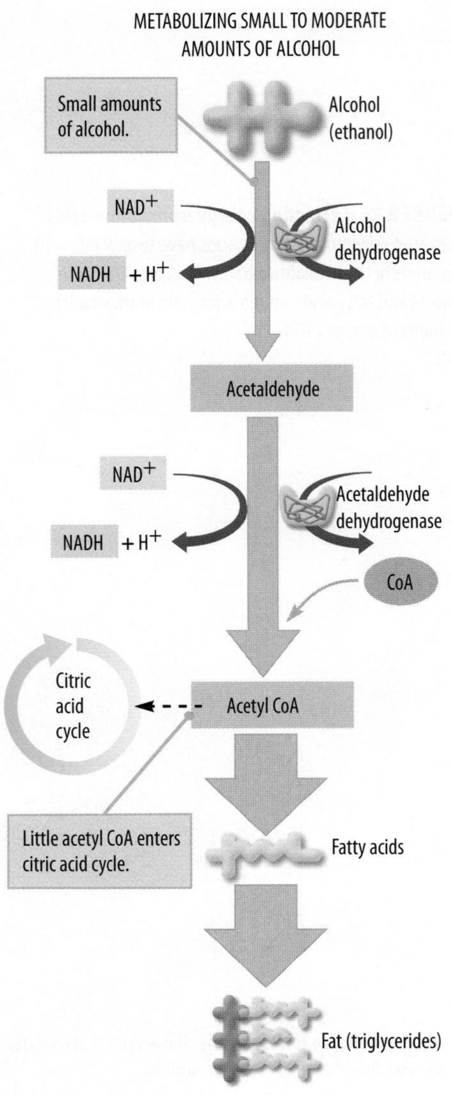

FIGURE 8.18 Metabolizing alcohol. The metabolism of alcohol inhibits the citric acid cycle and primarily forms fat.

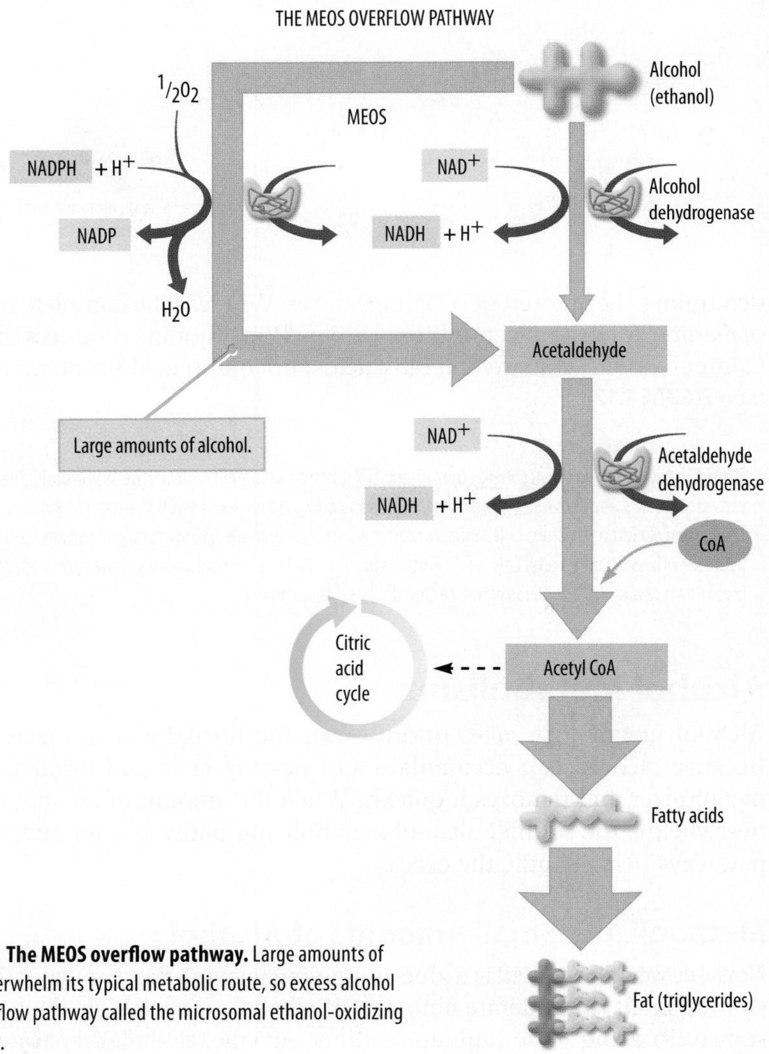

FIGURE 8.19 The MEOS overflow pathway. Large amounts of alcohol can overwhelm its typical metabolic route, so excess alcohol enters an overflow pathway called the microsomal ethanol-oxidizing system (MEOS).

MEOS bypass pathway to metabolize drugs and detoxify "foreign" substances. Chronic heavy drinking appears to activate MEOS enzymes, which might be responsible for transforming the pain reliever acetaminophen into chemicals that can damage the liver.

To transform alcohol into acetaldehyde, the MEOS pathway uses different enzymes than the alcohol dehydrogenase system. When repeatedly exposed to large doses of alcohol, the MEOS pathway increases its capacity and processing speed. Whether alcoholics metabolize alcohol differently from non-alcoholics is unknown. Clearly, chronic ingestion of alcohol leads to changes in the liver, and the alcohol abuser acquires an increased tolerance to alcohol and to drugs such as sedatives, tranquilizers, and antibiotics.

Key Concepts The liver is the alcohol processing center. The primary metabolic enzymes are alcohol dehydrogenase and aldehyde dehydrogenase. When large amounts of alcohol are consumed, some alcohol is metabolized by the MEOS pathway.

Quick Bite

Alcohol Aversion Therapy

In alcohol aversion therapy, the medication disulfiram (Antabuse) deliberately blocks the conversion of toxic acetaldehyde to acetate (acetic acid). Even small amounts of alcohol trigger the highly unpleasant Antabuse–alcohol reaction, which includes a throbbing headache, breathing difficulties, nausea, copious vomiting, flushing, vertigo, confusion, and a drop in blood pressure.

Biosynthesis and Storage

Uh-oh! Surveying the results of those holiday dinners and treats, you cringe with regret. Your clothes no longer fit, and you hate the idea of stepping on the scale. Your biosynthetic pathways have been hard at work, building fat stores from your excess intake of energy.

You head for the gym. After sweating through many workouts, your body begins to firm. You drop fat and add muscle. Now any problem with clothes fitting is due to muscle gain, not fat gain. To build muscle protein, different biosynthetic pathways have been busy making amino acids and assembling proteins.

Perhaps you've heard of "carb loading." This strategy uses high-carbohydrate meals to pack carbohydrate into your muscle glycogen stores before a race. Biosynthetic pathways assemble glucose into glycogen chains for storage. When needed, your body also can make glucose from certain amino acids and other precursors.

Both the breakdown and biosynthetic pathways are active at all times. While some cells are breaking down carbohydrate, fat, and protein to extract energy, other cells are busy building glucose, fatty acids, and amino acids. When your body needs energy, the breakdown pathways prevail. When it has an excess of nutrients, the biosynthetic pathways dominate. The activities in these pathways ebb and flow so they proceed at just the right rate, not too rapidly and not too slowly. **FIGURE 8.20** illustrates the interconnections among the metabolic pathways.

Making Carbohydrate (Glucose)

Your body sets a high priority on maintaining an adequate amount of glucose circulating in the bloodstream. **TABLE 8.2** shows the amount of energy, in kilocalories, that a typical 70-kilogram man has available. Blood glucose is the primary source of energy for your brain, central nervous system, and red blood cells. In fact, while you're at rest, your brain consumes about 60 percent of the energy consumed by your entire body.

The brain stores little glucose—only about 8 kilocalories. About 140 kilocalories of glucose circulate in the blood or are stored in adipose tissue. Your primary carbohydrate stores are in the form of glycogen. Muscle tissue holds about 1,200 kilocalories of glycogen, and the liver stores another 400 kilocalories.

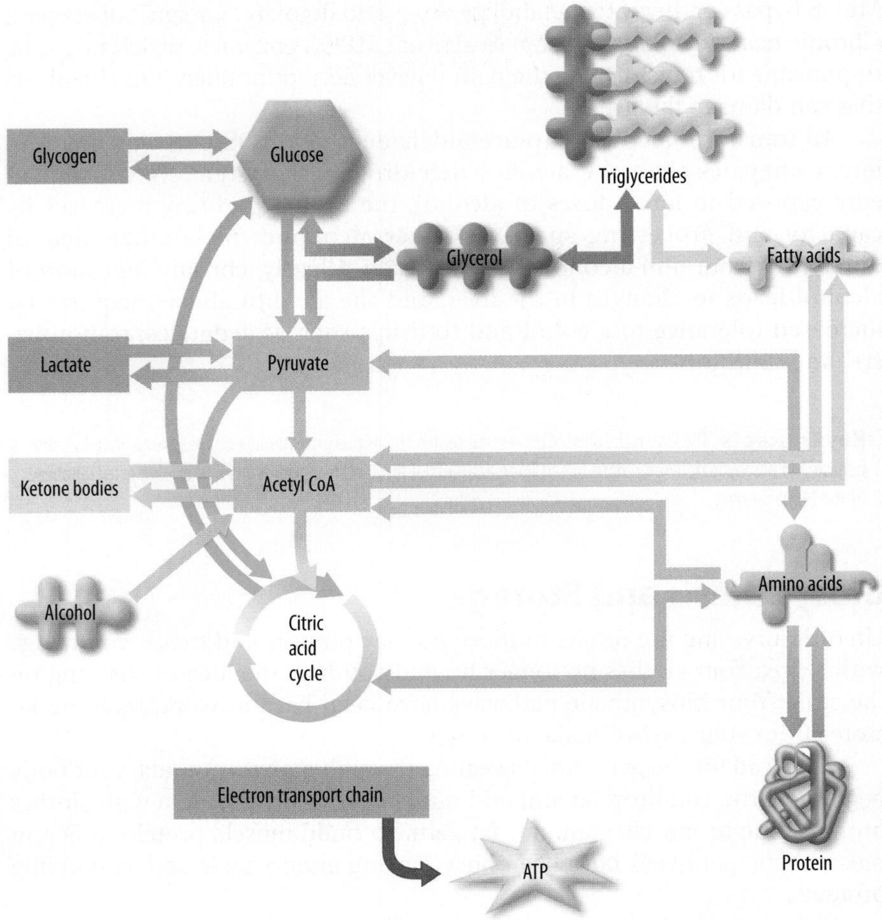

FIGURE 8.20 Overview of metabolic pathways. As if they were traveling through a maze of city streets, molecules move through a network of breakdown and biosynthetic pathways. Not all pathways are available to a molecule. Just as traffic lights and one-way streets regulate traffic flow, cellular mechanisms control the flow of molecules in metabolic pathways. These mechanisms include hormones, irreversible reactions, and the location of the reactions in the cell.

Gluconeogenesis: Pathways to Glucose

When you are exercising intensely or when you aren't taking in enough carbohydrate, such as a typical overnight fast, your body can remake glucose from pyruvate by using a clever strategy called **gluconeogenesis** (see **FIGURE 8.21**). Your liver is the major site of gluconeogenesis, accounting for about 90 percent of glucose production. Your kidneys make the rest.

▶ **gluconeogenesis** [gloo-ko-nee-oh-JEN-uh-sis] Synthesis of glucose within the body from noncarbohydrate precursors such as amino acids, lactate, and glycerol. Fatty acids cannot be converted to glucose.

Gluconeogenesis and glycolysis share many—but not all—reactions. During gluconeogenesis, however, reactions flow in the opposite direction as they do during glycolysis. But because some reactions of glycolysis flow only one way, gluconeogenesis must use energy-consuming detours to bypass them. Thus, gluconeogenesis is *not* simply a reversal of glycolysis.

TABLE 8.2
Available Energy (in kcal) in a Typical 70-Kilogram Man

Organ	Glucose or Glycogen	Triglycerides	Mobilizable Proteins
Blood	60	45	0
Liver	400	450	400
Brain	8	0	0
Muscle	1,200	450	24,000
Adipose tissue	80	135,000	40

Modified from Berg JM, Tymoczko JL, Stryer L. *Biochemistry*. 5th ed. New York: WH Freeman; 2002.

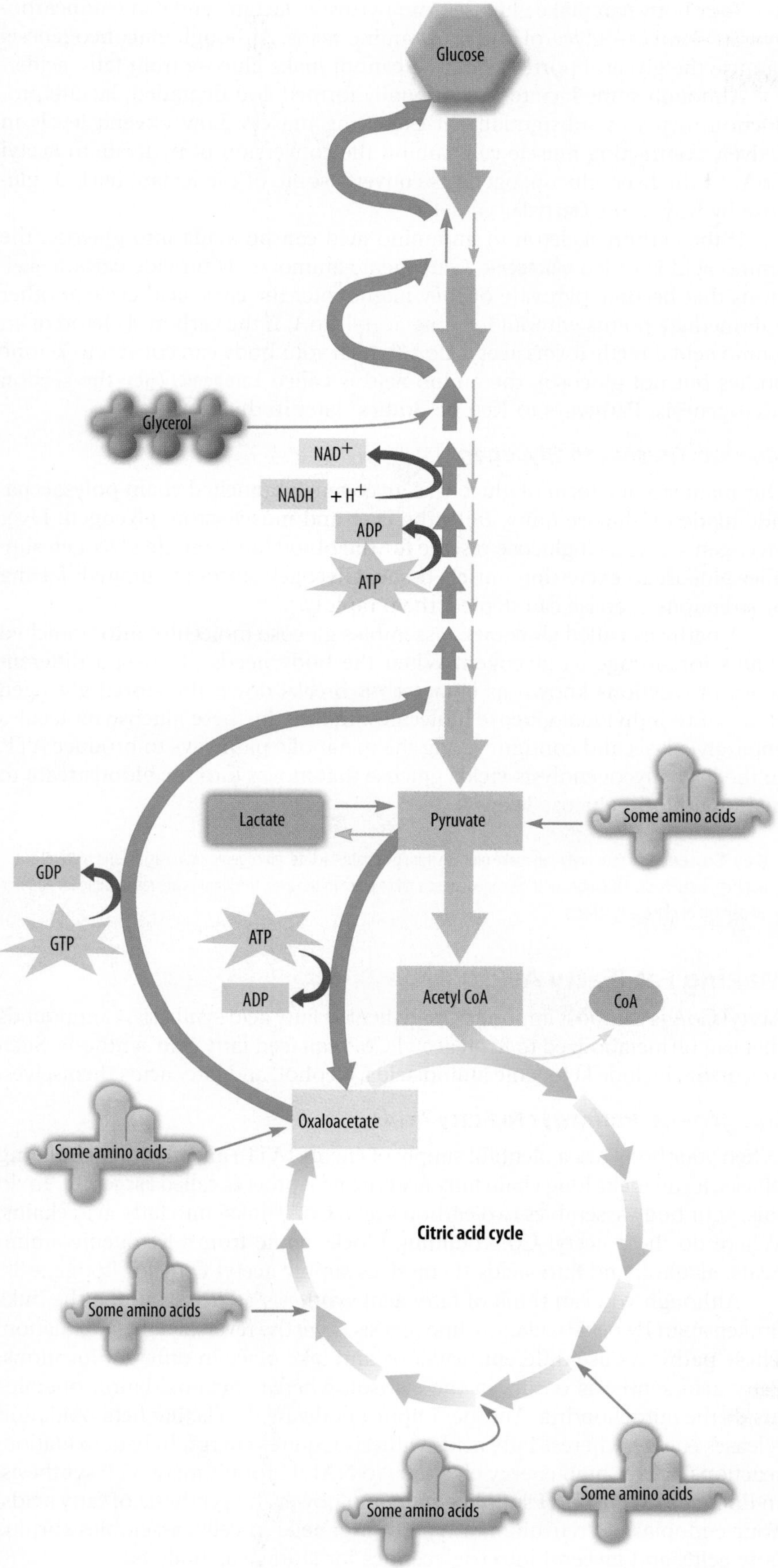

FIGURE 8.21 Gluconeogenesis. Liver and kidney cells make glucose from pyruvate by way of oxaloacetate. Gluconeogenesis is *not* a simple reversal of glycolysis. Although these pathways share many reactions, albeit in the reverse direction, gluconeogenesis must detour around the irreversible steps in glycolysis.

Your body can make glucose from pyruvate, lactate, and some noncarbohydrate sources—glycerol and most amino acids. Although gluconeogenesis can use the glycerol portion of fat, it cannot make glucose from fatty acids.

Although some lactate is continually formed and degraded, lactate production increases substantially in exercising muscle. Low oxygen levels in actively contracting muscle cells inhibit the conversion of pyruvate to acetyl CoA. In the liver, gluconeogenesis converts some of the lactate back to glucose by way of the **Cori cycle**.

▶ **Cori cycle** The circular path that regenerates NAD^+ and glucose when oxygen is low and lactate and NADH build up in excess in muscle tissue.

If the carbon skeleton of an amino acid can be made into glucose, the amino acid is called **glucogenic**. Glucogenic amino acids provide carbon skeletons that become pyruvate or they might enter the citric acid cycle at other intermediate points without forming acetyl CoA. If the carbon skeleton of an amino acid directly forms acetyl CoA (which your body can convert to ketone bodies but not glucose), the amino acid is called **ketogenic**. (See the section "Ketogenesis: Pathways to Ketone Bodies" later in this chapter.)

▶ **glucogenic** In the metabolism of amino acids, a term describing an amino acid broken down into pyruvate or an intermediate of the citric acid cycle; that is, any compound that can be used in gluconeogenesis to form glucose.

▶ **ketogenic** In the metabolism of amino acids, a term describing an amino acid broken down into acetyl CoA (which can be converted into ketone bodies).

Storage: Glucose to Glycogen

Our main storage form of glucose is glycogen, a branched-chain polysaccharide made of glucose units. Both the liver and muscle store glycogen. Liver glycogen serves as a glucose reserve for the blood, and muscle glycogen supplies glucose to exercising muscle tissue. Glycogen stores are limited; fasting or strenuous exercise can deplete them rapidly.

A pathway called **glycogenesis** assembles glucose molecules into branched chains for storage as glycogen. When the body needs glucose, a different series of reactions known as **glycogenolysis** breaks down the stored glycogen chains into individual glucose molecules. In muscle, these glucose molecules enter glycolysis and continue along the metabolic pathways to produce ATP. In the liver, glycogenolysis yields glucose that moves into the bloodstream to maintain blood glucose levels.

▶ **glycogenesis** The formation of glycogen from glucose.

▶ **glycogenolysis** The breakdown of glycogen to glucose.

Key Concepts Your body can make glucose from pyruvate, lactate, glucogenic amino acids, and glycerol but not from fatty acids. Although most gluconeogenesis takes place in the liver, the kidneys are responsible for about 10 percent of glucose synthesis.

Making Fat (Fatty Acids)

Acetyl CoA is the most important ingredient in fatty acid synthesis. Compounds that can be metabolized to form acetyl CoA can feed fatty acid synthesis. Such precursors include ketogenic amino acids, alcohol, and fatty acids themselves.

Lipogenesis: Pathways to Fatty Acids

When your body has a plentiful supply of energy (ATP) and abundant building blocks, it can make long-chain fatty acids using a process called **lipogenesis**. To do this, your body assembles two-carbon acetyl CoA "links" into fatty acid chains. Where do these acetyl CoA building blocks come from? Ketogenic amino acids, alcohol, and fatty acids themselves supply acetyl CoA for lipogenesis.

▶ **lipogenesis** [lye-poh-JEN-eh-sis] Synthesis of fatty acids, primarily in liver cells, from acetyl CoA derived from the metabolism of alcohol and some amino acids.

Although you can think of fatty acid synthesis as reassembling the links broken apart by beta-oxidation, lipogenesis is *not* the reversal of beta-oxidation. These pathways use different reactions and take place in different locations: Fatty acid synthesis occurs in the cytosol, whereas beta-oxidation operates inside the mitochondria. Another important distinction is that beta-oxidation releases energy, whereas fatty acid synthesis requires energy. In beta-oxidation, reactions deliver high-energy electrons to NADH for ultimate ATP synthesis. In lipogenesis, NADPH supplies energy to power the synthesis of fatty acids. Your endoplasmic reticulum, a type of organelle in cells, assembles surplus fatty acids and glycerol into triglycerides for storage as body fat.

Quick Bite

Sweet Origins

The word *gluconeogenesis* is derived from the Greek words *glykos*, meaning "sweet," *neo*, meaning "new," and *genesis*, meaning "origin" or "generation."

TABLE 8.3
Summary of Energy Yield and Interconversions

Dietary Nutrient	Yields Energy?	Convertible to Glucose?	Convertible to Amino Acids and Body Proteins?	Convertible to Fat?
Carbohydrate (glucose, fructose, galactose)	Yes	Yes	Yes, can yield certain amino acids when amino groups are available	Insignificant
Fat (triglycerides)				
Fatty acids	Yes, large amounts	No	No	Yes
Glycerol	Yes, small amounts	Yes, small amounts	Yes (see carbohydrate)	Insignificant
Protein (amino acids)	Yes, generally not much (see Fasting in Special States section)	Yes, from most amino acids, if insufficient carbohydrate is available	Yes	Yes, from some amino acids
Alcohol (ethanol)	Yes	No	No	Yes

Storage: Dietary Energy to Stored Triglyceride

When you overeat, your body uses body fat as a long-term energy storage depot. When you eat an excess of fat, most extra dietary fatty acids head straight to your fat stores. If you eat more protein than your tissues can use, your body converts most of the excess protein to body fat. Interestingly, excess carbohydrate does not readily become fat. In research studies, massive overfeeding of carbohydrate in normal men caused only minimal amounts of fat synthesis. (See the FYI feature "Do Carbohydrates Turn into Fat?") So, are carbohydrate calories "free"? Unfortunately, no. The first law of thermodynamics—the law of conservation of energy—still holds. Although excess carbohydrate does not dramatically increase fat synthesis, it shifts your body's fuel preferences toward burning more carbohydrate and fewer fatty acids.[12] Thus, eating excess carbohydrates still can make you fat by allowing the fat you eat to go directly to storage rather than to make ATP. (See **TABLE 8.3**.)

Key Concepts When ATP is plentiful and the diet supplies an excess of energy, your cells make fatty acids and triglycerides. Energy carried by NADPH powers the synthesis of fatty acids from acetyl CoA building blocks. Glycerol and fatty acids are assembled into triglycerides on the endoplasmic reticulum. Although excess dietary carbohydrate is not readily converted to fat, it does shift the body's selection of fuel and encourages the accumulation of dietary fat in body fat stores.

Making Ketone Bodies

Ketone bodies (sometimes incorrectly called **ketones**) include three compounds: acetoacetate, beta-hydroxybutyrate, and acetone. Acetoacetate and beta-hydroxybutyrate are acids, so they are sometimes referred to as keto acids. You might recognize the term *acetone* because this chemical is a common solvent. In fact, you can smell the strong odor of acetone on the breath of people with high levels of ketone bodies in their blood: Their breath smells sweet, like some nail polish removers.

Your body makes and uses small amounts of ketone bodies at all times. Although long considered to be just an emergency energy source or the result of an abnormal condition such as starvation or uncontrolled diabetes, small amounts of ketone bodies are normal, everyday fuels for tissues such as cardiac muscle, skeletal muscle, and the brain.[13]

Ketogenesis: Pathways to Ketone Bodies

During the breakdown of fatty acids, not all acetyl CoA enters the citric acid cycle. Your body converts some acetyl CoA to ketone bodies, a process called **ketogenesis** (see **FIGURE 8.22**).

▶ **ketones** [KEE-tones] Organic compounds that contain a chemical group consisting of C=O (a carbon–oxygen double bond) bound to two hydrocarbons.

▶ **ketogenesis** The process in which excess acetyl CoA from fatty acid oxidation is converted into the ketone bodies acetoacetate, beta-hydroxybutyrate, and acetone.

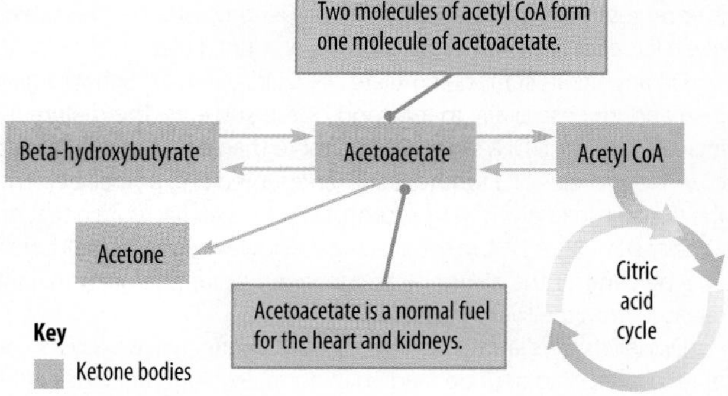

FIGURE 8.22 Ketogenesis. For acetyl CoA from fatty acid oxidation to enter the citric acid cycle, fat and carbohydrate metabolism must be synchronized. When acetyl CoA cannot enter the citric acid cycle, it is shunted to form ketone bodies, a process called ketogenesis.

Ketogenesis is highly active when fatty acid oxidation in the liver produces such an abundance of acetyl CoA that it overwhelms the available supply of oxaloacetate. Unable to enter the citric acid cycle, the excess acetyl CoA is shunted to ketone body production. When a person has uncontrolled diabetes or is actually starving, ketone bodies help provide emergency energy to all body tissues, especially the brain and the rest of the central nervous system (CNS). Other than glucose, ketone bodies are your central nervous system's only other effective fuel.[14] (See the section "Special States" for more details on starvation and diabetes mellitus.) After the liver makes ketone bodies from acetyl CoA molecules, the ketone bodies travel to other tissues in the bloodstream. Tissue cells can convert the ketone bodies back to acetyl CoA for ATP production by way of the citric acid cycle and electron transport chain.[15]

FYI For Your Information

Do Carbohydrates Turn into Fat?

Marc Hellerstein, MD, PhD

Forty years ago, Jules Hirsch and his colleagues addressed this question indirectly. They found that the composition of fatty acids in adipose tissue closely resembled a person's dietary fat intake. Moreover, when people were put on controlled diets of different fatty acid composition, after about six months their adipose fatty acids reflected the new dietary fatty acid composition. The conclusions were that "we are what we eat" with regard to body fat and that new fatty acid synthesis must therefore be minimal in healthy people.

The body's ability to make fat from carbohydrate is called *de novo lipogenesis (DNL)*. Concurrent DNL and burning of fatty acids is called *futile cycling*. About 25 to 28 percent of the energy in carbohydrates is lost if converted to fatty acids before being used as fuel. So, the futile cycle (fat synthesis/fat oxidation) could potentially waste a large number of calories. But does this costly conversion really happen?

Numerous studies using the technique of indirect calorimetry have shown that net DNL is typically absent or very low in humans under most dietary conditions, even after a large carbohydrate meal. This technique cannot answer, however, whether there is concurrent synthesis and burning of fat. Stable isotopic methods have helped to answer this question.

Direct Evidence

Direct evidence from stable isotopic labeling methods shows that DNL is minimal in normal (nonobese, nondiabetic, nonoverfed) men. DNL by the liver represents less than 5 grams of fat per day, whether the subjects are given large meals, intravenous glucose, or a liquid diet.

Do any circumstances stimulate DNL? Dr. Jean-Marc Schwarz gave fructose and glucose orally to lean and obese subjects. The dietary fructose increased hepatic DNL up to 20-fold more than equal calorie loads of glucose. Nevertheless, fat synthesis still represented only a small percentage of the fructose load given (< 5 percent). Dr. Scott Siler has shown that drinking alcohol stimulates DNL in the liver. Again, however, only a small percentage (< 5 percent) of the alcohol was converted to fat; the great majority was released from the liver as acetate.

Dr. Hellerstein's laboratory also studied the effect of five days of carbohydrate overfeeding or underfeeding in normal-weight men. Fat synthesis by the liver was highly sensitive to the degree of dietary carbohydrate excess. In fact, they could determine exactly which diet a person was eating by measuring DNL. Even so, the absolute amount of fat synthesis remained low, even on massively excessive carbohydrate intakes, for example, less than 5 grams of DNL out of more than 1,500 kilocalories of surplus carbohydrate in the diet. Rather than being converted to fatty acids, surplus carbohydrates replaced dietary fat in the whole-body fuel mixture. Hepatic DNL might be a sensitive *signal* of excess carbohydrate in the diet, but it is not a quantitatively important route for excess carbohydrate disposal.

Other conditions have revealed similar findings. Very-low-fat diets (10 percent of energy as fat; 70 percent as carbohydrate) stimulate lipogenesis, but, again, not a large amount. In young women, hepatic lipogenesis increases during the follicular phase of the menstrual cycle, but the amount is small, representing only 1 to 2 pounds of extra fat per year.

Adipose tissue DNL is slightly higher than liver DNL; approximately 20 percent of new adipose palmitate is from DNL. Hyperinsulinemia in obesity appears to stimulate adipose DNL, but the vast majority of adipose triglycerides still ultimately derive from diet, not DNL.

A high rate of DNL has been documented in humans only under conditions of massive carbohydrate overfeeding—for example, 5,000 to 6,000 carbohydrate calories per day for more than a week. Thus, only when total body glycogen stores are expanded to their maximum and intake of carbohydrate calories exceeds the daily rate of total energy expenditure is DNL substantially stimulated.

Are Carbohydrate Calories "Free"?

Does this mean that excess carbohydrate calories won't cause you to add body fat? Alas, we still become fatter if we overeat carbohydrate. At rest, our bodies normally burn fat as our primary fuel source. An excess of dietary carbohydrate energy causes a fat-sparing shift in fuel selection, markedly reducing the use of fat to fuel the body. Dietary fat makes a beeline for body fat storage rather than being burned to release energy. Excess dietary carbohydrate is not "free" when the diet also contains fat because the carbohydrate spares fat use.

Dr. Hellerstein is professor of medicine at the University of California, San Francisco, and professor of nutritional sciences at the University of California at Berkeley.

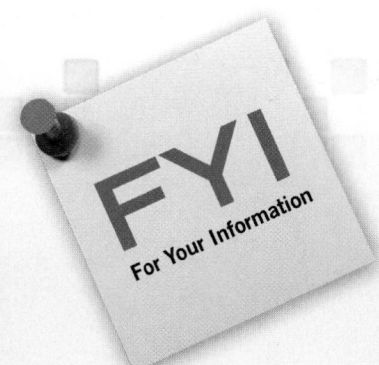

To dispose of excess ketone bodies, your kidneys excrete them in urine and your lungs exhale them. If this removal process cannot keep up with the production process, ketone bodies accumulate in the blood—a condition called ketosis. There are two types of ketosis: normal ketosis that occurs with fasting, and the medically dangerous hyperketonemia of diabetic **ketoacidosis**.[16] During even a brief fast, the catabolism of fat and protein increases the production of ketone bodies. Hyperketonemia can occur in uncontrolled type 1 diabetes mellitus. In this situation, blood acidity rises quickly, leading to ketoacidosis, which can cause brain damage, coma, and eventually death if untreated.[17] During a short fast, ketoacidosis rarely occurs.

Because "fat burns in a flame of carbohydrate," a very high-fat, low-carbohydrate diet promotes ketosis. The lack of carbohydrate inhibits formation of oxaloacetate, slowing entry of acetyl CoA into the citric acid cycle and rerouting acetyl CoA to form ketone bodies. Given time, however, the body can adapt to a very high-fat, low-carbohydrate diet and avoid ketosis. Inuit peoples, for example, sometimes live almost entirely on fat but do not develop ketosis.[18]

Quick Bite

Why Didn't My Cholesterol Levels Drop?

Your body can make cholesterol from acetyl CoA by way of ketone bodies. In fact, all 27 carbons in synthesized cholesterol come from acetyl CoA. The rate of cholesterol formation is highly responsive to cholesterol levels in cells. If levels are low, the liver makes more. If levels are high, synthesis decreases. This is why dietary cholesterol in the absence of dietary fat often has little effect on blood cholesterol levels.

▶ **ketoacidosis** Acidification of the blood caused by a buildup of ketone bodies. It is primarily a consequence of uncontrolled type 1 diabetes mellitus and can be life threatening.

Key Concepts Three types of ketone bodies—acetoacetate, beta-hydroxybutyrate, and acetone—can be made from any precursor of acetyl CoA: pyruvate, fatty acids, glycerol, and certain amino acids. Ketone bodies become an important fuel source during starvation because they are able to be used in place of glucose by the brain. In uncontrolled type 1 diabetes mellitus, an accumulation of ketone bodies can acidify the blood, a dangerous condition known as ketoacidosis.

Making Protein (Amino Acids)

Your body rebuilds proteins from a pool of amino acids in your cells. But how is that amino acid pool replenished? Your diet supplies some amino acids, the breakdown of body proteins supplies some, and cells make some. During protein synthesis, your cells can make nonessential (dispensable) amino acids and retrieve essential (indispensable) amino acids from the bloodstream. Your cells cannot make indispensable amino acids, however. If a cell lacks an indispensable amino acid and your diet doesn't supply it, protein synthesis comes to a stop. The cell breaks down this incomplete protein into its constituent amino acids, which are returned to the bloodstream.

▶ **transamination** [TRANS-am-ih-NAY-shun] The transfer of an amino group from an amino acid to a carbon skeleton to form a different amino acid.

Biosynthesis: Making Amino Acids

Your body uses many different pathways to synthesize dispensable amino acids. Each pathway is short, involving just a few steps, and builds amino acids from carbon skeletons. Pyruvate, along with intermediates of glycolysis and the citric acid cycle, supplies the carbon skeletons.

To make dispensable amino acids, the body transfers the amino group from one amino acid to a new carbon skeleton, a process called **transamination** (see **FIGURE 8.23**). To make the amino acid alanine, for example, pyruvate swipes an amino group from the amino acid glutamic acid to yield alanine and alpha-ketoglutaric acid. Transamination requires several enzymes. One group of enzymes, known as the aminotransferases, is derived from the B vitamin pyridoxine (B_6). Although vitamin B_6 deficiency is rare, a lack of B_6 will inhibit amino acid synthesis and impair protein formation.

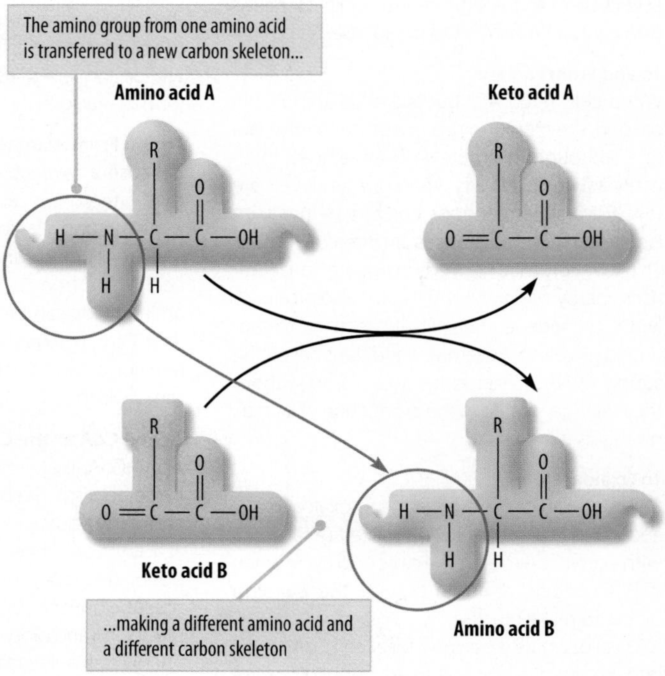

FIGURE 8.23 Transamination. A transamination reaction transfers the amino group from one amino acid to form a different amino acid.

Key Concepts Proteins are made from combinations of indispensable and dispensable amino acids. The body synthesizes dispensable amino acids from pyruvate, other glycolytic intermediates, and compounds from the citric acid cycle. To form amino acids, transamination reactions transfer amino groups to carbon skeletons.

Regulation of Metabolism

Just as the cruise control on your car regulates the vehicle's speed within a narrow range, your body tightly controls the reactions of your metabolic pathways. Whether highly or minimally active, each pathway proceeds at just the right speed, not too fast and not too slow. How does your body achieve this remarkable control? Although a number of strategies operate simultaneously, certain hormones are the master regulators.

FYI For Your Information

Key Intersections Direct Metabolic Traffic

Pyruvate Is Pivotal

Pyruvate is a pivotal point in the metabolic pathways. How does it select a path? What determines its destination? When ATP levels are low, cellular energy is in short supply, so the metabolic pathways flow toward the production of ATP. Depending on oxygen availability, low ATP routes pyruvate to acetyl CoA or lactate. When ATP is abundant, cells have ample energy, so the biosynthetic pathways prevail as pyruvate is converted to oxaloacetate or the amino acid alanine; oxaloacetate is converted to glucose and stored as glycogen.

To Acetyl CoA

When cells need ATP and have readily available oxygen, they rapidly convert pyruvate to acetyl CoA. This irreversible reaction commits the carbons of carbohydrates to oxidation by the citric acid cycle or to the biosynthesis of lipids. Acetyl CoA cannot be converted to glucose.

To and From Lactate

When cells need ATP but lack readily available oxygen, they reroute most pyruvate to form lactate. Although this route is always at least minimally active, it prevails when oxygen levels are low. Reversible reactions convert pyruvate to lactate, so these substances are interconvertible. The reaction that converts pyruvate to lactate uses energy carried by NADH, so it also produces NAD^+. This regeneration of NAD^+ is critical to continued glycolysis. Anaerobic conditions cut off the supply of NAD^+ from other sources, so without the NAD^+ generated in the production of lactate, glycolysis would stop.

To Oxaloacetate

Cells also can convert pyruvate to oxaloacetate, another pivotal molecule. Oxaloacetate can react with acetyl CoA to start the citric acid cycle when ATP is needed, or it can provide the building blocks to make glucose.

Oxaloacetate is essential for acetyl CoA's entry into the citric acid cycle. A steady supply of oxaloacetate is critical to the citric acid cycle's efficient extraction of energy from fatty acids. Carbohydrate feeds the pool of oxaloacetate as reactions break down carbohydrate to pyruvate and irreversibly convert the pyruvate to oxaloacetate. Cells also can make glucose from this oxaloacetate and store energy in the branched glucose chains of glycogen.

When cells have abundant ATP, they restrict the activities of certain enzymes, thus slowing the entry of acetyl CoA into the citric acid cycle. This reroutes the acetyl CoA into energy-storage pathways to form fatty acids so as to store energy as fat.

To and From Alanine

Because a reversible process converts pyruvate to the amino acid alanine, pyruvate and alanine are interconvertible. Although alanine is the only amino acid made from pyruvate, many other amino acids can be converted to pyruvate. Thus, pyruvate is located at a major junction of amino acid and carbohydrate metabolism.

Acetyl CoA at the Crossroads

Acetyl CoA, like pyruvate, stands at a pivotal point in metabolism. The breakdown pathways for glucose, fatty acids, and some amino acids converge at acetyl CoA. Once formed, what are acetyl CoA's options? It cannot return to pyruvate or make glucose, but acetyl CoA can enter major energy-producing and biosynthetic pathways. The body's energy status determines the predominant route.

To Energy Production

When cells need ATP and have oxaloacetate available, acetyl CoA enters the citric acid cycle for the ultimate production of ATP by the electron transport chain.

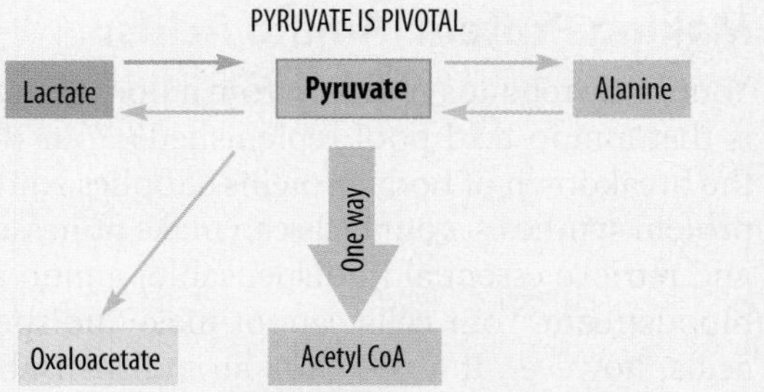

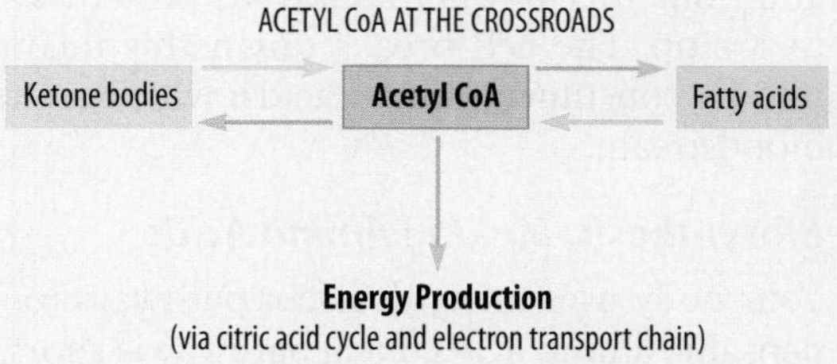

To and From Ketone Bodies

When the production of oxaloacetate does not match acetyl CoA production, acetyl CoA cannot enter the citric acid cycle, so the metabolic pathways shunt acetyl CoA to form ketone bodies.

To and From Fatty Acids

When energy is abundant, acetyl CoA molecules become building blocks for fatty acid chains. The body assembles these fatty acid chains into triglycerides and stores them in adipose tissue.

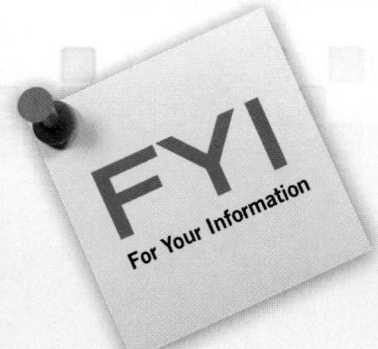

Hormones of Metabolism

Hormones are chemical messengers that help determine whether metabolic processing favors catabolic (breakdown) or anabolic (building) pathways. The major regulatory hormones are insulin, glucagon, cortisol, and epinephrine.

The pancreas secretes insulin, the leader of the storage (anabolic) team. Its mission is to decrease the amount of glucose in the blood, so it promotes carbohydrate use and storage (as glycogen). Because insulin stimulates the use of glucose over fat, its actions are said to be *fat-sparing*. In addition, insulin promotes fat storage in adipose tissue, cellular uptake of amino acids, and assembly of these amino acids into proteins. It also inhibits the breakdown of body proteins.

The pancreas also secretes glucagon, the leader of the breakdown (catabolic) team. Glucagon's mission is to increase the amount of glucose in circulation; it stimulates the breakdown of liver glycogen. The adrenal glands secrete two other members of the breakdown team—the hormones cortisol and epinephrine. Cortisol promotes the breakdown of amino acids for gluconeogenesis and helps increase the activity of the enzymes that drive gluconeogenic reactions.[19] Epinephrine stimulates the conversion of glycogen to glucose in muscle, increasing the amount of glucose available.

The actions of each team respond to the levels of available nutrients. Although both the storage and the breakdown teams are always active, storage dominates in times of plenty, and breakdown dominates in times of need.

Key Concepts Hormones and other factors regulate the balance of anabolic and catabolic pathways in energy metabolism. The hormone insulin stimulates glycogen, protein, and triglyceride synthesis. The hormones glucagon, cortisol, and epinephrine stimulate breakdown of glycogen and triglycerides.

Special States

Now you can put your new knowledge of metabolism to work by evaluating case studies of special physiological states: feasting and fasting. What happens to your metabolism under each situation? Read on to find out which states stimulate breakdown and which stimulate biosynthesis.

Feasting

You're stuffed. You just ate a huge holiday dinner: two servings of turkey with a big ladle of gravy and ample servings of dressing, mashed potatoes, caramelized sweet potatoes, green peas, and two bread rolls. To top it off, you ate a piece of pumpkin pie with whipped cream. You meant to stop there; you loudly proclaimed, "I'm so full, I can't eat another bite!" But eventually your grandmother convinced you to taste her special pecan pie. Gosh, that was good! But now you are lying on the couch, uncomfortable and bloated, with your belt loosened. Your feasting might be finished for now, but your body's work has just begun.

Your meal led to a huge influx of carbohydrate, fat, and protein—a plentiful supply for your tissues and far more energy than you need for life as a couch potato. The influx of food triggers the rapid secretion of the storage hormone insulin and inhibits the release of the breakdown hormones glucagon, cortisol, and epinephrine. Insulin is sometimes called the "hormone of plenty" because when energy is abundant, it promotes the replenishment of energy stores (glycogen and fat), the synthesis of protein, and the maintenance and repair of tissues. Its suppression of glucagon and cortisol reduces the rate of breakdown.

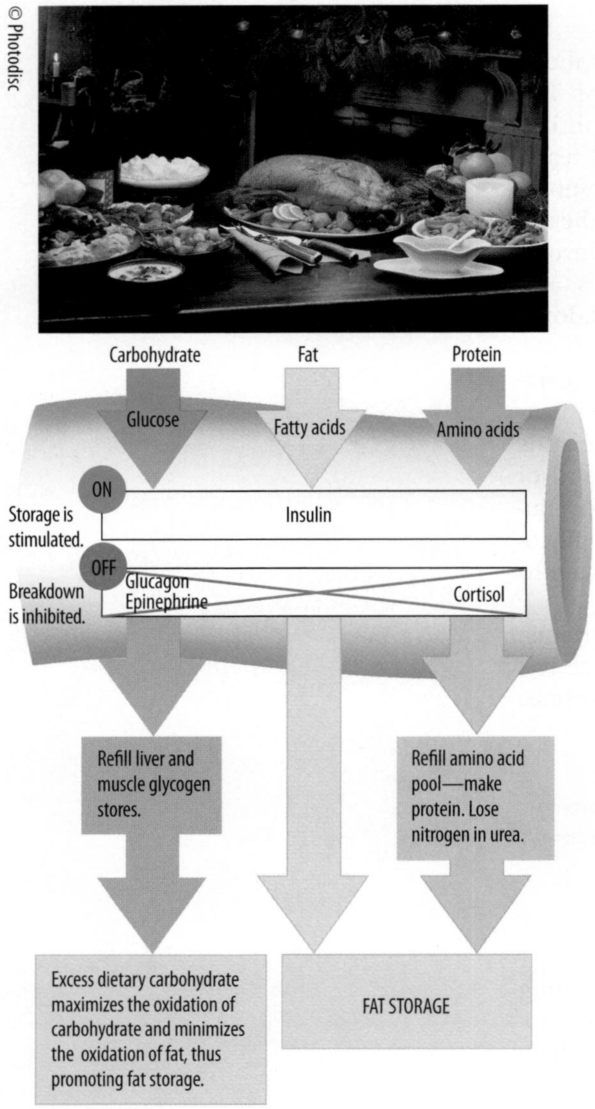

FIGURE 8.24 Feasting. Your body deals with a large influx of energy-yielding nutrients by increasing cellular uptake of glucose and promoting fat storage.

The storage hormone insulin signals your cells to "store, store, store!" Consequently, much of your holiday dinner will wind up stored as fat. The surplus carbohydrate first enters glycogen stores, filling their limited capacity. In the short term, excess carbohydrate primarily readjusts your body's fuel preferences to maximize its use of carbohydrate and minimize its use of fat. Although your body tends to burn off incoming carbohydrate, consumption in excess of calorie expenditures still promotes fat storage. What happens to the surplus fat and protein? Fat tissue is the perfect energy storage package for both. Although some ATP is produced from dietary fat, nearly all excess dietary fat becomes body fat. Excess protein, beyond what's needed to replenish the overall body pool of amino acids, also heads to fat storage (see **FIGURE 8.24**).

The Return to Normal

After this frenzied bout of storage, the amount of glucose and triglyceride circulating in the bloodstream drops to the fasting level. The level of amino acids in the blood also returns to baseline, and the secretion of insulin slows.

Hours later, after a nap and perhaps a game of touch football, a further decline in blood glucose levels signals the pancreas to secrete the breakdown hormone glucagon. Glucagon broadcasts the order "Release the glucose!" and your body swings into action to counteract falling blood glucose levels. The body breaks down liver glycogen to glucose, which is released into the bloodstream. Glucagon also stimulates the production of glucose from amino acids and slows the synthesis of glycogen and fatty acids. If blood glucose levels continue to fall, the adrenal glands secrete epinephrine, which signals the liver to further increase its release of glucose into the bloodstream. Epinephrine also stimulates the breakdown of muscle glycogen to form glucose that muscles can use. This glucose does not enter the bloodstream and is immediately available for muscle tissue to mount a fight-or-flight response to danger.

If low blood glucose levels persist for hours or days, the pituitary and adrenal glands join the battle by secreting growth hormone and cortisol, respectively. These hormones cause most cells to shift their fuel usage from glucose to fatty acids. Cortisol also promotes the breakdown of amino acids, and gluconeogenesis begins to ramp up and make glucose from circulating amino acids.[20] All breakdown hormones work in concert to maintain blood glucose levels and ensure a constant supply of glucose for the central nervous system and red blood cells[21]—until it is time to attack the leftovers!

> **Key Concepts** Feasting, or taking in too many calories, stimulates anabolic processes such as glycogen and triglyceride synthesis. Insulin is the key hormone that promotes synthesis and storage of glycogen and fat. Your body resists making fat from excess carbohydrate but shifts its fuel preferences. This shift still leads to the accumulation of fat stores.

Fasting

Feasting on a holiday dinner floods your body with excess energy that is stored for future use. In contrast, fasting and starvation deprive you of energy, so your body must employ an opposing strategy—the mobilization of fuel (see

FIGURE 8.25). Whether starvation occurs in a child during a famine, a young woman with anorexia nervosa, a patient with AIDS wasting syndrome, or a person who is intentionally fasting, the body responds in the same way.

Survival Priorities and Potential Energy Sources

Starvation confronts your body with several dilemmas. Where will it get energy to fuel survival needs? Which should it burn first—fat, protein, or carbohydrate? Can it conserve its energy reserves? Which tissues should it sacrifice to ensure survival?

THINK About It 4

Your body's first priority is to preserve glucose-dependent tissue: red blood cells, brain cells, and the rest of the central nervous system. Your brain will not tolerate even a short interruption in the supply of adequate energy. Once your body depletes its carbohydrate reserves, it begins sacrificing readily available circulating amino acids to make glucose and ATP.

Your body's second priority is to maintain muscle mass. In the face of danger, we rely upon our ability to mount a fight-or-flight response. This survival mechanism requires a large muscle mass, allowing us to move quickly and effectively. Your body grudgingly uses muscle protein for energy and breaks it down rapidly only in the final stages of starvation.

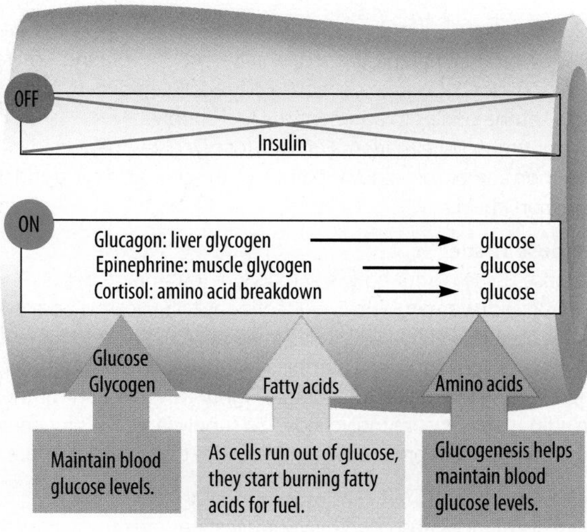

FIGURE 8.25 Fasting. During a short fast, cells first break down liver glycogen to maintain blood glucose levels. They also burn fatty acids and ramp up the production of glucose from amino acids.

FYI For Your Information

Metabolic Profiles of Important Sites

Brain

What powers your brain? Glucose! But brain cells cannot store glucose, so they need a constant supply. Your brain uses about 120 grams of glucose daily, which corresponds to a dietary energy intake of about 420 kilocalories. When your body's at rest, your brain accounts for about 60 percent of your glucose use.[a]

What happens during starvation? When glucose is in short supply, the liver comes to the rescue by converting fatty acids to ketone bodies. Ketone bodies are a critical source of replacement fuel that augments the supply of glucose to the brain.

Still, some brain cells can use only glucose. These cells survive by breaking down amino acids to make glucose through gluconeogenesis.[b]

Muscle

Muscle can use a variety of fuels: lactate, fatty acids, ketone bodies, glucose, and pyruvate. Unlike your brain, muscle stores large amounts of carbohydrate fuel—about 1,200 kilocalories—in the form of glycogen. This represents about three-fourths of the glycogen in your body. To fuel bursts of activity, muscle cells readily obtain glucose from glycogen.[c]

When your muscles actively contract, they rapidly deplete available oxygen, thus inhibiting the production of ATP through the aerobic breakdown pathways. ATP formed during glycolysis becomes the primary fuel. Muscle cells use the pyruvate from glycolysis to form lactate. The lactate travels to the liver, which converts it to glucose. The glucose returns to your muscle cells and undergoes anaerobic glycolysis. Known as the Cori cycle, this pathway rapidly produces ATP while shifting part of the metabolic burden from your muscles to your liver.

Whereas fatty acids are the primary fuel for muscles at rest, glycogen and glucose fuel short, intense activity, such as when you are sprinting to arrive at

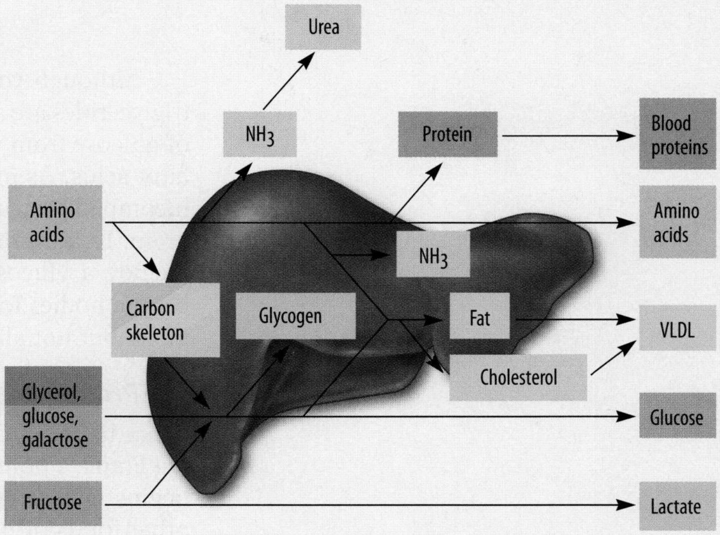

class on time. During prolonged exercise, such as running a marathon, fatty acid oxidation kicks in to help out. Fatty acids can directly supply energy or form ketone bodies to augment the fuel supply.

Your muscle cells are major sites for glycolysis, beta-oxidation, and the common aerobic breakdown pathways: the citric acid cycle and the electron transport chain.

Adipose Tissue

Adipose tissue is your body's primary energy storage depot. A 55-kilogram (121-pound) woman with 25 percent body fat (a healthy body composition) stores about 105,000 kilocalories in adipose tissue, enough energy to run 40 marathons! Your liver assembles fatty acids into triglycerides and sends them to adipose tissue for storage. Eighty to 90 percent of the volume of an adipose cell is pure triglyceride.[d] To supply fatty acids for energy production, adipose cells break down triglycerides to glycerol and free fatty acids.

Liver

Most substances absorbed by your intestines eventually pass through the liver, the body's main metabolic factory. This versatile organ performs glycolysis, gluconeogenesis, beta-oxidation, lipogenesis, ketogenesis, and cholesterol synthesis. Your liver can store up to 400 kilocalories of glucose as glycogen. When blood glucose levels are low, the liver breaks down stored glycogen to glucose or makes glucose from noncarbohydrate precursors. Several sources pitch in to provide glucose building blocks: Muscle supplies lactate and the amino acid alanine; adipose tissue supplies glycerol; and your diet supplies glucogenic amino acids.

The liver is the traffic cop for lipid metabolism. When energy is abundant, the liver directs fatty acids to storage. When energy is scarce, the liver breaks down fatty acids to form ATP. If an inadequate amount of carbohydrate blocks the entry of acetyl CoA into the citric acid cycle, the liver redirects fatty acids to ketone bodies.

Kidneys

Your kidneys are important disposal systems of metabolic wastes. Without rapid elimination, these wastes can build up to toxic levels. When your liver deaminates amino acids (removes amino groups), a cooperative effort eliminates the released nitrogen. Your liver captures the nitrogen in urea, which it releases into the bloodstream. The kidneys filter out the urea and excrete it in urine.

The kidneys can make glucose (gluconeogenesis) from amino acids and other precursors. During prolonged starvation, the kidneys produce glucose in amounts that rival production by the liver![e]

Heart

Your heart relies on an interesting mix of fuels. Rather than glucose, which it uses in only small amounts, your heart relies on free fatty acids, lactate, and ketone bodies.[f] When glucose is in short supply, your heart makes a special effort to spare its use. It uses ketone bodies, then free fatty acids, and finally glucose as its fuel source.[g] During heavy exercise, your body releases large amounts of lactate into the bloodstream. Compared with other types of tissue, your heart is particularly capable of using lactate to supply the energy it needs.[h]

Red Blood Cells

Just like the brain, red blood cells rely primarily on glucose for fuel. In these cells, glycolysis and the pentose phosphate pathway (an alternative energy-producing pathway) extract energy from glucose. Because red blood cells have no mitochondria, they do not contain the pathways for beta-oxidation, the citric acid cycle, or the electron transport chain.

The pentose phosphate pathway generates the NADPH that is critical for a red blood cell's health. Energy carried by NADPH helps maintain cell membrane pliability and ion transport capabilities. NADPH also helps preserve iron in the cell's hemoglobin and prevent premature breakdown of the cell's proteins.[i]

[a] Berg JM, Tymoczko JL, Stryer L. *Biochemistry.* 7th ed. New York: WH Freeman; 2010.

[b] Guyton AC, Hall JE. *Textbook of Medical Physiology.* 11th ed. Philadelphia: Elsevier Health Sciences; 2010.

[c] Berg JM, Tymoczko JL, Stryer L. *Biochemistry.* Op cit.

[d] Guyton AC, Hall JE. *Textbook of Medical Physiology.* Op cit.

[e] Ibid.

[f] Murray RK, et al. *Harper's Illustrated Biochemistry.* 28th ed. New York: McGraw–Hill; 2009.

[g] Ibid.

[h] Guyton AC, Hall JE. *Textbook of Medical Physiology.* Op cit.

[i] Ibid.

Although your body stores most of its energy reserve in adipose tissue, triglycerides are a poor source of glucose. Your body can make a small amount of glucose from the glycerol backbone, but it cannot make any glucose from fatty acids. As a consequence, your body's primary energy stores—fat—are incompatible with your body's paramount energy priority—glucose for your brain. To meet this metabolic challenge, your body's antistarvation strategies include a glucose-sparing mechanism. Your body shifts to fatty acids and ketone bodies for its primary fuel needs. In time, even your brain adapts, as most, but not all, brain cells come to rely on ketone bodies for fuel.

The Prolonged Fast: In the Beginning

What happens during the fasting state? Let's take a metabolic look at Fasting Frank, a political activist determined to make a dramatic statement. Frank begins fasting at sundown, planning to drink only water and consume no other foods or liquids.

The first few hours are no different from your nightly fast between dinner and breakfast. As blood glucose drops to fasting baseline levels, the liver breaks down glycogen to glucose. Gluconeogenesis becomes highly active and begins churning out glucose from circulating amino acids. The liver pours glucose into the bloodstream to supply other organs and shifts to fatty acids for its own energy needs. Muscle cells also start burning fatty acids. After about 12 hours, the battle to maintain a constant supply of blood glucose exhausts nearly all carbohydrate stores.[22]

The First Few Days

During the next few days, fat and protein are the primary fuels. To preserve structural proteins, especially muscle mass, Frank's body first turns to easily metabolized amino acids. It uses some to produce ATP and others to make glucose. Glucogenic amino acids, especially alanine, furnish about 90 percent of the brain's glucose supply. Glycerol from triglyceride breakdown supplies the remaining 10 percent. After a couple of days, production of ketone bodies ramps up, augmenting the fuel supply (see **FIGURE 8.26**).

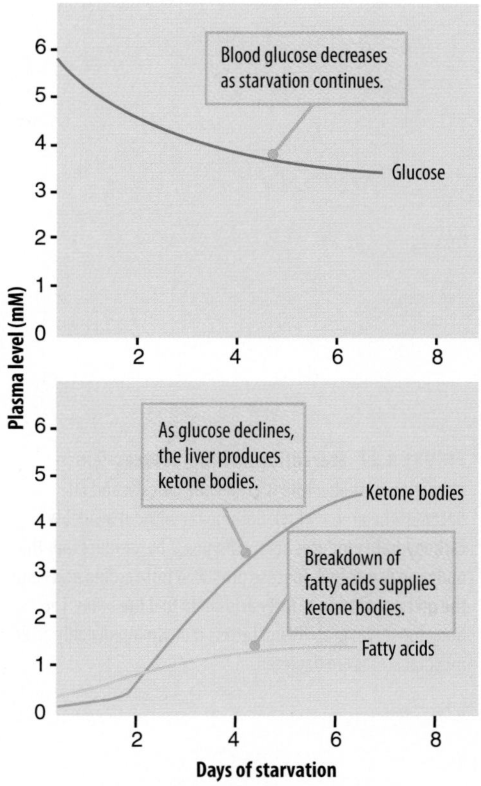

FIGURE 8.26 Shifting fuel selection during starvation. To fuel its needs as blood glucose levels decline, the body shifts from glucose to fatty acids and ketone bodies.

The Early Weeks

As starvation continues, Frank's body initiates several energy-conservation strategies. It ratchets down its energy use by lowering body temperature, pulse rate, blood pressure, and resting metabolism. Frank becomes lethargic, reducing the amount of energy expended in activity. He will also begin to have detectable signs of mild vitamin deficiencies as his body depletes its small reserves of vitamin C and most B vitamins.

If Frank's body continued to rapidly break down protein, he would survive less than three weeks. To avoid such a quick demise, protein breakdown slows drastically and gluconeogenesis drops significantly.[23] To pick up the slack, Frank's body doubles the rate of fat catabolism to supply fatty acids for fuel and glycerol for glucose. Ketone bodies pour into the bloodstream and provide an important glucose-sparing energy source for the brain and red blood cells. After about 10 days of fasting, ketone bodies meet most of the nervous system's energy needs. Some brain cells, however, can use only glucose. To maintain a small, but essential, supply of blood glucose, protein breakdown crawls along, supplying small amounts of amino acids for gluconeogenesis.

Several Weeks of Fasting

During prolonged fasting, the main determinant of survival is the amount of body fat at the start of the fast. The average adult has about two months' worth of stored fat.[24] As the later stages of starvation exhaust the final fat stores, the body turns again to protein, its sole remaining fuel source. Normally, Frank's body breaks down about 30 to 55 grams of protein each day, but now it accelerates the rate to several hundred grams daily (see **FIGURE 8.27**). You can see some of the effects of accelerated protein breakdown in starving children suffering from kwashiorkor. The loss of blood proteins causes the swollen limbs and bulging stomachs that typify this type of protein-energy malnutrition (PEM).

The End Is Near

In the final stage of protein depletion, the body deteriorates rapidly. You can see the severe muscle atrophy and emaciation in photos of Holocaust victims. Their bodies sacrificed muscle tissue in attempts to preserve brain tissue. Even organ tissues were not spared. The final stage of starvation attacks the liver and intestines, greatly depleting them. It moderately depletes the heart and kidneys, and even mounts a small attack on the nervous system. Amazingly, starving people can cling to life until they lose about half their body proteins, after which death generally occurs.

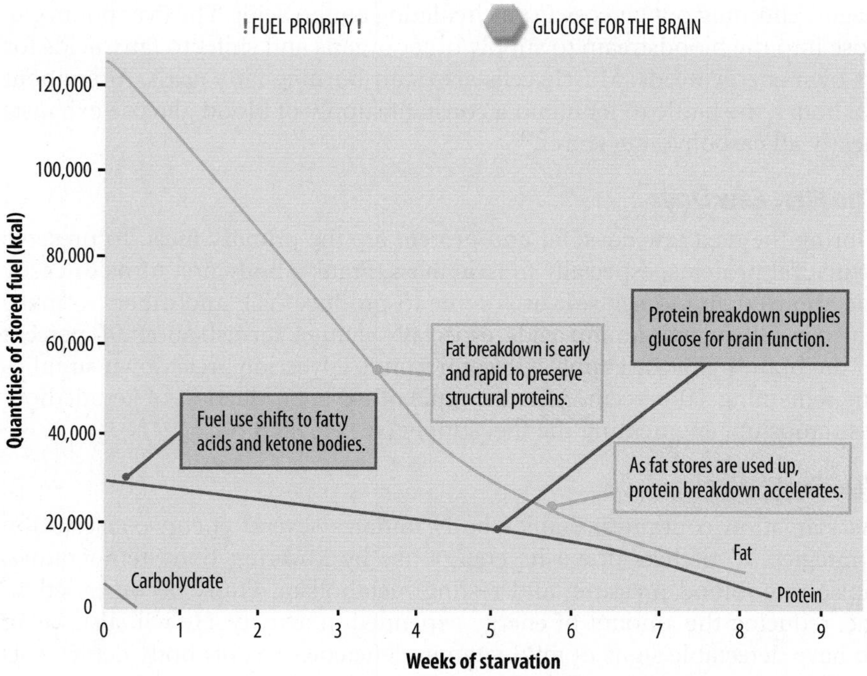

FIGURE 8.27 Starvation and fuel sources. During starvation, carbohydrate is exhausted quickly, and fat becomes the primary fuel. Burning fat without available carbohydrate produces ketone bodies, a by-product that the body can use as fuel. Glucose produced from amino acids and the glycerol portion of fatty acids help fuel the brain. The body conserves protein and breaks it down rapidly only after most fat stores are depleted.

How long can a person survive total starvation? Years ago, some Irish prisoners starved themselves to death—the average time was 60 days.[25] Most people survive total starvation for one to three months. Starvation survival factors include the following:

- *Starting percentage of body fat:* Ample adipose tissue prolongs survival.
- *Age:* Middle-aged people survive longer than children and older adults.
- *Sex:* Women fare better because of their higher proportion of body fat.
- *Energy expenditure levels:* Increased activity leads to an earlier demise.

Key Concepts Fasting, or underconsumption of energy (calories), favors catabolic pathways. The body first obtains fuel from stored glycogen, and then from stored fat and functional proteins, such as muscle. Over time, the body adapts to using increasing amounts of ketone bodies as fuel because limited carbohydrate is available. Larger stores of fat in adipose tissue extend survival time during starvation. In prolonged starvation, the body catabolizes muscle tissue to continue minimal production of glucose from amino acids.

Nutrition Science *in Action*

Energy Intake and Expenditure During Video Games and Television Watching

Background

Positive energy balance (energy surplus) occurs when energy intake is greater than energy expenditure. This can lead to weight gain over time. Sedentary activities such as watching television and playing hand-controlled video games burn little energy and are associated with higher energy intakes. Video games that are motion-controlled may be a healthier alternative to these traditional screen-based activities because they promote energy expenditure. However, little is known about how motion-controlled games affect energy intake.

Hypothesis

Motion-controlled games will be associated with a lower energy intake, higher energy expenditure, and lower energy surplus as compared to watching television or playing traditional video games.

Experimental Plan

Young adults aged 18–35 years were recruited through a university mailing list and local television advertisement. Subjects who weighed less than 300 pounds, had played video games three or more times in the past year, were willing to fast for two hours prior to their appointment, and agreed to be videotaped were included in the study. Participants were randomly assigned to watch television, play traditional video games, or play motion-controlled games during the one-hour study period. Snacks and beverages were provided to participating subjects. Energy intake, expenditure, and appetite were measured.

Results

There was no significant difference in energy intake among the three groups, although there was a trend toward lower energy intake in the motion-controlled group. There was a significantly higher energy expenditure and lower energy surplus in the motion-controlled group than in the sedentary television and video game groups. All conditions produced an energy surplus. (See **TABLE A**.)

Conclusion and Discussion

Motion-controlled games might be a healthier alternative to sedentary screen time such as television watching and traditional video games playing because they lead to a lower energy surplus. However, like those in the sedentary screen time groups, the participants in the motion-controlled group were still in positive energy balance after one hour of play. It should not be assumed that motion-controlled games produce a benefit on weight or health.

Data from Lyons EJ, Tate DF, Ward DS, Wang X. Energy intake and expenditure during sedentary screen time and motion-controlled video gaming. *Am J Clin Nutr.* 2012;96:234–239.

TABLE A
Outcomes Across Groups and Sexes[a]

	Men	Women	Total	Men	Women	Total	Men	Women	Total
Soda intake (kcal)	73 ± 89	54 ± 76	63 ± 82	114 ± 107	28 ± 67	71 ± 98	73 ± 93	29 ± 68	51 ± 84
Total intake (kcal)	764 ± 424	669 ± 396	716 ± 407	1,013 ± 504	481 ± 442	747 ± 540	769 ± 571	336 ± 290	553 ± 498
Energy expenditure (kcal × (kg – 1) × (h – 1)	1.08 ± 0.13	1.06 ± 0.11	1.07 ± 0.12[b]	1.36 ± 0.22	1.24 ± 0.22	1.30 ± 0.29[b]	2.72 ± 0.76	2.29 ± 0.73	2.50 ± 0.77
Energy surplus (kcal/hr)	676 ± 431	603 ± 431	638 ± 408[b]	906 ± 505	404 ± 442	655 ± 533[b]	565 ± 564	187 ± 305	376 ± 487

[a] All values are means ± standard deviations. Differences were tested using nonparametric analysis of covariance (ANCOVA) adjusted for sex and pairwise comparisons with Bonferroni adjustment as necessary. Significant differences between sexes are shown for all variables, $P < 0.01$.

[b] Significantly less than for motion-controlled video games, $P < 0.05$.

Reproduced from Lyons EJ, Tate DF, Ward DS, Wang X. Energy intake and expenditure during sedentary screen time and motion-controlled video gaming [Table 2, p. 238]. *Am J Clin Nutr.* 2012;96:234–239.

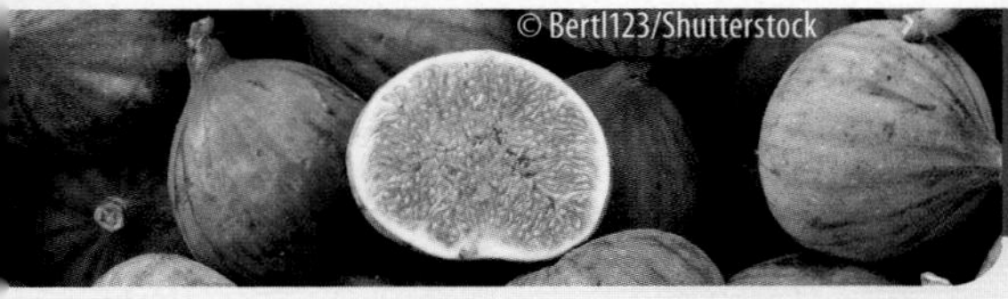

Learning Portfolio

Key Terms

acetyl CoA	293	guanosine triphosphate (GTP)	290
adenosine diphosphate (ADP)	289	hydrogen ions	290
adenosine monophosphate (AMP)	289	ketoacidosis	309
adenosine triphosphate (ATP)	289	ketogenesis	307
aerobic	293	ketogenic	306
alcohol dehydrogenase (ADH)	301	ketones	307
aldehyde dehydrogenase (ALDH)	301	Krebs cycle	294
anabolism	287	lactate	293
anaerobic	291	lipogenesis	306
beta-oxidation	297	metabolic pathway	287
biosynthesis	289	metabolism	285
carnitine	297	metabolites	287
catabolism	287	microsomal ethanol-oxidizing system (MEOS)	302
cells	288	mitochondria (mitochondrion)	289
chemical energy	285	mitochondrial membrane	295
citric acid cycle	293	NADH	289
coenzyme A	293	NADPH	289
coenzymes	289	nicotinamide adenine dinucleotide (NAD^+)	290
cofactors	289	nucleus	288
Cori cycle	306	organelles	288
cytoplasm	288	oxaloacetate	293
cytosol	288	oxidative phosphorylation	295
electron transport chain	295	photosynthesis	285
$FADH_2$	289	pyrophosphate (P_i)	289
flavin adenine dinucleotide (FAD)	291	pyruvate	291
glucogenic	306	transamination	309
gluconeogenesis	304	tricarboxylic acid (TCA) cycle	294
glycogenesis	306		
glycogenolysis	306		
glycolysis	291		

Study Points

- Energy is necessary to do any kind of work. The body converts chemical energy from food sources—carbohydrates, proteins, and fats—into a form usable by cells.
- Anabolic reactions (anabolism) build compounds. These reactions require energy.
- Catabolic reactions (catabolism) break compounds into smaller units. These reactions produce energy.
- Adenosine triphosphate (ATP) is the energy currency of the body.
- NADH, $FADH_2$, and NADPH are important carriers of hydrogen and high-energy electrons. NADH and $FADH_2$ are used in making ATP, whereas NADPH is used in biosynthetic reactions.
- Cells extract energy from carbohydrate by four main pathways: glycolysis, conversion of pyruvate to acetyl CoA, the citric acid cycle, and the electron transport chain. The citric acid cycle and electron transport chain require oxygen. Glycolysis does not. The electron transport chain produces more ATP than do other catabolic pathways.
- To extract energy from fat, first triglycerides are separated into glycerol and fatty acids. Next, beta-oxidation breaks down the fatty acids to yield acetyl CoA, NADH, and $FADH_2$. The acetyl CoA enters the citric acid cycle, producing more NADH and $FADH_2$. The NADH and $FADH_2$ molecules deliver their high-energy electrons to the electron transport chain to make ATP.
- To extract energy from an amino acid, first it is deaminated (the amino group is removed). Depending on the structure of the remaining carbon skeleton, it enters the catabolic pathways as pyruvate, acetyl CoA, or a citric acid cycle intermediate. The citric acid cycle and the electron transport chain complete the production of ATP.
- The liver converts the nitrogen portion of amino acids to urea, which the kidneys excrete.
- The liver metabolizes alcohol before metabolizing macronutrients. When large amounts of alcohol are consumed, the microsomal ethanol-oxidizing system (MEOS) helps metabolize the excess.
- Tissues differ in their preferred source of fuel. The brain, nervous system, and red blood cells rely primarily on glucose, whereas other tissues use a mix of glucose, fatty acids, and ketone bodies as fuel sources.
- When carbohydrate is available, glucose can be stored as glycogen in liver and muscle tissue. Glucose can be produced from the noncarbohydrate precursors glycerol and some (glucogenic) amino acids but not from fatty acids.

- The hormone insulin regulates metabolism by favoring anabolic pathways. It promotes the uptake of glucose by cells, thus removing it from the bloodstream.
- Glucagon, cortisol, and epinephrine stimulate catabolic pathways. These hormones promote the breakdown of glycogen to glucose and of amino acids to make glucose by way of gluconeogenesis. The breakdown of liver glycogen increases the amount of glucose in the blood.
- Feasting, or overconsumption of energy, leads to glycogen and triglyceride storage.
- Fasting, or underconsumption of energy, leads to the mobilization of liver glycogen and stored triglycerides. Starvation, the state of prolonged fasting, leads to protein breakdown as well and can be fatal.

Study Questions

1. What is the "universal energy currency"? Where is most of it produced?
2. Name the two energy-equivalent molecules that contain three phosphates as part of their structure. What makes these two molecules different? How many high-energy phosphate bonds do they contain?
3. In the catabolic pathways, which two molecules are major electron acceptors? After they accept electrons, which electron carriers do they become? What is the primary function of the electron carriers?
4. How many pyruvate molecules does glycolysis produce from one glucose molecule? What does the oxidative step after glycolysis produce? What does the citric acid cycle produce from a single glucose molecule?
5. Which two-carbon molecules does beta-oxidation form as it "clips" the links of a fatty acid chain? Which other molecules important to the production of ATP does beta-oxidation produce?
6. What dictates whether an amino acid is considered ketogenic or glucogenic?
7. What are ketone bodies, and when are they produced?
8. Name the three tissues where energy is stored. Which contains the largest store of energy?
9. Define gluconeogenesis and lipogenesis. Under what conditions do they predominantly occur? What are their primary inputs and outputs?

Try This

Comparing Fad Diets

The purpose of this exercise is to have you evaluate two fad diets in regard to their metabolic consequences. The two diets, Cabbage Soup and Super Protein, are described here. Once you've reviewed them, answer the following questions: Will these diets result in weight loss? Why or why not? On the seventh day of each diet, which of the following metabolic pathways will be highly active?

- Glycogen breakdown
- Fat breakdown
- Gluconeogenesis
- Ketogenesis

Diet 1: The Cabbage Soup Diet

A person following the Cabbage Soup diet eats only a water-based soup made out of cabbage and a few other vegetables. Three to four meals per day of this restricted diet supply approximately 500 kilocalories per day. The diet is devoid of protein and fat and gets its calories from the small amount of carbohydrate in the vegetables. Think about what happens during starvation.

Diet 2: The Super Protein Diet

In the Super Protein diet, a person can eat an unlimited amount of protein-rich foods such as meat, poultry, eggs, and seafood, but no added fats or carbohydrates are allowed. The average person can consume about 1,400 kilocalories if he or she eats three or four small meals each day. Think about what happens when little carbohydrate is available as a person metabolizes fat and protein.

Fasting for Ketones

The purpose of this experiment is to see whether a day without eating will cause your body to produce measurable ketones in your urine. Before starting your fast, check with your physician to be sure this won't pose any health risks. Go to your local pharmacy and ask the pharmacist for urine ketone strips (often called Ketostix). Bring them

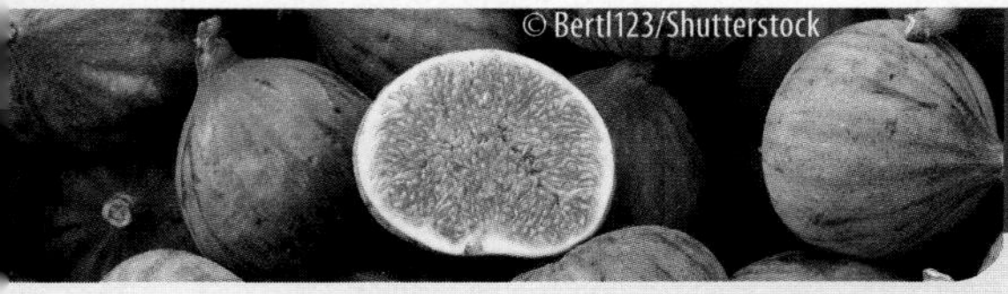
© Bertl123/Shutterstock

Learning Portfolio (continued)

home and read the directions. Before you start your one-day fast, test your urine to see whether it has a detectable amount of ketones. Start a 24-hour fast (or fast for as long as you can go without food or calorie-containing fluids but no longer than 24 hours), and test your urine at 6-hour intervals. Do you detect a color change on the strips as the day goes on? Why? What has happened metabolically as the day progresses?

Remember to drink lots of water!

References

1. Gropper SS, Smith JL. *Advanced Nutrition and Human Metabolism*. 6th ed. Belmont, CA: Wadsworth; 2012.
2. Butte NF, Caballero B. Energy needs: assessment and requirements. In: Ross AC, Caballero B, Cousins RJ, Tucker KL, Ziegler TR, eds. *Modern Nutrition in Health and Disease*. 11th ed. Philadelphia: Lippincott Williams & Wilkins; 2012:88–101.
3. Stipanuk MH, Caudill MA. *Biochemical and Physiological Aspects of Human Nutrition*. 3rd ed. Philadelphia: WB Saunders; 2012.
4. Nelson DL, Cox MM. *Principles of Biochemistry*. 6th ed. New York: WH Freeman and Co.; 2012.
5. Berg JM, Tymoczko JL, Stryer L. *Biochemistry*. 7th ed. New York: WH Freeman; 2010.
6. Gropper SS, Smith JL. *Advanced Nutrition and Human Metabolism*. Op cit.
7. Devlin TM. *Textbook of Biochemistry with Clinical Correlations*. 7th ed. Hoboken, NJ: Wiley; 2011.
8. Kleiner S, Greenwood-Robinson M. *Power Eating*. Champaign, IL: Human Kinetics; 2014.
9. Cederbaum AI. Alcohol metabolism. *Clin Liver Dis*. 2012;16(4):667–685.
10. Ibid.
11. Ibid.
12. Gropper SS, Smith JL. *Advanced Nutrition and Human Metabolism*. Op cit.
13. Devlin TM. *Textbook of Biochemistry*. Op cit.

14. Ibid.
15. Nelson DJ, Cox MM. *Principles of Biochemistry*. Op cit.
16. Devlin TM. *Textbook of Biochemistry*. Op cit.
17. Oh S, Kalyani RR, Dobs A. Nutritional management of diabetes mellitus. In: Ross AC, Caballero B, Cousins RJ, Tucker KL, Ziegler TR, eds. *Modern Nutrition in Health and Disease*. 11th ed. Philadelphia: Lippincott Williams & Wilkins; 2012:1043–1066.
18. Guyton AC, Hall JE. *Textbook of Medical Physiology*. 11th ed. Philadelphia: Elsevier Health Sciences; 2010.
19. Nelson DJ, Cox MM. *Principles of Biochemistry*. Op cit.
20. Ibid.
21. Martini FH, Nath JL. *Fundamentals of Anatomy and Physiology*. 9th ed. San Francisco: Benjamin Cummings; 2011:23.
22. Gropper SS, Smith JL. *Advanced Nutrition and Human Metabolism*. Op cit.
23. Ibid.
24. Hoffer LJ. Metabolic consequences of starvation. In: Ross AC, Caballero B, Cousins RJ, Tucker KL, Ziegler TR, eds. *Modern Nutrition in Health and Disease*. 11th ed. Philadelphia: Lippincott Williams & Wilkins; 2012:660–677.
25. Barrett KE, Barmanv SM, Boitano S, Brooks H. *Ganong's Review of Medical Physiology*. 24th ed. New York: McGraw-Hill; 2012.

Chapter 9

Energy Balance and Weight Management: Finding Your Equilibrium

Revised by Don Ross

THINK About It

1. How often do you reject dessert after a big meal?
2. When it comes to body fat distribution, what is your body shape? Are you an apple or a pear?
3. What does it mean to be metabolically fit?
4. How much time do you spend talking with your friends about weight?

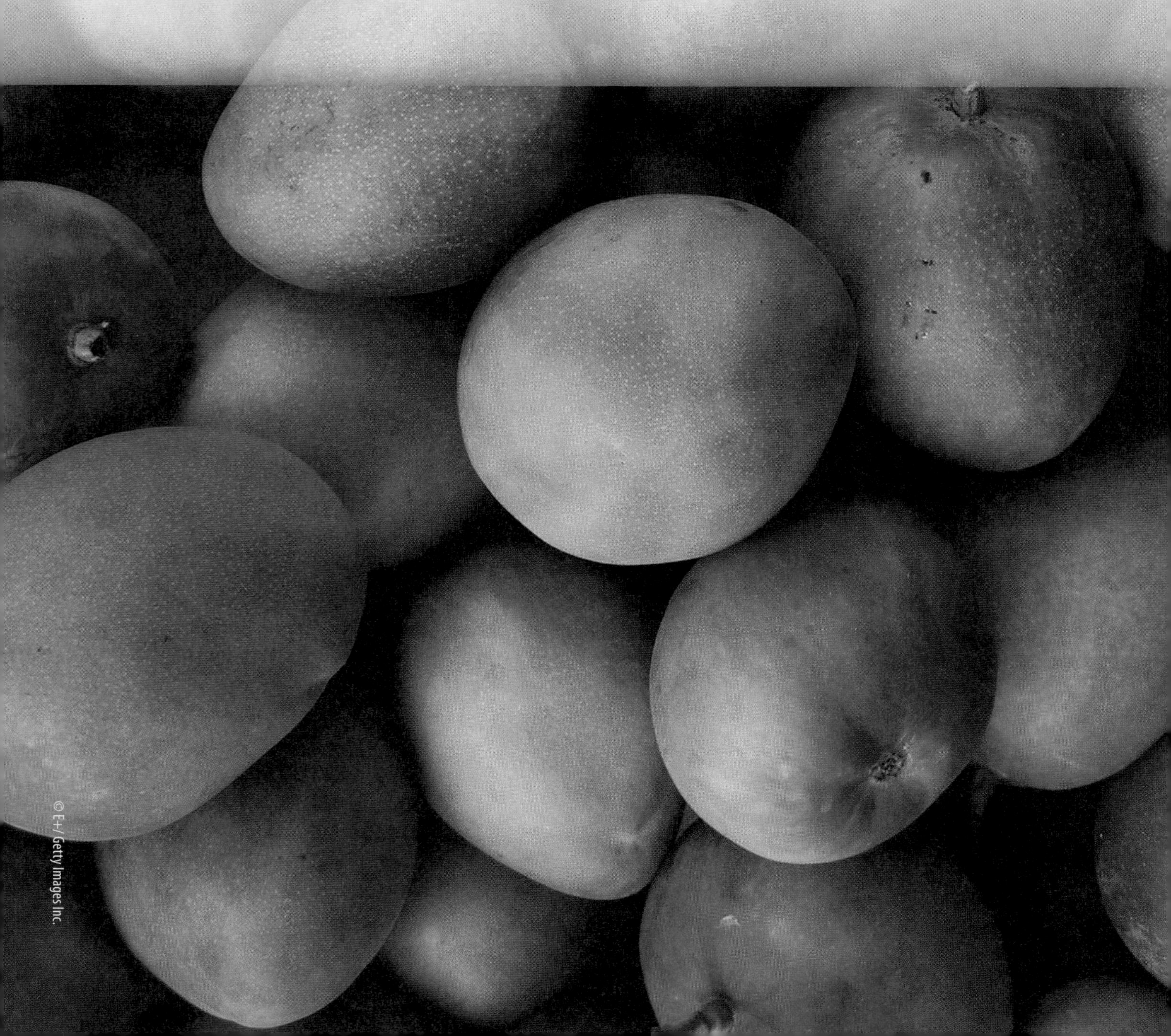

CHAPTER Menu

LEARNING Objectives

- Predict energy balance in the body.
- Determine BMI and total energy expenditure using standard equations.
- Determine the corresponding disease risks associated with body fat distribution.
- Recommend weight management strategies to overcome the risks of overweight, underweight, and obesity.

Your body is in the energy exchange business. Here's how it works. You balance the energy you expend with energy from the food in your diet. If you do a fairly good job of equalizing input and output, your body does the rest—maintaining energy equilibrium and keeping your weight steady. But what happens if you bring in more energy than your body can handle? It banks the excess energy as fat, and you gain weight. If your "account" grows too big, you become obese. Losing that extra weight—withdrawing the fat from your account—is not always easy.

Energy intake is the amount of fuel (calories) you take in through consumption of carbohydrate, protein, fat, and alcohol. **Energy output** is the amount you expend—primarily for basic body functions, physical activity, and the processing of food. An average adult consumes 1,800 to 3,000 kilocalories per day. In one year, that adds up to 657,000 to 1,095,000 kilocalories! Amazingly, despite such a huge intake of energy over time, many people maintain roughly the same weight during their adult lives.

People who maintain a relatively constant weight are in **energy equilibrium**. Within limits, your body automatically regulates your weight, thanks to its ability to balance intake and expenditure. Your body can be in energy equilibrium even if your energy intake is very high, as long as your expenditure also is high. Conversely, your body can be in energy equilibrium when you don't expend much energy, as long as your intake also is low.

When you take in more energy than you need, you have a **positive energy balance**. You store the surplus as fat—the major energy reserve—and as glycogen, the short-term carbohydrate energy reserve. Pregnant women and growing children need a positive energy balance to increase energy stores. But the positive energy balance that results from overeating and inactivity, a common occurrence around major holidays, leads to unneeded weight gain. When you take in less energy than you need, you have a **negative energy balance**. Reduced energy intake can be the result of illness, or it can be an intentional change for weight loss. To obtain fuel, your body uses stores of glycogen and fat (and breaks down body protein too, if the deficit is extreme), and body weight goes down. Thus, body weight change reflects overall **energy balance**. **FIGURE 9.1** shows different ratios of energy intake to energy expenditure.

▶ **energy intake** The caloric or energy content of food provided by the sources of dietary energy: carbohydrate (4 kcal/g), protein (4 kcal/g), fat (9 kcal/g), and alcohol (7 kcal/g).

▶ **energy output** The use of calories or energy for basic body functions, physical activity, and processing of consumed foods.

▶ **energy equilibrium** A balance of energy intake and output that results in little or no change in weight over time.

▶ **positive energy balance** Energy intake exceeds energy expenditure, resulting in an increase in body energy stores and weight gain.

▶ **negative energy balance** Energy intake is lower than energy expenditure, resulting in a depletion of body energy stores and weight loss.

▶ **energy balance** The balance in the body between amounts of energy consumed and expended.

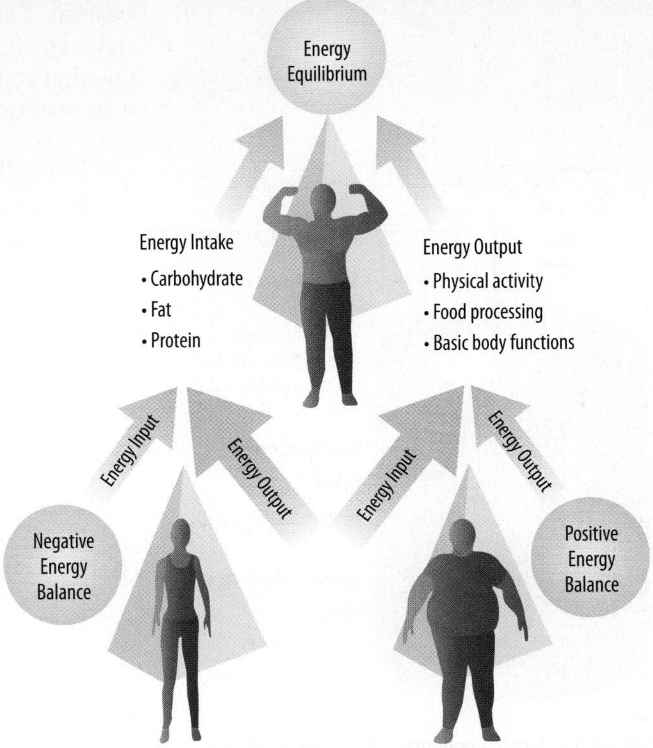

FIGURE 9.1 **Energy balance.** Most people balance energy intake and output and stay in energy balance. People in negative energy balance lose weight, and those in positive energy balance gain weight.

Key Concepts Energy balance is the relationship between energy intake and energy output. Energy intake comes from the calories in food and beverages. Energy output is the amount of fuel used mainly for basic body functions, the processing of food, and physical activity.

Energy In

▶ **bomb calorimeter** A device that uses the heat of combustion to measure the energy content of a food.

We can measure the energy content of a food with a **bomb calorimeter**, like that shown in **FIGURE 9.2**. Inside a sealed chamber, the food is completely burned and sensors measure the amount of heat produced by its combustion. Your body is not as efficient as a bomb calorimeter. It does not completely digest all food and is unable to oxidize nitrogen. When calculating the amount of energy your body can extract from food, the number of kilocalories released by complete combustion in a bomb calorimeter is adjusted downward as follows:

4 kilocalories per gram of pure carbohydrate
4 kilocalories per gram of pure protein
9 kilocalories per gram of pure fat
7 kilocalories per gram of pure alcohol

If we know a food's carbohydrate, fat, and protein content, we can use these numbers to estimate its calorie content.

Regulation of Food Intake

▶ **hunger** The internal, physiological drive to find and consume food. Unlike appetite, hunger is usually experienced as a negative sensation, often manifesting as an uneasy or painful sensation.

We know that energy intake is the number of calories consumed. But how does the body recognize how much energy it needs? A complex interaction between internal and external cues helps the body regulate food consumption and maintain energy equilibrium. Internal cues involve interactions and feedback mechanisms among hormones and hormone-like compounds and organ systems. External cues are stimuli in the eating environment and include the sight, smell, and taste of food. Although these internal and external cues work together to ensure that we eat enough to survive, they can be readily overridden, resulting in overeating and weight gain, or undereating and weight loss.

Hunger, Satiation, and Satiety

We experience internal cues as three different sensations that influence our eating behaviors (see **FIGURE 9.3**). The first, **hunger**, prompts eating

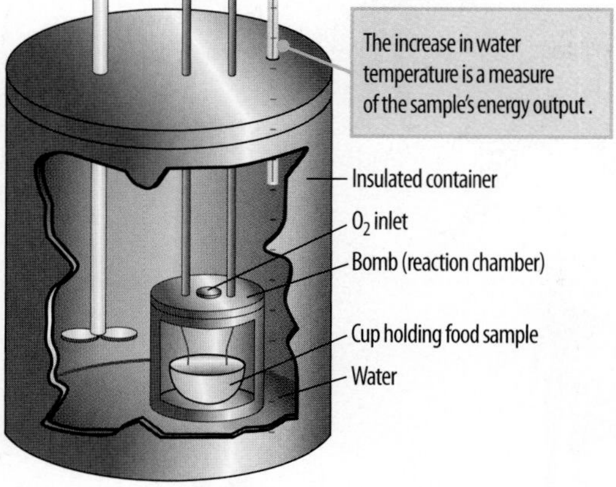

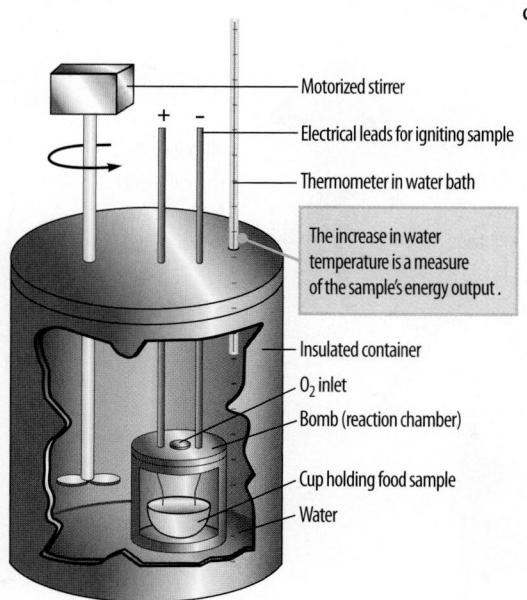

FIGURE 9.2 Bomb calorimeter. When a sample of food is completely burned inside the sealed chamber of a bomb calorimeter, it causes the temperature of the water surrounding the chamber to rise. This rise in temperature is a measure of the energy content of the food.

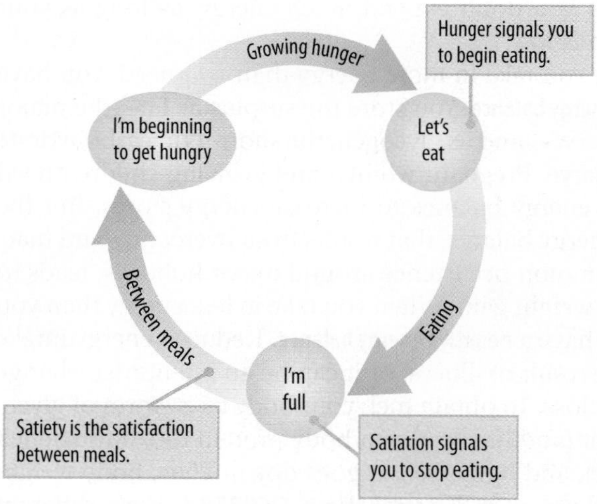

FIGURE 9.3 Hunger, satiation, and satiety. Hunger helps initiate eating. Satiation brings eating to a halt. Satiety is the state of nonhunger that determines the amount of time until eating begins again.

("I'm hungry"). Hunger is a physical sensation that includes the gnawing feeling in your stomach and signals the physiological need to eat. The second, **satiation**, tells you to stop eating ("I'm full"). The third, **satiety**, determines the interval between meals ("I'm not ready to eat again"). Satiety means not being hungry; it is influenced in part by how many calories you ate at your last meal.

▶ **satiation** Feeling of satisfaction and fullness that terminates a meal.

▶ **satiety** The effects of a food or meal that delay subsequent intake. A feeling of satisfaction and fullness following eating that quells the desire for food.

▶ **appetite** A psychological desire to eat that is related to the pleasant sensations often associated with food.

Appetite

Internal and external cues can stimulate **appetite**, which complicates the workings of hunger, satiation, and satiety. To ensure adequate nourishment, appetite and hunger work in tandem. Appetite is the psychological desire to eat and is related to pleasant sensations associated with food. Hunger is the physiological need for food. In this sense, whereas appetite reflects our eating experiences, hunger is a basic drive. When you are truly hungry, any food will do, but appetite can trigger your desire for a specific food or type of food, even though you might not be hungry. For example, after a big meal of steak, potato, salad, and bread, you probably wouldn't want a second helping. But you might be tempted by the dessert cart! That's appetite. Even when we are hungry, illness and medication can cause loss of appetite and a lack of interest in food.

THINK About It 1

Quick Bite

Early Energy Balance Experiments

Erasistraus of Chios performed the first recorded experiment on energy balance in 280 B.C.E. Seeking to balance intake with output, he used a jar to fashion a kind of respiration apparatus. He then put two birds in the jar, weighing them and their excreta before and after feeding.

Key Concepts Food intake is regulated by sensations of hunger, a physiological drive to eat; satiation, feelings of satisfaction that lead to ending a meal; and satiety, continued feelings of fullness that delay the start of the next meal. Appetite is the psychological urge to eat and often has no relation to hunger.

Control by Committee

What, then, stimulates hunger, satiation, satiety, and appetite? As you will see, multiple players are involved. What you eat, the amount that you eat, and responses in the digestive tract, central nervous system, and general circulation influence your eating behavior. Sites throughout the body monitor energy status and send reports to the brain. Even the temperature of our environment affects how much we eat.

Quick Bite

Why Do We Have Hunger Pangs?

When the stomach has been without food for at least three hours, intense stomach contractions can begin, sometimes lasting two to three minutes. Healthy young people have the strongest contractions because of good muscle tone in the gastrointestinal (GI) tract. After 12 to 24 hours, contractions of an empty stomach can cause painful hunger pangs.

Diet Composition

The energy density (kcal/g), balance of energy sources (carbohydrates, lipids, and protein), and the form (liquid vs. solid) of your foods affect the amount you eat. Regardless of its nutrient value, people tend to eat a fairly constant amount of food. Therefore, if your overall diet includes a lot of energy-dense foods (generally high-fat, high-sugar, low-fiber), your overall diet will likely result in excess energy consumption, and in turn, weight gain.

Dietary protein and fiber can help control energy intake. Protein consumption appears to increase satiety more than eating fats or carbohydrates.[1] Some types of fiber enhance satiation by slowing the rate at which the stomach empties, whereas others seem to enhance satiation by creating bulk.[2] Adding fiber to low-energy-dense foods can be an effective way to suppress appetite and control food intake.[3]

Simple carbohydrates and added sugars generally have low satiety value and can be a significant source of calories. People eating low carbohydrate diets tend to have higher energy expenditures than those eating low fat diets, and epidemiological studies have linked consumption sugar-sweetened beverages (such as soda) to the growing obesity rates in the United States.[4] In young children, research indicates that regular consumption of sugar-sweetened beverages increases risk for becoming overweight.[5] The current upward trend in consumption of sugar-sweetened beverages parallels the increase in childhood obesity rates. In general, liquid foods are less satiating than solid foods. One exception is soup, which despite its liquid form, has relatively high satiety value.

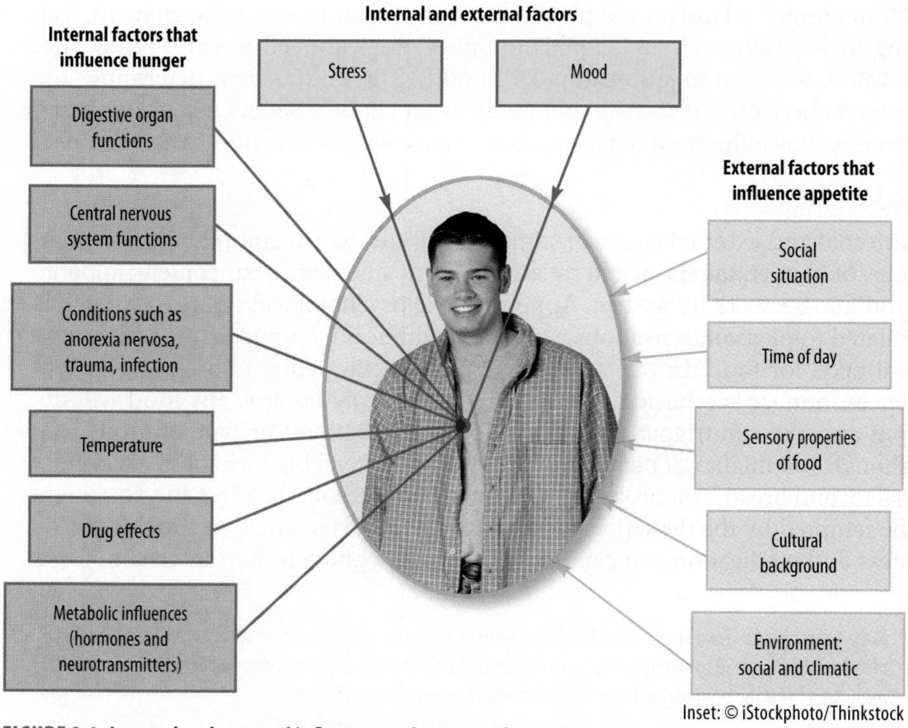

FIGURE 9.4 Internal and external influences on hunger and appetite.

Sensory Properties

The aroma of freshly baked bread or the warmth and chewiness of chocolate chip cookies right out of the oven encourage us to eat more than our hunger dictates. Food's sensory properties—flavor, texture, color, temperature, and presentation—influence its appeal, and such external cues affect food intake.[6] (See **FIGURE 9.4**.) Taste often is the reason why people choose a particular food, and unsurprisingly, we are more likely to overeat a food that tastes good.

Portion Size

Portion size plays a role in how much we eat, with large portions generally leading to an increase in energy intake. Over the past two decades, portion sizes have increased for virtually all foods and beverages prepared for immediate consumption, including fast food, individually packaged food, and ready-to-eat prepared food (see **TABLE 9.1**).

TABLE 9.1
Comparison of Common Portion Sizes 20 Years Ago Versus Today

	20 Years Ago		Today	
Food Item	**Portion**	**Calories**	**Portion**	**Calories**
Bagel	3-inch diameter	140	6-inch diameter	350
Cheeseburger	1	333	1	590
Spaghetti with meatballs	1 cup sauce and 3 small meatballs	500	2 cups sauce and 3 large meatballs	1,020
Soda	6.5 oz	82	20 oz	250
Blueberry muffin	1.5 oz	210	5 oz	500

Reproduced from National Heart, Lung, and Blood Institute; National Institutes of Health, U.S. Department of Health and Human Services. Portion distortion. http://www.nhlbi.nih.gov/health/educational/wecan/eat-right/portion-distortion.htm. Accessed January 6, 2016.

Several studies have documented a "portion distortion" phenomenon. Rather than paying attention to internal feelings of satiation, we tend to respond to the visual stimulation of the amount of food on a plate or the serving size and consider that to be "normal." In a study of 110 undergraduate students, the group offered a larger plate of cookies consumed more than the group presented with a smaller plate of cookies.[7] Another study looked at serving snack foods from different-sized containers. The results suggest that serving food in larger containers stimulates increased food intake.[8]

Children also are tempted by big portions. In a study of cereal consumption, children presented with a large bowl requested almost twice as much cereal as when presented with a smaller bowl.[9,10] In another study, children ate less when served smaller portions.[11] The ability of children to self-regulate energy intake at a meal is heavily influenced by portion size. A study of preschoolers found that the amount of food a child was served was highly predictive of the amount that they consumed.[12]

Americans are living in a "super-size" culture in which portion sizes keep getting larger. Buffets, fast-food restaurants, and convenience stores offer "value meals" providing more food for less money. Consumers indicate that value for money is important when purchasing food, and that large portion sizes offer more value for money than small portion sizes.[13] The dramatic increase in portion sizes eaten both at home and at restaurants may be a major contributing factor to excess energy intake and weight gain.

Does the idea of people eating more simply because they are served more always have to be associated with a negative consequence? The answer is no. For both children and adults, studies have found that serving more vegetables is an effective strategy to increase vegetable intake at a meal without influencing total meal energy intake, thus leading to more healthy eating overall.[14,15]

Environmental and Social Factors

We tend to eat more in cold weather and less in hot weather. Systems in the **hypothalamus** that regulate body temperature and food intake probably interact to link temperature and eating behavior. In cold temperatures, increased food intake helps us survive by supporting an increased metabolic rate, which helps generate heat, and an increase in fat stores, which provide insulation to reduce heat loss.[16]

▶ **hypothalamus** [high-po-THAL-ah-mus] A region of the brain involved in regulating hunger and satiety, respiration, body temperature, water balance, and other body functions.

Plate size, lighting, and socializing are other factors that influence consumption.[17] Any change in our surroundings that inhibits our self-monitoring of consumption tends to increase the volume that we eat. Larger plates and bowls encourage larger servings. We tend to eat more in dimly lit situations than when the lights are brighter, perhaps because we are less inhibited and self-conscious.[18]

In today's fast-paced society, many young adults eat alone with little advanced planning and while engaged in other activities. A shrinking proportion eats regularly in a traditional meal setting (eating at home with others in the absence of multitasking). When a person eats alone, his or her food choices often consist of highly processed, energy-dense, convenience products, and the overall intake of whole grains, fruits, and vegetables is low.[19]

Multitasking, such as watching television while eating, can increase food intake. The distraction of the television draws attention away from the amount of food being consumed.[20] Your friends also can influence your energy intake. Eating while talking with friends can increase energy intake. However, studies have shown that eating while talking with strangers does not increase intake.[21-23]

Emotional Factors

Many people use food to cope with stress and negative feelings. Eating can provide a powerful distraction from loneliness, anger, boredom, anxiety, shame, sadness, and inadequacy. To combat low moods, low energy levels, and low self-esteem, people often turn to the refrigerator. When we use food and eating to cope with our emotions, binge eating or other disturbed eating patterns can develop.

Gastrointestinal Sensations

As food fills your stomach and small intestine, they stretch and trigger signals to the brain. Your sense of fullness suppresses your urge to eat.[24] Just passing a reasonable amount of food through the mouth can satisfy hunger temporarily—even if the food never reaches the stomach. When researchers fed large amounts of food to a person with a hole in the esophagus, hunger decreased, even though the food never reached the stomach. As we taste, salivate, chew, and swallow, the brain probably measures the passage of food, much as a water meter measures the flow of water. After a certain amount of food passes through the mouth, hunger diminishes for 20 to 40 minutes.[25]

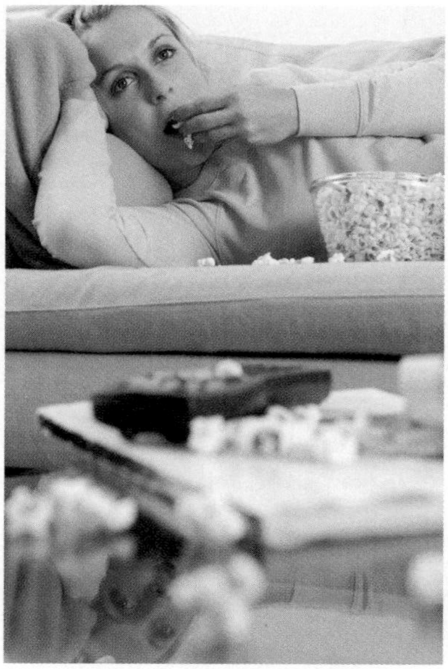

© Adam Gault/Digital Vision/Thinkstock

Neurological and Hormonal Factors

More than 50 different chemicals are thought to be involved in the regulation of feeding. Determining the way these chemical factors work is an active research area that may lead to improved therapies for those either overweight or underweight.

Hormones, hormone-like factors, and some drugs (including appetite suppressants) influence eating behavior through their direct or indirect effects on the brain.[26] **Neuropeptide Y (NPY)** is a hormone-like factor in the brain that powerfully stimulates appetite.[27] Although a number of signals can affect NPY activity, opposing signals from the hormones **ghrelin** and **leptin** link NPY secretion to daily feeding patterns.[28]

- **neuropeptide Y (NPY)** A neurotransmitter widely distributed throughout the brain and peripheral nervous tissue. NPY activity has been linked to eating behavior, depression, anxiety, and cardiovascular function.
- **ghrelin** A peptide hormone produced by the stomach that stimulates feeding; sometimes called the "hunger hormone."
- **leptin** A hormone produced by adipose cells that signals the amount of body fat content and influences food intake; sometimes called the "satiety hormone."

Ghrelin, sometimes called the "hunger hormone," is produced in the stomach. Ghrelin levels rise prior to a meal and fall quickly after food is consumed. The rise in ghrelin levels appears to stimulate NPY, thus encouraging feeding. As you might expect, ghrelin levels increase in people who are undereating and decrease in those who are overeating.

Leptin, sometimes called the "satiety hormone," is produced in fat cells in direct proportion to the amount of fat stored and helps regulate fat storage.[29] Thus, leptin levels are lower in thin people than in obese people. But unfortunately, many obese people have built up a resistance to the appetite-suppressing effects of leptin.[30] In normal-weight people, a rise in leptin levels appears to inhibit NPY, thus suppressing appetite.[31] A diet low in carbohydrates can lower leptin resistance, and a diet rich in whole grains or high in protein can suppress the "hunger hormone" ghrelin.[32]

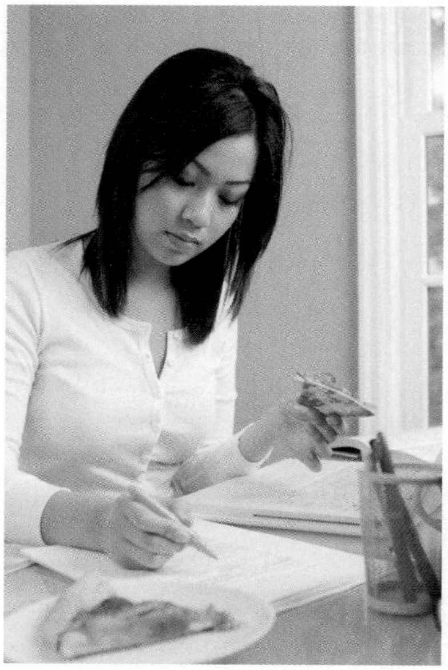

© YinYang/iStockphoto.com

Disruptions in the satiety signaling system can lead to consuming more calories, gaining weight, and storing fat. Stress-induced sleep loss, but not sleep loss per se, may result in decreased leptin levels, increased hunger, and a desire for "comfort foods."[33]

Key Concepts Diet composition and factors in the digestive tract and central nervous system influence eating behavior. The brain, especially the hypothalamus, receives signals from all over the body about energy status. External factors, such as portion size, social circumstances, and environmental conditions, as well as the food itself, can enhance or suppress appetite.

Energy Out: Fuel Uses

Our bodies use fuel (expend energy) for three primary purposes:

- To maintain basic physiological functions such as breathing and blood circulation

- To process the food we eat
- To power physical activity

We also expend energy to support growth, stay warm in cold environments, metabolize drugs, and deal with physical trauma, fever, and psychological stress. The sum of all energy expended is the **total energy expenditure (TEE)**. **FIGURE 9.5** illustrates the major components of energy expenditure.

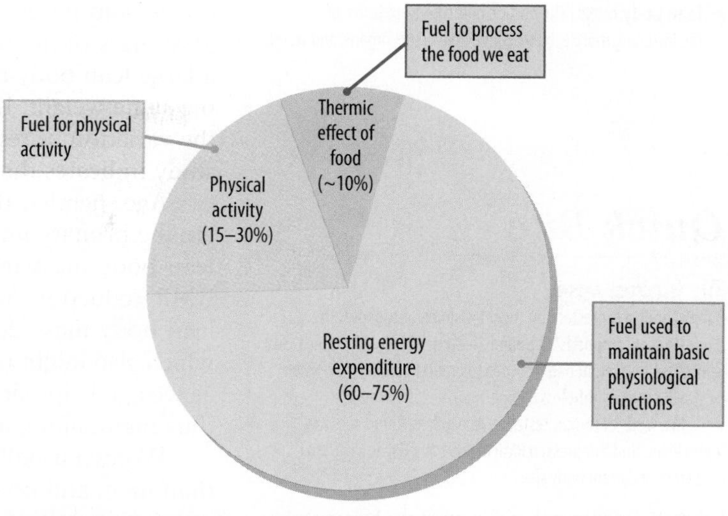

FIGURE 9.5 Major components of energy expenditure. You expend most of your energy to maintain basic body functions. Energy expended in physical activity can be significant and is the most variable component of total energy expenditure. The thermic effect of food is the energy needed to digest, absorb, transport, metabolize, and store ingested food.

Major Components of Energy Expenditure

Energy Expenditure at Rest

We generally expend most of our energy on the basic body functions needed to sustain life. This **basal energy expenditure (BEE)**, or **resting energy expenditure (REE)**, maintains heartbeat, respiration, nervous function, muscle tone, body temperature, and so on. Resting energy expenditure accounts for 60 to 75 percent of total energy expenditure. BEE and REE refer to energy expended in a 24-hour period. The rate of energy expended at rest (kcal/hour) is measured as either the **basal metabolic rate (BMR)** or the **resting metabolic rate (RMR)**. Researchers measure BMR under the following conditions:

- The person is lying at rest.
- The person has just awoken from a normal overnight sleep.
- Ten to 12 hours have elapsed since the person's last meal.
- No physical activity has taken place—usually for 12 to 18 hours.

The RMR differs slightly from the BMR. Researchers usually measure RMR three to four hours after a person eats or does significant physical work. RMR tends to be somewhat higher than BMR and is a more practical concept because the ideal conditions for measuring BMR are more difficult to meet. For this reason, we use the terms *resting metabolic rate* and *resting energy expenditure*.

Factors That Affect Resting Metabolic Rate

Although your RMR typically varies less than 5 percent over time, RMR can vary by as much as 25 percent among different people—mostly due to individual differences in muscle and organ mass. Because organs and resting muscles have greater metabolic activity than other tissues such as fat, they are the greatest contributors to RMR (see **TABLE 9.2**). Muscles, organs,

- **total energy expenditure (TEE)** The total of the resting energy expenditure (REE), energy used in physical activity, and energy used in processing food (TEF); usually expressed in kilocalories per day.
- **resting energy expenditure (REE)** The minimum energy needed to maintain basic physiological functions (e.g., heartbeat, muscle function, respiration). The resting metabolic rate (RMR) extrapolated to 24 hours. Often used interchangeably with BEE.
- **basal energy expenditure (BEE)** The basal metabolic rate (BMR) extrapolated to 24 hours. Often used interchangeably with REE.
- **basal metabolic rate (BMR)** A clinical measure of resting energy expenditure performed upon awakening, 10 to 12 hours after eating, and 12 to 18 hours after significant physical activity. Often used interchangeably with RMR.
- **resting metabolic rate (RMR)** A clinical measure of resting energy expenditure performed three to four hours after eating or performing significant physical activity. Often used interchangeably with BMR.

TABLE 9.2
Approximate Energy Expenditure of Organs in Adults

Organ	Percentage of RMR
Liver	29
Brain	19
Heart	10
Kidneys	7
Skeletal muscles (at rest)	18
Remainder (including bone)	17
	100

Modified from Mahan LK, Escott-Stump S. *Krause's Food, Nutrition and Diet Therapy.* 10th ed. Philadelphia: WB Saunders; 2000:20. Reprinted by permission of Elsevier.

Quick Bite

Supersize Me!

Morgan Spurlock wrote, directed, produced, and is the lead character in *Supersize Me!*, a film that documented Spurlock's consumption of a 30-day McDonald's-only diet. Whenever offered the option to "supersize" his order, Spurlock always selected the larger portion size. Starting at 185 pounds, the 6-foot, 2-inch Spurlock packed on 25 pounds and weighed 210 pounds by the end of his experiment. His total cholesterol shot up from 165 to 230, his libido flagged, and he suffered headaches and depression.

▶ **lean body mass** The portion of the body exclusive of stored fat, including muscle, bone, connective tissue, organs, and water.

bones, and fluids make up most of what is known as the **lean body mass**—the total mass of the body that isn't fat. An exceptionally muscular person with a large lean body mass typically has a higher RMR than an obese person of the same weight. Differences in lean body mass explain 70 to 80 percent of the variation in resting metabolic rate among individuals, although a recent study indicates that extreme weight loss can depress RMR significantly.[34]

Age, gender, degree of muscle development, and, of course, body size are the primary influences on a person's lean body mass. In the aging adult, lean body mass tends to decrease while body fatness rises, resulting in an RMR reduction of about 2 to 3 percent per decade.[35] However, declining lean body mass does not account fully for the age-related decline in RMR, which also might reflect declining organ function.[36] Keeping physically active as we age helps slow loss of lean tissue and discourages accumulation of fat, thus maintaining a higher RMR.

Women usually have lower RMRs than men. Women tend to be smaller than men, and pound for pound they generally have less lean body mass. A woman's RMR also varies during the menstrual cycle, fluctuating from the low point about one week before ovulation to the high point just before the onset of menstruation.[37]

Other factors that influence metabolic rate may be less consistent, of shorter duration, or limited to individual situations. During sleep, RMR falls about 10 percent. RMR relative to lean body mass rises during periods of rapid growth, such as in infancy and adolescence. Hormones, especially thyroxine (thyroid hormone) and norepinephrine, help regulate metabolic rate. Inadequate thyroxine production (hypothyroidism) can slow the metabolic rate; excess thyroxine (hyperthyroidism) can increase the metabolic rate. Physical stress increases the metabolic rate, probably in response to changes in norepinephrine levels. Fever increases RMR by about 7 percent for each degree of temperature over 98.6°F. Environmental temperature also affects the metabolic rate. During exposure to cold, RMR increases. As ambient temperatures rise above normal, RMR first decreases and then plateaus. At much higher temperatures, RMR increases. During starvation, the metabolic rate declines as the body slows basic functions to conserve energy and prolong survival. **FIGURE 9.6** shows the factors that affect RMR.

Quick Bite

The Biggest Loser

Danny Cahill, a contestant on the television reality show "The Biggest Loser," dropped 239 pounds—from 430 to 239 pounds. Six years later, his weight had returned to greater heights than when he started the weighht loss competition—450 pounds.

In a study of the contestants, researchers found very low leptin levels and a depressed RMR of 499kcals/day lower than expected for current body size.

Fothergill E, Guo J, Howard L, et al. Persistent metabolic adaptation 6 years after "The Biggest Loser" competition. Obesity. Early view online version May 2, 2016. http://onlinelibrary.wiley.com/doi/10.1002/oby.21538/full Accessed May 21, 2016.

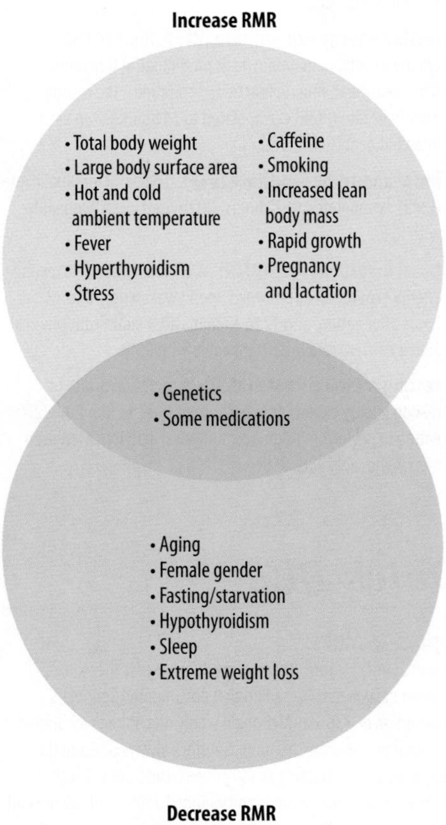

FIGURE 9.6 Factors that affect RMR. Inherited traits determine whether you have a generally high or low RMR. Many environmental and physiological factors can temporarily raise RMR, and other factors can temporarily lower it.

Key Concepts We use energy to fuel basic body functions, process the food we eat, and support physical activity. The energy used in these basic functions is called the resting energy expenditure, or REE. Factors that affect resting energy expenditure include body composition, age, gender, fitness, genetics, stage of growth, hormone levels, fever, and environmental temperatures.

Energy Expenditure for Physical Activity

Physical activity is more than just exercise and sport. It includes work, leisure activities, and other everyday activities—even fidgeting. Depending on whether a person is mostly sedentary or a top athlete in training, energy expended on physical activity accounts for 15 to 30 percent of total energy expenditure.[38] The energy cost of an activity depends on its type (whether it is walking, running, or typing, for example), duration, and intensity. **TABLE 9.3** shows the amounts of energy expended in specific activities.

Body size affects energy cost, too—it takes more energy to move a bigger mass, so a large person expends more calories per minute than a smaller person doing the same activity. Fitness level has an effect as well. A fit person exercises more efficiently, with lower energy costs. However, fit people also can exercise with greater intensity and duration, burning more calories overall.

Mental activity—such as studying for an exam—uses little energy. But if you fidget when you study, you may expend a significant amount of energy.

TABLE 9.3
Amount of Energy Expended in Specific Activities

			kcal/hr at Different Body Weights				
	kcal/hr/kg	kcal/hr/lb	50 kg (110 lb)	57 kg (125 lb)	68 kg (150 lb)	80 kg (175 lb)	91 kg (200 lb)
Aerobics							
Light	3.0	1.36	150	170	205	239	273
Moderate	8.0	2.27	250	284	341	398	455
Heavy	8.0	3.64	400	455	545	636	727
Bicycling							
Leisurely (< 10 mph)	4.0	1.82	200	227	273	318	364
Light (10–11.9 mph)	6.0	2.73	300	341	409	477	545
Moderate (12–13.9 mph)	8.0	3.64	400	455	545	636	727
Fast (14–15.9 mph)	10.0	4.55	500	568	682	795	909
Racing (16–19 mph)	12.0	5.45	600	682	818	955	1,091
BMX or mountain	8.5	3.86	425	483	580	676	773
Daily Activities							
Sleeping	1.2	0.55	60	68	82	95	109
Studying, reading, writing	1.8	0.82	90	102	123	143	164
Cooking, food preparation	2.5	1.14	125	142	170	199	227
Home Activities							
House painting, outside	4.0	1.82	200	227	273	318	364
General gardening	5.0	2.27	250	284	341	398	455
Shoveling snow	6.0	2.73	300	341	409	477	545
Running							
Jogging	7.0	3.18	350	398	477	557	636
Running 5 mph	8.0	3.64	400	455	545	636	727
Running 6 mph	10.0	4.55	500	568	682	795	909
Running 7 mph	11.5	5.23	575	653	784	915	1,045
Running 8 mph	13.5	6.14	675	767	920	1,074	1,227
Running 9 mph	15.0	6.82	750	852	1,023	1,193	1,364
Running 10 mph	16.0	7.27	800	909	1,091	1,273	1,455
Sports							
Frisbee, ultimate	3.5	1.59	175	199	239	278	318
Hacky sack	4.0	1.82	200	227	273	318	364
Wind surfing	4.2	1.91	210	239	286	334	382
Golf	4.5	2.05	225	256	307	358	409
Skateboarding	5.0	2.27	250	284	341	398	455
Rollerblading	7.0	3.18	350	398	477	557	636
Soccer	7.0	3.18	350	398	477	557	636
Field hockey	8.0	3.64	400	455	545	636	727
Swimming, slow to moderate laps	8.0	3.64	400	455	545	636	727
Skiing downhill, moderate effort	6.0	2.73	300	341	409	477	545
Skiing cross country, moderate effort	8.0	3.64	400	455	545	636	727
Tennis, doubles	6.0	2.73	300	341	409	477	545
Tennis, singles	8.0	3.64	400	455	545	636	727
Walking							
Strolling (< 2 mph), level	2.0	0.91	100	114	136	159	182
Moderate pace (~3 mph), level	3.5	1.59	175	199	239	278	318
Moderate pace (~3 mph), uphill	6.0	2.73	300	341	409	477	545
Brisk pace (~3.5 mph), level	4.0	1.82	200	227	273	318	364
Very brisk pace (~4.5 mph), level	4.5	2.05	225	256	307	358	409

Adapted from Nieman DC. *Exercise Testing and Prescription.* 7th ed. New York: McGraw-Hill; 2010.

▶ **nonexercise activity thermogenesis (NEAT)** The output of energy associated with fidgeting, maintenance of posture, and other minimal physical exertions.

The acronym **NEAT** stands for **nonexercise activity thermogenesis**, which is the energy associated with activities other than exercise, including fidgeting, maintenance of posture, occupational activities, and similar contributors to energy expenditure.[39]

Energy Expenditure to Process Food

▶ **thermic effect of food (TEF)** The energy used to digest, absorb, and metabolize energy-yielding foodstuffs. It constitutes about 10 percent of total energy expenditure but is influenced by various factors.

Our bodies expend energy to digest, absorb, and metabolize the nutrients we take in, and these processes generate heat. This energy output is collectively called the **thermic effect of food (TEF)**. TEF peaks about one hour after eating and normally dissipates within five hours. It is lowest for fat and highest for protein. Converting excess protein and carbohydrate to energy stores (fat and glycogen) requires more energy than the efficient process of simply storing excess dietary fat as body fat. Although altering macronutrient composition can alter TEF, observed changes are small—only about 50 kilocalories or so daily—and within normal day-to-day variations.[40] For a typical mixed diet, TEF accounts for approximately 10 percent of total energy expenditure and declines in older adults.[41] Although some research suggests that TEF is lower in obese people, other studies report no differences.[42] A cause-and-effect relationship between TEF and obesity has not been fully established and remains unclear.

Key Concepts An individual's fitness level, weight, and the type, duration, and intensity of activity affect the amount of energy expended in physical activity. The thermic effect of food is the energy needed to process the food we eat and is influenced by the amount and mix of nutrients in the diet.

The Measurement of Energy Expenditure

▶ **calorimetry** [kal-oh-RIM-eh-tree] The measurement of the amount of heat given off by an organism. It is used to determine total energy expenditure.

Calorimetry, the measurement of energy expenditure, helps us understand individual differences in energy expenditure and the effects of environmental conditions, as well as age, gender, exercise, and other factors.

A Brief History of Calorimetry

Antoine Lavoisier, an eighteenth-century French chemist, was the first to study food combustion in the body. He theorized that just as a burning candle needs oxygen and releases heat, organisms need oxygen to live and release heat as they combust food.

▶ **calorimeter** [kal-oh-RIM-eh-ter] A device used to measure quantities of heat generated by various processes.

Lavoisier built the first **calorimeter**, quite an achievement at that time. A calorimeter consists of a chamber within a chamber. The inner chamber is large enough to house an animal or human; the outer chamber is sensitive to temperature changes that occur in the inner one. Lavoisier packed ice into a sealed pocket around the inner chamber (his studies were possible only in winter, when ice was plentiful) and then placed it inside the outer chamber, which was insulated to shield it from the outside environment. As the animal in the inner chamber used energy, it produced heat that melted the ice. By collecting the resulting water and measuring its volume, Lavoisier could accurately calculate the amount of heat produced by the animal.

Quick Bite

Brr! Shivering Away Calories

Cold weather increases energy needs. Shivering alone can increase the RMR by 2.5 times. Although shivering bodies use both fat and carbohydrate, carbohydrates are the preferred fuel. In addition, people with less body fat shiver more in the cold.

Direct and Indirect Calorimetry

▶ **direct calorimetry** Determination of energy use by the body by measuring the heat released from an organism enclosed in a small insulated chamber surrounded by water. The rise in the temperature of the water is directly related to the energy used by the organism.

Lavoisier's technique illustrates the principles of **direct calorimetry**. When your body combusts food, it captures some energy while losing the rest as heat. This heat loss is proportional to the body's total energy use and can be measured directly using a chamber like that constructed by Lavoisier. Modern chambers measure the temperature change in a surrounding layer of water.

Direct calorimetry is expensive and complex. The chamber must be large enough to accommodate a person, yet maintain the precision to measure the relatively small changes in temperature. Since the advent of alternative methods, direct calorimetry is no longer widely used.

Indirect calorimetry is easier and less expensive than direct calorimetry. It is "indirect" because energy production (as heat) is not measured directly. Instead, energy expenditure is estimated from a person's oxygen consumption and carbon dioxide production. Burning (oxidizing) fuel consumes oxygen and produces carbon dioxide in proportion to the amount of fuel burned and the amount of energy released.

For indirect calorimetry, a technician collects respiratory gases. During short periods of rest or exercise, expired air can be collected using a face mask, mouthpiece, or canopy system (see **FIGURE 9.7**). This cumbersome apparatus makes indirect calorimetry impractical for use during physically demanding activities or normal living conditions.

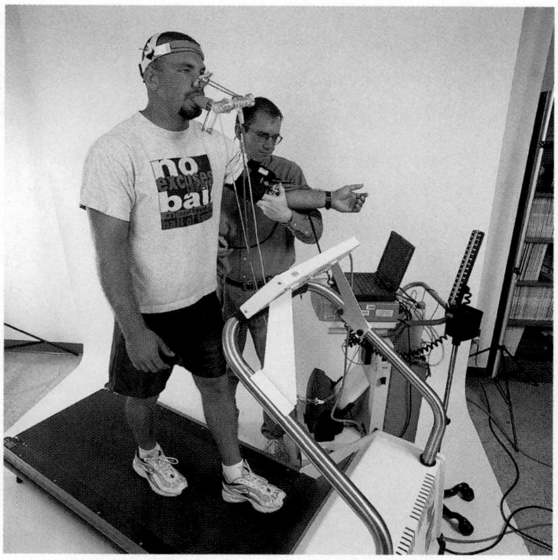

FIGURE 9.7 Indirect calorimetry. A technician collects respiratory gases and then calculates energy expenditure.

Doubly Labeled Water

An easier technique to measure total energy expenditure is **doubly labeled water** (see **FIGURE 9.8**). Rather than measuring respiratory gases, this indirect calorimetry technique relies on measuring the **isotopes** (typically a form of an element with a higher than usual atomic mass but the same characteristics as the usual element) of hydrogen and oxygen in excreted water and carbon dioxide. A person drinks a small quantity of two kinds of water, one labeled with the hydrogen isotope deuterium (^2H) and the other labeled with an isotope of oxygen (oxygen-18, or ^{18}O). Both isotopes occur naturally and are nonradioactive. The body excretes oxygen-18 as part of water ($H_2{}^{18}O$) and carbon dioxide ($C^{18}O_2$). It excretes deuterium only as part of water (^2H_2O). Scientists use the difference between the rate of deuterium loss and oxygen-18 loss to calculate carbon dioxide output and determine the total energy expenditure.

The doubly labeled water technique is noninvasive and unobtrusive. Subjects can stay in their normal environment and perform normal activities during the testing period, which typically lasts 7 to 14 days or longer. This method is emerging as the gold standard against which other energy expenditure measurement methods are compared. For best accuracy, doubly labeled water studies should last at least 14 days. Unfortunately, the doubly labeled water technique is not widely available, and it's expensive—the ^{18}O

▶ **indirect calorimetry** Determination of energy use by the body without directly measuring the production of heat. Methods include gas exchange, the measurement of oxygen uptake and/or carbon dioxide output, and the doubly labeled water method.

▶ **doubly labeled water** A method for measuring daily energy expenditure over extended time periods, typically 7 to 14 days, while subjects are living in their usual environments. Small amounts of water that is isotopically labeled with deuterium and oxygen-18 (^2H_2O and $H_2{}^{18}O$) are ingested. Energy expenditure can be calculated from the difference between the rates at which the body loses each isotope.

▶ **isotopes** [EYE-so-towps] Forms of an element in which the atoms have the same number of protons but different numbers of neutrons.

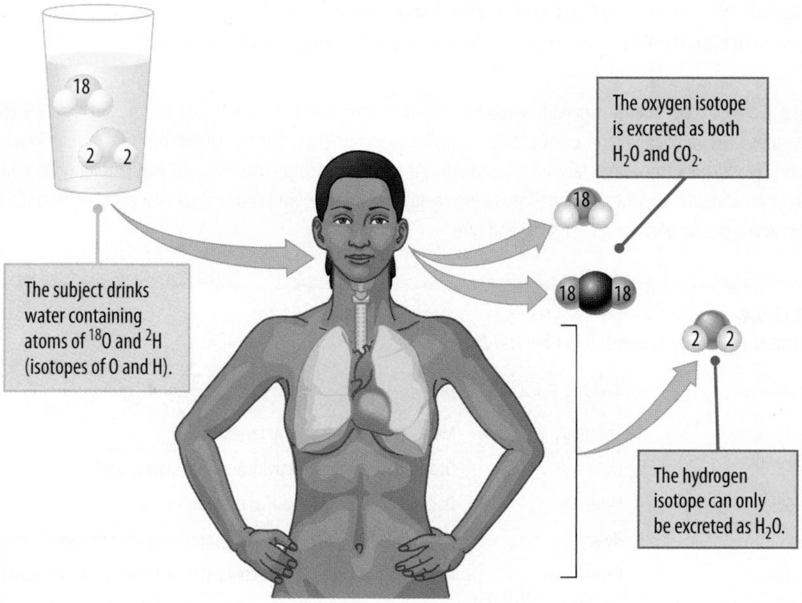

FIGURE 9.8 Doubly labeled water. When using doubly labeled water, scientists measure the excretion rates of the two isotopes to calculate carbon dioxide output and determine total energy expenditure.

Quick Bite

Magic Underwear

James Levine, the endocrinologist and professor of medicine at the Mayo Clinic who coined the term *NEAT*, uses what he calls "magic underwear," which contains sensors to measure the research subject's movements and body postures 120 times each minute.

isotope costs about $500 for a 70-kilogram (154-pound) adult, and the analytic equipment is costly. Therefore, the technique is not suited to large-scale studies. It has other limitations as well: It cannot give information about individual days, individual activities, or day-to-day variability.

Estimating Total Energy Expenditure

Directly measuring a person's total energy expenditure requires sophisticated equipment that is inaccessible to all but a few people in research settings. To determine the energy needs of most people, health professionals must rely on calculated estimates.

An adult's REE can be estimated using an abbreviated method (see margin). The 1.0 and 0.9 factors for kilocalories per kilogram reflect the differences in body composition between men and women. Men have proportionally more lean body mass and, therefore, burn more calories per kilogram of body weight. This abbreviated method dramatically underestimates children's REE, however, and somewhat overestimates the REE of older adults.

Abbreviated Method to Estimate REE

For adult men

REE = weight (kg) × 1.0 kcal/kg × 24 hr/day

REE = weight (kg) × 1.0 × 24

For adult women

REE = weight (kg) × 0.9 kcal/kg × 24 hr/day

REE = weight (kg) × 0.9 × 24

The abbreviated method estimates only REE. To determine total energy expenditure (TEE), energy for physical activity and the thermic effect of food must be included. Energy expended in physical activity can be estimated as a percentage of REE based on a person's general activity level (see **TABLE 9.4**). Most adults in the United States and Canada have a light or moderate activity level. The thermic effect of food can be estimated as roughly 10 percent of the sum of REE plus energy expended in physical activity. Summing the three estimated components—REE, physical activity, and TEF—delivers the estimated total energy expenditure. See the FYI feature "How Many Calories Do I Burn?" for an example of these estimates in action.

DRIs for Energy: Estimated Energy Requirements

Just as there are Dietary Reference Intakes (DRIs) for nutrients, there are also DRIs for energy, called Estimated Energy Requirements (EERs).[43] The EER is defined as the energy intake predicted to maintain energy balance in a healthy person of normal weight. The EER equations for adults (see **TABLE 9.5**) predict total energy expenditure from age, height, weight, gender, and physical activity level. Separate equations have been developed for infants, children, and teens, and adjustments are made for pregnancy and lactation.

Key Concepts Energy expenditure can be measured using direct or indirect calorimetry. Direct calorimetry measures heat production by the body, whereas indirect calorimetry measures oxygen consumption and carbon dioxide production. The doubly labeled water method is becoming accepted as the gold standard for determining energy expenditure. In most situations, measuring energy expenditure is not practical, so a variety of equations have been developed for predicting energy expenditure.

TABLE 9.4
Estimating Energy Expended in Physical Activity

Percentage of REE	Activity Level	Description
20–30	Sedentary	Mostly resting with little or no activity
30–45	Light	Occasional unplanned activity (e.g., going for a stroll)
45–65	Moderate	Daily planned activity, such as brisk walks
65–90	Heavy	Daily workout routine requiring several hours of continuous exercise
90–120	Exceptional	Daily vigorous workouts for extended hours; training for competition

Data from Institute of Medicine, Food and Nutrition Board. *Dietary Reference Intakes for Energy, Carbohydrate, Fiber, Fat, Fatty Acids, Cholesterol, Protein, and Amino Acids (Macronutrients)*. Washington, DC: National Academies Press; 2005.

TABLE 9.5
Estimated Energy Requirements (EER) for Adults

Males		
EER = 662 − 9.53 × Age [yr] + PA × (15.91 × Weight [kg] + 539.6 × Height [m])		
PA =	1.0	Sedentary
	1.11	Low active
	1.25	Active
	1.48	Very active
Females		
EER = 354 − 6.91 × Age [yr] + PA × (9.36 × Weight [kg] + 726 × Height [m])		
PA =	1.0	Sedentary
	1.12	Low active
	1.27	Active
	1.45	Very active

Reproduced from Institute of Medicine, Food and Nutrition Board. *Dietary Reference Intakes for Energy, Carbohydrate, Fiber, Fat, Fatty Acids, Cholesterol, Protein, and Amino Acids (Macronutrients).* © 2005 by the National Academy of Sciences, courtesy of the National Academies Press, Washington, DC.

FYI For Your Information

How Many Calories Do I Burn?

You can estimate the amount of energy you use each day by using some simple equations. Remember that there will be quite a lot of individual variation in actual energy output, so these calculated values are just estimates.

1. Convert your weight in pounds to weight in kilograms. For example, Carol is a 120-pound female. Her weight is 54.5 kilograms (54.5 = 120 ÷ 2.2).

$$\underset{\text{weight (lbs)}}{\underline{\qquad\qquad}} \div 2.2 = \underset{\text{weight (kg)}}{\underline{\qquad\qquad}}$$

2. Estimate your personal REE.

For adult women

$$REE = \underset{\text{weight (kg)}}{\underline{\qquad\qquad}} \times 0.9 \times 24$$

For adult men

$$REE = \underset{\text{weight (kg)}}{\underline{\qquad\qquad}} \times 1.0 \times 24$$

For example, Carol has an estimated REE of 1,177 kilocalories (1,177 = 54.5 × 0.9 × 24).

3. Estimate your energy expended in physical activity (see Table 9.4).

$$energy_{\text{physical activity}} = \underset{\text{from Table 9.4}}{\underline{\qquad\qquad\qquad}} \times EE$$

For example, Carol has a light to moderate physical activity level. She expends about 530 kilocalories in physical activity (530 = 0.45 × 1,177).

4. Estimate your thermic effect of food (TEF).

$$TEF = 0.1 \times (\underset{energy_{\text{physical activity}}}{\underline{\qquad\qquad}} + \underset{EE}{\underline{\qquad\qquad}})$$

For our example, Carol's thermic effect of food is about 171 kilocalories (171 = 0.1 × [530 + 1,177]).

5. Estimate your personal total energy expenditure (TEE).

$$TEE = \underset{REE}{\underline{\qquad}} + \underset{energy_{\text{physical activity}}}{\underline{\qquad\qquad}} + \underset{TEF}{\underline{\qquad\qquad}}$$

For our example, Carol's total energy expenditure is about 1,878 kilocalories (1,177 + 530 + 171).

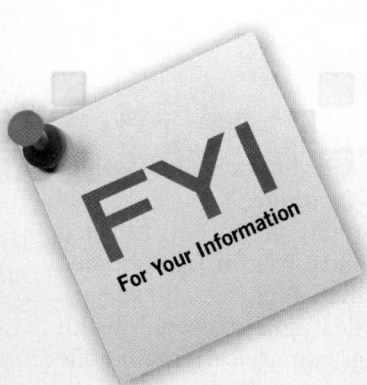

Body Composition: Understanding Fatness and Weight

Stepping onto a scale provides quick and easy feedback about your body weight. Yet many people have a distorted notion of their weight—thinking they're too fat when they aren't or thinking their weight is just fine when it isn't. In terms of your health risks, **body composition** is more important than body weight.

▶ **body composition** The chemical or anatomical composition of the body. Commonly defined as the proportions of fat, muscle, bone, and other tissues in the body.

Body composition is the relative amount of fat and lean body mass. Excess body fatness is linked with increased risk for heart disease, hypertension, cancer, diabetes, and other chronic diseases. Two people with the same height and high weight might have very different health risks. Whereas one might be obese and have many weight-related health risks, the other could be very fit and muscular, with no increased disease risk.

Assessing Body Weight

Body mass index (BMI) has become the accepted method for assessing body weight for height. This index, which is a ratio of weight to height squared, correlates reasonably well with body fatness and health risks. To determine your BMI, accurately measure your height without shoes and your weight with minimal clothing. Then, plug these numbers into the BMI equations in the margin. For adults, the National Heart, Lung, and Blood Institute (NHLBI) defines **underweight**, normal weight, **overweight**, and **obesity** as follows[44]:

▶ **body mass index (BMI)** Body weight (in kilograms) divided by the square of height (in meters), expressed in units of kg/m^2. Also called Quetelet index.

▶ **underweight** BMI less than 18.5 kg/m^2.

▶ **obesity** BMI at or above 30 kg/m^2.

▶ **overweight** BMI at or above 25 kg/m^2 and less than 30 kg/m^2.

- *Underweight:* BMI < 18.5 kg/m^2
- *Normal weight:* 18.5 kg/m$^2 \leq$ BMI < 25 kg/m^2
- *Overweight:* 25 kg/m$^2 \leq$ BMI < 30 kg/m^2
- *Obese:* BMI ≥ 30 kg/m^2

To Calculate BMI

$$\text{BMI} = \frac{\text{weight (kg)}}{\text{height (m)}^2}$$

or

$$\text{BMI} = \frac{\text{weight (lb)}}{\text{height (in)}^2} \times 04.5$$

TABLE 9.6 can help you determine whether your weight is a healthy weight according to the *National Heart, Lung, and Blood Insititute.*

As **FIGURE 9.9** shows, correlating BMI with mortality produces a *J*-shaped curve. Studies indicate that underweight (BMI less than 18.5 kg/m^2) is associated with increased mortality, as is obesity (BMI greater than or equal to 30 kg/m^2).

Although your BMI can give you a general idea of your overall health risks, it still doesn't tell you enough about whether you are carrying muscle weight or excess fat. A classic example is the heavy football player or bodybuilder with a large muscle mass who has a BMI greater than 30 kg/m^2 but is not overfat. For someone who has lost muscle mass, perhaps an older adult, BMI can underestimate health risks associated with excess body fat. BMI measurements should be interpreted cautiously when used for people who are petite, who have large body frames, or who are highly muscular.[45]

For children and teens, height and weight measurements can be compared with standard growth charts to see if the child is growing and gaining weight at an appropriate rate.

For children and teens (2 to 20 years old), pediatric growth charts include age- and sex-specific percentile curves for BMI.[46] A BMI-for-age at or above the 95th percentile indicates overweight and the need for further evaluation and possible treatment. Further evaluation also might be indicated if the child's BMI-for-age is at or above the 85th percentile and is accompanied by other risk factors such as high blood pressure, high blood cholesterol, diabetes, and family history of obesity-related disease.[47] A BMI-for-age below the 5th percentile suggests that the child is underweight.

Quick Bite

Is Tom Brady Too Fat?

Although BMI has become the standard reference for determining overweight and obesity, it has limitations at the extremes of body size and composition. Consider Tom Brady, quarterback for the New England Patriots. At 6 feet, 4 inches and 225 pounds, Tom has a BMI of 27.4, which puts him in the category of "Overweight." This star athletes does not have too much body fat!

Key Concepts Body composition is a key element in determining energy expenditure and is an important factor in disease risk. Weight and height measures can be used to calculate BMI, which is correlated with body fatness and health risks. Elevated BMI in adults or children can increase health risks.

TABLE 9.6
Adult BMI Chart

BMI	19	20	21	22	23	24	25	26	27	28	29	30	31	32	33	34	35
Height	**Weight in Pounds**																
4′10	91	96	100	105	110	115	119	124	129	134	138	143	148	153	158	162	167
4′11	94	99	104	109	114	119	124	128	133	138	143	148	153	158	163	168	173
5′	97	102	107	112	118	123	128	133	138	143	148	153	158	163	158	174	179
5′1	100	106	111	116	122	127	132	137	143	148	153	158	164	169	174	180	185
5′2	104	109	115	120	126	131	136	142	147	153	158	164	169	175	180	186	191
5′3	107	113	118	124	130	135	141	146	152	158	163	169	175	180	186	191	197
5′4	110	116	122	128	134	140	145	151	157	163	169	174	180	186	192	197	204
5′5	114	120	126	132	138	144	150	156	162	168	174	180	186	192	198	204	210
5′6	118	124	130	136	142	148	155	161	167	173	179	186	192	198	204	210	216
5′7	121	127	134	140	146	153	159	166	172	178	185	191	198	204	211	217	223
5′8	125	131	138	144	151	158	164	171	177	184	190	197	203	210	216	223	230
5′9	128	135	142	149	155	162	169	176	182	189	196	203	209	216	223	230	236
5′10	132	139	146	153	160	167	174	181	188	195	202	209	216	222	229	236	243
5′11	136	143	150	157	165	172	179	186	193	200	208	215	222	229	236	243	250
6′	140	147	154	162	169	177	184	191	199	206	213	221	228	235	242	250	258
6′1	144	151	159	166	174	182	189	197	204	212	219	227	235	242	250	257	265
6′2	148	155	163	171	179	186	194	202	210	218	225	233	241	249	256	264	272
6′3	152	160	168	176	184	192	200	208	216	224	232	240	248	256	264	272	279
	Healthy Weight						**Overweight**						**Obese**				

Adapted from U.S. Department of Agriculture and U.S. Department of Health and Human Services, National Heart, Lung, and Blood Institute. *Aim for a healthy weight: body mass index table 1*. http://www.nhlbi.nih.gov/health/educational/lose_wt/BMI/bmi_tbl.htm Accessed March 26, 2016. Also see the online BMI calculator at http://www.nhlbi.nih.gov/health/educational/lose_wt/BMI/bmicalc.htm Accessed March 26, 2016.

▶ **densitometry** A method for estimating body composition from measurement of total body density.

▶ **underwater weighing** Determining body density by measuring the volume of water displaced when the body is fully submerged in a specialized water tank. Also called hydrostatic weighing.

▶ **hydrostatic weighing** See *underwater weighing.*

Assessing Body Fatness

Fat is stored in the adipose tissue that lies directly under the skin. Fat tissue also surrounds internal organs. Healthy adult females typically have 20 to 35 percent body fat; for men, the range is 8 to 24 percent. Risk of chronic disease rises dramatically when body fat exceeds these levels.

Densitometry is the measure of body density (body mass divided by body volume). Because fat and lean tissues have different densities, if we know the person's volume and weight, we can calculate the ratio of fat to lean body mass. The density of fat doesn't vary, but hydration status, age, gender, and ethnicity all influence the density of lean body mass. For example, bone loss in older adults leads to a lower density of lean body mass.

Densitometry and Underwater Weighing

Underwater weighing, also called **hydrostatic weighing**, is an accurate densitometry method that is used in research settings and some sports programs. Because fat is less dense than muscle, a person with more body fat will have a lower underwater weight than a person with the same body

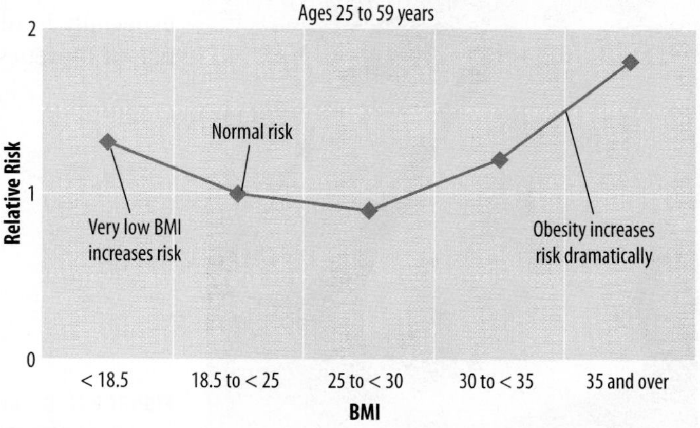

FIGURE 9.9 BMI and mortality. People with a high or very low BMI have a higher relative mortality rate.

Adapted from Flegal KM, Graubard BI, Williamson DF, Gail MH. Excess deaths associated with underweight, overweight, and obesity. JAMA. 2005;293:1861–1867.

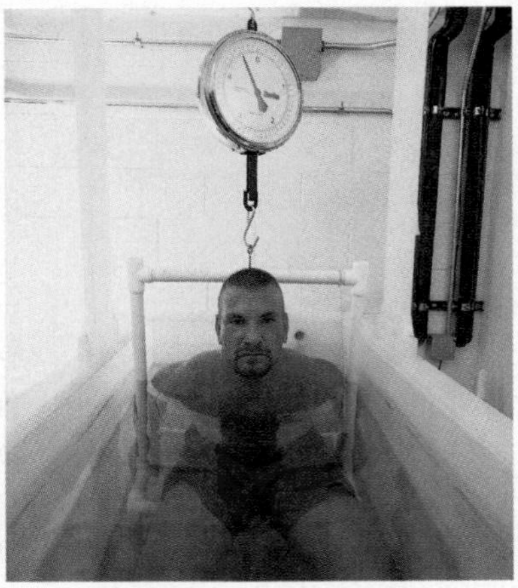

FIGURE 9.10 Underwater weighing. During underwater weighing, the subject must exhale completely, submerge without taking a breath, and remain motionless until the water is still and the scale is steady.

weight but less fat. With this technique, a seated person is submerged fully in water and weighed, as **FIGURE 9.10** illustrates. Body density is calculated using the above-water weight, the submerged weight, and the quantity of water displaced during submersion. Underwater weighing often is impractical because it requires a special water tank and other nonportable, expensive equipment. The subject must exhale completely, submerge without taking a breath, and remain motionless until the water is still and the scale is steady—clearly not a comfortable experience for everyone!

Densitometry and Air Displacement

The **BOD POD** measures displacement of air to determine relative amounts of fat and fat-free mass for calculating body density. With this technique, a person sits in a sealed chamber of known volume and displaces a certain volume of air. Air displacement uses the same principles as underwater weighing, but it is much faster and easier. **FIGURE 9.11** shows an air displacement chamber.

Dual-Energy X-Ray Absorptiometry

Dual-energy x-ray absorptiometry (DEXA), used to measure bone density, can also be used to analyze body composition by differentiating bone, other lean tissue, and fat.[48] A person undergoing a DEXA scan lies on a padded table while an x-ray detector above scans from head to foot, producing a two-dimensional image of tiny dots, or pixels. (See **FIGURE 9.12**.) Although the DEXA scan is an excellent technique, its accuracy in obese people and the effects of tissue thickness and hydration status on scan accuracy are unclear. The instrument is expensive but is becoming more widely available in medical settings.

Isotope Dilution

Researchers can directly measure **total body water** and use this quantity to estimate lean body mass. With this technique, the subject swallows a known quantity and concentration of isotopically labeled water. Unlike the doubly labeled water method, which compares two isotopes, this technique uses a single isotope to label the water. After three or four hours, it is assumed that the labeled water is fully mixed in the body's water pool. The researcher takes a sample of body water (e.g., from plasma, saliva, or urine), measures the concentration of the isotope, and calculates the total volume of body water. Based on the assumption that lean body mass is 73 percent water, researchers can estimate the total lean body mass. Unfortunately, this assumption does not hold true for all people; the amount of water in lean body mass can vary, especially in older adults. Obesity and dehydration from severe exercise and use of diuretics or laxatives also can influence the results.

- ▶ **BOD POD** A device used to measure the density of the body based on the volume of air displaced as a person sits in a sealed chamber of known volume.
- ▶ **dual-energy x-ray absorptiometry (DEXA)** A body composition measurement technique originally developed to measure bone density.
- ▶ **total body water** All of the water in the body, including intracellular and extracellular water, and water in the urinary and GI tracts.

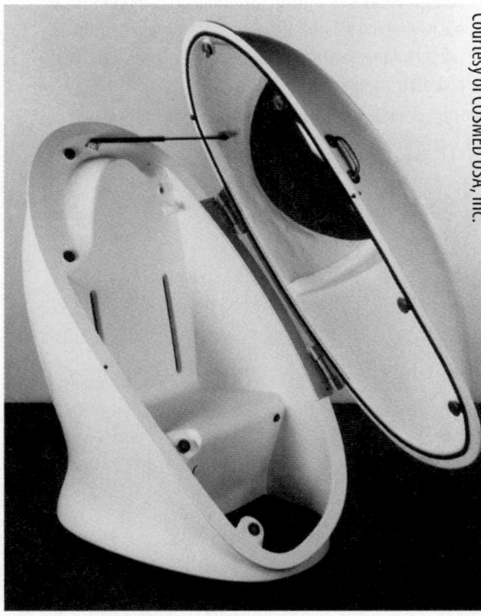

FIGURE 9.11 BOD POD. By using air displacement, the BOD POD provides an alternative to underwater weighing that is easier, cheaper, and of similar accuracy.

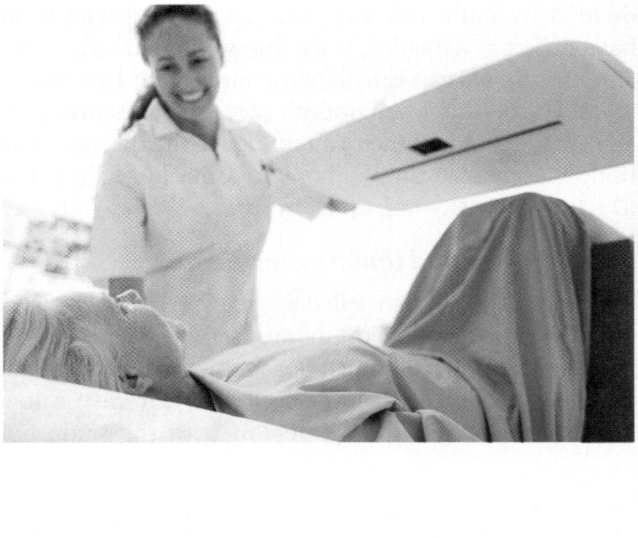

FIGURE 9.12 Dual-energy x-ray absorptiometry (DEXA) scan. The two-dimensional image produced from a DEXA scan can be used to assess body composition.

Skinfold Thickness

Skinfold measurements are a low-tech method for assessing body fatness. A special caliper is used to measure the thickness of fat deposits directly underneath the skin at several locations around the body. Skinfold measures are widely used in large population studies. When done correctly, body composition estimates from skinfolds correlate well with those from underwater weighing, but an inexperienced or careless measurer can easily make large errors. Skinfold thickness is especially useful in tracking changes in subcutaneous fat distribution in an individual over time. They usually work better for assessing malnutrition than for identifying overweight and obesity.

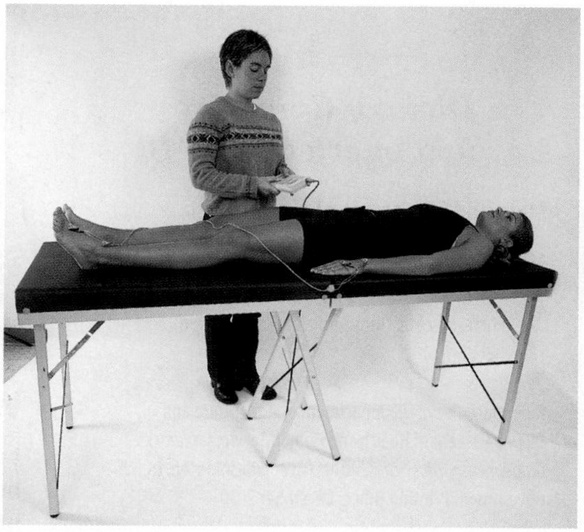

FIGURE 9.13 Bioelectrical impedance analysis (BIA). The measured resistance to a small electrical current passed through the body is used to estimate body composition.

Bioelectrical Impedance Analysis

Bioelectrical impedance analysis (BIA) measures the rate at which a small electric current flows through the body between electrodes placed on the wrist and ankle. (See **FIGURE 9.13**.) Because lean tissue contains more water than fat tissue, it is a better conductor of electricity. Fat is more resistant to electric current (has more "impedance"). Measurements of impedance are used to determine the amounts of lean and fat mass. Unfortunately, hydration status has a large effect on the results. For example, dehydration elevates impedance, leading to an overestimation of body fatness. Thus, the many factors that can affect hydration status (e.g., exercise, eating, drinking, medication) also can make BIA unreliable and inaccurate.

Despite its limitations, bioelectrical impedance is accepted as a valuable tool for measuring body composition in field studies. The equipment is easily portable and only moderately expensive ($2,500–$8,000), making the technique popular at upscale health clubs and weight-loss centers. Similar to BIA, total body electrical conductivity (TOBEC) is an acceptably accurate measure of conductivity but is less widely used because the equipment is expensive.

- **bioelectrical impedance analysis (BIA)** Technique to estimate amounts of total body water, lean tissue mass, and total body fat. It uses the resistance of tissue to the flow of an alternating electric current.
- **body fat distribution** The pattern of fat distribution on the body.
- **gynoid obesity** Excess storage of fat located primarily in the hips and thighs.
- **android obesity** [AN-droyd oh-BEE-sih-ty] Excess storage of fat located primarily in the abdominal area.
- **waist circumference** The waist measurement, as a marker of abdominal fat content; can be used to indicate health risks.

Body Fat Distribution

Measurements of body fatness tell you more about your health risks than your weight does, but they still don't tell the whole story. Where the fat is located—**body fat distribution**—can be an independent risk factor in both children and adults.[49,50] The "pear shape," or **gynoid obesity**, which is more common in women, has excess fat distributed predominantly around the hips and thighs. The "apple shape," or **android obesity**, typical of men, has extra fat distributed higher up, around the abdomen. **FIGURE 9.14** shows the gynoid and android distributions of body fat.

THINK About It 2

Excess abdominal fat appears to raise blood lipid levels, which in turn interferes with insulin function. Consequently, android obesity has been linked to high blood lipids, glucose intolerance and insulin resistance, and high blood pressure; it increases the risk of heart disease and diabetes mellitus. These risks exist for both men and women who have excess abdominal fat. In fact, android obesity can indicate an increased breast cancer risk for women.[51,52]

If your **waist circumference** increases, you are probably gaining abdominal fat. Clinical guidelines from the National Institutes of Health (NIH) suggest that for people with a BMI of 25 kg/m^2 to 34.9 kg/m^2, a waist circumference greater than 40 inches (102 centimeters) in men or greater than 35 inches (88 centimeters) in women is a sign of increased health risk.

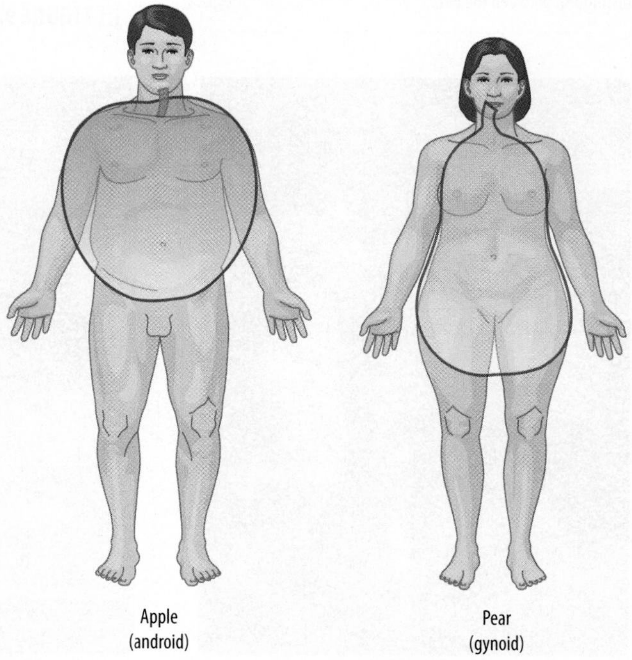

FIGURE 9.14 Differences in body fat distribution. Men tend to carry excess fat around their abdomen (android obesity). Women tend to accumulate excess fat in their hips and thighs (gynoid obesity).

Combining measures of BMI and waist circumference is more predictive of cardiovascular disease risk than either measure alone.[53] When BMI is 35 kg/m^2 or higher, however, waist circumference measures do not predict health risks accurately.

Key Concepts Excess body fatness is associated with increased risk for chronic diseases, including heart disease and diabetes. Researchers use a number of different methods to assess body fatness. High cost limits the usefulness of more sophisticated techniques. Distribution of body fat is important in evaluating risk of disease. Excess body fat around the abdomen is associated with higher disease risk than is excess fat around the hips and thighs. Waist circumference can be used to assess body fat distribution.

Dietary Guidelines for Americans, 2010

Main and Overarching Concepts

- Maintain calorie balance over time to achieve and sustain a healthy weight.
- Focus on consuming nutrient-dense foods and beverages.

Reproduced from US Department of Agriculture and US Department of Health and Human Services. *Dietary Guidelines for Americans, 2010*. 7th ed. Washington, DC: US Government Printing Office; December 2010.

Weight Management

Each person has a unique set of interrelated factors that lead to changes in body weight. Approaches to weight management are just as complex, and to be effective, they must be tailored to the individual. As you continue reading, keep in mind the following definition of **weight management** from the Academy of Nutrition and Dietetics; note that there is no mention of weight loss or ideal weight:

▶ **weight management** The adoption of healthful and sustainable eating and exercise behaviors that reduce disease risk and improve well-being.

Weight management is the adoption of healthful and sustainable eating and exercise behaviors indicated for reduced disease risk and improved feelings of energy and well-being.[54]

The Perception of Weight

The weights of celebrity models often mold popular notions about desirable weight. In the early 1960s, as today, thin was "in." (In the 1960s, the trendsetter was supermodel Twiggy, who at 5 feet, 7 inches weighed only 98 pounds; her BMI was a mere 15.4 kg/m^2!) Since then, the number of diet and exercise articles in women's magazines has escalated, and diet books have become best-sellers. Dieting has become an institution with its own magazines, television shows, camps and resorts, and weight-loss gurus. However, the images in **FIGURE 9.15** show that beauty has not always been associated with thinness.

Quick Bite

Where's the Fat?

The location of excess abdominal fat can hold information about health risks. Within the abdomen, visceral fat (fat surrounding the organs) might be more harmful than subcutaneous fat (fat under the skin). Only sophisticated imaging techniques, such as computed tomography (CT) scans and magnetic resonance imaging (MRI), can distinguish between the two.

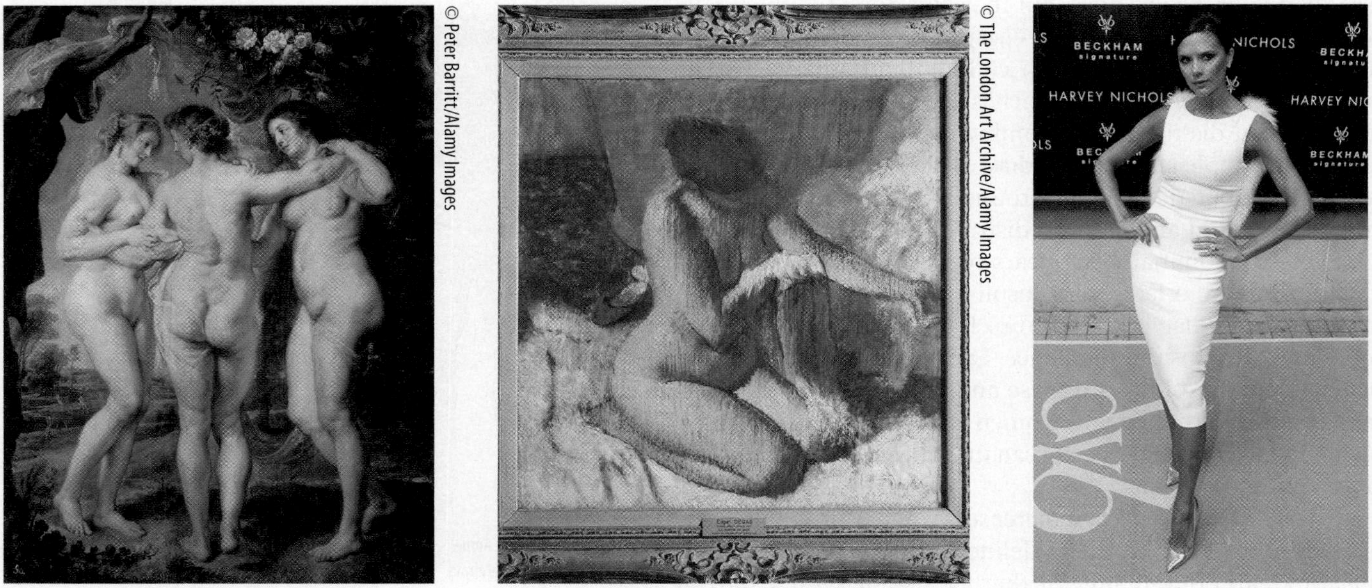

© Peter Barritt/Alamy Images

© The London Art Archive/Alamy Images

© Paul Thomas/AP Photos

(A) (B) (C)

FIGURE 9.15 Society's changing standards of beauty. Over time, society has increasingly valued thinness. (A) Ruben's *The Three Graces*, 1639. (B) Degas's *After the Bath*, 1896. (C) Celebrity Victoria Beckham.

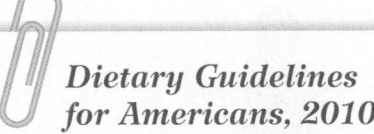

Although today's society and media glamorize thinness, obesity rates are at an all-time high. Health professionals now treat obesity as a complex disorder with multiple contributing factors. (See **FIGURE 9.16**.) They emphasize overall health and fitness rather than a number on the bathroom scale. Dietary recommendations emphasize moderation and a balanced diet that promotes consumption of healthful foods such as fruits, vegetables, and whole grains. Behavior change is still an important part of weight management, but change is seen as an ongoing process that requires new skills for maintaining a healthy lifestyle over the long run. Although vigorous exercise isn't required, moderate exercise is needed for long-term weight management, and physical activity appears to be crucial in the prevention of weight regain.[55]

There are limitations as to what each of us can look like or what we can healthfully weigh. Although we shouldn't abandon efforts to achieve good health, we should balance our desire to lose weight with self-acceptance. If we engage in futile attempts to achieve an "ideal" body shape and weight, we can undermine our self-esteem and be harmed emotionally or even physically.

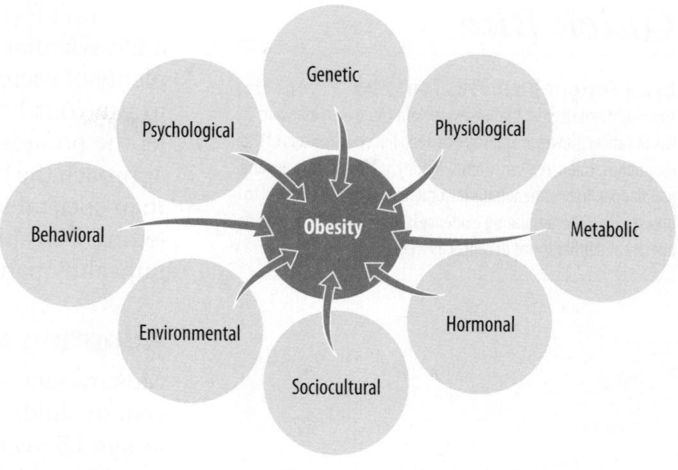

FIGURE 9.16 Multiple factors contribute to obesity. Obesity is a complex disorder that is not easy to treat.

Key Concepts Many factors contribute to the complex disorder of obesity. Currently, experts suggest that the best way to manage weight is to improve health by establishing healthy eating and exercise patterns and accepting the limitations of heredity.

▶ **metabolically healthy obesity** Obesity accompanied by normal metabolic features such as lipid profile, glucose tolerance, blood pressure, and waist circumference.

What Goals Should I Set?

What is a reasonable goal for weight management? Health professionals recommend targeting the following behavior changes to manage body weight:

1. Prevent and/or reduce overweight and obesity through improved eating and physical behavior.
2. Control total calorie intake to manage body weight.
3. Increase physical activity and reduce time spent in sedentary behaviors.
4. Maintain appropriate calorie balance during each stage of life.

If you are overweight, it doesn't take major weight loss to improve health. A modest weight loss of roughly 10 percent is sufficient to produce health benefits and might encourage continued effort and success. A key initial goal is to prevent or stop weight gain. Small changes in energy intake and expenditure—for example, an intake reduction of 100 kilocalories per day—can theoretically prevent weight gain in 90 percent of the U.S. adult population.[56,57] For success, goals must be realistic and attainable (see **FIGURE 9.17**).

THINK About It 3

When you are metabolically fit, you don't have any of the metabolic or biochemical risk factors associated with obesity—such as high low-density lipoprotein (LDL) cholesterol, low high-density lipoprotein (HDL) cholesterol, high levels of triglycerides, elevated blood glucose, insulin resistance, and high blood pressure. Obese people who are metabolically fit are described as having **metabolically healthy obesity**. Still, when compared with metabolically healthy normal-weight persons, metabolically healthy obese individuals are at increased risk for all-cause mortality and cardiovascular events over the long term (10 years).[58] Often, you can reduce metabolic risk factors or even bring them within normal ranges through modest weight loss (5 to 10 percent of initial body weight) achieved by a small reduction in calorie intake and a moderate increase in physical activity (e.g., walking 30 minutes per day, no fewer than five days per week).

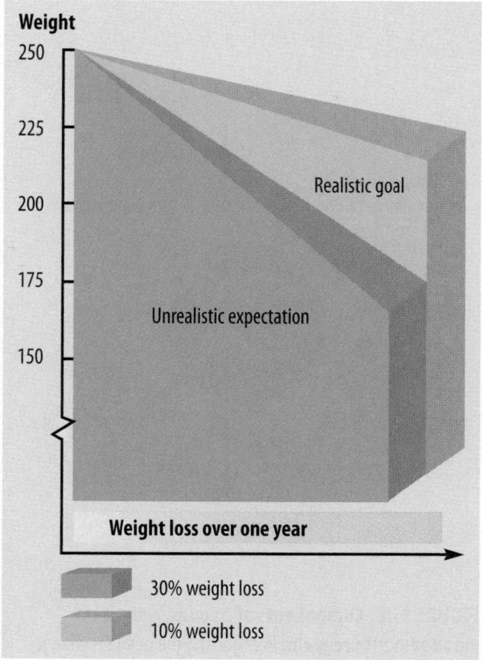

FIGURE 9.17 Expectations and reasonable weight goals. People who establish moderate rather than aggressive goals are more likely to succeed in their weight-loss program.

Quick Bite

Extra Weight Increases Your Risk of Cancer

You might not suspect that excess weight could increase your risk of cancer. However, obesity has been linked to cancers of the esophagus, colon, rectum, uterus, kidney, pancreas, thyroid, and gallbladder. In postmenopausal women obesity also is linked to breast cancer. Accumulating evidence is showing links between obesity and other forms of cancer as well.

Don't focus on a particular weight as your goal. Instead, focus on living a lifestyle that includes eating moderate amounts of healthful foods, getting plenty of exercise, thinking positively, and learning to cope with stress. Learn to use your body's hunger and satiation signals to regulate eating and then let the pounds fall where they may. Most people who follow this advice will approach the healthy BMI ranges discussed earlier. Some will still weigh more than societal standards call for—but their weight will be right for them. By letting a healthy lifestyle determine your weight, you can avoid developing unhealthy patterns of eating and a negative body image.

Adopting a Healthy Weight-Management Lifestyle

Most weight problems are lifestyle problems. It has been shown that 80 percent of children who were overweight at age 10 to 15 years are obese adults at age 25 years. Even though more and more young people are developing weight problems, many arrive at early adulthood with the advantage of having a "normal" body weight—neither too fat nor too thin. In fact, many young adults get away with terrible eating and exercise habits and don't develop a weight problem. But as the rapid growth of adolescence slows and family and career obligations increase, maintaining a healthy weight becomes a greater challenge. If you develop a lifestyle for successful weight management during early adulthood, healthy behavior patterns have a better chance of taking firm hold.

Permanent weight management is not something you start and stop. You need to adopt healthful behaviors that you can maintain throughout your life. People who have long-term success share common behavioral strategies that include eating a diet low in fat, frequent self-monitoring of body weight and food intake, and high levels of regular physical activity.[59] To maintain your weight over the long term, focus on healthy behaviors and develop coping strategies to deal with the stresses and challenges in your life. **FIGURE 9.18** shows the necessary components of an effective weight-management program.

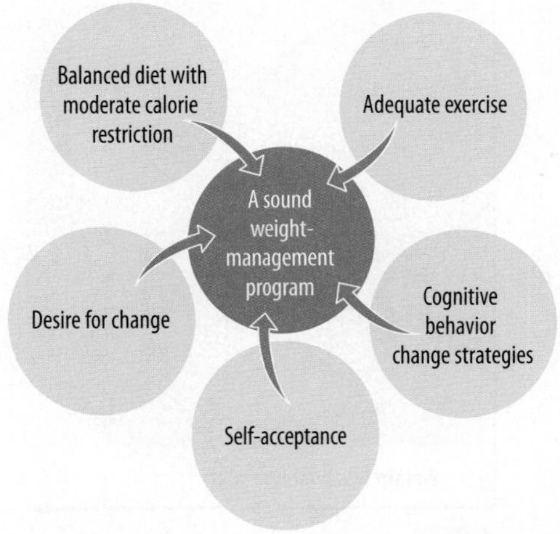

FIGURE 9.18 Components of a sound weight-management program. Recognizing the need for change, establishing reasonable goals, adopting goal-directed activities and self-monitoring them, and rewarding goal attainment can help successfully implement the components of a sound weight-management program.

Key Concepts Healthy weight management means focusing on metabolic fitness—healthy levels of blood lipids and blood pressure—rather than on achieving a specific weight. Permanent healthy behaviors are necessary for a long-term weight-management lifestyle.

Diet and Eating Habits

In contrast to "dieting," which involves some form of food restriction, "diet" refers to your daily food choices. Everyone has a diet, but not everyone is dieting. You need to develop a balanced diet of moderate caloric intake that includes foods you enjoy and that enables you to maintain a healthy body composition.

Total Calories

If you want to lose weight, you must take in fewer calories than you expend. Over the long term, you are more likely to control your weight successfully by cutting 200 to 300 kilocalories per day rather than drastically restricting your diet to only 1,000 to 1,200 kilocalories per day. Simply eliminating one can of regular soda from your daily routine would reduce your energy intake by about 150 kilocalories. You don't need to make major diet changes; just make small, sustainable changes and focus on the balance of food groups suggested by MyPlate. The ChooseMyPlate website has several interactive tools including:

- MyPlate Daily Checklist. The Checklist shows your food group targets—what and how much to eat within your calorie allowance. Your food plan is personalized based on your age, sex, height, weight, and physical activity level. (http://www.choosemyplate.gov/MyPlate-Daily-Checklist)
- SuperTracker's MyPlan. With this tool you can create a more advanced personal daily food plan. You will be asked to create a profile, and you can register and save it if you want. You can then use some or all of the SuperTracker's other features (https://www.supertracker.usda.gov/createprofile.aspx)

Most of us significantly underestimate the amount of food we eat, and large portion sizes are closely tied to overconsumption of calories. Limiting portion sizes to those recommended in MyPlate is critical for weight management. You'll probably find it easier to monitor and manage your total food intake if you concentrate on portion sizes rather than counting calories.

Crash Diets Don't Work

Don't go on a "crash diet" that contains only minimal calories. You need to consume enough food to meet your need for essential nutrients. Very low calorie intake promotes rapid loss of water, reduced RMR, and potential nutrient deficiencies. Once you lose weight, you probably won't maintain it unless you continue some degree of calorie restriction. So, it is important that you adopt a level of food intake that you can live with. A highly restricted diet just won't work over the long term.

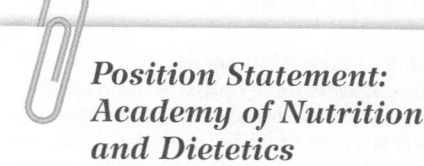

Position Statement: Academy of Nutrition and Dietetics

Weight Management

It is the position of the Academy of Nutrition and Dietetics that successful treatment of overweight and obesity in adults requires adoption and maintenance of lifestyle behaviors contributing to both dietary intake and physical activity. These behaviors are influenced by many factors; therefore, interventions incorporating more than one level of the socioecological model and addressing several key factors in each level may be more successful than interventions targeting any one level and factor alone.

Reproduced from Raynor HA and Champagne CM, Position of the Academy of Nutrition and Dietetics: interventions for the treatment of overweight and obesity in adults, *J Acad Nutr Diet.* 2016;116:129–147.

Going Green

Salad Days

When Christina graduated from high school four years ago she was an active, lithe 121 pounds. She now tips the scale at 140 and is heading north. Many of her conversations are about those "promising" weight-management plans that fail to work for you. She jokes with you that she is looking for the "Eat More, Weigh Less" diet. One of your friends who also is studying nutrition suggests that the plan already exists. It's called the low-energy-dense foods meal plan or the calorie-in, calorie-out diet. Foods with a lower energy density, such as lettuce, provide fewer calories than foods such as french fries. But, who wants to substitute lettuce for french fries? At the end of a meal you want to feel satisfied and not heading for the fridge for a midnight snack. Here's how it works: Satiety, that feeling of fullness and satisfaction, can be achieved by starting the meal with a low-energy-dense salad with lots of lettuce, veggies, and low-calorie dressing.

A number of studies have shown that eating lower-energy-dense meals can be effective in controlling hunger while reducing calories.[a] Adding extra vegetables to meals, for example, can lead to reduced calorie intake. Despite a reduced overall calorie intake, this helps people feel full and satisfied.

In a study by Williams and associates[b] over four weeks, three methods of reducing energy density (decreasing fat, increasing fruits and vegetables, and adding water) were compared for their impact on energy intake throughout the day. Reducing the energy density of entrées significantly decreased daily energy intake compared to the 2,667 kcal/day intake with standard entrées. Among the three methods, decreasing fat lowered energy intake by nearly 400 kcal, increasing fruits and vegetables saved about 300 kcal, and adding water saved about 230 kcal.

Did our "starting with salad" friend succeed in getting back to high school trim? Not exactly, but it was a good start. Also increasing physical activity, perhaps by routinely walking to the store rather than driving a car, will help accelerate weight loss and reduce one's carbon footprint.

[a] Karl JP, Roberts SB. Energy density, energy intake, and body weight regulation in adults. *Adv Nutr.* 2014;5(6):835–850.

[b] Williams RA, Roe LS, Rolls BJ. Comparison of three methods to reduce energy density: effects on daily energy intake. *Appetite.* 2013;66:75–83.

Quick Bite

Double-Checking Dietary Recall

When researchers checked the validity of food diaries and self-reports, they found that obese people underreported their energy intake by 20 to 50 percent and lean people underreported by 10 to 30 percent. Energy expenditure in the obese subjects was normal relative to their body size.

American Heart Association

Commercial Weight Reduction Programs

Being overweight, even by just 10 to 15 pounds, can lead to health problems. And obesity is a risk factor for cardiovascular disease. That's why the American Heart Association encourages people to achieve and maintain a healthy weight. Effective weight loss programs should include:

- Participant or patient information (informed consent)
- Screening of all persons beginning a weight management program by use of an appropriate medical history form to identify people who require a physician's supervision
- Guidelines for who needs to be evaluated by a physician before beginning a weight management program
- Staffing by individuals qualified by education, training, and experience to provide these services
- Identification of reasonable weight-loss goals
- Individualized nutritional, exercise, and behavioral components
- A maintenance program for at least two years
- Evaluation of the long-term effectiveness and safety of the program by review of weight loss and health status of all participants after completion of the program and at one, two, and five years after program completion
- Participants in most weight-loss programs meet once a week during the initial phase, which generally lasts from 12 to 24 weeks; because participants should be followed up for a full year, 12 contacts during the first year appears to be a reasonable minimum number of contacts

Balancing Energy Sources: Carbohydrates

In addition to balancing energy intake with energy output, achieving a balanced intake of energy sources is important for successful weight management. Foods rich in the complex carbohydrates and fiber, such as vegetables, legumes, and other grain products, can help you achieve and maintain a healthy body weight. Fiber-rich foods help provide a feeling of satiation, or fullness, that can keep you from overeating. Carbohydrates should make up 45 to 65 percent of your total daily calories. Avoid foods with added sugars and foods rich in simple carbohydrates, such as bread made with refined flour and potatoes.

Diets high in added sugars tend to reduce satiation and encourage overeating. Also, high-sugar foods usually provide few nutrients to accompany their high caloric content. You should consume high-sugar foods sparingly, and choose fresh fruits and whole grains instead of candy and sugary cereals. To choose a healthful cereal, the food label is a useful guide. Look for cereals with little sugar and high fiber per serving.

Balancing Energy Sources: Fat

Because fat is the most concentrated source of calories, limiting fat in the diet can help you limit your total calories. If you reduce your reliance on meats and processed foods and add whole grains, fresh fruits, and vegetables to your diet, you will reduce fat and total calorie consumption while increasing dietary fiber. Watch out for processed foods labeled "fat-free" or "reduced-fat"; they can be high in calories and added sugars despite their lower fat content.

Balancing Energy Sources: Protein

Most authorities recommend diets high in complex carbohydrates and moderate in protein consumption. (See the FYI feature "Learning Weight Management from Some of the 'Biggest' Weight Experts: Sumo Wrestlers.") Although protein promotes a sense of fullness, animal foods high in protein often are high in saturated fat. Vegetarian sources of protein (such as tofu, soymilk, beans, and lentils) and plant-based fats are healthy choices. Including some lean protein in each meal is a good idea, but stick to the recommended intake: 10 to 35 percent of total daily calories.

Eating Habits

Equally important to weight management is eating small, frequent meals—three or more per day plus snacks—on a dependable, regular schedule. If you skip meals, you are apt to feel excessively hungry and deprived, and you will be more likely to snack or binge on high-calorie, high-fat, or sugary foods. A person who eats on a regular schedule is more likely to reduce total energy intake and improve lipid levels than a person who eats irregularly.[60] Also, a regular meal pattern usually includes breakfast—a benefit when trying to manage weight. Research shows that morning intake is much more satiating than late-night eating and will help reduce overall energy intake.[61] Also, in a study of healthy, lean women, skipping breakfast lowered insulin sensitivity, raised LDL and total cholesterol, and led to higher energy intake.[62]

If you follow a regular pattern of eating and set up some "decision rules" that govern your food choices, you will be able to handle the many details that go into a healthful diet. Decision rules governing breakfast, for example, might be as follows:

- Most of the time, choose a low-sugar, high-fiber cereal with nonfat milk.

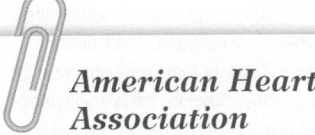

- Once in a while, have an egg that's prepared without added fat (e.g., hard-boiled, scrambled).
- Save pancakes and waffles for special occasions.

You don't have to give up your favorite comfort food. Healthy eating is all about balance. Even if your favorite foods are high in calories, fat or added sugars, you can enjoy them. The key is eating them only once in a while, controlling portions, and balancing them out with healthier foods and more physical activity. Eat high-calorie comfort foods less often and in smaller amounts. If you normally eat a comfort food every day, cut back to once a week or once a month. If your favorite high-calorie snack is a chocolate bar, have a smaller size or only half a bar. Also, try a lower calorie version but watch out for increases in added sugars.

When you proclaim some foods "off-limits," you are setting up a rule to be broken. Instead, adopt the principle of "everything in moderation." Troublesome foods might be placed off-limits temporarily until you regain control. If you can learn to eat in moderation, you can achieve a healthy diet and manage your weight successfully; no foods need to be entirely off-limits, though some should be eaten prudently. Making the healthier choice more often than not is the essence of moderation.

Key Concepts Balancing energy sources and controlling portion sizes can help reduce overall energy consumption. Reducing fat intake is a major step toward lowering calorie intake. Fiber-rich foods provide a feeling of fullness that can help prevent overeating. When planning a diet, avoid foods with added sugars or eat them sparingly.

Physical Activity

Regular physical activity is a vital component of weight management and promotes fitness and good health. At the same time, it discourages overeating by reducing stress; it produces positive feelings that reinforce self-worth and a sense of accomplishment; and it often includes pleasant socialization. To prevent weight gain and maximize health benefits, adults should aim for 2 hours and 30 minutes of moderate-intensity aerobic activity every week and muscle-strengthening activities on two or more days a week.[63] Even if you cannot meet these recommendations, some activity is better than nothing.

Look for ways to incorporate more physical activity into your daily life (see **FIGURE 9.19**). You might not think you have an hour each day to devote to moderate-intensity physical activity, but you don't have to get this exercise all at once; you can break it up throughout the day.[64] Walk the dog for an extra half-hour daily, for example. Use a stairway instead of an elevator. Walk briskly instead of using transportation. Take up an active hobby such as bicycling. Increasing your activity level by just a small amount can help you maintain your current weight or lose a moderate amount of weight. Regular exercise of moderate intensity—any activity that expends 4 to 7 kilocalories per minute (240 to 420 kilocalories per hour; see Table 9.3)—provides substantial health benefits.

Once you have increased your everyday activity level, consider beginning a formal exercise program that includes cardiorespiratory endurance exercise, resistance training, and stretching exercises. Regular, moderate cardiorespiratory endurance exercise, sustained for 45 minutes to 1 hour, can help trim body fat permanently. Strength training helps increase fat-free mass, which results in more calorie burning even outside of exercise periods.

One thing is clear: Regular exercise, maintained throughout life, makes weight management easier. The sooner you establish good habits, the better. You will succeed in maintaining your weight if you make exercise an integral part of the lifestyle you enjoy now and in the future.

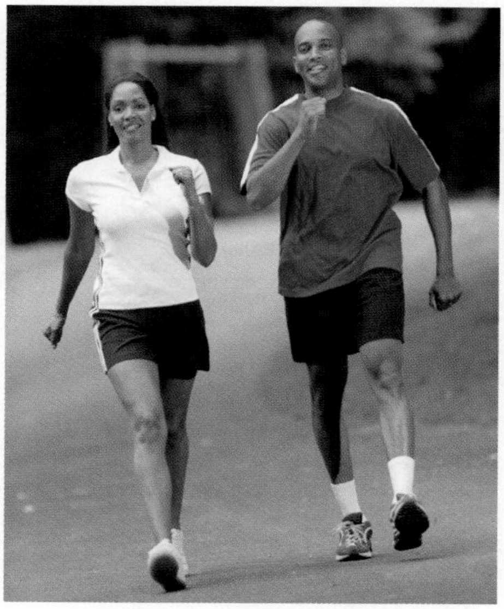

FIGURE 9.19 Weight management through lifetime habits. To achieve long-term weight management, healthy habits must become part of one's daily routine.

Quick Bite

The Fletcherism Fad

At the turn of the twentieth century, a retired businessman named Horace Fletcher started a dietary craze known as "Fletcherism." Calling the mouth "Nature's Food Filter," he believed that the sense of taste and the urge to swallow are perfect guides to nutrition. Although he recommended chewing food at least 50 times before swallowing, preferably until tasteless, he far exceeded this by once chewing a piece of onion 722 times. His philosophy did lead to some weight loss; people adhering to Fletcherism cut back on energy intake as a result of the additional mechanical effort of chewing.

Key Concepts Successful weight management involves regular physical activity as well as healthful food choices. Small increases in activity have significant health benefits and help weight loss and maintenance. To prevent weight gain and maximize health benefits, you should include at least 60 minutes of moderate physical activity in your daily routine.

Thinking and Emotions

What goes on in your head is another factor in a healthy lifestyle and successful weight management. The way you think about yourself and your world influences, and is influenced by, how you feel and how you act. Certain kinds of thinking produce negative emotions, which can undermine a healthy lifestyle.

When we compare ourselves to an internally held picture of an "ideal self," we are more likely to have low self-esteem and feel negative emotions. The ideal self we envision is often the result of having adopted perfectionistic goals and beliefs about how we "should" be. You might know someone who believes, "If I don't do things perfectly, I'm a failure" or "It's terrible if I'm not thin." When we accept these irrational beliefs, we can actually cause ourselves stress and emotional conflict. The remedy is to challenge such beliefs and replace them with more realistic ones.

The beliefs and attitudes you hold give rise to self-talk, an internal dialogue you carry on with yourself about events that happen to and around you. When you talk yourself through the steps of a job and then praise yourself when it's successfully completed, you are engaging in **positive self-talk**. When you make self-deprecating remarks or angry and guilt-producing comments and when you blame yourself unnecessarily, you are engaging in **negative self-talk**. Negative self-talk can undermine efforts at self-control and lead to feelings of anxiety and depression.

Your beliefs and attitudes influence how you interpret what happens to you and what you can expect in the future, as well as how you feel and react. Realistic beliefs and goals combined with positive self-talk and problem-solving efforts support a healthy lifestyle.

▶ **positive self-talk** Constructive mental or verbal statements made to one's self to change a belief or behavior.

▶ **negative self-talk** Mental or verbal statements made to one's self that reinforce negative or destructive self-perceptions.

▶ **ABC model of behavior** A behavioral model that includes the external and internal events that precede and follow the behavior. The A stands for antecedents, the events that precede the behavior (B), which is followed by consequences (C) that positively or negatively reinforce the behavior.

Stress Management

Stress management can be an important part of weight management, and you can use the **ABC model of behavior** (see **FIGURE 9.20**) to help cope with daily stresses and their effects on eating behavior.

The ABC model helps you manage the events that trigger behaviors and the factors that reinforce them. *Antecedents*, the A part of the model, are the events that precede the behavior and trigger it. Overeating is one possible *behavior*, the B part of the model. The *consequences*, or C, follow and reinforce the B. The C might be desirable, such as relief from stress, or undesirable, such as guilt or weight gain. Consequences can be immediate or, like weight gain, occur in the future; consequences that occur immediately have the greatest influence.

Identifying the cues (A) that trigger overeating is the first step to changing or avoiding these triggers. You might remove problem foods from the house or avoid the grocery store's candy aisle. You can sometimes manipulate antecedents to trigger positive behaviors (for example, putting exercise clothes by the door to prompt exercise).

You can change the behavior of overeating (B) by using positive self-talk to encourage a new behavior and avoiding excuses and rationalizations to eat something inappropriate. Positive consequences (C) help to reinforce new behaviors. You could sign a contract with a friend that rewards you for deciding not to overeat. Rewards such as time for physical activity not only reinforce behavior, but also develop fitness. **TABLE 9.7** summarizes cognitive-behavioral tools for changing habits and behavior patterns.

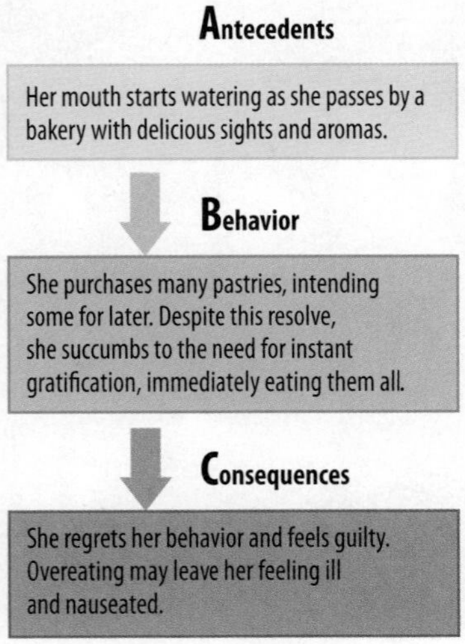

Antecedents
Her mouth starts watering as she passes by a bakery with delicious sights and aromas.
Behavior
She purchases many pastries, intending some for later. Despite this resolve, she succumbs to the need for instant gratification, immediately eating them all.
Consequences
She regrets her behavior and feels guilty. Overeating may leave her feeling ill and nauseated.

FIGURE 9.20 The ABC model of eating behavior. Conquering overeating often requires a psychological strategy for changing ingrained habits and other behaviors.

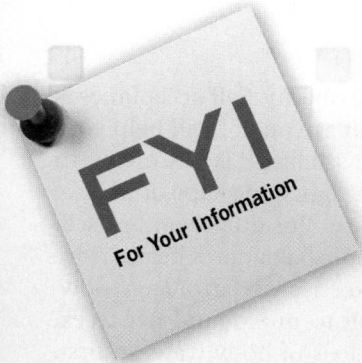

FYI
For Your Information

Learning Weight Management from Some of the "Biggest" Weight Experts: Sumo Wrestlers

Is it possible to work out three to five hours a day, seven days a week, eat a relatively low-fat diet, and still gain weight? Yes! This is the training way of Sumo wrestlers, and a way of life that allows them to pack on the pounds. The world's biggest people are experts at putting on fat, which means that the lessons they've learned can help teach us how to keep the weight off. If you do not want to gain weight, follow these tips. The wrestlers, of course, will be doing just the opposite.

- *Make your workouts slow and steady, not fast and frantic.* Sustained moderate workouts lasting 30 to 60 minutes are more helpful at burning calories than exerting yourself in a brief, intense burst of exercise. Sumo wrestlers train to win at a sport whose rules are simple: One of two wrestlers loses when he is forced out of the wrestling ring or if anything other than his feet touches the playing surface. The average sumo wrestler stands about 6 feet tall and weighs 336 pounds. Their training is focused on being powerful enough to push over something the size of a refrigerator. Going for a 3-mile run or riding a bicycle for 60 minutes is not a priority for sumo wrestler workouts.
- *Don't skip breakfast.* Try not to go longer than four to five hours without eating. Your body will adapt to the threat of starvation and decrease your metabolism so that you can survive on fewer calories. Most sumo wrestlers eat only twice a day.
- *Eat small meals and snacks throughout the day.* Split up your daily calories among breakfast, lunch, dinner, and a couple of snacks. You're less likely to put on weight eating small meals and never overeating, rather than letting yourself get too hungry and then eating too much. Sumo wrestlers eat about one-half of their overall daily food calories at one meal. For a person the size of a sumo wrestler, that can be more than 3,000 calories every day just for lunch!
- *Choose a well-balanced diet with a lot of variety.* Remember that balance, variety, and moderation are cornerstones of good nutrition. Sumo wrestlers eat a relatively low-fat diet but tend to have a diet heavy in complex carbohydrates, protein, and vegetables, with little fruit.

Data from Anderson J, Christensen N, Hoffman E, et al. *Eat Right! Healthy Eating in College and Beyond.* San Francisco: Pearson Benjamin Cummings; 2007:67–79.

TABLE 9.7
Cognitive-Behavioral Tools for Changing Behavior

Self-monitoring	Prospectively recording information about behavior to identify the antecedents (what precedes and elicits a particular action), the behaviors of interest (usually eating behavior), and the consequences (the thoughts, feelings, and reactions that accompany the behavior of interest)
Environmental management	Avoiding or changing cues that trigger undesirable behavior (e.g., not driving by the doughnut shop, putting the cookie jar out of sight), or instituting new cues to elicit new behaviors (e.g., putting your walking shoes by the door as a reminder to exercise); also called "stimulus control"
Alternate behaviors	Learning new ways of responding to old cues or circumstances that can't be changed or avoided (e.g., taking a walk when you get upset instead of getting something to eat)
Reward	Giving yourself, or arranging to be given, rewards for engaging in desired behaviors
Negative reinforcement	Arranging to give up something desirable (e.g., money) or to endure something undesirable (e.g., wash your friend's car) for engaging in unwanted behaviors
Social support	Getting others to participate in or otherwise provide emotional and physical support of your weight-management efforts
Cognitive coping	Reducing negative self-talk, increasing positive self-talk, and challenging beliefs that undermine your resolve and contribute to negative emotions; setting reasonable goals and avoiding "thinking traps"
Managing emotions	Using reframing, disengagement, imagery, and self-soothing to reduce or manage negative emotions
Relapse prevention and recovery	Identifying high-risk situations that pose a hazard for relapsing, and learning to recover from small indiscretions before they become major relapses

Adapted from Nash JD. *Maximize Your Body Potential.* 3rd ed. Palo Alto, CA: Bull; 2003.

Quick Bite

The Raw Foods Diet

The raw foods diet advocates eating only uncooked, unprocessed, mostly organic food. When beginning the diet, many raw food dieters experience an unpleasant side effect: diarrhea.

TABLE 9.8
Basic Tenets of Size Acceptance

- Human beings come in a variety of sizes and shapes. We celebrate this diversity as a positive characteristic of the human race.
- There is no ideal body size, shape, or weight that every individual should strive to achieve.
- Every body is a good body, whatever its size or shape.
- Self-esteem and body image are strongly linked. Helping people feel good about their bodies and about who they are can help motivate and maintain healthy behaviors.
- Appearance stereotyping is inherently unfair to the individual because it is based on superficial factors over which the individual has little or no control.
- We respect the bodies of others even though they might be quite different from our own.
- Each person is responsible for taking care of his or her body.
- Good health is not defined by body size; it is a state of physical, mental, and social well-being.

Note: People of all sizes and shapes can reduce their risk of poor health by adopting a healthy lifestyle.

Data from *Basic Tenets of Health at Every Size*, developed by dietitians and nutritionists who are advocates of size acceptance; their efforts coordinated by Joanne P. Ikeda, MA, RD, Nutrition Education Specialist, Department of Nutritional Sciences, University of California, Berkeley.

Balancing Acceptance and Change

It's not enough to change your behavior to manage obesity. Self-acceptance is equally necessary (see **TABLE 9.8**). Accepting yourself as you are will help your self-esteem and improve your general satisfaction with life. It is destructive to be overly concerned with the importance of body weight and shape or to have unattainable goals of idealized physical appearance. But don't confuse self-acceptance with complacency or a do-nothing attitude that ignores health risks.

If you must diet, do so in combination with exercise, and avoid very-low-calorie diets. Don't try to lose more than one-half to one pound per week. Realize that most low-calorie diets cause a rapid loss of body water at first. When this phase passes, weight loss declines. As a result, dieters often are misled into believing that their efforts are not working. They then give up, not realizing that smaller losses later in the diet actually are better than the initial big losses. In fact, the later loss is mostly fat loss, whereas the initial loss is primarily fluid loss.

Key Concepts Identifying cues that precede overeating can help a person make behavior changes. Long-term weight management should include self-acceptance and enhanced self-esteem. Goals of idealized body size and shape should be replaced with goals that promote good health and a lifetime of fitness.

Weight-Management Approaches

Do certain weight-loss diets have adverse health consequences? Is it unhealthy to lose weight quickly? Will the weight stay off? What motivates people to lose weight and to maintain weight? What are the barriers to losing weight and/or to maintaining weight?

In a study of popular weight-loss diets, 160 participants with an average BMI of 35 kg/m^2 were randomly assigned to one of four weight-loss diets: Weight Watchers (restriction of portion sizes and calories; 1,200 to 1,600 calories daily), Atkins (low carbohydrate—less than 20 grams daily at onset, gradual increase to 50 grams), Zone (40–30–30 balance of percentage of calories from carbohydrate, fat, and protein, respectively), and Ornish (vegetarian, less than 10 percent of calories from fat).[65] Subjects lost weight on all four diets, but no one diet was more effective than any of the others. Compliance was a key factor. Only about 25 percent of subjects in each group maintained the diet at a level of 6 on a 10-point scale (1 = no adherence, 10 = perfect adherence), and dietary adherence was strongly associated with weight loss. Those who stuck to the diets best lost on average 7 percent of body weight, a meaningful start in reducing health risks.

A wide range of weight-management approaches is available to the consumer. It's important to investigate your options thoroughly to find the approach best suited to your personal needs.

Self-Help Books and Manuals

Some people respond well to information provided in an easy-to-understand format. They are able to change their behavior by referring to good, well-researched self-help manuals and books, and even Internet-based resources. The proliferation of diet books is nothing short of phenomenal, however, and each year dozens of dubious weight-loss diet books reach the market. When evaluating a diet book or website diet plan, be alert to the following warning flags:

- *Unbalanced diet patterns:* The recommended pattern should not stray too far from that of MyPlate.
- *Claims of a "scientific breakthrough" or promises of "quick and easy" weight loss:* There is no quick fix when it comes to weight management.

- *Irrational food instructions, such as food restrictions (e.g., no fruits), illogical overemphasis of some foods (e.g., five grapefruits daily), and irrational food patterns (e.g., don't eat meat and bread at the same meal):* Such restrictions set the stage for feelings of deprivation and binge eating.
- *The promise of a cure for some disease along with weight loss:* That's not only a waste of money, but also potentially dangerous.

FYI For Your Information

Behaviors That Will Help You Manage Your Weight

Set the Right Goals

Setting the right goals is an important first step. Most people trying to lose weight focus just on weight loss; however, you'll be more successful if you focus on dietary and exercise changes that lead to long-term weight change. Successful weight managers select no more than two or three goals at a time.

Effective goals are (1) specific, (2) attainable, and (3) forgiving. "Exercise more" is a commendable ideal, but it's not specific. "Walk five miles every day" is specific and measurable, but is it attainable if you're just starting out? "Walk 30 minutes every day" is more attainable, but what happens if you're held up at work or there's a thunderstorm? "Walk 30 minutes, five days each week" is specific, attainable, and forgiving. In short, a great goal!

Nothing Succeeds Like Success

Select a series of short-term goals that get you closer and closer to the ultimate goal (for example, consider reducing fat intake from 40 percent of calories to 35 percent and later to 30 percent). Nothing succeeds like success. This strategy employs two important behavioral principles: (1) consecutive goals that move you ahead in small steps are the best way to reach a distant point, and (2) consecutive rewards keep the overall effort invigorated.

Reward Success (But Not with Food)

You're more likely to keep working toward your goal if you are rewarded—especially when goals are difficult to reach. An effective reward is something that is desirable, timely, and contingent on meeting your goal. Your rewards might be tangible (e.g., a movie, CD, payment toward buying a more costly item) or intangible (e.g., an afternoon off from studying, an hour of quiet time away from the daily demands of school). As you meet small goals, give yourself numerous small rewards; don't wait to meet your ultimate goal for a single reward. The long, difficult effort might lead you to give up.

Balance Your (Food) Checkbook

Keeping track of your behavior—observing and recording calorie intake, servings of fruits and vegetables, exercise frequency and duration, or any other wellness behavior—can help alter that behavior. Self-monitoring usually changes a behavior in the desired direction and can produce "real-time" records for you and your health care provider. For example, you can track your exercise progress. A record of increasing exercise encourages you to keep up the good work. If the record shows little or no progress, you know that a change of strategy is needed. Some people find that specific self-monitoring forms make it easier, whereas others prefer to use their own recording system.

Although you don't need to step on the scale every day, monitoring your weight regularly (once a week) can help you maintain your lower weight. Use a graph rather than a list or calendar notations so that you have a picture of cumulative progress. Changes in your body's water content, rather than fat content, are responsible for most of the up-and-down fluctuations from day to day. A long-term downward trend reflects fat losses.

Avoid a Chain Reaction

Identify the social or environmental cues that seem to encourage undesirable eating, and then change those cues. For example, you may learn from reflection or self-monitoring that you're more likely to overeat while watching television, when treats are on display at the campus café, or when you're around a certain friend. You might then try to break the association between eating and the cue (don't eat while watching television), avoid or eliminate the cue (avoid sitting near the display counter), or change the circumstances surrounding the cue (plan to meet with your friend in nonfood settings). In general, visible and accessible food items often are cues for unplanned eating.

Get the (Fullness) Message

Changing the way you eat can make it easier to eat less without feeling deprived. It takes 15 or more minutes for your brain to get the message you've been fed. Slowing the rate of eating can allow satiation (fullness) signals to begin by the end of the meal. Eating lots of vegetables also can make you feel fuller. Another trick is to use smaller plates so that moderate portions do not appear meager. Changing your eating schedule, or setting one, can be helpful, especially if you tend to skip or delay meals and overeat later.

The Backsliding Phenomenon

You've just signed a contract with yourself to avoid high-fat desserts for one month when you're presented with an array of your favorite "to die for" desserts. You say to yourself, "just this once" and satisfy your craving. Most of us have experienced the *backsliding phenomenon* in which we have lost our resolve and slipped back into a former bad habit. When it happens, be prepared for it and move on with your resolve. You're most apt to backslide when you're tempted by something unexpected and your self-control is threatened. You can remove high-fat snacks from your home but not from other places you eat. Imagine tempting situations in your mind's eye and practice coping with them successfully. If you do slip, don't waste time with self-blame. Learn from the experience and get back on track.

Adapted from National Heart, Lung, and Blood Institute. Guide to behavior change. http://www.nhlbi.nih.gov/health/public/heart/obesity/lose_wt/behavior.htm. Accessed January 6, 2016.

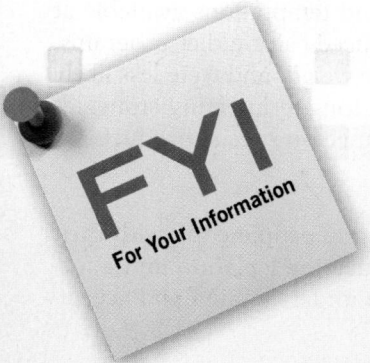

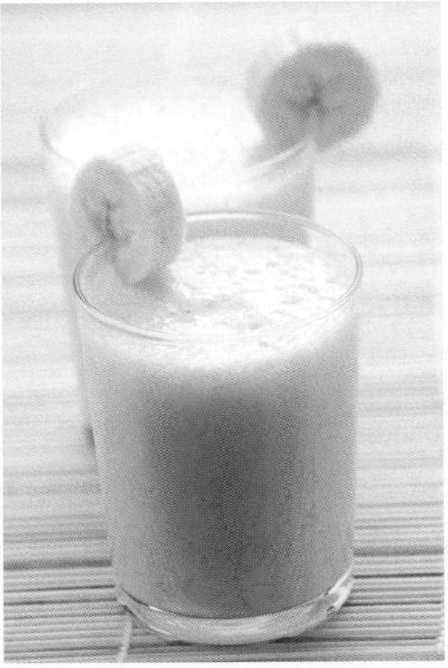

Should you decide on the do-it-yourself route, develop specific goals for your diet, exercise, and maintenance plans. (See the FYI feature "Behaviors That Will Help You Manage Your Weight.") Keep tabs on your habits and become more involved in activities other than eating, especially fitness activities.

Long-term success depends on maintaining the lifestyle changes that helped you lose the weight in the first place.

Meal Replacements

Some people turn to meal replacements—shakes and bars, for example—to help lose weight. Meal replacements are convenient, often contain added vitamins and minerals, and reduce the choices and temptations available at mealtime. When compared with traditional, reduced-calorie diet programs, people using meal replacements lost slightly more weight and were less likely to stop the program.[66] The challenge is to learn long-term eating strategies that will allow weight management without reliance on special products.

Self-Help Groups

Self-help groups, often led by laypeople, help many people cope with their weight. Such groups can share experiences, reduce the isolation and alienation felt by many obese people, and provide an understanding and accepting community.

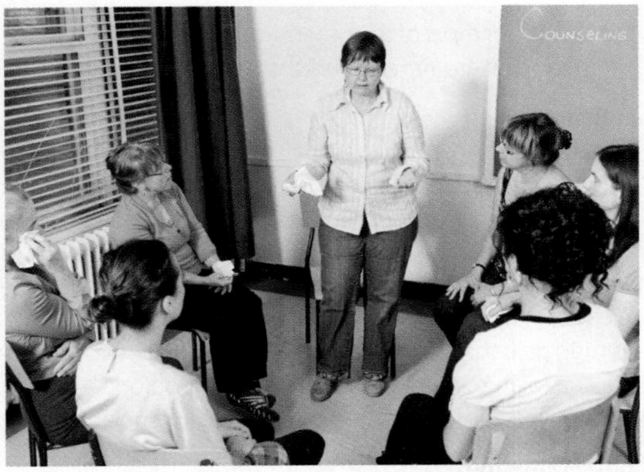

Commercial Programs

Commercial weight-loss programs provide group or individual counseling and group support. Some sell prepackaged foods or nutritional supplements. Some companies employ dietitians, health educators, psychologists, or physicians to develop and guide the program at the corporate level. The Federal Trade Commission (FTC) encourages commercial programs to release the following information to potential clients:

- Staff training and education
- Risks of overweight and obesity
- Risks of their products or program
- Cost
- Program outcomes: success and failure rates

Be sure to obtain this information before you register for a weight-loss program, and think twice about any program that does not willingly provide it.

Several commercial programs, such as Optifast and Health Management Resources (HMR), use **very-low-calorie diets (VLCDs)** containing only 400 to 800 kilocalories per day as the initial phase of treatment. When such diets were first introduced in the 1970s, several deaths resulted from cardiac abnormalities. As a result, VLCDs should be undertaken only with close medical supervision.

▶ **very-low-calorie diets (VLCDs)** Diets supplying 400 to 800 kilocalories per day, which include adequate high-quality protein, little or no fat, and little carbohydrate.

Digital Programs and Private Counselors

Private counselors can be physicians, psychotherapists, or registered dietitians/registered dietitian nutritionists. They provide individualized approaches to weight management and the support and attention that some obese people might need. Some programs use the Internet rather than face-to-face counseling sessions and have seen positive results. The Internet has shown potential for use in many areas of health behavior, including self-motivation and weight loss.

For the first time in its history, the Centers for Disease Control and Prevention recognized three digital programs—Omada Health, Noom Health, and DPS Health—as meeting evidence-based standards for the agency's National

Quick Bite

Letter on Corpulence

Published in the early 1800s, *Bantry's Letter on Corpulence* was the first popular diet book in the United States. The book advocated restricting intake of carbohydrates.

Diabetes Prevention Program.[67] The programs help people make lifestyle changes that lead to weight loss associated with reduced risk of chronic disease.

Food and Drug Administration–Approved Weight-Loss Medications

The pharmaceutical industry has long searched for a "magic bullet" to battle obesity, but so far a cure has failed to emerge. With the recognition that obesity involves multiple factors, the focus is shifting to drugs with multiple mechanisms and drugs used in conjunction with proper diet and exercise. When combined with changes to eating and physical activity, prescription drugs may help some people lose weight (usually less than 10 percent of their body weight). Results vary by drug and by person. Most weight loss takes place in the first 6 months of starting the medicine. After that time, the patient may lose weight more slowly or begin to regain weight.

One should never take a weight loss medicine only for cosmetic benefit. The chance that side effects may outweigh benefits is of great concern. In the past, some drugs for obesity treatment were linked to serious health problems. For example, sibutramine (sold as Meridia), was recalled because of concerns related to heart disease and stroke.

Antiobesity medications generally fall into one of two categories: appetite suppressants and lipase inhibitors. Most FDA-approved weight-loss medications are appetite suppressants and are approved for short-term use (a few weeks) only. Appetite suppressants work by limiting the desire for food by either decreasing appetite or increasing the feeling of fullness following eating. By increasing one or more brain chemicals that affect mood and appetite, appetite suppressants make you less hungry. Phentermine is the most common prescribed appetite-suppressant in the United States.

Xenical (orlistat) is approved by the FDA for long-term use (up to two years). This medication is a lipase inhibitor, which works by reducing the body's ability to absorb dietary fat. Orlistat blocks the enzyme lipase, which is responsible for breaking down dietary fat. Because the body cannot absorb fat that has not been broken down, the body eliminates it along with its calories. Orlistat must be accompanied by a low-fat diet, or the unabsorbed fat can produce diarrhea and flatulence. The drug also blocks fat-soluble nutrient absorption, so it's necessary to take a vitamin supplement as well.[68]

Belviq (lorcaserin) and Saxenda (liraglutide, a daily injectable) are appetite suppressants approved for use in patients who have a BMI over 30, or a BMI over 27 and at least one weight-related health condition, such as high blood pressure, type 2 diabetes, or high cholesterol.[69,70] Because Belviq can cause hallucinations at higher-than-approved doses, the U.S. Drug Enforcement Agency has classified it as a drug with potential for abuse.

Qsymia (pronounced kyoo-sim-EE-uh) combines two FDA-approved drugs: the appetite suppressant phentermine and the anti-seizure medication topiramate. After 1 year of treatment with Qsymia, 62 percent of patients who were prescribed the recommended dose lost at least 5 percent of their weight. If a patient has not lost 5 percent after only 12 weeks, it is unlikely that further use will produce weight loss. The drug label contains warnings for increased heart rate, suicidal behavior and ideation, glaucoma, mood and sleep disorders, creatine elevation, and metabolic acidosis. Qsymia also must not be used during pregnancy because it may cause harm to the baby.[71]

The FDA has approved the use of antiobesity drugs only in combination with calorie-restricted diets and regular physical activity. Most antiobesity drugs are addictive and have the potential for abuse. Antiobesity agents shouldn't be used in combination with each other or with other drugs for appetite control because the safety of such combinations has not been evaluated. A lesson from the withdrawal of previous anti-obesity drugs is that uncommon but serious adverse effects may become apparent only when a drug is used in larger populations or for longer periods of time than in preapproval trials.[72]

In using any medications for weight loss, one needs to understand that prescription medications alone, without behavior modification, are not effective for long-term weight-loss maintenance. In addition, long-term use of these drugs is limited by significant side effects and lack of long-term safety and efficacy data.[73]

Over-the-Counter Drugs and Dietary Supplements

> ## Quick Bite
> **The Fattest Mammals**
> Among mammals, humans carry the largest percentage of weight as body fat.

Although dietary supplement use is common among adults trying to lose weight, it actually can be counterproductive. Taking weight-loss supplements can create the illusion of protection against weight gain and loosen a dieter's self-control. In a recent study, participants with more positive attitudes toward weight loss supplements were more susceptible to the liberating effect of taking weight loss supplements on food intake.[74]

Nonprescription (over-the-counter, or OTC) weight-loss pills sometimes contain caffeine, benzocaine, or fiber. Caffeine is a stimulant and diuretic. Benzocaine numbs the tongue, which reduces taste sensations and discourages eating. Pills with fiber are designed to fill the stomach and provide a feeling of fullness. Although moderately effective, fiber pills can lead to dehydration; much of the lost weight is water, which is easily regained when the pills are stopped.

Numerous dietary supplements are marketed for weight loss, with names such as "Weight Away." Common ingredients include chromium picolinate, chitosan, hydroxycitric acid (HCA), glucomannan, and pyruvate. More and more studies are finding that over-the-counter products marketed for weight loss often contain potentially harmful substances.[75] These products are no substitute for exercise and healthful eating and, if used, should be used with caution.

Surgery

- **extreme obesity** Obesity characterized by body weight exceeding 100 percent of normal; a condition so severe it often requires surgery.
- **morbid obesity** See *extreme obesity.*

Sometimes, surgery can successfully treat **extreme obesity** (also called **morbid obesity**), defined as a BMI of 40 kg/m^2 or higher. Surgery should be a last-ditch effort, taken only when all legitimate, less-invasive methods have failed. The most common procedures are gastric banding, gastric bypass, and the gastric sleeve. Gastric banding reduces stomach size by creating a smaller upper stomach, or "pouch," thus limiting intake to only a few calories at one time.[76] Gastric bypass also creates a smaller stomach pouch and then connects that pouch to a shortened section of small intestine (see **FIGURE 9.21**). The gastric sleeve, also known as sleeve gastrectomy, is a surgery that reduces the size of the stomach and makes it into a narrow tube. Reducing the size of the stomach reduces food intake, and bypassing the upper part of the small intestine reduces digestion and absorption of caloric foods. The absorption of some micronutrients is also reduced—an obvious drawback. Such surgeries are growing in popularity, not only in the adult population, but also among adolescents.[77]

Although the results of surgery are impressive, long-term success is highly variable. Surgical patients lose substantially more weight initially than those who try diet and exercise or weight-loss medications. Although weight loss tends to plateau by 18 to 24 months after surgery, it is not unusual for patients to have maintained a 50-percent loss of initial body weight after five years.[78]

The long-term effectiveness of gastric surgery depends on how patients manage their eating and is more successful for those with more frequent physician visits (six to seven times) during the first year following the procedure.[79] Patients can defeat the procedure easily by consuming high-calorie drinks

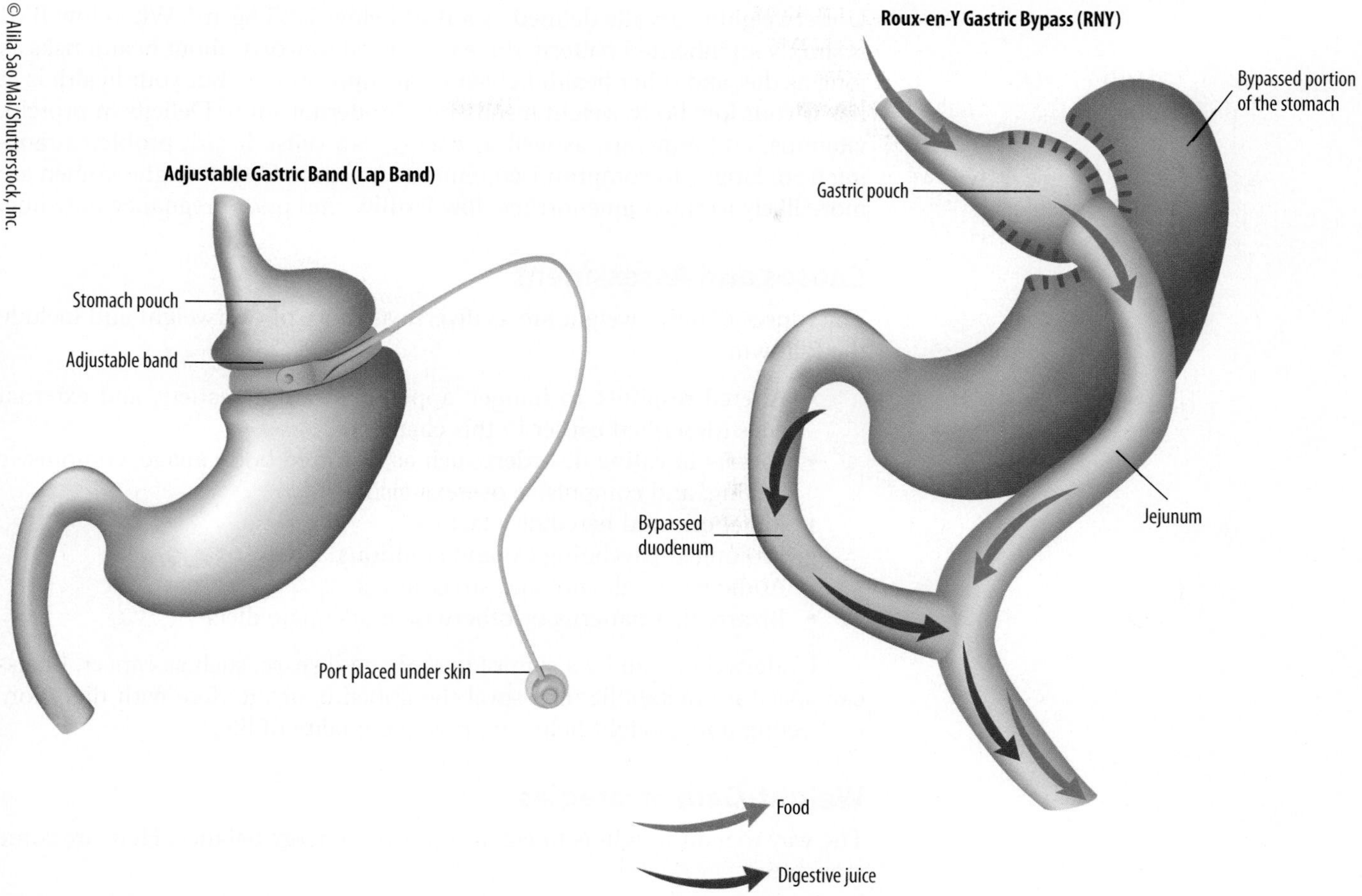

FIGURE 9.21 Gastric surgery in obesity treatment. In gastric banding, surgery reduces the size of the stomach. The band can be adjusted by an infusion of saline through a port that lies just beneath the skin. In gastric bypass, an alternate route carries food to the jejunum, bypassing the duodenum and most of the stomach.

or semisolid foods that overcome the restricted stomach size. With time the pouch stretches, allowing more solid foods, but by then, doctors hope that the patient has established healthy eating habits. After gastric surgery, lean body mass is lost and resting metabolic rate can decline significantly, thus exercise is important to include with diet modifications.[80]

Liposuction is a cosmetic surgical procedure that reshapes the body by removing fat. Although the procedure removes some fat cells, the body still has billions of other fat cells ready to store extra fat. Thus, liposuction is not effective for significant or long-term weight loss. It should not be undertaken casually. Risks include blood clots, perforation injuries, skin and nerve damage, and unfavorable drug reactions.

Key Concepts Books, Internet resources, and commercial programs can help some individuals lose weight. However, consumers should always proceed with caution before spending money. Drugs have potential side effects and must be used with caution and medical supervision. For those who are extremely obese, surgical intervention is an aggressive, last-resort approach to weight management. Liposuction removes fat cells from specific parts of the body but is not considered an effective approach to weight control.

Underweight

From a public health standpoint, underweight is much less of a problem than obesity, but those who are underweight can find it troublesome and frustrating.

Underweight is usually defined as a BMI below 18.5 kg/m^2. When low BMI is simply an inherited pattern, there is no need to worry about health risks as long as diet and other health behaviors are appropriate. But your health is at risk if your low body weight results from undernutrition. Deficits in protein, vitamins, and minerals, as well as energy, can cause health problems ranging from fatigue to compromised immune function. Underweight women are more likely to suffer amenorrhea, low fertility, and poor pregnancy outcome.

Causes and Assessment

The causes of underweight are as diverse as those of overweight and include the following:

- Altered response to hunger, appetite, satiation, satiety, and external cues (described earlier in this chapter)
- Factors in eating disorders such as distorted body image, compulsive dieting, and compulsive overexercising
- Metabolic and hereditary factors
- Prolonged psychological and emotional stress
- Addiction to alcohol and street drugs
- Bizarre diet patterns or otherwise inadequate diets

Underweight can be a sign of underlying disease, such as cancer. Illness can speed up metabolic rate, spoil the appetite, or interfere with digestion. Correcting underweight helps improve the quality of life.

Weight-Gain Strategies

The way to gain weight is to create a positive energy balance. Here are some strategies:

- Have small, frequent meals consisting of nutrient-dense and energy-dense foods and beverages.
- Drink fluids at the end of the meal or, better yet, between meals to avoid filling the stomach with liquids of low nutrient density.
- Try high-calorie weight-gain beverages and foods.
- Use timers or other cues (similar to the ABC model in Figure 9.20 but with a different goal) to prompt eating.
- Take a balanced vitamin/mineral supplement to ensure that poor appetite isn't a result of nutritional deficiency.

Sometimes prescription drugs, such as appetite stimulants, are helpful. Medication also can speed stomach emptying, improving appetite for the next meal. Digestive enzyme replacements help people who are underweight resulting from poor digestion or absorption.

Exercise has a role in weight gain as well. Simple anaerobic or isometric exercise encourages weight gain as lean body mass rather than fat.

Key Concepts Underweight is not as common as overweight. Gaining weight can be difficult, but the basic concepts of energy balance apply. Changes in diet along with regular physical activity are important strategies for gaining weight.

Label to Table

Do you believe that by choosing cookies or chips labeled "low-fat" or sticking with certain brand names associated with "diet foods" you are automatically making the right decisions? It might surprise you to know that many low-fat or fat-free products have nearly the same amount of calories as the full-fat versions! After reading this chapter you now know that when it comes to weight loss, total calories are just as important as calories from fat. If you eat a fat-free food, but eat so much of it that your calories are excessive, you will still gain weight. To illustrate this point, let's compare the nutrition labels from some leading cookie manufacturers. The lower-fat cookie label (on the right) claims they are "better for you" and have "50% less fat" compared to the regular cookies. Here are the key facts from the labels:

Regular Cookie	Lower-Fat Cookie
Serving:	Serving:
2 cookies (29 g)	2 cookies (26 g)
Calories: 140	Calories: 110
Calories from	Calories from
fat: 50	fat: 25
Total fat: 6 g	Total fat: 3 g

True, there is a 50 percent reduction in fat content (6 grams vs. 3 grams), which is an important part of the picture. However, take a look at the Total Calories. The lower-fat cookies only have 30 fewer kilocalories than the regular cookies, which can be a surprise to those who think they are saving more.

There is another interesting piece of information on these labels: the serving size. At first glance, you might think the serving size of the cookies is the same, two cookies. However, after further inspection you can see that the lower-fat cookies are slightly smaller. A 10 percent reduction in size/weight is certainly worth noting when you are trying to explain how a product can have fewer calories.

The next time you are in the cookie aisle debating whether you should settle a craving with a low-fat product or its full-fat version, be a smart consumer and read the label before you buy!

Regular cookie

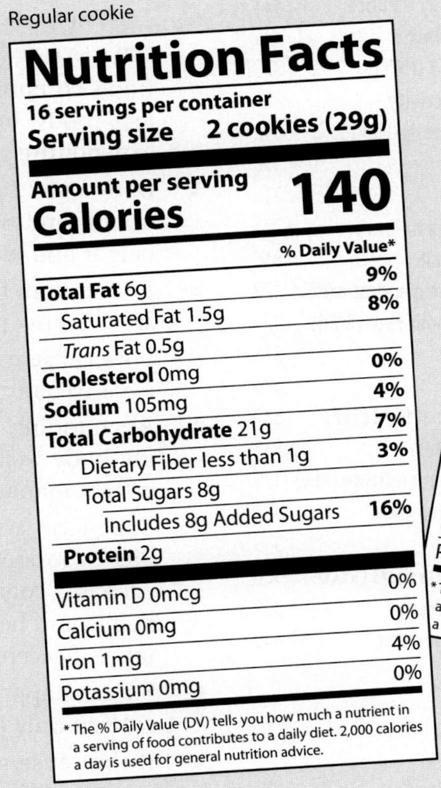
Nutrition Facts
16 servings per container
Serving size 2 cookies (29g)
Amount per serving
Calories 140
% Daily Value*
Total Fat 6g 9%
Saturated Fat 1.5g 8%
Trans Fat 0.5g
Cholesterol 0mg 0%
Sodium 105mg 4%
Total Carbohydrate 21g 7%
Dietary Fiber less than 1g 3%
Total Sugars 8g
Includes 8g Added Sugars 16%
Protein 2g
Vitamin D 0mcg 0%
Calcium 0mg 0%
Iron 1mg 4%
Potassium 0mg 0%
* The % Daily Value (DV) tells you how much a nutrient in a serving of food contributes to a daily diet. 2,000 calories a day is used for general nutrition advice.

Lower fat cookie

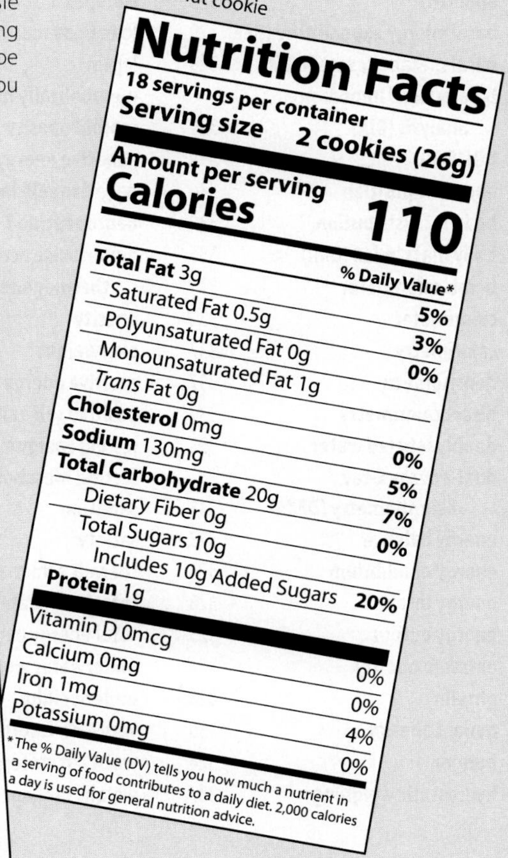
Nutrition Facts
18 servings per container
Serving size 2 cookies (26g)
Amount per serving
Calories 110
% Daily Value*
Total Fat 3g 5%
Saturated Fat 0.5g 3%
Polyunsaturated Fat 0g
Monounsaturated Fat 1g
Trans Fat 0g
Cholesterol 0mg 0%
Sodium 130mg 5%
Total Carbohydrate 20g 7%
Dietary Fiber 0g 0%
Total Sugars 10g
Includes 10g Added Sugars 20%
Protein 1g
Vitamin D 0mcg 0%
Calcium 0mg 0%
Iron 1mg 4%
Potassium 0mg 0%
*The % Daily Value (DV) tells you how much a nutrient in a serving of food contributes to a daily diet. 2,000 calories a day is used for general nutrition advice.

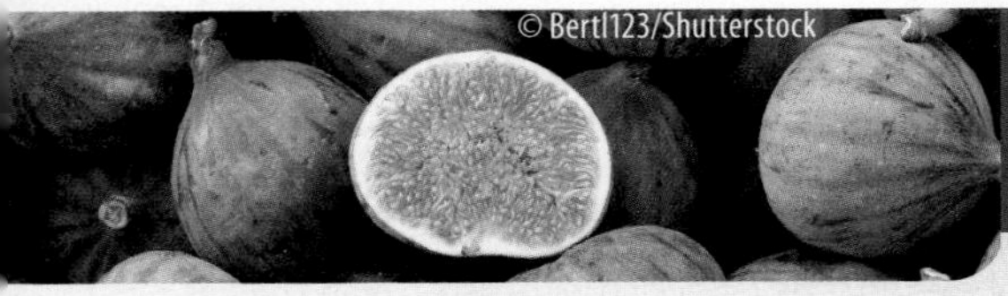
© Bertl123/Shutterstock

Learning Portfolio

Key Terms

Study Points

- Energy balance is the relationship between energy intake and energy output.
- The energy content in food can be measured directly using a bomb calorimeter or estimated using the following factors: 4 kilocalories per gram for carbohydrate and protein, 9 kilocalories per gram for fat, and 7 kilocalories per gram for alcohol.
- Food intake is regulated by hunger, satiation, satiety, and appetite, which are influenced by complex factors. Hunger is the physiological need to eat. Satiation is the feeling of fullness that leads to termination of a meal. Satiety determines the interval until the next meal. Appetite is a desire to eat that is influenced by external factors such as flavors and smells and environmental and cultural factors.
- Gastrointestinal stimulation, circulating nutrients, neurotransmitters, and hormones signal the brain to regulate food intake.
- The major components of energy expenditure are resting energy expenditure, the thermic effect of food, and energy for physical activity.
- Calorimetry is the measurement of energy use, either directly by measuring heat production or indirectly by determining oxygen intake and carbon dioxide production.
- Body composition, age, gender, genetics, and hormonal activity affect the amount of energy used for resting metabolism.
- The energy cost of physical activity is affected by a person's size and the intensity and duration of the activity.
- Body composition—the relative amounts of fat and lean body mass—has a major influence on energy expenditure and risk of chronic disease.
- Body mass index—a ratio correlated with total body fatness and risk of chronic disease—is calculated with height and weight measurements.
- Rather than focus on ideal body weight, many professionals now promote health and fitness goals.
- Physical activity improves fitness and helps achieve the negative energy balance needed for weight reduction.
- Abandoning unrealistic ideas of thinness and accepting body weight and shape are important elements in weight management.
- Long-term weight management includes a balanced diet of moderately restricted calorie intake, adequate exercise, cognitive-behavioral strategies for changing habits and behavior patterns, and attention to balancing self-acceptance and the desire for change.
- Surgical approaches to weight control should be considered only as a last resort for the morbidly obese.
- If the cause is not hereditary, being underweight can pose health problems.
- Gaining weight can be difficult for individuals who are underweight.

Study Questions

1. Explain the concept of energy balance.
2. List and describe the three main components of energy expenditure.
3. Explain the three main factors that determine energy expenditure in activity.
4. List the techniques for measuring body composition.
5. Describe the concept of metabolically healthy obesity.
6. What are the components of a sound approach to weight management?
7. Explain how the ABCs of behavior modification can assist with weight control.
8. Define underweight.

Try This

A One-Week Energy Balance Check

The purpose of this exercise is to see if you're in energy balance by monitoring your body weight for one week. Measure your weight on a Monday morning soon after you wake up. Record your weight. Don't change your normal routine of exercise and food intake. One week later weigh yourself again (on Monday morning just after waking). Did your weight change? If not, your energy intake closely matched your energy output. If so, did you gain or lose weight? What factors do you think contributed to your body weight change? Try repeating this exercise over a longer period of time. Measure and record your weight every Monday morning for six months. What happens?

Increasing Your Energy Output

Physical activity is the part of your energy output that varies the most. The purpose of this exercise is to increase your energy expenditure by committing to daily exercise for one week. Make each exercise session about 30 minutes long, and remember that the longer the duration, the harder the intensity, and the larger the muscle groups involved, the greater the energy expenditure. Choose an exercise you enjoy—such as walking, jogging, cycling, swimming, or inline skating. Once your week is complete, ask yourself these questions: How did this week's daily exercise affect my energy balance? Have I gained or lost weight during the week? Did I compensate for the extra energy expenditure by increasing my calorie intake?

Changing Your Energy Input

Would you like to change your weight by a pound or two? The purpose of this exercise is to increase or decrease your energy input (calorie intake) so that you gain or lose 1 pound by the end of a week. How? Make only minor adjustments in your usual diet but try to change the energy content for each of your meals by a small amount. Keep a food log and use EatRight Analysis Software or Nutritionist Pro software to estimate your calorie total for each of the days. Your goal is to change your calorie total by approximately 500 kilocalories per day. You should not consume fewer than 1,500 kilocalories (for women) or 1,800 kilocalories (for men) per day. Weigh yourself at the start of your week and at the end. What change, if any, do you see?

What About Bobbie?

Bobbie is a 20-year-old college sophomore who weighs 155 pounds and is 5 feet, 4 inches tall. She gained 10 pounds her freshman year and would like to lose it because she feels healthier when her weight is closer to 145 pounds. She exercises infrequently but likes to walk with her friends and occasionally goes to an aerobics class. How would you suggest she lose the extra 10 pounds? Let's start by reducing her calorie intake slightly. Some small changes in portion sizes that will save some calories.

As you can see in the right-hand column, small changes in Bobbie's diet can result in a 500-kilocalorie deficit, which will translate to approximately 1 pound per week of weight loss. This doesn't take into account any extra exercise she might do. So, if she starts to work out more regularly, she can make fewer changes in her calorie intake and still lose 1 pound per week.

Typical Day	Alternative	Kcal
Breakfast		
1 cinnamon-raisin bagel		70 saved
3 Tbsp. light cream cheese	1 Tbsp. light cream cheese	
Coffee, 2 Tbsp. 2% milk, 2 tsp. sugar		
Snack		
1 banana		
Lunch		
2 slices sourdough bread		
2 ounces turkey lunch meat		
2 tsp. regular mayo, 2 tsp. mustard, 1 slice tomato, dill pickle, lettuce leaf		
12 oz. diet cola		
Salad		
2 cups iceberg lettuce with	1 Tbsp. Italian dressing	55 saved
2 Tbsp. each shredded carrot, chopped egg, croutons, kidney beans, Italian dressing		
1 chocolate chip cookie		
Snack		
1½ oz. tortilla chips, ½ cup salsa	1 oz. tortilla chips	70 saved
Dinner		
1½ cups pasta	1 cup pasta	100 saved
3 oz. meatballs, 3 oz. spaghetti sauce, 2 Tbsp. Parmesan		
cheese	Delete garlic bread	185 saved
1 slice garlic bread	1 cup green beans	25 added
½ cup green beans	Delete butter	30 saved
1 tsp. butter		
12 oz. diet cola		
Snack		
1 slice cheese pizza		
Total **500 saved**		

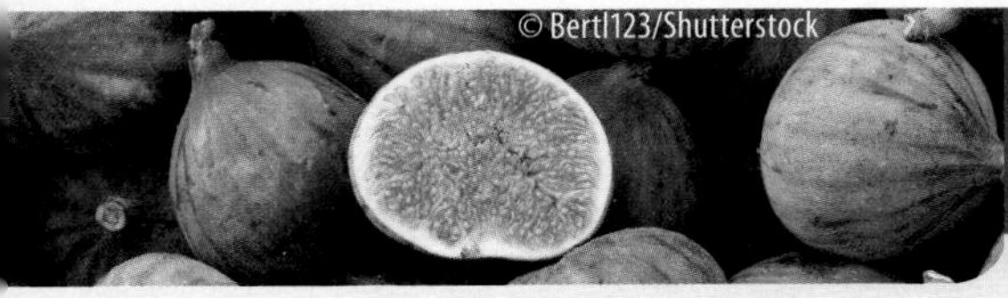

Learning Portfolio (continued)

References

1. Blatt AD, Roe LS, Rolls BJ. Increasing the protein content of meals and its effect on daily energy intake. *J Am Diet Assoc*. 2011:111(2):290–294.
2. Higgins JA. Resistant starch and energy balance: impact on weight loss and maintenance. *Crit Rev Food Sci Nutr*. 2014;54:1158–1166.
3. Wanders AJ, Feskens EJ, Jonathan MC, et al. Pectin is not pectin: a randomized trial on the effect of different physicochemical properties of dietary fiber on appetite and energy intake. *Physiol Behav*. 2014;128:212–219.
4. Park S, Blanck HM, Sherry B, Brener N, O'Toole T. Factors associated with sugar-sweetened beverage intake among United States high school students. *J Nutr*. 2012;142(2):306–312; and Ebbeling CB, Swain JF, Feldman HA, et al. Effects of dietary composition on energy expenditure during weight-loss maintenance. *JAMA*. 2012;307(24):2627–2634.
5. Bray GA, Popkin BM. Dietary sugar and body weight: have we reached a crisis in the epidemic of obesity and diabetes?: health be damned! Pour on the sugar. *Diabetes Care*. 2014;37(4):950–956.
6. Spahn JM, Reeves RS, Keim KS, et al. State of the evidence regarding behavior change theories and strategies in nutrition counseling to facilitate health and food behavior change. *J Am Diet Assoc*. 2010;110(60):879–891.
7. Marchiori D, Papies EK. A brief mindfulness intervention reduces unhealthy eating when hungry, but not the portion size effect. *Appetite*. 2014;75:40–45.
8. Marchiori D, Corneille O, Klein O. Container size influences snack food intake independently of portion size. *Appetite*. 2012;58(3):814–817.
9. Wansink B, Van Ittersum K, Payne CR. Larger bowl size increases the amount of cereal children request, consume, and waste. *J Pediatr*. 2014;164(2):323–326.
10. van Kleef E, Shimizu M, Wansink B. Serving bowl selection biases the amount of food served. *J Nutr Educ Behav*. 2012;44(1):66–70.
11. Marchiori D, Waroquier L, Klein O. "Split them!" Smaller item sizes of cookies lead to a decreased energy intake in children. *J Nutr Educ Behav*. 2012;44(3):251–255.
12. Johnson SL, Hughes SO, Li X, et al. Portion sizes for children are predicted by parental characteristics and the amounts parents serve themselves. *Am J Clin Nutr*. 2014;99(4):763–770.
13. Vermeer WM, Steenhauis IH, Seidell JC. Portion size: a qualitative study of consumers' attitudes toward point-of-purchase interventions aimed at portion size. *Health Educ Res*. 2010;25(1):109–120.
14. Mathias KC, Rolls BJ, Birch LL, et al. Serving larger portions of fruits and vegetables together at dinner promotes intake of both foods among young children. *J Am Diet Assoc*. 2011;112(2):266–270.
15. Rolls BJ, Roe LS, Meengs JS. Portion size can be used strategically to increase vegetable consumption in adults. *Am J Clin Nutr*. 2010;91(4):913–922.
16. Hall JE, Guyton AC. *Guyton and Hall Textbook of Medical Physiology*. 12th ed. Philadelphia: Saunders Elsevier; 2011.
17. Wansink B. From mindless eating to mindlessly eating better. *Physiol Behav*. 2010:100(5):454–463.
18. Ibid.
19. Laska MN, Graham D, Moe SG, Lytle L, Fulkerson J. Situational characteristics of young adults' eating occasions: a real-time data collection using personal digital assistants. *Public Health Nutr*. 2010, December 8:1–8.
20. Hetherington MM, Anderson AS, Norton GN, Newson L. Situational effects on meal intake: a comparison of eating alone and eating with others. *Physiol Behav*. 2006;88(4–5):498–505.
21. Ibid.
22. de Castro JM, Brewer E. The amount eaten in meals by humans is a power function of the number of people present. *Physiol Behav*. 1992;51:121–125.
23. Stroebele N, de Castro JM. Influence of physiological and subjective arousal on food intake in humans. *Nutrition*. 2006;22:996–1004.
24. Guyton JE, Hall AC. *Textbook of Medical Physiology*. Op cit.
25. Ibid.
26. Kalafatakis K, Triantafyllou K. Contribution of neurotensin in the immune and neuroendocrine modulation of normal and abnormal enteric function. *Regul Pept*. 2011;170(1–3):7–17.
27. Bartness TJ, Keen-Rhinehart E, Dalley MJ, Teubner BJ. Neural and hormonal control of food hoarding. *Am J Physiol Regul Integr Comp Physiol*. 2011:301(3):R641–R655.
28. Karatas Z, Durmus Aydogdu S, Dinleyici EC, et. al. Breastmilk ghrelin, leptin, and fat levels changing foremilk to hindmilk: is that important for self-control of feeding? *Eur J Pediatr*. 2011;170(10):1273–1280.
29. Rosenbaum M, Leibel RL. Adaptive thermogenesis in humans. *Int J Obes*. 2010;34(suppl):S47–S55.
30. Ozkan Y, Timurkan ES, Aydin S, et al. Acylated and deacylated ghrelin, preptin, leptin, and nesfatin-1 peptide changes related to the body mass index. *Int J Endocrinol*. 2013;2013:1–7.
31. Rosenbaum M, Leibel RL. Adaptive thermogenesis in humans. Op cit.
32. Magee E. Your 'hunger hormones.' WebMD. http://www.webmd.com/diet/features/your-hunger-hormones. Accessed January 6, 2016; and Ebbeling CB, Swain JF, Feldman HA, et al. Effects of dietary composition on energy expenditure during weight-loss maintenance. Op cit.
33. Pejovic S, Vgontzas AN, Basta M, et al. Leptin and hunger levels in young healthy adults after one night of sleep loss. *J Sleep Res*. 2010;19(4):552–558.
34. Institute of Medicine, Food and Nutrition Board. *Dietary Reference Intakes for Energy, Carbohydrate, Fiber, Fat, Fatty Acids, Cholesterol, Protein, and Amino Acids*. Washington, DC: National Academies Press; 2005; and Fothergill E, Guo J, Howard L, et al. Persistent metabolic adaptation 6 years after "The Biggest Loser" competition. Obesity. Early view online version May 2, 2016. http://onlinelibrary.wiley.com/doi/10.1002/oby.21538/full Accessed May 21, 2016.
35. Manini TM, Everhart JE, Anton SC, et al. Activity energy expenditure and change in body composition in late life. *Am J Clin Nutr*. 2009;90(5):1336–1342.
36. Mahan LK, Raymond JL. *Krause's Food, Nutrition and Diet Therapy*. 13th ed. Philadelphia: WB Saunders; 2011.
37. Ibid.
38. Kenny WL, Wilmore JH, Costill DL. *Physiology of Sport and Exercise*. 6th ed. Champaign, IL: Human Kinetics; 2015.
39. Alahmadi MA, Hills AP, King NA, Byrne NM. Exercise intensity influences nonexercise activity thermogenesis in overweight and obese adults. *Med Sci Sports Exerc*. 2011;43(4):624–631.
40. Galgani JE, Ravussin E. Effect of dihydrocapsiate on resting metabolic rate in humans. *Am J Clin Nutr*. 2010;92(5):1089–1093.
41. Du S, Rajjo T, Santosa S, Jensen MD. The thermic effect of food is reduced in older adults. Horm Metab Res. 2014;46(5):365–369.
42. Piaggi P, Krakoff J, Bogardus C, Thearle MS. Lower "awake and fed thermogenesis" predicts future weight gain in subjects with abdominal adiposity. *Diabetes*. 2013;62(12):4043–4051.
43. Institute of Medicine, Food and Nutrition Board. *Dietary Reference Intakes for Energy, Carbohydrate*. Op cit.
44. National Heart, Lung, and Blood Institute. Calculate your body mass index. https://www.nhlbi.nih.gov/health/educational/lose_wt/BMI/bmicalc.htm. Accessed January 6, 2016.
45. Garrido-Chamorro RP, Sirvent-Belando JE, Gonzalez-Lorenzo M, et al. Correlation between body mass index and body composition in elite athletes. *J Sports Med Phys Fitness*. 2009;49(3):278–284.
46. National Center for Health Statistics. 2000 CDC growth charts: United States. http://www.cdc.gov/growthcharts. Accessed January 6, 2016.
47. Mahan LK, Raymond JL. *Krause's Food and Nutrition Therapy*. Op cit.
48. Nana A, Slater GR, Hopkins WG, Burke LM. Effects of daily activities on DXA measurements of body composition in active people. *Med Sci Sports Exerc*. 2012;44(10):180–189.
49. Heymsfield SB, Baumgartner RN. Body composition and anthropometry. In: Shils ME, Shike M, Ross AC, et al., eds. *Modern Nutrition in Health and Disease*. 10th ed. Philadelphia: Lippincott Williams & Wilkins; 2006:751–770.
50. Dencker M, Wollmer P, Karlsson MK, Liden C, Andersen LB, Thorsson O. Body fat, abdominal fat and body fat distribution related to cardiovascular risk factors in prepubertal children. *Acta Paediatr*. 2012;101(8):852–857.
51. Ziegler RG. Anthropometry and breast cancer. *J Nutr*. 1997;127(suppl 5):924S–928S.

52. Pichard C, Plu-Bureau G, Neves-e-Castro M, Gompel A. Insulin resistance, obesity and breast cancer risk. *Maturitas*. 2008;60:19–30.
53. McAuley PA, Artero EG, Sui X, et al. The obesity paradox, cardiorespiratory fitness, and coronary heart disease. *Mayo Clin Proc*. 2012;87(5):443–451.
54. Position of the American Dietetic Association: weight management. *J Am Diet Assoc*. 2009;109(2):330–346.
55. Ibid.
56. Hill JO, Thompson H, Wyatt H. Weight maintenance: what's missing? *J Am Diet Assoc*. 2005;105:S63–S66.
57. Hill JO, Peters JC, Wyatt HR. Using the energy gap to address obesity: a commentary. *J Am Diet Assoc*. 2009;109(11):1848–1853.
58. Kramer CK, Zinman B, Retnakaran R. Are metabolically healthy overweight and obesity benign conditions? *Ann Intern Med*. 2013;159:758–769.
59. National Weight Control Registry. NWCR facts. http://www.nwcr.ws/Research/default.htm. Accessed January 6, 2016.
60. Larso NI, Neumark-Sztainer D, Hannan PJ, Story M. Family meals during adolescence are associated with higher diet quality and healthful meal patterns during young adulthood. *J Am Diet Assoc*. 2007;107(9):1502–1510.
61. Deshmukh-Taskar PR, Nicklas TA, O'Neil CE, et al. The relationship of breakfast skipping and type of breakfast consumption with nutrient intake and weight status in children and adolescents: the National Health and Nutrition Examination Survey, 1999–2006. *J Am Diet Assoc*. 2010:111(6):869–878.
62. Ibid.
63. Centers for Disease Control and Prevention. Physical activity: how much physical activity do adults need? December 2011. http://www.cdc.gov/physicalactivity/everyone/guidelines/adults.html. Accessed January 6, 2016.
64. Ibid.
65. Spahn J, Reeves R, Keim K. State of the evidence regarding behavior change theories and strategies in nutrition counseling to facilitate health and food behavior change. *J Am Diet Assoc*. 2010;110(6):879–891.
66. Smith TJ, Sigrist LD, Bathalo GP, et al. Efficacy of a meal-replacement program for promoting blood lipid changes and weight and body fat loss in US Army soldiers. *J Am Diet Assoc*. 2010;111(2):268–273.
67. Verel D. CDC recognizes digital health platforms that help prevent chronic diseases. MedCity News. March 9, 2015. http://medcitynews.com/2015/03/omada/. Accessed January 6, 2016.
68. WebMD. Drugs and medications: Xenical. http://www.webmd.com/drugs/2/drug-17218/xenical+oral/details#uses. Accessed January 6, 2016.
69. Food and Drug Administration. FDA approves Belviq to treat some overweight or obese adults. FDA News Release. June 27, 2012. http://www.fda.gov/newsevents/newsroom/pressannouncements/ucm309993.htm. Accessed January 6, 2016.
70. Food and Drug Administration. FDA approves weight-management drug Saxenda. FDA News Release. December 23, 2014. http://www.fda.gov/NewsEvents/Newsroom/PressAnnouncements/ucm427913.htm. Accessed January 6, 2016.
71. WebMD. Drugs and medications: Qsymia. http://www.webmd.com/drugs/2/drug-162311/qsymia+oral/details. Accessed January 6, 2016.
72. Lauer MS. Lemons for obesity. *Ann Intern Med*. 2012;157(2):139–140.
73. Yanovski SZ, Yanovski JA. Long-term drug treatment for obesity: a systematic and clinical review. *JAMA*. 2014;311(1):74–86.
74. Chang YY, Chiou WB. The liberating effect of weight loss supplements on dietary control: a field experiment. *Nutrition*. 2014;30(9):10071010. doi: 10.1016/j.nut.2014.02.002. Epub February 20, 2014.
75. Tang MH, Chen SP, Ng SW, Chan AY, Mak TW. Case series on a diversity of illicit weight-reducing agents: from the well known to the unexpected. *Br J Clin Pharmacol*. 2011;71(2):250–253.
76. Brethauer SA, Harris JL, Kroh M, Schauer PR. Laparoscopic gastric plication for treatment of severe obesity. *Surg Obes Relat Dis*. 2011;7(1):15–22.
77. Nguyen NT, Karipineni F, Masoomi H, et al. Increasing utilization of laparoscopic gastric banding in the adolescent: data from academic medical centers, 2002–2009. *Am Surg*. 2011;77(11):1510–1514.
78. Alexandrou A, Athanasiou A, Michalinos A, et al. Laparoscopic sleeve gastrectomy for morbid obesity: 5-year results. *Am J Surg*. 2015;209(2):230-234.
79. Beitner M, Kurian MS. Laparoscopic adjustable gastric banding. *Abdom Imaging*. 2012;37(5):687–689.
80. Forbush SW, Nof L, Echternach J, Hill C. Influence of activity on quality of life scores after RYGBP. *Obes Surg*. 2011;21(8):1296–1304.

Spotlight on Obesity: The Growing Epidemic

Revised by Don Ross

THINK About It

1. Do you think the problem of obesity is evidence of a genetic predisposition or simply the influence of lifestyle and more related to environment?
2. With portion sizes of foods getting larger and larger, what factors explain why people choose to eat such large food portions?
3. Why do you think that being overweight or obese as a child increases the likelihood of being an overweight adult?
4. What actions do you think people can take to help decrease the rising rate of obesity?

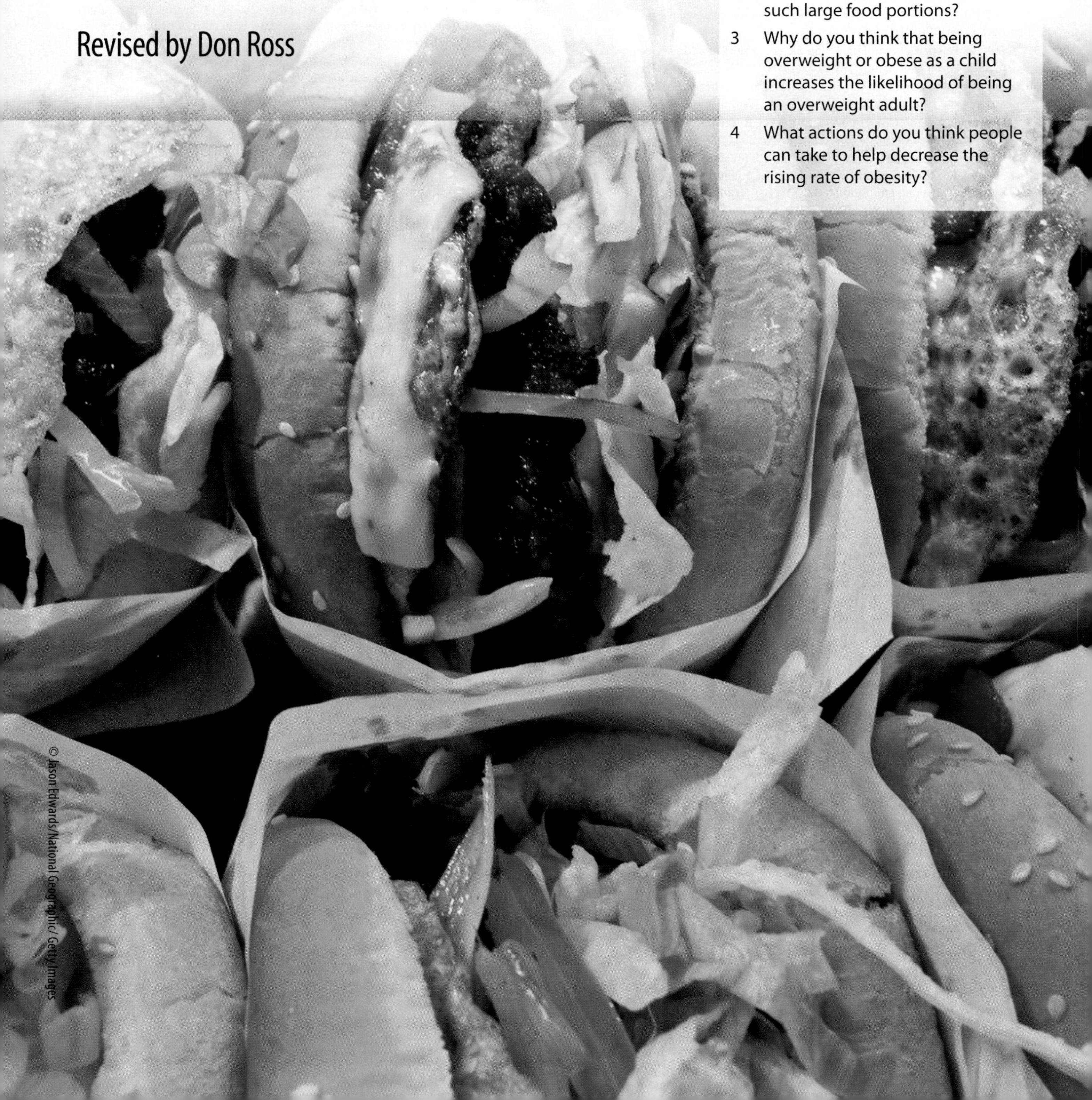

© Jason Edwards/National Geographic/ Getty Images

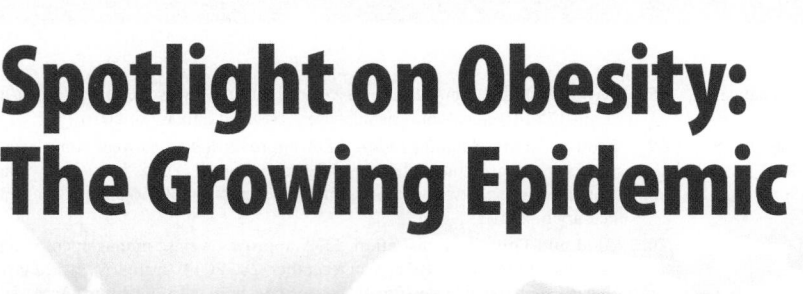

CHAPTER Menu

LEARNING Objectives

- Describe the biological, lifestyle, and behavioral factors that contribute to the development of obesity.
- Describe the factors involved in the development of overweight in childhood.
- Identify the causes of the obesity epidemic in children.
- Discuss approaches or solutions for the growing obesity epidemic.

Amanda, a college sophomore, is late for her usual Thursday night date with her boyfriend at the Pasta Palace near her dorm. She is annoyed because the new jeans she bought just a few months ago no longer fit. She is dating Dan, an overweight fire fighter who gets a letter from his chief that warns him of medical suspension unless he loses weight and brings down his blood pressure. He shares the letter with Amanda, who becomes worried, thinking that she might have a similar problem.

They discuss the problem and she suggests that maybe they should find a healthier diet. Her action plan is to make an appointment at the campus health clinic on Monday. Nevertheless, they order their usual: large plates of pasta with garlic bread and colas. Amanda feels stressed by this encounter with Dan and his lack of concern about his weight and high blood pressure. She meets with her girlfriends Maria and Anna, who are also overweight, and attempts to discuss her anxiety. They meet at the snack counter at the student union and Maria complains there are too many snack choices. Smiling, she says, "Apples or garlic fries?" Laughing, Anna announces, "Fries, of course."

Amanda makes her appointment at the health clinic and gets her test results back a couple days later. In some sense, Amanda's action plan paid off, but with news much more startling than she expected. The report shows she has an elevated blood pressure of 145/80 mm Hg, a body mass index (BMI) of 30, and a diagnosis of pre-diabetes and hypertension. The clinic recommends she make an appointment with the campus physician and registered dietitian as soon as possible. Amanda is obese. And she knows it. The campus dietitian suggests that Amanda is not just dealing with a metabolism problem, an exercise problem, or an eating problem.

Obesity is a behavioral problem. It is idiosyncratic; that is, people respond differently to different strategies and different situations. Behavior, for example, is shaped by the social environment. Some people are strongly influenced by their friends and colleagues, whereas others independently change their behaviors. In this spotlight, we examine some possible causes of this serious epidemic and suggest how people can tailor strategies to meet their own idiosyncratic needs.

Amanda's problem is not unique. Obesity has become a major global epidemic and a burden to society and health care systems[1] (see **FIGURE SO.1**). Worldwide, 1.5 billion people are obese, and obesity has emerged as the most important contributor to ill health, displacing undernutrition and infectious diseases.[2] Obesity not only is prevalent in North America and Europe,[3]

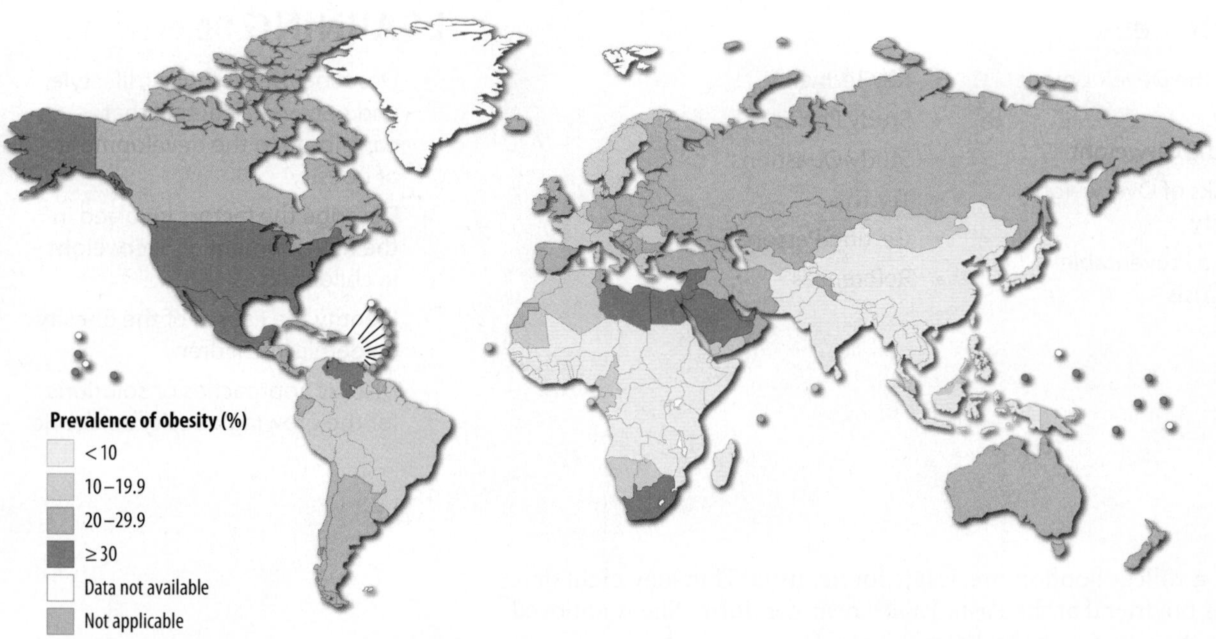

FIGURE SO.1 Prevalence of obesity, ages 20+, age-standardized, both sexes, 2008.

Note: BMI ≥ 30 kg/m^2.

but also is on the rise in Southeast Asia, especially China, India, and Japan. One-half of the children in Beijing are obese, and the rate of obesity in India is growing so quickly that it threatens to slow India's economic growth.[4] In North Africa and the Middle East, overweight and obesity are common, with Kuwait having the highest rates—79 percent of adults are overweight and nearly 43 percent are obese.[5]

Public health campaigns and food advertisements have promoted low-fat diets, which unintentionally led to high carbohydrate diets that often are high in simple sugars. With advancements in nutrition research, we've learned that highly processed carbohydrates are a significant contributor to obesity.

In the United States, the prevalence of overweight and obesity has increased dramatically over the past three decades, jumping from less than half of the adult population to about two-thirds![6] (See **FIGURE SO.2**.) What has caused this alarming increase? There are no simple answers. This spotlight discusses some possible answers and suggested solutions. Being overweight often is a stepping stone to becoming obese. Obesity not only is a threat to health and physical appearance, but also is a huge burden on society's wallets, leading to higher health care costs and reduced work productivity.

Perhaps most disconcerting is the rapidly increasing prevalence of overweight and obesity among U.S. youth. Approximately 17 percent of children and teens (ages 2 to 19) are obese.[7] This escalating problem is blamed on the overconsumption of energy-dense, sugar-laden foods that are easily accessible, convenient, widely available, and inexpensive (see **FIGURE SO.3**). This overconsumption, in combination with an increasingly sedentary lifestyle and decreased exercise and physical activity, paves a path toward obesity. There is a glimmer of good news. The prevalence of obesity among children ages 2 to 5 years has decreased significantly, from nearly 14 percent in 2004 to 8.4 percent in 2012.[8]

As the prevalence of overweight and obesity has increased, so has society's emphasis on thinness, as well as efforts at weight management. Every year, the diet industry rakes in more than $59 billion from weight-loss programs, diet soft drinks, diet books, pills, videos, and supplements.[9] Nearly half of Americans worry about their weight, and among those who consider themselves overweight, about two-thirds are preoccupied with their weight.[10] Children and

Quick Bite

BMI Distribution

If all countries had the BMI distribution of the United States, 58 million tons of human biomass would be added—equivalent to an extra 935 million people of average body mass—and the additional energy requirements would be equivalent to those of 473 million adults.

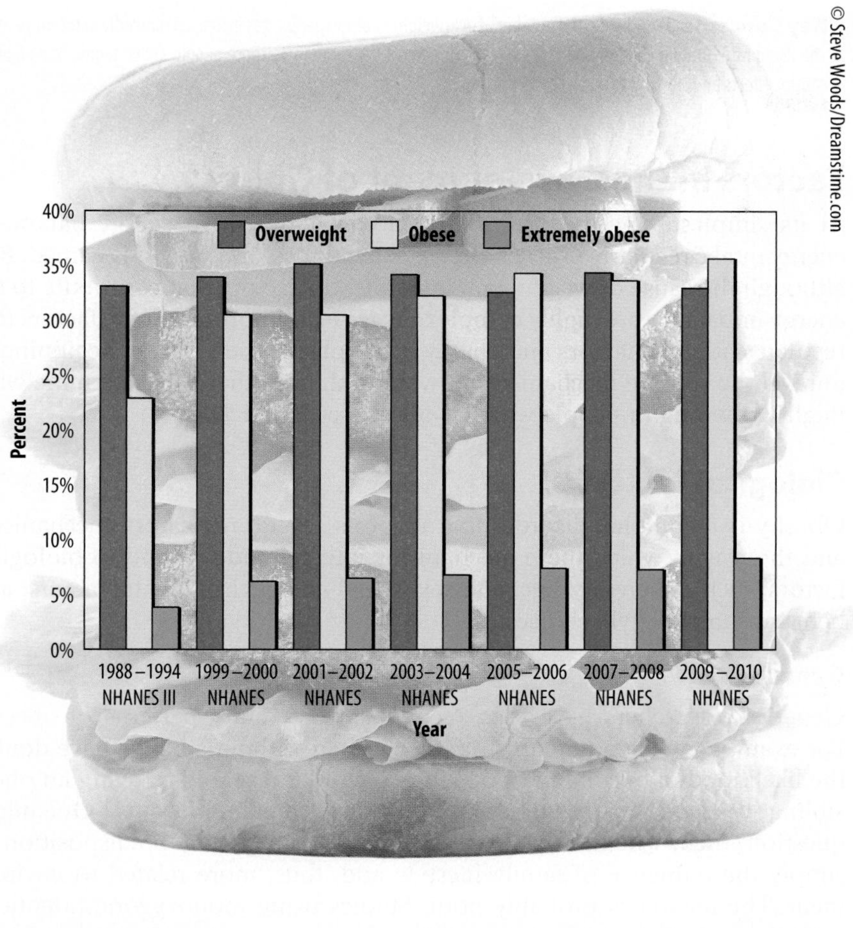

FIGURE SO.2 Age-adjusted prevalence of overweight, obesity, and extreme obesity among U.S. adults aged 20 and over.

Data from Fryar CD, Caroll MD, Ogden CL. *Prevalence of Overweight, Obesity, and Extreme Obesity Among Adults: United States, Trends 1960–1962 Through 2009–2010* [Table 1]. Washington, DC: Centers for Disease Control and Prevention, National Center for Health Statistics; 2012. http://www.cdc.gov/nchs/data/hestat/obesity_adult_09_10/obesity_adult_09_10.htm#table1. Accessed January 28, 2016.

adolescents also are concerned about weight. In studies of grade-school girls from various socioeconomic backgrounds, 68 percent reported that they have attempted to lose weight because they very often worried about being fat.[11]

Even when people lose weight, maintaining that loss is difficult. About one-third of the lost weight typically is regained within the first year. By the fifth year, half the people return to their previous baseline weight. Among overweight and obese adults, a mere one in six report maintaining weight loss of at least 10 percent for at least 1 year, at any point in their lives.[12]

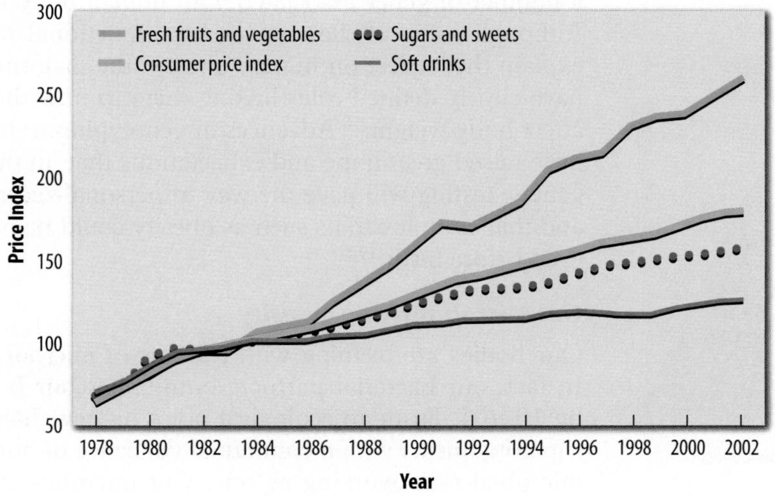

FIGURE SO.3 The rising cost of food.

Reproduced from Sturm R. Childhood obesity: what we can learn from existing data on societal trends, part 2. *Prev Chronic Dis.* April 2005. http://www.cdc.gov/pcd/issues/2005/apr/04_0039.htm. Accessed January 28, 2016.

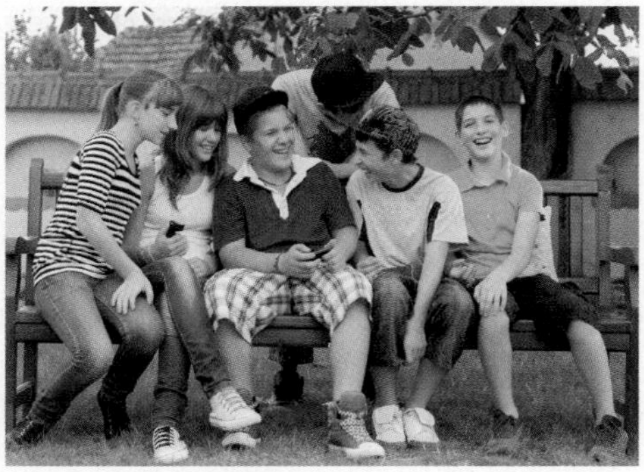

Key Concepts Worldwide, the number of overweight or obese people has increased markedly in recent years. The rising rates among children are especially disturbing. At the same time, more people are engaging in weight-control efforts and starting to do so at younger ages.

Factors in the Development of Obesity

At its simplest, obesity results from a chronic positive energy balance—energy intake regularly exceeds energy expenditure, and weight is gained. But, although the cause of weight gain is simple, the factors that contribute to the energy imbalance are highly complex. As we learn more about the factors that regulate eating behaviors and energy metabolism, scientists are beginning to unravel the specific mechanisms at work and, from there, to determine what might go wrong in people who are obese (see **FIGURE SO.4**).

Biological Factors

Obesity is a complex disorder that involves several regulatory mechanisms and the way in which these mechanisms interact and respond to biological factors, such as heredity, age, and sex; social and environmental factors; and behavior and lifestyle choices.

Genetics

Genetics researchers have long recognized hereditary patterns of obesity. For example, when a parent is obese, children without siblings have double the likelihood of becoming obese. In two-child households, having an obese sibling was an even stronger association than parental obesity.[14] One might question, then, whether this is truly evidence of a genetic predisposition or simply the influence of family lifestyle and, thus, more related to environment. The answer is probably both. Studies using monozygotic (identical) and dizygotic (fraternal) twins confirm that gene–environment interactions do influence energy balance. Researchers estimate that genes alone generally account for 50 to 90 percent of variations in the amount of stored body fat.[15]

THINK About It 1

Advances in genomics technologies are rapidly leading to new understandings of the roles that genetic variations play in obesity. Scientific advances, such as the identification of particular genes associated with regulating adipogenesis and adipocyte development in humans, suggest that genes have an effect on obesity.[16] Various studies have identified a number of genes associated with human body weight.[17] Although some of these genes have functional roles that explain their effect on human obesity, the majority do not have clearly defined roles linking them to how they might affect body weight.[18] Advances in genotyping technologies have raised great hope and expectations that, in the future, genetic testing will pave the way to personalized medicine and that complex traits such as obesity could be prevented even before birth.[19,20]

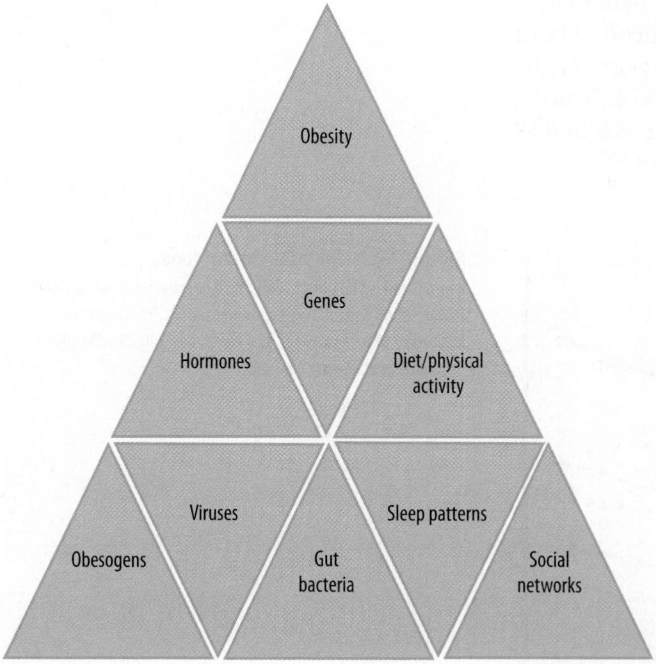

FIGURE SO.4 What influences obesity? Innovative views into individual and environmental interactions that contribute to obesity.

Gut Microbiota and Obesity

Our bodies are teeming with trillions of microorganisms. In fact, our bacterial partners outnumber our body cells by 10 to 1. From an ecological point of view, humans are superorganisms with a communal collective of human and microbial cells working as one. Gut microbes coevolved with their human host and affect digestion, production of vitamins B and K, energy metabolism, and immune function. For example, human gut microbes contribute 36 percent of the small molecules found in human blood.[21] In essence, our gut microbes function as a virtual, but vital, organ.

Accumulating evidence strongly suggests that gut microbes play an important role in the regulation of energy balance and weight, and they may influence the development of obesity and type 2 diabetes.[22] Changes in diet are accompanied by rapid changes in the composition of our gut microbes, suggesting that our microbial populations are influenced by both environmental and genetic factors. In addition, the composition of gut microbes differs among lean and obese individuals.[23]

Although not a substitute for diet and exercise, manipulation of the gut microbial population represents a novel approach to treating obesity. How to best manage our gut microbes is hotly debated. Probiotics are well advertised, and manufacturers tout the virtues of "good bacteria." However, probiotic trials have failed to show a consistent preventive effect, and their use as a medical therapy has not been approved in the United States or Europe.[24]

Fat Cell Development

The number and size of fat cells in the body help determine how easily a person gains or loses fat. People with **hypercellular obesity**, an above-average number of fat cells, might have been born with them or might have developed them at certain critical times in their lives because of overeating. In **hypertrophic obesity**, fat cells are larger than normal. Fat cells continue to expand as they fill with more fat; when their capacity is reached, the body generates more cells (see **FIGURE SO.5**). Once body fat reaches three to five times the normal amount, fat tissue is likely to have both bigger fat cells and more of them, a condition called **hyperplastic obesity (hyperplasia)**.

Even with weight loss, the number of fat cells does not decline (though presumably some could be removed by liposuction). Fat cells do become smaller, but beyond a certain point they resist further shrinking and the body strives to refill them with fat, making it difficult to maintain weight loss.

Sex and Age

The prevalence of obesity among men and women in the United States is similar at about 36 percent.[25] Despite the similarities in obesity statistics, men and women seem to set different weight standards for themselves. Beginning in grade school, boys are less likely than girls to consider themselves overweight; in fact, males of all ages accept some degree of overweight. Boys typically are more concerned about becoming taller and more muscular. As adolescents and young adults, most of us begin to worry about body weight and appearance.

By early adulthood, about the same percentage of men wants to lose or gain weight, whereas significantly more women want to lose weight. As adults, males tend to see themselves as overweight at higher weights, whereas females describe themselves as overweight even when they are closer to a healthy body weight (see **FIGURE SO.6**). Adult women feel thin only when they weigh less than 90 percent of desirable body weight, whereas men rate themselves as thin even when they are above a healthy body weight.[26]

As we get older, we become more concerned with our weight as it also relates to health. Both men and women gain the most weight between 25 and 34 years of age. After that, adults generally gain weight more slowly except during menopause, when many women will gain additional weight. Weight maintenance or slow gain often continues through adulthood until we reach old age, when frailty, disability, illness, and unintentional weight loss predict morbidity and mortality.

Quick Bite

Can You Pick Your Partners?

Liping Zhao, a professor of microbiology at Shanghai Jiao Tong University, adopted a dietary regimen involving Chinese yam, bitter melon, and whole grains. The yam and melon are fermented prebiotic foods believed to affect bacteria in the digestive system. After two years, Dr. Zhao had an increase in a particular gut microbial species with anti-inflammatory properties. He had lost 20 kilograms (44 pounds) and had lower blood pressure, heart rate, and cholesterol. These changes persuaded him to focus his research on the gut microbiome.

Quick Bite

Your Microbiota and You

The gut microbiota is the microbe population living in your intestines. It is composed of tens of trillions of microbes, can weigh up to 2 kilograms (4.4 pounds), and includes at least 1,000 different species with more than 3 million genes (150 times more than the number of human genes).

- **hypercellular obesity** Obesity due to an above average number of fat cells.
- **hypertrophic obesity** Obesity due to an increase in the size of fat cells.
- **hyperplastic obesity** (hyperplasia) Obesity due to an increase in both the size and number of fat cells.

Quick Bite

Island Obesity

Some of the most obese people in the world live on the islands of Micronesia. Among these populations, the Nauruans are the most obese.

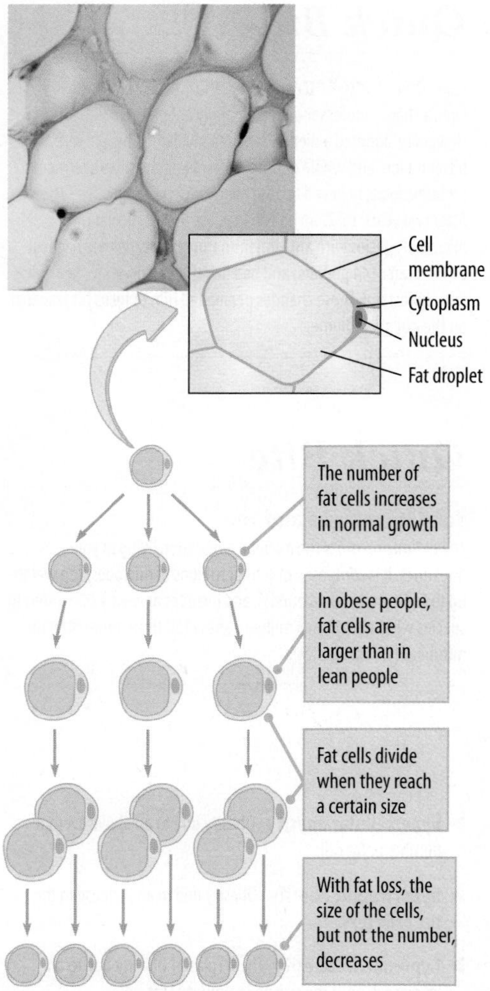

FIGURE SO.5 The formation of fat cells. As body fat accumulates, fat cells enlarge and divide. Fat loss reduces the size of fat cells but not their number.

Photo: © Donna Beer Stolz, Ph.D., Center for Biologic Imaging, University of Pittsburgh Medical School.

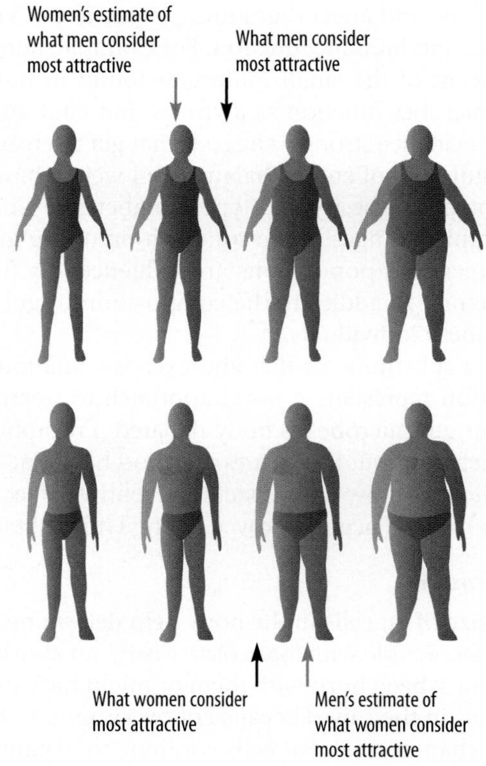

FIGURE SO.6 What men and women consider attractive. Compared with men, women perceive slimmer shapes to be more attractive.

Data from Bully P, Elosua P. Changes in body dissatisfaction relative to gender and age: the modulating character of BMI. *Span J Psychol.* 2011;14(1):313–322.

Race and Ethnicity

In the United States, the prevalence of obesity and attitudes about weight differ among racial and ethnic groups. African American and Hispanic women are more likely to be overweight than non-Hispanic white women (see **FIGURE SO.7**).[27] Rates of overweight are similar for African American, Hispanic, and white men. Because of cultural factors, African Americans, Hispanic Americans, Native Americans, and Pacific Islanders typically value thinness less than white Americans do.[28]

Social and Environmental Factors

Socioeconomic Status

Americans are more likely to become obese if they have low socioeconomic status. Just as in some racial and ethnic groups, overweight and obesity are more socially acceptable in some lower socioeconomic settings. Compared to those with low socioeconomic status, people with higher socioeconomic status have better nutrition- and health-related psychosocial factors, such as more nutrition knowledge, aptitude for making better food choices, and more awareness of nutrition-related health risks.[29] In general, they also have better and more convenient access to fresh foods.

Lower socioeconomic status and food insecurity are associated with being overweight or obese.[30] The relationship between obesity and food insecurity might be related to the low cost of energy-dense foods and reinforced by the satisfying taste of sugar and fat. Periods of overeating when food is available,

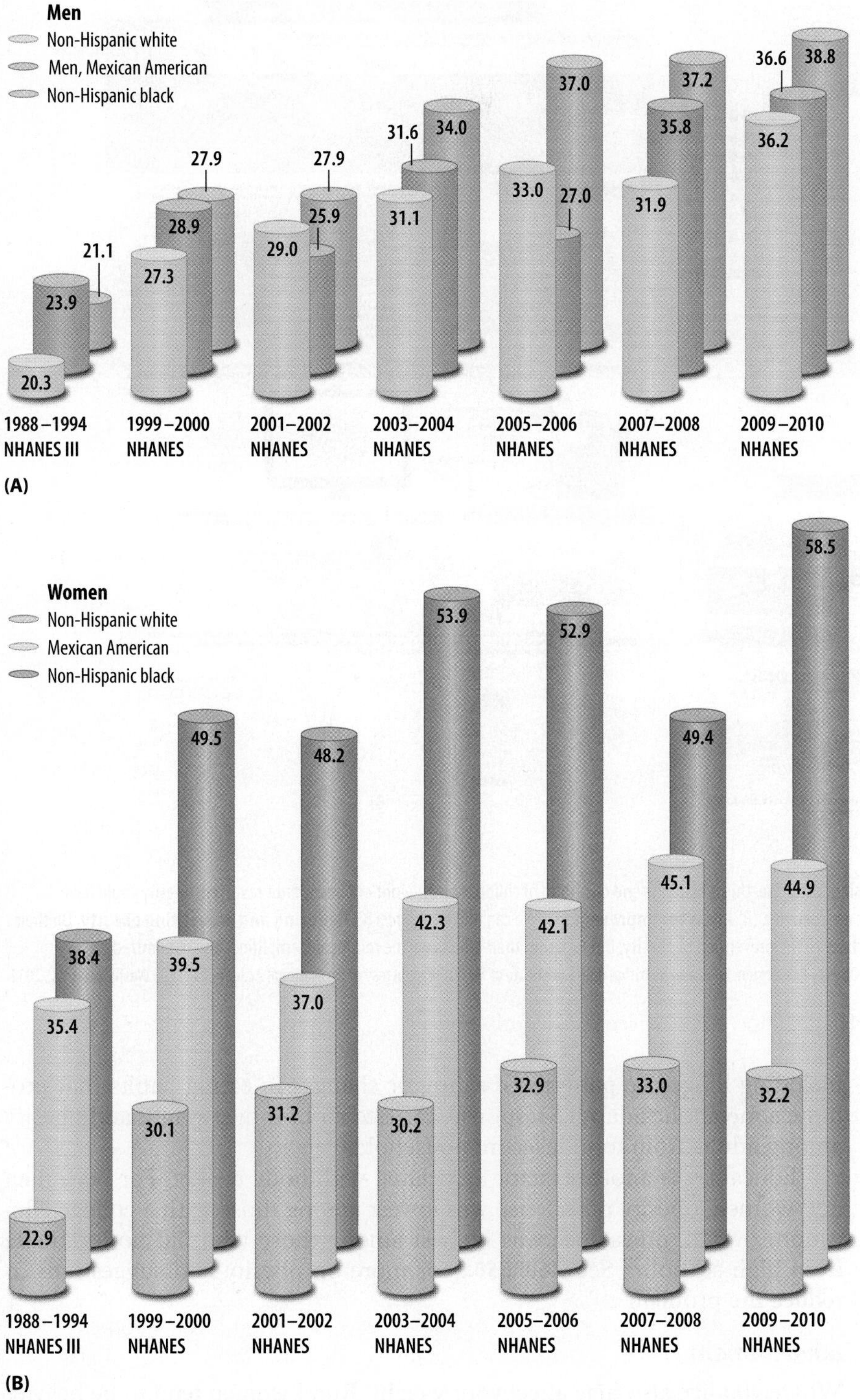

FIGURE SO.7 Rising obesity rates. The NHANES data show that the prevalence of obesity differs among men and women as well as among different racial and ethnic groups.

Data from Fryar CD, Caroll MD, Ogden CL. *Prevalence of Overweight, Obesity, and Extreme Obesity Among Adults: United States, Trends 1960–1962 Through 2009–2010* [Table 3]. Washington, DC: Centers for Disease Control and Prevention, National Center for Health Statistics; 2012. #http://www.cdc.gov/nchs/data/hestat/obesity_adult_09_10/obesity_adult_09_10.htm#table3. Accessed January 28, 2016.

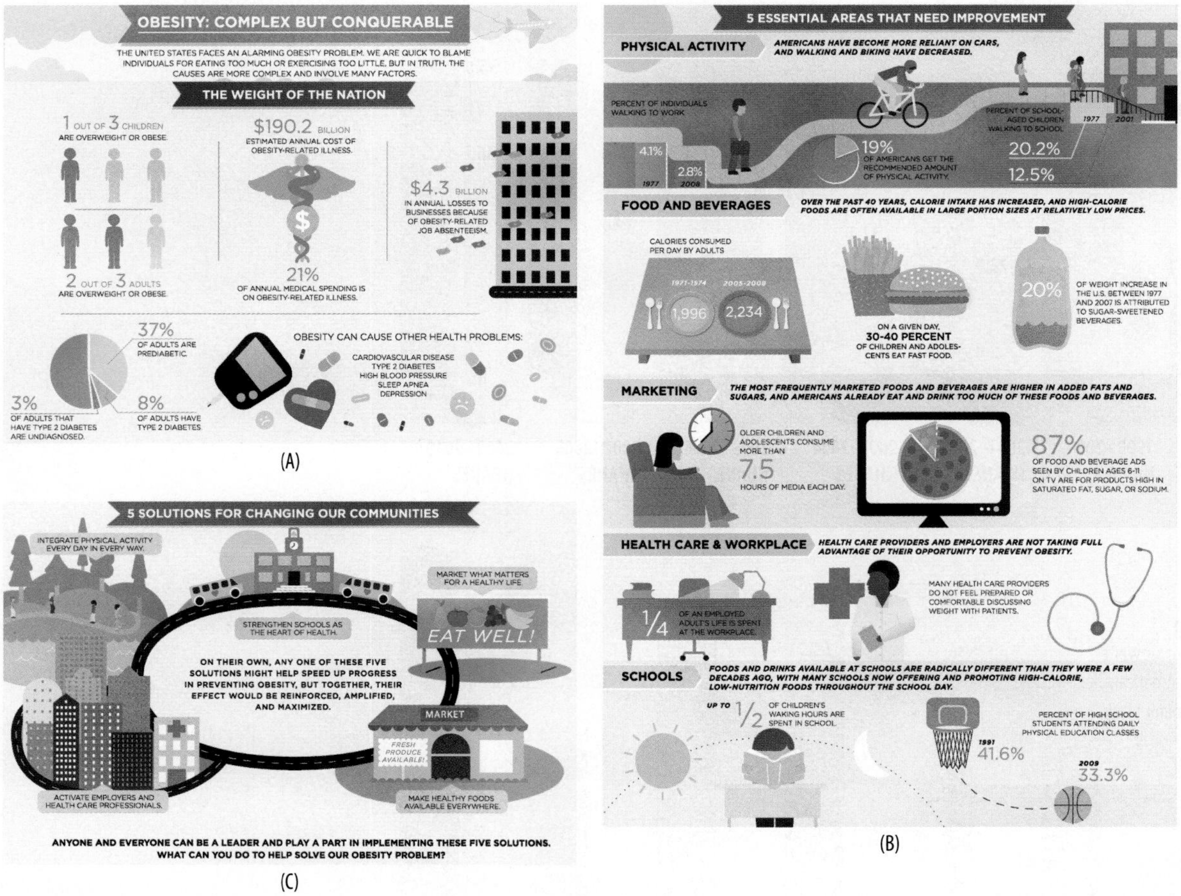

FIGURE SO.8 (A) **Sounding the alarm.** The rate of obesity is rising, with two-thirds of adults and one-third of children overweight or obese. If not reversed, obesity could have catastrophic effects on health, health care costs, and our economic productivity. (B) **Areas for improvement.** We can make changes! (C) **Reducing and preventing obesity.** On their own, any one of the goals for changing our communities can contribute to the prevention of obesity, but together their effects will be reinforced, amplified, and maximized.
Reproduced with permission from Committee on Accelerating Progress in Obesity Prevention, Food and Nutrition Board, Institute of Medicine. Courtesy of the National Academies Press, Washington, DC, 2012.

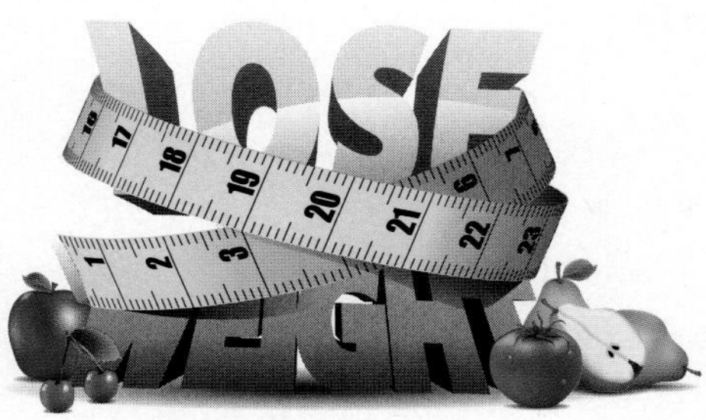

including binge-like patterns of eating or changes in eating habits that promote a metabolic-adaptive response, can account for overweight and obesity among adults from food-insecure households.[31]

Education is another factor associated with body weight. For both men and women, obesity prevalence was lowest among those with a college education; overall, prevalence was highest among those who did not graduate from high school.[32] See **FIGURE SO.8** for more on obesity and suggestions to reduce the problem.

Environment

Where you live also may affect your weight. Rural women tend to be heavier than women living in metropolitan areas.[33] Among the U.S. states, the prevalence of adult obesity in 2014 ranged from about 21 percent in Colorado to more than 35 percent in Mississippi. A total of 45 states had a prevalence of obesity greater than or equal to 25 percent, of which 19 states had prevalences from 30 to 35 percent and 3 (Arkansas, Mississippi and West Virginia) exceeded 35 percent.[34] All states continued to have high obesity rates, and none were below 20 percent. (See the FYI feature, "U.S. Obesity Trends: A Relentless Increase" for more information.)

FYI
For Your Information

U.S. Obesity Trends: A Relentless Increase

During the past decades, obesity in the United States has been increasing dramatically, and rates remain high. The maps in **Figure A** illustrate the trend from 1990 to 2010 by showing the increased prevalence of obesity across each of the states. Refer to the Centers for Disease Control and Prevention website for a complete slide show of each year during this time period: www.cdc.gov/obesity/data/prevalence-maps.html.

In 2011, the CDC initiated changes in its methodology for data collection, including using both landlines and cell phones to reach households and a new weighting methodology to better match samples to the general population.

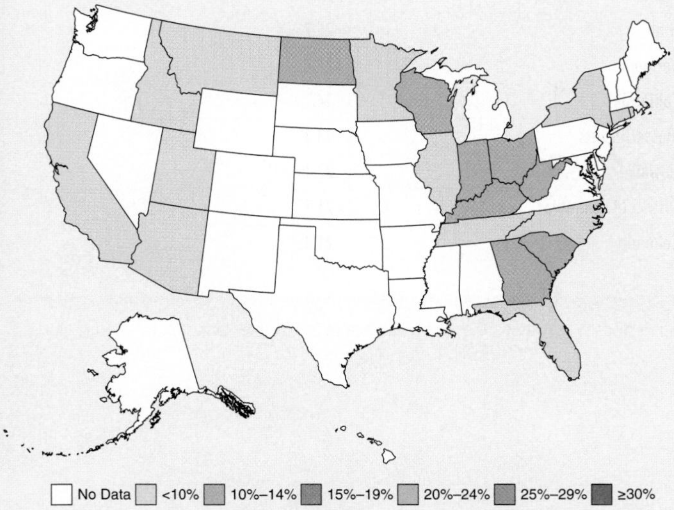

FIGURE A Trends in obesity (BMI ≥ 30) in U.S. adults, 1990–2010.

Reproduced from Centers for Disease Control and Prevention. Obesity trends among U.S. adults between 1985 and 2010. http://www.cdc.gov/obesity/downloads/obesity_trends_2010.ppt. Accessed June 25, 2015.

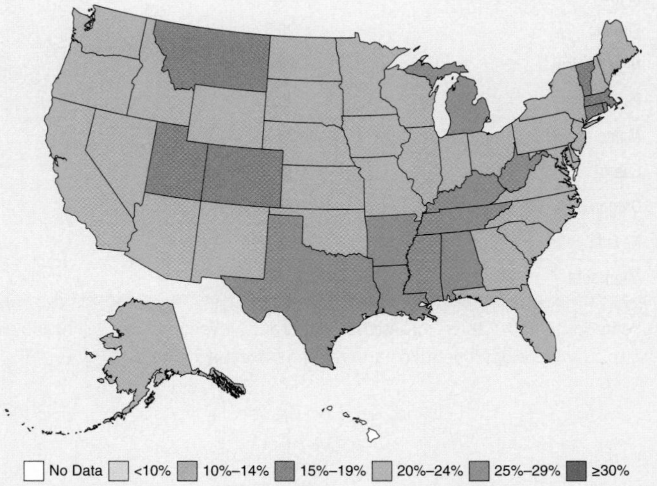

FIGURE B Percentage of obesity (BMI ≥ 30) in U.S. adults, 2013. Prevalence estimates reflect BRFSS methodological changes started in 2011. These estimates should not be compared to prevalence estimates before 2011.

Source: Reproduced from Centers for Disease Control and Prevention. Obesity prevalence maps: prevalence of self-reported obesity among U.S. adults by state and territory, BRFSS, 2013. http://www.cdc.gov/obesity/data/prevalence-maps.html. Accessed January 28, 2016.

Due to these methodological changes, prevalence estimates from 2011 and later should not be compared to prevalence estimates before 2011.

Figure B illustrates the adult obesity rates in 2014. No state had a prevalence of obesity less than 20 percent. Three states (Arkansas, Mississippi and West Virginia) had a prevalence of obesity of 35 percent or greater. Nineteen states had a prevalence of obesity between 30 percent and 35 percent. Twenty-three states had a prevalence of obesity between 25 percent and 30 percent. Five states and the District of Columbia had a prevalence of obesity between 20 percent and 25 percent. See **Table A**.

TABLE A
2014 State Adult Obesity Rates

Arkansas	35.9	Kentucky	31.6
West Virginia	35.7	Kansas	31.3
Mississippi	35.5	Tennessee	31.2
Louisiana	34.9	Wisconsin	31.2
Alabama	33.5	Iowa	30.9
Oklahoma	33.0	Delaware	30.7
Indiana	32.7	Michigan	30.7
Ohio	32.6	Georgia	30.5
North Dakota	32.2	Missouri	30.2
South Carolina	32.1	Nebraska	30.2
Texas	31.9	Pennsylvania	30.2

(continues)

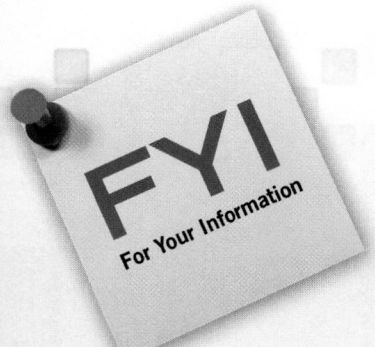

TABLE A
2014 State Adult Obesity Rates (Continued)

South Dakota	29.8	New Hampshire	27.4
Alaska	29.7	Washington	27.3
North Carolina	29.7	New York	27.0
Maryland	29.6	Rhode Island	27.0
Wyoming	29.5	New Jersey	26.9
Illinois	29.3	Montana	26.4
Arizona	28.9	Connecticut	26.3
Idaho	28.9	Florida	26.2
Virginia	28.5	Utah	25.7
New Mexico	28.4	Vermont	24.8
Puerto Rico	28.3	California	24.7
Maine	28.2	Massachusetts	23.3
Guam	28.0	Hawaii	22.1
Oregon	27.9	District of Columbia	21.7
Nevada	27.7	Colorado	21.3
Minnesota	27.6		

Reproduced from Centers for Disease Control and Prevention. Overweight and obesity. Adult obesity statistics. Obesity prevalence in 2013 varies across states and regions. http://www.cdc.gov/obesity/data/trends.html. Accessed June 26, 2015.

Where you shop also may affect your weight. Obesity rates have been linked to the supermarket that people typically use, and food cost was found to be more important than proximity.[35] The prevalence of obesity is markedly lower, just 9 percent, among those who shop at higher-priced supermarkets, compared to 27 percent at lower-cost stores.[36] Over the past 40 years, the actual cost of food has fallen. In the 1930s, Americans spent almost a quarter of their disposable income on food. Today it's less than 10 percent.[37]

In addition, dietary behaviors are, in large part, the consequence of automatic responses to a particular situation with food, many of which lead to increased caloric consumption and poor dietary choices.[38] Individuals are subject to inherent cognitive limitations and mostly lack the capacity to consistently recognize, ignore, or resist contextual cues that encourage eating. Take, for example, going to the movies. For many, a night at the movies also means sharing popcorn, candy, and soda. People often cannot resist this learned indulgence and are encouraged by the environment to eat a particular food. Another example is eating potato chips or peanuts that have been set out during a friendly card game or conversation with others. Individuals often consume snacks not because they are hungry, but because they are prompted by the social environment, which encourages them to eat. Grocery stores and restaurants have discovered the profits in suggestive selling, a sales technique where the customer is encouraged to make an additional purchase by taking advantage of a two-for-one sale or special discount. Grocery stores often use placement of items (candy bars at the checkout counter or higher-priced snack foods at children's eye level on the shelves) to encourage impulse buying.

FYI
For Your Information

Does Our Environment Make Us Fat?

Colors affect our moods. Crowding can increase stress. Environment psychologists have long known that elements of the built environment can influence our behaviors and physiology. For example, more than 600 rigorous studies have linked the built environment of hospitals to stress, staff effectiveness, patient safety and recovery, and overall health care quality.[a]

Does the environment also contribute to the rise in the rate of obesity? The answer is yes. Both the social and built environments in which we live, work, and play influence both sides of the energy balance equation. An obesogenic environment promotes overconsumption of calories and discourages physical activity and caloric expenditure.

At the same time, our choices about the types and amounts of food we eat and which physical activities we prefer can be limited. In some neighborhoods, restaurants and stores offer mostly high-fat, high-salt foods. Often, the neighborhood offers few options for walking or parks for play and other activities. When the built environment lacks readily available healthful foods and restricts options for physical activity, it supports the development of obesity.

The social-ecological model illustrates the forces that shape our eating and activity choices (see **Figure A**).

- *Individual factors* include personal genetics, physical characteristics, knowledge, beliefs, and attitudes.
- *Environmental settings* provide the context where we regularly make decisions and include schools, workplaces, recreational facilities, and food retail establishments.
- *Sectors of influence*, such as government, health care systems, agriculture, industry, and media, strongly affect the accessibility of healthful food.
- *Social and cultural norms* are based on societal values and include religious dietary laws, personal expectations, expectations of friends and family, lifestyles, and beliefs.
- *Cultural norms* shape choices for what, when, and how food and beverages are consumed. Cultural norms influence expectations for acceptable body weights and how much physical activity is a normal part of life.

Understanding the interactions among social-ecological factors can form the foundation for system-wide interventions to improve diet quality and increase physical activity. Nutritionists and public health experts expect this approach to have great potential in promoting a societal shift toward coping with the growing epidemic of obesity.

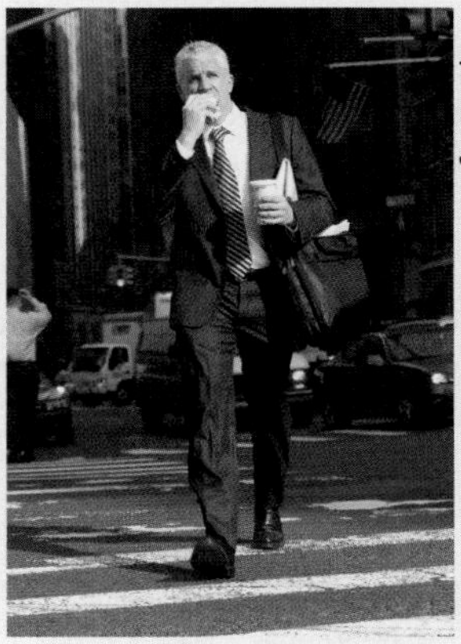
© Jupiterimages/Photos.com/Thinkstock

[a]Ulrich R, Zimring C, Quan X, et al. The role of the physical environment in the hospital of the 21st century: a once-in-a-lifetime opportunity. September 2004. https://www.healthdesign.org/sites/default/files/Role%20Physical%20Environ%20in%20the%2021st%20Century%20Hospital_0.pdf. Accessed February 28, 2016.

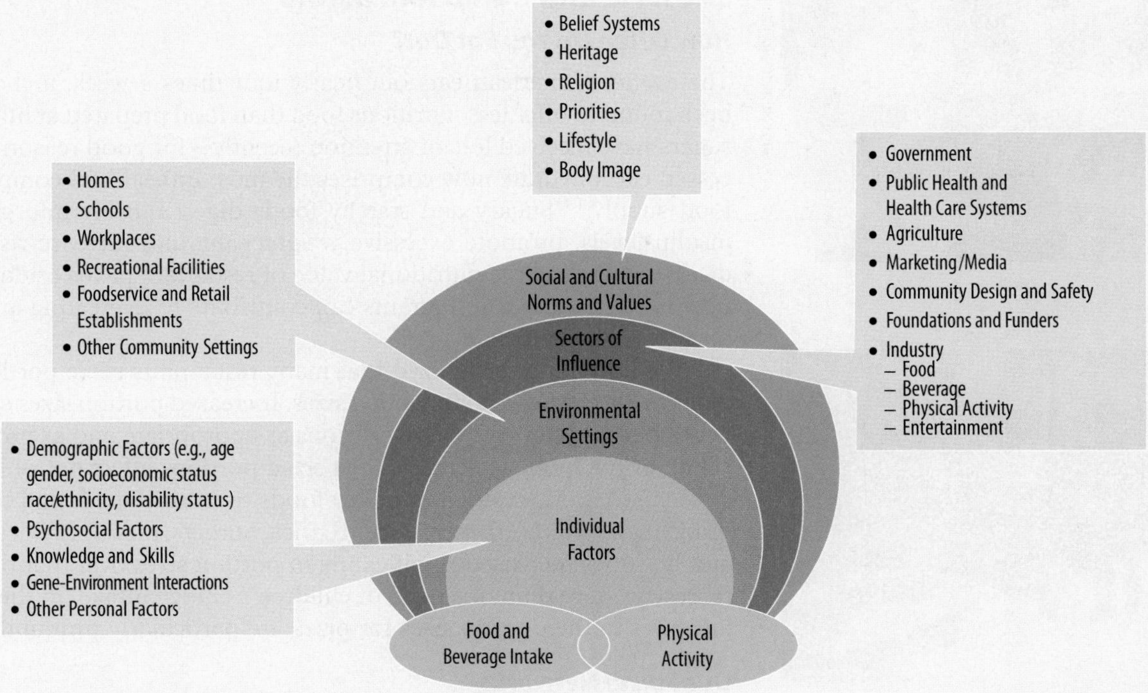

FIGURE A A social-ecological framework for nutrition and physical activity decisions.

Reproduced from U.S. Department of Health and Human Services and U.S. Department of Agriculture. *Dietary Guidelines for Americans, 2010.* 7th ed. Washington, DC: U.S. Government Printing Office; 2010:56.

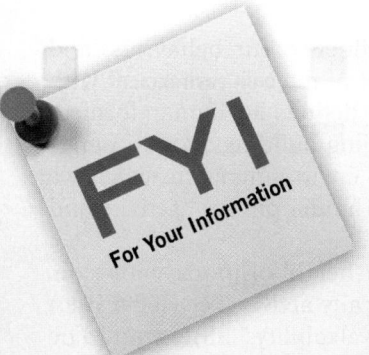

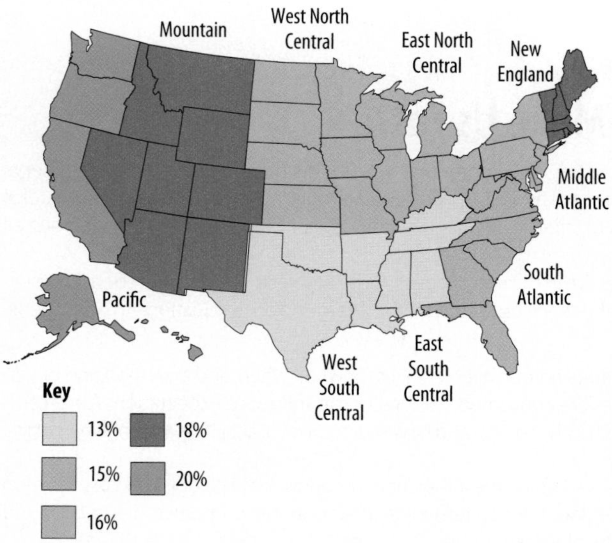

FIGURE SO.9 Percentage of people 15 years and older who engaged in sports or exercise activity on an average day by region.
Courtesy of U.S. Bureau of Labor Statistics.

▶ **built environment** Any human-formed, developed, or structured areas, including the urban environment that consists of buildings, roads, fixtures, parks, and all other human developments that form the area's physical character.

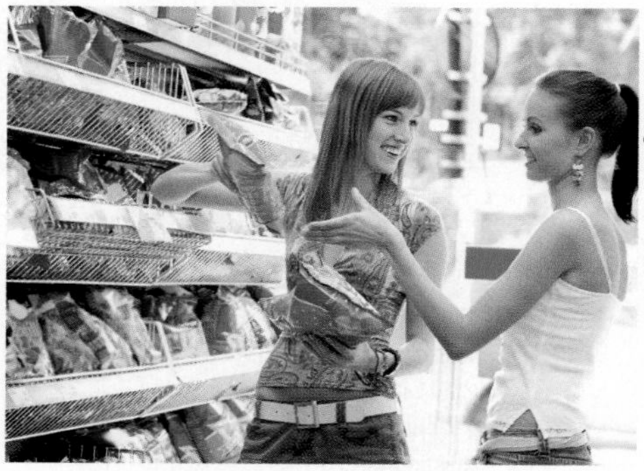

© Franz Pfluegl/Dreamstime.com

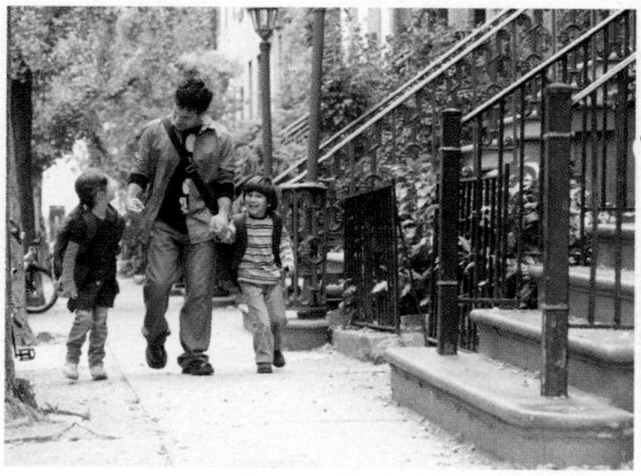

© Jupiterimages/Photos.com/Thinkstock

Our immediate surroundings influence our behaviors, and researchers have begun to link aspects of the **built environment** with obesity. The built environment can be defined as "human-formed, developed, or structured areas, including buildings, roads, parks, and transportation systems."[39] These environments in which we live and work can either encourage or hinder physical activity and healthful eating.

People who live in and work in neighborhoods with sidewalks and safe streets are more physically active. (See **FIGURE SO.9**.) But when neighborhoods have low "walkability," BMIs tend to be higher. Socioeconomic factors are at work, too—lower-income neighborhoods have fewer recreational facilities and healthful eating options. Fast food restaurants and convenience stores are more prevalent in low-income neighborhoods, a characteristic that is associated with higher obesity rates.[40] The number of supermarkets triples in wealthier neighborhoods.[41]

Many adults spend half (or more) of their day in sedentary activities, which often includes long hours at a computer or desk. Creating work environments that support and facilitate physical activity can have a large impact on health and body weight. Companies are beginning to feel the financial burden of obesity as well in terms of decreased worker productivity, number of lost workdays, and higher health insurance premiums. Many companies are now employing strategies such as the use of health and wellness coordinators or lifestyle coaches, gym facilities, organized fitness classes, running groups and walking tracks, and financial incentives for workers to make measureable improvements in their health such as weight loss or quitting tobacco use. Improvements in cafeteria and vending machine choices also are priorities for companies looking to reduce obesity in the workplace.

Lifestyle and Behavior Factors

How Often Do You Eat Out?

The average American eats out nearly four times a week, a choice that has been found to offer less nutritious food than food prepared at home.[42] Added sugars have received lots of attention recently—for good reason. Highly processed carbohydrate now comprises the most unhealthful component of the food supply.[43] Sugary and starchy foods digest quickly into glucose, raise insulin levels, promote excessive weight gain, and increase risk of chronic disease.[44] Putting the nutritional value of restaurant meals aside, let's look at how portion sizes at restaurants can contribute to overeating and ultimately to the obesity epidemic.

We have long recognized that many restaurants serve portions of foods that greatly exceed recommended sizes. Increased portion sizes can be a magnet to people who view large portions as appropriate and as providing more value for the money spent.[45] Super-sized portions affect not only adults, but also children. An evaluation of key foods over 30 years found that soft/fruit drinks, salty snacks, desserts, French fries, burgers, pizzas, Mexican fast foods, and hot dogs increased significantly in portion sizes over that time and now represent more than one-third of children's energy intake. In the last decade, increases in the portion sizes for pizza are particularly pronounced.[46]

THINK About It 2

Our Social Networks

Social factors also influence the development of obesity (see **TABLE SO.1**). Abundant high-calorie, highly palatable foods; pervasive advertising promoting

FYI For Your Information

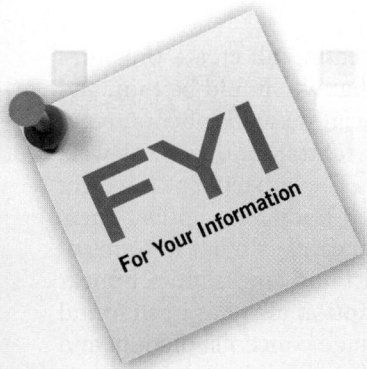

Is Food Addiction Real?

Palatable foods, which are typically associated with high energy content, lead to overeating, and it is almost a foregone conclusion that this is also an important contributor to the current obesity epidemic. How many of us are addicted to particular foods?[a] The tendency to indulge in unhealthy eating and overconsumption of palatable food appear to be crucial determinants, in the rising prevalence of obesity.[b] This tendency to consume food in quantities that exceed energy requirements has been linked to an addiction-like process.[c] The existence of food addiction has not been conclusively proven, but as seen in drug addiction, evidence points to alterations in the brain-reward circuitry induced by overconsumption of palatable foods.[d]

There is evidence that bingeing on sugar-dense, palatable foods increases extracellular dopamine in part of the forebrain called the striatum, suggesting addictive potential.[e] Moreover, elevated blood glucose levels cause tryptophan to be absorbed and converted into the mood-elevating chemical serotonin.[f] Are there biological and psychological similarities between food addiction and drug dependence? What about loss of control? In some individuals, palatable foods even have palliative properties and can be viewed as a form of self-medication.[g] In food environments where highly palatable foods are generally low in price and easy to obtain, and where increased portion size is routine, addictive-like behaviors seem to be encouraged.[h]

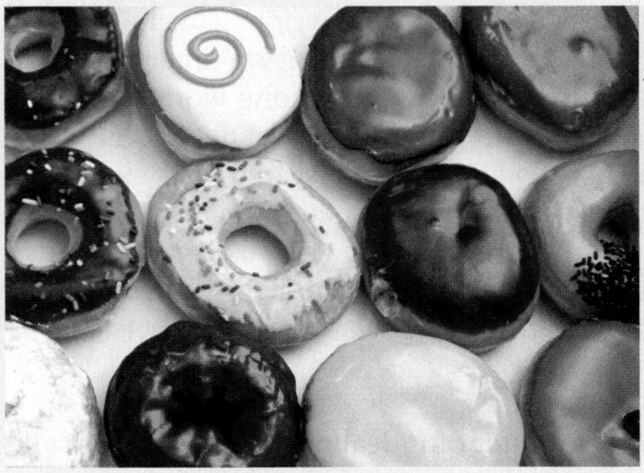
© iStockphoto/Thinkstock

[a]Berthoud HR, Zheng H. Modulation of taste responsiveness and food preference by obesity and weight loss. *Physiol Behav.* 2012;107(4):527–532.
[b]Pandit R, Mercer JG, Overdium J, et al. Dietary factors affect food reward and motivation to eat. *Obes Facts.* 2012;5(2):221–242.
[c]Ibid.
[d]Ibid.
[e]Fortuna JL. The obesity epidemic and food addiction: clinical similarities to drug dependence. *J Psychoactive Drugs.* 2012;44(1):56–63.
[f]Ibid.
[g]Ibid.
[h]Allen PJ, Batra G, Geiger BM. Rationale and consequences of reclassifying obesity as an addictive disorder: neurobiology, food environment and social policy perspectives. *Physiol Behav.* 2012;107(1):126–137.

TABLE SO.1
Sociocultural Influences on Obesity

Social Contexts	
Culture	People in developed societies have more body fat than those in developing societies.
History	Fatness is increasing in the United States, but idealized weights are decreasing.
Social Characteristics	
Age and lifestyle	Fatness increases during adulthood and declines in older adults.
Gender	Obesity is more prevalent in women than in men.
Race and ethnicity	Obesity is more prevalent in African American, Hispanic, Native American, and Pacific Islander women.
Socioeconomic Status	
Income	Obesity is more prevalent in lower-income women.
Education	Less-educated women have a higher incidence of obesity.
Occupational prestige	Obesity is more prevalent in women in less prestigious jobs.
Employment	Women who are unemployed have a higher incidence of obesity.
Household	Older adults who live with others have a higher incidence of obesity.
Marriage	Married men have a higher incidence of obesity.
Residence	Rural women have a higher incidence of obesity.
Region	People residing in the South have a higher incidence of obesity.

Adapted from Sobal J. Social and cultural influences on obesity. In: Bjorntorp P, ed. *International Textbook of Obesity.* Copyright © 2001 John Wiley & Sons Ltd.

their consumption; and the social enjoyment of eating all create pressures to overeat. At the same time, our culture tells us that we should be thin, and we might feel unhealthy pressures to diet. The social network phenomenon appears to be relevant to the biologic and behavioral trait of obesity as well, and obesity appears to spread through social ties.[47] The impact of peer weight is larger among females and adolescents with high body mass index. There is consistent evidence that school friends are significantly similar in terms of their body mass index, and friends with the highest body mass index appear to be most similar. Frequency of fast food consumption also has been found to cluster within groups of boys, as have body image concerns, dieting, and eating disorders among girls.[48] School friends can be critical in shaping young people's eating behaviors and body weight. This suggests the potential that social networks are likely to have a powerful influence on health promotion interventions in schools.[49]

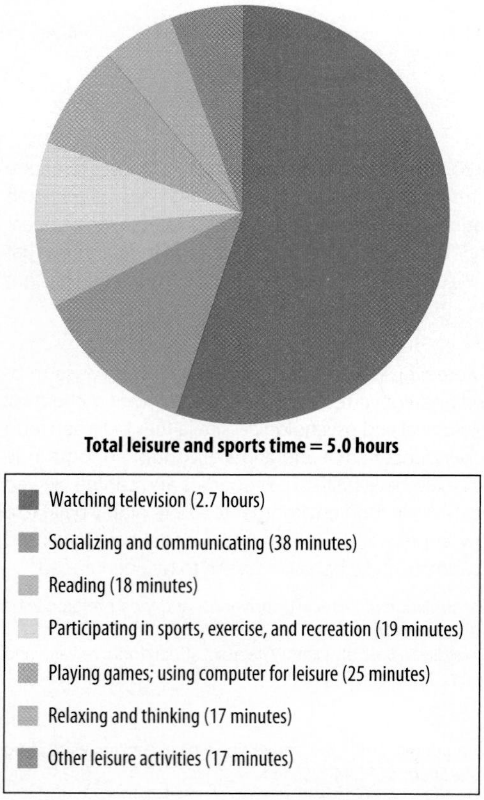

FIGURE SO.10 Time spent on leisure activities by persons 15 years and older on an average day.
Reproduced from U.S. Bureau of Labor Statistics. American time use survey. 2010. http://www.bls.gov/tus/charts/chart9.pdf. Accessed January 28, 2016.

Lack of Physical Activity

Lack of exercise is a major contributing factor to weight gain and obesity. Still, 26 percent of adults never engage in any type of leisure-time physical activity (see **FIGURE SO.10**).[50] Inactivity is more common among women, older adults, less-affluent adults, and African American and Hispanic adults.[51] Children also exercise less. In both children and adults, research links excessive television viewing and computer use to overweight and obesity.[52] Habits can start at an early age, and 80 percent of low-income 2- to 5-year-olds watch more than 2 hours of television daily.[53] For all ages, obesity itself can lead to physical inactivity, although the strength of this relationship is unclear.

Psychological Factors

Some people adopt eating as a strategy for dealing with the stresses and challenges of life. (Others use drugs, alcohol, smoking, shopping, or gambling.) There's also a pleasure in eating that alleviates boredom. Some people use eating as a pick-me-up when fatigued, and some use eating to distract themselves from difficult problems or as a means of punishing themselves or others for real or imagined transgressions.

Emotional Eating

▶ **restrained eaters** Individuals who routinely avoid food as long as possible, and then gorge on food.

▶ **binge eaters** Individuals who routinely consume a very large amount of food in a brief period of time (e.g., two hours) and lose control over how much and what is eaten.

Emotional eaters have a dysfunctional relationship with food, as illustrated by **restrained eaters** and **binge eaters**. Restrained eaters try to reduce their calorie intake by fasting or avoiding food as long as possible. They skip meals, delay eating, or severely restrict the types of food they eat. Then, like a dam that bursts, they overeat when environmental or emotional stress triggers a complete release of inhibitions toward eating. Although not all obese binge eaters follow this pattern, the "fast, then binge" behavior is common in obese people who chronically attempt to lose weight.[54] This pattern also occurs in women of normal weight who perceive themselves as fat. These restrained eating patterns appear to be passed on from mother to daughter.[55] In adolescents, dieting predicts binge eating, decreased physical activity, and decreased breakfast consumption, and is also associated with increased BMI.[56] Therefore, in part, dieting during adolescence can lead to weight gain.

People with a healthy lifestyle have more effective ways to meet their personal needs. They communicate assertively and manage interpersonal conflict effectively, so they don't shrink from problems or overreact. The person with a healthy lifestyle is better suited to create and maintain relationships with others and often has a solid network of friends and loved ones. Food is used appropriately—to fuel life's activities and gain personal satisfaction, not to manage stress.

Key Concepts Obesity tends to run in families. Sex, age, and social and environmental factors are related to weight. Lifestyle choices and behavioral factors also affect weight. Overly restrained eating can result in episodes of overeating and weight gain. Binge eating is common among people in weight-loss programs.

Childhood Overweight

In the United States, overweight and obesity are not concerns for only the adult population; childhood obesity also is increasing at an alarming rate. Approximately one-third of children ages 2 to 19 years are overweight (BMI from the 85th to 94th percentile) or obese (BMI greater than the 95th percentile).[57] An overweight child is likely to reach maturity earlier than a child of normal weight, but perhaps at the expense of height. Some overweight children already deal with the cardiovascular consequences of obesity, such as lipid abnormalities and hypertension, and many overweight children develop type 2 diabetes prior to their teen years. This public health problem is so drastic that many experts are saying this might be the first generation of people with shorter life expectancies than their parents. (See the FYI feature "Childhood and Teenage Obesity: 'The First Generation That Does Not Outlive Its Parents.'")

THINK About It 3

Overweight children are more likely to have social and academic difficulties[58] and experience the psychological trauma associated with obesity in our culture. In addition, obese children are more likely to become obese adults, and obesity in adulthood is likely to be more severe.[59] Factors involved in the development of overweight in childhood include genetics, environment, behavior, and activity levels (see **FIGURE SO.11**).

The good news is that childhood obesity is preventable and treatable. Programs designed to treat childhood obesity are generally multifactorial and provide behavior modification to help children adopt healthier eating patterns, suggestions to increase physical activity, psychological support or therapy, and family counseling including family meal planning and exercise guidance. In some early stages the goal is not weight loss but rather to allow the child's height to catch up with his or her weight. Instead of restricting caloric intake or food choices, the strategy is to increase activity and improve food choices.

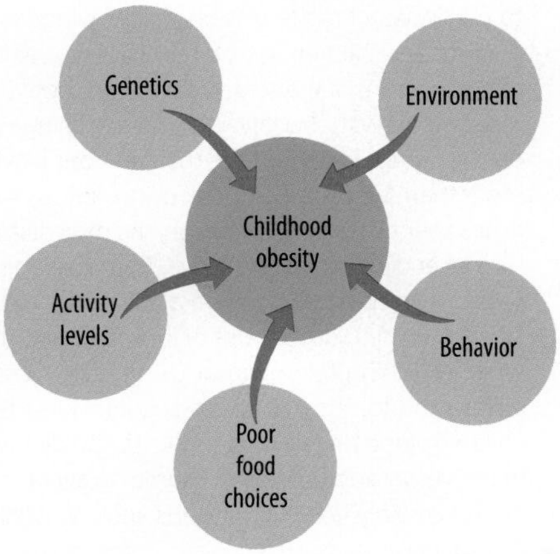

FIGURE SO.11 Factors that contribute to childhood obesity. Childhood obesity is on the rise and predisposes children to health problems when they become adults.

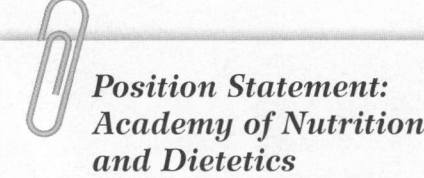

Position Statement: Academy of Nutrition and Dietetics

Weight Management

It is the position of the Academy of Nutrition and Dietetics that successful weight management to improve overall health for adults requires a lifelong commitment to healthful lifestyle behaviors emphasizing sustainable and enjoyable eating practices and daily physical activity.

Reproduced from Seagle HM, Strain GW, Makris A, et al. Position of the American Dietetic Association: weight management. *J Am Diet Assoc.* 2009;109(2):330–346.

Quick Bite

Rising Rates of Childhood Obesity: Kids and Car Seats

A *Pediatrics* article, "Tipping the Scales: Obese Children and Child Safety Seats," found that, based on National Health and Nutrition Examination Survey (NHANES) data, 285,305 children ages 6 and younger would have a difficult time fitting into most child safety seats because of their overweight status. More than half of these children are age 3 and weigh more than 40 pounds. The researchers found only four car seats on the market that could both accommodate these children and keep them safe.

Position Statement: American Heart Association

Overweight in Children

Overweight children are more likely to become overweight adults. Successfully preventing or treating overweight in childhood may reduce the risk of adult overweight. This may help reduce the risk of heart disease and other diseases.

Reproduced from American Heart Association, Inc.

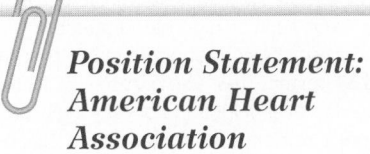

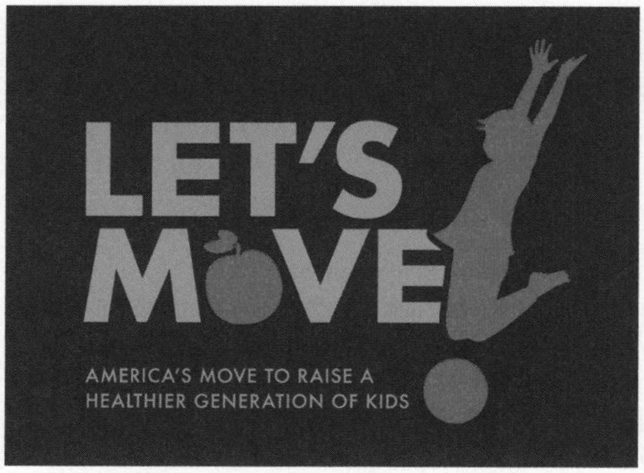
LET'S
MOVE
AMERICA'S MOVE TO RAISE A
HEALTHIER GENERATION OF KIDS

FIGURE SO.12 Let's Move!
Courtesy of Let's Move!

Let's Move!

To meet the challenge of childhood obesity and direct children toward healthy, active lifestyles, the White House Task Force on Childhood Obesity launched a campaign called Let's Move! (See **FIGURE SO.12**.) The primary goal of Let's Move! is to end childhood obesity within a generation. Comprehensive strategies of Let's Move! include providing parents with helpful information; creating environments that support healthy choices; providing healthier foods in schools; ensuring that every family has access to healthy, affordable foods; and helping children become more physically active.[60]

Health Risks of Overweight and Obesity

Overweight and obesity are major public health challenges. Obese people are at higher risk for heart disease, the leading cause of death in the United States and Canada, and for stroke, diabetes, hypertension, abnormal blood lipids, metabolic syndrome, some forms of cancer,

Childhood and Teenage Obesity: "The First Generation That Does Not Outlive Its Parents"

The most recent data on childhood obesity are frightening. Obesity affects 18 percent of all children and adolescents (ages 2–19 years) in the United States, triple the rate from just about one generation ago.[a] To meet the objective of promoting high-quality and longer lives free of preventable disease, disability, injury, and premature death, the Healthy People 2020 agenda calls for a 10 percent reduction in the percentage of children and adolescents considered obese in the United States.[b]

Compared to their normal-weight counterparts, obese children and adolescents are more likely to have risk factors associated with cardiovascular disease (CVD), such as high blood pressure, high cholesterol, and dyslipidemia. Seventy percent of obese children have at least one CVD risk factor, and 39 percent have two or more risk factors.[c] Other health problems connected to overweight and obesity in children and adolescents include sleep apnea, asthma, liver damage, type 2 diabetes, and an increased risk for becoming obese in adulthood. These additional challenges compound the risk for health problems through adulthood. In addition to the burden of physical health problems, overweight/obese children and adolescents also are likely to be plagued with emotional challenges from teasing, harassment, and decreased self-esteem.

What's Causing the Epidemic?

The causes of childhood obesity are numerous and far-reaching but can be narrowed down to a few main contributors:

- *Meals consumed away from home:* What used to be a weekly treat—eating out—has become an almost daily occurrence in this country. The number of meals consumed away from home has increased from 16 percent in 1978 to more than 30 percent in recent years. Intake of fruits, vegetables, and whole grains has decreased, whereas the quantity of saturated fat, sodium, and sugar consumed has increased.[d] Americans spend approximately 42 percent of their food budget paying for foods consumed away from home, which have been found to be less nutritious than foods prepared at home.[e]
- *Physical inactivity:* Only 29 percent of high school students met the *Physical Activity Guidelines for Americans.* Boys were more than twice as likely as girls to meet the *Guidelines* (38 percent vs. 19 percent).[f] Children and adolescents spend approximately 7.5 hours per day using entertainment media that promote a sedentary lifestyle.[g]
- *Screen time:* For many of us, it takes a real effort to get ourselves away from overusing our screens—this includes television screens, computer monitors, and even the handheld devices we use for checking email, listening to music, watching television, and playing video games. According to researchers, children ages 8 to 18 years spend the following amounts of time in front of the screen each day: about 7.5 hours using entertainment media with roughly 4.5 hours watching television, about 1.5 hours on the computer, and more than an hour playing video games.[h] This is more than 53 hours per week using various forms of media. The more hours spent watching television, the more likely children are to be both heavier and less physically active.[i] To make matters worse, it is not just the decrease in physical activity associated with screen use but that television advertising drives sales of junk food and that people tend to snack while watching television or using other screens.[j] In addition, media advertising for unhealthy foods contributes to obesity by influencing children's food preferences, requests, and diet.[k] While watching one hour of television, adolescents consume on average about 156 calories, with choices mainly from snack foods and soft drinks.[l]
- *"Competitive" foods:* In the United States, more than half of middle and high schools allow the advertisement of less healthy foods and offer access to sugary drinks throughout the day from vending machines, school canteens, fund-raising events, and parties.[m] On any given day, 80 percent of all children and adolescents in the United States consume sugary beverages.[n]

- *Food deserts:* Many rural, unsafe, lower-income, and minority neighborhoods have inadequate access to stores and supermarkets that offer healthy, reasonably priced food items such as fruits and vegetables. Adding to the food problem is the reality that in some neighborhoods, children do not have a safe place to play outside. Fifty percent of U.S. children do not have parks, community centers, or sidewalks in their neighborhood.[o]
- *Acceptance of obesity in social circles:* Close friends and associates of obese people are at higher risk of becoming obese themselves. A person's risk of becoming obese increases by 57 percent if he or she has obese friends, 40 percent if he or she has an obese sibling, and 37 percent if he or she has an obese spouse. However, the same is not true among neighbors in similar geographic areas, which indicates that obesity within a given social circle might influence overweight and obesity environments.[p]

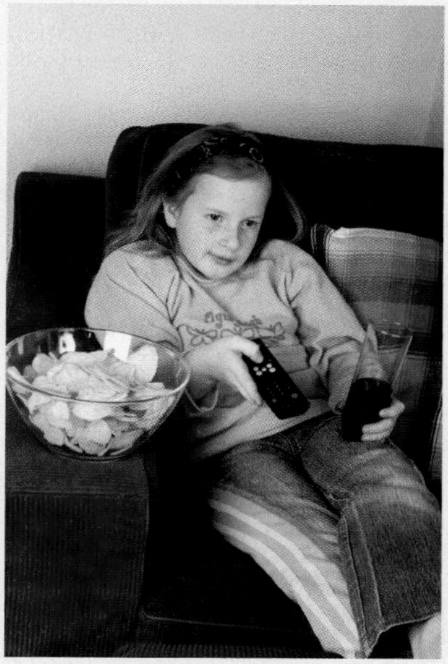

© Ivonne Wierink/ShutterStock, Inc.

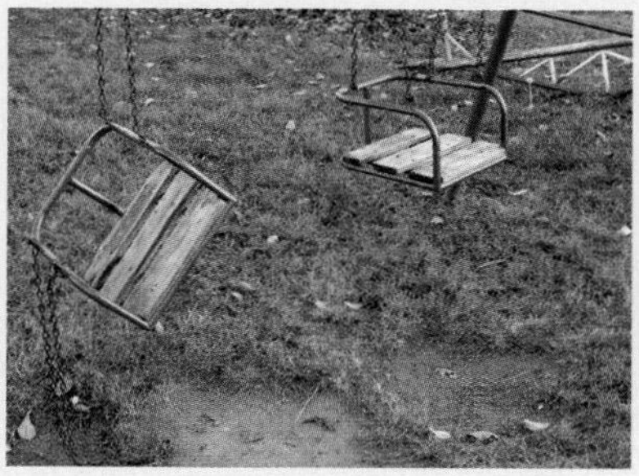

© Peter Gudella/ShutterStock, Inc.

What Can Be Done?

The approach or solution to the childhood obesity epidemic in this country is not a simple one. This generation has been referred to as "the first generation not expected to outlive their parents."[q] The severity of the problem has increased over the past 30 years. Until now, the focus to reduce childhood overweight and obesity has concentrated mainly on school-age children, with only slight consideration to children under age 5. The Institute of Medicine now recommends that efforts be shifted to preventing childhood obesity before children enter the school system.[r]

During their first years of life, children develop the eating patterns that can influence health and well-being throughout their life cycle. Childhood obesity predisposes individuals to become obese adults and increases the risks for obesity-related diseases and conditions (see **Table A**). Health care agencies should encourage pediatricians and other health care providers to emphasize to parents and caregivers the risks to their children's health, especially when they notice a trend toward unhealthy weight status.

TABLE A
Health Problems That May Result from Childhood Obesity

Heart disease, caused by:
• High cholesterol and/or
• High blood pressure
Type 2 diabetes
Asthma
Sleep apnea
Social discrimination

Reproduced from Centers for Disease Control and Prevention. Tips for parents: ideas to help children maintain a healthy weight. http://www.cdc.gov/healthyweight/children. Accessed January 27, 2016.

At the government level, legislators in some states are considering adding a 1-cent-per-ounce tax on sugar-sweetened sodas and other sugary drinks that contain less than 10 percent fruit juice. The tax is intended to raise money for projects to tackle childhood obesity, such as for sports programs and health education for children and adolescents. Drawing on data from the National Health and Nutrition Examination Survey (NHANES), one report found that increasing the price of sugary sodas by 20 percent could cause an average reduction of 37 calories per day, equivalent to 3.8 pounds of body weight over a year for adults, and an average of 43 calories per day, or 4.5 pounds over a year, for children.[s] Another study determined that taxes on soda do not substantially affect overall levels of soda consumption or obesity rates; however, obesity prevention efforts created from these revenues do have an important impact.[t]

Mexico and the city of Berkeley, California have instituted a tax on sugar-sweetened beverages. After one year of the new 10% tax in Mexico, sales of sugar-sweetened beverages have dropped by 6% compared to sales that would have been expected without the tax.[u]

The complexity of childhood obesity requires states, communities, and parents to work together toward "helping children make the healthy choice the easy choice." (See **Figure A**.) The Centers for Disease Control and Prevention offers the following recommendations for reducing obesity in children and adolescents[v]:

States and communities:

- Assess the retail food environment to determine the availability and accessibility of healthier foods.
- Develop incentive programs for supermarkets and farmers markets to establish and maintain their businesses in low-income areas and to sell healthier foods.
- Increase the number of programs that provide local fruits and vegetables and increase the number of salad bars in schools.
- Implement regulations/licensing requirements for child-care providers to decrease the availability of less healthy foodstuffs and sugary beverages and to limit screen time in support of daily physical activities.
- Encourage schools to partake in programs such as the U.S. Department of Agriculture's Healthier U.S. School Challenge (HUSSC), increase free drinking water while limiting the sale of sugary beverages, support breastfeeding programs in schools and workplaces, and promote safe neighborhoods that encourage physical activity by improving access to parks and playgrounds.

(continues)

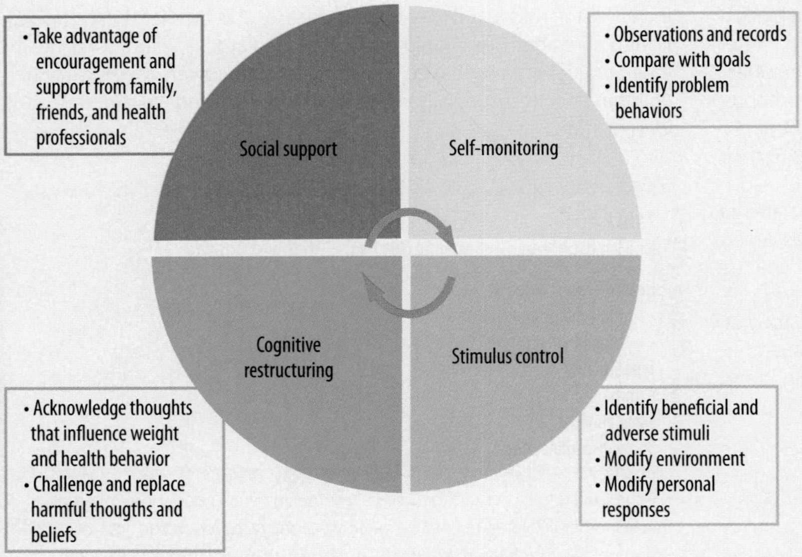

FIGURE A Behavior modification techniques to reduce obesity.

Parents:

- Limit screen time to no more than one to two hours per day.
- Monitor the foods provided in school and child-care settings to ensure that healthier foods and beverages are provided and that physical activity is part of the curriculum.
- In the home, provide plenty of fruits and vegetables, limit foods high in fat and sugar (including sugary beverages), and promote physical activities.

[a]Ogden C, Carroll M. Prevalence of obesity among children and adolescents: United States, trends 1963–1965 through 2007–2008. Division of Health and Nutrition Examination Surveys. NCHS Health E-Stat. July 2010. http://www.cdc.gov/nchs/data/hestat/obesity_child_07_08/obesity_child_07_08.htm. Accessed January 27, 2016.
[b]HealthyPeople.gov. About Healthy People. http://www.healthypeople.gov/2020/about/default.aspx. Accessed January 27, 2016.
[c]Freedman DS, Mei Z, Srinivasan SR, Berenson GS, Dietz WH. Cardiovascular risk factors and excess adiposity among overweight children and adolescents: the Bogalusa Heart Study. *J Pediatr.* 2007:150(1):12–17.
[d]Todd JE, Mancino L, Lin BH. The impact of food away from home on adult diet quality. U.S. Department of Agriculture, Economic Research Center. 2010. http://uhs.berkeley.edu/facstaff/pdf/healthmatters/FoodAwayFromHome.pdf. Accessed January 27, 2016.
[e]Ibid.
[f]U.S. Department of Health and Human Services, Subcommittee of the President's Council on Fitness, Sports and Nutrition. *Physical Activity Guidelines for Americans Midcourse Report: Strategies to Increase Physical Activity Among Youth.* Washington, DC: U.S. Department of Health and Human Services; 2012.
[g]Kaiser Family Foundation. Generation M2: media in the lives of 8- to 18-year-olds. January 2010. http://www.kff.org/entmedia/mh012010pkg.cfm. Accessed January 27, 2016.
[h]Ibid
[i]Boulos R, Vikre EK, Oppenheimer S, Chang H, Kanarek RB. ObesiTV: How television is influencing the obesity epidemic. *Physiol Behav.* 2012;107:146–153.
[j]Smith M. *Screen Time Driving Youth Obesity Epidemic* [presentation]. School of Medicine, University of Pennsylvania; June 27, 2011.
[k]Hingle M, Kunkel D. Childhood obesity and the media. *Pediatr Clin North Am.* 2012;59(3):677–692.
[l]Van den Bulck J, Van Mierlo J. Energy intake associated with television viewing in adolescents: cross-sectional study. *Appetite.* 2004;43(2):181–184.
[m]Centers for Disease Control and Prevention. Op cit.
[n]Ibid.
[o]Ibid.
[p]Christakis NA, Fowler JH. The spread of obesity in a large social network over 32 years. *N Engl J Med.* 2007;357:370–379.
[q]Bost EM. Testimony of Eric M. Bost, Under Secretary, Food, Nutrition, and Consumer Services, Before the House Committee on Government Reform Subcommittee on Human Rights and Wellness. U.S. Department of Agriculture. September 2004. http://www.gpo.gov/fdsys/pkg/CHRG-108hhrg98212/html/CHRG-108hhrg98212.htm. Accessed January 27, 2016.
[r]Birch LL, Parker L, Burns A. *Early Childhood Obesity Prevention Policies.* Washington, DC: National Academies Press; 2011.
[s]Scott-Thomas C. Calorie. Soda tax heads for November ballot in Richmond, CA. http://mobile.foodnavigator-usa.com/Regulation/Soda-tax-heads-for-November-ballot-in-Richmond-CA/?utm_source=newsletter_weekly&utm_medium=email&utm_campaign=Newsletter%2BWeekly&c=zALVolnqfd8MZ4eirfXZ%2F0P1z3G0HHGZ. Accessed January 27, 2016.
[t]Sturm R, Powell LM, Chriqui JF, Chaloupka FJ. Soda taxes, soft drink consumption, and children's body mass index. *Health Aff (Millwood).* 2010;29(5):1052–1058.
[u]Colchero MA, Popkin BM, Rivera JA, et al. Beverage purchases from stores in Mexico under the excise tax on sugar sweetened beverages: observational study. BMJ 2016;352:h6704 doi: 10.1136/bmj.h6704. http://press.psprings.co.uk/bmj/january/sugartax.pdf Accessed 2/28/16.
[v]Centers for Disease Control and Prevention. Overweight and obesity. Strategies and solutions. Op cit.

sleep apnea, gallbladder and joint diseases, and psychosocial problems.[61] The longer obesity persists, the higher the risks. **TABLE SO.2** lists the effects that excess weight could have on your health. Scientists speculate that rising rates of obesity will soon reverse the increases in life expectancy that occurred throughout the twentieth century as a result of improved living conditions, advances in public health, and medical interventions.[62] The costs of obesity-related diseases are staggering. In the United States and Canada, estimates for the total economic cost of overweight and obesity were approximately $300 billion annually. These costs included excess mortality, disability, and medical costs. The global economic impact is roughly

TABLE SO.2
What Are the Risks of Being Overweight?

Hypertension	Overweight people are more likely to have high blood pressure, a major risk factor for heart disease and stroke, than are people who are not overweight.
Heart disease and stroke	Hypertension and very high blood levels of cholesterol and triglycerides (blood fats) can lead to heart disease and often are linked to being overweight. Being overweight also contributes to angina (chest pain caused by decreased oxygen to the heart) and sudden death from heart disease or stroke without any signs or symptoms.
Diabetes	Overweight people are twice as likely to develop type 2 diabetes as are people who are not overweight. Type 2 diabetes is a major cause of early death, heart disease, kidney disease, stroke, and blindness.
Cancer	Several types of cancer are associated with being overweight. In women, these include cancer of the uterus, gallbladder, cervix, ovary, breast, and colon. Overweight men are at greater risk for developing cancer of the colon, rectum, and prostate. For some types of cancer, such as colon or breast, it is not clear whether the increased risk is the result of the extra weight or a high-fat and high-calorie diet.
Sleep apnea	Sleep apnea is a serious condition that is closely associated with being overweight. Sleep apnea can cause a person to stop breathing for short periods during sleep and to snore heavily. Sleep apnea can cause daytime sleepiness and even heart failure. The risk for sleep apnea increases with higher body weights. Weight loss usually improves sleep apnea.
Osteoarthritis	Extra weight appears to increase the risk of osteoarthritis by placing extra pressure on weight-bearing joints and wearing away the cartilage (tissue that cushions the joints) that normally protects them. Weight loss can decrease stress on the knees, hips, and lower back and can improve the symptoms of osteoarthritis.
Gout	Gout is a joint disease caused by high levels of uric acid in the blood. Uric acid sometimes forms into solid stone or crystal masses that become deposited in the joints. Gout is more common in overweight people, and the risk of developing the disorder increases with higher body weights. *Note:* Over the short term, some weight-loss diets can lead to an attack of gout in people who have high levels of uric acid or who have had gout before. People who have a history of gout should check with their doctors or other health professionals before trying to lose weight.
Gallbladder disease	Gallbladder disease and gallstones are more common if you are overweight. Your risk of disease increases as your weight increases. It is not clear how being overweight causes gallbladder disease. Weight loss itself, particularly rapid weight loss or loss of a large amount of weight, can actually increase your chances of developing gallstones. Modest, slow weight loss of about 1 pound a week is less likely to cause gallstones.

Source: Data from NIH Publication No. 07-4098; US DHHS. Weight-control Information Network. Do you know some of the health risks of being overweight?; December 2012.

$2 trillion—nearly equal to the global impact of smoking or of armed violence, war, and terrorism. [63]

The blood lipid levels that typically accompany obesity—high serum triglycerides, low high-density lipoprotein (HDL), and a high low-density lipoprotein (LDL)/HDL ratio—increase the risk for atherosclerosis.[64] A person who is only mildly to moderately obese has an elevated risk of coronary heart disease. However, even modest weight loss (about 10 percent of body weight) reduces risk.

Type 2 diabetes, the most common form of diabetes in the United States and Canada, is three times more likely to develop in people who are obese, especially if they have abdominal obesity ("apple"-shaped body). Obesity increases insulin resistance and compromises the ability of body cells to take up glucose. Diabetes, in turn, is a risk factor for heart disease, kidney disease, and vascular problems. Again, even modest levels of weight reduction can improve glucose tolerance.[65]

Being overweight or obese increases the risk of hypertension, probably because of increased resistance in the peripheral blood vessels, changes in the way the kidneys handle sodium, and other changes in kidney function. Weight loss lowers blood pressure in overweight people with hypertension.

Metabolic syndrome has become increasingly common and is linked to the rising incidence of obesity.[66] Metabolic syndrome is characterized by the combination of three or more metabolic risk factors that include elevated triglycerides, low levels of HDL ("good") cholesterol, elevated blood pressure, insulin resistance, and abdominal obesity.

Being overweight or obese also raises the risk for colon, breast, endometrial, and gallbladder cancers. The same food pattern that contributes to obesity (a diet high in calories and fat, plus low in fiber, fruits, and vegetables) also can be a cancer risk. Similarly, inactivity not only encourages obesity, but also increases cancer risk. Sedentary women, for example, have a higher risk of breast cancer compared to physically active women.[67]

▶ **sleep apnea** Periods of absence of breathing during sleep.

Obese people are also more likely to have obstructive **sleep apnea**, a condition in which the airway collapses during sleep and breathing briefly stops. As the body struggles for air, blood pressure spikes upward. Typically, the individual wakes up, gasps for air, begins breathing again, and then falls asleep until the airway collapses again and the cycle repeats. This pattern not only interrupts and prevents a good night's sleep, but also increases the risk of heart attack and stroke. Modest weight loss can alleviate sleep apnea, improve sleep quality, and reduce daytime drowsiness.[68]

Weight Cycling

▶ **weight cycling** Repeated periods of gaining and losing weight. Also called *yo-yo dieting*.

Weight cycling (or yo-yo dieting) is a pattern of losing and regaining weight, over and over again. In national surveys, approximately 10 to 40 percent of adult women have a history of weight cycling.[69] The pattern of weight cycling often results when a person has success with rapid weight loss but regains the weight. This up-and-down pattern of weight changes over time has negative effects on health risks, body composition, body fat distribution, and energy expenditure. In addition, weight cycling has been associated with increased risk for metabolic syndrome, coronary heart disease, all-cause mortality, and reduced quality of life, even if BMI is at a healthy range. Obese individuals with large fluctuations in body weight have greater taste preference for fat and are prone to future weight gain.[70]

Key Concepts Obesity is a risk factor for many chronic diseases, including heart disease, cancer, hypertension, and diabetes. In many cases, a modest amount of weight loss (about 10 percent) can improve symptoms and disease management.

Obesity Is a Preventable National Crisis

THINK About It 4

Although more than two-thirds of the U.S. population is overweight or obese, much can be done to turn this epidemic around. Dietary interventions, physical activity, behavior and environmental modifications, and surgical and pharmacological treatments are the most widely accepted methods for weight loss and management.

Dietary interventions aimed at obesity prevention and treatment should focus on the development of healthy food choices and behaviors. The bottom line is that if you want to lose weight, you must take in fewer calories than you expend; however, a low-calorie diet is not necessarily a healthy diet. Following a healthy food plan such as MyPlate serves as a guide to including all food groups in a calorie-controlled diet. Commercial weight reduction programs should offer individualized nutrition, physical activity, and behavioral components and recommend slow and steady weight loss and maintenance.

Physical activity is a necessary component of any weight management program and essential for a healthy lifestyle. All adults should aim to be physically active on most, if not all, days of the week. Weight loss also is aided by reducing the amount of time each day spent in sedentary activities such as screen time in front of computers, televisions, and video games each day. In addition to the numerous benefits of the exercise itself, regular physical activity makes it easier to maintain a healthier weight.

Behavioral and environmental modification techniques can successfully help with weight loss and management. Identification of internal or environmental cues that trigger poor food choices or overeating should first be identified. Appropriate strategies to deal with challenging situations and encourage behavior changes that lead to lifelong weight management begin with appropriate and realistic goal setting. Goals should be both short term and long term and be specific, attainable, and forgiving to increase their effectiveness. Altering environmental cues so they prompt healthy behaviors and elicit positive self-worth is a valuable part of successful weight reduction.

Pharmaceutical treatment and surgery have received much media attention. Pharmaceutical treatments, combined with eating changes and increased physical activity, have helped people to lose weight. Surgical procedures, again combined with eating changes and exercise, are another option that has treated morbidly or extremely obese adults successfully. Common surgical procedures for weight management include bypassing some of the stomach or small intestine or gastric banding to reduce the amount of contents that can be held in the stomach.

FYI For Your Information

Can Medicines Lead to Obesity?

After taking a steroid for asthma called prednisone for several months, 20-year-old Martha became painfully aware of a substantial weight gain. She immediately blamed her additional 20 pounds on increased snacking between meals, so she began exercising more. But her effort to exercise more wasn't working and she decided to curb her appetite. But this didn't work either. She felt depressed because she gained an additional 20 pounds and realized her BMI was now over 30: She was considered obese.

But, maybe it wasn't just the increased snacking that made Martha pack on the pounds. Obesogenic drugs also can cause weight gain. Although no one knows precisely how many prescription drugs promote weight gain, doctors suggest that there might be 40 or more of these common offenders. They can be found among drugs used to treat inflammation, diabetes, depression, psychosis, and other conditions. The effects of drugs are idiosyncratic; that is, they have different effects on different people. If you think your weight gain might be caused by a drug you are taking, work with your doctor—and your body—to find the drug that works best for you.

Martha's doctor thought her weight gain might be caused by the prednisone, an obesogenic drug, and substituted an inhaled steroid, which seemed to work. In the next few months, Martha lost most of the weight she had gained and felt that her normal optimism and positive attitude were back.

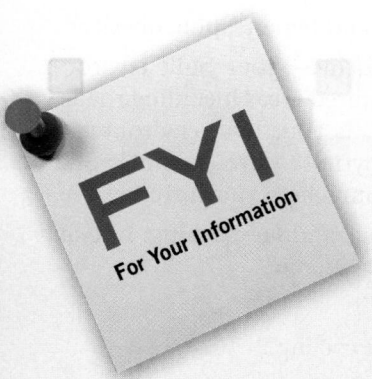

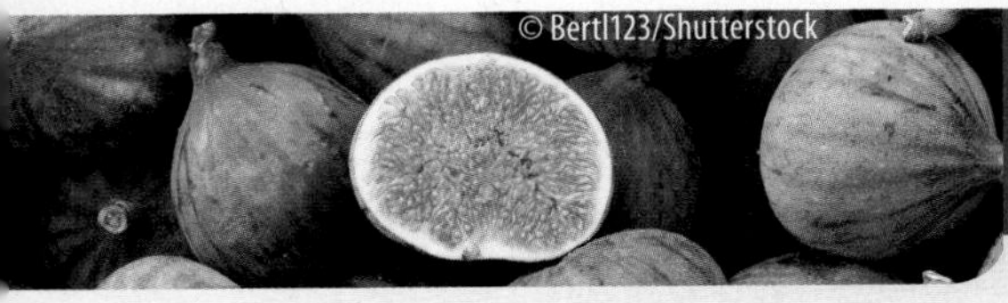
© Bertl123/Shutterstock

Learning Portfolio

Key Terms

binge eaters	374
built environment	372
hypercellular obesity	365
hyperplastic obesity	365
hypertrophic obesity	365
restrained eaters	374
sleep apnea	380
weight cycling	380

Study Points

- The prevalence of obesity and overweight is escalating worldwide, creating an epidemic responsible for numerous chronic diseases.
- The factors that cause obesity are not completely understood, but a complex interaction of hormonal and metabolic factors is believed to play a role, along with genetic, social, environmental, lifestyle, behavior, and psychological factors.
- In the United States, overweight and obesity are not concerns for only the adult population; childhood obesity also is increasing at an alarming rate.
- Compared to their normal-weight counterparts, obese children and adolescents are more likely to have risk factors associated with various chronic diseases.
- Eating meals away from home, physical inactivity, screen time, "competitive" foods, food deserts, and acceptance of obesity in social circles are all considered main contributors to childhood obesity.
- During the first years of life, children develop the eating patterns that can influence health and well-being throughout the life cycle.
- Obesity is a risk factor for many chronic diseases, including heart disease, cancer, hypertension, and diabetes. In many cases, a modest amount of weight loss can improve symptoms and disease management.

Study Questions

1. Obesity is seen as a complex disorder with multiple contributing factors. Give examples of each of the following factors: biological, social and environmental, lifestyle, and behavioral.
2. What is the difference between hyperplastic and hypertrophic obesity?
3. Think about the environment in which you live—your built environment, the human-formed, developed, or structured areas including roads, parks, sidewalks, and transportation system. Is your built environment conducive to a healthy lifestyle? Why or why not? Give examples of a built environment that would be different from where you currently live.
4. The causes of childhood obesity are numerous and far-reaching. List six main contributors to the childhood obesity epidemic.
5. List and identify the risks of being overweight.
6. Identify the negative consequences of weight cycling.
7. Discuss the four most widely accepted methods for weight loss and management.

Try This

Watch Your Screen Time

Monitor your screen time for a day. Keep track of the total amount of time you spend in any and all of the following activities: watching television;

using a computer; playing video games; checking email; and using or playing games on handheld devices such as smartphones, MP3 players, or tablets. In a 24-hour period, how many hours of screen time did you accrue? How does your use compare to the averages discussed earlier in this chapter? If your screen time is too high, identify ways you can improve it.

Tracking Your Activity

Physical activity is a necessary component of a healthy lifestyle. All adults should aim to be physically active (30–60 minutes/day) on most, if not all, days of the week. Keep track of the amount of physical activity you get this week. Try to be more physically active in your everyday routine, such as walking short distances that you normally would drive and taking the stairs instead of the elevator. Do you notice a difference in your overall feeling of well-being on the days that you are physically active compared to the days that you are not?

References

1. Bahia L, Coutinho ES, Barufaldi LA, et al. The costs of overweight and obesity-related diseases in the Brazilian public health system: cross-sectional study. *BMC Public Health*. 2012;12(1):440.
2. McCrady-Spitzer SK, Levine JA. Keynote: nonexercise activity thermogenesis: a way forward to treat the worldwide obesity epidemic. *Surg Obes Rel Dis*. 2012;8:501–506.
3. Lien N, Henriksen HB, Nymoen LL, et al. Availability of data assessing the prevalence and trends of overweight and obesity among European adolescents. *Public Health Nutr*. 2010;13(10A):1680–1687.
4. McCrady-Spitzer SK, Levine JA. Keynote. Op cit.
5. Abdul Rahim HF, Sibai A, Hwalla N, et al. Non-communicable diseases in the Arab world. *Lancet*. 2014;383(9914):356–367.
6. Merchant A, Vatanparast H, Barlas S, et al. Carbohydrate intake and overweight and obesity among healthy adults. *J Am Diet Assoc*. 2009;109(7):1165–1172.
7. Centers for Disease Control and Prevention. Childhood obesity facts. Prevalence of childhood obesity in the United States, 2011-2012 http://www.cdc.gov/obesity/data/childhood.html. Accessed June 26, 2015.
8. HealthyPeople.gov. 2020 topics and objectives: nutrition and weight status: objectives. http://www.healthypeople.gov/2020/topicsobjectives2020/objectiveslist.aspx?topicId=29. Accessed January 28, 2016.
9. MarketData Enterprises. *The U.S. Weight Loss Market: 2015 Status Report & Forecast*. January 28, 2015. http://www.giiresearch.com/report/md323535-us-weight-loss-market-status-report-forecast.html. Accessed January 28, 2016.
10. Wilke J. Nearly half in U.S. remain worried about their weight. Gallup Wellbeing. July 25, 2014. http://www.gallup.com/poll/174089/nearly-half-remain-worried-weight.aspx. Accessed January 28, 2016.
11. DeVault N, Kennedy T, Hermann J, et al. It's all about kids: preventing overweight in elementary school children in Tulsa, OK. *J Am Diet Assoc*. 2009;109(4):680–687.
12. Blomain ES, Dirhan DA, Valentino MA, Kim GW, Waldman SA. Mechanisms of weight regain following weight loss. *ISRN Obesity*. April 16, 2013. http://www.ncbi.nlm.nih.gov/pmc/articles/PMC3901982/. Accessed January 28, 2016.
13. Pachucki MC, Lovenheim MF, Harding M. Within-family obesity associations: evaluation of parent, child, and sibling relationships. *Am J Prev Med*. 2014;47(4):382–391.
14. Llewellyn CH, Trzaskowski M, Plomin R, Wardle J. From modeling to measurement: developmental trends in genetic influence on adiposity in childhood. *Obesity*. 2014;22(7):1756–1761.
15. Lippa NC, Sanderson SC. Impact of information about obesity genomics on the stigmatization of overweight individuals: an experimental study. *Obesity*. 2012;20(12):2367–2376.
16. Yan H, Guo Y, Yang TL, et al. A family-based association study identified *CYP17* as a candidate gene for obesity susceptibility in Caucasians. *Genet Mol Res*. 2012;11(3):1967–1974.
17. Williams MJ, Almen MS, Fredriksson R, Schilth HB. What model organisms and interactomics can reveal about the genetics of human obesity. *Cell Mol Life Sci*. 2012;69(22):3819–3834.
18. Ibid.
19. Manco M, Dallapiccola B. Genetics of pediatric obesity. *Pediatrics*. 2012;130(1):123–133.
20. Hood L. Tackling the microbiome. *Science*. 2012;336(6086):1209.
21. Moreno-Indias I, Cardona F, Tinahones FJ, et al. Impact of the gut microbiota on the development of obesity and type 2 diabetes mellitus. *Front Microbiol*. 2014;5(190):1–10.
22. DiBaise JK, Frank DN, Mathur R. Impact of the gut microbiota on the development of obesity: current concepts. *Am J Gastroenterol*. 2012;1(suppl):22–27.
23. Litonjua AA. Fat-soluble vitamins and atopic disease: what is the evidence? *Proc Nutr Soc*. 2012;71:67–74.
24. National Institute of Diabetes and Digestive and Kidney Diseases. Overweight and obesity statistics. October 2012. http://win.niddk.nih.gov/statistics/. Accessed January 28, 2016.
25. Acevedo P, Lopez-Ejeda N, Alferez-Garcia I, et al. Body mass index through self-reported data and body image perception in Spanish adults attending dietary consultation. *Nutrition*. 2014;30(6):679–684.
26. An R. Prevalence and trends of adult obesity in the US 1999–2012. *ISRN Obesity*. January 6, 2014. doi: 10.1155/2014/185312.
27. Vaughan CA, Sacco WP, Beckstead JW. Racial/ethnic differences in body mass index: the roles of beliefs about thinness and dietary restrictions. *Body Image*. 2008;5(3):291–298.
28. Wang Y, Chen X. Between-group differences in nutrition- and health-related psychosocial factors among US adults and their associations with diet, exercise, and weight status. *J Acad Nutr Diet*. 2012;112(4):486–498.
29. Walker RE, Kawachi I. Use of concept mapping to explore the influence of food security on food buying practices. *J Acad Nutr Diet*. 2012;112(5):711–717.
30. Castillo DC, Ramsey NL, Yu SS, et al. Inconsistent access to food and cardiometabolic disease: the effect of food insecurity. *Curr Cardiovasc Risk Rep*. 20112;6(3):245–250.
31. Fryar CD, Carroll MD, Ogden CL. NCHS health e-stat. Prevalence of overweight, obesity, and extreme obesity among adults: United States, trends 1960–1962 through 2009–2010. Centers for Disease Control and Prevention. http://www.cdc.gov/nchs/data/hestat/obesity_adult_09_10/obesity_adult_09_10.htm. Accessed January 28, 2016.
32. Befort CA, Nazir N, Perri MG. Prevalence of obesity among adults from rural and urban areas of the United States: finding from NHANES (2005–2008). *J Rural Health*. 2012;28(4):392–397.
33. Centers for Disease Control and Prevention. Obesity prevalence maps. http://www.cdc.gov/obesity/data/prevalence-maps.html. Accessed January 28, 2016.
34. Drewnowski A, Aggarwal A, Monsivais P, Moudon AV. Obesity and supermarket access: proximity or price? *Am J Public Health*. 2012;102(8):e74–e80.
35. Ibid.
36. Desilver, D. Chart of the week: is food too cheap for our own good? Pew Research Center. May 23, 2014. http://www.pewresearch.org/fact-tank/2014/05/23/chart-of-the-week-is-food-too-cheap-for-our-own-good/ Accessed 2/28/16; and Strum F, Ruopeng A. Obesity and economic environments. CA CANCER J CLIN 2014;64:337–350. http://onlinelibrary.wiley.com/doi/10.3322/caac.21237/pdf. Accessed 2/28/16.
37. Cohen DA, Babey SH. Contextual influences on eating behaviors: heuristic processing and dietary choices. *Obes Rev*. 2012;13(9):766–779.

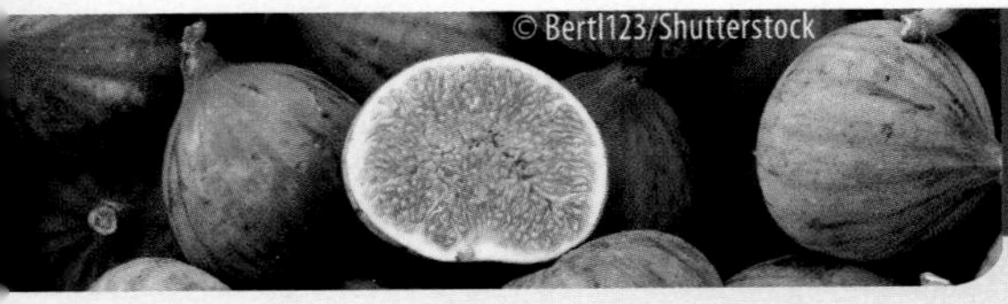

Learning Portfolio (continued)

38. Durand CP, Andalib M, Dunton GF, et al. A systematic review of built environment factors related to physical activity and obesity risk: implications for smart growth urban planning. *Obes Rev*. 2011;12(5):e173–e182.
39. He M, Tucker P, Irwin JD, et al. Obesogenic neighbourhoods: the impact of neighbourhood restaurants and convenience stores on adolescents' food consumption behaviours. *Public Health Nutr*. 2012;15(12):2331–2339.
40. Safron M, Cislak A, Gasper T, Luszczynska A. Micro-environmental characteristics related to body weight, diet, and physical activity of children and adolescents: a systematic umbrella review. *Int J Environ Health Res*. 2011;27:1–25.
41. Todd JE. Changes in eating patterns and diet quality among working-age adults, 2005–10. ERR-161. U.S. Department of Agriculture, Economic Research Service; January 2014.
42. Wu H, Sturm R. What's on the menu? A review of the energy and nutritional content of US chain restaurant menus. *Public Health Nutr*. May 11, 2012:1–10.
43. Phates EH. Dr. David Ludwig clears up carbohydrate confusion. The Nutrition Source: Ask the Expert. Harvard School of Public Health. December 16, 2015.
44. Ibid.
45. Piernas C, Popkin BM. Food portion patterns and trends among U.S. children and the relationship to total eating occasion size, 1977–2006. J Nutr. 2011;141(6):1159–1164.
46. Zhang J, Tong L, Lamberson PJ, Durazo-Arvizu RA, Luke A, et al. Leveraging social influence to address overweight and obesity using agent-based models: the role of adolescent social networks. *Social Sci Med*. 2015;125:203–213.
47. Fletcher A, Bonell C, Sorhaindo A. You are what your friends eat: systematic review of social network analysis of young people's eating behaviors and bodyweight. *J Epidemiol Community Health*. 2011;65(6):548–555.
48. Ibid.
49. Centers for Disease Control and Prevention. Nutrition, physical activity and obesity: data, trends and maps. https://nccd.cdc.gov/NPAO_DTM/. Accessed January 28, 2016.
50. Centers for Disease Control and Prevention. Facts about physical activity. May 23, 2014. http://www.cdc.gov/physicalactivity/data/facts.html. Accessed January 28, 2016.
51. Gilbert-Diamond D, Li Z, Adachi-Mejia AM, McClure AC, Sargent JD. Association of a television in the bedroom with increased adiposity gain in a nationally representative sample of children and adolescents. *JAMA Ped*. 2014;168(5):427–434.
52. Centers for Disease Control and Prevention. Nutrition, physical activity and obesity. Op cit.
53. Mason TB, Robin JL. Profiles of binge eating: the interaction of depressive symptoms, eating styles and body mass index. *Eating Disord J Treat Prevent*. 2014;1:1–11.
54. Allen KL, Gibson LY, McLean NJ, Davis EA, Byrne SM. Maternal and family factors and child eating pathology: risk and protective relationships. *J Eating Disord*. 2014;2:11.
55. Lowe MR, Doshi SD, Katterman SN, Feig EH. Dieting and restrained eating as prospective predictors of weight gain. *Frontiers Psychol*. 2013;4:577.
56. Ogden CL, Carroll MD, Kit BK, Flegal KM. Prevalence of childhood and adult obesity in the United States, 2011–2012. *JAMA*. 2014;311(8):806–814.
57. Latzer Y, Stein D. A review of the psychological and familial perspectives of childhood obesity. *J Eating Disord*. 2013;1:7. Epub February 25, 2013. doi: 10.1186/2050-2974-1-7.
58. Centers for Disease Control and Prevention. Health effects of childhood obesity. http://www.cdc.gov/healthyschools/obesity/facts.htm Accessed 2/28/16.
59. Let's Move! Home page. http://www.letsmove.gov. Accessed January 28, 2016.
60. National Heart, Lung, and Blood Institute. What are the health risks of overweight and obesity? http://www.nhlbi.nih.gov/health/health-topics/topics/obe/risks.html. Accessed January 28, 2016.
61. Kitahara CM, Flint AJ, Berrington de Gonzalez A, et al. Association between class III obesity (BMI of 40–59 kg/m^2) and mortality: a pooled analysis of 20 prospective studies. *PLOS Med*. 2014;11(7):e1001673.
62. Behan D, Cox S. Obesity and its relation to mortality and morbidity costs. Society of Actuaries. December 2010. http://www.soa.org/research/research-projects/life-insurance/research-obesity-relation-mortality.aspx. Accessed January 28, 2016; and Dobbs R, Sawers C, Thompson F, et al. How the world could better fight obesity. McKinsey Global Institute.

November 2014. http://www.mckinsey.com/industries/healthcare-systems-and-services/our-insights/how-the-world-could-better-fight-obesity. Accessed February 28, 2016.

63. Kuller L. The great fat debate: reducing cholesterol. *J Am Diet Assoc.* 2011;111(5):663–664.

64. Franz M, Powers M, Leontos C, et al. The evidence for medical nutrition therapy for type 1 and type 2 diabetes in adults. *J Am Diet Assoc.* 2010;110(12):1852–1889.

65. National Heart, Lung, and Blood Institute. What is metabolic syndrome? November 2011. http://www.nhlbi.nih.gov/health/health-topics/topics/ms/. Accessed January 28, 2016.

66. Land SR, Liu Q, Wickerham DL, Costantino JP, Gonz PA. Cigarette smoking, physical activity, and alcohol consumption as predictors of cancer incidence among women at high risk of breast cancer in the NSABP P-1 trial. *Cancer Epidemiol Biomarkers Prev.* 2014;23(5):823–832.

67. Dobrosielski DA, Patil S, Schwartz AR, Bandeen-Roche K, Stewart KJ. Effects of exercise and weight loss in older adults with obstructive sleep apnea. *Med Sci Sports Exerc.* 2015;47(1):20–26.

68. Mason C, Foster-Schubert KE, Imayama I, et al. History of weight cycling does not impede future weight loss or metabolic improvements in postmenopausal women. *Metabolism.* 2013;62(1):127–136.

69. Ibid.

Chapter **10**

Fat-Soluble Vitamins

Revised by Melissa Bernstein

THINK About It

1. How do you feel about taking vitamin supplements?
2. How likely are you to get vitamin toxicity from the food you eat?
3. Which food group, if any, supplies most of your vitamin needs?
4. From a well-lighted area, you step into a dark room. Over time, you see details. What's going on?
5. Your grandmother is a strict vegetarian and she seldom goes outdoors. What can you tell her about vitamin D intake?

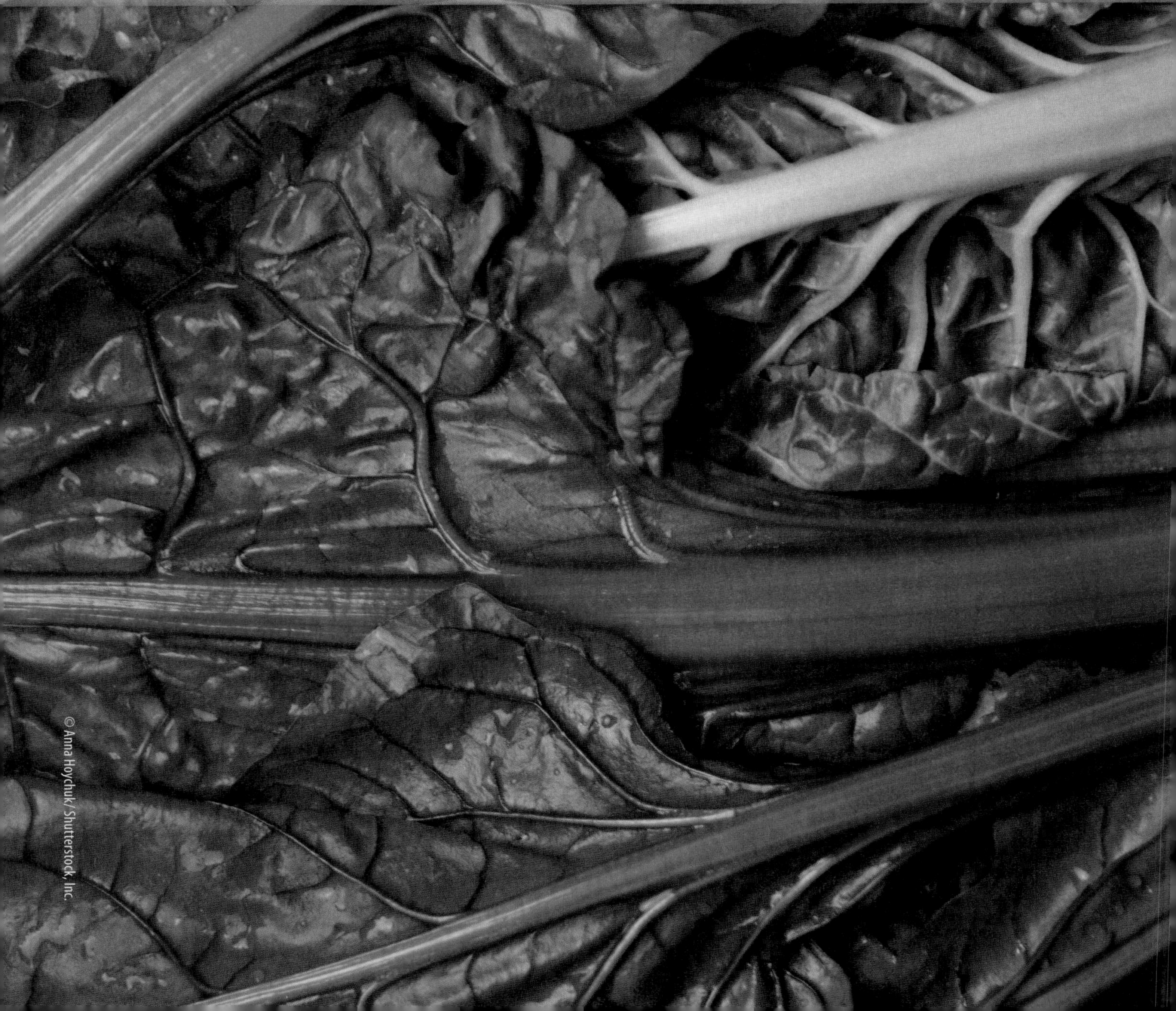

CHAPTER Menu

LEARNING Objectives

- Describe the key features of the fat-soluble vitamins.
- Identify the different forms of vitamins A, D, E, and K.
- Explain the absorption, storage, and transport of vitamins A, D, E, and K.
- List the major functions of vitamins A, D, E, and K.
- Identify major food sources of vitamins A, D, E, and K.
- Specify the major symptoms and diseases associated with deficiencies of vitamins A, D, E, and K.
- Discuss why fat-soluble vitamins have greater toxicity than water-soluble vitamins do.

You get a panicky call from your sister-in-law: Her 9-month-old baby is turning orange! She and her husband have done everything the pediatrician told them to do about feeding; just last month, they started giving the baby infant cereal, and now they have started him on strained baby food. They introduced just one food at a time. In fact, they have only fed him one food other than cereal—carrots. Yes, the baby liked them, so much that he eats two to three jars at each meal! Do you think that could be the problem?

Vegetables are healthful foods, and carrots are an important source of many nutrients. Carrots are probably best known as a source of beta-carotene, a vitamin A precursor and the pigment that gives carrots their orange color. Your sister-in-law's baby is eating large quantities of carrots, and the excess beta-carotene circulating in his blood gives the skin a yellow-orange cast. This condition is known as **carotenodermia** and is completely harmless. But it has probably given at least one or two new parents a scare!

▶ **carotenodermia** A harmless yellow-orange cast to the skin caused by high levels of carotenoids in the bloodstream resulting from consumption of extremely large amounts of carotenoid-rich foods, such as carrot juice.

Understanding Vitamins

Vitamins. Just the word probably makes you think of health and well-being! Children can quickly tell you that fruits and vegetables are good sources of vitamins and can recite some of the best food sources: oranges for vitamin C, carrots for vitamin A, and so on. For many people, however, vitamins have become something to purchase and take in supplement form, rather than a criterion for choosing foods. Americans spend huge amounts of money, billions of dollars each year, on vitamin supplements. Their reasons for taking vitamins are almost as varied as the vitamins themselves. Some people take supplements because they "don't eat right." Some take them for extra "insurance," whereas others look to vitamins to prevent and cure a whole host of conditions, from colds to cancer. Is all this money well spent?

To answer this question, you need to consider several aspects of vitamin supplementation. First, survey data indicate few widespread nutrient deficiencies in the United States among healthy people. From that perspective, many people may be taking supplements unnecessarily. A second aspect is the common sentiment that "if a little is good, more must be better." This misguided belief can lead to problems, especially when applied to fat-soluble vitamin supplementation. Although high doses of some vitamins cause no ill effects, others can have serious, lifelong consequences. A third consideration is that research continues to identify relationships between vitamins and reduced risk of some diseases, so some supplementation can be warranted.

THINK About It 1

TABLE 10.1
Summary of Fat-Soluble Vitamins

Vitamin	Important Dietary Sources	Major Functions	Signs/Symptoms of Deficiency	Toxic Effects of Megadoses	Special Considerations
A	Liver, fish liver oil, milk fat, carrots, spinach, broccoli, squash, sweet potatoes, cantaloupes, peaches, apricots, mangos, margarine, cereals, low-fat milk	Vision, cell differentiation, immunity, reproduction, bone health	Growth retardation, xerophthalmia/vision loss/night blindness/blindness, hyperkeratosis, reduced sperm production, infertility in women, loss of taste and smell	Fatigue, vomiting, abdominal pain, bone and joint pain, loss of appetite, skin disorders, headache, blurred or double vision, liver damage, birth defects (cleft palate, heart abnormalities, brain malfunction), spontaneous abortion	Increased risk for deficiency with medications that alter fat absorption, alcohol abuse/liver disease, protein-energy malnutrition, infancy/premature birth, and fat-malabsorptive disorders
D	Vitamin D–fortified foods such as milk, breakfast cereal, orange juice, margarine, yogurt, grains/breads	Regulation of blood calcium, bone health, regulation of cell differentiation and growth	Rickets, osteomalacia, osteoporosis	Hypercalcemia (causing nausea, vomiting, loss of appetite), bone loss, kidney stones	Increased risk for deficiency in children, girls, non-Hispanic blacks, Mexican Americans, those born outside the U.S., low-income households, obese children, those who watch more TV/play more video games/use computers
E	Wheat germ oil, safflower oil, cottonseed oil, sunflower seed oil, foods made from oils (margarine, salad dressing), sunflower seeds, almonds, spinach, fortified cereals	Protection and maintenance of cellular membranes through antioxidant capacity	Premature hemolysis, hemolytic anemia, neurological problems	Inhibition of platelet adhesion and countering vitamin K's blood clotting mechanism	Increased risk for deficiency with fat-malabsorptive disorders
K	Spinach, greens, broccoli, Brussels sprouts, vegetable oils (soybean, cottonseed, canola, olive)	Blood clotting, bone health/sustaining bone mineral density	Reduced bone density, bone fractures, bleeding	Hemolytic anemia	Increased risk for deficiency with fat-malabsorptive disorders, long-term antibiotic use (due to antibiotics destroying the intestinal bacteria that produce vitamin K)

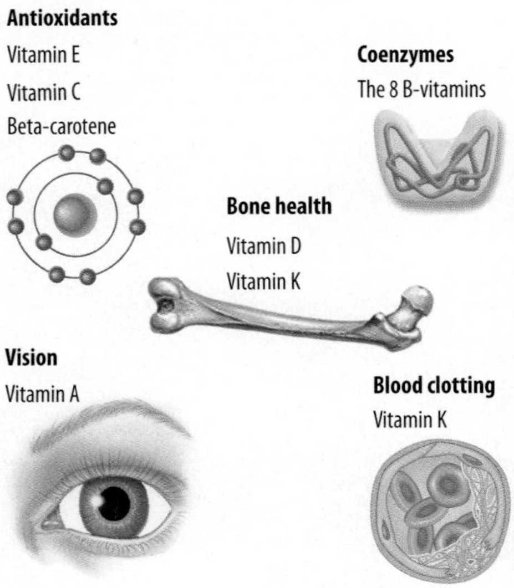

FIGURE 10.1 Major roles of vitamins. Vitamins are crucial for normal functioning, growth, and maintenance of body tissues. Compared to carbohydrate, fat, and protein, the body needs tiny amounts of vitamins.

This chapter on vitamins explores some of the implications of too much or too little of a vitamin in the diet and explains the facts about fat-soluble vitamins: what they are, what they do in the body, and which foods contain them. (See **TABLE 10.1** for a summary.) Armed with this information, you will be able to make wise decisions about food and whether to take supplements.

Anatomy of the Vitamins

Vitamins differ from fat, protein, and carbohydrate in many important ways. For one, the body requires large amounts of the macronutrients, carbohydrates, proteins, and fats—amounts measured in grams. By comparison, the daily needs for vitamins are small—a mere microgram or two in some cases. In addition, unlike fat, protein, and carbohydrate, vitamins are not a source of energy. However, many vitamins play crucial roles in regulating the chemical reactions that allow us to extract energy from those nutrients. Another difference is structural: Vitamins are individual units rather than long chains of smaller units.

Like fat, carbohydrate, and protein, however, vitamins are organic (carbon-containing) compounds essential for normal functioning, growth, and maintenance of the body. The functions of vitamins can be interrelated (see **FIGURE 10.1**), so a deficiency of just one can cause profound health problems.

Fat-Soluble Versus Water-Soluble Vitamins

Scientists classify vitamins as *fat-soluble* or *water-soluble*. Vitamins A, D, E, and K are lipid-like molecules that are soluble in fat. The B vitamins and vitamin C, on the other hand, are soluble in water. This difference in solubility affects the way the body absorbs, transports, and stores vitamins. **TABLE 10.2** provides

TABLE 10.2
A Comparison of Fat-Soluble and Water-Soluble Vitamins

Characteristic	Fat-Soluble Vitamins (Vitamins A, D, E, and K)	Water-Soluble Vitamins (B Vitamins and Vitamin C)
Solubility	Soluble in fat	Soluble in water
Digestion	Digestion begins in the mouth to break foods into small pieces, helping to release vitamins. In the stomach, digestive enzymes work to release vitamins from food. Bile is required to emulsify fat and aid digestion and absorption.	Digestion begins in the mouth to break foods into small pieces, helping to release vitamins. In the stomach, digestive enzymes work to release vitamins from food.
Absorption	Absorption occurs in the small intestine and is similar to that of dietary fats, with incorporation into micelles. Inside the intestinal cells, fat-soluble vitamins are packaged in chylomicrons and move to lymphatic circulation before being transported to the blood.	Absorption from the small intestine is similar to that of glucose and amino acids, directly into the blood.
Transport	Transported by protein carriers (lipoproteins) through watery compartments in the body.	Travel freely in the watery compartments of the body.
Storage	Liver or fatty tissue such as adipose tissue.	Not stored in the body, with the exception of vitamin B_{12} in the liver.
Excretion	Tend to build up in tissues because they are not readily excreted.	Readily excreted in urine.
Dietary requirement	Daily intake is not required because of body storage.	Regular intake is required and varies by vitamin because the body does not usually store significant amounts.

a general comparison of fat-soluble vitamins and water-soluble vitamins. **FIGURE 10.2** illustrates the body's absorption of vitamins.

Intestinal cells absorb fat-soluble vitamins along with dietary fat. The amount absorbed typically varies from 40 to 90 percent of the vitamin amount consumed; efficiency of absorption generally falls as the dietary intake rises

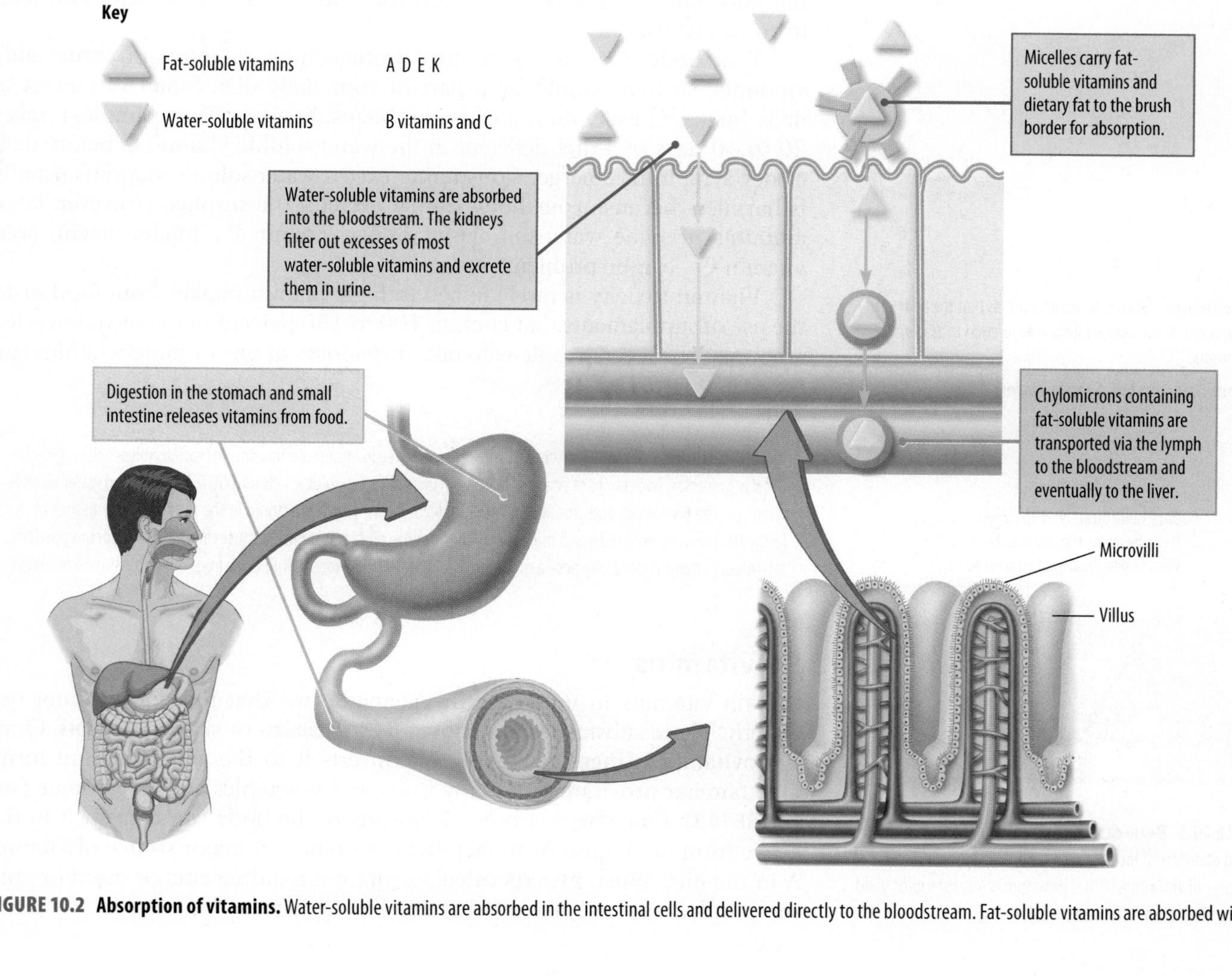

FIGURE 10.2 Absorption of vitamins. Water-soluble vitamins are absorbed in the intestinal cells and delivered directly to the bloodstream. Fat-soluble vitamins are absorbed with fat.

above the body's needs. Just like triglycerides and other dietary lipids, lipoproteins carry absorbed fat-soluble vitamins on their journey through the lymph and bloodstream. As chylomicrons move through the blood, cells take up most of the triglycerides and leave behind chylomicron remnants that contain the fat-soluble vitamins. The liver picks up these remnants and either stores the vitamins for future use or repackages them for delivery by way of the bloodstream to other tissues.

Water-soluble vitamins are dissolved in the watery compartments of foods. Once absorbed, these nutrients travel directly into the bloodstream and then move independently in and around the cells of the body. Unlike fat-soluble vitamins, water-soluble vitamins do not need lipoprotein carriers. Their storage and excretion differ too. Whereas most fat-soluble vitamins accumulate and can be stored indefinitely, the kidneys filter out excess amounts of most water-soluble vitamins and excrete them in urine. Two vitamins are exceptions to this general rule: Water-soluble vitamin B_{12} is stored more readily than the other water-soluble vitamins, and fat-soluble vitamin K is excreted more readily than the other fat-soluble vitamins.

Storage and Toxicity

Fat-soluble vitamins accumulate in the liver and adipose tissues, where they can be drawn upon in times of need. Once these vitamin stores are established, you can go for days, weeks, or even months without consuming more and suffer no ill effects. On the other hand, excessive intake of the fat-soluble vitamins can exceed the body's storage capacity and lead to toxic effects.

Your body does not store most water-soluble vitamins in appreciable amounts, so they should be a part of your daily diet. Small variations in daily intake typically do not cause problems, however. For example, it takes 20 to 40 days of a diet deficient in the water-soluble vitamin C before deficiency symptoms emerge. Consuming excess water-soluble vitamins usually is harmless because your body simply excretes the surplus. However, large amounts of some water-soluble vitamins—vitamin B_6, folate, niacin, even vitamin C—can be problematic.

Vitamin toxicity is rarely linked to high vitamin intakes from food or to the use of supplements that contain 100 to 150 percent of the recommended amounts. However, people who take megadoses of one or more vitamins run the risk of toxicity.

THINK About It 2

Key Concepts Vitamins are organic substances needed in minuscule amounts for various roles in the regulation of body processes. Two classes of vitamins have been identified: fat-soluble vitamins (A, D, E, and K) and water-soluble vitamins (the B vitamins and vitamin C). Fat-soluble vitamins, which are stored in the liver and fatty tissues of the body, are generally excreted much more slowly than water-soluble vitamins. Because they are stored for long periods, fat-soluble vitamins generally pose a greater risk of toxicity than water-soluble vitamins when consumed in excess.

▶ **provitamins** Inactive forms of vitamins that the body can convert into active usable forms. Also referred to as *vitamin precursors*.

▶ **vitamin precursors** See *provitamins*.

Provitamins

Certain vitamins in foods are in inactive forms that the body cannot use directly. These substances are known as **provitamins**, or **vitamin precursors**. Once a provitamin is ingested, the body converts it to the active vitamin form. One familiar provitamin in many fruits and vegetables is beta-carotene (see **FIGURE 10.3**). Once beta-carotene is absorbed, the body can convert it to the active form of vitamin A. In fact, beta-carotene is a major source of vitamin A in the diet. When experts calculate vitamin requirements or monitor consumption, they must take provitamins into account.

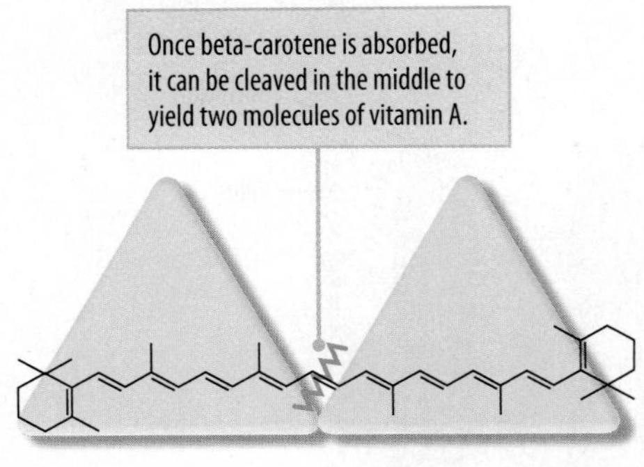

Once beta-carotene is absorbed, it can be cleaved in the middle to yield two molecules of vitamin A.

FIGURE 10.3 Beta-carotene. Beta-carotene can be cleaved at different locations, so it might yield fewer than two molecules of vitamin A. Other provitamin A carotenoids yield less vitamin A than beta-carotene does.

Vitamins in Foods

What foods do you think of as good sources of vitamins? As mentioned, even very young children know that fruits and vegetables are important in the diet because "they give you vitamins." In fact, vitamins are found in every food group, including the fats and oils that most of us are trying to eat less of. One more reason to include variety in your diet is that no one food group, or one choice within a food group, is a good source of all vitamins.

THINK About It 3

The amounts of specific vitamins in a food depend on several factors. For plant foods—whether fruits, vegetables, or grains—sunlight, soil and growing conditions, and the plant's maturity at harvest all affect the vitamin content. Although an animal's diet can have some impact on animal-derived food, its capacity for absorption and storage keeps the vitamin content fairly consistent. Packaging and storage can affect a food's vitamin content. Exposure to light damages vitamins A and the B vitamin riboflavin, for example, whereas exposure to air damages vitamins E and C.

Generally, the more a food is processed and cooked, the more vitamins it loses. Most food processing (e.g., cooking, milling grains, canning vegetables, drying fruit) reduces vitamin content. Eating a variety of foods and using different preparation techniques help ensure that your diet supplies plenty of vitamins.

Key Concepts All types of foods contain vitamins. Provitamins are vitamin precursors that the body can convert to the active vitamin form. Growing conditions, storage, processing, and cooking all affect the amounts of vitamins in foods.

Vitamin A: The Retinoids and Carotenoids

Vitamin A is best known for its role in vision, but it is also crucial for proper growth, reproduction, immunity, and cell differentiation. It helps maintain healthy bones as well as skin and mucous membranes. Vitamin A deficiency not only can destroy vision, but also disrupts numerous functions throughout the body.

Forms of Vitamin A

The body uses three active forms of vitamin A, known collectively as the **retinoids**. These compounds are **retinol**, the alcohol form of vitamin A; **retinal**, the aldehyde form of vitamin A; and **retinoic acid**, the acid form of vitamin A (see **FIGURE 10.4**). Although all three forms have essential functions, retinol is the key player in the vitamin A family. In fact, the standard unit for quantifying the biologic activity of the various forms of vitamin A and its precursors is known as a retinol activity equivalent (RAE).

Your body can easily convert retinol, which is required for reproduction and bone health, to retinal, the form of vitamin A essential for night and color vision. In turn, retinal can re-form retinol or it can irreversibly form retinoic acid, which is important for cell growth and differentiation. The interconvertible nature of retinol and retinal allows them to support all the activities of the vitamin A family. **FIGURE 10.5** shows the interconversions of the three active forms of vitamin A.

Colorful plant pigments called **carotenoids** are precursors of vitamin A. The body converts some carotenoids, the **provitamin A** compounds, to vitamin A with varying degrees of efficiency. The yellow-orange pigment beta-carotene can be cleaved into two molecules of retinal and thus has the highest potential vitamin A activity of the provitamin A family. Of all the provitamin A carotenoids, beta-carotene yields the most vitamin A.

- **retinoids** Compounds in foods that have chemical structures similar to vitamin A. Retinoids include the active forms of vitamin A (retinol, retinal, and retinoic acid) and the main storage forms of retinol (retinyl esters).
- **retinol** The alcohol form of vitamin A. It is one of the retinoids, and thought to be the main physiologically active form of vitamin A. It is interconvertible with retinal.
- **retinal** The aldehyde form of vitamin A. One of the retinoids, it is the active form of vitamin A in the photoreceptors of the retina. It is interconvertible with retinol.
- **retinoic acid** The acid form of vitamin A. One of the retinoids, it is formed from retinal but not interconvertible. It helps growth, cell differentiation, and the immune system, but does not have a role in vision or reproduction.
- **carotenoids** A group of yellow, orange, and red pigments in plants, including foods. Many of these compounds are precursors of vitamin A.
- **provitamin A** Carotenoid precursors of vitamin A in foods of plant origin, primarily deeply colored fruits and vegetables.

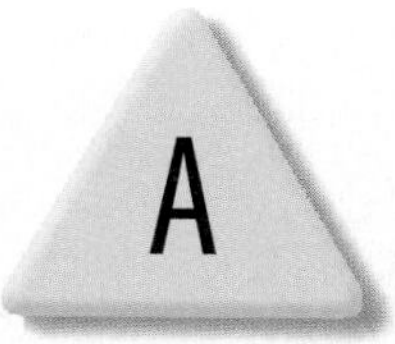

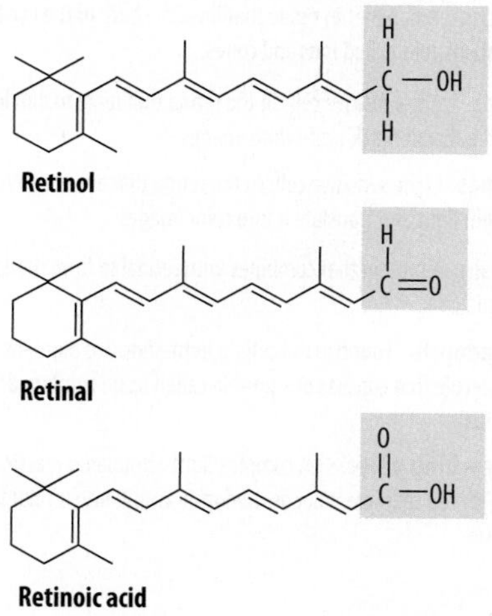

FIGURE 10.4 Forms of vitamin A. Retinol is the alcohol form of vitamin A, retinal is the aldehyde form, and retinoic acid is the acid form.

Courtesy of Joe Valbuena/USDA.

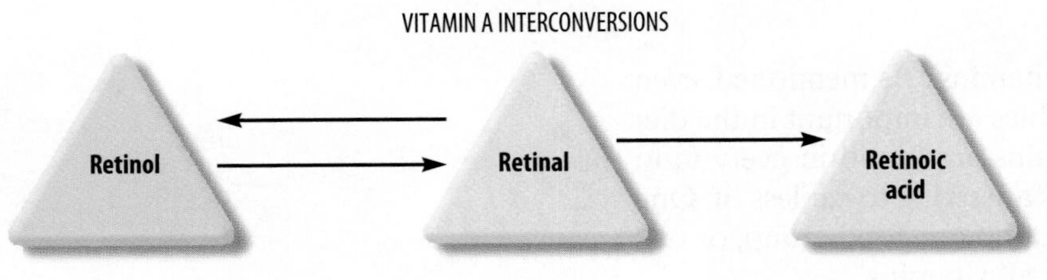

FIGURE 10.5 Vitamin A interconversions. Whereas retinol and retinal are interconvertible, the reaction that forms retinoic acid is irreversible.

Storage and Transport of Vitamin A

The liver stores over 90 percent of the vitamin A in the body, with the rest found in fatty tissues, the lungs, and the kidneys.[1] The body stores vitamin A primarily as **retinyl esters**—retinol linked to a fatty acid, usually palmitic acid. Your liver gradually accumulates vitamin A reserves, which reach their peak in adulthood. The liver releases retinol in just the right amounts to maintain normal retinol blood levels. A healthy liver can store up to a year's supply of vitamin A, but taking large doses of vitamin A supplements can exceed this capacity and lead to toxicity.

Many fat-soluble vitamins need carrier proteins to ferry them in the blood to where the body needs them. For instance, **retinol-binding protein (RBP)** carries retinol released by the liver. Once the RBP drops off the retinol to a target cell, the cell can convert retinol to retinal or retinoic acid as needed. Continued production of RBP requires zinc and adequate intake of protein.

▶ **retinyl esters** The main storage form of vitamin A. It is one of the retinoids. Retinyl esters are retinol combined with fatty acids, usually palmitic acid. Also known as preformed vitamin A.

▶ **retinol-binding protein (RBP)** A carrier protein that binds to retinol and transports it in the bloodstream from the liver to destination cells.

Key Concepts Vitamin A occurs in three forms in the body: retinol, retinal, and retinoic acid. Each form of the vitamin has specific roles in the body. Most vitamin A is stored by the liver in the form of retinyl esters. Retinol-binding protein carries vitamin A in the bloodstream.

Functions of Vitamin A

Vitamin A is crucial for vision, for maintaining healthy cells (particularly skin cells), for fighting infections and bolstering immune function, and for promoting growth and development (see **FIGURE 10.6**). In addition, the provitamin A carotenoids might play a role in the prevention of cancer and other chronic diseases.

Vitamin A and Vision

When light enters the eye, it passes through the **cornea**, a transparent membrane, and hits the **retina**, the paper-thin tissues that line the back of the eye. The retina contains millions of light-sensitive cells called **rods** and **cones**. The rods react to dim light and process black-and-white images. The cones respond to bright light and translate it into color images. Within both rods and cones, a cascade of reactions converts light into a nerve signal the brain can process so we experience sight.

How does retinol become a functioning part of the retina? Retinol is carried in the blood to the retina, where it is converted to retinal (see **FIGURE 10.7**). Retinal, in turn, combines with the protein **opsin** to form a pigment known as **rhodopsin**. Rhodopsin is abundant in rod cells and makes it possible to see in dim light. When light strikes the retina, rod cells undergo a **bleaching process**, causing the color of the rod cells to fade. In this transformation, retinal separates from the opsin and undergoes a structural shift, from a "bent," or *cis*, configuration, to a "straightened," or *trans*, configuration. As the retinal detaches, the opsin changes shape as well, disrupting the activities in the cell membrane and generating an electrical impulse. This impulse is relayed to the brain, and you see a black-and-white image. Most of the retinal released in this process is quickly converted back to *trans*-retinol, and then to *cis*-retinal, which spontaneously recombines with opsin. The re-formed rhodopsin can respond to light again and begin another cycle.

▶ **cornea** The transparent outer surface of the eye.

▶ **retina** A paper-thin tissue that lines the back of the eye and contains cells called rods and cones.

▶ **rods** Light-sensitive cells in the retina that react to dim light and transmit black-and-white images.

▶ **cones** Light-sensitive cells in the retina that are sensitive to bright light and translate it into color images.

▶ **opsin** A protein that combines with retinal to form rhodopsin in rod cells.

▶ **rhodopsin** Found in rod cells, a light-sensitive pigment molecule that consists of a protein called opsin combined with retinal.

▶ **bleaching process** A complex light-stimulated reaction in which rod cells lose color as rhodopsin is split into retinal and opsin.

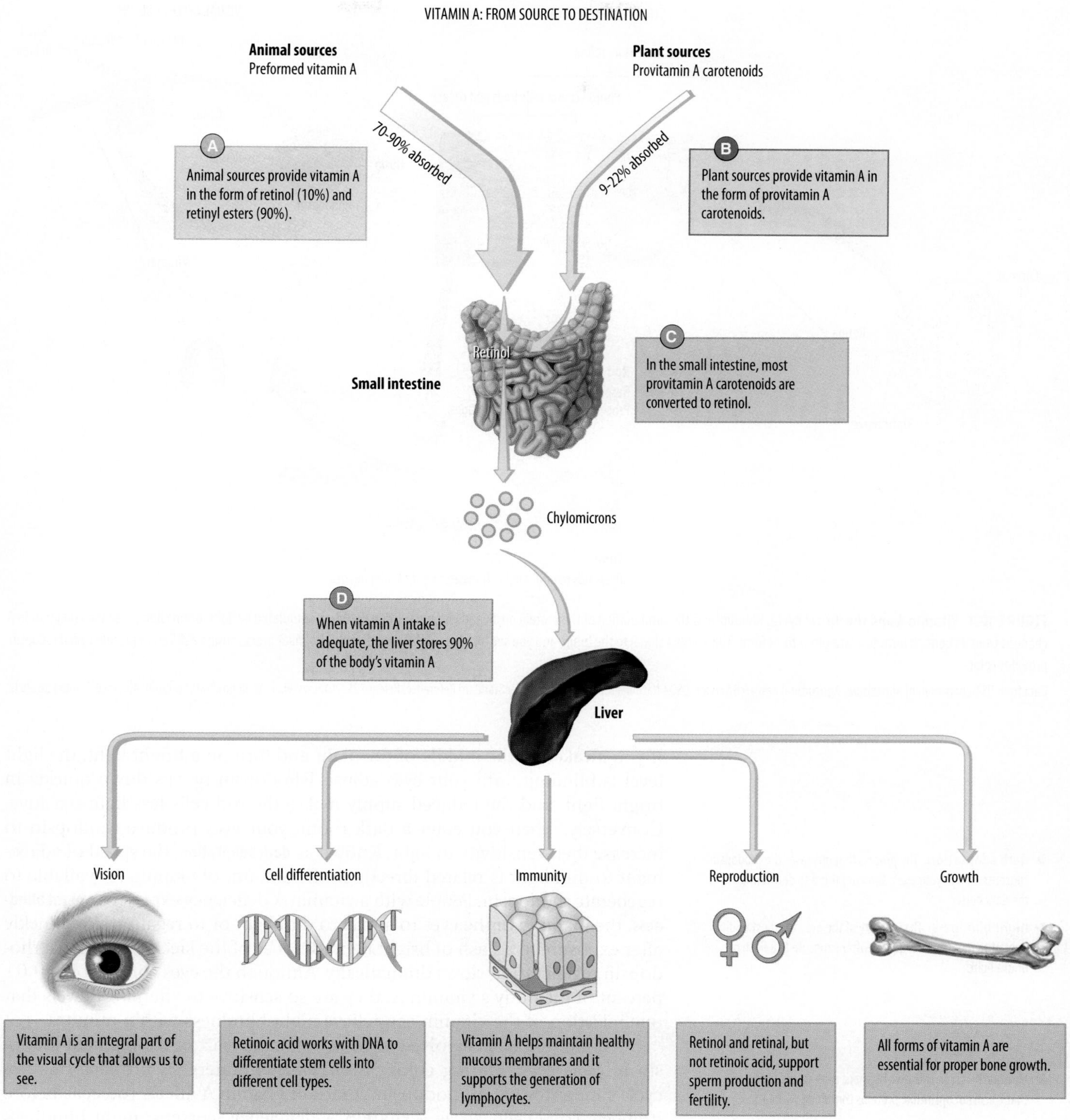

FIGURE 10.6 Vitamin A: from source to destination. Retinoids from animal foods and carotenoids from plant foods are absorbed from the small intestine and carried by chylomicrons to the liver. Vitamin A plays a crucial role in vision and is essential for proper cell synthesis, reproduction, and bone growth.

You've probably had the experience of stepping into a dark room and being unable to see until your eyes adjust. The familiar explanation for this, that you must wait for your pupils to dilate and let in more light, is only part of the story. Your eyes also adapt by changing the amount of available rhodopsin.

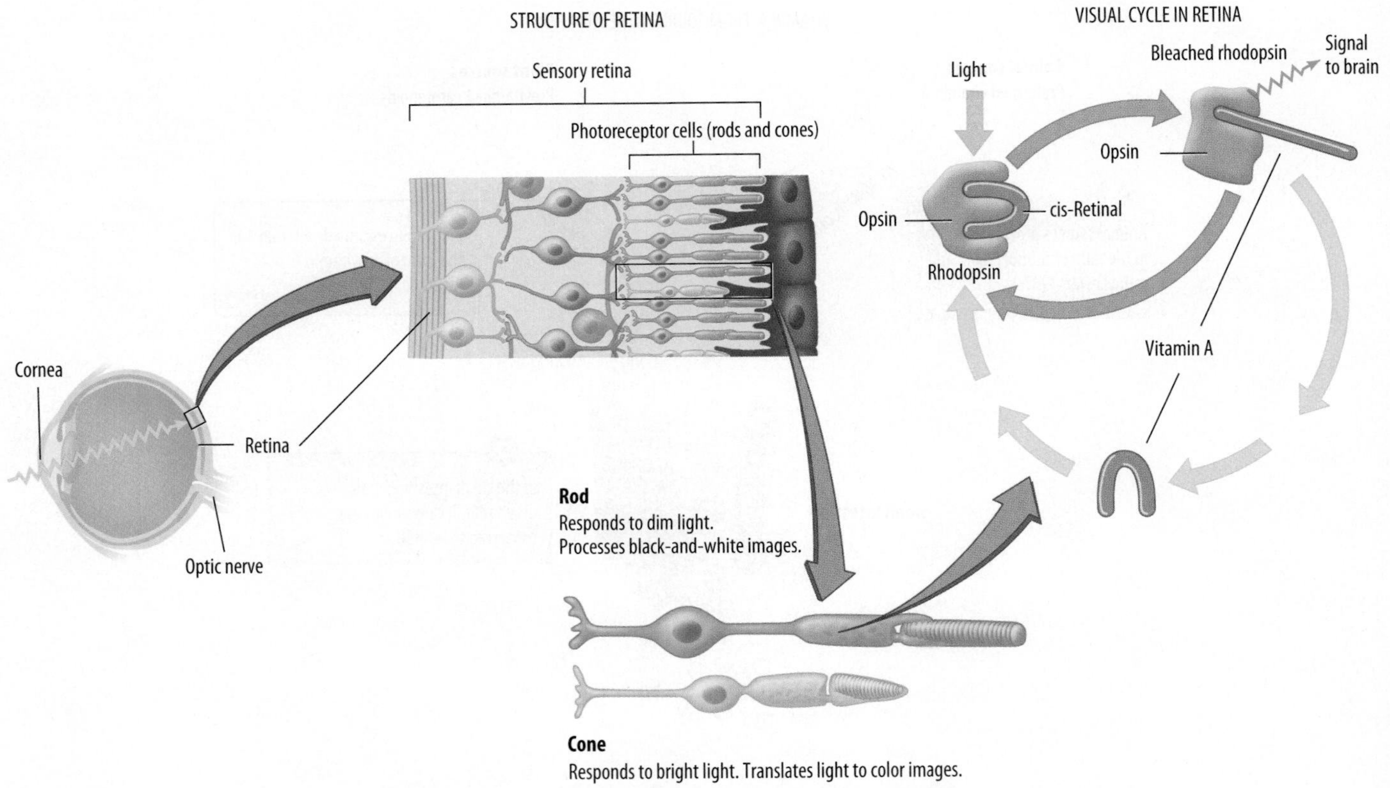

FIGURE 10.7 Vitamin A and the visual cycle. Rhodopsin is the combination of the protein opsin and vitamin A (retinal). When stimulated by light, opsin changes shape and vitamin A changes from its bent *cis* form to a straighter *trans* form. This sends a signal to the brain, and you see an image in black and white. A similar process using a different protein called iodopsin provides color.

Data from US Department of Agriculture, Agricultural Research Service. USDA National Nutrient Database for Standard Reference, Release 25. 2012. www.ars.usda.gov/ba/bhnrc/ndl. Accessed October 26, 2012.

If you awaken in the middle of the night and turn on a bright light, the light level is blinding until your eyes adjust. Rhodopsin breaks down quickly in bright light, and the reduced supply makes the rod cells less light-sensitive. Conversely, when you enter a dark room, your eyes produce rhodopsin to increase their sensitivity to light. Known as **dark adaptation**, the speed of adjustment to dim light is related directly to the amount of vitamin A available to regenerate rhodopsin. People with a vitamin A deficiency experience **night blindness**, the inability of the eyes to adjust to dim light or to regain vision quickly after exposure to a flash of bright light. Because of the lack of vitamin A, rhodopsin regeneration slows dramatically. Although the eyes contain only 0.01 percent of the body's vitamin A, they are so sensitive to vitamin A levels that one injection of the vitamin can relieve night blindness within minutes.[2]

THINK About It 4

▶ **dark adaptation** The process that increases the rhodopsin concentration in your eyes, allowing them to detect images in the dark better.

▶ **night blindness** The inability of the eyes to adjust to dim light or to regain vision quickly after exposure to a flash of bright light.

Vitamin A also is involved in color vision, as part of the pigment iodopsin in cone cells. During color vision, **iodopsin** undergoes a transformation cycle similar to that of rhodopsin. A lack of vitamin A affects rod cells before it affects cone cells, so as a vitamin A deficiency worsens, night blindness emerges before color blindness.

▶ **iodopsin** Color-sensitive pigment molecules in cone cells that consist of opsin-like proteins combined with retinal.

Vitamin A in Cell Differentiation

Vitamin A's role in vision is crucial, but this function uses only a small fraction of the body's vitamin A supply. A much larger proportion, in the form of retinoic acid, is put to work in normal **cell differentiation**, the process through which **stem cells** develop into highly specific types of cells with unique functions. Retinoic acid interacts with receptor sites on a cell's DNA—the genetic

▶ **cell differentiation** The process by which an immature cell develops into a specific type of mature cell.

▶ **stem cells** A formative cell whose daughter cells can differentiate into other cell types.

FYI For Your Information

A Short History of Vitamins

From roughly 1500 B.C.E. to 1900 C.E., there was an empirical understanding that some diseases (which we now call vitamin deficiency diseases) could be cured by eating certain foods. In about 400 B.C.E., the Greek physician Hippocrates, following the practice of Arab and Egyptian physicians, prescribed beef liver to people who were unable to see certain stars in the night sky. His maxim was "Let food be thy medicine," but he did not know that beef liver is a rich source of vitamin A, a fat-soluble vitamin necessary for vision.

Similarly, Native Americans knew empirically that extracts of pine needles could prevent or cure scurvy, a condition that includes bleeding gums and loss of energy. In 1753, James Lind, a Scottish surgeon, urged the British navy to include lemon juice in the diet of sailors to prevent scurvy. The navy finally adopted this practice 40 years later. In 1865, they substituted limes, which gave British sailors their nickname "limeys." We now know that the pine needles and citrus fruits provide vitamin C, a water-soluble vitamin whose deficiency causes scurvy.

Many scientists began systematically studying deficiency diseases in the late nineteenth century. They induced "deficiency states" in animals or humans by depriving them of certain foods. The subjects were restored to health when they ate the withheld food. In 1880, the Dutch scientist Christiaan Eijkman, for instance, produced beriberi in chickens by feeding them only polished (white) rice. When he restored their normal food of unpolished (brown) rice, the chickens quickly recovered. We now know that thiamin, which is removed during polishing, is essential for the health of both man and bird.

In the early twentieth century, scientists began to use chemistry to isolate and identify the critical factors in food that relieved "deficiency states." In 1912, for instance, Casimir Funk isolated a nitrogen-containing compound (an amine) in rice hulls. When given to thiamin-deprived chickens in its pure form, this amine restored the birds to health. Because this compound was required for life (*vita*) and was nitrogen-containing (*amine*), Funk coined the term *vitamines* to describe these essential growth factors. Other vitamines, or vitamins, as they later came to be called, continued to be discovered, purified, and eventually synthesized.

The discovery and naming of vitamins did not proceed without false starts. Some candidate substances did not meet the test of time, and thus we have no vitamins F, G, H, I, or J. On the other hand, vitamin B turned out to be a group of water-soluble vitamins rather than a single vitamin, so today we have eight B vitamins. The last vitamin to be discovered was vitamin B_{12}, and it was not completely synthesized until 1972.

As the vitamins were being isolated and characterized, it became clear that many Americans were not getting enough vitamins, so the National Academy of Sciences established recommended vitamin intakes. Many foods, especially flour and breads, are now fortified or enriched with vitamins.

Today we are exploring the health effects of vitamins beyond simply preventing deficiency diseases. This phase started in 1955, when large doses of niacin were found to lower cholesterol levels. Intense research is exploring the potential of the antioxidant vitamins C and E and provitamin A carotenoids to slow aging and reduce risks for cancer, heart disease, age-related macular degeneration, and cataract formation. Several B vitamins are under investigation for their role in heart disease. Vitamins B_6, folate, and vitamin B_{12} affect the body's levels of the amino acid homocysteine, which was identified as an independent risk factor for coronary heart disease. The roles of vitamins D and K in bone density and cancer are also areas of current nutrition research.

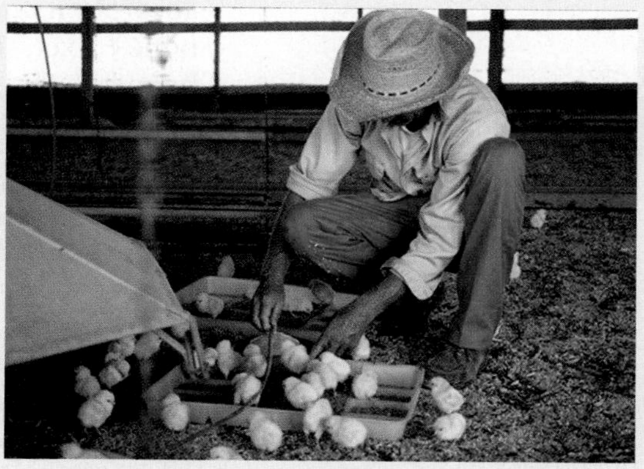

© Zoonar/Thinkstock

material that spurs production of particular proteins. Vitamin A, retinoic acid in particular, is required to turn on cell differentiation of many cells.

This retinoic acid–dependent differentiation can be seen in **epithelial cells**, the millions of cells that cover and protect the external and internal surfaces of the body as part of our skin and internal body tracts such as the respiratory system and the gastrointestinal tract[3] (see **FIGURE 10.8**). When epithelial cells differentiate, some develop into mucus-secreting cells (**goblet cells**). Mucous membranes provide lubrication where needed—for example, along bronchial tubes and the digestive tract. Epithelial cells are on the front line protecting your body, and they are destroyed and replaced relatively quickly. Replacing these

▶ **epithelial cells** The millions of cells that line and protect the external and internal surfaces of the body. Epithelial cells form epithelial tissues such as skin and mucous membranes.

▶ **goblet cells** One of the many types of specialized cells that produce and secrete mucus. These cells are found in the stomach, intestines, and portions of the respiratory tract.

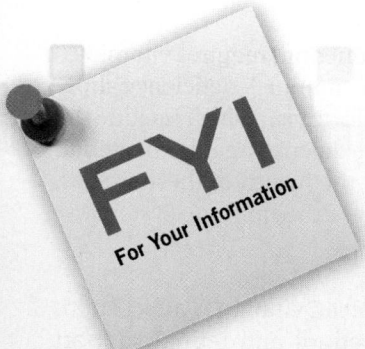

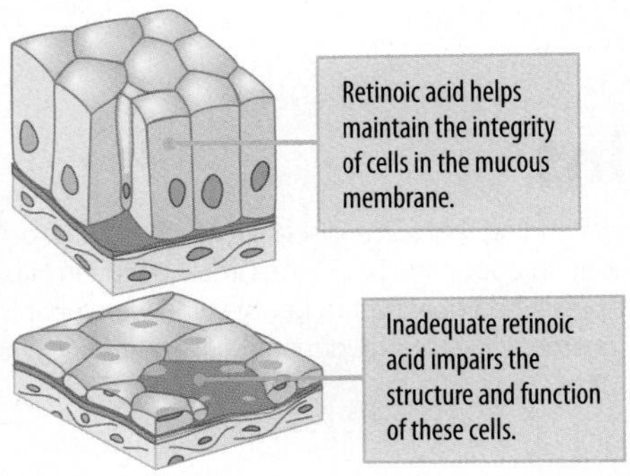

Retinoic acid helps maintain the integrity of cells in the mucous membrane.
Inadequate retinoic acid impairs the structure and function of these cells.

FIGURE 10.8 Mucous membrane integrity. Mucous membranes contain a higher percentage of goblet cells. Without retinoic acid, fewer stem cells become goblet cells, and these surfaces become hard and scaly.

▶ **epithelial tissues** Closely packed layers of epithelial cells that cover the body and line its cavities.

cells, as well as maintaining normal structure and function, requires vitamin A. Because the turnover of skin cells is rapid, signs of vitamin A deficiency show up early in the skin and mucous membranes. **Epithelial tissues**, which include the skin and mucous membranes, are the first line of defense against bacterial, parasitic, and viral attack. By helping to maintain the health of these tissues, vitamin A plays an important role in the integrity of the immune system.

Vitamin A and Reproduction

Although the exact biochemical mechanism is unclear, vitamin A affects both male and female reproductive processes. Both retinol and retinal support reproduction, but retinoic acid does not. In men, vitamin A supports the production of sperm; in women, it helps maintain fertility, possibly by supporting the production of reproductive tract secretions.

Vitamin A and Bone Health

Vitamin A (retinol, retinal, and retinoic acid) is needed for both bone growth and bone remodeling. As with the reproductive system, the exact mechanism is unclear, but a lack of vitamin A causes bones to weaken, although they also become thicker than normal. This may be the result of a disruption of the bone remodeling process and the failure of immature bone cells to develop properly. In a growing child, a lack of vitamin A disrupts bone remodeling and interferes with the development of immature bone cells, resulting in weak, poorly formed bones. On the other end of the spectrum, too much vitamin A has been linked to bone loss and an increased risk of fracture. Excessive amounts of vitamin A can interfere with the ability of vitamin D to promote calcium absorption and can trigger an increase in cellular activity that breaks down bone.[4] Excessive vitamin A intake also has been linked to increased risk of bone loss and hip fracture.[5]

Key Concepts Vitamin A plays a crucial role in vision as part of the compound rhodopsin in the rod cells of the retina. When light hits the retina, rhodopsin separates, changes shape, and sends a nerve impulse to the brain. When vitamin A is inadequate, the lack of rhodopsin makes it difficult to see in dim light. Vitamin A also is involved in cell differentiation, growth and development, immune function, reproduction, and bone health.

▶ **retinol activity equivalents (RAEs)** A unit of measurement of the vitamin A content of a food. One RAE equals 1 microgram (μg) of retinol.

▶ **preformed vitamin A** Retinyl esters, the main storage form of vitamin A. About 90 percent of dietary retinol is in the form of esters, mostly found in foods from animal sources.

Dietary Recommendations for Vitamin A

Similar amounts of dietary retinoids and carotenoids do not provide the same amount of vitamin A. To develop dietary recommendations, scientists reconciled this difference by creating a standardized measurement based on retinol, called **retinol activity equivalents (RAEs)**. One RAE is the amount of a given form of vitamin A equal to the activity of 1 microgram (1/1,000,000 of a gram) of retinol. Using this standard, 12 micrograms (μg) of beta-carotene equals 1 RAE, and 24 micrograms of other carotenoids yield 1 RAE[6] (see **FIGURE 10.9**).

Most Americans take in adequate amounts of vitamin A and have large stores of the vitamin in their livers. The RDA for vitamin A for males aged 14 years and older is 900 micrograms RAE. For females aged 14 years and older, the vitamin A RDA is 700 micrograms RAE. Pregnant women should consume slightly more vitamin A (770 micrograms), and lactating women are advised to consume 1,300 micrograms RAE.[7]

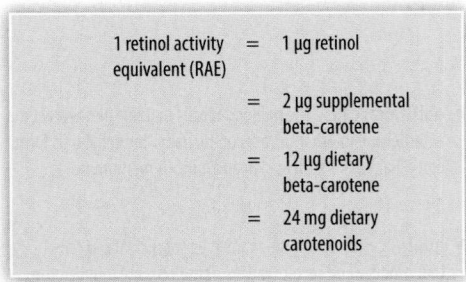

1 retinol activity equivalent (RAE)	=	1 μg retinol
	=	2 μg supplemental beta-carotene
	=	12 μg dietary beta-carotene
	=	24 mg dietary carotenoids

FIGURE 10.9 Retinol equivalents conversion.

Sources of Vitamin A

Most dietary vitamin A comes from animal food sources as **preformed vitamin A**, the retinoids (including retinyl esters, which are the main storage form

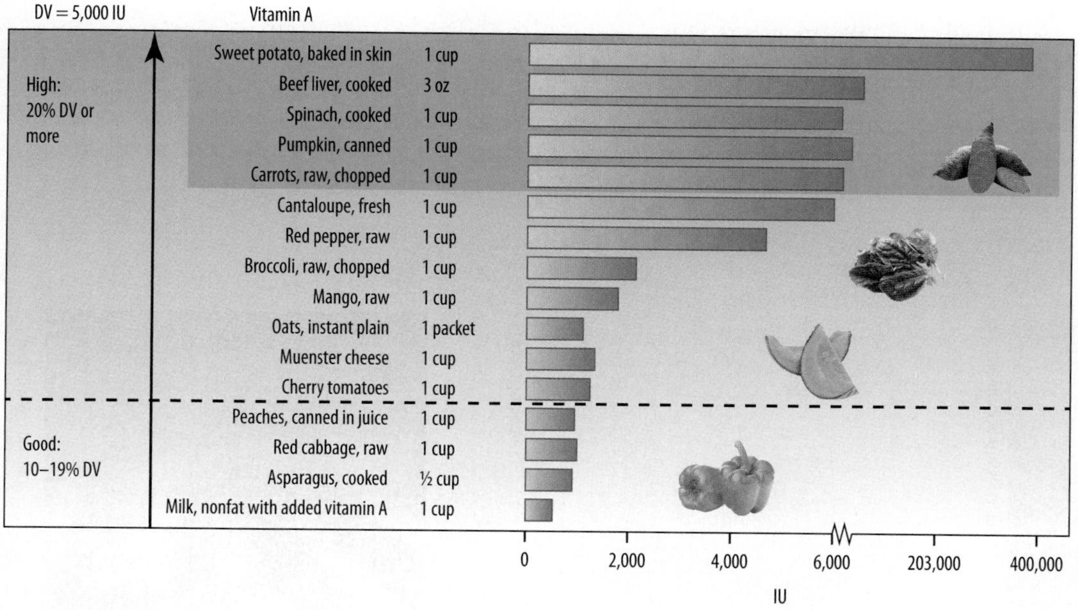

FIGURE 10.10 Food sources of vitamin A. Vitamin A is found as retinol in animal foods and as beta-carotene and other carotenoids in plant foods. Some of the best sources are liver, orange and deep-yellow vegetables, and dark-green leafy vegetables. This figure and others like it reference the Daily Value standard used on food labels. By law, a food may be labeled a "Good Source" of a nutrient if it contains 10 to 19 percent of the Daily Value for that nutrient, and it is a "High Source" if it contains 20 percent or more of the Daily Value. Units are IU to be consistent with Daily Value definitions.

Data from US Department of Agriculture, Agricultural Research Service, Nutrient Data Laboratory. USDA National Nutrient Database for Standard Reference, Release 28. Version Current: September 2015. Internet: http://www.ars.usda.gov/nea/bhnrc/ndl.

Photos (from top to bottom): (sweet potoato) © Kroeger/Gross/Getty Images; (spinach leaves) © dionisvero/Getty Images Inc.; (fresh cantaloupe) © Ursula Alter/Getty images, Inc.; (red pepper) © Nattika/Shutterstock, Inc.

of vitamin A). One-quarter to one-third of our dietary vitamin A intake comes from fruits and vegetables in the form of provitamin A carotenoids, especially beta-carotene.[8] **FIGURE 10.10** shows foods that are good sources of vitamin A.

Retinoids are found naturally only in animal foods. About 10 percent of vitamin A content is in the form of retinol, and the remaining 90 percent is retinyl esters. Liver and fish liver oils (e.g., cod liver oil) are among the top sources. Milk fat (as in whole milk, butter, and other dairy products) also contains vitamin A. Foods fortified with vitamin A (in the form of retinyl palmitate or retinyl acetate) include margarine, some breakfast cereals, and reduced-fat milks. Reduced-fat milks that are not fortified vary greatly in vitamin A content (e.g., unfortified nonfat milk contains no vitamin A). Products that are made from reduced-fat or skim milk, such as yogurt, are not generally fortified with vitamin A. The body absorbs about 75 percent of dietary retinol and retinyl esters.

The best sources of provitamin A carotenoids are dark-green and yellow-orange vegetables, such as carrots, spinach, broccoli, squash, sweet potatoes, and some orange-colored fruits such as cantaloupes, peaches, apricots, and mangos. In a varied diet, beta-carotene supplies about one-third the total vitamin A, even though the body absorbs this provitamin less efficiently than it can absorb retinol or retinyl esters. For more information about carotenoids, see "The Carotenoids" section later in this chapter.

Quick Bite

Vitamin A Isn't Just for Eyes

A study conducted in Nepal showed that women who took vitamin A supplements during pregnancy had a much lower risk of maternal mortality than those who took a placebo. The researchers concluded that regular and adequate intake of vitamin A or beta-carotene can reduce the risk of pregnancy-related death in areas where vitamin A deficiency is common.

Key Concepts Intake recommendations for vitamin A are expressed in RAEs (retinol activity equivalents) to account for the differences in bioavailability between retinoids and carotenoids. Current recommendations suggest that adult men consume 900 micrograms RAE each day; the recommendation for adult women is 700 micrograms RAE. Retinol is available from a few animal foods such as liver, fish liver oils, milk fat, and egg yolks. Vitamin A can also be formed from precursor compounds called carotenoids, which are found in some yellow-orange fruits and in dark-green and yellow-orange vegetables.

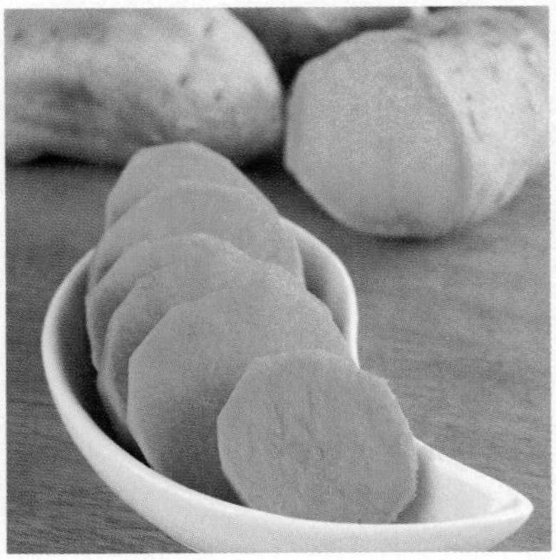

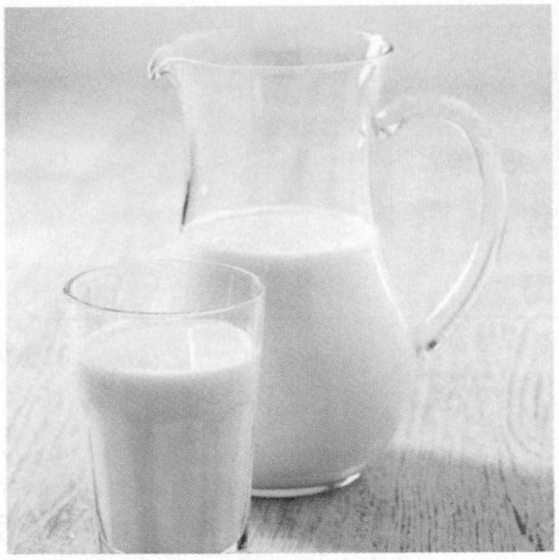

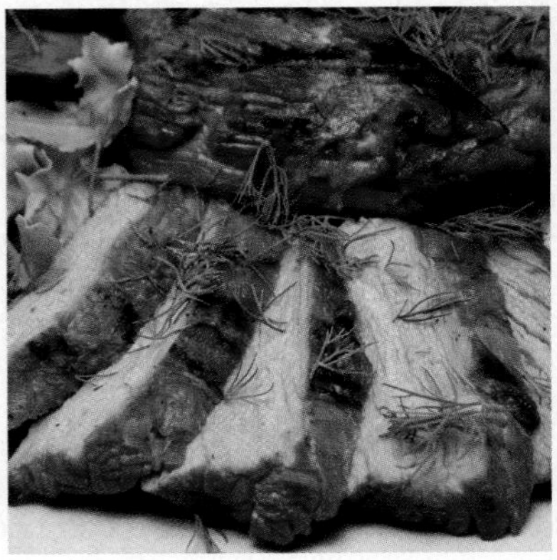

Vitamin A Deficiency

Although dietary deficiency of vitamin A is rare in North America and western Europe, it is the leading cause of childhood blindness worldwide, especially in Southeast Asia, parts of Africa, India, and Central and South America. In these regions, vitamin A deficiency typically occurs alongside general protein-energy malnutrition in infants and young children. It is estimated that 500,000 preschool-aged children worldwide become blind each year as a result of vitamin A deficiency (see **FIGURE 10.11**). Vitamin A deficiency retards growth and development and leads to bone deformities.

Although few Americans suffer from a vitamin A deficiency, certain groups are at risk. Newborns, especially premature infants, are at risk because their liver stores of vitamin A are low. Because their diets lack vitamin A–rich foods, impoverished people, particularly children and older adults, can suffer marginal vitamin A status. People with alcoholism or liver disease are at risk because their damaged livers might be incapable of storing much vitamin A. Medicines that alter lipid absorption inhibit vitamin A absorption, too. People who have chronic diarrhea, celiac disease, Crohn's disease, cystic fibrosis, or pancreatic insufficiency and other fat-malabsorption conditions can develop vitamin A deficiency over time. In the United States, vitamin A deficiency occurs most often in people who suffer from fat-malabsorption syndromes or severely restricted diets as seen in anorexia nervosa.

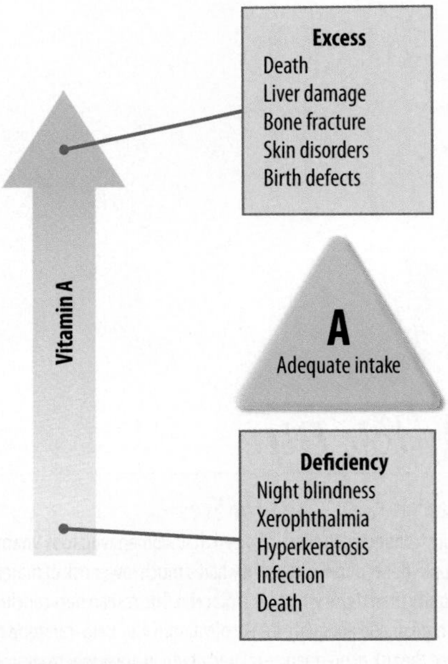

FIGURE 10.11 Vitamin A intake. A broad range of vitamin A intake is adequate and provides for normal function. Too much or too little vitamin A can have serious consequences.

Eyes

Night blindness is an early symptom of vitamin A deficiency and can be corrected completely with early treatment. As the deficiency worsens, the lack of retinoic acid interferes with the normal differentiation of epithelial cells and reduces the formation of mucus-secreting goblet cells. As mucus production drops, the cornea and conjunctiva (the outer surface of the eye) and the mucous membrane lining the inner surface of the eyelid become extremely dry. The lack of mucus prevents the eye from washing away dirt and bacteria, thus increasing the likelihood of infection. As the cornea deteriorates, foamy, white triangular patches known as Bitot's spots develop. Eventually, irreversible scars form on the cornea, which also develops ulcers and sometimes liquefies during the final stages of deterioration. Collectively, these symptoms that progress toward total blindness are known as **xerophthalmia**. Unlike night blindness, which can be reversed with a single dose of vitamin A, corneal drying and scarring usually are permanent.

▶ **xerophthalmia** A condition caused by vitamin A deficiency that dries the cornea and mucous membranes of the eye.

Skin

A lack of retinoic acid shifts the differentiation of epithelial cells toward the production of skin cells. This increased supply packs the skin with extra cells, increasing the density and making the skin hard and scaly. An early symptom of vitamin A deficiency is follicular **hyperkeratosis**, or "goose flesh." In this condition, the hair follicles on the skin become plugged with keratin, a protein normally present only on the outermost surface of the skin. As a result, the skin becomes rough and bumpy. Sweat glands lose their ability to secrete perspiration. Typically, hyperkeratosis causes thickening of the palms and soles, as well as attacking the flexure areas (elbows, knees, wrists, and ankles) of the skin. In advanced stages, the entire body can be involved.

▶ **hyperkeratosis** Excessive accumulation of the protein keratin that produces rough and bumpy skin, most commonly affecting the palms and soles, as well as flexure areas (elbows, knees, wrists, ankles). It can affect moist epithelial tissues and impair their ability to secrete mucus. Also called hyperkeratinization.

Other Epithelial Cells

Hyperkeratosis affects other types of epithelial cells and disrupts their ability to secrete mucus. This particularly affects the mouth, respiratory tract, urinary tract, female genital tract, seminal vesicles of the testes, and glands of the eyes, making them vulnerable to infection. In men, a vitamin A deficiency halts the production of sperm. Women can become infertile, possibly as a result of disruptions in the production of reproductive tract secretions. Hyperkeratinization near sensory receptors causes a loss of taste and smell, which in turn can cause loss of appetite and weight.

Immune Function

Vitamin A deficiency leaves a person especially vulnerable to infection as the damaged epithelium allows microorganisms to breach this first line of defense. Invading microorganisms attack the weakened respiratory tract, mucous membranes, and skin.

Under ordinary circumstances, entry of these enemy invaders would then trigger protective immune cells to quickly multiply. But immune cells need vitamin A to multiply. With too few immune cells to mount an effective counterattack, the invading microorganisms can cause severe, even fatal, diarrhea or respiratory infection.

Children with mild vitamin A deficiencies run a high risk of diarrhea, respiratory tract infections, and measles. When a child is deficient in vitamin A, a relatively harmless infection such as measles can be fatal.[9]

Vitamin A Toxicity

For adults, including adult women who are pregnant or breastfeeding, the Tolerable Upper Intake Level (UL) for vitamin A is 3,000 micrograms RAE as retinol. Vitamin A toxicity occurs infrequently, but as more people take megadoses of nutritional supplements, the potential for toxic overdoses increases. With the exception of a sustained diet of large amounts of liver or fish oils, food alone generally cannot supply massive amounts of vitamin A. Children are more vulnerable to toxicity, and overenthusiastic supplementation of vitamin A is dangerous and can be fatal. Consumption of large amounts of fish liver oil has been found to cause vitamin A toxicity in children.[10]

Vitamin A toxicity has a wide range of symptoms, both subtle and overt, including fatigue, vomiting, abdominal pain, bone and joint pain, hip fracture, loss of appetite, skin disorders, headache, blurred or double vision, and liver damage, which in turn leads to jaundice. Toxicity symptoms can often be corrected when intake levels are lowered.

▶ **teratogen** Any substance that causes birth defects.

Preformed vitamin A, taken in excess, is a known **teratogen**. Birth defects associated with vitamin A toxicity include cleft palate, heart abnormalities, and brain malfunction.[11] Excess vitamin A is most hazardous when taken during the two weeks prior to conception and the first two months of pregnancy. The embryo is undergoing a great deal of cell differentiation, and excess amounts of vitamin A appear to interfere with the vitamin's normal support of this process. An acute excess intake of vitamin A as retinol during pregnancy also can cause spontaneous abortions. Pregnant women should avoid prenatal supplements that contain retinol and instead use those that have beta-carotene as the vitamin A source. Although large doses of beta-carotene (provitamin A) can cause the harmless condition carotenodermia, yellowing of the skin from carotenoids, they do not seem to cause any serious side effects. Conversion of beta-carotene to retinol occurs relatively slowly, and its absorption decreases as dietary intake increases.

Acne Treatment

Up to 90 percent of boys and up to 80 percent of girls experience acne during adolescence, making it the most common skin ailment seen by physicians. The disease has a wide spectrum, ranging from just a few transient pimples to large, chronic, painful nodules that scar when healing.

Retinoic acid is the most commonly prescribed treatment to reduce the formation of blackheads and whiteheads. Retin-A (all-*trans*-retinoic acid) is available for topical use (applied to the skin). Accutane (13-*cis*-retinoic acid) is taken orally. These medications, like any large dose of vitamin A, cause birth defects, so any woman who might become pregnant should not take them. Because retinoids accumulate in fat stores, even from topical administration, these medications should be discontinued at least two years before becoming pregnant.

Quick Bite

Avoid Polar Bear Liver

Liver and onions might be your favorite meal, but don't use polar bear liver. Polar bear liver is so rich in vitamin A that a single serving can be toxic for humans.

Key Concepts Deficiency of vitamin A results in progressive vision loss from temporary night blindness, to reversible blindness, and finally to permanent blindness. In addition, the lack of mucus secretions and reduced immune function make the person with vitamin A deficiency vulnerable to infections. Vitamin A toxicity can result from the use of supplements, even with dosages just a few times higher than the RDA. The consequences of vitamin A toxicity during pregnancy are potentially devastating, and pregnant women should avoid both retinol-containing supplements and medications made from retinoids, such as Accutane and Retin-A.

The Carotenoids

Carotenoids are naturally occurring compounds that give the deep yellow, orange, and red colors to fruits and vegetables such as apricots, carrots, and tomatoes. Carotenoids also are abundant in dark-green vegetables, such as spinach, but the carotenoid colors are hidden by the plentiful green pigment chlorophyll. Although researchers have identified hundreds of carotenoids, only a small portion are typically found in the U.S. diet, and even less are found in blood samples and human milk.[12] The major carotenoids are alpha-carotene, beta-carotene, lutein, zeaxanthin, cryptoxanthin, and lycopene. The yellow-orange pigment beta-carotene, which lends its color to cantaloupe, carrots, and squash, is the most common carotenoid. The body can convert alpha-carotene, beta-carotene, and beta-cryptoxanthin to retinol, so they are

TABLE 10.3
Common Carotenoids

Class/Components	Source[a]	Potential Benefits	Tips for Including Healthful Components in the Diet
Beta-carotene	Carrots, pumpkin, sweet potato, cantaloupe	Neutralizes free radicals, which may damage cells; bolsters cellular antioxidant defenses; can be made into vitamin A in the body	For beta-carotene–rich french fries: thinly slice sweet potatoes and coat with olive oil or fat-free cooking spray, add spices to taste (pepper, rosemary, thyme), and bake in a 425°F oven until golden brown on both sides (10–15 minutes). Time-saver: buy precut sweet potatoes in the frozen foods section.
Lutein, zeaxanthin	Kale, collards, spinach, corn, eggs, citrus	May contribute to maintenance of healthy vision	Freezing kale can bring out a sweeter, more flavorful taste. For an easy sautéed side dish, try this simple recipe: add kale to a skillet with oil and garlic, slivered almonds, and red pepper flakes. If kale doesn't top your list of food preferences, spinach, which provides the same health benefits, can be an easy substitute. Did you know that many multivitamin and -mineral dietary supplements include lutein?
Lycopene	Tomatoes and processed tomato products, watermelon, red/pink grapefruit	May contribute to maintenance of prostate health	Research shows lycopene is best absorbed by the body when consumed from tomatoes that have been cooked using a small amount of oil. This includes products such as tomato sauce and tomato paste. Try adding 1 cup tomato sauce to sautéed zucchini for a fun and colorful side dish! Don't like the bitter taste of grapefruit? Try sprinkling on a little sugar or a low-calorie sweetener, or even a pinch of salt before eating one to bring out the rich natural sweetness within.

[a] Examples are not an all-inclusive list.

Note: Preformed vitamin A is found in foods that come from animals. Provitamin A carotenoids are found in many darkly colored fruits and vegetables and are a major source of vitamin A for vegetarians.

Data from International Food Information Council Foundation. Functional foods component chart. 2009. http://www.foodinsight.org/Content/6/FINAL-IFIC-Fndtn-Functional-Foods-Backgrounder-with-Tips-and-changes-03-11-09.pdf. Accessed January 7, 2016.

called provitamin A carotenoids. Other carotenoids, such as lycopene, lutein, and zeaxanthin, have no vitamin A activity, so they are called nonprovitamin A carotenoids. See **TABLE 10.3**, which details the common carotenoids.

FUNCTIONS OF CAROTENOIDS

Although carotenoids have diverse biological functions independent of their conversion to vitamin A, there is no evidence that carotenoids are essential nutrients in the technical sense. Because no other specific nutrient functions have been identified for any of the carotenoids, the Food and Nutrition Board has not established Dietary Reference Intakes (DRIs) for carotenoids.[13] However, carotenoids have roles in fighting free radicals, bolstering immune function, enhancing vision, and preventing cancer.

Carotenoids as Antioxidants Beta-carotene and other carotenoids function as potent antioxidants—substances that can interfere with the damaging effects of free radicals, which are highly unstable, reactive compounds.

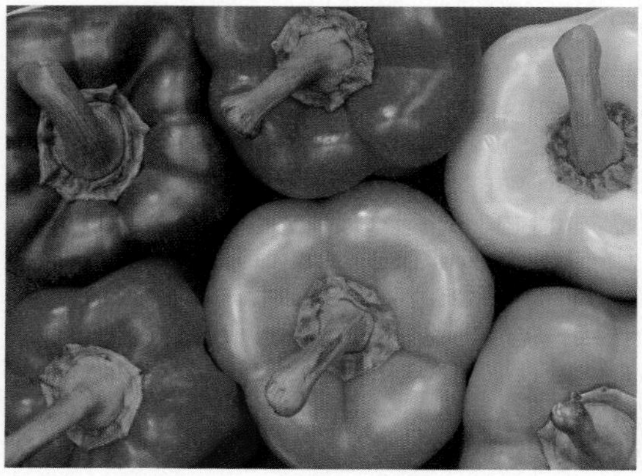

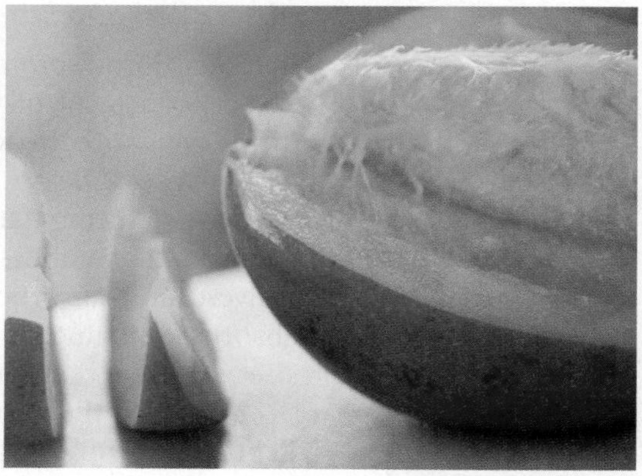

Free radicals can damage both the structure and function of cell membranes, nucleic acids, and electron-dense regions of proteins. There is an ongoing demand for dietary antioxidants to prevent and reduce the oxidative damage from free radicals.[14] This damage may form the biological basis of several diseases associated with aging. People who eat generous amounts of foods rich in carotenoids reduce their risk of many major degenerative conditions such as premature aging, cancer, atherosclerosis, cataracts, age-related macular degeneration (AMD), bone loss, and diabetes.[15] Carotenoids are potent antioxidants, which might explain their beneficial effects. For more information about free radicals and antioxidants, see the section titled "Vitamin E" later in this chapter.

Carotenoids and Vision Macular degeneration is the leading cause of age-related blindness and affects approximately 50 million people worldwide.[16] Higher intake of carotenoids, especially lutein and zeaxanthin, from foods or supplements may play an important role in protecting vision.[17] Lutein and its close relative zeaxanthin are found in the macula, the central portion of the retina that is responsible for sharp and detailed vision. One theory is that carotenoids protect the eyes by inhibiting the oxidative damage that contributes to age-related blindness.[18] Studies have found that a supplement combination containing carotenoids and other antioxidants can slow the progression of AMD[19] and that people with the highest intakes of lutein and zeaxanthin also have a decreased risk of cataracts.[20] Although the precise mechanism of action by which nutrients function in preventing AMD remains unclear, an overall healthy diet is widely supported as the best strategy for reducing the risk of its development.[21]

Carotenoids and Cancer In addition to providing antioxidant protection from free-radical cell membrane and DNA damage, certain carotenoids, including lycopene and beta-carotene, can strengthen growth-regulatory signals between cells and help prevent damaged cells from reproducing and forming tumors. People with the highest intakes of carotenoid-rich fruits and vegetables and/or high blood levels of specific carotenoids usually have the lowest risk for certain types of cancer. Tomato products, for example, are excellent sources of lycopene, and research suggests that a diet rich in tomato products reduces the risk of heart disease, osteoporosis, and several cancers.[22]

The beneficial effects of carotenoids on health generally reflect food intake, rather than isolated carotenoid supplementation. To date, trials of beta-carotene supplements for cancer prevention have been disappointing; paradoxically, megadose supplements are associated with increased lung cancer among smokers or those exposed to asbestos.[23]

Quick Bite

And They Called It Cantaloupe

The word *cantaloupe* comes from a papal garden in a small town near Rome named Cantaloupo. One-half of a medium cantaloupe has 466 RAE as beta-carotene.

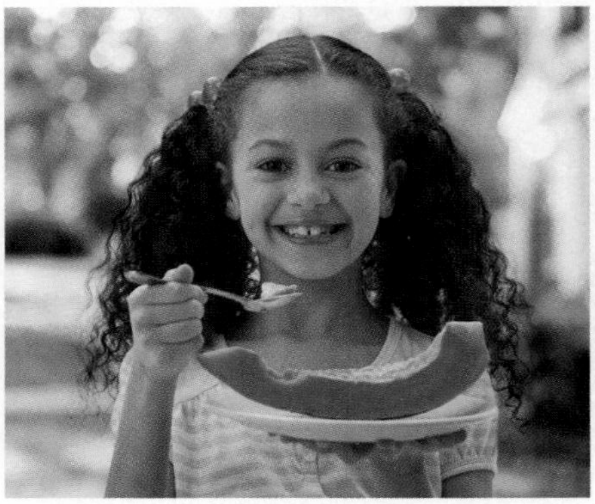

© Amble Design/Shutterstock, Inc.

Absorption and Storage of Carotenoids

In foods, fibrous proteins tightly bind carotenoids, so your body absorbs only 20 to 40 percent of what you consume (see **FIGURE 10.12**). This proportion drops even further—to 10 percent or less—as the amount of carotenoids you eat increases. Dietary fat, protein, and vitamin E enhance carotenoid absorption. When dietary fat enters the small intestine, bile is secreted, which helps emulsify the fat and enhances the absorption of carotenoids. Intestinal cells convert most absorbed carotenoids to vitamin A and deliver the remaining absorbed and unchanged carotenoids to the lymph and eventually the bloodstream, where they circulate bound to lipoproteins.

Although the liver and adipose tissue are the primary carotenoid storage depots, the kidneys, adrenal glands, and other fatty tissues throughout the body also contain carotenoids.[24] Extremely large intakes of carotenoid-rich

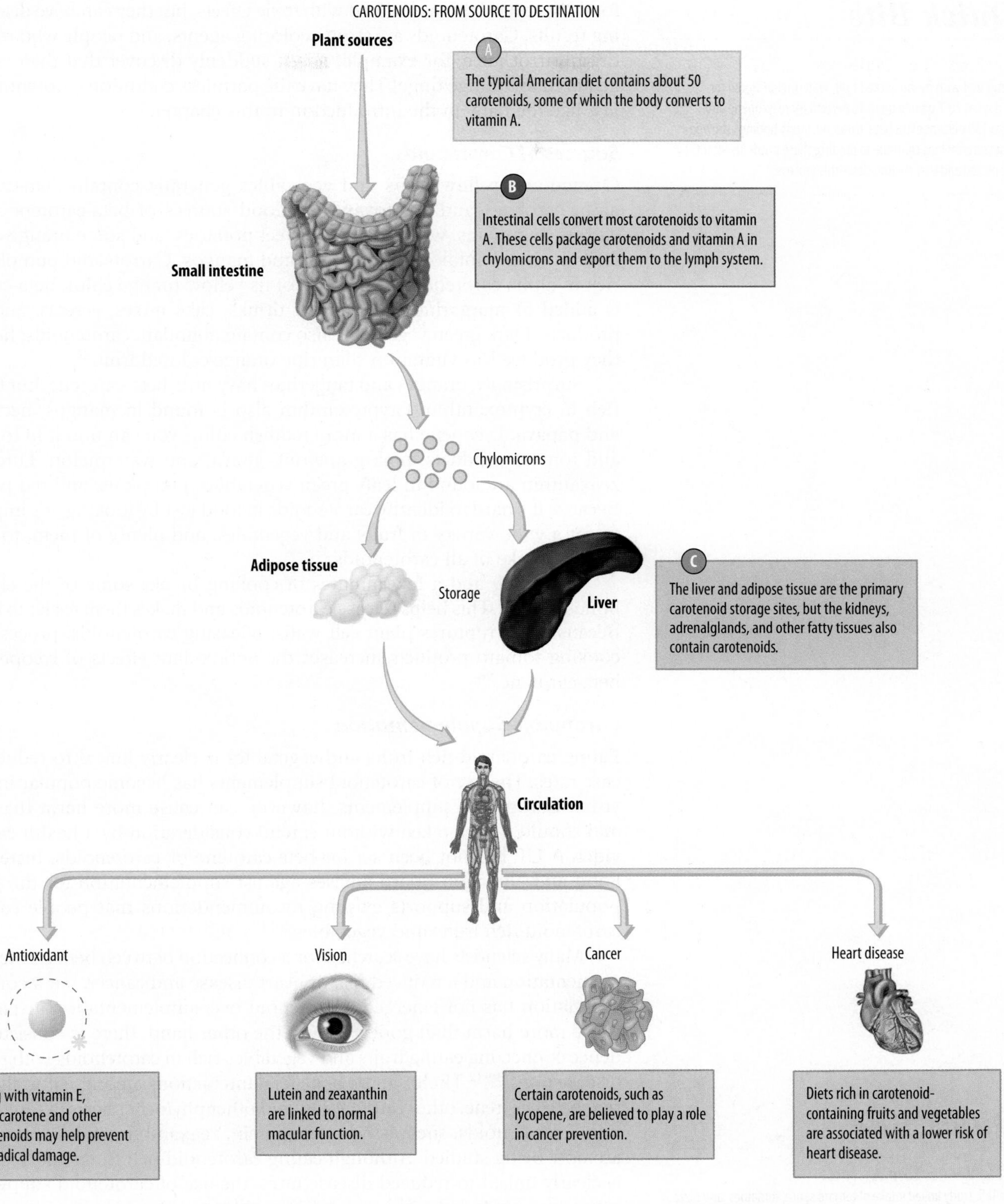
CAROTENOIDS: FROM SOURCE TO DESTINATION
Plant sources
A
The typical American diet contains about 50 carotenoids, some of which the body converts to vitamin A.
B
Intestinal cells convert most carotenoids to vitamin A. These cells package carotenoids and vitamin A in chylomicrons and export them to the lymph system.
Small intestine
Chylomicrons
Adipose tissue
Storage
Liver
C
The liver and adipose tissue are the primary carotenoid storage sites, but the kidneys, adrenalglands, and other fatty tissues also contain carotenoids.
Circulation
Antioxidant
Vision
Cancer
Heart disease
Along with vitamin E, beta-carotene and other carotenoids may help prevent free radical damage.
Lutein and zeaxanthin are linked to normal macular function.
Certain carotenoids, such as lycopene, are believed to play a role in cancer prevention.
Diets rich in carotenoid-containing fruits and vegetables are associated with a lower risk of heart disease.

FIGURE 10.12 Carotenoids: from source to destination. In the body, the provitamin A carotenoids alpha-carotene, beta-carotene, and beta-cryptoxanthin can be converted to retinol. The nonprovitamin A carotenoids lycopene, lutein, and zeaxanthin have no vitamin A activity. Independent of vitamin A activity, carotenoids can function as antioxidants and may be involved in normal macular function and reduced risk of heart disease and cancer.

Quick Bite

The Production Continues

Compared with freshly picked fruit, watermelon stored for 14 days at 70°F gained up to 40 percent more lycopene and 50 to 139 percent extra beta-carotene. Study findings showed that watermelons continue to produce these nutrients after they are picked and that chilling slows this process.

foods have not been associated with toxic effects, but they can have disconcerting results. Carotenoids are strong coloring agents, and people who regularly drink carrot juice, for example, might suddenly discover that their skin has acquired an orange tinge! They have the harmless condition carotenodermia, just like the baby in the introduction to this chapter.

Sources of Carotenoids

Orange and yellow fruits and vegetables generally contain beta-carotene, alpha-carotene, and cryptoxanthin. Good sources of beta-carotene include carrots, pumpkins, winter squash, sweet potatoes, and some orange-colored fruits such as cantaloupes, apricots, and mangos. Carrots and pumpkins are rich in alpha-carotene, too. Because of its yellow-orange color, beta-carotene is added to margarine, gelatin, soft drinks, cake mixes, cereals, and other products. Dark-green vegetables also contain abundant carotenoids; however, they produce less vitamin A than ripe orange-colored fruit.[25]

Surprisingly, oranges and tangerines have little beta-carotene, but they are rich in cryptoxanthin. Cryptoxanthin also is found in mangos, nectarines, and papaya. Lycopene has a more reddish color; you can find it in tomatoes and tomato products, pink grapefruit, guava, and watermelon. Lutein and zeaxanthin are found in leafy green vegetables, pumpkins, and red peppers. Because it's hard to identify carotenoids in food just by looking, it's important to eat a wide variety of fruits and vegetables, and plenty of them, to ensure a good intake of all carotenoids.

Chopping and a few minutes of cooking breaks some of the chemical bonds in food. This helps release carotenoids and makes them easier to absorb. Because heat ruptures plant cell walls, releasing carotenoids, processing or cooking tomato products increases the antioxidant effects of lycopene and beta-carotene.[26]

Carotenoid Supplementation

Eating carotenoid-rich fruits and vegetables is clearly linked to reduced disease rates. The use of carotenoid supplements has become popular in recent years. Carotenoid supplements, however, can cause more harm than good and should not be taken without careful consideration by a health care provider. A UL has not been set for beta-carotene or carotenoids. Instead, the Food and Nutrition Board advises against supplementation for the general population and supports existing recommendations that people eat more carotenoid-rich fruits and vegetables.[27]

Many scientists have searched for a connection between beta-carotene supplementation and a reduced risk of heart disease and cancer, but a consistent association has not emerged. Carotenoid oversupplementation actually can cause more harm than good.[28,29] On the other hand, there is consistent evidence connecting eating fruits and vegetables rich in carotenoids with reduced disease rates.[30-32] There can be beneficial interactions among naturally occurring beta-carotene, other carotenoids, and other phytochemicals in foods. Additional carotenoids, such as lycopene, lutein, zeaxanthin, and cryptoxanthin, are now being studied. Although eating carotenoid-rich fruits and vegetables is clearly linked to reduced disease rates, the use of carotenoid supplements is not recommended without careful consideration by a health care provider.

Quick Bite

Pizza Versus Tomato Juice

One U.S. study linked intake of tomato sauce, tomatoes, and pizza to lowered risk of prostate cancer. Tomato juice, however, was not protective. That's not surprising. According to John Erdman, PhD, of the University of Illinois at Urbana–Champaign, the cancer-fighting carotenoid found in tomatoes (lycopene) is a fat-soluble substance, so it needs some fat like that found in pizza and most pasta sauces to be absorbed. The lycopene in tomato juice, however, seems to be especially poorly absorbed.

Vitamin D

Sometimes called the sunshine vitamin, vitamin D is unique because, given sufficient sunlight, your body can synthesize all it needs of this fat-soluble nutrient. In fact, it could be argued that vitamin D is technically not a nutrient—it is synthesized and functions like a hormone, and it is not always necessary in the diet. When the ultraviolet rays of the sun strike the skin, they alter a precursor derived from cholesterol, converting it into vitamin D. Although fortified milk and other foods supply vitamin D, your body can make plenty as long as it gets regular exposure to sunlight.

Vitamin D is essential for bone health, and it protects against certain cancers, heart disease, and other chronic diseases. In children, it promotes bone development and growth. In adults, it is necessary for bone maintenance. In older adults, vitamin D and calcium supplementation helps prevent bone loss and fractures.[33] Desirable blood levels of vitamin D are currently under investigation to understand its role in the prevention of cardiovascular disease, type 2 diabetes, and cancer, and its role in immunity and muscular disorders.[34,35] Vitamin D may even help to reduce the risk of death in elderly people.[36] Although severe vitamin D deficiency in children and adults is rare, groups at risk for vitamin D deficiency include exclusively breastfed infants, patients with fat malabsorption, obese people, individuals with limited sunlight exposure, those with dark skin, and older adults.[37]

Forms and Formation of Vitamin D

Vitamin D can be considered either a vitamin or a hormone. Like other vitamins, a lack of dietary vitamin D (coupled with minimal sun exposure) causes a deficiency. The active form of vitamin D is like a hormone because it is made in one part of the body and regulates activities in other parts (see **FIGURE 10.13**).

Ten compounds, called vitamin D_1 through D_{10}, exhibit **antirachitic** properties; that is, they prevent a childhood bone disease called rickets. The most important of these compounds are D_2 (ergocalciferol) and D_3 (cholecalciferol). Ergocalciferol is found exclusively in plant foods. Cholecalciferol is found in animal foods (eggs and fish oils), but most is synthesized in the skin.

In the skin, ultraviolet (UV) radiation from the sun converts a cholesterol derivative (7-dehydrocholesterol) to cholecalciferol, which then enters the bloodstream and travels to the liver. The liver also receives dietary cholecalciferol and ergocalciferol from chylomicrons. In the liver, cholecalciferol and ergocalciferol are converted into calcidiol and then sent to the kidneys. The kidneys perform the final step—the formation of **1,25-dihydroxyvitamin D_3 [1,25$(OH)_2D_3$]**, also called **calcitriol**. 1,25$(OH)_2D_3$ is the active form of vitamin D.[38]

▶ **antirachitic** Pertaining to activities of an agent used to treat rickets.

▶ **1,25-dihydroxyvitamin D_3 [1,25$(OH)_2D_3$]** The active form of vitamin D. It is an important regulator of blood calcium levels.

▶ **calcitriol** See *1,25-dihydroxyvitamin D_3 [1,25$(OH)_2D_3$]*.

Functions of Vitamin D

Vitamin D is considered both a vitamin and a hormone. Many simply regard vitamin D as a vitamin that keeps bones healthy, but first and foremost vitamin D is a regulatory compound. Although its primary role is to regulate blood calcium levels, vitamin D also is important for regulating cell differentiation and growth. Because vitamin D made in one part of the body regulates activities in other parts, scientists consider it a hormone. Vitamin D has a role in preventing cancer cells from dividing and has anti-inflammatory properties. As such, it might play a role in preventing cancer and cardiovascular disease, an area of considerable research activity.[39] Vitamin D also is involved in the regulation of insulin formation and secretion, which suggests a role in blood sugar maintenance and the development of type 2 diabetes mellitus—another area of current research interest.[40]

Regulation of Blood Calcium Levels

The liver and adipose tissues store vitamin D. In times of need, the liver and kidneys convert stored vitamin D to 1,25$(OH)_2D_3$, the biologically active form in the body. The 1,25$(OH)_2D_3$ helps maintain calcium and phosphorus

Quick Bite

A Fishy Cure

Cod liver oil was well known in the early nineteenth century as a treatment for rickets, a bone disease common in children. It wasn't until the early 1900s, however, that vitamin D was identified as the "antirachitic" (antirickets) substance in cod liver oil.

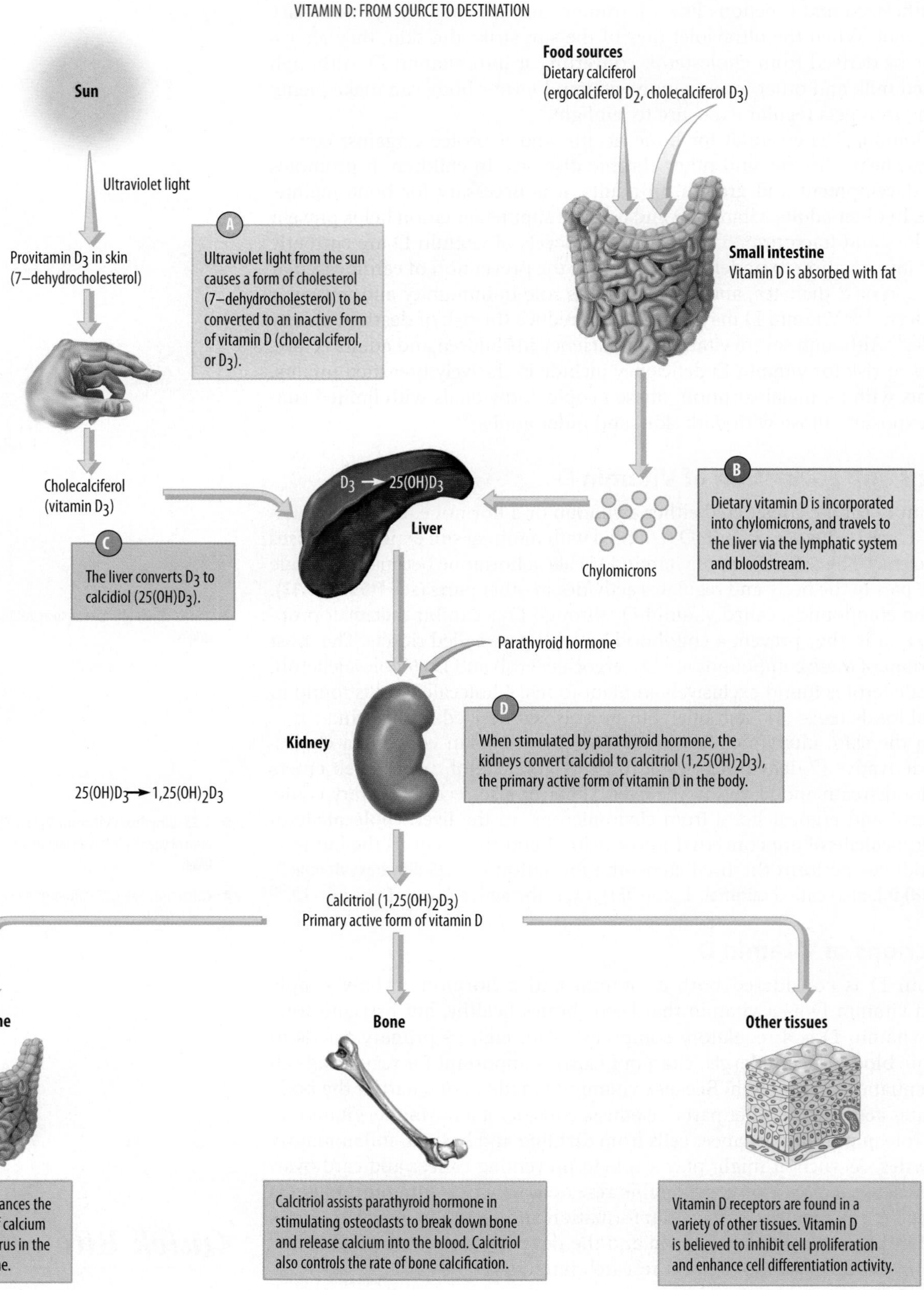

VITAMIN D: FROM SOURCE TO DESTINATION
Sun
Ultraviolet light
Provitamin D3 in skin (7–dehydrocholesterol)
A
Ultraviolet light from the sun causes a form of cholesterol (7–dehydrocholesterol) to be converted to an inactive form of vitamin D (cholecalciferol, or D3).
Cholecalciferol (vitamin D3)
C
The liver converts D3 to calcidiol (25(OH)D3).
Food sources
Dietary calciferol (ergocalciferol D2, cholecalciferol D3)
Small intestine
Vitamin D is absorbed with fat
D3 → 25(OH)D3
Liver
Chylomicrons
B
Dietary vitamin D is incorporated into chylomicrons, and travels to the liver via the lymphatic system and bloodstream.
Parathyroid hormone
Kidney
25(OH)D3 → 1,25(OH)2D3
D
When stimulated by parathyroid hormone, the kidneys convert calcidiol to calcitriol (1,25(OH)2D3), the primary active form of vitamin D in the body.
Calcitriol (1,25(OH)2D3)
Primary active form of vitamin D
Intestine
Bone
Other tissues
Calcitriol enhances the absorption of calcium and phosphorus in the small intestine.
Calcitriol assists parathyroid hormone in stimulating osteoclasts to break down bone and release calcium into the blood. Calcitriol also controls the rate of bone calcification.
Vitamin D receptors are found in a variety of other tissues. Vitamin D is believed to inhibit cell proliferation and enhance cell differentiation activity.

FIGURE 10.13 Vitamin D: from source to destination. Vitamin D is unique because, given sufficient sunlight, your body can synthesize all it needs. Both dietary and endogenous vitamin D must be activated by reactions in the kidneys and liver. Active vitamin D [$1,25(OH)_2D_3$, or calcitriol] is important for calcium balance and bone health and may have a role in cell differentiation.

Going Green

Vitamin Buddies

When our early ancestors first moved from the rainforest onto the East African savannah they had to cope with an entirely new environment. The hot sun beat down mercilessly, forcing them back into the shade. To survive in the open they needed to develop a better way of fending off the sun—find something that would absorb or disperse ultraviolet light. The solution was melanin, the dark pigment in skin cells.

Biologists first thought that this pigmentation arose to protect against skin cancer. But skin cancers mostly develop after reproductive age and therefore could not have exerted the evolutionary pressure necessary to account for darker skin colors.

An alternative theory emerged when investigators showed that light-skinned people who had been exposed to strong sunlight had abnormally low levels of folate in their blood. In the laboratory, they found that subjecting human blood serum to simulated strong sunlight destroyed half its folate content within one hour. Scientists suggested that protection against the breakdown of folate was the evolutionary pressure selecting for dark skin.

Because folate status during the early stages of pregnancy is strongly linked with birth defects, adequate folate levels confer a reproductive advantage. So, why don't we all have dark skin? The answer lies in another vitamin—vitamin D.

As long as your skin gets regular exposure to sunlight, your body can make plenty of vitamin D. But as you move away from the equator, the intensity of the sunlight decreases. Because light skin absorbs more UV sunlight than dark skin does, light skin confers a reproductive advantage as you move toward the poles. Data from NASA on worldwide UV exposure levels on the earth's surface enabled scientists to map the world into three vitamin D zones, which correlate strongly with variations in skin color. Evolution struck a balance. Human populations evolved to have skin light enough to make sufficient vitamin D, yet dark enough to protect their stores of folate.

But What About the Inuits?

The Inuits are dark-skinned people who live in arctic regions where sunlight is poor. How can they have good vitamin D stores without good vitamin D synthesis in their dark skin? The answer lies in their diet, which is very high in fat from fish and whale blubber. Because vitamin D is found in oily fish (e.g., herring, salmon, and sardines) as well as in cod liver oil and other fish oils, the Inuits do not need sunlight to maintain good vitamin D status. Do you?

blood levels within a normal range. The $1,25(OH)_2D_3$ acts directly and in concert with two other hormones: **parathyroid hormone** (parathormone) from the parathyroid gland and **calcitonin** from the thyroid gland. These hormones regulate activity in the bones, kidneys, and small intestine to adjust blood calcium levels. Much as a thermostat monitors temperature, receptors in the parathyroid gland monitor the blood levels of calcium.

When blood calcium levels drop, the parathyroid gland releases parathyroid hormone (PTH). PTH stimulates the activity of **osteoclasts** (bone cells that digest the bone matrix), releasing calcium ions from bone into the bloodstream. Parathyroid hormone also raises blood calcium levels by signaling the kidneys to slow calcium excretion. In addition, PTH stimulates the kidneys to activate vitamin D. The kidneys release $1,25(OH)_2D_3$, which enhances the action of PTH on bone cells. The $1,25(OH)_2D_3$ then stimulates the intestinal cells to make more carrier proteins for calcium transport, enhancing the absorption of calcium from food and thereby helping to elevate blood levels of calcium.

When blood calcium levels are too high, the thyroid gland releases calcitonin and the parathyroid gland decreases its release of PTH. Calcitonin inhibits the activity of osteoclasts, shifting the balance toward the activity of **osteoblasts** (bone-building cells). This net bone-building activity removes calcium

- **parathyroid hormone** A hormone secreted by the parathyroid glands in response to low blood calcium. It stimulates calcium release from bone and calcium absorption by the intestines, while decreasing calcium excretion by the kidneys. It acts in conjunction with $1,25(OH)_2D_3$ to raise blood calcium. Also called parathormone.
- **calcitonin** A hormone secreted by the thyroid gland in response to elevated blood calcium. It stimulates calcium deposition in bone and calcium excretion by the kidneys, thus reducing blood calcium.
- **osteoclasts** Bone cells that promote bone resorption and calcium mobilization.
- **osteoblasts** Bone cells that promote bone deposition and growth.

Quick Bite

"Children's Disease of the English"

In the seventeenth century, vitamin D deficiency was so common in British children that rickets was called the "children's disease of the English." Diets provided little vitamin D, and the lack of sun during many months of the year inhibited vitamin D synthesis in the skin.

ions from the bloodstream and deposits them in new bone. Calcitonin promotes bone growth in children and helps maintain bone health during pregnancy and lactation. High levels of calcium in the blood inhibit parathyroid hormone, which allows the kidneys to excrete calcium and reduces intestinal calcium absorption.

Key Concepts The best-known function of vitamin D, in the active form of $1,25(OH)_2D_3$, is to help regulate blood calcium levels. $1,25(OH)_2D_3$ works with two other hormones, parathyroid hormone and calcitonin, to alter the amount of calcium in the bone, the amount excreted from the kidneys, and the amount absorbed from the small intestine to keep blood levels in a normal range. It is known that $1,25(OH)_2D_3$ has effects on other tissues, but these functions have not been well established.

Dietary Recommendations for Vitamin D

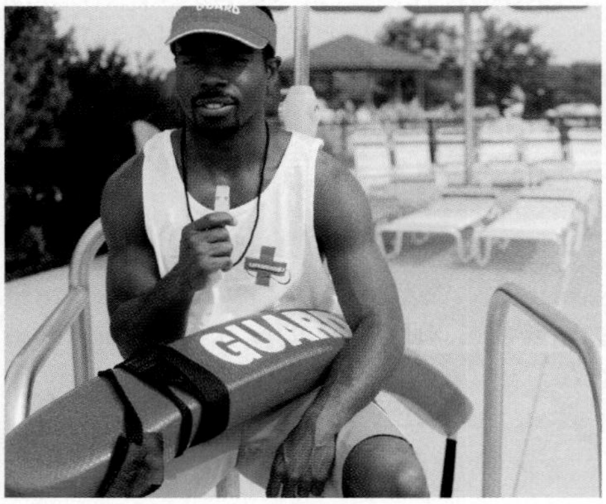

Although the body can synthesize vitamin D, scientists still recognize vitamin D as an essential nutrient for most people. The Dietary Reference Intake for vitamin D is based on skeletal health and assumes only minimal sunlight exposure. When updating the recommendations, the Food and Nutrition Board recognized that sunlight availability varies throughout the year and some people have limited exposure.[41] The expert panel considered the role of vitamin D in conditions such as cancer, cardiovascular disease, diabetes, infections, and autoimmune disorders, but the evidence was insufficient to make additional intake recommendations.[42] The panel also cautions against exceeding recommendations for calcium and vitamin D: "Higher levels of both nutrients have not been shown to confer greater benefits, and in fact, they have been linked to other health problems, challenging the concept that 'more is better.'"[43] Because infants and children have inadequate vitamin D intakes and limited direct sun exposure, the panel recommends that all infants, children, and adolescents consume a minimum of 400 IU of daily vitamin D beginning soon after birth.[44] For people between the ages 1 and 70 years, the RDA for vitamin D is 600 International Units (IU) per day.[45] Vitamin D skin synthesis decreases markedly with age; RDA recommendations therefore increase to 800 IU per day for men and women older than age 70 years.[46] Many nutritionists recommended for all adults to increase their vitamin D intake because most people do not reach optimal blood vitamin D levels with current dietary levels.

Sources of Vitamin D

We get vitamin D from exposure to sunlight, our diets, and dietary supplements. Sensible sun exposure can provide an adequate amount of vitamin D, which is stored in body fat during the winter, when vitamin D production is low.

Sunlight and Vitamin D Synthesis

How much exposure to the sun is needed for an adequate supply of vitamin D? Brief exposure to direct sunlight for as little as 15 minutes for a fair-skinned person to a few hours for a person with darker skin can produce as much vitamin D as your body can make in a day.[47] Controversy exists between appropriate sun exposure as a source of vitamin D synthesis versus the risk of skin cancer. The exact amount of sun exposure depends on several factors, including time of day, season, location, sunscreen use, and skin type. The sun's rays are more intense at latitudes closer to the equator and during midday and summertime (see **FIGURE 10.14**). Topical sunscreens (those with sun protection factor [SPF] of 8 or greater) block UV light. People with dark skin do not absorb UV rays as well as light-skinned people do. UV rays can penetrate the atmosphere, but ordinary window glass blocks the UVB light needed for Vitamin D synthesis. Pollution and smog can reduce UV rays.

Dietary Sources of Vitamin D

Few foods naturally contain vitamin D, so the major dietary sources of the nutrient are fortified foods such as vitamin D–fortified milk. Other fortified foods, such as breakfast cereal, orange juice, margarine, yogurt, grains, and breads, are also available in the United States.

THINK About It 5

Vitamin D is found in oily fish (e.g., herring, salmon, sardines) as well as in cod liver oil and other fish oils. Egg yolk, butter, and liver supply various amounts of vitamin D depending on the vitamin D content of the foods consumed by the source animals. Plants are a poor source, so strict vegetarians must get their vitamin D through exposure to sunlight. If sun exposure is not possible, nutritionists might recommend dietary supplements. (See the Nutrition Science in Action feature "Vitamin D Supplements: D_2 Versus D_3.") **FIGURE 10.15** shows some foods that are sources of vitamin D. Among older adults who live on their own, usual dietary intake from food alone is approximately one-third of the AI for vitamin D.[48]

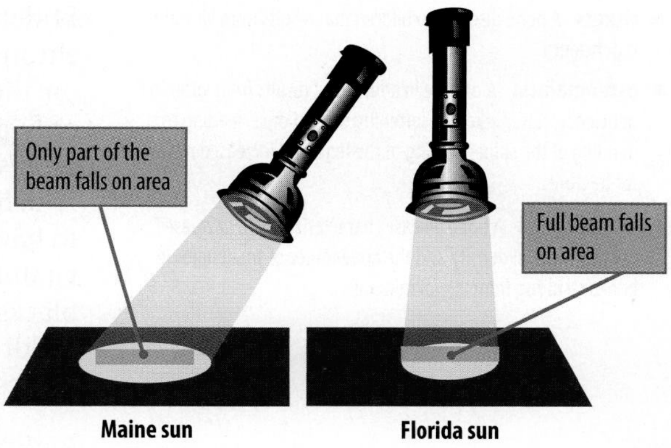

FIGURE 10.14 Sunlight in Maine and Florida.

Key Concepts Intake recommendations for vitamin D are very small: only 5 micrograms per day for young adults. Needs from the diet increase with age as the ability of the skin to synthesize vitamin D declines. Few foods are naturally good sources of vitamin D, and so most of the dietary intake comes from fortified milk and other fortified foods.

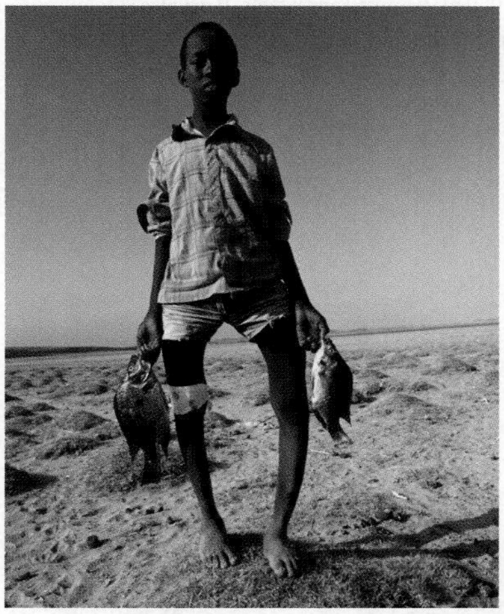

© Jeff Rotman/Science Source

Vitamin D Deficiency

Approximately 1 billion people worldwide in all age and ethnic groups have inadequate levels of vitamin D in their blood,[49,50] including up to 80 percent of U.S., Canadian, and European men and women.[51] Experts believe that the increase in the incidence of obesity, a decrease in milk consumption, and an increase in sun protection are major contributors to the high number of children and adults in the United States with low vitamin D levels.[52] Vitamin

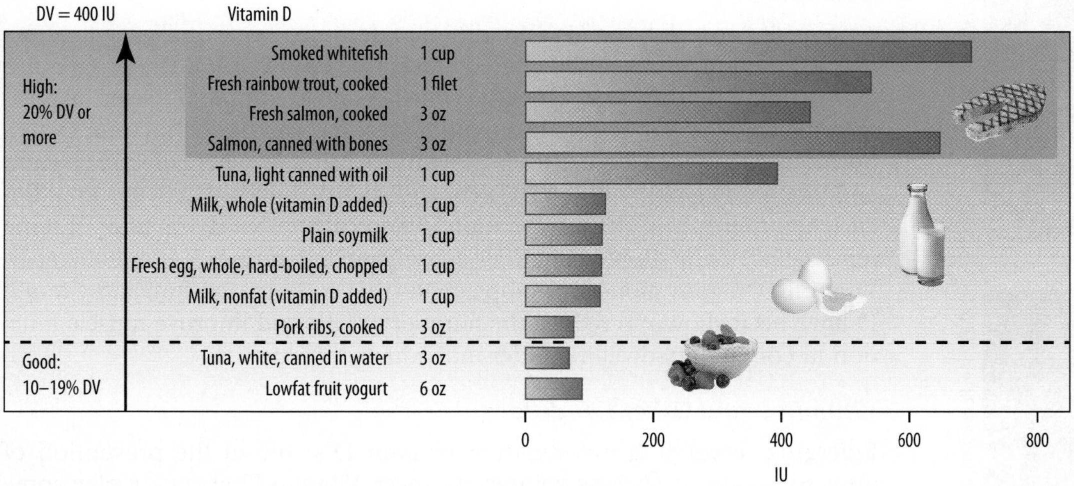

FIGURE 10.15 Food sources of vitamin D. Only a few foods are naturally good sources of vitamin D. Therefore, fortified foods such as milk and ready-to-eat cereals are important, especially for people with limited exposure to the sun. Units are IU to be consistent with Daily Value definitions.

Data from US Department of Agriculture, Agricultural Research Service, Nutrient Data Laboratory. USDA National Nutrient Database for Standard Reference, Release 28. Version Current: September 2015. Internet: http://www.ars.usda.gov/nea/bhnrc/ndl.

Photos (from top to bottom): (grilled salmon steak) © indigolotos/Shutterstock, Inc.; (bottle/glass of milk) © pjohnson1/Getty Images, Inc.; (boiled eggs) © eventina/Getty Images, Inc.; (yogurt) © Volosina/Getty Images.

- **rickets** A bone disease in children that results from vitamin D deficiency.
- **osteomalacia** A disease in adults that results from vitamin D deficiency; it is marked by softening of the bones, leading to bending of the spine, bowing of the legs, and increased risk for fractures.
- **osteoporosis** A bone disease characterized by a decrease in bone mineral density and the appearance of small holes in bones resulting from loss of minerals.

Quick Bite

Do You Know Vitamin D When You See It?

The general terms *vitamin D* and *calciferol* are used to refer to both vitamin D_2 (ergocalciferol) and vitamin D_3 (cholecalciferol), and to any combination of these two compounds.

D deficiency damages bones and contributes to a wide range of acute and chronic conditions. Long-term deficiency of vitamin D takes a profound toll on the skeleton. When vitamin D is in short supply, the intestines absorb only about 10 to 15 percent of dietary calcium, so bones don't get enough of this bone-building mineral. U.S. children and adolescents who are vitamin D deficient are predisposed to the development of rickets and are more likely to have hypertension and lower calcium and HDL cholesterol levels.[53] Lower vitamin D levels are found more often in older children, girls, non-Hispanic blacks, Mexican Americans, those living in low-income households, obese children, and those who spend more time watching television, playing video games, or using computers.[54]

Rickets and Osteomalacia

In children with vitamin D deficiency, the bones weaken and the skeleton fails to harden. This condition, called **rickets**, is characterized by "bow legs," "knock-knees," and other skeletal deformities. In the United States and Canada, nutritional rickets has been all but eliminated by vitamin D–fortified milk, infant vitamin supplements, and vitamin supplements for children with fat malabsorption conditions. Still, rickets from inadequate vitamin D intake and decreased sunlight exposure continues to occur in infants who are exclusively breastfed and infants with darker skin.[55] Twenty to 80 percent of U.S., Canadian, and European men and women are estimated to be vitamin D deficient, with a high prevalence estimated in the Middle East, Asia, and Australia as well.[56]

In adults, vitamin D deficiency causes a similar skeletal problem called **osteomalacia**, or "soft bones." Osteomalacia increases the risk for fractures in the hip, spine, and other bones. In addition to preventing adequate calcium absorption, osteomalacia alters the function of the parathyroid gland, boosting calcium losses from the bones. Risk of osteomalacia is high in people who have diseases that affect the stomach, kidneys, gallbladder, liver, or intestines—organs that are involved with the absorption or activation of vitamin D.

Osteoporosis

Osteoporosis, "porous bone," is a condition of declining bone quality that affects over 40 million adults in the United States (see **FIGURE 10.16**). The progressive loss of bone density and strength, which is most commonly seen in postmenopausal women, results in fragile bones that can easily fracture. Osteoporosis, like other chronic diseases, begins early in life, where dietary calcium and vitamin D along with lifestyle choices such as physical activity can influence its progression. Because vitamin D and calcium work together in bone remodeling, many supplement trials investigate both nutrients simultaneously. Vitamin D therapy alone and supplements that combine calcium and vitamin D have been shown to reduce the number of falls and improve muscle function in community-dwelling older individuals.[57,58]

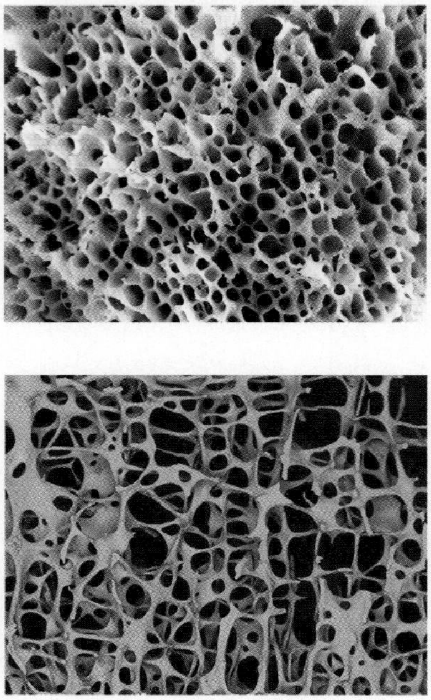

FIGURE 10.16 Osteoporosis. Normal (top) and osteoporotic bone (bottom). The osteoporotic bone is noticeably less dense.

Vitamin D and Other Conditions

Emerging research is investigating vitamin D's role in the prevention of numerous cancers such as colorectal cancer. Vitamin D also may play some role in the prevention and treatment of autoimmune diseases such as type 1 diabetes, multiple sclerosis, and rheumatoid arthritis, as well as hypertension and other medical conditions.[59] Supplementation with Vitamin D has been the subject of much recent scientific investigation and is still hotly debated. The level of vitamin D supplementation is likely to be health and disease specific to optimize preventative and therapeutic goals.

Nutrition Science *in Action*

Vitamin D Supplements: D_2 Versus D_3

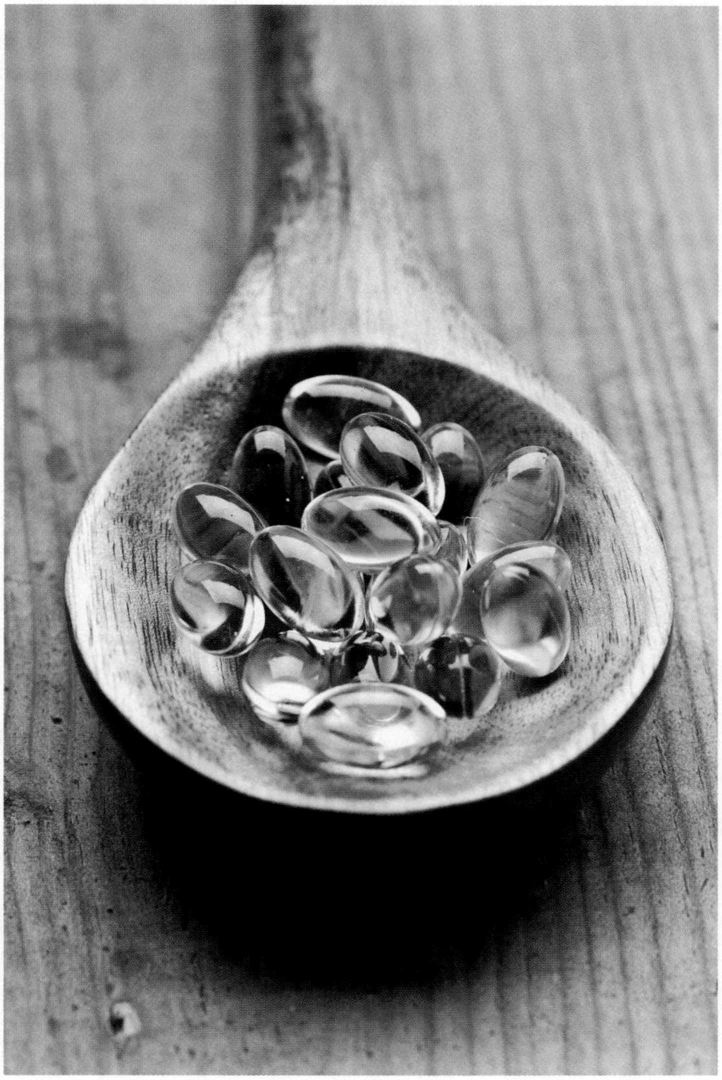
© R_Szatkowski/Shutterstock

Background

The clinical measure of vitamin D status is blood levels of 25-hydroxyvitamin D [25(OH)D]. At the present time, it remains unclear which form of supplemental vitamin D (D_2 or D_3) is more effective at raising 25(OH)D levels. The current widespread thought is that ergocalciferol (vitamin D_2) and cholecalciferol (vitamin D_3) are equally efficacious in their ability to raise blood 25(OH)D levels. Interestingly, most vitamin D–fortified foods are fortified with vitamin D_2. If a difference is found between the ability of vitamin D_2 and D_3 to raise serum 25(OH)D levels, this could potentially lead to changes in the food industry's fortification process as well as consumers' supplement choices.

Hypothesis

There is a difference in the efficacy of vitamin D_2 compared with vitamin D_3 in raising blood levels of 25(OH)D.

Experimental Plan

Scientific research databases were systematically searched for relevant randomized intervention trials from January 1950 to November 2011 in adult men and women that compared vitamin D_2 with vitamin D_3. All articles were screened and assessed for quality prior to inclusion. Ten studies were included in the systematic review, and seven in the meta-analysis.

Results

The meta-analysis of seven randomized controlled trials found that vitamin D_3 had a significant positive effect in raising serum 25(OH)D concentrations when compared to vitamin D_2.

Conclusion and Discussion

This meta-analysis showed that vitamin D_3 is more efficacious at raising blood levels of 25(OH)D than is vitamin D_2. However, there were important differences among studies including the dose, frequency, and method of administration of vitamin D. For example, all studies included in the meta-analysis used doses higher than the current Recommended Dietary Allowance (RDA), which is 600 IU per day for males and females aged 1 to 70 years. Therefore, there is still a need for further research on the effect of lower doses of vitamin D. Low doses of vitamin D are more realistic in terms of what individuals can consume in their diet, gain from sunlight exposure, and get through consumption of vitamins available commercially. Additionally, large, high-quality studies are needed to examine dose, frequency, and administration methods, as well as metabolic studies to determine why vitamin D_3 is more effective than vitamin D_2 at raising serum 25(OH)D levels.

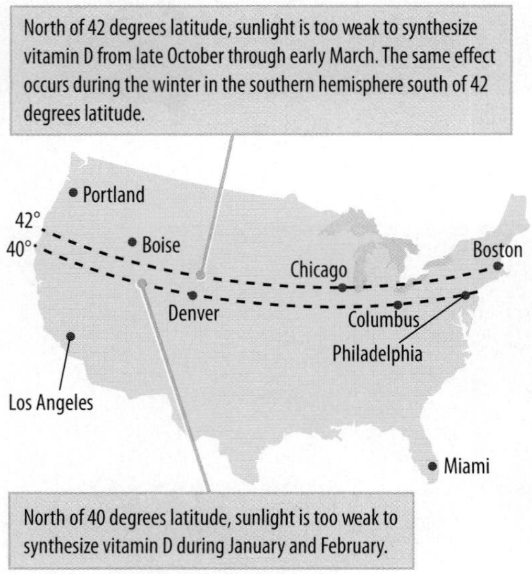

North of 42 degrees latitude, sunlight is too weak to synthesize vitamin D from late October through early March. The same effect occurs during the winter in the southern hemisphere south of 42 degrees latitude.
Portland
42°
40°
Boise
Chicago
Boston
Denver
Columbus
Philadelphia
Los Angeles
Miami
North of 40 degrees latitude, sunlight is too weak to synthesize vitamin D during January and February.

FIGURE 10.17 Mapping vitamin D synthesis. Vitamin D synthesis halts for part of the winter if sunlight is too weak. In Los Angeles and Miami, the sunlight is strong enough to synthesize vitamin D year-round, even in January.

Who Is Most at Risk for Vitamin D Deficiency?

Infants are born with stores of vitamin D that last about nine months. Beyond that, they must obtain vitamin D through exposure to sunlight, formula, or a supplement administered under the guidance of a physician. Breast milk contains very little vitamin D and is unlikely to meet a baby's needs beyond infancy. Exclusively breastfed infants who receive little exposure to sunlight need supplemental vitamin D.

In 1998, a pivotal study was published suggesting that many more people are deficient in vitamin D than had been suspected. The investigation of nearly 300 patients hospitalized in Boston showed that almost three of five people had too little vitamin D to maintain optimal levels of calcium in their bones.[60]

One explanation for the vitamin D shortfall may be that more people are protecting their skin with sunscreen, which might help prevent skin cancer but reduces vitamin D synthesis. Any sunscreen with a sun protection factor (SPF) of 8 or more blocks vitamin D synthesis in the skin. The problem worsens with age. Adults older than 70 years have a four-fold reduction in their ability to produce vitamin D_3 from the sun compared with younger adults.[61]

Living in a northern region compounds the problem. During the dead of winter, daylight hours are so short and the sunlight is so weak that vitamin D synthesis halts (see **FIGURE 10.17**). Fortunately, the skin of most people younger than 50 years can make sufficient amounts of vitamin D with just the amount of skin on the hands exposed for 10 to 15 minutes per day during warmer months. Most younger people make and store enough vitamin D during the summer to last through the winter months.

Individuals with a high body mass index (BMI) have also been found to be at increased risk of vitamin D deficiency.[62] There is an inverse relationship between BMI and plasma 25(OH)D levels. Because vitamin D is fat soluble, it is thought that the vitamin gets "trapped" in the subcutaneous fat tissue and is not as readily released into circulation.[63]

Vitamin D Toxicity

Sun exposure does not cause vitamin D toxicity, but high supplement doses can be highly toxic. The UL for adults older than 19 years is 4,000 IU per day.[64] Before consuming supplements that contain more than the RDA, people should consult a physician.

The hallmark of vitamin D toxicity is hypercalcemia—a high concentration of calcium in the blood. This condition affects numerous tissues in the body and can result in bone loss and kidney stones. Initially, it hampers the kidneys' ability to concentrate urine, causing excessive urination and thirst. Prolonged hypercalcemia can cause the excess calcium in the bloodstream to leave deposits in the soft tissues of the body, including the kidneys, blood vessels, heart, and lungs. Hypercalcemia also seems to affect the central nervous system, causing a severe depressive illness as well as nausea, vomiting, and loss of appetite. Vitamin D toxicity is severe but unlikely in healthy people with intake levels lower than 10,000 IU per day.

Key Concepts Because vitamin D's primary function is to regulate the level of calcium in the blood, which affects storage of calcium in bone, a deficiency of the nutrient affects the skeletal system. In children, vitamin D deficiency leads to rickets; in adults, lack of the nutrient causes osteomalacia and contributes to osteoporosis. Vitamin D is toxic when consumed in excess, and large doses should be taken only under a physician's supervision. Exposure to sun does not cause vitamin D toxicity.

Quick Bite

Too Much Cover

Many Arab women are clothed so that only their eyes are exposed to sunlight. Even though these women live in sunny climates near the equator, many suffer from osteomalacia.

Vitamin E

Consumers have long embraced the practice of taking large amounts of vitamin E, once touted as having the ability to boost sexual prowess and to prevent gray hair, wrinkles, and other signs of aging. Although many of these rumored benefits of vitamin E have never been supported by science, a growing body of research suggests that the nutrient may, in fact, be an important protector against chronic diseases associated with aging.

Forms of Vitamin E

In 1922, researchers discovered that an unknown substance in vegetable oils was necessary for reproduction in rats. It was given the chemical name **tocopherol**, from the Greek word *tokos*, meaning "childbirth," added to the verb *phero*, meaning "to bring forth." The ending *ol* reflects the alcohol nature of the molecule. It was a full 40 years after discovery, however, before scientists gathered evidence showing that humans also need this substance, which they labeled vitamin E. In 1968, the Food and Nutrition Board of the National Academy of Sciences officially recognized vitamin E as an essential nutrient.

▶ **tocopherol** The chemical name for vitamin E. There are four tocopherols (alpha, beta, gamma, and delta), but only alpha-tocopherol is active in the body.

Vitamin E is not a single compound. It is actually two sets of four compounds each: the tocopherols (alpha, beta, gamma, and delta) and the chemically related **tocotrienols** (alpha, beta, gamma, and delta). Although all are absorbed, only alpha-tocopherol contributes to meeting the human vitamin E requirement. Alpha-tocopherol is the most common form of vitamin E in food.

▶ **tocotrienols** Four compounds (alpha, beta, gamma, and delta) chemically related to tocopherols. The tocotrienols and tocopherols are collectively known as vitamin E.

As with all fat-soluble vitamins, absorption of vitamin E requires adequate absorption of dietary fat. Like the other fat-soluble vitamins, it travels by way of chylomicrons and other lipoproteins for distribution throughout the body (see **FIGURE 10.18**). The gastrointestinal (GI) tract absorbs 20 to 80 percent of dietary alpha-tocopherol, and the percentage declines as the amount of vitamin E consumed increases. Unabsorbed vitamin E is excreted in fecal matter.

Unlike the fat-soluble vitamins A and D, vitamin E does not accumulate in the liver. Adipose tissue contains about 90 percent of the vitamin E in the body. The remaining vitamin E is found in virtually every cell membrane in every tissue.

Functions of Vitamin E

Vitamin E's most well-known function is as an antioxidant. Its activity is enhanced by other nutrients involved in antioxidant pathways, such as vitamin C and selenium (a mineral). During normal metabolic processes, oxygen often reacts with other compounds to generate free radicals—highly unstable, toxic molecules that contain one unpaired electron. These unpaired electrons make free radicals highly reactive. Typically, a free radical attacks a nearby compound and steals an electron from it. Although that stabilizes the original free radical "thief," it turns the "robbed" molecule into a free radical, sparking a chain reaction capable of instantly producing a flood of free radicals.

Under normal circumstances, your body generates free radicals to help eliminate unwanted molecules. If various enzymes and antioxidants fail to control free radical activity, these highly reactive compounds attack cell membranes and cell constituents, including DNA. This unleashing of free radicals sets the stage for chronic diseases such as cancer and atherosclerosis.

A form of free radical damage that promotes atherosclerosis is **lipid peroxidation**—the production of unstable lipid molecules that contain an excess of oxygen. In this process, the cleavage of a carbon–carbon double bond in a fatty acid yields an intermediate compound that reacts with oxygen to form peroxides or free radicals. To stop lipid peroxidation, vitamin E acts

▶ **lipid peroxidation** Production of unstable, highly reactive lipid molecules that contain excess amounts of oxygen.

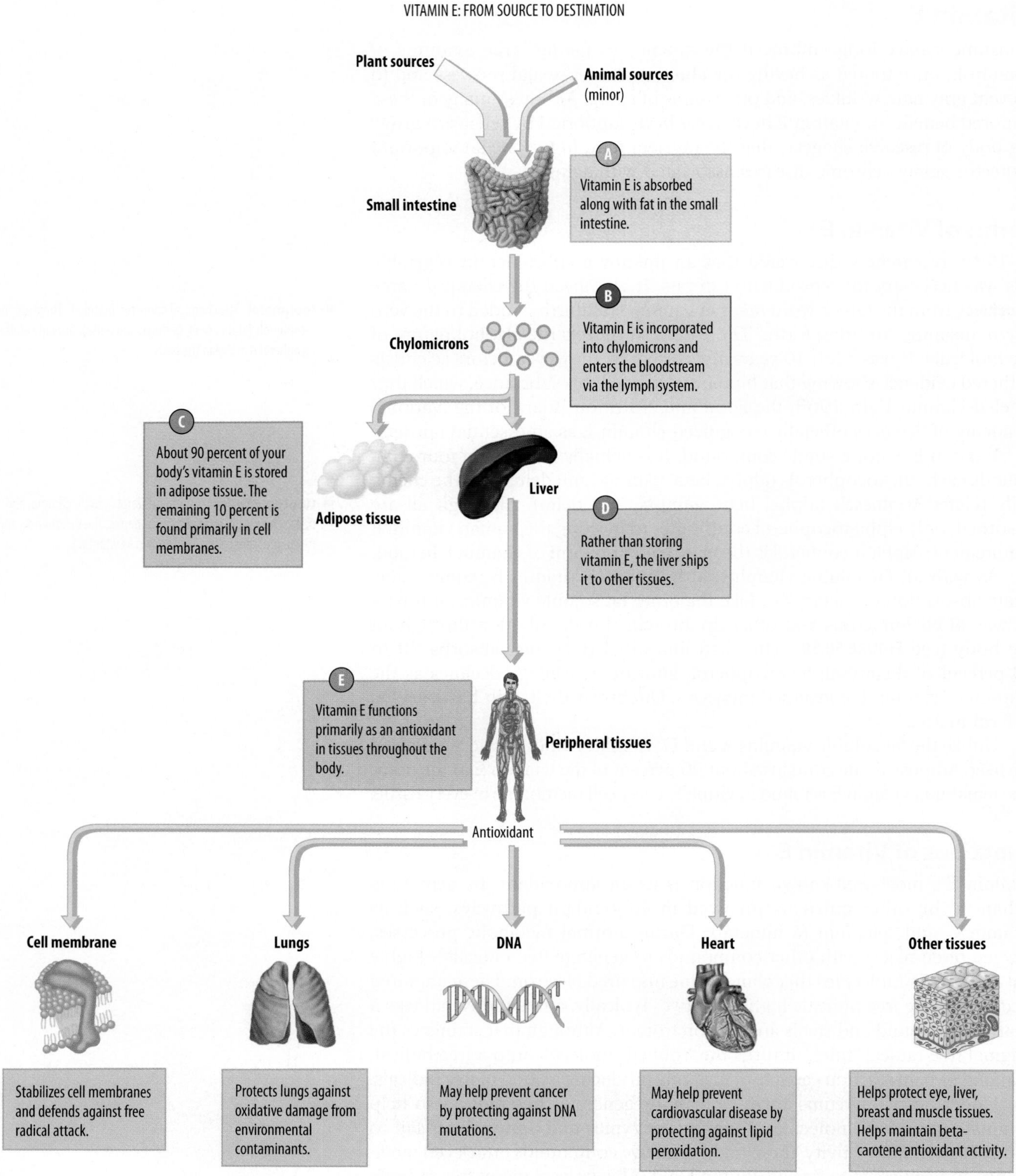

FIGURE 10.18 Vitamin E: from source to destination. Vitamin E is absorbed in the small intestine and carried to the liver by chylomicrons. The antioxidant activity of vitamin E helps stabilize cell membranes, protects tissues from oxidative damage, and reduces the risk of cancer and heart disease.

as a potent antioxidant and interrupts the cascade of free radical formation. Vitamin E donates an electron to the electron-seeking free radical, thus preventing the free radical from finding an electron somewhere else and causing more damage. This makes vitamin E itself a free radical, but not a very reactive one. The body excretes some of this altered vitamin E and recycles the rest by adding an electron from another antioxidant, such as vitamin C. This vitamin C radical can regain its antioxidant form by swiping an electron from **glutathione**. The enzyme glutathione reductase restores glutathione to its antioxidant form.

▶ **glutathione** A tripeptide of glycine, cysteine, and glutamic acid that is involved in protection of cells from oxidative damage.

The polyunsaturated fatty acids (PUFAs) in cell membranes are especially vulnerable to assault by free radicals. Vitamin E resides in cell membranes and other phospholipid-rich tissues, where it serves as one of the body's chief defenses against damage by free radicals (see **FIGURE 10.19**).

Numerous studies have suggested that dietary factors such as high intakes of antioxidant vitamins, including vitamin E, lower the risk of some chronic diseases, especially heart disease.[65] However, results from large clinical trials generally do not support routine use of vitamin E supplementation for the prevention of cardiovascular disease or reduction in related morbidity and mortality.[66] Although antioxidant food sources, especially plant foods, whole grains, and vegetable oils, are recommended, current evidence is insufficient to recommend supplemental vitamin E for heart disease or cancer prevention in the general population.[67]

What about other age-related diseases? Nutritionists have investigated a possible preventive role for vitamin E and found promising results in numerous conditions, including cancer, eye disorders such as age-related macular degeneration and cataracts, immune function, cognitive declines, and Alzheimer's disease.[68] In general, however, research regarding vitamin E supplementation does not support large-scale supplementation for the prevention or treatment of these conditions.

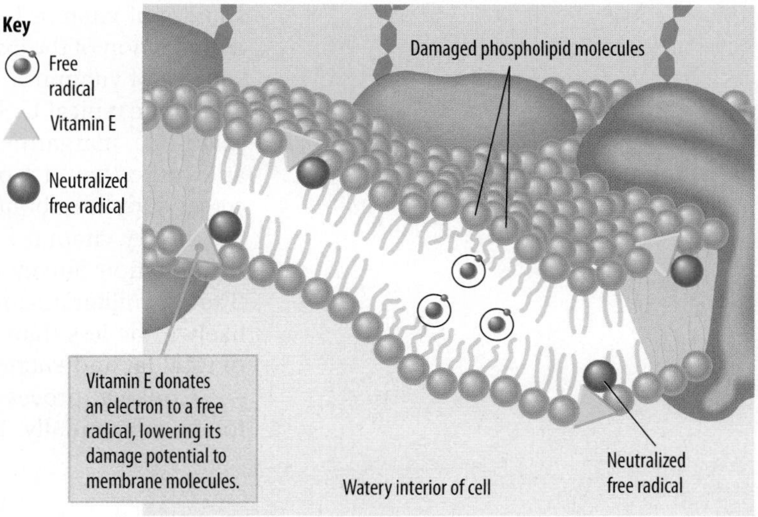

FIGURE 10.19 Free radical damage. Vitamin E helps prevent free radical damage to polyunsaturated fatty acids in cell membranes.

Key Concepts Vitamin E is really a set of compounds called tocopherols and tocotrienols. Alpha-tocopherol is the only form of vitamin E that meets the vitamin E requirement. Vitamin E functions as an antioxidant, protecting cell membranes in all parts of the body from the damaging effects of oxidation. Vitamin E has been connected to reduction of risk for many degenerative diseases, such as heart disease and cancer.

Dietary Recommendations for Vitamin E

To prevent vitamin E deficiency, the intake requirement must be related to body size and to polyunsaturated fatty acid intake. When PUFA intake is minimal, small amounts of vitamin E prevent symptoms of deficiency. As PUFA intake increases, the concentration of PUFA in tissues also rises and more vitamin E is needed to prevent oxidation. Because the vitamin E content of oils tends to parallel the PUFA concentration, balancing the two is usually not a problem; however, when people limit fat intake, they also may limit vitamin E intake.

The RDA for vitamin E accommodates generous PUFA intake. It is set at 15 milligrams per day of alpha-tocopherol for adults (including pregnant women) and 19 milligrams per day for women who are breastfeeding.

Sources of Vitamin E

Vitamin E is found in many different foods from both plant and animal sources. Wheat germ oil contains the highest concentration of usable vitamin E. Vegetable and seed oils, such as safflower, cottonseed, and sunflower seed oils, also are rich sources. Although soybean and corn oils contain much vitamin E, only about 10 percent is the active form, alpha-tocopherol.[69] Foods made from vegetable oils, such as margarine and salad dressings, as well as nuts and seeds, also are good sources. Although substantial amounts of vitamin E are found in strawberries and some green leafy vegetables, most fruits and vegetables contribute only small amounts. Animal products are medium to poor sources of vitamin E and vary widely in their content depending on the fat composition of the given animal's diet. **FIGURE 10.20** shows foods that are good sources of vitamin E.

In the typical U.S. diet, about 20 percent of vitamin E intake comes from salad oils, margarine, and shortening. Vegetables supply about 15 percent, and more than 12 percent comes from meat, poultry, and fish. Breakfast cereal supplies about 10 percent and fruit contributes about 9 percent of the dietary vitamin E.[70] Data from the third National Health and Nutrition Examination Survey (NHANES III) suggest that American adults consume 8 to 12 milligrams of vitamin E per day from foods. However, this value is likely to be less than actual consumption because of typical underreporting of total fat and energy intake.[71]

Cooking, processing, and storage can reduce the vitamin E content of foods substantially. During the milling of wheat to make white flour, for

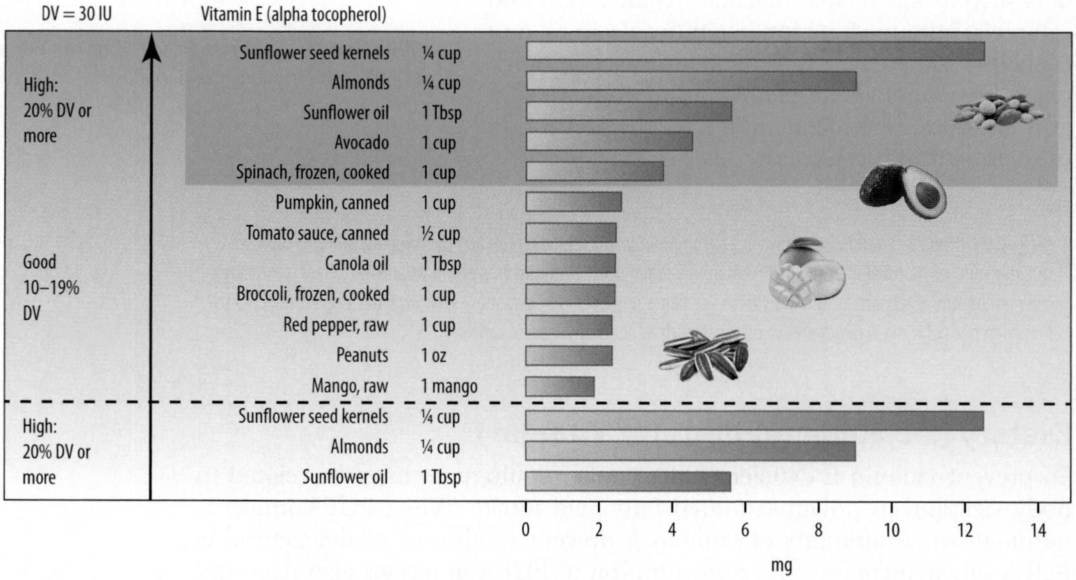

FIGURE 10.20 Food sources of vitamin E. Nuts and seeds, vegetable oil, and products made from vegetable oil, such as margarine, are among the best sources of vitamin E. Units are IU to be consistent with Daily Value definitions.

Data from US Department of Agriculture, Agricultural Research Service, Nutrient Data Laboratory. USDA National Nutrient Database for Standard Reference, Release 28. Version Current: September 2015. Internet: http://www.ars.usda.gov/nea/bhnrc/ndl.

Photos (from top to bottom): (almonds) © Africa Studio/Shutterstock, Inc.; (avocados) © masa44/Shutterstock, Inc.; (mango fruit) © Maks Narodenko/Shutterstock, Inc.; (sunflower seeds) Shutterstock, Inc.

instance, vitamin E–rich wheat germ is removed, and if chloride dioxide is used for the bleaching process, all vitamin E is lost. Refining and purifying vegetable oils takes a substantial toll on their vitamin E content. In fact, the by-products of the refining process contain so much vitamin E that they are used to make supplements. Oxygen is the destructive culprit that attacks vitamin E, and both light and heat accelerate oxidation.

Key Concepts The RDA for vitamin E is 15 milligrams of alpha-tocopherol for both men and women. Vitamin E is found in wheat germ, vegetable and seed oils, and products made from these oils, such as salad dressing and margarine. Processing foods can reduce their vitamin E content.

Vitamin E Deficiency

Because of the widespread use of vegetable oils and other sources in the food supply, overt vitamin E deficiency is rare in North America. Most deficiencies occur in people with fat-malabsorption syndromes such as cystic fibrosis. One feature of vitamin E deficiency is premature **hemolysis**—the breakdown of red blood cells. Without vitamin E to protect the cells against oxidation, destruction of cell membranes is rampant, causing red blood cells to burst. Hemolysis, and the associated anemia (called hemolytic anemia), is most often seen in infants born prematurely, before vitamin E has been transferred from mother to fetus in the last weeks of pregnancy. Special formulas and supplemental vitamin E are administered to premature babies to help correct the problem.

▶ **hemolysis** The breakdown of red blood cells that usually occurs at the end of a red blood cell's normal life span. This process releases hemoglobin.

In children and adults, fat-malabsorption disorders and subsequent vitamin E deficiency usually cause neurological problems that affect the spinal cord and peripheral nerves. In adults, malabsorption is usually prolonged, from 5 to 10 years, before signs of deficiency surface.

Vitamin E Toxicity

The antioxidant effects of vitamin E along with its inhibitory effects on platelet adhesion make it a logical choice for reducing heart disease risk. For a fat-soluble vitamin, vitamin E is surprisingly nontoxic; adverse effects have not been found from consuming foods rich in vitamin E.[72] However, it is not totally safe, and large supplement amounts can cause an increased risk of bleeding, especially in people with vitamin K deficiency and in those taking anticoagulant medication or aspirin.[73] For adults, the UL is 1,000 milligrams per day of supplemental alpha-tocopherol. Some large studies have found that vitamin E supplementation led to a small increase in the risk of death, although other evidence does not support those findings.[74]

Key Concepts Deficiencies of vitamin E are rare in adults, occurring primarily in people with fat-malabsorption syndromes. Preterm infants also run a high risk of vitamin E deficiency because they are delivered before the nutrient has a chance to move from the mother to the infant. Hemolysis is the hallmark of such a deficiency. Vitamin E is relatively nontoxic, although large doses interfere with blood clotting.

Vitamin K

In 1929, Danish researcher Henrik Dam discovered a nutrient that plays a crucial role in blood clotting. He named it vitamin "K" for "koagulation." Although most people give little thought to consuming enough of this nutrient, vitamin K stands between life and death. Without vitamin K to promote blood clotting, a single cut would eventually lead to death by blood loss.

▶ **phylloquinone** The form of vitamin K that comes from plant sources. Also known as vitamin K_1.

▶ **menaquinones** Forms of vitamin K that come from animal sources. Also produced by intestinal bacteria, they are collectively known as vitamin K_2.

▶ **menadione** A medicinal form of vitamin K that can be toxic to infants. Also known as vitamin K_3.

Vitamin K is a family of compounds known as quinones. It includes **phylloquinone** (K_1) from plant sources, **menaquinones** (collectively known as K_2) from animal sources and synthesized by our intestinal bacteria, and the synthetic substances **menadione**, sold under the trade name Synkavite (also known as K_3). Phylloquinone is the major form in the diet and the most biologically active. Menaquinones are only 70 percent as active, and the synthetics drop to 20 percent.

Phylloquinone, menaquinones, and the synthetic compound menadione are fat-soluble and primarily stored in the liver. These stores are relatively small and used up rapidly. The synthetic compound menadione is water-soluble. These forms are well suited to the treatment of vitamin K deficiency caused by fat-malabsorption disorders. Menadione is considered an unsafe supplemental form of vitamin K.

Functions of Vitamin K

When you get a cut, small or large, and start to bleed, a series of reactions forms a clot that stops the flow of blood. This cascade of reactions involves the production of a series of proteins, and ultimately the protein fibrin (see **FIGURE 10.21**). Four of the procoagulation proteins in the cascade are vitamin K dependent, and all require calcium for activation. For example, vitamin K converts the precursor protein preprothrombin to prothrombin by adding carbon dioxide to glutamic acid (an amino acid) in the protein. This change imparts a calcium-binding capacity, which allows prothrombin to be changed to thrombin. These reactions are integral to the formation of a blood clot.

In addition to promoting the formation of blood clots, vitamin K assists bone formation.[75] The vitamin is thought to work by facilitating a process needed to allow the protein osteocalcin to strengthen the skeleton. Vitamin K is important to the carboxylation of osteocalcin, which allows osteocalcin to become saturated with carboxyl groups (see **FIGURE 10.22**). Low dietary levels of vitamin K are associated with increased risk of fractures and age-related bone loss.[76] For the purpose of improving bone health, however, the evidence is currently mixed and not strongly supportive of vitamin K supplementation in older adults.[77] Other vitamin K–dependent proteins have been isolated in bone, underscoring the vitamin's importance to bone health.

Key Concepts Vitamin K was named for the Danish word *koagulation* because the nutrient works to promote the formation of blood clots. Vitamin K also is involved in bone health.

Dietary Recommendations for Vitamin K

Dietary intake of vitamin K varies with age; however, typical diets easily meet the dietary recommendations for vitamin K. The AI for vitamin K for adult males is 120 micrograms. Recommendations for women are slightly lower: 90 micrograms per day. The AI doesn't change with age or for women who are pregnant or lactating.[78] As with other fat-soluble vitamins, vitamin K absorption depends on normal consumption and digestion of dietary fat. Absorption is poor in people with fat-malabsorption syndromes. Even under normal conditions, absorption of dietary vitamin K might be as low as 40 percent (see **FIGURE 10.23**).

Typical diets easily support vitamin K's role in blood clotting; however, a higher amount of dietary vitamin K may be necessary to facilitate its role in bone health.[79]

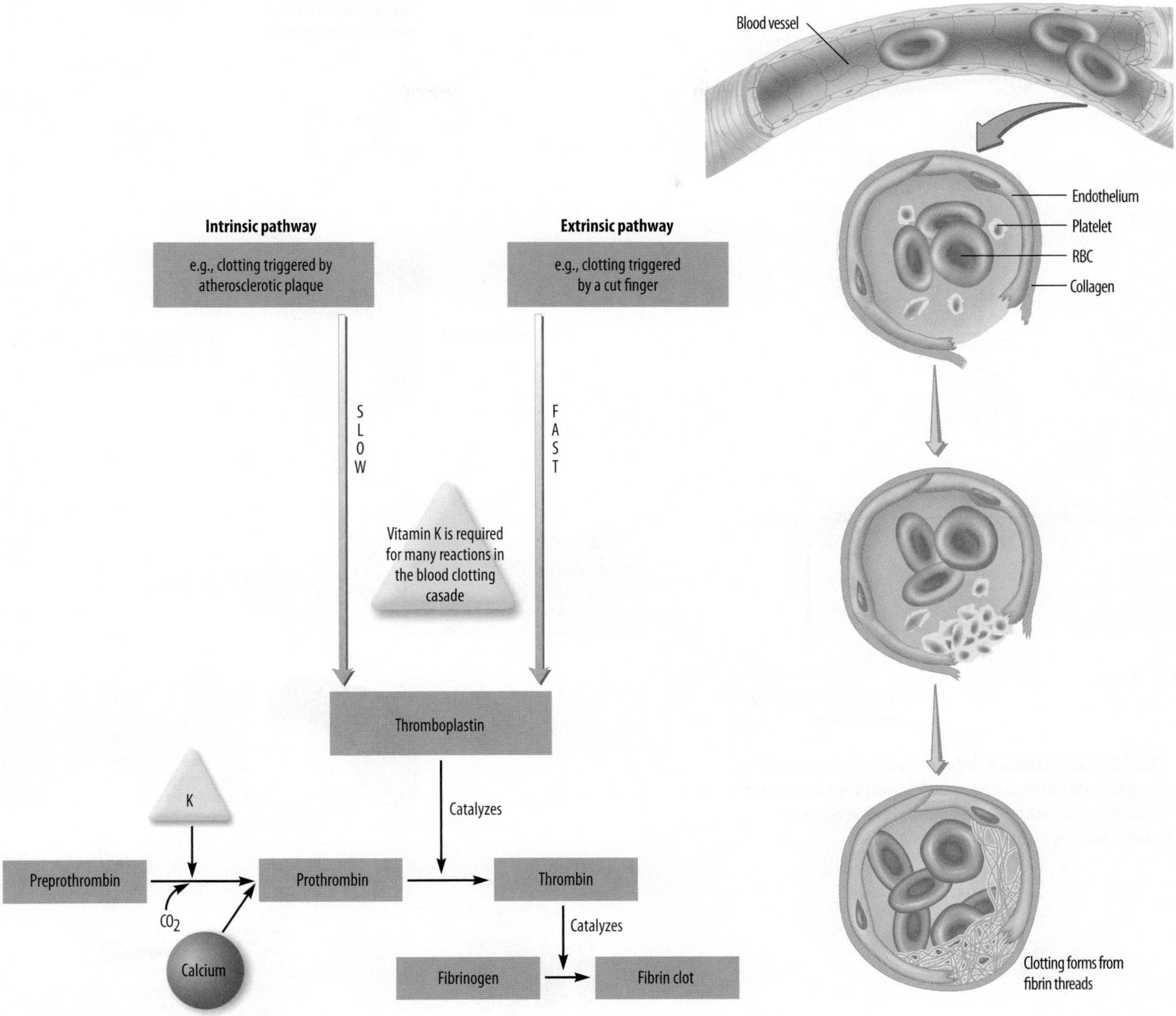

FIGURE 10.21 Blood clotting and vitamin K. The extrinsic and intrinsic pathways share the final steps in forming a clot. Vitamin K has a key role at several points—four of the procoagulation proteins in the cascade are vitamin K dependent.

Sources of Vitamin K

We obtain vitamin K from two sources: food (mostly plant food) and bacteria living in our colons. Dietary vitamin K is absorbed in the small intestine, and vitamin K produced by bacteria is absorbed in the colon.[80]

Phylloquinone is the primary form of dietary vitamin K. Green leafy vegetables, especially spinach, turnip greens, broccoli, and Brussels sprouts, supply substantial amounts of phylloquinone. Certain vegetable oils (soybean, cottonseed, canola, and olive) also are good sources.[81] Exposure to light degrades vitamin K, so the phylloquinone content of oils varies not only with brand

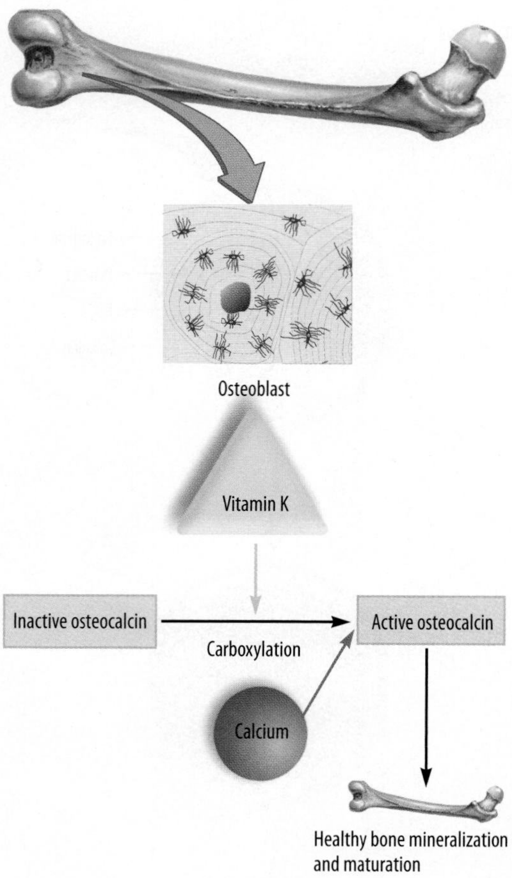

FIGURE 10.22 Vitamin K and bone health. Osteocalcin is an abundant bone protein that is required for bone mineralization and maturation. Vitamin K helps in the carboxylation of osteocalcin, greatly enhancing its calcium-binding properties.

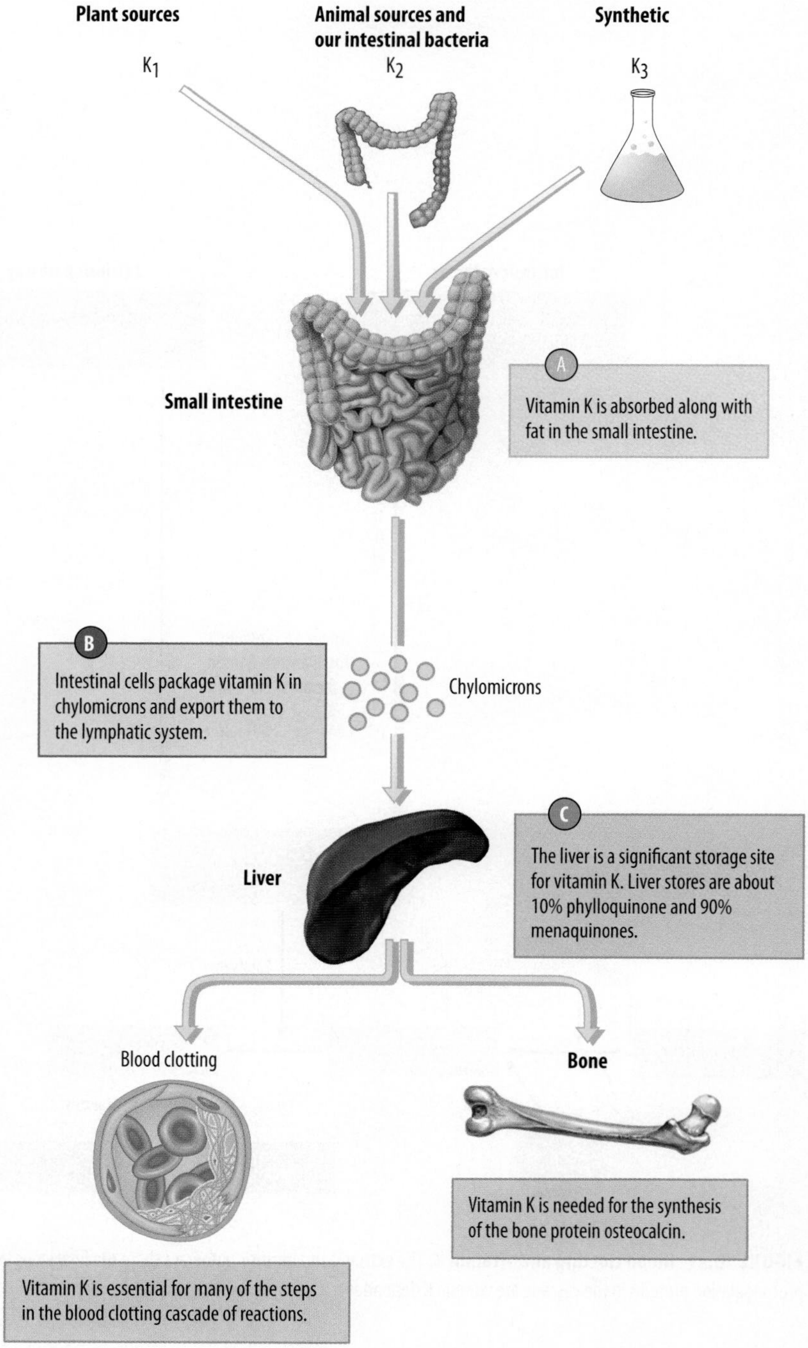

FIGURE 10.23 Vitamin K: from source to destination. Green leafy vegetables are rich sources of vitamin K. Intestinal bacteria produce 10 to 15 percent of our vitamin K, much less than previously believed. Vitamin K is important in both blood clotting and bone health.

and batch, but also with storage time if the oils are bottled in transparent containers. Therefore, vegetable oils may not be a reliable source of vitamin K.

In general, animal products contain limited amounts of vitamin K. Small amounts of menaquinones are found in egg yolks and butter, and various cheeses contain moderate amounts. Soybean products such as tofu contain substantial amounts of menaquinones. Liver contains moderate amounts of

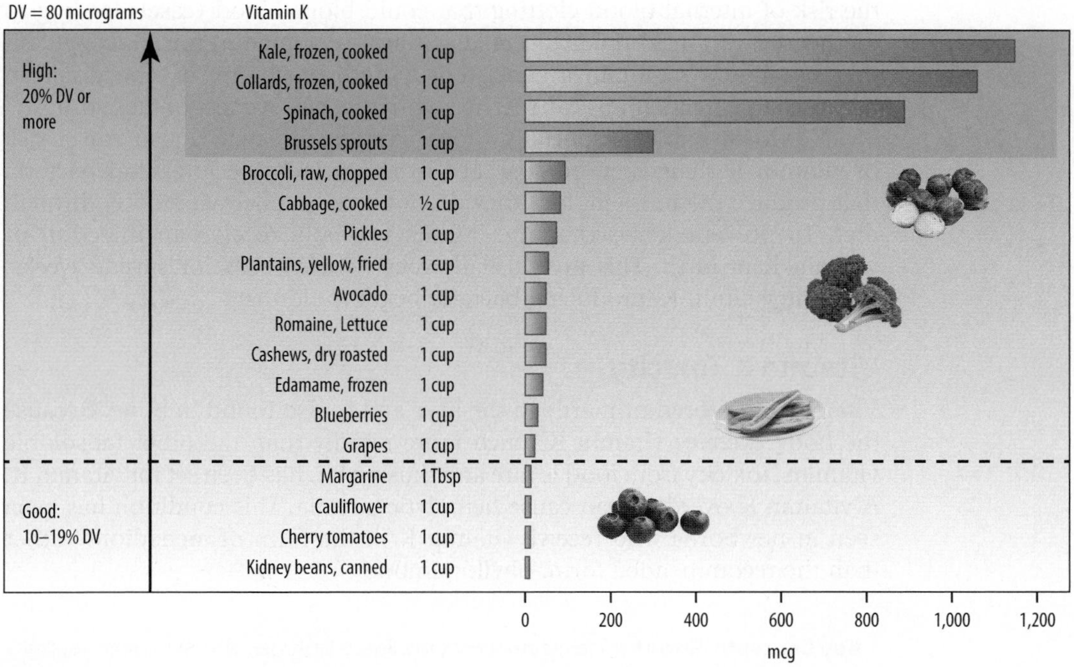

FIGURE 10.24 Food sources of vitamin K. The best sources of vitamin K are vegetables, especially leafy greens and those in the cabbage family.

Data from US Department of Agriculture, Agricultural Research Service, Nutrient Data Laboratory. USDA National Nutrient Database for Standard Reference, Release 28. Version Current: September 2015. Internet: http://www.ars.usda.gov/nea/bhnrc/ndl.

Photos (from top to bottom): (brussel sprouts) © Brigitte Sporrer/Getty Images, Inc.; (broccoli florets) © Antonova Anna/Shutterstock, Inc.; (fried plantain banana) © bonchan/Getty Images, Inc.; (fresh blueberries) © photastic/Shutterstock, Inc.

menaquinones, but because most people rarely eat liver, it is unlikely to contribute much to the general consumption of vitamin K. **FIGURE 10.24** shows foods that contain vitamin K.

Key Concepts Dietary recommendations for vitamin K intake are small; the AI for adult men is 120 micrograms, and for adult women it is 90 micrograms. Vitamin K is found primarily in green vegetables and in some vegetable oils. Animal foods, in general, contain limited amounts of vitamin K.

Vitamin K Deficiency

Although vitamin K has a crucial role in blood clotting, the body needs only small amounts. This makes vitamin K deficiency rare in healthy adults. On the other hand, preliminary research suggests that typical diets are supplying less than optimal amounts for bone health. People who suffer fat-malabsorption syndromes, such as celiac disease, cystic fibrosis, ulcerative colitis, and Crohn's disease, can develop vitamin K deficiency. Prolonged use of antibiotics can cause a deficiency because the drugs can destroy the intestinal bacteria that produce vitamin K. Prior to surgery, a patient's vitamin K status often is tested to assess the risk for hemorrhaging because antibiotics are frequently part of the treatment regimen.

Megadoses of vitamins A and E counteract the actions of vitamin K. Vitamin A appears to hamper intestinal absorption of vitamin K, and excess vitamin E seems to decrease the vitamin K–dependent clotting factor, thus promoting bleeding. Physicians prescribe anticoagulant medications to reduce the risk of internal blood clotting that could block blood vessels leading to the heart or brain. People who take warfarin (Coumadin) for anticoagulant therapy should maintain a consistent pattern of vitamin K consumption because large fluctuations can interfere with the effectiveness of these drugs.[82]

Newborn babies, especially those who are breastfed, also run a risk of vitamin K deficiency because at birth they lack the intestinal bacteria that produce the nutrient, and they do not receive much vitamin K through diet. To prevent hemorrhaging, infants typically receive an injection of vitamin K at birth. This dose usually meets their needs for several weeks, until the vitamin K–producing bacteria begin to flourish.

Vitamin K Toxicity

Vitamin K is stored primarily in the liver and is also found in bone. Because the body excretes vitamin K much more rapidly than the other fat-soluble vitamins, toxicity from food is rare and thus no UL has been set for vitamin K. A vitamin K overdose can cause hemolytic anemia. This condition has been seen in newborns who receive vitamin K in the form of menadione rather than the recommended form, phylloquinone.

Key Concepts Vitamin K deficiencies are extremely rare. Because it takes several weeks before the intestinal bacteria that produce vitamin K begin to flourish in the intestine, newborns are routinely given injections of vitamin K at birth. Vitamin K toxicity is rare because the body excretes the nutrient more readily than the other fat-soluble vitamins.

Label to Table

It is well known that milk is an excellent source of calcium, but did you know that milk also contains three of the four fat-soluble vitamins? Let's take a look at the Nutrition Facts from a carton of nonfat milk.

Milk contains the fat-soluble vitamins A and D. Vitamin A is found naturally in whole milk and is added to reduced-fat milks. All milks are fortified with vitamin D. Although it is true that fat-soluble vitamins can be toxic in large doses because they are stored in the body, the amounts added to milk are not of concern. Vitamin K is not listed on the label, but milk is a good source of this fat-soluble vitamin as well. (Each cup of milk provides 10 micrograms, which is 12.5 percent of the Daily Value.)

A one-cup serving of fortified milk provides 10 percent of the 5,000 IU Daily Value of vitamin A. If you drank three cups of milk per day, you would get about one-third of your recommended amount of vitamin A. That's good news because dietary vitamin A is not always easy to obtain. One form, retinol, is found mainly in liver and fish liver oil, which are not staples of the typical American diet. The provitamin forms of vitamin A, the carotenoids, are found in green leafy and dark-orange vegetables.

Vitamin D is important because it helps with the absorption of calcium and phosphorus, both important for bone health. Canned tuna, salmon, and sardines, and some fortified cereals, also are good sources of vitamin D. As shown in the nutrition label, just one cup of milk gives you one-quarter of the vitamin D Daily Value. That's 25 percent of 10 micrograms, or 2.5 micrograms.

The new food labels will include a declaration of Vitamin D that will include the actual gram amount, in addition to the %DV. Vitamin D is a nutrient that some people are not getting enough of, which puts them at higher risk for chronic disease. The %DV for calcium will continue to be required, along with the actual gram amount. Vitamin A will no longer be required because deficiencies of this vitamin are rare, but this nutrient can be included on a voluntary basis.

Keep in mind when selecting milk that nonfat (skim) milk contains vitamins A and D just like the higher-fat 2% and whole milk. Don't let the large banner "Vitamin A and D" printed on containers of whole milk trick you into thinking it contains more. It doesn't!

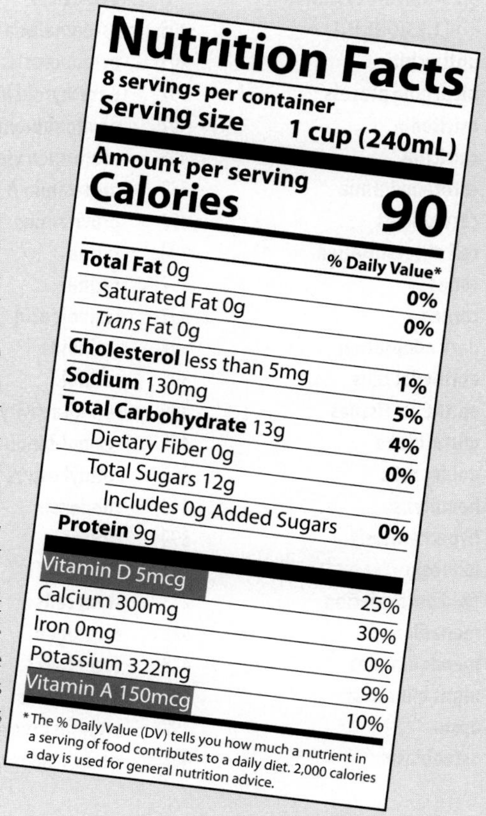

Nutrition Facts
8 servings per container
Serving size 1 cup (240mL)

Amount per serving	
Calories	**90**
	% Daily Value*
Total Fat 0g	**0%**
Saturated Fat 0g	**0%**
Trans Fat 0g	
Cholesterol less than 5mg	**1%**
Sodium 130mg	**5%**
Total Carbohydrate 13g	**4%**
Dietary Fiber 0g	**0%**
Total Sugars 12g	
Includes 0g Added Sugars	**0%**
Protein 9g	
Vitamin D 5mcg	25%
Calcium 300mg	30%
Iron 0mg	0%
Potassium 322mg	9%
Vitamin A 150mcg	10%

*The % Daily Value (DV) tells you how much a nutrient in a serving of food contributes to a daily diet. 2,000 calories a day is used for general nutrition advice.

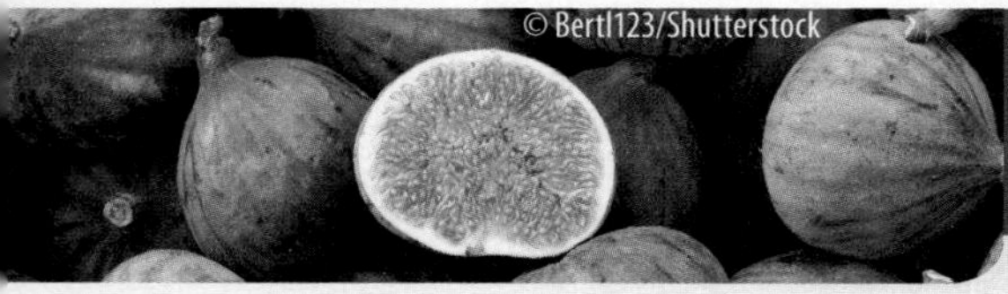

© Bertl123/Shutterstock

Learning Portfolio

Key Terms

Study Points

- Vitamins are organic substances the body needs in minuscule amounts.
- Two classes of vitamins exist: fat-soluble vitamins (A, D, E, and K) and water-soluble vitamins (B vitamins and vitamin C).
- Vitamin A comes from preformed retinoids and the precursor carotenoids.
- Vitamin A functions in vision, cell differentiation, growth and development, and immune function.
- Sources of vitamin A include milk fat, liver, and fortified foods. Good sources of provitamin A carotenoids are green leafy and yellow-orange vegetables and yellow-orange fruits.
- Night blindness is an early symptom of vitamin A deficiency that, if not treated, can result in permanent blindness.
- Vitamin A is toxic when taken in large doses, causing liver damage and other problems.
- Carotenoids naturally occur in fruits and vegetables and function as important antioxidants.
- The provitamin A carotenoids alpha-carotene, beta-carotene, and beta-cryptoxanthin can be converted to retinol.
- Vitamin D functions like a hormone and the body can synthesize it, but it is still considered a vitamin.
- A vitamin D precursor is produced from cholesterol when UV light hits the skin. Reactions in the liver and kidneys are needed to produce a fully active vitamin D molecule.
- Vitamin D in foods is available mainly from fortified milk and other fortified products.
- The primary function of vitamin D is the regulation of blood levels of calcium.
- Vitamin D deficiency contributes to skeletal problems.
- Vitamin D toxicity from sun exposure is unlikely, but high supplement doses can be toxic.
- Vitamin E is an important antioxidant in the body and may help reduce the risk of chronic diseases such as heart disease and cancer.
- Vitamin E is found in vegetable oils and foods made from those oils.
- Deficiency and toxicity of vitamin E are relatively rare.
- Vitamin K is an important factor in blood coagulation.
- Although synthesized by intestinal bacteria, most of the vitamin K in the body comes from dietary sources, especially green vegetables.
- Vitamin K deficiency is rare, but newborns are susceptible if not given an injection of vitamin K at birth.
- Because the body excretes vitamin K easily, toxicity is unlikely.

Study Questions

1. List at least three characteristics of fat-soluble vitamins.
2. List the four fat-soluble vitamins by their general names and specific active forms.
3. What are the main roles of vitamin A in the body?
4. What vitamin deficiency is associated with night blindness?

5. What antioxidant is responsible for the yellow-orange color of cantaloupes?
6. Which fat-soluble vitamin is considered a hormone? Which organs does this hormone affect?
7. From what precursor can vitamin D be synthesized?
8. What are the toxicity and deficiency symptoms of vitamin E?
9. How does a vitamin K deficiency lead to the inability to form a blood clot?
10. Which two fat-soluble vitamins are most toxic? Least toxic?

Try This

The PUFA Protection Challenge: Vitamin E Versus Oxygen

The object of this experiment is to see if vitamin E protects polyunsaturated fats (PUFAs) from oxidation. You'll need two glasses, one bottle of either safflower or corn oil, and some liquid vitamin E gel caps (which can be purchased at any pharmacy). Pour equal amounts of oil in each of the glasses. Poke a hole in 10 of the vitamin E gel caps and squeeze their contents into *one* of the glasses. Mark this glass with tape and write the letter E on it. Let the glasses sit uncovered on a countertop for several days or weeks. Check the freshness or rancidity of the oils by smelling them and noting whether they look clear or cloudy. Over time, one will become more rancid than the other. Which glass container won the challenge—the one with or without vitamin E? Why?

Getting Personal

List all of the foods and drinks that you consume in a 24-hour period, ideally a day where your schedule is fairly predictable and you are eating what is considered normal for you.

Let's check out your intake of the fat-soluble vitamins.

1. Which foods provided you with high amounts of fat-soluble vitamins?
2. Which foods provided you with little fat-soluble vitamins?
3. Is your intake meeting your needs?
   - What are your best vitamin A sources?
   - How can you improve your vitamin A intake?
   - What are your best carotenoid sources?
   - How can you improve your carotenoid intake?
   - What are your best vitamin D sources?
   - How can you improve your vitamin D intake?
   - What are your best vitamin E sources?
   - How can you improve your vitamin E intake?
   - What are your best vitamin K sources?
   - How can you improve your vitamin K intake?
4. Choosing more of what foods would help increase your intake of fat-soluble vitamins?
5. Select two processed foods from your diet and suggest fruits or vegetables that you would consider as substitutions. What will this do to the overall vitamin content of your diet?

References

1. Mahan KL, Escott-Stump S, Raymond JL, eds. *Krause's Food and the Nutrition Care Process*. 13th ed. Philadelphia: WB Saunders; 2011.
2. Guyton AC, Hall JE. *Textbook of Medical Physiology*. 13th ed. Philadelphia: WB Saunders; 2013.
3. Gropper SS, Smith JL. *Advanced Nutrition and Human Metabolism*. 6th ed. Belmont, CA: Cengage Learning; 2012.
4. National Institutes of Health Osteoporosis and Related Bone Diseases National Resource Center. Vitamin A and bone health. http://www.niams.nih.gov/Health_Info/Bone/Bone_Health/Nutrition/vitamin_a.asp. Accessed January 7, 2016.
5. Ibid.
6. Institute of Medicine, Food and Nutrition Board. *Dietary Reference Intakes for Vitamin A, Vitamin K, Arsenic, Boron, Chromium, Copper, Iron, Manganese, Molybdenum, Nickel, Silicon, Vanadium, and Zinc*. Washington, DC: National Academies Press; 2001.
7. Ibid.
8. Ibid.
9. Gropper SS, Smith JL. *Advanced Nutrition and Human Metabolism*. Op cit.
10. Hayman RM, Dalziel SR. Acute vitamin A toxicity: a report of three paediatric cases. *J Paediatr Child Health*. 2012;48(3):E98–E100.
11. Institute of Medicine, Food and Nutrition Board. *Dietary Reference Intakes for Vitamin A, Vitamin K, Arsenic, Boron, Chromium, Copper, Iron, Manganese, Molybdenum, Nickel, Silicon, Vanadium, and Zinc*. Op cit.
12. Institute of Medicine, Food and Nutrition Board. *Dietary Reference Intakes for Vitamin C, Vitamin E, Selenium, and Carotenoids*. Washington, DC: National Academies Press; 2000.
13. Ibid.
14. Bouayed J, Bohn T. Exogenous antioxidants—double-edged swords in cellular redox state: health beneficial effects at physiologic doses versus deleterious effects at high doses. *Oxid Med Cell Longev*. 2010;3(4):228–237.
15. Liu RH. Health-promoting components of fruits and vegetables in the diet. *Adv Nutr*. 2013;4:384S–392S.
16. Weikel KA, Chui CJ, Taylor A. Nutritional modulation of age-related macular degeneration. *Mol Aspects Med*. 2012;33(4):318–375.
17. Linus Pauling Institute Micronutrient Information Center. Alpha-carotene, beta-carotene, beta-cryptoxanthin, lycopene, lutein, and zeaxanthin. http://lpi.oregonstate.edu/infocenter/phytochemicals/carotenoids. Accessed January 7, 2016.
18. Gropper SS, Smith JL. *Advanced Nutrition and Human Metabolism*. Op cit.
19. Olson JH, Erie JC, Bakri SJ. Nutritional supplementation and age-related macular degeneration. *Semin Ophthalmol*. 2011;26(3):131–136.

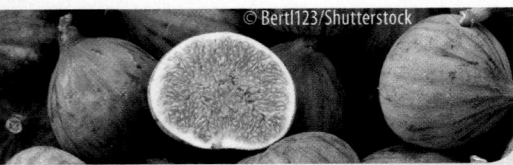

Learning Portfolio (continued)

20. Liu XH, Yu RB, Liu R, Hao ZX, Han CC, Zhu ZH, Ma L. Association between lutein and zeaxanthin status and the risk of cataract: a meta-analysis. *Nutrients*. 2014;6(1):452–465. doi: 10.3390/nu6010452.
21. Zampatti S, Ricci F, Cusumano A, Marsella LT, Novelli G, Giardina E. Review of nutrient actions on age-related macular degeneration. *Nutr Res*. 2014;34(2):95–105.
22. Raiola A, Rigano MM, Calafiore R, Frusciante L, Barone A. Enhancing the health-promoting effects of tomato fruit for biofortified food. *Mediators Inflamm*. 2014;2014:139873. doi: 10.1155/2014/139873. Epub March 12, 2014.
23. Institute of Medicine, Food and Nutrition Board. *Dietary Reference Intakes for Vitamin C, Vitamin E, Selenium, and Carotenoids*. Op cit.
24. Ibid.
25. Institute of Medicine, Food and Nutrition Board. *Dietary Reference Intakes for Vitamin A, Vitamin K, Arsenic, Boron, Chromium, Copper, Iron, Manganese, Molybdenum, Nickel, Silicon, Vanadium, and Zinc*. Op cit.
26. Capanoglu E, Beekwilder J, Boyacioglu D, et al. The effect of industrial food processing on potentially health-beneficial tomato antioxidants. *Crit Rev Food Sci Nutr*. 2010;50(10):919–930.
27. Institute of Medicine, Food and Nutrition Board. *Dietary Reference Intakes for Vitamin A, Vitamin K, Arsenic, Boron, Chromium, Copper, Iron, Manganese, Molybdenum, Nickel, Silicon, Vanadium, and Zinc*. Op cit.
28. Wang XD. Carotenoids. In: Ross AC, Caballero B, Cousins RJ. et al., eds. *Modern Nutrition in Health and Disease*. 11th ed. Philadelphia: Wolters Kluwer/Lippincott Williams & Wilkins; 2014.
29. American Institute for Cancer Research. Recommendations for cancer prevention. http://www.aicr.org/reduce-your-cancer-risk/recommendations-for-cancer-prevention/recommendations_08_supplements.html. Accessed January 7, 2016.
30. World Health Organization. Global strategies on diet, physical activity and health. Promoting fruit and vegetable consumption around the world. http://www.who.int/dietphysicalactivity/fruit/en/index2.html. Accessed January 7, 2016.
31. Boeing H, Bechthold A, Bub A, et al. Critical review: vegetables and fruit in the prevention of chronic diseases *Eur J Nutr*. 2012;51:637–663.
32. Wang X, Ouyang Y, Liu J, Zhu M, Zhao G, Bao W, Hu FB. Fruit and vegetable consumption and mortality from all causes, cardiovascular disease, and cancer: systematic review and dose-response meta-analysis of prospective cohort studies. *BMJ*. 2014;349:g4490. doi: 10.1136/bmj.g4490. http://www.bmj.com/content/bmj/349/bmj.g4490.full.pdf. Date accessed March 20, 2016
33. Avenell A, Mak JC, O'Connell D. Vitamin D and vitamin D analogues for preventing fractures in post-menopausal women and older men. *Cochrane Database Syst Rev*. 2014;4:CD000227. doi: 10.1002/14651858.CD000227.pub4.
34. Wacker M, Holick MF. Vitamin D—effects on skeletal and extraskeletal health and the need for supplementation. *Nutrients*. 2013;5(1):111–148. doi: 10.3390/nu5010111.
35. Battault S, Whiting SJ, Peltier SL, Sadrin S, Gerber G, Maixent JM. Vitamin D metabolism, functions and needs: from science to health claims. *Eur J Nutr*. 2013;52(2):429–441. Epub August 12, 2012.
36. Bjelakovic G, Gluud LL, Nikolova D, et al. Vitamin D supplementation for prevention of mortality in adults. *Cochrane Database Syst Rev*. 2014;1:CD007470. doi: 10.1002/14651858.CD007470.pub3.
37. National Institutes of Health, Office of Dietary Supplements. Vitamin D: fact sheet for health professionals. http://ods.od.nih.gov/factsheets/vitamind.asp. Accessed January 7, 2016.
38. Gropper SS, Smith JL. *Advanced Nutrition and Human Metabolism*. Op cit.
39. Manson JE, Mayne ST, Clinton SK. Vitamin D and prevention of cancer—ready for prime time? *N Engl J Med*. 2011;364(15):1385–1387.
40. Shapses SA, Manson JE. Vitamin D and prevention of cardiovascular disease and diabetes: why the evidence falls short. *JAMA*. 2011;305(24):2565–2566.
41. Institute of Medicine, Food and Nutrition Board. *Dietary Reference Intakes for Calcium and Vitamin D*. Washington, DC: National Academies Press; 2010.
42. Ibid.
43. Institute of Medicine of the National Academies of Science. Dietary reference intakes for calcium and vitamin D. March 2011. http://www.iom.edu/~/media/Files/Report%20Files/2010/Dietary-Reference-Intakes-for-Calcium-and-Vitamin-D/Vitamin%20D%20and%20Calcium%202010%20Report%20Brief.pdf. Accessed January 7, 2016.
44. Wagner CL, Greer FR, and Section on Breastfeeding and Committee on Nutrition. Prevention of rickets and vitamin D deficiency in infants, children, and adolescents. *Pediatrics*. 2008;122(5):1142–1152.
45. Institute of Medicine, Food and Nutrition Board. *Dietary Reference Intakes for Calcium and Vitamin D*. Op cit.
46. Ibid.
47. Vitamin D Council. How do I get the vitamin D my body needs? http://www.vitamindcouncil.org/about-vitamin-d/how-do-i-get-the-vitamin-d-my-body-needs/. Accessed January 7, 2016.
48. Bailey RL, Dodd KW, Goldman JA, et al. Estimation of total usual calcium and vitamin D intakes in the United States. *J Nutr*. 2010;140:817–822.
49. Lips P. Worldwide status of vitamin D nutrition. *J Steroid Biochem Mol Biol*. 2010;121:297–300.
50. Holick MF. Vitamin D deficiency. *N Engl J Med*. 2007;357:266–281.
51. Hossein-nezhad A, Holick MF. Vitamin D for health: a global perspective. *Mayo Clin Proc*. 2013;88(7):720–755. http://www.mayoclinicproceedings.org/article/S0025-6196(13)00404-7/pdf. Accessed January 7, 2016.
52. Ibid.
53. Kumar J, Muntner P, Kaskel FJ, et al. Prevalence and associations of 25-hydroxyvitamin D deficiency in US children: NHANES 2001–2004. *Pediatrics*. 2009;124(3):e362–e370.
54. Ibid.
55. Jones G. Vitamin D. In: Ross AC, Caballero B, Cousins RJ et al *Modern Nutrition in Health and Disease*. 11th ed. Philadelphia: Wolters Kluwer/Lippincott Williams & Wilkins; 2014.
56. Hossein-nezhad A, Holick MF. Vitamin D for health: a global perspective. Op cit.
57. Kalyani RR, Stein B, Valiyil R, et al. Vitamin D treatment for the prevention of falls in older adults: systematic review and meta-analysis. *J Am Geriatr Soc*. 2010;58(7):1299–1310.
58. Pfeifer M, Begerow B, Minne HW, et al. Effects of a long-term vitamin D and calcium supplementation on falls and parameters of muscle function in community-dwelling older individuals. *Osteoporos Int*. 2009;20:315–322.
59. Linus Pauling Institute Micronutrient Information Center. Vitamin D. November 2014. http://lpi.oregonstate.edu/infocenter/vitamins/vitaminD/index.html#lpi_recommend. Accessed January 7, 2016.
60. Thomas MK, Lloyd-Jones DM, Thadhani RF, et al. Hypovitaminosis D in medical inpatients. *N Engl J Med*. 1998;338:777–783.
61. Saffel-Shier S. Vitamin status and requirements of the older adult. In: Bernstein M, Munoz N, eds. *Nutrition for the Older Adult*. 2nd ed. Burlington, MA: Jones and Bartlett; 2015 pages 73-86.
62. Jones G. Vitamin D. Op cit.
63. Ibid.
64. Institute of Medicine, Food and Nutrition Board. *Dietary Reference Intakes for Calcium and Vitamin D*. Op cit.
65. Mente A, de Koning L, Shannon HS, Anand SS. A systematic review of the evidence supporting a causal link between dietary factors and coronary heart disease. *Arch Intern Med*. 2009;169(7):659–669.
66. National Institutes of Health, Office of Dietary Supplements. Vitamin E: fact sheet for health professionals. http://ods.od.nih.gov/factsheets/vitamine. Accessed January 7, 2016.
67. U.S. Preventive Services Task Force. Final recommendation statement. Vitamin supplementation to prevent cancer and CVD: counseling, February 2014. http://www.uspreventiveservicestaskforce.org/Page/Document/RecommendationStatementFinal/vitamin-supplementation-to-prevent-cancer-and-cvd-counseling. Accessed January 7, 2016.

68. Traber MG. Vitamin E. In: Ross AC, Caballero B, Cousins RJ, Tucker KL, Ziegler TR, eds. *Modern Nutrition in Health and Disease*. 11th ed. Philadelphia: Lippincott Williams & Wilkins; 2014 pages 293-304.
69. Institute of Medicine, Food and Nutrition Board. *Dietary Reference Intakes for Vitamin C, Vitamin E, Selenium, and Carotenoids*. Op cit.
70. Ibid.
71. Ibid.
72. Otten JJ, Hellwig JP, Meyers LD. Vitamin E. In: Institute of Medicine. *DRI, Dietary Reference Intakes: The Essential Guide to Nutrient Requirements*. Washington, DC: National Academies Press; 2006:234–244.
73. Mayo Clinic. Vitamin E. http://www.mayoclinic.com/health/vitamin-e/NS_patient-vitamine. Accessed January 7, 2016.
74. National Institutes of Health, Office of Dietary Supplements,. Vitamin E: fact sheet for health professionals. Op cit.
75. Devlin TM, ed. *Textbook of Biochemistry with Clinical Correlations*. 7th ed. Hoboken, NJ: Wiley; 2011.
76. Hamidi MS1, Cheung AM. Vitamin K and musculoskeletal health in postmenopausal women. *Mol Nutr Food Res*. 2014;58(8):1647–1657. doi: 10.1002/mnfr.201300950. Epub June 23, 2014.
77. Shah K, Gleason L, Villareal DT. Vitamin K and bone health in older adults. *J Nutr Gerontol Geriatr*. 2014;33(1):10–22.
78. Institute of Medicine, Food and Nutrition Board. *Dietary Reference Intakes for Vitamin A, Vitamin K, Arsenic, Boron, Chromium, Copper, Iodine, Iron, Manganese, Molybdenum, Nickel, Silicon, Vanadium, and Zinc*. Op cit.
79. Hamidi MS, Cheung AM. Vitamin K and musculoskeletal health in postmenopausal women. Op cit.
80. Institute of Medicine, Food and Nutrition Board. *Dietary Reference Intakes for Vitamin C, Vitamin E, Selenium, and Carotenoids*. Op cit.
81. U.S. Department of Agriculture, Agricultural Research Service, Nutrient Data Laboratory. USDA National Nutrient Database for Standard Reference, Release 27 (revised). May 2015. http://www.ars.usda.gov/ba/bhnrc/ndl. Accessed January 7, 2016.
82. Li RC, Finkelman BS, Chen J, Booth SL, Bershaw L, Brensinger C, Kimmel SE. Dietary vitamin K intake and anticoagulation control during the initiation phase of warfarin therapy: a prospective cohort study. *Thromb Haemost*. 2013;110(1):195–196.

Chapter 11

Water-Soluble Vitamins

Revised by Melissa Bernstein

THINK About It

1 When cooking vegetables, how often do you think about vitamin loss?

2 Because of a friend's suggestion, you take a vitamin pill, and it causes intense flushing and itching. What has she probably given you, and what does your reaction tell you?

3 You decide to follow a vegetarian lifestyle. What vitamin deficiency should you watch out for?

4 Do you know anyone who takes vitamin C to prevent colds? What do you think of this strategy?

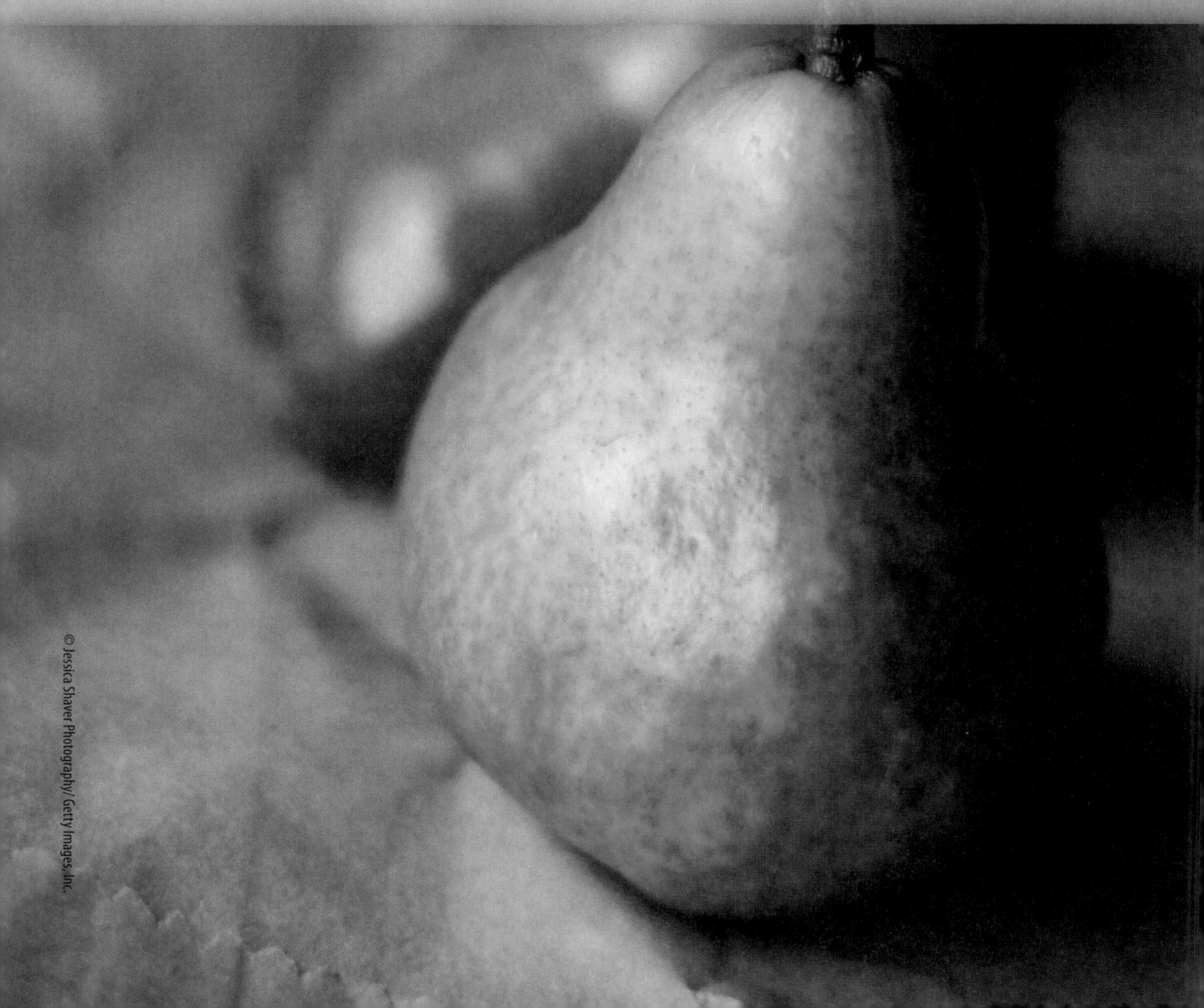

CHAPTER Menu

LEARNING Objectives

- Identify the key features of the water-soluble vitamins.
- Discuss the reasons behind enrichment and fortification programs.
- List ways to select, prepare, and store foods to maximize vitamin content.
- Describe the absorption, storage, and transport of the B vitamins and vitamin C.
- List major functions of the B vitamins and vitamin C.
- Identify major food sources of the B vitamins and vitamin C.
- Specify the major symptoms and diseases associated with deficiencies of the B vitamins and vitamin C.

Feeling tired, run down, stressed out? Burning the candle at both ends? Too many workouts wearing you out? You've heard that vitamins give you energy. So, a lack of energy must be a signal that you need more vitamins, right? Well, probably not.

First, the facts: Although many people like to think of vitamins as energy boosters, in truth, vitamins do not supply calories for the body—a fact that distinguishes them from fat, carbohydrate, and protein. However, many B vitamins (water-soluble vitamins) facilitate the metabolic reactions that release energy. So, in a sense, vitamins help you *get* energy by allowing carbohydrate, fat, and protein to become cellular fuel.

In times of stress, you need more energy than normal and therefore more vitamins, so a supplement is in order, right? Well, not necessarily. First, we need to consider *stress.* Certainly physical stress (e.g., injury and illness) increases the body's need for energy, protein, and many vitamins and minerals, to aid healing. But emotional stress (e.g., anxiety, fear) does not. It might seem that you expend a lot of mental energy studying for finals, but studying requires no more energy than sitting and chatting with your friends.

But surely if you do more physical exercise, you should take a vitamin, right? Again, not necessarily. Physical activity requires energy and therefore vitamins to help extract energy from food. But the food you consume to meet your energy needs for physical activity contains vitamins too, unless you meet your extra energy needs with chips and sodas! In most cases, healthful food choices—whole grains, fruits, vegetables, lean meats or meat substitutes, and low-fat dairy products—provide all the vitamins you need. So, check out your diet before you check out the vitamin supplements.

The Water-Soluble Vitamins: Eight Bs and a C

Water-soluble vitamins consist of the eight B vitamins and vitamin C. Scientists first viewed vitamin B as a single compound. However, after further study, they discovered that "it" was actually several vitamins. To differentiate the various B vitamins, scientists initially added numbers to the letter B—vitamins B_6 and B_{12}, for example. Today, with the exception of B_6 and B_{12}, we usually refer to the B vitamins by their names: thiamin (B_1), riboflavin (B_2), niacin (B_3), pantothenic acid, biotin, and folate. **TABLE 11.1** shows a summary of the water-soluble vitamins.

Although fat-soluble vitamins tend to accumulate in the body, the kidneys generally remove and excrete excess water-soluble vitamins. The exception is vitamin B_{12}, which the liver stores in large amounts. Because your body does not store other water-soluble vitamins in appreciable amounts,

TABLE 11.1
Summary of Water-Soluble Vitamins

Vitamin	Important Dietary Sources	Major Functions	Signs/Symptoms of Deficiency	Toxic Effects of Megadoses	Special Considerations
Thiamin	Pork, legumes, types of nuts and seeds, types of fish and seafood, fortified foods including bread, pasta, rice, and ready-to-eat cereals	Important participant in energy-yielding reactions (as part of the coenzyme thiamin pyrophosphate), nerve function	Beriberi (symptoms include muscle wasting, mental confusion, anorexia, enlarged heart, nerve changes), and Wernicke–Korsakoff syndrome (alcohol-induced deficiency with symptoms including mental confusion, staggering, rapid eye movements, paralysis of the eye muscles)	n/a	Increased risk for deficiency with alcohol abuse and for the poor and the elderly (due to consumption of inadequate energy and nutrient-poor foods)
Riboflavin	Milk, milk drinks, yogurt, fortified bread products, and ready-to-eat cereals	Energy metabolism; maintenance of the integrity of skin, mucous membranes, and nervous system structures	Shiny, smooth, inflamed tongue (glossitis), painful mouth, cracks at the corners of the mouth (angular stomatitis), inflamed lips (cheilosis)	n/a	Increased risk for deficiency with alcohol abuse, long-term barbiturate use, cancer, heart disease, diabetes
Niacin	Meat, poultry, fish, seafood, peanuts, liver, mushrooms, enriched and whole grain breads, grain products, and ready-to-eat cereals	Transformation of carbohydrates, fats, and protein into usable forms of energy	Redness around the neck, dermatitis, dementia, diarrhea	Flushing of the face and upper body, itching and tingling, liver toxicity	Increased risk for deficiency with diets primarily consisting of corn, and for people with limited protein in their diet
B_6	Fortified and ready-to-eat cereals; mixed foods that contain primarily meat, fish, or poultry; white potatoes and other starchy vegetables; noncitrus fruits; organ meats; soy-based meat substitutes; bananas; sunflower seeds	Supports protein metabolism, blood cell synthesis, carbohydrate metabolism, and neurotransmitter synthesis	Microcytic hypochromic anemia, seborrheic dermatitis, depression, confusion, convulsions	Irreversible nerve damage affecting the ability to walk and causing numbness in the extremities	Increased risk for deficiency with alcohol abuse
Folate	Fortified cereals, flour, and grain products; dark green leafy vegetables; asparagus; broccoli; orange juice; wheat germ; liver; sunflower seeds; legumes	Supports DNA synthesis and cell division, amino acid metabolism, maturation of red blood cells and other cells, and embryonic development	Anemia, atherosclerosis development, neural tube defects, adverse pregnancy outcomes, neuropsychiatric disorders	Masks B_{12} deficiency; hives and/or respiratory distress	Increased risk for deficiency with poor nutrition status, advanced age, alcohol abuse, intestinal malabsorption, medications that interfere with folate metabolism, certain types of anemia, pregnancy, leukemia, lymphoma, psoriasis, and with prolonged diarrhea
B_{12}	Mixed foods with the main ingredient of fish, meat, or poultry; liver; crab; fortified cereals; milk/milk products; and beef	Plays a key role in folate metabolism, the conversion of homocysteine to methionine, maintaining the myelin sheath, and preparation of fatty acid chains for entry into the citric acid cycle	Anemia, brain abnormalities and spinal cord degeneration, neurological symptoms including tingling and numbness in the extremities, abnormal gait, cognitive changes	n/a	Increased risk for deficiency with pernicious anemia, strict vegetarianism, advanced age, and impaired absorption (e.g., after gastric bypass surgery)
Pantothenic acid	Chicken, beef, potatoes, oats, tomato products, liver, kidney, yeast, egg yolk, broccoli, and whole grains	Metabolism of fats, carbohydrate, and protein	Irritability, restlessness, fatigue, apathy, malaise, sleep disruption, nausea/vomiting, numbness, tingling, muscle cramps, staggering gait, hypoglycemia	n/a	Increased risk for deficiency with administration of substances that prevent pantothenic acid metabolism
Biotin	Cauliflower, liver, peanuts, cheese	Coenzyme for dozens of reactions including the reactions of gluconeogenesis, fatty acid synthesis, release of energy from fatty acids, and DNA synthesis	Hair loss, rash, neurologic disorders (convulsions), delay of growth and development	n/a	Increased risk for deficiency with the consumption of raw egg whites over a long period of time (months to years), long-term anticonvulsant drug therapy, and in infants born with biotinidase deficiency
Vitamin C	Potatoes, citrus fruits, tomatoes, fortified juice drinks, broccoli, strawberries, kiwi, cabbage, spinach, leafy greens, green peppers	Antioxidant activity; the synthesis of collagen, carnitine, norepinephrine, epinephrine, serotonin, thyroxine, bile acids, steroid hormone, and purine bases; the absorption of nonheme iron; participant in immune function	Connective tissue breakdown, inflammation/bleeding of the gums and joints, fatigue/weakness, hemorrhage, bone pain and fracture, diarrhea, depression	Nausea, abdominal cramping, diarrhea, nose bleeds, formation of oxalate-containing kidney stones, and possible free radical damage	Increased risk for deficiency with alcohol/drug abuse, limited fruit and vegetable consumption, and restrictive diets

they should be a part of your daily diet. Small variations in daily intake typically do not cause problems, however. For example, symptoms of vitamin C deficiency do not emerge until after 20 to 40 days of a diet deficient in this water-soluble vitamin.

In general, water-soluble vitamins are more fragile than fat-soluble vitamins, and some cooking practices are particularly harmful. Vitamin C, thiamin, and riboflavin are especially vulnerable to heat and alkalinity, which can break chemical bonds. Water-soluble vitamins are hydrophilic by nature and will leach from vegetables into water during cooking. Cooking only partially destroys the vitamin content of a food, and some cooking methods are less destructive than others. To preserve vitamin content in foods, the best cooking methods are steaming, stir-frying, and microwaving using minimal amounts of water.

THINK About It 1

The B Vitamins

B vitamins act primarily in energy metabolism as coenzymes, or as parts of coenzymes (compounds that enable specific enzymes to function) (see **FIGURE 11.1**). The B vitamin part of a coenzyme helps catalyze the workings of metabolic pathways in cells. All B vitamins function in energy-producing metabolic reactions, and some also participate in other aspects of cellular metabolism.

Varied diets contain significant amounts of many vitamins, and vitamins often are added to foods such as cereals and other grain products. In the 1940s, the U.S. government mandated enrichment of bread and cereal products made from milled grains. Milling or refining grains removes the bran and germ to make white flour, white rice, refined cornmeal, flour for pasta, and most breakfast cereals. Processing grains also removes most B vitamins, vitamin E, and minerals such as iron, magnesium, and zinc. The loss of these nutrients from such staple foods could be devastating. In fact, during the nineteenth and early twentieth centuries, widespread adoption of these milling techniques left a wake of vitamin-deficiency diseases such as beriberi and pellagra. To prevent overt deficiencies, food manufacturers now return iron and B vitamins to the grains they process. Replacing lost nutrients is called "enrichment." Most countries now require enrichment of staple grain products.

Food processors also fortify foods. Fortification is the process of adding extra nutrients to foods where they wouldn't be found naturally in consistently significant amounts. Iodized table salt (salt with added iodine) is a fortified food. Read the labels on some breakfast cereals: The ones with the long list of added vitamins and minerals are fortified foods. Because most breakfast cereals are fortified, they usually are good sources of vitamins and minerals. Fortification is sometimes required by law, as in the addition of vitamins A and D to milk and, more recently, the addition of folic acid to enriched cereal and grain products. Because of a 1998 Food and Drug Administration (FDA) requirement, all enriched bread, flour, cornmeal, pasta, rice, and other grain products must be fortified with folic acid.[1] Food manufacturers also fortify foods with dietary supplements and other ingredients to make functional foods with a variety of health benefits beyond basic nutrition.

Enrichment and mandatory fortification programs helped eliminate most overt deficiency diseases in the United States and many other countries. However, mandatory enrichment replaces only some of the many nutrients lost in milling. Moreover, the American diet contains lots of highly refined foods that are not fortified or enriched—foods that have calories but relatively few micronutrients.

During the production of highly refined grain products, processing also removes vitamin B_6, magnesium, and zinc. To ensure a good balance of nutrients, experts recommend that people regularly eat whole-grain products such as whole-wheat bread, brown rice, and oatmeal.

Quick Bite

What Do You Believe?

More than half of adults in the United States use dietary supplements. Improving health and maintaining overall health are the most commonly reported reasons given by supplement users, yet less than 25 percent of supplements are recommended by a health care provider.

Quick Bite

Is It a Fruit or a Vegetable?

In the eighteenth century, botanists defined fruits as the organ surrounding the seeds. This definition considers cucumbers, eggplants, peppers, pea pods, and corn kernels as fruits. Legally, though, they are all vegetables. In the late 1800s, the U.S. Supreme Court, while trying the case of a tomato importer, established a definition based on linguistic custom and usage. The importer had to pay the vegetable tax.

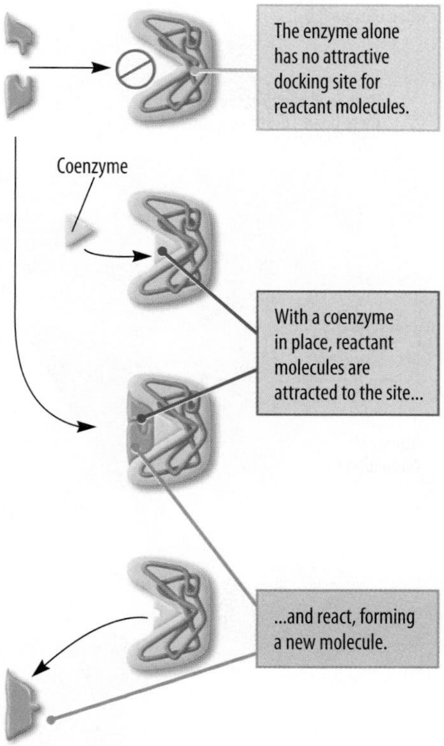

The enzyme alone has no attractive docking site for reactant molecules.
Coenzyme
With a coenzyme in place, reactant molecules are attracted to the site...
...and react, forming a new molecule.

FIGURE 11.1 The coenzyme–enzyme partnership. The B vitamins form coenzymes that enable specific enzymes to catalyze reactions.

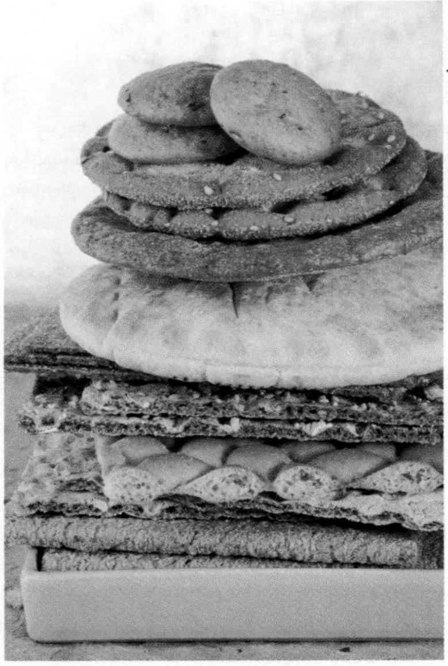

© iStockphoto/Thinkstock

Thiamin

Although mentioned in ancient Chinese writings from 2600 B.C.E., the thiamin-deficiency disease **beriberi** remained largely unknown until the nineteenth century, when milling and refining grains became popular. In 1885, Dr. K. Takaki, director general of the Japanese Naval Medical Services, demonstrated beriberi's dietary origins when he cured afflicted sailors by supplementing their diets with meat, milk, and whole grains.[2] Some years later, Christian Eijkman, a Dutch medical officer, induced beriberi in birds by feeding the birds only white rice, and then cured them by adding bran to their diet.[3] This led to the discovery of an "anti-beriberi" factor—thiamin.

Isolated in 1926, thiamin (also known as vitamin B_1) gets its name from *thio*, meaning "sulfur," and *amine*, the nitrogen-containing group in the vitamin. As **FIGURE 11.2** shows, thiamin consists of a sulfur-containing ring and a nitrogen-containing ring attached to a carbon atom. Heat easily breaks the bonds between the two rings and the carbon atom, so cooking reduces a food's thiamin content.

- **beriberi** Thiamin-deficiency disease. Symptoms include muscle weakness, loss of appetite, nerve degeneration, and in some cases, edema.
- **thiamin pyrophosphate (TPP)** A coenzyme of which the vitamin thiamin is a part. It plays a key role in decarboxylation and helps drive the reaction that forms acetyl CoA from pyruvate during metabolism.
- **decarboxylation** Removal of a carboxyl group (–COOH) from a molecule. The carboxyl group is then released as carbon dioxide (CO_2).

Functions of Thiamin

Along with other B vitamins, thiamin is an important participant in many energy-yielding reactions. Specifically, thiamin is the vitamin portion of the coenzyme **thiamin pyrophosphate (TPP)**, shown in **FIGURE 11.3**. TPP participates in a vital reaction known as **decarboxylation**, which removes a carboxyl group (–COOH) and releases it as carbon dioxide (CO_2). During glucose metabolism, for example, decarboxylation removes one carbon from the three-carbon substance pyruvate to form the two-carbon molecule acetyl CoA (see **FIGURE 11.4**). TPP also is involved in a decarboxylation step in the citric acid cycle.

Cells also use TPP in the pentose phosphate pathway, an alternative pathway to glycolysis. This series of reactions metabolizes glucose to make, among other products, the five-carbon monosaccharide deoxyribose for DNA synthesis, the five-carbon monosaccharide ribose for RNA synthesis, and the energy-rich molecule NADPH to help power biosynthesis. Thiamin pyrophosphate also plays a role in nerve function and helps synthesize and regulate neurotransmitters—chemicals that act as messengers between nerve cells.[4]

Dietary Recommendations for Thiamin

The small difference in the RDA for adult men and women reflects the differences in their average size and energy use. The RDA for adult men aged 19 years and older is 1.2 milligrams; for adult women of the same age, the RDA is 1.1 milligrams per day. Pregnancy and lactation increase energy requirements, so thiamin requirements rise during these life stages. Thiamin intake recommendations are 1.4 milligrams per day during pregnancy and 1.5 milligrams per day during lactation.[5] If a person's diet supplies adequate energy and includes thiamin-rich foods, it generally contains adequate amounts of thiamin.

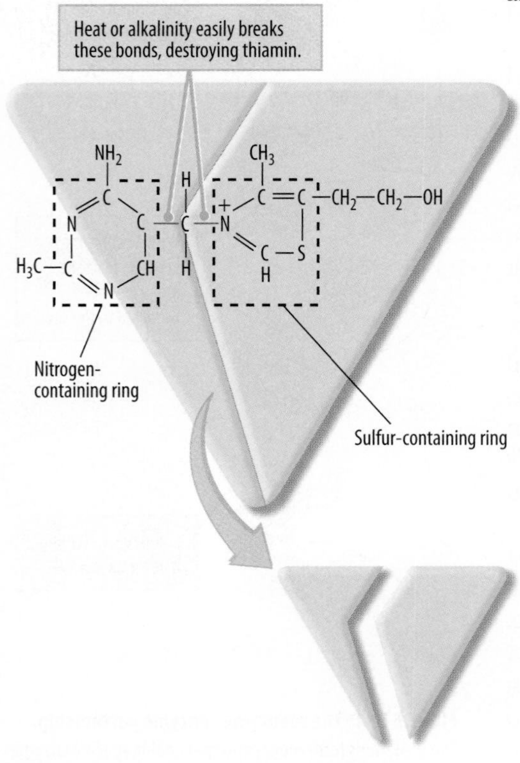

FIGURE 11.2 Thiamin structure and vulnerability. Water-soluble vitamins, especially thiamin, riboflavin, and vitamin C, are vulnerable to heat and alkalinity.

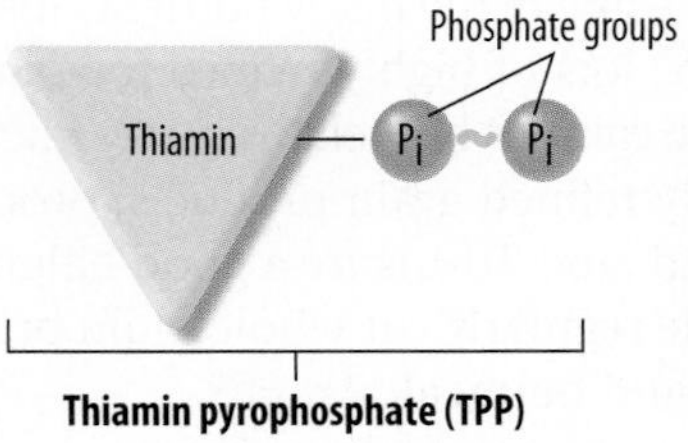

FIGURE 11.3 Thiamin pyrophosphate (TPP). Thiamin pyrophosphate contains the B vitamin thiamin and two phosphate groups.

Sources of Thiamin

Thiamin is found throughout the food supply, although most foods contain only small amounts. Pork is one of the richest food sources of thiamin. Legumes (mature beans and peas), some nuts and seeds, and some types of fish and seafood are good sources. Typically, however, most of our dietary thiamin comes from enriched or whole-grain products such as bread, pasta, rice, and ready-to-eat cereals.[6] **FIGURE 11.5** shows some foods that provide thiamin.

Meat (except pork and organ meats), dairy products, seafood, and most fruits contain very little thiamin. Eating a wide variety of foods is the best way to ensure adequate thiamin consumption.

There are few data from studies of humans on the bioavailability of thiamin from food.[7] Refer to the later section on thiamin toxicity for details about absorption of thiamin from supplements.

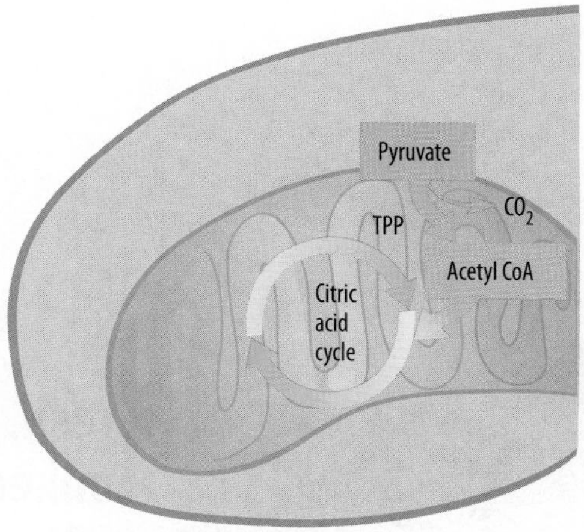

FIGURE 11.4 TPP helps convert pyruvate to acetyl CoA. In addition to coenzyme A and NAD$^+$, three other catalytic cofactors—TPP, α-lipoic acid, and FAD—help convert pyruvate to acetyl CoA.

Thiamin Deficiency

In industrialized countries, thiamin deficiency usually is related to heavy alcohol consumption combined with limited food consumption. Alcoholics are at risk for thiamin deficiency for two reasons: (1) alcohol contributes calories without contributing nutrients, and (2) alcohol interferes with absorption of thiamin and many other vitamins. Poor people and older adults also can be at risk of deficiency as a result of inadequate energy intake or consumption of nutrient-poor foods. Eating mostly highly processed but unenriched foods and empty-calorie items such as alcohol, sugar, and fat can lead to a deficiency. A genetic defect that affects thiamin's transport and metabolism has been described in patients with other inborn errors of metabolism that can often be overcome with high concentrations of thiamin.[8]

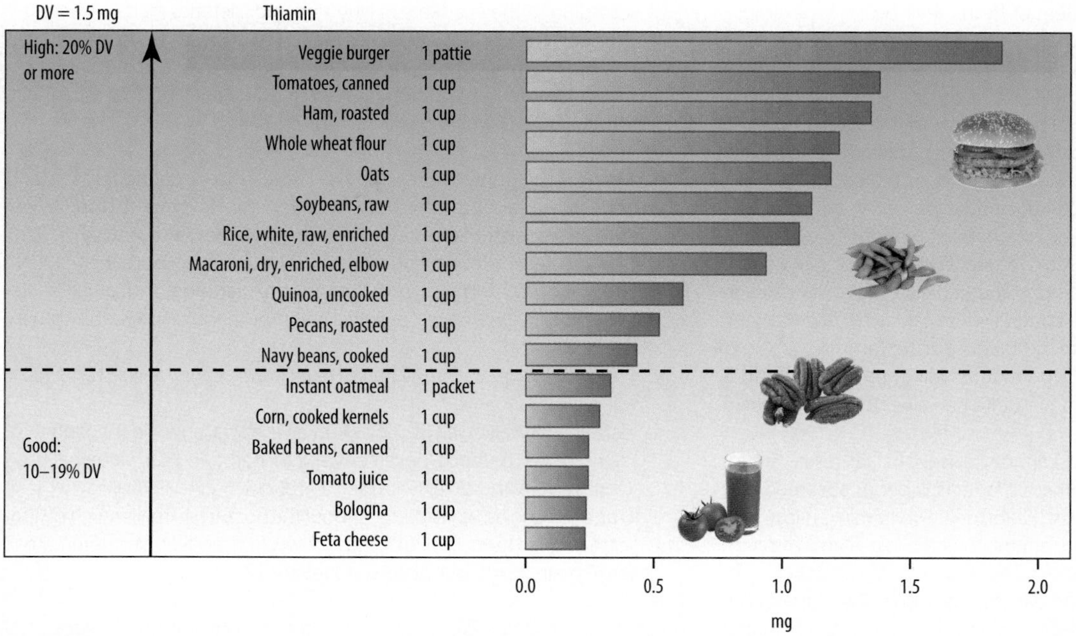

FIGURE 11.5 Food sources of thiamin. Pork, whole and enriched grains, and fortified cereals are rich in thiamin. Most animal foods contain little thiamin.

Data from US Department of Agriculture, Agricultural Research Service, Nutrient Data Laboratory. USDA National Nutrient Database for Standard Reference, Release 28. Version Current: September 2015. Internet: http://www.ars.usda.gov/nea/bhnrc/ndl.

Beriberi

Beriberi is a term from the Singhalese language (spoken in Sri Lanka) that means "I can't, I can't." The phrase describes how doctors long ago diagnosed the disease: Their patients were unable to rise from a squatting position. In fact, overall profound muscle weakness combined with nerve destruction

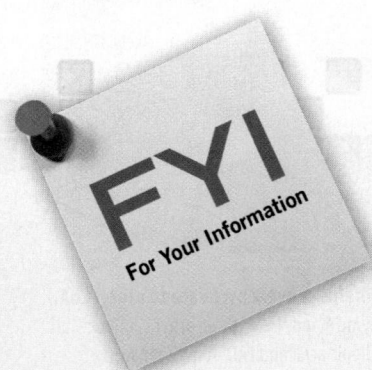

FYI For Your Information

Fresh, Frozen, or Canned? Raw, Dried, or Cooked? Selecting and Preparing Foods to Maximize Nutrient Content

A food's vitamin content depends first on the original amount in the plant or animal while it is alive and growing. Although grazing materials and feed have a minor impact on vitamin content, animal products tend to have fairly consistent levels. This reflects the animal's ability to concentrate and store vitamins. The vitamin content of plants, however, depends more on soil and growing conditions such as available moisture and sunlight. The maturity of a fruit or vegetable at the time it is harvested also influences its vitamin content.

Light, heat, air, acid, alkali, and cooking fluids can attack vitamins, so proper storage, processing, and cooking are important. Ideally, you should shop for produce as the Europeans do: Choose fresh fruits and vegetables daily to minimize nutrient losses associated with prolonged storage. Barring that, choose clean, undamaged produce at each of your regular shopping trips. When storing foods, avoid temperature extremes, and minimize exposure to light and air with refrigeration or covered storage. It's best to eat fruits and vegetables soon after purchase; normal storage can decrease their vitamin content. The vitamin C content of fresh green beans, for example, drops by half after six days at home.

What about frozen and canned foods? Their vitamin content is much better than you might guess. Vegetables are frozen immediately after they are picked, so that their nutritional value and flavor are preserved.[a] Choose fruits and plain vegetables instead of those in a sauce, fried, or breaded, and use nutrition labeling to compare products and control calories.[b]

Although canning uses destructive heat, the processor typically uses fresh-picked produce, which is higher in vitamins than fresh food transported to faraway markets. The thiamin content of canned meats and beans is comparable to home-prepared versions. Vegetable sources of folate, such as spinach, retain most of their folate content when canned or frozen. When using canned vegetables, incorporate the liquid from the can into soups and stews to get the benefit of any vitamins that remain in the liquid. Recipes prepared with canned foods have similar nutritional values to those prepared with fresh or frozen ingredients.[c]

Carotenoids are stable during the canning process. In fact, research suggests the lycopene in processed tomato products is better absorbed into the body than that from raw tomatoes.[d] Unfortunately, vitamin C is lost from fruits and vegetables during canning, but much of the lost vitamin remains in the canning liquid or juice.

Dried fruits also are a good way to eat your daily fruit. The biggest concern is portion size because when fruits are dried, their nutrient, calorie, and sugar content becomes concentrated, and it is easy to eat too much. Dried fruits have a low to moderate glycemic index and a glycemic response that is comparable to fresh fruits. They are a good source of nutrients such as potassium and fiber.[e] Data from the National Health and Nutrition Examination Survey (NHANES) 1999–2004 show that dried fruit consumption is associated with lower body mass index (BMI), reduced waist circumference, reduced abdominal obesity, improved nutrient intake (higher vitamin A, vitamin K, potassium, iron, magnesium, and fiber), more fruit servings per day, and healthier overall diets for both adults and children.[f,g]

Once fruits and vegetables are home and stored carefully, what is the best way to cook them? To maximize the vitamin content, think minimal—minimal amounts of heat, minimal amounts of cooking water, and minimal exposure to air. Try to minimize handling the food before and during cooking. Although dicing a food such as a potato reduces cooking time, it also exposes more surface area to vitamin-destroying influences. So, cut if you must, but not too small.

Steaming and microwaving are the best cooking methods for preserving vitamin content because they minimize cooking time and water use. If you boil foods, try to use the cooking water for sauces, stews, or soups because it contains many of the water-soluble vitamins lost from the food during cooking.

According to the Academy of Nutrition and Dietetics, fruits and vegetables are good-for-you foods that can be enjoyed at any time, no matter what form they take—fresh, frozen, canned, or dried.[h] To retain the most nutrients in your food, be gentle with storage, handling, and cooking. Minimize (heat, water, and air exposure) to maximize!

a. Fruit and Veggies: More Matters. Fresh, frozen, canned, dried and 100% juice: all forms of fruits and vegetables matter! http://www.fruitsandveggiesmorematters.org/?page_id=47. Accessed January 28, 2016.
b. Duffy R. Frozen foods: convenient and nutritious. February 14, 2014. http://www.eatright.org/resource/food/planning-and-prep/smart-shopping/frozen-foods-convenient-and-nutritious. Accessed February 24, 2016.
c. Fruit and Veggies: More Matters. Fresh, frozen, canned, dried and 100% juice. Op cit.
d. Carlsen MH, Halvorsen BL, Holte K, et al. The total antioxidant content of more than 3100 foods, beverages, spices, herbs and supplements used worldwide. *Nutr J.* 2010; 9:3. doi: 10.1186/1475-2891-9-3.
e. Fruit and Veggies: More Matters. About the buzz: fresh fruit is much healthier than dried fruit? July 2011. http://www.fruitsandveggiesmorematters.org/?page_id=18744. Accessed January 28, 2016.
f. Ibid.
g. Keast DR, O'Neil CE, Jones JM. Dried fruit consumption is associated with improved diet quality and reduced obesity in US adults: National Health and Nutrition Examination Survey, 1999–2004. Nutr Res. 2011 Jun; 31(6): 460–467. doi: 10.1016/j.nutres.2011.05.009.
h. Denny S. Fresh, canned, or frozen: get the most from your fruits and vegetables. November 11, 2014. http://www.eatright.org/resource/food/nutrition/nutrition-facts-and-food-labels/fresh-canned-or-frozen-get-the-most-from-your-fruits-and-vegetables. Accessed February 24, 2016.

ultimately leaves the victim of beriberi almost unable to move. This deficiency disease occurs in people whose major source of energy is polished rice, which is common in Southeast Asia. Polishing removes the rice hulls and thus their major source of thiamin.

An inadequate supply of this essential nutrient affects the cardiovascular, muscular, nervous, and gastrointestinal systems, which all rely on thiamin to help fuel their activities. The brain and nervous system rely on glucose for energy, and thiamin, as part of TPP, is crucial in glucose metabolism. The first signs of thiamin deficiency are weakness, irritability, headache, fatigue, and depression—functions associated with the brain and nervous system. These disturbances can appear after only 10 days on a thiamin-free diet.

As symptoms progress, "dry" beriberi (beriberi without edema) causes nerve degeneration, loss of nerve transmission leading to tingling sensations throughout the body, muscle wasting, poor arm and leg coordination, and deep pain in the calf muscles. "Wet" beriberi has additional symptoms, including an enlarged heart, heart failure, and severe edema (see **FIGURE 11.6**). Because many B vitamins are in the same foods as thiamin, thiamin deficiency and other B vitamin deficiencies often go hand in hand.

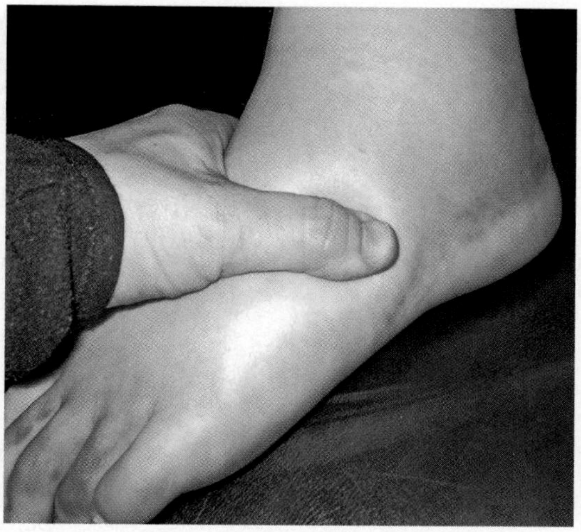
Courtesy of Scott Landis, Bryan College.

FIGURE 11.6 Edema, especially in the feet and legs, is a symptom of wet beriberi.

Wernicke-Korsakoff Syndrome

Alcohol-induced malnutrition is the most common cause of Wernicke-Korsakoff syndrome, another thiamin-deficiency disease. Symptoms include mental confusion, staggering, and constant rapid eye movements or paralysis of the eye muscles. Although the syndrome most often is associated with the stereotypical alcoholic, it can occur in any heavy drinker, especially an aging alcoholic.

Thiamin Toxicity

Supplements, which are cheap to produce, often include up to 200 times the Daily Value for thiamin. The Food and Nutrition Board has not set a Tolerable Upper Intake Level (UL) for this nutrient. The kidneys rapidly excrete excess thiamin in urine.[9]

Riboflavin

At first, riboflavin and thiamin were considered the same vitamin. Scientists then discovered that heating the "anti-beriberi factor" destroyed its anti-beriberi properties but left its growth-promoting properties unscathed. The factor actually contained two active compounds: heat-vulnerable thiamin and a heat-stable component. In 1917, scientists identified the heat-stable component as another vitamin—called vitamin B_2 in England and vitamin G in the United States. This naming confusion ended when the new vitamin was finally dubbed riboflavin.

Riboflavin is named for its yellow color (*flavin* means "yellow" in Latin). In foods, though, it can give a green or bluish cast. You'll notice the color in uncooked egg whites and some brands of fat-free milk.

Functions of Riboflavin

The vitamin accepts and donates electrons with ease, so it participates in many oxidation-reduction reactions. Riboflavin is a part of two coenzymes: flavin mononucleotide (FMN) and flavin adenine dinucleotide (FAD). These coenzymes participate in numerous metabolic pathways, including the citric acid cycle and the beta-oxidation pathway that breaks down fatty acids. FMN and FAD act first as electron and hydrogen acceptors. In the citric acid cycle, for instance, FAD accepts hydrogen and electrons, forming the reduced form, $FADH_2$ (see **FIGURE 11.7**). Later, this coenzyme delivers its high-energy electrons

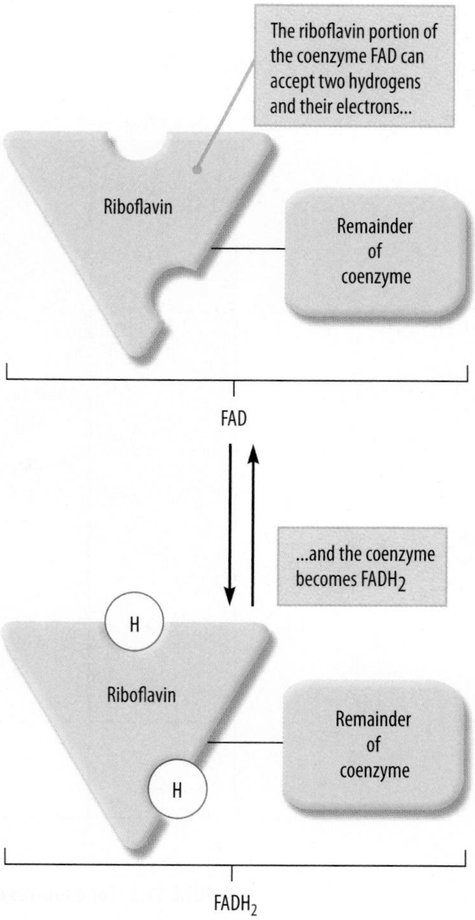

FIGURE 11.7 Riboflavin coenzymes easily transfer hydrogens. The riboflavin coenzyme flavin adenine dinucleotide (FAD) accepts hydrogens and electrons to become $FADH_2$.

to the mitochondrial electron transport chain to produce ATP. Another riboflavin coenzyme, FMN, also accepts hydrogen and electrons, forming $FMNH_2$. FMN works in the electron transport chain to move electrons. Both coenzymes are crucial in energy metabolism.

Riboflavin-containing coenzymes participate in reactions that remove ammonia during the deamination of some amino acids.[10] Riboflavin also is associated with the antioxidant activity of the glutathione reductase, **glutathione peroxidase**, and xanthine oxidase enzymes.

▶ **glutathione peroxidase** A selenium-containing enzyme that promotes the breakdown of fatty acids that have undergone peroxidation.

Dietary Recommendations for Riboflavin

For adults aged 19 years and older, the RDA is 1.1 milligrams per day for women and 1.3 milligrams per day for men. Intake recommendations for riboflavin, like those for thiamin, reflect the higher energy needs of males. Pregnancy and lactation increase energy needs, so the RDA for women rises to 1.4 milligrams per day during pregnancy and to 1.6 milligrams per day during lactation.[11]

Sources of Riboflavin

Although most plant and animal foods contain some riboflavin, milk, milk drinks, and yogurt supply about 15 percent of the riboflavin in the U.S. diet. Bread and bread products contribute approximately 10 percent, and ready-to-eat cereals add nearly as much.[12] Riboflavin is one of the four vitamins (thiamin, riboflavin, niacin, and folic acid) and one mineral (iron) that are added to enriched grain products. Organ meats such as liver and kidney are good sources of riboflavin, as are mushrooms and cottage cheese.[13] **FIGURE 11.8** shows some foods that provide riboflavin.

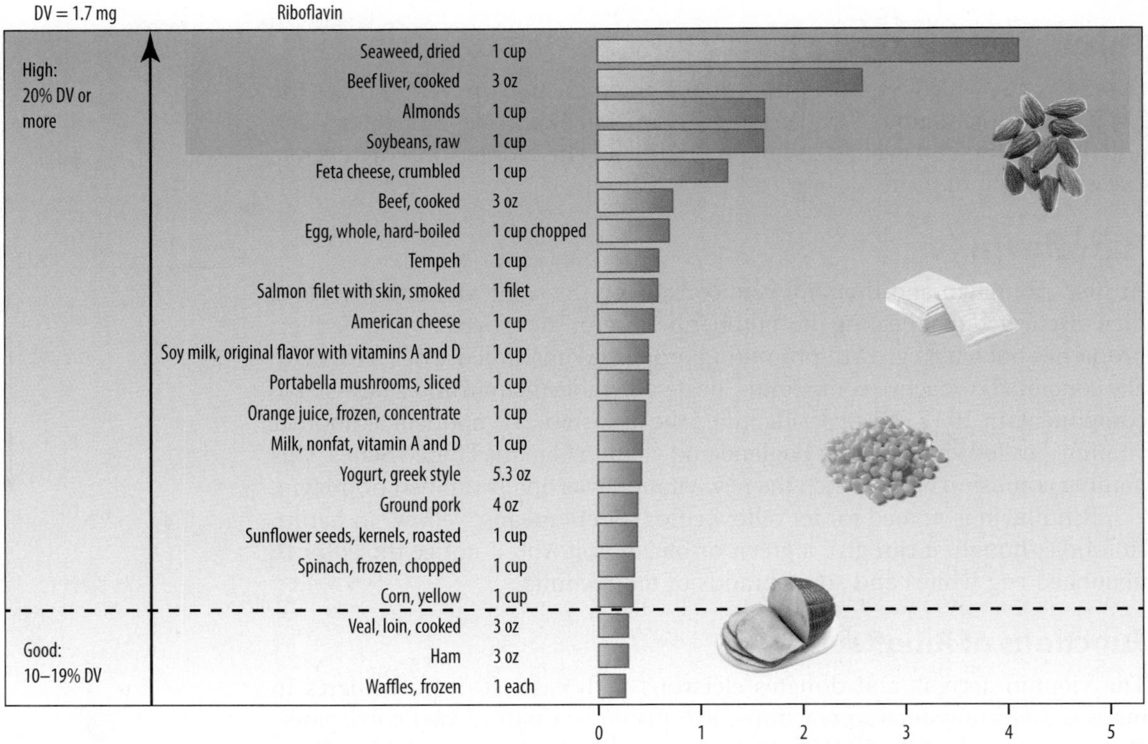

FIGURE 11.8 Food sources of riboflavin. The best sources of riboflavin include milk, liver, whole and enriched grains, and fortified cereals.

Data from US Department of Agriculture, Agricultural Research Service, Nutrient Data Laboratory. USDA National Nutrient Database for Standard Reference, Release 28. Version Current: September 2015. Internet: http://www.ars.usda.gov/nea/bhnrc/ndl. Accessed January 29, 2016.

Photos (from top to bottom): (almonds) © vkbhat/Getty Images, Inc.; (cheese slices) © Binh Thanh Bui/Shutterstock, Inc.; (corn kernels) © Renee Comet Photography/Getty Images, Inc.; (ham) © Paul Poplis/Getty Images.

Riboflavin is more stable than thiamin and is resistant to acid, heat, and oxidation. On the other hand, light easily breaks it down. Riboflavin-rich foods should be stored in opaque packages. For example, packaging milk in paper or plastic cartons rather than clear glass better protects milk's riboflavin content (see **FIGURE 11.9**). Approximately 95 percent of riboflavin from food is absorbed.[14]

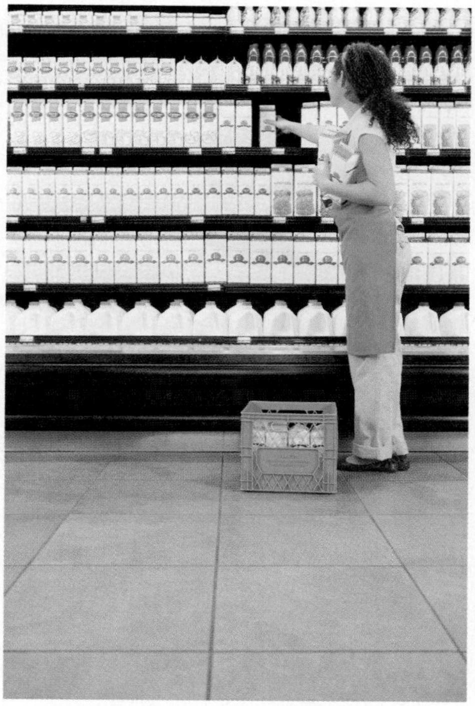

FIGURE 11.9 Packaging affects riboflavin content in milk. Light breaks down riboflavin easily, so foods high in riboflavin (e.g., milk) are best stored in opaque containers.

Riboflavin Deficiency

Riboflavin deficiencies are rare. Several large surveys suggest that, in the United States, men take in about 2 milligrams of riboflavin per day, and women consume about 1.5 milligrams per day. Some people, however, consume only marginal amounts. Because people with alcoholism tend to have poor diets, for example, they risk riboflavin deficiency.

Riboflavin deficiency (**ariboflavinosis**) shows up first around the mouth. The tongue gets shiny, smooth, and inflamed (**glossitis**); the mouth becomes painful and sore; the skin at the corners of the mouth cracks (**angular stomatitis**); and the lips become inflamed and split (**cheilosis**). The oil-producing glands of the skin become clogged (**seborrheic dermatitis**). As the deficiency becomes severe, a characteristic anemia develops. Riboflavin deficiency usually exists along with other nutrient deficiencies. In fact, because riboflavin is involved in the metabolism of other B vitamins such as vitamin B_6, folate, and niacin, severe riboflavin deficiency can make other deficiencies even worse.

- ▶ **ariboflavinosis** Riboflavin deficiency.
- ▶ **glossitis** Inflammation of the tongue; a symptom of riboflavin deficiency.
- ▶ **angular stomatitis** Inflammation and cracking of the skin at the corners of the mouth; a symptom of riboflavin deficiency.
- ▶ **cheilosis** Inflammation and cracking of the lips; a symptom of riboflavin deficiency.
- ▶ **seborrheic dermatitis** Disease of the oil-producing glands of the skin; a symptom of riboflavin deficiency.

Riboflavin Toxicity

Riboflavin toxicity has not been reported. Because the body readily excretes excess riboflavin, even large doses appear to pose no risk of harm. A UL has not been set for riboflavin.

Niacin

In 1867, scientists first produced a substance called nicotinic acid by oxidizing the nicotine from tobacco. Nicotinic acid is not, however, the same as or even closely related to the nicotine molecule. Seventy years later, Conrad Elvehjem at the University of Wisconsin demonstrated that nicotinic acid cured dogs of a canine version of the human niacin-deficiency disease pellagra. In the early 1940s, the vitamin was renamed *niacin*, an acronym of "nicotinic acid vitamin," so people would not confuse it with nicotine.

Niacin actually is the name for two similarly functioning compounds: nicotinic acid and nicotinamide (also known as niacinamide). Like the other B vitamins, niacin is a coenzyme component (see **FIGURE 11.10**) and participates in at least 200 metabolic pathways.

Functions of Niacin

The niacin coenzymes, nicotinamide adenine dinucleotide (NAD^+) and nicotinamide adenine dinucleotide phosphate ($NADP^+$), play key roles in oxidation-reduction reactions. NAD^+ accepts electrons and hydrogen (i.e., is reduced) to form NADH. Under aerobic conditions, NADH carries high-energy electrons to the electron transport chain to help produce ATP. When you need energy in anaerobic conditions (say, during vigorous activity that pushes the body beyond its aerobic capacity), NADH powers the conversion of pyruvate to lactate as it loses electrons and a hydrogen (i.e., is oxidized) to become NAD^+. (See **FIGURE 11.11**.) This regenerated NAD^+ helps power the continued operation of glycolysis. Without it, glycolysis would halt, shutting off the supply of energy from glucose.

Quick Bite

Are You Smoking That Bread?

In the 1940s, anti-tobacco forces were confused about the differences between niacin and nicotine. They mistakenly warned that niacin-enriched bread could cause an addiction to cigarettes!

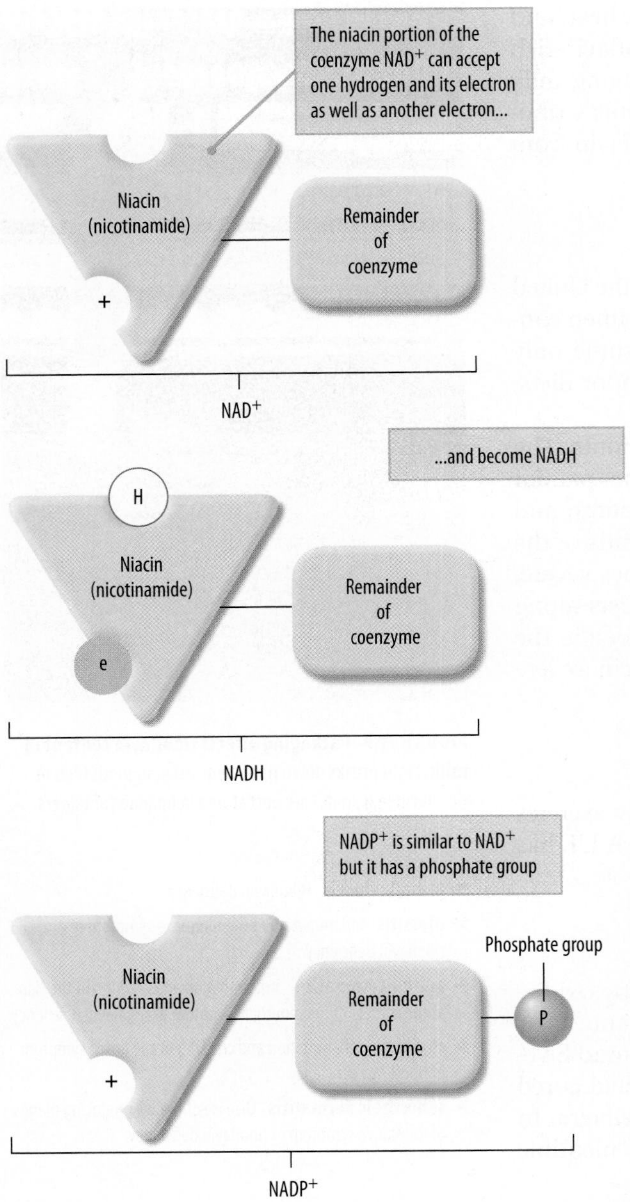

FIGURE 11.10 Niacin is part of the coenzymes NAD^+ and $NADP^+$. Niacin, as nicotinamide, is an integral part of coenzymes critical to several metabolic reactions. NAD^+ is crucial to the formation of ATP, and $NADP^+$ is crucial to biosynthesis.

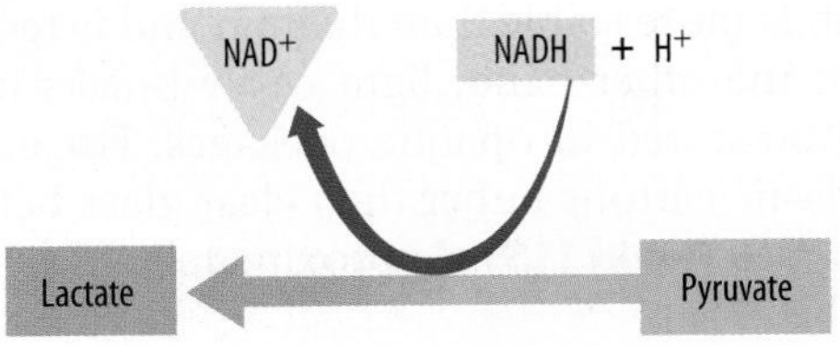

FIGURE 11.11 Niacin helps convert pyruvate to lactate. As a component of the coenzymes NAD^+ and NADH, niacin participates in many metabolic reactions.

Many metabolic pathways that promote the synthesis of new compounds, such as fatty acids, rely on NADPH, the reduced form of $NADP^+$. NADPH is concentrated in cells (such as liver cells) that make large amounts of fatty acids.

Dietary Recommendations for Niacin

Niacin is unique among the B vitamins because your body can make it from the amino acid **tryptophan** as well as obtain it from foods. Intake recommendations are expressed as **niacin equivalents (NE)**, a measure that includes both preformed dietary niacin and niacin derived from tryptophan. The RDA for adult men of all ages is 16 milligrams of NE per day, and the RDA for adult women of all ages is 14 milligrams of NE. It increases to 18 milligrams of NE for pregnancy and 17 milligrams of NE for lactation.[15]

Sources of Niacin

Most of the preformed niacin in the U.S. diet comes from meat, poultry, fish, enriched and whole-grain breads and grain products, and fortified ready-to-eat cereals.[16] Other good sources of niacin include mushrooms, peanuts, liver, and seafood. In a typical U.S. diet, beef and processed meats are substantial contributors.[17] **FIGURE 11.12** shows some foods that provide niacin. Because the vitamin is stable when heated, little niacin is lost during cooking.

The niacin precursor tryptophan is found in protein-rich animal foods, with the exception of gelatin. To convert tryptophan to niacin, your body needs other nutrients: riboflavin, vitamin B_6, and iron. Sixty milligrams of tryptophan yield about 1 milligram of niacin, or 1 niacin equivalent (NE).

Because riboflavin, vitamin B_6, and iron affect the conversion of tryptophan to niacin, a deficiency of any one of these nutrients decreases tryptophan conversion. Certain rare metabolic disorders disrupt tryptophan conversion pathways. Pregnancy, on the other hand, increases the efficiency of converting tryptophan to niacin.

Tryptophan supplies about half of the average American's niacin intake. When estimating niacin consumption, remember that tables of food composition list only preformed niacin and therefore underestimate the amount of niacin some foods contribute by way of tryptophan.

Niacin Deficiency

First documented in 1735 by a Spanish physician named Gaspar Casal, the niacin-deficiency disease pellagra was originally named *mal de la rosa*, or "red sickness," for the telltale redness that appears around the necks of people with the disease. Severely roughened skin is another hallmark, and

▶ **tryptophan** An amino acid that serves as a niacin precursor in the body. In the body, 60 milligrams of tryptophan yield about 1 milligram of niacin, or 1 niacin equivalent (NE).

▶ **niacin equivalents (NEs)** A measure that includes preformed dietary niacin as well as niacin derived from tryptophan; 60 milligrams of tryptophan yield about 1 milligram of niacin.

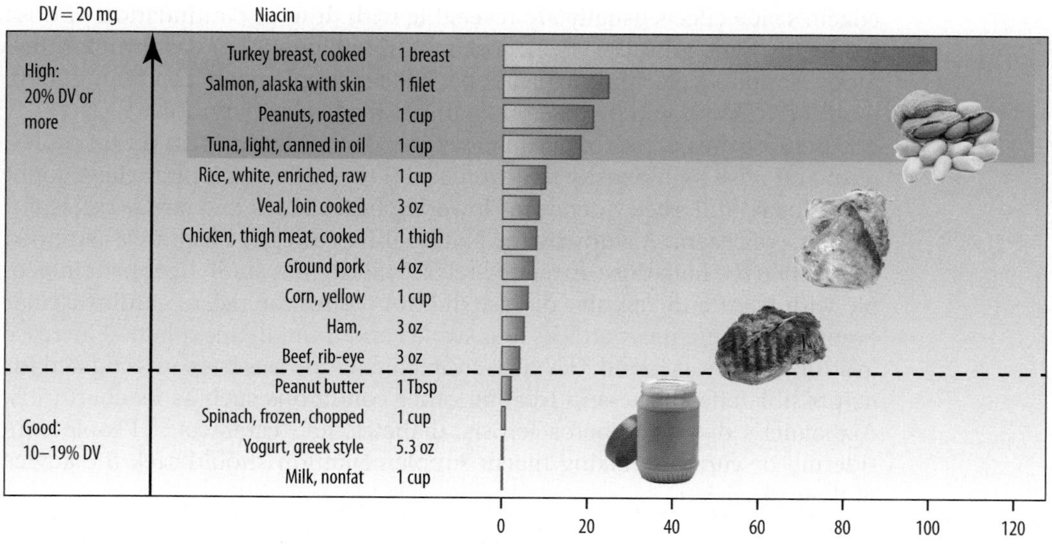

FIGURE 11.12 Food sources of niacin. Niacin is found mainly in meats and grains. Enrichment adds niacin as well as thiamin, riboflavin, folic acid, and iron to processed grains.

Data from US Department of Agriculture, Agricultural Research Service, Nutrient Data Laboratory. USDA National Nutrient Database for Standard Reference, Release 28. Version Current: September 2015. Internet: http://www.ars.usda.gov/nea/bhnrc/ndl. Accessed January 29, 2016.

Photos (from top to bottom): (dried peanuts) © Hong Vo/Shutterstock, Inc.; (grilled chicken thighs) © Yury Smelov/Shutterstock, Inc.; (rib eye steak) © JoeGough/Getty Images, Inc.; (peanut butter) © Andrea Bricco/Getty Images Inc.

the condition was later dubbed *pellagra* for the Italian *pelle*, or "skin," and *agra*, or "rough." Because the niacin coenzymes NAD^+ and $NADP^+$ are involved in just about every metabolic pathway, niacin deficiency wreaks havoc throughout the body. The primary symptoms of pellagra are known as the three Ds: dementia, diarrhea, and dermatitis. In severe cases, a fourth D—death—is the final outcome. Deficiencies of iron and vitamin B_6 also contribute to pellagra.

During the early 1900s, as corn became a staple in the southern United States, pellagra emerged in epidemic proportions.[18] Because a protein in corn binds niacin tightly, it dramatically reduces niacin's bioavailability. Corn is also low in the amino acid tryptophan, limiting the availability of niacin and further contributing to the development of pellagra. We now know, however, that soaking corn in a solution of lime (calcium hydroxide) releases that bound niacin (see **FIGURE 11.13**). This disease was common among the rural poor, who subsisted on a diet of corn (maize), molasses, and salt pork, which is mostly fat. Between the end of World War I and the end of World War II, pellagra afflicted some 200,000 Americans. The incidence of pellagra started to decline during World War II because of the mandatory enrichment of bread flour and other cereal grains with niacin. After World War II, the enrichment program, combined with the postwar affluence that allowed people to purchase more protein-rich meat, poultry, and fish, finally curbed the disease. Sadly, pellagra continues to plague people whose diets lack sufficient niacin and protein.

Calculation of NE for an 80-kg (176-lb) Man

His protein RDA is

80 kg × 0.8 g/kg = 64 g protein

Let us assume his diet contains 94 g of high-quality protein so that

94 g dietary protein
– 64 g protein (his protein RDA)

30 g protein in excess of needs

Tryptophan makes up about 1% of the protein so that

30 g protein × 0.01 = 0.3 g tryptophan (300 mg tryptophan)

60 mg tryptophan × 1 mg niacin (1 NE) so that

300 mg tryptophan ÷ 60 = 5 mg niacin (5 NE)

Shortcut Method

30 g excess protein ÷ 6 = 5 mg niacin (5 NE)

Niacin Toxicity and Medicinal Uses of Niacin

THINK About It 2

Although niacin has shown little severe toxicity, its side effects discourage widespread use. The principal side effects are flushing (a feeling of prickly heat on the face and upper body), related itching, and tingling. Serious side effects of higher niacin levels are rare, but include liver toxicity and impaired glucose tolerance.[19]

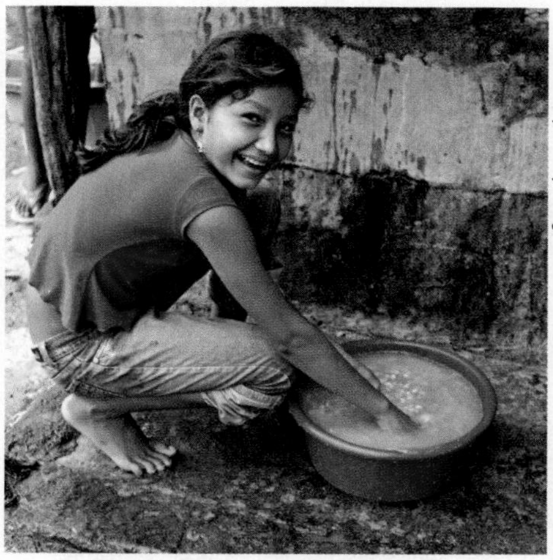

© Tina Manley/Alamy Images

FIGURE 11.13 Soaking corn in a solution of lime (calcium hydroxide) releases bound niacin.

Niacin's side effects usually are reversible with drug discontinuation or dose reduction. For adults, the UL for niacin is 35 milligrams per day from fortified foods, supplements, and medications. Niacin supplements containing more than the RDA should be taken only under medical supervision.

Because megadoses of niacin lower low-density lipoprotein (LDL) cholesterol and raise high-density lipoprotein (HDL) cholesterol, physicians might prescribe it. Still, the evidence for lowering heart attack and stroke risk is not entirely consistent. A study by the National Institutes of Health was stopped early when the high-dose, extended-release niacin plus statin treatment in people with heart and vascular disease did not reduce the risk of cardiovascular events, including heart attacks and stroke, and a small, unexplained increase in stroke rates was found.[20] Niacin supplementation has been investigated for its possible effectiveness in treating other conditions such as osteoarthritis, Alzheimer's disease, atherosclerosis, diabetes, and cataracts.[21] People considering or currently taking niacin supplementation should seek the advice of their physician.

Key Concepts Thiamin, riboflavin, and niacin are all incorporated in coenzymes that catalyze energy-yielding reactions. All three B vitamins participate in pathways that metabolize carbohydrate, protein, and fat. Enriched grains are a major source of these B vitamins, with pork ranking as a good source of thiamin, milk as a major source of riboflavin, and high-protein foods as sources of niacin. Deficiencies of these vitamins are rare in the United States. People with alcoholism have the highest risk of deficiencies. High doses of thiamin and riboflavin appear to be harmless, but megadoses of niacin should be taken only under medical supervision.

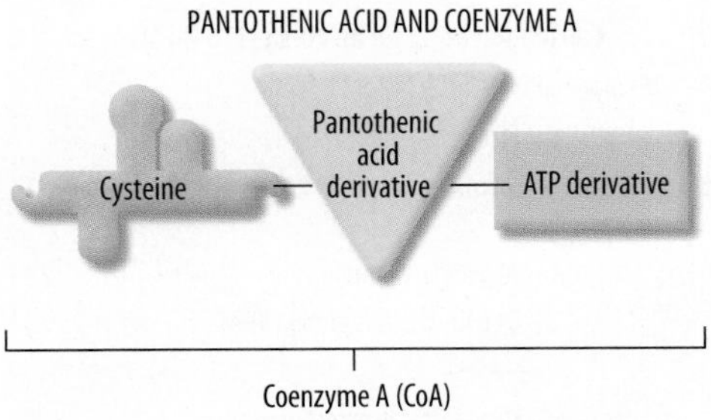

FIGURE 11.14 Pantothenic acid and coenzyme A. Pantothenic acid forms part of coenzyme A, which in turn is a component of acetyl CoA. Through coenzyme A, pantothenic acid is involved in many metabolic reactions.

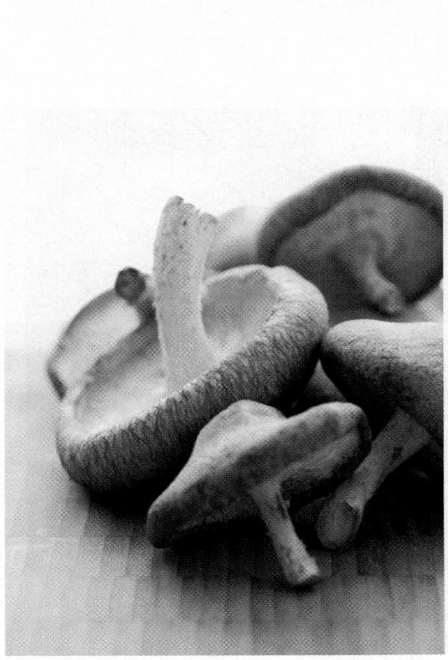

Pantothenic Acid

In the 1930s, a chemist named Roger J. Williams discovered that yeast requires a certain nutrient, which he called pantothenic acid. He suggested that if yeast needed this nutrient, humans might need it, too. First isolated in 1938, the chemical structure of pantothenic acid was identified by scientists in 1940.

The name *pantothenic acid* is derived from the Greek word *pantothen*, meaning "from every side." This B vitamin is widespread in the food supply, so it is well named. Despite marketers promoting pantothenic acid supplements for a long list of uses, in most cases there is not enough scientific evidence to determine its effectiveness.[22]

Functions of Pantothenic Acid

Pantothenic acid is a component of coenzyme A (CoA), which in turn is a component of acetyl CoA (see **FIGURE 11.14**). Acetyl CoA sits at the crossroads of a number of metabolic pathways—both energy-generating pathways and biosynthetic pathways. It is formed from pyruvate (see **FIGURE 11.15**), starts the citric acid cycle, is a key building block of fatty acids, and is a precursor of ketone bodies.

Fatty acids also are known as acyl groups, and pantothenic acid is a component of the acyl carrier protein. During fatty acid synthesis, the acyl carrier protein binds fatty acids and carries them through a series of reactions that increases their chain length.

Dietary Recommendations for Pantothenic Acid

There are few data upon which to base dietary recommendations for pantothenic acid. When the data are insufficient to set an Estimated Average Requirement (EAR) for a nutrient, an RDA cannot be established. In these cases, and thus for pantothenic acid, an Adequate Intake (AI) level is set instead. For adults aged 19 to 50 years, the AI for pantothenic acid is 5 milligrams per day.[23]

Sources of Pantothenic Acid

Pantothenic acid is widely available in the food supply. Food sources known to contain this vitamin include chicken, beef, potatoes, oats, tomato products, liver, kidney, yeast, egg yolk, broccoli, and whole grains.[24] **FIGURE 11.16** shows foods that are good sources of pantothenic acid.

Pantothenic acid is damaged easily. Freezing and canning appear to decrease the pantothenic acid content of vegetables, meat, fish, and dairy products. Processing and refining grains can reduce their pantothenic acid content by nearly 75 percent.[25]

Pantothenic Acid Deficiency

Pantothenic acid deficiencies are virtually nonexistent in the general population. The only observed cases of pantothenic acid deficiency are in people who were fed diets that completely lacked the nutrient or who were given a substance that prevents metabolism of pantothenic acid. These people suffered symptoms that included irritability, restlessness, fatigue, apathy, malaise, sleep disturbances, nausea, vomiting, numbness, tingling, muscle cramps, staggering gait, and hypoglycemia.

Pantothenic Acid Toxicity

High intakes of pantothenic acid have not caused adverse effects. Risk of toxicity appears to be extremely low, and therefore a UL has not been established.

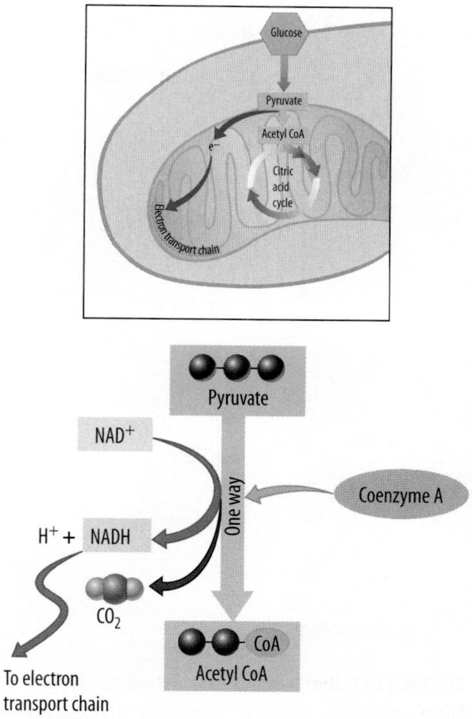

FIGURE 11.15 Pantothenic acid helps convert pyruvate to acetyl CoA. As part of coenzyme A, pantothenic acid helps form acetyl CoA from pyruvate. Niacin participates in this reaction as part of the coenzyme NAD$^+$.

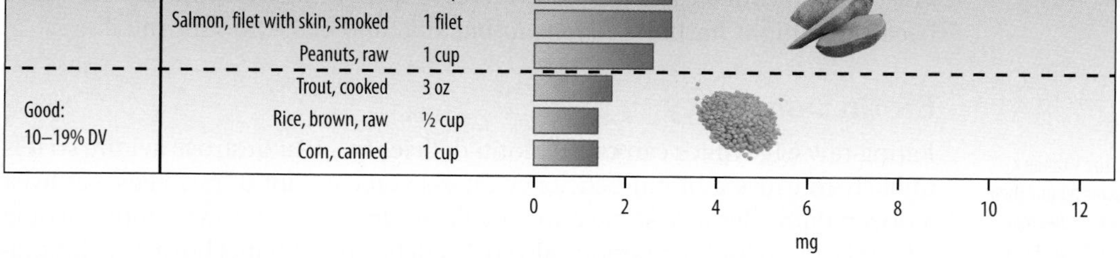

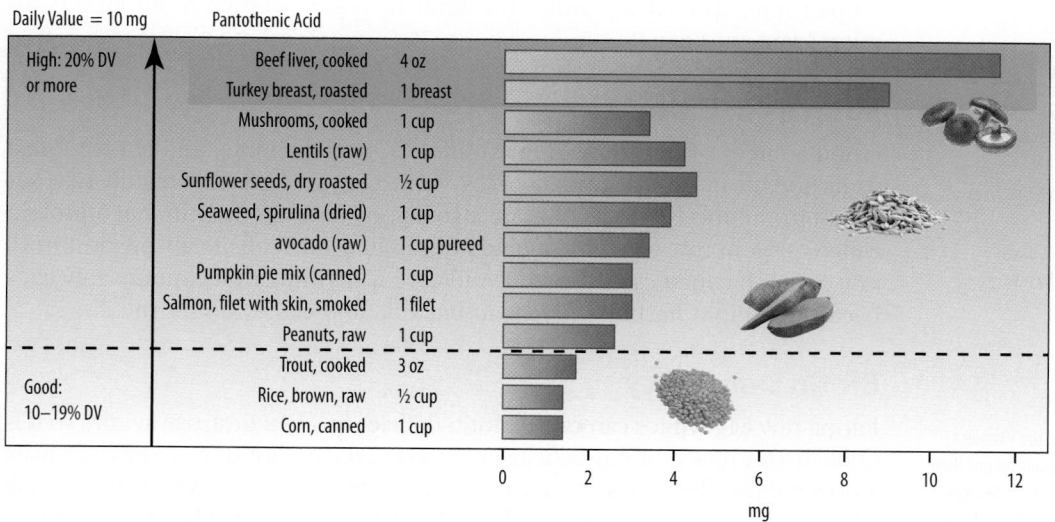

FIGURE 11.16 Food sources of pantothenic acid. Pantothenic acid is found widely in foods but is abundant in only a few sources, such as liver.

Data from US Department of Agriculture, Agricultural Research Service, Nutrient Data Laboratory. USDA National Nutrient Database for Standard Reference, Release 28. Version Current: September 2015. Internet: http://www.ars.usda.gov/nea/bhnrc/ndl.

Photos (from top to bottom): (mushrooms) © Hiroshi Higuchi/ Getty Images, Inc.; (sunflower seeds) © Alasdair Thomson/ Getty images; (sweet potato) © uliedeshaies/ Getty Images, Inc.; (red lentils) © Marcel Jancovic/ Shutterstock, Inc.

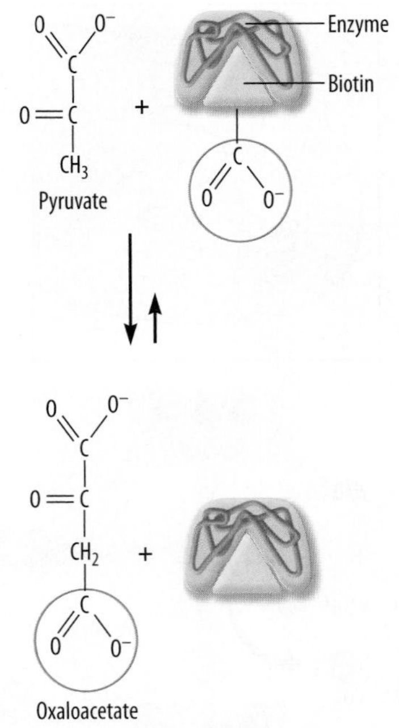

FIGURE 11.17 Biotin aids carboxylation reactions. Biotin is a coenzyme for several carboxylase enzymes. These enzymes transfer carboxyl groups, such as in the conversion of pyruvate to oxaloacetate.

Biotin

In 1924, three factors were identified as necessary for the growth of microorganisms. They were called "bios II," "vitamin H," and "coenzyme R." It soon became clear that all three were the same water-soluble, sulfur-containing vitamin—biotin. In food, biotin is found both free and bound to protein. When proteins are digested, a biotin–lysine complex called **biocytin** is released.

Functions of Biotin

Like the other B vitamins, biotin acts as a coenzyme in dozens of reactions. Among these reactions are amino acid metabolism, including the conversion of amino acids to glucose (gluconeogenesis); fatty acid synthesis; release of energy from fatty acids; and DNA synthesis.

Biotin-containing enzymes mainly catalyze **carboxylation** reactions, in which carbon dioxide is added to a substrate (see **FIGURE 11.17**). Some of the reactions that rely on biotin-containing enzymes include the following:

- Adding carbon dioxide to three-carbon pyruvate to yield four-carbon oxaloacetate. This process is one of the first steps in gluconeogenesis.
- Entry of three-carbon fatty acids into the citric acid cycle to yield energy.
- Elongating fatty acid chains during fatty acid synthesis.
- Breaking down leucine to the ketone body acetoacetate.
- Breaking down isoleucine, methionine, threonine, and valine for entry into the citric acid cycle.
- Synthesizing DNA.

Dietary Recommendations for Biotin

Just like pantothenic acid, there are not enough data on biotin to establish an EAR or an RDA. In fact, we know so little about human biotin requirements that the Adequate Intake value for adults is mathematically determined from the AI level for infants. The infant value is based on the amount of biotin in human milk. The AI for biotin for adult men and women of all ages is 30 micrograms per day.[26]

Sources of Biotin

Good sources of biotin include cauliflower, liver, peanuts, and cheese. Most fruits and meats rank as poor sources.[27] The enzyme **biotinidase** readily releases biotin from biocytin. Egg yolks are also a good source of biotin, but a protein called **avidin** in raw egg whites binds biotin and prevents its absorption from raw eggs. Of course, you should avoid eating anything that contains raw eggs because it might harbor *Salmonella* bacteria and cause foodborne illness.

Biotin Deficiency

Eating raw egg whites can cause biotin deficiency. Heat destroys avidin, so it is unlikely to cause a biotin deficiency unless you eat a lot of raw eggs—at least a dozen daily. Because some anticonvulsant drugs break down biotin, people who take them for long periods also risk a deficiency. Infants born with biotinidase deficiency suffer from a rare genetic defect that leads to biotin depletion. Symptoms progress from initial hair loss and rash to convulsions and other neurological disorders. The deficiency also can delay growth and development. Early diagnosis and daily high doses of biotin (e.g., 10 milligrams per day) usually clear up symptoms. If not treated, biotin deficiency causes changes in blood pH that can lead to coma and death.

- **biocytin** A biotin–lysine complex released from digested protein.
- **carboxylation** A reaction that adds a carboxyl group (–COOH) to a substrate, replacing a hydrogen atom.
- **biotinidase** An enzyme in the small intestine that releases biotin from biocytin.
- **avidin** A protein in raw egg whites that binds biotin, preventing its absorption. Avidin is destroyed by heat.

Quick Bite

Busy Bacteria

You may be aware that bacteria in the colon synthesize vitamin K, but did you know that colonic bacteria also make some biotin? Then again, when synthesizing this B vitamin these busy microbes may be pursuing a futile effort. Because the colon is downstream from the small intestine, the site of most biotin absorption, the bacteria's biotin may not be absorbed efficiently. Bacterial synthesis of biotin probably does not make an important contribution to your body's supply of biotin.

Biotin Toxicity

Biotin does not appear to be toxic at high doses. Children with biotinidase deficiency have been given as much as 200 milligrams of biotin daily without adverse side effects. A UL for biotin has not been established.

Vitamin B_6

Vitamin B_6 is a group of six compounds: pyridoxal (PL), pyridoxine (PN), pyridoxamine (PM), and their phosphorylated forms (PLP, PNP, and PMP), in which a phosphate group has been added (see **FIGURE 11.18**). Food contains the phosphorylated forms PLP, PNP, and PMP, but digestion strips off the phosphate groups. PL, PN, and PM then travel to the liver, which converts them to PLP (pyridoxal phosphate), the primary active coenzyme form.[28]

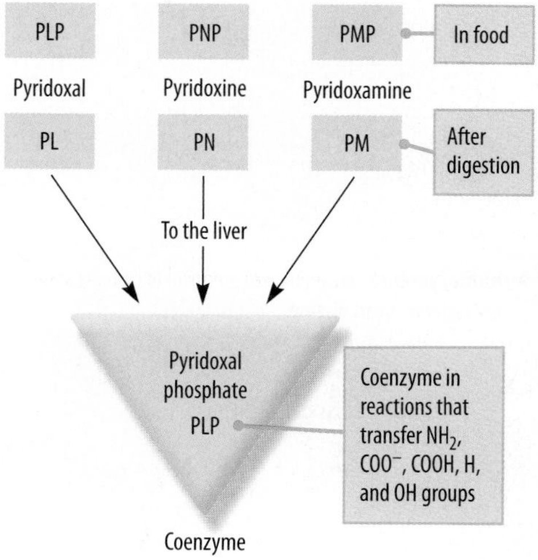

FIGURE 11.18 The vitamin B_6 family and coenzyme form. Vitamin B_6 is a group of six compounds: pyridoxal (PL), pyridoxine (PN), pyridoxamine (PM), and their phosphorylated forms PLP, PNP, and PMP. Digestion removes the phosphate groups and the liver converts PL, PN, and PM to PLP (pyridoxal phosphate), the active coenzyme form.

Functions of Vitamin B_6

The vitamin B_6 coenzyme PLP supports more than 100 different enzymes involved in reactions that include the transfer of amino groups (NH_2), carboxyl groups (COO– or –COOH), or water (as H and OH). These enzymes support protein metabolism, blood cell synthesis, carbohydrate metabolism, and neurotransmitter synthesis.

Protein Metabolism

One of the primary tasks of PLP is to help metabolize amino acids and other nitrogen-containing compounds. As **FIGURE 11.19** shows, PLP plays a key role in transamination reactions, helping transfer an amino group from an amino acid to a keto acid and produce a new amino acid. Transamination, catalyzed by PLP, enables the body to make the 11 nonessential amino acids. Without adequate supplies of vitamin B_6, all amino acids become "essential," meaning the body cannot synthesize them and must obtain them from the diet. Over time, vitamin B_6 deficiency impairs protein synthesis and cell metabolism.

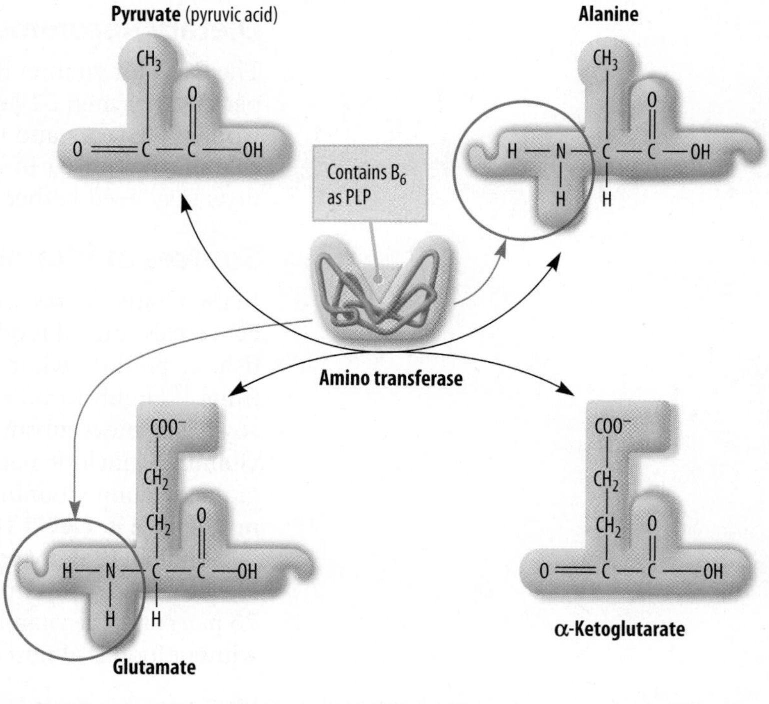

FIGURE 11.19 Vitamin B_6 aids transamination reactions. Vitamin B_6, as part of PLP, helps transfer an amino group from an amino acid to a keto acid and produce a new amino acid.

Blood Cell Synthesis

PLP supports the synthesis of the white blood cells of the immune system and is crucial for the synthesis of the red blood cells' hemoglobin rings, which carry oxygen. PLP also helps bind oxygen to hemoglobin. Inadequate vitamin B_6 disturbs this binding process, causing **microcytic hypochromic anemia**. In this type of **anemia**, red blood cells are smaller than normal and lack sufficient hemoglobin to carry oxygen. Iron deficiency also can cause microcytic hypochromic anemia.

Carbohydrate Metabolism

Through its role in transamination reactions, PLP participates in gluconeogenesis—producing glucose from amino acids. In addition, PLP facilitates glycogen breakdown.

▶ **microcytic hypochromic anemia** Anemia characterized by small, pale red blood cells that lack adequate hemoglobin to carry oxygen; can be caused by deficiency of iron or vitamin B_6.

▶ **anemia** Abnormally low concentration of hemoglobin in the bloodstream; can be caused by impaired synthesis of red blood cells, increased destruction of red cells, or significant loss of blood.

Neurotransmitter Synthesis

PLP helps produce a number of neurotransmitters, including serotonin, gamma-amino butyric acid (GABA), dopamine, and norepinephrine. A vitamin B_6 deficiency can cause neurological symptoms—depression, headaches, confusion, and convulsions.

Vitamin B_6, Folate, and Heart Disease

▶ **homocysteine** An amino acid precursor of cysteine and a risk factor for heart disease.

Moderately high blood levels of the amino acid **homocysteine** are associated with fatal cardiovascular events. Homocysteine blood levels are influenced by dietary intake of vitamin B_6, folate, and vitamin B_{12}. Low intake of vitamin B_6 or folate can increase homocysteine levels, and high homocysteine levels can be a marker for heart disease.[29] Because the body accumulates large vitamin B_{12} stores to draw on when needed, variations in B_{12} intake seldom affect homocysteine levels. The body lowers homocysteine levels in one of two ways: (1) two PLP-dependent enzymes help convert homocysteine to cysteine, or (2) folate and vitamin B_{12}–dependent enzymes help convert homocysteine to methionine. An increase in fruit and vegetable intake also can affect homocysteine levels. Interestingly, although diets high in fruits and vegetables can offer protection against heart disease, using folic acid supplementation to reduce homocysteine has not been proven to reduce risk.[30] A healthy dietary pattern, such as one that includes fruits and vegetables, fish, and whole grains, has consistently been shown to have considerable cardioprotective effects for the primary prevention of heart disease.[31]

Dietary Recommendations for Vitamin B_6

The RDA for vitamin B_6 for men and women aged 19 to 50 is 1.3 milligrams per day. For men 51 years and older, the RDA is 1.7 milligrams per day; for women 51 years and older, the RDA is 1.5 milligrams per day. Due to the role of vitamin B_6 in amino acid metabolism, people on very-high-protein diets may need higher intakes.[32]

Sources of Vitamin B_6

In the United States, the primary sources of vitamin B_6 are fortified, ready-to-eat cereals; mixed foods (including sandwiches) that contain primarily meat, fish, or poultry; white potatoes and other starchy vegetables; and noncitrus fruits.[33] Highly fortified cereals, beef liver and other organ meats, and fortified soy-based meat substitutes are especially rich sources. Other good sources of vitamin B_6 include bananas, potatoes, and sunflower seeds. Although whole grains contain vitamin B_6, refining removes vitamin B, and enrichment does not replace it. **FIGURE 11.20** shows foods that provide vitamin B_6.

Vitamin B_6 is not particularly stable and is especially sensitive to temperature. Heat can destroy as much as 50 percent of a food's vitamin B_6 content. About 75 percent of the vitamin B_6 in a varied diet is bioavailable, and vitamin B_6 taken without food is almost completely absorbed, even when taken in megadoses.[34]

Vitamin B_6 Deficiency

Vitamin B_6 deficiencies are rare. When one does occur, the deficiency leads to microcytic hypochromic anemia, seborrheic dermatitis, and neurological symptoms such as depression, confusion, and convulsions. Even small deficits of vitamin B_6 can disrupt homocysteine metabolism, leading to increased blood levels of homocysteine.

Alcoholism boosts the risk of vitamin B_6 deficiency because alcohol decreases absorption of the nutrient and hampers synthesis of the coenzyme PLP. A breakdown product of alcohol metabolism also interferes with the functioning of vitamin B_6 coenzymes. In addition, two conditions frequently

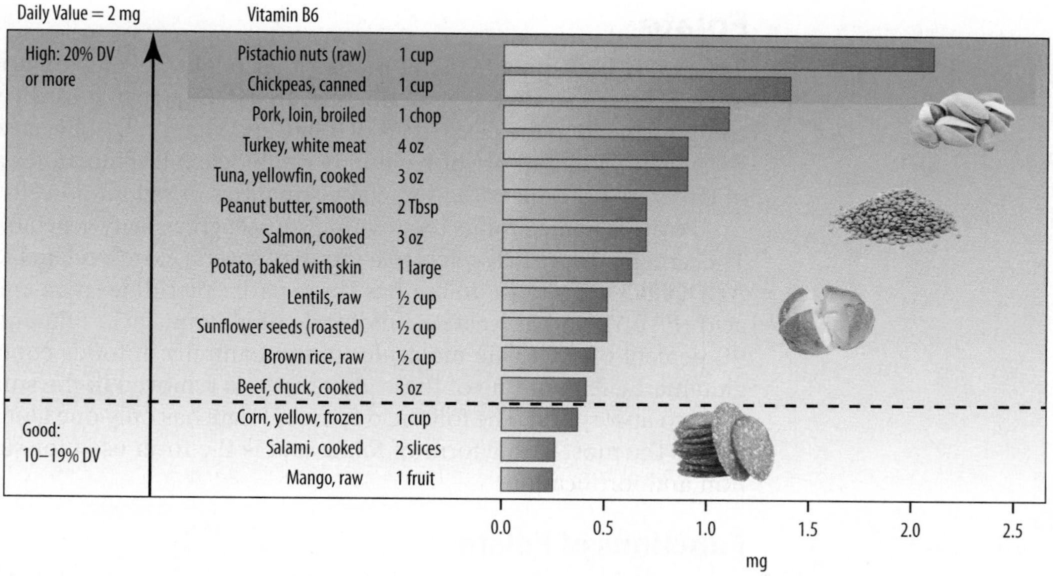

FIGURE 11.20 Food sources of vitamin B_6. Meats are generally good sources of vitamin B_6 along with certain fruits (e.g., bananas) and vegetables (e.g., potatoes, carrots).

Data from US Department of Agriculture, Agricultural Research Service, Nutrient Data Laboratory. USDA National Nutrient Database for Standard Reference, Release 28. Version Current: September 2015. Internet: http://www.ars.usda.gov/nea/bhnrc/ndl.

Photos (from top to bottom): (dried pistachio) © Dionisvera/Shutterstock, Inc.; (baked potato) © Joe Gough/Shutterstock, Inc.; (lentils) © Imageman/Shutterstock, Inc.; (fresh salami) © Sergiy Kuzmin/Shuttterstock, Inc.

suffered by people with alcoholism—cirrhosis and hepatitis—damage liver tissue, preventing the liver from metabolizing vitamin B_6 to its coenzyme form.

Vitamin B_6 Toxicity and Medicinal Uses of Vitamin B_6

Megadoses of supplemental vitamin B_6 can cause irreversible nerve damage that affects the ability to walk and causes numbness in the extremities. Other side effects include upset stomach, headache, sleepiness, and a tingling, prickling, or burning sensation. Some women self-prescribe large doses of vitamin B_6 as an antidote to treat premenstrual syndrome (PMS)—the headache, bloating, irritability, and depression that can occur during the week or so before the onset of menstruation. Women have taken vitamin B_6 for PMS and to reduce symptoms of morning sickness during pregnancy with some promising results; however, current scientific evidence of these benefits is unclear, and additional research is needed to confirm its safety and effectiveness. Women should not take supplemental vitamin B_6 without consulting their physician.[35]

Despite the risk of toxicity, some people have recommended high doses of vitamin B_6 as a treatment for carpal tunnel syndrome—a repetitive strain injury characterized by painful tingling in the wrist and fingers. Most well-designed scientific studies have found no evidence that vitamin B_6 improves carpal tunnel syndrome.[36]

The reasons for the nerve damage associated with B_6 excess are unclear, but modification of proteins by PLP might be involved. The UL for vitamin B_6 intake is 100 milligrams per day, a common amount in over-the-counter vitamin supplements. Because of the potential hazards, vitamin B_6 megadoses should be taken only under medical supervision.

Key Concepts Pantothenic acid and biotin are widespread in the food supply. Deficiencies of these B vitamins are rare because most people consume adequate amounts. Like the other B vitamins, pantothenic acid and biotin are parts of coenzymes involved in the metabolism of fat, carbohydrate, and protein. Vitamin B_6 is found in animal and plant foods and participates in protein metabolism, synthesis of neurotransmitters, and other metabolic pathways. Prolonged megadoses of vitamin B_6 can cause nerve damage.

Folate

Eating raw liver, unappetizing though that might be, has long been known to cure a degenerative type of anemia. In 1945, a search for liver's curative component led to the discoveries of folate and vitamin B_{12}. Because folate and B_{12} work together to perform a number of biochemical functions, a deficiency of either one produces the same abnormalities in red blood cells.

Folate is named for its best natural source: green leafy vegetables (foliage). The term *folate* actually refers to a group of several closely related folate forms. As **FIGURE 11.21** shows, folate has three parts: pteridine, para-aminobenzoic acid (PABA), and at least one molecule of glutamic acid (glutamate). About 90 percent of the folate molecules found naturally in foods contain 3 to 11 glutamates. All but one of these glutamates is removed in the small intestine prior to absorption. The folic acid form of folate has only one glutamate. Folic acid is the most stable form of folate and is the form used for supplementation and fortification.

Functions of Folate

As a coenzyme, folate is crucial to DNA synthesis and cell division, amino acid metabolism, and the maturation of red blood cells and other cells. This involvement in basic cell reproduction and growth makes folate essential for healthy embryonic development. Good folate status in early pregnancy greatly reduces the risk of birth defects called neural tube defects.[37] However, many women do not realize they have become pregnant or don't seek prenatal care until it's too late. That is why experts recommend folic acid supplements before pregnancy to all women who might become pregnant, and it is why the government mandated folic acid fortification.

The body converts folate to a coenzyme called tetrahydrofolic acid (THFA). (See **FIGURE 11.22**.) THFA has five active forms, all of which can accept and donate one-carbon units during metabolic reactions. Folate functions with

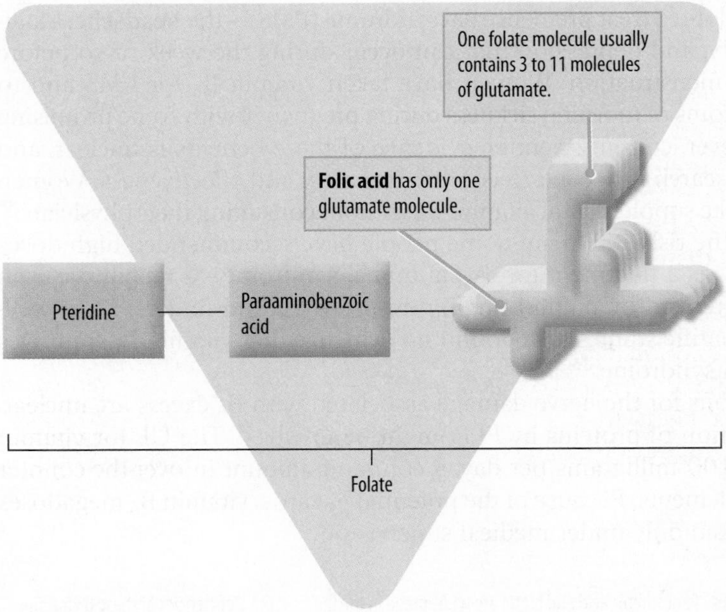

FIGURE 11.21 Folate and its major components. Folate is made up of pteridine, para-aminobenzoic acid (PABA), and at least one molecule of glutamic acid (glutamate).

vitamins B_6 and B_{12}. All three support red blood cell synthesis and help control homocysteine levels.

Dietary Recommendations for Folate

The bioavailability of folate varies depending on stomach contents and the folate source. The body absorbs nearly 100 percent of folic acid in supplements and fortified foods, but only about half to two-thirds of the folate naturally present in food.[38,39] To account for these differences, RDA values are expressed as **dietary folate equivalents (DFEs)**.

The RDA for folate for males and females aged 19 years and older is 400 micrograms of DFE per day. The folate RDA for women increases significantly during pregnancy and lactation: 600 micrograms of DFE per day for pregnant women and 500 micrograms of DFE per day while a woman is breastfeeding.[40]

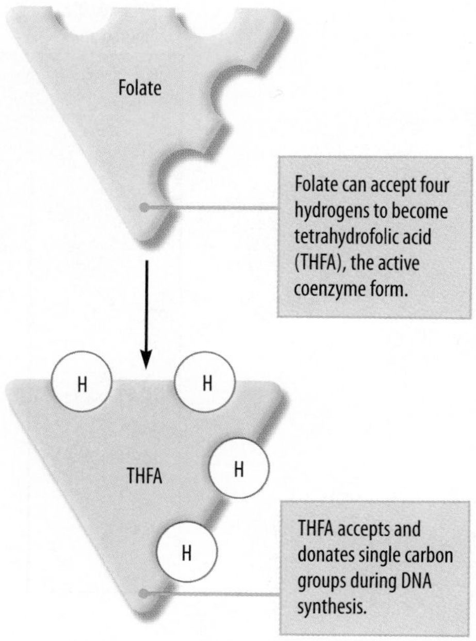

Folate
Folate can accept four hydrogens to become tetrahydrofolic acid (THFA), the active coenzyme form.
H
H
THFA
H
H
THFA accepts and donates single carbon groups during DNA synthesis.

FIGURE 11.22 Folate, THFA, and DNA. Five forms of tetrahydrofolic acid (THFA) are the active coenzyme forms of folate.

DRI Values and Bioavailability of Folate
1 μg DFE = 1 μg food folate
= 0.5 μg folic acid taken on an empty stomach
= 0.6 μg folic acid consumed with meals

Sources of Folate

Fortified breakfast cereals supply dietary folate. Some provide 400 micrograms in a moderate-size serving.[41] Since 1998, folic acid fortification of enriched flour (including that used by commercial bakers) and enriched grain products has been mandatory in the United States and Canada.[42] This mandate calls for a fortification level of 1.4 milligrams of folic acid per kilogram of grain. A serving of enriched pasta, for example, typically provides 30 percent of the folate RDA. Dark-green leafy vegetables, asparagus, broccoli, orange juice, wheat germ, liver, sunflower seeds, and legumes are other good sources. Although vegetables other than dark-green leafy ones are less rich in folate, we eat foods such as green beans and vegetable soup so often that they make major contributions to our total folate intake.[43] **FIGURE 11.23** shows some foods that provide folate.

Similar to other water-soluble vitamins, folate is extremely vulnerable to heat, ultraviolet light, and oxygen. Cooking and other food-processing and preparation techniques can destroy up to 90 percent of a food's folate. Experts recommend eating folate-rich fruits and vegetables raw or cooking them quickly in minimal amounts of water by steaming, stir-frying, or microwaving. Vitamin C in foods also helps protect folate from oxidation.

Low folate status during the early stages of pregnancy is strongly linked with birth defects, specifically neural tube defects. According to the Centers for Disease Control and Prevention, 50 to 70 percent of **neural tube defects (NTDs)** could be prevented by taking 400 micrograms of folate daily before and during pregnancy.[44] Scientists estimate that folate fortification increases folic acid intake by about 100 micrograms per day (an amount provided by slightly more than one-half cup of enriched pasta or one slice of bread), with the goal being to boost daily consumption by women of childbearing age to 400 micrograms of folic acid. Because most U.S. women are not eating enough foods fortified with folic acid to optimally reduce the risk of birth defects, the U.S. Preventative Services Task Force recommends that all women who are capable of becoming pregnant take a daily supplement containing 400–800 micrograms of folic acid.[45]

▶ **dietary folate equivalents (DFEs)** A measure of folate intake used to account for the high bioavailability of folic acid taken as a supplement compared with the lower bioavailability of the folate found in foods.

▶ **neural tube defect (NTD)** A birth defect resulting from failure of the neural tube to develop properly during early fetal development.

Folate Deficiency

Approximately 10 percent of the U.S. population may have insufficient folate stores. Many scientists believe that folate deficiency is the most prevalent of all vitamin deficiencies. In developed countries, folate deficiency has been associated with those who have poor nutrition, such as older adults or those with alcoholism. Others have increased risk as a result of intestinal malabsorption,

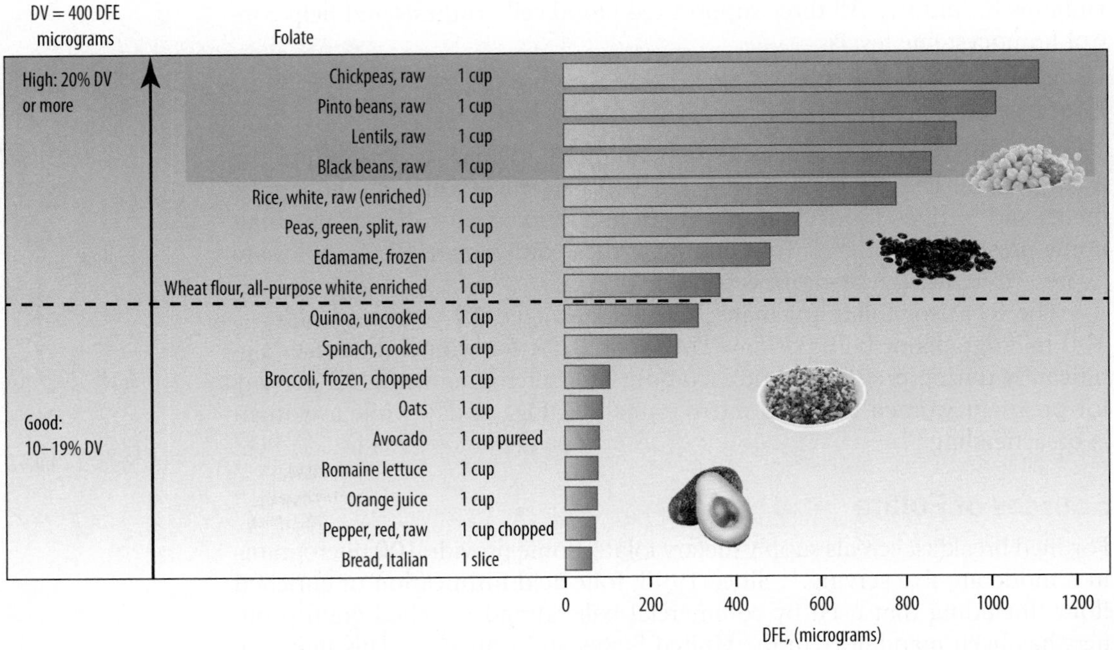

FIGURE 11.23 Food sources of folate. Good sources of folate are a diverse collection of foods: liver, legumes, leafy greens, and orange juice. Enriched grains and fortified cereals are other ways to include folic acid in the diet.

Data from US Department of Agriculture, Agricultural Research Service, Nutrient Data Laboratory. USDA National Nutrient Database for Standard Reference, Release 28. Version Current: September 2015. Internet: http://www.ars.usda.gov/nea/bhnrc/ndl.

Photos: (from top to bottom): (chickpea isolated) © margouillatphotos/Getty Images; (black beans) © ALEAIMAGE/Getty Images, Inc.; (cooked quinoa) © DebbiSmirnoff/Getty Images, Inc. (two avocados) © Joff Lee/Getty Images.

certain anemias, and the use of medications that interfere with folate absorption or activity. Folate deficiency appears to play an important role in the development of anemia, atherosclerosis, neural tube defects, adverse pregnancy outcomes, and neuropsychiatric disorders.

When your folate reserves are good, your body normally can store enough folate to last two to four months without additional intake. Abnormal cell reproduction resulting from folate deficiency can be corrected within 24 hours by vitamin replacement. Deficiency can result from the following conditions:

- *Inadequate folate consumption:* General malnutrition, often resulting from famine or poverty, causes folate deficiency. Cultural cooking methods that destroy folate, eating habits that avoid raw folate-rich vegetables, alcoholism, excessive dieting, and anorexia nervosa and bulimia nervosa can severely limit folate intake. Infirm or neglected older adults and institutionalized psychiatric patients also are at risk.
- *Inadequate folate absorption* resulting from abnormalities in the mucosal cells lining the GI tract.
- *Increased folate requirements* caused by pregnancy and lactation or other conditions. Certain diseases, such as blood disorders, leukemia, lymphoma, and psoriasis, can increase folate needs.
- *Impaired folate utilization*, typically associated with a vitamin B_6 deficiency.
- *Altered folate metabolism* arising from use of alcohol or certain prescription drugs such as barbiturates. Sulfa drugs and anticonvulsants probably impair folate absorption.
- *Excessive folate excretion* caused by prolonged diarrhea.

Folate and Heart Disease

Research suggests that folate has an important role in preventing heart disease. Folate works with vitamin B_{12} and vitamin B_6 to reduce elevated homocysteine, which is a risk factor for cardiovascular disease.[46,47] (See **FIGURE 11.24.**) When folate intake is inadequate, homocysteine levels rise. (During folate deficiency, homocysteine levels are markedly elevated.) As folate intake increases, homocysteine levels drop. The Food and Nutrition Board used homocysteine levels as a primary factor in estimating the folate RDA, and the recommended folate intakes help maintain homocysteine at reduced levels. The role of folate in protecting against heart disease contributed to the FDA decision to fortify grain products. Since the FDA mandated folic acid fortification of the grain supply, blood folate levels have increased and homocysteine levels have decreased in the United States.[48] The role of folate supplementation for the prevention or treatment of cardiovascular disease, stroke, and all-cause mortality is currently under investigation.

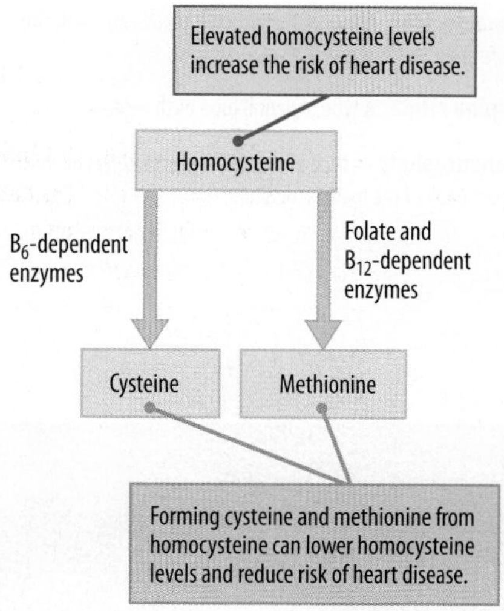
Elevated homocysteine levels increase the risk of heart disease.
Homocysteine
B_6-dependent enzymes
Folate and B_{12}-dependent enzymes
Cysteine
Methionine
Forming cysteine and methionine from homocysteine can lower homocysteine levels and reduce risk of heart disease.

FIGURE 11.24 Homocysteine and heart disease. Elevated homocysteine levels are linked to an increased risk of heart disease. B_6-, B_{12}-, and folate-dependent enzymes help lower the amount of homocysteine by converting it to cysteine and methionine.

Megaloblastic Anemia

Both folate and vitamin B_{12} are required for DNA synthesis and normal cell growth. A deficiency shows up soonest in cells that are reproducing the fastest, such as rapidly dividing red blood cells. The immature red blood cells cannot grow and mature normally (see **FIGURE 11.25**) and instead develop into large, fragile, immature cells, called **megaloblasts**, which are a hallmark of **megaloblastic anemia**.

▶ **megaloblasts** Large, immature red blood cells produced when precursor cells fail to divide normally because of impaired DNA synthesis.

▶ **megaloblastic anemia** Excess amounts of megaloblasts in the blood caused by deficiency of folate or vitamin B_{12}.

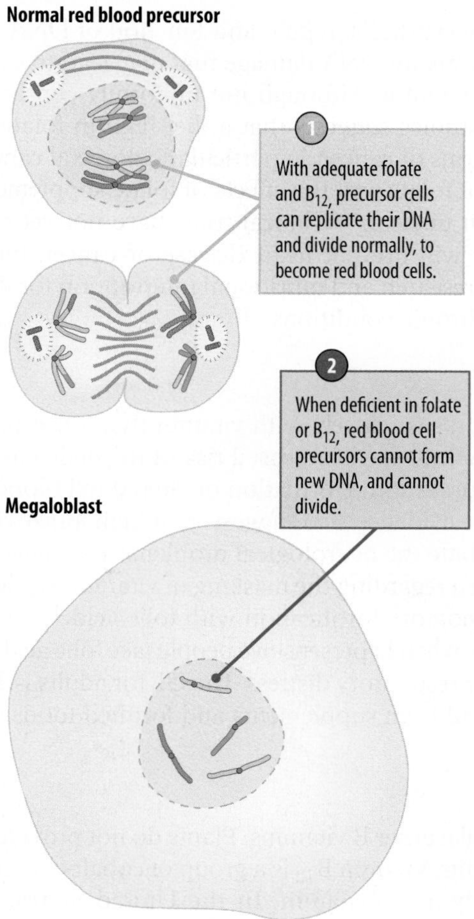
Normal red blood precursor
1
With adequate folate and B_{12}, precursor cells can replicate their DNA and divide normally, to become red blood cells.
2
When deficient in folate or B_{12}, red blood cell precursors cannot form new DNA, and cannot divide.
Megaloblast

FIGURE 11.25 Megaloblastic anemia. When red blood cell precursors in the bone marrow cannot form new DNA, they cannot divide normally. These precursor cells continue to grow and become large, fragile, immature cells called megaloblasts. Megaloblasts displace red blood cells, resulting in megaloblastic anemia.

▶ **macrocytes** Abnormally large red blood cells with short life spans.

▶ **spina bifida** A type of neural tube birth defect.

▶ **anencephaly** A type of neural tube birth defect in which part or all of the brain is missing.

Megaloblasts can mature into **macrocytes**—abnormally large red blood cells with bizarre shapes and short life spans. As megaloblasts and macrocytes proliferate and the number of normal red blood cells decreases, the blood's ability to carry oxygen drops, causing weakness and fatigue. Folate-deficiency anemia commonly causes depression, irritability, forgetfulness, and disturbed sleep.

Impaired DNA synthesis caused by folate deficiency also affects the rapidly dividing cells lining the gastrointestinal tract, interfering with absorption and interfering with the synthesis of white blood cells, which are vital to the immune response.

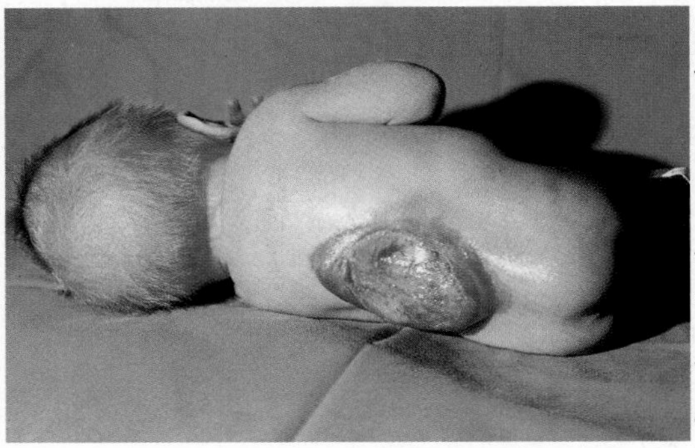

Courtesy of Leonard V. Crowley, MD, Century College.

FIGURE 11.26 Neural tube defects. Poor folate status during the early stages of pregnancy, even before a woman might realize she is pregnant, increases the risk of a neural tube defect.

Neural Tube Defects

Poor folate status during the early stages of pregnancy is linked to an increased risk of a birth defect known as a neural tube defect. In this type of birth defect, the neural tube fails to encase the spinal cord during early fetal development. This causes a number of disorders, including **spina bifida** and **anencephaly** (see **FIGURE 11.26**). These defects in the central nervous system occur within the first 30 days after conception.[49] Worldwide, NTDs afflict between 1 and 9 of every 1,000 infants born. The FDA's mandate to fortify enriched grains with folic acid has been estimated to have reduced the incidence of spina bifida by 26 percent.[50] Folate also might be important in the prevention of other undesirable birth outcomes such as low-birth-weight babies, premature deliveries, and congenital birth defects such as cleft lip and palate.[51]

Folate and Cancer

Folate's role in the synthesis, repair, and function of DNA and RNA has led researchers to investigate DNA damage that may lead to cancer as a result of deficiency of this vitamin. Although not uniformly consistent, a large body of observational studies suggests that a diet high in folate offers protection against various forms of cancer, in particular colorectal cancer.[52,53] However, the precise roles of folate and the effects of folate supplementation in cancer prevention remain unclear.[54] Clinical trials have not yet conclusively determined that folate will prevent heart disease or cancer, but these are active areas of scientific research and nutritional intervention for the prevention and management of chronic conditions.[55]

Quick Bite

Can Folate Prevent Cancer?

When women took multivitamins containing folate for at least 15 years, they had a 75 percent reduction in colon cancer risk, according to the Harvard Nurses' Health Study. Folate intakes of more than 600 micrograms per day reduced breast cancer risk by 50 percent.

Folate Toxicity

Because folate works so closely with vitamin B_{12}, it can mask a vitamin B_{12} deficiency. Older adults have increased risk of B_{12} deficiency, and consuming excess folate can prevent the formation of altered red blood cells that signals a lack of B_{12}. Some evidence also suggests that high intakes of folic acid might prompt or exacerbate the neurological problems associated with vitamin B_{12} deficiency. Concern regarding the masking of vitamin B_{12} deficiency escalated following the mandatory fortification with folic acid.[56]

Although rare, when hypersensitive people take folic acid supplements, they may suffer hives or respiratory distress. The UL for adults is 1,000 micrograms per day of folic acid from supplements and fortified foods.

Vitamin B_{12}

Vitamin B_{12} is unlike other B vitamins. Plants do not provide it, and your body stores large amounts. Vitamin B_{12} is a group of cobalt-containing compounds, known collectively as cobalamin. In the United States, cyanocobalamin,

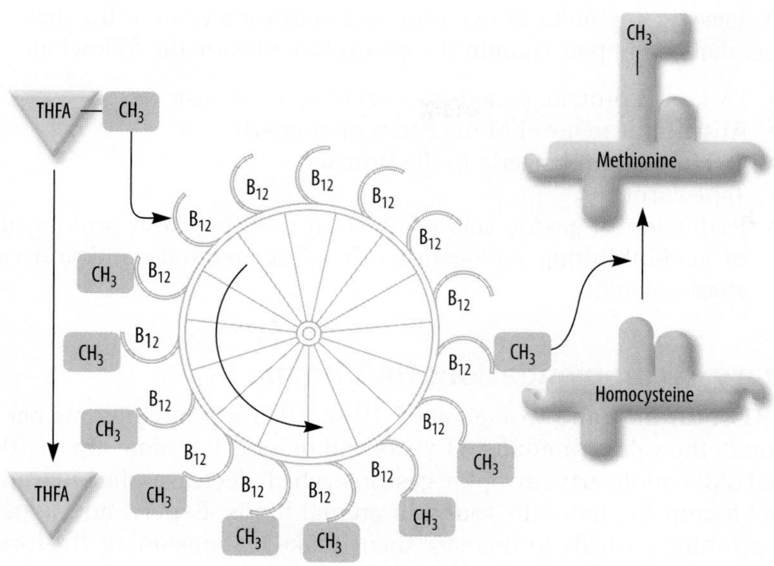

FIGURE 11.27 Vitamin B_{12} helps transfer methyl groups. Vitamin B_{12} helps transfer a methyl group ($-CH_3$) from the folate coenzyme THFA. One destination for the methyl group is the reaction that converts homocysteine to methionine. This conversion reduces homocysteine blood levels, thereby lowering the risk of heart disease.

▶ **myelin sheath** The protective coating that surrounds nerve fibers.

▶ **R-protein** A protein produced by the salivary glands that might protect vitamin B_{12} as it travels through the stomach and into the small intestine.

hydroxocobalamin, and methylcobalamin are forms of vitamin B_{12} commercially available in supplements.

Functions of Vitamin B_{12}

Vitamin B_{12} plays a key role in folate metabolism by transferring a methyl group ($-CH_3$) from the folate coenzyme THFA, as **FIGURE 11.27** shows. Without vitamin B_{12}, THFA cannot change into its methylene form—the active form in many important metabolic pathways. For instance, a deficiency of the methylene form of THFA inhibits DNA synthesis. The partnership between vitamin B_{12} and folate coenzyme THFA means that a vitamin B_{12} deficiency can lead to a folate deficiency, and a lack of either B_{12} or folate can precipitate megaloblastic anemia. Vitamin B_{12}–dependent enzymes also work with THFA to convert homocysteine to methionine, thereby reducing homocysteine blood levels and lowering the risk of heart disease.

Vitamin B_{12} also helps maintain the **myelin sheath**, the protective coating that surrounds nerve fibers. In addition, by helping to rearrange carbon atoms in fatty acid chains, vitamin B_{12} helps prepare them to enter the citric acid cycle.

Absorption of Vitamin B_{12}

Unless you're a vegan, it's easy to get enough vitamin B_{12} from your diet. But absorbing it is a complex process that requires several factors (see **FIGURE 11.28**). In the stomach, vitamin B_{12} binds with **R-protein**, a protein produced by the salivary glands that might protect vitamin B_{12} as it travels through the stomach and into the small intestine. Once there, pancreatic proteases such as trypsin cleave vitamin B_{12} from R-protein. Vitamin B_{12} then binds to intrinsic factor, a substance produced by the parietal cells of the stomach, the same cells that produce hydrochloric acid. Together, the two substances journey to the ileum of the small intestine and attach to receptor cells on the organ's brush border. The receptor cells absorb vitamin B_{12} and transfer it to transcobalamin II, a protein carrier in the blood. Transcobalamin II enters the bloodstream and delivers vitamin B_{12} to the liver, bone marrow, and developing blood cells.

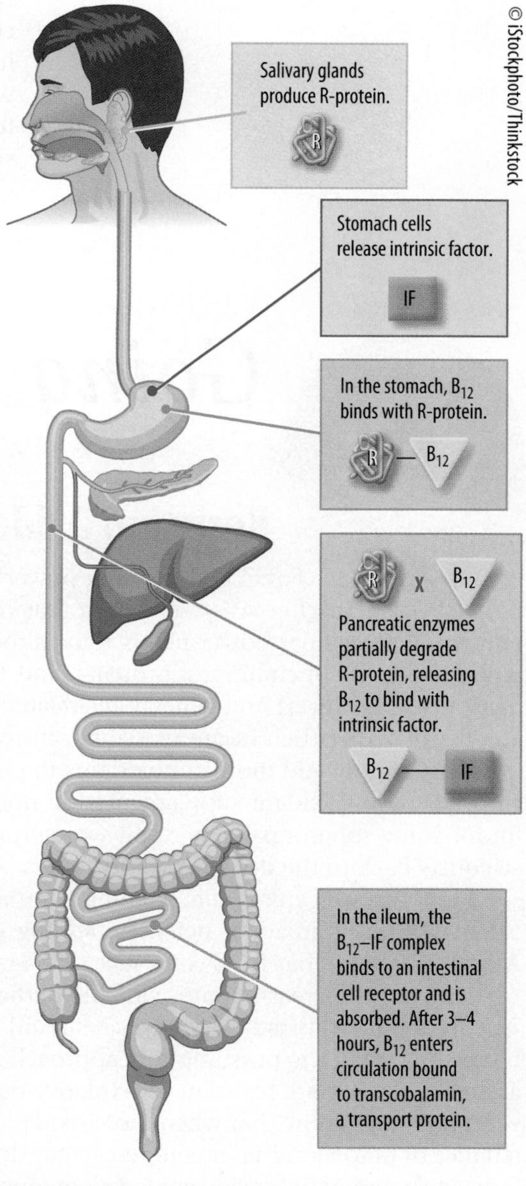

Salivary glands produce R-protein.
R
Stomach cells release intrinsic factor.
IF
In the stomach, B_{12} binds with R-protein.
R — B_{12}
R X B_{12}
Pancreatic enzymes partially degrade R-protein, releasing B_{12} to bind with intrinsic factor.
B_{12} — IF
In the ileum, the B_{12}–IF complex binds to an intestinal cell receptor and is absorbed. After 3–4 hours, B_{12} enters circulation bound to transcobalamin, a transport protein.

FIGURE 11.28 Absorption of vitamin B_{12}. Absorption of B_{12} is a complex process that involves many factors and sites in the GI tract. Defects in this process, especially a lack of intrinsic factor, impair B_{12} absorption and can lead to B_{12} deficiency.

A defect at any point in this process can cause a vitamin B_{12} deficiency. Factors that can impair vitamin B_{12} absorption include the following:

- Lack of R-protein, pancreatic enzymes, or intrinsic factor
- Absence or removal of the ileum or stomach
- Overgrowth of bacteria in the stomach
- Tapeworm
- Reduction of gastric acid production resulting from prolonged use of acid-inhibiting medications or an age-related condition called **atrophic gastritis**

▶ **atrophic gastritis** An age-related condition in which the stomach loses its ability to secrete acid. In severe cases, ability to make intrinsic factor is also impaired.

Dietary Recommendations for Vitamin B_{12}

The RDA for men and women aged 19 to 50 is 2.4 micrograms per day. Although the value for adults 51 years and older is the same, up to 30 percent of older adults have atrophic gastritis, which decreases the bioavailability of vitamin B_{12} naturally found in animal foods. Experts advise people with atrophic gastritis to increase their intake by consuming B_{12}-fortified foods or supplements. Our bodies efficiently absorb vitamin B_{12} from these sources.[57]

Going Green

Resisting Oxidative Stress

Fossil fuel–burning power plants pump out a steady stream of essential energy, but they also produce reactive waste products that can damage the environment. Like coal-fired power plants that pollute the environment, cellular power plants (our mitochondria) produce reactive oxygen species (ROS) that slowly oxidize lipids and damage cell membranes, proteins, and DNA. Such oxidative stress has been implicated in diseases of aging (e.g., heart disease, cancer) and general age-related declines.

Because diets rich in antioxidants can reduce the incidence of age-related diseases, a dietary solution once seemed possible: Simply add more antioxidants to our diet, and there should be fewer ROS to cause harm. However, large clinical trials of antioxidant supplementation not only failed to show clinically significant benefits, but were actually harmful for some subgroups. This result was surprising. It illustrates that we still have a lot to learn about aging, and it sent scientists back to the drawing board.

How can we explain this seeming contradiction? Some scientists suggested that our cells are already stuffed to near capacity with antioxidant defenses; adding even more antioxidants could compromise intricate molecular machinery. Also, it might be that ROS can cause damage even before encountering the neutralizing antioxidants.

Instead of increasing antioxidants, perhaps we could make biomolecules intrinsically more resistant to oxidation? At a minimum, this radical approach should tell us something about antioxidants and aging. Retrotope, a Silicon Valley biotech company, is pursuing this approach using a stable isotope of hydrogen to construct variants of fatty acids and amino acids that are resistant to oxidative damage. (Tiny amounts of these variants already occur in nature.) Studies in yeast and mice show that when these oxidation-resistant variants replace oxidation-prone fatty acids critical to the maintenance of mitochondrial membranes, they do in fact provide protection from oxidative stress. It is hoped that when these fatty acids and amino acids are fed to mammals, similar resistance to oxidation will occur.

Sources of Vitamin B_{12}

All naturally occurring vitamin B_{12} originates with bacteria. Bacteria produce it, and animals obtain it from bacteria on their food or from their intestinal bacteria. Animals concentrate and store vitamin B_{12}, mainly in the liver. Consequently, animal-derived foods are our only good natural source of vitamin B_{12}, and liver is the richest source. Other sources are fortified foods, such as ready-to-eat cereals and some soy products.

Blue-green algae (cyanobacteria) are sometimes promoted as a vitamin B_{12} plant source, but their cobalamin is an inactive and biologically unavailable form. For vegans (vegetarians who avoid eggs and dairy as well as meats), the most reliable food sources are fortified breakfast cereals, fortified soy products, and other foods fortified with vitamin B_{12}.

Mixed foods, including sandwiches whose main ingredient is meat, fish, or poultry, contribute most of our dietary vitamin B_{12}. The next most important sources are milk and milk products for women and beef for men. Although shellfish, liver and other organ meats, some game meat, and some kinds of fish are the richest sources of vitamin B_{12}, few people regularly eat these foods.[58] **FIGURE 11.29** shows foods that provide vitamin B_{12}.

Although definitive data are lacking, scientists conservatively estimate that about 50 percent of dietary vitamin B_{12} is bioavailable. That percentage can drop when a person consumes foods particularly high in vitamin B_{12}.

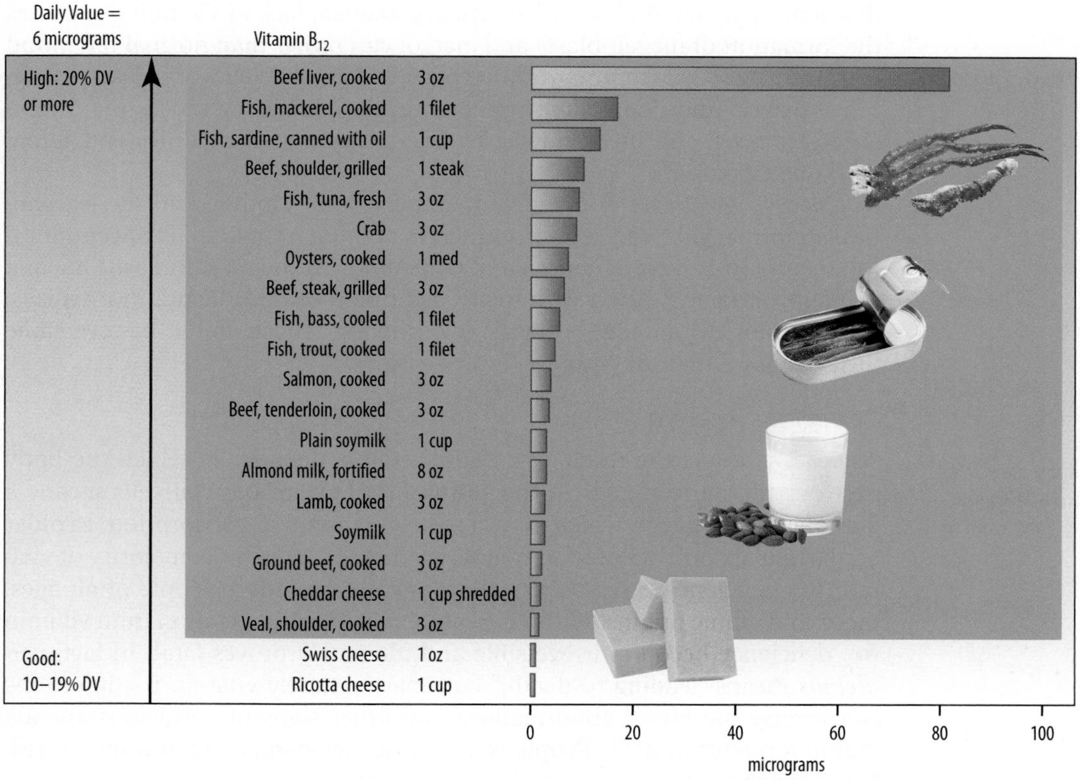

FIGURE 11.29 Food sources of vitamin B_{12}. Vitamin B_{12} is found naturally only in foods of animal origin such as liver, meats, and milk. Some cereals are fortified with vitamin B_{12}.

Note: The DV for vitamin B_{12} is substantially higher than the current (1998) RDA of 2.4 micrograms for those age 14 and older.

Data from US Department of Agriculture, Agricultural Research Service, Nutrient Data Laboratory. USDA National Nutrient Database for Standard Reference, Release 28. Version Current: September 2015. Internet: http://www.ars.usda.gov/nea/bhnrc/ndl.

Photos (from top to bottom): (King crab legs) © supermimicry/Getty Images; (anchovies) Jiri Hera/Shutterstock, Inc.; (almond milk) 5 second Studio/Shutterstock, Inc.; (piece of cheese) Binh Thanh Bui/Shutterstock, Inc.

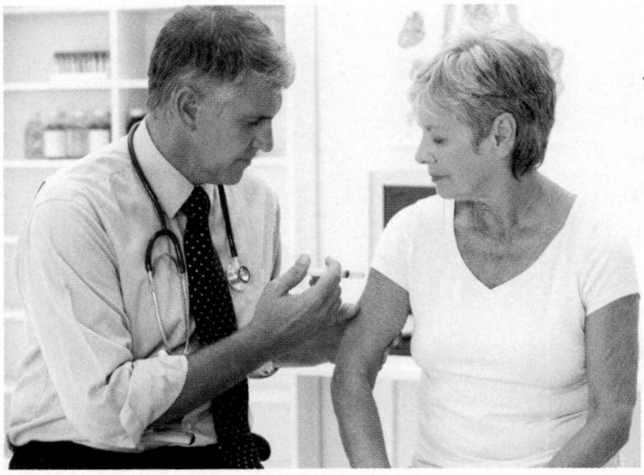
© iStockphoto/Thinkstock

Vitamin B_{12} Deficiency

We can store enough vitamin B_{12} in the liver to last more than 2 years, and symptoms of deficiency might not appear for up to 12 years. Vegetarians who eat neither meat nor dairy products are at risk of vitamin B_{12} deficiency unless they take vitamin B_{12} supplements or regularly eat fortified cereals. Strict vegetarian (vegan) mothers who breastfeed can put their infants at risk of long-term neurological problems unless they include supplemental vitamin B_{12} in their diets.

THINK About It 3

Researchers report that 3.2 to 12 percent of older adults are vitamin B_{12} deficient; however, the true prevalence of vitamin B_{12} deficiency is difficult to estimate due to a lack of standard criteria.[59] Most vitamin B_{12} deficiency, especially in older people, is caused by inadequate intake or impaired absorption. To circumvent malabsorption, vitamin B_{12} injections deliver the vitamin directly to the bloodstream. Because the liver stores a substantial amount of vitamin B_{12}, monthly shots usually are sufficient. Other treatments include taking megadoses of vitamin B_{12} supplements (300 times the RDA) that overwhelm impaired absorption, and using a nasal spray containing vitamin B_{12}. Fortified bread products are effective in improving vitamin B_{12} status; therefore, many experts suggest that foods that are fortified with folic acid should also include vitamin B_{12} to reduce deficiency.[60,61]

Symptoms of Vitamin B_{12} Deficiency

The major outcome of impaired vitamin B_{12} absorption is vitamin B_{12}–deficiency anemia. As in folate-deficiency anemia, lack of vitamin B_{12} causes the formation of megaloblasts and macrocytes rather than normal red blood cells. But there are important differences. Folate deficiency can lead to cognitive defects and depression, but vitamin B_{12} deficiency causes the myelin sheath to swell and break down, leading to brain abnormalities and spinal cord degeneration.

Neurological symptoms include tingling and numbness in the extremities, abnormal gait, and cognitive changes ranging from loss of concentration to memory loss, disorientation, and dementia.[62] If the megaloblastic anemia is inappropriately treated with folate, red blood cell production normalizes, but neurological damage worsens. Neurological effects might be reversible, depending on their duration.

Pernicious Anemia

▶ **pernicious anemia** A form of anemia that results from an autoimmune disorder that damages cells lining the stomach and inhibits vitamin B_{12} absorption, leading to vitamin B_{12} deficiency.

Pernicious anemia is the result of an autoimmune disorder in which the body destroys the parietal cells in the stomach.[63] Loss of parietal cells means a loss of intrinsic factor, which in turn reduces vitamin B_{12} absorption. In older adults, malabsorption of food-bound vitamin B_{12} causes the majority of vitamin B_{12} deficiency cases.[64] Pernicious anemia can affect people of all ages, races, and ethnic origins. Without treatment, nerve degeneration from vitamin B_{12} deficiency becomes irreversible and ultimately proves fatal. In fact, *pernicious* means "leading to death." Fortunately, timely vitamin B_{12} injections can reverse the blood abnormalities and other signs of pernicious anemia within a matter of days. People with pernicious anemia are at a higher risk for stomach cancer.

Vitamin B_{12} Toxicity

High levels of vitamin B_{12} from food or supplements have not been shown to cause harmful side effects in healthy people. Monthly doses of 1,000 micrograms are routinely used to treat pernicious anemia with no ill effects. A UL for vitamin B_{12} has not been determined.

Key Concepts Folate and vitamin B_{12} work closely together. Fruits, vegetables, enriched grains, and fortified cereals contain folate, but only animal foods and fortified cereals contain bioavailable vitamin B_{12}. A deficiency of folate causes megaloblastic anemia and has been associated with neural tube defects. Deficiency of B_{12} causes a form of megaloblastic anemia and irreversible nerve damage. Vitamin B_{12} deficiency usually results from poor absorption because of either pernicious anemia or other GI problems, such as atrophic gastritis. Because vitamin B_{12} is found only in animal foods, strict vegetarians must find an alternate source. Folate, vitamin B_{12}, and vitamin B_6 all play roles in the metabolism of the amino acid homocysteine, which has been implicated in heart disease.

Vitamin C

For centuries, the insidious disease scurvy dogged humankind. Explorers and seafaring men especially feared this mysterious ailment that inflicted aching pain and made each journey a gamble with death. Writings that date back as far as 1500 B.C.E. describe their suffering in detail.

Although they did not know why, some travelers avoided this scourge. Unknowingly, they had eaten foods that contained vitamin C. The mystery began to be solved in 1746 by James Lind, a 30-year-old ship's surgeon in the British navy. In a controlled human nutrition clinical trial, he carefully evaluated six different therapies for scurvy and showed that only those patients who received lemons or oranges recovered.[65] In the mid-1800s in Great Britain, it was known that when potatoes were scarce, outbreaks of scurvy occurred.[66] When neither potatoes nor fruit were available, green vegetables were found to prevent scurvy. It was not until 1930 that scientists isolated the substance responsible for curing scurvy, the "antiscorbutic" factor, and named it vitamin C.

Vitamin C comes in two interchangeable, biologically active forms: a reduced form called ascorbic acid and an oxidized form called dehydroascorbic acid. Although most animals manufacture their own vitamin C, humans cannot, sharing this dubious distinction with fruit-eating bats, guinea pigs, and a few other isolated species. For some unknown reason, humans also appear to require much less vitamin C than most other animals.

Functions of Vitamin C

Vitamin C is an antioxidant—it acts as a **reducing agent** and participates in many reactions by donating electrons or hydrogen ions. It also is essential to the activity of many enzymes. Unlike the B vitamins, however, it is not a coenzyme, and only indirectly activates enzymes.

▶ **reducing agent** A compound that donates electrons or hydrogen atoms to another compound.

Collagen Synthesis

Vitamin C plays an important role in the formation of collagen, a fibrous protein that helps reinforce the **connective tissues** that hold together the structures of the body. Collagen is made up of individual, linear proteins that wrap around one another like a cord of rope, forming a triple helix that imparts strength and flexibility. It is the most abundant protein in our bodies and the main fibrous component of skin, bone, tendons, cartilage, and teeth. It also is the major protein in connective tissue, which binds cells and tissues together, and in scar tissue.

▶ **connective tissues** Tissues composed primarily of fibrous proteins such as collagen, and which contain few cells. Their primary function is to bind together and support various body structures.

Antioxidant Activity

Like vitamin E and beta-carotene, vitamin C works as an antioxidant and minimizes free radical damage in cells.[67] In addition to working independently as an antioxidant (see **FIGURE 11.30**), vitamin C helps recycle oxidized vitamin E for reuse in the cells and stabilizes the reduced form of the folate coenzyme.[68] Eating foods rich in vitamin C can reduce the risk of chronic

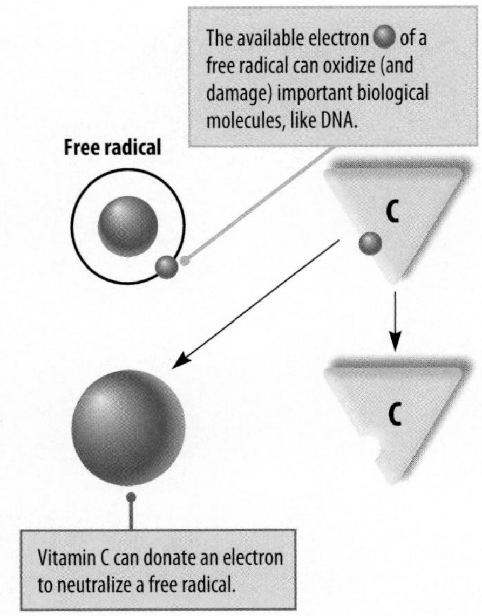

FIGURE 11.30 Vitamin C is an antioxidant. Vitamin C minimizes free radical damage by donating an electron. Vitamin C also indirectly activates many enzymes. Although essential to enzyme activity, unlike the B vitamins, vitamin C is not a coenzyme.

conditions such as heart disease, certain forms of cancer, and macular degeneration, and promote bone health; however, it remains unclear whether the protective effects are caused by vitamin C or fruit and vegetable consumption in general.[69]

Iron Absorption

As a reducing agent, vitamin C enhances the absorption of nonheme iron, which comes mainly from plant foods. (The small intestine absorbs nonheme iron better when it is reduced.)

Synthesis of Vital Cell Compounds

Vitamin C helps synthesize carnitine, a compound that carries fatty acids from the cytosol to the mitochondria for energy production. Vitamin C also helps synthesize norepinephrine, epinephrine, the neurotransmitter serotonin, the thyroid hormone thyroxine, bile acids, steroid hormones, and purine bases used in DNA synthesis.

Immune Function

Vitamin C enables lymphocytes and other cells of the immune system to function properly. Based in part on the vitamin's importance to immunity, vitamin C has been reputed to prevent or cure the common cold. Regular supplementation with vitamin C has been found to have a modest effect on shortening the duration of the common cold in the general population; however, it is particularly beneficial in individuals exposed to extreme physical stress.[70]

THINK About It 4

Quick Bite

Chili Peppers Are Hot Stuff

An estimated one-quarter of the world's adults eat chili peppers every day. By weight, chili peppers are one of the richest sources of vitamins A and C. In addition, capsaicin, the substance that causes your mouth to burn, jump-starts the digestive process by stimulating salivation.

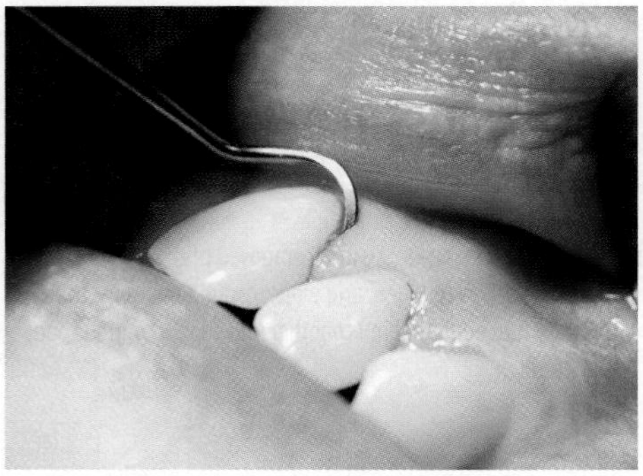

© LeggNet/iStockphoto.com

Dietary Recommendations for Vitamin C

For adults aged 19 years and older, the RDA for vitamin C is 90 milligrams per day for men and 75 milligrams per day for women. For women, the RDA rises to 85 milligrams per day during pregnancy and 120 milligrams per day during lactation. Because smoking increases the metabolic turnover of vitamin C, the Food and Nutrition Board estimates that smokers require 35 milligrams per day more than nonsmokers.[71]

Sources of Vitamin C

Many, but not all, fruits and vegetables are high in vitamin C. Particularly good sources of vitamin C include potatoes, citrus fruits, tomatoes, fortified juice drinks, broccoli, strawberries, kiwifruit, cabbage, spinach and other leafy greens, and green peppers.[72] Because vitamin C is highly vulnerable to heat and oxygen, fresh fruits and vegetables are the optimal sources. **FIGURE 11.31** shows some foods that provide vitamin C.

The more vitamin C you consume, the less efficiently your intestines absorb the vitamin. When people take in 30 milligrams to 120 milligrams daily, the intestines absorb about 80 to 90 percent of vitamin C. However, when vitamin C consumption exceeds 6,000 milligrams daily, absorption drops to about 20 percent. Most of the excess vitamin C is excreted in the urine.

Vitamin C Deficiency

Scurvy is the well-known vitamin C–deficiency disease. Its first symptoms surface after about a month on a vitamin C–free diet. As the body loses its ability to synthesize collagen, connective tissue starts breaking down and gums and joints begin to bleed. Weakness develops, and small hemorrhages appear around the hair follicles on the arms and legs. As the disease progresses,

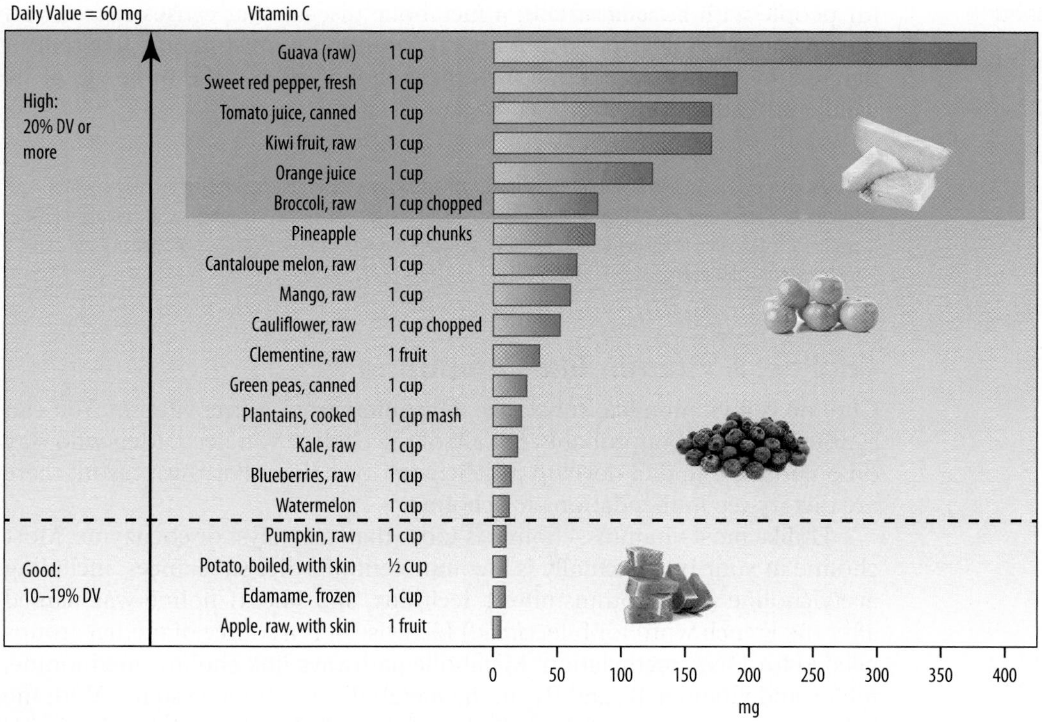

FIGURE 11.31 Food sources of vitamin C. Vitamin C is found mainly in fruits and vegetables. Although citrus fruits are notoriously good sources, many other popular fruits and vegetables are rich in vitamin C.

Data from US Department of Agriculture, Agricultural Research Service, Nutrient Data Laboratory. USDA National Nutrient Database for Standard Reference, Release 28. Version Current: September 2015. Internet: http://www.ars.usda.gov/nea/bhnrc/ndl.

Photos (from top to bottom): (pineapple pieces) © Maks Narodenko/Shutterstock, Inc.; (clementines) © Ewais/Shutterstock, Inc.; (blueberries) © Diana Taliun/Shutterstock, Inc.; (watermelon) © Nattika/Shutterstock, Inc.

previously healed wounds reopen, and bone pain, fractures, diarrhea, and psychological problems such as depression commonly emerge.

Scurvy is rare in developed countries but possible among those who eat few fruits and vegetables, follow extremely restricted diets, or abuse alcohol or drugs.[73] Less severe vitamin C deficiency can impair cellular functions without causing overt scurvy. The most common symptoms are inflammation of the gums and fatigue. Although much of the past research on vitamin C has centered on the prevention of scurvy, this vitamin has also undergone speculation for its role in the prevention of chronic disease. The use of vitamin C for prevention of coronary heart disease, stroke, cancer, cataracts, and lead toxicity and in the treatment of cardiovascular disease, hypertension, cancer, diabetes mellitus, and the common cold require additional investigation.

Vitamin C Toxicity

The UL for vitamin C is 2,000 milligrams per day. Although megadoses of vitamin C do not appear to be acutely toxic to most healthy people, taking more than 2,000 milligrams daily for a prolonged period can lead to nausea, abdominal cramps, diarrhea, and nosebleeds.[74] In healthy people, epidemiological studies do not support an association between excess vitamin C intake and kidney stones; however, in people with kidney disease, excess vitamin C might contribute to oxalate-containing kidney stones.[75] High vitamin C intakes also might bolster iron absorption—useful for some, but problematic

▶ **hemochromatosis** A metabolic disorder that results in excess iron deposits in the body.

for people with **hemochromatosis**, a metabolic disease that causes excess iron accumulation. Finally, large amounts of vitamin C can stimulate free-radical damage by enhancing oxidation (a pro-oxidant effect), the opposite of its usual antioxidant activity.[76]

Key Concepts Vitamin C, which is found in many fruits and vegetables, functions mainly in collagen synthesis. It also acts as an antioxidant. Vitamin C helps boost iron absorption and plays a part in hormone and neurotransmitter synthesis. A deficiency of vitamin C leads to scurvy, although this is rare today. Megadoses of vitamin C can cause gastrointestinal disturbances.

Choline: A Vitamin-like Compound

Choline is a vitamin-like substance, but differs from a true vitamin. You can synthesize most, but probably not all, of the choline you need. Men who stay on a choline-free diet develop a deficiency over time. For this reason, there are dietary recommendations for choline.

Unlike most vitamins, choline is more than a catalyst or coenzyme. Most choline in your body actually is a component of other substances, including acetylcholine (a neurotransmitter), lecithins, and bile. (Choline was named after the French word for bile, *chole*.) Likewise, it is a source of methyl groups needed for DNA methylation. Metabolic pathways link choline, methionine, folate, and vitamins B_6 and B_{12} in the metabolism of homocysteine. With the help of vitamin B_{12} and folate, the liver forms choline from the amino acids serine and methionine.

If you eat enough protein to provide the essential amino acid methionine, your body can manufacture choline. Because choline is widespread in the food supply, the risk of a deficiency is minimal in healthy people. Liver, eggs, beef, cauliflower, and peanuts are especially rich in choline. An AI for choline has been set at 550 milligrams per day for adult men, and 425 milligrams per day for adult women.[77]

High doses of choline can cause hypotension (low blood pressure), sweating, diarrhea, and fishy body odor. The UL for adults is 3,500 milligrams of choline per day.

Conditional Nutrients

Relatively speaking, there are few substances we need for life that our bodies cannot make. Although our bodies make countless essential substances, we must eat food to obtain nutrients such as vitamins. However, under some circumstances—illnesses or inherited metabolic errors—we cannot make enough of the essential substances our bodies need, so we must obtain them from our diets. These substances are conditional nutrients. Inositol, carnitine, taurine, and lipoic acid are examples of nutrients that are conditional. Inositol helps form cell membrane phospholipids and precursors of eicosanoids, substances that work like hormones. Carnitine transports fatty acids to sites in the cell where your body can break them down. Taurine, derived from the amino acids methionine and cysteine, seems to play a role in such diverse functions as vision, insulin activity, and cell growth. Lipoic acid is a potent antioxidant and a necessary cofactor in many energy-releasing reactions. You might see conditional nutrients in dietary supplements, and they might be prescribed medically.

Bogus Vitamins

Many dietary supplements contain unnecessary substances. Savvy marketers will often label these substances "essential" and tout their supposed benefits as health enhancers and disease treatments. The Internet is full of websites representing themselves as "nutrition sites" that endorse nutritional supplements that can prevent or cure almost any condition, despite ample scientific evidence to the contrary. Consumers should be wary of anything that sounds too good to be true and investigate the claims using reputable websites and resources. Think twice before you pay a premium price for supplements that contain bogus vitamins.

Key Concepts The body contains a number of vitamin-like compounds synthesized from glucose and amino acids and found in the food supply. Although deficiencies of these substances are unlikely, some people with certain medical conditions may benefit from supplemental amounts. Of course, supplements should be taken only with a physician's recommendation. Researchers are examining the needs for these substances and their effects on the body.

Label to Table

The FDA requires all manufacturers to add folic acid to enriched grain products such as bread, flour, rice, and pasta. Folic acid, the synthetic form of folate, has been shown to decrease risk of neural tube defects. Folic acid or folate (its natural form) might also be important in reducing risk of heart disease and colon cancer. Prior to the fortification of enriched grains, it was difficult for some people to get enough of this B vitamin, in part because it is destroyed easily during cooking and storage. The purpose of folic acid fortification is to ensure that most people, especially women of childbearing age, can meet their needs for this B vitamin. Look at the Nutrition Facts label on a pasta package. Note how much folic acid is in a serving of pasta.

Some vegetables and legumes also contain folate, so combining pasta with vegetables, or enriched rice with black beans, would provide substantial amounts of folate. The next time you are at the grocery store, pay close attention to the food labels on grain products to see just how much folate you could consume from different grain products.

Looking again at this food label, what other water-soluble vitamins do you see? In addition to folic acid, this pasta contains substantial amounts of thiamin, niacin, and riboflavin. These are the "enrichment" vitamins, and one serving of pasta provides 15 to 35 percent of the Daily Value of each.

Some people are not getting enough potassium, which puts them at higher risk for chronic disease. The new food labels will include a declaration of potassium that will include the actual gram amount, in addition to the %DV. The %DV for iron will continue to be required, along with the actual gram amount.

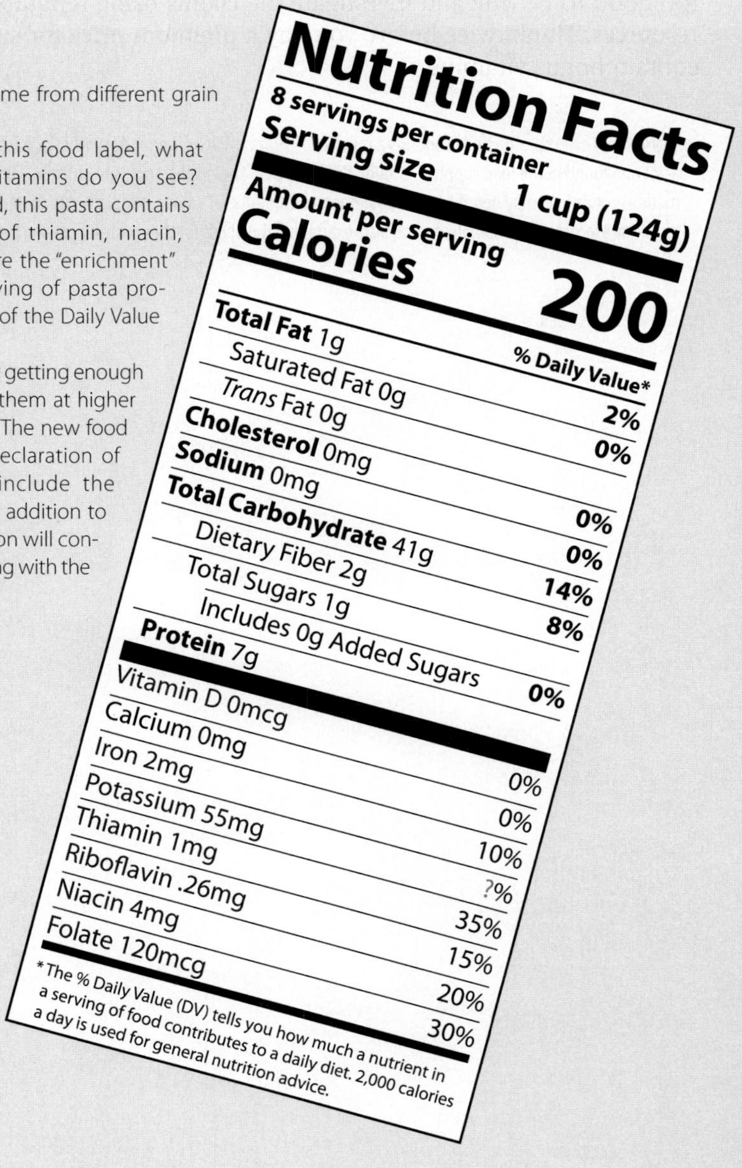
Nutrition Facts
8 servings per container
Serving size 1 cup (124g)
Amount per serving
Calories 200
% Daily Value*
Total Fat 1g 2%
Saturated Fat 0g 0%
Trans Fat 0g
Cholesterol 0mg 0%
Sodium 0mg 0%
Total Carbohydrate 41g 14%
Dietary Fiber 2g 8%
Total Sugars 1g
Includes 0g Added Sugars 0%
Protein 7g
Vitamin D 0mcg 0%
Calcium 0mg 0%
Iron 2mg 10%
Potassium 55mg ?%
Thiamin 1mg 35%
Riboflavin .26mg 15%
Niacin 4mg 20%
Folate 120mcg 30%
*The % Daily Value (DV) tells you how much a nutrient in a serving of food contributes to a daily diet. 2,000 calories a day is used for general nutrition advice.

Learning Portfolio

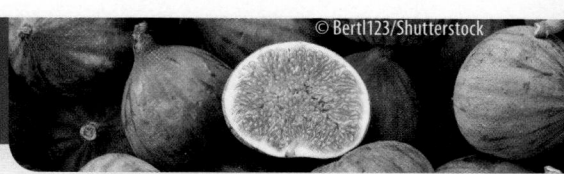

Key Terms

anemia	443	**hemochromatosis**	458
anencephaly	450	**homocysteine**	444
angular stomatitis	437	**macrocytes**	450
ariboflavinosis	437	**megaloblastic anemia**	449
atrophic gastritis	452	**megaloblasts**	449
avidin	442	**microcytic hypochromic anemia**	443
beriberi	432	**myelin sheath**	451
biocytin	442	**neural tube defect (NTD)**	447
biotinidase	442	**niacin equivalents (NE)**	438
carboxylation	442	**pernicious anemia**	454
cheilosis	437	**R-protein**	451
connective tissues	455	**reducing agent**	455
decarboxylation	432	**seborrheic dermatitis**	437
dietary folate equivalents (DFE)	447	**spina bifida**	450
glossitis	437	**thiamin pyrophosphate (TPP)**	432
glutathione peroxidase	436	**tryptophan**	438

Study Points

- The water-soluble vitamins include the eight B vitamins and vitamin C.
- Thiamin (vitamin B_1) functions as the coenzyme thiamin pyrophosphate (TPP) in energy metabolism.
- Thiamin deficiency results in the classic disease beriberi. In industrialized countries, thiamin deficiency most often is associated with alcoholism. There is no known danger of toxicity related to high intakes of thiamin.
- Riboflavin (vitamin B_2) forms part of the coenzymes FAD and FMN, which function in energy metabolism as hydrogen and electron carriers.
- Ariboflavinosis (riboflavin deficiency) is characterized by inflammation of the mouth and tongue.
- Niacin (vitamin B_3) participates in energy metabolism as part of the coenzymes NAD^+ and $NADP^+$.
- Niacin deficiency results in pellagra, a disease characterized by the 4 Ds: diarrhea, dermatitis, dementia, and death.
- High doses of niacin, such as in the treatment of high blood cholesterol, can have toxic side effects, including liver damage.
- Pantothenic acid is a part of coenzyme A, a critical player in energy metabolism.
- Biotin-containing enzymes catalyze carboxylation reactions, which are important in many pathways involving energy-yielding nutrients.
- The coenzyme form of vitamin B_6 (pyridoxine) is called pyridoxal phosphate (PLP); it participates in a variety of reactions, primarily involving amino acid metabolism.
- Megadoses of vitamin B_6 can cause permanent nerve damage.
- Folate and vitamin B_{12} work closely together in a number of metabolic pathways, including reactions in cell division, DNA synthesis, and to control blood levels of homocysteine.
- Deficiency of either folate or vitamin B_{12} results in megaloblastic anemia, but vitamin B_{12} deficiency also causes irreversible nerve damage.
- Poor maternal folate status is associated with development of neural tube defects during pregnancy. Therefore, women of childbearing age are advised to take 400 micrograms of folic acid each day from supplements in addition to fortified foods and other dietary folate.
- Vitamin C (ascorbic acid) functions in the synthesis of collagen and other vital compounds and also works as an antioxidant.
- Vitamin C deficiency can cause scurvy, which is characterized by bleeding gums and small hemorrhages on the skin.
- A number of vitamin-like compounds have been identified, including choline, inositol, and taurine. These compounds are synthesized by the body and are not dietary essentials.

Study Questions

1. List the nine water-soluble vitamins and give one main function of each.
2. Which water-soluble vitamin can be made from an amino acid?
3. Name the diseases and/or characteristic symptoms of deficiency of each water-soluble vitamin.
4. A lack of which three B vitamins can cause anemia? Describe the differences among these anemias.
5. List the water-soluble vitamins demonstrated to be toxic in large doses. What signs indicate toxic levels of each vitamin?

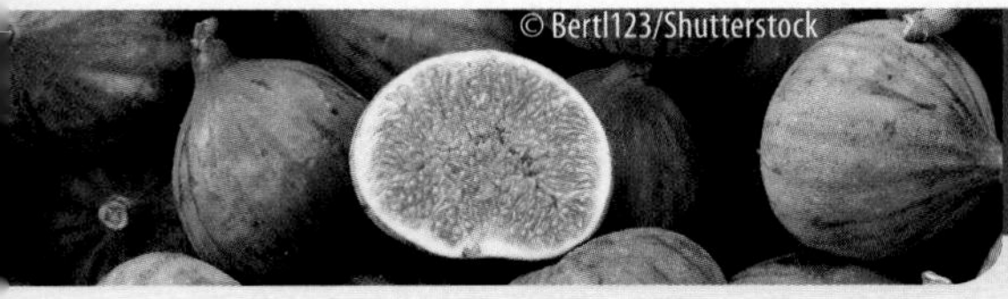

Learning Portfolio (continued)

Try This

The Antioxidant and the Apple

This experiment will help you see how vitamin C acts as an antioxidant. You need an apple and a lemon. Slice the apple into eight pieces. Put four on one plate and four on another. Slice open the lemon and squeeze its juices over the apple slices on one plate. Leave the lemon on this plate to remind you which apple slices have been coated with lemon juice. Let both plates sit for 30 minutes. Do the apple slices look any different after 30 minutes? What is the difference? Why?

Supplemental Income

The object of this exercise is to critically review vitamin supplements. Go to the drug store and look at a few multivitamin supplements and "stress" formulas. Look at the %DV for the water-soluble vitamins. Do you see any that have more than 1,000% of the DV? Compare prices. Is it more expensive to buy supplements with more of these vitamins? Considering what you learned in this chapter, would it benefit you to take supplements that contain such a high amount of these vitamins? Why do you think supplements contain such large quantities of these vitamins?

References

1. Junod SW. Folic acid fortification: fact and folly. April 2009. http://www.fda.gov/aboutfda/whatwedo/history/productregulation/selectionsfromfdliupdateseriesonfdahistory/ucm091883.htm. Accessed January 29, 2016.
2. Carpenter KJ. A short history of nutritional science: part 2 (1885–1912). *J Nutr*. 2003;133:975–984.
3. Ibid.
4. Manzetti S1, Zhang J, van der Spoel D. Thiamin function, metabolism, uptake, and transport. *Biochemistry*. 2014;53(5):821–835. doi: 10.1021/bi401618y. Epub January 31, 2014.
5. Institute of Medicine, Food and Nutrition Board. *Dietary Reference Intakes for Thiamin, Riboflavin, Niacin, Vitamin B_6, Folate, Vitamin B_{12}, Pantothenic Acid, Biotin, and Choline*. Washington, DC: National Academies Press; 1998.
6. U.S. Department of Agriculture, Agricultural Research Service, Nutrient Data Laboratory. USDA National Nutrient Database for Standard Reference, Release 27 (revised). May 2015. http://www.ars.usda.gov/ba/bhnrc/ndl. Accessed January 29, 2016.
7. Institute of Medicine, Food and Nutrition Board. *Dietary Reference Intakes for Thiamin, Riboflavin, Niacin, Vitamin B_6, Folate, Vitamin B_{12}, Pantothenic Acid, Biotin, and Choline*. Op cit.
8. Brown G. Defects of thiamine transport and metabolism. *J Inherit Metab Dis*. 2014 Jul;37(4):577–85.
9. Institute of Medicine, Food and Nutrition Board. *Dietary Reference Intakes for Thiamin, Riboflavin, Niacin, Vitamin B_6, Folate, Vitamin B_{12}, Pantothenic Acid, Biotin, and Choline*. Op cit.
10. Rodwell VW, Bender D, Botham KM, et al. *Harper's Illustrated Biochemistry*. 30th ed. New York: McGraw-Hill Education/Medical; January 8, 2015.
11. Institute of Medicine, Food and Nutrition Board. *Dietary Reference Intakes for Thiamin, Riboflavin, Niacin, Vitamin B_6, Folate, Vitamin B_{12}, Pantothenic Acid, Biotin, and Choline*. Op cit.
12. Ibid.
13. U.S. Department of Agriculture, Agricultural Research Service, Nutrient Data Laboratory. USDA National Nutrient Database for Standard Reference. Op cit.
14. Said HM, Ross AC. Riboflavin. In: Ross AC, Caballero, B, Cousins RJ, et al., eds. *Modern Nutrition in Health and Disease*. 11th ed. Wolters Kluwer/Lippincott Williams & Wilkins; Philadelphia, PA 2014 pages 325–330.
15. Institute of Medicine, Food and Nutrition Board. *Dietary Reference Intakes for Thiamin, Riboflavin, Niacin, Vitamin B_6, Folate, Vitamin B_{12}, Pantothenic Acid, Biotin, and Choline*. Op cit.
16. U.S. Department of Agriculture, Agricultural Research Service, Nutrient Data Laboratory. USDA National Nutrient Database for Standard Reference. Op cit.
17. Institute of Medicine, Food and Nutrition Board. *Dietary Reference Intakes for Thiamin, Riboflavin, Niacin, Vitamin B_6, Folate, Vitamin B_{12}, Pantothenic Acid, Biotin, and Choline*. Op cit.
18. Kirkland JB. Niacin. In: Ross AC, Caballero, B, Cousins RJ et al., eds. *Modern Nutrition in Health and Disease*. 11th ed. Wolters Kluwer/Lippincott Williams & Wilkins; Philadelphia, PA 2014 pages 331–340.
19. Ibid.
20. National Institutes of Health. NIH stops clinical trial on combination cholesterol treatment. [Press release]. May 26, 2011. http://www.nih.gov/news/health/may2011/nhlbi-26.htm. Accessed January 29, 2016.
21. U.S. National Library of Medicine. Niacin and niacinamide (vitamin B3). MedlinePlus. http://www.nlm.nih.gov/medlineplus/druginfo/natural/924.html. Accessed January 29, 2016.
22. U.S. National Library of Medicine. Pantothenic acid (vitamin B5). MedlinePlus. http://www.nlm.nih.gov/medlineplus/druginfo/natural/853.html. Accessed January 29, 2016.
23. Institute of Medicine, Food and Nutrition Board. *Dietary Reference Intakes for Thiamin, Riboflavin, Niacin, Vitamin B_6, Folate, Vitamin B_{12}, Pantothenic Acid, Biotin, and Choline*. Op cit.
24. U.S. Department of Agriculture, Agricultural Research Service, Nutrient Data Laboratory. USDA National Nutrient Database for Standard Reference. Op cit.
25. Institute of Medicine, Food and Nutrition Board. *Dietary Reference Intakes for Thiamin, Riboflavin, Niacin, Vitamin B_6, Folate, Vitamin B_{12}, Pantothenic Acid, Biotin, and Choline*. Op cit.
26. Ibid.
27. U.S. Department of Agriculture, Agricultural Research Service, Nutrient Data Laboratory. USDA National Nutrient Database for Standard Reference. Op cit.
28. Gropper SS, Smith JL. *Advanced Nutrition and Human Metabolism*. 6th ed. Belmont, CA: Wadsworth; June 1, 2012.
29. Ciaccio M, Bellia C. Hyperhomocysteinemia and cardiovascular risk: effect of vitamin supplementation in risk reduction. *Curr Clin Pharmacol*. 2010;5(1):30–36.
30. Eilat-Adar S, Goldbourt U. Nutritional recommendations for preventing coronary heart disease in women: evidence concerning whole foods and supplements. *Nutr Metab Cardiovasc Dis*. 2010;20(6):459–466.
31. Bhupathiraju SN, Tucker KL. Coronary heart disease prevention: nutrients, foods, and dietary patterns. *Clin Chim Acta*. 2011;412(17–18):1493–1514.
32. Institute of Medicine, Food and Nutrition Board. *Dietary Reference Intakes for Thiamin, Riboflavin, Niacin, Vitamin B_6, Folate, Vitamin B_{12}, Pantothenic Acid, Biotin, and Choline*. Op cit.
33. U.S. Department of Agriculture, Agricultural Research Service, Nutrient Data Laboratory. USDA National Nutrient Database for Standard Reference. Op cit.
34. Institute of Medicine, Food and Nutrition Board. *Dietary Reference Intakes for Thiamin, Riboflavin, Niacin, Vitamin B_6, Folate, Vitamin B_{12}, Pantothenic Acid, Biotin, and Choline*. Op cit.
35. National Institutes of Health, Office of Dietary Supplements. Vitamin B6: dietary supplement fact sheet. http://ods.od.nih.gov/factsheets/VitaminB6-HealthProfessional/. Accessed January 29, 2016.
36. LeBlanc KE, Cestia W. Carpal tunnel syndrome. *Am Fam Phys*. 2011;83(8):952–958.
37. Centers for Disease Control and Prevention. Folic acid. April 28, 2015. www.cdc.gov/ncbddd/folicacid/index.html. Accessed January 29, 2016.

38. Institute of Medicine, Food and Nutrition Board. *Dietary Reference Intakes for Thiamin, Riboflavin, Niacin, Vitamin B_6, Folate, Vitamin B_{12}, Pantothenic Acid, Biotin, and Choline*. Op cit.
39. Suitor CW, Bailey LB. Dietary folate equivalents: interpretation and application. *J Am Diet Assoc*. 2000;100:88–94.
40. Institute of Medicine, Food and Nutrition Board. *Dietary Reference Intakes for Thiamin, Riboflavin, Niacin, Vitamin B_6, Folate, Vitamin B_{12}, Pantothenic Acid, Biotin, and Choline*. Op cit.
41. US Department of Agriculture, Agricultural Research Service, Nutrient Data Laboratory. USDA National Nutrient Database for Standard Reference. Op cit.
42. Crider KS, Bailey LB, Berry RJ. Folic acid food fortification—its history, effect, concerns, and future directions. *Nutrients*. 2011;3:370–384.
43. Institute of Medicine, Food and Nutrition Board. *Dietary Reference Intakes for Thiamin, Riboflavin, Niacin, Vitamin B_6, Folate, Vitamin B_{12}, Pantothenic Acid, Biotin, and Choline*. Op cit.
44. Centers for Disease Control and Prevention. Folic acid: data and statistics. http://www.cdc.gov/ncbddd/folicacid/data.html. Accessed January 29, 2016.
45. U.S. Preventive Services Task Force. Folic acid for the prevention of neural tube defects: U.S. Preventive Services Task Force recommendation statement. *Ann Intern Med*. 2009;150(9):626–631.
46. Stover P. Folic acid. In: Ross AC, Caballero, B, Cousins RJ et al., eds. *Modern Nutrition in Health and Disease*. 11th ed. Wolters Kluwer/Lippincott Williams & Wilkins; Philadelphia, PA 2014 pages 358–368.
47. Stipanuk MH. Cysteine, taurine and homocysteine. In: Ross AC, Caballero, B, Cousins RJ et al., eds. *Modern Nutrition in Health and Disease*. 11th ed. Wolters Kluwer/Lippincott Williams & Wilkins; Philadelphia, PA 2014 pages 447–463.
48. Ganji V, Kafai MR. Demographic, lifestyle, and health characteristics and serum B vitamin status are determinants of plasma total homocysteine concentration in the post-folic acid fortification period, 1999–2004. *J Nutr*. 2009;139(2):345–352.
49. National Institutes of Health, National Institute of Neurological Disorders and Stroke. Spina bifida fact sheet. February 23, 2015. http://www.ninds.nih.gov/disorders/spina_bifida/detail_spina_bifida.htm. Accessed January 29, 2016.
50. Centers for Disease Control and Prevention. Spina bifida and anencephaly before and after folic acid mandate—United States, 1995–1996 and 1999–2000. *MMWR*. 2004;53(17):362–365.
51. Greenberg JA, Bell SJ, Guan Y, Yu Y-H. Folic acid supplementation and pregnancy: more than just neural tube defect prevention. *Rev Obstet Gynecol*. 2011;4(2):52–59.
52. Lee JE, Willett WC, Fuchs CS, et al. Folate intake and risk of colorectal cancer and adenoma: modification by time. *Am J Clin Nutr*. 2011;93(4):817–825.
53. Kennedy DA, Stern SJ, Moretti M, et al. Folate intake and the risk of colorectal cancer: a systematic review and meta-analysis. *Cancer Epidemiol*. 2011;35(1):2–10.
54. Mason JB. Folate, cancer risk, and the Greek god, Proteus: a tale of two chameleons. *Nutr Rev*. 2009;67(4):206–212.
55. Stover P. Folic acid. Op cit.
56. Refsum H, Smith AD. Are we ready for mandatory fortification with vitamin B-12? *Am J Clin Nutr*. 2008;88(2):253–254.
57. National Institutes Health, Office of Dietary Supplements. Dietary supplement fact sheet: vitamin B12. http://ods.od.nih.gov/factsheets/VitaminB12-HealthProfessional. Accessed January 29, 2016.
58. U.S. Department of Agriculture, Agricultural Research Service, Nutrient Data Laboratory. USDA National Nutrient Database for Standard Reference. Op cit.
59. Langan RC, Zawistoski KJ. Update on vitamin B_{12} deficiency. *Am Fam Physician*. 2011;83(12):1425–1430. http://www.aafp.org/afp/2011/0615/p1425.html. Accessed January 29, 2016.
60. Allen LH, Rosenberg IH, Oakley GP, Omenn GS. Considering the case for vitamin B12 fortification of flour. *Food Nutr Bull*. 2010;31(1 suppl):S36–S46.
61. Selhub J, Paul L. Folic acid fortification: why not vitamin B12 also? *Biofactors*. 2011;37(4):269–271. doi: 10.1002/biof.173. Epub June 14, 2011.
62. Institute of Medicine, Food and Nutrition Board. *Dietary Reference Intakes for Thiamin, Riboflavin, Niacin, Vitamin B_6, Folate, Vitamin B_{12}, Pantothenic Acid, Biotin, and Choline*. Op cit.
63. Ibid.
64. Carmel R. Cobalamin (vitamin B12). In: Ross AC, Caballero, B, Cousins RJ et al., eds. *Modern Nutrition in Health and Disease*. 11th ed. Wolters Kluwer/Lippincott Williams & Wilkins; Philadelphia, PA 2014 pages 369–389.
65. Carpenter KJ. A short history of nutritional science: part 1 (1785–1885). *J Nutr*. 2003;133:638–645.
66. Ibid.
67. Gropper SS, Smith JL. *Advanced Nutrition and Human Metabolism*. Op cit.
68. Levine M, Padayatty SJ. Vitamin C. In: Ross AC, Caballero, B, Cousins RJ et al., eds. *Modern Nutrition in Health and Disease*. 11th ed. Wolters Kluwer/Lippincott Williams & Wilkins; Philadelphia, PA 2014 pages 399–415.
69. Ibid.
70. Douglas RM, Hemilä H, Chalker E, Treacy B. Vitamin C for preventing and treating the common cold. *Cochrane Database Syst Rev*. 2013;1: CD000980. doi: 10.1002/14651858.CD000980.pub4.
71. Institute of Medicine, Food and Nutrition Board. *Dietary Reference Intakes for Vitamin C, Vitamin E, Selenium, and Carotenoids*. Washington, DC: National Academies Press; 2000.
72. U.S. Department of Agriculture, Agricultural Research Service, Nutrient Data Laboratory. USDA National Nutrient Database for Standard Reference. Op cit.
73. Institute of Medicine, Food and Nutrition Board. *Dietary Reference Intakes for Vitamin C, Vitamin E, Selenium, and Carotenoids*. Op cit.
74. Ibid.
75. Ibid.
76. Gropper SS, Smith JL. *Advanced Nutrition and Human Metabolism*. Op cit.
77. Institute of Medicine, Food and Nutrition Board. *Dietary Reference Intakes for Thiamin, Riboflavin, Niacin, Vitamin B_6, Folate, Vitamin B_{12}, Pantothenic Acid, Biotin, and Choline*. Op cit.

Chapter **12**

Water and Major Minerals

Revised by Veronica Oates

THINK About It

1. How much water does it usually take to quench your thirst?
2. Does drinking caffeinated beverages make you feel dehydrated?
3. How often do you salt your food before tasting it?
4. What's your primary source of calcium?

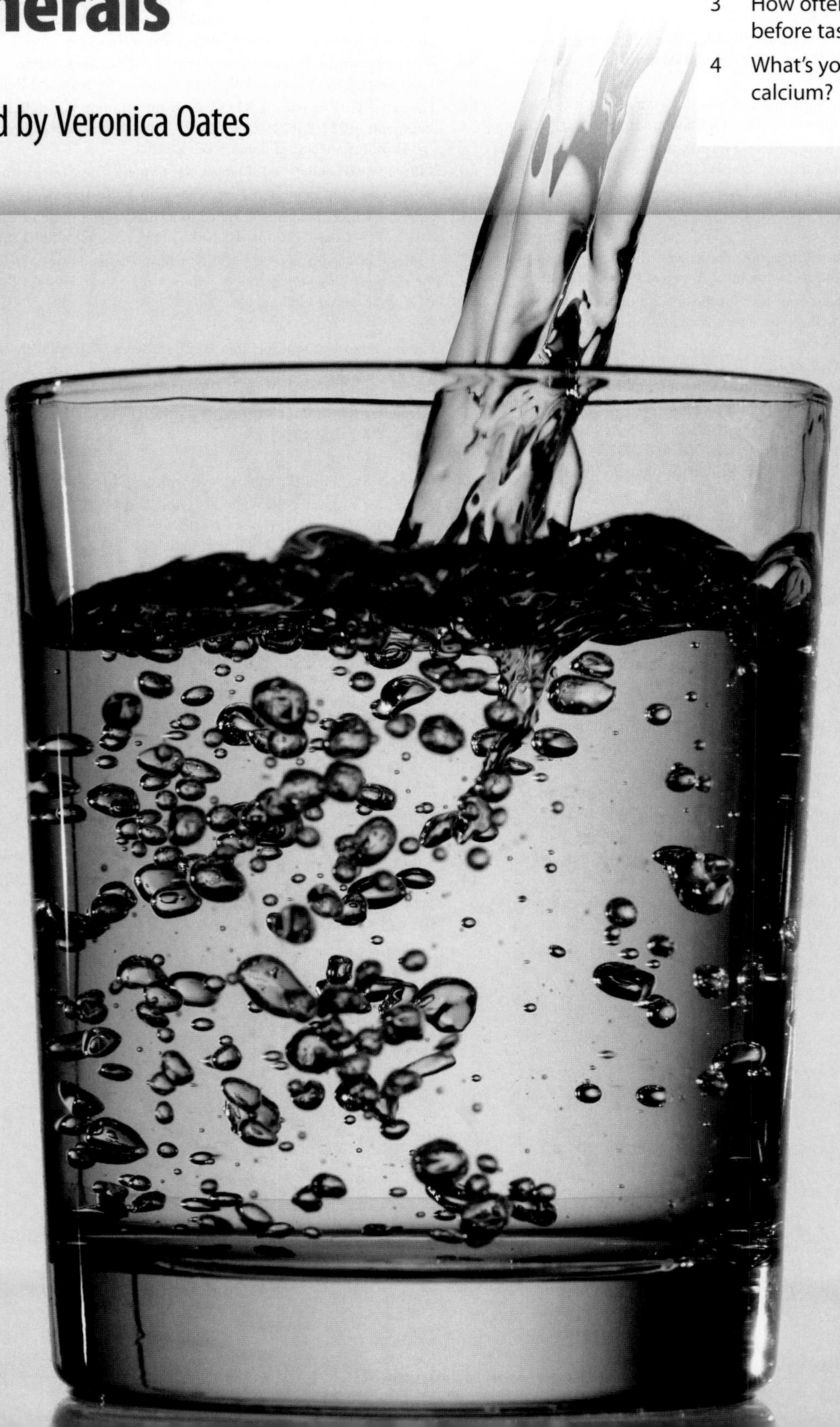

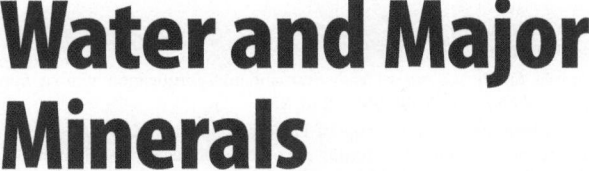

CHAPTER Menu

- Water: The Essential Ingredient for Life
- Intake Recommendations: How Much Water Is Enough?
- Major Minerals
- Sodium
- Potassium
- Chloride
- Calcium
- Phosphorus
- Magnesium
- Sulfur
- Key Terms
- Study Points
- Study Questions
- Try This
- References

LEARNING Objectives

- State the functions of water.
- Identify the factors that affect mineral bioavailability.
- Describe the absorption, storage, and transport of minerals.
- List the major functions of minerals.
- Identify major food sources of minerals.
- Specify the major symptoms and diseases associated with mineral deficiency and toxicity.
- Discuss the risks and benefits of mineral supplementation.
- Discuss the role of major minerals in health and disease.

On your coast-to-coast flight with your father and your brother, you observe your father drinking water frequently throughout the flight, whereas your brother rejects the beverages offered. When you arrive at your destination, your brother complains of feeling utterly exhausted. In contrast, your father is lively and feels good. How could you explain this?

First, it's important to know that the familiar beverage cart is not a random gesture of kindness by the airlines: Regular fluid intake on flights is necessary for health! Although you are unaware of it, water evaporates from the skin at an accelerated rate in the low-humidity, high-altitude, pressurized cabin of an airplane. Thus, drinking fluids during the flight helps prevent dehydration. But you must choose the fluids carefully. Alcohol is a diuretic. This means that alcoholic beverages increase fluid loss as urine and therefore are less effective than water, juice, and other caffeine-free beverages in replacing fluid losses.

Your brother's lack of energy can be a symptom of mild dehydration. Dad had the right idea—plenty of water along the way—and he feels just fine!

Water: The Essential Ingredient for Life

Water is absolutely essential. You could probably survive for weeks without food, but you can live only a few days without water. Humans have no capacity to store "spare" water, so we must quickly replace any that's lost.

Overall, water makes up between 45 and 75 percent of a person's weight (see **FIGURE 12.1**). Leaner people have proportionately more water because muscle tissue is nearly three-fourths water by weight, whereas adipose tissue is only about 10 percent water.

The one bit of chemistry that almost everyone can rattle off is the chemical formula for water: H_2O. Water is such a simple molecule (see **FIGURE 12.2**) that people often do not appreciate its extraordinary physical and chemical properties. Water's strong surface tension, high heat capacity, and ability to dissolve many substances result from **hydrogen bonds** between a hydrogen atom of one water molecule and the oxygen atom of another water molecule.

Water in your body contains numerous dissolved minerals, called **electrolytes**, that are kept in constant balance. To live, each cell must have just the right mix of water and electrolytes. Although intracellular and extracellular fluids have different mixes, the proportions in each must stay within a narrow range. Despite a continuous flow of molecules among intracellular fluid, extracellular fluid, and the outside environment, the body maintains its electrolyte balance through the intake and excretion of water and the movement of ions.

▶ **hydrogen bonds** Noncovalent bonds between hydrogen and an atom, usually oxygen, in another molecule.

▶ **electrolytes** [ih-LEK-tro-lites] Substances that dissociate into charged particles (ions) when dissolved in water or other solvents and thus become capable of conducting an electrical current. The terms *electrolyte* and *ion* often are used interchangeably.

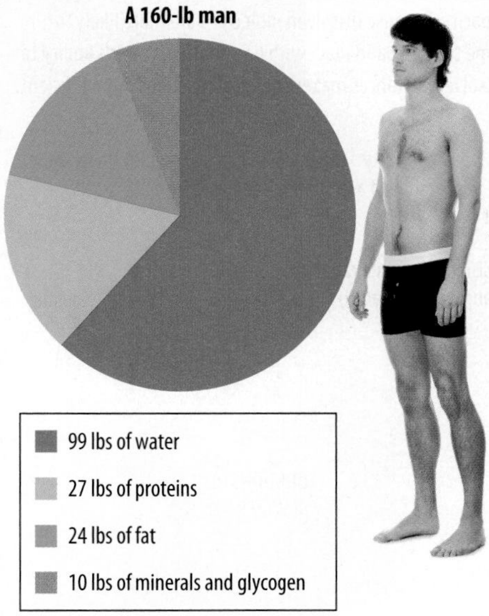

FIGURE 12.1 Body composition. The main constituent of the body is water. Adult males have more lean tissue and less fat than adult females do, and therefore have more body water. An adult male is approximately 62 percent water, 17 percent protein, 15 percent fat, and 6 percent minerals and glycogen.

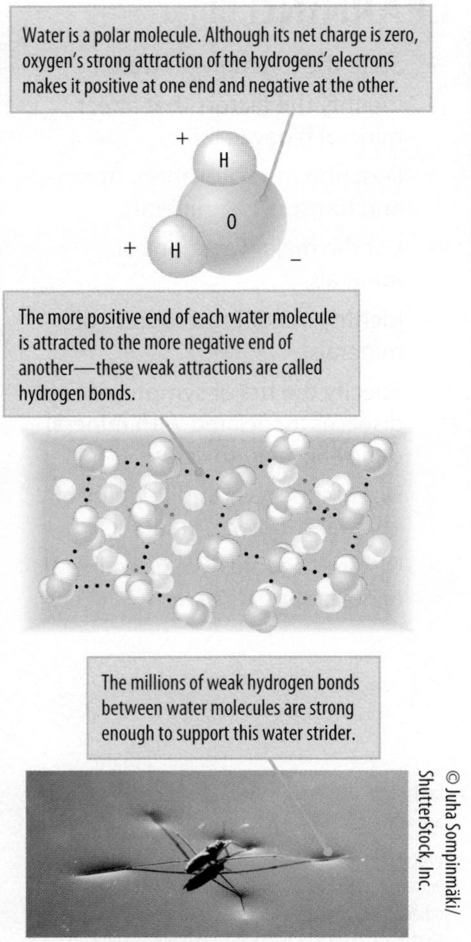

Water is a polar molecule. Although its net charge is zero, oxygen's strong attraction of the hydrogens' electrons makes it positive at one end and negative at the other.
+
H
O
+
H
–
The more positive end of each water molecule is attracted to the more negative end of another—these weak attractions are called hydrogen bonds.
The millions of weak hydrogen bonds between water molecules are strong enough to support this water strider.
© Juha Sompinmäki/ShutterStock, Inc.

FIGURE 12.2 Water—a simple, yet powerful, molecule. Water has a strong surface tension and high heat capacity. Because dissolved molecules are more likely to come together and react with one another, water's ability to dissolve substances makes chemical reactions more efficient.

▶ **heat capacity** The amount of energy required to raise the temperature of a substance 1 degree Celsius.

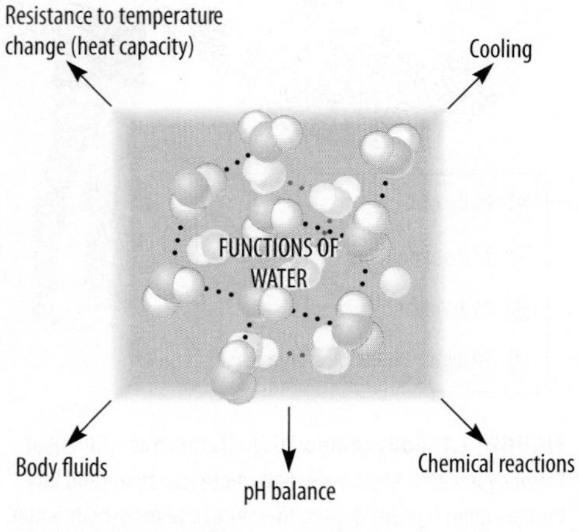

FIGURE 12.3 Functions of water. Water has many critical functions in the body.

Functions of Water

Water performs a wide variety of tasks in the body (see **FIGURE 12.3**). Water is the highway that moves nutrients and wastes between cells, tissues, and organs. It also carries waste out of your body in urine. What about nutrients and wastes that are not water-soluble? Your body either modifies them chemically so they dissolve in water or packages them with proteins (e.g., lipoproteins). Your body's watery fluids, such as the bloodstream, can easily transport these protein packages throughout the body.

Heat Capacity

The **heat capacity** of a substance is the amount of energy required to raise its temperature 1 degree Celsius. Raising the temperature of a substance with a high heat capacity requires more energy than raising the temperature of a substance with a low one. Water, for instance, has about three times the heat capacity of iron. Warming or cooling a substance with a high heat capacity requires a relatively large amount of energy. You might have noticed this property when heating items in a microwave oven. Watery foods such as soup take much longer to heat than foods that contain little water, such as pizza and butter. Because of water's high heat capacity, it takes a lot of heat to change the temperature of the body; body water dampens the effects of extreme environmental temperatures on conditions in cells.

Cooling Ability

A rise in body temperature, whether resulting from exercise, environmental conditions, or illness, triggers the body's cooling system. If you get too warm, blood vessels dilate and you begin to sweat. The perspiration evaporates from the skin, thereby cooling your body. Moisture readily evaporates in dry air, so perspiring is most effective for cooling when the humidity is low. When the humidity is high, such as in humid, tropical environments, sweat does not evaporate readily, so even profuse sweating might not cool the body effectively.

Participation in Metabolism

Nearly all the chemical reactions of metabolism involve water. Water is the solvent for many biologically essential molecules (e.g., glucose, vitamins, minerals, amino acids), and it is a product or reactant in many biochemical reactions.

pH Balance

Water is also an essential component of the body's mechanisms to maintain pH (acid–base) balance in the narrow range necessary for life. One of the major buffer systems involves carbonic acid and bicarbonate. Carbonic acid forms when dissolved carbon dioxide reacts with water ($CO_2 + H_2O \rightarrow H_2CO_3$). Carbonic acid can then dissociate to form H^+ and HCO_3^- (bicarbonate). The resulting H^+ helps increase acidity, lowering pH.

Body Fluids

Water is the major component of all body fluids. These fluids serve essential mechanical functions such as shock absorption, lubrication, cleansing, and protection. For example, amniotic fluid provides a gentle cushion that protects the fetus, synovial fluid allows joints to move smoothly, tears lubricate and cleanse the eyes, and saliva moistens food and makes swallowing possible.

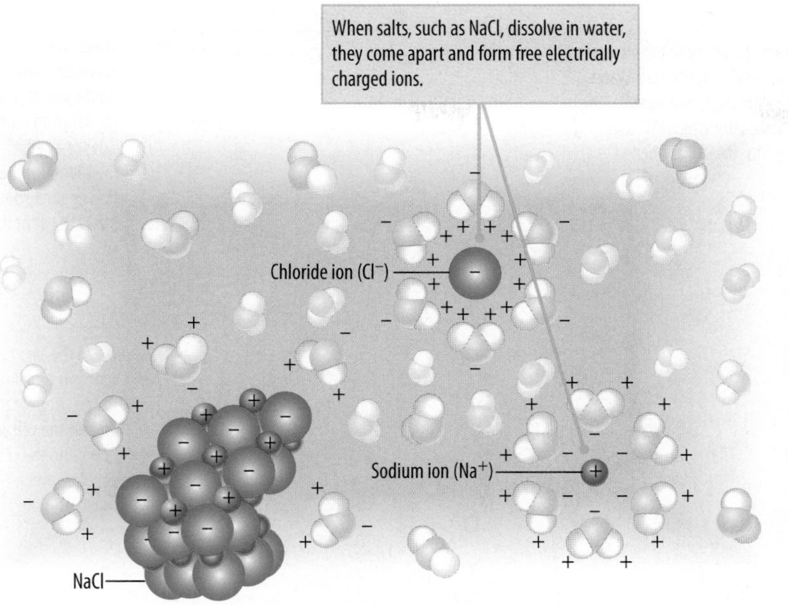

FIGURE 12.4 Dissolving salt in water. When dissolving salt, the oxygen atoms of the water molecules are attracted to the positively charged sodium ions. Water's hydrogen atoms are attracted to the negatively charged chloride ions.

Electrolytes and Water: A Delicate Equilibrium

Your body precisely controls and balances the concentration of electrolytes dissolved in its watery fluids. When **salts**, such as sodium chloride, dissolve in water (see **FIGURE 12.4**), they come apart and form free **ions**, which are positively (e.g., Na^+) and negatively (e.g., Cl^-) charged particles. In an electrolyte solution, the number of positive charges always equals the number of negative charges. The main positively charged ions (**cations**) in the body are sodium and potassium, and the main negatively charged ions (**anions**) are chloride and phosphate.

There are two major fluid compartments in the body. About two-thirds of body water is in intracellular fluid, and one-third is in extracellular fluid. The major components of extracellular fluid are interstitial fluid (the fluid between cells) and blood **plasma** (the fluid portion of blood) (see **FIGURE 12.5**).

▶ **salts** Compounds that result from the replacement of the hydrogen of an acid with a metal or a group that acts like a metal.

▶ **ions** Atoms or groups of atoms with an electrical charge resulting from the loss or gain of one or more electrons.

▶ **cations** Ions that carry a positive charge.

▶ **anions** Ions that carry a negative charge.

▶ **plasma** The fluid portion of the blood that contains blood cells and other components.

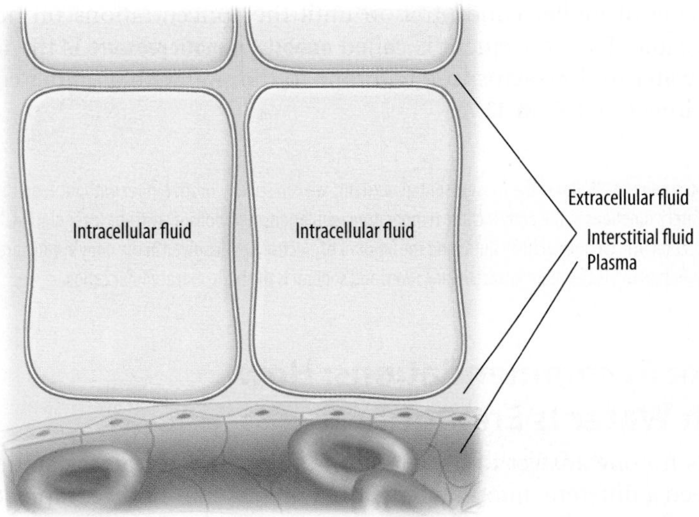

FIGURE 12.5 Intracellular and extracellular fluid. Extracellular fluids and their solutes (except for proteins) move across capillary membranes easily. Plasma (the fluid portion of the blood) has a higher concentration of proteins than interstitial fluid. Excluding protein, their compositions are roughly the same.

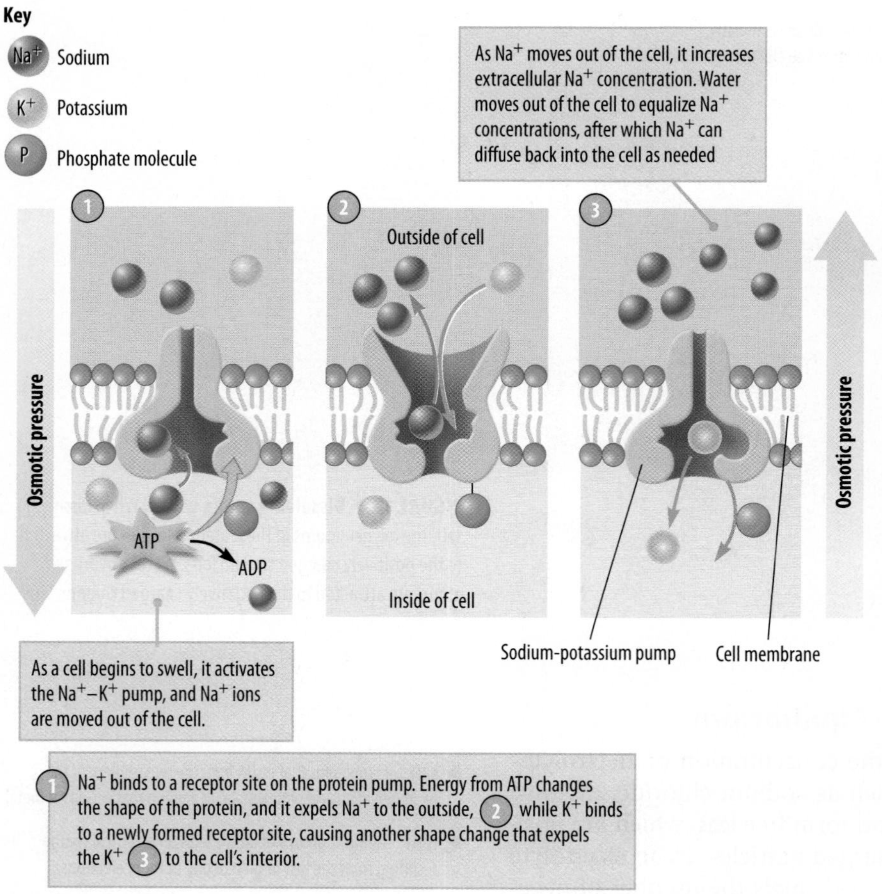

Na+ Sodium

Inside of cell

As a cell begins to swell, it activates the Na+–K+ pump, and Na+ ions are moved out of the cell.
1 Na+ binds to a receptor site on the protein pump. Energy from ATP changes the shape of the protein, and it expels Na+ to the outside, 2 while K+ binds to a newly formed receptor site, causing another shape change that expels the K+ 3 to the cell's interior.

FIGURE 12.6 Sodium–potassium pump. The movement of sodium and potassium into and out of cells helps maintain the proper volume of fluid in the cell.

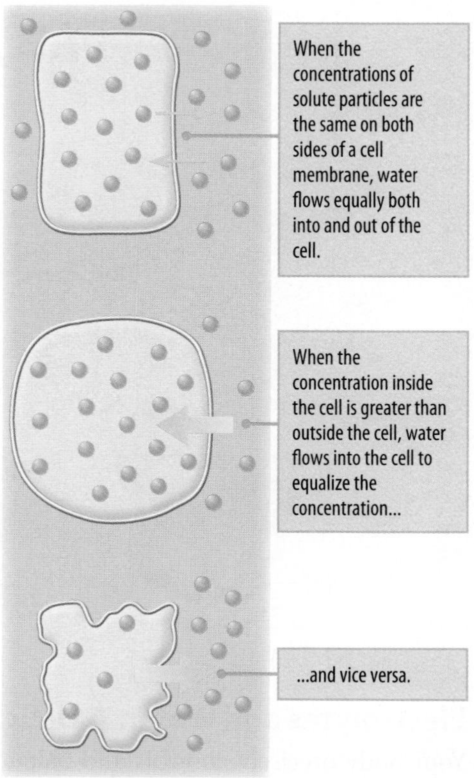

When the concentrations of solute particles are the same on both sides of a cell membrane, water flows equally both into and out of the cell.
When the concentration inside the cell is greater than outside the cell, water flows into the cell to equalize the concentration...
...and vice versa.

FIGURE 12.7 Osmosis. Water moves across cell membranes to equalize concentrations of dissolved particles.

- **sodium–potassium pumps** Mechanisms that pump sodium ions out of a cell, allowing potassium ions to enter the cell.
- **solutes** Substances that are dissolved in a solvent.
- **semipermeable membrane** Membrane that allows passage of some substances but blocks others.
- **osmosis** The movement of a solvent, such as water, through a semipermeable membrane from the low-solute to the high-solute solution until the concentrations on both sides of the membrane are equal.
- **osmotic pressure** The pressure exerted on a semipermeable membrane by a solvent, usually water, moving from the side of low-solute to the side of high-solute concentration.

Sodium is the main cation in extracellular fluid, whereas potassium is the predominant cation in intracellular fluid. To maintain the balance of sodium and potassium, all cell membranes incorporate **sodium–potassium pumps** (see **FIGURE 12.6**) that actively pump sodium out of the cell while allowing potassium back in. If **solutes** are more concentrated on one side of a **semipermeable membrane** (through which water, but not solutes, can pass easily), water flows to the side of higher concentration until the concentrations on both sides are the same. This movement is called **osmosis**; **osmotic pressure** is the force that causes water to flow across a membrane to the side with a higher concentration of ions (see **FIGURE 12.7**).

Key Concepts Water is the most essential nutrient; we can survive much longer without food than without water. Water's functions in the body include temperature regulation, metabolism, acid–base regulation, lubrication, and protection. The balance of body fluids and the amount of electrolytes dissolved in the body's water are controlled precisely. Potassium is the main intracellular cation, and sodium is the main extracellular cation.

Intake Recommendations: How Much Water Is Enough?

There is no one answer to the question of how much water is sufficient. We each need a different amount, depending on our size, body composition, and activity level as well as the temperature and humidity of the environment. Over

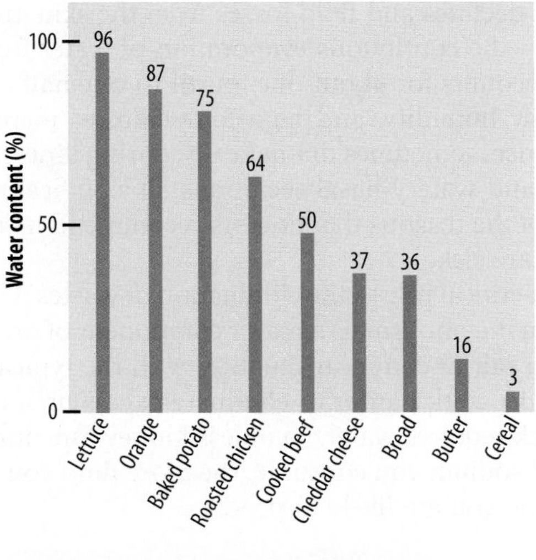

FIGURE 12.8 Water content of various foods. As you might expect, crunchy vegetables contain more water than dry cereal. But did you know that potatoes contain a high percentage of water?

the course of a few hours, body water deficits can occur as a result of reduced intake or increased water losses from physical activity and environmental (e.g., heat) exposure. However, on a day-to-day basis, fluid intake, driven by the combination of thirst and the consumption of food and beverages at meals, allows maintenance of hydration status and total body water at normal levels.

The Adequate Intake (AI) for total water, including drinking water, beverages, and food, is 3.7 liters per day for men and 2.7 liters per day for women.[1] Intake recommendations are higher during pregnancy (3.0 liters per day) and lactation (3.8 liters per day). Activity and sweating increase water needs, so athletes and active people need much more water, especially if they work and train in warm, humid climates.

Water intake comes from a combination of drinking water, beverages, and the water in foods. Approximately 81 percent of our total daily water intake comes from beverages, with the remaining 19 percent from foods.[2] Some foods, such as fruits and vegetables, contain a substantial amount of water, whereas others—grain products, for example—provide very little (see **FIGURE 12.8**). Our bodies also produce a small amount of water (about 250 to 350 milliliters per day) in metabolic reactions.

Drinking plenty of plain water and eating a healthful diet easily replaces the fluid and electrolytes a person loses during moderate exercise in pleasant weather. But, if you are involved in endurance activities or strenuous exercise in hot weather, consider using sports drinks instead of just plain water. Sports drinks contain glucose and electrolytes that improve the drink's taste, help maintain blood glucose levels, and enhance absorption.[3]

Water Excretion: Where Does the Water Go?

We continuously lose water from our bodies through various routes. In the lungs, water evaporates and exits in exhaled air. Water also departs through the skin by evaporation and perspiration. In the gastrointestinal (GI) tract, feces carry water out of the body. The kidneys excrete water in urine. **FIGURE 12.9** summarizes sources and amounts of fluid output and shows how these balance with fluid intake.

Depending on the amount of water, protein, and sodium consumed, the body loses about 1 to 2 liters of water each day through urine. During exercise,

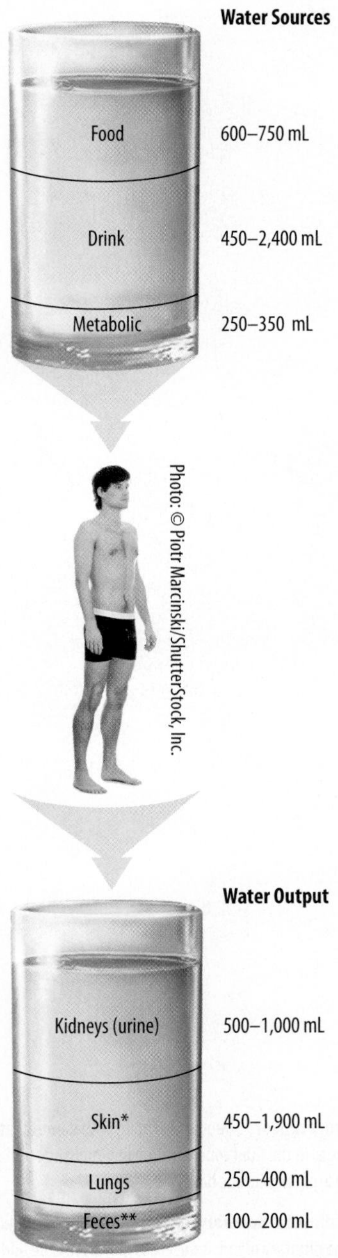

* (Insensible and perspiration)
The volume of perspiration is normally about 100 mL per day. In very hot weather or during heavy exercise, a person may lose 1 to 2 liters per hour.

** People with severe diarrhea can lose several liters of water per day in feces.

FIGURE 12.9 Typical daily fluid intake and output. To maintain fluid balance, your body regulates its fluid intake and output.

urine production declines and fluid losses from the skin and lungs increase. **Insensible water loss**—the continuous evaporation of water from the lungs and skin—typically accounts for about one-fourth to one-half of daily fluid loss. High altitude, low humidity, and high temperatures increase these losses. Insensible losses rise, sometimes dramatically, during illness. Fever, coughing, rapid breathing, and watery nasal secretions all significantly increase water loss. This is one of the reasons that doctors recommend increasing your fluid intake when you are sick.

▶ **insensible water loss** The continual loss of body water by evaporation from the respiratory tract and diffusion through the skin.

Water plays a critical role in the elimination of wastes. Urea, a breakdown product of protein metabolism, is a major component of urine. If we overconsume protein and salt (a common situation with the typical American diet), the kidneys have to work harder to eliminate excess urea and sodium from the body. This task requires water, so unless kidney function is impaired, the more protein and sodium you consume, the more fluid you need to consume and the more urine you are likely to produce.

Key Concepts The AI for fluid intake is 3.7 liters per day for men and 2.7 liters per day for women. Water intake comes from a combination of foods, fluids, and water produced in normal metabolism. The main method of water excretion is in urine. In addition, fluid is lost through the skin and lungs, and in the feces. Losses are higher when a person perspires heavily or is ill. Water is critical in eliminating the body's waste products.

Water Balance

Our bodies maintain water balance by mechanisms that control water intake (e.g., thirst) and water excretion. Because of water's critical roles, the body works not only to balance fluid between compartments, but also to closely regulate total body water.

Regulation of Fluid Excretion

Our kidneys adjust the amount and concentration of urine in response to the body's hydration status. The kidneys can excrete a small volume of concentrated urine or a large volume of dilute urine while maintaining a relatively constant excretion of solutes such as sodium and potassium. This ability to regulate water excretion without major changes in solute excretion is an important survival mechanism, especially when water is in short supply.

When water intake is low, the kidneys conserve water. While continuing to excrete solutes, they reabsorb water, thus decreasing urine volume and concentrating the urine. When the body has an excess of water, the kidneys form and excrete a large volume of dilute urine.

How do the kidneys know when to conserve water? **Osmoreceptors**, special cells in the hypothalamus of the brain, are exquisitely sensitive to very small increases in extracellular sodium concentration and thus sense the body's need for water. If the sodium concentration rises, these receptors signal the pituitary gland to release **antidiuretic hormone (ADH)**. ADH decreases water loss by causing the kidneys to reabsorb water rather than excrete it in the urine (see **FIGURE 12.10**).

▶ **osmoreceptors** Neurons in the hypothalamus that detect changes in the fluid concentration in blood and regulate the release of antidiuretic hormone.

▶ **antidiuretic hormone (ADH)** A peptide hormone secreted by the pituitary gland. It increases blood pressure and prevents fluid excretion by the kidneys. Also called *vasopressin*.

▶ **vasoconstrictor** A substance that causes blood vessels to constrict.

▶ **vasopressin** See *antidiuretic hormone.*

▶ **osmolarity** The concentration of dissolved particles (e.g., electrolytes) in a solution expressed per unit of volume.

The presence of ADH signals the kidneys to conserve water. In higher concentrations, ADH is a potent **vasoconstrictor**, which is why it also is called **vasopressin**. Although ADH is far less sensitive to blood volume than to plasma **osmolarity** (concentration of electrolytes), a severe loss of blood also triggers its release. A loss of 15 to 25 percent of blood volume will cause up to a 50-fold increase in ADH levels. Nausea is also a potent trigger. ADH levels increase 100-fold after vomiting. Some drugs (e.g., nicotine and morphine) stimulate the release of ADH, but others (e.g., alcohol and caffeine) inhibit it.[4]

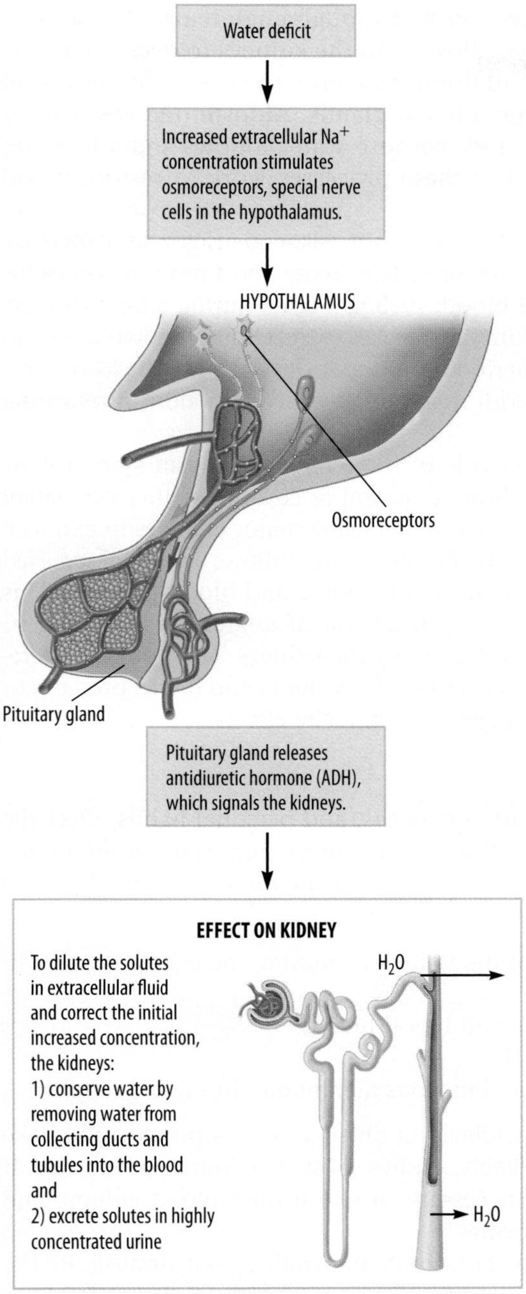

FIGURE 12.10 Antidiuretic hormone regulates excretion. In response to a water deficit, the osmoreceptor—ADH feedback system regulates solute concentrations in extracellular fluid.

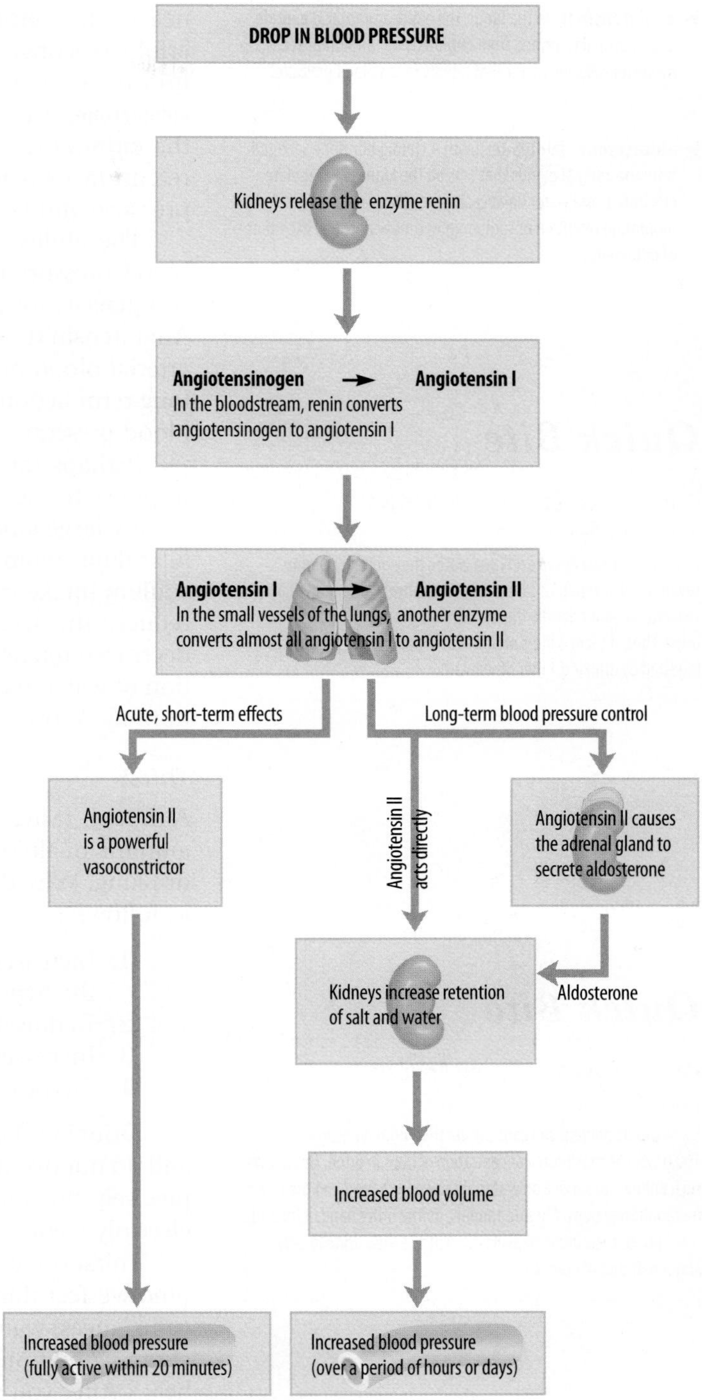

FIGURE 12.11 Regulating blood volume and pressure. Within minutes after severe hemorrhage, the renin-angiotensin vasoconstrictor mechanism is powerful enough to cause a life-saving rise in blood pressure. Malfunctions in the long-term blood pressure control mechanism can cause persistently high blood pressure (hypertension).

Regulation of Blood Volume and Pressure

The kidneys themselves have sensors that detect falling blood pressure (see **FIGURE 12.11**). In response, the kidneys release **renin**, an enzyme that splits off a small protein, **angiotensin I**, from the blood protein **angiotensinogen**. Within seconds, enzymes in the small blood vessels of the lungs convert

- ▶ **renin** An enzyme, produced by the kidney, that affects blood pressure by catalyzing the conversion of angiotensinogen to angiotensin I.
- ▶ **angiotensin I** [an-jee-oh-TEN-sin one] A 10-amino-acid peptide that is a precursor of angiotensin II.
- ▶ **angiotensinogen** A circulating protein produced by the liver from which angiotensin I is cleaved by the action of renin.

▶ **angiotensin II** In the lungs, the eight-amino-acid peptide angiotensin II is formed from angiotensin I. Angiotensin II is a powerful vasoconstrictor that rapidly raises blood pressure.

▶ **aldosterone** [al-DOS-ter-own] A steroid hormone secreted from the adrenal glands that acts on the kidneys to regulate electrolyte and water balance. It raises blood pressure by promoting retention of sodium (and thus water) and excretion of potassium.

nearly all angiotensin I to **angiotensin II**. Although angiotensin II is a powerful vasoconstrictor, it also acts directly on the kidneys to decrease excretion of sodium and water. In addition, this protein causes the release of **aldosterone**, a hormone from the adrenal glands. Aldosterone also causes the kidneys to retain sodium, and, because water follows sodium, water retention increases as well. All of these processes work to restore blood pressure and volume.

The ability of angiotensin II to act as a vasoconstrictor and increase blood pressure is a life-saving measure. This acute short-term action helps compensate for a severe loss of blood, such as occurs during a hemorrhage. Angiotensin II's effect on the kidneys increases extracellular fluid volume and arterial blood pressure over a period of hours or days. Although slower, this long-term action is more powerful than acute vasoconstriction in returning blood pressure to normal.

Perhaps the most important role of the renin-angiotensin system is its response to dietary sodium. It allows a person to consume either very small or very large amounts of sodium without causing major changes in extracellular fluid volume or blood pressure. Because water follows sodium, increased sodium intake increases extracellular fluid volume and blood pressure. This reduces the secretion of renin and production of angiotensin, leading to decreased retention of sodium and water by the kidneys. The resulting excretion of water and sodium returns extracellular volume and blood pressure to normal. A low sodium intake triggers the opposite effects.

Quick Bite

Water, Water Everywhere and Not a Drop to Drink!

When people lost at sea drink sea water, they quickly become severely dehydrated. This is because the concentration of salt in seawater is about double the maximum concentration of salt in urine. Thus, it takes 2 liters of urine to rid the body of the solutes ingested by drinking 1 liter of seawater.

Thirst

Although taste, availability, cultural patterns, and personal habits affect the amount of fluids we consume, thirst is our most important stimulus for drinking. Why do we become thirsty? The four major stimuli for thirst are as follows[5]:

1. Increased osmolarity of the fluid surrounding the osmoreceptors in the hypothalamus
2. Reduced blood volume and blood pressure
3. Increased angiotensin II
4. Dryness of the mouth and mucous membranes lining the esophagus

Drinking fluids temporarily alleviates thirst, so we stop our fluid intake and do not overhydrate. Remarkably, studies show that animals drink almost precisely the amount of water necessary to return their blood volume and electrolyte concentrations to normal.[6]

Quick Bite

How Do Desert-Dwelling Animals Avoid Dehydration?

Some desert animals can concentrate their urine to nearly 100 times the maximum concentration of human urine. This allows such animals to survive on water obtained from food and their own metabolic reactions. Aquatic animals, on the other hand, minimally concentrate their urine. Beavers concentrate their urine to only about half that of humans.

Thirst on its own is an unreliable guide to avoiding dehydration. By the time we feel thirsty, our fluids already can be depleted. Under normal circumstances, water losses in adults can range from 0.3 liters per hour in sedentary conditions to 2.0 liters per hour during high physical activity in the heat.[7] After you drink water, your body can take 30 to 60 minutes to absorb and distribute it throughout the body. For example, imagine you are hiking or playing soccer in the hot sun and after an hour you pause momentarily to quench your thirst with a 0.5-liter bottle of water. That's not enough—you still have a deficit of 0.5 to 1.5 liters of water, and you'll continue to lose water while your body absorbs and distributes the water you just drank. To avoid dehydration in hot weather or when exercising, you need to drink fluids early and often. THINK About It 1

Quick Bite

Why Do Salty Foods Make You Thirsty?

The thirst mechanism is highly sensitive to extracellular sodium concentration. Even a tiny rise in sodium crosses the thirst threshold and triggers the desire to drink.

Because heavy activity easily can cause dehydration, athletes also must be careful to drink adequate amounts of fluid. Athletic performance improves if athletes anticipate their water needs well before they begin to feel thirst.

Water Reabsorption in the Gastrointestinal Tract

The gastrointestinal tract manages many liters of fluid each day. If all the secretions from the salivary glands, stomach, small intestine, pancreas, and gallbladder passed through the GI tract and out in the feces, we would dehydrate very rapidly! Fortunately, the small and large intestines reabsorb almost all of the water that enters them, so little water actually is lost in feces.

Key Concepts The body has mechanisms that balance water among compartments and regulate total body water. Antidiuretic hormone (ADH) stimulates water reabsorption in the kidneys, whereas aldosterone stimulates the kidneys to reabsorb sodium. Thirst is not a reliable indicator to avoid dehydration when fluid losses are high, such as during hot weather or heavy exercise.

Alcohol, Caffeine, and Common Medications Affect Fluid Balance

Anyone who regularly consumes alcohol probably realizes that it is a diuretic—a substance that increases fluid loss through increased urination. Alcohol suppresses ADH production (see **FIGURE 12.12**), and excessive alcohol consumption can cause dehydration, with symptoms of thirst, weakness, dryness of mucous membranes, dizziness, and light-headedness—all common side effects of a hangover.

THINK About It 2

A cup of coffee can provide a morning pick-me-up, but the caffeine is a mild diuretic. A typical pattern of many busy Americans is a few cups of coffee in the morning, a caffeinated soda with lunch, another in the afternoon, and maybe a glass of wine or a beer with dinner. Studies of the effects of caffeinated beverages on overall hydration status have produced inconsistent results.[8] Although some suggest that a fondness for caffeinated beverages can cause chronic mild dehydration, the Dietary Reference Intakes (DRIs) committee examining water and electrolyte requirements concluded that caffeinated beverages contribute to the total water intake in a manner similar to noncaffeinated beverages.[9] Most Americans seem to consume a sufficient quantity and variety of fluids from foods and beverages to maintain fluid balance.[10]

Doctors often prescribe diuretic medications to help lower blood pressure or decrease swelling caused by fluid retention. Because these medications can disrupt sodium and potassium balance, doctors typically monitor the patient's blood electrolyte levels and may prescribe potassium supplements to maintain a proper balance.

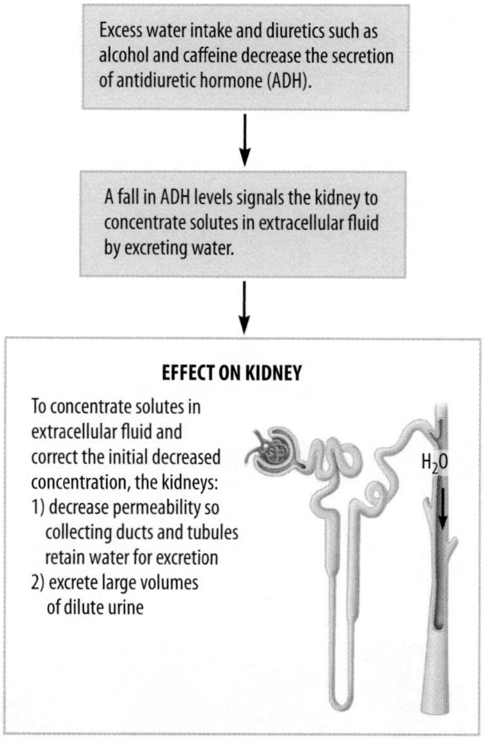
Excess water intake and diuretics such as alcohol and caffeine decrease the secretion of antidiuretic hormone (ADH).
A fall in ADH levels signals the kidney to concentrate solutes in extracellular fluid by excreting water.
EFFECT ON KIDNEY
To concentrate solutes in extracellular fluid and correct the initial decreased concentration, the kidneys:
1) decrease permeability so collecting ducts and tubules retain water for excretion
2) excrete large volumes of dilute urine
H2O

FIGURE 12.12 Effects of decreased ADH level on kidney output. Alcohol and caffeine increase water excretion by slowing the release of antidiuretic hormone (ADH).

Dehydration

Dehydration, or too little water, is a major killer worldwide. Gastrointestinal infections are primarily responsible. These infections cause diarrhea and prolonged vomiting, leading to excessive water loss. Unless treated rapidly, a person who loses an amount of water equal to 20 percent of body weight is likely to become comatose and die. Burns also can cause deadly dehydration. Extensively damaged skin cannot protect the body and prevent excessive fluid loss.

Dehydration diminishes physical and mental performance (see **FIGURE 12.13**). Chronic mild dehydration—a fluid deficit of as little as 1 to 2 percent of body weight—can cause declines in alertness, physical performance, and the ability to concentrate, while increasing feelings of tiredness and headache.[11] Such low levels of dehydration also impair decision making and reaction times. This can be important for tasks that involve judgment and skill, such as driving a car. Chronic dehydration plays a role in the development of many conditions such as constipation, hypertension, coronary heart disease, glaucoma, and complications of diabetes.[12]

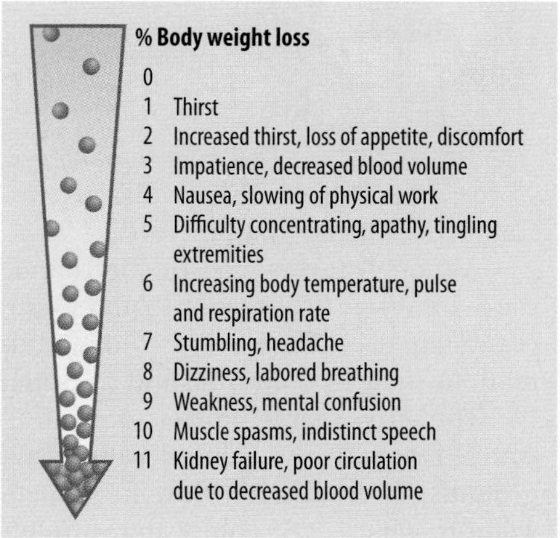
% Body weight loss
0
1 Thirst
2 Increased thirst, loss of appetite, discomfort
3 Impatience, decreased blood volume
4 Nausea, slowing of physical work
5 Difficulty concentrating, apathy, tingling extremities
6 Increasing body temperature, pulse and respiration rate
7 Stumbling, headache
8 Dizziness, labored breathing
9 Weakness, mental confusion
10 Muscle spasms, indistinct speech
11 Kidney failure, poor circulation due to decreased blood volume

FIGURE 12.13 Effects of progressive dehydration. Dehydration leads to symptoms such as nausea, headache, dizziness, and even death.

Early signs of dehydration include fatigue, dry mouth, headache, and dark urine with a strong odor. Change in urine color reflects the body's attempt to conserve water by increasing water reabsorption in the kidneys. You may have noticed that your urine becomes darker when you haven't had much to drink, whereas your urine is almost colorless when you've had plenty to drink.

Older adults and infants are particularly vulnerable to dehydration. The sense of thirst often diminishes with age, which can lead to decreased fluid intake. Older adults often take diuretic medications, which increases urine output. For a variety of reasons, older adults also might stop or reduce eating and drinking. The resulting physical and mental deterioration creates a vicious cycle, with food and fluid intake continuing to worsen.

Because infants can lose water rapidly through their skin, they need ample fluid relative to their size. Breast milk or infant formula generally provides all the fluid a baby needs. Severe diarrhea can cause swift and deadly dehydration, especially in older adults and infants. Normally, the intestines reabsorb nearly all the fluid secreted by digestive organs, but when intestinal disease causes diarrhea or prolonged vomiting, dehydration can occur. Worldwide, dehydration is a major killer of babies and young children, with infection the underlying culprit.

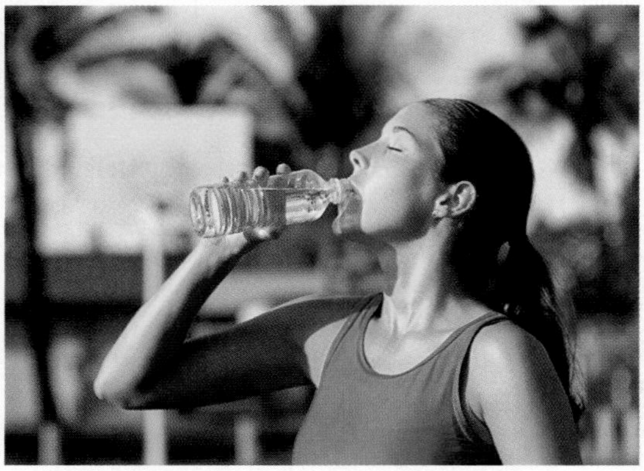

Water consumption, of course, is the primary treatment for dehydration. Oral rehydration solutions also can be used; typically these consist of simple ingredients including clean water, sugar, and table salt. Oral rehydration can be sufficient for mild dehydration, but intravenous fluids and hospitalization might be necessary for moderate to severe dehydration. Diarrhea and prolonged vomiting, which cause heavy fluid and electrolyte losses, can be fatal unless the person is rapidly rehydrated with electrolyte solutions.

Water Intoxication

Because drinking fluids temporarily alleviates thirst, we rarely drink to the point of overhydration and dilution of body fluids. Acute water toxicity has been reported to result from rapid consumption of large

Going Green

The Thirst for Water Resources

The nets remained on deck and the boats stayed in the harbor. In 2008, in one of the worst man-made fishery disasters in the nation, low levels of salmon stocks caused the closure of salmon fisheries in California for the first time ever.

Although several causes contributed to the decline, one of the most significant—and reversible—is the operation of the State Water Project (SWP) and Central Valley Project. These projects manage water for drinking, agriculture, urban, and ecosystem uses. The SWP provides a portion of the drinking water to 25 million Californians. Water has long been a contentious issue in California and the semiarid West. Population growth and climate change promise to worsen the problem.

The most visible impacts of California's water projects are the dams that have been constructed to store and divert water. Dams in the Central Valley have entirely cut off access to more than 80 percent of historic salmon spawning grounds. Alterations in flow have increased water temperatures and reduced the survival and reproductive success of salmon, which need cold water throughout their life cycle.

In 2015, California adopted emergency regulation to ensure a minimum flow of water into river tributaries to protect self-sustaining populations of threatened fish. Such regulation is necessary to promote and restore healthy salmon runs during the long-term drought the state is currently experiencing. Fish-friendly strategies include water conservation, better efficiency, improved groundwater management, water recycling, and urban stormwater management.

FYI For Your Information

Tap, Filtered, or Bottled: Which Water Is Best?

Everywhere you look, it seems like more and more people are carrying and sipping on bottles of water. Theme parks even sell shoulder holsters for you to carry your bottle around with you. What's with the water craze? And what's wrong with the good old water fountain?

During the mid-to-late 1980s, the growth in use of bottled water began. Initially, bottled mineral waters, such as Perrier, were associated with wealth and glamour. But like many trends adopted by the wealthy (white bread, for instance), bottled water soon became desirable to a wider range of people. It is estimated that Americans drink approximately 11 billion gallons of bottled water each year.[a] In 2014, the U.S. per capita consumption of bottled water was 34.2 gallons.[b] U.S. residents now drink more bottled water annually than any other beverage except carbonated soft drinks. Soft drink consumption, at 12.6 billion gallons in 2014, is just a little more than bottled water consumption.[c] Soft drink consumption has been declining steadily over the last seven years and is predicted to be less than bottled water by 2017 if the decline continues.[d] Major soft drink companies, such as Coca-Cola and PepsiCo, sell their own brands of bottled water.

Several factors are fueling the growth of the bottled-water industry. Baby boomers are seeking natural, low-calorie beverages, and fitness consciousness has reemphasized the importance of hydration. Media reports of contamination of tap water in major metropolitan areas sparked concerns about the safety and quality of tap water, with the lead contamination crisis in Flint, Michigan, being one of the most recent examples. Most Americans choose bottled water for what they think is *not* in it rather than for what it contains.

Some bottled water companies now add dietary supplements such as vitamins to their water. Other companies make powdered dietary supplements that are designed to be added to your water. In addition to vitamins and minerals, these products may contain other ingredients such as herbs. Being aware of the ingredients and the effect they can have on your body can help you make informed decisions about what to drink.

When choosing among vitamin waters, powdered supplements, or plain water, consider the following[e]:

- *Sugar and calories:* Look at the Nutrition Facts or ingredient label to know if the product has added sugar. Sugar adds calories to water, which can lead to unwanted weight gain. Remember, plain water has zero calories.
- *Vitamins at 100% DV:* The best way to get your daily value of vitamins and minerals is by eating a variety of foods in the appropriate amounts. Vitamins and minerals from food are much better absorbed.
- *Herbals and botanicals:* Many bottled waters advertise that they contain plant extracts like echinacea or ginseng; however, most of these extracts are in relatively small amounts in the water and have little to no effect on your body.

From a nutritional perspective, it's important to drink plenty of fluids. Water is one of the best ways to replace lost fluids, and, at the simplest level, the source of the water doesn't really matter. Standards for municipal water systems are enforced by the Environmental Protection Agency (EPA), which requires regular testing and monitoring. In most places, tap water can be considered a safe, clean source of water. Many municipal water systems add fluoride to tap water, an important weapon in the prevention of tooth decay. However, home-installed filtration systems for removing chlorine might also remove added fluoride, and most bottled waters do not contain fluoride. Some people don't like the taste of their local water supply and don't want to bother with maintaining a filtration system. In this case, or if you want your water "to go," bottled water can be the choice. The bottled-water industry offers:

- High-volume, returnable containers from suppliers who stock the water coolers for offices or supermarkets
- The familiar brands (e.g., Evian, Dasani, Aquafina) that are sold as alternatives to soft drinks
- Bottled water in vending machines

The bottled-water industry is regulated by the Food and Drug Administration (FDA), which, in 1995, published Standards of Identity for bottled water, set maximum allowable standards for contaminants, and established Current Good Manufacturing Practices (CGMPs) for bottling plants. Keep in mind that the FDA regulates bottled waters that are sold interstate, and not those sold only in a particular area or state. Individual states can have their own quality standards for locally distributed waters.

Look beyond terms such as *artesian*, *mineral*, *spring*, or *purified* (see **TABLE A**). The labels on most bottled water list the source of the water. Some consumers are surprised to find that their favorite brand of water is really from a municipal source, not an underground spring! Nutrition Facts labels

TABLE A
Definitions of Bottled Water Terms

- Mineral water must contain at least 250 parts per million (ppm) of dissolved minerals and come from a geologically and physically protected underground water source.
- Purified water is tap or ground water that has been treated by distillation, deionization, or reverse osmosis. This may be labeled "distilled water" if produced by steam distillation and condensation.
- Spring water comes from an underground formation from which water flows naturally to the surface; it is collected either at the spring or from a borehole to the underground formation.
- Artesian water comes from tapping a confined underground aquifer that is below the natural water table. Generally, the artesian well is located in a depression where the water table of the surrounding hills is higher. The "head" of pressure from the water table forces the water up through the tap line.
- Ground water comes from a subsurface saturated zone and is not under the direct influence of surface water.
- Well water comes from a drilled hole that taps the water of an aquifer and is pumped to the surface.

Data from International Bottled Water Association. Labeling. http://www.bottledwater.org/content/labeling-0. Accessed January 29, 2016.

[a] International Bottled Water Association. Bottled water market. http://www.bottledwater.org/economics/bottled-water-market. Accessed January 29, 2016.

[b] International Bottled Water Association. Bottled water sales and consumption projected to increase in 2014. http://www.bottledwater.org/bottled-water-sales-and-consumption-projected-increase-2014-expected-be-number-one-packaged-drink. Accessed April 28, 2016.

[c] Esterl M. Soft drinks hit 10th year of decline. *The Wall Street Journal.* March 26, 2015. http://www.wsj.com/articles/pepsi-cola-replaces-diet-coke-as-no-2-soda-1427388559. Accessed January 29, 2016.

[d] Sanger-Katz M. The decline of 'big soda.' *The New York Times.* October 2, 2015. http://www.nytimes.com/2015/10/04/upshot/soda-industry-struggles-as-consumer-tastes-change.html. Accessed January 29, 2016.

[e] Oates VJ. Vitamin water and powdered multivitamin supplements in water. January 5, 2011. http://www.extension.org/pages/32335/vitamin-water-and-powdered-multivitamin-supplements-in-water#.VdKzLINViko. Accessed January 29, 2016.

(continues)

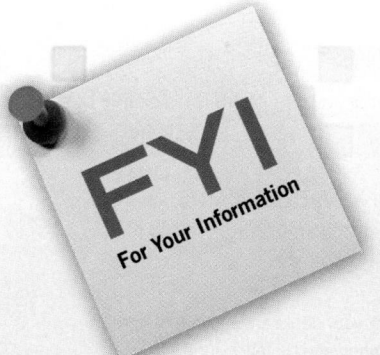

are required if the manufacturer makes a claim (e.g., sodium free) or adds minerals. These labels often do not show the natural mineral content of the water, which is really the only other nutritional aspect that could be expected.

The Academy of Nutrition and Dietetics suggests the following five factors be considered when choosing between bottled and tap water: the environment, safety, cost, taste, and fluoride.[f] The bottom line, according to the Academy, is that both tap and bottled water are safe, and that bottled water offers no nutritional advantage unless it is fortified. Bottled water might encourage fluid consumption by making water more accessible; however, this can come at an environmental cost by contributing to additional waste.[g] Drinking sufficient water is the primary objective, especially when it replaces high-calorie, low-nutrient beverages. The amount of water needed daily depends on gender, size, and physical activity level.[h]

Ultimately, the choice is up to the consumer—there is no clearly best choice of water.

[f] Academy of Nutrition and Dietetics. Bottled water: is bottled water a better choice than tap water? May 2008. http://www.eatright.org/cps/rde/xchg/ada/hsxsl/nutrition_17382_ENU_HTML.htm. Accessed May 24, 2012.

[g] Ibid.

[h] Academy of Nutrition and Dietetics. Rethink your drinks and hydrate right this summer with tips from the Academy of Nutrition and Dietetics. June 24, 2014. http://www.eatrightpro.org/resource/media/press-releases/new-in-food-nutrition-and-health/rethink-your-drinks-and-hydrate-right-this-summer-with-tips-from-the-academy. Accessed January 29, 2016.

quantities of fluids that greatly exceeded the kidneys' maximal excretion rate of approximately 0.7 to 1.0 liters per hour.[13] Overhydration first causes headaches and then seizures and can be fatal.

Replacement of fluid losses following intensive or prolonged exercise with plain water (and no electrolytes) can result in overhydration and hyponatremia (low blood sodium) in athletes, which can cause changes in mental status, difficulty breathing, seizures, coma, and death.[14,15] A fraternity hazing ritual, for example, caused fatal water intoxication in a California State University student who was forced to drink large quantities of water while exercising vigorously.[16]

Overhydration also can occur in people with untreated glandular disorders that cause excessive water retention or with mental disorders that cause a compulsion to drink huge quantities of water. Fortunately, their kidneys usually can keep up with the increased fluid intake; normal kidneys can excrete 15 to 20 liters of urine per day. But the kidneys' ability to excrete excess fluid can be overwhelmed. Several years ago, some dieters overenthusiastically followed a fad weight-reduction diet calling for massive water intake and suffered seizures from overhydration.

Quick Bite

Is Airline Drinking Water Safe?

Concerned that drinking water on airplanes can become unsanitary, the Environmental Protection Agency launched the Aircraft Drinking Water Rule (ADWR) to ensure the availability of safe and reliable drinking water during flight travel. The rule provides protection for the public against disease-causing organisms that sometimes are found in airline drinking water. The ADWR requires airlines to sample for bacteria, follow best management practices, take corrective action, notify the public, train operators, and follow guidelines for reporting and recordkeeping to improve public health protection.[17]

Key Concepts Diuretic medications increase urinary fluid losses. Alcohol and caffeine have mild diuretic effects. Dehydration occurs when fluid loss exceeds fluid intake; it is a potential consequence of gastrointestinal disease, burns, and heavy sweating. Treatment involves replacing fluids, along with electrolytes if the condition is severe. Water intoxication is rare; normal kidneys can excrete many liters of fluid each day.

Major Minerals

Unlike the nutrient molecules you have studied so far, minerals are inorganic elemental atoms or ions. Unlike carbohydrate, protein, and fat, minerals are not changed during digestion or when the body uses them. Unlike many vitamins, minerals are not destroyed by heat, light, or alkalinity. Calcium remains calcium, be it in seashells, milk, or bones. Iron remains iron, whether it is part of a cast-iron skillet or carried in the bloodstream as part of hemoglobin. This is true for all minerals.

Minerals play many essential roles in the body. Some minerals are needed in larger quantities (macrominerals) and some in smaller or trace amounts (microminerals), but all essential minerals are important to health. Some minerals, such as magnesium, participate in the catalytic activity of enzymes.

Others serve a structural function; for example, calcium and phosphorus are among the minerals that make our bones hard. Minerals are categorized as major or trace minerals based on the amount needed in the diet and the amount of the mineral in the body. The body requires more than 100 milligrams per day of each **major mineral**, whereas the dietary need for each trace mineral is less than 100 milligrams daily. **FIGURE 12.14** shows the relative amounts of the major and trace minerals in the body. This classification of minerals is unrelated to the mineral's biological importance. For example, iron is a trace mineral, but it plays a critical role in many major metabolic reactions.

▶ **major mineral** A mineral required in the diet and present in the body in large amounts compared with trace minerals.

Minerals in Fluid Balance

The macrominerals sodium, calcium, potassium, chlorine, phosphate, and magnesium are electrolytes—minerals that carry an electrical charge. Electrolytes are important not only in maintaining fluid balance, but also in maintaining blood pH, nerve transmission, and muscle function. Electrolytes are lost through urination, sweating, vomiting, and diarrhea. Small losses are easily replaced through a balanced diet. Excessive losses, however, may require the use of oral rehydration therapy or sports recovery drinks designed to restore electrolyte balance. Fluid may leak from cells and capillaries and become trapped in tissues. This swelling, called edema, can be caused by diseases such as heart failure, kidney disease, or cirrhosis. Pregnancy and some medications can also cause edema.

Minerals in Foods

Foods from both plants and animals are sources of minerals. Generally speaking, animal tissue contains minerals in the proportion that the animal needs, so animal-derived foods are more reliable mineral sources.

Plant foods can be excellent sources of several minerals, but the mineral content of plants can vary dramatically depending on the minerals in the soil where the plants are found. Even the maturity of a vegetable, fruit, or grain can influence its mineral content. Because actual mineral content varies so much, the values published in food composition tables can be misleading. Like plant foods, drinking water has variable mineral content. Nevertheless, it sometimes can be a significant source of minerals such as sodium, magnesium, and fluoride.

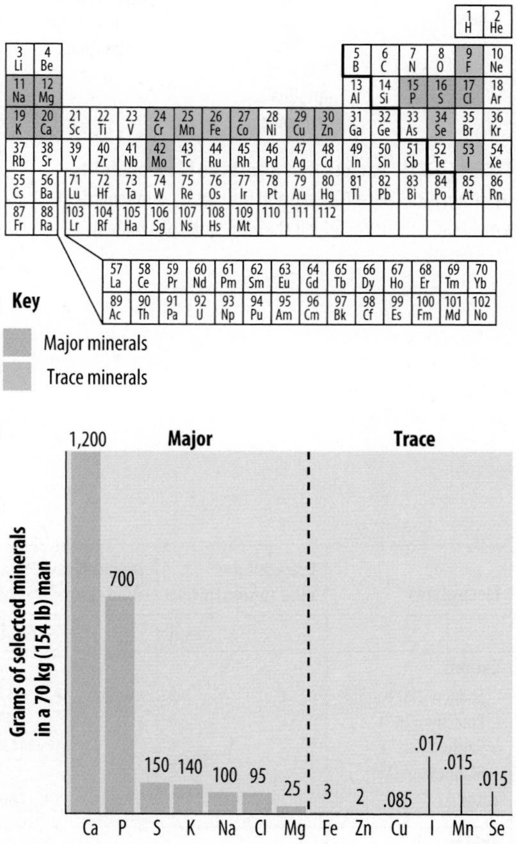

FIGURE 12.14 Minerals in the human body. Dietary minerals also are elements in the periodic table. Based on the amount of a mineral needed in the diet and the amount in the body, nutritionists categorize a mineral as major or trace.

Data from Gropper SS. Smith JL, Groff JL. Advanced Nutrition and Human Metabolism. 5th ed. Belmont, CA: Wadsworth/ Cengage Learning; 2009; and Stipanuk MH. Biochemical and Physiological Aspects of Human Nutrition. 2nd ed Philadelphia: WB Saunders; 2006. Data from Gropper SS. Smith JL, Groff JL. Advanced Nutrition and Human Metabolism. 5th ed. Belmont, CA: Wadsworth/Cengage Learning; 2009; and Stipanuk MH. Biochemical and Physiological Aspects of Human Nutrition. 2nd ed Philadelphia: WB Saunders; 2006.

Bioavailability

Your GI tract absorbs a much smaller proportion of minerals than vitamins—and probably for good reason. Once absorbed, excess minerals often are difficult for the body to flush out. In many cases, the body adjusts mineral absorption in relation to needs. For example, a calcium-deficient person absorbs calcium more readily than does a person with normal calcium status.

Megadosing with single-mineral supplements can hamper the absorption of other minerals. Minerals such as calcium, iron, zinc, and magnesium, for example, all have similar chemical properties and compete for absorption.

Fiber and other components of food also affect mineral bioavailability (see **FIGURE 12.15**). High-fiber diets reduce absorption of iron, calcium, zinc, and magnesium. **Phytate** (a component of whole grains) binds minerals and carries them out of the intestines unabsorbed. **Oxalate** (found in spinach and rhubarb) binds calcium, markedly reducing calcium absorption.

▶ **phytate (phytic acid)** A phosphorus-containing compound in the outer husks of cereal grains that binds with minerals and inhibits their absorption.

▶ **oxalate (oxalic acid)** An organic acid in some leafy green vegetables, such as spinach, that binds to calcium to form calcium oxalate, an insoluble compound the body cannot absorb.

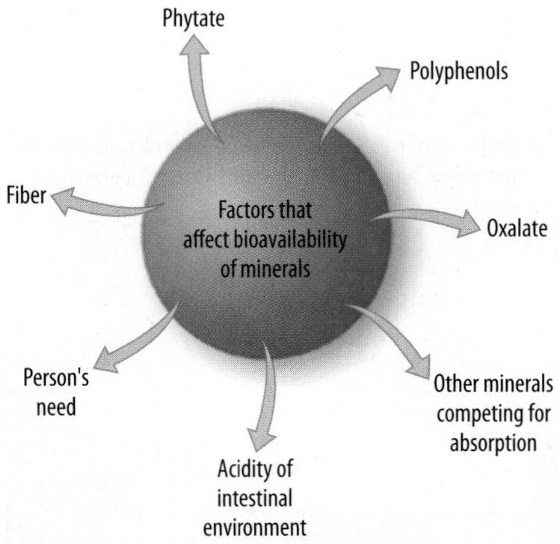

FIGURE 12.15 Factors that affect the bioavailability of minerals. A person's need and the dietary components of a meal can enhance or inhibit the absorption of a mineral.

Key Concepts Minerals are essential inorganic elements. Those that we need and store in larger amounts are called major minerals, and those that we need in very small quantities are called trace minerals. A wide variety of foods contain minerals. Physiological needs, competition with other minerals, and the fiber content of food all affect mineral bioavailability.

Sodium

Many people do not realize that sodium (Na) is an essential nutrient. We know sodium best as a component of sodium chloride (table salt is about 40 percent sodium), and we have heard for years that we shouldn't eat too much salt. The *Dietary Guidelines* recommend that we reduce daily sodium intake to less than 2,300 milligrams (mg).[18] It may be healthful to further reduce intake to 1,500 mg among persons who are 51 and older and those of any age who are African American or have hypertension, diabetes, or chronic kidney disease.[19] Nevertheless, some sodium in the diet is essential for normal body function.

Functions of Sodium

Sodium is the major cation in extracellular fluid and a critical electrolyte in the regulation of body fluids. It acts in concert with potassium, the major cation in intracellular fluid, and chloride, the major anion in extracellular fluid, to maintain proper body water distribution and blood pressure (see **FIGURE 12.16**). Nerve transmission and muscle function require sodium. Sodium also helps control the body's acidity and aids the absorption of some nutrients, such as glucose.

Electrolytes	Extracellular* fluid concentration	Intracellular** fluid concentration
	meq/L	meq/L
Cations		
Sodium (Na^+)	140	13
Potassium (K^+)	5	140
Calcium (Ca^{2+})	5	Minimal
Magnesium (Mg^{2+})	2	7
Total	**151**	**160**
Anions		
Chloride (Cl^-)	104	3
Bicarbonate (HCO_3^-)	24	10
Sulfate (SO_4^{2-})	1	---
Phosphate (HPO_4^{2-})	2	107
Proteins	15	40
Organic anions	5	---
Total	**151**	**160**

* Values are for plasma. Interstitial fluid concentration vary slightly (about 4 percent).
** Values are for cell water in muscle.

FIGURE 12.16 Cations and anions in intracellular and extracellular fluid. Potassium, magnesium, phosphate, and proteins are the main solutes inside a cell. Sodium, chloride, and bicarbonate are the main solutes outside the cell.

Modified from Shils ME, Shike M, Ross AC, et al., eds. *Modern Nutrition in Health and Disease*. 10th ed. Philadelphia: Lippincott Williams & Wilkins; 2005:149–193.

Dietary Recommendations for Sodium

We rarely eat too little sodium; in fact, most of us eat substantially more than we need. Actual sodium *requirements* by the body are relatively small—only a few hundred milligrams daily. To make sure that the diet contains adequate amounts of all nutrients, however, the Food and Nutrition Board set the AI for sodium for adults at 1,500 milligrams per day.[20] This suggested AI level is similar to the American Heart Association's recommendation to limit sodium to less than 1,500 milligrams per day.[21] Further, the Tolerable Upper Intake Level (UL) for sodium is 2,300 milligrams per day (the approximate amount in about 1 teaspoon of table salt) and the level at which all Americans regardless of risk factors should try to stay below. The Daily Value on food labels is similar—2,400 milligrams per day.

Sources of Sodium

The typical American diet contains 3,000 to 5,000 milligrams of sodium daily. Surprisingly, processed foods—not table salt—contribute the most sodium to the diets of Americans (see **TABLE 12.1**). THINK About It 3

FIGURE 12.17 shows a breakdown of the sources of sodium in our diets. Most of the sodium in the American diet comes from processed foods.[22] In addition to being higher in sodium, these foods are often lacking in many other nutrients such as fiber and antioxidants. Soy sauce and other sauces; pickled foods; salty or smoked meats, cheese, and fish; salted snack foods; bouillon cubes; and canned and instant soups are all high-sodium foods. Seasonings based on salt (such as lemon salt and seasoning salt) and those containing the flavor enhancer monosodium glutamate (MSG) also are high in sodium.

Your intestinal tract absorbs nearly all dietary sodium, which then travels throughout the body in the bloodstream. Your kidneys, those remarkable organs, retain the exact amount of sodium the body needs and excrete the excess sodium in the urine along with water.

Taking in too much sodium and not enough water can worsen dehydration. The old practice of giving athletes salt tablets before or after exercise is unnecessary and possibly harmful. On the other hand, radical sodium restriction is not a good idea either. Even though most Americans consume too much sodium, severe sodium restriction can lead to an unpalatable diet or limit the availability of other essential nutrients.

TABLE 12.1
Sodium Content of Various Foods

Food	Serving Size	Sodium (mg)
Cucumber, with peel, raw	1 large (301 g)	6
Pickles, cucumber, dill	1 large (135 g)	1,092
Pork, loin, roasted	3 oz (85 g)	42
Ham, cured	3 oz (85 g)	1,128
Whole-wheat bread	1 slice (28 g)	146
Biscuit from recipe	4″ biscuit (101 g)	586
Tomatoes, fresh	1 (123 g)	6
Spaghetti sauce, ready-to-serve	1/2 cup (132 g)	577
Milk, 2% milkfat	1 cup (244 g)	145
American cheese	1 oz (28.35 g)	468
Baked potato	1 (156 g)	8
Potato chips	1 oz (28.35 g)	148

Note: As food becomes more processed, the sodium content increases.

Data from U.S. Department of Agriculture, Agricultural Research Service. USDA National Nutrient Database for Standard Reference, Release 28. 2015. http://www.ars.usda.gov/Services/docs.htm?docid=8964. Accessed January 30, 2016.

Hyponatremia

Blood sodium concentration sometimes can drop too low, usually as a result of severe diarrhea, vomiting, or intense prolonged sweating with replacement of water but not sodium. Consuming only water without food or other mineral sources also can depress blood sodium levels. The primary symptoms of low blood sodium, **hyponatremia**, resemble dehydration symptoms, and the treatment is similar—replacement of fluid and minerals through liquids and foods or through intravenous solutions if necessary. If severe

▶ **hyponatremia** Abnormally low sodium concentrations in the blood resulting from excessive excretion of sodium (by the kidneys), prolonged vomiting, or diarrhea.

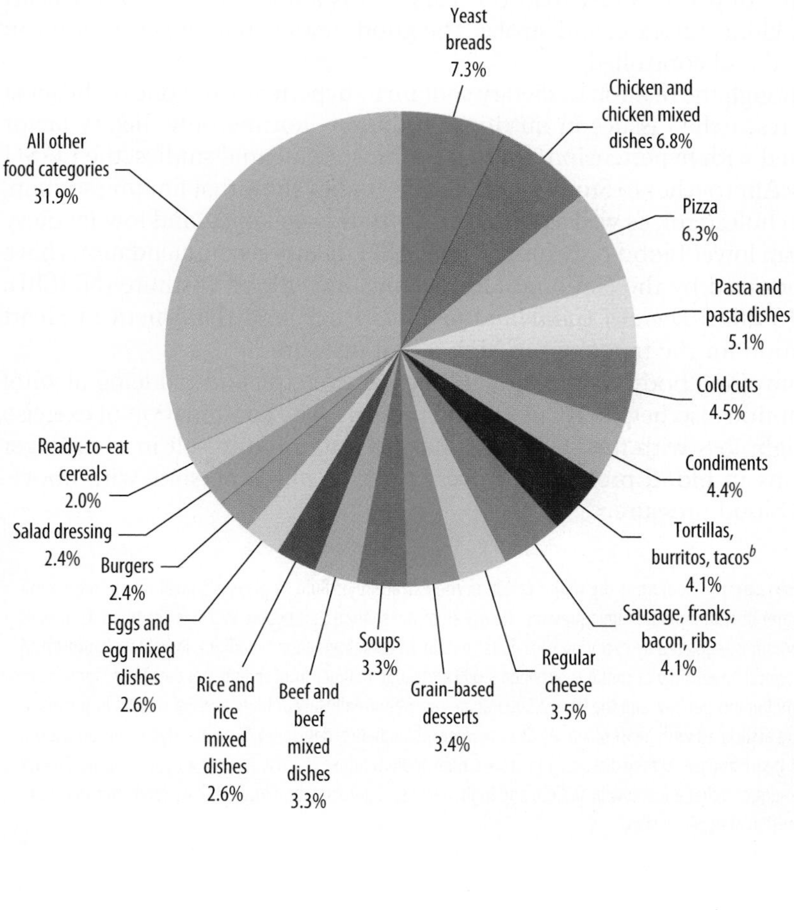

FIGURE 12.17 Sources of sodium in the diets of the U.S. population ages 2 years and older, NHANES, 2005–2006.[a]

[a] Data are drawn from analyses of usual dietary intake conducted by the National Cancer Institute. Foods and beverages consumed were divided into 97 categories and ranked according to sodium contribution to the diet. "All other food categories" represents food categories that each contributes less than 2% of the total intake of sodium from foods.

[b] Also includes nachos, quesadillas, and other Mexican mixed dishes.

Courtesy of USDA. Data from National Cancer Institute. Sources of Sodium in the Diets of the U.S. Population Ages 2 Years and Older, NHANES 2005–2006. Risk Factor Monitoring and Methods, Cancer Control and Population Sciences.

hyponatremia is not treated, extracellular fluid moves into cells, causing them to swell. As brain cells swell and malfunction, the afflicted person can experience headache, confusion, seizures, or coma. Many illnesses, including cancer, kidney disease, and heart disease, can cause low blood sodium concentration. In these situations, treatment usually targets the underlying condition that caused the electrolyte imbalance.

Hypernatremia

Rapid intake of large amounts of sodium (e.g., drinking seawater) can cause the retention of sodium and water. This causes **hypernatremia**, abnormally high concentration of sodium in the blood, and **hypervolemia**, an abnormal increase in blood volume. This leads to edema (swelling) and a rise in blood pressure. A healthy person with normal kidneys and ample water intake rapidly excretes excess sodium, so hypernatremia usually is seen only in patients with congestive heart failure or kidney disease. Eating too much sodium over a long period of time can contribute to high blood pressure (hypertension) in some people. For those with high blood pressure, lowering sodium intake is a useful dietary change that might lower blood pressure.[23] Excess dietary sodium can also contribute to osteoporosis by increasing calcium loss in the urine.

Hypertension

Hypertension, or persistent high blood pressure, often is called a "silent killer" because it usually has no specific symptoms or early warning signs. Hypertension affects approximately one in three American adults and more than two-thirds of people older than 65 years.[24] It is a major risk factor for heart disease, kidney disease, and stroke. The good news is that hypertension can be treated and controlled.

Although the relation of dietary sodium to hypertension is one of the most heavily researched issues in nutrition, sodium is not the only dietary factor associated with hypertension. Among the most influential studies, the DASH (Dietary Approaches to Stop Hypertension) studies show that limiting sodium, fat, and cholesterol, as well as eating more fruits, vegetables, and low-fat dairy foods, can lower blood pressure.[25] The DASH dietary recommendations have been endorsed by the National Heart, Lung, and Blood Institute (NHLBI), the *2015-2020 Dietary Guidelines for Americans*, and the American Heart Association for the treatment of high blood pressure.[26]

Controlling body weight, getting regular exercise, and reducing alcohol consumption also help to reduce blood pressure. The combination of exercise and weight loss with the DASH diet has been found to result in even larger reductions in blood pressure for overweight or obese persons with above-normal blood pressure.[27]

Key Concepts Sodium is the major cation in the extracellular fluid; it plays a critical role in regulating proper water distribution and blood pressure. Nearly all of the sodium that people ingest is absorbed. Control of serum sodium is regulated by excretion. Our diets contain an overabundance of sodium, largely from processed foods. A typical American diet contains between 3,000 and 5,000 milligrams of sodium per day. The AI for sodium is 1,500 milligrams per day, and the UL is 2,300 milligrams. Abnormally low or high levels of sodium in the blood usually are associated with heart or kidney disease rather than dietary deficiency or excess. Hypertension is a risk factor for heart disease, kidney disease, and stroke. High sodium intake is a risk factor for hypertension. Dietary evidence suggests that a diet low in sodium and high in fruits, vegetables, and low-fat dairy foods contributes to the prevention of hypertension.

2015-2020 Dietary Guidelines for Americans

Key Recommendations

Key Elements of Healthy Eating Patterns

Healthy eating patterns limit sodium to less than 2,300 mg per day for adults and children ages 14 years and older and to the age- and sex-appropriate Tolerable Upper Intake Levels (UL) of sodium for children younger than 14 years... The recommendation for adults and children ages 14 years and older to limit sodium intake to less than 2,300 mg per day is based on evidence showing a linear dose-response relationship between increased sodium intake and increased blood pressure in adults.

Adults with prehypertension and hypertension would particularly benefit from blood pressure lowering. For these individuals, further reduction to 1,500 mg per day can result in even greater blood pressure reduction.

Reproduced from U.S. Department of Health and Human Services and U.S. Department of Agriculture. 2015–2020 Dietary Guidelines for Americans. 8th Edition. December 2015. Available at http://health.gov/dietaryguidelines/2015/guidelines/.

▶ **hypernatremia** Abnormally high sodium concentrations in the blood resulting from increased kidney retention of sodium or rapid ingestion of large amounts of salt.

▶ **hypervolemia** An abnormal increase in the circulating blood volume.

Quick Bite

Sacred Salt

The physiological need for salt played an important role in shaping human history. Population groups tended to congregate where salt could be found, and civilizations in Africa, India, the Middle East, and China developed around rich salt deposits. At times, salt was traded at a value twice that of gold.

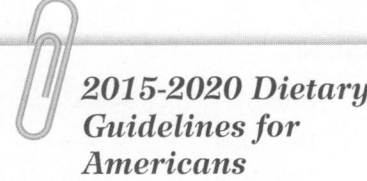

Nutrition Science *in Action*

Calcium and Vitamin D and Abdominal Fat in Overweight and Obese Adults

Background

Calcium and vitamin D may play a role in the regulation of abdominal fat mass and body weight (see **FIGURE A**). Overweight, obesity, and abdominal fat (central adiposity) have been linked to several metabolic disorders and diseases. In mice, it has been suggested that increasing dietary calcium lowers adipose intracellular calcium, reducing fatty acid synthesis and increasing the breakdown (lipolysis) of adipose tissue. Other investigators suggest that increased calcium intake is associated with increased oxidation of fat and thermogenesis. Calcium also might increase fecal fat excretion and suppress hunger to prevent weight gain. Vitamin D intake affects weight status and total fat mass. Low circulating levels of vitamin D have been independently associated with increased body mass index (BMI) and fat mass. In addition, one study found that overweight and obese premenopausal women lost more body fat on a hypocaloric diet when their baseline vitamin D concentrations were higher. Interestingly, the results of prospective studies that have examined both calcium and vitamin D intake on body weight and/or abdominal fat mass have been inconclusive.

Hypothesis

In overweight and obese adults, calcium and vitamin D supplementation will lead to a greater loss of body weight and visceral adipose tissue in 16 weeks when compared to placebo supplementation.

Experimental Plan

Healthy overweight and obese men and women, ages 18–65 years, with a BMI of 25 to 35 were recruited for the study. Two parallel, double-blind, placebo-controlled trials were conducted using either regular or reduced energy (lite) orange juice (OJ). Participants were randomly assigned to treatment versus control. For each 16-week trial, the treatment group consumed three 240-milliliter glasses of OJ (regular vs. lite) fortified with 350 milligrams of calcium and 100 IU of vitamin D per serving. The control group consumed three 240-milliliter glasses of unfortified OJ (regular vs. lite).

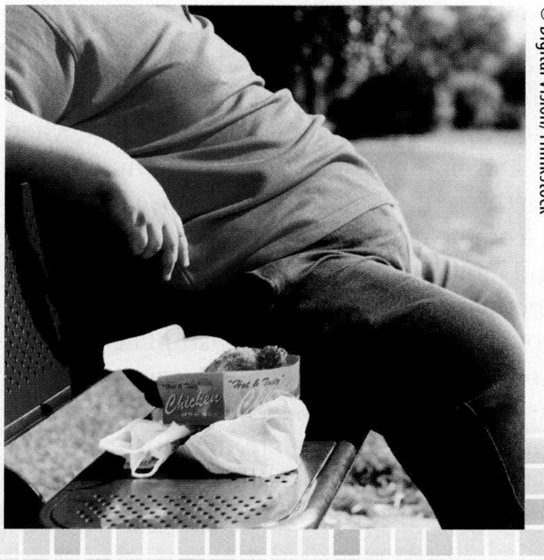

FIGURE A **Calcium and vitamin D may affect abdominal fat.**

Computed tomography was used to assess visceral and subcutaneous adipose tissue. In both trials, caloric reduction and physical activity were standardized to avoid masking any intervention effect of calcium and vitamin D supplementation on weight loss and changes in body fat. At the initial screening visit, participants met with a dietitian to establish a daily caloric goal. Study participants were instructed to limit dairy and dietary calcium intake to two or fewer servings per day and learned how to estimate calories consumed using a three-day food record. Subjects were given a pedometer to measure the number of steps taken daily. Monthly clinic visits involved a group lesson focused on healthy eating and exercise.

Results

In the regular OJ trial, the reduction of visceral adipose tissue was significantly greater in the calcium and vitamin D group than in the control group. In the lite OJ trial, the reduction of visceral adipose tissue also was significantly greater in the calcium and vitamin D group than in the control group, after controlling for baseline visceral adipose tissue (see **FIGURE B**). Weight loss did not differ significantly between groups.

Conclusion and Discussion

The results of this study suggest that in overweight and obese adults, a moderate reduction in energy intake and supplementation with calcium and vitamin D in juice beverages can lead to a reduction in visceral adipose tissue. These findings present a dietary modification that can help reduce visceral adipose tissue, a cause of metabolic disorder and disease. Future research is needed to clearly determine the roles that calcium and vitamin D play in fat metabolism.

Data from Rosenblum JL, Castro VM, Moore CE, Kaplan LM. Calcium and vitamin D supplementation is associated with decreased abdominal visceral adipose tissue in overweight and obese adults. *Am J Clin Nutr.* 2012;95:101-108.

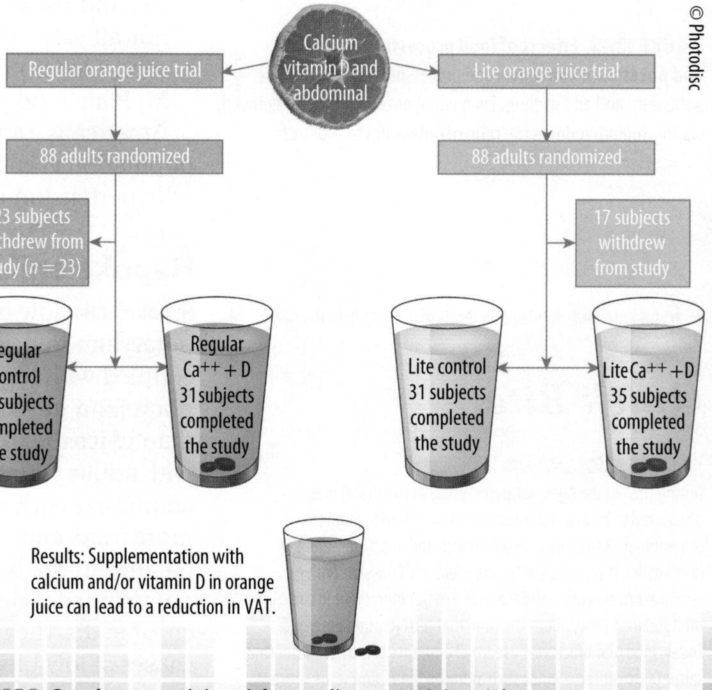

FIGURE B **Regular orange juice trial versus lite orange juice trial.**

Data from Rosenblum JL, Castro VM, Moore CE, Kaplan LM. Calcium and vitamin D supplementation is associated with decreased abdominal visceral adipose tissue in overweight and obese adults. Am J Clin Nutr. 2012;95:101–108.

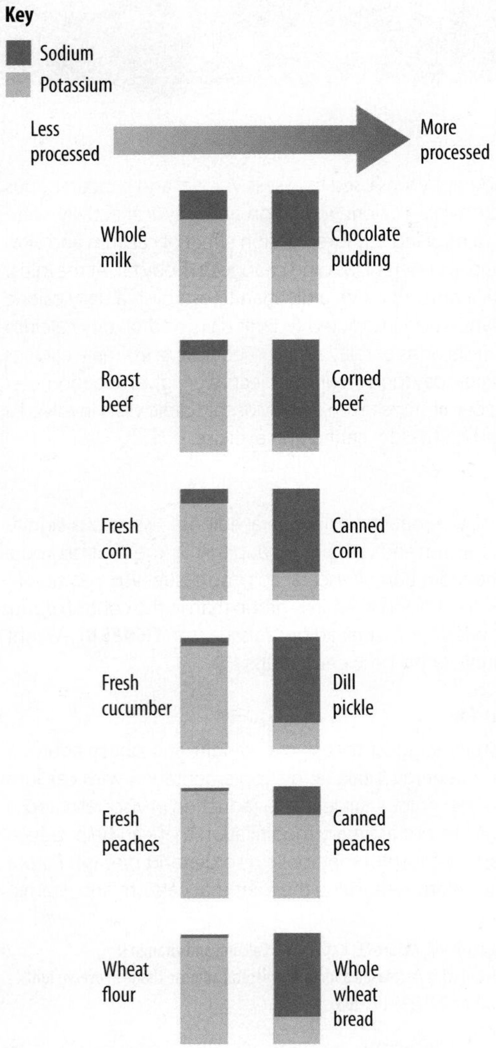

FIGURE 12.18 Effects of food processing on sodium and potassium content. Food processing tends to remove potassium and add sodium. Even when potassium is not removed, adding sodium reduces the ratio of potassium to sodium.

Potassium

Just as sodium is the major extracellular cation, potassium (K) is the key cation in cells. Potassium also can affect hypertension, but in a different way. If people with hypertension eat a diet rich in potassium-containing foods (such as fruits and vegetables), their blood pressure often improves.[28]

Functions of Potassium

Intracellular fluid contains about 95 percent of the body's potassium, with the highest amount in skeletal muscle cells. The flow of sodium and potassium into and out of cells is an important component of muscle contractions and the transmission of nerve impulses. The central nervous system (CNS) zealously protects its potassium—CNS potassium levels remain constant even in the face of falling levels in the muscle and blood. Potassium also helps regulate blood pressure.

Dietary Recommendations for Potassium

Although food manufacturers often add sodium to processed foods, they do not routinely add potassium. If a person's diet includes a lot of processed foods, it can fail to meet the potassium recommendations. Based on studies showing that potassium blunts the blood-pressure-raising effects of salt, the DRI Committee suggested a target intake level (AI) of 4,700 milligrams per day for adults.[29] This is higher than the current Daily Value of 3,500 milligrams and substantially more than most Americans eat (2,000 to 3,000 milligrams per day). **FIGURE 12.18** shows the effects that food processing has on the sodium and potassium levels in foods.

Sources of Potassium

Fresh vegetables and fruits, especially potatoes, spinach, melons, and bananas, are major dietary sources of potassium. Fresh meat, milk, coffee, and tea also contain significant potassium (see **FIGURE 12.19**). Many but not all salt substitutes contain potassium chloride—check the label to be sure. Generous intakes of fruits and vegetables, as recommended by the MyPlate food guidance system, will help increase potassium intake. African Americans can especially benefit from increased potassium intake—this population group typically has low intake of potassium and a high prevalence of hypertension and salt sensitivity.[30]

Hypokalemia

▶ **hypokalemia** Inadequate levels of potassium in the blood.

Hypokalemia, low blood potassium, results from potassium depletion. Moderate potassium deficiency is a likely factor in hypertension risk, especially when coupled with high sodium intakes. U.S. adults who eat more sodium and less potassium have a 50 percent higher risk of dying from any cause and more than twice the likelihood of dying from heart attacks over 15 years compared with adults who eat less sodium and more potassium.[31] These findings further emphasize current dietary recommendations to reduce sodium intake and eat more fruits and vegetables. Low potassium intake can also disrupt acid—base balance in the body and contribute to bone loss and kidney stones.[32] Severe potassium deficiency usually results from excessive losses. Prolonged vomiting, chronic diarrhea, laxative abuse, and use of diuretics are the most common causes of low blood potassium. Insufficient dietary potassium intake magnifies

Quick Bite

Versatile Potassium

During the Middle Ages, saltpeter (potassium nitrate) was discovered to be a useful substance. It was used to extract other minerals from rock, as a fertilizer, and as an ingredient in gunpowder. It wasn't used to cure meat until the sixteenth or seventeenth century. Saltpeter was a major ingredient in the curing mixture until 1940, about the time that refrigeration emerged. Today, food manufacturers use small amounts of nitrites rather than saltpeter to preserve foods such as bacon, ham, and some sausages.

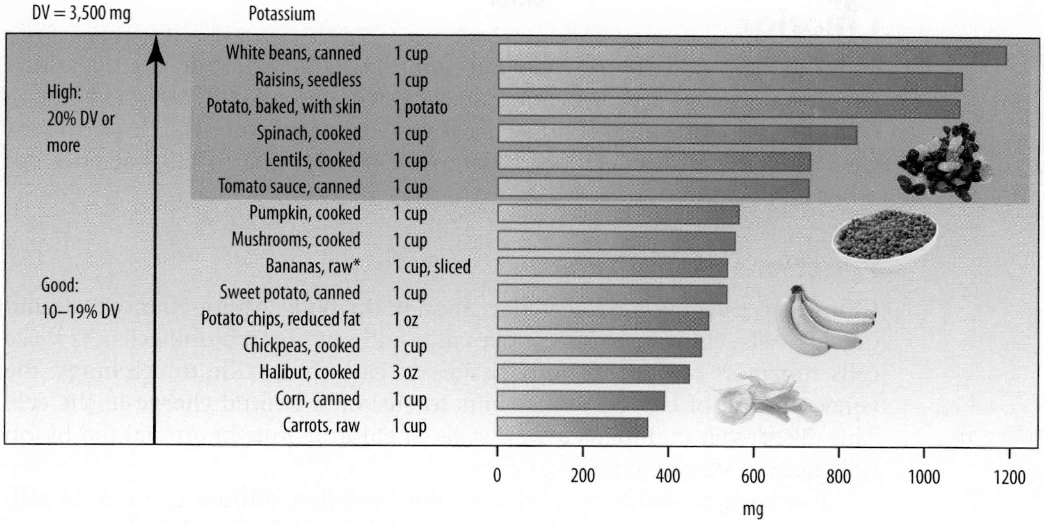

FIGURE 12.19 Food sources of potassium. The best food sources of potassium are fresh fruits and vegetables and certain dairy products and fish.

Data from US Department of Agriculture, Agricultural Research Service, Nutrient Data Laboratory. USDA National Nutrient Database for Standard Reference, Release 28. Version Current: September 2015. Internet: http://www.ars.usda.gov/nea/bhnrc/ndl.

the effects of excess potassium loss. Symptoms include muscle weakness, loss of appetite, and confusion. Severe or rapid potassium depletion can disrupt heart rhythms—a potentially fatal problem.

People with poor diets, such as alcoholics and individuals who suffer from anorexia nervosa or bulimia nervosa, are at highest risk of potassium deficiency. Hypokalemia also is possible in people who overuse strong laxatives. Some diuretics prescribed for hypertension cause increased excretion of both water and potassium. People taking these diuretics are at increased risk for hypokalemia and must pay special attention to their potassium intake. Their doctors might prescribe potassium supplements to counter losses. Athletes and people doing physical labor in high temperatures have high water losses, so they also risk potassium deficiency.

Hyperkalemia

The kidneys effectively remove excess potassium, so the risk of toxicity from dietary intake is usually low. However, malfunctioning kidneys or an excess of intravenous potassium can cause **hyperkalemia**, or a high concentration of potassium in the blood. Because severe hyperkalemia can slow and eventually stop the heart, people who suffer from kidney failure must monitor their potassium intake carefully. The "cocktail" of drugs administered during execution by lethal injection sometimes includes potassium.

▶ **hyperkalemia** Abnormally high potassium concentrations in the blood.

Key Concepts Potassium is the major cation in the intracellular fluid. With sodium, it regulates muscle contractions and nerve impulse transmissions. For healthy adults, the AI for potassium is 4,700 milligrams per day, substantially more than most Americans consume. The major sources of dietary potassium are vegetables and fruits. The symptoms of hypokalemia are loss of appetite, muscle cramps, and confusion. Severe hyperkalemia can cause cardiac arrest and death.

Quick Bite

Banana Facts

You might know that bananas are high in potassium, but did you also know that they have an unusually high carbohydrate content? Before ripening, a banana is almost entirely starch. After ripening, certain varieties are almost entirely sugar—as much as 20 percent by weight.

▶ **chloride shift** The movement of chloride ions into and out of red blood cells to maintain a lower level of chloride in red blood cells in the arteries than in the veins.

Chloride

Chloride (Cl^-) and chlorine (Cl_2) are not the same. Chloride is a negatively charged atom that people commonly eat as a component of table salt (NaCl). Chlorine, a highly reactive molecule composed of two atoms, is a poisonous gas. Water treatment facilities commonly use chlorine to kill bacteria and other germs.

Functions of Chloride

Chloride is the major extracellular anion in the body. Although mostly found outside cells, chloride readily moves into and out of red blood cells. As these cells transport oxygen to body tissues or carbon dioxide to the lungs, the concentration of chloride ions shifts to sustain a neutral charge in the cell. This **chloride shift** maintains lower levels of chloride ions in arterial red blood cells than in venous red blood cells.

You have probably noticed the salty taste that sodium chloride (NaCl) imparts to blood, sweat, and tears. Both sodium and chloride help maintain the body's fluid balance. Chloride also readily combines with hydrogen ions (H^+) to form hydrochloric acid (HCl). In the stomach, hydrochloric acid kills many disease-causing bacteria that have been ingested and helps prepare protein for enzymatic digestion. In the large intestine, bacterial activity forms acid products. To neutralize these acid products, the cells lining the large intestine absorb chloride ions and secrete alkaline bicarbonate ions.[33] During an immune response, white blood cells use chloride ions to form a powerful chemical weapon to kill invading bacteria. In neurons, the coordinated movements of chloride and the cations sodium, potassium, and calcium help transmit nerve impulses.

Dietary Recommendations for Chloride

Most of us consume much more chloride than the 2,300 milligrams per day that is the adult AI. Consumption of excess sodium and chloride can aggravate hypertension in salt-sensitive people. Because most chloride is consumed with sodium, limiting sodium to 2,300 milligrams as recommended by the American Heart Association would result in a chloride intake of about 3,450 milligrams. The Daily Value for chloride is 3,400 milligrams, just under the adult UL for chloride, which is 3,600 milligrams per day.

Sources of Chloride

Although some fruits and vegetables naturally contain chloride, most of our chloride intake comes from salt. (For dietary sources of salt, see the "Sodium" section earlier in this chapter.)

Reducing the use of salt, as recommended in the *2015-2020 Dietary Guidelines for Americans*, also will reduce chloride intake. The kidneys excrete excess chloride, and some chloride also is lost in sweat. The only known cause of high blood chloride levels is severe dehydration.

Quick Bite

Discouraging Discoloration

Cutting or bruising causes discoloration of many fruits and vegetables, such as apples, bananas, pears, eggplants, avocados, and raw potatoes. Chloride ions inhibit the responsible enzyme, so salt retards discoloration, although it also changes the flavor.

Hypochloremia

Because vomiting removes hydrochloric acid along with other stomach contents, frequent vomiting can cause a chloride deficiency. People with bulimia nervosa often use self-induced vomiting as a way to compensate for binge eating, and thus might have low levels of chloride and other critical electrolytes, such as potassium. A person who combines repeated vomiting with inadequate consumption of fluid and minerals can suffer dehydration and

metabolic alkalosis (high blood pH). Alkalosis can cause abnormal heart rhythm, a substantial drop in blood flow to the brain, decreased oxygen delivery to tissues, abnormal metabolic activity, and even death. To treat this problem, doctors administer oral or intravenous fluids containing the deficient minerals, which restores pH balance.

▶ **metabolic alkalosis** An abnormal pH of body fluids, usually caused by significant loss of acid from the body or increased levels of bicarbonate.

Key Concepts Chloride is involved in many important metabolic functions. It is used to form the hydrochloric acid secreted in the stomach and is important in the generation of nerve impulses as well as in immune function. For healthy adults, the AI for chloride is 2,300 milligrams per day; average chloride intake from salt is 4,500 milligrams per day. People with bulimia nervosa can develop chloride deficiency as a result of self-induced vomiting.

Quick Bite

Low-Calorie Chlorine?

Sucralose is a low-calorie sweetener made from sugar. During manufacture, a multistep process substitutes three chlorine atoms for three hydrogen–oxygen groups on the sugar molecule. This creates an exceptionally stable molecular structure that is 600 times sweeter than sugar. The sucralose molecule is chemically and biologically inert, so it passes through the body without being digested and is eliminated after consumption.

Calcium

Our bodies contain more calcium (Ca) than any other mineral, about 1.5 to 2 percent of our total weight. Adequate calcium intake over one's lifetime is essential for healthy bones and teeth that will remain strong into old age. Although we associate calcium primarily with bones, it plays many important roles in the body. Getting enough calcium in your diet not only maintains healthy bones, but also helps prevent hypertension, decreases your odds of getting colon or breast cancer, improves weight control, and reduces the risk of developing kidney stones.

Quick Bite

We All Scream for . . . Calcium?

The children's refrain, "I scream, you scream, we all scream for ice cream" could encourage better calcium consumption. "Calcium bioavailability in calcium-fortified ice cream is as high as milk, indicating that ice cream may be a good vehicle for delivery of calcium," according to researchers.

Functions of Calcium

Bones and teeth contain more than 99 percent of the body's calcium. This mineral makes bones hard and strong, able to withstand tremendous force without breaking—most of the time. The other 1 percent of body calcium is in blood and soft tissues, where it plays many equally crucial roles in such vital functions as muscle contraction, nerve impulse transmission, blood clotting, and cell metabolism. **FIGURE 12.20** shows the functions of calcium.

▶ **hydroxyapatite** A crystalline mineral compound of calcium and phosphorus that makes up bone.

▶ **linear growth** Increase in body length/height.

Bone Structure

Most of us think of bone as a simple structural framework for our bodies. We forget that bone is living tissue that changes in response to dietary intake and physical stresses. Bone also encases the marrow, the source of many types of blood and immune cells, and serves as the reserve site for minerals such as calcium and phosphorus.

Bone is made up of cells and an extracellular matrix. Two types of cells, osteoblasts and osteoclasts, continually remodel our bones—building them up and tearing them down. Osteoblasts are the construction team, and osteoclasts are the demolition team. Osteoblasts first secrete the collagen protein matrix that forms the initial framework for new bone. Then, these bone builders help move minerals from the extracellular fluid to the bone surface, where the minerals become a hard crystalline material that surrounds the collagen fibers. Most of the calcium in bone is in the form of **hydroxyapatite**, a crystalline mineral complex of calcium and phosphorus. By weight, bone is two-thirds mineral and one-third water and protein, primarily collagen. While osteoblasts continually deposit bone, osteoclasts perform the opposite function by resorbing bone. As they break down bone, they release calcium and phosphate, which enter the bloodstream.

The activities of osteoblasts and osteoclasts determine how bones grow and change over time. Mineralization of bone is favored during **linear growth** (growth in height) and for 5 to 10 years thereafter. It is thought that we achieve peak bone mass sometime around age 30.

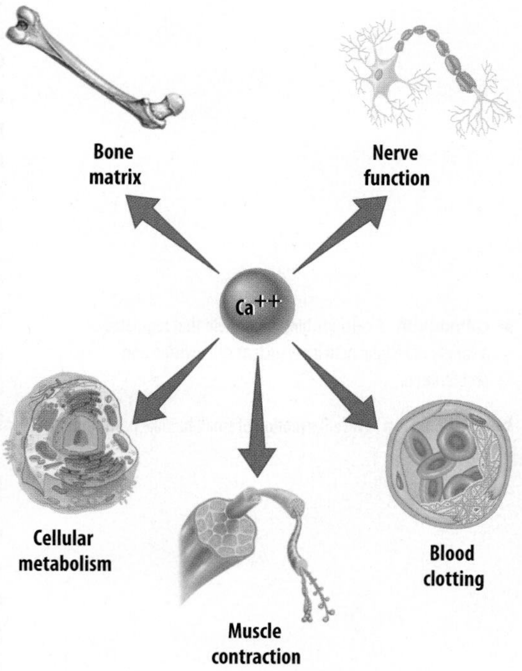

FIGURE 12.20 Functions of calcium. In addition to playing a key role in bone health, calcium in blood and soft tissues is essential for such diverse functions as blood clotting, muscle contractions, and nerve impulse transmission.

Throughout life, our bones change in response to our activities. The dynamic nature of bone allows it to be strengthened and rebuilt in areas under repeated stress—bone thickens when repeatedly subjected to loads. Even older adults can strengthen and rebuild their bones by performing weight-bearing exercise such as walking or weight lifting.[34]

The calcium in bones serves as a reservoir for calcium that is needed throughout the body. The body maintains a constant calcium blood level at all costs—at the expense of bone strength if necessary. Even if calcium intake is very low, the calcium concentration in the bloodstream remains steady because the body removes calcium from bone to sustain an adequate supply to other tissues. In the absence of kidney disease or hormonal abnormalities, your blood calcium level remains normal even if your diet is extremely deficient in calcium.

Nerve Function

Calcium is a key factor in normal transmission of nerve impulses. The movement of calcium into nerve cells triggers the release of neurotransmitters at the junction between nerves. The neuron releases neurotransmitters in direct proportion to the number of calcium ions that flow through the cell's calcium channels. Insufficient calcium can inhibit nerve transmissions.

Blood Clotting

▶ **fibrin** A stringy, insoluble protein that is the final product of the blood-clotting process.

Calcium is essential for the formation of **fibrin**, the fibrous protein that makes up the structure of blood clots. Calcium participates in nearly every step of the blood-clotting cascade. Blood will not clot in the absence of calcium, but calcium levels in the body seldom fall low enough to significantly impair blood clotting.

Muscle Contraction

Calcium has a central role in muscle contractions because the flow of calcium ions inside muscle cells is crucial for enabling muscles to contract and relax. Calcium sits at a critical location on the muscle fiber, facilitating the interaction of the muscle proteins myosin and actin. Stimulation of muscle fibers by nerve impulses, hormones, or stretch in the fiber increases the amount of calcium in the muscle cells and causes the muscle to contract. As the cells pump calcium ions back outside, the muscle relaxes. During exercise, one cause of muscle fatigue is the impaired activity of calcium in muscle cells.

Cellular Metabolism

▶ **calmodulin** A calcium-binding protein that regulates a variety of cellular activities, such as cell division and proliferation.

▶ **ciliary action** Wavelike motion of small hairlike projections on some cells.

Calcium also is a key player in regulation of cellular metabolism. When calcium enters a cell, it can bind to **calmodulin**, a regulatory protein. This binding activates calmodulin, which helps regulate a variety of enzymatic processes that affect cell secretions, **ciliary action**, cell division, and cell proliferation.

Regulation of Blood Calcium

Circulating calcium performs a myriad of functions that are so critical that the body will demineralize bone to prevent even minor dips in blood calcium levels. Three hormones—calcitriol (the active form of vitamin D), parathyroid hormone, and calcitonin—regulate calcium status. They control intestinal absorption of calcium, bone calcium release, and calcium excretion by the kidneys (see **FIGURE 12.21**). The hormone estrogen also affects calcium balance. Lower estrogen production, as seen with menopause in women, causes both an increase in bone resorption and a decrease in calcium absorption.[35]

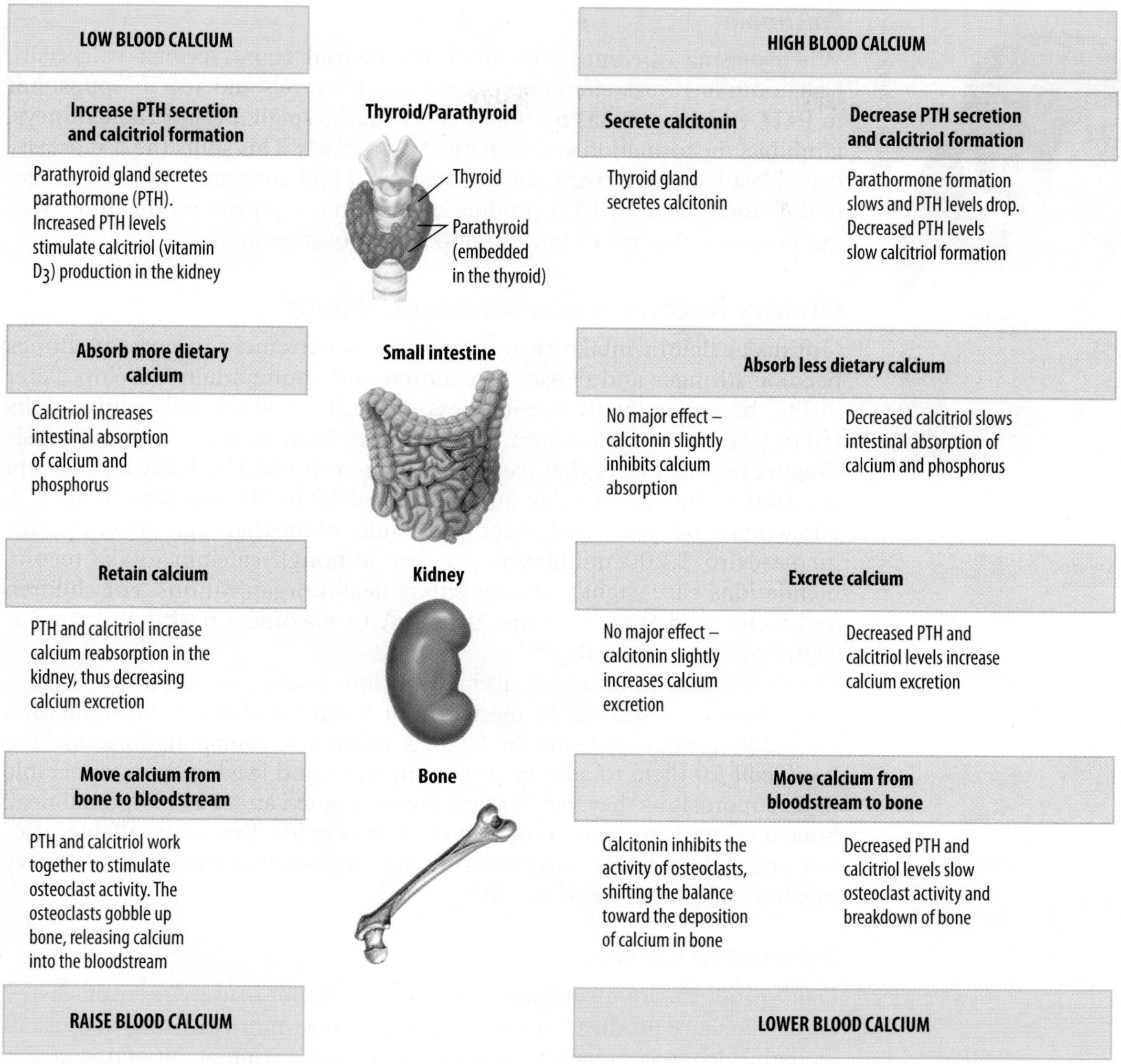

LOW BLOOD CALCIUM
Increase PTH secretion and calcitriol formation
Parathyroid gland secretes parathormone (PTH). Increased PTH levels stimulate calcitriol (vitamin D3) production in the kidney
Absorb more dietary calcium
Calcitriol increases intestinal absorption of calcium and phosphorus
Retain calcium
PTH and calcitriol increase calcium reabsorption in the kidney, thus decreasing calcium excretion
Move calcium from bone to bloodstream
PTH and calcitriol work together to stimulate osteoclast activity. The osteoclasts gobble up bone, releasing calcium into the bloodstream
RAISE BLOOD CALCIUM
Thyroid/Parathyroid
Thyroid
Parathyroid (embedded in the thyroid)
Small intestine
Kidney
Bone
HIGH BLOOD CALCIUM
Secrete calcitonin
Thyroid gland secretes calcitonin
Decrease PTH secretion and calcitriol formation
Parathormone formation slows and PTH levels drop. Decreased PTH levels slow calcitriol formation
Absorb less dietary calcium
No major effect – calcitonin slightly inhibits calcium absorption
Decreased calcitriol slows intestinal absorption of calcium and phosphorus
Excrete calcium
No major effect – calcitonin slightly increases calcium excretion
Decreased PTH and calcitriol levels increase calcium excretion
Move calcium from bloodstream to bone
Calcitonin inhibits the activity of osteoclasts, shifting the balance toward the deposition of calcium in bone
Decreased PTH and calcitriol levels slow osteoclast activity and breakdown of bone
LOWER BLOOD CALCIUM

FIGURE 12.21 Regulating blood calcium levels. Calcitonin has only a weak effect on calcium ion concentration. It is fast acting, but any decrease in calcium ion concentration triggers the release of PTH, which almost completely overrides the calcitonin effect. In prolonged calcium excess or deficiency, the parathyroid mechanism is the most powerful hormonal mechanism for maintaining normal blood calcium levels.

Vitamin D

Vitamin D increases calcium absorption by the intestines. Calcitriol, the active form of vitamin D, increases the production of calcium-binding proteins in the lining of the small intestine. The rate of calcium absorption seems to be directly proportional to the quantity of calcium-binding proteins.

Parathyroid Hormone

When plasma calcium levels are too low, the parathyroid gland secretes parathyroid hormone (PTH). PTH activates bone-resorbing osteoclasts that break down bone and release calcium and phosphorus into the blood. It also increases kidney reabsorption of calcium and stimulates calcitriol production, which then enhances intestinal calcium absorption. PTH greatly increases phosphorus excretion, so phosphorus blood levels actually drop in response to PTH despite an initial increase in supply from the breakdown of bone.

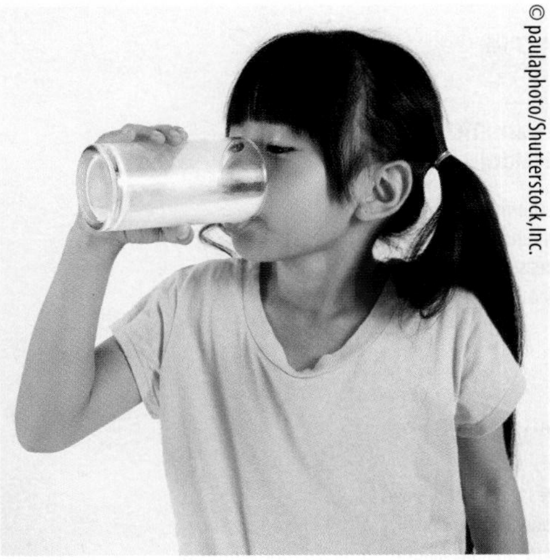

Calcitonin

When plasma calcium is too high, the thyroid gland secretes calcitonin. Calcitonin has weak effects on plasma calcium levels and acts in opposition to PTH. Although it has no major effects in the small intestine and kidneys, it inhibits the formation and activity of osteoclasts. This shifts the osteoclast–osteoblast balance toward bone deposition. High concentrations of calcium in the blood decrease PTH production, and thus calcitriol production, slowing processes that move calcium into the bloodstream.

Dietary Recommendations for Calcium

Optimal calcium intake throughout life is extremely important. Bones become stronger and denser as children and young adults develop. Later in life, bones gradually become less dense. If children and young adults fail to take in enough calcium, they are more likely to develop osteoporosis (fragile, porous bones that easily break) later in life. The RDA for calcium is 1,000 milligrams per day for adults aged 19 to 50, and men to age 70. For women 51 years and older and adults older than age 70 years, this increases to 1,200 milligrams per day, although calcium intake recommendations vary slightly among public health organizations. For children and teens aged 9 to 18 years, the RDA to maximize peak bone mass is 1,300 milligrams per day.[36]

Unfortunately, although average calcium intake has increased slightly, most Americans still fail to meet current recommendations. Most children and adolescents worldwide fail to meet calcium recommendations, making it difficult for them to achieve peak bone mass and leaving them vulnerable to osteoporosis as they age.[37] Many young women attain a suboptimal peak bone mass and are prone to osteoporosis later in life. Excessive caffeine, alcohol, and sodium intake and misuse of diuretics—factors that increase urinary calcium—make bone loss worse.[38]

Sources of Calcium

THINK About It 4

Dairy products are a substantial source of calcium in the American diet.[39] Of all the dairy products, nonfat milk is the most nutrient dense because of its high calcium content and lower fat and calorie content. Nonfat yogurt is another excellent source of calcium. Cottage cheese has the least calcium of the dairy foods because processing removes much of its calcium. Ice cream and cheese are good sources of calcium, but they should be eaten only in moderation because of their high fat content.

Green leafy vegetables such as spinach have high levels of calcium, but most of the calcium is bound to oxalate and therefore cannot be absorbed. Chinese cabbage, kale, turnip greens, and calcium-processed tofu contain significant amounts of bioavailable calcium. Canned fish with bones, such as sardines, provides lots of calcium as long as you eat the bones. **FIGURE 12.22** shows food sources of calcium.

Some brands of orange juice, cereal, bread, and yogurt products are now fortified with calcium, making them good sources. Check labels carefully, because only a few of the many products on grocery shelves are fortified with calcium.

Although eating a variety of healthful foods is always the best way to obtain nutrients, some people, especially those with limited dairy intake, might need to take supplements to ensure adequate calcium intake. Flavored, chewable, calcium-containing antacids are an inexpensive and easy-to-take source of extra calcium. For more information, see the FYI feature "Calcium Supplements: Are They Right for You?"

Quick Bite

Paleolithic Calcium Intake

Hunter-gatherer populations during the late Paleolithic period did not drink milk or consume dairy products. Nonetheless, they do not appear to have suffered from calcium deficiency. Researchers estimate that the calcium intake by these populations was almost 1,600 milligrams per day, mostly from wild plants and nectars.

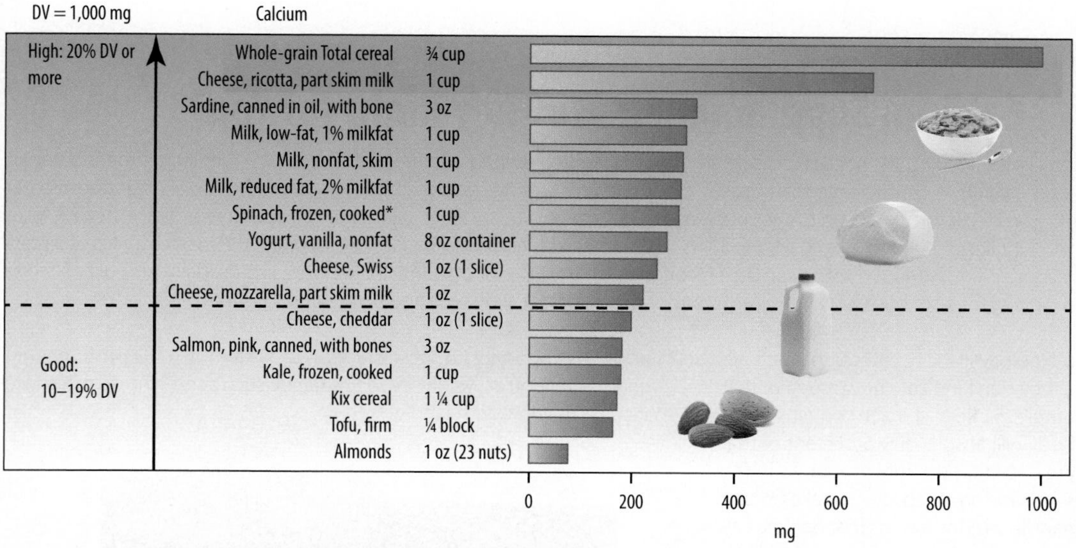

* In spinach, oxalate binds calcium and prevents absorption of all but about 5 percent of the plant's calcium.

FIGURE 12.22 Food sources of calcium. Calcium is found in milk and dairy products, certain green leafy vegetables, and canned fish with bones. In spinach, oxalate binds calcium and prevents absorption of all but about 5 percent of the plant's calcium.

Data from US Department of Agriculture, Agricultural Research Service, Nutrient Data Laboratory. USDA National Nutrient Database for Standard Reference, Release 28. Version Current: September 2015. Internet: http://www.ars.usda.gov/nea/bhnrc/ndl.

Photos (from top to bottom): (bowl of sugar-coated corn flakes) © Oliver Hoffmann/Shutterstock, Inc.; (ripe with Mozzarella di Bufala, Italian water buffalo milk cheese) © Dorling Kindersley/ Getty Images; (milk bottle) © Mega Pixel/ Shutterstock, Inc.; (dried almonds) © Dionisvera/Shutterstock, Inc.

Calcium Absorption

Calcium absorption is relatively inefficient, and we usually absorb only 25 to 35 percent of the calcium we eat.[40] Calcium absorption can vary because of a number of factors, including age, presence of adequate vitamin D, the body's need for calcium, and calcium intake. For example, if a child and a healthy elderly person eat the same meal, the child may absorb 60 percent of the calcium in the food, whereas the elderly person might absorb only 15 percent. Calcium absorption is particularly high during pregnancy and infancy and is at its lowest in old age.

Calcium absorption is inversely related to calcium intake. The body adjusts the percentage it absorbs based on the amount in the diet: An increase in dietary calcium reduces absorption, and a decrease in dietary calcium enhances absorption.[41] In the absence of vitamin D, calcium absorption can drop dramatically. Phytates (in nuts, seeds, and grains) depress calcium absorption, as do oxalates and high levels of phosphorus and magnesium from supplements.

Dietary fiber, except for wheat bran, has little effect on calcium absorption. High intakes of wheat bran have been found to depress calcium absorption from milk. Low estrogen levels, as seen in postmenopausal women, can lower calcium absorption to about 20 percent. Many women take estrogen supplements after menopause to maintain calcium absorption and lower the risk of osteoporosis. Calcium from supplements is absorbed most efficiently when taken between meals at individual doses of 500 milligrams or less.[42]

Hypocalcemia

A lower than normal level of calcium in the blood is called **hypocalcemia**. Because the body uses bone calcium to maintain normal blood calcium

▶ **hypocalcemia** A deficiency of calcium in the blood.

FYI For Your Information

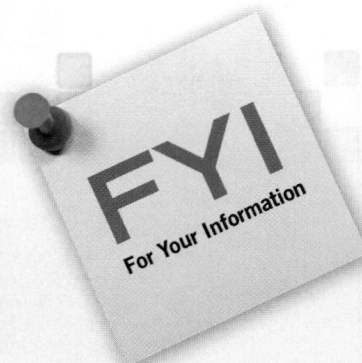

Calcium Supplements: Are They Right for You?

After reading the section on calcium, you may be wondering whether you need a calcium supplement. After all, calcium is critical for so many bodily functions, and getting enough calcium reduces the risk of osteoporosis later in life. Before you head to the supplement aisle at the grocery store, take a critical look at your diet, especially your intake of milk and other dairy products. In the United States and Canada, dairy foods are the major sources of dietary calcium; without them, it can be difficult to reach the RDA for calcium. People who exclude dairy products, such as vegans and those with milk allergy, must choose foods carefully to find rich calcium sources.

Calcium sources vary widely in their bioavailability. Although labels are required to list the %DV for calcium, they don't indicate how much of that calcium the body will absorb. For example, ½ cup of spinach contains about 120 milligrams of calcium, but the body will absorb only 5 percent of that calcium! Intake recommendations are based on the mix of sources in the typical American diet. Other cultures manage on much lower intakes in part because they do not consume the many food constituents that deplete calcium or reduce its absorption. Vegetarians can, in fact, need less calcium than meat-eaters. If you are considering spinach as your sole source of calcium, however, you will need to eat almost 8 cups to equal the calcium available from 1 cup of milk. (About 30 percent of the 300 milligrams of calcium in 1 cup of milk is bioavailable.)

The amount of bioavailable calcium varies quite a bit among green leafy vegetables. The calcium in kale, Chinese cabbage, and mustard greens, for example, is significantly more bioavailable than in spinach. Tofu is also a good vegetarian source of bioavailable calcium. If your diet is low in calcium, try adding some of the higher-calcium foods. Incorporating calcium-rich and calcium-fortified foods into the diet adds other important vitamins and minerals.

Even armed with more information about calcium in the diet, you might still decide to investigate the supplement market. Again, there is a variety of choices: calcium carbonate, calcium citrate, calcium lactate, calcium phosphate, coral calcium … how to decide? First, it's important to know that the absorption of calcium from most supplements is about equal—roughly 30 percent. The calcium citrate malate that is used in some brands of fortified juice and a limited number of supplements is absorbed a little better—35 percent. However, a typical calcium citrate malate tablet has less calcium than a tablet of another type, such as calcium carbonate. Calcium carbonate is usually the most concentrated per tablet, so taking fewer pills per day will supply enough; also, this type of supplement tends to be less expensive. Chelated calcium supplements can improve absorption a bit, but the extra expense is probably not worth it.

Other factors to consider are that calcium supplements might be absorbed better if taken between meals. Also, you need to get plenty of vitamin D, either through casual exposure to the sun, in fortified milk, or as part of a supplement (many calcium supplements have added vitamin D). Vitamin D is important for the absorption of calcium. In addition, bones get stronger with regular, weight-bearing exercise such as walking, so make sure to include that in your healthful lifestyle.

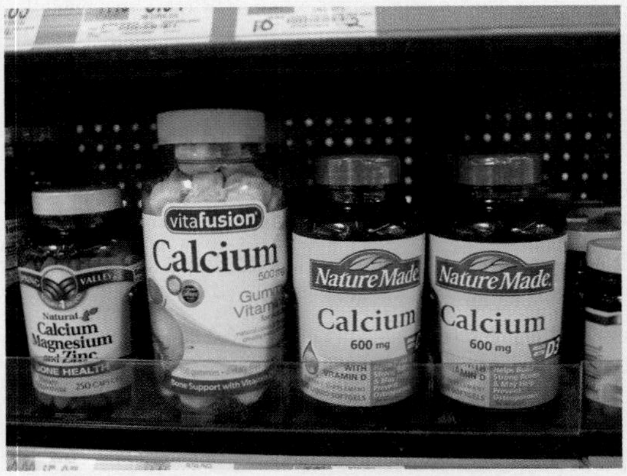

© picturelibrary/Alamy

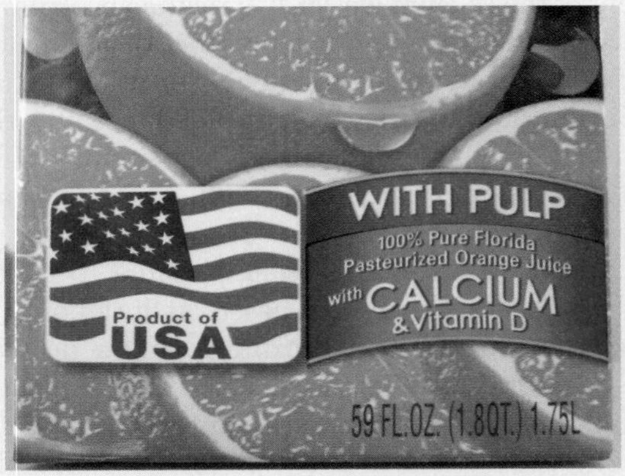

© Jones & Bartlett Learning. Photo by Amy Rathburn.

levels, hypocalcemia is relatively uncommon. The causes of hypocalcemia include kidney failure, parathyroid disorders, and vitamin D deficiency. Significant hypocalcemia can cause muscle spasms, facial grimacing, and convulsions.

A chronic dietary calcium deficiency can result in osteoporosis due to either suboptimal bone growth in childhood and adolescence or increased rate of bone loss after menopause. Low calcium intake has been linked to an increased risk of cardiovascular disease, hypertension, obesity, and certain types of cancer including colon cancer.[43]

Hypercalcemia

Although certain illnesses can cause high blood calcium, dietary calcium intake does not. The two major causes of **hypercalcemia** are cancer and the overproduction of PTH by the parathyroid gland. Hypercalcemia can result in fatigue, confusion, loss of appetite, and constipation. Calcium can be deposited in the soft tissues, where it can impair organ function. Very high levels of blood calcium can lead to coma and cardiac arrest.

▶ **hypercalcemia** Abnormally high concentrations of calcium in the blood.

Excess calcium supplementation usually does not result in hypercalcemia but can cause mineral imbalances by interfering with the absorption of other minerals, such as iron, magnesium, and zinc. Although calcium supplements can dramatically affect absorption of other minerals, dietary calcium intake has not been shown to cause a deficiency for any of these minerals.[44] Calcium supplements that contain citrate and ascorbic acid enhance iron absorption, but other forms can cut iron absorption in half. Calcium supplements also can interfere with absorption of some medications. The Food and Nutrition Board has established a UL for calcium of 2,500 milligrams per day for adults aged 19–50 years.

Osteoporosis

Osteoporosis means "porous bone." It's a good description. In osteoporosis, bone mass or density declines and bone quality deteriorates, leaving the bones fragile and vulnerable to fractures. Osteoporosis is the major cause of bone fractures in older adults, primarily postmenopausal women. The U.S. Surgeon General estimates that by 2020, one in two Americans aged 50 years or older will be at risk for fractures from osteoporosis or low bone mass.[45,46] Although 80 percent of those with osteoporosis are women, by age 75 one-third of all men have osteoporosis.

Calcium is an important factor in bone health, but it is not the only nutritive factor. Normal development and mineralization of bone requires calcium, phosphorus, fluoride, magnesium, vitamin D, vitamin A, vitamin K, and protein. Lifestyle factors including regular weight-bearing exercise and not smoking are also important for bone health.

Key Concepts Calcium is a major component of bones and teeth. In addition, calcium is required for muscle contraction, nerve impulse transmission, blood clotting, and regulation of cell metabolism. For adults, 1,000 milligrams per day is recommended; a greater amount is suggested for adolescents and older adults. Dairy foods and fortified foods are major dietary sources of calcium. Calcium status is regulated by hormones that control intestinal absorption, bone calcium release, and kidney excretion. Lack of dietary calcium contributes to the development of osteoporosis. Osteoporosis is a progressive loss of bone mass, resulting in fragile bones that are susceptible to fracture. Several minerals, including calcium, phosphorus, magnesium, and fluoride, are important for bone health.

Phosphorus

Phosphorus (P), like calcium, serves many roles in the biochemical reactions of cells and has a critical role in bone as part of the mineral complex hydroxyapatite. Phosphorus intake typically exceeds that of calcium because it is so widespread in the food supply. Most phosphorus in the body is in the form of the phosphate ion (PO_4^{3-}). In fact, phosphate is the most abundant intracellular anion.

▶ **phosphorylation** The addition of phosphate to an organic (carbon-containing) compound. Oxidative phosphorylation is the formation of high-energy phosphate bonds (ADP + P_i = ATP) from the energy released by oxidation of energy-yielding nutrients.

Functions of Phosphorus

Bones are the major storehouse of phosphorus, holding nearly 85 percent of the body's supply. The remaining phosphorus is found in cells of soft tissues (approximately 15 percent) and extracellular fluid (approximately 0.1 percent). It helps activate and deactivate enzymes in a process called **phosphorylation**.

Dietary Recommendations for Phosphorus

The phosphorus RDA for adults is 700 milligrams per day. Adolescents need more, about 1,250 milligrams per day, to support growth. The average adult intake is between 1,000 and 1,500 milligrams per day, so phosphorus deficiencies resulting from dietary insufficiency are rarely seen.

Sources of Phosphorus

Phosphorus is abundant in our food supply. In general, foods rich in protein (milk, meat, and eggs) also are rich in phosphorus. Food additives, especially those in processed meat and soft drinks, supply up to 30 percent of our phosphorus. **FIGURE 12.23** shows selected food sources of phosphorus. Food manufacturers often add phosphate salts to processed foods to improve moisture retention and smoothness.

Soft drinks often contain phosphoric acid, although the phosphorus level is not high—about 50 milligrams in a 12-ounce cola, compared with 370 milligrams in 12 ounces of fat-free milk. However, among heavy cola drinkers who consume five or more per day, soda is an important contributor to phosphorus intake.[47] Dairy products have phosphorus plus calcium (460 milligrams in 12 ounces), whereas sodas have phosphorus but virtually no calcium (10 milligrams or less in a 12-ounce can)—an important distinction.

Generally, we absorb between 55 and 70 percent of dietary phosphorus, and the kidneys excrete any excess in the urine. Unlike calcium absorption, phosphorus absorption does not increase as dietary intake decreases.[48] On the other hand, the body's phosphorus needs can drive phosphorus absorption efficiency.

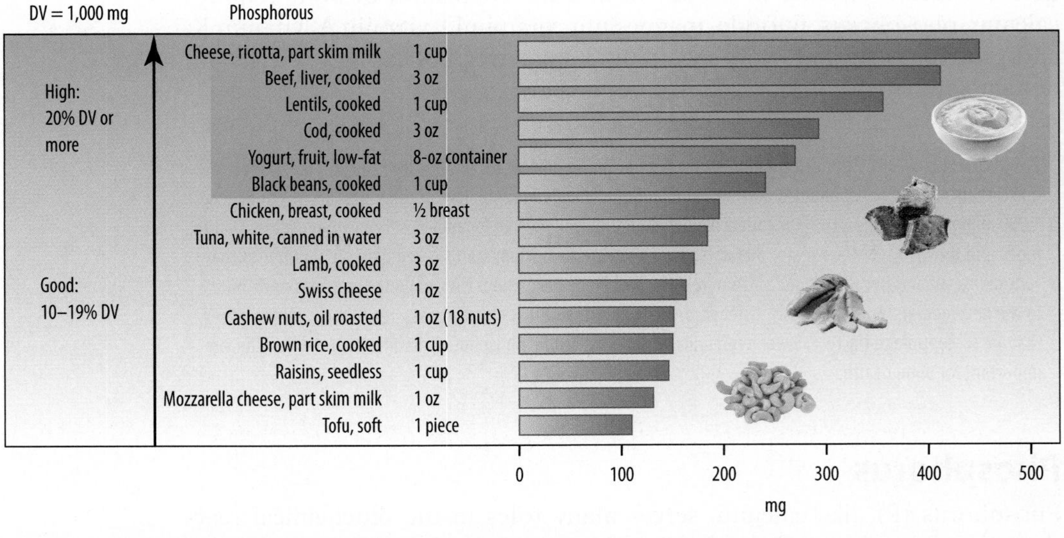

FIGURE 12.23 Food sources of phosphorus. Phosphorus is abundant in the food supply. Meats, legumes, nuts, dairy products, and grains tend to have more phosphorus than fruits and vegetables.

Data from US Department of Agriculture, Agricultural Research Service, Nutrient Data Laboratory. USDA National Nutrient Database for Standard Reference, Release 28. Version Current: September 2015. Internet: http://www.ars.usda.gov/nea/bhnrc/ndl.

Photos (from top to bottom): (pink yogurt) © MaraZe/Shutterstock, Inc.; (beef liver) © nadi555/ Shutterstock,Inc.; (chicken breasts) © Viktor1 /Shutterstock, Inc.; (cashew nuts) © SOMMAI/Shutterstock, Inc.

In the intestines, calcitriol enhances both calcium and phosphorus absorption. Parathyroid hormone, on the other hand, has opposite effects on calcium and phosphorus levels. PTH not only maintains calcium levels by stimulating the kidneys to reabsorb calcium, but also causes rapid loss of phosphorus in the urine. The two most important regulators of urinary phosphorus excretion are PTH and the amount of phosphorus in the diet.[49]

Quick Bite

The Double Helix Depends on Phosphorus
The backbone of DNA's twisting, ladderlike structure contains alternating molecules of phosphoric acid and deoxyribose.

Hypophosphatemia

Phosphorus is so common in foods that only near-total starvation will cause a dietary phosphorus deficiency. Rather, an underlying disorder typically causes **hypophosphatemia**, low blood phosphate, either by restricting absorption or enhancing excretion. Physicians commonly encounter hypophosphatemia, and about 1 percent of patients admitted to general hospitals suffer from it.[50,51] Some of its more common causes include **hyperparathyroidism** (excessive secretion of PTH, often because of a parathyroid tumor), vitamin D deficiency, and overuse of aluminum-, magnesium-, or calcium-containing antacids that bind phosphate. Common symptoms of hypophosphatemia include anorexia, dizziness, bone pain, muscle weakness, and a waddling gait. Chronic hypophosphatemia affects primarily the musculoskeletal system, causing muscle weakness and damage, including respiratory problems caused by poor diaphragm function. Long-standing hypophosphatemia can cause rickets and osteomalacia.

▶ **hypophosphatemia** Abnormally low phosphate concentration in the blood.

▶ **hyperparathyroidism** Excessive secretion of parathyroid hormone, which alters calcium metabolism.

Hyperphosphatemia

Physicians also frequently see **hyperphosphatemia**, high blood phosphate, which most commonly is a consequence of kidney disease. Other causes include an underactive parathyroid gland, taking too many vitamin D supplements, and overuse of phosphate-containing laxatives. Excess phosphorus can bind calcium, and, because low calcium concentrations can cause nerve fibers to discharge repeatedly without provocation, this can lead to severe muscle spasms and convulsions.

▶ **hyperphosphatemia** Abnormally high phosphate concentration in the blood.

If your diet contains excessive phosphorus and not enough calcium, you might be at risk for increased bone loss. However, a high phosphorus intake alone is unlikely to have an adverse effect on bone health.[52] Replacing milk as a beverage with cola, a common practice among adolescents and Americans of all ages, increases phosphates in the diet (from cola) while reducing calcium intake. Some experts believe that this practice is a significant factor in the development of osteoporosis later in life. The UL for phosphorus is 4,000 milligrams per day for people aged 9 to 70 years.

Key Concepts Phosphorus is common in many crucial metabolic systems. It is used to activate and deactivate enzymes and is an essential component of ATP, the energy source of the cell. Phosphorus is found in the phospholipids of cell membranes and is part of the hydroxyapatite in bone. About 85 percent of phosphorus is found in bone. Milk and meat are major sources of dietary phosphorus, and up to 30 percent of dietary intake comes from food additives. The RDA for adults is 700 milligrams per day, increasing to 1,250 milligrams per day for teens. Diets high in phosphorus and low in calcium can contribute to bone loss.

Magnesium

Magnesium (Mg) is the fourth most abundant cation in the body and is about one-sixth as plentiful in cells as potassium. About 50 to 60 percent of the body's magnesium is in bone, with the remainder distributed equally between muscle and other soft tissue. The magnesium in bone provides a large reservoir

Quick Bite

Magnesium Says: "Let the Competition Begin!"

The pigment chlorophyll, which is responsible for the deep green color of vegetables, contains a magnesium atom at its molecular center. Heat easily displaces this magnesium, and in acidic cooking water, hydrogen ions rush in to replace it. The altered chlorophyll is grayish-green. This replacement of magnesium by hydrogen is the most common cause of the dull, olive-green color of many cooked vegetables. On the other hand, if the acidic cooking water also contains zinc or copper ions, these minerals beat out hydrogen in the race for the central spot in the chlorophyll. This combination makes cooked vegetables bright green.

in case deficiencies in soft tissue magnesium occur. Most magnesium resides in cells, with only 1 percent in extracellular fluid.

Functions of Magnesium

Magnesium participates in more than 300 types of enzyme-mediated reactions in the body, including those in DNA and protein synthesis. In the mitochondria, magnesium is essential for the production of ATP by way of the electron transport chain. Because ATP is the universal energy source for all cells, an absence of magnesium would quickly halt cellular activity. In the glycolysis pathway alone, seven key enzymes require magnesium. Magnesium also participates in muscle contraction and blood clotting.

Dietary Recommendations for Magnesium

Because of the large amount of magnesium in bone, blood magnesium levels might not be indicative of total body status. Therefore, assessing deficiency and setting intake recommendations are difficult. The RDA for magnesium in adults aged 19 to 30 years is 400 milligrams per day for men and 310 milligrams per day for women. This value rises slightly in adults aged 31 to 70 to 420 milligrams for men and 320 milligrams for women. The average adult diet in the United States contains only about three-fourths of the magnesium RDA, and slightly less than the Estimated Average Requirement (EAR) for magnesium. However, overt symptoms of low magnesium are relatively uncommon in healthy people.[53] This is because so much magnesium is stored in bone that levels in cells and body fluids remain constant even if intake is somewhat less than optimal.

Sources of Magnesium

Magnesium is ubiquitous in foods, but the amount varies widely depending on the food source. This mineral enters our diet mostly from plants. Whole grains and vegetables such as spinach and potatoes are good sources of magnesium, as are legumes, tofu, and some types of seafood. **FIGURE 12.24** shows food sources of magnesium.

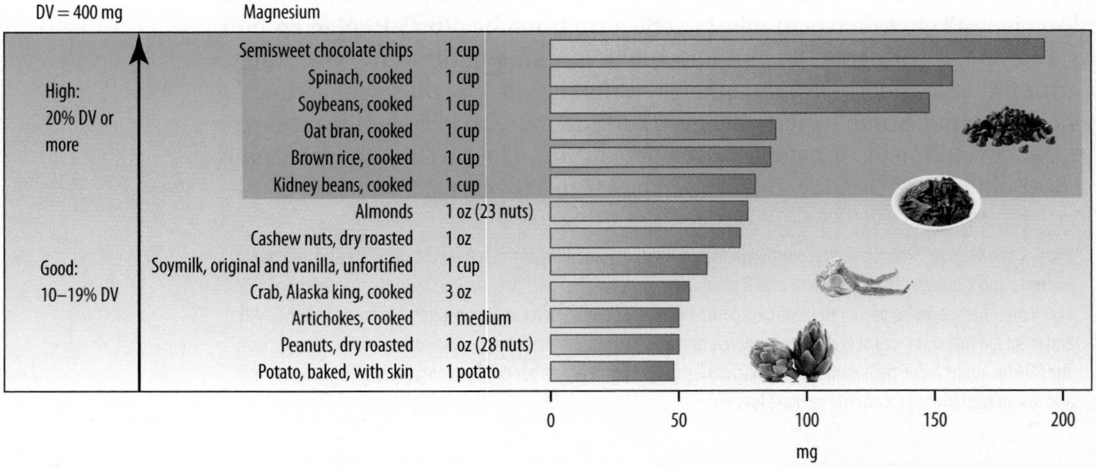

FIGURE 12.24 Food sources of magnesium. Most of the magnesium in the diet comes from plant foods such as grains, vegetables, and legumes.

Data from US Department of Agriculture, Agricultural Research Service, Nutrient Data Laboratory. USDA National Nutrient Database for Standard Reference, Release 28. Version Current: September 2015. Internet: http://www.ars.usda.gov/nea/bhnrc/ndl.

Photos (from top to bottom): (chocolate chips) © masa44/Shutterstock, Inc.; (steamed spinach) © Smneedham/ iStockphoto; (king crab legs) © Jason Lugo/ iStock /Getty Images Plus; (two artichokes) © MidoSemsem/Shutterstock, Inc.

Refined foods are low in magnesium content. Processed grains lose up to 80 percent of their magnesium, and enrichment does not replace it. Chocolate contains modest amounts of magnesium, but unfortunately not enough to compensate for its high fat and calorie content. Tap water can also be a significant source of the mineral in some communities with "hard" water. Total magnesium intake usually is proportional to calorie intake, so young people and adult men have higher intakes than women and older adults.

We generally absorb about 50 percent of dietary magnesium. Although high-fiber diets often have a negative effect on mineral absorption, high-fiber foods containing fermentable carbohydrates (e.g., resistant starch, oligosaccharides, pectin) actually improve magnesium absorption. High calcium intake, usually in the form of supplements, can interfere with magnesium absorption. This is another reason why food is a better source of nutrients than supplements. People who must take calcium supplements should be sure to regularly eat foods with high magnesium content.

Hypomagnesemia

Low magnesium intake typically goes hand in hand with poor intake of other nutrients; magnesium deficiency by itself is unusual.[54] Poor magnesium status also can occur with certain chronic illnesses such as diabetes mellitus, renal disease, and cardiovascular disease and is worsened by diarrhea and vomiting.[55] **Hypomagnesemia**, or magnesium deficiency, is associated with chronically poor diets, alcoholism, and use of certain diuretic drugs. Nearly all chronic alcoholics have symptoms of hypomagnesemia resulting from a combination of poor diets and alcohol's diuretic effect that increases urinary excretion of magnesium.

► **hypomagnesemia** An abnormally low concentration of magnesium in the blood.

In research studies, healthy people whose diets are deficient in magnesium usually have no symptoms for a few weeks because of the large supply of magnesium stored in bone. Gradually, loss of appetite, nausea, and weakness develop. After more time, muscle cramps, irritability, and confusion occur. The heart rhythm can become disturbed. If hypomagnesemia becomes extreme, death can result, usually as a result of heart rhythm problems.

Hypermagnesemia

Hypermagnesemia, an abnormally high concentration of magnesium in the blood, is uncommon in the absence of kidney disease. People with kidney failure, especially if they use magnesium-containing antacids or laxatives, are most likely to suffer from hypermagnesemia. Magnesium toxicity causes diarrhea, nausea, weakness, paralysis, and cardiac and respiratory failure.[56] The UL established by the Food and Nutrition Board recommends that healthy people not take more than 350 milligrams of magnesium per day as a supplement or in medicines. Physicians sometimes intentionally administer high doses of magnesium during pregnancy to stop premature labor. This requires frequent monitoring to avoid toxicity that can lead to respiratory paralysis and death.

► **hypermagnesemia** An abnormally high concentration of magnesium in the blood.

Key Concepts Magnesium is a cofactor for more than 300 enzymes. Magnesium is required for cardiac and nerve function, and it helps form ATP. Sixty percent of magnesium is stored in bone. The RDA for magnesium in adults is 400 milligrams per day for men and 310 milligrams per day for women. Whole grains and vegetables are good sources of magnesium. People who suffer from chronic diarrhea or vomiting can be at risk for magnesium deficiency. Alcoholism is associated with magnesium deficiency because alcoholics are often malnourished and because alcohol stimulates urinary loss of magnesium.

Quick Bite

Do Onions Make You Cry?

The cabbage and onion families have sulfur-based compounds that are transformed into odiferous compounds when their tissues are broken. Cutting into a raw onion mixes the contents of its cells, bringing enzymes into contact with an odorless precursor substance apparently derived from the sulfur-containing amino acid cysteine. The volatile result, a powerful sulfur-containing irritant, causes most people's eyes to water, apparently by dissolving in fluids that surround the eye and forming sulfuric acid.

Sulfur

Sulfur (S) is different from the other minerals discussed in this chapter because it is not used alone as a nutrient. In the body, sulfur primarily is a component of organic compounds, such as the vitamins biotin and thiamin and the amino acids methionine and cysteine. Sulfur in these amino acids is especially important to protein structure. Disulfide bridges that form when sulfur atoms bind to each other cause proteins to fold in specific ways as sulfur atoms along the protein are pulled together. A protein's folding and shape are critical for its function. Sulfur also is important in some of the liver's drug-detoxifying pathways. In its ionic form, sulfate (SO_4^{2-}), sulfur helps maintain acid–base balance.

Sulfur-containing amino acids provide ample sulfur for anyone who consumes adequate amounts of protein. Deficiency of sulfur is unknown in humans.

Key Concepts Sulfur is a component of the amino acids methionine and cysteine, as well as of the vitamins biotin and thiamin. Sulfur is important in drug detoxification and in maintaining acid–base balance. Because sulfur is a component of all proteins, a diet sufficient in protein contains adequate sulfur.

Label to Table

After reading this chapter, you should have a greater appreciation of the importance of calcium in your diet. If you don't consume dairy products, or consume them infrequently, getting enough calcium can be difficult. Today, soft drinks have become significantly more popular than milk. To combat your potential lack of calcium and vitamin D, more and more food products are being fortified with these nutrients. Did you know that many brands of orange juice now provide as much calcium per serving as a glass of milk? Check out the following Nutrition Facts label from a calcium and vitamin D-fortified orange juice.

This orange juice contains 35 percent of the Daily Value for calcium (1,000 mg). That's 350 milligrams of the 1,000 milligrams you need. That's a pretty good hit of calcium for just one 8-ounce glass of OJ. Surprisingly, it's slightly more calcium than an 8-ounce cup of milk. You can see from the comparison at the bottom of the label that this fortified juice increases the calcium %DV from 2 percent (in regular orange juice) to 35 percent.

Look at the label again. How much fiber can you get from this juice? That's right; fiber isn't listed on the label, because most juices don't contain fiber. Because the majority of Americans need more fiber in their diets, it's a good idea not to go overboard on juices; choose whole pieces of fruit as well.

In addition to being a great source of calcium, this orange juice contains folate and Vitamin D (nutrients often insufficient in diets), lots of vitamin C, other B vitamins, potassium, and phytochemicals. As part of a breakfast or even with a snack, this juice packs a lot of nutrients in its 110 calories.

% of Daily Value of Calcium:
Calcium-Fortified Orange Juice
Calcium-Fortified Orange Juice 35%
Regular Orange Juice 2%
% of Daily Value of Vitamin C 180%
Regular Orange Juice 120%
Regular OJ has 0 Vitamin D
Calcium and Vitamin D fortified has 2mcg 10%DV

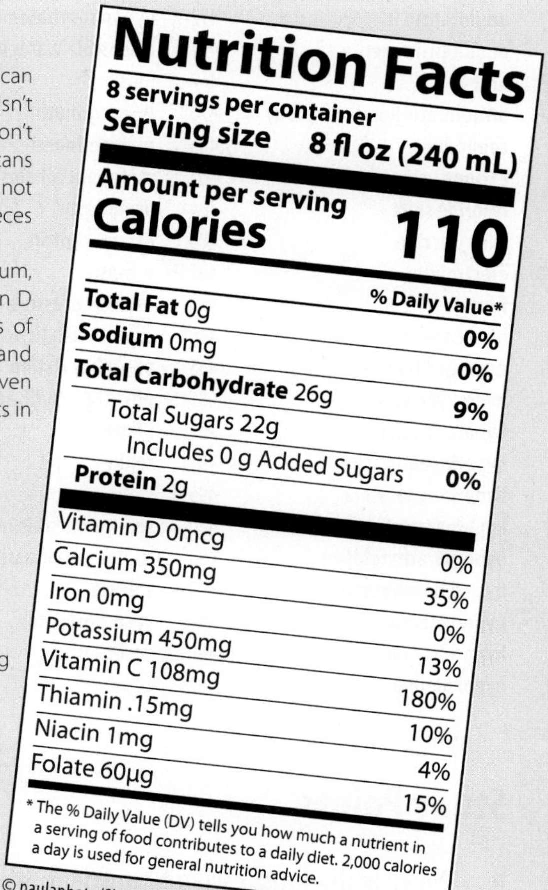
Nutrition Facts
8 servings per container
Serving size 8 fl oz (240 mL)
Amount per serving
Calories 110
% Daily Value*
Total Fat 0g
Sodium 0mg 0%
Total Carbohydrate 26g 0%
Total Sugars 22g 9%
Includes 0 g Added Sugars
Protein 2g 0%
Vitamin D 0mcg
Calcium 350mg 0%
Iron 0mg 35%
Potassium 450mg 0%
Vitamin C 108mg 13%
Thiamin .15mg 180%
Niacin 1mg 10%
Folate 60µg 4%
15%
* The % Daily Value (DV) tells you how much a nutrient in a serving of food contributes to a daily diet. 2,000 calories a day is used for general nutrition advice.

© paulaphoto/Shutterstock, Inc.

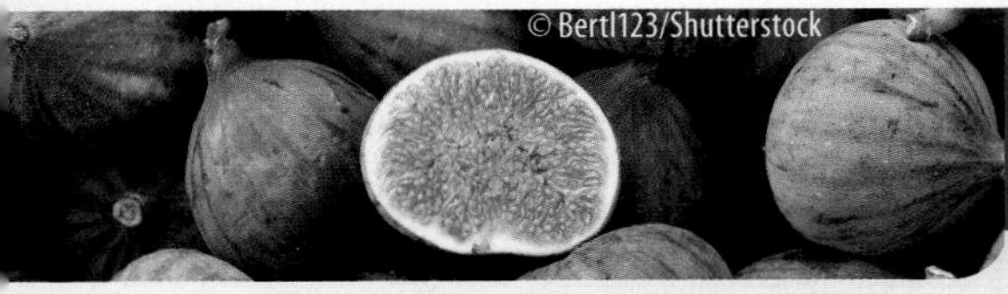
© Bertl123/Shutterstock

Learning Portfolio

Key Terms

aldosterone	472	**hypomagnesemia**	495
angiotensin I	471	**hyponatremia**	479
angiotensin II	472	**hypophosphatemia**	493
angiotensinogen	471	**insensible water loss**	470
anions	467	**ions**	467
antidiuretic hormone (ADH)	470	**linear growth**	485
calmodulin	486	**major mineral**	477
cations	467	**metabolic alkalosis**	485
chloride shift	484	**osmolarity**	470
ciliary action	486	**osmoreceptors**	470
electrolytes	465	**osmosis**	468
fibrin	486	**osmotic pressure**	468
heat capacity	466	**oxalate (oxalic acid)**	477
hydrogen bonds	465	**phosphorylation**	492
hydroxyapatite	485	**phytate (phytic acid)**	477
hypercalcemia	491	**plasma**	467
hyperkalemia	483	**renin**	471
hypermagnesemia	495	**salts**	467
hypernatremia	480	**semipermeable membrane**	468
hyperparathyroidism	493	**sodium—potassium pumps**	468
hyperphosphatemia	493	**solutes**	468
hypervolemia	480	**vasoconstrictor**	470
hypocalcemia	489	**vasopressin**	470
hypokalemia	482		

Study Points

- Water is the most essential nutrient; we can live much longer without food than without water. The AI for water is 3.7 liters per day for men and 2.7 liters per day for women.
- Water is important for the movement of nutrients and waste, cellular reactions, temperature regulation, and acid–base balance. Moreover, fluids in the body lubricate and cushion joints, cleanse the eyes, and moisten the food we eat.
- Dissolved ions, or electrolytes, help to maintain normal fluid balance.
- Fluid is lost from the body through the urine, skin, feces, and lungs. The hormones ADH and aldosterone regulate fluid excretion from the kidneys.
- The thirst response stimulates fluid intake. Alcohol and diuretic medications increase fluid excretion. Dehydration results when fluid intake is less than losses; it can seriously impair physical and mental performance.
- Minerals are inorganic elements and are categorized as major or trace depending on the amount in the body and the amount needed in the diet.
- The bioavailability of minerals can be affected by excess intake of single-mineral supplements, phytate, oxalate, fiber in plant foods, and mineral status in the body.
- Sodium, the major extracellular cation, helps regulate water distribution and blood pressure. The adult AI for sodium is 1,500 milligrams per day, and the UL is 2,300 milligrams—less than average intakes (3,000 milligrams to 5,000 milligrams per day).
- Hypertension increases risk for heart disease, stroke, and kidney disease. Sodium has long been linked to hypertension, but only some individuals are salt sensitive. Other dietary factors linked to hypertension include high chloride intake and low potassium, calcium, and magnesium intake.
- Potassium, the major cation in the intracellular fluid, is necessary for nerve and muscle function. It is provided in the diet mainly from unprocessed foods, including fruits and vegetables. The adult AI for potassium is 4,700 milligrams per day, substantially more than what most Americans eat (2,000 to 3,000 milligrams per day).
- Chloride is the major extracellular anion and a component of stomach acid. Chloride deficiency is most often associated with prolonged vomiting. Most Americans consume much more chloride than the AI, which is 2,300 milligrams per day.
- Calcium, the most abundant mineral in the body, is found in bones. It also functions in blood clotting, nerve and muscle function, and cellular metabolism. Major dietary sources of calcium are dairy products, calcium-fortified foods, and certain vegetables.
- Osteoporosis results from excessive bone loss. Postmenopausal women are at highest risk for osteoporosis. Adequate dietary calcium, vitamin D, and physical activity throughout the life span reduce the risk for osteoporosis.

- Phosphorus is a key component of ATP, DNA, RNA, phospholipids, and lipoproteins. Because phosphorus is widespread in foods, dietary phosphorus intake is rarely inadequate.
- Plant foods such as whole grains and vegetables are important sources of magnesium, which is a cofactor for hundreds of enzymes. Low levels of magnesium are associated with kidney disease, alcoholism, and use of diuretics.
- Sulfur does not function alone as a nutrient, but as a component of certain amino acids and the vitamins biotin and thiamin.

Study Questions

1. What are the two main factors that affect absorption of a mineral?
2. What functions does chloride perform in the human body?
3. What is the role of aldosterone in the body, and how is it released?
4. Name four of the main biological functions of water.
5. What is the recommended intake level for sodium?
6. What three major minerals affect bone health?
7. What are the major functions of calcium, other than its relation to bone health?
8. How does the body compensate for low calcium intake?
9. Which people have a high risk of hypomagnesemia?
10. How does the body use sulfur? What is its role in protein function?

Try This

Calcium Food Diary

The purpose of this exercise is to see how much calcium you consume in a typical day. Start by keeping a food diary for three days (two weekdays and one weekend day). While keeping the diary, try not to change your eating habits. (Altering the way you eat would reduce the accuracy of your project.) After completing the diary, add up the amounts of calcium you consume using EatRight Analysis or Nutritionist Pro software. The calcium RDA value for adults between the ages of 19 and 50 is 1,000 milligrams. How does your average calcium intake compare? If your calcium intake is not meeting the AI, how can you include more calcium in your diet?

Osmosis Experiment

Purchase some celery and let it sit for a week or two until it becomes limp. When the celery looks limp and lifeless, fill your sink with cold water and soak the celery. When it has soaked for several hours, take the celery out and examine its appearance. Notice anything different? Because the crispness of celery is the result of osmotic pressure, when you soaked the limp celery, it absorbed water into its cells and became crisp again.

What Does This Mean to Me?

Keep a log of everything you eat for 24 hours. Go to www.choosemyplate.gov/tools-supertracker to analyze your intake of calcium, magnesium, and sodium. How did you do?

References

1. Institute of Medicine, Food and Nutrition Board. *Dietary Reference Intakes for Water, Potassium, Sodium, Chloride, and Sulfate*. Washington, DC: National Academies Press; 2005.
2. Campbell SM. Hydration needs throughout the lifespan. *J Am Coll Nutr.* 2007;26:585S–587S.
3. Sawka MN, Burke LM, Eichner ER, et al. American College of Sports Medicine position stand: exercise and fluid replacement. *Med Sci Sports Exerc.* 2007;39:377–390.
4. Guyton AC, Hall JE. *Textbook of Medical Physiology*. 12th ed. Philadelphia: Elsevier Saunders; 2010.
5. Ibid.
6. Ibid.
7. Popkin BM, D'Anci KE, Rosenberg IH/ Water, hydration, and health. *Nutr Rev.* 2010;68(8):439–458.
8. Institute of Medicine, Food and Nutrition Board. *Dietary Reference Intakes for Water, Potassium, Sodium, Chloride, and Sulfate.* Op cit.
9. Ibid.
10. Popkin BM, D'Anci KE, Rosenberg IH. Water, hydration, and health. Op cit.
11. Shirreffs SM. Conference on "Multidisciplinary approaches to nutritional problems." Symposium on "Performance, exercise and health." Hydration, fluids and performance. *Proc Nutr Soc.* 2009;68(1):17–22.
12. Manz F. Hydration and disease. *J Am Coll Nutr.* 2007;26(5):535S–541S.
13. Institute of Medicine, Food and Nutrition Board. *Dietary Reference Intakes for Water, Potassium, Sodium, Chloride, and Sulfate.* Op cit.
14. Cosca DD, Navazio F. Common problems in endurance athletes. *Am Fam Phys.* 2007;76:237–244.

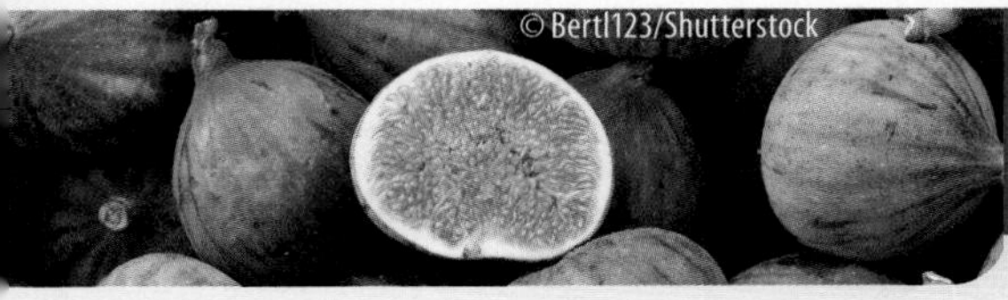

Learning Portfolio (continued)

15. Stuempfle KJ. Exercise-associated hyponatremia during winter sports. *Phys Sportsmed.* 2010;38(1):101–106.
16. Nevius CW. In hazing, dumb stunts can be fatal. *San Francisco Chronicle.* February 8, 2005. http://www.sfgate.com/bayarea/nevius/article/In-hazing-dumb-stunts-can-be-fatal-3313417.php. Accessed January 30, 2016.
17. Environmental Protection Agency. Aircraft drinking water rule (ADWR). http://water.epa.gov/lawsregs/rulesregs/sdwa/airlinewater/index.cfm. Accessed January 30, 2016.
18. U.S. Department of Health and Human Services and U.S. Department of Agriculture. *2015–2020 Dietary Guidelines for Americans.* 8th Edition. December 2015. Available at http://health.gov/dietaryguidelines/2015/guidelines/. Accessed April 28, 2016.
19. Ibid.
20. Institute of Medicine, Food and Nutrition Board. *Dietary Reference Intakes for Water, Potassium, Sodium, Chloride, and Sulfate.* Op cit.
21. American Heart Association. The American Heart Association's diet and lifestyle recommendations. May 2010. http://www.heart.org/HEARTORG/GettingHealthy/Diet-and-Lifestyle-Recommen-dations_UCM_305855_Article.jsp. Accessed January 30, 2016.
22. U.S. Department of Health and Human Services and U.S. Department of Agriculture. *2015–2020 Dietary Guidelines for Americans.* Op cit.
23. American Heart Association. The American Heart Association's diet and lifestyle recommendations. Op cit.
24. National Center for Health Statistics. *Health, United States, 2008.* Hyattsville, MD: Author; 2008.
25. The Dash Diet Eating Plan. http://dashdiet.org/default.asp. Accessed January 30, 2016.
26. American Heart Association. Your high blood pressure questions answered: potassium. http://www.americanheart.org. Accessed May 21, 2012.
27. Blumenthal JA, Babyak MA, Hinderliter A, et al. Effects of the DASH diet alone and in combination with exercise and weight loss on blood pressure and cardiovascular biomarkers in men and women with high blood pressure: the ENCORE study. *Arch Intern Med.* 2010;170(2):126–135.
28. Guyton AC, Hall JE. *Textbook of Medical Physiology.* Op cit.
29. Institute of Medicine, Food and Nutrition Board. *Dietary Reference Intakes for Water, Potassium, Sodium, Chloride, and Sulfate.* Op cit.
30. U.S. Department of Health and Human Services and U.S. Department of Agriculture. *2015–2020 Dietary Guidelines for Americans.* Op cit.
31. Yang Q, Liu T, Kuklina EV, et al. Sodium and potassium intake and mortality among US adults: prospective data from the Third National Health and Nutrition Examination Survey. *Arch Intern Med.* 2011;171(13):1183–1191.
32. Institute of Medicine, Food and Nutrition Board. *Dietary Reference Intakes for Water, Potassium, Sodium, Chloride, and Sulfate.* Op cit.
33. Guyton AC, Hall JE. *Textbook of Medical Physiology.* Op cit.
34. Howe TE, Shea B, Dawson LJ, et al. Exercise for preventing and treating osteoporosis in postmenopausal women. *Cochrane Database Syst Rev.* 2011;(7):CD000333.
35. National Institutes of Health, Office of Dietary Supplements. Calcium: dietary supplement fact sheet. http://ods.od.nih.gov/factsheets/calcium.asp. Accessed January 30, 2016.

36. National Academy of Science, Food and Nutrition Board. *Dietary Reference Intakes for Calcium and Vitamin D.* Washington, DC: National Academies Press; 2011.

37. Yang YJ, Martin BR, Boushey CJ. Development and evaluation of a brief calcium assessment tool for adolescents. *J Am Diet Assoc.* 2010;110:111–115.

38. National Institutes of Health, Office of Dietary Supplements. Calcium: dietary supplement fact sheet. Op cit.

39. National Academy of Science, Food and Nutrition Board. *Dietary Reference Intakes for Calcium and Vitamin D.* Op cit.

40. Rafferty K, Heaney RP. Nutrient effects on the calcium economy: emphasizing the potassium controversy. *J Nutr.* 2008;138(1 suppl):166S–171S.

41. National Academy of Science, Food and Nutrition Board. *Dietary Reference Intakes for Calcium and Vitamin D.* Op cit.

42. National Institutes of Health, Office of Dietary Supplements. Calcium: dietary supplement fact sheet. Op cit.

43. Ibid.

44. National Academy of Science, Food and Nutrition Board. *Dietary Reference Intakes for Calcium and Vitamin D.* Op cit.

45. Centers for Disease Control and Prevention. Nutrition for everyone: calcium and bone health. April 2011. http://www.cdc.gov/nutrition/everyone/basics/vitamins/calcium.html. Accessed January 30, 2016.

46. U.S. Department of Health and Human Services. *Bone Health and Osteoporosis: A Report of the Surgeon General.* Rockville, MD: U.S. Department of Health and Human Services, Office of the Surgeon General; 2004.

47. Institute of Medicine, Food and Nutrition Board. *Dietary Reference Intakes for Calcium, Phosphorus, Magnesium, Vitamin D, and Fluoride.* Washington, DC: National Academies Press; 1997.

48. Ibid.

49. Ibid.

50. Stein JH, Sande MA, Zvaifler NJ, et al. *Internal Medicine.* 5th ed. St. Louis: Mosby; 1998.

51. Lederer E, Ouseph R, Mittal D, et al. Hypophosphatemia: treatment and medication. Medscape. http://emedicine.medscape.com/article/242280-treatment. Accessed January 30, 2016.

52. Institute of Medicine, Food and Nutrition Board. *Dietary Reference Intakes for Calcium, Phosphorus, Magnesium, Vitamin D, and Fluoride.* Op cit.

53. Ibid.

54. Longo D, Fauci A, Kasper D, et al. *Harrison's Principles of Internal Medicine.* 18th ed. New York: McGraw-Hill; 2011.

55. Gropper SS, Smith JL, Groff JL. *Advanced Nutrition and Human Metabolism.* 5th ed. Belmont, CA: Wadsworth Cengage Learning; 2009.

56. Ibid.

Chapter 13

Trace Minerals

Revised by Diane K. Tidwell

THINK About It

1 You disclose to a friend that you tend to be low in iron. She knows you are a vegetarian and suggests you drink milk. What false assumption might she be making?

2 You know that a number of people in your family have had goiter or take thyroxine. You also notice that none of these people like fish or seafood. Any relationship?

3 Some people argue that fluoridation is overdone. What is your position? Would you vote for fluoridating all water supplies?

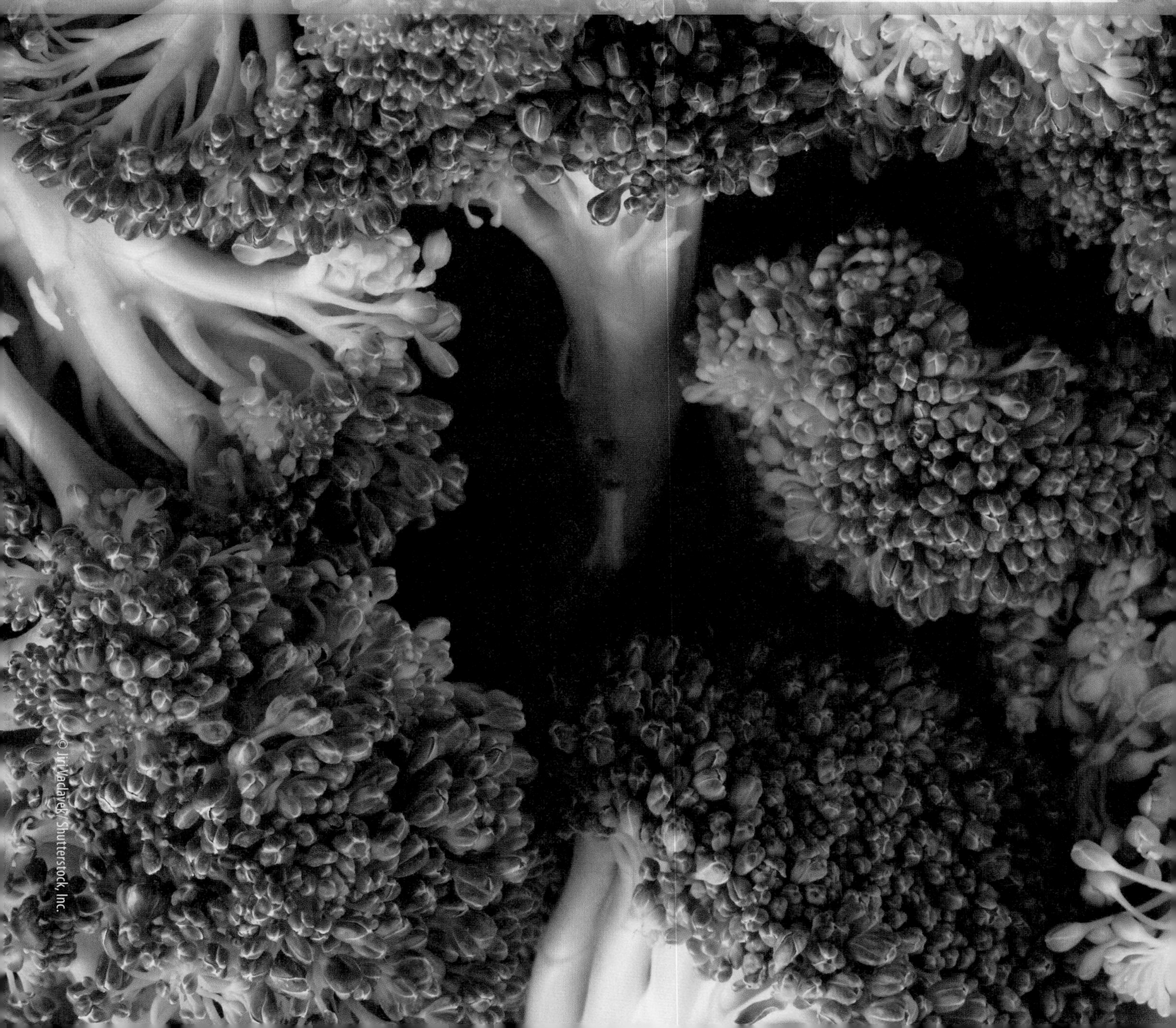

CHAPTER Menu

LEARNING Objectives

- Describe how diet can affect the bioavailability of trace minerals.
- Identify important sources of iron, zinc, selenium, iodine, manganese, fluoride, chromium, molybdenum, and copper in the diet.
- Identify situations in which trace mineral deficiency and toxicity can occur.
- Discuss the functional impact of marginal or inadequate intake of trace minerals on metabolism, body composition, and immune function.
- Describe trace mineral deficiency symptoms.
- Discuss positive effects and negative consequences of fluoridation of a water supply.
- Differentiate between trace and ultratrace minerals.

One of your "meat-and-potatoes" friends argues that animal foods are the best sources of minerals because animals concentrate the minerals they eat from plants. Your vegetarian friend disagrees, saying that minerals are plentiful in plant foods, but processing removes them. Another friend contends that American agricultural practices have stripped the mineral content from the soil, so supplements are really the only way to obtain adequate mineral intake. Who's right?

Protein-rich animal foods are good sources of some minerals such as calcium, phosphorus, and sulfur. Other major minerals (e.g., potassium, magnesium) are plentiful in plant foods. This chapter focuses on trace minerals—that is, minerals present in the body in small quantities, and therefore needed by the body in small amounts. Meats are the best food sources for some of these minerals—iron and zinc, for instance. Whole grains are also good sources of several minerals, including iron, copper, selenium, and manganese. Water is a major source of fluoride, a mineral that often occurs naturally in water or is added during municipal water treatment. But what about the mineral content of soil? (See **FIGURE 13.1**.) The mineral content of soil certainly influences the nutrient value of the plants that grow in it. This is especially true for the trace minerals selenium and iodine. How important is this to our dietary intake? Is the soil's mineral content depleted, as some supplement suppliers claim? Adequate nutrition is as important for healthy plants as it is for healthy livestock and people. If soil lacks a nutrient the plant needs, the plant will not grow properly. Fertilization adds nutrients to the soil, and so does the natural degradation of rocks, plants, and animals. There is little evidence for specific nutritional claims based on the mineral content of the soil. A varied diet typically includes foods from many different locales and thus from a wide variety of soils.

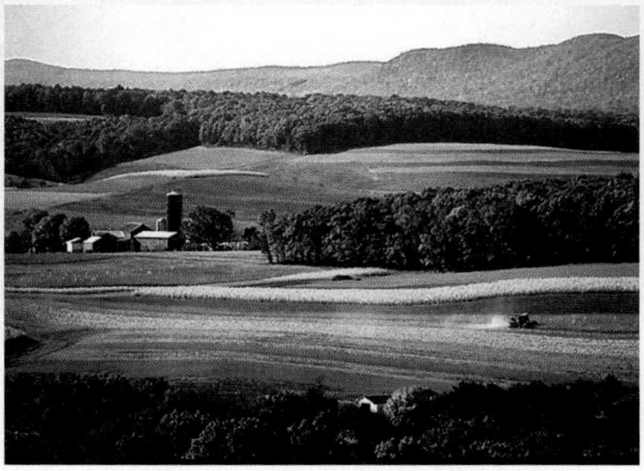

FIGURE 13.1 Mineral content of soil influences the nutrient value of plants. The mineral content of plants reflects the mineral content of the soil in which they are grown.

What Are Trace Elements?

Trace elements are essential minerals found in a large variety of animal and plant foods; these nutrients have both regulatory and structural functions in the body. Trace elements differ from the major minerals (e.g., calcium, phosphorus, magnesium) in two ways. First, the dietary requirements for each of the trace elements are less than 100 milligrams per day. For example, iron and zinc intake recommendations for adults range from 8 milligrams to 18 milligrams per day, whereas the adult daily calcium recommendation is

Quick Bite

Hair Analysis Is a Misguided Measure

Although discredited as a measure of trace mineral status in individuals, hair analysis is promoted with the claim that it can reveal mineral deficiencies. This measure lacks sensitivity and is unreliable. The color, diameter, and rate of growth of a person's hair, the season of the year, the geographic location, and the person's age and sex can affect the levels of minerals in hair. It is possible for hair concentration of an element (zinc, for example) to be high even though deficiency exists in the body. Hair dyes, perming agents, and certain shampoos also alter the mineral content of hair.

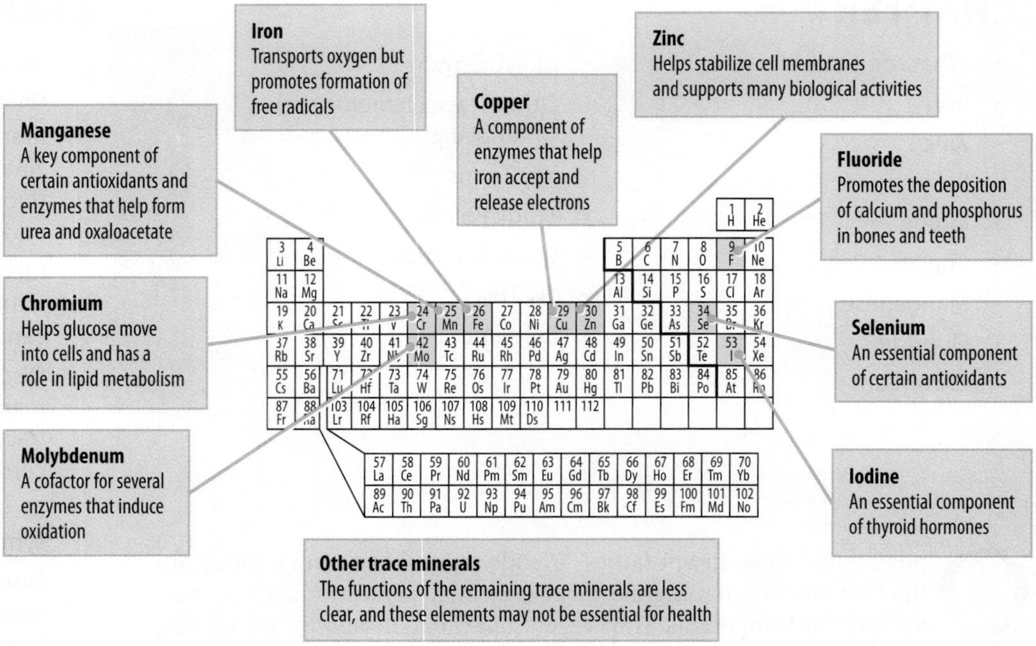

Iron
Transports oxygen but promotes formation of free radicals
Zinc
Helps stabilize cell membranes and supports many biological activities
Copper
A component of enzymes that help iron accept and release electrons
Manganese
A key component of certain antioxidants and enzymes that help form urea and oxaloacetate
Fluoride
Promotes the deposition of calcium and phosphorus in bones and teeth
Chromium
Helps glucose move into cells and has a role in lipid metabolism
Selenium
An essential component of certain antioxidants
Molybdenum
A cofactor for several enzymes that induce oxidation
Iodine
An essential component of thyroid hormones
Other trace minerals
The functions of the remaining trace minerals are less clear, and these elements may not be essential for health

FIGURE 13.2 Trace elements on the periodic table. Trace minerals are found in the body and required in the diet in small amounts, but they play important roles in the body.

1,000 milligrams per day. Second, the total amount of each trace element found in the body is small, less than 5 grams. For example, the total amount of iron in the body is 2 to 4 grams, or about the amount of iron in a small nail. In contrast, a typical adult body contains more than 1,000 grams of calcium. **FIGURE 13.2** shows the trace elements on the periodic table.

Why Are Trace Elements Important?

Despite the minuscule amounts in the body, trace elements are crucial to many body functions, including metabolic pathways. Trace elements serve as cofactors for enzymes, components of hormones, and participants in oxidation-reduction reactions. They are essential for growth and for normal functioning of the immune system. Deficiencies can cause delayed sexual maturation, poor growth, mediocre work performance, faulty immune function, tooth decay, and altered hormonal function.

Technological advances in recent years have triggered an explosion of exciting new research because scientists can now track trace elements throughout the body more effectively. Working together, nutritionists, biochemists, biologists, immunologists, geneticists, and epidemiologists are uncovering the mysteries behind many of these fascinating elements and finding new links between trace elements and a variety of diseases and genetic disorders.

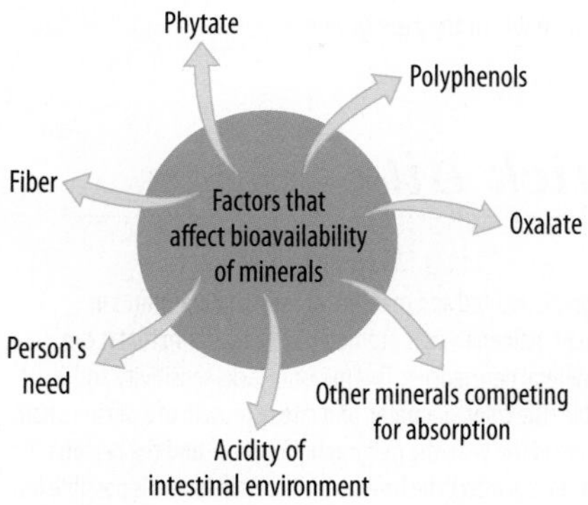

FIGURE 13.3 Factors that affect the bioavailability of minerals.

Other Characteristics of Trace Elements

Foods from animal sources, particularly liver, are good sources of many trace minerals. Amounts in plant foods can differ dramatically from region to region, depending on the soil's mineral content. Even the maturity of a vegetable, fruit, or grain can influence its mineral content.

The bioavailability of trace minerals is affected by the same factors that affect bioavailability of the major minerals (see **FIGURE 13.3**), including fiber, phytate, polyphenols, oxalate, the acidity of the intestinal environment, and the person's need for that mineral. High doses of some minerals can compete with trace minerals and inhibit their absorption. Treatment for mineral toxicity sometimes exploits these antagonistic interactions between minerals. For example, high doses of zinc might be given to patients with a genetic disorder of copper overload (Wilson disease) because zinc inhibits copper absorption.

Iron

Iron (Fe) is the fourth most abundant mineral in the earth's crust, yet iron deficiency is the most common nutrient deficiency in the world. Not only does iron deficiency affect a large number of children and women in developing countries, it is the only mineral deficiency that is significantly prevalent in industrialized countries.[1] On the other hand, hemochromatosis, a disease of excess iron absorption, is one of the most common inherited disorders. If not detected early, this disorder can damage organs severely, causing premature death.[2]

Why is iron useful? Iron has a special property. It easily changes between two of its oxidation states—**ferrous iron (Fe^{2+})** and **ferric iron (Fe^{3+})**—by transferring electrons to other atoms. This property makes iron essential for numerous oxidation-reduction reactions and allows it to bind reversibly with oxygen, nitrogen, and sulfur. The ability to shift easily between oxidative states also endows iron with its "dark side"—the ability to promote formation of destructive free radicals.

▶ **ferrous iron (Fe^{2+})** The reduced form of iron most commonly found in food.

▶ **ferric iron (Fe^{3+})** The oxidized form of iron able to be bound to transferrin for transport.

Functions of Iron

Iron is well known for its role in the body's use of energy; it is required for oxygen transport and is an essential component of hundreds of enzymes, many of which are involved in energy metabolism. In addition, iron plays a role in brain development and in the immune system.

Oxygen Transport

Iron's ability to carry oxygen is crucial. As a component of two **heme** proteins—hemoglobin and **myoglobin**—iron transports oxygen in the body. **FIGURE 13.4** shows the structures of heme and hemoglobin. With iron at the center, heme proteins have the unique chemical property of easily loading and unloading oxygen, and they give blood its red color. Hemoglobin in red blood cells transports oxygen in the blood, delivering it through the capillary beds to the tissues. Myoglobin in muscle facilitates the movement of oxygen into muscle cells.

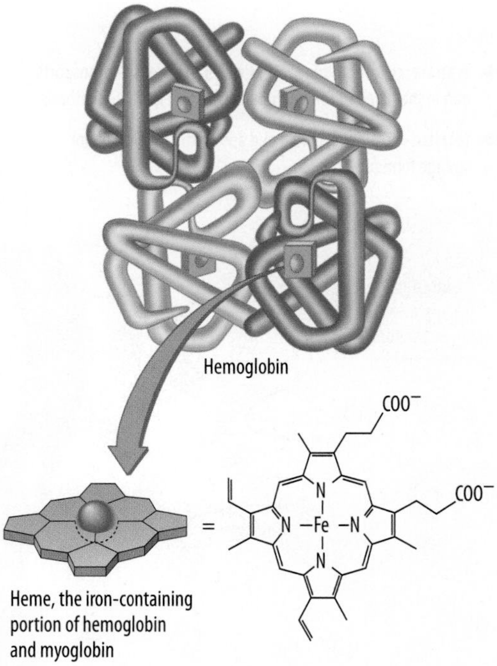

FIGURE 13.4 Heme in hemoglobin. Iron in the heme portion of hemoglobin and myoglobin binds and releases oxygen easily. Hemoglobin in red blood cells transports oxygen in the blood and gives blood its red color.

Enzymes

Hundreds of enzymes have iron as a constituent or need it as a cofactor in reactions. One of iron's best-known roles is as a component of enzymes involved in energy metabolism. **Cytochromes**, for example, are heme-containing compounds critical to the electron transport chain.

The rate-limiting enzyme in gluconeogenesis requires iron. Iron also is a cofactor for antioxidant enzymes that protect against damaging free radicals. Interestingly, excess iron can also catalyze the formation of these highly reactive and potentially destructive substances.

▶ **heme** A chemical complex with a central iron atom (ferric iron Fe^{3+}) that forms the oxygen-binding part of hemoglobin and myoglobin.

▶ **myoglobin** The oxygen-transporting protein of muscle that resembles blood hemoglobin in function.

▶ **cytochromes** Heme proteins that transfer electrons in the electron transport chain through the alternate oxidation and reduction of iron.

Energy Metabolism

Iron-containing enzymes play a vital role in reactions widespread in energy metabolism. Iron-containing proteins in the citric acid cycle and the electron transport chain are required for ATP production. Changes in the oxidation state of iron allow for transfer of electrons.

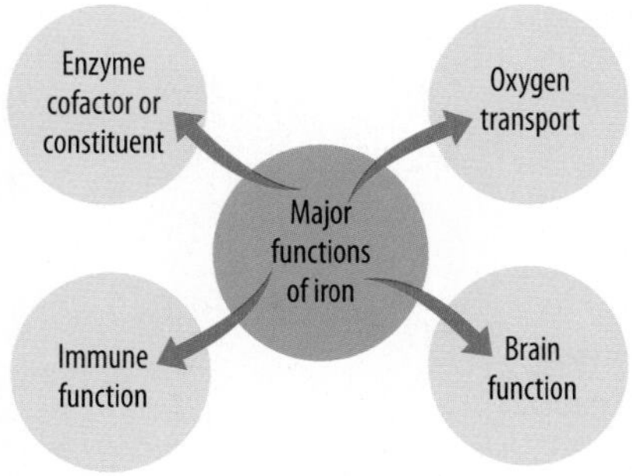

FIGURE 13.5 Major functions of iron. Well known for its role in transporting oxygen in the blood, iron also is essential for optimal immune function and nerve health. In addition, it is a cofactor in numerous reactions.

Immune Function

Optimal immune function requires iron, which creates a treatment dilemma in areas of the world with rampant disease and iron deficiency. Because iron nourishes certain bacteria, iron supplementation can worsen an infection. In the absence of an infection, iron supplementation is appropriate for treating iron deficiency (see **FIGURE 13.5**).

Regulation of Iron in the Body

Total body iron averages about 4 grams in men and a little more than 2 grams in women.[3] When the body has sufficient iron to meet its needs, most iron (greater than 70 percent) can be classified as functional iron; the remainder is storage or transport iron. The majority of the iron in the body, more than two-thirds, can be found in hemoglobin, and the rest is found in myoglobin and enzymes (e.g., cytochromes).[4] The body regulates its iron status by balancing absorption, transport, storage, and losses.[5]

Iron Absorption

The body controls its iron levels by regulating intestinal absorption.[6] When the absorptive mechanism operates normally, a person maintains functional iron and tends to establish iron stores. The body's capacity to absorb dietary iron depends on the body's iron status and need, normal gastrointestinal (GI) function, the amount and type of iron in the diet, and dietary factors that enhance or inhibit iron absorption.

▶ **transferrin** A protein synthesized in the liver that transports iron in the blood to the erythroblasts for use in heme synthesis.

▶ **ferritin** A complex of iron and apoferritin that is a major storage form of iron.

Process of Iron Absorption and Avoiding Iron Toxicity The body has a mechanism to avoid iron toxicity. (See **FIGURE 13.6**.) Intestinal cells act as gatekeepers, forming an initial barrier that turns away excess (and potentially harmful) iron. Once admitted into the intestinal cell, iron has three potential fates:

- It can be used by the cell itself.
- It can be released into the blood and carried to other tissues by **transferrin**, the major iron-transporting protein in the body.
- It can be stored as **ferritin**.

The body's need for iron determines its fate: The greater the need, particularly for synthesis of red blood cells, the more transferrin binds iron and transports it to bone marrow and other tissues. If iron stores are high, the extra iron remains in the cell and is excreted along with mucosal cells that are sloughed off at the end of their life cycle. In cells lining the small intestine, ferritin stores iron. These cells have a major role in regulating the amount of iron in the body and help prevent toxic accumulations.

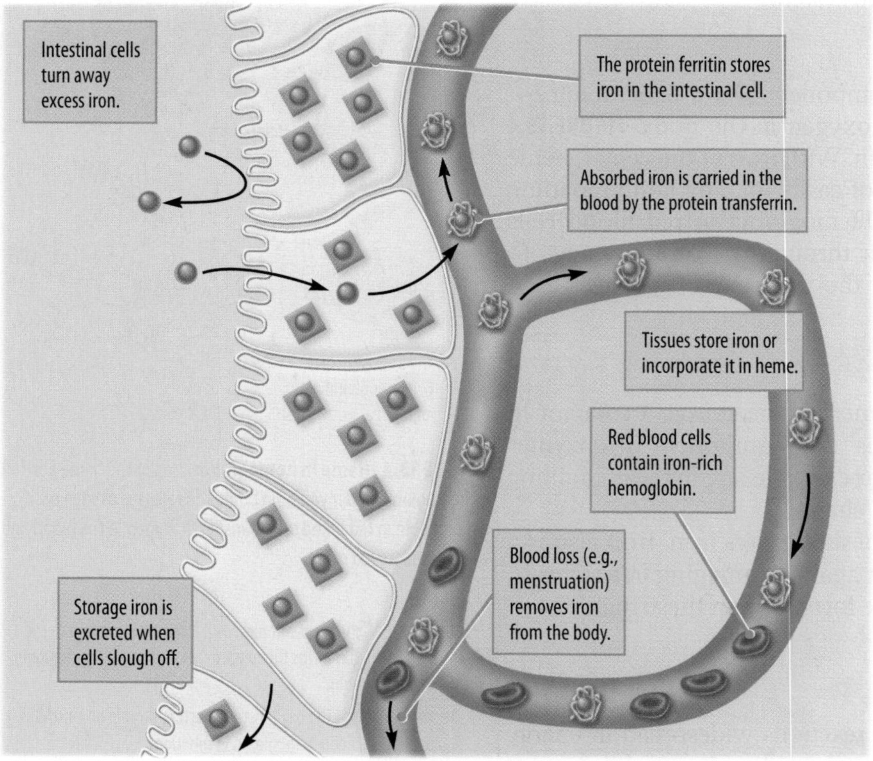

FIGURE 13.6 Iron absorption. The amount of iron absorbed depends on several factors: normal GI function, need for iron, the amount and kind of iron consumed, and dietary factors that enhance or inhibit iron absorption.

Effect of the Body's Iron Status on Iron Absorption Iron status is the primary factor in determining how much iron a person will absorb from food.[7] Depending on the size of the body's iron stores, absorption of dietary iron (i.e., iron bioavailability) can vary from less than 1 percent to greater than 50 percent. The GI tract increases iron absorption when the body's iron stores are low and decreases absorption when stores are sufficient. The body also gives priority to red blood cell production; an increased production rate, such as during pregnancy or after blood loss, can trigger a several-fold increase in iron uptake.[8]

Among adults, men absorb approximately 6 percent of dietary iron, and nonpregnant women of childbearing age absorb approximately 13 percent. Women's higher absorption rate primarily reflects their lower iron intake and higher iron losses as a result of menstruation. Iron absorption also is high among iron-deficient persons.

Effect of GI Function on Iron Absorption Although most iron absorption occurs in the duodenum and jejunum of the small intestine, the stomach also has an important role. Gastric acid facilitates the solubilization of iron and promotes the conversion of ferric iron (Fe^{3+}) to ferrous iron (Fe^{2+}), the form that most easily enters the absorptive intestinal cells. The stomach's retention and mechanical mixing of food also maximize iron's bioavailability. Gastric acid production generally declines with age, reducing iron absorption in older adults.

Effect of the Amount and Form of Iron in Food Food contains two types of iron—**heme iron** and **nonheme iron**. Heme iron is a part of hemoglobin and myoglobin, so it is found only in animal tissue. Heme iron is much more absorbable than nonheme iron. Although meat, fish, and poultry contain various amounts of heme iron and nonheme iron, the mix averages about 50 percent heme iron and 50 percent nonheme iron.[9] In contrast, plant-based and iron-fortified foods contain only nonheme iron (see **FIGURE 13.7**). Vegetarian diets, by definition, contain little to no heme iron.

Heme iron is much more bioavailable than nonheme iron.[10] Depending on the body's iron stores, heme iron absorption ranges from 15 to 35 percent of the amount ingested.[11] As the amount of iron ingested increases, the proportion absorbed decreases.

Dietary Factors That Enhance Iron Absorption Heme iron absorption is relatively independent of meal composition. However, meal composition strongly influences nonheme iron absorption. **TABLE 13.1** lists factors that inhibit or enhance absorption of iron. The two most important dietary factors that boost absorption of nonheme iron are organic acids, especially vitamin C (ascorbic acid), and meat, including fish and poultry. Organic acids maintain the iron in a soluble, bioavailable form as the stomach contents enter the duodenum. To exert this effect, ascorbic acid must be present in the same meal as the nonheme iron. Other organic acids (e.g., citric, malic, and tartaric acids) appear to have effects comparable to those of ascorbic acid. It is unclear exactly how meat enhances absorption of nonheme iron, but the presence of meat, fish, or poultry increases absorption efficiency.

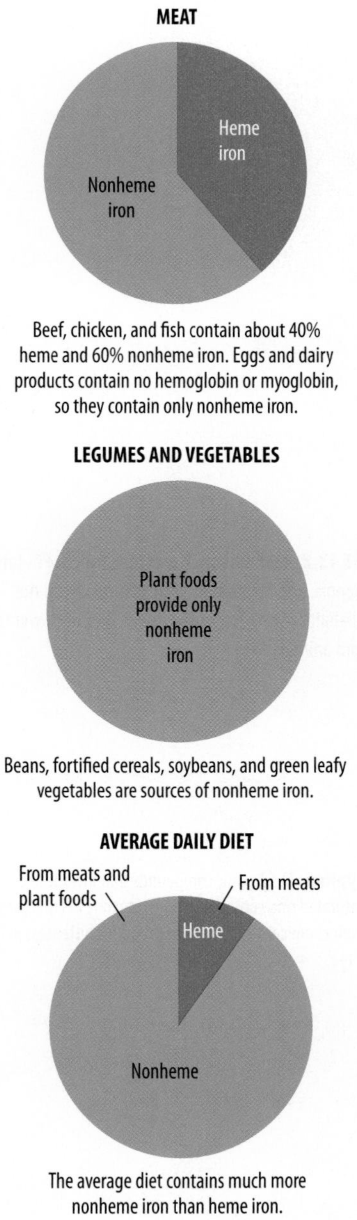
MEAT
Heme iron
Nonheme iron
Beef, chicken, and fish contain about 40% heme and 60% nonheme iron. Eggs and dairy products contain no hemoglobin or myoglobin, so they contain only nonheme iron.
LEGUMES AND VEGETABLES
Plant foods provide only nonheme iron
Beans, fortified cereals, soybeans, and green leafy vegetables are sources of nonheme iron.
AVERAGE DAILY DIET
From meats and plant foods
From meats
Heme
Nonheme
The average diet contains much more nonheme iron than heme iron.

FIGURE 13.7 Sources of heme and nonheme iron. Heme iron is found only in meats. Nonheme iron is found in both plant and animal foods. Eggs and dairy products contain only small amounts of nonheme iron.

▶ **heme iron** The iron found in the hemoglobin and myoglobin of animal foods.

▶ **nonheme iron** The iron in plants and the iron in animal foods that is not part of hemoglobin or myoglobin.

TABLE 13.1
Factors That Affect Iron Absorption

Inhibitors	Enhancers
• Fiber and phytate	• Vitamin C (ascorbic acid)
• Calcium and phosphorus (milk/dairy)	• Meat, poultry, and fish
• Tannins, found in tea and coffee	• Hydrochloric acid (HCl) secreted in the stomach
• Polyphenols	• Citric, malic, and tartaric acids
• Oxalate	

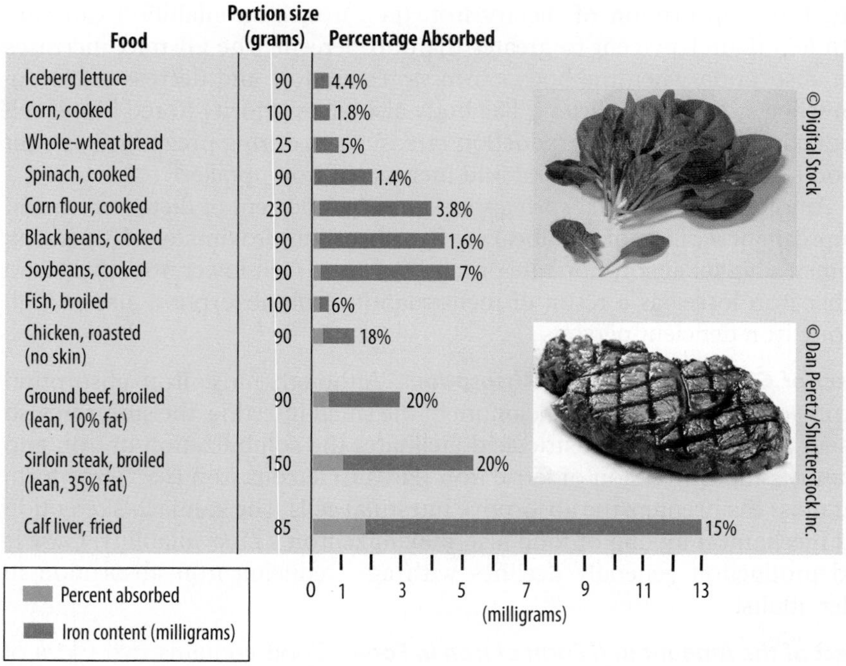

Food
Portion size (grams)
Percentage Absorbed
Iceberg lettuce 90 4.4%
Corn, cooked 100 1.8%
Whole-wheat bread 25 5%
Spinach, cooked 90 1.4%
Corn flour, cooked 230 3.8%
Black beans, cooked 90 1.6%
Soybeans, cooked 90 7%
Fish, broiled 100 6%
Chicken, roasted (no skin) 90 18%
Ground beef, broiled (lean, 10% fat) 90 20%
Sirloin steak, broiled (lean, 35% fat) 150 20%
Calf liver, fried 85 15%
Percent absorbed
Iron content (milligrams)
0 1 3 5 7 9 11 13
(milligrams)
© Digital Stock
© Dan Peretz/Shutterstock Inc.

FIGURE 13.8 Iron absorption from foods. Phytates, polyphenols, and fiber inhibit iron absorption, so the bioavailability of iron from plant foods is much lower than that from animal foods.

▶ **polyphenols** Organic compounds that include an unsaturated ring containing more than one OH group as part of their chemical structures; they produce bitterness in coffee and tea.

Dietary Factors That Inhibit Iron Absorption The most significant inhibitors of iron absorption are phytic acid (phytate), which is found in whole grains and legumes, and **polyphenols**, which are in tea, coffee, other beverages such as cola soft drinks, and many plants (see **FIGURE 13.8**). Even though minute amounts of these substances can reduce iron absorption, eating foods rich in vitamin C at the same meal counteracts this effect. The benefits of eating whole grains, which are nutrient dense and rich in fiber, outweigh the negative impact on iron absorption. Rather than cut back on whole grains, include small amounts of meat and/or generous amounts of vitamin C–rich fruits and vegetables with meals to improve iron absorption.

Other inhibitors of nonheme iron absorption include soy, calcium, zinc, oxalates, tannins (found in tea and coffee), and fiber. The long-term significance of these inhibitory factors on iron status is unclear. Calcium, zinc, and iron compete for absorption, and each can inhibit absorption of the other.[12] Many women take calcium supplements to reduce their risk of osteoporosis. To minimize interference with iron absorption, calcium supplements should be taken alone at bedtime rather than with meals.

Iron Absorption and Vegetarianism

When evaluating the nutritional value of a vegetarian or vegan diet, iron and zinc are key concerns. Even though total dietary iron intake meets recommended levels, vegetarians absorb less dietary iron and zinc than nonvegetarians. Factors include elimination of meat, reliance on less-well-absorbed nonheme iron, and increased intake of legumes and whole grains containing phytate, which inhibits absorption. Thus, vegetarians might need more dietary iron than those who eat animal products.[13] In developed countries with ample and varied food supplies, vegetarians generally consume sufficient iron. Although vegetarians tend to have lower iron stores than nonvegetarians, they appear to have no greater incidence of iron deficiency.

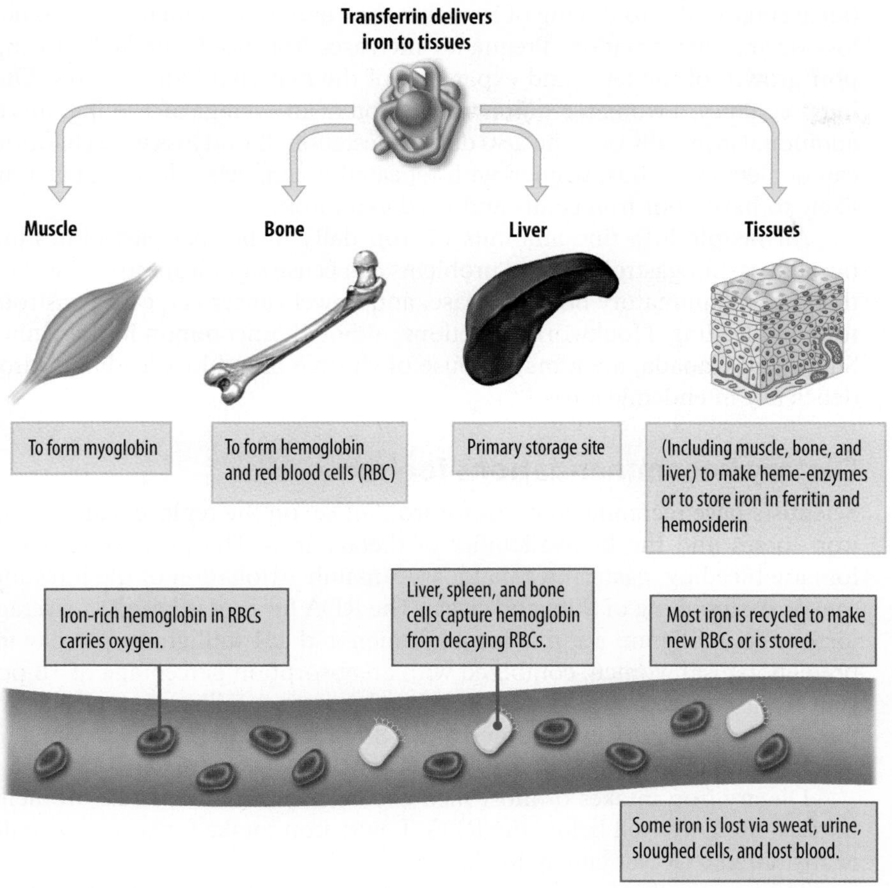
Transferrin delivers iron to tissues
Muscle
Bone
Liver
Tissues
To form myoglobin
To form hemoglobin and red blood cells (RBC)
Primary storage site
(Including muscle, bone, and liver) to make heme-enzymes or to store iron in ferritin and hemosiderin
Iron-rich hemoglobin in RBCs carries oxygen.
Liver, spleen, and bone cells capture hemoglobin from decaying RBCs.
Most iron is recycled to make new RBCs or is stored.
Some iron is lost via sweat, urine, sloughed cells, and lost blood.

FIGURE 13.9 Iron in the body. Transferrin transports iron to tissues for the synthesis of heme or storage in ferritin and hemosiderin.

Iron Transport and Storage

Transferrin delivers iron from the intestines to the tissues and redistributes iron from storage sites to various body compartments. Individual cells take up the iron transported on transferrin by way of **transferrin receptors** on the cell membranes.[14] The number of transferrin receptors varies with the cell's need for iron; tissues with the highest iron need (e.g., bone marrow, liver, placenta) have the highest concentration of transferrin receptors (see **FIGURE 13.9**).

The body stores surplus iron either as part of the soluble protein complex ferritin or as the insoluble protein complex **hemosiderin**. The liver, bone marrow, spleen, and skeletal muscle harbor most of the body's ferritin and hemosiderin, and small amounts of ferritin circulate in the bloodstream. In healthy people, ferritin contains most of the stored iron. When long-term negative iron balance depletes iron stores, iron deficiency begins.

▶ **transferrin receptors** Specialized receptors on the cell membrane that bind transferrin.

▶ **hemosiderin** An insoluble form of storage iron.

Iron Turnover and Loss

The body tightly regulates its iron content to ensure adequate stores while protecting against toxicity. It recycles iron and adjusts absorption and excretion as needed.

Red blood cell formation and destruction are responsible for most iron turnover. In adult men, for example, the breakdown of older red blood cells supplies approximately 95 percent of the iron required to produce new red blood cells. Dietary sources supply only 5 percent. In contrast, this balance is 70/30 in infants, whose growth needs tend to outstrip the recycled supply.

Adults lose about 1 milligram of iron daily in feces and sloughed-off mucosal and skin cells. Women of childbearing age require additional iron

Quick Bite

But It Worked in the Lab . . .

The evidence is clear from carefully conducted clinical trials that supplements reduce iron deficiency during pregnancy. However, public health supplementation programs in communities often are unsuccessful. Why the discrepancy? Although clinical trials support the distribution and consumption of iron pills, programs in the "real world" have several limiting factors: inadequate supply of iron tablets, limited access to care, poor or nonexistent nutrition counseling, lack of knowledge, and the uncomfortable side effects experienced by some women. These factors are important causes of noncompliance. However, with adequate resources and nutrition counseling, iron supplementation can be successful for improving iron status.

(an average of 0.3 to 0.5 mg of iron absorbed daily) to compensate for blood loss during menstruation. Pregnancy increases iron needs markedly to support growth of the fetus and expansion of the maternal blood supply. During pregnancy, a woman requires absorption of an average of 4 milligrams of additional iron daily over the 280 days of gestation. Blood loss with childbirth can deplete iron; thus, women with repeated pregnancies close together are likely to have poor iron status and need extra iron.

All people lose tiny amounts of iron daily in normal gastrointestinal blood loss, but gastrointestinal problems can cause significant iron loss. Peptic ulcer, inflammatory bowel disease, and bowel cancer can cause gastrointestinal bleeding. Hookworm infections, although uncommon in the United States and Canada, are a major cause of chronic blood loss leading to iron deficiency in endemic areas.[15]

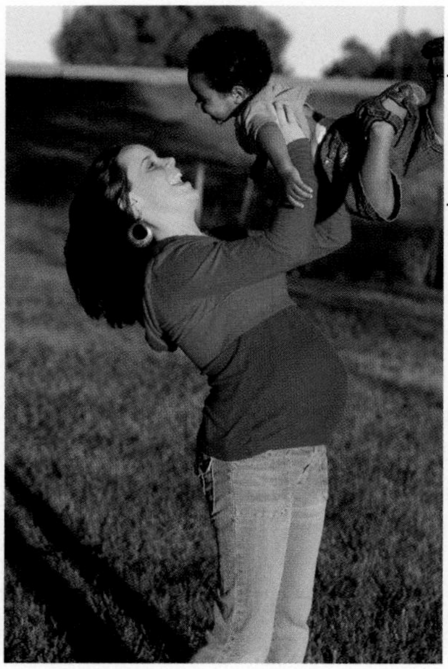

Dietary Recommendations for Iron

Scientists base recommendations for iron intake on the replacement of daily iron losses and the bioavailability of dietary iron. The primary routes of loss are bleeding, gastrointestinal losses (mainly exfoliation of the intestinal mucosa), sloughing of skin, and sweat. The RDA for iron is based on average losses of 1 milligram per day for adult men and 1.4 milligrams per day for premenopausal women, combined with an absorption percentage of 18 percent from a mixed diet. The RDAs for adults are 8 milligrams per day for men and postmenopausal women and 18 milligrams per day for women of childbearing age.[16]

Dietary iron intakes of most men exceed their RDA, whereas women's intakes often are well below the RDA. Lower iron intake for women usually is attributed to lower energy intake.

The iron needs of infants are a special concern. During the final weeks of pregnancy, fetuses ideally store enough iron in the liver, bone marrow, spleen, and hemoglobin-rich blood to see them through their first six months of life. However, if the mother's iron nutrition is poor or the baby is born early, the baby's iron stores are smaller and do not last. To help ensure that babies have adequate iron, pregnant women are urged to meet the RDA of 27 milligrams per day. Baby cereal and many infant formulas are fortified with iron.

Sources of Iron

Beef is an excellent dietary source of iron, in terms of both amount and bioavailability. Other excellent sources include clams, oysters, and liver. Poultry, fish, pork, lamb, tofu, and legumes are also good sources. Whole-grain and enriched-grain products contain less bioavailable iron than meat but are significant sources of iron because they constitute a major part of our diets. Fortified cereals also make an important contribution to iron intake in the United States. Dairy products are low in iron. **FIGURE 13.10** shows the iron content of some foods.

A varied diet (adequate in calories, rich in fruits and vegetables, and with small amounts of lean animal flesh) generally provides adequate iron. Vegetarians who consume no animal tissue can maximize iron bioavailability from other sources by consuming vitamin C–rich fruits and vegetables with every meal. THINK About It 1

Iron Deficiency and Measurement of Iron Status

Iron deficiency is the most common nutritional deficiency worldwide. Although significantly more prevalent in developing countries than in the rest of the world, it remains a public health concern in the United States. Infants and

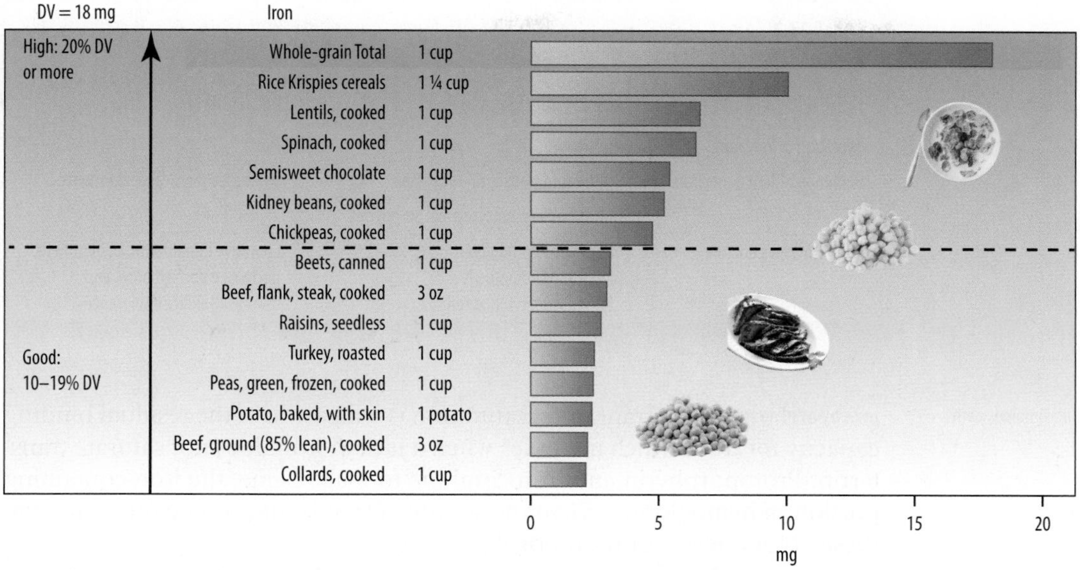

FIGURE 13.10 Food sources of iron. Iron is found in red meats, certain types of seafood, vegetables, and legumes and is added to enriched grains and breakfast cereals.

Data from US Department of Agriculture, Agricultural Research Service, Nutrient Data Laboratory. USDA National Nutrient Database for Standard Reference, Release 28. Version Current: September 2015. Internet: http://www.ars.usda.gov/nea/bhnrc/ndl.

toddlers, adolescent girls, women of childbearing age, and pregnant women are particularly vulnerable.

Iron deficiency is most prevalent in 6- to 24-month-old children, who are in a period of rapid brain growth and development of cognitive and motor skills. Iron stores from fetal development have been depleted, and a major source of energy in the young child's diet is milk, a poor source of iron. If iron stores are not replaced before the child passes critical developmental milestones, developmental deficits from iron deficiency can be irreversible.

Significant and potentially irreversible alterations in brain and central nervous system development can occur in infants who experience iron deficiency during the early stages of life.[17] Children with low iron levels also are more likely to have sleep disturbance and attention-deficit/hyperactivity disorder.[18] Research in this area is still evolving and complicated by the difficulty of separating the roles of iron deficiency and other environmental factors (e.g., generalized malnutrition, poverty, and low parental education) that also impair psychomotor and mental development.

Progression of Iron Deficiency

Iron deficiency progresses through three distinct stages, shown in **TABLE 13.2**.

Depletion of iron stores is the first stage of iron deficiency, which causes no physiological impairments. Because serum ferritin is proportional to the body's total iron stores, a test of serum ferritin is a good way to assess iron deficiency.

Depletion of functional and transport iron is the second stage of iron deficiency—the stage between iron depletion and actual anemia. This intermediate stage is measured by the serum level of transferrin receptors (TfRs). As the body's iron status falls, TfR levels increase in proportion to the iron deficit. Other blood values used to detect this stage are **transferrin saturation** and

▶ **transferrin saturation** The extent to which transferrin has vacant iron-binding sites (e.g., low transferrin saturation indicates a high proportion of vacant iron-binding sites).

TABLE 13.2
Stages of Iron Deficiency

Stage	Biochemical Sign	Functional Implications
Depletion of iron stores	Decreased ferritin	None
Depletion of functional iron	Decreased transferrin saturation	Decreased physical performance
	Increased erythrocyte protoporphyrin	
Iron-deficiency anemia	Decreased hemoglobin Decreased hematocrit Decreased red blood cell size	Cognitive impairment, poor growth, decreased performance, and decreased exercise tolerance

▶ **protoporphyrin** A chemical complex that combines with iron to form heme.

▶ **hematocrit** Percentage volume occupied by packed red blood cells in a centrifuged sample of whole blood.

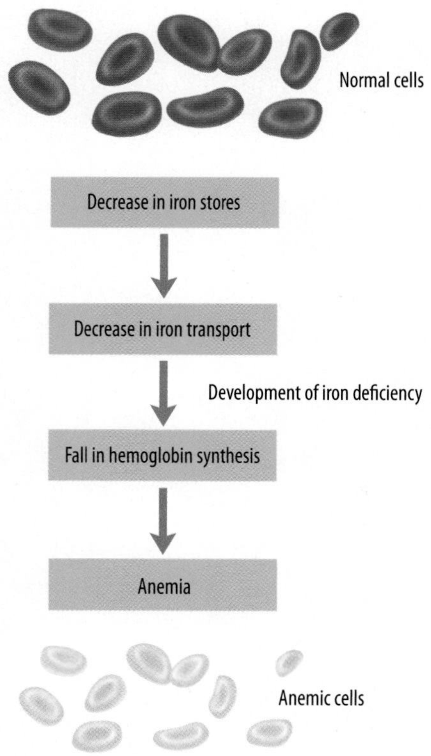

FIGURE 13.11 Normal and anemic red blood cells. Iron deficiency can progress to iron-deficiency anemia, a severe form of iron deficiency that is accompanied by low hemoglobin levels.

protoporphyrin levels. Transferrin saturation is a measure of the residual binding capacity for iron, which increases when a lack of iron does not saturate transferrin. Protoporphyrin and iron combine to make heme, the iron-containing portion of hemoglobin. When the supply of iron is inadequate for heme synthesis, blood levels of protoporphyrin rise.

Because second-stage iron depletion impairs the function of iron-requiring enzymes needed for aerobic energy production, an iron-depleted person might be unable to work at full capacity. The impact of mental and physical performance impairments in iron deficiency even without anemia is a cause for concern for women in roles such as the military. Prevalence rates of almost 30 percent for iron deficiency and 13 percent for iron-deficiency anemia have been found among active female recruits.[19] More human studies are required to determine whether iron depletion affects other physiological processes.

The third and most severe stage of iron deficiency is anemia—a disease characterized by insufficient or defective red blood cells, or both. A lack of iron inhibits production of normal red blood cells, while normal cell turnover continues to deplete the red blood cell population. Red blood cell production falters, producing red blood cells that are pale and smaller than normal. Hemoglobin and **hematocrit** (concentration of red blood cells in the blood) levels also are low. This type of anemia, known for its small, pale red blood cells, is called microcytic hypochromic anemia. Inadequate vitamin B_6 also can cause microcytic hypochromic anemia. Another type of anemia, megaloblastic anemia, is known for its abnormally large, immature red blood cells and is caused by inadequate folate or vitamin B_{12}. **FIGURE 13.11** shows normal and anemic blood cells.

The symptoms of microcytic hypochromic anemia vary according to its severity and the speed of its development. They include fatigue, pallor, breathlessness with exertion, decreased tolerance of cold, behavioral changes, deficits in immune function, cognitive impairment, decreased work performance, and impaired growth. In children, iron deficiency is associated with apathy, short attention span, irritability, and reduced ability to learn.[20]

Iron Toxicity

The Tolerable Upper Intake Level (UL) for iron is based on the level that causes gastrointestinal distress. For adults, the UL for iron is 45 milligrams per day.

Iron Poisoning in Children

Accidental iron overdose is a leading cause of poisoning deaths in young children in the United States.[21] Parents who are cautious about keeping medications out of reach often do not realize that over-the-counter iron tablets and even iron-containing multivitamin/mineral supplements for children can be toxic. Just a few pills can cause the death of a small child. Symptoms of iron toxicity include nausea, vomiting, diarrhea, rapid heartbeat, dizziness, and confusion. Death can occur within hours of ingestion. If iron poisoning is suspected, the child should receive immediate emergency medical care.

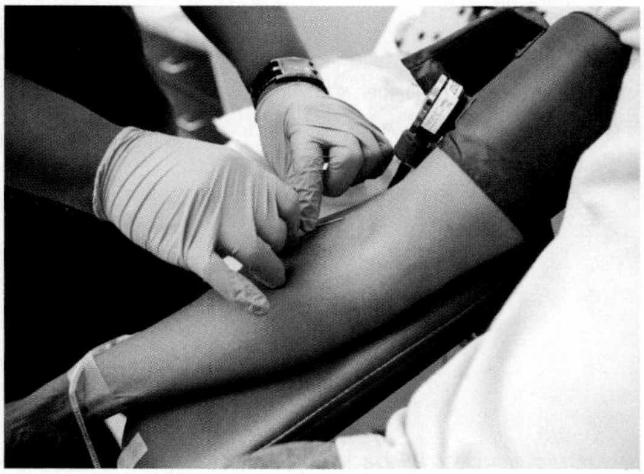

Hereditary Hemochromatosis

Hereditary hemochromatosis is a form of chronic **iron overload**. Although it was once believed to be rare, scientists now know that mild forms are quite common and estimated to affect 1 to 6 people per 100 in the United States.[22] A genetic defect causes excessive iron absorption. Over the years, iron can build up in many parts of the body, leading to severe organ damage and even death. Diabetes, heart disease, cirrhosis, liver cancer, and arthritis can all be consequences of hemochromatosis. Serious complications of hemochromatosis are 5 to 10 times more common in men than in women, primarily because of women's blood loss associated with menstruation and pregnancy. Treatment of hemochromatosis includes minimizing iron intake and frequent phlebotomy (removal of blood) to withdraw some of the iron that blood carries in cells. With early diagnosis and treatment, a person with hemochromatosis can avoid organ damage and other complications and have a normal life span.

▶ **iron overload** Toxicity from excess iron.

Key Concepts Iron is essential for life but highly toxic in excess. Iron is a key component of the oxygen transporters hemoglobin and myoglobin and of many enzymes involved in energy metabolism. Heme iron is absorbed more efficiently than nonheme iron. The body carefully regulates iron absorption; iron can be bound to transferrin for transport or stored as ferritin or hemosiderin. The best dietary source of iron is red meat. Iron deficiency develops gradually, with anemia being the most severe manifestation of deficiency. Iron poisoning is potentially deadly, especially for young children. Hereditary hemochromatosis is a common genetic disease that causes iron overload.

Quick Bite

Grandma's Cast-Iron Skillet Helped Her Avoid Iron Deficiency

Iron deficiency is the most common form of malnutrition in the United States. However, this is a relatively recent phenomenon. Americans used to cook using cast-iron pots and pans. A study showed that using these utensils to cook acidic foods like spaghetti sauce and apple butter increases the iron content of such foods by a factor of 30- to 100-fold. Our preference for stainless steel, aluminum, and enamelware does not allow this fortification.

Zinc

It's hard to believe that a nutrient so important to health could go unnoticed until as recently as 50 years ago, but that is the case with zinc (Zn). Some people think of zinc only in connection with the "zinc oxide" cream used topically as a sunscreen or with zinc lozenges promoted as a treatment for colds; few students realize that dietary zinc is absolutely essential for health.

Scientists first recognized human zinc deficiency in 1961.[23] They found severe zinc deficiencies in young, severely growth-retarded Iranian men. In

Going Green

Could Iron Help Cool Global Warming?

Recent experimentation, as well as geological records, suggest that iron deficiency is limiting phytoplankton production. Researchers studying ocean sediment cores suggest that ice ages were preceded by high levels of ocean iron. They inferred that this iron, derived from terrestrial environments, balanced the natural oceanic iron deficit and resulted in the eruption of plant and phytoplankton life. From the surface waters, phytoplankton drew down carbon dioxide from the atmosphere. Scientists believe that this drawdown of the greenhouse gas led to global cooling and ice ages.

▶ **hypogonadism** Decreased functional activity of the gonads (ovaries or testes) with retardation of growth and sexual development.

▶ **geophagia** Ingestion of clay or dirt.

addition to suffering from dwarfism, these men were anemic and extremely lethargic and had **hypogonadism** (poorly developed genitals), and some could not see well in the dark. Their diets consisted mainly of wheat bread and were almost devoid of animal protein. These men also were known to eat clay (**geophagia**). Scientists hypothesized that the high phytate content of their diet, along with the geophagia, impaired absorption of both zinc and iron. Six years later, a study in Egypt confirmed zinc's role; zinc supplementation improved growth and genital development.[24]

Functions of Zinc

▶ **galvanized** Iron or steel with a thin layer of zinc plated onto it to protect against corrosion.

The body contains a small amount of zinc—between 1.5 and 2.5 grams, or about the same amount of zinc as is in a **galvanized** nail, which has a thin layer of zinc to protect it from corrosion. Zinc is a component of every living cell. The functions of zinc fall into three categories: catalytic, structural, and regulatory. Zinc is best known for its participation in enzyme structure and function, but it also supports many other diverse biological activities through a role in controlling gene regulation. **FIGURE 13.12** illustrates the functions of zinc in the body.

Zinc and Enzymes

▶ **metalloproteins** Proteins with a mineral element as an essential part of their structure.

Zinc is critical to the proper function of more than 70 and possibly more than 200 enzymes.[25] As a component of **metalloproteins**, which are proteins that have a mineral as an essential part of their structure, zinc is essential for their structural integrity and function, regulation of their activities, and their ability to catalyze reactions. In the cytoplasm, zinc and copper are key components of superoxide dismutase, an enzyme that speeds antioxidant reactions and helps protect cells from free radical damage.

Zinc's Role in Nucleic Acid Metabolism

Zinc also is inextricably linked to gene expression. In severe zinc deficiency, cells fail to replicate. This may be why zinc is so important for the normal growth of children and the sexual maturation of adolescents. Furthermore, certain tissues with high turnover rates, such as cells lining the GI tract, skin cells, immune cells, and blood cells, are particularly vulnerable to a zinc deficiency. As a result, zinc-deficient people often have diarrhea, dermatitis, and depressed immunity.

Zinc and the Immune System

Zinc is vital to a vigorous immune response and is essential to the proper development and maintenance of the immune system. Without zinc, your body could not fight off invading viruses, bacteria, and fungi. Even mild deficiency can increase the risk of infection.

Zinc and Gene Regulation

Zinc enables certain small proteins to fold and form a stable "zinc-finger" structure. This structure interacts with a region of DNA. Without zinc, that area of a gene will not function.[26] This function of zinc can explain how it influences the immune system. Discovery and characterization of zinc-finger protein families are active areas of nutrition research.

Zinc and Vision

Zinc-deficient people can show signs of night blindness or other classic signs of vitamin A deficiency. Zinc is a key component of the enzyme that activates vitamin A in the retina. Thus, a lack of zinc interferes with vitamin A activity in the eye.

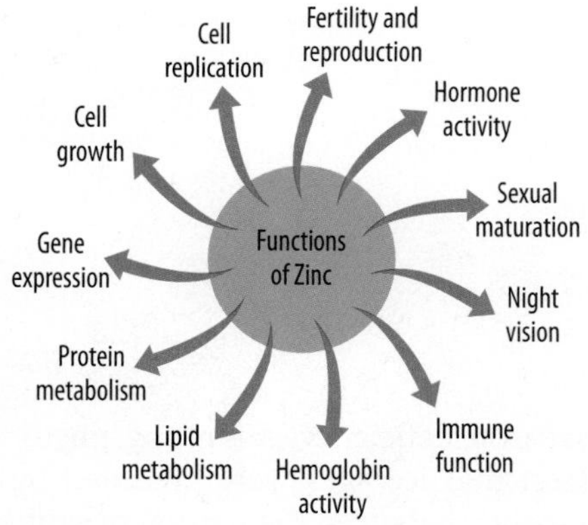

FIGURE 13.12 Functions of zinc in the body. Because zinc is involved in so many different functions, it is fortunate that overt zinc deficiency is rare.

Other Zinc Functions

Zinc is essential for a number of other diverse biological functions:

- *Hormonal:* Zinc interacts with a number of hormones, including insulin and its influence on carbohydrate metabolism.
- *Growth and reproduction:* Zinc plays an important role in pregnancy outcome, fetal development, and bone health.
- *Hemoglobin activity:* Zinc increases the affinity of hemoglobin for oxygen and indirectly influences hemoglobin synthesis.
- *Taste and smell:* Zinc participates in taste perception, smell or olfactory function, and appetite regulation.
- *Cell death:* Zinc can induce as well as inhibit the process of apoptosis, also known as programmed cell death.[27]
- *Wound healing:* Since ancient Egyptian times, zinc has been used to enhance wound healing.[28] Zinc participates in the maintenance of skin and mucosal membrane integrity.[29] Skin ulcers are frequently treated with zinc supplementation.

Regulation of Zinc in the Body

Zinc Absorption

The body absorbs small amounts of zinc more effectively than large doses, and absorption ranges between 10 and 35 percent—a range similar to heme iron absorption. The degree of zinc absorption depends on the person's zinc status and zinc needs, the zinc content of the meal, and the presence of competing minerals. People with zinc deficiency absorb zinc more thoroughly than those with optimal zinc status. Absorption increases during times of increased need, such as growth spurts, pregnancy, and lactation. On the other hand, certain dietary factors, such as phytate and fiber, can impair absorption of zinc. **FIGURE 13.13** shows the zinc absorption process.

▶ **albumin** A protein that circulates in the blood and functions in the transport of many minerals and some drugs.

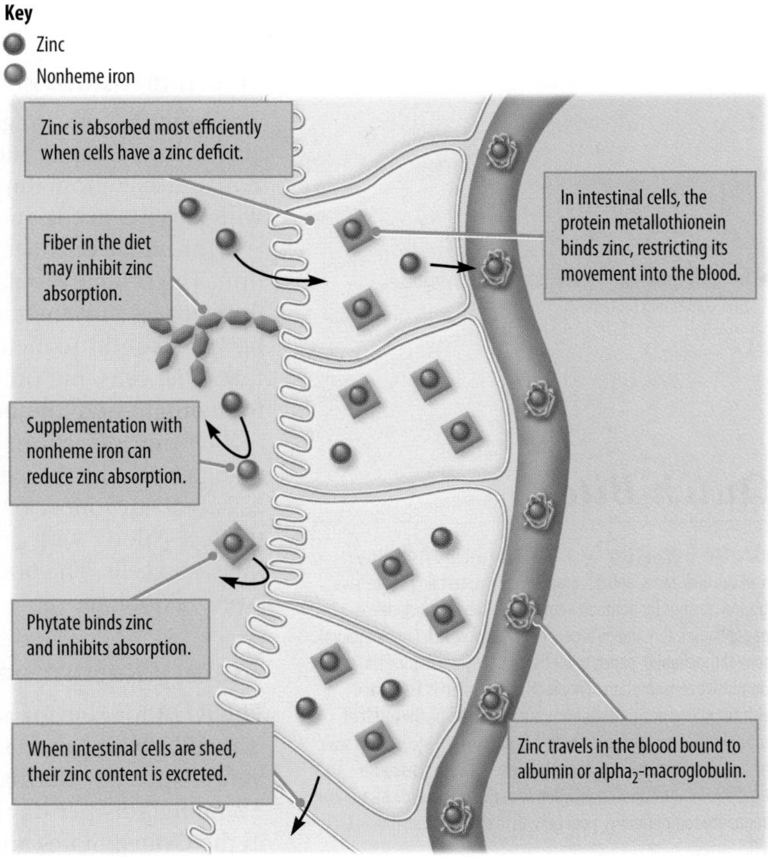

Key
Zinc
Nonheme iron
Zinc is absorbed most efficiently when cells have a zinc deficit.
Fiber in the diet may inhibit zinc absorption.
Supplementation with nonheme iron can reduce zinc absorption.
Phytate binds zinc and inhibits absorption.
When intestinal cells are shed, their zinc content is excreted.
In intestinal cells, the protein metallothionein binds zinc, restricting its movement into the blood.
Zinc travels in the blood bound to albumin or alpha$_2$-macroglobulin.

FIGURE 13.13 Zinc absorption. Intestinal cells act as temporary buffers that help regulate zinc absorption.

Dietary Factors That Inhibit Zinc Absorption

Phytate from whole grains is the main dietary factor that inhibits zinc absorption.[30] For vegetarians whose diet consists of mainly phytate-rich unrefined grains and legumes, zinc requirements can exceed the RDAs.[31] Although calcium supplements can interfere with the absorption of zinc, dietary calcium does not appear to reduce zinc absorption.[32,33] Nonheme iron in the form of iron supplements also depresses zinc absorption.[34] Iron from food, whether heme iron (from meat) or nonheme iron, does not have the same effect.[35]

Zinc Transport and Distribution

Zinc circulates in the bloodstream loosely bound to **albumin** and more tightly bound to another protein, alpha-2-macroglobulin. Zinc travels to the liver and to the tissues where it is most needed. Muscle and bone contain 90 percent of the body's zinc; the remainder is divided primarily among the liver, kidneys, pancreas, brain, skin, and prostate. **FIGURE 13.14** shows zinc in the body.

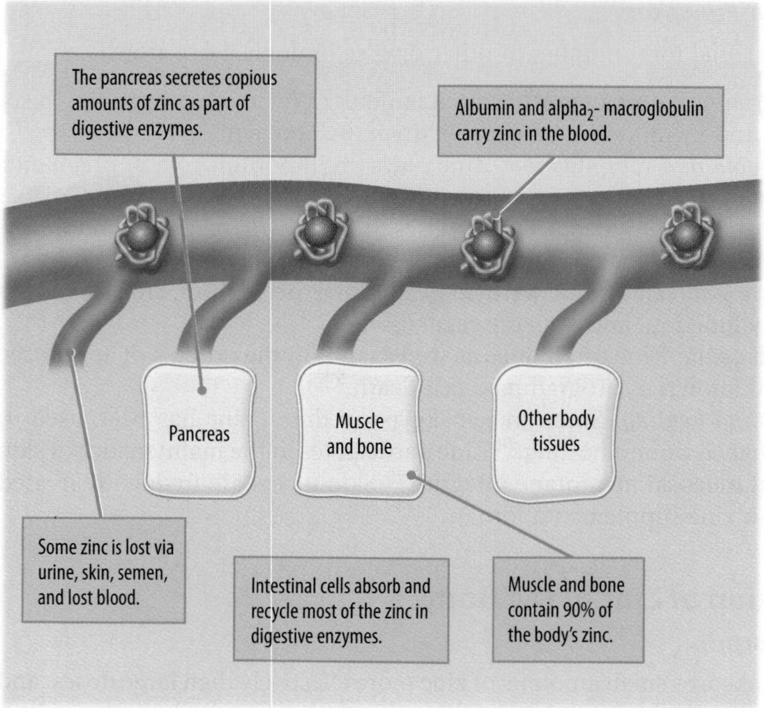

The pancreas secretes copious amounts of zinc as part of digestive enzymes.
Albumin and alpha2- macroglobulin carry zinc in the blood.
Pancreas
Muscle and bone
Other body tissues
Some zinc is lost via urine, skin, semen, and lost blood.
Intestinal cells absorb and recycle most of the zinc in digestive enzymes.
Muscle and bone contain 90% of the body's zinc.

FIGURE 13.14 Zinc in the body. Zinc is a component of every living cell and helps stabilize cell membranes. More than 80 enzymes contain zinc.

Zinc Homeostasis and Excretion

The body has no long-term storehouse of zinc to draw upon when dietary zinc is low. Despite the lack of zinc storage, the body balances zinc absorption and excretion, thus maintaining zinc homeostasis even when confronted with varying needs and dietary conditions.

Intestinal cells act as temporary buffers that help regulate zinc absorption. The protein **metallothionein** binds zinc in the intestinal mucosal cells and impedes its movement into the bloodstream. When zinc intake is high, the body makes more metallothionein to retain more zinc in the intestinal cells. Intestinal cells and other cells produce zinc transporter proteins, which help to maintain body homeostasis.[36]

▶ **metallothionein** An abundant, nonenzymatic, zinc-containing protein.

During digestion, the pancreas secretes as much as 4.0 milligrams of zinc per day in the pancreatic juice. When the body needs zinc, intestinal cells reabsorb most of this secreted zinc. Otherwise, the body excretes it in the feces along with unabsorbed dietary zinc and sloughed, zinc-containing intestinal cells. The body also excretes zinc in minor amounts through urine, sweat, skin, hair, semen, and menstrual fluids.

Dietary Recommendations for Zinc

The RDA for zinc for adult males is 11 milligrams per day, and for females it is 8 milligrams per day. Experts recommend increasing zinc intake to 11 milligrams per day during pregnancy to provide for the growing fetus, and to 12 milligrams per day during lactation. Although most children and adults in the United States and Canada consume more than the RDA, a significant number of older adults eat less than recommended levels.[37]

Quick Bite

Bizarre Behavior or Nutritional Deficiency?

In all cultures, races, and geographic regions, certain people have strange cravings for nonfood items. These cravings include ice (pagophagia), clay and dirt (geophagia), cornstarch (amylophagia), stone (lithophagia), paper, toilet tissue, soap, and foam. Pica, the compulsive consumption of nonfood items, often is associated with either iron or zinc deficiency, but it can also be the result of cultural beliefs or a response to family stresses. Whatever the cause, the behavior is not benign. It can injure teeth as well as cause constipation, intestinal obstruction or perforation, lead poisoning, pregnancy complications, poor growth in children, and mineral deficiencies.

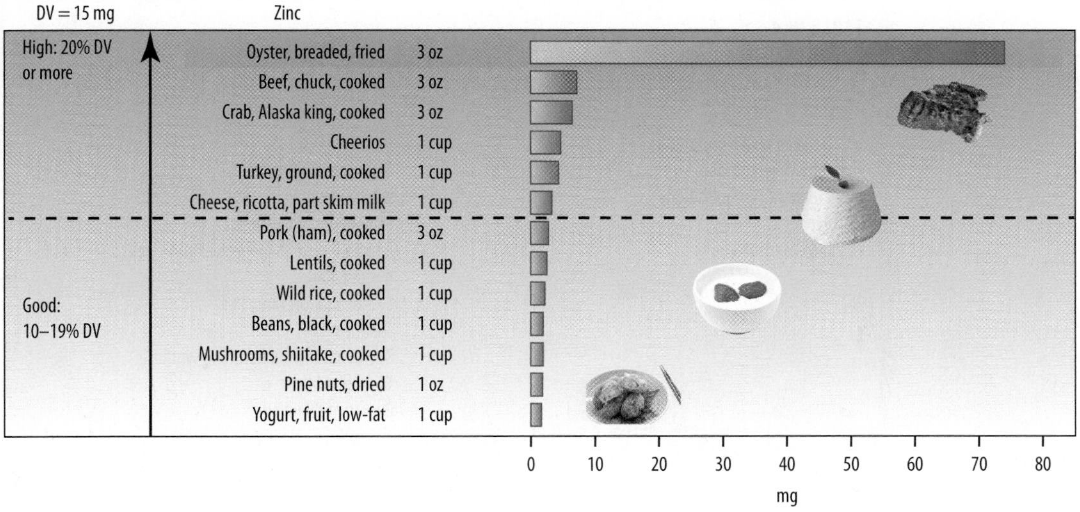

FIGURE 13.15 Food sources of zinc. Meats, organ meats, and seafood are the best sources of zinc.

Data from US Department of Agriculture, Agricultural Research Service, Nutrient Data Laboratory. USDA National Nutrient Database for Standard Reference, Release 28. Version Current: September 2015. Internet: http://www.ars.usda.gov/nea/bhnrc/ndl.

Photos (from top to bottom): (chuck roast) © MSPhotographic/Shutterstock, Inc.; (fresh ricotta) © BrunoRosa/Shutterstock, Inc.; (strawberry yogurt) © Watthano/Shutterstock, Inc.; (Japanese food) © jreika/Shutterstock.com.

Sources of Zinc

Zinc usually is abundant in foods that are good sources of protein, especially red meat and seafood such as oysters and clams. For poultry, dark meat is a richer source than white meat. The zinc in animal foods is generally well absorbed. Conversely, whole grains have a relatively high amount of zinc, but it is poorly absorbed. Fruits and vegetables generally are poor zinc sources. Adequate zinc intake is of special concern for vegetarians because they do not eat many of the foods that are the best sources of this mineral. **FIGURE 13.15** shows the zinc content of some foods.

Zinc Deficiency

In the United States and Canada, zinc deficiency is uncommon and usually occurs in people with illnesses that impair absorption. In other parts of the world, zinc deficiency is most prevalent in populations that subsist on cereals and little else. Diarrhea and chronic infections such as pneumonia can cause excessive zinc excretion. These diseases are commonplace in developing countries, where zinc deficiency is widespread. In some of these areas, zinc supplementation has decreased the incidence of acute lower respiratory infection, diarrhea, and attacks of malaria in children.

As **TABLE 13.3** shows, the primary culprits in marginal zinc deficiency are increased needs, poor intake, poor absorption, and excessive losses. During pregnancy, zinc deficiency contributes to complications and low birth weight.[38] Malabsorption syndromes such as cystic fibrosis and **Crohn's disease** impair zinc absorption. Symptoms of moderate to severe zinc deficiency include poor growth, delayed or abnormal sexual development, diarrhea, severe skin rash and hair loss, impaired immune response, and impaired taste and smell acuity (see **TABLE 13.4**).

TABLE 13.3
Risk Factors for Zinc Deficiency

Dietary Deficiency
• IV feeding without zinc • Protein-energy malnutrition • Poor food choices • Vegan diets
Increased Requirements
• Chronic infection • Burn patients • Growth spurts • Pregnancy and lactation
Malabsorption
• Acrodermatitis enteropathica • Celiac disease, Crohn's disease • Chronic iron supplementation • Cystic fibrosis • Geophagia or pica • High-phytate diets
Increased Losses
• Burns and surgery • Chronic diarrhea • Diabetes • Renal disease • Sickle cell disease

▶ **Crohn's disease** A disease that causes inflammation and ulceration along sections of the intestinal tract.

TABLE 13.4
Effects of Zinc Deficiency

Moderate Deficiency	Severe Deficiency
• Delayed sexual maturation • Growth retardation • Pregnancy complications • Acne • Increased infections	• Hypogonadism • Cessation of growth • Patchy loss of hair • Skin lesions and rashes • Impaired taste (hypogeusia) and smell (olfactory dysfunction) • Loss of appetite/anorexia • Diarrhea • Decreased thyroid hormone synthesis • Night blindness • Recurrent infections

Zinc Toxicity

Isolated accounts reported acute zinc toxicity in people who consumed large amounts of acidic foods or beverages that had been stored in galvanized containers. Although toxicity from high dietary zinc intake is rare, chronic supplementation with too much zinc has adverse effects. High doses of zinc can cause acute gastrointestinal distress, nausea, vomiting, and cramping. The UL for zinc is 40 milligrams per day.

► **Wilson disease** Genetic disorder of increased copper absorption, which leads to toxic levels in the liver and heart.

Chronic doses of zinc (100 to 150 mg/day) for prolonged periods can interfere with copper metabolism and cause low blood copper levels and impaired immunity.[39] Doctors use the interaction of zinc and copper to treat people with **Wilson disease**, a genetic disorder of hyperabsorption and accumulation of copper. Zinc works by blocking copper absorption and increasing its excretion, thus preventing its accumulation in the body. For those who cannot tolerate drug treatment, zinc supplements of 150 milligrams daily can help prevent copper accumulation.[40]

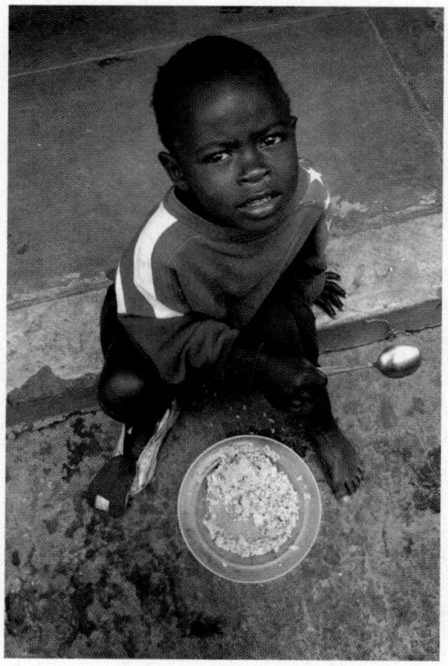

Key Concepts Zinc is important for normal growth and development, immune function, and the function of many enzymes. Zinc homeostasis is maintained by regulating intestinal absorption. Iron, zinc, and copper all compete for absorption, but problems do not usually occur if these minerals are coming from balanced dietary rather than supplemental sources. The best food sources for zinc are beef, oysters, crab, legumes, and unrefined whole grains. Zinc deficiency is most prevalent in populations that subsist on cereal protein.

Selenium

► **Keshan disease** Selenium-deficiency disease that impairs the structure and function of the heart.

The story of selenium (Se) is a recent one and becomes more complex as scientists explore its role at the molecular level. Historically, because animals grazing on selenium-rich soils suffered selenium poisoning, scientists focused on its toxicity. This changed in 1957, when researchers first demonstrated selenium's nutritional benefits in vitamin E–deficient animals. But not until 1979 did evidence emerge that selenium is essential for humans. Chinese scientists reported an association between low selenium status and **Keshan disease**, a heart disorder that strikes children in the Keshan province of China. The Chinese scientists demonstrated that selenium supplements could prevent the disease. Although selenium deficiency does not cause the disease, it predisposes a child to heart damage after a particular type of viral infection. When selenium intake is adequate, the virus apparently does not cause Keshan disease.

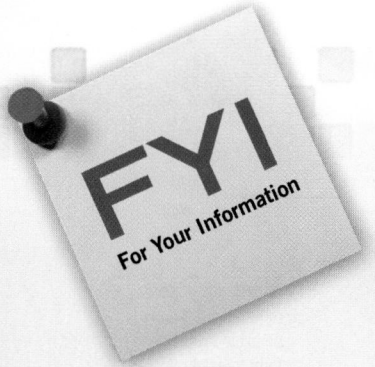

FYI For Your Information

Zinc and the Common Cold

The common cold, one of our most common illnesses, affects American adults 2 to 4 times per year and children 6 to 10 times per year.[a] Colds are even more frequent in young children in day care settings and preschools. Because of missed work and decreased productivity, colds can be economically costly as well as a physical nuisance. A cure for the common cold would be of great benefit, and scientists have long pursued this goal.

Although scientists have suggested several hypotheses, the mechanism underlying a person's vulnerability to contracting a cold remains unclear. Zinc deficiency is known to impair immune function, but could all these people have been zinc deficient? This is doubtful. Some speculate that zinc can reduce the severity and duration of cold symptoms by inhibiting viral replication. This is why products such as zinc lozenges and zinc syrups are under investigation.

Although overall zinc supplementation can be beneficial under certain circumstances, studies of zinc and colds have produced conflicting results. One older study with positive results gained considerable attention from the press, and as a result, zinc lozenges are on nearly every pharmacy shelf in the United States. In this study, colds resolved in an average of four days for participants in the zinc group, as compared to seven days for the control group.[b] The same researchers then studied children who took zinc gluconate lozenges at the first sign of cold symptoms but found no difference for all cold symptoms to resolve—a median of nine days.[c]

Research continues to provide mixed results, with some studies finding a benefit of lozenges[d] and others finding no effect of zinc supplementation.[e] Review studies also have reported inconclusive findings.[f]

A large systematic review of scientific literature reported benefits and concluded that "zinc (lozenges or syrup) is beneficial in reducing the duration and severity of the common cold in healthy people, when taken within 24 hours of onset of symptoms. People taking zinc are also less likely to have persistence of their cold symptoms beyond seven days of treatment."[g]

High doses of zinc could have harmful effects beyond mild side effects and cost of lozenges. People taking zinc lozenges (not syrup or tablet form) are more likely to experience adverse events, including bad taste and nausea.[h] Long-term use of high doses of zinc also could induce copper deficiency. In addition, loss of smell from the use of nasal zinc sprays prompted the FDA to issue a warning in 2009 instructing consumers to discontinue their use.[i]

Research to determine the effects of zinc for the treatment of the common cold is ongoing. Before a general recommendation can be made for using zinc in the treatment of the common cold, additional research is needed to determine the best formulation, dose, and treatment duration that provide a clinical benefit with minimal adverse effects.[j] Until there is more scientific agreement and standardized treatments, we should regard zinc as we would any other medical therapy and think twice before routinely giving children (and ourselves) zinc lozenges every time a cold strikes.

[a] National Institute of Allergy and Infectious Diseases. Common colds: protect yourself and others. http://www.niaid.nih.gov/topics/commoncold/Pages/default.aspx. Accessed January 8, 2016.

[b] Mossad SB, Macknin ML, Medendorp SV, Mason P. Zinc gluconate lozenges for treating the common cold: a randomized, double-blind placebo-controlled study. *Ann Intern Med*. 1996;125:81–88.

[c] Macknin ML, Piedmonte M, Calendine C, et al. Zinc gluconate lozenges for treating the common cold in children: a randomized controlled trial. *JAMA*. 1998;279:1962–1967.

[d] Prasad AS, Beck FW, Bao B, et al. Duration and severity of symptoms and levels of plasma interleukin-1 receptor antagonist, soluble tumor necrosis factor receptor, and adhesion molecules in patients with common cold treated with zinc acetate. *J Infect Dis*. 2008;197:795–802.

[e] Eby GA, Halcomb WW. Ineffectiveness of zinc gluconate nasal spray and zinc orotate lozenges in common-cold treatment: a double-blind, placebo-controlled clinical trial. *Altern Ther Health Med*. 2006;12:34–38.

[f] Caruso TJ, Prober CG, Gwaltney JM Jr. Treatment of naturally acquired common colds with zinc: a structured review. *Clin Infect Dis*. 2007;45:569–574.

[g] Marshall I. Zinc for the common cold. *Cochrane Database Syst Rev*. 2011;(2):CD001364.

[h] Ibid.

[i] U.S. Department of Agriculture and U.S. Food and Drug Administration. Warnings on three Zicam intranasal zinc products. http://www.fda.gov/ForConsumers/ConsumerUpdates/ucm166931.htm. Accessed January 8, 2016.

[j] Marshall I. Zinc for the common cold. Op cit.

Functions of Selenium

Although scientists have identified nearly 50 selenium-containing proteins, two amino acid derivatives—**selenomethionine**, a methionine derivative, and **selenocysteine**, a cysteine derivative—contain most of the body's selenium. Selenomethionine is a selenium "storage compartment," and selenocysteine is selenium's biologically active form. As selenocysteine, selenium is a component of enzymes involved in antioxidant protection and thyroid hormone metabolism.

Selenium is best known as a component of glutathione peroxidases, a family of antioxidant enzymes. The discovery of these enzymes resolved a puzzling overlap in the functions of selenium and vitamin E. Both nutrients play a role in preventing lipid peroxidation and membrane damage. Glutathione peroxidases promote the breakdown of fatty acids that have

▶ **selenomethionine** A selenium-containing amino acid derived from methionine that is the storage form of selenium.

▶ **selenocysteine** A selenium-containing amino acid that is the biologically active form of selenium.

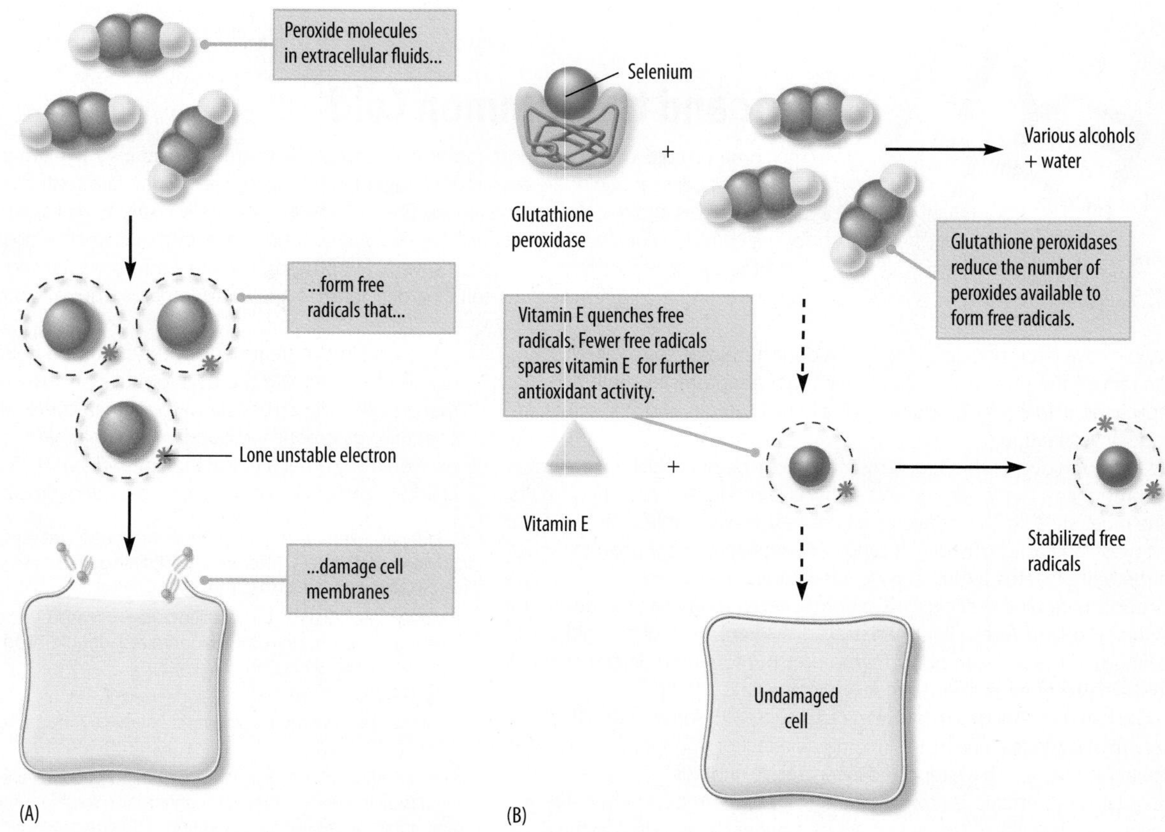

FIGURE 13.16 Free radicals. (a) Peroxides form free radicals that damage cell membranes and have been implicated in heart disease. (b) Selenium and vitamin E help combat free radicals. Because glutathione peroxidases require selenium, dietary selenium indirectly spares vitamin E.

undergone peroxidation, thus eliminating highly reactive free radicals (see **FIGURE 13.16A**). This reduction in free radicals spares vitamin E, making it available to stop other chain reactions of free radicals (see **FIGURE 13.16B**). Because glutathione peroxidases require selenium, dietary selenium indirectly spares vitamin E.

▶ **hypothyroidism** The result of a lowered level of circulating thyroid hormone, with slowing of mental and physical functions.

▶ **cretinism** A congenital condition often caused by severe iodine deficiency during gestation, which is characterized by arrested physical and mental development.

Scientists have identified selenium as a component of enzymes involved in the metabolism of iodine and thyroid hormone. Iodine deficiency alone causes **hypothyroidism**, and a combined deficiency of selenium and iodine increases the severity of the disease. There also is some evidence that a combined deficiency of both minerals during pregnancy is involved in some forms of **cretinism** in newborns.

Selenium is important in the immune system and its response to infections. Research suggests that selenium might have some anticancer benefits, but more investigation is needed.[41] Ongoing population research and large-scale trials are working to determine selenium's relationship to cancer. Small increases in selenium intake can be toxic, and selenium supplements for cancer prevention are not recommended. Selenium is also under investigation for its role in heart disease, arthritis, and HIV.[42]

Regulation of Selenium in the Body

Selenomethionine and selenocysteine are the principal dietary forms of selenium. The body efficiently absorbs these selenoamino acids, with estimates ranging from 50 to 90 percent.[43] The presence of vitamins A, C, and E and reduced glutathione enhance selenium absorption, but phytates and heavy metals such as mercury interfere with its bioavailability.

The selenium regulatory process maintains a low concentration of highly reactive free selenocysteine and achieves homeostasis through excretion of excess mineral. The major routes of selenium excretion are the urine and the feces. When intake is excessive, the skin and lungs serve as additional excretory routes.

Selenium status, like the status of many trace minerals, is difficult to evaluate. There are no sensitive tests that can readily distinguish between adequate and suboptimal levels of selenium.

Quick Bite

On Your Next Moonlit Stroll, Think Selenium!

Selenium takes its name from the Greek word *Selênê*, "moon," because it has a pasty white color. In mythology, Selene is the Greek goddess of the moon. Ancient Greeks often blamed Selene and her brother Helios (god of the sun) for pestilent diseases and death.

Dietary Recommendations for Selenium

Selenium is one of the "youngest" nutrients for which an RDA exists. The first RDA for selenium was established in 1989. The RDA was based on data from Chinese scientists who conducted repletion experiments in selenium-depleted subjects living in areas where Keshan disease was endemic. The RDA for selenium was revised in 2000. For both men and women, the selenium RDA is 55 micrograms per day.[44]

Sources of Selenium

Selenium levels are quite variable in plant foods and generally reflect the selenium content of the soil in which the plant was grown. Because animals accumulate selenium in their tissues, the selenium content of food from animal sources generally is more consistent than the selenium content of plants. Organ meats and seafood are consistently good selenium sources. Other meats contain somewhat lower amounts of the mineral. The typical American diet provides adequate selenium. **FIGURE 13.17** shows some food sources of selenium.

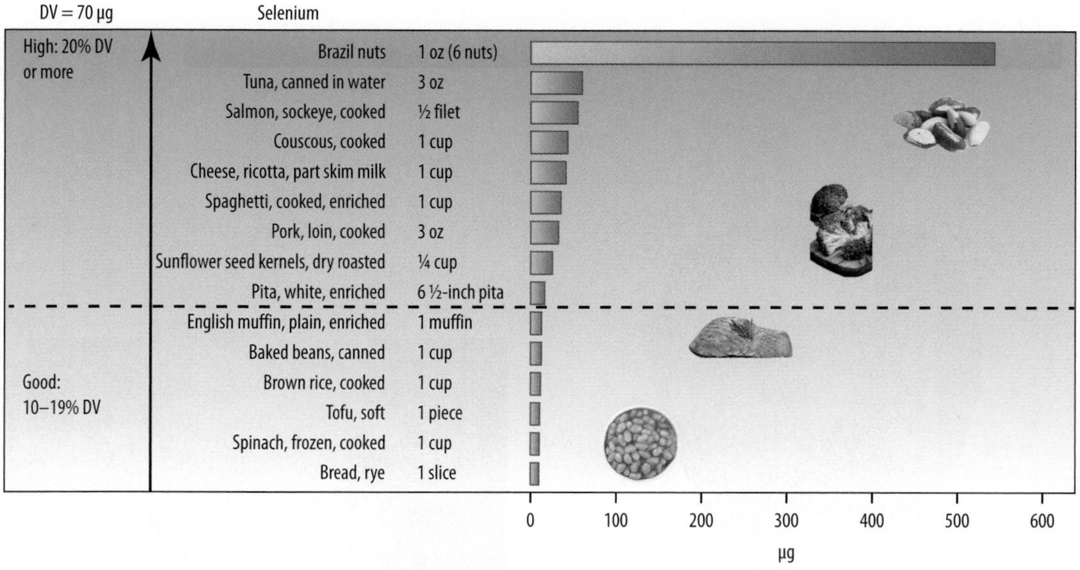

FIGURE 13.17 Food sources of selenium. Selenium is found mainly in meats, organ meats, seafood, and grains. Brazil nuts are exceptionally high in selenium.

Data from US Department of Agriculture, Agricultural Research Service, Nutrient Data Laboratory. USDA National Nutrient Database for Standard Reference, Release 28. Version Current: September 2015. Internet: http://www.ars.usda.gov/nea/bhnrc/ndl.

Photos (from top to bottom): (Brazil nuts) © Leonid Shcheglov/Shutterstock, Inc.; (raw organic broccoli) © poplasen/ iStock/Getty Images Plus; (grilled salmon) © amenic181/Shutterstock, Inc.; (baked beans) © Paul_Brighton/Shutterstock, Inc.

Selenium Deficiency

Selenium deficiency is rare, although it can be seen where soil selenium concentrations are low. Chronic selenium deficiency interferes with immune function. Three conditions have been associated with selenium deficiency: Keshan disease, which occurs in selenium-deficient children and results in an enlarged heart and poor heart function; Kashin-Beck disease, which results in diseases of the joints and bones; and cretinism, which results in mental retardation.[45]

Doctors have found selenium deficiency in people who receive long-term **total parenteral nutrition (TPN)**. Although after several years of TPN these patients might suffer heart problems and muscle weakness, no specific visible symptoms have been defined for selenium deficiency.

▶ **total parenteral nutrition (TPN)** Feeding a person by giving all essential nutrients intravenously.

Selenium Toxicity

Chronic consumption of excess selenium can cause brittle hair and nails, and their eventual loss. Although typical dietary intakes are unlikely to exceed safe amounts, selenium supplements can cause problems. Overenthusiastic media reports of research on selenium and cancer, coupled with easy access to selenium supplements, might cause some people to consume unhealthful quantities. The UL is set at 400 micrograms per day for adults.[46]

Key Concepts Selenium is best known for its role as an essential component of the antioxidant enzymes glutathione peroxidases. Selenium interacts with vitamin E in antioxidant systems and with iodine in thyroid hormone metabolism. It also is important for good immune function. Good dietary sources for selenium are organ meats and seafood. A deficiency of selenium can predispose a child to Keshan disease, a rare heart disease caused by a virus. New research also links marginal selenium status to cancer risk.

Iodine

Ancient Chinese writings first recorded descriptions of what we now know to be the iodine-deficiency diseases cretinism and **goiter** (see **FIGURE 13.18**).

▶ **goiter** A chronic enlargement of the thyroid gland, visible as a swelling at the front of the neck; usually associated with iodine deficiency.

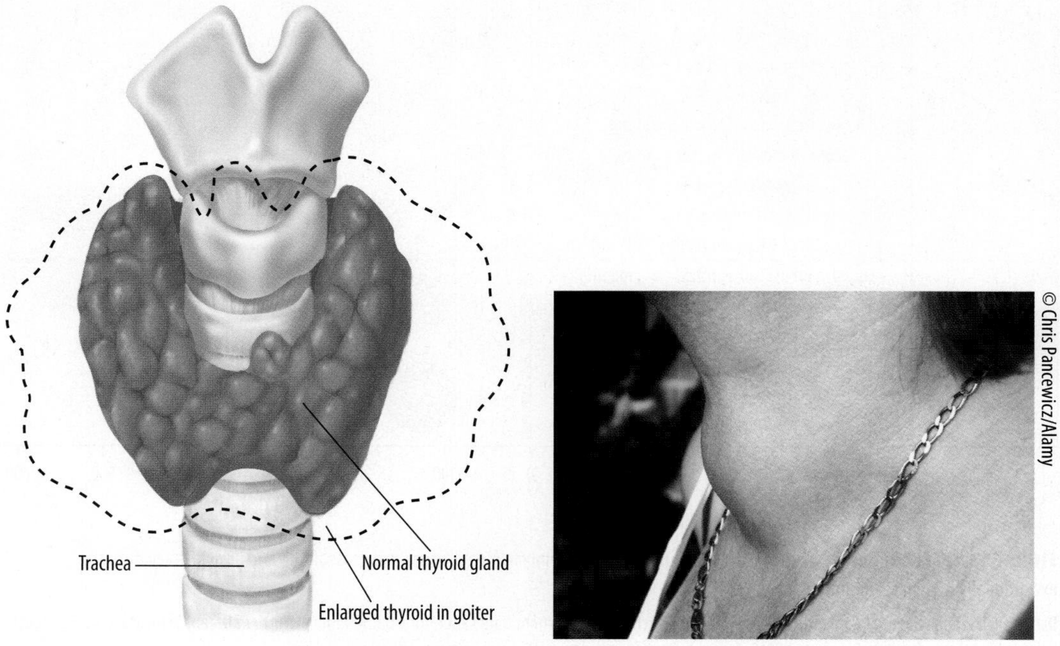

FIGURE 13.18 Enlargement of the thyroid gland in goiter. Iodine deficiency results in goiter. Use of iodized salt dramatically reduces goiter rates. This finding led to the widespread fortification of table salt with iodine.

Cretins were described as feeble-minded dwarfs with puffy facial features and a stumbling gait. In the Middle Ages, European paintings commonly depicted cretins as angels or demons.[47] As late as the early 1900s, goiter was common in certain parts of the United States, particularly the upper Midwest. In 1922, scientists demonstrated that the use of iodized salt by 50,000 schoolchildren dramatically reduced goiter rates. In the United States, these findings led to the widespread fortification of table salt with iodine (I). Iodine deficiency remains a significant nutritional problem in some parts of the world, and its eradication is an important goal of the World Health Organization, which promotes universal salt iodization.[48]

Functions of Iodine

Iodine is an essential component of the two thyroid hormones: **triiodothyronine (T3)** and **thyroxine (T4)**. Thyroid hormones control the regulation of body temperature, basal metabolic rate, reproduction, and growth. Although the thyroid hormones released by the thyroid gland are about 93 percent thyroxine and only 7 percent triiodothyronine, triiodothyronine is about four times more potent than thyroxine.[49] Within a few days of secretion, the body converts most of the thyroxine to the more active triiodothyronine.

▶ **triiodothyronine (T3)** An iodine-containing thyroid hormone with several times the biologic activity of thyroxine (T4).

▶ **thyroxine (T4)** An iodine-containing hormone secreted by the thyroid gland to regulate the rate of cell metabolism; known chemically as tetraiodothyronine.

Iodine Absorption and Metabolism

Much of the iodine in foods is in the form of iodide (the reduced form) and iodates. The intestine absorbs nearly all of it, from 95 to 100 percent. The entire body contains between 15 and 20 milligrams, 70 to 80 percent of which resides in the thyroid gland. Each day the thyroid gland "traps" between 60 and 120 micrograms of iodide for eventual incorporation into the thyroid hormones. Enzymes oxidize the iodide, and then other enzymes bind it to **thyroglobulin**, the storage form of thyroid hormones.

Thyroid-stimulating hormone (TSH) signals the thyroid gland to cleave T3 and T4 from thyroglobulin and release them into the bloodstream. In various body organs, three different enzymes convert most of the T4 to T3. Research reveals that all three of these converting enzymes are selenium dependent. Therefore, a deficiency in selenium can lead to inefficient use of iodine in thyroid hormones.

The kidneys excrete most excess iodine in urine, but some is lost in sweat, especially in hot, humid climates.

▶ **thyroglobulin** The storage form of thyroid hormone in the thyroid gland.

▶ **thyroid-stimulating hormone (TSH)** Secreted from the pituitary gland at the base of the brain, a hormone that regulates synthesis of thyroid hormones.

Dietary Recommendations for Iodine

To replace losses and prevent deficiency of iodine, the thyroid gland needs at least 60 micrograms daily. Because iodine absorption is very efficient, intakes of 75 micrograms per day should be sufficient for adults. To provide a margin of safety, however, the RDA is set at 150 micrograms per day for both men and women.

Sources of Iodine

THINK About It 2

Because the ocean is the best source of iodine, the best food source is seafood. Saltwater fish have higher concentrations of iodine than freshwater fish. The dairy industry adds iodide to cattle feed and uses sanitizing solutions that contain iodine. These measures add substantial amounts of iodine to milk and dairy products. Natural iodine levels in plants reflect soil levels. For many people, iodized salt used in cooking and at the table is their primary source of iodine. In the United States, iodized salt contains an average of 76 micrograms of iodine per gram of salt. In addition to common iodized table salt,

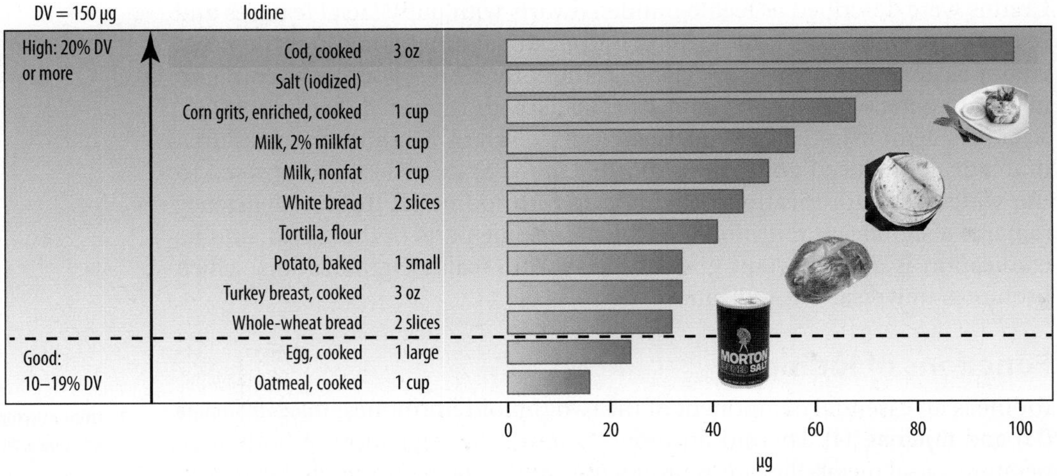

FIGURE 13.19 Food sources of iodine. Few foods are rich in iodine; it is found mainly in milk, seafood, and some grain products.

Data from Pennington JAT. Bowes and Church's Food Values of Portions Commonly Used. 17th ed. Philadelphia, PA: Lippincott-Raven Publishers; 1998.

Photos (from top to bottom): (baked cod) © finaeva_i/Shutterstock Inc.; (homemade whole wheat flour) © Africa Studio/Shutterstock, Inc.; (baked potato) © Joe Gough/Shutterstock, Inc.; (iodized table salt) © GIPhotoStock/Getty Images, Inc.

specialty sea salts are available that are usually not iodized. However, sea salts naturally contain trace amounts of iodine and other minerals because these salts are derived from evaporated sea water.

Excluding iodized salt, the average U.S. diet contains between 230 and 400 micrograms of iodine per day. After salt, dairy products supply most of our dietary iodine, followed by 10 to 15 percent from meat, fish, and poultry and 5 to 15 percent from grains and cereals. Salt added during cooking and at the table contributes 35 to 70 micrograms of iodide to the average adult's daily diet. **FIGURE 13.19** shows the iodine content of some foods.

Quick Bite

Iodine or Iodide: What's in a Name?

Iodine (I_2) is a bluish-black solid that gives off a purple vapor, which gives the element its name. The word *iodine* stems from the Greek word *iôdês*, meaning "violet-colored." Iodide (I^-) is the colorless negative ion of iodine. Iodine circulates in the body either bound to protein or as free iodide ions. Sodium iodide and potassium iodide are iodide salts commonly used in medicines.

▶ **goitrogens** Compounds that can induce goiter.

Iodine Deficiency

As early as 1830, iodine deficiency was linked to the presence of goiter. We now understand that a deficiency of iodine inhibits the synthesis of thyroid hormones. As the body senses the lack of thyroid hormones, it produces more and more TSH. TSH causes the thyroid gland to grow, eventually resulting in a goiter. Goiter causes the usual symptoms of hypothyroidism—cold intolerance, weight gain, sluggishness, and a decreased body temperature. Severe iodine deficiency during pregnancy increases prenatal death and can result in birth defects, cretinism, and infant mortality.[50] Most people with cretinism have stunted growth and are deaf, mute, and mentally retarded.

Raw cabbage, turnips, rutabagas, and cassava contain compounds known as **goitrogens**, which are compounds that block the body's absorption and use of iodine. Consuming large amounts of these foods in their raw form can cause problems; cooking inactivates the goitrogens. Iodine-deficiency disorders are common in developing countries where iodine consumption is low and raw cassava and similar vegetables are a major part of the diet.

Iodine Toxicity

Because high amounts of iodine inhibit synthesis of thyroid hormones and stimulate growth of the thyroid gland, iodine toxicity also can cause goiter. Overzealous supplementation is the most common cause of iodine toxicity. A successful program of iodine fortification must be balanced against the risk of iodine-induced hyperthyroidism, especially in areas of severe iodine deficiency. The UL for iodine is 1,100 micrograms per day.

Key Concepts Iodine is an essential component of thyroid hormones. Iodine deficiency causes overstimulation of the thyroid gland and eventual goiter. The best food source of iodine is seafood. Many people around the world are still at risk for iodine deficiency, but iodization of salt is a powerful preventive measure.

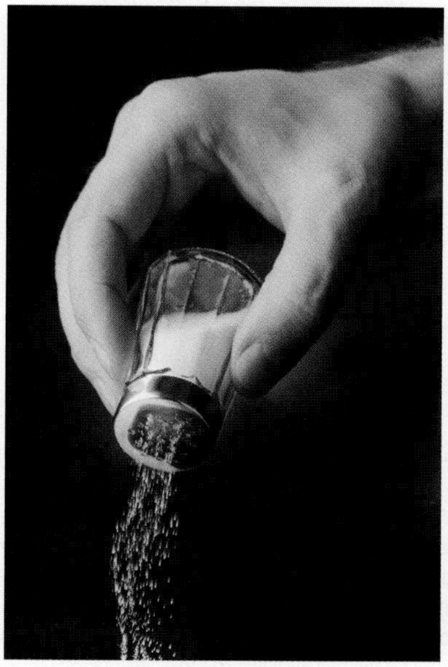

©iStockphoto/Thinkstock

Copper

Researchers first recognized the essential nature of copper (Cu) for experimental animals in 1928, but not until the 1960s did evidence emerge that copper deficiency occurs in humans. Cloning of the genes for two genetic disorders of copper metabolism—Wilson disease (copper toxicity) and **Menkes syndrome** (copper deficiency)—has fueled interest in copper and led to exciting new discoveries about its metabolism and physiological role. Although simple dietary copper deficiency is not a significant public health concern, excessive supplementation with other trace minerals can cause a secondary copper deficiency.

▶ **Menkes syndrome** A genetic disorder that results in copper deficiency.

Functions of Copper

Copper-containing enzymes have many functions, including acting as an antioxidant, participating in the electron transport chain, and aiding the biosynthesis of the pigment melanin and the connective tissue proteins collagen and elastin. Perhaps the most important function of copper is as a component of **ceruloplasmin**, the enzyme that catalyzes the oxidation of ferrous (Fe^{2+}) to ferric (Fe^{3+}) iron for incorporation into transferrin. The absence of ceruloplasmin leads to accumulation of iron in the liver, similar to what is seen in iron overload or hemochromatosis. Copper is an important component of the superoxide dismutases, enzymes involved in antioxidant reactions. Copper also plays a role in various other activities, including **myelinization** of nervous tissue, immune function, and cardiovascular function.

▶ **ceruloplasmin** A copper-dependent enzyme responsible for the oxidation of ferrous iron (Fe^{2+}) to ferric iron (Fe^{3+}), enabling iron to bind to transferrin. Also known as ferroxidase I.

▶ **myelinization** Development of the myelin sheath, a substance that surrounds nerve fibers.

Copper Absorption, Use, and Metabolism

Depending on the amount of copper in the meal and other dietary factors, the intestine absorbs approximately 50 percent of dietary copper. Amino acids, particularly histidine, enhance copper absorption. On the other hand, a number of minerals, most notably iron and zinc, can interfere with copper absorption. Because high-dose iron supplementation is more common than zinc supplementation, the iron–copper interaction is of greater concern. Dietary phytates do not appear to inhibit copper absorption. Because copper is best absorbed in an acidic environment, antacids can reduce copper absorption.

Albumin transports copper from the intestinal cells to the liver, where about two-thirds is incorporated into ceruloplasmin. The average healthy adult body contains approximately 100 milligrams of copper at any time, mainly distributed among the liver, brain, blood, and bone marrow. The body stores relatively little copper, and excretes nearly all excess copper in feces and a minor amount in the urine. Copper excreted in the feces includes unabsorbed dietary copper, copper released in bile, and copper in cells sloughed from the intestinal wall.

Quick Bite

A Penny for Your . . .

How do the amounts of zinc and copper in a U.S. penny compare to the amounts in your body? Today's penny is mostly zinc (2.4 grams), covered with some copper plating (62.5 milligrams). A penny's zinc is in the upper range of the body's zinc content, but the amount of copper falls short. The copper in about 1½ pennies is equal to the amount of copper in your body.

Dietary Recommendations and Food Sources for Copper

There is no single reliable index of copper status. Balance studies have been previously used to estimate copper needs. However, balance studies in humans are problematic, so a combination of plasma, serum, and blood cell measures were used to develop the copper RDA.[51] The RDA for both men and women is 900 micrograms per day.

Copper is widely distributed in foods. The richest food sources include organ meats (e.g., liver), shellfish, nuts and seeds, legumes, peanut butter, and chocolate (see **FIGURE 13.20**). Dietary surveys in the United States suggest that adults consume an average of about 1.0 to 1.6 milligrams of copper per day.[52]

Copper Deficiency

Overt copper deficiency is relatively rare in humans. Copper deficiency occurs most commonly in preterm infants. These babies have low copper stores at birth and a rapid growth rate, which elevates needs. Because cow's milk has little copper and it is poorly bioavailable, infants who are inappropriately fed unmodified cow's milk are more likely to develop a deficiency than are breastfed infants.

Copper deficiency most commonly causes anemia, hypercholesterolemia, and bone abnormalities.[53] In copper-deficiency anemia, low ceruloplasmin activity causes defective iron mobilization. Copper-deficient young children often suffer bone abnormalities. Probably caused by poor synthesis of connective tissue, these abnormalities mimic the changes observed in scurvy. In experimental settings, copper deficiency causes elevated blood cholesterol, impaired glucose tolerance, and heart-related abnormalities. Copper deficiency during pregnancy can have adverse consequences for fetal growth and development.[54]

Menkes syndrome is an extremely rare (approximately 1 in 50,000 live births) genetic copper disorder in which there is a failure to absorb copper into the bloodstream and therefore a lack of functional copper-containing proteins such as ceruloplasmin.[55] Serum copper and ceruloplasmin levels are low, but copper accumulates in the intestinal mucosal cells and in the muscle,

Quick Bite

Egg Whites? Please Stand Up!

Although cooking food in a copper pot is inadvisable, copper mixing bowls can be a plus. Meringues made in ceramic or steel bowls tend to be snowy white and drier than those made in copper bowls. Making meringue in a copper bowl leads to a creamier, yellowish foam that is harder to overbeat into a lumpy liquid. The copper bowl contributes copper ions to conalbumin, a metal-binding egg protein, thus stabilizing the whipped egg whites.

Quick Bite

Cooking in Copper

Because the copper imparted a bright green color to cooked green vegetables, cooking vegetables in uncoated copper pans was once encouraged. This practice often led to decreased liver and brain function. The Swedish military recognized copper toxicity and banned copper cooking utensils in 1753.

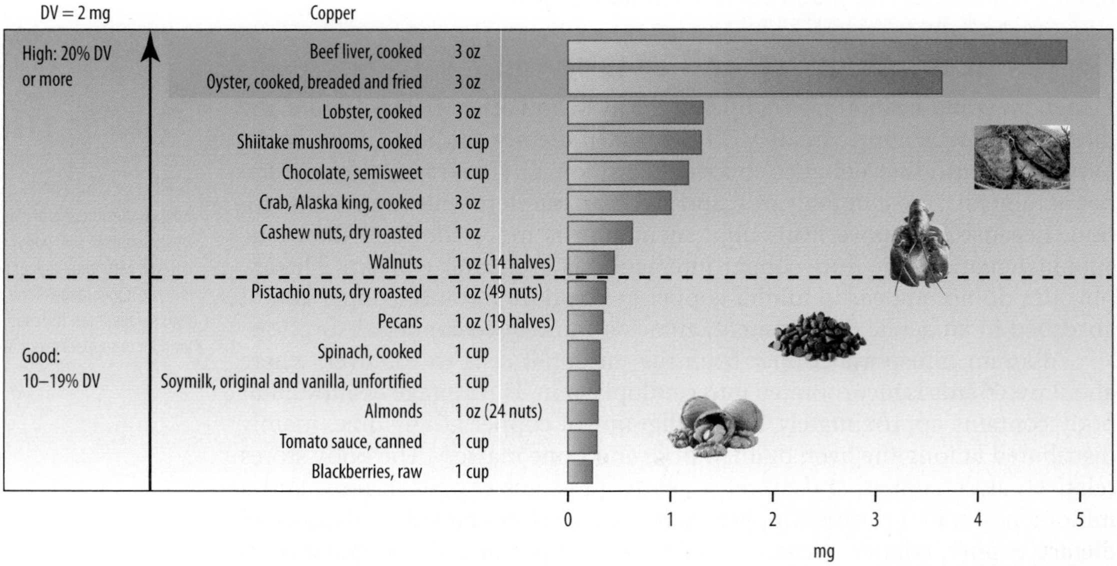

FIGURE 13.20 Food sources of copper. Copper is found in a limited variety of foods. The best sources are beef, seafood, legumes, and nuts.

Data from US Department of Agriculture, Agricultural Research Service, Nutrient Data Laboratory. USDA National Nutrient Database for Standard Reference, Release 28. Version Current: September 2015. Internet: http://www.ars.usda.gov/nea/bhnrc/ndl.

Photos (from top to bottom): (liver) © MauMar70/Shutterstock, Inc.; (lobster) © Alena Haurylik/Shutterstock, Inc.; (chocolate chips) © bonchan/Shutterstock, Inc.; (walnut) © oriori/Shutterstock, Inc.

spleen, and kidneys.[56] Menkes syndrome causes neurological degeneration, peculiar kinky hair, abnormal connective tissue development, osteoporosis, and poor growth. Although this syndrome is usually fatal in infancy or early childhood, copper-histidine treatment within the first few days of life can prevent irreversible damage.

Copper Toxicity

Compared with other trace elements, copper is relatively nontoxic. The UL for copper is 10,000 micrograms per day. Wilson disease is a rare (1 in 200,000) genetic copper toxicity disorder that impairs copper excretion in bile, causing toxic accumulation in the liver, brain, kidneys, and eyes. As copper accumulates in red blood cells, it causes anemia. People with Wilson disease frequently appear healthy until adolescence or early adulthood. Without treatment, they develop serious liver and neurological problems. Copper toxicity can be treated either by **chelation therapy** to bind and remove copper or with zinc supplementation to decrease copper absorption. Lifelong treatment can prevent many complications of Wilson disease.

▶ **chelation therapy** Use of a chelator (e.g., EDTA) to bind metal ions to remove them from the body.

Key Concepts The most important function of copper is as a component of ceruloplasmin, the enzyme that catalyzes the oxidation of iron for transport in transferrin. Food sources for copper include organ meats, shellfish, nuts and seeds, legumes, peanut butter, chocolate, and dried fruits. Copper deficiency is relatively rare in humans. Usual copper intakes fall below the current safe and adequate level.

Manganese

Recognized for centuries, manganese (Mn) derives its name from a Greek term for magic. Although its many functions are not magical, they are unique. Manganese is essential not only in biological systems, but also in iron and steel production. It has many industrial uses in such diverse products as dry-cell batteries, glass, ceramics, paints, varnishes, inks, dyes, and fertilizers. Industrial exposure, rather than excessive intake, is the more frequent cause of manganese toxicity.

Functions of Manganese

The body contains between 10 and 20 milligrams of manganese, which is concentrated primarily in the bone, liver, pancreas, and brain. Despite this limited quantity, manganese is a key component of several enzymes:

- *Mn-superoxide dismutase*, located in the mitochondria of cells, is an antioxidant that prevents tissue damage caused by lipid oxidation.
- *Arginase* helps form urea in the urea cycle.
- *Pyruvate carboxylase* helps convert pyruvate to oxaloacetate.

Manganese also activates numerous enzymes involved in the formation of cartilage in bone and skin.

Manganese Absorption, Use, and Homeostasis

Absorption of manganese is poor, only 1 to 15 percent. This low absorption rate can protect against toxicity. Some research suggests that high levels of iron, calcium, and phosphorus inhibit absorption. Fiber and phytate also can limit manganese absorption, but to a lesser degree than they affect the absorption of most other trace minerals. Following absorption, transferrin binds manganese and transports it in the bloodstream.

Excretion, rather than absorption, regulates the body's manganese. Bile is the main excretory route. Should the small intestine absorb excess manganese,

Quick Bite

Highway Harvest

Oil companies often add a type of manganese to modern gasoline as an antiknock compound to increase the octane rating for high-compression engines. It is now evident that plants along highways accumulate manganese from passing cars.

the body can quickly dump this excess back into the small intestine as part of bile. There is no storage form of manganese. As with zinc, there does not appear to be a reliable indicator of manganese status in adults.

Dietary Recommendations and Food Sources for Manganese

The AI for manganese is 2.3 milligrams per day for men and 1.8 milligrams per day for women.[57] Tea, nuts, cereals, and some fruits are the best food sources of manganese. Some estimates suggest that coffee or tea supplies as much as 20 to 30 percent of our daily manganese intake. Meat, dairy products, poultry, fish, and refined foods are poor sources; they contain little manganese. **FIGURE 13.21** shows the manganese content of some foods.

Manganese Deficiency

Although people who consume normal varied diets do not appear to be at risk for manganese deficiency, certain disorders can cause suboptimal status. Manganese deficiency has been shown to lead to bone demineralization and impaired growth in children, decreased serum cholesterol levels and a transient skin rash in young men, and mildly abnormal glucose tolerance in young women.[58] In animal studies, manganese deficiency has dramatic effects: impaired growth, skeletal abnormalities, impaired glucose tolerance, impaired reproductive system, and altered carbohydrate and fat metabolism.[59]

Manganese Toxicity

Manganese toxicity is a greater threat than manganese deficiency. Foundry workers exposed to airborne manganese dust have experienced severe manganese toxicity. Their symptoms included irritability, hallucinations, and severe lack of coordination. Lower doses of airborne manganese can impair memory

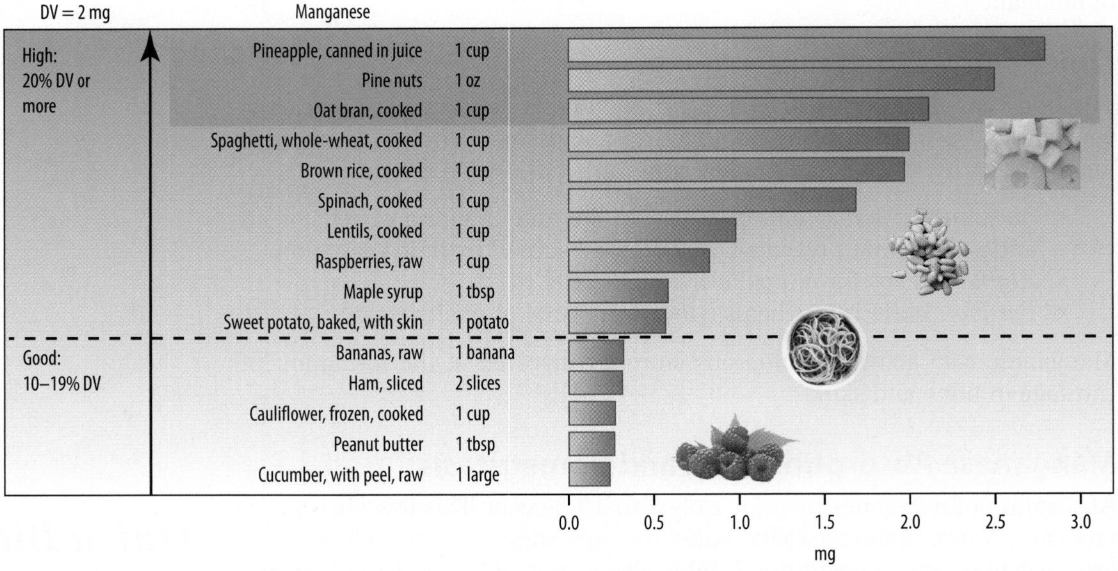

FIGURE 13.21 Food sources of manganese. Manganese is found mainly in plant foods such as grains, legumes, vegetables, and some fruits.

Data from US Department of Agriculture, Agricultural Research Service, Nutrient Data Laboratory. USDA National Nutrient Database for Standard Reference, Release 28. Version Current: September 2015. Internet: http://www.ars.usda.gov/nea/bhnrc/ndl.

Photos (from top to bottom): (canned slices of pineapple) © Africa Studio/Shutterstock, Inc.; (pine nuts) © Jiri Hera/Shutterstock, Inc.; (organic whole grain spaghetti) © Anna Hoychuk/Shutterstock, Inc.; (raspberry) © Nattika/Shutterstock, Inc.

and cause impaired motor coordination similar to that experienced in Parkinson's disease. The UL for manganese is 11 milligrams per day.

Key Concepts Manganese is important to the functioning of several enzymes in the human body. Our usual intake of manganese falls within the currently recommended intake range. Food sources for manganese are tea, coffee, cereals, and some fruits. Toxicity is more a threat than deficiency is, primarily in people who are exposed industrially to high levels of manganese dust.

Fluoride

Fluoride (F), the ionized form of fluorine, has the unique ability to prevent dental caries. Although people first observed this beneficial effect in the early 1800s, scientific proof did not emerge until the time of World War II. In 1945, many U.S. water suppliers began voluntarily fluoridating water to improve the dental health of children. Now that use of fluoridated toothpaste and mouthwash is widespread, some experts are raising concerns about potential harm from excessive fluoride intake.

Functions of Fluoride

Bones and teeth contain nearly 99 percent of the body's fluoride. Fluoride supports the **mineralization** of bones and teeth by promoting the deposition of calcium and phosphorus.

Fluoride's cavity-prevention activity is an effect localized in the mouth. Bacteria in the mouth cause dental caries. When a person eats food, especially carbohydrate foods, these oral bacteria multiply and produce organic acids that eat away tooth enamel, especially beneath plaque. When food leaves the mouth, remineralization begins. If remineralization does not keep pace with demineralization, your teeth become pitted with dental caries. Fluoride decreases the demineralization of tooth enamel and accelerates the subsequent remineralization process. It also inhibits bacterial activity in dental plaques. These cavity-fighting actions can help make your next trip to the dentist a more pleasant one.

Regular ingestion of fluoride is especially important during the eruption of new teeth in children. When administered topically, fluoride's support of tooth enamel remineralization can benefit people of all ages.

Fluoride also may play a role in preventing bone loss,[60] and fluoride supplements have been used along with calcium and other medications to treat osteoporosis. Although the risk of fracture is reduced, proper dosage is not clear, and fluoride is not an approved treatment for osteoporosis.

▶ **mineralization** The addition of minerals, such as calcium and phosphorus, to bones and teeth.

Quick Bite

Accidental Discovery

In the early 1900s, people noticed that inhabitants of towns with naturally high levels of fluoride in their water had healthier teeth. To test the correlation between fluoride and tooth decay, in 1945 four cities in the United States and one in Canada took part in a controlled study of water fluoridation. The results were impressive, establishing that fluoride helps to prevent tooth decay.

Fluoride Absorption and Excretion

Your body absorbs almost all the fluoride in water and other liquid beverages. The bioavailability of fluoride in food ranges between 50 and 80 percent. After absorption, the body distributes fluoride in "hard" tissues, mainly the bones and teeth. Excess fluoride is excreted mainly in the urine.

Dietary Recommendations for Fluoride

The AI for fluoride is 4 milligrams per day for adult men and 3 milligrams per day for women. The AI is 0.01 milligram per day for infants through 5 months, 0.5 milligram for those aged 6 to 11 months, 0.7 milligram for ages 1 to 3 years old, and 1.0 milligram for those aged 4 to 8 years.[61] Dental caries is the most common chronic disease in children, and the American Dental Association recommends fluoride supplements beginning with children

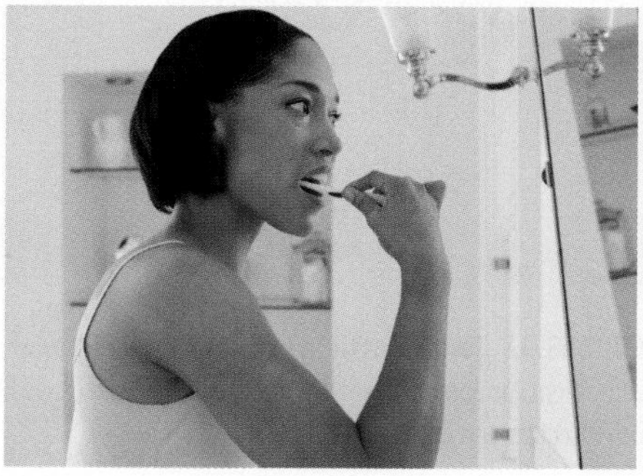

© Jupiterimages/Comstock/Thinkstock

6 months of age whose drinking water supplies less than 0.3 milligram fluoride per liter.[62,63]

Sources of Fluoride

Water is the main source of fluoride. Water might contain fluoride naturally, or fluoride can be added to produce fluoridated water. Fluoride naturally present in drinking water varies from less than 0.1 milligram to more than 10 milligrams per liter. Where naturally occurring fluoride levels are low, many water companies add fluoride.

The U.S. Department of Health and Human Services (DHHS) recommends 0.7 milligram of fluoride per liter of water, based on an assessment by the Environmental Protection Agency and DHHS of the benefits versus side effects.[64] The Environmental Protection Agency requires public drinking water systems to remove excess fluoride so it does not exceed 4.0 milligrams per liter.[65]

The Centers for Disease Control and Prevention named the fluoridation of drinking water one of the 10 great public health achievements of the twentieth century.[66] Almost three-quarters of the U.S. population receive the benefit of optimally fluoridated public water.[67] Since we first began fluoridating water supplies, other fluoride sources have emerged. Today, fluoride sources include ready-to-feed infant formulas, fluoride supplements, mouthwash, toothpaste, and some beverages. In any given week, almost one-quarter of U.S. children younger than 12 years of age and 30 percent of 2-year-olds use supplemental vitamins, fluoride, and iron.[68] The combination of fluoride sources can put children at increased risk for excessive fluoride intake and **fluorosis**.

▶ **fluorosis** Mottled discoloration and pitting of tooth enamel caused by prolonged ingestion of excessive fluoride.

Position Statement: Academy of Nutrition and Dietetics

The Impact of Fluoride on Health

It is the position of the Academy of Nutrition and Dietetics to support optimal systemic and topical fluoride as an important public health measure to promote oral health and overall health throughout life.

Reproduced from Palmer C, Gilbert JA. Position of the Academy of Nutrition and Dietetics: the impact of fluoride on health. *J Acad Nutr Diet.* 2012;112(9):1443–1453.

The balance between the positive effects of just enough fluoride and the negative effects of too much fluoride has caused fluoridation to become hotly debated. When fluoridation was first instituted in 1945, it served as the exclusive source of fluoride for children. Now, however, because there are so many sources of fluoride, it is difficult to determine the current effectiveness of artificial fluoridation of the water supply. Yet the dramatic decline in dental carries since fluoridation was initiated is undeniable. Opponents argue that fluoridation is outdated and involuntary. The Canadian Medical Association stated, "If you administer fluoride by fluoridating the tap water in the community then you have no control of the dose an individual gets per day."[69] To retain the benefits yet avoid overconsumption, the American Dental Association supports the fluoridation of all water supplies and monitoring of other fluoride sources.[70,71]

THINK About It 3

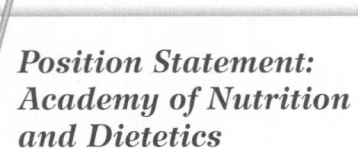

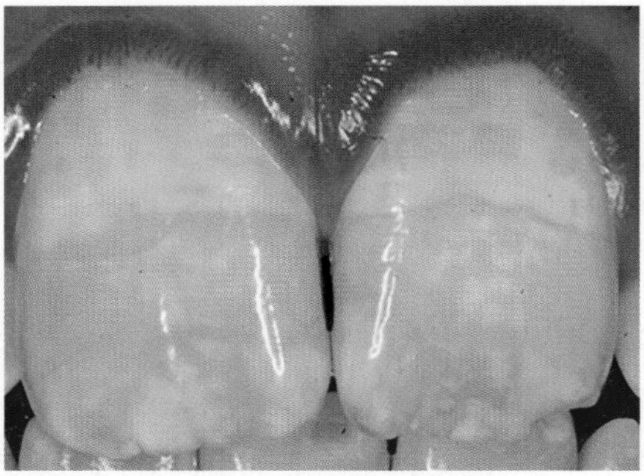

Centers for Disease Control

FIGURE 13.22 Tooth mottling in fluorosis. During tooth development, prolonged excessive fluoride intake can cause fluorosis, which discolors and damages teeth.

Fluoride Deficiency, Toxicity, and Pharmacological Applications

Low fluoride intake increases the risk for dental caries and can hamper the integrity of bone. Adequate fluoride intake in childhood can decrease the incidence of tooth decay by 30 to 60 percent. During tooth development, prolonged excessive fluoride intake can cause fluorosis (see **FIGURE 13.22**). In mild fluorosis, white specks form on the teeth. Severe fluorosis can cause permanent brownish stains and weakened teeth. Consumption of water naturally high in fluoride is the main cause of fluorosis, but children who chronically swallow large amounts of fluoridated toothpaste are also at risk. For children younger than 6 years old, parents should supervise the use of fluoride-containing products to prevent consumption. The UL for fluoride is 10 milligrams per day. Bone health can also benefit from adequate fluoride intake.

Researchers have studied fluoride for the treatment of osteoporosis in postmenopausal women. Although fluoride treatment appears to increase bone density, it also seems to make them more brittle and susceptible to fracture, despite their higher density.[72]

Key Concepts Bones and teeth contain 99 percent of body fluoride. Fluoride supports remineralization, and its major function is the prevention of dental caries. Fluoride is unique in that the main dietary source is water, not food. The majority of our nation's municipal water supplies are artificially fluoridated. Excess fluoride can cause fluorosis. Mild fluorosis with mottling of the teeth is primarily a cosmetic problem; severe fluorosis can weaken teeth.

Chromium

The chromium (Cr) content of the body is approximately 4 to 6 milligrams, mostly in the liver, spleen, and bone; the remainder is widely dispersed at very low concentrations.[73] Chromium plays an important but poorly understood role in moving glucose into cells and in lipid metabolism. Although researchers established chromium's essential role in glucose tolerance during the late 1950s and early 1960s, the development of reliable analytical methods took another 20 years.

Quick Bite

Conspiracy Theory

Although the U.S. Public Health Service and the World Health Organization officially endorsed the fluoridation of water in the 1950s, some groups continue to oppose the practice. Objectors claim that water fluoridation violates civil rights, that fluoride is a nerve poison, and that fluoride is unwanted compulsory medication that can have dangerous side effects. Some groups even claim that fluoridation is a component of a conspiracy for national destruction. So far, objectors have been unable to substantiate their claims, and the courts have upheld the constitutionality of fluoridation.

Functions of Chromium

Chromium enhances the effects of insulin and is important for proper metabolism of carbohydrates and lipids. It also plays a role in metabolism of nucleic acids and immune function and growth. Athletes are especially interested in chromium because of its purported effects on body composition.

Chromium Absorption, Transport, and Excretion

Little is known about chromium absorption. Uptake of the inorganic form is thought to be low (about 1 to 2 percent); absorption of organic chromium (a combination of chromium and an organic acid such as chromium picolinate) might be higher (10 to 25 percent). Absorption increases with need and decreases with higher amounts in the diet. Other dietary factors also can influence chromium absorption. Vitamin C and niacin, for example, can increase chromium absorption, and diets high in sugar decrease it.[74] Transferrin and albumin transport chromium in the bloodstream. The body excretes excess chromium in the urine.

Dietary Recommendations and Food Sources for Chromium

For adults aged 19 to 50 years, the AI for chromium is 35 micrograms per day for men and 25 micrograms per day for women. The AI for older adults is 5 micrograms less. More data on actual requirements for chromium and the chromium content of foods are needed for more specific dietary recommendations.

The chromium content of foods varies widely. Good sources include broccoli, whole grains, grape juice, brewer's yeast, lean meats, green beans, potatoes, and spices. Cooking acidic foods in stainless steel containers leaches some chromium into the food.

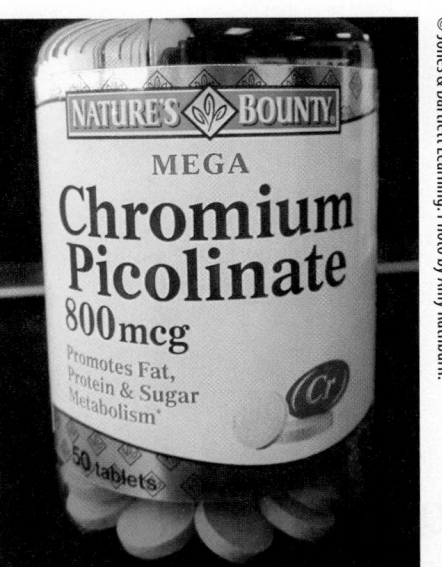

© Jones & Bartlett Learning. Photo by Amy Rathburn.

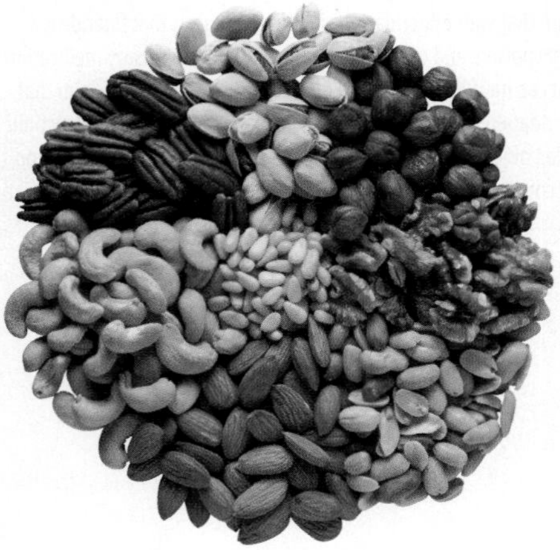

© Photodisc

Chromium Deficiency

The difficulty of assessing chromium status makes it hard to determine the effects of deficiency. Nevertheless, studies in animals and humans point to the following signs of chromium deficiency: decreased insulin-mediated glucose uptake by cells, decreased insulin sensitivity, elevated blood glucose and insulin levels, and blood lipid abnormalities. Patients who subsist on long-term intravenous feedings inadequate in chromium can suffer brain and nerve disorders.[75]

Chromium Toxicity

The only known cases of chromium toxicity occurred in people exposed to airborne chromium compounds in industrial settings. Because inorganic chromium is so poorly absorbed, extremely high oral intakes would be necessary to attain toxic levels. Numerous experiments show 200 micrograms of inorganic chromium to be a safe dose for supplementation. However, studies of chromium picolinate supplements showed DNA damage in animal cells, which has raised safety concerns about this supplemental form. (See the FYI feature "Chromium, Exercise, and Body Composition.") To date, no UL has been set for chromium.

The role of chromium supplements remains controversial. Supplementation with chromium has been shown to reduce risk factors for type 2 diabetes and cardiovascular disease.[76] However, the current body of evidence does not support chromium supplementation as a tool for diabetes management.[77] Based on perceived but unfounded beneficial effects on body composition, chromium supplements are popular among many athletes and bodybuilders. However, there is little evidence from well-designed studies that chromium increases lean body mass or decreases body fat.[78]

Key Concepts The primary function of chromium in the body is to potentiate the effects of insulin. Sources of chromium include broccoli, whole grains, grape juice, brewer's yeast, lean meats, green beans, potatoes, and spices. Reliable assessment of chromium status is difficult.

Molybdenum

Molybdenum (Mo) is essential to both plants and animals. In humans, molybdenum functions as a cofactor for several enzymes that induce oxidation.

Molybdenum Absorption, Use, and Metabolism

The small intestine absorbs molybdenum efficiently—some studies suggest up to 80 to 90 percent of the amount consumed. However, the body excretes it rapidly in urine and in bile. Fiber and phytate have no effect on its absorption.

Dietary copper is the only significant inhibitor of molybdenum absorption. The body contains about 2 milligrams of molybdenum, 90 percent of which is located in the liver.

Dietary Recommendations and Food Sources for Molybdenum

For adults, the molybdenum RDA is 45 micrograms per day. Although data are limited, typical intakes in the United States exceed the RDA. Peas, beans, and some breakfast cereals are the richest food sources for molybdenum.

Quick Bite

Chrome-Plated Cars

The cars of the 1950s sported fins and loads of chrome. The chromium in your body is the same metal used for electroplating hard chrome. Using electric current, chromium ions bond with the original surface, creating a bond between the metals so hard it will remain intact even when subjected to extreme force.

FYI
For Your Information

Chromium, Exercise, and Body Composition

Chromium's role in carbohydrate and lipid metabolism, as well as its purported effects on body composition, have made it a popular supplement among both recreational and professional athletes. Chromium's advertised role to increase lean body mass (LBM) and decrease body fat during resistance training has generated a great deal of popular interest. Yet study results are contradictory, and chromium's influence on body composition is controversial. Previous studies examining the effects of chromium on body composition and body mass, including gains in lean mass and help with weight loss, have found negligible or mixed results. In overweight adults, supplemental chromium alone, and in combination with nutritional education, did not affect weight loss over 24 weeks.[a] Based on available research, the evidence behind chromium's fat metabolism–enhancing properties is lacking, and supplement sales are driven by industry marketing, not scientific evidence.[b]

Differences in experimental design could explain many of these inconsistent results. One of the limitations of any chromium study is the inability to assess the initial status of the subjects. Additionally, in some studies the sample size might be too small, the dosage might have been too low, and the time period might have been too short to show any effect. Whether the supplement was given alone or in combination with an energy-restricted diet or increased exercise expenditure are additional factors that can confound research results.[c]

What are the issues raised by these studies and how are we to understand the contradictory findings? After researchers reported the initial positive results, the press and supplement advertisers overstated the benefits of chromium supplementation, thereby creating unrealistic expectations. In 1996, the Federal Trade Commission (FTC) ordered the makers of chromium picolinate supplements to stop making unsubstantiated claims of weight loss and health benefits. Despite the FTC's intervention, sales of chromium supplements continue to grow.[d]

Scientific evidence currently does not support that a specific nutritional supplement will produce significant or long-term weight loss.[e] Additionally, there is no evidence that chromium supplements provide a "quick fix" for athletes, and long-term chromium intake probably has a minimal effect on body composition and body weight. Because chromium can interact with iron and zinc, chromium supplementation raises concern about adverse effects. As is the case with many trace minerals, only further investigation will clarify the role of chromium in human health.

The best advice for achieving a healthy, fit body? A varied diet and regular exercise—not reliance on supplements.

[a] Yazaki Y, Faridi Z, Ma Y, et al. A pilot study of chromium picolinate for weight loss. *J Altern Complement Med.* 2010;16(3):291–299.

[b] Jeukendrup AE, Randell R. Fat burners: nutrition supplements that increase fat metabolism. *Obes Rev.* 2011;12(10):841–851.

[c] Manore MM. Dietary supplements for improving body composition and reducing body weight: where is the evidence? *Int J Sport Nutr Exerc Metab.* 2012;22(2):139–154.

[d] Vincent JB. *The Nutritional Biochemistry of Chromium* (III). Amsterdam: Elsevier; 2007.

[e] Manore MM. Dietary supplements for improving body composition and reducing body weight. Op cit.

Organ meats such as liver and kidney also are fairly rich sources, but other meats tend to be poor sources.

Molybdenum Deficiency and Toxicity

Molybdenum deficiency does not occur in people who eat a normal diet. People on total parenteral nutrition who do not receive molybdenum can suffer weakness, mental confusion, and night blindness. People with a rare congenital disorder have deficient amounts of sulfite oxidase, a molybdenum-dependent enzyme. These people suffer from neurological problems similar to those of severe molybdenum deficiency.

Scientists first recognized the interaction between dietary copper and molybdenum in sheep and cattle that grazed on grass grown on soil either

Quick Bite

Molybdenum Takes a Stand Against the Elements

Molybdenum is a silvery-gray metal that is not found free in nature. It has properties similar to tungsten and is used as an alloy to strengthen and protect metal from corrosion.

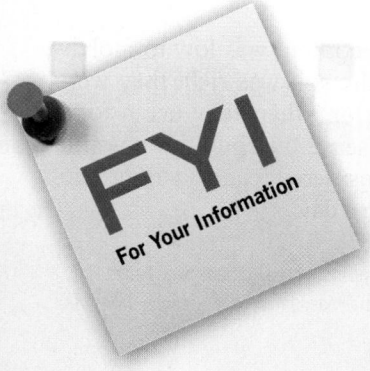

very poor or very rich in molybdenum. If the soil content was low in molybdenum, the animals suffered copper toxicity; if the soil was rich, they were deficient in copper. Doctors exploit this interaction when they use a form of molybdenum to treat patients with Wilson disease. Despite the possible interaction with copper, molybdenum salts are considered relatively nontoxic. The UL for molybdenum is 2,000 micrograms per day.

Key Concepts Several important enzymes require molybdenum. Good food sources include peas, beans, and some breakfast cereals. Healthy people with normal diets do not suffer molybdenum deficiency. High intakes of molybdenum can inhibit absorption of copper.

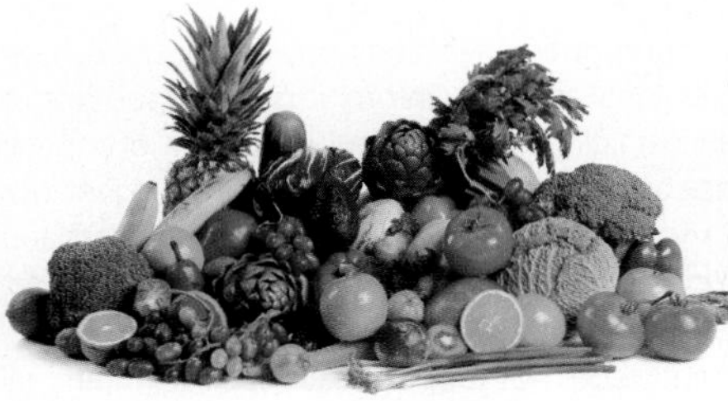

Other Trace Elements and Ultratrace Elements

The body contains minuscule amounts of *ultratrace* minerals and might require less than 1 milligram per day of each. At least 19 minerals could be considered ultratrace: aluminum, arsenic, boron, bromide, cadmium, chromium, fluoride, germanium, iodine, lead, lithium, manganese, molybdenum, nickel, rubidium, selenium, silicon, tin, and vanadium. Dietary recommendations are fairly clear, and there is substantial research on five of these minerals: iodine, fluoride, manganese, molybdenum, and selenium (all discussed previously). The functions of the remaining minerals are less clear. Although new evidence and media coverage have focused on arsenic, boron, nickel, silicon, and vanadium, data do not exist for the establishment of AIs or RDAs for these minerals. ULs have been set for boron, nickel, and vanadium (see **TABLE 13.5**).

TABLE 13.5
Tolerable Upper Intake Levels (UL) for Ultratrace Elements

Arsenic	No UL set
Boron	20 mg/day
Nickel	1 mg/day
Silicon	No UL set
Vanadium	1.8 mg/day

Arsenic

Although arsenic (As) has been an infamous poison for centuries, inorganic arsenic might actually be an essential ultratrace element.[79] As a colorless, tasteless toxin, arsenic trioxide can be fatal in a dose as low as 2 milligrams.

On the other hand, arsenic-deprived laboratory animals have poor growth and abnormal reproduction. Arsenic might also participate in methionine metabolism. For adults, median intake of arsenic was 2.0 to 2.9 micrograms per day in men and 1.7 to 2.1 micrograms per day in women.[80] Recently it has been of concern that many rice-based products contain high levels of arsenic, which can cause cancer and other adverse health conditions. Food sources with the highest concentrations of arsenic are rice, especially brown rice that contains the bran portion of the rice kernel; organic brown rice syrup, which is used as a natural sweetener in many organic food products; apples; seafood; and drinking water.[81] A UL has not been established for arsenic. Given arsenic's highly poisonous nature, much more careful research is required to establish recommended intake and UL levels.

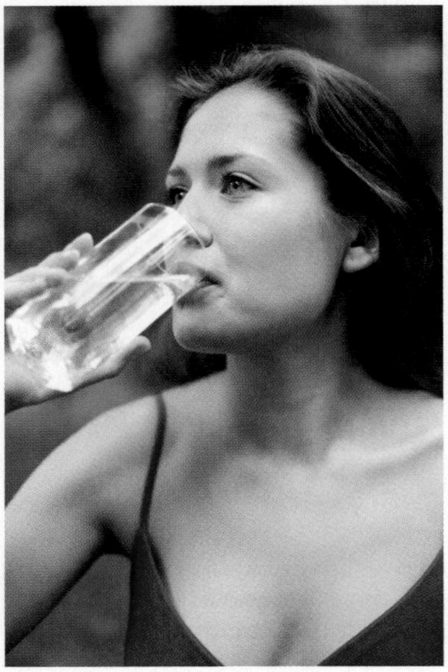

Boron

Boron (B) appears to play an important role in bone metabolism, probably in conjunction with other nutrients such as calcium, magnesium, and vitamin D. Studies indicate that boron also plays a role in promoting brain health and immunity.[82] Boron deficiency depresses growth and is worsened by a vitamin D deficiency. Conversely, boron supplementation lessens the bone abnormalities observed in vitamin D deficiency.

Fruits, nuts, vegetables, legumes, and, depending on geographic location, water are the main sources of boron. The body absorbs close to 90 percent of the amount consumed and then promptly excretes most of it in the urine. The usual dietary intake of boron is between 0.87 and 1.35 milligrams per day for adults.[83] Based on average consumption as well as supplementation studies, scientists estimate that the daily boron requirement is 1 milligram per day. Chronic boron toxicity symptoms include poor appetite, nausea, weight loss, and decreased sexual activity, seminal volume, and sperm count.[84] More research is needed to set safe lower limits for dietary intake. The UL for boron is 20 milligrams per day.

Nickel

Nickel (Ni) is widely distributed throughout the body in very low concentrations that add up to a total body content of approximately 10 milligrams. Most of the research on nickel has been conducted in animals; by extrapolation, scientists assume nickel is essential in humans.

The specific function of nickel in humans has not yet been determined. A few nickel-containing enzymes have been identified, and nickel can activate or inhibit a number of enzymes that usually contain other elements. Nickel alters the properties of cell membranes and affects oxidation-reduction systems in cells. Nickel also might function in vitamin B_{12} and folate metabolism.[85]

Nuts, legumes, grains, and vegetables are the best sources of nickel. Depending on the amount of plant foods consumed, dietary intake of nickel varies widely. Adults consume approximately 79 to 105 micrograms of nickel per day from dietary sources and supplements.[86] There is no known nickel deficiency in humans. Toxicity has occurred only in workers exposed to nickel dust or nickel carbonyl in industrial settings. The UL for nickel is 1 milligram per day.

Silicon

Silicon (Si) is the most common element in the earth's crust. The human body contains roughly 1.5 grams of silicon—less than the amount of magnesium, but about the same as iron and zinc. Connective tissues such as the aorta, trachea, tendons, bones, and skin contain much of the body's silicon. Silicon plays a role in bone formation and growth. Silicon also might have a role in preventing atherosclerosis in older adults. There are no known symptoms of silicon deficiency in humans. This element is relatively nontoxic when ingested orally, and no UL has been set for it. However, breathing airborne silicon particles can cause **silicosis**, a type of silicon toxicity.

▶ **silicosis** A disease that results from excess silicon exposure.

Unrefined grains, cereals, vegetables, and fruits supply most of our dietary silicon. Animal foods are poor sources. Determining a dietary recommendation is difficult because of the lack of human studies showing signs of deficiency.

Vanadium

In the body, vanadium (V) can exist in a form that is structurally similar to phosphate. Interestingly, in the late 1970s it was noted that in vitro vanadium inhibits ATP synthase, an enzyme required for ATP production. Presumably, vanadium replaces phosphate and blocks the reaction. In rats with experimentally induced diabetes, vanadium has also been shown to mimic insulin. However, a precise function for vanadium in humans has not been found, and given the tiny amounts that we consume, deficiencies have not been observed. The UL for vanadium is 1.8 milligrams per day.

Key Concepts Ultratrace minerals are elements with very low estimated requirements. Although specific biochemical functions have not been defined for the minerals arsenic, boron, nickel, silicon, and vanadium, they are thought to be essential for humans in very low amounts.

Label to Table

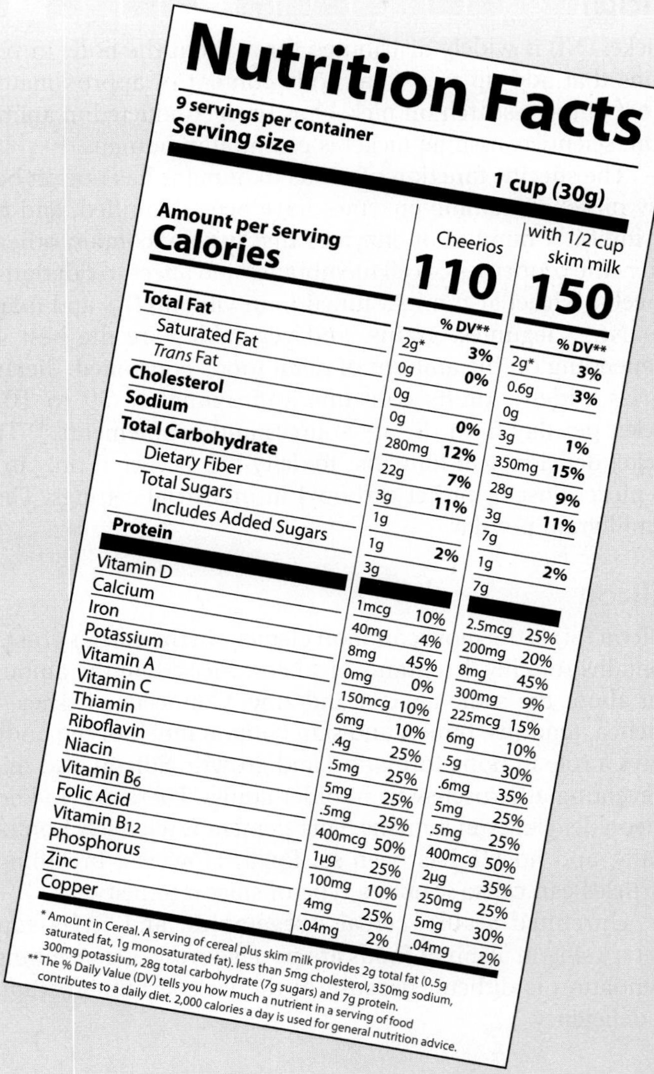

Amount per serving	Cheerios		with 1/2 cup skim milk	
Calories	110		150	
		% DV**		% DV**
Total Fat	2g*	3%	2g*	3%
Saturated Fat	0g	0%	0.6g	3%
Trans Fat	0g		0g	
Cholesterol	0g	0%	3g	1%
Sodium	280mg	12%	350mg	15%
Total Carbohydrate	22g	7%	28g	9%
Dietary Fiber	3g	11%	3g	11%
Total Sugars	1g		7g	
Includes Added Sugars	1g	2%	1g	2%
Protein	3g		7g	
Vitamin D	1mcg	10%	2.5mcg	25%
Calcium	40mg	4%	200mg	20%
Iron	8mg	45%	8mg	45%
Potassium	0mg	0%	300mg	9%
Vitamin A	150mcg	10%	225mcg	15%
Vitamin C	6mg	10%	6mg	10%
Thiamin	.4g	25%	.5g	30%
Riboflavin	.5mg	25%	.6mg	35%
Niacin	5mg	25%	5mg	25%
Vitamin B_6	.5mg	25%	.5mg	25%
Folic Acid	400mcg	50%	400mcg	50%
Vitamin B_{12}	1μg	25%	2μg	35%
Phosphorus	100mg	10%	250mg	25%
Zinc	4mg	25%	5mg	30%
Copper	.04mg	2%	.04mg	2%

* Amount in Cereal. A serving of cereal plus skim milk provides 2g total fat (0.5g saturated fat, 1g monosaturated fat). less than 5mg cholesterol, 350mg sodium, 300mg potassium, 28g total carbohydrate (7g sugars) and 7g protein.
** The % Daily Value (DV) tells you how much a nutrient in a serving of food contributes to a daily diet. 2,000 calories a day is used for general nutrition advice.

If you looked at a list of minerals, could you pick out the trace minerals? Let's see how well you do! Look at the accompanying Nutrition Facts label from a breakfast cereal and guess how many trace minerals are listed.

You should be able to spot three trace minerals on the label: iron, zinc, and copper. Looking at the "ingredients" and "vitamins and minerals" lists, you can see that the iron and zinc were added, but the copper appears to come naturally from the cereal. Why do you think these trace minerals are added to this cereal? Many people (especially children) eat marginal amounts of iron and zinc. The best sources of these minerals are meats, liver, and shellfish. Most children don't eat much shellfish or liver, so adding the minerals to cereals, which they do eat, is an easy way to make sure they get 45 percent and 25 percent of the Daily Values for iron and zinc, respectively.

The last mineral you see listed is copper. There is 2 percent of the Daily Value for copper in one serving of this cereal. That's 0.04 milligram (2% of 2 mg).

Learning Portfolio

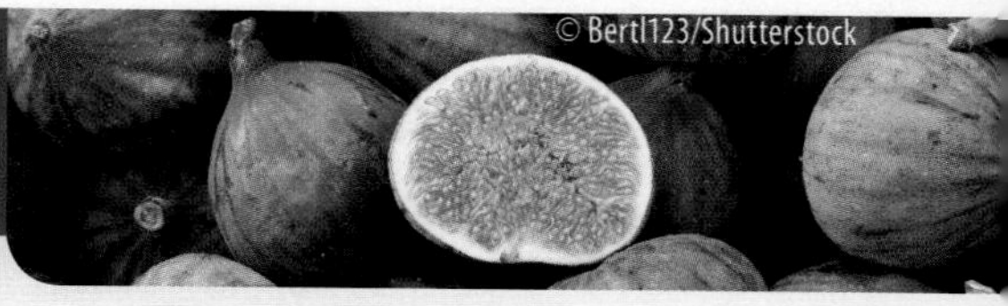

Key Terms

Study Points

- Trace elements are minerals that the body needs in small amounts. They are involved in a variety of structural and regulatory functions and are found in both animal and plant foods.
- Iron functions in oxygen transport as part of hemoglobin and myoglobin. It is also an enzyme cofactor, important for immune function, and involved in normal brain function.
- Iron balance is regulated through absorption; absorption increases when body status is low, and decreases when stores are normal. Meat, vitamin C, and stomach acid tend to increase nonheme iron absorption. Phytate, phenolic compounds, and high doses of other minerals tend to decrease iron absorption.
- Recommendations for iron intake consider the amount needed to replace daily losses and the bioavailability of iron from a typical mixed diet. Because of regular iron losses through menstrual bleeding, women of childbearing age need more iron than adult men do.
- The best sources of iron are meats. Enriched and whole grains are significant sources in the American diet.
- Iron deficiency is the most common nutritional deficiency worldwide. The most severe stage of deficiency, following reduction of iron stores and transport iron, results in anemia.
- Iron toxicity can result from acute ingestion of high doses or chronic excessive iron absorption. Accidental iron overdose is a leading cause of poisoning deaths of children younger than age 6 in the United States.
- Zinc is a cofactor for numerous enzymes and is crucial for normal growth, development, and immune function. It is found in protein-rich foods, particularly red meats.
- Zinc deficiency results in poor growth, impaired taste and smell, delayed wound healing, and impaired immune response.
- Selenium functions as part of the glutathione peroxidases, important antioxidant enzymes. Good sources of selenium are organ meats and seafood. Deficiency of selenium appears to be rare, but has been described in an area of China called the Keshan region.
- Iodine is necessary for the formation of thyroid hormones, which regulate metabolic rate and body temperature. Much of the iodide in the American diet comes from iodized salt. Iodine deficiency results in goiter. If severe deficiency occurs during pregnancy, the child can be born with cretinism.
- Copper functions in many enzyme systems, including those involved with antioxidant mechanisms, iron utilization, and immune function. The richest food sources of copper include organ meats, shellfish, nuts and seeds, peanut butter, and chocolate.
- Copper deficiency results in anemia, decreased numbers of white blood cells, and bone abnormalities.

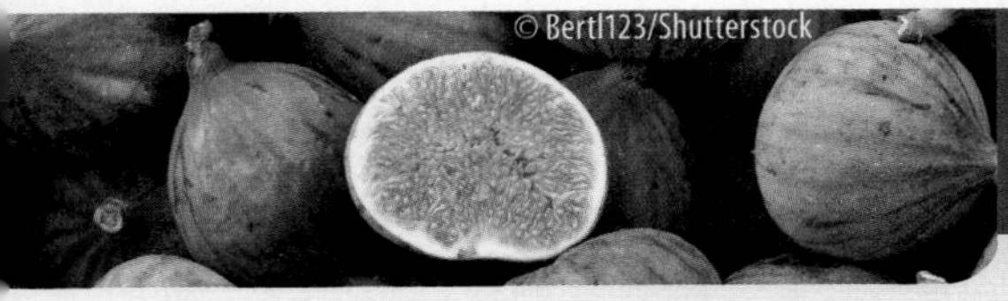

Learning Portfolio (continued)

- Manganese functions in conjunction with several enzyme systems. The best food sources include tea, coffee, nuts, cereals, and some fruits. Manganese deficiency and toxicity are uncommon; toxicity is usually associated with exposure through manganese mines.
- Fluoride promotes mineralization of bones and teeth and protects the teeth from caries. Water is a major source of fluoride, from either naturally high content or added fluoride. Fluorosis is the result of excessive fluoride intake and results in mottling of the teeth.
- Chromium functions in the normal use of insulin to promote glucose use. Rich sources of chromium are mushrooms, dark chocolate, prunes, nuts, asparagus, whole grains, wine, brewer's yeast, and some beers. Chromium deficiency in humans is difficult to assess, and toxicity of inorganic chromium is unlikely.
- Although the body contains only about 2 milligrams of molybdenum, it is an important enzyme cofactor. Good food sources are peas, beans, and some breakfast cereals. Molybdenum deficiency and toxicity are both rare.
- Ultratrace minerals are those required in extremely small amounts; the specific function of many of these nutrients is unknown. Some ultratrace minerals are arsenic, boron, nickel, silicon, and vanadium.

Study Questions

1. In what two ways do trace minerals differ from major minerals?
2. Name two ways that minerals differ from most vitamins.
3. List five factors that can affect a mineral's bioavailability.
4. Explain the differences between "heme" and "nonheme" iron. Which is absorbed better?
5. List the three stages of iron deficiency and the effects of each.
6. What are some of the main functions of zinc?
7. Describe the common causes of zinc deficiency.
8. What are the main functions of selenium?
9. Iodine is a component of which hormones? What are the functions of these hormones? How is selenium linked to these hormones?
10. What are goitrogens, and how are they related to goiter?
11. Define Wilson disease and Menkes syndrome.
12. What are the functions of manganese in the body?
13. How does fluoride prevent dental caries?
14. Which foods contain chromium, and why is chromium important?

Try This

A Simple Check on Your Zinc

Reported in the *Lancet* in the early 1980s, this simple test can provide a rough estimate of your zinc status. Buy some zinc sulfate at a health food store. Dissolve it in distilled water to make a 0.1 percent zinc sulfate solution (0.1 gram of zinc sulfate in 100 milliliters of distilled water). Refrain from eating, drinking, and smoking for at least an hour before the test. Then swish a teaspoon of the solution around your mouth for 10 seconds and spit it out. If it tastes unpleasant or metallic, your level of zinc is probably adequate. However, if the solution tastes like water, you might be consuming less zinc than you need.

References

1. World Health Organization. Micronutrient deficiencies: iron deficiency anemia. http://www.who.int/nutrition/topics/ida/en. Accessed January 8, 2016.
2. Gleason G, Scrimshaw NS. An overview of the functional significance of iron deficiency. In: Kraemer K, Zimmermann MB, eds. *Nutritional Anemia*. Basel, Switzerland: Sight and Life Press; 2007:45–58.
3. Institute of Medicine, Food and Nutrition Board. *Dietary Reference Intakes for Vitamin A, Vitamin K, Arsenic, Boron, Chromium, Copper, Iodine, Iron, Manganese, Molybdenum, Nickel, Silicon, Vanadium, and Zinc*. Washington, DC: National Academies Press; 2001.
4. National Institutes of Health, Office of Dietary Supplements. Iron: dietary supplement fact sheet. https://ods.od.nih.gov/factsheets/Iron-HealthProfessional/. Accessed January 8, 2016.
5. Institute of Medicine, Food and Nutrition Board. *Dietary Reference Intakes for Vitamin A, Vitamin K*. Op cit.
6. Gropper SS, Smith JL, Groff JL. *Advanced Nutrition and Human Metabolism*. 5th ed. Belmont, CA: Wadsworth Cengage Learning; 2009.
7. Hurrell R, Egli I. Iron bioavailability and dietary reference values. *Am J Clin Nutr*. 2010;91(suppl):1461S–1467S.
8. Institute of Medicine, Food and Nutrition Board. *Dietary Reference Intakes for Vitamin A, Vitamin K*. Op cit.
9. Otten JJ, Hellwig JP, Meyers JD, eds. *Dietary Reference Intakes: The Essential Guide to Nutrient Requirements*. Washington, DC: National Academies Press; 2006.
10. Hurrell R, Egli I. Iron bioavailability and dietary reference values. Op cit.
11. Gropper SS, Smith JL, Groff JL. *Advanced Nutrition and Human Metabolism*. Op cit.
12. Ibid.
13. Institute of Medicine, Food and Nutrition Board. *Dietary Reference Intakes for Vitamin A, Vitamin K*. Op cit.
14. Gropper SS, Smith JL, Groff JL. *Advanced Nutrition and Human Metabolism*. Op cit.

15. Pearson RD. Hookworm infection (ancylostomiasis). In: Porter RS, Kaplan JL, eds. *Merck Manual for Healthcare Professionals*. Whitehouse Station, NJ: Merck & Co; 2005. http://www.merckmanuals.com/professional/infectious_diseases/nematodes_roundworms/hookworm_infection.html. Accessed January 8, 2016.
16. Institute of Medicine, Food and Nutrition Board. *Dietary Reference Intakes for Vitamin A, Vitamin K*. Op cit.
17. Beard J. Why iron deficiency is important in infant development. *J Nutr*. 2008;138(12):2534–2536.
18. Cortese S, Konofal E, Bernardina BD, et al. Sleep disturbances and serum ferritin levels in children with attention-deficit/hyperactivity disorder. *Eur Child Adolesc Psychiatry*. 2009;18(7):393–399.
19. Israeli E, Merkel D, Constantini N, et al. Iron deficiency and the role of nutrition among female military recruits. *Med Sci Sports Exerc*. 2008;40(11 suppl):S685–S690.
20. Institute of Medicine, Food and Nutrition Board. *Dietary Reference Intakes for Vitamin A, Vitamin K*. Op cit.
21. Spanierman CS. Iron toxicity. Medscape. http://emedicine.medscape.com/article/815213-overview. Accessed January 8, 2016.
22. Centers for Disease Control and Prevention. Hemochromatosis (iron storage disease). http://www.cdc.gov/ncbddd/hemochromatosis/training/epidemiology/prevalence.html. Accessed January 8, 2016.
23. Prasad AS, Helstead JA, Nadami M. Syndrome of iron deficiency anemia, hepatosplenomegaly, hypogonadism, dwarfism and geophagia. *Am J Med*. 1961;31:532–546.
24. Sandstead HH, Prasad AS, Schubert AR, et al. Human zinc deficiency endocrine manifestations and response to treatment. *Am J Clin Nutr*. 1967;20;422–442.
25. Gropper SS, Smith JL, Groff JL. *Advanced Nutrition and Human Metabolism*. Op cit.
26. King JC, Cousins RJ. Zinc. In: Shils ME, Shike M, Ross AC, et al., eds. *Modern Nutrition in Health and Disease*. 10th ed. Philadelphia: Lippincott Williams & Wilkins; 2006:271–285.
27. Ibid.
28. Medline Plus. Zinc. http://www.nlm.nih.gov/medlineplus/druginfo/natural/patient-zinc.html. Accessed January 8, 2016.
29. Wintergerst ES, Maggini S, Hornig DH. Contribution of selected vitamins and trace elements to immune function. *Ann Nutr Metab*. 2007;51:301–323.
30. Hambidge KM, Miller LV, Westcott JE, Sheng X, Krebs NF. Zinc bioavailability and homeostasis. *Am J Clin Nutr*. 2010;91(5):1478S–1483S.
31. Craig WJ, Mangels AR, American Dietetic Association. Position of the American Dietetic Association: vegetarian diets. *J Am Diet Assoc*. 2009;109(7):1266–1282.
32. Norris J. RD resources for consumers: zinc in vegetarian diets. Vegetarian Nutrition Dietetic Practice Group of the American Dietetic Association. http://vegetariannutrition.net/docs/Zinc-Vegetarian-Nutrition.pdf. Accessed January 8, 2016.
33. Hunt JR, Beiseigel JM. Dietary calcium does not exacerbate phytate inhibition of zinc absorption by women from conventional diets. *Am J Clin Nutr*. 2009;89:839–843.
34. Hunt JR. Bioavailability of iron, zinc, and other trace minerals from vegetarian diets. *Am J Clin Nutr*. 2003;78(suppl):633S–639S.
35. Gropper SS, Smith JL, Groff JL. *Advanced Nutrition and Human Metabolism*. Op cit.
36. King JC, Cousins RJ. Zinc. Op cit.
37. Institute of Medicine, Food and Nutrition Board. *Dietary Reference Intakes for Vitamin A, Vitamin K*. Op cit.
38. Johnson LE. Zinc. In: Porter RS, Kaplan JL, eds. *Merck Manual for Healthcare Professionals*. Whitehouse Station, NJ: Merck & Co; 2005. http://www.merck.com/mmpe/sec01/ch005/ch005j.html. Accessed January 8, 2016.
39. Ibid.
40. Johnson LE. Copper. In: Porter RS, Kaplan JL, eds. *Merck Manual for Healthcare Professionals*. Whitehouse Station, NJ: Merck & Co; 2005. http://www.merck.com/mmpe/sec01/ch005/ch005c.html. Accessed January 8, 2016.
41. Dennert G, Zwahlen M, Brinkman M, et al. Selenium for preventing cancer. *Cochrane Database Syst Rev*. 2011;(5):CD005195.
42. National Institutes of Health, Office of Dietary Supplements. Selenium: dietary supplement fact sheet. http://ods.od.nih.gov/factsheets/selenium. Accessed January 8, 2016.
43. Institute of Medicine, Food and Nutrition Board. *Dietary Reference Intakes for Vitamin C, Vitamin E, Selenium, and Carotenoids*. Washington, DC: National Academies Press; 2000.
44. Ibid.
45. National Institutes of Health, Office of Dietary Supplements. Selenium: dietary supplement fact sheet. Op cit.
46. Institute of Medicine, Food and Nutrition Board. *Dietary Reference Intakes for Vitamin C, Vitamin E*. Op cit.
47. Hetzel BS. *The Story of Iodine Deficiency: An International Challenge in Nutrition*. Oxford, England: Oxford University Press; 1989.
48. World Health Organization. Micronutrient deficiencies: iodine deficiency disorders. http://www.who.int/nutrition/topics/idd/en/index.html. Accessed January 8, 2016.
49. Guyton AC, Hall JE. *Medical Textbook of Physiology*. 12th ed. Philadelphia: WB Saunders; 2010.
50. Johnson LE. Iodine. In: Porter RS, Kaplan JL, eds. *Merck Manual for Healthcare Professionals*. Whitehouse Station, NJ: Merck & Co; 2005. http://www.merck.com/mmpe/sec01/ch005/ch005e.html. Accessed January 8, 2016.
51. Institute of Medicine, Food and Nutrition Board. *Dietary Reference Intakes for Vitamin A, Vitamin K*. Op cit.
52. Ibid.
53. Harvey LJ, McArdle HJ. Biomarkers of copper status: a brief update. *Br J Nutr*. 2008;99(suppl 3):S10–S13.
54. Gambling L, Andersen HS, McArdle HJ. Iron and copper, and their interactions during development. *Biochem Soc Trans*. 2008;36(pt 6):1258–1261.
55. Johnson LE. Copper. Op cit.
56. Turnland JR. Copper. In: Shils ME, Shike M, Ross AC, et al., eds. *Modern Nutrition in Health and Disease*. 10th ed. Philadelphia: Lippincott Williams & Wilkins; 2006:286–299.
57. Institute of Medicine, Food and Nutrition Board. *Dietary Reference Intakes for Vitamin A, Vitamin K*. Op cit.
58. Linus Pauling Institute, Micronutrient Information Center. Manganese. http://lpi.oregonstate.edu/infocenter/minerals/manganese. Accessed January 8, 2016.
59. Ibid.
60. Everett ET. Fluoride's effects on the formation of teeth and bones, and the influence of genetics. *J Dent Res*. 2011;90(5):552–560.
61. Institute of Medicine, Food and Nutrition Board. *Dietary Reference Intakes for Calcium, Phosphorus, Magnesium, Vitamin D, and F luoride*. Washington, DC: National Academy of Sciences; 1997.
62. Benjamin RM. Oral health: the silent epidemic. *Public Health Rep*. 2010;125(2):158–159.
63. American Dental Association. Oral health topics: fluoride supplements: fluoride supplement dosing schedule—2010. http://www.ada.org/2684.aspx#dosschedule. Accessed January 8, 2016.
64. U.S. Department of Health and Human Services. HHS and EPA announce new scientific assessments and actions on fluoride. Press release. January 7, 2011.
65. Environmental Protection Agency. Questions and answers on fluoride. January 2011. https://www.epa.gov/sites/production/files/2015-10/documents/2011_fluoride_questionsanswers.pdf. Accessed March 21, 2016.
66. Environmental Protection Agency. EPA and HHS announce new scientific assessments and actions on fluoride/Agencies working together to maintain

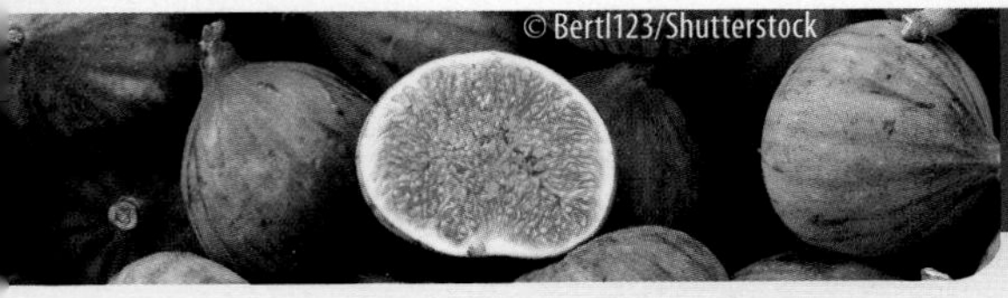
© Bertl123/Shutterstock

Learning Portfolio (continued)

benefits of preventing tooth decay while preventing excessive exposure. January 7, 2011. http://yosemite.epa.gov/opa/admpress.nsf/6427a6b7538955c585257359003f0230/86964af577c37ab285257811005a8417!OpenDocument. Accessed January 8, 2016.

67. American Dental Association. Fluoride in water. 2016. http://www.ada.org/en/public-programs/advocating-for-the-public/fluoride-and-fluoridation. Accessed March 21, 2016.
68. Vernacchio L, Kelly JP, Kaufman DW, Mitchell AA. Vitamin, fluoride, and iron use among US children younger than 12 years of age: results from the Slone Survey 1998–2007. *J Am Diet Assoc.* 2011;111(2):285–289.
69. Canadian Medical Association. Battle renewed over value of fluoridation. *CMAJ.* 2011;183(9):E531–E532.
70. American Dental Association. Fluoride and fluoridation. Op cit.
71. Berg J, Gerweck C, Hujoel PP, et al. Evidence-based clinical recommendations regarding fluoride intake from reconstituted infant formula and enamel fluorosis: a report of the American Dental Association Council on Scientific Affairs. *J Am Dental Assoc.* 2011;142(1):79–87.
72. Licata A. Bone density vs bone quality: what's a clinician to do? *Cleveland Clin J Med.* 2009;76(6):331–336.
73. Gropper, Smith, Groff. *Advanced Nutrition and Human Metabolism.*
74. National Institutes of Health, Office of Dietary Supplements. Chromium: dietary supplement fact sheet. http://ods.od.nih.gov/factsheets/chromium.asp. Accessed January 8, 2016.

75. Hummel M, Standt E, Schnell O. Chromium in metabolic and cardiovascular disorders. *Horm Metab Res*. 2007;39:743–751.
76. Sharma S, Agrawal RP, Choudhary M, et al. Beneficial effect of chromium supplementation on glucose, HbA(1)C and lipid variables in individuals with newly onset type-2 diabetes. *J Trace Elem Med Biol*. 2011;25(3):149–153.
77. Chehade JM, Sheikh-Ali M, Mooradian AD. The role of micronutrients in managing diabetes. *Diabetes Spectrum*. 2009;22(4):214–218.
78. Sarubin-Fragakis A, Thomson C. *The Health Professional's Guide to Popular Dietary Supplements*. 3rd ed. Chicago: American Dietetic Association; 2007.
79. Eckhert CD. Other trace elements. In: Shils ME, Shike M, Ross AC, et al., eds. *Modern Nutrition in Health and Disease*. 10th ed. Philadelphia: Lippincott Williams & Wilkins; 2006:338–350.
80. Institute of Medicine, Food and Nutrition Board. *Dietary Reference Intakes for Vitamin A, Vitamin K*. Op cit.
81. Yosim A, Bailey K, Fry RC. Arsenic, the "king of poisons," in food and water. *Am Scientist*. 2015;103:34–41.
82. Nielsen FH. Is boron nutritionally relevant? *Nutr Rev*. 2008;66(4):183–191.
83. Institute of Medicine, Food and Nutrition Board. *Dietary Reference Intakes for Vitamin A, Vitamin K*. Op cit.
84. Eckhert CD. Other trace elements. Op cit.
85. Gropper SS, Smith JL, Groff JL. *Advanced Nutrition and Human Metabolism*. Op cit.
86. Institute of Medicine, Food and Nutrition Board. *Dietary Reference Intakes for Vitamin A, Vitamin K*. Op cit.

Chapter 14

Sports Nutrition: Eating for Peak Performance

Revised by Don Ross

THINK About It

1. How much importance do you place on being physically active?
2. How often do you suffer from muscle fatigue? What do you think causes it?
3. How often do you think about food choices when you're planning a physical activity?
4. What kind of protein do you emphasize in your diet?

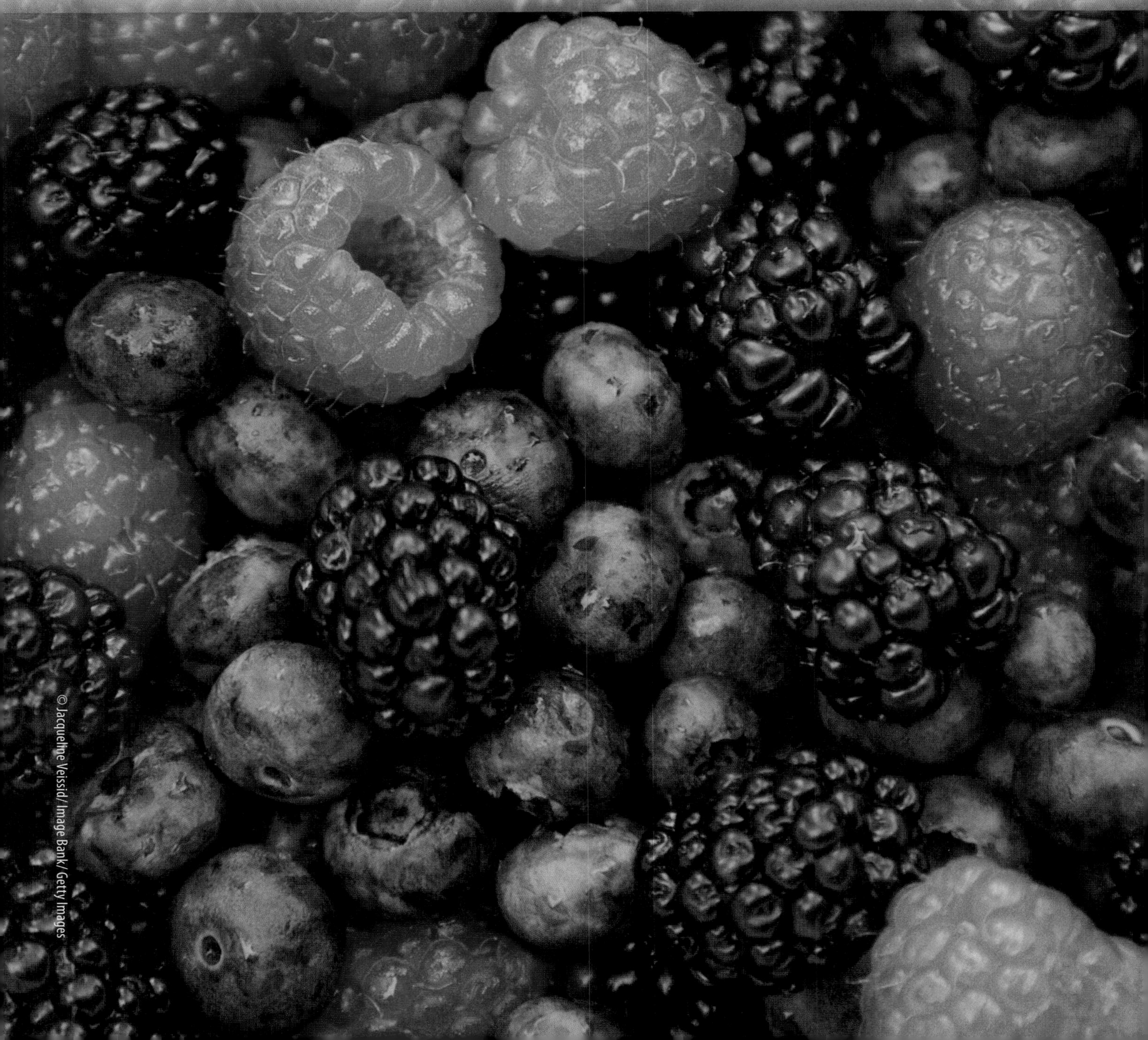

CHAPTER Menu

LEARNING Objectives

- State the components and guidelines to physical fitness.
- Trace the metabolic energy systems for ATP–CP, lactate, and oxygen, and apply each system to a specific sport type.
- Distinguish the types of muscle fibers.
- Apply nutrition concepts to a food plan for athletic performance.
- Evaluate nutrition supplements and ergogenic aids designed to enhance athletic performance.

Today is the big 10,000-meter race. You've trained for months. Fans in the crowd shade their eyes as they watch you and your competitors walk onto the track. "Ready," shouts the starter. "Get set." You toe the starting line and adrenaline increases your heart rate, diverting blood to your muscles and mobilizing energy stores in your liver, muscles, and fat. "Go!" Within a fraction of a second, a torrent of calcium flows into your muscle cells, causing your muscles to contract and launching you from the starting line.

How will you perform in this race? Will your breakfast help or hinder your performance? Will what you ate yesterday and the day before affect your stamina? Does it matter what you eat after you finish the race? Find the answers to these questions and learn about the links between nutrition and sports performance in this chapter.

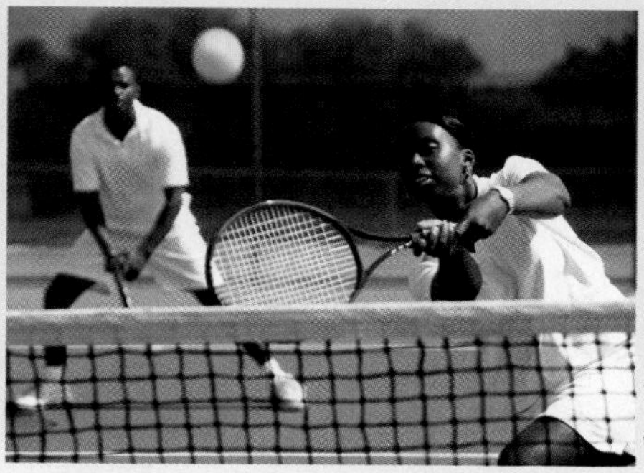

Nutrition and Physical Performance

THINK About It 1

Just how physically active do you need to be? (See **FIGURE 14.1**.) Both the National Institutes of Health (NIH) and Health Canada have found that small to moderate amounts of physical activity can produce substantial health benefits. Physically active people have a lower risk of developing many chronic diseases, such as coronary heart disease, diabetes, hypertension, osteoporosis, and obesity. Active people also experience an increased sense of well-being and are much better equipped to cope with stress.

"Exercise is Medicine" is an initiative focused on encouraging primary care physicians, nutritionists, and other healthcare providers to include exercise when designing treatment plans for patients. Launched by the American Medical Association (AMA) and the American College of Sports Medicine (ACSM), Exercise is Medicine is committed to making physical activity and exercise a standard part of disease prevention and treatment. The vision of Exercise is Medicine is to:

- Have healthcare providers assess every patient's level of physical activity at every clinic visit
- Determine if the patient is meeting the U.S. National Physical Activity Guidelines
- Provide patients with brief counseling to help him/her meet the guidelines and/or refer the patient to either healthcare or community-based resources for further physical activity (PA) counseling.[1]

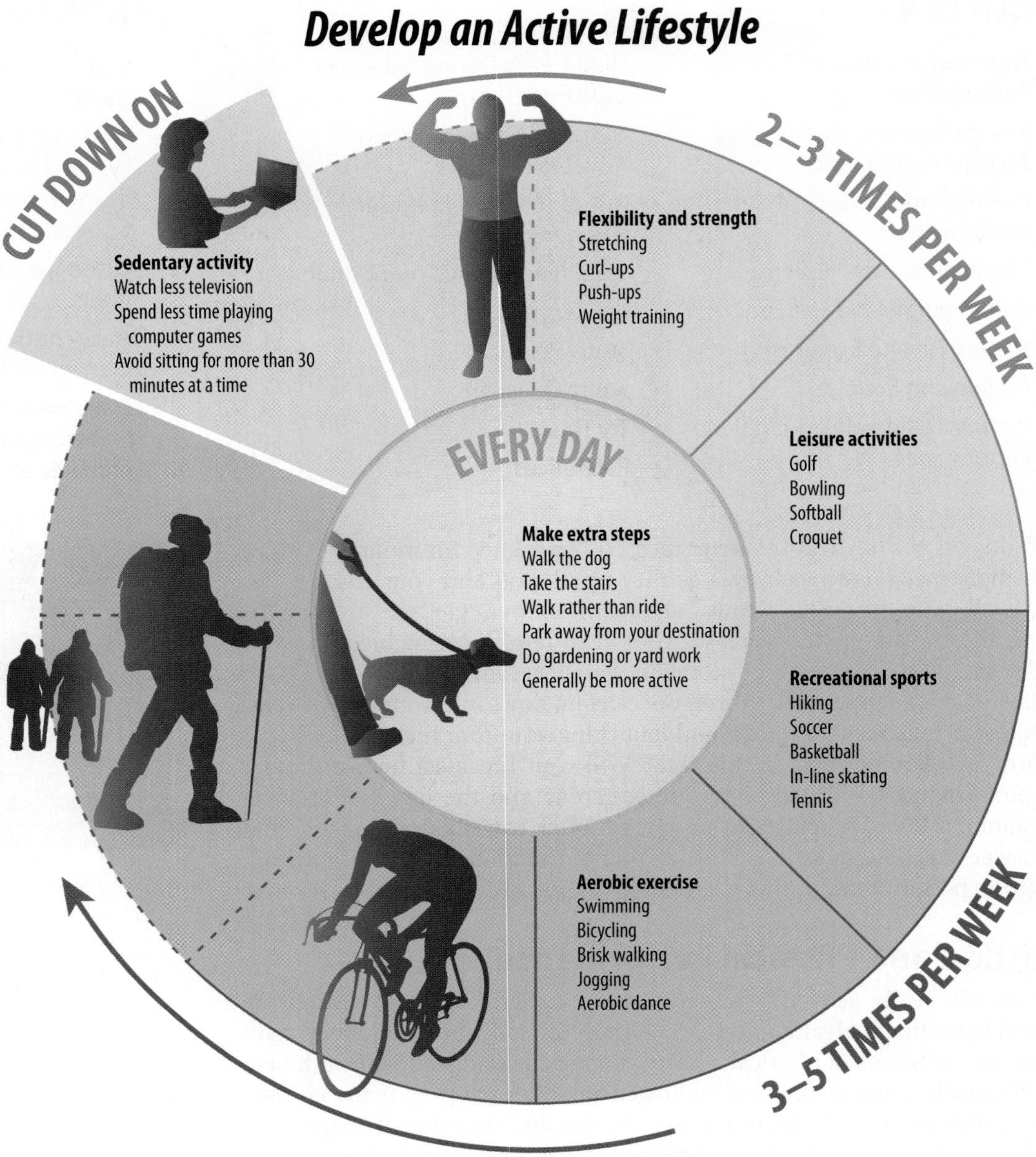

FIGURE 14.1 Be active. Perhaps the most important aspect of increasing physical activity is to have fun.

The ACSM notes an important distinction between physical activity as it relates to health and exercise for physical fitness.[2] According to the ACSM, the level of physical activity that can reduce the risk of various chronic diseases might not be enough—in quantity or quality—to improve physical fitness. The *Physical Activity Guidelines for Americans* recommends that children and adolescents should do at least 60 minutes of physical activity daily, and all adults should avoid inactivity. For substantial health benefits, adults should do at least 2 hours and 30 minutes a week of moderate-intensity or 1 hour and 15 minutes a week of vigorous-intensity aerobic activity.[3] Unfortunately, U.S. adults generally fall short of meeting the activity recommendations. In 48 states, less than 25 percent of adults meet the guidelines for aerobic and muscle-strengthening physical activity.[4]

What is physical fitness? The ACSM defines physical fitness as "the ability to perform moderate to vigorous levels of physical activity without undue fatigue and the capability of maintaining this level of activity throughout life."[5] In other words, it is more than being able to run a long distance or lift a lot of weight at the gym. Being fit is not defined only by what kind of activity you do, how long you do it, or at what level of intensity. Although these are important measures of fitness, they only address single areas. Overall fitness is made up of five main components:

1. *Cardiorespiratory fitness:* The ability of the body's circulatory and respiratory systems to supply fuel during sustained physical activity.
2. *Muscular strength:* The ability of the muscle to exert force during an activity.
3. *Muscular endurance:* The ability of the muscle to continue to perform without fatigue.
4. *Body composition:* The relative amounts of fat and lean body mass. Body composition is an important component to consider for health and weight management.
5. *Flexibility:* The range of motion around a joint. Good flexibility in the joints can help prevent injuries through all stages of life.

Exercise Intensity

Intensity is how hard your body is working during aerobic activity. For most people, light-intensity activities such as shopping, cooking, and doing the laundry don't provide health benefits. Why? Their bodies are not working hard enough to increase their heart rates. When you are working enough to raise your heart rate and break a sweat, you are performing a *moderate-intensity aerobic activity*. One way that you can tell is that you'll be able to talk, but not sing, during a moderate-intensity aerobic activity. Examples of moderate-intensity activities include brisk walking, doing water aerobics, riding a bike on level ground, playing doubles tennis, and pushing a lawnmower. Vigorous-intensity aerobic activity means that you are breathing hard and your heart rate has gone up quite a bit. At this level of activity, you will be able to say only a few words before pausing for a breath. Examples of vigorous activities include running, swimming laps, riding a bike fast or up hills, and playing singles tennis or basketball. To meet your activity goals for health, you can do moderate or vigorous activities or a combination of both. A rule of thumb is that 2 minutes of moderate-intensity activity is about the same as 1 minute of vigorous-intensity activity.

Muscle-Strengthening Exercises

Muscle-strengthening exercises (also called resistance training) should work all major muscle groups (legs, hips, back, abdomen, chest, shoulders, and arms). For maximal health benefits, these exercises should be done to the point where it's hard to do another repetition without assistance. A *repetition* is one complete movement, such as doing a sit-up or lifting a weight. A *set* is a minimum of 8–12 repetitions per activity. When exercising, try to do at least one set of muscle-strengthening activities; two or three sets is better. Strengthening activities include lifting weights, working with resistance bands, doing push-ups and sit-ups, digging and shoveling, and practicing yoga.

Flexibility and Neuromotor Exercises

Flexibility exercises improve joint range of motion and are most effective after the muscles are warmed by at least five minutes of light- to moderate-intensity

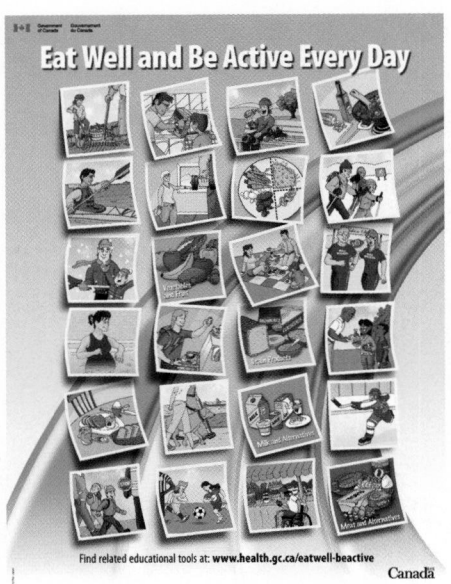

FIGURE 14.2 Eat well and be active every day.
Eat Well and Be Active Every Day Poster. Health Canada, 2011. Eat Well and Be Active Everyday. Health Canada, 2015. Adapted and reproduced with permission from the Minister of Health, 2016.

activities. Stretches should be to the point of feeling tightness or slight discomfort. Neuromotor exercises, such as yoga, improve balance, agility, coordination, and gait.

Some Is Better Than None

It's best to spread your activities throughout the week. You can even break sessions into smaller chunks of time during the day, as long as you're making a moderate or vigorous effort for at least 10 minutes at a time. You may wish to use digital devices to monitor your activity. A study of healthy adults found that bestselling smartphone applications and wearable devices are generally accurate for tracking step counts.[6] These applications and devices have the potential to better engage people in their health. **TABLE 14.1** shows the levels of physical activity needed to promote health and to achieve and maintain body weight (see also **FIGURE 14.2**).

Nutrition has taken its rightful place as a vital component of any program that seeks to enhance health, fitness, and athletic performance. In a joint position paper, the Academy of Nutrition and Dietetics, the Dietitians of Canada,

TABLE 14.1
Guidelines for Physical Activity: Health and Fitness

For Important Health Benefits
Aerobic activities:* • 5 or more days per week (preferably every day) • 30–60 minutes per day; 2 hours and 30 minutes (150 minutes) per week • Moderate-intensity activities Muscle-strengthening activities: • 2 or more days per week • 8–12 repetitions to improve strength and power • 2–4 sets to improve muscular endurance Flexibility exercises: • 2 or more days per week • A series of flexibility exercise for each major muscle group • Hold a static stretch for 30–60 seconds, longer in older adults Neuromotor exercises: • 2 or more days per week • Effective intensity and duration have not been determined All healthy adults should reduce total time engaged in sedentary activities. When sedentary, even people who generally are physically active should intersperse frequent, short bouts of standing and physical activity. Your exercise program can be modified according to your habitual physical activity, physical function, health status, exercise responses, and stated goals. Engaging in amounts of exercise less than recommended still will provide benefits.
For Weight Loss
Increase your aerobic activities. With moderate diet restrictions, 150 to 250 minutes per week of moderate-intensity activity supports clinically significant weight loss (> 5 percent reduction in body weight).
For Weight Maintenance After Weight Loss
After weight loss, weight maintenance (< 3 percent change in body weight) is improved with moderate-intensity activity for more than 250 minutes per week.

*Moderate-intensity activities may be replaced with vigorous-intensity activities for 1 hour and 15 minutes (75 minutes) per week. An equivalent mix of moderate- and vigorous-intensity activities also meets the guidelines.

Garber CE, Blissmer B, Deschenes MR, et al. American College of Sports Medicine position stand. Quantity and quality of exercise for developing and maintaining cardiorespiratory, musculoskeletal, and neuromotor fitness in apparently healthy adults: guidance for prescribing exercise. *Med Sci Sports Exerc*. 2011; 43(7):1334–1359; Donnelly JE, Blair SN, Jakicic JM, et al. American College of Sports Medicine position stand. Appropriate physical activity intervention strategies for weight loss and prevention of weight regain for adults. *Med Sci Sports Exerc*. 2009; 41(2):459–471; Centers for Disease Control and Prevention. How much physical activity do adults need? http://www.cdc.gov/physicalactivity/everyone/guidelines/adults.html. Accessed February 9, 2016.

American Heart Association

Physical Activity
Physical inactivity is a major risk factor for developing coronary artery disease. Even moderately intense physical activity such as brisk walking is beneficial when done regularly for a total of 30 minutes or longer on most days.

and the ACSM state that "physical activity, athletic performance, and recovery from exercise are enhanced by optimal nutrition."[7] But just what is "optimal nutrition?" Is it the same for a child who plays recreational softball and for a senior citizen who takes daily walks to reduce the risk of type 2 diabetes? What about the competitive athlete who strives to maximize athletic performance and uses nutrition to gain a competitive edge? To understand the relationship between physical activity and nutrition, you first need to appreciate how we use energy during exercise.

Key Concepts Exercise provides numerous health benefits, including reduced risk of chronic disease. Physical fitness includes strength, endurance, and flexibility. For optimal physical performance, nutrition is an essential part of all athletic training programs.

Position Statement: Academy of Nutrition and Dietetics

Nutrition and Athletic Performance

It is the position of the Academy of Nutrition and Dietetics (Academy), Dietitians of Canada (DC), and the American College of Sports Medicine (ACSM) that the performance of, and recovery from, sporting activities are enhanced by well-chosen nutrition strategies. These organizations provide guidelines for the appropriate type, amount, and timing of intake of food, fluids, and supplements to promote optimal health and performance across different scenarios of training and competitive sport.

Reproduced from Thomas DT, Erdman KA, Burke LM, et al. Position of the American Dietetic Association, Dietitians of Canada, and the American College of Sports Medicine: nutrition and athletic performance. *Journal of the Academy Nutrition and Diet*. 2016;116(3):501–528.

Energy Systems, Muscles, and Physical Performance

Let's return to your race. As you leave the starting line, your body immediately ramps up energy production to meet the increased demand. Just as a rocket uses different fuel systems and stages to power its leap into space, your body uses three different energy systems to launch, accelerate, and maintain the exercise you are performing (endurance).

ATP–CP Energy System

As you launch yourself from the starting line, it takes less than a second for your contracting muscles to burn their entire reserve of adenosine triphosphate (ATP), the immediate energy source for cells. Luckily, your body has a small reservoir of **creatine phosphate** (also called **phosphocreatine**) that your muscles can convert quickly to ATP (see **FIGURE 14.3**). Together, your available ATP and creatine phosphate, the **ATP–CP energy system**, can power an all-out effort for

- **creatine phosphate** An energy-rich compound that supplies energy and a phosphate group for the formation of ATP. Also called *phosphocreatine*.
- **phosphocreatine** See *creatine phosphate*.
- **ATP–CP energy system** A simple and immediate anaerobic energy system that maintains ATP levels. Creatine phosphate is broken down, releasing energy and a phosphate group, which is used to form ATP.

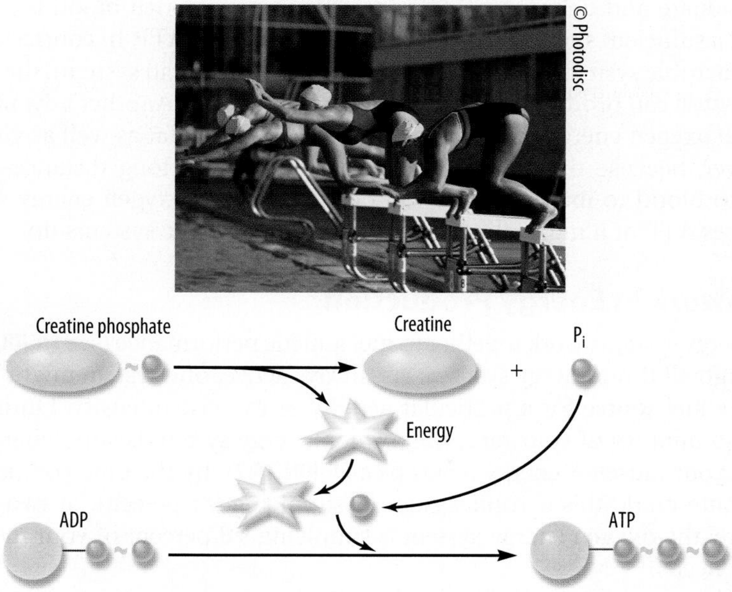

FIGURE 14.3 ATP–CP energy system. To maintain relatively constant ATP levels during an initial explosive burst of high-intensity activity, your body uses its ATP–CP energy system to generate ATP from creatine phosphate.

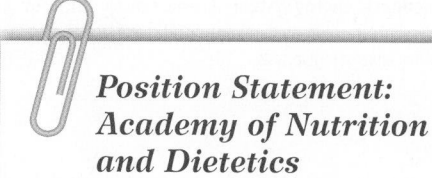

▶ **lactic acid energy system** Anaerobic energy system; using glycolysis, it rapidly produces energy (ATP) and lactate. Also called anaerobic glycolysis.

▶ **oxygen energy system** A complex energy system that requires oxygen. To release ATP, it completes the breakdown of carbohydrate and fatty acids through the citric acid cycle and electron transport chain.

only 3 to 15 seconds.[8] To continue the race, you must enlist carbohydrate stored as glycogen in your muscles and liver. Your cells rapidly disassemble glycogen to glucose, from which they can extract ATP.

Lactic Acid Energy System

For the next minute or two, the acceleration stage, your body uses the simplest and speediest chemical pathways to produce ATP from glucose: the **lactic acid energy system** (see **FIGURE 14.4**). The term *lactic acid energy system* is a misnomer. Although "lactic acid" and "lactate" are used interchangeably, they are different chemically, and lactic acid is not produced in the body.

Like the ATP–CP energy system, these pathways are anaerobic—they do not require oxygen. The raw material, glucose, is much more plentiful than creatine phosphate, but its breakdown also produces a by-product: lactate. The rapid extraction of energy from ATP molecules produces ADP molecules and protons. During aerobic metabolism, these protons are used by cells, but during anaerobic metabolism these protons accumulate and make the cells acidic. A rise in acidity impairs the breakdown of glucose and inhibits calcium binding. Without calcium, muscles cannot contract. For years, coaches and athletes have blamed lactic acid for muscle fatigue, but it's actually the change in pH due to excess protons that is the primary culprit.[9] To continue running beyond the first few minutes, your body employs a sophisticated, oxygen-based system to process lactate and squeeze out much more ATP from glucose. THINK About It 2

creatine phosphate + ADP + H^+ = ATP + creatine

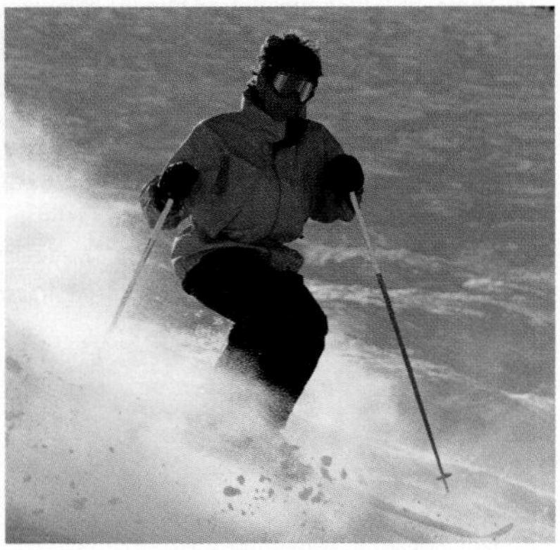

© Photodisc

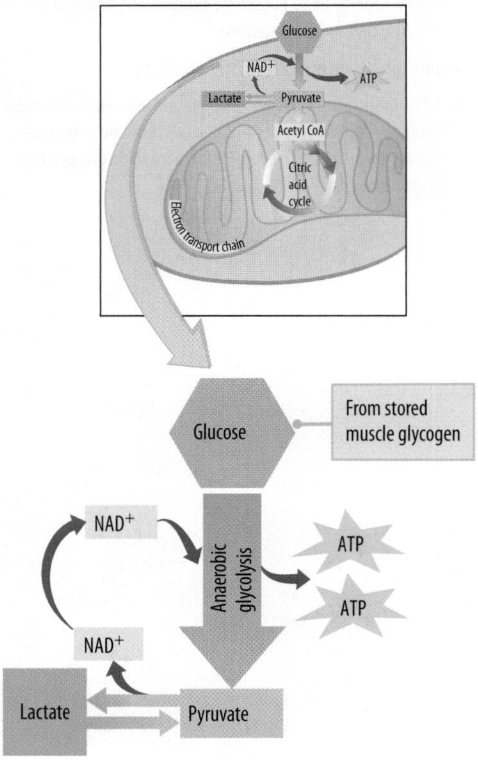

FIGURE 14.4 Lactic acid energy system. During short events requiring power and speed, the lactic acid energy system supplies much of the energy. Because the lactic acid system does not require oxygen, these events are anaerobic activities.

Oxygen Energy System

For the endurance stage, cells can use lengthy, complex chemical pathways in their mitochondria—small units within cells that function as power-generating plants—to convert food and oxygen to ATP (see **FIGURE 14.5**). These reactions are aerobic—they require abundant oxygen. In contracting muscle, blood vessels dilate and deliver a 20-fold increase in oxygen-rich blood to muscle cells,[10] a sufficient supply for mitochondria to produce ATP. In contrast to the two anaerobic systems (the ATP–CP system and lactic acid system), the **oxygen energy system** can produce a tremendous amount of ATP. Another advantage is that the oxygen energy system can extract energy from fat as well as glucose. However, because the required oxygen must travel a long distance—from lungs to blood to muscle cells to mitochondria—the oxygen energy system produces ATP at a much slower rate than the anaerobic systems do.

Teamwork in Energy Production

The energy systems work together to fuel athletic performance (see **FIGURE 14.6**). Although all three energy systems are always active, one system might be the primary fuel source for a particular activity or exercise intensity. During the first two minutes of your race, the oxygen energy system is supplying about half of your muscles' energy needs (see **FIGURE 14.7**). By the time you pass the 30-minute mark, this aerobic system is supplying 95 percent; at two hours or more, the oxygen energy system is supplying 98 percent of your muscles' energy needs.[11]

As long as ATP production by the mitochondria meets energy needs, you are exercising aerobically; highly trained athletes can sustain such exercise for hours. If the exercise rate exceeds your body's ability to supply oxygen to your muscles, you are exercising anaerobically, rapidly depleting your creatine phosphate and glycogen reserves. Once these are exhausted, if available oxygen cannot support the oxygen energy system, performance plummets.

Carbohydrate stores are limited. A 68-kilogram (150-pound) man with 10 to 20 percent body fat, for example, has carbohydrate stores of 1,800 to 2,000 kilocalories in muscle glycogen, liver glycogen, and blood glucose. Compare this with the energy he stores in fat. His fat tissue holds roughly 63,000 to 120,000 kilocalories.[12] Although the body can burn protein for energy, in well-fed people protein probably provides no more than 5 percent of energy expended in exercise.[13]

Glycogen Depletion

At the beginning of the race, your body rapidly uses muscle glycogen. But as the race grinds on, the rate of glycogen use markedly slows. During the first one and a half hours, glycogen stores drop steadily to about one-third their starting levels. About three hours into the run, as glycogen stores become almost entirely depleted, you might "hit the wall." Your muscles become weak and heavy, your legs shake, and you become confused. Marathon runners commonly experience a sudden onset of exhaustive fatigue around the 18- to 20-mile mark. Drinking fluids that contain glucose can partially compensate for glycogen depletion and soften its effects. Dehydration can cause an even faster onset of fatigue, so drinking plenty of fluids is essential during endurance events.

As exercise intensity increases, glycogen depletion accelerates. Sprinting, for example, uses muscle glycogen 35 to 40 times faster than walking does.[14] **FIGURE 14.8** illustrates how the sensation of fatigue relates to the depletion of muscle glycogen.

Endurance Training

In untrained people, endurance training can increase endurance by as much as 500 percent.[15] To increase endurance, training enhances aerobic capacity by increasing the number of mitochondria and improving the body's ability to deliver oxygen to them. This decreases the reliance on anaerobic energy systems, extending the availability of glycogen reserves and delaying fatigue.

Key Concepts Muscle cells use three different energy systems to produce ATP: the ATP–CP energy system, the lactic acid energy system, and the oxygen aerobic system. The ATP–CP and lactic acid energy systems rely on carbohydrates and do not require oxygen. The oxygen energy system requires oxygen and relies on carbohydrates and fats. During the early minutes of high-intensity exercise, the anaerobic systems are the predominant source of ATP. During lower-intensity endurance events, the aerobic system supplies ATP, although at a much slower rate. Dehydration and depletion of glycogen stores are major factors in fatigue. Training increases the efficiency of oxygen delivery to muscle and increases the number of muscle mitochondria available for aerobic metabolism.

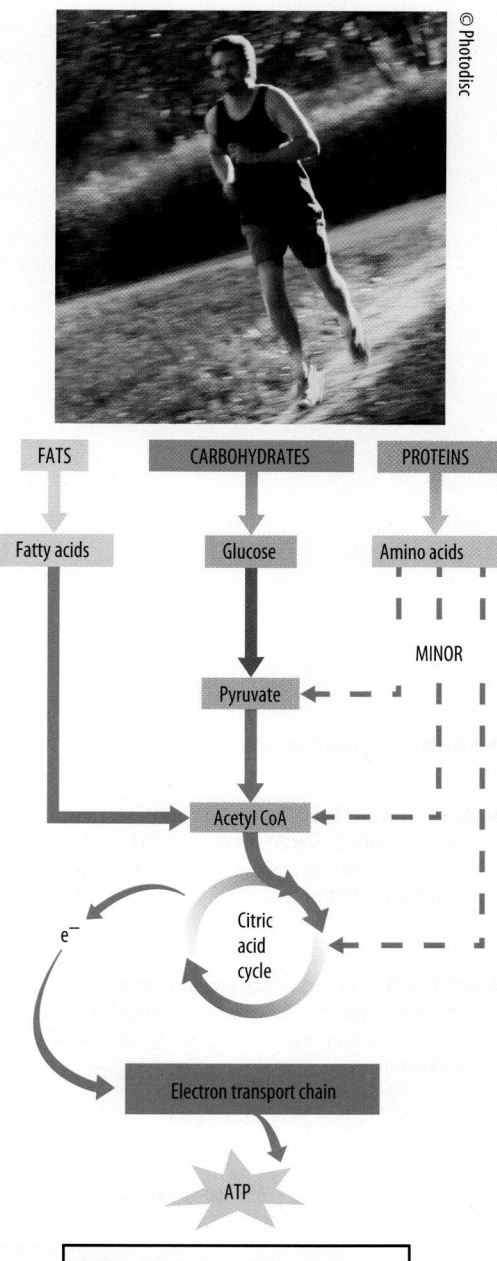

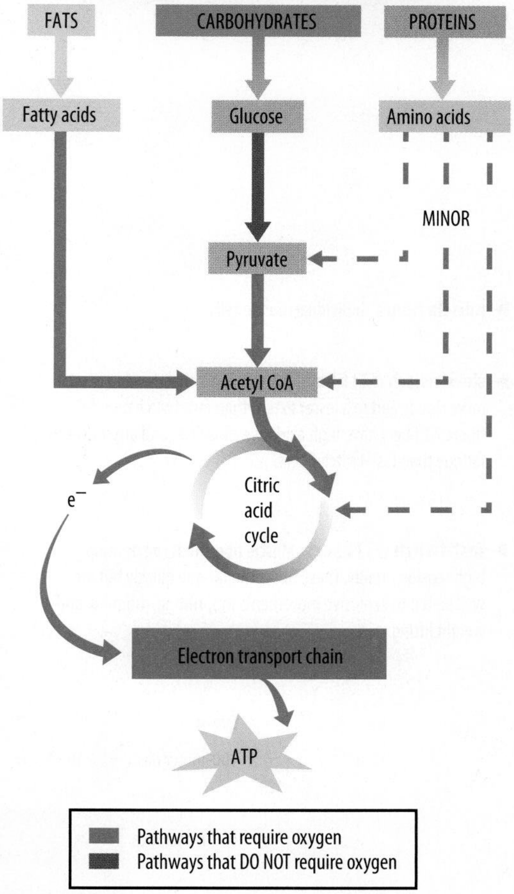

FIGURE 14.5 Oxygen energy system. During longer endurance events (aerobic events), the oxygen energy system supplies most of the energy. This energy system requires oxygen and primarily relies on carbohydrate and fat as fuels.

Muscles and Muscle Fibers

Your body contains hundreds of muscles that help control a myriad of functions, from regulating blood pressure to climbing stairs. **Skeletal muscles** are bundles of parallel, striated fibers attached to your skeleton (see **FIGURE 14.9**). These muscles are responsible for your physical movement and are under your conscious control. If you decide to bend your arm, for example, you consciously contract your biceps. Your body contains more than 600 skeletal muscles and uses 9 of them just to control your thumb!

▶ **skeletal muscles** Muscles composed of bundles of parallel, striated muscle fibers under voluntary control. Also called voluntary muscle or striated muscle.

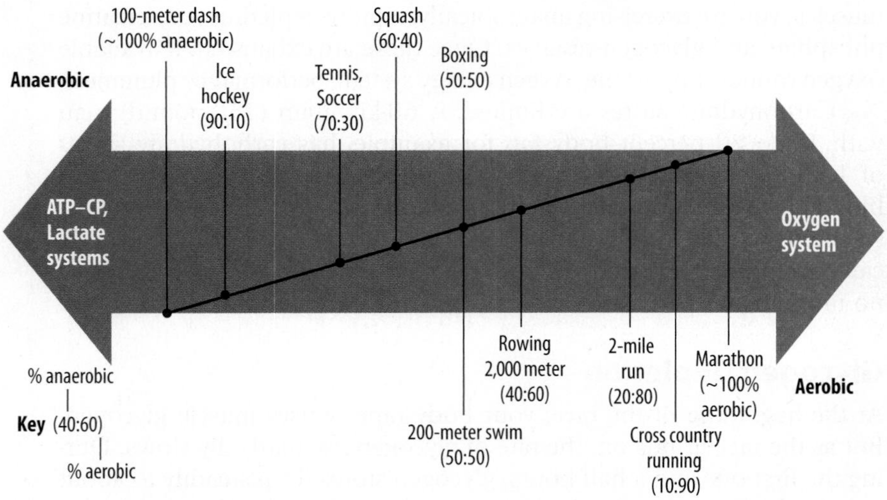

FIGURE 14.6 The anaerobic–aerobic continuum. Most activities use ATP from both anaerobic and aerobic energy systems. However, the 100-meter dash is considered completely anaerobic, and the marathon is considered completely aerobic.

▶ **muscle fibers** Individual muscle cells.

▶ **slow-twitch (ST) fibers** Muscle fibers that develop tension more slowly and to a lesser extent than fast-twitch muscle fibers. ST fibers have high oxidative capacities and are slower to fatigue than fast-twitch fibers.

▶ **fast-twitch (FT) fibers** Muscle fibers that can develop high tension rapidly. These fibers can fatigue quickly but are well suited to explosive movements in sprinting, jumping, and weight lifting.

Individual muscle cells are called **muscle fibers**; skeletal muscle has two primary types:

- **Slow-twitch (ST) fibers**
- **Fast-twitch (FT) fibers**

They derive their names from the difference in their speed of action. One type of fast-twitch fiber can contract 10 times faster than slow-twitch fibers.[16]

Slow-Twitch Fibers

To power their activity, slow-twitch fibers efficiently produce energy by breaking down carbohydrate and fat by way of aerobic pathways—metabolic

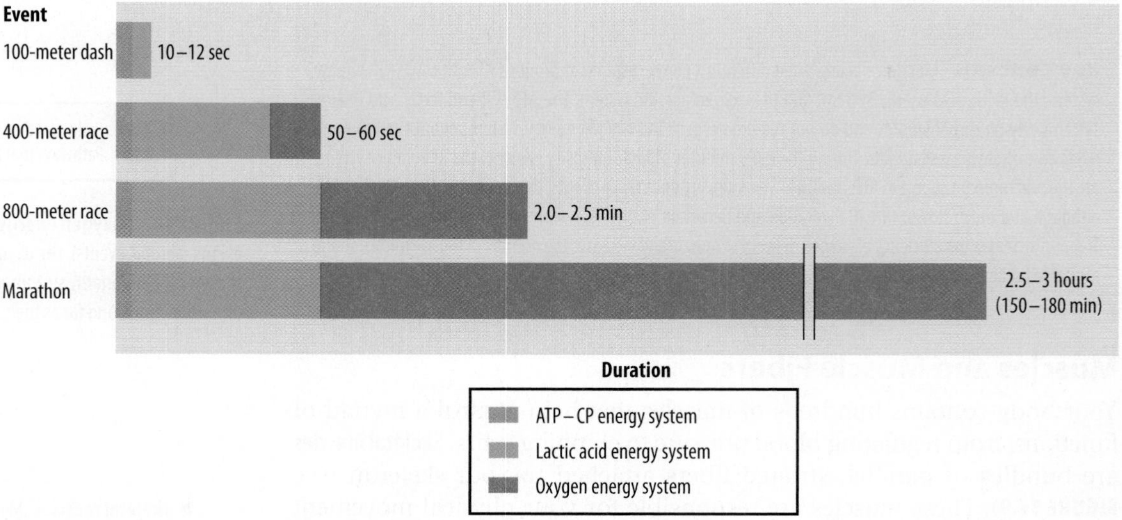

FIGURE 14.7 Sports events and energy systems. Short-term, explosive events rely on the ATP–CP and lactic acid energy systems. For longer events, your body turns to the oxygen energy system. During endurance events, your body uses this system to burn fat as well as glucose.

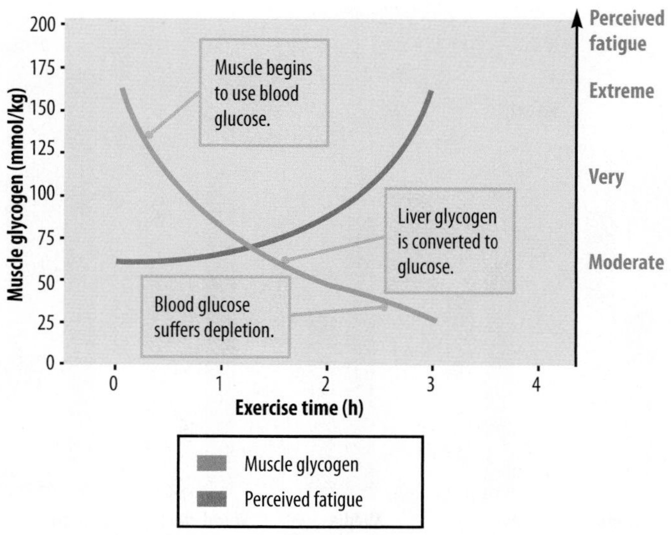

FIGURE 14.8 Glycogen depletion and the sensation of fatigue. As muscle glycogen levels decline, fatigue and eventually exhaustion set in.

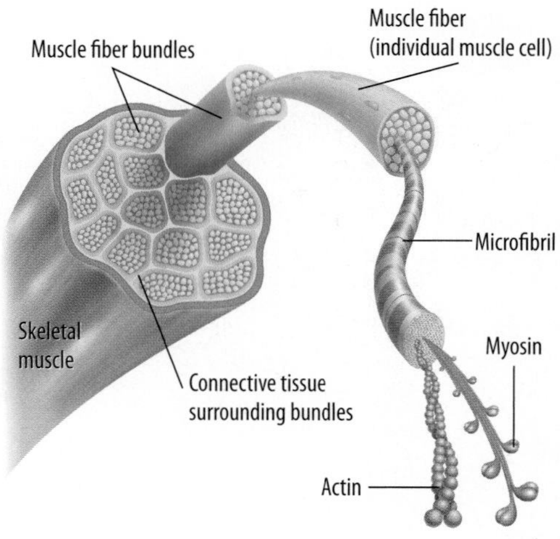

FIGURE 14.9 Basic structure of skeletal muscle. A muscle fiber is an individual muscle cell that usually extends the entire length of the muscle. Each muscle fiber contains hundreds to thousands of microfibrils. Each microfibril contains thousands of actin and myosin filaments, large protein molecules responsible for muscle contractions.

reactions that require oxygen. As long as the aerobic pathways are active, ST fibers can produce energy to sustain their movement. With a sufficient supply of oxygen, ST fibers can maintain muscular activity for a prolonged time. This ability is known as **aerobic endurance**.

Because ST fibers have high aerobic endurance, your body predominantly relies on them during low-intensity endurance events, such as long-distance running, and during everyday activities, such as walking.

► **aerobic endurance** The ability of skeletal muscle to obtain a sufficient supply of oxygen from the heart and lungs to maintain muscular activity for a prolonged time.

Fast-Twitch Fibers

Compared with ST fibers, fast-twitch fibers have poor aerobic endurance. They are optimized to perform anaerobically (when the oxygen supply is limited). FT fibers can efficiently produce energy for their use by metabolic pathways that do not require oxygen. Bundles of FT fibers exert considerably more force than bundles of ST fibers; because of their limited endurance, however, FT fibers tire quickly.

The body recruits both ST and FT fibers during shorter, higher-intensity endurance events, such as the mile run or the 400-meter swim. During highly explosive events, such as the 100-meter dash and the 50-meter sprint swim, the body still recruits both types, but FT fibers contribute most of the muscle power.

Fiber Type and the Athlete

Genes determine the relative proportion of muscle fiber types in athletes. Although distance runners who have a high percentage of ST fibers are well suited for endurance events, they will not succeed as elite sprinters. Conversely, sprinters who have predominantly FT fibers are better equipped for explosive events, but they will not become competitive marathon runners (see **FIGURE 14.10**).

Key Concepts A muscle cell is called a muscle fiber. The two main types of skeletal muscle fibers are slow-twitch and fast-twitch fibers. Slow-twitch fibers generate fuel through aerobic pathways, whereas fast-twitch fibers produce energy using anaerobic pathways. Fast-twitch fibers can exert more force but have limited endurance.

Quick Bite

Use It or Lose It!

The benefits of training begin to disappear after only two weeks of inactivity. Muscular endurance—the ability of a muscle to avoid fatigue—declines, and activities of certain oxidative enzymes drop by as much as 40 percent. By the fourth week, muscle glycogen levels also can drop by 40 percent. Flexibility is quickly lost, and inactivity can substantially decondition the heart muscle and cardiovascular system.

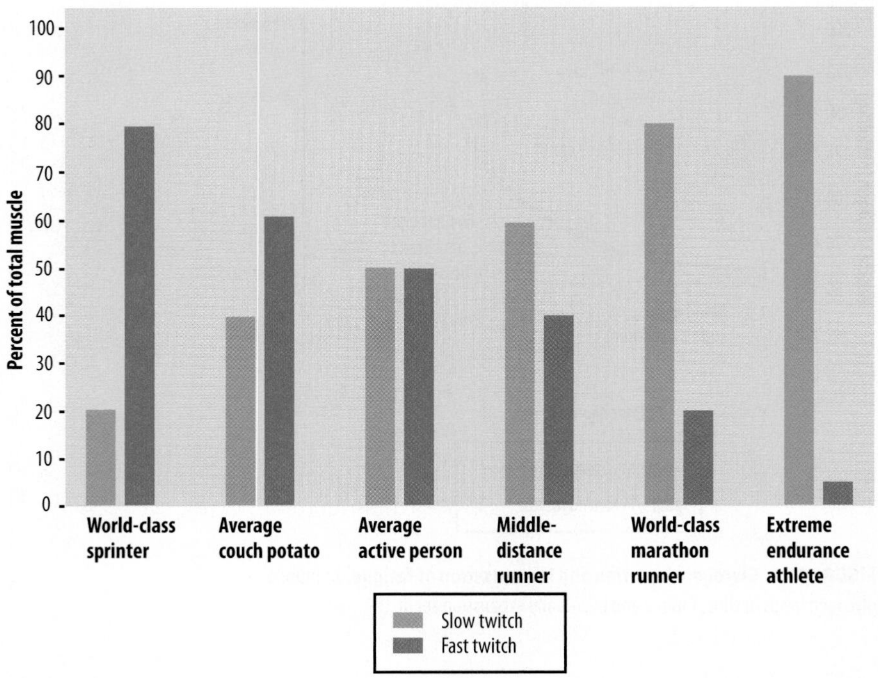

FIGURE 14.10 What's your mix of muscle fibers? If you are best at events requiring explosive movements, you may have a greater percentage of fast-twitch muscle fibers. If endurance events are your specialty, you may have more slow-twitch fibers.

Adapted from Andersen JL, Scherling P, Saltin B. Muscle, genes and athletic performance. *Sci. Am.* 2000;283(3):49.

Optimal Nutrition for Athletic Performance

The one-minute video "We Are All Athletes" showcases U.S. Olympians, Paralympians, and recreational athletes of various backgrounds, including different genders, races and ethnicities, religions, sexual orientations, and abilities.[17] While promoting diversity, social inclusion, sportsmanship, and teamwork, it delivers the important message that each and every one of us is an athlete, albeit with different capabilities. Although there is no sharp dividing line between recreational athletes and competitive athletes, competitive athletes typically train at higher intensity levels and focus on specific events.

The optimal diet for most physically active people—from the college student who plays recreational basketball to the 50-year-old woman who enjoys walking during her lunch break—includes a variety of nutrient-dense foods. Food choices should be high in carbohydrate (more than 60 percent of calories), low in fat (less than 30 percent of calories), and moderate in protein. When energy needs are met by eating a variety of foods, micronutrient (vitamin and mineral) needs are often met as well.

Athletes, coaches, and scientists have long recognized that training and good nutrition go hand in hand when it comes to improving performance. Nutrition can profoundly influence the molecular and cellular processes that occur in muscle during exercise and recovery. Optimal nutrition is an essential part of every athlete's training program and can make a difference when winning is measured in fractions of seconds or inches. General recommendations for competitive athletes include the following[18]:

- Consume adequate energy (calories) during periods of high-intensity and/or long-duration training to maintain body weight and health and to maximize training effects.

- Body weight and composition should not be a sole criterion for participation in sports; daily weigh-ins are discouraged.
- Carbohydrate recommendations for athletes range from 6 to 10 grams per kilogram body weight per day.
- Protein recommendations for endurance and strength-trained athletes range from 1.2 to 1.7 grams per kilogram body weight per day.
- Fat intake should range from 20 to 35 percent of total energy intake.
- At greatest risk of micronutrient deficiencies are athletes who restrict energy intake or use severe weight-loss practices, eliminate one or more food groups from their diet, or consume high- or low-carbohydrate diets of low micronutrient density. (Examples of athletes who may be at risk include ballet dancers and wrestlers.)
- Adequate fluid intake before, during, and after exercise is important for health and optimal performance.
- In general, no vitamin and mineral supplements are required if an athlete is consuming adequate energy from a variety of foods to maintain body weight.

The underlying foundations of a training diet are similar to the basic principles incorporated in the *Dietary Guidelines for Americans* and Canada's *Guidelines for Healthy Eating*. The primary differences are increased fluid needs to cover an athlete's sweat losses and increased energy needs to fuel physical activity. Let's take a closer look at the nutritional needs of athletes.

Energy Intake and Exercise

Adequate energy intake is the first nutrition priority for athletes. Meeting energy needs is critical for athletic performance and for maintaining or increasing lean body mass. Sports nutritionists recommend eating small, frequent meals to maintain energy metabolism, improve nutrient intake, achieve desired body composition, support a training schedule, and reduce injuries.[19] During times of high physical activity, energy and macronutrient needs—especially carbohydrate and protein intake—must be met to maintain body weight, replenish glycogen stores, and provide adequate protein for building and repairing tissues.[20]

World-class athletes who train strenuously three to four hours each day can almost double their energy needs. The energy demand can be so high that some athletes have trouble consuming enough calories.[21] In contrast, athletes who compete in sports where they are judged by build and in sports with weight classifications often restrict energy intake to avoid weight gain. Energy intakes that are too low can lead to a loss of muscle mass, menstrual dysfunction, lower bone density, and increased risk of fatigue, injury, and illness.[22]

Carbohydrate and Exercise

Guidelines for athletes recommend high carbohydrate intakes during training.[23] A high-carbohydrate diet helps increase glycogen stores and extend endurance (see **FIGURE 14.11**). For endurance athletes, carbohydrate should supply a minimum of 60 percent of total calories.[24] A high-carbohydrate diet also can prevent mental as well as physical fatigue and is important for stop-and-go sports such as basketball, football, and soccer.[25]

For all athletes, dietary carbohydrates should come mainly from complex carbohydrates, which provide many of the B vitamins necessary for energy metabolism, along with iron (if enriched) and fiber (if whole grain). Although added sugars should be minimized, some athletes might need to include more simple sugars to meet energy requirements.

Quick Bite

Pound for Pound?

Women's muscles have smaller muscle fiber cross sections and less muscle mass than men's muscles. For a given amount of muscle, however, there is no difference in strength between men and women.

Quick Bite

Fast-Twitch Fish

A large percentage (40 to 60 percent) of a fish's body weight is muscle tissue. Although it spends much of its life slowly cruising, a fish must be able to execute occasional quick bursts of high speed to escape predators or catch a meal. Thus, fish muscle is composed of approximately 75 to 90 percent fast-twitch fibers, and fish flesh often is white. The slow-twitch fibers generally are concentrated just under the skin or near fins that are used during slow or high speeds. This arrangement is possible only because fish are buoyant. Land animals could not survive dragging around a large mass of muscle that they used only occasionally in extreme situations.

Quick Bite

The Weaker Sex?

Prior to the 1960s, women were banned from running any race longer than 800 meters, and they could not officially participate in marathon competitions until 1970. The race authorities mistakenly believed that women could harm themselves and were unsuited to distance running. Imagine their amazement during the 1984 Olympic Games when Joan Benoit won the gold medal for the women's marathon with a time of 02:24:52—a time that would have won 11 of the previous 20 men's Olympic marathons!

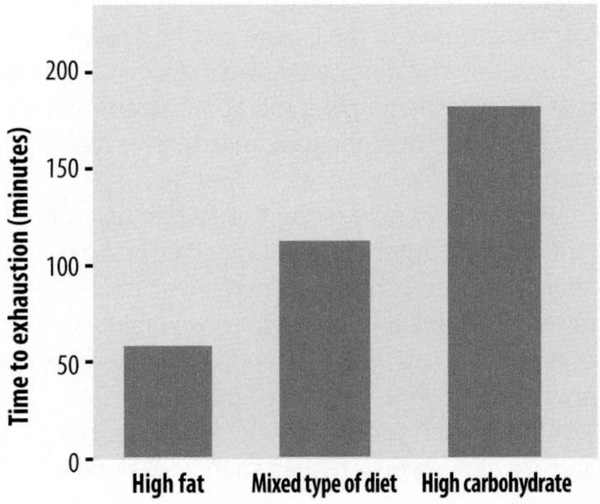

FIGURE 14.11 Diet composition and endurance.
Athletes can exercise longer when eating a high-carbohydrate diet.

FYI For Your Information

Lactate Is Not a Metabolic Dead-End

Today's race is 200 meters, and you are in the lead. The crowd roars with excitement and your coach screams as your feet slam over and over on the hard, gray cinder track. Other runners are close behind, and you can feel them breathing and pounding at your heels. Air whistles in and out of your wheezing lungs as you doggedly push to stay ahead. Your muscles are screaming, but they carry you across the finish line. A winner!

As you slump in exhaustion, you wonder how your limp muscles carried you through to the end. Each leg seemed to weigh a thousand pounds. As your muscles tire, lactate levels rise and the pH in your muscle cells drops.

Scientists, coaches, and athletes have long believed that lactate was a useless, even toxic, dead-end substance. Research proves otherwise. It is the overall acidification of the muscle tissue, rather than a buildup of lactate, that primarily causes muscle fatigue. Also, lactate is now recognized as a fuel in its own right. In addition to acting as a metabolic shunt, lactate is a useful fuel produced and consumed under all conditions of oxygen availability, while exercising or at rest.

Without the energy supplied by the lactic acid energy system, you would never have crossed the finish line. While your body anaerobically burned muscle glycogen, it produced large amounts of lactate. Where does this lactate come from, and how does your body handle it?

Cori Cycle

During vigorous exercise, your contracting muscle cells quickly extract small amounts of ATP from glucose. This simple pathway, called glycolysis, splits glucose into pyruvate molecules faster than the oxygen energy system can accept them for further processing. Cells divert excess pyruvate to lactate to help alleviate the backup.

Lactate accumulates rapidly in muscle cells, which receive a boost of energy by burning some lactate with oxygen—a strategy that yields far more energy than glycolysis alone.[a] Most lactate easily diffuses through muscle cell membranes into the bloodstream. The liver picks up the circulating lactate and converts it back to pyruvate. Using energy-demanding reactions, the liver transforms pyruvate to glucose. Glucose enters the bloodstream and travels back to the skeletal muscle cells, where it reenters energy-producing pathways.

This recurring circular pathway is called the *Cori cycle* (see **Figure A**). When pyruvate is backed up in muscle cells, the Cori cycle buys time with a detour through the liver. When oxygen becomes readily available, the oxygen energy system becomes the main pathway.

Lactate Shuttle

The pathways of the Cori cycle are an important, but incomplete, part of the lactate picture. The use of the Cori cycle as a holding pattern led to the mistaken belief that lactate was simply a metabolic dead-end. More recent studies describe a more extensive role for this long-maligned substance.

Researchers now recognize lactate as an important means of distributing carbohydrate energy sources after a meal and during sustained physical exercise. Lactate's advantage is its ability to move rapidly between cells. It is a small molecule and, unlike glucose, does not need insulin to cross a cell membrane.

Under resting conditions of plentiful carbohydrate and oxygen, diverse tissues such as skeletal muscle, liver, and skin produce lactate.[b] In these conditions, the supply of raw materials, rather than limited oxygen, drives the formation of lactate.

According to the lactate shuttle hypothesis, lactate formed in muscle cells becomes an energy source at other sites, either adjacent or remote. Skeletal muscle, once thought simply to produce lactate, also directly uses lactate as a fuel. At times, skeletal muscle actually removes more lactate than it produces. The heart muscle is fully aerobic, but it both produces and consumes lactate. Studies suggest that during exercise lactate is the major fuel for the heart and the preferred fuel for certain muscle fibers.[c]

The next time you complain about sore, tired muscles, don't blame lactate. Instead, think about the daily usefulness of lactate and how this little-respected substance helped power you to the finish.

[a] van Hall G, Lundby C, Araoz M, et al. The lactate paradox revisited in lowlanders during acclimatization to 4100 m and in high-altitude natives. *J Physiol.* 2009;587(Pt 5):1117–1129.

[b] van Hall G. Lactate kinetics in human tissues at rest and during exercise. *Acta Physiol (Oxf).* 2010;199(4):499–508.

[c] Cruz RS, de Aguiar RA, Turnes T, et al. Intracellular shuttle: the lactate aerobic metabolism. *Sci World J.* 2012;2012:420984.

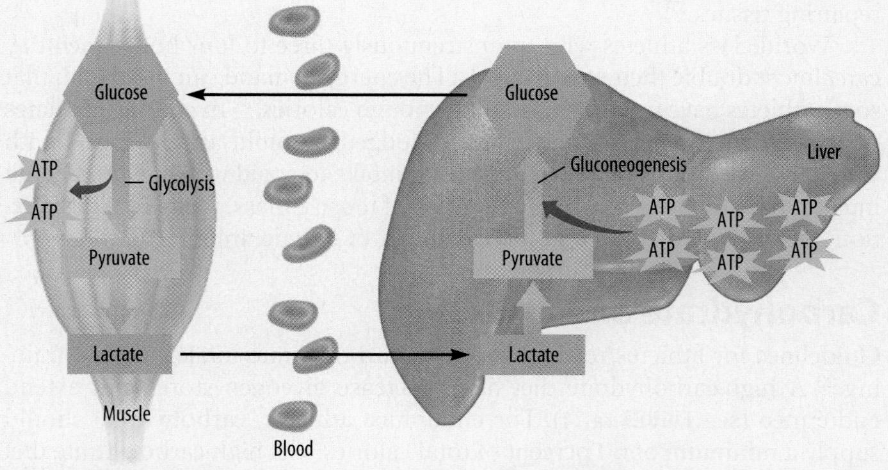

FIGURE A The Cori cycle. The Cori cycle shifts some of the metabolic burden of contracting muscle to the liver. Lactate formed in contracting muscle travels to the liver, which uses it to form glucose. This glucose returns to the muscle to fuel further contractions.

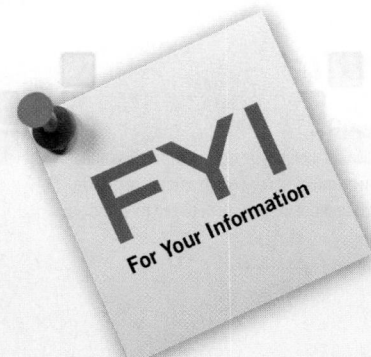

Going Green

Exercise High

You and your friend are off to Denver, Colorado, a mile-high city surrounded by beautiful mountains and tons of greenery. Like other outdoor athletes, you are environmentally conscious, vocal, and passionate about maintaining a pristine environment. You can't wait for that invigorating 5-mile run in the fresh mountain air as you try out your new running shoes. Your friend, however, warns that what you easily can do at home is more difficult at 5,000 feet and suggests a less strenuous hike for that first day in Denver. Although you recognize that your friend is offering sound advice, your immediate exuberance makes you feel invulnerable and up to the challenge. Then, you remember that you got sick running in the mountains several years ago and instead agree to take another day to acclimate yourself and read about exercising at high altitudes. Here are some tips about exercising at high altitudes:

- *Acclimate*. Allow time for your body to acclimate. Thin air at high altitudes makes exercising more difficult by reducing the oxygen available to your lungs. Your body adjusts within a day or two.
- *Hydrate*. Another difficulty in high-altitude exertion is dehydration stopping body processes. Mountain air is cool and dry, so drink lots of water to keep hydrated. At least for the first few days, avoid caffeine and don't drink alcohol. Both caffeine and alcohol are diuretics and can quickly cause dehydration and hinder performance.
- *Attend to physical symptoms*. Be aware of the symptoms of acute mountain sickness, such as nausea, dizziness, and headache. If you experience any of these symptoms, it's a good idea to descend to a lower level. If that doesn't help, you should seek medical attention.
- *Eat appropriately*. A diet high in carbohydrate and low in salt offers a better adaptation to high-altitude exercising and reduces the risk of acute mountain sickness.

Greening Your Exercise Routine

In addition to practicing good nutrition, sports enthusiasts and athletes can contribute to a green planet by using reusable water bottles or a hydration system instead of single-use disposable plastic bottles, and by picking up bottles, cans, and paper along the running and walking trails.

Carbohydrate Loading

Just as you might top off the gas tank in a car before a long trip, athletes can fill their glycogen stores prior to training or competing. In a process called **carbohydrate loading**, or **glycogen loading**, athletes manipulate their carbohydrate intake and exercise regimen to maximize muscle glycogen stores (see **FIGURE 14.12**).

Recommendations for carbohydrate loading include an intake of 60 to 70 percent of total calories from carbohydrate, along with a decrease in exercise intensity and duration prior to competition.[26] Carbohydrate loading is most beneficial for endurance athletes, such as marathon runners, swimmers, or cyclists who are preparing for an event that will last 90 minutes or more. In athletes who "carbo-load," the glycogen content of muscles can double and improve performance. For example, distance runners who carbohydrate load might be able to keep a faster pace for a longer time and finish a race sooner.[27]

Even though "extra" glycogen prior to competition sounds like a perfect plan, there is a downside to carbohydrate loading. For each gram of glycogen stored in muscle tissue, the body also stores about 3 grams of water. Many athletes who carbohydrate load complain about this weight gain and subsequent sluggishness. Some opt to train and compete without carbohydrate loading because, for them, the risk of physical discomfort outweighs the benefit of a greater carbohydrate store.

▶ **carbohydrate loading** Changes in dietary carbohydrate intake and exercise regimen before competition to maximize glycogen stores in the muscles. It is appropriate for endurance events lasting 60 to 90 consecutive minutes or longer. Also known as *glycogen loading*.

▶ **glycogen loading** See *carbohydrate loading*.

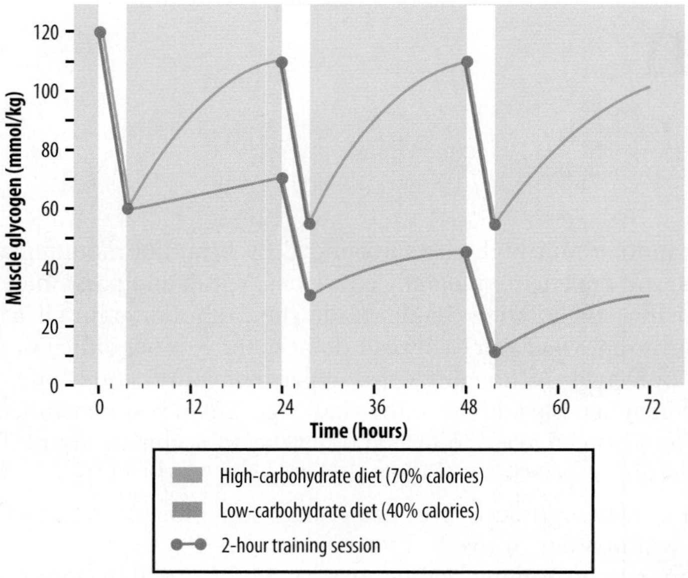

FIGURE 14.12 Diet composition, training, and muscle glycogen. A high-carbohydrate diet replenishes glycogen stores better than a low-carbohydrate diet.

Data from Ferguson-Stegall L, McCleave EL, Ding Z, et al. Postexercise carbohydrate-protein supplementation improves subsequent exercise performance and intracellular signaling for protein synthesis. *J Strength Cond Res.* 2011;24(5):1210–1224.

For an aerobic activity lasting fewer than 60 to 90 consecutive minutes, carbohydrate loading probably will provide no benefit. Instead, experts recommend that you taper your training program a few days before competition and eat a diet that provides 70 percent of its calories from carbohydrate for one or two days before the event.[28]

Carbohydrate Intake Before Extensive Exercise

Eating carbohydrate two to four hours before morning exercise helps replenish glycogen stores and improve endurance. To minimize problems with gastrointestinal (GI) distress, the carbohydrate and caloric content of the meal should be smaller when eaten closer to a workout. Although some athletes can tolerate solid foods, others prefer liquids to avoid GI distress. Because protein and fat take longer to digest and absorb, preexercise meals should contain no more than 10 to 15 percent of the total calories as protein and less than 20 percent of calories from fat. **TABLE 14.2** offers guidelines for timing of meals before an event.

Many athletes are confused about whether to eat less than an hour before exercise. To decrease hunger, delay fatigue, and improve performance, athletes who cannot fully refuel several hours prior to a workout must rely on "last-minute" carbohydrate intake. Although early research suggested that consuming carbohydrate within one hour before activity could cause low blood glucose levels and early fatigue, later studies report no effect or no improved performance.[29]

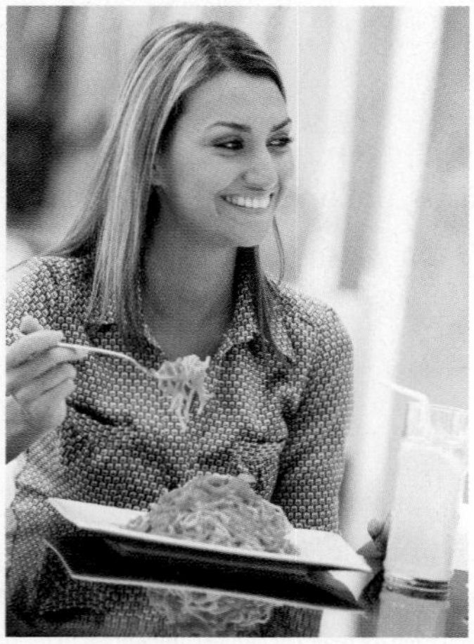

Preexercise Meals and the Glycemic Index

Individual foods have different effects on blood glucose levels independent of carbohydrate content. The glycemic index of foods is a measure of this effect and has attracted recent interest in relation to the diets of athletes. Current studies have produced mixed results, so it remains unclear whether the glycemic index of carbohydrate in preexercise meals affects performance.[30]

Carbohydrate Intake During Extensive Exercise

During exercise, athletes can maintain their carbohydrate supply to exercising muscle by consuming beverages with low to moderate amounts of simple carbohydrate.[31] When an event lasts one hour or more, drinking fluids with 4 to 8 percent carbohydrate, the amount in sports drinks, enables athletes to exercise longer and sprint harder at the finish. Although sports drinks also are suitable during events lasting less than one hour, plain water is adequate for maintaining hydration during these shorter events.[32] Consuming carbohydrate before and during an event improves performance more than either strategy alone.

Carbohydrate Intake Following Extensive Exercise

The timing and type of carbohydrates are important factors in the refueling process that replenishes glycogen stores. When athletes ingest 1.5 grams of carbohydrate per kilogram body weight within 30 minutes after exercise, they have a greater rate of muscle glycogen synthesis compared to waiting for two hours.

TABLE 14.2
Timing Meals Before Events

Time: 8:00 a.m. event, such as a road race, swim meet, or intense spin (stationary cycling) class	Meals: The day before, eat a carbohydrate-rich dinner, and drink extra water. On the morning of the event, about 6:00 or 6:30, have a light 200- to 400-calorie meal (depending on your tolerance), such as yogurt and a banana or a granola bar and a latte, and extra water. Eat familiar foods. If you want a larger meal, consider getting up to eat between 5:00 and 6:00. If your body cannot handle any breakfast before early-morning exercise, eat your breakfast before going to bed the night before. A bowl of cereal, bagel with peanut butter, or packets of oatmeal will help boost liver glycogen stores and prevent low blood sugar the next morning.
Time: 10:00 a.m. event, such as a bike race or soccer game	Meals: The day before, eat a carbohydrate-based dinner such as chicken stir-fry with extra rice, and drink extra water. On the morning of the event, eat a familiar breakfast by 7:00 to allow three hours for the food to digest. This meal will prevent the fatigue that results from low blood sugar. Popular choices are oatmeal with nuts and raisins, a bagel with peanut butter and a banana, and yogurt with Grape-Nuts and berries.
Time: 11:00 a.m. event, such as lightweight crew race, wrestling match, or other weight-class sport that requires a weigh-in one to two hours beforehand	Meals: Athletes who have crash dieted and dehydrated themselves to reach a specific weight for their sport have only a few hours after weigh-in to prepare for the competition. They need to replace water, carbohydrate, and sodium. An ideal target for a 150-pound (68-kg) depleted athlete would be 700 calories (primarily from carbohydrate), 2,200 milligrams of sodium, and 2 quarts (2 L) of water. The intake will vary greatly depending on the athlete's tolerance for food. Too many wrestlers end up vomiting on the mat after having pigged out after the weigh-in. The following are good food choices: • Chicken noodle soup, bread, and lots of water • Salted boiled potatoes, broth, salted crackers, and water • Ginger ale or cola, a ham and mustard sandwich, and water • Gatorade Endurance plus baked potato chips
Time: 2:00 p.m. event, such as a football or lacrosse game	Meals: An afternoon game allows time for you to have either a hearty, carbohydrate-based breakfast, such as French toast, and a light lunch or a substantial brunch by 10:00, allowing four hours for digestion. As always, eat a carbohydrate-based dinner the night before, and drink extra fluids the day before and up to noon. Popular brunch choices include French toast, pancakes, cereal, scrambled eggs, poached eggs on toast, Canadian bacon, bagels, fresh fruit salad, 100 percent fruit juice, fruit yogurt, and fruit smoothies.
Time: 8:00 p.m. event, such as a basketball game	Meals: You can thoroughly digest a hefty carbohydrate-based breakfast and lunch by evening. Plan for an early dinner, as tolerated, by 5:00 p.m., and you might even want a pregame snack at 7:00 p.m. Drink extra fluids all day. Two popular dinner choices are pasta with tomato sauce and meatballs, and chicken with a large serving of rice or potato, plus rolls, fruit salad, and low-fat frozen yogurt.
Time: All-day event, such as a hard hike, 100-mile (160-km) bike ride, triathlon training, or a day of cross-country skiing	Meals: Two days before the event, cut back on your exercise. The day before, take a rest to allow your muscles the chance to replace depleted glycogen stores. Eat carbohydrate-rich meals at breakfast, lunch, and dinner. Drink extra fluids. On the day of the event, eat a tried-and-true breakfast depending on your tolerance. Bagels with a little peanut butter are a favorite. While exercising, plan to eat carbohydrate-based foods (energy bars, dried fruit, sports drinks, gels) every 60 to 90 minutes to maintain normal blood sugar. If you stop at lunchtime, eat a comfortable-sized meal, but in general try to distribute your calories evenly throughout the day. Foods with fat, such as peanut butter, nuts, and cheese, can offer sustained energy; dietary fat takes a few hours to be converted into fat used for fuel. Drink fluids before you get thirsty; you should need to urinate at least three times throughout the day.

Reprinted by permission from Clark N. *Nancy Clark's sports nutrition guidebook*. 5th ed. Champaign, IL: Human Kinetics; 2014:184–187.

The increased glycogen synthesis is due largely to a greater sensitivity of muscle to insulin immediately after exercise.[33] Some research shows that the first 15 minutes are critical.[34]

The best way to replenish glycogen stores after intense exercise is to consume 1 to 1.5 grams of carbohydrate per kilogram of body weight during the first 30 minutes after a workout, and again every two hours for four to six hours.[35] A 70-kilogram (154-pound) athlete who exercises vigorously for 90 minutes or more, for example, would consume 70 to 100 grams of carbohydrate immediately after exercise, followed by another 70 to 100 grams every two hours for four to six hours. Consuming high-glycemic-index foods enhances glycogen synthesis. Among simple sugars, glucose and sucrose appear equally effective in replenishing glycogen, but fructose alone is not as effective.[36]

Carbohydrate intake after exercise also benefits protein metabolism, and consuming three times more carbohydrate than protein is recommended.[37]

Several researchers have shown that the levels of carbohydrates taken immediately or one hour after resistance exercise decrease protein breakdown and enhance protein retention.[38]

Key Concepts Energy intake is the most important element of the athlete's diet, and the major source of energy should be carbohydrates. Foods rich in complex carbohydrates, which also can provide fiber, iron, and B vitamins, are best. A high-carbohydrate diet prior to competition helps maximize glycogen stores and endurance. Carbohydrate loading is a process of adjusting carbohydrate intake and training intensity to maximize glycogen stores just before an event. Consuming carbohydrates soon after exercise enhances the rebuilding of glycogen stores.

Dietary Fat and Exercise

During exercise, carbohydrates and fats are the two main fuel sources. Endurance (aerobic) training increases the capacity of your oxygen energy system, enhancing your body's ability to use fat as a fuel. Exercise intensity also affects fuel use. During low- to moderate-intensity exercise, fatty acids are the major fuel source. During high-intensity exercise, the predominant energy source is glucose.

This does not mean that endurance athletes should consume diets high in fat. High-fat diets usually are lower in carbohydrate, thus limiting muscles' ability to replenish glycogen stores. High-fat diets often are high in calories, saturated fat, and cholesterol; your body also digests fat more slowly than carbohydrate.

Fat Intake and the Athlete

Fat intake should not be overly restricted. There is no performance benefit in consuming a diet with less than 15 percent of energy from fat.[39] Extreme fat restriction limits food choices, especially sources of protein, iron, zinc, and essential fatty acids. In addition, athletes with high caloric needs (greater than 5,000 kilocalories per day) can find it difficult to eat enough food without consuming more than 20 to 35 percent of their calories from fat, the range recommended for the general population. Sports nutritionists recommend that any extra fat calories come from monounsaturated and polyunsaturated sources. Saturated fat intake should be limited to less than 10 percent of energy, and trans fats should be avoided as much as possible.

Protein and Exercise

Historically, many athletes believed that the best diets to help build muscle mass were based on foods from animal sources, such as steak and eggs. The idea was that meat-eating athletes were stronger, more muscular, and more aggressive. Today, we know that strength and muscles are built with exercise (not extra protein) and that carbohydrate provides the fuel needed for muscle-building exercise. Although the body uses protein to rebuild and repair damaged muscles, athletes require only slightly higher protein intakes than sedentary people.

Protein Recommendations for Athletes

The adult Recommended Dietary Allowance (RDA) for protein is 0.8 gram of protein per kilogram of body weight per day, which is sufficient for sedentary people and those engaging in low-intensity exercise. Adults training for endurance events may require 1.2 to 1.7 grams of protein per kilogram of body weight per day, and resistance training may may require up to 1.6 to 1.7 grams per kilogram of body weight. Even with maximal training for extreme events,

FYI
For Your Information

Nutrition Periodization: Tailoring Nutrition Intake to Exercise Goals

Athletes, competitive as well as recreational, adjust their training schedules based on desired performance outcomes. Athletes are not constantly "in season," and their training during a 12-month period can be broken down into three phases: preparation, competition, and transition. This concept is referred to as exercise periodization.[a]

Let's take a look at each training phase more closely:

- *Preparation:* Also called the macrocycle, this phase leads up to the competition phase. Training is both general and specific, with goals to improve aerobic endurance, strength, and flexibility.
- *Competition:* Also called the mesocycle, the performance goals during this phase are to improve strength and speed.
- *Transition:* Also called the microcycle, this phase is the time spent between competition and the next preparation cycle. Workouts in this phase, also referred to as the "off-season" or "active recovery," are generally less structured and are intended for the athlete to improve on his or her weaknesses.

During exercise periodization, an athlete's nutrition needs change. Adjusting macronutrient (carbohydrate, fat, and protein) intake to enhance the training cycle enables athletes to provide the best combination of fuel for their bodies all year long.[b] This process is referred to as nutrition periodization, and it goes hand in hand with exercise periodization:

- *Preparation:* This is the one phase where, if needed, athletes should focus on changing their weight or body fat percentage or on building muscle. This is a time when habits regarding diet can be changed and an in-depth evaluation of regular dietary habits can occur. Adjustments are made within the diet to work toward a desired competition weight or body composition.
- *Competition:* During this phase, a routine for eating during the competition season should be well established. The focus should not be on changing weight or experimenting with different food choices. Recovery after exercise is an important focus.
- *Transition:* This is a time to focus on calorie control and good nutrition. It is a time to experiment with and enjoy different types of foods.

The information in the accompanying tables can be used by athletes as guidelines for successful nutrition periodization.

[a]Seebohar B. *Nutrition Periodization for Endurance Athletes*. Boulder, CO: Bull Publishing; 2004.

[b]Block O, Kravitz L. Tailoring nutrient intake to exercise goals. *IDEA Fitness J*. 2006;3:48–55.

Daily Needs: No Weight Loss

Training Phase	Carbohydrate (g/kg)	Protein (g/kg)	Fat (g/kg)	Hydration (color of urine)
Preparation	5–12+	1.2–1.7	0.8–1.0	Lemonade
Prerace	7–13	1.4–2.0	0.8–2.0	Lemonade
Race	7–19	1.4–2.0	0.8–3.0	Diluted lemonade
Transition	5–6	1.2–1.4	0.8–1.0	Lemonade

Reproduced from Seebohar B. *Nutrition Periodization for Endurance Athletes*. Boulder, CO: Bull Publishing; 2004. Reprinted with permission of Bull Publishing.

Daily Needs: Summary

Training Phase	Daily Kilocalorie Difference
Preparation	—
Prerace	620–1,007
Race	0–2,322
Transition	−620–5,101

Reproduced from Seebohar B. *Nutrition Periodization for Endurance Athletes*. Boulder, CO: Bull Publishing; 2004. Reprinted with permission of Bull Publishing.

Example: 155-Pound Male

Training Phase	Carbohydrate (g)/Kilocalories	Protein (g)/Kilocalories	Fat (g)/Kilocalories	Total Daily Kilocalories
Preparation	352–845+/1,408–3,380	85–120/340–480	56–70/504–630	2,252–4,490+
Prerace	493–916/1,972–3,664	99–141/396–564	56–141/504–1,269	2,872–5,497
Race	493–1,339/1,972–5,356	99–151/396–564	56–211/504–1,899	2,872–7,819
Transition	352–453/340–396	85–99/340–396	56–70/504–630	2,252–2,718

Reproduced from Seebohar B. *Nutrition Periodization for Endurance Athletes*. Boulder, CO: Bull Publishing; 2004. Reprinted with permission of Bull Publishing.

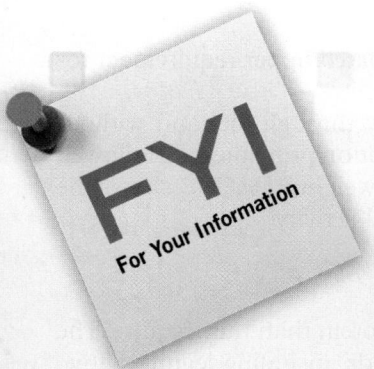

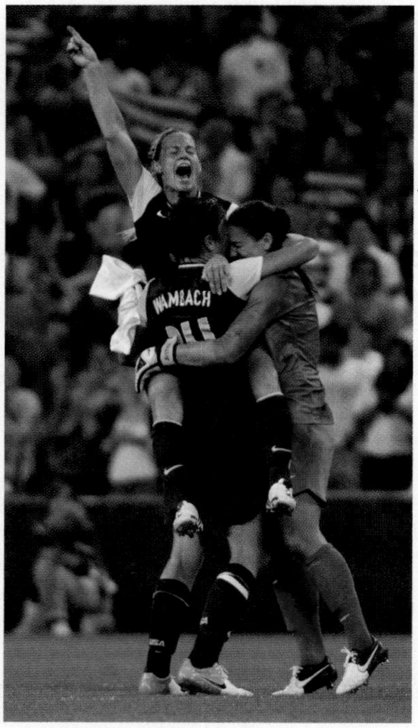

© ZUMA Press, Inc./Alamy

FIGURE 14.13 Optimal nutrition. Nutrition is an important component of the USA Women's soccer team training program — a program that helped them to win the 2012 Summer Olympics Gold medal.

such as the Olympics (see **FIGURE 14.13**), the estimated upper requirement for adults is 2.0 grams per kilogram of body weight.[40]

An athlete's protein needs can be met easily through diet and without the use of supplements, provided that sound nutrition principles are followed and energy intake is adequate to maintain body weight. **TABLE 14.3** shows the protein requirements of various levels of physical activity.

Protein Intake and the Athlete

THINK About It 4

Hungry adults generally eat meals with more protein than they require. The best protein sources are high-quality protein foods, including legumes, low-fat dairy products, egg whites, lean beef and pork, chicken, turkey, and fish. Protein powders and amino acid supplements are not needed.

Vegetarian athletes and weekend warriors can achieve adequate protein intake and meet their energy needs by eating a variety of protein-rich foods from plant sources such as grains, nuts, beans, and seeds. Because plant proteins are less digestible than animal foods, the total amount of protein consumed may need to be higher.

Protein Intake After Extensive Exercise

Protein combined with carbohydrate in a postexercise meal increases glycogen synthesis more than carbohydrate alone.[41] Researchers suggest athletes consume 4 grams of protein for every 10 grams of carbohydrate (grams protein = 40% grams carbohydrate).[42] For example, using postexercise recommendations of 1.5 grams of carbohydrate per kilogram of body weight, a 55-kilogram (121-pound) female athlete would need 82.5 grams of carbohydrate ($55 \times 1.5 = 82.5$ g) and 33 grams of protein ($82.5 \times 0.40 = 33$ g). How does this translate to food? A small bagel, 2 ounces of string cheese, and 8 ounces of low-fat yogurt would be a portable snack to enjoy after a hard workout (provides 86 grams of carbohydrate and 33 grams of protein). Another food that provides ample amounts of carbohydrate and protein is low-fat milk. Low-fat milk has been shown to be at least as effective as commercially available sports drinks as a rehydration beverage, if not more effective.[43] Milk is more nutrient-dense than traditional sports drinks and thus can be a better beverage choice for individuals who partake in strength and endurance activities.

Dangers of High Protein Intake

▶ **diuresis** The formation and secretion of urine.

Excessive protein intake from food or supplements enhances **diuresis** (loss of body water) as the body attempts to excrete excess nitrogen through the urine. This increases the risk for dehydration and can contribute to mineral losses. High-protein diets often are high in saturated and total fat and can contribute to obesity, osteoporosis, heart disease, and certain types of cancer.

TABLE 14.3
Protein Requirements of Sedentary and Active People

Activity Level	Protein Requirements (g protein/kg body weight)
Sedentary	0.8
Endurance athlete	1.2–1.4
Strength athlete	1.6–1.7
Maximum estimated requirement for adults	2.0

Adapted from Fink HH, Burgoon LA, Mikesky AE. *Practical Applications in Sports Nutrition.* 3rd ed. Burlington, MA: Jones & Bartlett Learning; 2011.

High intakes of single-amino-acid supplements can impair absorption of other amino acids. Further, the amount of amino acids contained in supplements is very small compared with the amount in food. For example, one pill may contain 500 milligrams of an amino acid, but 1 ounce of meat, poultry, or fish provides more than 7,000 milligrams of indispensable and dispensable amino acids! And, the cost of supplements is higher.

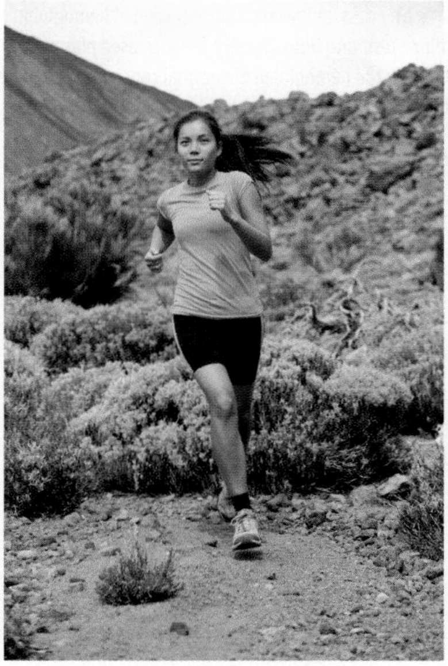
© iStockphoto/Thinkstock

Key Concepts Although fat is an important fuel for exercise, a high-fat diet is not necessary. General recommendations that fat not exceed 20 to 35 percent of total energy intake are appropriate for athletes. Dietary protein is a source of energy and also a source of amino acids for body protein synthesis. The protein requirements of athletes are slightly higher than those of sedentary adults but still within the normal range of protein consumption. High-protein diets are neither recommended nor necessary. Low-fat dairy products, egg whites, lean beef and pork, chicken, turkey, fish, and legumes are good sources of protein.

Vitamins, Minerals, and Athletic Performance

Many reactions that support exercise and physical activity require vitamins and minerals. They help extract energy from nutrients, transport oxygen, and repair tissues. Researchers have long debated whether physically active people have greater vitamin and mineral needs than sedentary people.

B Vitamins

Because B vitamins are essential for energy metabolism, wouldn't athletes, with their high energy needs, require more B vitamins? Not necessarily. B vitamins are needed for chemical reactions that release energy. But if athletes consume adequate calories and ample complex carbohydrates, fruits, and vegetables, they eat plenty of B vitamins. However, if overall diet quality is poor, with too-few calories or mostly refined sugars in lieu of complex carbohydrates, B-vitamin intake can be compromised.

Vegan athletes who do not include fortified foods, such as some soy products and ready-to-eat cereals, can have a problem with vitamin B_{12} intake. They should consult a medical advisor or registered dietitian to determine whether they need B_{12} supplements.

Calcium

Calcium is essential for normal muscle function and strong bones. Adequate calcium intake coupled with regular exercise slows skeletal deterioration that occurs with age and can reduce the risk of osteoporosis.

Inadequate calcium increases the risk of stress fractures in athletes. This is of particular concern for women of reproductive age who exercise heavily and are not menstruating (see the "Female Athlete Triad" section later in this chapter). Athletes should strive to meet the Adequate Intake (AI) for calcium from a variety of low-fat dairy products and other calcium-rich foods. This is especially true for teens, whose calcium needs (1,300 mg/day) are higher than those of adults (1,000 mg/day).

Iron

Iron is vital to oxygen delivery for aerobic energy production during endurance exercise and may be the most critical mineral with implications for sports performance. As an essential part of hemoglobin and myoglobin, iron helps deliver oxygen to active muscle cells. It is also a key component of several enzymes vital to the production of ATP by the oxygen energy system.

▶ **sports anemia** A lowered concentration of hemoglobin in the blood resulting from dilution. The increased plasma volume that dilutes the hemoglobin is a normal consequence of aerobic training.

Because of menstrual losses and lower dietary iron intakes, female athletes have a greater risk of iron deficiency than male athletes. In endurance athletes, the impact of running can cause mechanical trauma to capillaries in the feet and increase the breakdown of red blood cells. The increased breakdown can contribute to low iron status. Some studies suggest that athletes involved in heavy training need 30 to 70 percent more iron than nonathletes.[44]

Endurance training also increases the volume of plasma in the blood without initially changing the amount of hemoglobin. This dilutes the hemoglobin, even though training typically maintains or increases the amount of total hemoglobin. This condition, called **sports anemia**, is a false anemia for most athletes and can be remedied with a few days of rest.

Although many elite athletes, especially females, have depleted iron stores (low serum ferritin), the incidence of iron-deficiency anemia in this population is similar to that of the nonathletic female population.[45] Anemia can seriously impair a person's capacity to perform activities, but there is disagreement about the impact of mild iron deficiency. Still, most authorities suggest iron supplementation for athletes who have documented iron deficiency without anemia.[46] A recent study found that iron supplementation improved energetic efficiency in iron-depleted female endurance athletes.[47]

Quick Bite

Lost in Space

Vigorous weight training can double or triple a muscle's size, whereas the lack of use during space travel can shrink it by 20 percent in two weeks.

TABLE 14.4
A Sample Training Diet

Athlete performs prolonged daily training Body weight = 70 kilograms Energy intake = 3,400 kilocalories		
Macronutrients		
Carbohydrate	**Protein**	**Fat**
535 g	128 g	83 g
63% kcal	15% kcal	22% kcal
7.5 g/kg body weight[a]	1.8 g/kg body weight[b]	
Breakfast	**Postexercise**	
8 oz orange juice	1 bagel	
2 cups Cheerios cereal	2 oz string cheese	
8 oz 1% milk	16 oz apple juice	
1 large bran muffin		
Lunch	**Dinner**	
2 slices whole-wheat bread	3 oz chicken breast	
2 oz turkey	1 lg baked potato with	
2 slices tomato	2 Tbsp low-fat sour cream	
Lettuce leaf	2 whole-wheat dinner rolls	
2 tsp mayonnaise	1 tsp margarine	
1 med apple	1 cup cooked broccoli	
12 oz cranberry juice	1 cup salad greens with 2 Tbsp Italian salad dressing 8 oz 1% milk 1 cup low-fat frozen yogurt	
Pre-exercise		
8 oz Gatorade		
1 cereal bar		

[a] Recommended carbohydrate intake goals for prolonged daily training.

[b] Recommended protein intake goals up to 2 g/kg body weight for extreme training loads.

Other Trace Minerals

Strenuous exercise taxes the body's reserves of copper (essential for red blood cell synthesis) and zinc (vital to the work of many enzymes involved in energy production). During endurance events, increased fluid loss increases mineral losses—zinc in urine and relatively high amounts of both zinc and copper in sweat.

Although these losses can cause marginal deficiencies, supplementation is not necessarily recommended. High-dose supplements of iron, copper, or zinc can interfere with the normal absorption of these and other minerals, so an excess of one can cause a deficiency of the others. **TABLE 14.4** is an example of a training diet that would meet an athlete's needs for vitamins and minerals through food, which is preferable to taking supplements.

Key Concepts Vitamins and minerals are important components of athletes' diets. B vitamins are necessary for normal energy metabolism. Adequate calcium intake can help protect against stress fractures and, coupled with exercise, delays the onset of osteoporosis. Iron is needed to carry oxygen. Strenuous exercise can tax the body's reserves of both copper and zinc.

Fluid Needs During Extensive Exercise

Exercise generates heat, and heavy exercise can increase heat production 15- to 20-fold (see **FIGURE 14.14**). The increase in body heat triggers sweating, and sweat cools your body as it evaporates on your skin. The body of a well-trained athlete begins to cool itself soon after exercise begins. Even before core body temperature rises, the athlete's body starts to produce sweat. Sweat rate is affected by environmental temperature (extreme heat or extreme cold), humidity (higher humidity increases the rate of sweat production but reduces the efficiency of evaporation), type of clothing, fitness level, and initial fluid balance. During exercise in hot weather, the risk of dehydration and heat injury increases dramatically. Depending on temperature, humidity, exercise intensity, and

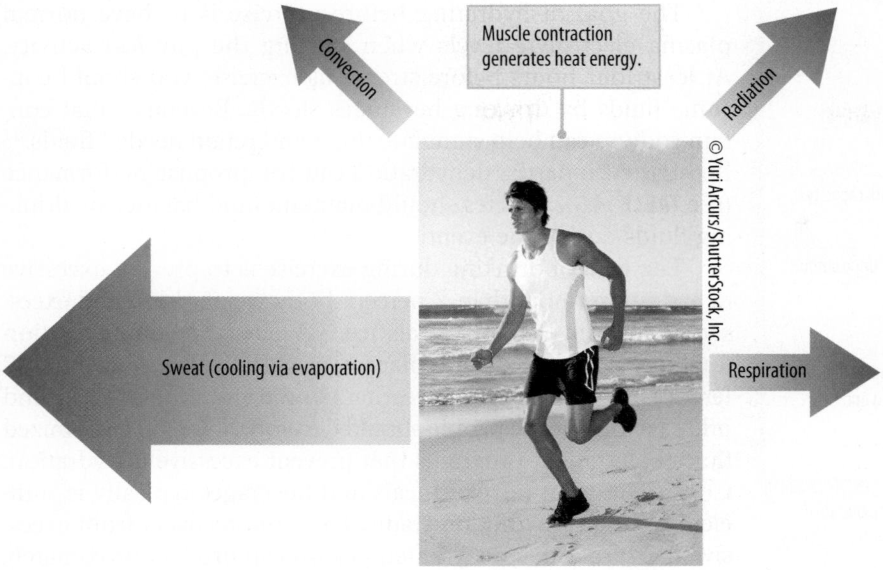

FIGURE 14.14 Dissipation of heat during exercise. During exercise, radiation, convection, and respiration are responsible for some heat loss, but evaporation of sweat dissipates more than 80 percent of the heat generated by increased physical activity.

the individual's sweat response to exercise, normal sweat rates for athletes range from 0.5 to 2.0 liters per hour.[48]

To keep the body from overheating, blood must flow to the skin, where evaporating sweat can dissipate heat. During exercise, the cooling demand for blood flow to the skin can compete with the cardiovascular demand for blood to deliver fuel to working muscles. Dehydration stresses both systems, making each less efficient. Without fluid replacement during heavy exercise, athletes can become dehydrated quickly, and a water deficit of 2 percent of body weight degrades athletic performance.[49] Signs of dehydration include the following:

- Elevated heart rate at a given exercise intensity
- Increased rate of **perceived exertion** during activity
- Decreased performance
- Lethargy
- Concentrated urine
- Infrequent urination
- Loss of appetite

Drinking fluid during exercise helps offset fluid loss, minimize cardiovascular changes, reduce perception of effort, and maintain a supply of fuel to working muscles. When possible, athletes should drink fluid at rates that most closely match their sweating rates.[50] Because exercise inhibits the body's thirst signal, you must begin drinking fluids before you feel thirsty to keep up with your losses.

Hydration

Active people must train themselves to consume adequate amounts of fluid before, during, and after exercise. Because each person has different water electrolyte losses based on factors such as body weight, genetic makeup, and metabolism, hydration strategies must be personalized.

▶ **perceived exertion** The subjective experience of how difficult an effort is.

Quick Bite

Sweating a World Record

When Alberto Salazar ran the Olympic marathon in 1984, he went down in the record books for sweat production. He lost 12 pounds during the 26.2-mile race, despite drinking about 2 liters. His sweat rate was approximately 3.7 liters per hour.

TABLE 14.5
Adverse Effects of Dehydration on Exercise and Performance

Percentage of Body Weight Loss	Adverse Effects on Performance
1	The thirst threshold. Leads to decrease in physical work capacity.
2	Stronger thirst, vague discomfort, loss of appetite.
3	Dry mouth, increasing hemoconcentration, reduction in urine output.
4	Decrease of 20% to 30% in physical work capacity.
5	Difficulty concentrating, headache, sleepiness.
6	Severe impairment in ability to regulate body temperature during exercise; increased respiratory rate, leading to tingling and numbness of extremities.
7	Collapse is likely if combined with heat and exercise.

Reproduced from Fink HH, Burgoon LA, Mikesky AE. Practical Applications in Sports Nutrition. 2nd ed. Burlington, MA: Jones & Bartlett Learning; 2009.

The goal of hydrating before exercise is to have normal plasma electrolyte levels when starting the physical activity. At least four hours before strenuous exercise, you should consume fluids by drinking beverages slowly. Beverages that contain sodium can help stimulate thirst and retain needed fluids.[51] Because even partial dehydration can compromise performance (see **TABLE 14.5**), athletes should maintain fluid balance by drinking fluids during the event.

The goal of drinking during exercise is to prevent excessive dehydration (more than 2 percent body weight loss) and excessive changes in electrolyte balance.[52] A general recommendation for fluid and electrolyte replacement is difficult due to the differences in exercise tasks, weather conditions, fitness levels, and other factors. Active people should develop their own customized fluid-replacement programs that prevent excessive dehydration. Consumption of normal meals and beverages typically is sufficient to restore hydration status. For rapid recovery from excessive dehydration, a dehydrated person can drink approximately 1.5 liters of fluid for each kilogram of body weight lost.[53]

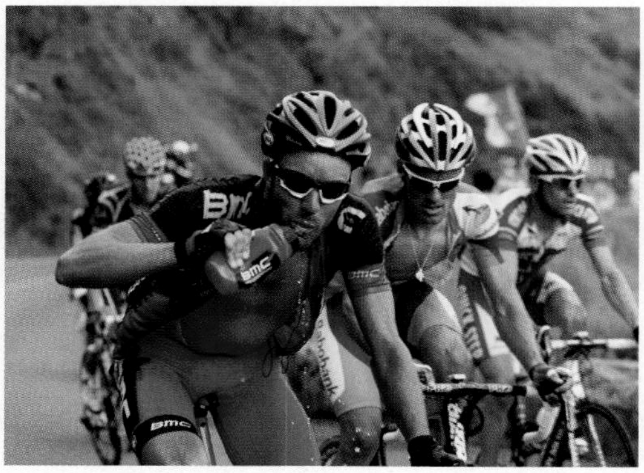

© Radu Razvan/Shutterstock, Inc.

Sports Drinks

Water is now a designer beverage. On store shelves, you can find fortified water, fitness water, herbal water, electrolyzed water, and coconut water. Although some taste great, watch out for unsubstantiated claims and sugar content. Some sweetened waters have as much sugar as soda.

For rehydration, should you choose water, sports drinks, or other beverages? During activities that last fewer than 60 continuous minutes, water is your best sports drink. Drinking water can replace fluid lost in sweat and help offset the rise in core temperature. During exercise that lasts longer than 60 continuous minutes, electrolytes and glycogen stores become depleted. Consuming fluids that contain carbohydrate and sodium can delay fatigue (see **FIGURE 14.15**), enhance palatability of fluids, and promote fluid retention.

▶ **palatable** Pleasant tasting.

Optimal sports drinks provide energy (from glucose, glucose polymers, or sucrose) and electrolytes in a **palatable** solution that promotes rapid absorption (less than 10 percent carbohydrate concentration) (see **TABLE 14.6**).The palatability of beverages containing electrolytes and 4 to 8 percent carbohydrate may increase the voluntary intake of fluid. Beverages such as fruit juices and soft drinks are concentrated sources of carbohydrates (more than 10 percent)

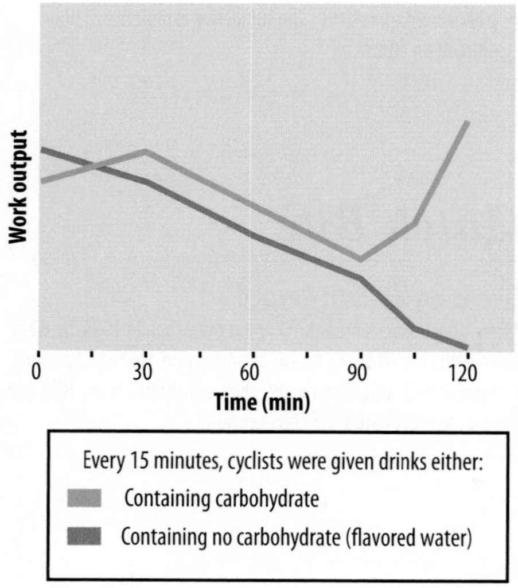

FIGURE 14.15 Sports drinks and performance.
Consuming carbohydrate drinks dramatically increases power output after 90 minutes.

TABLE 14.6
Desirable Composition of Sports Beverages

Characteristic	Comment
Fuel source	Contains carbohydrate: glucose, sucrose, and glucose polymers (maltodextrin). Goal intake is 60–70 g/hour (approximately 1 liter of a 6–8 percent carbohydrate drink).
Electrolytes	Contains sodium (70–165 mg per 240 mL) and potassium (30–75 mg per 240 mL) to replace sweat electrolyte loss when exercise is longer than 3–4 hours. Electrolytes also enhance palatability.
Rapid absorption	Contains 6–8 percent carbohydrate. Higher carbohydrate concentration slows gastric emptying and intestinal absorption.
Palatability	Flavored beverages enhance consumption. Electrolytes enhance flavor. Carbonation can decrease the amount of fluid consumed.

Reproduced from Fink HH, Burgoon LA, Mikesky AE. *Practical Applications in Sports Nutrition*. 2nd ed. Burlington, MA: Jones & Bartlett Learning; 2009.

and can slow gastric emptying. Coconut water contains no added sugars and is rich in potassium, vitamin C, antioxidants, and phytochemicals. Claims for coconut water beyond rehydration are unsubstantiated and not backed by scientific studies. In juices and many soft drinks, the main carbohydrate is fructose, which is associated with slower stomach emptying and abdominal cramps. Carbonated soft drinks can decrease the volume of fluid consumed and delay stomach emptying.

Athletes should avoid beverages that contain alcohol. Some athletes use alcohol for psychological benefits—calming nerves, improving self-confidence, and reducing anxiety, pain, and muscle tremor. This misguided effort fails to recognize alcohol's negative influence on physical performance. Alcohol slows reaction time, impairs coordination, and upsets balance. Its diuretic action contributes to dehydration and impairs regulation of body temperature.

For endurance events that last longer than four to five hours (or shorter events in high heat and humidity), athletes who do not replace electrolytes put themselves at risk for abnormally low levels of blood sodium. This life-threatening condition is associated with an excessive loss of electrolytes in sweat and with the excessive consumption of fluid, such as plain water, that does not replace electrolytes. See **TABLE 14.7** for a summary of the American College of Sports Medicine's position on the amount and type of fluid to consume before, during, and after activity.

Muscle Cramps

A muscle cramp is excruciatingly painful and often associated with dehydration. Although massage and stretching may provide immediate relief, the causes of a cramp are not well understood. Likely related to overexertion, other contributing factors may include fluid loss, inadequate conditioning, and electrolyte imbalance. Lack of water, sodium, calcium, magnesium, and potassium, individually or together, may trigger a cramp during exercise. Before exercising, drink plenty of fluids and make certain that your diet is rich in these minerals.

Quick Bite

Training: Young at Heart or Skeletal Old Age?
With endurance training, younger athletes largely achieve improvements as a result of increased cardiac output. Older athletes show greater improvement in the activities of the oxidative enzymes in their skeletal muscles.

TABLE 14.7
American College of Sports Medicine Position on Fluid Replacement

Before activity or competition	Drink adequate fluids during the 24 hours before an event, especially during the meal before exercise, to promote proper hydration before exercise or competition. Drink about 500 milliliters (~17 ounces) of fluid about two hours before exercise to promote adequate hydration and allow time for excretion of excess ingested water.
During activity or competition	Start drinking early and at regular intervals to consume fluids at a rate sufficient to replace all the water lost through sweating or consume the maximal amount that can be tolerated. Fluids should be cooler than ambient temperature and flavored to enhance palatability and promote fluid replacement.
During competition that lasts more than one hour	To maintain blood glucose concentration and delay the onset of fatigue, the fluid replacement should contain 4 to 8 percent carbohydrate. Electrolytes (primarily salt) are added to make the solution taste better and reduce the risk of low blood levels of sodium. About 0.5 to 0.7 gram of sodium per liter of water replaces sodium lost by sweating.
Following activity or competition	Complete restoration of the extracellular fluid compartment cannot be sustained without replacement of lost sodium. For each pound (0.45 kilogram) of body weight lost, consume at least 2 cups (0.47 liter) of fluid. Thirst sensation is not an adequate gauge of dehydration, and postexercise consumption stimulates obligatory urine losses. Research shows that drinking an amount of liquid that is 125 to 150 percent of fluid loss is usually enough to promote complete rehydration.

Modified from American College of Sports Medicine. Position stand: exercise and fluid replacement. *Med Sci Sports Exerc*. 2007;39:377–390.

Nutrition Needs of Young Athletes

Young athletes (younger than 19 years) should place a higher priority on nutritional needs for growth and development than on athletic performance.[54] Young athletes often consume insufficient calories; the consequences of chronic low energy intake include[55]:

- Short stature and delayed puberty
- Nutrient deficiencies and dehydration
- Menstrual irregularities
- Poor bone health
- Increased incidence of injuries
- Increased risk of developing eating disorders

Parents and youth must understand the energy and nutrient demands of growth and training, and many need help in planning meals and snacks to meet those needs. Many sport activities for this age group take place after school, and some schools serve lunch as early as 10:45 a.m. To provide energy for the activity and nutrients for recovery, young people should have meals and snacks before and after exercise. Easily portable snacks include fruit, pretzels, dry cereal, cereal bars, yogurt, sports drinks, sandwiches, and milk. Young athletes must drink adequate fluids during the day as well as at practice and competition. This is especially important because youth have a high tolerance for exercising in heat, which puts them at increased risk for heat exhaustion and heatstroke.

Key Concepts Exercise of any type increases fluid losses through sweat. Evaporation of sweat from the skin allows the body to cool itself. Fluid losses must be replaced to avoid dehydration. Athletes need to drink plenty of fluid before, during, and after exercise. Fluid choices depend on the duration of activity and the preferences of the athlete. Optimal sports drinks provide energy and electrolytes in a solution that promotes rapid absorption. Nutrient intakes by young athletes must support both competition and continued growth.

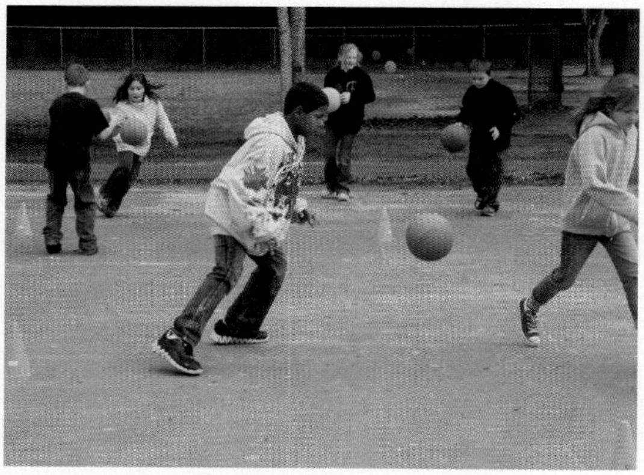

Nutrition Supplements and Ergogenic Aids

The pressure to win contributes to the search for a competitive edge, and the use of dietary supplements in an attempt to enhance athletic performance is increasing. A study of young Canadian athletes found that 98 percent were taking at least one dietary supplement. Whereas athletes 11–17 years old focused on vitamin and mineral supplements, athletes 18–25 years old took **ergogenic aids** with the expectation of improved performance.[56] (See **TABLE 14.8** for a review of the different types of ergogenic aids.) In a study of nearly 22,000 American high school students, about 30 percent reported using energy drinks or shots.[57] Nutrition supplements and ergogenic aids include products and practices that:

- Provide calories (e.g., liquid supplements, energy bars)
- Provide vitamins and minerals (including multivitamin supplements)
- Contribute to performance during exercise and enhance recovery after exercise (e.g., sports drinks, carbohydrate supplements)
- Are believed to stimulate and maintain muscle growth (e.g., purified amino acids)
- Contain micronutrient, herbal, and/or cellular components that are promoted as ergogenic aids to enhance performance (e.g., caffeine, chromium picolinate, creatine)
- Are used for nutritional, physiological, psychological, biomechanical, or pharmacological reasons

▶ **ergogenic aids** Substances that can enhance athletic performance.

TABLE 14.8
Types of Ergogenic Aids

Type of Ergogenic Aid	Description	Examples
Nutritional	Any supplement, food product, or dietary manipulation that enhances work capacity or athletic performance	Carbohydrate loading; amino acid and vitamin supplements
Physiological	Any practice or substance that enhances the functioning of the body's various systems (e.g., cardiovascular, muscular) and thus improves athletic performance	Any type of physical training (e.g., endurance, strength), blood doping through transfusions, warming up and/or stretching
Psychological	Any practice or treatment that changes mental state and thereby enhances sport performance	Visualization, hypnosis, pep talks, relaxation techniques
Biomechanical	Any device, piece of equipment, or external product that can be used to improve athletic performance during practice or competition	Weight belts, knee wraps, oversize tennis rackets, body suits (swimming/track)
Pharmacological	Any substance or compound classified as a drug or hormonal agent that is used to improve work output and/or sport performance	Hormones (e.g., growth hormones, anabolic steroids), caffeine

Quick Bite

Climbing with Age

Aging does not seem to impair a healthy person's ability to perform activities at a high altitude. However, aging reduces our ability to sweat. Our ability to regulate body temperature declines, thus reducing our ability to exercise safely in hot environments.

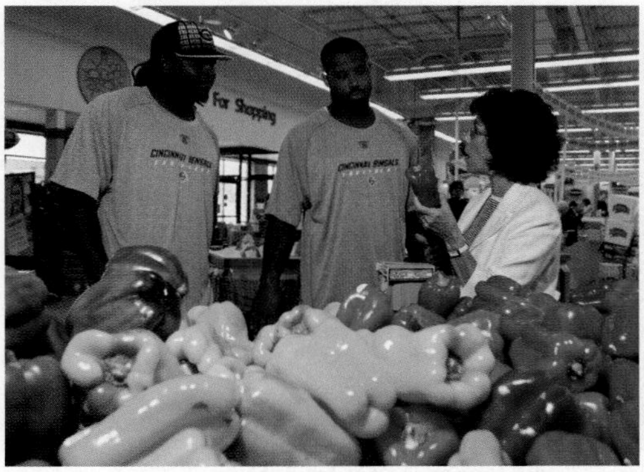

Most nutritional supplements are unnecessary for athletes who select a variety of foods and meet their energy needs. However, iron and calcium supplements may be recommended for female athletes if their diets are low in these nutrients. Liquid supplements and sports bars that contain carbohydrates, proteins, and fats can provide an easy way to increase energy intake. Sports drinks, gels, and recovery drinks also can contribute to needed fluids and carbohydrates before, during, and after exercise.

Dietary supplements marketed as performance enhancers are another matter. Herbals, glandulars, enzymes, hormones, and other compounds aimed at athletes carry many attractive claims. Although some products have been well researched, most lack vigorous clinical trials to evaluate efficacy, apply to only one gender (usually males), or are relevant to only one sport (e.g., weight lifting). (See the Nutrition Science in Action feature "Elite Adolescent Athletes' Use of Dietary Supplements.")

Regulation and Concerns About Dietary and Herbal Supplements

All prescription and over-the-counter drugs and food additives must meet the Food and Drug Administration's safety and effectiveness requirements; however, dietary supplements bypass these regulations. Before 1994, when the Dietary Supplement Health and Education Act (DSHEA) was signed into law, dietary supplements were regulated in the same manner as other foods. Prior to DSHEA, many people felt that the U.S. Food and Drug Administration (FDA) was too restrictive in regulating dietary supplements. As a result, DSHEA was passed and dietary supplements were placed in a special category of "foods." Currently, dietary supplement manufacturers must adhere to a number of federal regulations before a product can go on the market, they must have evidence that the ingredients sold in their supplements are generally safe if required to do so by the FDA, and they must follow Good Manufacturing Practice Guidelines.

Manufacturers themselves have the responsibility to determine and communicate product safety, as well as defend any representations or claims made about the product and show that the claims are not false or misleading.[58] For supplements that make structure/function claims, DSHEA requires supplement manufacturers to include the following information on the label: "This statement has not been evaluated by the FDA. This product is not intended to diagnose, treat, cure, or prevent any disease."[59] To abide by the DSHEA requirements and follow the Good Manufacturing Practice Guidelines, a number of supplement companies have employed teams of researchers (many of whom are MS- or PhD-prepared exercise physiologists or sports nutrition specialists) to help educate the public about nutrition and exercise, provide input on product development, conduct research on products, and assist in coordinating research trials.

Despite ongoing improvements to regulatory and manufacturing guidelines, the potential for contaminated nutritional supplements to cause a failed doping test for an athlete remains a concern. Several surveys of supplements available through the Internet and at retail stores have confirmed that many are contaminated with steroids and stimulants that are prohibited for use in elite sport.[60]

High-performing athletes are generally advised to stay away from supplements because their purity and safety are not guaranteed. This recommendation should not, however, be confused with responsible and educated use of supplements, if and when indicated. A joint position statement by the Academy of Nutrition and Dietetics, the Dietitians of Canada, and the American College of Sports Medicine indicates that physical performance and recovery are enhanced by optimal nutrition and that although supplementation is normally not necessary for athletes with an adequate diet, it can be needed if energy intake is restricted or groups of food are eliminated from their diet.[61]

The federal government has been concerned about possible underreporting of adverse events by the supplement industry. As of 2014, the FDA is accepting online submission of voluntary and mandatory dietary supplement adverse event reports (www.safetyreporting.hhs.gov). Manufacturers, packers, and distributors are required to report to the FDA any serious adverse events received regarding their dietary supplement products.[62]

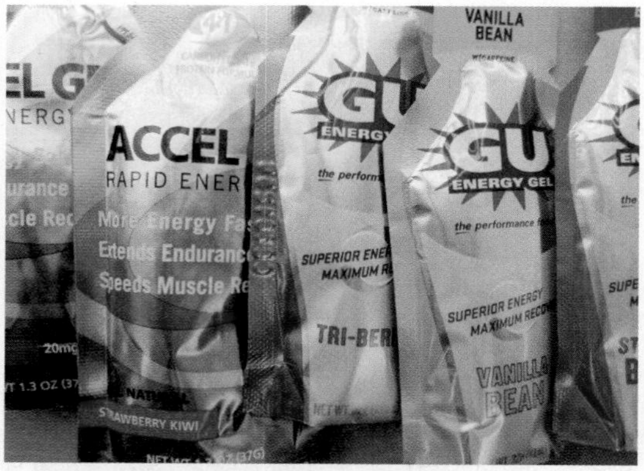

© Jones & Bartlett Learning. Photo by Amy Rathburn.

Convenience Supplements

Convenience supplements represent the largest segment of the supplement industry and include meal-replacement powders, ready-to-drink supplements, energy bars, and energy gels. Most are fortified with one-third to one-half of the RDA for vitamins and minerals, but differ on the amount of carbohydrate, protein, and fat they contain. For the endurance cycler, marathoner, and triathlete, convenience supplements can quickly provide energy, carbohydrate, protein, and other nutrients. Still, they are most appropriately used to improve availability of macronutrients, not as a replacement for a day of good eating. All active people should maintain a foundation of wholesome foods in their day-to-day diets.

Weight-Gain Powders

One common way athletes try to increase muscle mass is to add extra calories from protein to their diet. Adding an extra 500 to 1,000 kilocalories per day to your diet will promote significant weight gain, and protein powders are a relatively easy way to do just that. However, weight gained on a high-calorie

Elite Adolescent Athletes' Use of Dietary Supplements

Background

The Dietary Supplement Health and Education Act of 1994 (DSHEA) defines dietary supplements as any product taken to supplement the diet. These products may contain vitamins, minerals, botanicals, herbs, amino acids, enzymes, or metabolites. Current literature shows that dietary supplements are widely used among young athletes, and that supplement users often consume more than one supplement. Young athletes often use various supplements in an attempt to gain an advantage over their opponent. However, dietary supplements are not well regulated or sufficiently tested, especially for use in children and adolescent populations. According to one report, approximately 25 percent of dietary supplements are contaminated. Common contaminants include anabolic androgenic steroids, caffeine, and ephedrine. Unfortunately, most adolescent athletes seem to know very little about dietary supplements. Few studies have examined supplement use among elite adolescent athletes, specifically, the prevalence of supplement use, opinions surrounding supplement use, sources of information regarding supplements, and how supplements are obtained by users.

Study Purpose

The purpose of this study was to investigate the use of dietary supplements among adolescent athletes. There were four primary objectives of this study: First, to examine the prevalence of supplement use with respect to demographics and a wide range of sport-specific characteristics in young athletes; second, to analyze the differences among nonusers, users, and daily users; third, to study the association between athletes' opinions on the need for supplements and supplement use; and fourth, to identify sources of information and supply.

Experimental Plan

The data were collected from the cross-sectional GOAL study, a nationwide study of elite German adolescent athletes. Athletes who engaged in one sport in the 2010 Winter Olympics or the 2012 Summer Olympics, who were born between 1992 and 1995, and who had competed in at least the lowest national squad level were included. A total of 1,138 athletes from 51 sports answered a self-administered questionnaire between February 2010 and January 2011. Dietary supplements were categorized into three groups (short-term function, long-term function, and medium-term muscle-building function), and statistical analysis was completed to establish which supplement group was used and how often and what type of athletes used supplements from each group. Athletes' sociodemographic information, sport-specific characteristics, and opinions on the need for supplement use also were examined.

Results

The study found that 91.1 percent of elite German adolescent athletes consumed one supplement at least one time per month (see **Figure A**). More than 25 percent of athletes were daily users of dietary supplements. Male athletes were more frequent users than were female athletes. The highest frequency of daily users was found in endurance and power sports; the lowest frequency of daily users was found in technical sports. The highest proportion of nonusers was found to be aesthetic athletes. As expected, athletes who were obligated by their sporting organization to consume supplements were more frequent users and daily users than were athletes having no requirements concerning supplementation. The highest daily

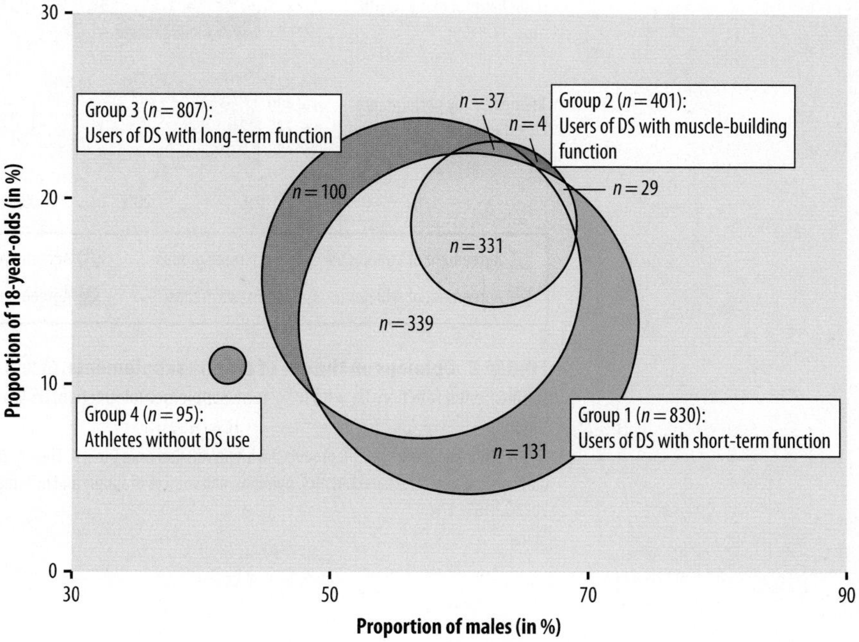

FIGURE A **Distribution of dietary-supplement groups (*N* = 1,066).** DS with short-term supplemental function: dextrose and energy drinks; DS with long-term supplemental function: complex carbohydrates, vitamins C and E, multivitamins, iron, magnesium, calcium, and zinc; DS with medium-term muscle-building function: protein and creatine.

consumption was found for supplements with long-term supplemental function. Intake of dietary supplements with muscle-building function was nearly two times as frequent among daily users than among nondaily users. The most common supplements consumed (at least once per month) were magnesium, dextrose, energy drinks, vitamin C, and calcium.

Male athletes were significantly more likely to use supplements with short- and medium-term muscle-building function than were females. Supplements with muscle-building function were used mostly by endurance athletes, and supplements with long-term supplemental function were used mostly by ball game athletes and endurance athletes.

Coaches were the main source of information about dietary supplements (36.5 percent), followed by family (29.7 percent), physicians (29.3 percent), and, last, nutritionists (13.9 percent). The study found that 15.6 percent of athletes learned about supplements from the media. Parents were the most frequent supplier of supplements. Athletes had strong positive opinions regarding the use of dietary supplements (see **Figure B**).

Conclusion and Discussion

The large number of participants in this study allowed for the determination of new associations and confirmation of previous study findings on dietary supplement use, opinions, characteristics, sources, and supply. The high prevalence of dietary supplement use, newly identified sources of supply and information, and the finding that certain sport federations require young athletes to take supplements confirm a need for education surrounding the appropriate use of dietary supplements. Education programs should focus on providing athletes, coaches, and parents with reliable sources of information about supplement use and the potential consequences of overuse.

Data from Diehl K, Thiel A, Zipfel S, et al. Elite adolescents' use of dietary supplements: characteristics, opinions, and sources of supply and information. *Int J Sport Nutr Exerc Metab*. 2012;22:165–174.

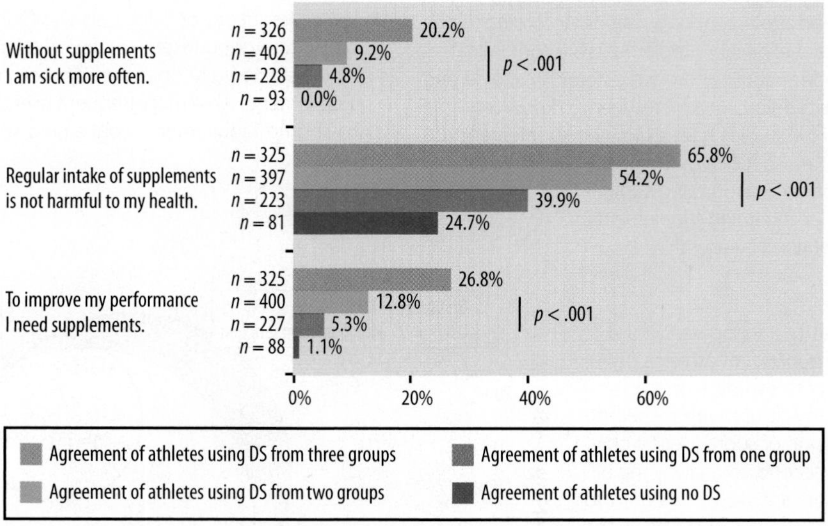

FIGURE B Opinions on the use of dietary supplements. Groups of DS: DS with short-term supplemental function, DS with long-term supplemental function, DS with medium-term muscle-building function.

diet is only about 30 to 50 percent muscle; the rest of the gain is fat. Although protein intake above recommended levels does not improve muscle growth, protein supplements may help athletes meet protein requirements when their dietary protein intake is inadequate. Remember, muscle formation results from resistance training fueled by sufficient calorie intake, along with adequate rest between training sessions, not protein intake alone. Because the extra calories in high-protein diets can increase body fat, this approach to weight gain should be used with caution.

Amino Acids

Researchers have studied the use of individual amino acids to enhance performance and have not found obvious benefits.

Branched-chain amino acids (BCAAs) compete with the amino acid tryptophan for uptake in the brain. Tryptophan is a precursor of serotonin, which may produce symptoms of fatigue. Some researchers have proposed that increasing intake of BCAAs will inhibit the uptake of tryptophan, but studies are inconclusive.[63] A small study suggests that BCAA supplementation before exercise may reduce delayed-onset muscle soreness.[64] Because safety and effectiveness have not been established, BCAA supplements are not recommended.

HMB, also known as beta-hydroxy beta-methylbutyrate, is a metabolite of the essential branched-chain amino acid leucine. It is found in foods such as catfish, citrus fruits, and breast milk. HMB is thought to increase strength and lean body mass in adults who exercise, including elderly exercisers. However, the evidence is inconsistent and inconclusive. More study is needed.

Glutamine, the dispensable amino acid, is a popular supplement for strength athletes. Some proponents of glutamine supplements note the transient decrease in glutamine levels after acute exercise and chronic overtraining. Others suggest the glutamine supplementation would improve immune function during exercise. However, glutamine is a byproduct of many metabolic reactions and is synthesized easily in the body. Supplementation has not been shown to be beneficial.[65]

Creatine

Creatine, a nitrogenous compound in meats and fish, is synthesized by the liver, pancreas, and kidneys. Muscles store creatine mainly as creatine phosphate, which functions as part of the ATP–CP energy system. Creatine is one of the most popular nutritional supplements, and it has been shown to increase muscle performance in short-duration, high-intensity resistance exercises, such as weight lifting, that rely on the ATP–CP energy system.[66] Creatine has been studied extensively, with more than 5,000 studies to date. Of these, about 300 looked at performance enhancement; 70 percent reported positive effects.[67]

▶ **creatine** An important nitrogenous compound found in meats and fish and synthesized in the body from amino acids (glycine, arginine, and methionine).

When combined with heavy resistance training, supplementation with creatine has regularly been shown to increase strength, fat-free mass, and muscle cross-sectional area more than resistance training alone. Creatine also may be of benefit in other types of exercise, such as high-intensity sprints or endurance training. However, it appears that the effects of creatine diminish as the length of time spent exercising increases. The most common adverse effect is temporary water retention during early stages of supplementation. High doses and combining creatine with certain other supplements can lead to liver and kidney complications. Creatine supplements are considered safe and ethical to ingest. Still, long-term safety is yet to be proven in different populations (athletes, sedentary individuals, active adults, the young, or the elderly).[68]

Quick Bite

Placebo Power!

Athletes involved in a heavy weight-lifting program volunteered to participate in a study in which they would take what they thought were anabolic steroids. The results were dramatic: During four weeks of treatment, these experienced weightlifters had a nearly 7.5-fold increase in the rate of their strength gain. However, they were taking a placebo—an inactive substance identical in appearance to the genuine drug. Because there was no pharmacological effect, gains were solely due to the result of their belief in the treatment.

Antioxidants

As we exercise, our muscles consume more oxygen than when we are at rest. Increased oxygen consumption leads to increased production of free radicals. Free radicals can damage cell membranes and DNA, leading to conditions such as cancer, aging, and a number of degenerative diseases. So, exercise promotes health, but it also may increase cell damage.

Antioxidants, which are compounds that seek out and neutralize free radicals, can protect muscles and cells from the damage that can result from exercise. Antioxidants come in different forms, such as vitamins, minerals, enzyme complexes, and herbs. Vitamin C, vitamin E, and beta-carotene are well-known antioxidants. Antioxidants can be obtained through food or supplements. Examples of good food sources of antioxidants include deep orange- and green-colored vegetables, citrus fruits, whole grains, and green tea.

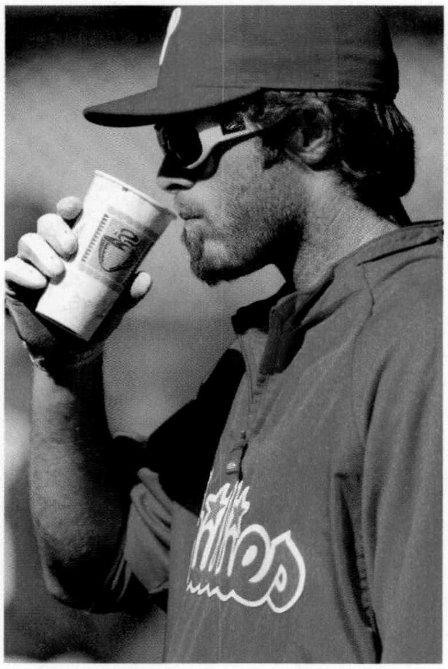

© Aspen Photo/Shutterstock, Inc.

People who exercise infrequently or sporadically, as well as those who exercise intensely and for long periods of time, have higher risk for damage than those who exercise regularly and on a more moderate schedule. Regular, moderate exercise enhances the antioxidant defense system and protects against exercise-induced free-radical damage. In contrast, intense exercise in untrained individuals overwhelms the body's defenses, resulting in increased free-radical damage.

Does supplementing with antioxidants or eating foods rich in antioxidants repair free-radical damage after exercise? The answer is a bit complex. Nutrition deficiencies can create difficulties in training and recovery (possibly because of free-radical damage); however, the role of antioxidant supplementation in a well-nourished athlete is controversial. It is not necessary, or advisable, for a well-nourished athlete to take antioxidant supplements.

Regarding antioxidants and exercise, the best recommendation goes back to the basics: Follow a balanced training program that emphasizes regular exercise, and eat five servings of fruits or vegetables each day. These practices ensure that you are developing your antioxidant systems and that your diet is providing the necessary components.

Caffeine

Caffeine naturally occurs in plants and is a stimulant. For more than a century, caffeine has been used to enhance sports performance, and during the last four decades, a robust body of research has emerged. Caffeine appears to improve exercise capacity and performance by affecting the central nervous system. These effects reduce the perception of fatigue, allowing the athlete to maintain optimal pacing, skills, and intensity for a longer period. Caffeine's effects can enhance performance for a wide range of sports[69]:

- Endurance sports (> 60 minutes)
- Brief, sustained, high-intensity sports (1–60 minutes)
- Team and intermittent sports

Caffeine consumption before and during exercise can enhance performance. Because the amount that enhances performance is indistinguishable from everyday caffeine use (and testing was unreliable), the World Anti-Doping Agency removed caffeine from its Prohibited List.

Because caffeine doses as low as 2–3 mg/kg are effective, the "standard" protocol for caffeine use (6 mg/kg body mass taken an hour prior to exercise) is outdated. Most studies of caffeine and performance have been in laboratory settings, and studies that investigate performance effects outside the laboratory or during real-life sporting events are scarce. Individuals vary widely in their response to caffeine intake. Although caffeine may enhance sports performance in most people, some are nonresponders, and others may respond negatively.

For caffeine, more is not better. The effects of the acute intake of caffeine follow a U-shaped curve. Although low to moderate doses produce positive effects and a sense of well-being, higher doses can increase heart rate, impair fine motor control, and cause anxiety. These may have health consequences as well as interfering with sports performance. Even at low levels of intake caffeine can affect sleep, which may interfere with the ability to recover between training sessions or during multiday competitions. Discontinuing caffeine also may cause withdrawal side effects including headaches and listlessness. It is important to find the lowest effective dose of caffeine that can be used to achieve performance enhancement. Before specific recommendations for caffeine supplementation can be made, real-world studies of sports performance enhancement must be done.

Ephedrine

Ephedrine was a popular ergogenic supplement until its sale in the United States was banned by the FDA in 2004.[70] Despite its ban by the FDA, National Football League (NFL), National Collegiate Athletic Association (NCAA), and International Olympic Committee (IOC), athletes continued to use ephedrine, either as a weight-loss aid or to gain a performance edge. More than a decade after the ban, ephedrine supplements still are available via the Internet despite the drug's dangers. Ephedrine stimulates the central nervous system and is an effective bronchodilator. In addition, it raises both heart rate and blood pressure. Athletes hoped its stimulatory effects would improve performance, suppress appetite, and promote weight loss.

Found in many products as either the herbal ma huang (ephedra) or the synthetic ephedrine, ephedrine was one of the most controversial supplements on the market. Ephedra use was linked to the heatstroke-related death of Major League Baseball pitcher Steve Bechler, and a government-sponsored review concluded that the use of ephedrine, ephedra-containing dietary supplements, or ephedrine plus caffeine is associated with two to three times the risk of nausea, vomiting, psychiatric symptoms such as anxiety and change in mood, autonomic hyperactivity, and palpitations.[71] Studies such as this led to the FDA's conclusion that ephedrine posed an unreasonable risk of illness and injury.

Sodium Bicarbonate

Some athletes consume sodium bicarbonate (baking soda) in the belief that it will help neutralize the acidity (buildup of protons) in muscles. Whether **soda loading** actually produces an ergogenic effect is controversial. Sodium bicarbonate ingestion has been shown to improve performance in single-bout, high-intensity events, probably because of an increase in buffering capacity.[72] Likewise, studies that evaluate events lasting from 2 to 10 minutes, where proton buildup is most likely, have shown some positive results related to interval training performance.[73]

▶ **soda loading** Consumption of bicarbonate (baking soda) to raise blood pH. The intent is to increase the capacity to buffer acids, thus delaying fatigue. Also known as bicarbonate loading.

Bicarbonate loading also can produce negative effects. Athletes who follow this regimen report side effects such as intestinal discomfort, stomach distress, nausea, cramping, diarrhea, and water retention. Although bicarbonate loading is not banned, it does have serious health-related consequences. Bicarbonate loading increases blood alkalinity and influences

Quick Bite

Ouch! But I Felt Fine Yesterday . . .

After a bout of heavy exercise, a person may not feel muscle soreness for a day or two. We do not fully understand this painful phenomenon, which is called delayed-onset muscle soreness. Activities that lengthen muscles seem to be the primary cause. The muscles suffer damage, with micro-tears in their structure. This leads to an inflammatory response, causing localized muscle pain, swelling, and tenderness.

blood pressure. Anyone with high blood pressure (hypertension) should not bicarbonate load.

Chromium

The trace mineral chromium appears to assist the movement of glucose into cells. The theory is that by enhancing insulin action, chromium increases amino acid uptake, which then increases protein synthesis and promotes a gain in muscle mass.

Among mineral supplements, chromium supplements (typically chromium picolinate) have become so popular for purported weight loss and muscle development that sales are second only to calcium.[74] However, chromium has been shown not to have beneficial effects on body mass or composition. A review of the evidence also finds no improvements in fasting glucose levels or relevant effects on body weight.[75] Due to the lack of evidence and concerns over safety, this supplement cannot be recommended.

Iron

Iron supplements are used commonly by athletes. Exercise-induced iron-deficiency anemia (also known as sports anemia) is prevalent in athletic populations, particularly those with heavy training loads. It leads to a decline in performance and other physiological problems.[76] For sports anemia, iron supplementation is relatively safe but may be ineffective in raising hemoglobin concentrations due to an exercise-induced decrease in iron absorption and increase in iron retention by liver cells and macrophages. Athletes who have used long-term supplementation have increased iron stores, putting them at risk for iron overload.[77]

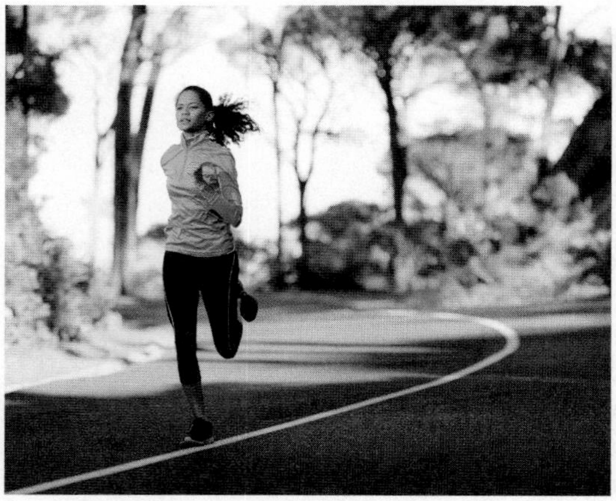

© Daxiao Productions/Shutterstock

Beta-Alanine

Research has shown that beta-alanine (β-alanine) supplementation can increase levels of carnosine, an intramuscular buffer.[78] During bouts of high-intensity exercise that are likely limited by muscle acidosis, increased carnosine has been linked to performance improvements.[79] But when this idea was tested with sprinting athletes, β-alanine supplementation was ineffective for increasing endurance.[80]

Key Concepts Numerous dietary supplements, such as caffeine, beta-alanine, creatine, and antioxidants, are marketed for performance-enhancing effects. However, few have been subjected to rigorous clinical trials or long-term safety evaluation. Athletes should consult a physician before adding dietary supplements to their training regimen.

Quick Bite

The Burn to the Finish

The pain a runner feels when approaching the finish line and immediately after the event is called acute muscle soreness. The culprits include a buildup of metabolic by-products and tissue edema caused by fluid seeping from the bloodstream into surrounding tissues. The pain and soreness usually disappear within minutes or hours.

Weight and Body Composition

Pete, a bodybuilder, wants to bulk up by gaining 15 pounds of muscle and not fat. Sarah, on the other hand, wants to compete as a lightweight rower and needs to lose 7 pounds. Some athletes struggle to lose weight, but others find it nearly impossible to gain weight and muscle mass. Whether intentionally gaining or losing weight, weight change should be accomplished slowly—during the off-season or at the beginning of the season before competition starts.

Body composition and body weight are just two of many factors that affect exercise performance. Body composition can affect strength, agility, and appearance. Body weight can influence speed, endurance, and power. Because body fat adds weight without adding strength, many sports emphasize low body fat percentages. Yet, by themselves, body composition and body weight do not predict athletic performance accurately.

Weight Gain: Build Muscle, Lose Fat

Weight gain is influenced by genetics, stage of adolescent development, gender, body mass, diet, training program, prior resistance training, motivation, and use of supplements and anabolic steroids, among other factors. Complex interactions among these factors make it difficult to predict an athlete's ability to meet a weight goal. However, experience tells us the following:

- Untrained male athletes can gain approximately 3 to 4 pounds of lean body mass per month in the early stages of a rigorous resistance-training program.[81,82] Because of their smaller muscle mass and lean tissue, young women can achieve only 50 to 75 percent of the gains seen in male counterparts, but with the same relative strength.
- Approximately 20 percent of the increase in lean body mass occurs in the first year of resistance training, tapering to 1 to 3 percent in subsequent years. Scientists believe that the rate declines as muscle mass approaches the maximum potential amount determined by genetics.
- Some male athletes of high school age have difficulty gaining muscle mass. These athletes might be in the early stages of the adolescent growth spurt and can lack sufficient levels of the male hormones to stimulate muscle development.

Nutrition plays an important role in increasing lean body mass. Athletes must consume enough calories, along with adequate carbohydrate and protein, to gain the desired muscle mass.

Key Concepts Athletes often seek to improve their power and strength by increasing muscle mass. Weight gain as muscle requires increased dietary calories, primarily as carbohydrate, combined with strength training.

Weight Loss: The Panacea for Optimal Performance?

As the pressure to win increases, many coaches and athletes come to believe that weight loss and lower body fat composition will provide that competitive edge. Athletes strive for lower body weight and lower body fat for three reasons: (1) to improve appearance, especially in aesthetic sports (e.g., diving, figure skating, gymnastics), (2) to enhance performance where lower body weight can increase speed (e.g., race walking, running, pole vaulting, jumping, cross-country skiing), or (3) to qualify in a lower weight category (e.g., wrestling, boxing, rowing).[83] **FIGURE 14.16** illustrates the key factors in a successful weight-loss program.

As healthy young adults, men average 15 percent body fat, and women average 25 percent.[84] Although these averages provide starting points, recommendations for individual athletes must account for genetic background, age, gender, sport, health, and weight history. Male athletes should not go below 5 to 7 percent body fat. For female athletes, at least 13 to 17 percent body fat is needed to maintain normal menstrual function, which in turn is important for maintaining bone health.

Keeping accurate food and training records provides information on energy intake and expenditure. The best way for athletes to sustain a safe and sensible loss of body fat is to reduce calorie intake moderately and modify their training program. A combination of resistance training and aerobic activity is best for weight loss because it helps maintain or even increase lean body mass while simultaneously decreasing fat mass.

Beware of fad weight-loss methods such as ketogenic diets, high-protein diets, and semistarvation diets. These practices can compromise energy reserves, body composition, and psychological well-being, leading to decreased

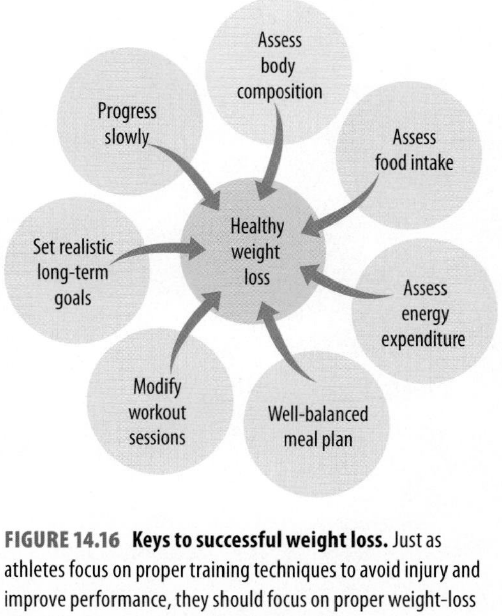

FIGURE 14.16 Keys to successful weight loss. Just as athletes focus on proper training techniques to avoid injury and improve performance, they should focus on proper weight-loss strategies to lose weight and maintain health.

performance and increased health risks. Athletes often are alert to the latest supplements to hit the market. Many claim to raise metabolism, accelerate the burning of body fat, and augment weight loss. In reality, most "fat burners" are ineffective or associated with only very modest weight loss in obese people. Despite patient perceptions that herbal remedies are more "natural" and thus free of adverse effects, some herbal supplements are associated with severe liver damage.[85]

Key Concepts Before embarking on a weight-loss program, athletes should carefully evaluate their goals and set a realistic plan for weight loss and maintenance. Safe weight-loss practices include modest changes in food intake accompanied by gradual increases in aerobic activity.

Weight Loss: Negative Consequences for the Competitive Athlete?

Changing body size and shape can have detrimental effects. An unrealistic perception of optimal body weight and a belief that weight loss is necessary for improved performance can contribute to unhealthy weight-loss practices. Athletes risk medical problems when dieting goes awry.

Making Weight

▶ **pathogenic** Capable of causing disease.

Wrestlers, weight lifters, boxers, jockeys, rowers, and coxswains face competitive pressures to "make weight" to compete or to be certified in a lower weight classification. Such athletes often resort to the **pathogenic** weight-control behaviors summarized in **TABLE 14.9**. Repeated cycles of rapid weight loss and subsequent regain increase the risk of disordered eating, fatigue, psychological distress (e.g., anger, anxiety, depression), dehydration, and sudden death.

Studies show that wrestlers, in attempts to gain a competitive advantage, will try to reduce weight a few days before or on the day of competition.[86] Often, extreme measures are taken to lose a significant amount of weight.

TABLE 14.9
Pathogenic Weight-Loss Practices

Behavior	Consequences
Fasting	Loss of lean body mass and decreased metabolic rate
Diet pills	Medical side effects and weight regained when discontinued
Fat-free diets	Deficiency in macronutrients and micronutrients; difficult to maintain
Diuretics	Dehydration and electrolyte imbalance; no fat loss
Laxatives	Dehydration; no fat loss; may develop tolerance
Sweating	Dehydration; heat injury; no fat loss
Excessive exercise	Risk of injury and overtraining; no fat loss
Enemas	Dehydration and GI problems; no fat loss
Fluid restriction	Dehydration; heat injury; no fat loss
Self-induced vomiting	Dehydration; acid–base and electrolyte imbalances; esophageal tears and GI bleeding; erosion of dental enamel and swollen parotid glands

Data from Otis CL. Too slim, amenorrheic, fracture-prone: the female athlete triad. *ACSM Health Fitness.* 1998;2:2–25; Turocy PS, DePalma BF, Horswill CA, et al. National Athletic Trainers Association position statement: safe weight loss and maintenance practices in sport and exercise. *J Athl Train.* 2011;46(3):322–336. http://www.ncbi.nlm.nih.gov/pmc/articles/PMC3419563/. Accessed February 10, 2016.

In the process, body water loss can be extensive and dangerous. A fluid loss of only 2 percent of initial body weight (3 pounds for a 150-pound individual) can decrease athletic performance by elevating heart rate and lowering **cardiac output**. Moderate to severe dehydration (more than 3 to 5 percent of body weight) can be dangerous because of increased core body temperature, electrolyte imbalances, and cardiac and kidney changes. These conditions can result in heat illness, including heat cramps, heat exhaustion, or heatstroke.

▶ **cardiac output** The amount of blood expelled by the heart.

▶ **hyperthermia** A much higher than normal body temperature.

Rapid weight loss can have serious health consequences. A tragic example occurred in 1998, when three previously healthy collegiate wrestlers died trying to make weight.[87] These athletes had not only dropped significant weight preseason—more than 20 pounds (9 kilograms)—but also lost between 3.5 and 9 pounds (1.6 and 4 kilograms) in the one to nine hours before their deaths. The wrestlers restricted food and fluid intake. To maximize sweat losses, they wore vapor-impermeable suits under cotton warm-up suits and exercised vigorously in hot environments. Dehydration and **hyperthermia** (elevated body temperature) led to their demise.

Today, the NCAA has better guidelines for monitoring weight-loss practices and weigh-in procedures (see **FIGURE 14.17**). These include educating coaches and athletic trainers about healthy weight-control strategies and limiting the amount of preseason and precompetition weight loss.[88] The NCAA weigh-in format requires athletes to have a season minimum weight, established at the start of the year. This format attempts to prevent the use of techniques and tools that have been used in the past for rapid dehydration that results in rapid weight loss.[89]

Quick Bite

What's the Best "Fat-Burning" Exercise?

It's a common misconception that low-intensity exercise is superior for "fat burning." Aerobic activities do use a greater percentage of fat as fuel, but it is the total amount of calories expended during exercise that supports increased mobilization of fat in response to a caloric deficit. In terms of actual energy expenditure, higher-intensity exercise requires more calories for a given time period than exercise at a lower intensity. Thus, to lose body fat, the fuel (source of calories) is not as important as the amount of energy expended.

Female Athlete Triad

Although the majority of female athletes benefit from increased physical activity, there are those who go too far and risk developing a trio of medical problems. In 1991, the American College of Sports Medicine coined the term *female athlete triad* to describe the interaction of disordered eating, amenorrhea, and premature osteoporosis.[90] Female athletes who compete in endurance sports such as long-distance running, aesthetic sports such as gymnastics, antigravitational sports such as indoor rock climbing, and sports with weight classifications such as karate are at the greatest risk.[91]

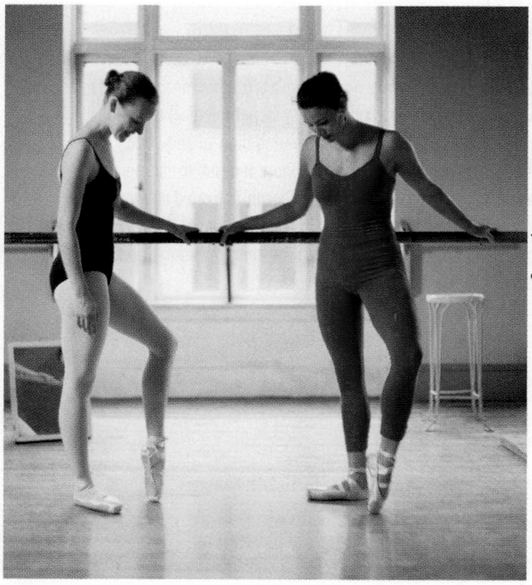

Disordered Eating

Female athletes who compete in endurance events, such as long-distance running, or in sports where appearance is important (e.g., gymnastics, figure skating, diving) are at higher risk for disordered eating behaviors. In some cases, disordered eating can progress to an eating disorder. Anorexia nervosa appears to be no more prevalent among female athletes than among nonathletes. However, the prevalence of eating disorders is increasing in elite athletes and for those individuals who start dieting because of (1) perception of appearance in the specific sport, (2) perceived performance improvements, or (3) sociocultural pressures for thinness or an "ideal" body.[92] Data suggest that lean-sport athletes are at greater risk for disordered eating than are athletes in nonlean sports.[93]

Amenorrhea

In the general population, 2 to 5 percent of women have amenorrhea. However, the prevalence is much higher in athletes.[94] Amenorrhea in athletic women is related to the combined effects of increased physical activity, weight loss, low body fat levels, and insufficient energy intake.

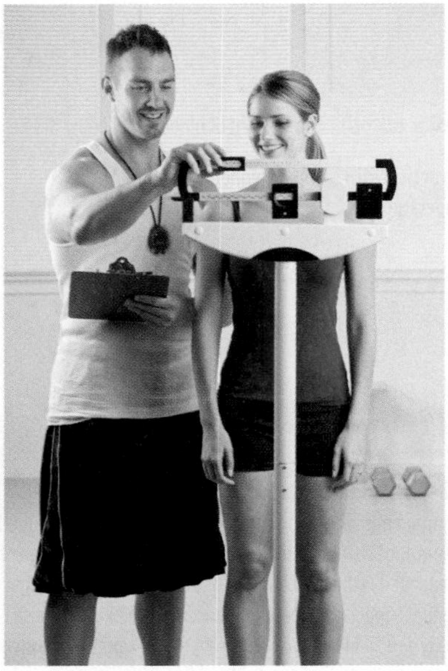

© AVAVA/ShutterStock, Inc.

FIGURE 14.17 Weighing in. The NCAA discourages athletes from reducing their weight through intentional dehydration, a dangerous and potentially deadly practice.

Premature Osteoporosis

Health consequences of amenorrhea include premature osteoporosis. Amenorrheic athletes experience rapid loss of bone mineral density in the spine, which can spread to other parts of the skeleton if amenorrhea continues for a long time.

Treatment involves replacing estrogen, which is low in amenorrheic females. Oral contraceptives are the most common method of estrogen replacement and also can serve as a reliable form of birth control. Calcium supplementation also is recommended. Although bone mineralization might never return to normal in amenorrheic athletes, studies indicate that reducing the intensity of training, improving dietary intake, and increasing body weight can help restore menstruation and increase bone density.[95]

Breaking the Triad

Female athletes at risk are perfectionists, driven to excel in a given sport, who believe that a specific athletic body image is required to excel as an athlete.

Some reports estimate as many as 60 percent of female athletes in aesthetic sports (e.g., dance, skating, diving, gymnastics) and weight-dependent sports (e.g., rowing, martial arts, horse racing) can be at risk.[96]

Screening, referral, and education are keys to preventing the female athlete triad. Prevention and treatment are most successful when they are multidisciplinary efforts carried out by a team of medical, athletic, nutrition, and mental health experts. Proactive sports education includes reducing the emphasis on body weight, eliminating group weigh-ins, treating each athlete individually, and facilitating healthy weight management (see **TABLE 14.10**).

Quick Bite

Too Much of a Good Thing ...

Many athletes adhere to rigid dietary habits, which could lead to eating disorders or *orthorexia nervosa*, a term that means literally "fixation on righteous eating." This psychopathological condition is characterized by an obsession for eating high-quality food. Although the behavior starts as an innocent desire to eat more healthfully, a person with orthorexia becomes fixated on food purity. The person adheres to such a rigid diet that health can suffer. Coaches should be alert not only to symptoms of eating disorders, but also to those of orthorexia nervosa.

Key Concepts Pathogenic weight-control practices increase the risk of dehydration and compromise performance; they can have long-term serious consequences for athletes. The female athlete triad—disordered eating, amenorrhea, and premature osteoporosis—results from excessive weight loss. Often weight loss is driven by unrealistic ideas of appropriate body weight and shape for competition. Education of coaches and athletes is essential to prevent the female athlete triad.

TABLE 14.10
Combating Disordered Eating in Athletes

Deemphasize body weight.	Do not view the athlete's weight as the primary contributor to, or detractor from, athletic performance. Research indicates that athletes can achieve appropriate weight and fitness when the focus is on physical conditioning and strength development, as well as the cognitive and emotional aspects of performance.
Eliminate group weigh-ins.	Often viewed as a way to motivate the team, the practice of group weigh-ins can be destructive to people who are struggling with their body image and disordered eating. If there is a legitimate reason for weighing an athlete, explain the reason and weigh the athlete privately.
Treat each athlete individually.	Many athletes have an unrealistic perception of what an ideal body weight is, especially in sports for which leanness is considered important. Additionally, athletes might strive for weight and body composition that is realistic in only a few genetically endowed people. It is important to understand that genetic and biological processes, rather than one's willpower to control food intake, affect a person's weight.
Facilitate healthy weight management.	Be sensitive to issues related to weight control and dieting. Because many athletes have limited knowledge of sports nutrition, they resort to pathogenic weight-loss practices. Athletes can benefit from nutrition counseling by a sports nutritionist or a registered dietitian who has experience in working with athletes and disordered eating.

Based on Thompson RA, Sherman RT. Reducing the risk of eating disorders in athletics. *Eating Disorders: J Treatment Prevent.* 1993;1:65–78. Retrieved from: http://www.tandf.co.uk/journals.

Label to Table

Sports drinks often are recommended instead of plain water for those who engage in vigorous physical activity. Their proponents claim that they quickly replenish the body's supply of nutrients, particularly electrolytes. Let's take a look at the Nutrition Facts panel from a popular sports drink, Gatorade.

First, look closely at the serving size—it's not the whole container. This is worth noting because many people might drink the whole container and assume they were getting 50 kilocalories. Not true! The whole container has 200 kilocalories (50 × 4 servings). It's always a good idea to look at the serving size when you are studying a nutrition label.

So, what makes this sports drink different from plain (and inexpensive) water? This one has added carbohydrate, sodium, and potassium. Replacing carbohydrate during long workouts prevents complete depletion of glycogen stores. Most sports drinks have between 6 and 8 percent simple sugar. Higher amounts would limit water absorption, and replacement of water is more critical than replacement of glucose.

Sodium and potassium are added to sports drinks to improve taste and help replace electrolytes that are lost during exercise. Gatorade contains 110 milligrams of sodium and 30 milligrams of potassium. For many athletes, and certainly for recreational exercisers, water really is the best fluid replacer. Although both sodium and potassium are lost in sweat, water is lost in greater quantities. Sports drinks have been shown to benefit only athletes who are strenuously exercising for longer than an hour. With prolonged exercise and sweat losses, large losses of electrolytes can make a person dizzy and weak and can even lead to heat exhaustion or heatstroke.

The next time you head out for a bike ride, consider how long you'll be gone and how strenuous your ride will be, and then consider whether you'll need a sports drink. Also consider your personal taste—if a flavored sports drink will encourage you to replace fluids more than plain water will, that can be an important advantage. Just don't forget to read the label!

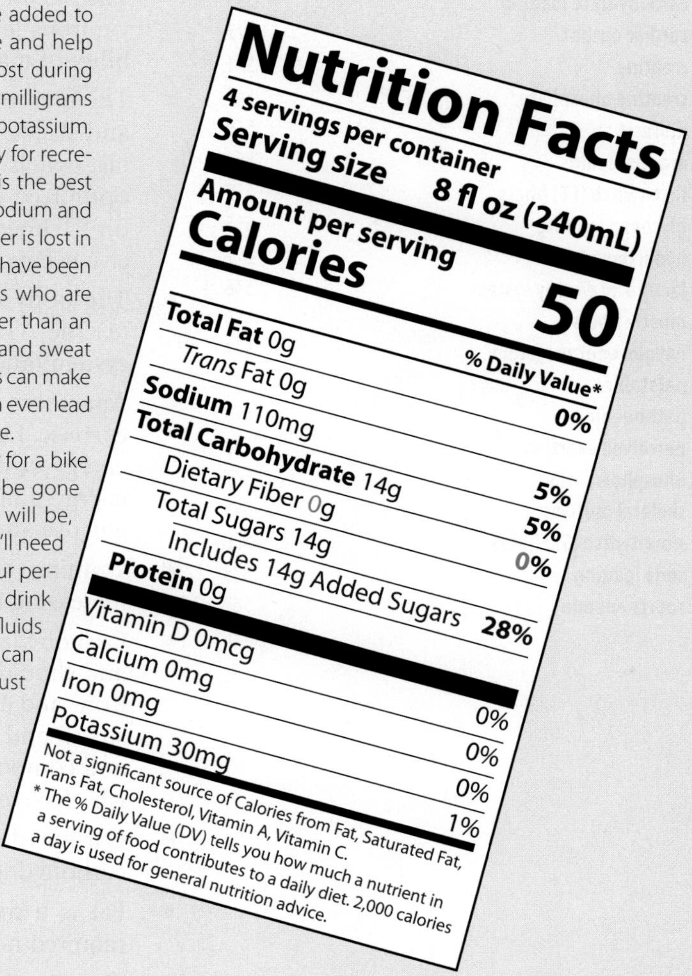
Nutrition Facts
4 servings per container
Serving size 8 fl oz (240mL)

Amount per serving	
Calories	**50**
	% Daily Value*
Total Fat 0g	0%
Trans Fat 0g	
Sodium 110mg	5%
Total Carbohydrate 14g	5%
Dietary Fiber 0g	0%
Total Sugars 14g	
Includes 14g Added Sugars	28%
Protein 0g	
Vitamin D 0mcg	0%
Calcium 0mg	0%
Iron 0mg	0%
Potassium 30mg	1%

Not a significant source of Calories from Fat, Saturated Fat, Trans Fat, Cholesterol, Vitamin A, Vitamin C.
* The % Daily Value (DV) tells you how much a nutrient in a serving of food contributes to a daily diet. 2,000 calories a day is used for general nutrition advice.

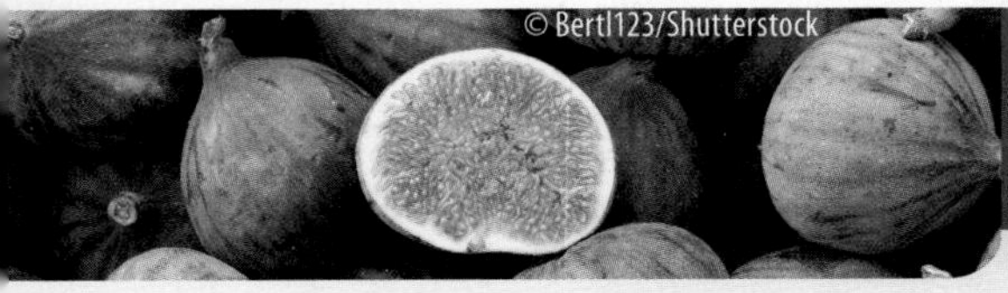
© Bertl123/Shutterstock

Learning Portfolio

Key Terms

Study Points

- Exercise promotes health and reduces risk of chronic diseases.
- The ACSM defines physical fitness as "the ability to perform moderate to vigorous levels of physical activity without undue fatigue and the capability of maintaining this level of activity throughout life."
- The muscular system contains three types of muscles: smooth, cardiac, and skeletal. There are two types of muscle fibers: slow-twitch (ST) and fast-twitch (FT). ST fibers have high aerobic endurance; FT fibers are optimized to perform anaerobically. Your body depends predominantly on ST fibers for low-intensity events and on FT fibers for highly explosive events.
- The body uses three systems to produce energy for physical activity: (1) the ATP–CP energy system (anaerobic), (2) the lactic acid energy system (anaerobic), and (3) the oxygen energy system (aerobic).
- Anaerobic and aerobic metabolism work together to fuel all types of exercise. During the early minutes of high-intensity exercise, the ATP–CP energy system and the lactic acid energy system provide most of the energy. Endurance activities are fueled primarily by the metabolism of glucose and fatty acids in the oxygen energy system.
- Training improves use of fat as a fuel by enhancing oxygen delivery and increasing the number of mitochondria in muscle.
- Carbohydrates should be the major source of energy in the athlete's diet and should come from complex carbohydrates, which can provide fiber, iron, and B vitamins. Athletes need carbohydrates so muscle glycogen stores and blood glucose concentrations will be adequate for training and competitive events. Likewise, carbohydrates are necessary to replenish glycogen stores after intense exercise.
- Carbohydrate loading is a process of reducing activity while increasing carbohydrate intake to maximize glycogen stores.
- Fat is a major fuel source for exercise, but high fat intake is neither required nor recommended.
- The protein needs of athletes are higher than for sedentary individuals, but generally athletes who consume adequate amounts of energy get enough protein. High-protein foods include low-fat dairy products, egg whites, lean beef and pork, chicken, turkey, fish, and legumes.
- Other nutrients important to the athlete's diet include B vitamins, iron, zinc, and calcium.
- Water is the most essential nutrient and is easily lost from the body with heavy sweating. Replacing fluid with water or sports drinks is important to prevent dehydration. Optimal sports drinks provide energy and electrolytes in a palatable solution that is rapidly absorbed.
- Athletes who are still growing have even higher energy and nutrient needs to support both physical activity and normal growth.
- Many dietary supplements are promoted as ergogenic aids—substances that enhance performance. Few well-controlled studies on their efficacy and safety have been done, however.

- Many athletes strive to either gain or lose weight so as to improve performance. In both cases, realistic goals and gradual changes are necessary for long-term success. Gains in muscle mass require increased calorie intake and weight training. Successful weight loss requires modest reductions in energy intake and increases in aerobic activity.
- Weight-control efforts that involve fasting, excessive sweating, purging, diuretics, or laxatives are detrimental to health.
- Disordered eating accompanied by amenorrhea and premature osteoporosis is known as the female athlete triad.

Study Questions

1. List the three different energy systems that your body uses to generate energy during exercise. When is each active during exercise?
2. What are muscle fibers, and what are the two major types?
3. What are the general recommendations for the balance of carbohydrate, fat, and protein in an athlete's diet?
4. What is carbohydrate loading?
5. How do protein recommendations for athletes vary from those for nonathletes?
6. Name three minerals that are of concern for athletes because they may not consume enough.
7. What is sports anemia and why does it happen? How does it compare with other anemias?
8. Define the term *ergogenic aid*. Is there a clear, research-based answer to whether ergogenic supplements work?
9. List the three components of the female athlete triad.

Try This

The Popularity of Ergogenic Aids

Take a trip to a health food store to see just how popular (and expensive!) ergogenic aids are. Try to locate each of the supplements listed in this chapter. Are they all available? What are their prices? Ask a salesperson what he or she knows about each of them. Do the answers match what you read in the text?

Commit to Get Fit

Do you meet the American College of Sports Medicine's definition of fitness? Answer the following questions with a yes or no:

1. Do you exercise consistently three to five days per week?
2. When you exercise, does it include 20 to 60 minutes (20 minutes for intense activity and 60 minutes for less intense activity) of continuous aerobic activity?
3. Does your type of exercise use large muscle groups? Can you maintain it? Is it rhythmical and aerobic?
4. Does part of your activity include strength training of a moderate intensity (a minimum of one set of 8 to 12 repetitions of 8 to 10 exercises) at least two days per week?

If you answered no to any of these questions, you are not following the ACSM's suggestions to develop and maintain cardiorespiratory and muscular fitness. Choose a question to which you answered no and set a specific goal to include that factor in your exercise routine.

References

1. American College of Sports Medicine (ACSM). About Exercise is Medicine. http://http://exerciseismedicine.org/support_page.php?p=113. Accessed February 29, 2016.
2. Jonas S, Phillips E. *ACSM'S Exercise Is Medicine: A Clinician's Guide to Exercise Prescription*. Philadelphia: Lippincott Williams & Wilkins; 2009.
3. U.S. Department of Health and Human Services. *2008 Physical Activity Guidelines for Americans*. http://www.health.gov/paguidelines/guidelines/default.aspx. Accessed February 10, 2016.
4. Centers for Disease Control and Prevention. *State Indicator Report on Physical Activity, 2014*. Atlanta, GA: U.S. Department of Health and Human Services; 2014.
5. Jonas S, Phillips E. *ACSM'S Exercise Is Medicine*. Op cit.
6. American Dietetic Association, Dietitians of Canada, American College of Sports Medicine. Position statement: nutrition and athletic performance. *J Am Diet Assoc*. 2009;109(3):509–527.
7. Maughan R, Shirreffs S. Physiology of Exercise. In: Rosenbloom C, Coleman E, eds. Sports Nutrition: *A practice Manual for Professionals*. 5th ed. Chicago: Academy of Nutrition and Dietetics; 2012:4–14.
8. Fink HH, Burgoon LA, Mikesky AE. *Practical Applications in Sports Nutrition*. 3rd ed. Sudbury, MA: Jones & Bartlett; 2011.
9. McArdle WD, Katch FI, Katch VL. *Exercise Physiology: Nutrition, Energy, and Human Performance*. 8th ed. Philadelphia: Lippincott Williams & Williams; 2014.
10. Brown GC. Speed limits. *The Sciences*. 2000;40(5):32–37.
11. McArdle WD, Katch FI, Katch VL. *Exercise Physiology*. Op cit.
12. Ibid.
13. American Dietetic Association, Dietitians of Canada, American College of Sports Medicine. Position statement: nutrition and athletic performance. Op cit.

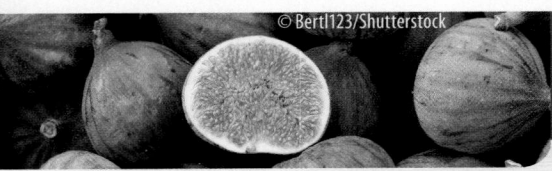

Learning Portfolio (continued)

14. Wilmore JH, Costill D, Kenney WL. *Physiology of Sport and Exercise*. 5th ed. Champaign, IL: Human Kinetics; 2011.
15. Jeukendrup A, Gleeson M. *Sport Nutrition: An Introduction to Energy Production and Performance*. 2nd ed. Champaign, IL: Human Kinetics; 2010.
16. Ibid.
17. U.S. Department of State. Sochi Olympics 2014: we are all athletes [Video]. January 31, 2014. https://www.youtube.com/watch?v=sv40xrvIOlw&list=UU6ZhpmNnLxlOYipqh8wbM3A&feature=share&index=5 http://goo.gl/C4qpzR. Accessed February 10, 2016.
18. American Dietetic Association, Dietitians of Canada, American College of Sports Medicine. Position statement: nutrition and athletic performance. Op cit.
19. Mota J, Fidalgo F, Silva R, et al. Relationships between physical activity, obesity, and meal frequency in adolescents. *Ann Hum Biol*. 2008;35(1):1–10.
20. American Dietetic Association, Dietitians of Canada, American College of Sports Medicine. Position statement: nutrition and athletic performance. Op cit.
21. Sundgot-Borg J, Garthe I. Elite athletes in aesthetic and Olympic weight class sports and the challenges of body weight and body composition. *J Sports Sci*. 2011;29(S1):1–14.
22. American Dietetic Association, Dietitians of Canada, American College of Sports Medicine. Position statement: nutrition and athletic performance. Op cit.
23. Maughan RJ, Burke LM. Practical nutritional recommendations for the athlete. *Nestle Nutr Inst Workshop Ser*. 2011;69:131–149.
24. Donaldson DM, Perry TL, Ross MC. Glycemic index and endurance performance. *Int J Sport Nutr Exer Metab*. 2010;20(2):154–165.
25. Dunford M. *Fundamentals of Sport and Exercise Nutrition*. Champaign, IL: Human Kinetics; 2010.
26. Sedlock DA. The latest on carbohydrate loading; a practical approach. *Curr Sports Med Rep*. 2008;7(4):209–213.
27. Coleman EJ. Carbohydrate and exercise. In: Rosenbloom C, ed. *Sports Nutrition: A Practice Manual for Professionals*. 5th ed. Chicago: Academy of Nutrition and Dietetics; 2012 p 469.
28. Sedlock DA. The latest on carbohydrate loading. Op cit.
29. American Dietetic Association, Dietitians of Canada, American College of Sports Medicine. Position statement: nutrition and athletic performance. Op cit.
30. Ibid.
31. O'Reilly J, Wong S, Chen Y. Glycemic index, glycemic load, and exercise performance. *Sports Med*. 2010;40(1):27–39.
32. American Dietetic Association, Dietitians of Canada, American College of Sports Medicine. Position statement: nutrition and athletic performance. Op cit.
33. Kirksick C, Harvey T, Stout J, et al. International Society of Sports Nutrition position stand: nutrition timing. *J Int Soc Sports Nutr*. 2008;5:17.
34. Coleman EJ. Carbohydrate and exercise. Op cit.
35. Ibid.
36. American Dietetic Association, Dietitians of Canada, American College of Sports Medicine. Position statement: nutrition and athletic performance. Op cit.
37. Clark N. *Nancy Clark's sports nutrition guidebook*. 5th ed. Champaign, IL: Human Kinetics; 2014:184–187.
38. Moore DR, Camera DM, Areta JL, Hawley JA. Beyond muscle hypertrophy: why dietary protein is important for endurance athletes. *Appl Physiol Nutr Metab*. 2014;39:987–997. doi: 10.1139/apnm-2013-0591.
39. Position of the American Dietetic Association, Dietitians of Canada, and the American College of Sports Medicine: nutrition and athletic performance. Op cit.
40. Clark N. *Nancy Clark's sports nutrition guidebook*. Op cit.
41. Aragon AA, Schoenfeld BJ. Nutrient timing revisited: is there a post-exercise anabolic window? *J Int Soc Sports Nutr*. 2013;10:5. http://www.jissn.com/content/10/1/5. Accessed February 10, 2016.
42. Storlie J. From fork to muscle. *Train Condition*. 1998;8:26, 28–29, 32–33.
43. Lunn WR, Pasiakos SM, Colletto MR, Karfonta KE, Carbone JW, Anderson JM, Rodriguez NR. Chocolate milk and endurance exercise recovery: protein balance, glycogen, and performance. Med Sci Sports Exerc. 2012;44(4):682–691.
44. American Dietetic Association, Dietitians of Canada, American College of Sports Medicine. Position statement: nutrition and athletic performance. Op cit.
45. Ibid.
46. Rowland T. Iron deficiency in athletes: an update. *Am J Lifestyle Med*. 2012;6(4):319–327.
47. DellaValle DM, Haas JD. Iron supplementation improves energetic efficiency in iron-depleted female rowers. *Med Sci Sports Exerc*. 2014;46(6):1204–1215.
48. Kreider RB, Wilborn DC, Taylor L, Campbell B. Exercise and sport nutrition review: research and recommendations. *J Int Soc Sports Nutr*. 2010;7:7.
49. Ibid.
50. Williams MH, Anderson DE, Rawson ES. *Nutrition for Health, Fitness, and Sport*. 10th ed. Boston: McGraw-Hill; 2012.
51. American College of Sports Medicine, Sawka MN, Burke LM, et al. American College of Sports Medicine position stand. Exercise and fluid replacement. *Med Sci Sports Exerc*. 2007;39:377–390.
52. Ibid.
53. Ibid.
54. Armstrong N, McManus AM, eds. The elite young athlete. *Med Sport Sci*. 2011;56:47–58.
55. Brown JE. *Nutrition Through the Life Cycle*. 4th ed. Belmont, CA: Wadsworth Cengage Learning; 2011.
56. Wiens K, Erdman KA, Stadnyk M, Parnell JA. Dietary supplement usage, motivation, and education in young Canadian athletes. *Int J Sport Nutr Exerc Metab*. 2014. Epub ahead of print.
57. Terry-McElrath YM, O'Malley PM, Johnston LD. Energy drinks, soft drinks, and substance use among United States secondary school students. *J Addict Med*. 2014;8(1):6.
58. U.S. Food and Drug Administration. Dietary supplements. http://www.fda.gov/Food/DietarySupplements/default.htm. Accessed February 10, 2016.
59. U.S. Food and Drug Administration. Questions and answers on dietary supplements. http://www.fda.gov/Food/DietarySupplements/UsingDietarySupplements/ucm480069.htm#wording. Accessed February 29, 2016.
60. Judkins C, Prock P. Supplements and inadvertent doping—how big is the risk to athletes? *Med Sport Sci*. 2012;59:143–152.
61. American Dietetic Association, Dietitians of Canada, American College of Sports Medicine. Position statement: nutrition and athletic performance. Op cit.
62. U.S. Food and Drug Administration. FDA initiates new online reporting method for dietary supplement adverse events to facilitate reporting. January 13, 2014. http://www.fda.gov/Food/NewsEvents/ConstituentUpdates/ucm381317.htm. Accessed February 10, 2016.
63. Fragakis AS, Thomson C. *The health professional's guide to dietary supplements*. 3rd ed. American Dietetic Association. Chicago, IL; 2007.
64. Shimomura Y, Inaguma A, Watanabe S, et al. Branched-chain amino acid supplementation before squat exercise and delayed-onset muscle soreness. *Int J Sport Nutr Exerc Metab*. 2010;20(3):236–244.
65. Nogied CD, Kasif S. To supplement or not to supplement: a metabolic network framework for human nutritional supplements. *PLoS One*. 2013;8(8):e68751.
66. Hall M, Trojian TH. Creatine supplementation. *Curr Sports Med Rep*. 2013;12(4):240–244.
67. Kleiner S, Greenwood-Robinson M. *Power Eating*. Champaign, IL: Human Kinetics; 2014.
68. Cooper R, Naclerio F, Allgrove J, Jimenez A. Creatine supplementation with specific view to exercise/sports performance: an update. *J Int Soc Sports Nutr*, 2012;9(1):33.
69. American College of Sports Medicine. Vitamin and mineral supplements and exercise. https://www.acsm.org/docs/current-comments/vitaminandmineralsupplementsandexercise.pdf. Accessed February 10, 2016.
70. U.S. Food and Drug Administration. FDA issues regulation prohibiting sale of dietary supplements containing ephedrine alkaloids and reiterates its advice that consumers stop using these products. *FDA News*. February 6, 2004. http://www.fda.gov/NewsEvents/Newsroom/PressAnnouncements/2004/ucm108242.htm. Accessed February 10, 2016.

71. Shekelle PG, Hardy ML, Morton SG, et al. Efficacy and safety of ephedra and ephedrine for weight loss and athletic performance: a meta-analysis. *JAMA.* 2003;289:1537–1545.
72. Peart DJ, Kirk RJ, Hillman AR, et al. The physiological stress response to high-intensity sprint exercise following the ingestion of sodium bicarbonate. *Eur J Appl Physiol.* 2013 Jan;113(1):127–134.
73. Joyce S, Minahan C, Anderson M, Osborne M. Acute and chronic loading of sodium bicarbonate in highly trained swimmers. *Eur J Appl Physiol.* 2012 Feb;112(2):461–469.
74. Vincent JB. Chromium: Is it essential, pharmacologically relevant, or toxic? *Met Ions Life Sci.* 2013;13:171–198.
75. Landman GW, Bilo HJ, Wouweling ST, Kleefstra N. Chromium does not belong in the diabetes treatment arsenal: Current evidence and future perspectives. *World J Diabetes.* 2014;5(2):160–164.
76. Reinki S, Taylor WR, Duda GN, et al. Absolute and functional iron deficiency in professional athletes during training and recovery. *Int J Cardiol.* 2012;156(2):186–191.
77. Mettler S, Zimmermann MB. Iron excess in recreational marathon runners. *Eur J Clin Nutr.* 2010;4:490–494.
78. Stellingwerff T, Decombaz J, Harris RC, Boesch C. Optimizing human in vivo dosing and delivery of p-alanine supplements for muscle carnosine synthesis. *Amino Acids.* 2012;43(1):57–65.
79. Jagim AR, Wright GA, Brice AG, Doberstein ST. Effects of beta-alanine supplementation on sprint endurance. *J Strength Cond Res.* 2013 Feb;27(2):526–532.
80. Ibid.
81. Houtkooper LB. Body composition. In: Manore MM, Thompson JL, eds. *Sport Nutrition for Health and Performance.* Champaign, IL: Human Kinetics; 2000:199–219.
82. Garcia-Pallares J, Lopez-Gullon JM, Muriel X, et al. Physical fitness factors to predict male Olympic wrestling performance. *Eur J Appl Physiol.* 2011;111(8):1747–1758.
83. McArdle WD, Katch FI, Katch VL. *Exercise Physiology.* Op cit.
84. Ibid.
85. Yellapu RK, Mittal V, Grewal P, Fiel M, Schiano T. Acute liver failure caused by "fat burners" and dietary supplements: a case report and literature review. *Can J Gastroenterol.* 2011;25(3):157–160.
86. Marttinen RH, Judelson DA, Wiersma LD, Coburn JW. Effects of self-selected mass loss on performance and mood in collegiate wrestlers. *J Strength Cond Res.* 2011;25(4):1010–1015.
87. Centers for Disease Control and Prevention. Rapid weight loss in wrestlers results in death. *MMWR.* 1998;47(6):105–108.
88. Kundrat S. Sport nutrition for coaches. *J Nutr Educ Behav.* 2010;42(6):430.
89. Loenneke J, Wilson J, Barnes J, Pujol T. Validity of the current NCAA minimum weight protocol: a brief review. *Ann Nutr Metab.* 2011;58:245–249.
90. Gibbs, JC, Williams NI, De Souza NJ. Prevalence of individual and combined components of the female athlete triad. *Med Sci Sports Exerc.* 2013;45(5):985–996.
91. Sundgot-Borgen J, Torstveit MK. Aspects of disordered eating continuum in elite high-intensity sports. *Scand J Med Sci Sports.* 2010;20(Suppl 2):112–121.
92. Ibid.
93. Ibid.
94. Coelho GM, Soares Ede A, Ribeiro BG. Are female athletes at increased risk for disordered eating and its complications? *Appetite.* 2010;55(3):379–387.
95. Arends JC, Cheung MY, Barrack MT, Nattiv A. Restoration of menses with nonpharmacologic therapy in college athletes with menstrual disturbances: a 5-year retrospective study. *Int J Sport Nutr Exerc Metab.* 2012;22(2):98–108.
96. Otis CL, Drinkwater B, Johnson M, et al. American College of Sports Medicine position stand: the female athlete triad. *Med Sci Sports Exerc.* 1997;29:i–ix.

Spotlight on Eating Disorders

Revised by Paul Insel

THINK About It

1 What's your view of the ideal female body?
2 When should you be concerned that you—or someone you know—is dieting obsessively?
3 Given the right situation, what foods are you likely to binge on?
4 How many magazines do you read that promote dieting or encourage thinness?

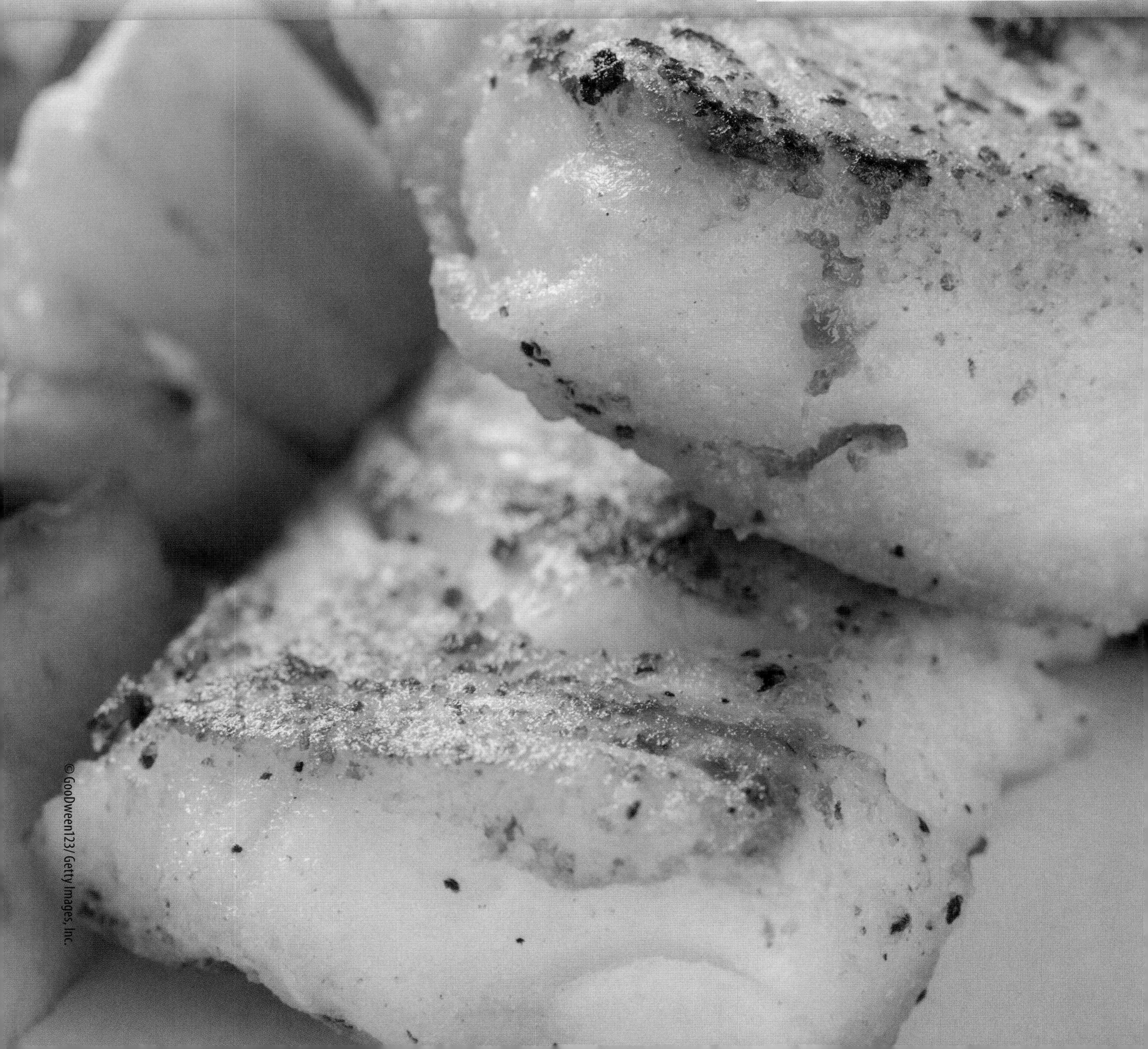

CHAPTER Menu

- The Eating Disorder Continuum
- No Simple Causes
- Anorexia Nervosa
- Bulimia Nervosa
- Binge-Eating Disorder
- Body Dysmorphic Disorder
- Night-Eating Syndrome
- Males: An Overlooked Population
- Anorexia Athletica
- The Female Athlete Triad
- Pregorexia
- Infantile Anorexia
- Combating Eating Disorders
- Key Terms
- Study Points
- Study Questions
- Try This
- References

LEARNING Objectives

- Describe the eating disorder continuum from anorexia nervosa to binge-eating disorder.
- Identify common causes of eating disorders.
- List causes, warning signs, and treatment of anorexia nervosa and bulimia nervosa.
- Discuss what often triggers binge-eating disorder and describe its treatment.
- Identify characteristics of body dysmorphic disorder and night-eating syndrome.
- Describe eating disorders in males.
- Discuss each component of the female athlete triad.

A gaunt, hollow-cheeked college freshman confides to her roommate that she feels chubby. After an enormous lunch, a secretary works her way through a bag of cookies and polishes off a box of chocolates. A swimming champion who obsesses over every calorie becomes concerned that she hasn't had a period in two months. Disordered eating? Very likely. Eating disorder? Possibly.

Eating disorders and **disordered eating** are not the same. An eating disorder such as anorexia nervosa, bulimia nervosa, or binge eating is an illness that can seriously interfere with daily activities. Disordered eating is usually a temporary or mild change in eating patterns. Although it can occur after an illness or stressful event, it often is related to a dietary change intended to improve one's health or appearance. Unless disordered eating persists, it rarely requires professional intervention. Disordered eating, however, can become an eating disorder.

▶ **eating disorders** A spectrum of abnormal eating patterns that eventually can endanger a person's health or increase the risk for other diseases. Generally, psychological factors play a key role.

▶ **disordered eating** An abnormal change in eating pattern related to an illness, a stressful event, or a desire to improve one's health or appearance. If it persists, it can lead to an eating disorder.

Most of us take much pleasure in eating. For people with an eating disorder, however, food is a source of continual stress and anxiety (see **FIGURE SED.1**). Eating disorders include a spectrum of emotional illnesses ranging from self-imposed starvation to chronic binge eating. These illnesses stem from severe distortions of the eating process and produce physical consequences that often threaten life and require professional intervention.[1]

On particular occasions most of us have eaten to the point of discomfort. (Thanksgiving dinner comes to mind.) And many of us have cut out desserts at one time or another, hoping to fit into a special outfit or to lose weight for an athletic event or job interview. But stuffing yourself at a holiday meal or going on an occasional diet does not constitute an eating disorder. According to the *Manual of Clinical Dietetics*, a defining characteristic of an eating disorder is a persistent inability to eat in moderation.[2] The range of eating disorder categories has been expanded to include attitudes and behaviors that previously didn't meet the criteria for an "official" eating disorder, and modified so that the diagnoses more accurately describe and reflect the experiences of individuals who have eating issues.

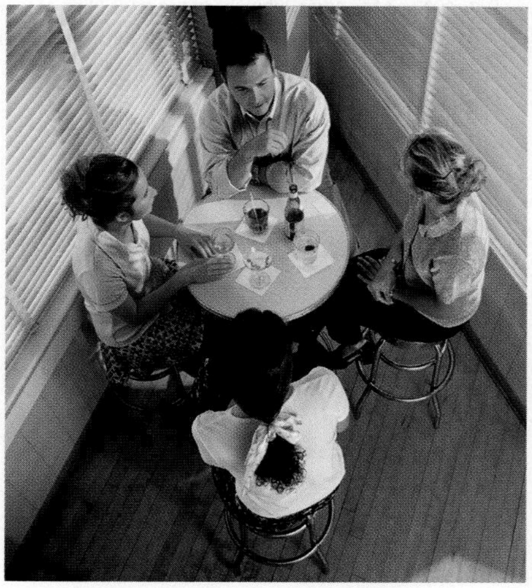

FIGURE SED.1 Can you identify the person with the eating disorder? Some people with eating disorders have normal body weights and are difficult to spot.

The Eating Disorder Continuum

The American Psychiatric Association's *Diagnostic and Statistical Manual of Mental Disorders* (DSM-5) assigns eating disorders to categories that form a continuum, with self-starvation at one end and compulsive overeating at the

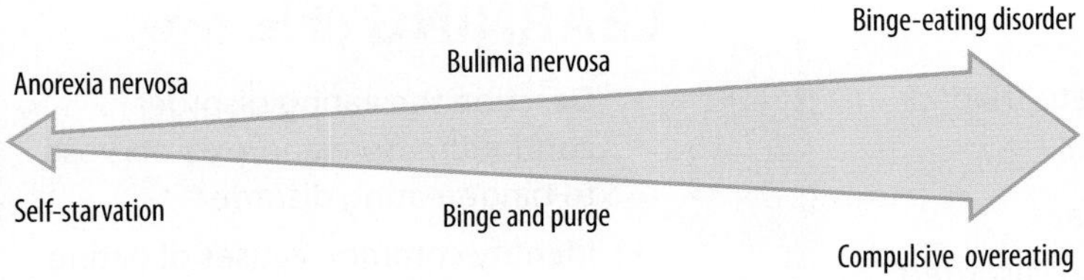

FIGURE SED.2 The eating disorder continuum.

other (see **FIGURE SED.2**). **Anorexia nervosa** occurs at the self-starvation end of the continuum. Anorexia is a self-imposed starvation syndrome that is triggered by a severely distorted **body image**.

What is perceived as beautiful can vary with cultural and individual preferences. Fashion designers, for example, view beauty as sinewy women who line the fashion catwalks and fill fashion magazines and appear in stark contrast to the majority of U.S. women, whose average dress size has grown to size 14. In contrast to the Western preference for bony beauty, some cultures do not view obesity negatively but instead prize large, corpulent bodies.

▶ **anorexia nervosa** [an-or-EX-ee-uh ner-VOH-sah] An eating disorder marked by prolonged decrease of appetite and refusal to eat, leading to self-starvation and excessive weight loss. It results in part from a distorted body image and intense fear of becoming fat, often linked to social pressures.

▶ **body image** A person's mental concept of his or her physical appearance, constructed from many different influences.

People with anorexia are at war with their bodies. Even when they are dangerously underweight, people with anorexia typically see themselves as fat. Severely restricting food intake is another symptom of anorexia nervosa. It can also involve purging (self-induced vomiting) and exercising excessively. Anorexia is most prevalent among adolescent females.

At the opposite end of the continuum is **binge-eating disorder**, formerly known as **compulsive overeating**. People with this disorder chronically consume massive quantities of food. Sufferers are typically obese; however, not all obese people binge eat. Diagnosis of binge-eating disorder is based on a person having an average of two binge-eating episodes per week for six months. These episodes often are triggered by frustration, anger, depression, and anxiety.[3]

▶ **binge-eating disorder** An eating disorder marked by repeated episodes of binge eating and a feeling of loss of control. The diagnosis is based on a person's having an average of at least two binge-eating episodes per week for six months.

▶ **compulsive overeating** See *binge-eating disorder.*

▶ **bulimia nervosa** [bull-EEM-ee-uh ner-VOH-sah] An eating disorder marked by consumption of large amounts of food at one time (binge eating) followed by a behavior such as self-induced vomiting, use of laxatives, excessive exercise, fasting, or other practices to avoid weight gain.

In the middle of the continuum is **bulimia nervosa**. Like those with binge-eating disorder, people with bulimia nervosa compulsively gorge themselves. Like those with anorexia, people with bulimia desperately want to be thin and resort to purging to reach this goal. After gorging, people with bulimia often become disgusted with themselves and terrified of getting fat. To compensate, people with bulimia make themselves vomit, use laxatives, exercise excessively, and take other action to avoid gaining weight.

Few people who suffer from eating disorders are purely anorexic, bulimic, or binge eaters. Many swing from one disordered eating pattern to another, alternately starving and gorging themselves. People may suffer from binge-eating disorder at one point in their lives, and anorexia or bulimia at another.[4] Studies also find that during adolescence people with disordered eating behaviors are at increased risk for dieting and disordered eating behaviors 10 years later.[5] **TABLE SED.1** shows some criteria used to diagnose eating disorders.

TABLE SED.1
Some Criteria for Eating Disorders

Anorexia Nervosa
• BMI of less than 17.5 kg/m^2 in adults • Intense fear of gaining weight • Disturbance in the way in which body size or weight is perceived • Purposive avoidance of food and a steadfast and implacable attitude in pursuing a low body weight and then maintaining it • Relentless pursuit of thinness
Bulimia Nervosa
• Recurrent episodes of binge eating • Recurrent purging behavior • Excessive exercise or fasting • Excessive concern about body weight or shape, and absence of anorexia nervosa • Self-evaluation unduly influenced by body shape and weight
Criteria for Binge Eating

• Recurrent episodes of binge eating associated with at least three behavioral and attitudinal characteristics, such as:
  • Eating large amounts when not physically hungry
  • Feeling disgusted or guilty after overeating
  • Eating much more rapidly than normal
• Occurs, on average, at least two days a week for six months
• The regular use of purging, fasting, and excessive exercise

Data from Schweiger U, Fichter M. Eating disorders: clinical presentation, classification and aetiological models. *Baillieres Clin Psychol.* 1997;3:199–216; Coulston A, Rock C, Monsen E. *Nutrition in the Prevention and Treatment of Disease.* New York: Academic Press; 2001.

Although eating disorders are not an exclusively modern malady, it's clear that eating disorders have become increasingly common in the past four decades. A British model named Twiggy, nicknamed for her sticklike appearance, ushered in the epidemic in the early 1960s. Fashion magazine stories reported that she subsisted on water, lettuce, and a single daily serving of steak and that she had learned to suppress her hunger pangs. Rather than condemn these clearly dangerous eating habits, the magazines held Twiggy up as a model of self-control for girls and young women (see **FIGURE SED.3**).

Our national denial regarding the dangers of semistarvation ended abruptly and dramatically in 1983 with the highly publicized death of 32-year-old pop singer Karen Carpenter from complications of anorexia. Widespread media coverage of her death highlighted the lethal potential of eating disorders and made the terms *anorexia* and *bulimia* household words.

Other stars of film, television, sports, and the fashion world—Princess Diana, Demi Lovato, Janet Jackson, Lady Gaga, Calista Flockhart, Ke$ha, Zina Garrison, Felicity Huffman, Lindsay Lohan, Mary-Kate Olsen, and Kate Beckinsale, to mention a few—have spoken about their eating disorders. Some have described the physical, emotional, and social damage these diseases caused in their own lives. But, ironically, increased visibility and knowledge have not stemmed the tide of eating disorders. The overall incidence rate for anorexia nervosa has remained stable over the past decade; however, there has been an increase in the high-risk group of 15- to 19-year-old girls.[6] The age of onset of anorexia nervosa and bulimia nervosa is decreasing.

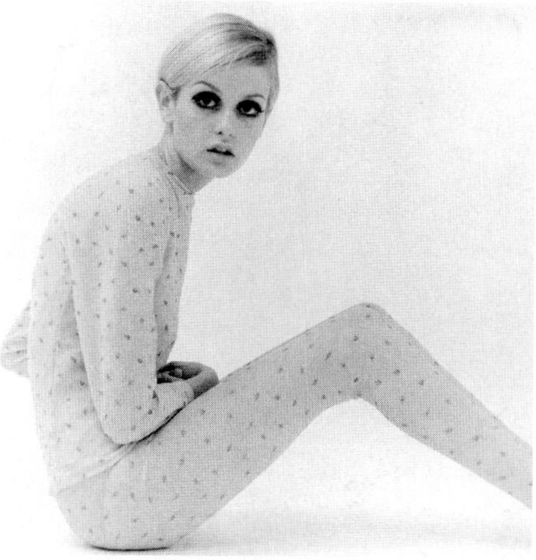

FIGURE SED.3 Eye of the beholder. In the 1960s, Twiggy became the new role model for young women who wanted to be thin and glamorous.

Key Concepts Eating disorders are unhealthy behavioral conditions known to exist from ancient times. Today, they have become alarmingly common in industrialized countries, particularly the United States. Eating disorders range from the self-starvation of anorexia nervosa to the compulsive overeating of binge-eating disorder.

No Simple Causes

Certain people appear to have a predisposition to eating disorders that might be rooted in psychological, biological, or cultural causes. A person who suffers from depression or **obsessive-compulsive disorder**, for example, can have an increased risk of developing an eating disorder. The vulnerability also may be biological. Indeed, some evidence suggests that genetic factors create an increased risk for eating disorders. Another important factor in the development of eating disorders is society's emphasis on extreme thinness. It is clear that eating disorders are complex problems, with multiple causes. Social, psychological, and biological factors all play roles.

▶ **obsessive-compulsive disorder** A disorder in which a person attempts to relieve anxiety by ritualistic behavior and continuous repetition of certain acts.

THINK About It 1

Eating disorders can develop when people, especially women, feel social pressure to achieve an unrealistic standard of thinness. Modern Western culture would have women weigh less than what is considered healthy. This means that most women cannot attain what society considers the "ideal" female form without significant food deprivation. These pressures affect even very young girls, starting with their first Barbie doll and her attenuated, unnatural shape (see **FIGURE SED.4**), if not before.[7] Studies also suggest that television programing provides a media outlet that negatively affects body image of young girls.[8]

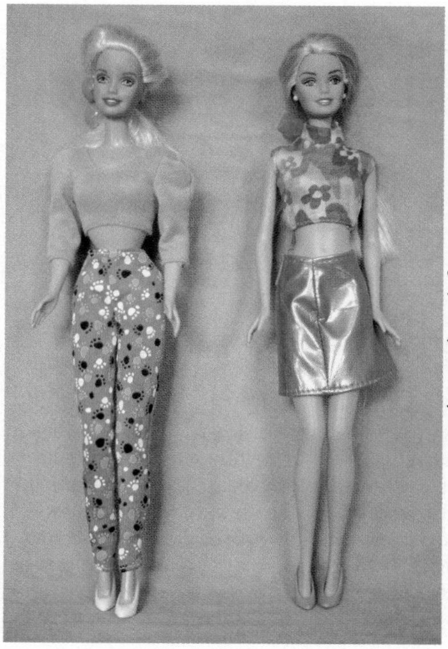

FIGURE SED.4 Thin is in. In 1998, Mattel overhauled Barbie's look for the millennium, giving her slimmer hips, a wider waist, and smaller breasts. Barbie's periodic overhauls are meant to fit the fashion of the times. Does this updated Barbie (right) represent a realistic role model for today's young girls?

How individuals feel about themselves can also be a strong predictor of disordered eating patterns. Body dissatisfaction, which is linked to the development of eating disorders, is a common problem among adolescent girls, and self-esteem is a relevant variable for helping to identify middle-adolescent girls who may be at risk for subsequent increases in body dissatisfaction.[9] Psychological factors are important as well. These encompass everything from peer relationships to relationships with parents. Studies have shown that adolescent girls who were teased about their weight by peers had a more negative image of their bodies and lower self-esteem, regardless of their actual weight.[10,11] In addition, children who were subjected to weight-based teasing did not perform as well in school as those who had not suffered such teasing.[12] Findings were similar for adolescent boys and for teens of varied racial and ethnic backgrounds. Studies also have linked more severe forms of emotional trauma to disordered eating. For example, trauma exposure and distress have been linked to eating for psychological reasons, and ultimately to binge eating.[13] One study found that more than 50 percent of bulimic and anorexic patients suffered from **post-traumatic stress disorder (PTSD)**.[14] PTSD occurs in people who have endured a significant trauma, such as child abuse or rape. Eating disorders also can be associated with dysfunctional family

▶ **post-traumatic stress disorder (PTSD)** An anxiety disorder characterized by an emotional response to a traumatic event or situation involving severe external stress.

relationships. Some psychologists believe that people with anorexia and bulimia are trying to fulfill unrealistic parental expectations of perfection, in part by succumbing to societal pressure to be very thin. Another strong predictor of dieting behavior is a woman's recollection of how much physical appearance was valued by her family members.[15] In addition, cross-sectional research suggests that friends are an important influence, especially among females. In this study, friends' dieting was positively associated with chronic dieting, unhealthy weight control behaviors, extreme weight control behaviors, and binge eating five years later among females, and with extreme weight control behaviors five years later among males.[16]

Overall, factors that increase the risk for the onset of eating disorders in adolescents are genetics, body changes during puberty, the vulnerability of adolescents to the ideals of thinness, social pressures to be thin, body image dissatisfaction, restrictive diet, depression, and low self-esteem.[17]

Scientists have made major advances in understanding the biological foundation of eating disorders, and studies have linked abnormal levels of neurotransmitters, especially serotonin, in people to their eating disorders.[18] Researchers, for example, have shown that bulimia patients experience spontaneous improvement in eating habits when taking antidepressant medication that increases brain levels of serotonin.[19] Many antiobesity drugs also affect serotonin levels.[20]

Neurotransmitters are just one focus of research into the biology of eating disorders. Another line of investigation focuses on genes. Recently, researchers have confirmed that eating disorders run in families. For some women, social characteristics within the family, such as having highly educated parents and grandparents, as well as achieving higher grades in school, have been found to increase the risk for developing an eating disorder.[21] In addition, eating disorders occur most frequently in families with a history of obsessive-compulsive disorders, anxiety disorders, and depression.[22] Both depression and obsessive-compulsive behavior have been linked to atypical levels of serotonin and norepinephrine in the brain.[23]

It's likely that a number of genes are involved in the development of eating disorders. Two genes in particular, *leptin* and *orexin*, have gained a lot of attention for their possible contribution to body weight. The leptin gene regulates the body's production of leptin, a hormone that causes rapid weight loss in genetically obese mice. (Unfortunately, leptin has not stimulated the same reaction in humans.) The **orexin** gene regulates production of two appetite-stimulating hormones: orexin A and orexin B (after the Greek word *orexis*, meaning "appetite"). Rodents injected with either leptin or orexin have been shown to increase their food consumption 8- to 10-fold.[24]

▶ **orexin** A class of hormones in the brain that may affect human food consumption.

The discoveries of leptin and orexin genes significantly advance our understanding of brain chemistry and eating disorders and may eventually lead to new classes of more effective drugs. Drugs that mimic orexins, for example, might help patients with anorexia or other wasting syndromes by increasing their appetites. Conversely, drugs that block orexins might help patients struggling with obesity and binge eating. Or a leptin-like drug may eventually be used to stimulate weight loss. At the very least, discovery of these genes supports the idea that biological factors probably contribute to the development of eating disorders in vulnerable people.

Quick Bite

Magazine Manipulations

When researchers studied fifth- through twelfth-grade girls in a working-class suburb in the northeastern United States, nearly 50 percent reported that they wanted to lose weight because of pictures in magazines. Frequent readers of fashion magazines were two to three times more likely to be influenced to diet or exercise to lose weight. Seventy percent of the girls reported that magazine pictures influenced their conception of the perfect body.

Quick Bite

A Skinny Trend

In 1970, the average *Playboy* Playmate weighed 11 percent below the national average. Only 8 years later, in 1978, the average weight of *Playboy* Playmates was 17 percent below average. Today, the average model is 22 to 23 percent leaner than the average American woman.

Key Concepts The precise causes of eating disorders remain obscure. Researchers have debated whether eating disorders are primarily psychological or genetic in origin. The current view is that eating disorders are a result of the complex interaction of social, biological, and psychological factors. In other words, eating disorders occur in biologically susceptible individuals exposed to particular types of environmental stimuli.

Anorexia Nervosa

Although they learned about the condition in medical school, until the 1960s few doctors saw a case of anorexia nervosa. By the mid-1970s, however, physicians were reporting many cases of anorexia, particularly among young women. Today this serious disorder occurs in about 1 in 200 women, usually starting in adolescence. More than 90 percent of cases occur in women, and the death rate from anorexia nervosa is about 10 times the death rate of women without anorexia.[25]

The term *anorexia nervosa*, which translates to "nervous loss of appetite," is misleading. People diagnosed with anorexia don't lose their appetite except in the final stages of the disorder. Instead, they are obsessed with food. But their obsession with thinness is even greater. The German term for the disorder, *pubertätsmagersucht*, or "mania for leanness," more accurately reflects the nature of the disease. The hallmark of anorexia nervosa is dramatic loss of weight, usually to less than 85 percent of the expected weight for height or a body mass index (BMI) of less than or equal to 17.5 kg/m^2 (see **FIGURE SED.5**).

Anorexia is more prevalent in industrialized societies that have an abundance of food and an attitude that equates beauty, particularly feminine beauty, with thinness. Nine of 10 anorexia sufferers are female—probably because Western society emphasizes thinness more for women than for men.[26] Studies show that the peak age of onset is between 15 and 19 years old,[27] and the typical anorexia sufferer has been an upper-class Caucasian female adolescent. Unfortunately, during the past decade, anorexia has become more of an equal-opportunity disorder. Physicians have reported cases of the disorder in young women from all social and ethnic backgrounds; it is especially prevalent in women who participate in activities that emphasize leanness, including modeling, ballet, and gymnastics. In addition, anorexia has increased significantly among African-American women.[28]

Causes of Anorexia Nervosa

On the surface, anorexia nervosa usually seems to result from a weight-loss program gone awry. A high school freshman may go on a diet after her boyfriend or gymnastics coach tells her she is too heavy. An eighth-grader may

Quick Bite

Fashion Designers and Weight Guidelines for Models

The fashion industry sells women an ideal of beauty embodied in the models who walk the runways and appear in fashion magazines. Spurred by the deaths of several South American models—one reportedly trying to live on lettuce and Diet Coke—fashion designers in Spain and Italy issued regulations to raise weight limits for fashion models. They require a BMI of at least 18, which means that models must weigh at least 56 kilograms (123 pounds) if their height is greater than or equal to 1.75 meters (5 feet, 9 inches). These figures are in sync with World Health Organization (WHO) standards of the minimum healthy weight. Designers excluded super-skinny models who did not meet the minimum requirements from performing in a Madrid fashion show.

The U.S. fashion industry has not followed suit. It has no plans to require models to achieve an objective measure of health, such as a height-to-weight ratio, despite a poll on *Elle* magazine's website in which two-thirds of respondents indicated they wished that American designers would follow the examples of fashion show organizers in Milan and Madrid in banning overly skinny models. However, at a meeting of the Council of Fashion Designers of America, the industry introduced guidelines for designers aimed at promoting healthier behavior among its models and at educating designers on how to recognize eating disorders.

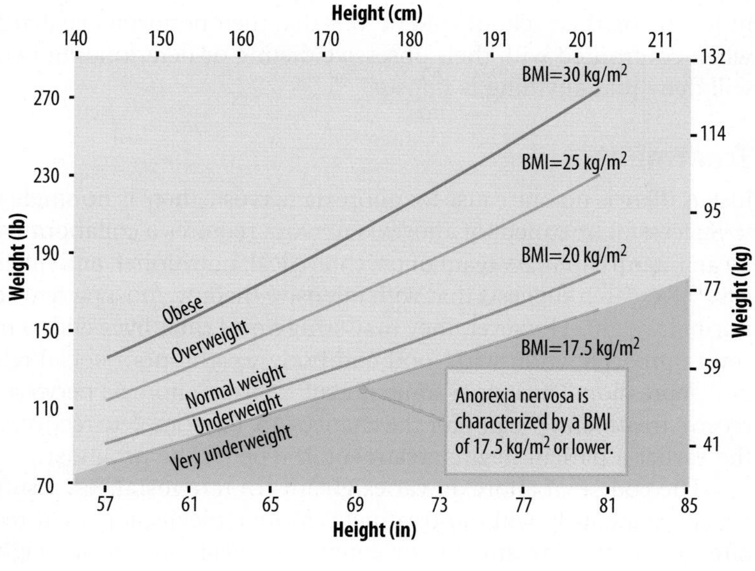

FIGURE SED.5 BMI and underweight. When managing eating disorders, BMI can help guide decisions about nutrition, medications, and psychotherapy.

Data from *Diagnostic and Statistical Manual of Mental Disorders*, 5th ed., text rev. Copyright © 2013. American Psychiatric Association.

TABLE SED.2
Warning Signs of Anorexia

Anorexia nervosa is a disorder in which preoccupation with dieting and thinness leads to excessive weight loss. The person with anorexia may not acknowledge that weight loss and restricted eating are problems. Family and friends can help by recognizing that the following are warning signs:

- Loss of a significant amount of weight
- Continuing to diet (although thin)
- Pretending to eat or lying about eating
- Feeling fat, even after losing weight
- Fear of weight gain
- Cessation of monthly menstrual periods
- Preoccupation with food, calories, nutrition, and/or cooking
- Strange or secretive food rituals
- Harshly critical of appearance
- Exercising compulsively
- Bingeing and purging

want to lose weight to be more popular at a new school. The diet may start out just fine, but it never stops.

Psychologists report that anorexia sufferers tend to be rigid, perfectionistic, all-or-nothing thinkers. Sufferers tend to lack a sense of independence and control. Parents can enable this syndrome by being overly protective or rigid or by holding a child to excessively high standards of achievement,[29] and the child may feel a significantly lower emotional connectedness, contributing to onset of an eating disorder.[30] Additional risk factors commonly associated with onset of anorexia include extremely high levels of exercise, distorted body image, obsessive-compulsive disorders, and negative self-esteem.[31]

Warning Signs

Parents and friends of people with anorexia often miss early signs of the disease. Avoidance of particular foods, unconventional food choices, or a rigorous exercise routine can easily be mistaken as determination to lose a few pounds, rather than the underlying issue, an obsession with food and dieting. Many eating disorders start with a simple diet. Stress and a lack of appropriate coping mechanisms, dysfunctional family relationships, and drug abuse can cause dieting to get out of control.[32]

Initially, someone with anorexia has a feeling of power. Sufferers enjoy a feeling of control as they learn to deny their hunger and limit their food intake. Early warning signs include obsessively counting calories; developing lists of "safe" foods and foods to avoid; cutting foods, even peas, into small pieces; and spending a great deal of time rearranging food on a plate. To suppress hunger, a person with anorexia may drink up to 30 cups of water or diet soda a day. Anorexia sufferers also may channel their obsessions with food into the preparation of elaborate meals for others without eating any of the food themselves.[33] **TABLE SED.2** shows the warning signs of anorexia.

THINK About It 2

As the disease progresses, anorexia sufferers become increasingly disillusioned, withdrawn, and hostile. Success always seems beyond their grasp. No matter how thin they are, they see themselves as overweight (see **FIGURE SED.6**). When they eat more than they think they should, they may induce vomiting or use **emetics**, **enemas**, **diuretics**, or **laxatives**. Or they might exercise relentlessly. Eventually, their efforts to avoid obesity take over their lives. They start to avoid social situations that could expose their behaviors and so withdraw more and more from friends and family. Groggy and irritable from food deprivation and sleep disturbances, people with advanced anorexia spend so little time on their schoolwork or jobs that their performance deteriorates. Yet when confronted with their obsessive dieting or deteriorating behavior, they will deny that anything is unusual.[34]

▶ **emetics** Agents that induce vomiting.

▶ **enemas** Infusions of fluid into the rectum, usually for cleansing or other therapeutic purposes.

▶ **diuretics** [dye-u-RET-iks] Drugs or other substances that promote the formation and release of urine. Diuretics are given to reduce body fluid volume in treating such disorders as high blood pressure, congestive heart disease, and edema. Both alcohol and caffeine act as diuretics.

▶ **laxatives** Substances that promote evacuation of the bowel by increasing the bulk of the feces, lubricating the intestinal wall, or softening the stool.

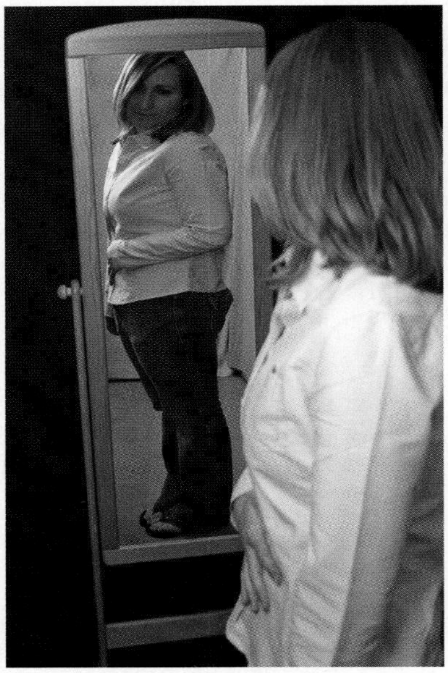

FIGURE SED.6 Distorted body image.

Treatment

Just as there is no one cause for anorexia nervosa, there is no single way to cure it. Successful treatment of anorexia nervosa requires a collaborative approach by an interdisciplinary team of psychological, nutritional, and medical specialists.[35] Research suggests that with intensive therapy, most patients can achieve normal weight. However, they may struggle all their lives with a moderate to severe preoccupation with food and body weight, poor social relationships, and depression. The longer someone suffers from anorexia nervosa before they receive treatment, the poorer the chances are for complete recovery; therefore, the earlier a patient begins treatment, the better the prognosis.

The course of anorexia varies greatly. In rare instances, a sufferer recovers spontaneously without treatment. More typically, a patient recovers only after a variety of treatments or enters a cyclical pattern of weight gain and relapse. Thirty to 50 percent of anorexia patients also have symptoms of bulimia, which can complicate diagnosis and treatment.[36] Tragically, in 6 to 18 percent of cases, the disease proves fatal (see **FIGURE SED.7**). Patients who have other emotional disorders, such as major depression or substance abuse, are the most likely to die from complications of the disease. Potentially fatal consequences of anorexia include heart attack, organ failure, starvation, and suicide.[37,38]

As with many other behavioral disorders, people with anorexia usually deny the danger of their situation, so family and friends must intervene to get sufferers to treatment—often by getting together and supportively confronting the person with evidence that something is seriously wrong. This common technique helps people accept the need for at least an initial medical screening. The complex and multifaceted nature of anorexia requires a team of experienced health care professionals, including physicians, clinical dietitians, and psychotherapists, so both the physical and psychological aspects of the disorder can be addressed. One of the best places to find an experienced team of therapists is at an eating disorder clinic associated with a major medical facility.[39] The first goal of treatment is to stabilize the patient's physical condition. The second is to convert the patient, who is typically reluctant, into a willing participant in the treatment plan. A combination of hospitalization, psychotherapy, and pharmacotherapy is often necessary.

Restoring the patient's nutritional status is of prime importance. Otherwise, dehydration, starvation, and electrolyte imbalances can lead to serious health problems and even death (see **TABLE SED.3**). If a patient has lost more than

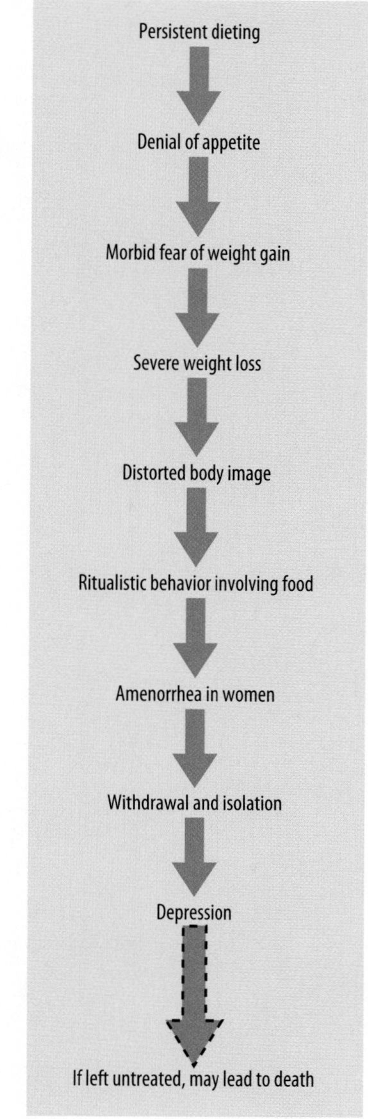

FIGURE SED.7 The progression of anorexia.

TABLE SED.3
Side Effects of Excessive Weight Loss in Anorexia Nervosa

Emaciation	• Loss of fat stores and muscle mass • Reduced thyroid metabolism • Cold intolerance • Difficulty maintaining core body temperature
Hematological	• Leukopenia (abnormal decrease of white blood cells) • Iron-deficiency anemia
Other	• Growth of lanugo (fine, babylike hairs) over the trunk • Osteopenia (mineral depletion in bone) • Premature osteoporosis
Neuropsychiatric	• Abnormal taste sensation • Depression • Impaired thought processes
Cardiac	• Loss of cardiac muscle, resulting in a smaller heart • Abnormal heart rhythm • Increased risk of sudden death
Gastrointestinal	• Delayed gastric emptying • Bloating • Constipation • Abdominal pain

30 percent of body weight over a three-month period or weighs 70 percent or less of the standard weight considered healthy for height, hospitalization is essential. Restoration of body weight and return of menses are primary therapeutic goals for treatment.[40] Once the patient's physical condition has stabilized and some physical symptoms of starvation have disappeared, psychotherapy can begin in earnest. Many therapists use a cognitive behavioral approach to help the patient challenge irrational beliefs and establish healthy attitudes and behaviors for gaining and maintaining weight.

The early phases of weight gain are fraught with challenges for both patient and clinician. Patients must gain a certain amount of weight to prevent death or permanent damage while the psychotherapeutic portion of their treatment is still in the very early phases. At first, the patient is encouraged to simply eat enough food to minimize or stop weight loss. Next, the patient is started on a very slow process of weight gain, all the while receiving intensive psychotherapy. The first sign of weight gain can precipitate a crisis. Phobia of obesity can return with renewed vengeance. Many patients refuse to eat. Others resist treatment in covert ways. If not restricted to bed and closely supervised, they may try to burn off calories through relentless exercise or by purging. To avoid detection, they adopt a series of behaviors to conceal their lack of weight gain. These include wearing concealing clothes or "bulking up" before weigh-ins by filling their pockets with coins or drinking large amounts of water or diet soda.[41]

Psychologists use a variety of psychotherapeutic techniques to help the patient deal with underlying emotional issues such as depression. Treatment programs generally use a combination of behavioral therapy, individual psychotherapy, patient education, family education, and family therapy. Frequently, therapists find family conflicts at the heart of the eating disorder. Ongoing therapy for the patient and family is key to successful recovery. As the patient's symptoms resolve, she or he must find new ways to relate to and communicate with family members. Family members must remain open and willing to change their behavior toward the person with the eating disorder.

Dietitians work closely with the psychotherapist to help patients develop a realistic view of food and to reshape their food selection and eating behaviors. Although no pharmaceutical agent has been developed specifically to treat anorexia, some antidepressants have proved useful.

Most patients with anorexia nervosa require continued intervention after discharge from the hospital or treatment program. Support groups for people with eating disorders and their families can be an important link in the recovery process. Support groups also can be a useful technique for easing a resistant patient into treatment. With expert help and ongoing therapy, patients with anorexia can develop new mechanisms for coping with life's stresses, eventually replacing their disordered relationship with food with new, healthier interpersonal relationships.

Key Concepts The hallmark symptoms of anorexia nervosa are a mania for thinness and self-imposed starvation. Sufferers manifest a body weight as much as 30 percent below normal, a severely distorted body image, withdrawal from family and friends, and various physical and psychological changes related to starvation.

Bulimia Nervosa

The behavior we now call bulimia was practiced as long ago as Greek and Roman times. Gerald Russell, a British psychiatrist, first coined the term *bulimia nervosa* in 1979 to describe a syndrome of bingeing and purging in young Caucasian women. The average patient with bulimia is an unmarried

Caucasian woman in her twenties or thirties with a normal or near-normal body weight (see **FIGURE SED.8**). People with bulimia are more likely to be sexually active than are those with anorexia and often are involved in destructive relationships. Almost anyone can be affected, however.

The relationships among dieting, bingeing severity, and alcohol use have been studied in samples of college-age women. Researchers have found a relationship among binge drinking, dieting, and maladaptive coping patterns, such as using substances and/or denial as coping mechanisms.[42] It also has been shown that girls who engage in binge eating, alcohol use, or both have higher levels of negative urgency, or the tendency to act rashly when distressed.[43]

People with bulimia nervosa tend to feel very disorganized. They report suffering from depression and low self-esteem. Many were sexually abused as children. Food was often a source of comfort, and eating gradually evolved into a tool for dealing with every unpleasant event, from boredom to major life crises.

It is estimated that between 1 and 3 percent of American adolescent and young adult females have bulimia. But bulimia, particularly in its milder forms, often goes undetected. This is because people with bulimia are very secretive about their behaviors, typically limiting their binge-and-purge episodes to the middle of the night or times when they are assured of privacy. Also, unlike patients with anorexia or binge-eating disorder, whose body weights can hint at their underlying psychiatric disorder, the body weight of a patient with bulimia is usually average or only slightly above average. Several studies have found that as many as 40 percent of college-age women occasionally binge and purge—often enough to raise concern but too infrequently for an official diagnosis of bulimia.[44]

The college environment itself could be conducive to overconsumption as a result of factors such as readily available energy-dense foods and academic pressures leading to sedentary activities, such as reading, studying, and sitting at a computer, while at the same time devaluing exercise and organized sports participation.[45] For example, a survey of college students found their priorities, in order of most to least important, to be going to class, studying, hanging out with friends, sleeping, exercising, dating or meeting partners, eating healthy foods, work, having an ideal body, surfing the Internet, and going to a great party.[46] Before entering college, healthful meals and regular exercise are generally part of a regular routine, but these positive health behaviors appear to decline in the transition from high school to college, an environment vulnerable to unhealthy eating patterns, which can start with occasional food binges.[47] **TABLE SED.4** lists the warning signs of bulimia.

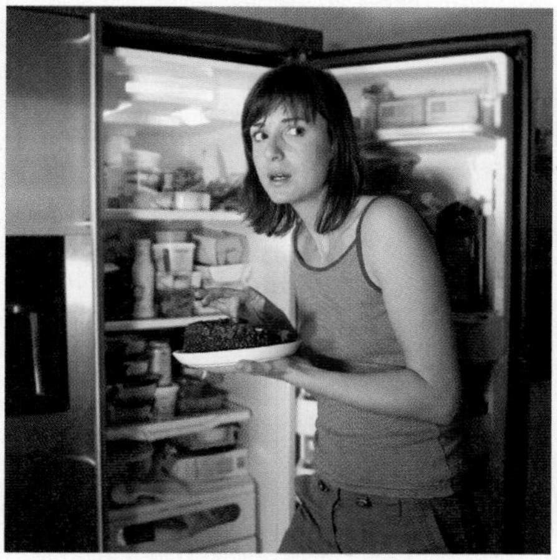

FIGURE SED.8 Bulimia nervosa. The typical person suffering from bulimia is an unmarried Caucasian woman in her twenties or thirties.

Quick Bite

I'm So Hungry I Could Eat an Ox!

The term *bulimia* is derived from the Greek words *bous*, meaning "ox," and *limos*, meaning "hunger."

Causes of Bulimia

Bulimia seems to occur most often in people who have an intense desire to nurture themselves with food but who are also strongly influenced by our societal obsession with thinness. One description of people with bulimia characterizes them as being obsessed with food but repulsed by fat. In contrast to people with anorexia, people with bulimia focus more on food than on thinness.

Psychologists who have treated patients with bulimia have found that they typically did not receive sufficient nurturing during their formative years. Whereas families of anorexic patients tend to have a lot of rigidly defined roles and rules, families of bulimic patients tend to lack structure. Roles may be loosely defined. Parents are often described as distant and judgmental. Significant family conflict usually exists. Patients often feel that their families failed to provide an adequate sense of security and protection.

TABLE SED.4
Warning Signs of Bulimia

Bulimia nervosa involves frequent episodes of binge eating, almost always followed by purging and intense feelings of guilt or shame. The sufferer feels out of control and recognizes that the behavior is not normal. The signs that a person may have bulimia include the following:

- Bingeing or eating uncontrollably
- Compensating for binges by strict dieting, fasting, vigorous exercise, vomiting, or abusing laxatives or diuretics in an attempt to lose weight
- Using the bathroom frequently after meals
- Preoccupation with body weight
- Depression or mood swings
- Irregular menstrual periods
- Dental problems, swollen cheeks or glands, heartburn, or bloating
- Personal or family problems with drugs or alcohol

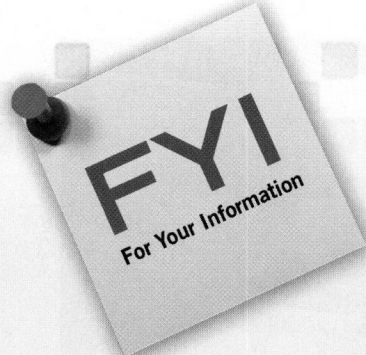

FYI For Your Information

Diary of an Eating Disorder

Every time I leave one of my sessions I feel better. We talk about stuff; I feel, express, and even cry. Today was the third time since I left her office to come home and throw up. I think things are getting better despite the fact that my mind focuses 80 percent of the time on food during the 55 minutes. But it's like the kitchen is a refuge for my mind. I always know it will be there, waiting to embrace me when I get home.

Alone is how I hope to find it. I have been thinking of what I will sink my teeth into first. Usually I go for the fat-free chocolate cake, then to the frozen yogurt (which makes it all come up much smoother). I don't think this is normal, though I am not really concerned. I feel like a million-pound weight has been swept away by the effortless flush of the toilet. The hardest thing is to look in the mirror after I have thrown up. Sometimes I wipe my face before I look. Other times I leave the spit, bile, and food on my mouth and hands. I just stand there holding my hands up, with my shoulders slumped over. I produce this expression of absolute helplessness—then I laugh. I guess I am amazed by the act I've just committed. I can't explain why, I can't believe that it is really me doing this. Why would I do something like throw up? I really have no reason to torture myself. Bulimia was always them—I can't possibly be like that. I throw up, but I am not a bulimic. I sure as hell don't have an eating disorder.

I am totally for this whole counseling thing because I feel sad a lot and I want to feel better. But I can't leave there and not feel that I have to get this crap out. All this stuff that we talk about.

Today, Dr. Tant asked me when this all began. My first thought was, "Oh this throwing up thing? I can't remember." But I do recall one time when my ex-boyfriend Matt and I had gone to a really nice dinner. My recollection of the evening was that it was perfect. I remember thinking about how this food was really fattening, though, and how it would make me fat if I kept it down. I didn't know or have the willpower to just not eat it. Over and over I tortured and berated myself about the effects this dinner would have on my body. I couldn't bear it. This dinner was no longer one meal; it was going to ruin my body and make me fat. I couldn't stand that food being inside me another moment. Looking back I can't imagine how I could have thrown up right there on the side of the road. It was like I had no couth. I told Matt to pull over, and I just stuck my hand down my throat. Rationalizing the act while engaging in it, I then jumped back in the truck to carry on with the night. We never discussed my vile act other than Matt saying, "I can't believe you just did that."

"I know," I responded, "but it just was making me feel so sick. I mean, my stomach was really nauseous [sic]." Basically I don't know when I began this war with myself, but I know it caused me to fear myself. The rest is a blur—its beginning, its incentive. I heard Dr. Tant's question. I just didn't have the answer.

—Chelsea Browning Smith

Reproduced from Smith CB. *Diary of an Eating Disorder.* Dallas, TX: Taylor Publishing; 1998. Reprinted by permission of Taylor Trade Publishing, an imprint of Rowman & Littlefield Publishing Group.

▶ **binges** Episodes of consuming a very large amount of food in a brief time (e.g., two hours) accompanied by a loss of control over how much and what is eaten.

▶ **purges** Episodes of emptying the gastrointestinal (GI) tract by self-induced vomiting and/or misuse of laxatives, diuretics, or enemas.

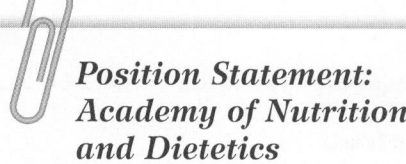

Position Statement: Academy of Nutrition and Dietetics

Nutrition Intervention in the Treatment of Eating Disorders

It is the position of the Academy of Nutrition and Dietetics that nutrition intervention, including nutritional counseling by a registered dietitian, is an essential component of the team treatment of patients with anorexia nervosa, bulimia nervosa, and other eating disorders during assessment and treatment across the continuum of care.

Reproduced from Position of the American Dietetic Association: nutrition intervention in the treatment of eating disorders. *J Am Diet Assoc.* 2011;111:1236–1241.

Obsessed by Thoughts of Food

A person with bulimia chronically **binges** and **purges**. To meet the official definition of the disorder, bingeing and purging occurs at least twice a week for at least three months. Purging may be accompanied or replaced by fasting, excessive exercise, or other behaviors that compensate for the binge episode. Between binges, people with bulimia typically restrict their dietary intake to a limited number of low-calorie foods they consider "safe." This dietary control is an illusion, however. The average bulimic sufferer is obsessed by thoughts of food and spends a great deal of time both planning the next binge and trying to resist the urge to binge.[48] **FIGURE SED.9** illustrates the binge-and-purge pattern of bulimia.

Just what triggers a binge is not clear. People with bulimia tend to be all-or-nothing thinkers. If they eat a single piece of food from their forbidden list, such as a cookie, they feel driven to consume the entire box. Some researchers believe that hunger caused by very restrictive dieting, combined with a buildup of everyday stresses, overwhelms the person's resolve and precipitates a binge.

During a binge, individuals with bulimia typically consume massive quantities of highly palatable, "forbidden" foods such as pastry, ice cream, and candy. This gorging takes place over a relatively short time span—say, an hour or two. Binges may contain up to 10,000 kilocalories. Afterward, feeling physically ill from overindulgence, sufferers use a variety of purging techniques, such as self-induced vomiting or excessive quantities of laxatives, to rid themselves of the food. Or they may follow a binge with a period of very strict fasting and heightened exercise.

Purging leads to a variety of physical symptoms. Over time, gastric acid in vomit burns the lining of the pharynx, esophagus, and mouth; erodes tooth enamel; and can even result in loss of teeth. Repeated vomiting also can enlarge the salivary glands and erode the lining of the stomach and esophagus.

Excessive self-induced vomiting and diarrhea can upset the body's delicate biochemical balance through loss of electrolytes and body water. Among other dangers, changes in electrolyte balance can trigger an irregular heartbeat and precipitate a life-threatening medical crisis.

Excessive use of emetics (drugs to induce vomiting) and laxatives carries its own risks. Repeated use of emetics is toxic to the liver and kidneys, and abuse of laxatives can damage the lining of the large intestine. **TABLE SED.5** describes the side effects of bulimic purging.

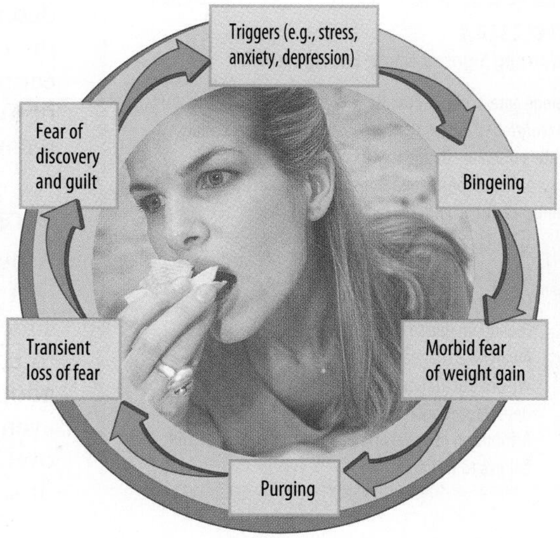

FIGURE SED.9 The binge-and-purge cycle of bulimia.

Treatment

Little research has been done on the long-term course of bulimia. It appears, however, that bulimia is easier to treat than anorexia, perhaps because bulimic patients tend to recognize that their behavior is abnormal. Following treatment, more than half of patients report an improvement in their binge-eating and coping behaviors. About 30 percent of patients eventually become symptom-free. The rest, however, struggle with the disorder to some degree throughout their lives. To reduce the risk of relapse, therapists encourage patients to stay involved in support groups after completing formal therapy.

Cognitive behavior therapy is key to helping patients reshape their attitudes about food and identify situations that trigger bingeing. The therapist's goal is to help patients let go of their need to categorize foods as safe or dangerous, good or bad. Patients must learn techniques for dealing with stress and uncomfortable or painful memories and feelings. Depression, which typically accompanies this disorder, must be treated as well. Many patients with bulimia also require treatment for substance abuse. A patient is hospitalized only when severely depressed or when purging is so frequent that physical damage has occurred or is imminent.

Medication can be an effective adjunct to psychotherapy. Serotonin-enhancing antidepressants have been used successfully to treat bulimia.

Key Concepts Key symptoms of bulimia nervosa are binge-eating episodes at least twice a week for three months, followed by behaviors that compensate for the binges, such as severe dieting, purging, or a combination of dieting and purging. The body weights of people with bulimia are typically close to or slightly above that considered healthy for their heights.

TABLE SED.5
Side Effects of Purging in Bulimia Nervosa

Side Effects of Purging in Bulimia Nervosa
Metabolic Effects
• Electrolyte abnormalities • Low blood magnesium
Gastrointestinal
• Inflammation of the salivary glands • Pancreatic inflammation and enlargement • Esophageal inflammation or ulcers • Gastric erosion • Dysfunctional bowel
Dental
• Erosion of dental enamel, particularly of front teeth, with corresponding decay
Neuropsychiatric
• Fatigue • Weakness • Impaired thought processes • Seizures (related to large fluid shifts and electrolyte disturbances) • Mild inflammation of peripheral nerves

Binge-Eating Disorder

Binge eating is the most common eating disorder in industrialized nations. It differs from bulimia in that the person with binge-eating disorder does not attempt to compensate for his or her binge by purging or other means. Overeating has been reported in the medical literature since scribes first put stylus to tablet. And over past generations, societies, including our own, have considered obesity a sign of good health, wealth, and even fertility. Binge eating is now recognized as an other specified feeding or eating disorder (OSFED).[49] OSFED comprises the largest category of eating disorders. This term is used to

TABLE SED.6
Warning Signs of Binge-Eating Disorder

Binge eaters, like bulimia sufferers, experience periods of uncontrolled eating that they usually keep secret. Binge eaters often are depressed and sometimes have other psychological problems. Signs that a person may have a binge-eating disorder include the following:

- Episodes of binge eating
- Eating when not physically hungry
- Frequent dieting
- Feeling unable to stop eating voluntarily
- Awareness that eating patterns are abnormal
- Weight fluctuations
- Depressed mood
- Attribution of social and professional successes and failures to weight

describe those conditions that meet the definition for eating disorders but not the criteria for anorexia or bulimia. Its precise causes are unclear, but binge eating seems to be related to an intense desire to nurture oneself with food or to reduce stress by eating.[50] In 1994, the American Psychiatric Association recognized binge-eating disorder as an emotional illness (see **TABLE SED.6**).[51]

Stress and Conflict Often Trigger Binge Eating

A person with binge-eating disorder consumes excessive quantities of food in a relatively short period of time at least twice a week. Unlike the bulimia sufferer, however, the person with binge-eating disorder does not attempt to compensate by purging or other means. In some instances, binge eaters adopt a grazing pattern. "Grazers" eat constantly for extended periods of time, eventually consuming an exceptionally large quantity of food. This pattern of overindulgence can be seen in people who restrict their food intake at work or school but seek solace in food at home.

Many binge eaters begin dieting in grade school and start bingeing during adolescence or in their early twenties. Typically, they try numerous weight-loss programs without long-term success. Research suggests that dieting during adolescence does not predict weight loss or even weight maintenance, but rather predicts weight gain and overweight status over time. In Project EAT (Eating Among Teens), a five-year longitudinal study of eating and weight in adolescents, adolescents who reported dieting were at nearly twice the risk for being overweight five years later.[52]

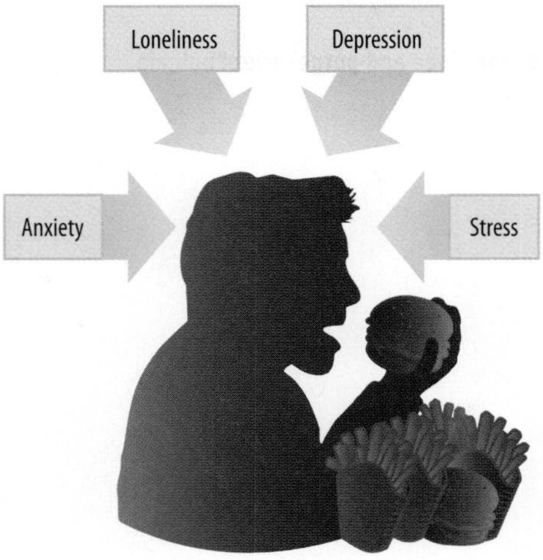

FIGURE SED.10 Emotions that can trigger binge eating. Feelings of loneliness, depression, anxiety, or stress can trigger a binge-eating episode.

Binge eaters exhibit many of the same characteristics as bulimic patients. More than 50 percent have clinical depression. Feelings of depression, loneliness, anxiety, or stress can precipitate a binge. Like other patients with eating disorders, those with binge-eating disorder are all-or-nothing thinkers. They tend to categorize foods as safe or dangerous. Eating even a small serving of a forbidden food can trigger a binge. Typical binge foods include sweets, pastries, ice cream, and high-fat snacks such as nuts and chips. However, if junk foods aren't handy, binge eaters might eat large quantities of starchy foods such as potatoes, bread, and pasta. **FIGURE SED.10** illustrates some factors that trigger binge eating.

THINK About It 3

Most binge eaters are people who have not learned to express or even acknowledge their feelings. During therapy sessions, many binge eaters report feeling helpless to influence the course of events or behaviors of others around them. Rather than acknowledge their feelings, they swallow them—aided by large quantities of food. They become addicted to the behavior itself because it is the only way they can get relief from stress (see **FIGURE SED.11**).

Binge eating often is a learned response to stress or conflict, passed down from one generation to the next. Parents may use food rather than affection and discussion to shape their children's behavior. Food is used for celebration and consolation, for reward and punishment. Children growing up in such environments learn to eat in response to emotions rather than hunger. As adults, they turn to food to satisfy all their emotional needs.

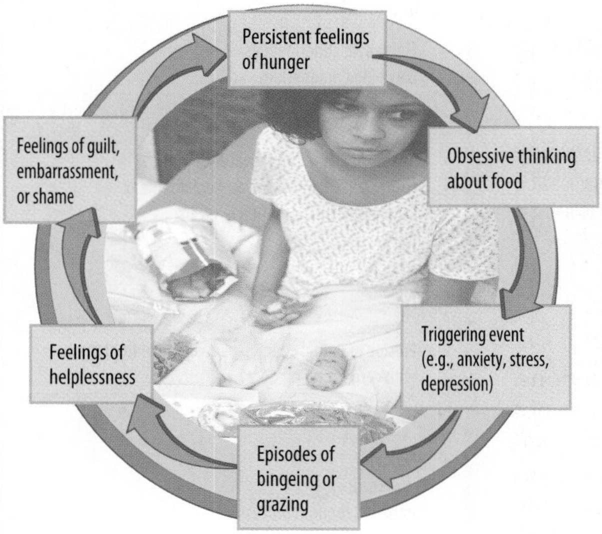

Photo © Jack Star/PhotoLink/Photodisc/Getty Images

FIGURE SED.11 The vicious cycle of binge eating. Binge-eating disorder is the most common eating disorder.

Treatment

Little is known about the course and prognosis of binge-eating disorder. However, people who become obese as a result of this disorder are at risk of developing weight-related health problems, including type 2 diabetes, hypertension, degenerative joint disease, heart disease, and even certain cancers.

People who have binge-eating disorder are rarely able to control the condition themselves. They usually require therapy to help them identify their long-buried emotions and learn techniques for giving voice to their feelings. Therapists experienced in treating this disorder discourage patients from trying to lose weight initially. Any attempts to restrict food intake can backfire by creating anxiety and provoking a binge. The major focus of therapy is to help patients identify their emotions and separate true biological hunger from emotional hunger. Once significant progress is made in these areas, the patient is better equipped psychologically to address weight issues.

Long-term support is key to keeping binge eaters from relapsing. Self-help groups such as Overeaters Anonymous are one source of support. These groups are organized according to the 12-step philosophy of Alcoholics Anonymous. In addition, many hospitals in large urban areas have support groups led by trained therapists.

Many patients with binge-eating disorder benefit from antidepressant medications. These drugs reduce the urge to binge, most likely by altering the brain's serotonin level. Various weight-management medications are now in development. These also can curb the urge to binge.

Key Concepts Binge-eating disorder is the most common eating disorder seen in people of all ages and backgrounds. Like people with bulimia, those with binge-eating disorder consume significantly more food than is typically eaten in a given period of time. Unlike people with bulimia, those with binge-eating disorder do not purge or fast. Not all binge eaters are obese, although many obese people binge.

Quick Bite

When Plumpness Was Valued

In centuries past, extra pounds displayed one's wealth and prosperity. The wealthy could afford abundant food and didn't perform physical labor.

Body Dysmorphic Disorder

People with **body dysmorphic disorder (BDD)** are preoccupied with an imagined or slight defect in appearance, worrying, for example, that their skin is scarred, they are balding, or their nose is too big. Such people may engage in long rituals of grooming, repeatedly combing hair, applying makeup, or picking at their skin. The condition's severity varies. Whereas some people can manage it, for others, the preoccupation causes significant distress and impairment: They may have few friends, avoid dating, miss school or work, and feel very self-conscious in social situations.

▶ **body dysmorphic disorder (BDD)** An eating disorder in which a distressing and impairing preoccupation with an imagined or slight defect in appearance is the primary symptom.

Many patients affected with BDD have coexisting conditions, such as obsessive-compulsive disorder (OCD), major depression, delusions, or social phobia. Approximately 2 to 7 percent of patients who undergo plastic surgery have BDD and are generally unhappy with the results.

BDD affects 1 to 2 percent of the general population; however, BDD frequently goes undiagnosed. Sufferers are ashamed of their problem and fail to report it to their physicians. Even though it is a serious and distressing condition, it is easily trivialized. In addition, even many health professionals are unaware that BDD is a psychiatric disorder that often responds to psychiatric treatment. Many people seek treatment from dermatologists, plastic surgeons, and other physicians, but these professionals often are ignorant of this disorder and thus are unhelpful.

Psychiatric treatment, including medication and cognitive-behavior therapy, can effectively decrease symptoms and suffering. The therapist helps the person with BDD resist compulsive BDD behaviors (e.g., mirror checking), face avoided situations (e.g., social situations), and develop a more realistic view of his or her appearance. Medications, including selective serotonin reuptake inhibitors (SSRIs), can relieve obsession and decrease distress and depression.[53]

Key Concepts Body dysmorphic disorder often coexists with other conditions such as obsessive-compulsive disorder, major depression, delusions, or social phobia. Patients with BDD magnify slight defects and are preoccupied with their appearance.

Night-Eating Syndrome

▶ **night-eating syndrome (NES)** An eating disorder in which a habitual pattern of interrupting sleep to eat is the primary symptom.

When a person grazes through the evening, finds herself plotting midnight refrigerator raids, and wakes at night to eat, she might have **night-eating syndrome (NES)**. A person with this disorder:

- Eats more than half of daily calories during and after the evening meal
- Wakes up at least once a night to eat, especially high-carbohydrate snacks
- Feels tense, anxious, worried, or guilty while eating
- Lacks appetite for breakfast and postpones it for hours
- Persists in this behavior for at least three months

Night-eating syndrome is a fairly uncommon eating disorder in the general population—perhaps only 1 to 2 percent of adults in the general population have this problem—but it affects up to a quarter of obese people. Although underlying causes are not fully understood, the disorder can result from a combination of biologic, genetic, and emotional factors. Researchers have noted several hormonal imbalances among NES sufferers, such as low levels of both melatonin (a sleep-inducing hormone) and leptin (an appetite-suppressing hormone). Cortisol—the so-called stress hormone that kicks in when we feel tense—appears higher at night in night eaters, perhaps arousing them to wake up and head for the kitchen. Stress, depression, and anxiety commonly affect mood among those with the condition.

Night-eating syndrome involves a disturbed food-intake circadian rhythm, which may be out of sync by as much as four to five hours with a person's normal sleep rhythm. It is possibly the first clinical disorder to manifest differing circadian rhythms of two biological systems.

The heavy preference for carbohydrates, which triggers the brain to produce "feel-good" neurochemicals, suggests that night eating may be an attempt to self-medicate mood problems. A dietitian can help develop meal plans that distribute intake more evenly throughout the day so a person is not as vulnerable to caloric loading in the evening. Stress-reduction programs, including psychological therapy, can be helpful.

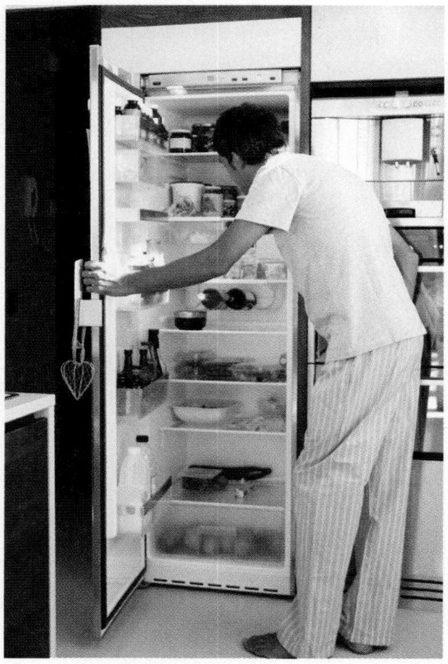
© Yuri Arcurs/ShutterStock, Inc.

Key Concepts Night-eating syndrome, though uncommon, affects up to a quarter of obese people. People with NES interrupt normal sleep to eat and often feel stressed, anxious, and depressed. They typically have hormonal imbalances. Psychotherapy and stress reduction therapy can be helpful.

Males: An Overlooked Population

As many as a million boys and men in the United States struggle with eating disorders.[54] Yet males with eating disorders have been "ignored, neglected or dismissed because of statistical infrequency of the disease, combined with the pervasive myth that eating disorders are a female disease," according to Arnold E. Andersen, former director of the Eating and Weight Disorders Clinic at Johns Hopkins University and scientific editor of the book *Males with Eating Disorders*.[55]

Women who develop eating disorders may feel fat, but they typically are near average weight. In contrast, most men who develop these diseases are overweight. Many were seriously teased about their weight as children. Whereas women are concerned primarily with weight, men are concerned with shape and muscle definition. Indeed, men often develop disordered eating habits while trying to improve their athletic performance. More men than women diet to prevent medical consequences associated with being overweight.

THINK About It 4

Why do fewer males than females develop full-blown eating disorders? Some researchers suggest that there is a "dose-response" relationship between the amount of sociocultural pressure to be thin and the probability of developing an eating disorder. Note that articles and advertisements that promote dieting usually target young women rather than young men. When men are exposed to activities that require leanness, such as wrestling, swimming, running, and horse racing, they exhibit a substantial increase in anorexic behavior. In fact, perceived pressure from social agents such as advertising, verbal messages, and social situations related to eating and dieting are strong predictors of eating disorders,[56] indicating that cultural conditions, rather than gender, are the contributing factor for developing an eating disorder.

Furthermore, the degree of thinness held up as desirable for women is 15 percent below a healthy body weight, whereas the degree of thinness held up as desirable for men is well within the healthy limits of normal weight. Thus, women are more likely than men to alter their eating habits to achieve the desired appearance.

TABLE SED.7
Signs of an Undisclosed Eating Disorder

People with eating disorders usually exhibit several of the following signs.

Physical

- Arrested growth
- Marked change or frequent fluctuations in weight
- Inability to gain weight
- Fatigue
- Constipation or diarrhea
- Susceptibility to fractures
- Delayed menarche
- Calcium or phosphorus imbalances, abnormal blood pH, or high serum amylase levels

Behavioral

- Change in eating habits
- Difficulty in social settings
- Reluctance to be weighed
- Depression
- Social withdrawal
- Repeated absence from school or work
- Deceptive or secretive behavior
- Stealing (e.g., to obtain food)
- Substance abuse
- Excessive exercise

Reproduced from Becker AE, Grinspoon SK, Klibanski A, Herzog DB. Eating disorders. *N Engl J Med.* 1999;340(14):1092–1098.

An Unrecognized Disorder

Like women, most men develop eating disorders during adolescence. But males can develop eating disorders during preadolescence and young adulthood as well. The diagnostic criteria for anorexia and bulimia in men and women are similar, but doctors are so conditioned to viewing eating disorders as a female phenomenon that they often miss eating disorders in males. Likewise, the patient, his family, and friends may not recognize disordered eating patterns (see **TABLE SED.7**). Because our culture accepts overeating among men more readily than in women, binge eating in particular can go unrecognized in men. In addition, anorexia can elude diagnosis in men more often than in women because malnourished men don't experience definitive symptoms, such as a woman's loss of menstrual periods, that can alert professionals and others to the problem.

Key Concepts Men also suffer from eating disorders, although at rates much lower than those of women. Like women, men typically develop eating disorders during adolescence and young adulthood, but they are more often overweight and striving for a particular body shape and muscularity. Although the diagnostic criteria are the same, with the exception of amenorrhea, eating disorders in men are often undiagnosed as a result of societal conditioning that views eating disorders as "female" diseases.

Anorexia Athletica

Regardless of social or ethnic background, participation in competitive athletics seems to be a common link in the development of eating disorders among males and females. Sports-related eating disorders are known as **anorexia athletica**.[57] Among those who participate in sports, and particularly team sports, there is a correlation between eating disorders and the excessive physical activity demanded during sports training.[58] Participation in lean sports (i.e., those that emphasize leanness or body image), such as distance running, swimming, gymnastics, dance, and diving, increases the risk for developing an eating disorder.[59] Athletes who have anorexia athletica want to achieve

▶ **anorexia athletica** Eating disorder associated with competitive participation in athletic activity.

- **female athlete triad** A syndrome in young female athletes that involves disordered eating, amenorrhea, and lowered bone density.
- **amenorrhea** [A-men-or-EE-a] Absence or abnormal stoppage of menses in a female; commonly indicated by the absence of three to six consecutive menstrual cycles.

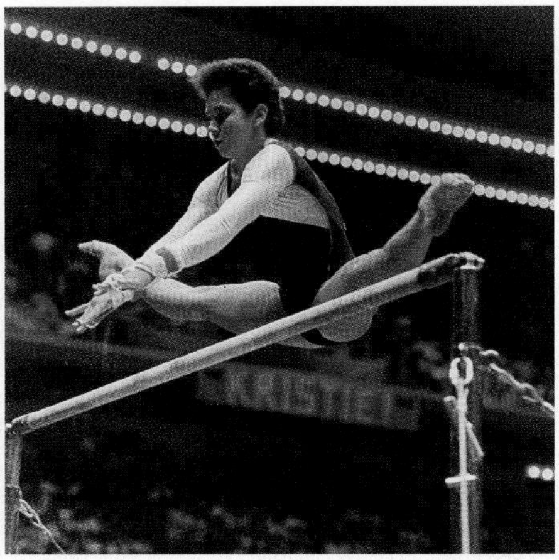
© AP Photos

FIGURE SED.12 Christy Henrich. Christy, a top Olympic gymnast, weighed less than 60 pounds when she died in 1994 at age 22 of multiple organ failure, a complication resulting from anorexia and bulimia.

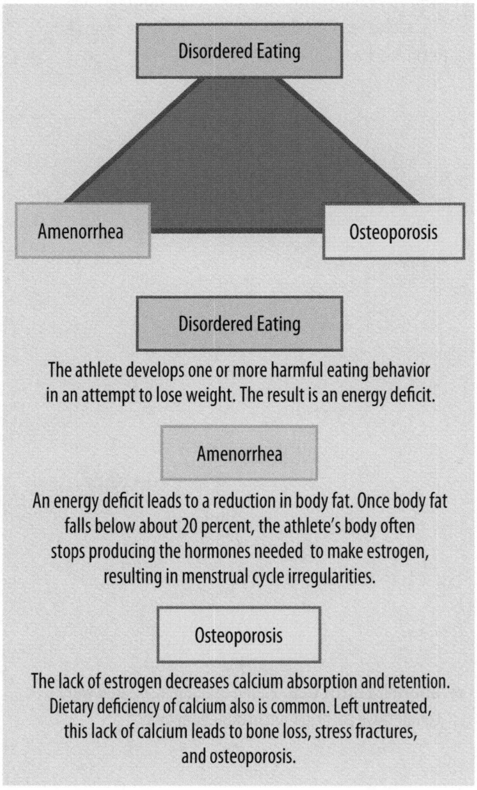

FIGURE SED.13 Female athlete triad. Disordered eating that results in excessive weight loss can lead to amenorrhea, which, in turn, can lead to osteoporosis.

an unrealistic body size that they consider desirable for competition. In many cases, athletes with mild eating disorders are able to disguise their disease as attention to fitness. People who are addicted to their exercise routine are at greater risk of developing eating disorders.[60]

The Female Athlete Triad

Although the majority of female athletes benefit from increased physical activity, there are those who go too far and risk developing a trio of medical problems (see **FIGURE SED.12**). Female athletes who fall prey to the "thin-at-any-cost" philosophy are at risk of developing a condition known as the **female athlete triad** (see **FIGURE SED.13**). This syndrome is characterized by problems with the interrelationship among energy availability, menstrual function, and bone mineral density, which can have clinical consequences including eating disorders, **amenorrhea**, and premature osteoporosis.[61] Research is now exploring a possible fourth component—endothelial dysfunction. Consequences of this include imbalance between vasodilating and vasoconstricting substances produced by (or acting on) the endothelium, which affects electrolyte volume and content and mediates coagulation. Athletic-associated amenorrhea combined with endothelial dysfunction is a concern for future cardiovascular risk, public health issues, and athletic performance.[62]

Who is at the greatest risk of suffering from the female athlete triad? They tend to be female athletes who compete in endurance sports such as long-distance running; aesthetic sports, such as gymnastics; antigravitational sports, such as indoor rock climbing; and sports with weight classifications, such as karate or wrestling.[63]

Triad Factor 1: Disordered Eating

Restrictive eating behaviors practiced by girls and women in sports or physical activities that emphasize leanness are of special concern. When these athletes try to lose weight as a way to improve their athletic performance, they may be putting themselves at risk for disordered eating. Research suggests that female athletes are at greater risk for disordered eating than females not involved with an athletics program.[64]

Triad Factor 2: Amenorrhea

Once body fat falls below 20 percent, a woman's estrogen levels often drop significantly. As a result, women's bodies enter a menopause-like state years ahead of time. Their periods become irregular or cease altogether. Bone loss accelerates, just as it would after natural menopause. Many female athletes who suffer from this triad have the decreased bone density of women in their fifties and sixties. Weakened bones are more likely to fracture during exercise or daily activities. Stress fractures can be a red flag for the female athlete triad. Because much of this bone loss is irreversible, women who suffer from the female athlete triad are at increased risk of developing osteoporosis.[65]

In the general population, 2 to 5 percent of women have amenorrhea. However, the prevalence is much higher in athletes.[66] Research indicates that amenorrhea in athletic women is related to the combined effects of increased physical activity, weight loss, low body fat levels, and insufficient energy intake.

Triad Factor 3: Premature Osteoporosis

Health consequences of amenorrhea often include premature osteoporosis. Research shows that amenorrheic athletes experience rapid loss of bone mineral density in the spine, which can spread to other parts of the skeleton if amenorrhea continues for a long time.

Treatment involves replacing estrogen, which is low in amenorrheic females. Calcium supplementation is also recommended. Although bone mineralization may never return to normal in amenorrheic athletes, studies indicate that reducing the intensity of training, improving dietary intake, and increasing body weight can help restore menstruation and increase bone density.[67]

To help combat this alarming trend, the American College of Sports Medicine and the National Collegiate Athletic Association (NCAA) have established an eating disorders awareness campaign aimed at coaches and trainers. The NCAA also has a three-part video series, *Nutrition and Eating Disorders*, to acquaint coaches and trainers with the causes and effects of eating disorders as well as the steps to take when they suspect an athlete has an eating disorder.

Screening, referral, and education are keys to preventing the female athlete triad. Prevention and treatment are most successful when they are interdisciplinary efforts provided by a team of medical, athletic, nutrition, and mental health experts. Proactive sports education includes reducing the emphasis on body weight, eliminating group weigh-ins, treating each athlete individually, and facilitating healthy weight management.

Key Concepts Athletics can be a gateway to eating disorders. Female athletes who develop restrictive eating habits are at risk for developing a severe syndrome known as the female athlete triad. Disordered eating, amenorrhea, and abnormally low bone density characterize this syndrome. If not corrected, the female athlete triad can hinder athletic performance and set the stage for lifelong health problems.

Pregorexia

In the summer of 2008, the mainstream media introduced us to a new term, **pregorexia**, to describe pregnant women who reduce calories and exercise in excess in an effort to control pregnancy weight gain.[68] However, many women gain too much weight while pregnant, which prompted the American College of Obstetricians and Gynecologists to encourage physicians to discuss appropriate weight gain with their pregnant patients.[69] But what about those women with a history of eating disorders who become pregnant? Women who struggled with body image prior to becoming pregnant can need special attention, care, and recommendations. The good news is that research shows that some women with eating disorders experience a reduction in the severity of their symptoms during pregnancy.[70] However it is viewed, the term *pregorexia* has given health care professionals an avenue into talking about eating disorders with women who are or who are trying to become pregnant.

▶ **pregorexia** A term used to describe pregnant women who reduce calories and exercise in excess in an effort to control pregnancy weight gain.

Infantile Anorexia

Can unwitting parents create disordered eating in infants, perhaps setting the stage for eating disorders later in life? Do maternal feeding patterns play a role?[71] Childhood nutrition specialist Ellyn Satter has analyzed videotapes of infant feedings. Satter examined whether parents responded to—or ignored—their babies' nonverbal eating readiness cues. She concluded that many parents fail to recognize their babies' body language: They feed their babies too rapidly or too slowly, they offer foods the baby doesn't care for, or they persist in trying to feed a clearly full baby who is turning away from food. These well-meaning parents may inadvertently teach their babies to ignore hunger and satiety (fullness) cues and, instead, to eat in response to outside influences.[72]

▶ **infantile anorexia** Severe feeding difficulties that begin with the introduction of solid foods to infants. Symptoms include persistent food refusal for more than one month, malnutrition, parental concern about the child's poor food intake, and significant caregiver–infant conflict during feeding.

Infantile anorexia is described as a feeding disorder of infancy characterized by extreme food refusal, growth deficiency, and an apparent lack of appetite.[73] It can result in acute and/or chronic malnutrition. In addition, the condition usually results in conflict in the mother–infant relationship over issues of autonomy, dependency, and control.[74] Symptoms include persistent food refusal for more than a month, malnutrition, parental concern about the child's poor food intake, and significant caregiver–infant conflict during feeding. The disorder typically starts or worsens during the transition from nursing to spoon-feeding and self-feeding, between ages 6 months and 3 years. Food refusal by the infant usually varies from meal to meal and among different caregivers, with the result being inadequate food intake in general.

Babies with infantile anorexia should not be confused with picky eaters. Picky eaters might initially refuse all foods but allow themselves to be coaxed into eating. Picky eaters have strong food likes and dislikes but are not malnourished. And the relationship between the picky eaters and their parents or caregivers lacks the element of frustration and conflict seen in infantile anorexia.

Infantile anorexia has many serious consequences. Malnutrition can impair the developing brain and adds special stress to the parent–infant relationship. Furthermore, early conflict around meals can herald a lifelong unhealthy relationship with food.

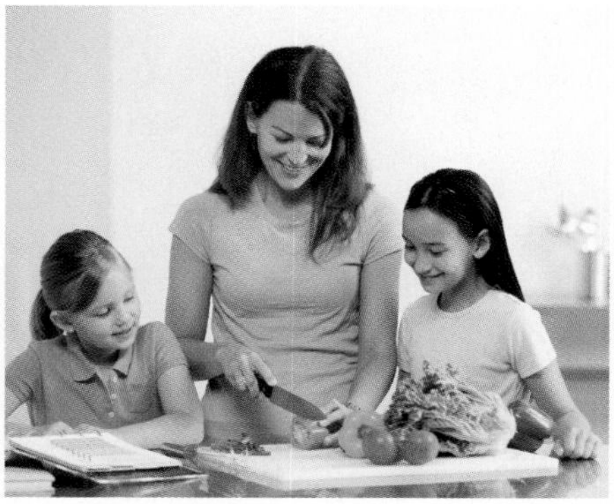

Key Concepts Researchers are continuously recognizing associations between eating disorders and behaviors such as vegetarianism. Even babies and young children can suffer from disordered eating patterns.

Combating Eating Disorders

Eating disorders are extremely difficult to treat, although advances in neurochemistry and scientific understanding of the mind–body connection provide new avenues of treatment. Most experts agree that emphasis should be placed on preventing eating disorders. See Table 14.11.

Preventing eating disorders depends on establishing appropriate mind–body–food relationships. Eating intuitively, an alternative approach to the diet mentality of our culture, suggests that we should trust ourselves and follow the body's signals. This approach might entail reframing our relationships to our body—for example, learning to distinguish physical from emotional feelings and gaining a sense of body wisdom. It's also a process of making peace with food and expunging constant "food worry" thoughts. One plan for learning to eat intuitively is presented in **TABLE SED.8**.

Although intuitive eating appears simple, it entails complex processes. For example, one basic principle of intuitive eating is the ability to respond to inner body cues. "Eat when you're hungry and stop when you're full" may sound like a no-brainer, but it requires developing sensitivity to your body's signals.

The National Institutes of Health (NIH) believes that healthcare professionals should lead the eating disorder prevention effort by learning to promote self-esteem in their patients and teaching patients that people can be healthy at every size. Ideally, this approach would have a ripple effect: Patients would transmit these beliefs to others. A variety of public information campaigns aimed at parents and people who work with children and adolescents have evolved over the past decade to help promote eating disorder awareness. (See **TABLE SED.9**.) One example is the "size acceptance" approach to obesity treatment, led by Joanne Ikeda at the University of California, Berkeley.

Quick Bite

Scary Statistics

About 5 million Americans have anorexia nervosa, bulimia, or binge-eating disorders. Researchers estimate that 15 percent of young women have disordered eating attitudes and behaviors. Every year an estimated 1,000 people die from anorexia nervosa.

TABLE SED.8
Intuitive Eating

1. Reject the Diet Mentality
Throw out the diet books and magazine articles that offer you false hope of losing weight quickly, easily, and permanently. Get angry at the lies that have led you to feel as if you were a failure every time a new diet stopped working and you gained back all of the weight. If you allow even one small hope to linger that a new and better diet might be lurking around the corner, it will prevent you from being free to rediscover *intuitive eating*.
2. Honor Your Hunger
Keep your body biologically fed with adequate energy and carbohydrates. Otherwise you can trigger a primal drive to overeat. Once you reach the moment of excessive hunger, all intentions of moderate, conscious eating are fleeting and irrelevant. Learning to honor this first biological signal sets the stage for rebuilding trust with yourself and food.
3. Make Peace with Food
Call a truce, stop the food fight! Give yourself unconditional permission to eat. If you tell yourself that you can't or shouldn't have a particular food, it can lead to intense feelings of deprivation that build into uncontrollable cravings and, often, bingeing. When you finally "give in" to your forbidden food, eating will be experienced with such intensity, it usually results in Last Supper overeating and overwhelming guilt.
4. Challenge the Food Police
Scream a loud "NO" to thoughts in your head that declare you're "good" for eating minimal calories or "bad" because you ate a piece of chocolate cake. The Food Police monitor the unreasonable rules that dieting has created. The police station is housed deep in your psyche, and its loudspeaker shouts negative barbs, hopeless phrases, and guilt-provoking indictments. Chasing the Food Police away is a critical step in returning to intuitive eating.
5. Respect Your Fullness
Listen for the body signals that tell you that you are no longer hungry. Observe the signs that show that you're comfortably full. Pause in the middle of a meal or food and ask yourself how the food tastes, and what is your current fullness level?
6. Discover the Satisfaction Factor
The Japanese have the wisdom to promote pleasure as one of their goals of healthy living. In our fury to be thin and healthy, we often overlook one of the most basic gifts of existence—the pleasure and satisfaction that can be found in the eating experience. When you eat what you really want, in an environment that is inviting and conducive, the pleasure you derive will be a powerful force in helping you feel satisfied and content. By providing this experience for yourself, you will find that it takes much less food to decide you've had "enough."
7. Honor Your Feelings Without Using Food
Find ways to comfort, nurture, distract, and resolve your issues without using food. Anxiety, loneliness, boredom, and anger are emotions we all experience throughout life. Each has its own trigger, and each has its own appeasement. Food won't fix any of these feelings. It may comfort for the short term, distract from the pain, or even numb you into a food hangover. But food won't solve the problem. If anything, eating for an emotional hunger will only make you feel worse in the long run. You'll ultimately have to deal with the source of the emotion as well as the discomfort of overeating.
8. Respect Your Body
Accept your genetic blueprint. Just as a person with a shoe size of 8 would not expect to realistically squeeze into a size 6, it is equally as futile (and uncomfortable) to have the same expectation with body size. But mostly, respect your body, so you can feel better about who you are. It's hard to reject the diet mentality if you are unrealistic and overly critical about your body shape.
9. Exercise—Feel the Difference
Forget militant exercise. Just get active and feel the difference. Shift your focus to how it feels to move your body, rather than the calorie burning effect of exercise. If you focus on how you feel from working out, such as energized, it can make the difference between rolling out of bed for a brisk morning walk or hitting the snooze alarm. If when you wake up, your only goal is to lose weight, it's usually not a motivating factor in that moment of time.
10. Honor Your Health—Gentle Nutrition
Make food choices that honor your health and taste buds while making you feel well. Remember that you don't have to eat a perfect diet to be healthy. You will not suddenly get a nutrient deficiency or gain weight from one snack, one meal, or one day of eating. It's what you eat consistently over time that matters; progress not perfection is what counts.

Courtesy of Evelyn Tribole and Elyse Resch. http://www.intuitiveeating.org.

TABLE SED.9
Preventing Eating Disorders

To join the effort to prevent eating disorders, follow these tips:

- Celebrate the diversity of human body shapes and sizes.
- Present accurate information about nutrition, weight management, and health.
- Discourage restrictive eating practices, including skipping meals.
- Encourage people to eat in response to hunger, not emotions.
- Reinforce messages about good eating and activity patterns at school and at home.
- Carefully phrase comments about a person's weight, body, or fitness level.
- Teach children and young people how to constructively express negative emotions.
- Encourage parents, teachers, coaches, and other professionals who work with children to do likewise.
- Encourage people of all ages to focus on personal qualities rather than physical appearance of themselves and others.
- Find and promote images of fit people of all sizes and shapes.

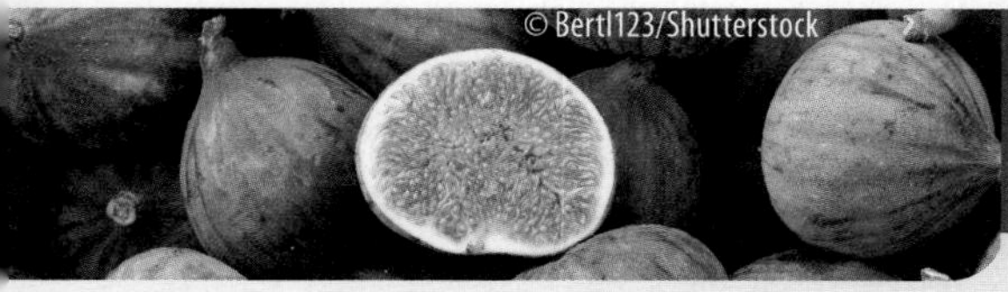
© Bertl123/Shutterstock

Learning Portfolio

Key Terms

Study Points

- An eating disorder is a complex emotional illness, the primary symptom of which is significantly altered eating habits. Eating disorders occur in susceptible people exposed to particular types of environmental stimuli.
- Although eating disorders existed even in ancient times, they have become alarmingly common in industrialized countries.
- Eating disorders involve highly restrictive eating patterns (seen in anorexia nervosa), a combination of compulsive overeating and purging (seen in bulimia nervosa), or unrestricted binge eating.
- Eating disorders are common in people who participate in body-conscious activities such as dance, wrestling, gymnastics, and bodybuilding.
- From 1 to 5 percent of people with eating disorders are male.
- Anorexia nervosa is an obsession with thinness manifested in self-imposed starvation.
- The typical person with anorexia nervosa is a young Caucasian woman from an upper-class, achievement-oriented family.
- Victims of anorexia nervosa have a body weight at least 15 percent below normal, a distorted body image, and physical and psychological symptoms related to starvation.
- The body weight of people with bulimia nervosa is close to or even slightly above that considered healthy for their height.
- Key symptoms of bulimia nervosa are binge-eating episodes occurring at least twice a week for three months, followed by severe dieting, purging, or a combination of dieting and purging.
- Binge-eating disorder is the most common eating disorder.
- Like those with bulimia, people with binge-eating disorder consume more food than is typically eaten in a given period of time.
- People with body dysmorphic disorder (BDD) are preoccupied with an imagined or slight defect in appearance.
- In night-eating syndrome, the food intake rhythm can be out of sync with a person's normal sleep rhythm by as much as four to five hours.
- Many competitive athletes, both male and female, have disordered eating behaviors.
- Disordered eating, amenorrhea, and abnormally low bone density characterize the female athlete triad.
- The best treatment for eating disorders is prevention. Once an eating disorder has become entrenched, intensive and prolonged treatment is typically required. Many people require lifelong support to maintain healthful eating and lifestyle habits.

Study Questions

1. List the diagnostic criteria for anorexia nervosa, bulimia nervosa, and binge-eating disorder.
2. What are the warning signs of anorexia nervosa?
3. What is the usual treatment for people with anorexia nervosa, and what do most experts say about their recovery?
4. What is the typical profile of a person with bulimia nervosa?
5. Describe an eating binge and all the behaviors that constitute purging.
6. How does binge-eating disorder differ from bulimia?

Try This

Is There Any Help Out There?

How much help is available in your community for people with eating disorders? Scan the telephone directory (Yellow Pages) and the Internet for eating disorder clinics, programs, and centers. Call them to inquire about their services. Do they have a psychologist, medical doctor, dietitian, nurse, and/or social worker on staff? Is it an inpatient or outpatient program? What is their philosophy of therapy? What is their success rate? What are their payment plans?

References

1. American Dietetic Association. Position of the American Dietetic Association: nutrition intervention in the treatment of eating disorders. *J Am Diet Assoc.* 2011;111:1236–1241.
2. American Dietetic Association. *Manual of Clinical Dietetics*. 6th ed. Chicago: American Dietetic Association; 2000.
3. Eat Right. Academy of Nutrition and Dietetics. 2015. http://www.eatright.org. Accessed February 11, 2016.
4. Neumark-Sztainer D, Wall M, Larson N, Eisenberg M, Loth K. Dieting and disordered eating behaviors from adolescence to young adulthood: findings from a 10-year longitudinal study. *J Am Diet Assoc.* 2011;111(7):1004–1011.
5. Ibid.
6. Smink FR, van Hoeken D, Hoek HW. Epidemiology of eating disorders: incidence, prevalence and mortality rates. *Curr Psychiatr Rep.* 2012;14(4):406–414.
7. Dittmar H, Halliwell E, Ive S. Does Barbie make girls want to be thin? The effect of experimental exposure to images of dolls on the body image of 5- to 8-year-old girls. *Dev Psychol.* 2006;42(2):283–292.
8. Cho JH, Han SN, Kim JH, Lee HM. Body image distortion in fifth and sixth grade students may lead to stress, depression, and undesirable dieting behavior. *Nutr Res Pract.* 2012;6(2):175–181.
9. Wojtowicz AE, von Ranson KM. Weighing in on risk factors for body dissatisfaction: a one-year prospective study of middle-adolescent girls. *Body Image.* 2012;9(1):20–30.
10. Yoo JJ, Jonson KK. Effects of appearance-related testing on ethnically diverse adolescent girls. *Adolescence.* 2007;42(166):353–380.
11. Heijens T, Janssens W, Streukens S. The effect of history of teasing on body dissatisfaction and intention to eat healthy in overweight and obese subjects. *Eur J Public Health.* 2012;22(1):121–126.
12. Krukowski RA, West S, Perez P, et al. Overweight children, weight-based teasing, and academic performance. *Int J Pediatr Obes.* 2009;4(4):274–280.
13. Harrington EF, Crowther JH, Shipherd JC. Trauma, binge eating, and the "strong Black woman." *J Consult Clin Psychol.* 2010;78(4):469–479.
14. Tagay S, Schlegl S, Senf W. Traumatic events, posttraumatic stress symptomatology and somatoform symptoms in eating disorder patients. *Eur Eat Disord Rev.* 2010;18(2):124–132.
15. Worobey J. Barbie at 50: maligned but benign? *Eat Weight Disord.* 2009;14(4):e219–e224.
16. Eisenberg ME, Neumark-Sztainer D. Friends' dieting and disordered eating behaviors among adolescents five years later: findings from Project EAT. *J Adolesc Health.* 2010;47(1):67–73.
17. Portela de Santana ML, da Costa Ribeiro H Jr, Mora Giral M, Raich RM. Epidemiology and risk factors of eating disorder in adolescence: a review. *Nurt Hosp.* 2012;27(2):391–401.
18. Lock J, Fitzpatrick KK. Anorexia nervosa. *Clin Evid* [Online]. 2009;2009:1011.
19. Flament MF, Bissada H, Spettigue W. Evidence-based pharmacotherapy of eating disorders. *Int J Neuropsychopharmacol.* 2012;15(2):189–207.
20. Redman LM, Ravussin E. Lorcaserin for the treatment of obesity. *Drugs Today (Barc).* 2010;46(12):901–910.
21. Ahren-Moonga J, Silverwood R, AF Klinteberg B, Koupil I. Association of higher parental and grandparental education and higher school grades with risk of hospitalization for eating disorders in females. The Uppsala Birth Cohort Multigenerational Study. *Am J Epidemiol.* 2009;170(5):566–575.
22. Perdereau F, Faucher S, Wallier J, Vibert S, Godart N. Family history of anxiety and mood disorders in anorexia nervosa: review of the literature. *Eat Weight Disord.* 2008;13(1):1–13.
23. Briley M, Moret C. Improvement of social adaptation in depression with serotonin and norepinephrine reuptake inhibitors. *Neuropsychiatr Dis Treat.* 2010;6:647–655.
24. Stice E, Yokum S, Zaid D, Dagher A. Dopamine-based reward circuitry responsivity, genetics, and overeating. *Curr Top Behav Neurosci.* 2011;6:81–93.
25. American Medical Association. JAMA patient page; anorexia nervosa. *JAMA.* 2006;295(22):2684.
26. Urquhart CS, Mihalynuk TV. Disordered eating in women: implications for the obesity pandemic. *Can J Diet Pract Res.* 2011;72(1):50.
27. Stice E, Marti CN, Shaw H, Jaconis M. An 8-year longitudinal study of the natural history of threshold, subthreshold, and partial eating disorders from a community sample of adolescents. *J Abnorm Psychol.* 2009;118(3):587–597.
28. Wood NA, Petrie TA. Body dissatisfaction, ethnic identity, and disordered eating among African American women. *J Couns Psychol.* 2010;57(2):141–153.
29. Ma JL. Eating disorders, parent–child conflicts, and family therapy in Shenzhen, China. *Qual Health Res.* 2008;18(6):803–810.
30. Huemer J, Haidvogl M, Mattejat F, et al. Perception of autonomy and connectedness prior to the onset of anorexia nervosa and bulimia nervosa. *Z Kinder Jugendpsychiatr Psychother.* 2012;40(1):61–68.
31. Position of the American Dietetic Association: nutrition intervention in the treatment of anorexia nervosa, bulimia nervosa, and other eating disorders. *J Am Diet Assoc.* 2006;109:2073–2082.

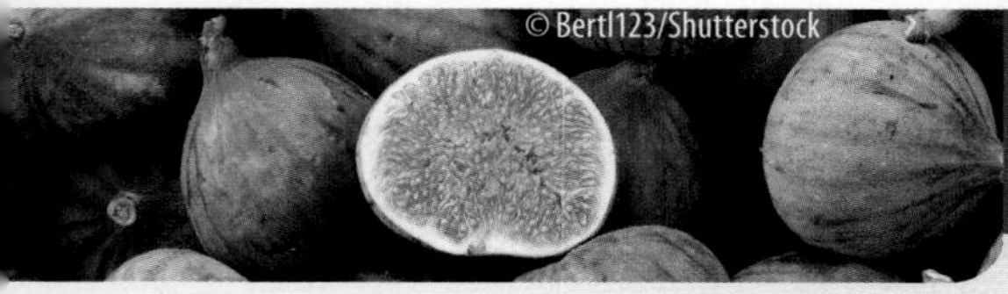

Learning Portfolio (continued)

32. Byrd-Bredbenner C, Moe G, Beshgetoor D, Bernign J. *Wardlaw's Perspectives in Nutrition*. 8th ed. New York: McGraw-Hill; 2009.
33. Smith M, Segal J. Anorexia nervosa: signs, symptoms, causes and treatment. Helpguide.org. http://www.helpguide.org/articles/eating-disorders/anorexia-nervosa.htm. Accessed February 11, 2016.
34. Position of the American Dietetic Association: nutrition intervention in the treatment of anorexia nervosa, bulimia nervosa, and other eating disorders. Op cit.
35. Ibid.
36. Monteleone P, Di Genio M, Monteleone AM, Di Filippo C, Maj M. Investigation of factors associated to crossover from anorexia nervosa restricting type (ANR) and anorexia nervosa binge-purging type (ANBP) to bulimia nervosa and comparison of bulimia nervosa patients with or without previous ANR or ANBP. *Compr Psychiatry*. 2011;52(1):56–62.
37. Mehler PS, Winkelman AB, Anderson DM, Gaudiani JL. Nutritional rehabilitation: practical guidelines for refeeding the anorectic patient. *J Nutr Metab*. 2010:2010. http://www.hindawi.com/journals/jnume/2010/625782/. Accessed February 11, 2016.
38. Forcano L, Alvarez E, Santamaria JJ, et al. Suicide attempts in anorexia nervosa subtypes. *Compr Psychiatry*. 2011;52(4):352–358.
39. Lock J, Fitzpatrick KK. Anorexia nervosa. Op cit.
40. Gentile MG, Manna GM, Pastorelli P, Oitolini A. Resumption of menses after 32 years in anorexia nervosa. *Eat Weight Disord*. 2011;16(3):e223–e225.
41. Keel PK, Dorer DJ, Eddy KT, et al. Predictors of mortality in eating disorders. *Arch Gen Psych*. 2003;60:179–183.
42. Khaylis A, Trockel M, Taylor CB. Binge drinking in women at risk for developing eating disorders. *Int J Eat Disord*. 2009;42(5):409–414.
43. Fischer S, Settles R, Collins B, Gunn R, Smith GT. The role of negative urgency and expectancies in problem drinking and disordered eating: testing a model of comorbidity in pathological and at-risk samples. *Psychol Addict Behav*. 2012;26(1):112–123.
44. Greene GW, Schembre SM, White AA, et al. Identifying clusters of college students at elevated health risk based on eating and exercise behaviors and psychosocial determinants of body weight. *J Am Diet Assoc*. 2011;111(3):394–400.
45. Strong KA, Parks SL, Anderson E, Winett R, Davy BM. Weight gain prevention: identifying theory-based targets for health behavior change in young adults. *J Am Diet Assoc*. 2008;108(10):1708–1715.
46. Ibid.
47. Ibid.
48. Kaye W. Neurobiology of anorexia and bulimia nervosa. *Physiol Behav*. 2008;94(1):121–135.
49. Position of the American Dietetic Association: nutrition intervention in the treatment of anorexia nervosa, bulimia nervosa, and other eating disorders. Op cit.
50. American Psychiatric Association. *Diagnostic and Statistical Manual of Mental Disorders*. 5th ed., text rev. Washington, DC: American Psychiatric Association; 2013.
51. Allen KL, Fursland A, Watson H, Byrne SM. Eating disorder diagnosis in general practice settings: comparison with structured clinical interview and self-report questionnaires. *J Ment Health*. 2011;20(3):270–280.

52. Neumark-Sztainer D, Wall M, Haines J, Story M, Eisenberg ME. Why does dieting predict weight gain in adolescents? Findings from Project EAT-II: a 5-year longitudinal study. *J Am Diet Assoc*. 2007;107(3):448–455.
53. Fenske JN, Schwenk TL. Obsessive compulsive disorder: diagnosis and management. *Am Fam Physician*. 2009;80(3):239–245.
54. Hudson JI, Hiripi E, Pope HG, Kessler RC. The prevalence and correlates of eating disorders in the National Comorbidity Survey Replication. *Biol Psychiatry*. 2007;61:348–358.
55. National Institute of Mental Health. The numbers count: mental disorders in America. 2015. http://www.nimh.nih.gov/health/statistics/prevalence/index.shtml.
56. Caqueo-Urizar A, Ferrer-Garcia M, Toro J, Gutierrez-Maldonado J, et al. Associations between sociocultural pressures to be thin, body distress, and eating disorder symptomatology among Chilean adolescent girls. *Body Image*. 2011;8(1):78–81.
57. Resch M. Eating disorders in sports—sport in eating disorders. *Orv Hetil*. 2007;148(40):1899–1902.
58. Ibid.
59. Sundgot-Borgen J, Torstveit MK. Aspects of disordered eating continuum in elite high-intensity sports. *Scand J Med Sci Sports*. 2010;20(Suppl 2):112–121.
60. Schaal K, Tafflet M, Nassif H, et al. Psychological balance in high level athletes: gender-based differences and sport-specific patterns. *PLoS One*. 2011;6(5):e19007.
61. Nattiv A, Loucks AB, Manore MM, Sanborn CF, Sundgot-Borgen J, Warren MP. American College of Sports Medicine position stand: the female athlete triad. *Med Sci Sports Exerc*. 2007;39(10):1867–1882.
62. Zach KN, Smith Machin A, Hoch AZ. Advances in management of the female athlete triad and eating disorders. *Clin Sports Med*. 2011;30(3):551–573.
63. Nattiv A, Loucks AB, Manore MM, et al. American College of Sports Medicine position stand. Op cit.
64. Hoch AZ, Pajewski NM, Moraski L, et al. Prevalence of the female athlete triad in high school athletes and sedentary students. *Clin J Sport Med*. 2009;19(5):421–428.
65. Ackerman KE, Misra M. Bone health and the female athlete triad in adolescent athletes. *Phys Sportsmed*. 2011;39(1):131–141.
66. Enea C, Boisseau N, Fargeas-Gluck MA, Diaz V, Dugue B. Circulating androgens in women: exercise-induced changes. *Sports Med*. 2011;41(1):1–15.
67. Ibid.
68. Mathieu J. What is pregorexia? *J Am Diet Assoc*. 2009;109(6):976–979.
69. Ibid.
70. Ibid.
71. Kroller K, Warschburger P. Problematic eating behavior in childhood: do maternal feeding patterns play a role? *Prax Kinderpsychol Kinderpsychiatr*. 2011;60(4):253–269.
72. Satter E. *Secrets of Feeding a Healthy Family: Orchestrating and Enjoying the Family Meal*. Madison, WI: Kelcy Press; 2008.
73. Ammaniti M, Lucarelli L, Cimino S, D'Olimpio F, Chatoor I. Feeding disorders of infancy: a longitudinal study to middle childhood. *Int J Eat Disord*. 2012;45(2):272–280.
74. Kroller K, Warschburger P. Problematic eating behavior in childhood. Op cit.

Chapter 15

Diet and Health

Revised by Don Ross

THINK About It

1. Is there a history of heart disease in your family?
2. Do you know your blood pressure?
3. Do you know how your current weight might influence your health later in life?
4. How often do you worry about your personal risk of cancer?

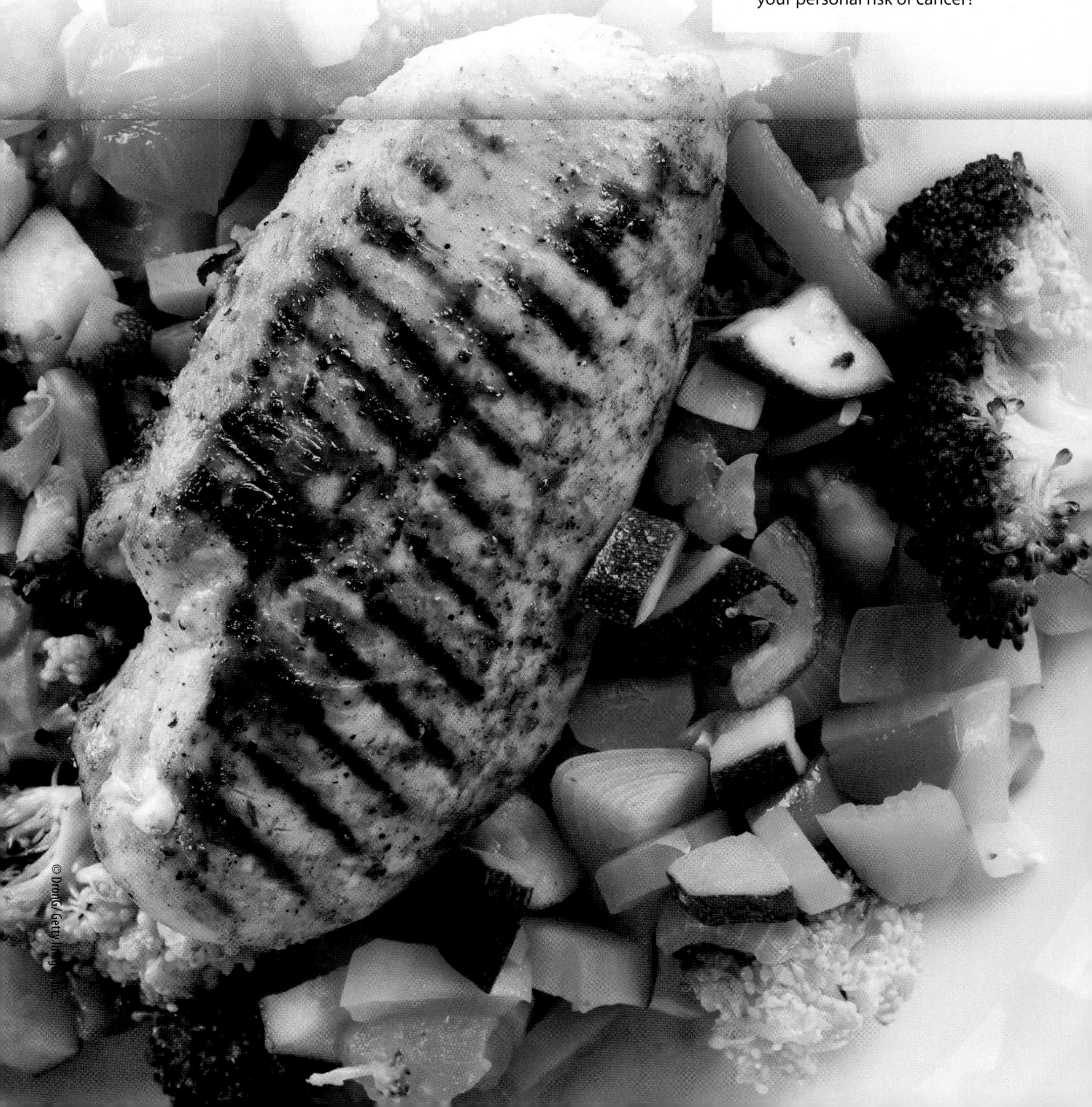

CHAPTER Menu

- Nutrition and Chronic Disease
- Obesity and Chronic Disease
- Physical Inactivity and Chronic Disease
- Genetics and Disease
- Cardiovascular Disease
- Hypertension
- Diabetes Mellitus
- Metabolic Syndrome
- Osteoporosis
- Key Terms
- Study Points
- Study Questions
- Try This
- Getting Personal
- References

LEARNING Objectives

- Describe how nutrition and other lifestyle factors influence the risk of developing chronic diseases.
- Define and describe cardiovascular disease and its risk factors, including dietary and lifestyle factors for reducing the risk of atherosclerosis.
- Identify risk factors for hypertension and describe dietary and lifestyle factors for reducing hypertension.
- Explain risk factors for developing cancer and the dietary and lifestyle factors for reducing cancer risk.
- Differentiate among the three major types of diabetes mellitus.
- Identify risk factors for diabetes and explain dietary and lifestyle factors for reducing diabetes risk.
- Describe osteoporosis, its risk factors, and dietary and lifestyle factors for reducing osteoporosis risk.

Why did Joel Smith have a heart attack at age 48? Not his age. Few men suffer heart attacks before age 50. What about his cholesterol? Possibly. Joel inherited the tendency to have high levels of both low-density lipoprotein (LDL) cholesterol and homocysteine, an amino acid that is a risk factor for heart disease. Could his diet have been a contributing factor? Joel was a meat and potatoes guy. Over his lifetime, Joel enjoyed plenty of hearty meals with lots of meat, gravy, pie, and ice cream. He never developed the habit or pleasure of eating many fruits or vegetables.

Back in high school, Joel was a star athlete. Yet despite his enjoyment of sports, his current physical activity was limited to an occasional weekend basketball game. In fact, just prior to his heart attack, Joel was playing a spirited game of basketball with his kids. Sometime before his heart attack, Joel developed a respiratory infection from bacteria called *Chlamydia pneumoniae* (thought to contribute to arterial damage and atherosclerosis).

All these factors may have contributed to Joel's heart attack. It is difficult to separate out the relative importance of each factor, but, taken collectively, they culminated in a potentially fatal event. With some changes in his lifestyle, could Joel have avoided his early heart attack? Possibly! Some changes in his lifestyle, eating more fruits and vegetables, and limiting intake of fat may have helped, as would shooting hoops on a more regular basis or taking a brisk, 60-minute walk each day. You cannot change the inherited tendency to develop a disease, but many of us can reduce our risk by modifying our lifestyle.

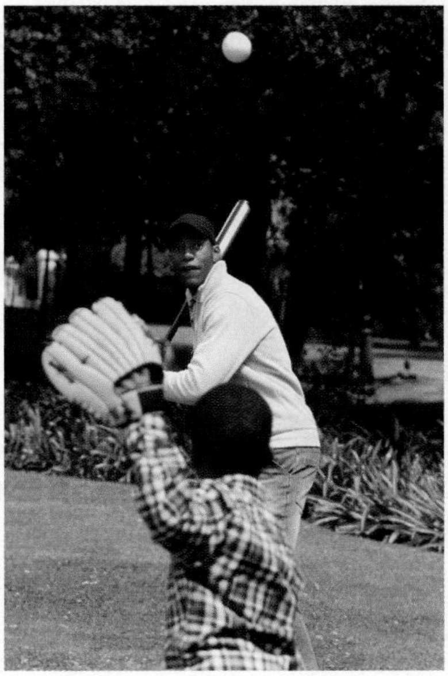
© Stockbyte/Thinkstock

Nutrition and Chronic Disease

What does it mean to be healthy? The World Health Organization (WHO) defines health as "a state of complete physical, mental, and social well-being and not merely the absence of disease or infirmity."[1] Although most of us focus on the last part of that definition, "the absence of disease or infirmity," the first part is equally important. As you have learned, nutrition is an important part of physical, mental, and social well-being. It also is important for preventing disease.

Disease can be defined as an impairment of the normal state of a living animal or one of its parts and can arise from environmental factors or specific infectious agents, such as bacteria or viruses.[2] Diseases can be acute (short-lived illnesses that arise and resolve quickly) or chronic (diseases with a slow onset and long duration). Although nutrition can affect our susceptibility to acute diseases—and contaminated food is certainly a source of acute disease—our food choices are more likely to affect our risk for developing chronic diseases such as heart disease, diabetes, or cancer. In its report *Diet, Nutrition, and the Prevention of Chronic Diseases*, the WHO states that "the diets people eat, in all their cultural variety, define to a large extent people's health, growth, and development."[3] Other lifestyle factors such as tobacco use and exercise, in addition to genetic factors, also determine who gets sick and who remains healthy.

Nutrition Informatics

▶ **nutrition informatics** According to the Academy of Nutrition and Dietetics, this is "the effective retrieval, organization, storage and optimum use of information, data and knowledge for food- and nutrition-related problem solving and decision-making. Informatics is supported by the use of information standards, processes and technology."

Nutrition informatics is the intersection of information, nutrition, and technology. With the U.S. healthcare system moving from a largely paper-based system to electronic records, dietitians will have new tools and opportunities for chronic disease management through evidence-based decision support, quality management, outcomes reporting, and other strategies. As valued members and decision makers of the healthcare team, dietitians practice in a wide variety of settings from private practice to corporate wellness to the hospital clinic. Each setting has unique information needs, but all require skills in finding, evaluating, and sharing accurate food and nutrition information.

Nutrition informatics represents the next evolution in the practice of dietetics, and the Academy of Nutrition and Dietetics has established a collaboration with the Health Information Management Systems Society (HIMSS).[4] The Academy has long been at the forefront of the exploration of biomedical informatics-related nutrition, and HIMSS is a global organization focused on better health through information technology. The collaboration will support nutrition informatics competencies for Registered Dietitians/Dietetic Technicians (RDs/DTRs) and the nutrition community.

Healthy People 2020

▶ **health disparities** Differences in health outcomes and their determinants between segments of the population, as defined by social, demographic, environmental, and geographic attributes.

Healthy People 2020, from the U.S. Department of Health and Human Services, is a comprehensive set of disease prevention and health promotion objectives for the nation.[5] Healthy People 2020's vision is to establish a society in which all people live long, healthy lives. The initiative includes four overarching goals: (1) attain high-quality, longer lives free of preventable disease, disability, injury, and premature death; (2) achieve health equity, eliminate disparities, and improve the health of all groups; (3) create social and physical environments that promote good health for all; and (4) promote quality of life, healthy development, and healthy behaviors across all life stages (see **FIGURE 15.1**).

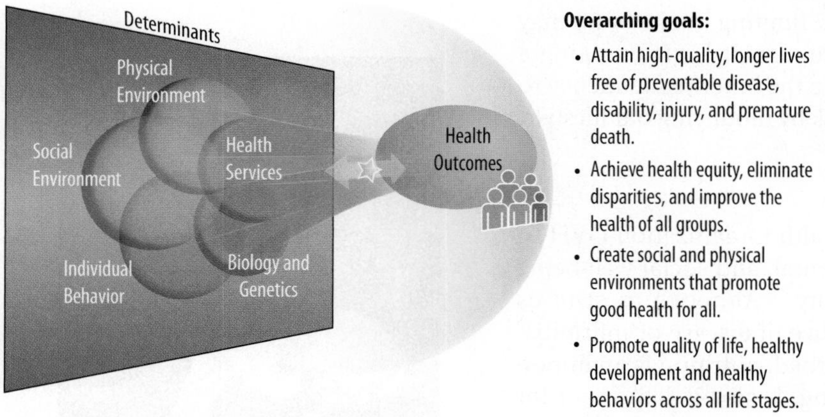
Determinants
Physical Environment
Social Environment
Health Services
Individual Behavior
Biology and Genetics
Health Outcomes
Overarching goals:
• Attain high-quality, longer lives free of preventable disease, disability, injury, and premature death.
• Achieve health equity, eliminate disparities, and improve the health of all groups.
• Create social and physical environments that promote good health for all.
• Promote quality of life, healthy development and healthy behaviors across all life stages.

FIGURE 15.1 Healthy People 2020. Healthy People 2020 is a comprehensive set of disease prevention and health promotion objectives for the United States to achieve over the first decade of this century. This graphic framework illustrates the fundamental degree of overlap among the social determinants of health, as well as emphasizes their collective impact and influence on health outcomes and conditions. For more on Healthy People 2020, visit www.healthypeople.gov.

Reproduced from U.S. Department of Health and Human Services, Office of Disease Prevention and Health Promotion. Healthy People 2020. http://healthypeople.gov/2020/about/GenHealthAbout.aspx. Accessed February 12, 2016.

Health Disparities

A key challenge is the disparities in health associated with race/ethnicity, gender, income, education, disability status, and geography. The *CDC Heath Disparities and Inequalities Report* documents these **health disparities** and provides a framework for comprehensive, community-driven approaches to reducing health disparities in the United States.[6,7]

Why are health and health outcomes so different among various groups? Beyond genetic susceptibility and traditional environmental factors are barriers to access found in our healthcare system. Consider for a moment the impact of cultural differences. Does your healthcare provider speak your language? Does your provider understand and respect your culture and beliefs? When the answers to these questions are "no," suspicion and mistrust often result. If you do not trust your provider, will you follow your provider's recommendations carefully? Usually the answer is no, and needed care is rejected.

Obesity and Chronic Disease

Once considered merely an aesthetic issue, obesity is now widely recognized as a major public health problem. It is a risk factor for the major chronic diseases of public health significance in the United States and Canada: coronary heart disease, cancer, diabetes, hypertension, and metabolic syndrome. Good health habits and proper weight management are key components of a healthy lifestyle that avoids or at least delays the onset of these diseases. Often, weight loss—or, at a minimum, no further weight gain—can improve health outcomes dramatically.

Physical Inactivity and Chronic Disease

A sedentary lifestyle also is a significant risk factor for chronic disease. Physically active people generally outlive those who are inactive, and inactivity is almost as significant a risk factor for heart disease as high blood pressure, smoking, or high blood cholesterol. Physical activity also plays a significant role in long-term weight management. The *Physical Activity Guidelines for Americans* states that "Physical activity is safe for almost everyone and the health benefits of physical activity far outweigh the risks. ... For all individuals, some activity is better than none."[8] Including at least 30 minutes per day of moderate physical activity such as brisk walking or cycling helps reduce chronic disease risk; weight-management efforts are enhanced by higher amounts of exercise—at least 60 minutes per day.

Genetics and Disease

In the last several years, knowledge has exploded regarding the relationship between our genetic makeup and disease. We now recognize that nearly all diseases have some genetic component. Most human illnesses occur because of the interaction of many genetic, environmental, nutritional, and lifestyle factors (see **FIGURE 15.2**). As the number one killer in the United States, cardiovascular disease is a good example of how genetic influences affect the development of disease.[9] A family history of heart disease indicates genetic vulnerability and is an important risk factor for developing the disease. Although some cancers, for example, breast cancer, have a genetic basis and affect many members of a given family, most cancers seem to be caused by a variety of factors.

Understanding how our **genes** influence our risk for disease has been a major goal of the **Human Genome Project**, an international effort spearheaded by the U.S. National Institutes of Health (NIH). The Human Genome Project is providing scientists with clues to the genetic variations that are responsible for common illnesses. Understanding the genetics of diseases will allow researchers to develop more effective medications and may lead to routine gene-based treatments.[10]

▶ **genes** Sections of DNA that contain hereditary information. Most genes contain information for making proteins.

▶ **Human Genome Project** An effort coordinated by the Department of Energy and the National Institutes of Health to map the genes in human DNA.

THINK About It 1

Quick Bite

Biological Blueprint
Nearly all 100 trillion cells in the human body contain a copy of the entire human genome, the complete set of genetic instructions necessary to build a human being.

The Workings of DNA and Genes

Our genetic instructions are carried by deoxyribonucleic acid (DNA), a molecule that can be visualized as an immensely long, corkscrew-shaped ladder—a

Chronic diseases	High-fat diet	Excessive alcohol intake	Low complex carbohydrate/fiber	Low vitamin and/or mineral intake	High sugar intake	High intake of salty or pickled foods	Genetics	Age	Sedentary lifestyle	Smoking and tobacco use	Stress	Environmental contaminants
	Dietary risk factors						**Nondietary risk factors**					
Cancers	X	X	X	X		X	X	X	X	X		X
Hypertension	X	X		X		in salt sensitive people	X	X	X	X	X	
Diabetes (type 2)	X		X				X	X	X			
Osteoporosis		X		X			X	X	X	X		
Atherosclerosis	X		X	X			X	X	X	X	X	
Obesity	X	X	X		X		X		X			
Stroke	X		X				X	X	X	X	X	
Diverticulosis	X		X	X				X	X			
Dental and oral diseases				X	X		X			X		

FIGURE 15.2 Risk factors for chronic diseases. Diet, lifestyle choices, and genetics interact to shape a person's risk profile.

▶ **nucleotides** Subunits of DNA or RNA consisting of a nitrogenous base (adenine, guanine, thymine, or cytosine in DNA; adenine, guanine, uracil, or cytosine in RNA), a phosphate molecule, and a sugar molecule (deoxyribose in DNA and ribose in RNA). Thousands of nucleotides are linked to form a DNA or RNA molecule.

double helix (see **FIGURE 15.3**). DNA is made of subunits called **nucleotides**. Each nucleotide contains one sugar molecule (deoxyribose—a five-carbon sugar), one phosphate molecule, and one base. The sugar and phosphate molecules make up the "side rails" of a DNA molecule, and the bases form the "rungs";

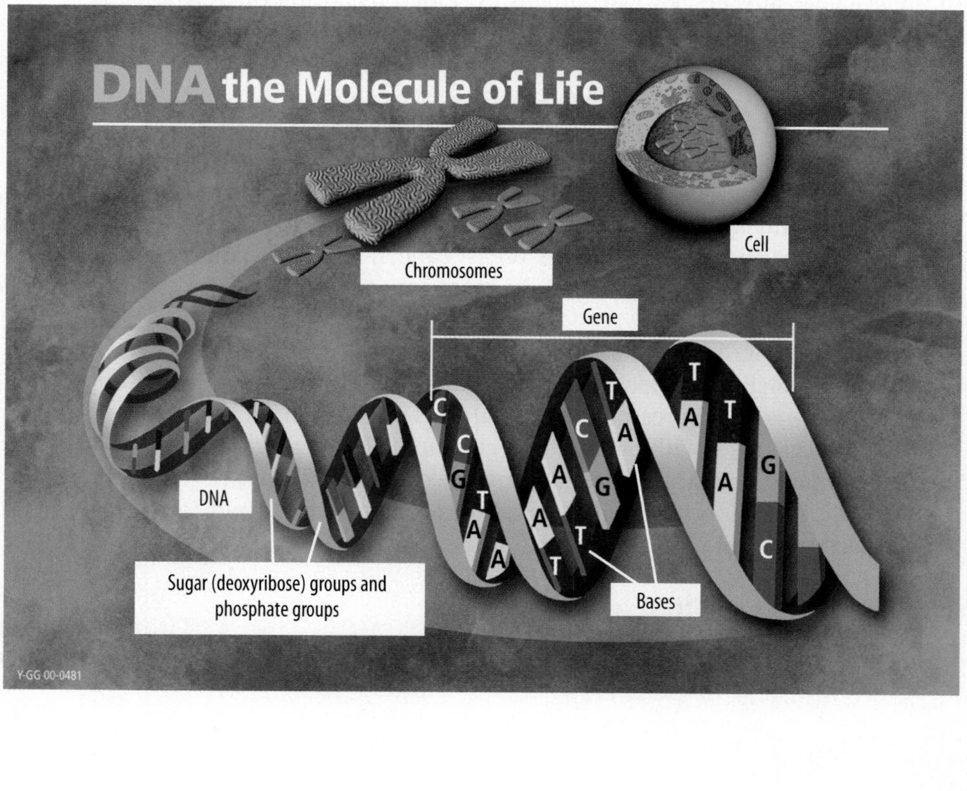

FIGURE 15.3 Structure of DNA. All the instructions needed to direct cellular activities are contained within the chemical DNA (deoxyribonucleic acid). The DNA sequence is the particular side-by-side arrangement of bases along the DNA strand (e.g., ATTCCGGA). This order spells out the exact instructions required to build proteins and create a unique person.

Courtesy of the Office of Biological and Environmental Research of the U.S. Department of Energy Office of Science. http://science.energy.gov/ber. Accessed February 12, 2016.

that is, the base in each nucleotide of one side rail joins with a base in a nucleotide on the opposite side rail. DNA has only four bases—adenine (A), thymine (T), guanine (G), and cytosine (C)—and each base is picky about its partner. To form a **base pair**, A always joins with T, and G always joins with C. Thus, the sequence of bases on one side of the ladder (for example, AGCGT) determines the **complementary sequence** on the other side (TCGCA). Using this "genetic alphabet," an enormous number of messages can be written.

Genes are sequences of DNA that carry the **genetic code** for making functional molecules, especially proteins. The genetic code combines the four "letters" of the genetic alphabet in various ways to spell out three-letter "words" that specify which amino acid is needed at each step in making a protein. Errors in the code can be harmless, or they can lead to serious disease. For example, people with sickle cell anemia have a mistake (called a **mutation**) in their genetic code for the amino acids making up the protein beta-globin. Beta-globin is part of the oxygen-carrying protein hemoglobin found in red blood cells. This mutated section of the genetic code in sickle cell anemia patients contains the sequence GTG (the code for valine) instead of GAG (the code for glutamate), so their cells manufacture beta-globin proteins with the wrong amino acid. Hemoglobin containing this faulty protein cannot carry a full load of oxygen and causes red blood cells to form a sickle shape.

Diet influences **gene expression**—the making of proteins. Components in the diet can enhance or inhibit gene expression, thereby increasing or decreasing protein synthesis. For example, folate status interacts with a genetic mutation that impacts the production of an enzyme that helps convert homocysteine to methionine. People with this particular DNA mutation have reduced enzyme activity and, as a result, higher homocysteine levels. When their folate status is low, their risk for heart disease is significantly elevated.[11] Scientists also are studying how folate status and this genetic mutation can influence cancer risk.

Nutritional genomics, which focuses on the influences of food components on gene expression and protection of the genome, is in its infancy. Nutrigenomics is the junction of health, diet, and genetics. The study of nutrigenomics will increase our understating of how nutrition affects normal body functioning and the development and prevention of diet-related diseases. As we learn more about the genetic causes of disease and the lifestyle factors that influence them, we will be able to better screen individuals for disease susceptibility, and then target appropriate lifestyle interventions to reduce their risk.[12]

Key Concepts Diseases can be acute or chronic. Nutrition and other lifestyle factors such as obesity and physical inactivity strongly influence the risk of developing chronic diseases. Our genetic makeup also influences disease risk. Genes are segments of DNA that contain the code for making proteins. Gene expression can be modified by diet. Understanding how our genes can affect the course of a disease can influence future population screening and produce targeted interventions to reduce disease risk.

Cardiovascular Disease

Cardiovascular disease (CVD) is the leading cause of death in the United States and Canada, claiming one life every 40 seconds. More people die from CVD than all forms of cancer combined. But not all the news is bad: Lifestyle changes and medical advances have led to significant progress in the fight against CVD.

CVD is significantly related to what some people call the American way of life. Too many Americans eat a high-fat diet, are overweight and sedentary, smoke cigarettes, manage stress ineffectively, do not manage their high blood pressure or high blood cholesterol levels, and do not know the signs of CVD. Of course, not all the risk factors for CVD are controllable—some

▶ **base pair** Two nitrogenous bases (adenine and thymine or guanine and cytosine), held together by weak bonds, that form a "rung" of the "DNA ladder." The bonds between base pairs hold the DNA molecule together in the shape of a double helix.

▶ **complementary sequence** Nucleic acid base sequence that can form a double-stranded structure with another DNA fragment by following base-pairing rules (A pairs with T, and C pairs with G). The complementary sequence to GTAC, for example, is CATG.

▶ **genetic code** The instructions in a gene that tell the cell how to make a specific protein. A, T, G, and C are the "letters" of the DNA code; they stand for the chemicals adenine, thymine, guanine, and cytosine, respectively, which make up the nucleotide bases of DNA. Each gene's code combines the four chemicals in various ways to spell out three-letter "words" that specify which amino acid is needed at every step in making a protein.

▶ **mutation** A permanent structural alteration in DNA. In most cases, DNA changes either have no effect or cause harm. Occasionally, a mutation can improve an organism's chance of surviving and passing the beneficial change on to its descendants. Certain mutations can lead to cancer or other diseases.

▶ **gene expression** The process by which proteins are made from the instructions encoded in DNA.

Quick Bite

Adaptation Gone Awry

Sickle-cell anemia is a hereditary blood disorder characterized by red blood cells that are a *C* or sickle shape. This disorder is a result of the human body adapting to resist malaria, a disease that attacks red blood cells, and is found primarily in people with sub-Saharan ancestry.

Quick Bite

Who Am I?

Our entire collection of genes, the human genome, contains about 19,000 genes. These genes consist of building blocks called base pairs. The human genome contains about 3 billion base pairs. Your mother supplied half of your genes and your father supplied the other half to create your unique combination. Unless you are an identical twin, no other person has your exact combination of genes.

▶ **cardiovascular disease (CVD)** Any abnormal condition characterized by dysfunction of the heart and blood vessels. CVD includes atherosclerosis (especially coronary heart disease, which can lead to heart attacks), cerebrovascular disease (e.g., stroke), and hypertension (high blood pressure).

people inherit a tendency toward persistent high blood pressure. But many factors can be changed, treated, or modified, so you have the power to significantly reduce your risk.

The Cardiovascular System and Cardiovascular Disease

The cardiovascular system consists of the heart and blood vessels (veins, arteries, and capillaries) (see **FIGURE 15.4**). Together, they pump and circulate blood throughout the body. A person weighing 150 pounds has about 5 quarts of blood, which circulates about once every minute.

What Is Atherosclerosis?

When we talk about diet and heart disease, we are usually referring to **coronary heart disease (CHD)**. CHD is caused by **atherosclerosis**, a slow, progressive hardening and narrowing of the arteries by deposits of fat, cholesterol, and other substances (see **FIGURE 15.5**). When serious, atherosclerosis can result in angina pectoris (chest pain) or myocardial infarction (heart attack). Atherosclerosis of the cerebral arteries leading to the brain can cause a stroke.

Atherosclerosis is one type of arteriosclerosis, which literally means "hardening of the arteries." As deposits, called **plaque**, accumulate along the artery walls, the arteries lose their elasticity and their ability to expand and contract, thereby restricting blood flow. Once narrowed in this way, an artery is vulnerable to plaque rupture and blockage by blood clots.

Plaque buildup begins when excess lipid particles collect beneath the cells that line an artery, called **endothelial cells** or the **endothelium**. High cholesterol, high blood pressure, smoking, and diabetes can all damage the endothelium and initiate atherosclerosis. Certain viral and bacterial infections also can damage blood vessels,[13] and a large number of infectious agents have been linked with an increased risk of vascular disease.[14] Infections contribute to atherosclerosis by direct infection of vascular cells and indirect effects of infection at "nonvascular" sites.[15]

Platelets, components of one of the body's protective mechanisms, collect at the damaged area and form a cap of cells, thereby isolating the plaque within the artery wall. The narrowed artery is vulnerable to blockage by clots that can

▶ **coronary heart disease (CHD)** A type of heart disease caused by narrowing of the coronary arteries that feed the heart, which needs a constant supply of oxygen and nutrients carried by the blood in the coronary arteries. When the coronary arteries become narrowed or clogged by fat and cholesterol deposits and cannot supply enough blood to the heart, CHD results.

▶ **atherosclerosis** A type of "hardening of the arteries" in which cholesterol and other substances in the blood build up in the walls of arteries. As the process continues, the arteries to the heart can narrow, cutting down the flow of oxygen-rich blood and nutrients to the heart.

▶ **plaque** A buildup of substances that circulate in the blood (e.g., calcium, fat, cholesterol, cellular waste, fibrin) on a blood vessel wall, making it vulnerable to blockage from blood clots.

▶ **endothelial cells** Thin, flattened cells that line internal body cavities in a single layer.

▶ **endothelium** See *endothelial cells*.

▶ **platelets** Tiny disk-shaped components of blood that are essential for blood clotting.

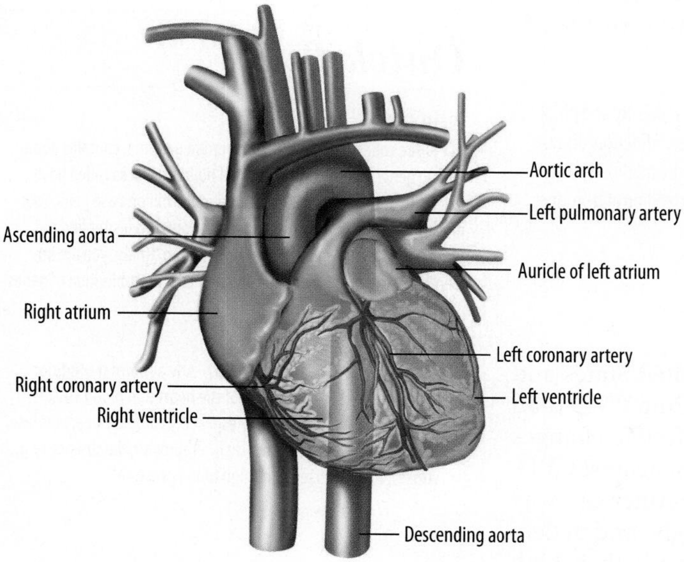

FIGURE 15.4 The heart and major arteries. Oxygenated blood is pumped through the arteries (red), and oxygen-depleted blood is returned to the heart through the veins (blue).

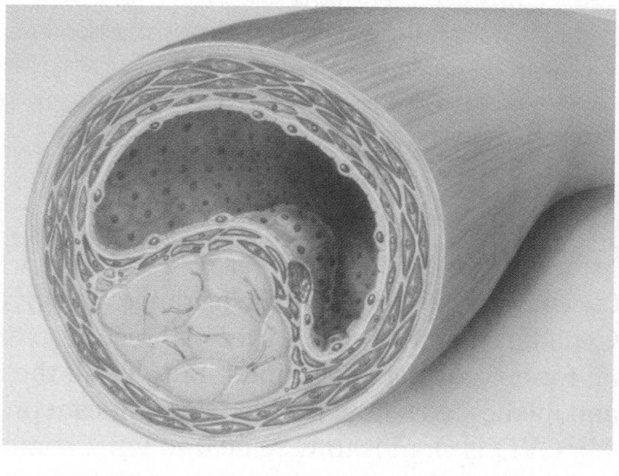

FIGURE 15.5 Development of atherosclerosis. Atherosclerotic plaque is formed by a buildup of fatty material in the wall of an artery. An artery narrowed by plaque is vulnerable to blockage by a blood clot, causing a heart attack or stroke.

form if the cap breaks and the fatty core of the plaque combines again with platelets and other clot-producing factors in the blood. If the heart, brain, or other organs are deprived of blood and the vital oxygen that blood carries, the effects of atherosclerosis can be deadly.

Cholesterol and Atherosclerosis

In the early 1960s researchers identified high blood cholesterol, or **hypercholesterolemia**, along with smoking and high blood pressure, as a principal risk factor for coronary heart disease. They understood that a high-fat, high-cholesterol diet tends to raise blood cholesterol, and high blood cholesterol levels promote atherosclerosis. Atherosclerosis leads to artery disease and often causes heart attacks or strokes.

▶ **hypercholesterolemia** The presence of greater than normal amounts of cholesterol in the blood.

Total cholesterol levels do not tell the entire story. The levels of low-density lipoprotein (LDL) and high-density lipoprotein (HDL) cholesterol predict a person's risk for developing atherosclerosis more accurately than the individual's total cholesterol levels. High LDL cholesterol is a greater risk than high total cholesterol, with some kinds of LDL being more dangerous than others. For example, high levels of **lipoprotein a [Lp(a)]**, a low-density lipoprotein, seem especially harmful. High levels of Lp(a) prevent the normal breakup of blood clots that cause heart attack or stroke. High levels of triglycerides and other blood lipids also increase the risk of cardiovascular disease, as do low HDL cholesterol levels.

▶ **lipoprotein a [Lp(a)]** A substance that consists of an LDL "bad cholesterol" part plus a protein (apoprotein a), whose exact function is currently unknown.

▶ **C-reactive protein (CRP)** A protein released by the body in response to acute injury, infection, or other inflammatory stimuli. CRP is associated with future cardiovascular events.

Deaths from coronary heart disease have fallen dramatically over the past two decades. That drop seems to be correlated with a drop in total cholesterol levels (see **FIGURE 15.6**) and reductions in smoking. These gains, however, are being threatened by substantial increases in obesity and diabetes mellitus.[16]

Experts recommend that patients who begin drug treatments to lower their cholesterol also make lifestyle changes to lower their risk in other ways and minimize medication use.[17] Although CHD can result from the interplay of genetic and environmental factors, modifiable lifestyle factors play a large role in the risk of disease. Multidimensional treatment of cholesterol and other heart disease risk factors that includes both lifestyle modifications and pharmacotherapy is likely the most beneficial way to prevent the vast majority of CHD events.[18]

Inflammation and Atherosclerosis

The idea that chronic infection can lead to unsuspected disease is not new. Bacterial infection, for example, is known to cause stomach ulcers. Infection caused by bacteria or viruses is suspected to be a factor in heart disease as well. *Chlamydia pneumoniae* bacteria have been shown to have a significant association with atherosclerotic plaque, and the herpes simplex virus also has been proposed as an infectious agent leading to inflammatory atherosclerosis.[19]

C-reactive protein (CRP), a protein released in response to acute injury, infection, or other inflammatory stimuli, indicates the presence of infection. Following a heart attack, high CRP levels are associated with adverse outcomes, such as an increased rate of death. Although CRP's association with atherosclerosis suggests that it is a risk factor for the development of arterial plaques, CRP may simply be an innocent bystander in inflammation with no causal relationship.[20]

Interleukin-6 (IL-6) is another inflammatory biomarker and can be used to predict coronary artery disease.[21] In addition, there is growing evidence that blood markers for HbA1c and DHEAS (dehydroepiandrosterone sulfate), along with organ-specific functional reserve

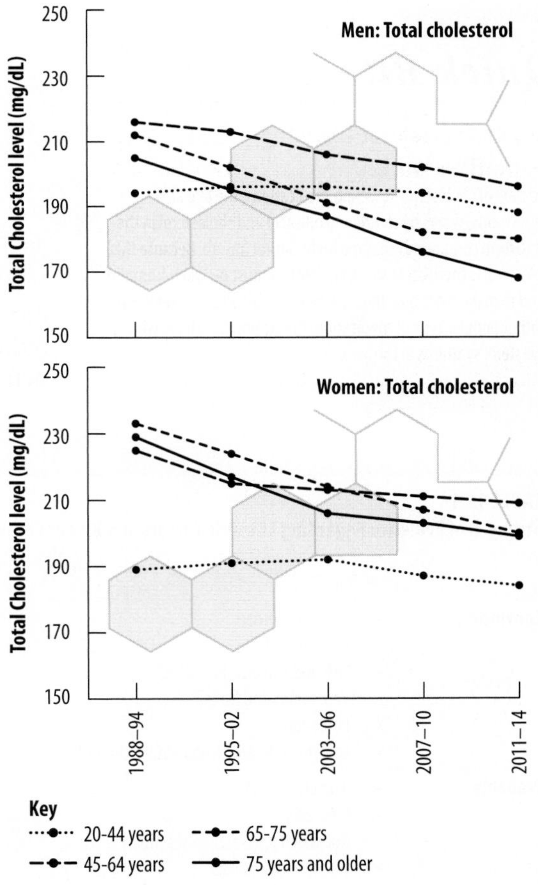

FIGURE 15.6 Trends in age-adjusted mean serum cholesterol. Mean cholesterol levels have been declining since the 1960s, along with a decline in death rates from coronary heart disease.

Reproduced from National Center for Health Statistics. Health, United States, 2015: With Special Feature on Racial and Ethnic Health Disparities. Hyattsville, MD. 2016. http://www.cdc.gov/nchs/data/hus/hus15.pdf#055 Accessed April 30, 2016 [Note: See page 207].

Quick Bite

Who Discovered Atherosclerosis?

Leonardo da Vinci offered the first detailed analysis of diseased blood vessels and was also the first to attribute this pathology to diet.

indicators (handgrip, walking speed, and pulmonary peak flow), are valuable tools for identifying elderly individuals who are vulnerable to heart disease.[22]

Key Concepts Cardiovascular disease is the leading cause of death in the United States and Canada. CVD is significantly related to unhealthy aspects of the North American lifestyle, such as smoking, overeating, lack of exercise, high cholesterol levels, and uncontrolled blood pressure. An infection caused by bacteria or viruses can also lead to heart disease. The body releases C-reactive protein (CRP) in response to acute injury, infection, or other inflammatory stimuli; CRP levels might be predictive of heart disease risk.

Risk Factors for Atherosclerosis

▶ **risk factors** Anything that increases a person's chance of developing a disease, including substances, agents, genetic alterations, traits, habits, or conditions.

Risk factors are conditions or behaviors that increase your likelihood of developing a disease. When you have more than one risk factor for atherosclerosis, your chance of having a heart attack or stroke greatly multiplies. Fortunately, most heart disease risk factors are largely within your control. Risk factors for atherosclerosis that are under your control include:

- High blood pressure
- High blood cholesterol
- Cigarette smoking
- Diabetes
- Overweight
- Physical inactivity

Risk factors beyond your control include:

- Age (45 or older for men; 55 or older for women)
- Family history of early heart disease (having a mother or sister who has been diagnosed with heart disease before age 65, or a father or brother diagnosed before age 55)

TABLE 15.1 shows not only factors associated with increased risk of cardiovascular disease, but also factors that can decrease risk. Focusing on risk reduction factors is an important public health strategy for reducing the burden of atherosclerosis in the United States and Canada.

Quick Bite

How Do Cholesterol-Lowering Medications Work?

One class of cholesterol-lowering medications, the bile acid sequestrants, works by combining bile acid and cholesterol in the gut to form compounds that the body cannot absorb. Because this cholesterol is then lost in feces, cholesterol must be taken from the blood to make more bile, thus lowering the blood cholesterol level. Another popular type of medication, the statins, interferes with cholesterol synthesis in the liver.

TABLE 15.1
Strength of Evidence Regarding Lifestyle Factors and Risk of Cardiovascular Disease

	Decreased Risk	No Relationship	Increased Risk
Convincing	• Regular exercise • Linoleic acid • Fish and fish oils (EPA, DHA) • Vegetables and fruits • Potassium • Low to moderate alcohol intake (for CHD)	• Vitamin E supplements	• Myristic and palmitic acid (saturated fatty acids) • Trans fatty acids • High sodium intake • Overweight • High alcohol intake (for stroke) • Smoking
Probable	• α-linolenic acid • Oleic acid • Nonstarch polysaccharides (fiber) • Whole-grain cereals • Nuts (unsalted) • Plant sterols/stanols • Folate	• Stearic acid	• Dietary cholesterol • Unfiltered boiled coffee

EPA: eicosapentaenoic acid
DHA: docosahexaenoic acid
CHD: coronary heart disease

Modified from Technical Report Series 916, *Diet, Nutrition and the Prevention of Chronic Diseases: A Report of a Joint WHO/FAO Expert Consultation.*

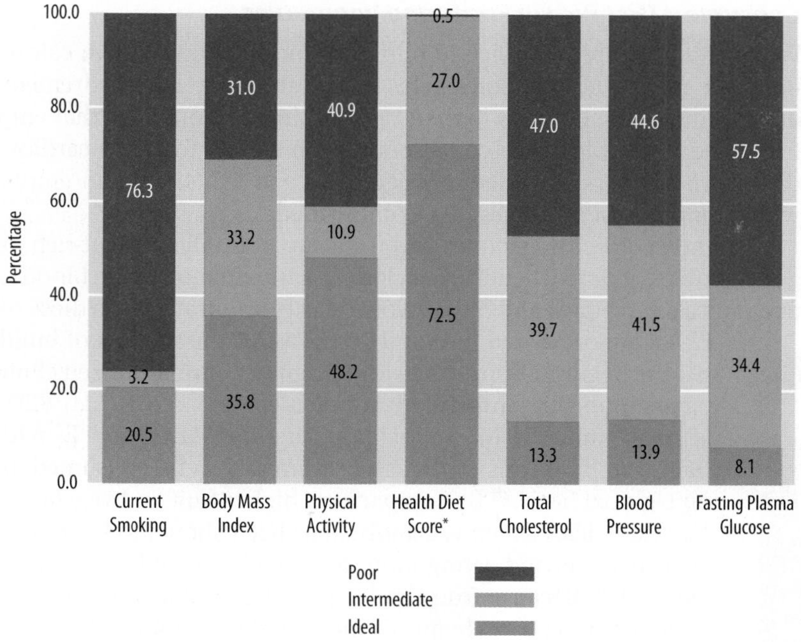

FIGURE 15.7 Life's Simple 7. Among the seven goals for cardiovascular health set by the American Heart Association, U.S. adults aged ≥ 20 years have the worst results for eating a healthy diet.

Go AS, Mozaffarian D, Roger V, et al. Heart Disease and Stroke Statistics—2014 Update *Circulation.* 2014;129:e28–e292.

Dietary and Lifestyle Factors for Reducing Atherosclerosis Risk

The diet and lifestyle recommendations of the American Heart Association (AHA) are part of a comprehensive plan to reduce the incidence of atherosclerosis and are appropriate for anyone over the age of 2 years. The AHA has proposed "The 2020 Impact Goal: By 2020, to improve the cardiovascular health of all Americans by 20 percent while reducing deaths from cardiovascular diseases and stroke by 20 percent." The AHA defines "ideal cardiovascular health" as the absence of disease and the presence of seven key health factors and behaviors called Life's Simple 7.[23] Unfortunately, U.S. adults have the poorest score on the factor for an overall healthy diet (Healthy Diet Score). See **FIGURE 15.7**.

The seven goals are (1) consuming an overall healthy diet, (2) aiming for a healthy body weight (defined as a body mass index [BMI] of 18.5 to 24.9 kg/m^2), (3) aiming for a desirable lipid profile as defined by the National Cholesterol Education Program (NCEP) of the National Heart, Lung, and Blood Institute (NHLBI) (see **TABLE 15.2**), (4) aiming for a normal blood pressure, (5) aiming for a normal blood glucose level, (6) being physically active, and (7) avoiding use of and exposure to tobacco products. Specific AHA recommendations, along with other diet and lifestyle factors related to cardiovascular disease risk reduction, are summarized in the following subsections.

Balance Calorie Intake and Physical Activity to Achieve or Maintain a Healthy Body Weight

Obesity is an independent risk factor for cardiovascular disease, and weight gain during the teen years and in adulthood is associated with increased risk of heart disease.[24] In an effort to avoid weight gain, calorie intake needs to match calorie output. Awareness of the calorie content of foods and beverages and control of portion sizes are major steps toward calorie control.

Physical activity helps reduce cardiovascular disease. Current recommendations suggest engaging in a minimum of 30 minutes of moderate-intensity activity on most days of the week; more activity would reduce heart disease risk further.

TABLE 15.2
Adult Blood Cholesterol and Triglyceride Levels

Total	
Cholesterol	**LDL Cholesterol**
Desirable	< 200
Optimal	< 100
Borderline high	200–239
Near or above optimal	100–129
High	≥ 240
Borderline high	130–159
High	160–189
Very high	≥ 190
Triglyceride	**HDL Cholesterol**
Normal	< 150
Low	< 40
Borderline high	150–199
High	≥ 60
High	200–499
Very high	≥ 500

Note: All units are mg/dL.

Data from National Cholesterol Education Program. *Third Report of the Expert Panel on Detection, Evaluation, and Treatment of High Blood Cholesterol in Adults (Adult Treatment Panel III), Final Report.* Washington, DC: U.S. Department of Health and Human Services; 2003. NIH publication 02-5215.

Consume a Diet Rich in Fruits and Vegetables

Fruits and vegetables are rich in nutrients and fiber and low in calories. Eating more fruits and vegetables helps meet nutrient intake requirements without overindulging in foods high in calories. In addition, diets that emphasize fruits and vegetables have consistently been shown to lower cardiovascular disease risk factors. A variety of vegetables and fruits, with an emphasis on whole, unprocessed sources, is recommended.

Brightly colored vegetables and fruits are not only nutrient-rich, but also good sources of phytochemicals, including antioxidants. In the blood, oxygen free radicals can attack and oxidize low-density lipoproteins; as these oxidized LDLs are deposited in blood vessel walls, the process of building up plaque begins. Despite the lack of significant randomized clinical trial data supporting antioxidant supplement use, more than $20 billion is spent annually on antioxidant vitamins A, C, and E, with more than 6 million tons of the latter estimated to be consumed annually on a global basis.[25] By comparison, higher fruit and vegetable intake, especially leafy green vegetables, has been shown to lower the risk of heart disease, and eating more fruits and vegetables is highly recommended.[26] Because fruits and vegetables contain so many vitamins, minerals, and phytochemicals that could be working alone or in combination, diets rich in a variety of fruits and vegetables—sources of antioxidant vitamins and other antioxidant compounds—continue to constitute a cornerstone of dietary recommendations.[27]

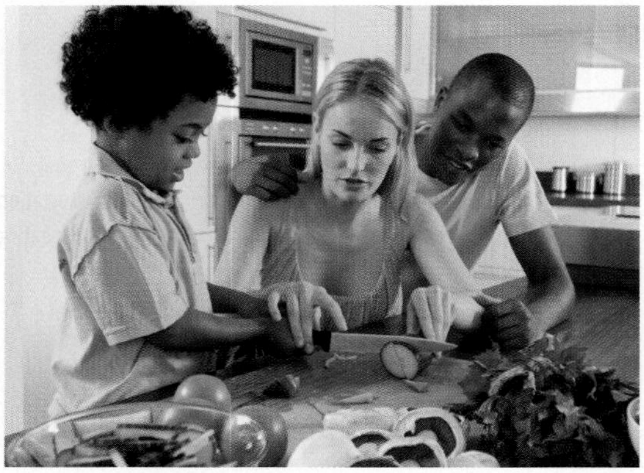

Choose Whole-Grain, High-Fiber Foods

Diets that emphasize whole grains and other foods rich in fiber have been linked to improved overall diet quality and reduced cardiovascular disease risk.[28] Certain types of fiber can bind to bile acids in the gastrointestinal tract. These bile acids are excreted in the feces rather than recycled and reused. Additional bile acids must then be made from cholesterol, lowering the total amount in the body. In the large intestine, intestinal bacteria partially digest fiber and then produce short-chain fatty acids, some of which may reduce cholesterol synthesis.[29] The Adequate Intake (AI) level for fiber (14 grams per 1,000 kilocalories) is based on the amount of fiber that has been shown to reduce CVD risk.[30] Despite U.S. Food and Drug Administration (FDA) approval of health claims for fiber supplements, whether these supplements can provide protection against CVD similar to that provided by whole-grain foods remains controversial.[31]

Consume Fish, Especially Oily Fish, at Least Twice a Week

In the 1970s, a study of the Inuits (Greenland Eskimos) focused attention on the beneficial effects of eicosapentaenoic acid (EPA) and docosahexaenoic acid (DHA), the omega-3 fatty acids in fish fats.[32] Researchers were puzzled: This group of people had a high intake of fat, saturated fat, and cholesterol from marine mammals and fish, yet they showed little evidence of atherosclerosis. The Inuits were compared with the Danes, among whom atherosclerosis was common and whose diet was similarly high in fat, but from meats and dairy products. It became clear that the high EPA and DHA content of fish in the Inuit diet protects against heart disease by discouraging blood cells from clotting and from sticking to artery walls, and by reducing inflammation. Studies of other groups have since shown similar results. The Japanese, for example, with their generous fish intake, have low rates of atherosclerosis. Many other studies point in the same direction; some show that as few as two or three servings of fish weekly can be protective.

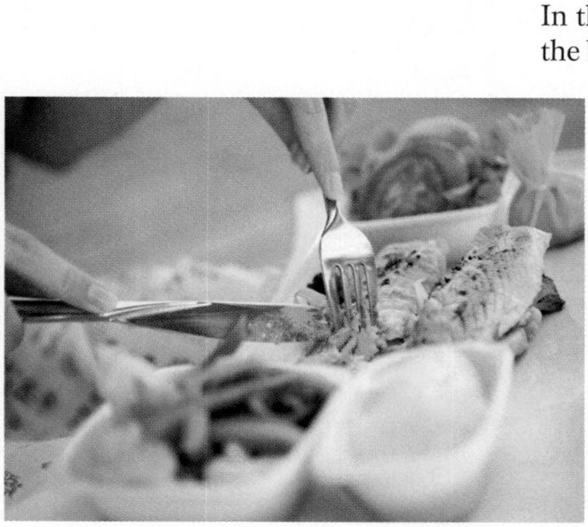

Nutrition Science *in Action*

Multi-Ethnic Study of Atherosclerosis

Background

Elevated blood cholesterol levels, specifically high levels of low-density lipoprotein cholesterol (LDL-C) have been associated with an increased risk of cardiovascular disease (CVD). High dietary intake of most saturated fatty acids is associated with elevated levels of blood total cholesterol and LDL-C. Clinical trials have shown that replacing saturated fatty acids with mono- and polyunsaturated fatty acids reduces cholesterol levels and therefore CVD risk. However, not all scientific literature supports a relationship between dietary saturated fatty acids intake and CVD risk. It is plausible that this is the result of differences in the dietary source of saturated fatty acids being examined.

Hypothesis

Meat saturated fatty acids will be positively associated with CVD, whereas dairy and plant saturated fatty acids will be unassociated or inversely associated with CVD.

Experimental Plan

Recruit healthy adults (ages 45–84 years) from various U.S. communities. Exclude participants with a clinical diagnosis of CVD or type 2 diabetes, daily energy intakes of less than 600 or more than 6,000 kilocalories per day, and who did not return for examination after baseline. Obtain average food consumption using a food frequency questionnaire, and use these data to calculate nutrient intake. Assess CVD incidents during follow-up visits conducted over a 10-year period (2000 to 2010).

Results

After adjustment for confounding variables, a higher intake of meat saturated fatty acids was associated with a greater CVD risk. In contrast, a higher intake of dairy saturated fatty acids was associated with a lower CVD risk. The substitution of 2 percent of energy from meat saturated fatty acids with energy from dairy saturated fatty acids was associated with a 25 percent lower CVD risk. No association was seen between plant or butter saturated fatty acids and CVD risk. This might have been related to relatively low consumption of saturated fatty acids from these food sources, which may have limited the statistical power to detect any association.

Conclusion and Discussion

Associations between saturated fatty acids and incident CVD depend on the food source. It is plausible that the difference in risk for CVD recognized among the meat, dairy, and plant sources of saturated fatty acids is related to the saturated fatty acid profile of these foods. It is also possible that the beneficial nutrients contained in dairy and plant foods might counterbalance the negative physiological effects of saturated fatty acids.

Data from De Oliveira Otto MC, Mozaffarian D, Kromhout D, et al. Dietary intake of saturated fat by food source and incident cardiovascular disease: the Multi-Ethnic Study of Atherosclerosis. *Am J Clin Nutr.* 2012;96:397–404.

Quick Bite

Hardy Hearts

By the end of a normal life span, the human heart has pumped more than 3 billion times. Despite this heavy use, heart failures are usually caused by heart attacks or problems with blood vessels and valves; heart muscle itself rarely wears out.

Fish is a good source of omega-3 fatty acids, which decrease risk of abnormal heartbeats that can lead to sudden deaths. Omega-3 fatty acids also decrease triglyceride levels, slow the rate of atherosclerosis, and slightly reduce blood pressure.[33] Although consumption of foods rich in omega-3 fatty acids reduces CVD risk, the potential benefits from consuming omega-3 fatty acid supplements is less clear. A large review of data from 20 trials that included more than 60,000 people and more than 6,000 major cardiovascular events questions the use of fish oil supplements for the prevention of CVD.[34]

All in all, there are certainly enough positive results to encourage further study and recommend regular consumption of cold-water fish (e.g., salmon, cod) for EPA and DHA as well as plant foods with alpha-linolenic acid.[35]

Controversy: Limiting Your Intake of Saturated and Trans Fat and Cholesterol

A major, but controversial, study questions the link between saturated fat and heart disease. The analysis included 27 clinical trials and 49 observational studies, totaling more than 600,000 participants. It concluded that "current evidence does not clearly support cardiovascular guidelines that encourage high consumption of polyunsaturated fatty acids and low consumption of total saturated fats."[36] The findings on omega-3 fatty acids and trans fats were mixed.

On the other hand, an extensive review and new guidelines released by the American College of Cardiology and the American Heart Association found strong evidence linking saturated fat and heart disease.[37] Still, modifying fat composition is less important than BMI, aging, and gender. In cross-sectional studies, differences in saturated fat intake accounted for only about 5 percent of the variance in blood cholesterol levels. The bottom line? Rather than focusing on a single dietary component, dietitians recommend that you "consume a heart-healthy diet that emphasizes vegetables, fruits and whole grains; includes low-fat dairy products, poultry, fish, legumes, nontropical vegetable oils and nuts; and limits intake of sweets, sugar-sweetened beverages and red meats."[38]

Although saturated fat can raise total and "bad" LDL cholesterol, it also *raises* "good" HDL cholesterol. By comparison, trans fats raise total and "bad" LDL cholesterol while *lowering* "good" HDL cholesterol. The American Heart Association recommends limiting saturated fat intake to less than 5 to 6 percent of total calories and trans fat intake to less than 1 percent.[39] (The *Dietary Guidelines* recommends keeping trans fat intake "as low as possible.")

Research shows that consuming monounsaturated fats, such as olive oil, lowers total and LDL cholesterol without lowering HDL.[40] This positive effect of olive oil may partially explain why Greeks, Turks, Italians, and others around the Mediterranean who eat a traditional diet higher in fat still have low rates of heart disease. The multicenter PREDIMED study found that a Mediterranean diet is linked to a reduced risk of heart disease and cognitive decline.[41] Defining a Mediterranean diet has been challenging. A meta-analysis of 41 prospective cohort studies with a total of 2.9 million participants attempted to calculate optimal daily intakes of most of the key components of a Mediterranean diet. This analysis identified the following average daily consumptions as optimal:[42]

- *Dairy products:* 5.8 oz for men, 7 oz for women
- *Fruit:* 5 oz for men, 4.4 oz for women
- *Vegetables:* 4.4 oz for men, 5 oz for women
- *Cereals/grains:* 4.6 oz for men, 4.4 oz for women
- *Meat:* 2.7 oz for men and women
- *Fish:* 0.7 oz for men, 0.9 oz for women
- *Legumes:* 0.35 oz for men and women

The overall diet pattern seems to model AHA recommendations. An average of 0.7 to 0.9 ounce of fish daily, for example, is about two 3-ounce servings per week (as is recommended by the AHA). Specific amounts were not identified for red wine, olive oil, or nuts, which also are important components of a Mediterranean diet. Moderate consumption of alcohol may account for about one-fourth or more of the positive health benefit.[43,44] Consistently favorable results from both epidemiological and intervention studies have made the Mediterranean diet popular.

What about cholesterol intake? Because our bodies can make all the cholesterol they need, cholesterol is not essential in the diet. According to the Dietary Guidelines for Americans 2015–2020: "More research is needed regarding the dose-response relationship between dietary cholesterol and blood cholesterol levels. Adequate evidence is not available for a quantitative limit for dietary cholesterol specific to the *Dietary Guidelines*."[45]

Minimize Your Intake of Beverages and Foods That Contain Added Sugars

Added sugar intake in the United States has risen dramatically in the last 20 years. Reducing consumption of added sugars helps to improve the nutrient quality of the diet and also reduces calorie intake. Paying attention to sources of added sugars will help individuals achieve weight goals.

Choose and Prepare Foods with Little or No Salt

Hypertension is a major risk factor for cardiovascular disease, and generally, blood pressure rises as salt intake rises. Further discussion of salt, sodium, other minerals, and blood pressure follows in the section "Hypertension" later in this chapter. The AHA suggests that reducing sodium intake to 2,300 milligrams (about 1 teaspoon of salt) per day or less is an achievable goal.

If You Consume Alcohol, Do So in Moderation

Moderate alcohol consumption is associated with a substantial decrease in heart disease risk.[46] However, alcohol is addictive, and high intake can have adverse effects on the body. So, the AHA recommends limiting alcohol intake to no more than one drink per day for women and two drinks per day for men, ideally with meals.

The positive effects of alcohol on heart disease risk provide at least a partial explanation for the "French paradox," the fact that the French eat rich cheeses and fatty meats, yet still have low rates of heart disease. They also have relatively high intakes of fruits, vegetables, and red wine—all rich sources of antioxidant phytochemicals. The active compound of the French paradox was recently identified to be a compound called resveratrol. In addition to its heart-protective effects, resveratrol also may have anticancer, anti-inflammatory, and antiaging benefits.

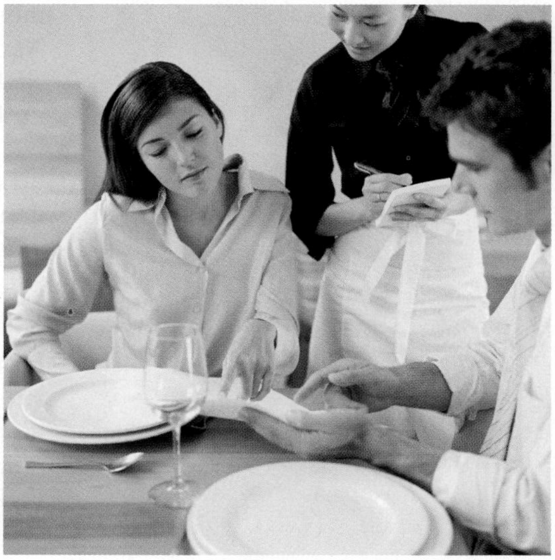
© Stockbyte/Thinkstock

When You Eat Food That Is Prepared Outside of the Home, Follow the AHA's Diet and Lifestyle Recommendations

More and more of our meals are either eaten away from home or brought home as takeout food. All too often, our choices away from home are high in fat, added sugars, and sodium and low in fiber, fruits, and vegetables. Also, portion sizes at restaurants are typically more than those recommended by MyPlate. Consumers need to make wise choices both at home and away from home. Splitting entrée portions with a companion, choosing steamed vegetables instead of a loaded baked potato, or substituting a salad with low-fat dressing for french

TABLE 15.3
Heart Healthy Tips for Dining Out

Are you able to stick to your low-saturated-fat, low-cholesterol diet when eating out? If not, you will be able to if you follow these tips:

- Choose restaurants that have low-saturated-fat, low-cholesterol menu choices. Don't be afraid to make special requests—it's your right as a paying customer.
- Control serving sizes by asking for a side-dish or appetizer-size serving, sharing a dish with a companion, or taking some home.
- Ask that gravy, butter, rich sauces, and salad dressing be served on the side. That way, you can control the amount of saturated fat and cholesterol that you eat.
- Ask to substitute a salad or baked potato for chips, fries, coleslaw, or other extras—or just ask that the extras be left off your plate.
- When ordering pizza, order vegetable toppings such as green pepper, onions, and mushrooms instead of meat or extra cheese. To make your pizza even lower in saturated fat and cholesterol, order it with half the cheese or no cheese.
- At fast food restaurants, go for salads, grilled (not fried or breaded) skinless chicken sandwiches, regular-sized hamburgers, or roast beef sandwiches. Go easy on the regular salad dressings and fatty sauces. Limit your consumption of jumbo or deluxe burgers, sandwiches, french fries, and other foods.

Reading the Menu

- Choose low-saturated-fat, low-cholesterol cooking methods. Look for terms such as the following: steamed, in its own juice (au jus), garden fresh, broiled, baked, roasted, poached, tomato juice, dry boiled (in wine or lemon juice), and lightly sautéed or lightly stir-fried.
- Be aware of dishes that are high in saturated fat and cholesterol. Watch out for terms such as the following: butter sauce, fried, crispy, creamed, in cream or cheese sauce, au gratin, au fromage, escalloped, Parmesan, hollandaise, béarnaise, marinated (in oil), stewed, basted, sautéed, stir-fried, casserole, hash, prime, pot pie, pastry crust.

Courtesy of National Heart, Lung, and Blood Institute.

fries will help individuals follow the AHA guidelines. For more tips for heart-healthy choices when dining out, see **TABLE 15.3**.

Other Dietary Factors

The B vitamins folate, and B_6 and B_{12} are involved in pathways that convert one amino acid, homocysteine, to another amino acid, methionine. As noted earlier, high levels of homocysteine can contribute to heart disease by promoting atherosclerosis, excessive blood clotting, or blood vessel rigidity. Folate and vitamins B_6 and B_{12} can help reduce destructive levels of homocysteine. Scientists believe that consuming a diet rich in fruits, vegetables, and low-fat dairy products—such as the DASH diet, which is also rich in these vitamins—helps lower blood homocysteine and therefore reduce risk of heart disease.[47]

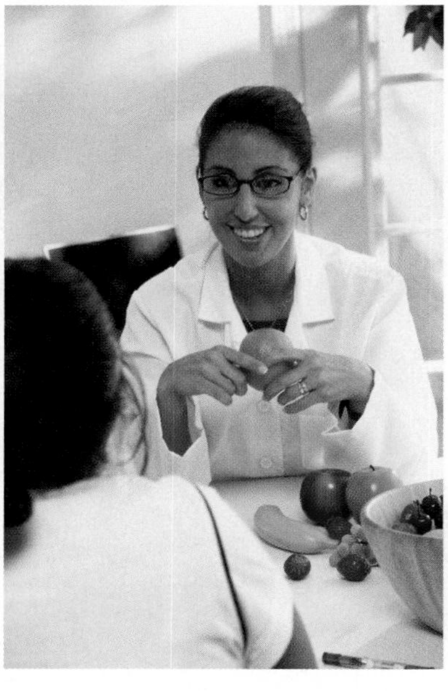

© LiquidLibrary/Thinkstock

Soy Soy-based foods, such as soy milks, soy burgers, tofu, and tempeh, have become popular items in grocery stores. In October 1999, the FDA approved labeling for foods containing soy protein as protective against coronary heart disease. Since then, many well-controlled studies on soy protein substantially added to our scientific knowledge base. The American Heart Association Nutrition Committee reevaluated the evidence on soy protein and found that the direct cardiovascular health benefit of soy protein is minimal at best.[48] In their assessment of 22 randomized trials, the AHA Nutrition Committee found that isolated soy protein with isoflavones (ISF) slightly lowered LDL cholesterol in hyperlipidemic people and had no effect on HDL cholesterol, triglycerides, lipoprotein a, or blood pressure.[49]

Other components in soybeans can provide favorable effects. Because many soy products have a high content of polyunsaturated fats, fiber, vitamins, and minerals and low content of saturated fat, these foods are part of a heart-healthy diet.

Putting It All Together

Healthy People 2020 objectives target reducing deaths from heart disease and stroke as well as reducing the number of adults with high blood cholesterol levels. To accomplish these goals, dietitians recommend lowering total fat intake, maintaining a healthy body weight, and exercising on a regular basis. Eating fruits, vegetables, legumes, and grains that contain fiber helps lower cholesterol levels, too. These foods contain antioxidants and B vitamins, such as B_6 and folate, that also may reduce the risk of heart disease. Substituting fish or soy foods for high-fat meats and cheeses and choosing low-fat dairy products can be beneficial as well.

Key Concepts To reduce your risk of heart disease, get regular exercise, control your weight, and don't smoke. Dietary changes you can make to reduce your heart disease risk include eating less fat and cholesterol while increasing intake of fruits, vegetables, and whole grains. Look for sources of omega-3 fatty acids and fiber in your food choices.

Hypertension

Persistent high blood pressure (**hypertension**) often is called a "silent killer" because, although it usually has no specific symptoms or early warning signs and appears as no threat, it can kill you. You can be hypertensive for years without realizing it. During those years, untreated hypertension can cause damage to vital organs, particularly the heart, the brain, the kidneys, and the eyes. It increases the risk of heart attack, congestive heart failure, stroke, and kidney failure. In 2011–2012, more than 7 percent of adults ages 18–39 and almost 33 percent of adults ages 40–59 were hypertensive; for those older than age 60, the prevalence of hypertension was 65 percent. Hypertension currently affects nearly 78 million adults in the United States.[50,51] The good news is that hypertension can be treated and controlled.

THINK About It 2

▶ **hypertension** When resting blood pressure persistently exceeds 140 mm Hg systolic or 90 mm Hg diastolic.

What Is Blood Pressure?

Blood pressure is the force exerted by the blood on the walls of the blood vessels, especially the arteries. This force is created by the pumping action of the heart. Every time the heart contracts, or beats (systole), blood pressure increases. When the heart relaxes between beats (diastole), the pressure decreases. Blood pressure can fluctuate considerably, depending on various factors. When you are excited, afraid, or exercising, for example, your heart pumps more blood into your arteries and your blood pressure rises. Blood pressure rises and falls during the day. When it stays elevated over time, it's called hypertension.

Blood pressure is measured using a **sphygmomanometer** (blood pressure cuff) (see **FIGURE 15.8**) and is expressed as two numbers. The **systolic** pressure is the higher number and represents pressure during the heart's contraction. The

▶ **blood pressure** The pressure of blood against the walls of a blood vessel or heart chamber. Unless there is reference to another location, such as the pulmonary artery or one of the heart chambers, this term refers to the pressure in the systemic arteries, as measured, for example, in the forearm.

▶ **sphygmomanometer** [sfig-mo-ma-NOM-eh-ter] An instrument for measuring blood pressure and especially arterial blood pressure.

▶ **systolic** Pertaining to a heart contraction. Systolic blood pressure is measured during a heart contraction, a time period known as systole.

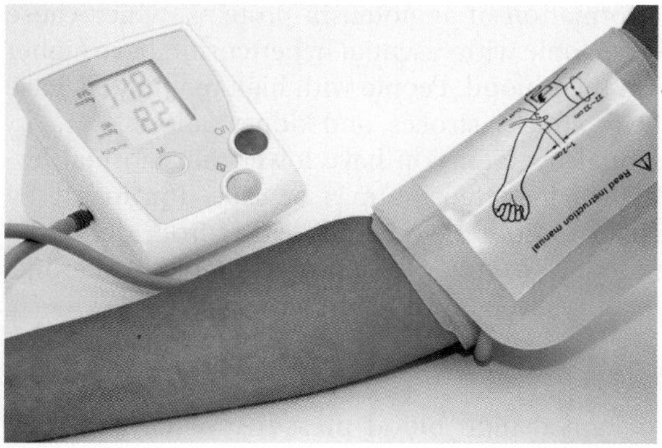

(A)

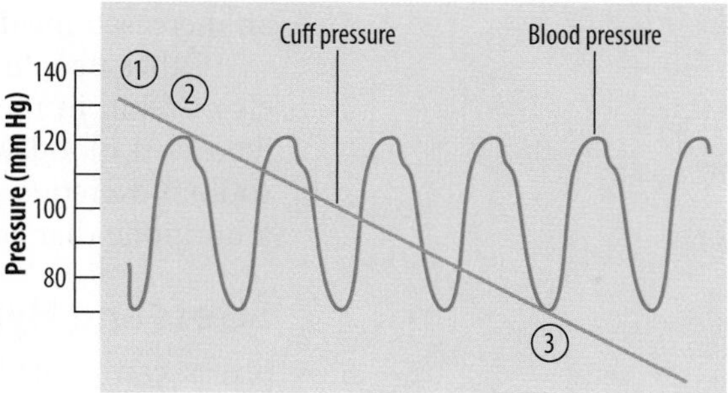

(B)

FIGURE 15.8 Blood pressure reading. (A) A sphygmomanometer (blood pressure cuff) is used to determine blood pressure. (B) As shown, the blood pressure rises and falls with each contraction of the heart.

1. When the pressure in the cuff exceeds the arterial peak pressure, blood flow stops. No sound is heard.
2. As cuff pressure is gradually released, a sound can be heard when pressure in the cuff falls below the peak arterial pressure. At this point, called systolic pressure, blood begins flowing through the artery again.
3. As cuff pressure continues to drop, the sound stops when the cuff pressure is equal to the lowest pressure in the artery. At this point, called the diastolic pressure, the artery is fully open.

TABLE 15.4
Blood Pressure Classifications for Adults

Blood Pressure Category	Systolic mm Hg (upper #)		Diastolic mm Hg (lower #)
Normal	less than **120**	and	less than **80**
Prehypertension	**120–139**	or	**80–89**
High Blood Pressure (Hypertension) **Stage 1**	**140–159**	or	**90–99**
High Blood Pressure (Hypertension) **Stage 2**	**160** or higher	or	**100** or higher
Hypertensive Crisis (Emergency care needed)	Higher than **180**	or	Higher than **110**

American Heart Association. Understanding blood pressure readings. http://www.heart.org/HEARTORG/Conditions/HighBloodPressure/AboutHighBloodPressure/Understanding-Blood-Pressure-Readings_UCM_301764_Article.jsp. Accessed February 11, 2016.

▶ **diastolic** Pertaining to the time between heart contractions, a period known as diastole. Diastolic blood pressure is measured at the point of maximum cardiac relaxation.

diastolic pressure is the lower number, measured during the heart's resting phase. Normal blood pressure is defined as a systolic pressure less than 120 mm Hg (millimeters mercury) and a diastolic pressure less than 80 mm Hg.

What Is Hypertension?

Hypertension is a medical condition with chronic high blood pressure (see **TABLE 15.4**). Hypertension is classified as either primary (essential) hypertension or secondary hypertension. Most cases of hypertension (about 90 percent) are **essential hypertension**, which is defined by the lack of an obvious cause. Essential hypertension most likely has many contributing factors, including diet, obesity, alcohol abuse, lack of exercise, physical and emotional stress, and psychological and genetic factors. When hypertension results from another problem, such as a kidney defect, it is called **secondary hypertension**. In secondary hypertension, blood pressure usually returns to normal when the underlying defect is corrected.

▶ **essential hypertension** Hypertension for which no specific cause can be identified. Ninety to 95 percent of people with hypertension have essential hypertension.

▶ **secondary hypertension** Hypertension caused by an underlying condition such as a kidney disorder. Once the underlying condition is treated, the blood pressure usually returns to normal.

Renin and Hypertension

The enzyme renin is associated with some cases of essential hypertension. This enzyme promotes the formation of angiotensin proteins, which cause the arteries to constrict. Some people with essential hypertension have higher than normal levels of renin in their blood. People with high renin levels have an increased incidence of heart attacks, strokes, and kidney failure.

Other people with essential hypertension have lower than normal levels of renin in their blood. Their hypertension may be caused primarily by increased blood volume. This condition could result either from decreased sodium excretion by the kidneys or from increased secretion of aldosterone, a hormone that causes the kidneys to retain sodium and water.

Stress and Hypertension

Stress can contribute to sustained high blood pressure. When stressors, either internal or external, activate the sympathetic nervous system, heart rate increases, arteries constrict, and the blood exerts greater force on the artery walls. Chronic stress has been implicated in heart disease.

Risk Factors for Hypertension

Even though the cause for most cases of hypertension is unknown, several factors clearly contribute to hypertension. As with heart disease risk, some hypertension risk factors are controllable and others are uncontrollable. Risk factors for hypertension under your control include the following:

- *Obesity:* People with a BMI of 30 kg/m^2 or higher are more likely to develop high blood pressure.
- *Eating too much salt:* High sodium intake increases blood pressure in some people.
- *Lack of physical activity:* A sedentary lifestyle is associated with overweight and increased blood pressure.
- *Drinking too much alcohol:* Heavy and regular use of alcohol increases blood pressure.

Risk factors for hypertension that are beyond your control include the following:

- *Race:* African Americans develop high blood pressure more often, at earlier ages, and with more severity than Caucasians do.[52]
- *Age:* Blood pressure risk rises with age; people with normal blood pressure at age 55 have a 90 percent lifetime risk of developing hypertension.[53]
- *Heredity:* Family history of hypertension is a strong predictive factor.

Dietary and Lifestyle Factors for Reducing Hypertension

The American Heart Association has guidelines for dietary approaches to prevent and treat hypertension.[54] They direct you to do the following:

- Maintain normal body weight for adults (BMI 18.5–24.9 kg/m^2).
- Reduce dietary sodium intake to no more than 3,800 milligrams of sodium chloride or 1,500 milligrams of sodium per day.
- Engage in regular aerobic physical activity, such as brisk walking, at least 30 minutes per day most days of the week.
- Limit alcohol consumption to no more than 2 drinks per day for most men and no more than 1 drink per day for most women.
- Consume a diet rich in fruits and vegetables (8–10 servings per day), low-fat dairy products (2–3 servings per day), and foods with a reduced content of saturated and total fat (DASH-like eating plan).

Sodium

Excess sodium can hold excessive fluid in the body, at least temporarily. These excesses can be burdensome on the kidneys, heart, and blood vessels. The consensus among heart disease experts is that too much sodium, ingested routinely over the years, plays a role in the underlying causes of hypertension in genetically predisposed or "salt-sensitive" people. The more salt they eat, the higher their blood pressure.

Population studies appear to confirm this conclusion. Rates of hypertension are higher in countries with high sodium intakes. On the other hand, indigenous people, whose diets contain very little sodium, seldom have hypertension. If they continue to eat their traditional diet, their blood pressure does not rise with age. If they adopt a "modern" (higher-sodium) diet, however, their blood pressure tends to rise, and they are more likely to become hypertensive. In a multiethnic sample, for those born outside the United States, each 10 years of living in the United States has been associated with a higher prevalence of hypertension.[55]

Other Dietary Factors

Sodium is not the only dietary factor associated with hypertension. Excess weight tends to raise blood pressure; regular exercise and weight loss help to

Quick Bite

The Salt Wars

Salt was so precious historically that battles were fought over access to it. Of warring German tribes, the Roman historian Tacitus wrote, "These Chatti and Hermanduri! They fight bloody wars over who shall possess a salt 'stream.'" In Roman times, soldiers were paid a special allowance to buy salt. This allowance was called a *salarium*, which gives us the word *salary*.

reduce blood pressure. Reducing consumption of alcohol also tends to reduce blood pressure and improves the effectiveness of antihypertensive medications. Eating a diet rich in calcium, magnesium, and potassium reduces blood pressure as well.[56] The mechanism by which these minerals act on hypertension in part reflects their interrelationship with sodium metabolism.

The DASH Diet

▶ **DASH (Dietary Approaches to Stop Hypertension)** An eating plan low in total fat, saturated fat, and cholesterol and rich in fruits, vegetables, and low-fat dairy products that has been shown to reduce elevated blood pressure.

The original **DASH (Dietary Approaches to Stop Hypertension)** study, a multicenter NHLBI-sponsored trial, tested the effects of different dietary patterns on blood pressure. After a control period, the 459 subjects in this study received one of three diets for an eight-week period[57]:

- *Control diet:* Macronutrient and fiber content equal to U.S. average; 4 servings of fruits and vegetables per day; 0.5 serving of dairy products per day; potassium, magnesium, and calcium levels close to the 25th percentile of U.S. consumption
- *Fruit and vegetable diet:* 8.5 servings of fruits and vegetables per day; potassium and magnesium levels at the 75th percentile of U.S. consumption; other nutrients similar to control diet
- *Combination diet:* 10 servings of fruits and vegetables per day; 2.7 servings of low-fat dairy products per day; less fat, saturated fat, and cholesterol than control diet; potassium, magnesium, and calcium levels at the 75th percentile of U.S. consumption

The sodium content of the diets averaged about 3,000 milligrams per day. The study excluded subjects who were taking antihypertensive medications, unless their physicians had given them permission to discontinue their medication for the course of the study.[58] **TABLE 15.5** shows sample meals from the three DASH diets used in the study.

Both the fruit and vegetable diet and the combination diet significantly lowered the systolic and diastolic blood pressure in all subjects and in

Quick Bite

What Smells in Blood Pressure?

A family of complex cell receptors, some of which play a role in the nose detecting odors, has been found to be involved in the kidneys' integration of signals from gut microbes and the regulation of blood pressure. This discovery identifies a previously unknown connection among the gut, kidneys, and cardiovascular systems.

TABLE 15.5
Sample Menus from the DASH Study

Meal	Control Diet	Fruit and Vegetable Diet	DASH Combination Diet
Breakfast	• Apple juice • Sugar-frosted flakes • White toast • Butter • Jelly • Whole milk	• Orange juice • Oat bran muffin • Raisins • Dried apricots • Butter	• Orange juice • Granola bar • Fat-free yogurt • 1% low-fat milk • Banana
Lunch	• Ham-and-chicken sandwich on white bread, with lettuce, pickles, mustard, and mayonnaise • Fruit cocktail	• Ham-and-Swiss cheese sandwich on whole-wheat bread • Banana	• Smoked turkey sandwich on whole-wheat bread with lettuce and mayonnaise • Fresh orange
Dinner	• Spiced cod • Scallion rice • Carrots • Butter • French rolls	• Spiced cod • Scallion rice • Lima beans • Butter • Dinner rolls • Melon balls	• Spiced cod • Scallion rice • Spinach • Margarine • Dinner rolls • Melon balls • 1% low-fat milk
Snack	• Graham crackers • Vanilla frosting • Tropical fruit punch	• Peanuts	• Peanuts • Dried apricots • Melon balls

Reproduced from Karanja NM, Obarzanek E, Lin P-H, et al. Descriptive characteristics of the dietary patterns used in the Dietary Approaches to Stop Hypertension trial. *J Am Diet Assoc*. 1999;99(Suppl 8):S19–S27.

subgroups analyzed by sex, ethnicity, and hypertensive/normotensive status. For hypertensive individuals, the DASH combination diet lowered blood pressure as much as antihypertensive drugs. Widespread adoption of the DASH eating plan could lead to a downward shift in the incidence and severity of the disease. The NHLBI recommends that all Americans—not just those with hypertension—follow the DASH eating plan.[59]

Results from a follow-up study, the DASH-Sodium trial, support both the DASH-style dietary changes and lower sodium intake. This study used different levels of daily sodium restriction (3,300 mg, 2,400 mg, and 1,500 mg) and two diet plans (a "typical" American diet and the DASH diet). Approximately 41 percent of the participants had hypertension. Reducing sodium intake lowered blood pressure for participants in both dietary treatment arms, but the DASH diet in combination with sodium restriction was more effective than the low-sodium control diet alone.[60]

To help keep blood pressure at healthy levels, the DASH eating plan is rich in potassium. A potassium-rich diet can help to reduce elevated or high blood pressure, but be sure to get your potassium from food sources, not from supplements. Many fruits and vegetables, some milk products, and fish are rich sources of potassium. Because of the additional fruits and vegetables—and therefore the antioxidant nutrients, phytochemicals, and fiber—that people consume while following the DASH diet, the eating plan has the potential to extend beyond cardiovascular benefits.

The major landmark studies on the DASH diet used feeding trials with all food provided to the participants. A review of nine studies found that compliance is generally low when only counseling services were provided without food supplies. Given the health benefits of the DASH diet, studies for improving adherence are warranted.[61]

Putting It All Together

As previously described, hypertension can be controlled and even prevented by making modifications in diet and lifestyle. Blood pressure can be unhealthy even if it stays only slightly above the cutoff level of 120/80 mm Hg. The higher that blood pressure rises above normal, the greater the health risk. Recognition and control of high blood pressure are essential for avoiding damage to vital organs. Checking your blood pressure on a regular basis is the key to detecting this silent killer. Following diet and lifestyle recommendations as suggested by the National High Blood Pressure Education Program, including the DASH eating plan, reducing dietary sodium, and engaging in regular physical activity, can be the key to prevention.

Key Concepts Hypertension is a risk factor for atherosclerosis, kidney disease, and stroke. Blood pressure tends to rise with age, and rates of hypertension are higher among African Americans. Sodium intake affects blood pressure, especially in those individuals who are salt sensitive. Low intake of potassium, calcium, and possibly magnesium also contribute to the development of hypertension. Eating a diet replete with fresh foods and avoiding processed foods will not only improve the balance of minerals in our diet, but also can reduce risk of disease.

Cancer

Cancer is the second leading cause of death in the United States.[62] In fact, one in every four deaths in this country can be attributed to cancer. Reducing both the number of new cancer cases and the death rates from cancer are key objectives of Healthy People 2020. Cancer comprises a group of more than 100 diseases that involve the uncontrolled division of the body's cells. Although it can develop in virtually any of the body's tissues, and each type

▶ **cancer** A term for diseases in which abnormal cells divide without control. Cancer cells can invade nearby tissues and can spread through the bloodstream and lymphatic system to other parts of the body.

of cancer has its unique features, the basic processes that produce cancer are quite similar in all forms of the disease. To understand cancer, it is helpful to know what happens when normal cells become cancerous.

What Is Cancer?

The body consists of many types of cells. Normally, cells grow and divide to produce more cells only when the body needs them. This orderly process helps keep the body healthy. Sometimes, however, cells keep dividing when new cells are not needed. These extra cells form a mass of **tissue**, called a growth or **tumor**.

- **tissue** A group or layer of cells that are alike and that work together to perform a specific function.
- **tumor** An abnormal mass of tissue that results from excessive cell division. Tumors perform no useful body function. They can be benign (not cancerous) or malignant (cancerous).
- **benign** [beh-NINE] Not cancerous; does not invade nearby tissue or spread to other parts of the body.
- **malignant** [ma-LIG-nant] Cancerous; a growth with a tendency to invade and destroy nearby tissue and spread to other parts of the body.
- **metastasis** [meh-TAS-ta-sis] The spread of cancer from one part of the body to another. Tumors formed from cells that have spread are called *secondary tumors* and contain cells that are like those in the original (primary) tumor. The plural is metastases.
- **leukemia** [loo-KEE-mee-a] Cancer of blood-forming tissue.
- **melanocytes** [mel-AN-o-sites] Cells in the skin that produce and contain the pigment called melanin.
- **melanoma** A form of skin cancer that arises in melanocytes, the cells that produce pigment. Melanoma usually begins in a mole.
- **lymphoma** [lim-FO-ma] Cancer that arises in cells of the lymphatic system.

Tumors can be **benign** or **malignant**. Benign tumors are not cancer. They can often be removed and, in most cases, they do not regrow. Cells from benign tumors do not spread to other parts of the body. Most important, benign tumors rarely pose a threat to life. In contrast, malignant tumors are cancerous. Cells in these tumors are abnormal and divide without control or order. As a result, they can invade and damage nearby tissues and organs. Also, cancer cells can break away from a malignant tumor and enter the bloodstream or the lymphatic system. In this way, cancer can spread from the original site to form new tumors in other organs. The spread of cancer is called **metastasis**.

Most cancers are named for the organ or type of cell in which they originate. Cancer that begins in the colon is colon cancer, for example, and cancer that begins in skin cells known as **melanocytes** is called **melanoma**. **Leukemia** and **lymphoma** are cancers that arise in blood-forming cells. The abnormal blood cells circulate in the bloodstream and lymphatic system. They also may invade (infiltrate) body organs and form tumors.

Cancer develops in a multistage process that can take many years. There are typically three phases of development.

1. *Initiation* occurs when something alters a cell's genetic structure and prepares it to act abnormally during later stages.
2. *Promotion*, a reversible stage, occurs when a chemical or other factor encourages initiated cells to become active.
3. *Progression* occurs when promoted cells multiply and perhaps invade surrounding healthy tissue.

When cancer spreads (metastasizes), cancer cells are often found in nearby or regional **lymph nodes** (sometimes called lymph glands). If the cancer has reached these nodes, it means that cancer cells may have spread to other organs, such as the liver, bones, or brain (see **FIGURE 15.9**). When cancer spreads from its original location to another part of the body, the new tumor has the same kind of abnormal cells and the same name as the primary tumor. If lung cancer spreads to the brain, for example, the cancer cells in the brain are actually lung cancer cells. The disease is called metastatic lung cancer (not brain cancer).

- **lymph nodes** [limf nodes] Rounded masses of lymphatic tissue that are surrounded by a capsule of connective tissue. Lymph nodes filter lymph (lymphatic fluid) and store lymphocytes (white blood cells). They are located along lymphatic vessels. Also called lymph glands.

Risk Factors for Cancer

The more we can learn about what causes cancer, the more likely we are to find ways to prevent it. Although doctors can seldom explain why one person gets cancer and another does not, they know that cancer is not caused by an injury, such as a bump or bruise. Also, although being infected with certain viruses can increase the risk of some types of cancer, cancer is not contagious; no one can "catch" cancer from another person.

Cancer usually develops over time. It results from a complex mix of factors related to lifestyle, heredity, and environment. Researchers have identified a number of factors that increase a person's chance of developing cancer.

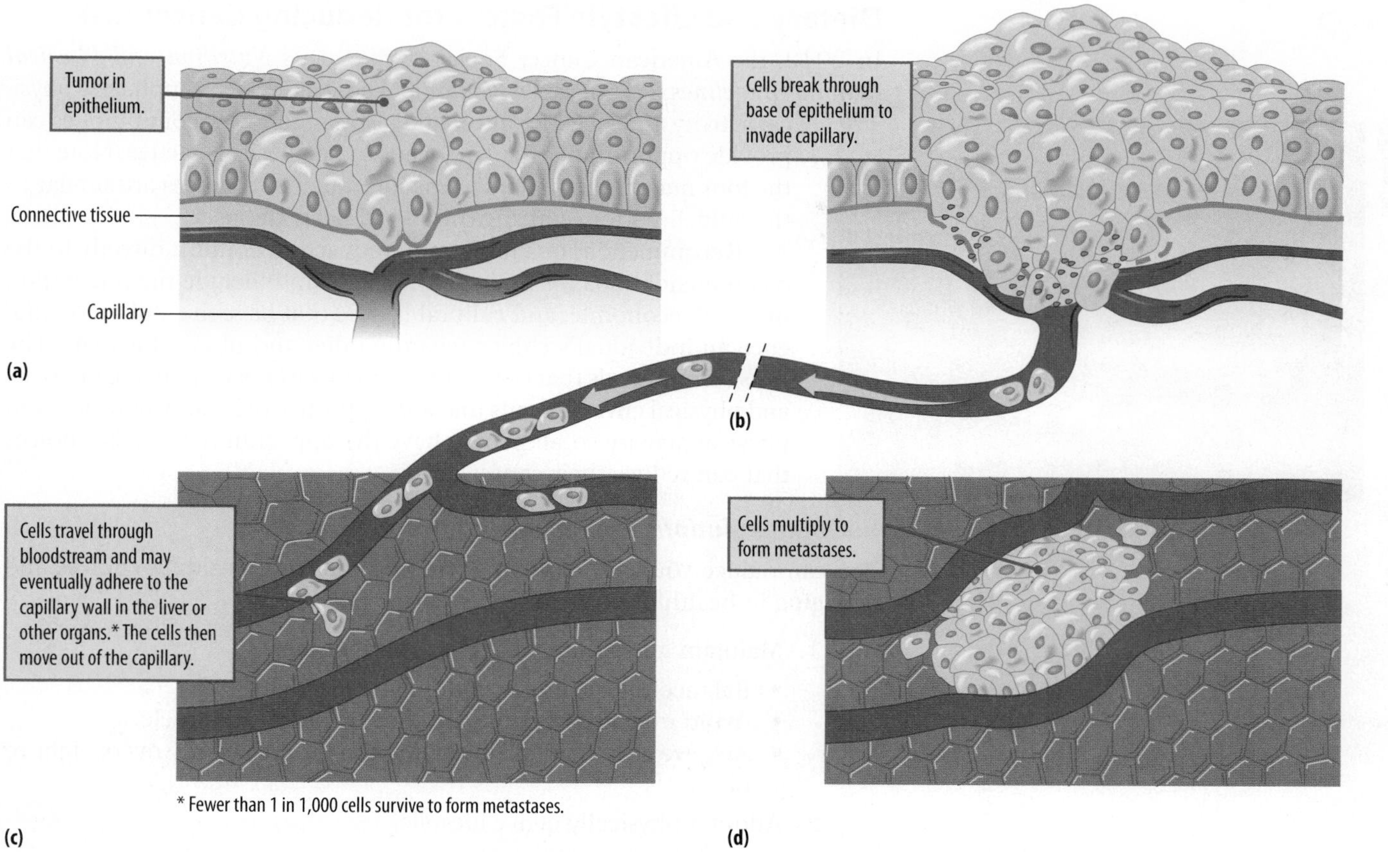
Tumor in epithelium.
Connective tissue
Capillary
(a)
Cells break through base of epithelium to invade capillary.
(b)
Cells travel through bloodstream and may eventually adhere to the capillary wall in the liver or other organs.* The cells then move out of the capillary.
Cells multiply to form metastases.
* Fewer than 1 in 1,000 cells survive to form metastases.
(c)
(d)

FIGURE 15.9 How cancer cells multiply and spread. Cancer cells can break away from a malignant tumor, enter the bloodstream or the lymphatic system, and travel to new sites to form new tumors in other organs.

Many types of cancer are related to the use of tobacco, items that people eat and drink, exposure to ultraviolet (UV) radiation from the sun, and exposure to cancer-causing agents (**carcinogens**) in the environment and the workplace. Some people are more sensitive than others to factors that cause cancer.

▶ **carcinogens** [kar-SIN-o-jins] Any substances that cause cancer.

Nevertheless, some people who develop cancer have none of the known risk factors. And some people who do have risk factors do not develop the disease. Researchers have learned that cancer is caused by changes (called mutations or alterations) in genes that control normal cell growth and cell death. Most cancer-causing gene changes are generated by factors in a person's lifestyle or the environment. However, some alterations that lead to cancer are inherited; that is, they are passed from parent to child. Having such an inherited gene alteration increases the risk of cancer, but it does not mean that the person is certain to develop cancer.

The Diet–Cancer Link

Although evidence suggests that between 20 and 30 percent of cancers result from poor food choices and physical inactivity, the role played by nutrition and diet in cancer development is complex.[63] Some dietary factors act as promoters; many others have protective roles, blocking the cellular changes in one of the developmental stages. Food choices interact with other lifestyle factors and also with genetics to affect cancer risk.[64] As the field of nutritional genomics evolves, it will enhance our ability to target dietary interventions for cancer prevention and treatment. Until that time, the general dietary guidelines from the American Cancer Society (ACS) can be used.

Dietary and Lifestyle Factors for Reducing Cancer Risk

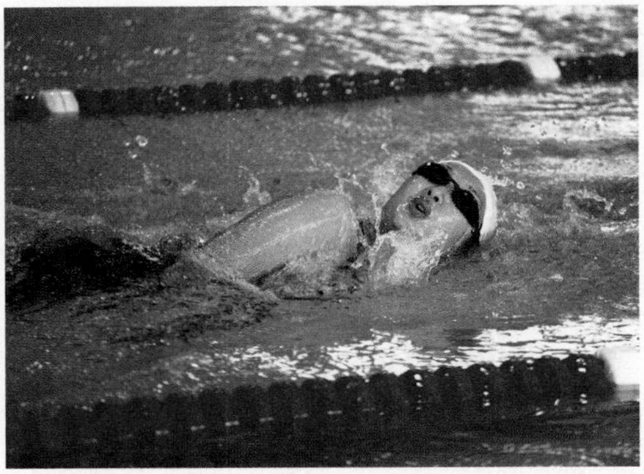
© Photos.com

In 2012, the American Cancer Society updated its *Nutrition and Physical Activity Guidelines for Cancer Prevention*.[65] These guidelines emphasize physical activity and weight control and also suggest how communities can provide opportunities for Americans to be physically active. Note that the four major recommendations for individual choices are similar to the guidelines for reducing the risk of heart disease.

Recommendations for community action connect directly to the recommendations for individual choices and include the integration of social, economic, and cultural factors that have the ability to influence an individual's choice regarding diet and physical activity. The ACS recommends that community organizations work to create social and physical environments that are supportive of healthy nutrition and physical activity so all people have the opportunity to make choices that can reduce their cancer risk.

Recommendations for Individual Lifestyle Choices

You can reduce your risk of getting cancer by making healthful choices and engaging in healthful behaviors.

1. Maintain a healthful weight throughout life.
   - Balance caloric intake with physical activity.
   - Avoid excessive weight gain throughout the life cycle.
   - Achieve and maintain a healthy weight if currently overweight or obese.
2. Adopt a physically active lifestyle.
   - *Adults:* Engage in at least 30 minutes of moderate to vigorous physical activity, above usual activities, on five or more days of the week. Forty-five to 60 minutes of intentional physical activity is preferable.
   - *Children and adolescents:* Engage in at least 60 minutes per day of moderate to vigorous physical activity at least five days per week.
3. Eat a healthy diet, with an emphasis on plant sources.
   - Choose foods and beverages in amounts that help achieve and maintain a healthy weight.
   - Eat five or more servings of vegetables and fruits each day.
   - Choose whole grains in preference to processed (refined) grains and sugars.
   - Limit consumption of processed meats and red meats.
4. If you drink alcoholic beverages, limit consumption.
   - People who drink alcohol should limit their intake: not more than two drinks per day for men and one drink per day for women.

Fat

High-fat diets have been associated with an increase in the risk of cancers of the colon and rectum, prostate, and endometrium. The association between high-fat diets and breast cancer appears to be much weaker. Several studies have evaluated the role of dietary fat on breast cancer risk, but the evidence has been inconclusive. Currently, the American Cancer Society considers the dietary fat recommendations for the general population for heart disease prevention appropriate for the population of cancer survivors due to shared risk factors between cancer and heart disease.[66]

Going Green

What Do Smokers Eat?

Is smoking bad for you? What about the health of the planet? We all know the answer: a loud and resounding *yes*. Smoking dramatically increases the risk for many diseases, including cancer and cardiovascular disease. But what about the dietary habits of smokers? Are they any different from nonsmokers?

Researchers analyzed 51 published nutritional studies from 15 different countries comparing 47,250 nonsmokers with 35,870 smokers. The studies showed that smokers have higher intakes of total fat, saturated fat, cholesterol, and alcohol. Compared with nonsmokers, smokers also have lower intakes of antioxidant vitamins and fiber. The researchers concluded that "the nutrient intakes of smokers differ substantially from those of nonsmokers." They also suggested that these differences may contribute to the already harmful effects of smoking on cancer and coronary heart disease.

Not only is smoking a serious health problem, but also the way in which smokers dispose of unsmoked remnants is a serious problem for the planet. Cigarette butt litter may be the world's greatest environmental litter problem, with about 4.3 trillion cigarette butts tossed onto roads, pavements, beaches, parks, forests, and waterways each year.

What can we do with this information? Perhaps public health prevention programs aimed at smokers as well as potential smokers should include promoting better nutritional habits as well as effective cigarette butt disposal.

High intake of red meat (e.g., beef, pork, lamb) and processed meat (e.g., bacon, sausage, hot dogs, lunch meat) is associated with some types of colorectal cancer; long-term consumption of poultry and fish is associated with reduced risk.[67,68]

Vegetables and Fruits

Evidence that vegetable and fruit consumption reduces cancer risk has led to attempts to isolate specific nutrients and to administer these in pharmacological doses to high-risk populations. Most attempts have failed to prevent cancer and, in some cases, have produced adverse effects.

It remains unclear which components of vegetables and fruits are most protective against cancer. Vegetables and fruits are complex foods, with each containing more than 100 potentially beneficial substances, including vitamins, minerals, and fiber. Specific phytochemicals, such as carotenoids, flavonoids, terpenes, sterols, indoles, and phenols, show benefit against certain cancers in experimental studies. In addition to having antioxidant effects, nutrients and other phytochemicals might inhibit multiplication of cancer cells, alter enzymes, inhibit the conversion of chemicals into toxins, and alter hormone metabolism. Until more is known about specific food components, however, the best advice is to eat five or more servings a day of a variety of vegetables and fruits.

Despite strong encouragement from numerous health agencies to eat at least five servings of vegetables and fruits each day, intake of these foods remains below recommended levels among both adults and children. Many states are attempting to increase fruit and vegetable consumption with improved access and policies that make it easier to get fruits and vegetables in communities, schools, and child care. California and Oregon are above the national average on access to a healthier food retailer, density of farmers markets, and acceptance of nutrition assistance programs. These and other factors explain why adults in California and Oregon eat more vegetables than adults in other states. They also are among the highest in fruit consumption.[69] On

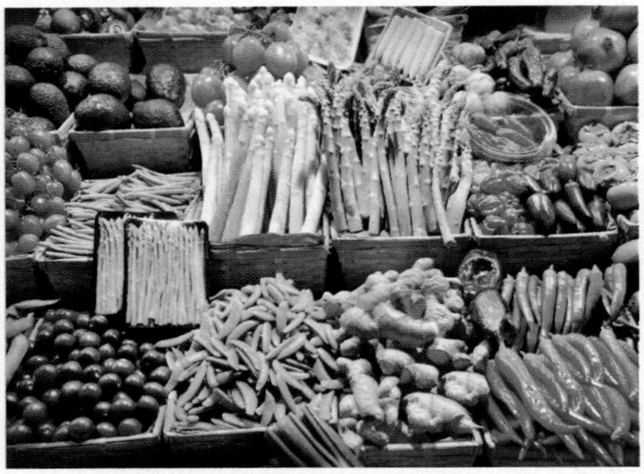

the national scene, Fruit & Veggies—More Matters is a public health campaign that encourages people to eat more fruits and vegetables. Recommended intake is based on individual calorie needs, ranging from 4 to 13 servings daily.[70]

Whole Grains and Legumes

Whole grains are higher in fiber, certain vitamins, and minerals than are processed (refined) flour products. The Black Women's Health Study, a prospective study of more than 59,000 African American women, suggests that a diet containing more whole grains, vegetables, fruit, and fish (the "prudent diet") is associated with lower risk of breast cancer when compared with a Western diet containing refined grains, processed meats, and sweets.[71] In another study, adherence to a Mediterranean diet and dietary patterns characterized by low intake of meat and starches and high intake of legumes was found to reduce risk of breast cancer in Asian-American women.[72]

Evidence for the association between fiber intake and cancer risk supports consumption of high-fiber foods.[73] Because the benefits that grain-based foods impart might derive from their other nutrients and phytochemicals, as well as from fiber, it is best to obtain fiber from whole grains—and vegetables and fruits—rather than from fiber supplements.

Beans and other legumes are excellent sources of many vitamins and minerals, protein, and fiber. Legumes, in particular soy, are especially rich in nutrients and phytochemicals that can protect against prostate cancer[74] and possibly breast cancer[75] and can be a useful low-fat, high-protein alternative to meat.

Putting It All Together

Some cancer risk factors can be avoided. Others, such as inherited factors, are unavoidable, but it is helpful to be aware of them. People can help protect themselves by avoiding known risk factors whenever possible. They can also talk with their doctors about regular checkups and the value of cancer screening tests (see **FIGURE 15.10**). Reducing both the number of new cancer cases and the death rates from cancer are key objectives of Healthy People 2020.

To reduce your cancer risk, eat a moderately low-fat diet and increase your consumption of fruits, vegetables, and whole grains. Maintain a healthy weight, exercise regularly, don't smoke, and don't use alcohol excessively. If these recommendations are beginning to sound like a broken record, you're right—the same lifestyle changes that reduce risk of atherosclerosis and hypertension can reduce risk of cancer.

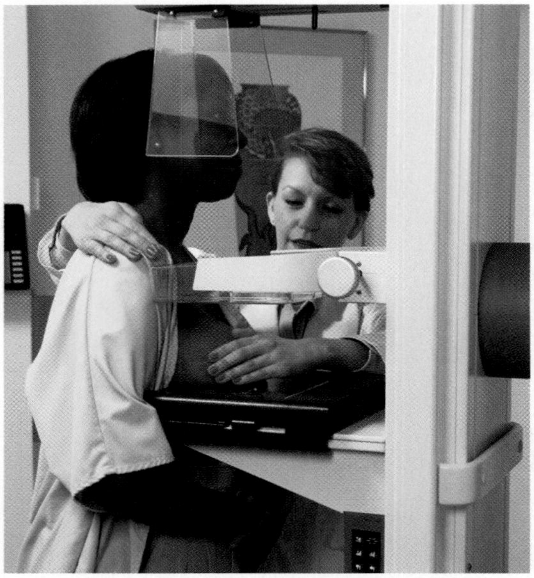

FIGURE 15.10 Cancer screening tests. Mammograms can detect breast cancer at an early stage and improve chances for successful treatment.

Key Concepts Cancer develops when something alters cellular DNA so cells divide and multiply uncontrollably. Both genetic factors and environmental factors, including diet, influence cancer risk. Although the evidence linking dietary fats with cancer is contradictory, many other dietary factors play key roles in reducing risk. Strategies for reducing cancer risk include eating more fruits, vegetables, and whole grains; increasing physical activity; maintaining a healthy weight; and limiting alcohol consumption.

Diabetes Mellitus

Almost everyone knows someone who has diabetes. An estimated 25.8 million people—8.3 percent of the population—in the United States have diabetes mellitus.[76] Although an estimated 18.8 million have been diagnosed, unfortunately 7.0 million people do not realize that they have this serious, lifelong condition.[77] If present trends continue, 1 in 3 American adults will have diabetes in 2050.[78] **FIGURE 15.11** shows the prevalence of obesity and diagnosed diabetes among U.S. adults.

What Is Diabetes?

Diabetes is a disorder of carbohydrate metabolism—the way our bodies use digested carbohydrates for growth and energy. Carbohydrates in food are digested and absorbed and end up as glucose in the blood. Glucose is a major source of fuel for the body. After digestion, glucose passes into the bloodstream and into cells, where it is used for growth and energy. For glucose to enter into most types of cells, insulin must be present. Insulin is a hormone produced by the pancreas.

When we eat carbohydrates, the pancreas should automatically produce the right amount of insulin to move glucose from blood into our cells. In people with diabetes, however, either the pancreas produces little or no insulin or the cells do not respond appropriately to the insulin that is produced. As a result, glucose builds up in the blood, causing **hyperglycemia**—an abnormally high blood glucose level that is the hallmark of diabetes mellitus.

Even though glucose in the blood is overabundant, it is unable to enter starving cells to fuel their needs. For this reason, diabetes often is called a disease of "starvation in the midst of plenty." In an ironic twist of fate, these starving cells signal the liver to make more glucose, worsening the hyperglycemia. The kidneys are taxed beyond their capacity to reabsorb glucose, and the excess spills into the urine, where it can be detected by urine glucose tests. Thus, even though the blood contains large amounts of glucose, the body loses access to its main source of fuel.

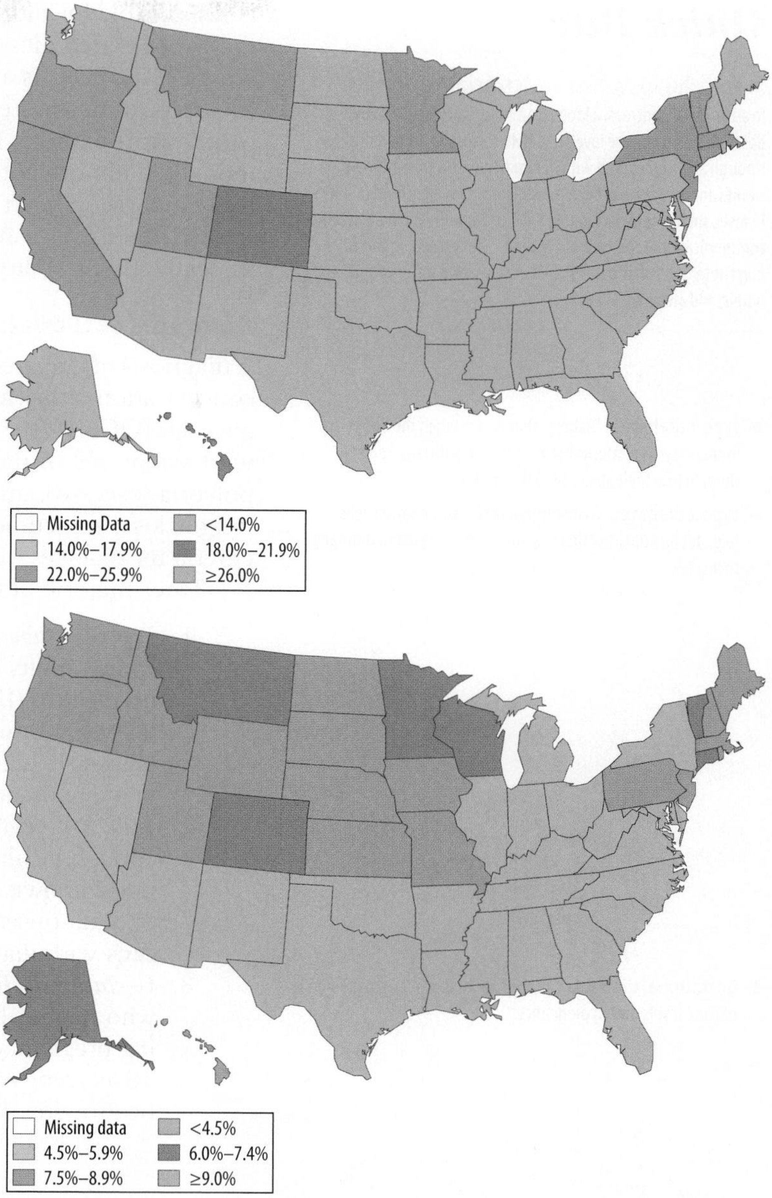

FIGURE 15.11 Prevalence of obesity and diagnosed diabetes among U.S. adults, 2009.

Reproduced from Centers for Disease Control and Prevention. National Diabetes Surveillance System. Data and statistics. http://www.cdc.gov/diabetes/statistics/index.htm. Accessed February 12, 2016.

Unable to use glucose, cells turn to other energy sources—fat and protein. But these options can lead to other problems. Excessive use of fat as an energy source, without available glucose in the cell, causes ketosis and acidosis, dangerously high acidity levels in the blood. Breaking down muscle proteins to fuel the cells causes muscle wasting and weakness. Alterations in fat and protein metabolism often accompany hyperglycemia.[79]

▶ **hyperglycemia** [HIGH-per-gly-SEE-me-uh] Abnormally high concentration of glucose in the blood.

Over time, abnormally high blood glucose levels increase the risk of high blood pressure, heart disease, and kidney disease. Excess glucose in the blood reacts with and damages body proteins and tissues, especially in the eyes, kidneys, nerves, and blood vessels. Complications of diabetes can contribute to degenerative conditions such as peripheral vascular disease (a disease of blood vessels that supply the feet and legs), deterioration of the eye and eventual blindness, kidney disease, and progressive nerve damage. Diabetes

Quick Bite

Smartphones Advance Artificial Pancreas

In an artificial pancreas, a laptop computer calculates insulin doses based on glucose levels and delivers insulin automatically through an insulin pump with minimal human input. Although significant progress has been made, laptops severely limit mobility. In tests, smartphone technology replaced laptops and had proper communication 98 percent of the time—far exceeding the 80 percent target. Participants stayed in real-world settings, such as hotels, and ate whatever they wanted.

is responsible for more than 60 percent of all nontraumatic amputations of the lower extremities and 44 percent of all new cases of kidney failure in adults.[80] Diabetes is also the leading cause of blindness in adults.[81] Diabetics are 40 times more likely to develop glaucoma.[82] Sixty-seven percent of people with diabetes have high blood pressure, and nearly all have one or more lipid abnormalities.[83] People with diabetes are two to four times more likely to develop heart disease or have a stroke than people without diabetes. In the United States and Canada, diabetes is one of the leading contributors to death and disability.

Diagnosis of Diabetes Mellitus

A diagnosis of diabetes mellitus is usually made by measuring plasma glucose concentration either after an overnight fast, as part of an oral glucose tolerance test (OGTT) (see **FIGURE 15.12**), or any time of the day if a patient presents with symptoms of diabetes. The classic symptoms of diabetes mellitus are polyuria (excessive urination), polydipsia (excessive thirst), and unexplained weight loss, sometimes with polyphagia (excessive eating). The diagnostic criteria for diabetes mellitus are shown in **TABLE 15.6**.

Three major types of diabetes exist:

1. *Type 1 diabetes:* **Type 1 diabetes** usually is diagnosed in children and young adults and was previously known as insulin-dependent diabetes mellitus (IDDM) or juvenile diabetes. In type 1 diabetes, the body fails to produce insulin, the hormone that "unlocks" cells, allowing glucose to enter and fuel them. Roughly 5 to 10 percent of Americans who are diagnosed with diabetes have type 1 diabetes.[84]
2. *Type 2 diabetes:* In **type 2 diabetes**, either the body does not produce enough insulin or cells ignore the insulin. Type 2 diabetes was previously known as non-insulin-dependent diabetes mellitus (NIDDM) or adult-onset diabetes. Approximately 90 to 95 percent of all Americans with diabetes mellitus have type 2 diabetes.[85]
3. *Gestational diabetes:* **Gestational diabetes** occurs in a pregnant woman who has never had diabetes, but who develops hyperglycemia during pregnancy. In the United States, gestational diabetes affects 7 to 18 percent of pregnancies, and the number of cases is thought to be growing.[86]

▶ **type 1 diabetes** Diabetes that occurs when the body's immune system attacks beta cells in the pancreas, causing them to lose their ability to make insulin.

▶ **type 2 diabetes** Diabetes that occurs when target cells (e.g., fat and muscle cells) lose the ability to respond normally to insulin.

▶ **gestational diabetes** A condition that results in high blood glucose levels during pregnancy.

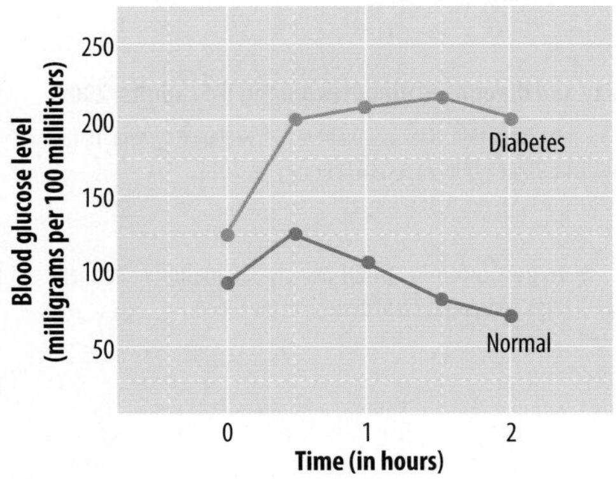

FIGURE 15.12 Glucose tolerance test. A glucose tolerance test measures the level of glucose in the blood following consumption of a standard dose of glucose. Glucose tolerance tests are used to diagnose diabetes.

TABLE 15.6
Diagnostic Criteria for Diabetes Mellitus

	A1C (percent)	Fasting plasma glucose (mg/dL)	Oral glucose tolerance test (mg/dL)
Diabetes	6.5 or above	126 or above	200 or above
Prediabetes	5.7 to 6.4	100 to 125	140 to 199
Normal	About 5	99 or below	139 or below

Reproduced from National Institute of Diabetes and Digestive and Kidney Diseases. Retrieved from: http://www.niddk.nih.gov/health-information/health-topics/Diabetes/diagnosis-diabetes-prediabetes/Pages/index.aspx.

Pre-diabetes (impaired glucose tolerance or impaired fasting glucose) is a condition in which a person's blood glucose levels are higher than normal but not high enough to warrant a diagnosis of type 2 diabetes. In 2012, an estimated 86 million American adults over the age of 20 had pre-diabetes, up from 79 million in 2010.[87]

▶ **pre-diabetes** Blood glucose levels higher than normal but not high enough to warrant a diagnosis of diabetes.

Type 1 Diabetes Mellitus

Type 1 diabetes usually occurs in people younger than 30 years and often develops suddenly. People with type 1 diabetes lack insulin, usually because an autoimmune response has destroyed insulin-producing cells of the pancreas. Symptoms include excessive thirst, frequent urination, rapid weight loss, and blurred vision.[88] When blood glucose levels rise, glucose spills into the urine, taking water with it and causing frequent urination and increased thirst. Although blood glucose levels are high, the lack of insulin prevents glucose from entering cells to be burned for energy. The result is weight loss and feelings of hunger.

People with type 1 diabetes require lifelong, daily insulin injections balanced with a healthful diet and regular exercise to maintain blood glucose levels in the normal range. Initiating good control of blood glucose levels early reduces kidney damage and reduces long-term risk of kidney disease by 50 percent.[89] Because exercise lowers blood glucose levels, individuals must consider the timing of exercise in addition to food intake and insulin injections to avoid lowering blood glucose levels excessively.

Type 2 Diabetes Mellitus

In type 2 diabetes, glucose has trouble entering body cells because either the pancreas cannot produce enough insulin or cells in the body become resistant to the action of insulin. Although obesity contributes to **insulin resistance** in many people with type 2 diabetes, genetic factors also play a role. Type 2 diabetes usually develops in overweight individuals aged 45 and older. However, with the rising prevalence of obesity, type 2 diabetes is occurring more frequently in adolescents.

The result is the same as for type 1 diabetes—glucose builds up in the blood, and the body cannot use its main source of fuel efficiently. Type 2 diabetes often is part of a metabolic syndrome that includes obesity, elevated blood pressure, and high levels of blood triglycerides. (See the "Metabolic Syndrome" section later in this chapter.)

In contrast to the sudden onset of type 1 diabetes, the symptoms of type 2 diabetes develop gradually, and some people may not show symptoms for many years. Symptoms of type 2 diabetes eventually include fatigue or nausea, frequent urination, unusual thirst, weight loss, blurred vision, frequent infections, and slow healing of wounds or sores.

Pre-diabetes

Before people develop type 2 diabetes, they usually have pre-diabetes—impaired glucose tolerance that results in a blood glucose level that is higher than normal yet not high enough to be diagnosed as diabetes. Some long-term damage to the body, especially to the heart and circulatory system, may already be occurring during the pre-diabetes stage.

People who have pre-diabetes are at increased risk for developing both type 2 diabetes and heart disease. Unless they take steps toward prevention, such as dietary changes, moderate weight loss, and regular exercise, many will develop type 2 diabetes within 10 years.

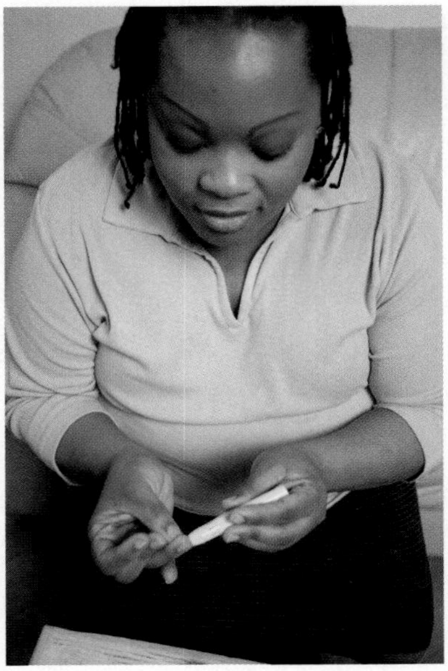

© Custom Medical Stock Photo/Alamy Images

Gestational Diabetes Mellitus

Pregnant women who have never had diabetes before but who develop impaired glucose tolerance during pregnancy are said to have gestational diabetes. Although the cause of gestational diabetes remains unknown, researchers have uncovered certain clues. The placenta produces hormones that help the baby develop. Unfortunately, these hormones also block the action of the mother's insulin in her body. This insulin resistance makes it difficult for the mother's body to use insulin and can triple the amount of insulin needed to get sufficient glucose into her cells. Gestational diabetes occurs more often in African Americans, Native Americans, and Hispanic Americans and is more common among obese women and women with a family history of diabetes.

In women with gestational diabetes, blood glucose levels usually decrease after pregnancy. Once a woman has had gestational diabetes, however, her chances are two in three that it will return in future pregnancies. In a few women, pregnancy reveals preexisting type 1 or type 2 diabetes that requires ongoing treatment after pregnancy. Forty to 60 percent of women who had gestational diabetes will develop type 2 diabetes later in life.[90] Both forms of diabetes involve insulin resistance.

Low Blood Glucose Levels: Hypoglycemia

▶ **hypoglycemia** [HIGH-po-gly-SEE-mee-uh] Abnormally low concentration of glucose in the blood; any blood glucose value below 40 to 50 mg/dL of blood.

▶ **reactive hypoglycemia** A type of hypoglycemia that occurs about one hour after eating carbohydrate-rich food.

▶ **fasting hypoglycemia** A type of hypoglycemia that occurs because the body produces too much insulin even when no food is eaten.

Excess insulin results in low blood sugar, or **hypoglycemia**. Too much glucose enters cells, lowering blood glucose levels too far. When blood glucose levels drop too low, nervousness, irritability, hunger, headache, shakiness, rapid heartbeat, and weakness can develop. A further drop in blood glucose levels can cause coma and death.

A person with diabetes can develop hypoglycemia in response to an overdose of insulin or vigorous exercise. In nondiabetic individuals, two types of hypoglycemia occur. **Reactive hypoglycemia** occurs about one hour after eating carbohydrate-rich food. The body overreacts and produces too much insulin in response to the food. Individuals can prevent reactive hypoglycemia by eating frequent, smaller meals to smooth out blood glucose responses to food. **Fasting hypoglycemia** occurs because the body produces too much insulin even when no food is eaten. Pancreatic tumors can cause fasting hypoglycemia.

Key Concepts Approximately 25.8 million people in the United States have diabetes mellitus, a leading cause of death and disability. Unfortunately, 7 million of these people are unaware that they have the disease. Three major types of diabetes have been identified: type 1, type 2, and gestational diabetes. Type 1, the most severe form, requires a daily regimen of insulin, careful diet control, and physical activity. In type 2 diabetes, the treatment focuses on diet and weight loss. Gestational diabetes occurs during pregnancy and usually goes away after delivery.

Risk Factors for Diabetes

Some people are at higher risk than others for developing diabetes. **TABLE 15.7** lists the risk factors for type 1 and type 2 diabetes. Anyone with a family history of diabetes has an increased risk. In most cases of type 1 diabetes, people must inherit risk factors from both parents, and whites have the highest rate of this disease.[91] Yet genes do not tell the complete story. When one identical twin has type 1 diabetes, for example, the other twin gets the disease at most only half the time.[92] Possible environmental triggers include certain viruses or other infectious agents that activate the immune system. Type 1 diabetes develops more often in winter than summer and is more common in countries with cold climates (Sweden, Finland). Early diet also can play a role. For

TABLE 15.7
Risk Factors for Diabetes Mellitus

Modifiable	Nonmodifiable
Physical inactivity	45+ years of age
CVD or other vascular disease	Family history of diabetes mellitus—first-degree relative
Overweight BMI ≥ 25 Obesity BMI ≥ 35 Waist circumference > 35 inches in females and 40 inches in males	Ethnicity: African American, Native American, Asian American, Pacific Islander
Blood pressure ≥ 140/90 mm Hg	Gestational diabetes mellitus
Triglycerides > 250 mg/dL (2.82 mmol/L)	Delivery of baby weighing ≥ 9 pounds
HDL cholesterol < 35 mg/dL (0.90 mmol/L)	Treatment for depression
Prediabetes: impaired fasting glucose (100 to 125 mg/dL) or impaired glucose tolerance (140–199 mg/dL) or ≥ 5.7%	If none of the risk factors are present: Screening for adults should begin at the age of 45 years.
Sleep apnea	Reevaluation every 3 years if normal blood glucose level.
Insulin resistance syndrome (MetS, acanthosis nigricans, or history of polycystic ovary syndrome)	

BMI = body mass index; CVD = cardiovascular disease; HDL = high-density lipoprotein; MetS = metabolic syndrome.

Data from: American Diabetes Association. Standards of medical care in diabetes—2014. *Diabetes Care.* 2014;37(1):S14–S80.

example, type 1 diabetes is less common in people who were breastfed and began eating solid food at older ages.[93]

A family history of type 2 diabetes is one of the strongest risk factors for getting the disease.[94] As with gestational diabetes, the ethnic groups at highest risk of type 2 diabetes are Native Americans, Hispanic Americans, and African Americans. An increased risk of type 2 diabetes seems to occur more frequently in people who follow a "Western" lifestyle characterized by too much fat; too few fruits, vegetables, and fiber; and not enough exercise.[95]

The risk of developing type 2 diabetes increases progressively as body fat increases, especially around the midsection. The dramatic surge in obesity rates in the United States is a major reason that the incidence of type 2 diabetes not only has increased dramatically in adults, but also has become a sizable and growing problem among U.S. children and adolescents.[96] Compared with a normal-weight person, an obese person has a significantly increased risk of developing type 2 diabetes.[97] Unfortunately, as more children and adolescents become overweight, type 2 diabetes is becoming more common in young people. Contrary to popular opinion, high sugar or high carbohydrate intake does not by itself cause diabetes as long as it does not contribute to excess energy intake and obesity.

Do other dietary factors make a difference? Dietary fat is of interest to researchers due to its influence on glucose metabolism by altering cell function, enzyme activity, insulin signaling, and gene expression. A review of the literature suggests that replacing saturated fats and trans fats with unsaturated (polyunsaturated and/or monounsaturated) fats improves insulin sensitivity and is likely to reduce the risk of type 2 diabetes. In dietary practice, foods rich in vegetable oils should replace meats and fat-rich dairy products.[98] Numerous studies have shown a protective effect of increased consumption of nonstarch polysaccharides (fiber). Conversely, drinking more sugar-sweetened beverages[99,100] or diet beverages[101] has been associated with an increased risk of type 2 diabetes. **TABLE 15.8** summarizes the evidence linking lifestyle factors and type 2 diabetes risk.

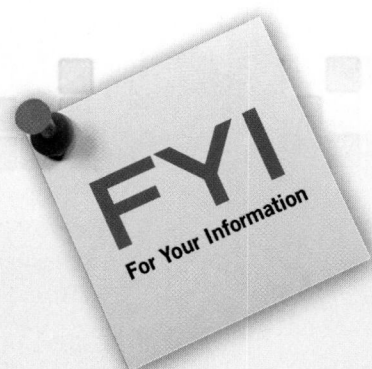

FYI For Your Information

The Pima Indians

The Pima Indians of Arizona, along with teams of scientists and doctors from the National Institutes of Health, have been responsible for unraveling some of the complex interactions among genetics, lifestyle, and disease. For five decades, Pima volunteers and scientists have been working together to try to understand why the Pimas have extremely high rates of obesity as well as the highest known rate of type 2 diabetes of any community in the world.[a] Half of all adult Pima Indians have diabetes, and 95 percent of those with diabetes are overweight.[b] Complications of diabetes such as kidney disease are common in the Pima community.

The ravages of diabetes were not always a problem for the Pimas. Hundreds of years ago, they developed a sophisticated irrigation system that allowed them to cultivate such crops as wheat, beans, squash, and cotton. Hard physical work and a low-fat, high-fiber diet were the norm. Obesity and diabetes were essentially nonexistent. The Pimas lived this traditional lifestyle until the late nineteenth century, when American farmers living upstream diverted their water supply. Their way of life was seriously disrupted, resulting in poverty and severe malnutrition. The U.S. government gave the Pimas lard, sugar, and flour to help them survive. Although life improved for the Pimas as the economy rebounded after World War II, the increasing prosperity was accompanied by high-fat and sugary foods, more leisure time, and less physical work, resulting in an epidemic of obesity and diabetes.

Modern Pima Indians are not much different from most Americans in their diet and exercise habits, but they have much higher rates of obesity and diabetes. Scientists have postulated that they have inherited "thrifty genes" that allow them to retain fat more easily than most people. After the first month of life, Pima children have higher BMI scores than the general U.S. population at all ages. Even during childhood, the diabetes that occurs in this population primarily consists of type 2 diabetes.[c]

This genetic trait (the "thrifty genes") helped the ancestors of modern Pima Indians survive the hard times when food was not plentiful. During times of plenty, the thrifty genes allowed them to store extra fat so they would not starve when famine struck. Unfortunately, the genetic traits that once helped them survive became a liability in modern times, when high-fat, high-calorie foods are readily available and the need for physical work is greatly diminished. In the 1890s, the traditional Pima Indian diet consisted of only about 15 percent fat; today, it is nearly 40 percent fat.[d] Genetically, this is a recipe for disaster.

Although the specific genes for the inheritance of type 2 diabetes have not yet been located, several genes that play a role in insulin resistance (a major factor in the development of type 2 diabetes) have been found to be much more common in Pima Indians than in the general U.S. population. Pima Indians with diabetes develop kidney failure more often and at a younger age than non–Native Americans with diabetes. Ongoing research seeks to identify the genetic reasons for the high rate of kidney disease among American Indians and their families.[e,f]

Further evidence for the effects of diet and exercise on health is seen when the Arizona Pimas are compared with a genetically similar population in Mexico. The Pimas who currently live in Arizona migrated there from the Sierra Madre of Mexico hundreds of years ago. A Pima community still exists in a remote part of those mountains. These Mexican Pimas live much as their ancestors did, farming mostly by hand and eating a traditional diet that is very low in fat and high in fiber. Although the people in this region are genetically similar to the Arizona Pimas, obesity and diabetes are rarely seen among them.[g]

The Diabetes Prevention Program, a nationwide, randomized, controlled clinical trial, included several American Indian communities. With modest changes, including eating a healthier diet, exercising 2½ hours per week, and losing at least 7 percent of body weight, risk of diabetes was reduced by a remarkable 58 percent in just 3 years.[h,i]

The challenge for the Arizona Pimas, as with the majority of Americans, is to incorporate some health practices of our ancestors into modern life. Until the last 100 years, most humans had to engage in heavy physical work on a daily basis to survive. Our bodies simply were not designed to handle the amount of high-fat, high-calorie foods that most Americans eat, especially when sedentary pursuits occupy the bulk of our time.

[a] Baier LJ. Research summary. http://www.niddk.nih.gov/about-niddk/staff-directory/intramural/leslie-baier/pages/research-summary.aspx. Accessed February 12, 2016.

[b] Schneider C. The frightening increase in diabetes rates. August 25, 2014. http://www.diabetescare.net/authors/clara-schneider/the-frightening-increase-in-diabetes-rates. Accessed February 12, 2016.

[c] Thearle MS, Muller YL, Hanson RL, et al. Greater impact of melanocortin-4 receptor deficiency on rates of growth and risk of type 2 diabetes during childhood compared with adulthood in Pima Indians. *Diabetes*. 2012;61(1):250–257.

[d] Schneider C. The frightening increase in diabetes rates. Op cit.

[e] Baier L. Research summary. Op cit.

[f] Thearle MS, Muller YL, Hanson RL, et al. Greater impact of melanocortin-4 receptor deficiency on rates of growth and risk of type 2 diabetes during childhood compared with adulthood in Pima Indians. Op cit.

[g] Schulz LO, Bennett PH, Ravussin E, et al. Effects of traditional and Western environments on prevalence of type 2 diabetes in Pima Indians in Mexico and the U.S. *Diabetes Care*. 2006;29(8):1866–1871.

[h] Diabetes Prevention Program Outcomes Study. About DPP. https://dppos.bsc.gwu.edu/web/dppos/dpp. Accessed February 12, 2016.

[i] National Institute of Diabetes and Digestive and Kidney Diseases. Message of hope: we can prevent diabetes in Native American communities. February 5, 2014. http://www.niddk.nih.gov/about-niddk/research-areas/diabetes/diabetes-prevention-program-dpp/message-hope-prevent-diabetes-native-american-communities/Pages/default.aspx. Accessed February 12, 2016.

TABLE 15.8
Strength of Evidence Related to Lifestyle and Type 2 Diabetes Risk

Evidence	Decreased Risk	Increased Risk
Convincing	• Voluntary weight loss in overweight/obese people • Physical activity	• Overweight and obesity • Abdominal obesity • Physical inactivity • Maternal diabetes
Probable	• Nonstarch polysaccharides	• Saturated fats • Intrauterine growth

Modified from Technical Report Series 916, *Diet, Nutrition and the Prevention of Chronic Diseases: A Report of a Joint WHO/FAO Expert Consultation.* Copyright 2003 World Health Organization.

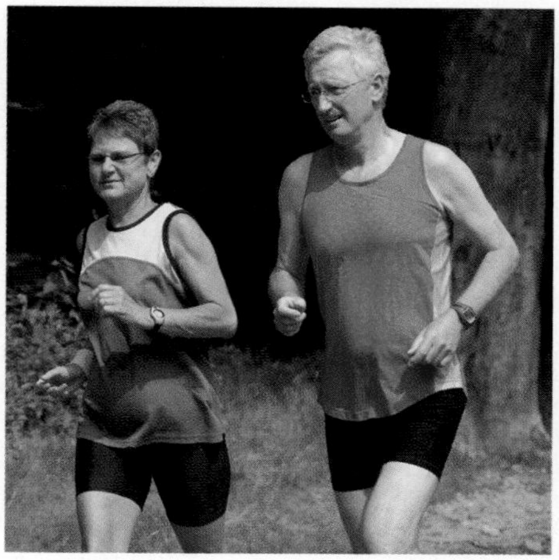
© M.G. Mooij/ShutterStock, Inc.

FIGURE 15.13 Exercise and diabetes. Regular physical activity improves glucose tolerance and helps reduce the risk of developing type 2 diabetes later in life.

Dietary and Lifestyle Factors for Reducing Diabetes Risk

Obesity is the single largest modifiable risk factor in the development of type 2 diabetes. Therefore, the best measures for preventing pre-diabetes and obesity-related type 2 diabetes are a healthful diet and regular exercise. Reducing excess body fat improves glucose tolerance and reduces related risk factors for heart disease. Regular exercise improves carbohydrate and lipid metabolism and increases insulin sensitivity (see **FIGURE 15.13**). As previously mentioned, exercise improves blood flow to the extremities, bringing blood pressure down to normal levels and reducing risk of heart disease.

The Diabetes Prevention Program, a study of more than 3,000 people, 45 percent of whom were minorities, found that people who received intensive lifestyle intervention were able to reduce their risk of developing type 2 diabetes by 58 percent. The lifestyle interventions included walking or other moderate physical exercise for about 30 minutes per day and weight reduction of 5 to 7 percent.[102]

Online social media can support diabetes prevention. Use of an online social network program based on the Diabetes Prevention Program (Prevent) has been validated against the Centers for Disease Control and Prevention outcome standards for weight loss and blood glucose control. Online delivery platforms such as Prevent offer an effective and scalable solution.[103]

Management of Diabetes

Before the discovery of insulin in 1921, everyone with type 1 diabetes died within a few years after diagnosis. Although insulin therapy is not a cure, its discovery represented the first major breakthrough in diabetes treatment.

Today, healthy eating, physical activity, and insulin delivery by injection (see **FIGURE 15.14**) or an insulin pump are the basic therapies for type 1 diabetes. The amount of insulin must be balanced with food intake and daily activities. Blood glucose concentrations must be closely monitored.

Healthy eating, physical activity, and blood glucose testing are the basic management tools for type 2 diabetes, and weight loss often restores normal glucose metabolism. Weight loss can decrease insulin resistance and improve blood glucose levels. Exercise increases the sensitivity of body cells to insulin, so the body needs less insulin to get glucose into cells. Small Steps, Big Rewards Prevent Type 2 Diabetes is a diabetes prevention campaign created by the National Diabetes Education Program based on the Diabetes Prevention Program.[104] Aimed at helping people lose a modest amount of weight, get 30 minutes of exercise five days a week, and make healthier food

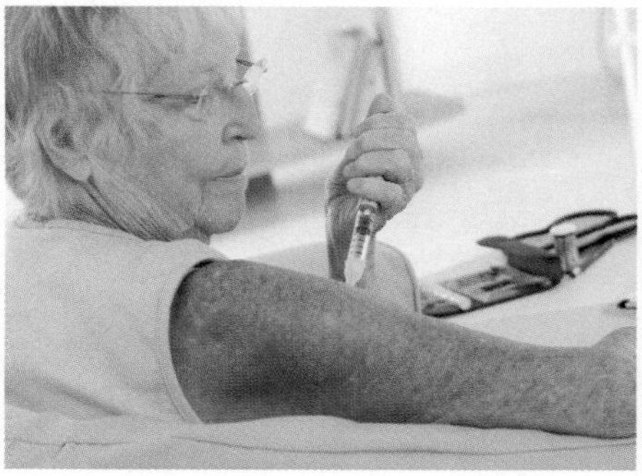
© CHASSENET/age fotostock

FIGURE 15.14 Insulin injections. In type 1 diabetes and some cases of type 2 diabetes, people need daily insulin injections to normalize blood glucose levels.

choices, the program enables people at risk to delay or prevent the onset of type 2 diabetes.

If diet and exercise fail to maintain blood glucose levels in the normal range, people with type 2 diabetes need medications to either increase insulin production or improve glucose uptake by cells. In some cases, insulin injections are needed to normalize blood glucose levels.

Nutrition

Although people with diabetes have the same nutritional needs as anyone else, good diabetes control requires that they monitor their food intake carefully.

By eating well-balanced meals in the correct amounts, people can keep their blood glucose levels as close to normal (nondiabetes level) as possible. The American Diabetes Association offers My Health Advisor, an online resource that helps with diabetes management and includes a database of foods, recipes, and nutrient information.[105]

Specific meal plans should be based on an individual's usual food intake. People with type 1 diabetes should eat at about the same time each day and should try to be consistent regarding the types of food they choose. Keeping calorie and carbohydrate intake consistent helps to prevent blood glucose levels from becoming too high or too low. People with type 2 diabetes should consume a diet that is well balanced, is low in fat, and promotes a healthy body weight. Dietary carbohydrates should come from fruits, vegetables, and whole grains.

Having diabetes once meant a lifetime of meals that lacked one of the most pleasant aspects of taste: sweetness. Although in the past dietary treatment of diabetes eliminated simple sugars from the diet, current recommendations allow individuals with diabetes to include moderate amounts of simple sugars in their diet as long as sugar intake does not contribute to excess energy intake and obesity.

Putting It All Together

Researchers continue to search for the cause or causes of diabetes and ways to prevent and cure it. Some genetic markers for type 1 diabetes have been identified, and it is now possible to screen relatives of people with type 1 diabetes to see whether they are at increased risk. In the future, it may be possible to administer insulin through inhalers, a pill, or a patch. Devices also are being developed that can monitor blood glucose levels without having to prick a finger to get a blood sample.

For now, the challenge is to slow the rate at which diabetes incidence is increasing. Healthy People 2020 objectives include a reduction in incidence of diabetes along with the economic burden it presents. Results from the Diabetes Prevention Program show that relatively modest changes in weight and exercise can be enough to reduce the incidence of diabetes. We turn, once again, to advice encouraging healthful eating (consumption of more fruits, vegetables, and fiber), regular physical activity, and lifelong weight management.

Key Concepts Family history is a risk factor for both type 1 and type 2 diabetes. For type 2 diabetes, additional risk factors include increasing age, overweight, sedentary lifestyle, and ethnicity. Risk reduction can be achieved through healthy eating, modest weight loss, and increases in physical activity.

Metabolic Syndrome

Thirty-four percent of adults in the United States meet the criteria for **metabolic syndrome**, a group of symptoms that occur together and promote the development of coronary artery disease, stroke, and type 2 diabetes. The prevalence will continue to grow because of the widespread tendency toward a sedentary lifestyle, according to the Centers for Disease Control and Prevention.[106] Metabolic syndrome is usually indicated by a cluster of at least three of the following signs[107]:

▶ **metabolic syndrome** A cluster of at least three of the following risk factors for heart disease: hypertriglyceridemia (high blood triglycerides), low HDL cholesterol, hyperglycemia (high blood glucose), hypertension (high blood pressure), and excess abdominal fat.

- *Abdominal obesity:* For most men, a 40-inch waist or greater; for women, a waist of 35 inches or greater
- *High fasting blood glucose:* At least 100 mg/dL
- *High serum triglycerides:* At least 150 mg/dL
- *Low HDL cholesterol:* Less than 40 mg/dL for men; less than 50 mg/dL for women
- *Elevated blood pressure:* 130 mm Hg or above, systolic; or 85 mm Hg or above, diastolic

Taken individually, these risk factors might not look particularly serious. When you put them together, however, the problems rise substantially. Individuals with metabolic syndrome are at increased risk for both cardiovascular disease and type 2 diabetes.[108,109] More studies are needed to understand the relationship among the risk factors embodied in metabolic syndrome, but researchers have identified people with metabolic syndrome as having the greatest risk of death from heart attack.

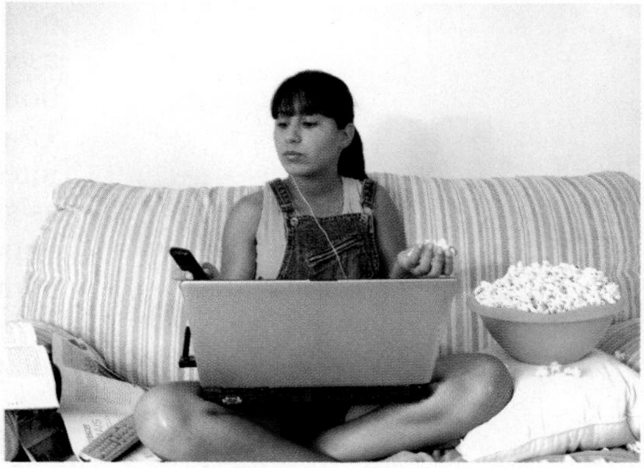

© Hemera/Thinkstock

Although some scientists think that metabolic syndrome is genetically based, it is unlikely that metabolic syndrome results from a single cause. The primary underlying diabetic and cardiac risk factors appear to be insulin resistance and abdominal obesity. For many people, poor diet and lack of physical activity combined with a genetic predisposition lead to the development of the syndrome. The high prevalence of metabolic syndrome underscores an urgent need to develop comprehensive efforts directed at controlling the obesity epidemic and improving physical activity levels.

People with metabolic syndrome should work with their doctors to

- Monitor blood glucose, lipoproteins, and blood pressure
- Achieve and maintain a healthy body weight and increase physical activity—both are time-tested methods of improving insulin sensitivity, blood pressure, and lipoprotein levels
- Treat diabetes and hyperlipidemia according to established guidelines
- Choose drug therapy for hypertension with care—different medications have different effects on insulin sensitivity

Key Concepts Metabolic syndrome, associated with an increased risk of death from heart attack, is a cluster including at least three of the following signs: abdominal fat, elevated blood glucose, elevated triglycerides and HDL cholesterol, and elevated blood pressure. A poor diet and sedentary lifestyle combined with a genetic predisposition are thought to be the underlying causes.

Osteoporosis

Osteoporosis is a major public health problem, and in the United States, more than 53 million people either already have osteoporosis or are at high risk because of low bone mass.[110] Although 80 percent of those with osteoporosis are women, up to one in four men over age 50 will break a bone due to osteoporosis.[111] However, women are most at risk for bone fractures related to osteoporosis. During their lifetime, 1 in 3 women will suffer an osteoporotic fracture, and the risk increases with age.[112] Although we often associate osteoporosis with being elderly, the stage for its emergence is actually set much earlier in life, much like other chronic diseases. Fortunately, diet and lifestyle changes can help to delay the onset of osteoporosis and prevent related fractures.

What Is Osteoporosis?

Osteoporosis means "porous bone." It's a good description because bone mass or density declines and bone quality deteriorates, leaving the bones fragile and vulnerable to fracture. The hip, spine, and wrist bones are especially vulnerable. Often called a "silent disease," osteoporosis develops over several years without outward symptoms. Eventually bone loss makes bones so weak that they break with a mild strain, bump, or fall. In fact, in some cases, the break may occur first and cause the fall!

Bone strength depends on two main features: bone density and bone quality. Bone density is determined by peak bone mass and amount of bone loss. Bone quality refers to architecture, turnover, damage accumulation (e.g., microfractures), and mineralization. Currently, no accurate measure of overall bone strength exists. Bone mineral density (BMD) is frequently used as a proxy measure and accounts for approximately 70 percent of bone strength.

Low bone mineral density is an important predictor of future bone fractures. Other predictors include a history of falls, low physical function such as slow gait speed and decreased leg muscle strength, impaired cognition, impaired vision, and the presence of environmental hazards (e.g., throw rugs). Some risks for fracture, such as age, low BMI, and low levels of physical activity, probably increase the rate of fractures through decreased bone density, increased propensity to fall, and inability to absorb impact.

Risk Factors for Osteoporosis

A common misperception is that osteoporosis always results from excessive bone loss. Bone loss commonly occurs as men and women age; however, a person who does not reach optimal (i.e., peak) bone mass during childhood and adolescence can develop osteoporosis without the occurrence of accelerated bone loss. Hence, suboptimal bone growth in childhood and adolescence is as important as bone loss to the development of osteoporosis. **TABLE 15.9** lists the risk factors for osteoporosis.

Bone mass typically peaks sometime around age 30. Starting in midlife, bone breakdown exceeds bone formation, and the progressive loss of bone begins. If you got enough calcium and vitamin D earlier in life so you maximized bone mass, then when bone loss begins you are likely to be a long way from low bone density and fractures.

Because declining estrogen levels accelerate bone loss, postmenopausal women have the highest risk of developing osteoporosis. By age 65, some women have lost half their skeletal mass, and they may show deformities of the upper spine, known as a "dowager's hump" (see **FIGURES 15.15** and **15.16**). Women who reach menopause with low bone mass have a greatly increased risk of fractures.

Many medical disorders, such as genetic disorders, endocrine disorders, congestive heart failure, kidney disease, and alcoholism, as well as administration of certain drugs such as steroids, also can lead to osteoporosis and increased fracture risk.

TABLE 15.9
Risk Factors for Osteoporosis

- Advanced age
- Female
- Thin and/or small frame
- Family history of osteoporosis
- Early menopause, whether natural or surgically induced
- Low testosterone levels in men
- Abnormal absence of menstrual periods (amenorrhea)
- Anorexia nervosa or bulimia nervosa
- Medical conditions, such as thyroid disease, rheumatoid arthritis, and problems that block intestinal absorption of calcium
- Use of certain medications, such as corticosteroids and anticonvulsants
- Insufficient dietary calcium
- Lack of weight-bearing exercise
- Cigarette smoking
- Excessive use of alcohol or caffeine

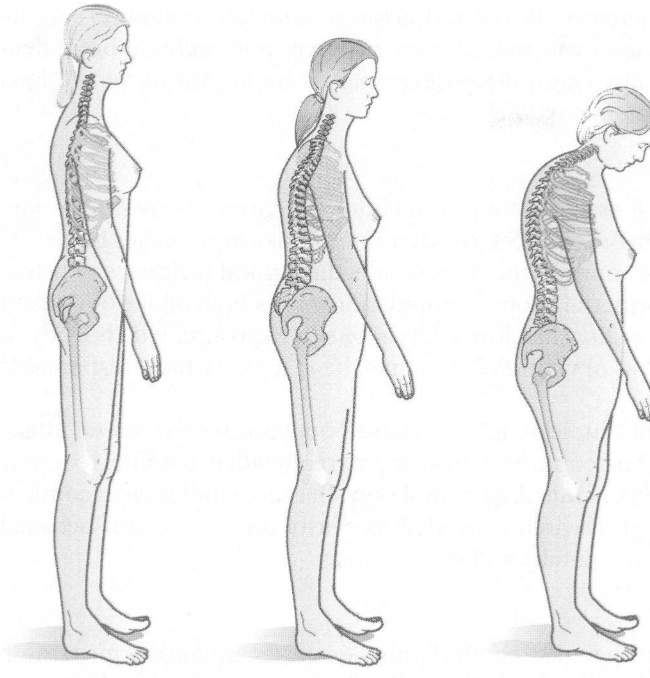

FIGURE 15.15 Progression of dowager's hump.

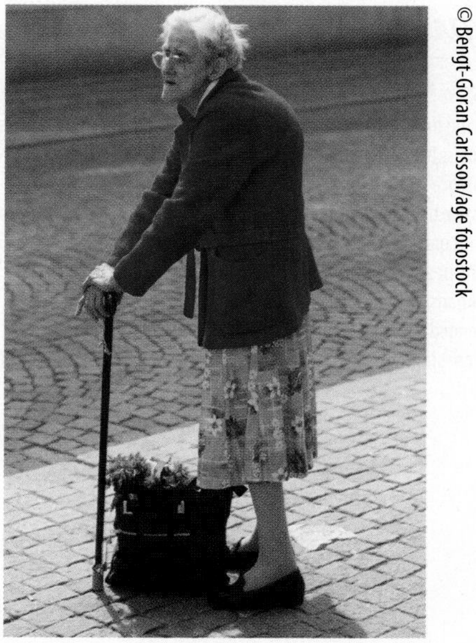

FIGURE 15.16 Dowager's hump. In people with osteoporosis, the bones in the upper spine develop small compression fractures. These bones heal into wedge shapes, and the upper spine assumes a deformed, curved shape known as a "dowager's hump."

Dietary and Lifestyle Factors for Reducing Osteoporosis Risk

The main factor in reducing risk of osteoporosis and related fractures is maximum peak bone mass. Dietary components such as calcium and vitamin D help to achieve and maintain bone mass. Engaging in physical activity, especially weight-bearing exercise, helps to increase peak bone mass early in life and helps to maintain muscle strength and coordination that will reduce risk for falls later in life.

Calcium

Calcium is important for attaining peak bone mass and for preventing and treating osteoporosis. Adequate calcium intake throughout life helps prevent osteoporosis, and good calcium intake during childhood and adolescence helps maximize peak bone mass. Even in adulthood, adequate calcium slows bone loss, and it reduces fracture rates in postmenopausal women.

Calcium is clearly an important nutrient in bone health, but it's not the only one. Normal mineralization and maintenance of bone also require vitamins D, A, and K; the minerals phosphorus, fluoride, and magnesium; and protein.

Vitamin D

You need vitamin D for calcium absorption and bone maintenance. Because aging limits the ability to manufacture active vitamin D, older people should use vitamin D–fortified foods such as milk or consider taking vitamin D supplements. Phytate and oxalate, caffeine, and smoking can reduce calcium absorption or increase excretion rates.

Vitamin D deficiency, which occurs more often in postmenopausal women and older Americans,[113] has been associated with a greater risk of hip fractures.

Quick Bite

Lost in Space

Knowing that stress on bones maintains their strength, what would you guess happens in the gravity-free environment of outer space? Experience with prolonged space travel has made it clear that extensive bone and mineral loss are one health hazard of living without gravity's constant pull. Interestingly, changes in non-weight-bearing bones were not seen in studies of space travelers. As humans spend longer periods in space, scientists will be challenged to discover how to preserve bone strength without the constant stimulation of gravity on weight-bearing bones.

Because bone loss increases the risk of fractures, moderate vitamin D supplementation (800 IU/day) can reduce bone turnover and increase bone density.[114] Because toxicity can quickly develop, it is important to be cautious with vitamin D supplements.

Vitamin A

Although vitamin A is essential for normal bone formation, some studies suggest an association between excessive vitamin A intake and weaker bones.[115] Researchers have also noticed that worldwide, the highest incidence of osteoporosis occurs in northern Europe, a population with a high intake of vitamin A.[116] However, this region has lower levels of sun exposure, which leads to decreased biosynthesis of vitamin D that may be at least partially responsible for these findings.

Evidence does not indicate an association between beta-carotene intake and increased risk of osteoporosis. Instead, current evidence points to a possible association with vitamin A as retinol only. Because studies yield conflicting results, additional research is needed to clarify the association between high levels of vitamin A intake and osteoporosis.

Exercise

Regular weight-bearing and strength-training exercises enhance bone remodeling and strength. Exercise helps maximize bone mass when you're young and will slow bone loss during your later years. In addition to getting enough calcium and vitamin D to promote bone health and slow the development of osteoporosis, fitness experts make the following suggestions:

- Exercise should include weight-bearing and resistance training and should put stress on bones. (Examples include walking and running.)
- For continued improvement, exercise intensity should increase progressively.
- There is a maximum achievable bone density. As this point is approached, greater efforts are needed to achieve smaller gains.
- Discontinuing an exercise program reverses the benefits.
- Don't smoke, and drink alcoholic beverages only in moderation.

Putting It All Together

Osteoporosis is a debilitating degenerative disease that contributes to poor quality of life in older adults. Although bone loss with age is a major contributor to osteoporosis, maximizing peak bone mass early in life can go a long way toward preventing or at least delaying osteoporosis. Reducing the proportion of adults with osteoporosis is one of the Healthy People 2020 objectives.

To improve your bone health, the U.S. Surgeon General suggests the following: Eat foods rich in calcium and vitamin D, be physically active every day, maintain a healthy body weight throughout your life, protect yourself from falls, avoid smoking, limit alcohol intake, and discuss increased risks with your doctor.[117] Postmenopausal women with low bone density might be advised to consider strength training to prevent or reduce bone loss.

Key Concepts Osteoporosis is the progressive loss of bone mass, resulting in fragile bones that break easily. Osteoporosis primarily affects postmenopausal women who have lower estrogen levels and accelerated rates of bone loss. Adequate calcium intake early in life helps maximize peak bone mass and reduces the risk of osteoporosis. Adequate amounts of vitamin D and regular exercise also are important for bone health.

Label to Table

Sodium is found naturally in many foods, but processed foods account for most of the salt and sodium Americans consume. Processed foods with high amounts of salt include regular canned vegetables and soups, frozen dinners, lunch meats, instant and ready-to-eat cereals, and salty chips and other snacks. You can use food labels to choose products lower in sodium.

Compare Labels

Which of these two items is lower in sodium? To tell, check the Percent Daily Value.

The frozen peas are lower in sodium, with just 5 percent of the DV per ½ cup serving. The canned peas have three times more sodium than the frozen peas: 16 percent of the DV in one serving.

Sodium is found in many foods that might surprise you, such as baking soda, soy sauce, and monosodium glutamate (MSG). Sodium is even found in some antacids—the range is wide.

Before trying salt substitutes, check with your doctor, especially if you have high blood pressure. Many salt substitutes contain potassium chloride and can be harmful for individuals who have certain medical conditions or who take diuretic medications.

Nutrition Facts

3 servings per container

Serving size	1/2 cup
Amount per serving	
Calories	**60**
	% Daily Value*
Total Fat 0g	**0%**
Saturated Fat 0g	**0%**
Trans Fat 0g	
Cholesterol 0mg	**0%**
Sodium 380mg	**16%**
Total Carbohydrate 12g	**4%**
Dietary Fiber 3g	**14%**
Total Sugars 4g	
Includes 4g Added Sugars	**8%**
Protein 4g	
Vitamin D 0mcg	0%
Calcium 20mg	2%
Iron 1.4mg	8%
Potassium 124mg	4%

* The % Daily Value (DV) tells you how much a nutrient in a serving of food contributes to a daily diet. 2,000 calories a day is used for general nutrition advice.

Nutrition Facts

3 servings per container

Serving size	1/2 cup
Amount per serving	
Calories	**60**
	% Daily Value*
Total Fat 0g	**0%**
Saturated Fat 0g	**0%**
Trans Fat 0g	
Cholesterol 0mg	**0%**
Sodium 125mg	**5%**
Total Carbohydrate 11g	**4%**
Dietary Fiber 6g	**22%**
Total Sugars 5g	
Includes 5g Added Sugars	**10%**
Protein 5g	
Vitamin D 0mcg	0%
Calcium 300mg	30%
Iron 1.1mg	6%
Potassium 87mg	2%

* The % Daily Value (DV) tells you how much a nutrient in a serving of food contributes to a daily diet. 2,000 calories a day is used for general nutrition advice.

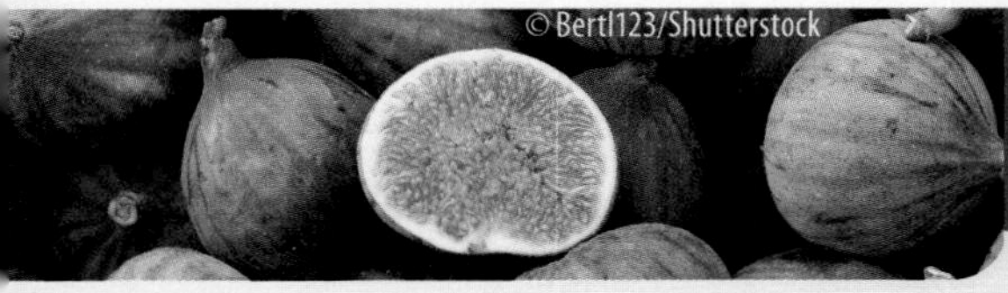
© Bertl123/Shutterstock

Learning Portfolio

Key Terms

atherosclerosis	614
base pair	613
benign	628
blood pressure	623
C-reactive protein (CRP)	615
cancer	627
carcinogens	629
cardiovascular disease (CVD)	613
complementary sequence	613
coronary heart disease (CHD)	614
DASH (Dietary Approaches to Stop Hypertension)	626
diastolic	624
endothelial cells	614
endothelium	614
essential hypertension	624
fasting hypoglycemia	636
gene expression	613
genes	611
genetic code	613
gestational diabetes	634
health disparities	610
Human Genome Project	611
hypercholesterolemia	615
hyperglycemia	633
hypertension	623
hypoglycemia	636
insulin resistance	635
leukemia	628
lipoprotein a [Lp(a)]	615
lymph nodes	628
lymphoma	628
malignant	628
melanocytes	628
melanoma	628
metabolic syndrome	641
metastasis	628
mutation	613
nucleotides	612
nutrition informatics	610
plaque	614
platelets	614
pre-diabetes	635
reactive hypoglycemia	636
risk factors	616
secondary hypertension	624
sphygmomanometer	623
systolic	623
tissue	628
tumor	628
type 1 diabetes	634
type 2 diabetes	634

Study Points

- Genetics plays a part in nearly all human diseases.
- Much of the prevalence of cardiovascular disease and cancer can be attributed to smoking, consumption of a high-fat diet, and a sedentary lifestyle.
- LDL and HDL cholesterol levels predict heart disease risks more accurately than do total cholesterol levels. Infection and the inflammatory process play a role in heart disease, and C-reactive protein might offer a new assessment of CVD risk.
- Ways to reduce risk for CVD include stopping smoking, exercising daily, managing weight, controlling blood pressure, and eating a healthful diet. Antioxidants, regular fish intake, and moderate alcohol consumption also can help protect against heart disease.
- Because hypertension usually has no specific symptoms or early warning signs, it is often called a silent killer.
- Added weight places greater demands on the cardiovascular system, so people who are overweight are at higher risk for hypertension. Rates of hypertension are higher in countries with high sodium intakes.
- The three phases in the development of cancer are initiation, promotion, and progression.
- Evidence shows that generous intake of vegetables and fruits reduces the risk of cancer.
- An estimated 25.8 million people—8.3 percent of the population—in the United States have diabetes mellitus, and just over one-third of these are unaware of their condition.
- Three major types of diabetes are type 1, type 2, and gestational diabetes.
- The dramatic surge in obesity rates in the United States is a major reason why the incidence of type 2 diabetes has tripled since 1970.
- Dietary recommendations for people with diabetes emphasize consuming diets rich in complex carbohydrates (including fiber) and low in fat.
- Often called a silent disease, osteoporosis develops over several years without outward symptoms or diagnosis. Osteoporosis affects more than 53 million Americans, making it a major public health problem.
- To promote bone health and slow the development of osteoporosis, fitness experts suggest that exercise should be weight-bearing and should put stress on bones. Examples include walking and running.

Study Questions

1. In what ways do diet and exercise affect your health?
2. What is the major goal of the Human Genome Project?
3. What are the diet-related guidelines for reducing heart disease risk?
4. How do high levels of homocysteine contribute to heart disease?
5. What are the risk factors for hypertension?

6. How can people with hypertension lower their blood pressure?
7. What is the difference between cancer initiation and cancer promotion?
8. What are the major types of diabetes? Describe the differences among them.
9. What is metabolic syndrome?
10. Which vitamin and mineral are most important for maximizing bone mass and reducing risk of osteoporosis?

Try This

Learn CPR!

The CPR (cardiopulmonary resuscitation) courses given by the American Red Cross, the American Heart Association, your local fire department, and other groups can help you save a life someday. Anyone can take these courses and become qualified to perform CPR. Investigate CPR courses in your community, and sign up to take one.

What's Your Family History?

Look into your family medical history. Is there cardiovascular disease in your family, as indicated by premature deaths from heart attack, stroke, or congestive heart failure? Are there any cases of cancer in your family, and has anyone died of cancer? How about diabetes, hypertension, or osteoporosis? Interview your parents and other relatives and develop a history of chronic disease in your family. These diseases might be risk factors for you. Keep that point in mind as you consider whether you need to make lifestyle changes to stay healthy and avoid chronic disease.

References

1. World Health Organization. WHO definition of health. In: *Preamble to the Constitution of the World Health Organization, 1948*. 45th ed., supplement. October 2006. http://www.who.int/governance/eb/who_constitution_en.pdf. Accessed February 12, 2016.
2. MedlinePlus. Medical dictionary: disease. http://www.merriam-webster.com/medlineplus/disease. Accessed February 12, 2016.
3. World Health Organization. *Diet, Nutrition, and Chronic Disease in Context*. http://www.who.int/nutrition/topics/4_dietnutrition_prevention/en/. Accessed February 12, 2016.
4. Health Information Management Systems Society. Our partnership: the Academy of Nutrition & Dietetics & HIMSS. http://www.himss.org/ResourceLibrary/ContentReg.aspx?ItemNumber=17147. Accessed February 12, 2016.
5. U.S. Department of Health and Human Services. The vision, mission, and goals of *Healthy People 2020*. https://www.healthypeople.gov/sites/default/files/HP2020Framework.pdf. Accessed February 12, 2016.
6. Centers for Disease Control and Prevention. CDC health disparities and inequalities report—United States, 2013. *MMWR*. 2013;62(Suppl. 3).
7. Centers for Disease Control and Prevention. CDC strategies for reducing health disparities—selected CDC-sponsored interventions, United States, 2014. *MMWR*. 2014;63(Suppl. 1).
8. U.S. Department of Health and Human Services. 2008 physical activity guidelines for Americans. http://www.health.gov/Paguidelines/pdf/paguide.pdf. Accessed February 12, 2016.
9. Centers for Disease Control and Prevention. Strong men put their heart first. February 10, 2016. http://www.cdc.gov/features/heartmonth. Accessed February 29, 2016.
10. U.S. Department of Energy, Office of Science. Genomic Science Program. http://genomicscience.energy.gov/index.shtml. Accessed February 12, 2016.
11. Singh PR, Lele SS, Mukheerjee MS. Gene polymorphisms and low dietary intake of micronutrients in coronary artery disease. *J Nutrigenet Nutrigenomics*. 2011;4(4):203–209.
12. Sales NMR, Pelegrini PB, Goersch MC. Nutrigenomics: definitions and advances of this new science. *J Nutr Metab*. 2014;2014:202759. Epub March 25, 2014. http://www.ncbi.nlm.nih.gov/pmc/articles/PMC3984860/. Accessed February 12, 2016.
13. Go A, Mozaffarian D, Roger V, et al. Heart disease and stroke statistics—2014 update: a report from the American Heart Association. *Circulation*. 2014;129:e28–e292. http://circ.ahajournals.org/content/129/3/e28. Accessed February 12, 2016.
14. Tufano A, Di Capua M, Coppola A, et al. The infectious burden in atherothrombosis. *Semin Thromb Hemost*. 2012;38(5):515–523.
15. Ibid.
16. Go A, Mozaffarian D, Roger V, et al. Heart disease and stroke statistics—2014 update. Op cit.
17. Yoon SS, Carroll MD, Johnson CL, Gu Q. Cholesterol management in the United States: the National Health and Nutrition Examination Survey, 1999 to 2006. *Ann Epidemiol*. 2011;21(5):318–326.
18. Hu FB. Diet and lifestyle influences on risk of coronary heart disease. *Curr Atheroscler Rep*. 2009;11(4):257–263.
19. Takaoka N, Campbell LA, Lee A, Rosenfeld ME, Kuo CC. Chlamydia pneumoniae infection increases adherence of mouse macrophages to mouse endothelial cells in vitro and to aortas ex vivo. *Infect Immun*. 2008;76(2):510–514.
20. Strang F, Schunkert H. Review article: C-reactive protein and coronary heart disease: All said—is not it? *Mediators Inflamm*. 2014;2014:757123. Epub April 7, 2014. http://www.ncbi.nlm.nih.gov/pmc/articles/PMC3997990/pdf/MI2014-757123.pdf. Accessed February 12, 2016.
21. Panichi V, Scatena A, Migliori M, et al. Biomarkers of chronic inflammatory state in uremia and cardiovascular disease. *Int J Inflamm*. 2012;2012:360147.
22. Rosero-Bixby L, Dow WH. Predicting mortality with biomarkers: a population-based prospective cohort study for elderly Costa Ricans. *Popul Health Metr*. 2012;10(1):111.
23. American Heart Association. The 2020 impact goal. http://www.heart.org/idc/groups/heart-public/@wcm/@swa/documents/downloadable/ucm_425189.pdf. Accessed February 12, 2016.
24. Raj M. Obesity and cardiovascular risk in children and adolescents. *Indian J Endocrinol Metab*. 2012;16(1):13–19.
25. Pashkow FJ. Oxidative stress and inflammation in heart disease: Do antioxidants have a role in treatment and/or prevention? *Int J Inflamm*. 2011; Article ID 514623. http://dx.doi.org/10.4061/2011/514623. Accessed February 12, 2016.
26. Riccioni G, Sblendorio V, Genello E, et al. Dietary fibers and cardiometabolic diseases. *Int J Mol Sci*. 2012;13(2):1524–1540.
27. Padayatty SJ, Levine M. Fruit and vegetables: think variety, go ahead, eat! *Am J Clin Nutr*. 2008;87(1):5–7.
28. Ye EQ, Chacko SA, Chou EL, Kugizaki M, Liu S. Greater whole-grain intake is associated with lower risk of type 2 diabetes, cardiovascular disease, and weight gain. *J Nutr*. 2012;142(7):1304–1313.

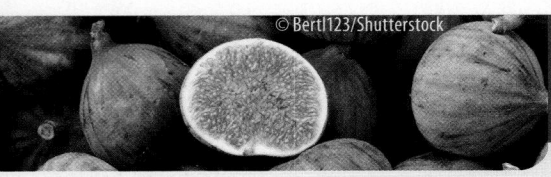

Learning Portfolio (continued)

29. Wong J, de Souza R, Kendall C, et al. Colonic health: fermentation and short chain fatty acids. *J Clin Gastroenterol*. 2006;40(3):235–243.
30. Institute of Medicine, Food and Nutrition Board. *Dietary Reference Intakes for Energy, Carbohydrate, Fiber, Fat, Fatty Acids, Cholesterol, Protein, and Amino Acids*. Washington, DC: National Academies Press; 2005.
31. Eilat-Adar S, Sinai T, Yosefy C, Henkin Y. Review: nutritional recommendations for cardiovascular disease prevention. *Nutrients*. 2013;5(9):3646–3683. http://www.ncbi.nlm.nih.gov/pmc/articles/PMC3798927/pdf/nutrients-05-03646.pdf. Accessed February 12, 2016.
32. Bang HO, Dyerberg J. The composition of food consumed by Greenlandic Eskimos. *Acta Med Scand*. 1973;200:69–73.
33. American Heart Association. Fish and omega-3 fatty acids. http://www.heart.org/HEARTORG/GettingHealthy/NutritionCenter/HealthyDietGoals/Fish-and-Omega-3-Fatty-Acids_UCM_303248_Article.jsp. Accessed February 12, 2016.
34. Kotwal S, Jun M, Sullivan D, et al. Omega 3 fatty acids and cardiovascular outcomes: systematic review and meta-analysis. *Circulation*. 2012;5:808–818. http://circoutcomes.ahajournals.org/content/5/6/808.full.pdf. Accessed February 12, 2016.
35. American Heart Association. Fish and omega-3 fatty acids. Op cit.
36. Chowdhury R, Warnakula S, Kunutsor S, et al. Association of dietary, circulating, and supplement fatty acids with coronary risk: a systematic review and meta-analysis. *Ann Intern Med*. 2014;160(6):398–406.
37. Eckel RH, Jakicic JM, Ard JD, et al. 2013 AHA/ACC guideline on lifestyle management to reduce cardiovascular risk. *Circulation*. 2014;129(suppl 2):S76–S99.
38. Tufts University. Does new study mean "butter is back"? Tufts Health and Nutrition Letter. June 2014. http://www.nutritionletter.tufts.edu/issues/10_6/current-articles/Does-New-Study-Mean-Butter-Is-Back_1467-1.html?ET=tuftshealthletter:e1955:1459886a:&st=email&s=p_update052714&t=tl1. Accessed February 12, 2016.
39. Eckel RH, Jakicic JM, Ard JD, et al. 2013 AHA/ACC guideline on lifestyle management to reduce cardiovascular risk. Op cit.
40. Baum SJ, Kris-Etherton PM, Lichtenstein AH, et al. Fatty acids in cardiovascular health and disease: a comprehensive update. *J Clin Lipidol*. 2012;6(3):216–234.
41. Ros E, Martinez-Gonzales MA, Estruch R, et al. Mediterranean diet and cardiovascular health: teaching of the PREDIMED study. *Adv Nutr*. 2014;5(3):330S–336S.
42. Fryxell DA. Forget pizza. TuftsNow. April 17, 2014. http://now.tufts.edu/articles/forget-pizza. Accessed February 12, 2016.
43. Arriola L, Martinez-Camblor P, Larranaga N, et al. Alcohol intake and the risk of coronary heart disease in the Spanish EPIC study. *Heart*. 2010;96(2):124–130.
44. Phend C. Mediterranean diet still being refined. Medpage Today. April 23, 2013. http://www.medpagetoday.com/MeetingCoverage/EuroPRevent/38621. Accessed February 12, 2016.
45. Dietary Guidelines for Americans 2015–2020. Key elements of healthy eating patterns. http://health.gov/dietaryguidelines/2015/guidelines/chapter-1/ Accessed February 29, 2016.
46. Arriola L, Martinez-Camblor P, Larranaga N, et al. Alcohol intake and the risk of coronary heart disease in the Spanish EPIC study. Op cit.
47. Clarke R, Halsey J, Bennett D, Lewinston S. Homocysteine and vascular disease: review of published results of the homocysteine-lowering trials. *J Inherit Metab Dis*. 2011;34(1):83–91.
48. Sacks FM, Lichtenstein A, Van Horn L, et al. Soy protein, isoflavones, and cardiovascular health: an American Heart Association science advisory for professionals from the nutrition committee. *Circulation*. 2006;113:1034–1044.
49. Xiao CW. Health effects of soy protein and isoflavones in humans. *J Nutr*. 2008;138(6):1244S–1249S.
50. Nwankwo T, Yoon S, Burt V, et al. Hypertension among adults in the United States: National Health and Nutrition Examination Survey, 2011-2012. October 2013. http://www.cdc.gov/nchs/data/databriefs/db133.pdf. Accessed February 12, 2016.
51. Go AS, Bauman MA, Coleman-King SM, et al. An effective approach to high blood pressure control: a science advisory from the American Heart Association, the American College of Cardiology, and the Centers for Disease Control and Prevention. *Hypertension*. 2014;63(4):878–885.
52. American Heart Association. High blood pressure and African Americans. April 4, 2014. http://www.heart.org/HEARTORG/Conditions/HighBloodPressure/UnderstandYourRiskforHighBloodPressure/High-Blood-Pressure-and-African-Americans_UCM_301832_Article.jsp. Accessed February 12, 2016.
53. National Heart, Lung, and Blood Institute. Your guide to lowering your blood pressure with DASH—What is high blood pressure? https://www.nhlbi.nih.gov/health/resources/heart/hbp-dash-what-blood-pressure-html. Accessed February 12, 2016.
54. Appel LJ, Brands MW, Daniels SR, et al. Dietary approaches to prevent and treat hypertension: a scientific statement from the American Heart Association. *Hypertension*. 2006;47:296–308.
55. Yi S, Elfassy T, Gupta L, Myers C, Kerker B. Nativity, language spoken at home, length of time in the United States, and race/ethnicity: associations with self-reported hypertension. October 7, 2013. http://ajh.oxfordjournals.org/content/27/2/237.short. Accessed February 12, 2016.
56. U.S. Department of Health and Human Services, National Heart, Lung and Blood Institute. *In Brief: Your Guide to Lowering Your Blood Pressure with DASH*. August 2015. NIH publication 06–5834. http://www.nhlbi.nih.gov/files/docs/public/heart/dash_brief.pdf. Accessed February 12, 2016.
57. Harsha DW, Lin PW, Obarzanek E, et al. Dietary Approaches to Stop Hypertension: a summary of study results. *J Am Diet Assoc*. 1999;99(8 Suppl):S35–S39.
58. Vogt TM, Appel LJ, Obarzanek E, et al. Dietary Approaches to Stop Hypertension: rationale, design, and methods. *J Am Diet Assoc*. 1999;99(8 Suppl):S12–S18.
59. National Heart, Lung, and Blood Institute. The DASH eating plan as part of a heart-healthy lifestyle. http://www.nhlbi.nih.gov/health/health-topics/topics/dash/lifestyle Accessed Feb ruary 29, 2016.
60. Ibid.
61. Kwan WM, Wong MC, Wang HH, et al. Compliance with the Dietary Approaches to Stop Hypertension (DASH) diet: a systemic review. *PloS One*. 2013;8(10):e78412. http://www.ncbi.nlm.nih.gov/pmc/articles/PMC3813594/#!po=3.57143. Accessed February 12, 2016.
62. National Center for Health Statistics. Leading causes of deaths. http://www.cdc.gov/nchs/fastats/leading-causes-of-death.htm. Accessed February 12, 2016.
63. Berretta M, Cappellani A, Lleshi A. The role of diet in gastric cancer: still an open question. *Front Biosci*. 2012;17:1640–1647.
64. National Cancer Institute. Causes of cancer. http://www.cancer.gov/research/areas/causes. Accessed February 12, 2016.
65. Kushi LH, Doyle C, McCullough M, et al., American Cancer Society 2010 Nutrition and Physical Activity Guidelines Advisory Committee. American Cancer Society guidelines on nutrition and physical activity for cancer prevention: reducing the risk of cancer with healthy food choices and physical activity. *CA Cancer J Clin*. 2012;62:30–67.
66. Makarem N, Chandran U, Bandera EV, Parekh N. Dietary fat in breast cancer survival. *Annu Rev Nutr*. 2013;33:319–348.
67. Rohmann S, Linseisen J, Nothlings U, et al. Meat and fish consumption and risk of pancreatic cancer: results from the European Prospective Investigation into Cancer and Nutrition. *Int J Cancer*. 2013;132(3):617–624.
68. Xu X, Yu E, Gao X, et al. Red and processed meat intake and risk of colorectal adenomas: a meta-analysis of observational studies. *Int J Cancer*. 2013;132(2):437–438.
69. Centers for Disease Control and Prevention. State indicator report on fruits and vegetables, 2013. http://www.cdc.gov/nutrition/downloads/State-Indicator-Report-Fruits-Vegetables-2013.pdf. Accessed February 12, 2016.
70. Fruits and Veggies—More Matters. http://www.fruitsandveggiesmorematters.org. Accessed February 12, 2016.
71. Agurs-Collins T, Rosenberg L, Makambi K, et al. Dietary patterns and breast cancer risk in women participating in the Black Women's Health Study. *Am J Clin Nutr*. 2009;90(3):621–628.
72. Wu AH, Yu MC, Tseng C-C, et al. Dietary patterns and breast cancer risk in Asian American women. *Am J Clin Nutr*. 2009;89(4):1145–1154.
73. Bradbury KE, Appleby PN, Key TJ. Fruit, vegetable, and fiber intake in relation to cancer risk: findings from the European Prospective Investigation into

Cancer and Nutrition (EPIC). *Am J Clin Nutr*. 2014;100(Suppl 1):394S–398S. http://ajcn.nutrition.org/content/100/Supplement_1/394S.short. Accessed February 12, 2016.

74. Kushi LH, Doyle C, McCullough M et al. American Cancer Society guidelines on nutrition and physical activity for cancer prevention. Op cit.
75. Messina M, Wu AH. Perspectives on the soy-breast cancer relation. *Am J Clin Nutr*. 2009;89:1673S–1679S.
76. Centers for Disease Control and Prevention, National Center for Chronic Disease Prevention and Health Promotion. National diabetes fact sheet, 2011. http://www.cdc.gov/diabetes/pubs/pdf/ndfs_2011.pdf. Accessed February 12, 2016.
77. Ibid.
78. Centers for Disease Control and Prevention, National Center for Chronic Disease Prevention and Health Promotion. Diabetes report card 2012. http://www.cdc.gov/diabetes/pubs/pdf/DiabetesReportCard.pdf. Accessed February 12, 2016.
79. Gropper SS, Smith JL, Groff JL. *Advanced Nutrition and Human Metabolism*. 6th ed. Belmont, CA: Wadsworth; 2012.
80. National Institute of Diabetes and Digestive and Kidney Diseases. National diabetes statistics, 2014. http://diabetes.niddk.nih.gov/DM/PUBS/statistics. Accessed February 29, 2016.
81. Ibid.
82. American Diabetes Association. Complications. http://www.diabetes.org/living-with-diabetes/complications/. Accessed February 12, 2016.
83. Ibid.
84. American Diabetes Association. Diagnosis and classification of diabetes mellitus. *Diabetes Care*. 2014;37(Suppl 1):S81–S90.
85. Ibid.
86. San Francisco General Hospital and Trauma Center, Center for Vulnerable Populations. The prevalence of gestational diabetes is growing. February 2013. http://cvp.ucsf.edu/docs/gdm_factsheet_format.pdf. Accessed February 12, 2016.
87. American Diabetes Association. Statistics about diabetes: data from the National Diabetes Statistics Report, 2014. http://www.diabetes.org/diabetes-basics/statistics. Accessed February 12, 2016.
88. Ibid.
89. National Institute of Diabetes and Digestive and Kidney Diseases. NIDDK: recent advances & emerging opportunities. March 2014. http://www.niddk.nih.gov/about-niddk/strategic-plans-reports/Documents/Feb%20Doc%202014/2014NIDDK_RecentAdvances_508c.pdf. Accessed February 12, 2016.
90. Centers for Diseases Control and Prevention, National Center for Chronic Disease Prevention and Health Promotion. National diabetes fact sheet, 2011. Op cit.
91. American Diabetes Association. Genetics of diabetes. http://www.diabetes.org/diabetes-basics/genetics-of-diabetes.html. Accessed February 12, 2016.
92. Ibid.
93. Frederiksen B, Kroehl M, Lamb MM, et al. Infant exposures and development of type 1 diabetes mellitus: the Diabetes Autoimmunity Study in the Young (DAISY). *JAMA Pediatr*. 2013;167(9):808–815.
94. American Diabetes Association. Genetics of diabetes. Op cit.
95. Ibid.
96. Centers for Disease Control and Prevention. Childhood obesity facts. http://www.cdc.gov/healthyschools/obesity/facts.htm. Accessed February 12, 2016.
97. Hunger M, Schunk M, Meisinger C, Peters A, Holle R. Estimation of the relationship between body mass index and EQ-5D health utilities in individuals with type 2 diabetes: evidence from the population-based KORA studies. *J Diabetes Complications*. 2012;26(5):413–418.
98. Risérusa U, Willett WC, Hu FB. Dietary fats and prevention of type 2 diabetes. *Prog Lipid Res*. 2009;48(1):44–51. http://www.ncbi.nlm.nih.gov/pmc/articles/PMC2654180/pdf/nihms91661.pdf. Accessed February 12, 2016.
99. Malik VS, Hu FB. Sweeteners and risk of obesity and type 2 diabetes: the role of sugar-sweetened beverages. *Curr Diabetes Rep*. 2012;12(2):195–203.
100. Lana A, Rodriquez-Artalejo F, Lopez-Garcia E. Consumption of sugar-sweetened beverages is positively related to insulin resistance and higher plasma leptin concentration in men and nonoverweight women. *J Nutr*. 2014 Jul;144(7):1099-1105.
101. Imamura F, O'Connor L, Ye Z, et al. Consumption of sugar sweetened beverages, artificially sweetened beverages, and fruit juice and incidence of type 2 diabetes: systematic review, meta-analysis, and estimation of population attributable fraction. *BMJ* 2015;351:h3576. http://www.bmj.com/content/351/bmj.h3576.full. Accessed February 12, 2016.
102. National Diabetes Information Clearinghouse. Diabetes prevention program. http://diabetes.niddk.nih.gov/dm/pubs/preventionprogram/#results. Accessed February 12, 2016.
103. Sepah SC, Jiang L, Peters AL. Translating the diabetes prevention program into an online social network: validation against CDC standards. *Diabetes Educ*. April 15, 2014. Epub ahead of print.
104. National Diabetes Education Program. Small steps big rewards. Prevent type 2 diabetes for life. Campaign overview. http://www.niddk.nih.gov/health-information/health-communication-programs/ndep/partnership-community-outreach/campaigns/small-steps-big-rewards/Pages/smallstepsbigrewards.aspx Accessed February 29, 2016.
105. American Diabetes Association. My health advisor. http://www.diabetes.org/are-you-at-risk/my-health-advisor/. Accessed February 12, 2016.
106. Bankoski A, Harris TB, McClain JJ, et al. Sedentary activity associated with metabolic syndrome independent of physical activity. *Diabetes Care*. 2011;34(2):497–503. doi: 10.2337/dc10-0987. http://www.ncbi.nlm.nih.gov/pubmed/21270206. Accessed February 12, 2016.
107. Ibid.
108. Novo S, Peritore A, Guameri FP, et al. Metabolic syndrome (MetS) predicts cardio and cerebrovascular events in a twenty year follow-up. A prospective study. *Atherosclerosis*. 2012;223(2):468–472.
109. Ogbera AO. Relationship between serum testosterone levels and features of the metabolic syndrome defining criteria in patients with type 2 diabetes mellitus. *West Afr J Med*. 2011;30(4):277–281.
110. NIH Osteoporosis and Related Bone Diseases National Resource Center. Osteoporosis overview. June 2015. http://www.niams.nih.gov/Health_Info/Bone/Osteoporosis/overview.asp. Accessed February 12, 2016.
111. National Osteoporosis Foundation. The man's guide to osteoporosis. 2011. http://nof.org/files/nof/public/content/file/252/upload/85.pdf. Accessed February 12, 2016.
112. Osteoporosis Canada. Osteoporosis facts & statistics. http://www.osteoporosis.ca/osteoporosis-and-you/osteoporosis-facts-and-statistics/. Accessed February 12, 2016.
113. National Institutes of Health, Office of Dietary Supplements. Vitamin D: fact sheet for health professionals. November 10, 2014. https://ods.od.nih.gov/factsheets/VitaminD-HealthProfessional/#h6. Accessed February 12, 2016.
114. Cândido FG, Bressan J. Review: vitamin D: link between osteoporosis, obesity, and diabetes? *Int J Mol Sci*. 2014;15:6569–6591.
115. Granados JM, Cuenca-Acevedo JR, Luque de Castro MD. Vitamin D insufficiency together with high serum levels of vitamin A increases the risk for osteoporosis in postmenopausal women. *Arch Osteoporos*. 2013;8(1–2):124.
116. Lippuner K. Epidemiology and burden of osteoporosis in Switzerland. *Ther Umsch*. 2012;69(3):137–144.
117. NIH Osteoporosis and Related Bone Diseases National Resource Center. The Surgeon General's report on bone health and osteoporosis. March 2012. NIH publication no. 12–7827. http://www.niams.nih.gov/Health_Info/Bone/SGR/surgeon_generals_report.asp. Accessed February 12, 2016.

Chapter 16

Life Cycle: Maternal and Infant Nutrition

Revised by Paul Insel

THINK About It

1. Saying she is eating for two, your pregnant friend can't seem to stop eating. What do you think about this?
2. Your best friend tells you she is pregnant. You know that she enjoys wine with dinner. What do you say to her?
3. Were you breastfed? Do you know of any benefits of breastfeeding?
4. At a fast food restaurant, you observe a man and woman giving a very young infant tiny pieces of french fries and a baby bottle filled with cola. Any thoughts?

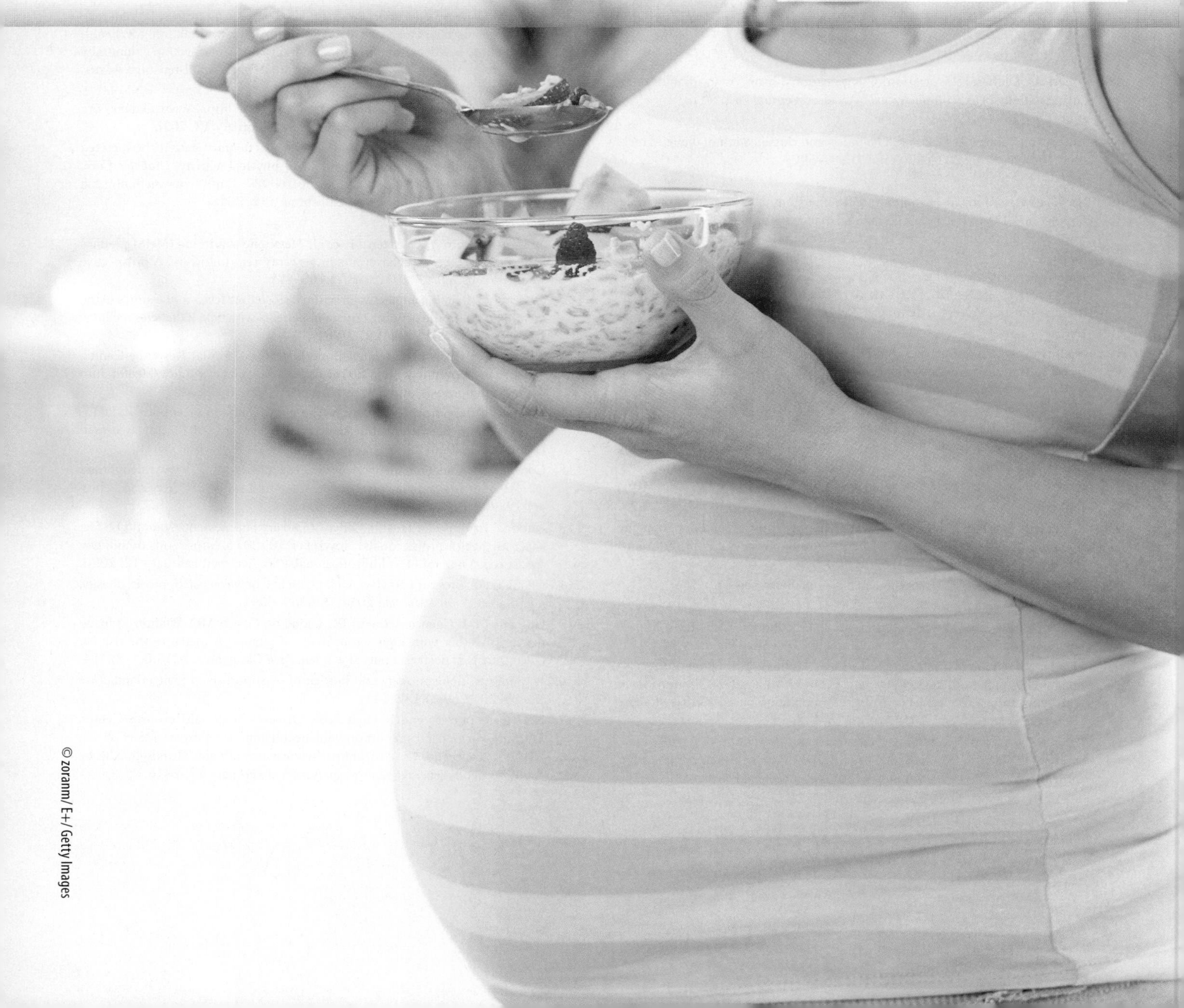

CHAPTER Menu

- Pregnancy
- Lactation
- Resources for Pregnant and Lactating Women and Their Children
- Infancy
- Key Terms
- Study Points
- Study Questions
- Try This
- References

LEARNING Objectives

- Discuss maternal physiological changes that occur during pregnancy, including the components of maternal weight gain and the corresponding nutritional needs.
- Identify benefits of breastfeeding for both infant and mother.
- Describe energy and nutrient needs during infancy.
- Summarize the appropriate steps for introducing solid foods into an infant's diet.
- Identify feeding problems during infancy and provide recommendations to overcome them.

Imagine waking up tomorrow and finding a newborn baby in the house! Play along for a moment with the idea that it's your baby. Would your current eating habits have been sufficient to support the nutritional demands of pregnancy? If not, what changes should you have made and why? What about other aspects of your lifestyle that you may need to modify before pregnancy, such as smoking, alcohol use, or exercise? How would you feed a new baby? Breastfeeding imposes nutritional demands on the mother but provides many benefits for the infant. If you've never shopped for infant formula or baby food before, you may be surprised at the variety of choices and confused as to which is best. So, although the likelihood of waking up to find an unexpected newborn in the house is remote, it's never too early to learn about the nutritional implications of pregnancy, breastfeeding, and infant feeding.

Pregnancy

In both mother and fetus, pregnancy is a time of tremendous physiological change that demands healthful dietary and lifestyle choices. Energy and nutrient needs both increase, but the need for calories increases by a smaller percentage than the need for most vitamins and minerals. As a result, food choices during pregnancy must be nutrient-dense.

What about tobacco and alcohol? Research clearly shows that both tobacco and alcohol inflict damaging effects on a developing fetus, and it's essential to abstain from both during pregnancy. Although research about the effects of caffeine is less conclusive, most healthcare professionals also recommend limiting caffeine intake during pregnancy.

Nutrition Before Conception

THINK About It 1

Once she becomes pregnant, a woman needs to focus on a healthful diet. But her nutritional status at the moment of conception also is important. Vitamin status at conception, for example, can determine the difference between a healthy baby and one with a devastating birth defect. In addition, a woman's weight at conception can influence her pregnancy and delivery as well as the baby's health.

For these reasons, it's important for a woman to get health care and guidance before she gets pregnant. Many experts recommend extending prenatal care—the routine, professional health care that a woman receives during her pregnancy—to include the preconception period as well (see **FIGURE 16.1**).

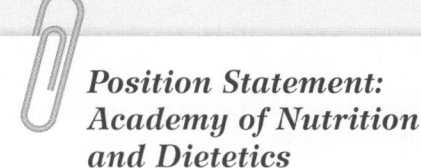

Position Statement: Academy of Nutrition and Dietetics

Nutrition and Lifestyle for a Healthy Pregnancy Outcome

It is the position of the Academy of Nutrition and Dietetics that women of childbearing age should adopt a lifestyle optimizing health and reduce the risk of birth defects, suboptimal fetal development, and chronic health problems in both mother and child. Components leading to healthy pregnancy outcomes include healthy prepregnancy weight, appropriate weight gain and physical activity during pregnancy, consumption of a variety of foods, appropriate vitamin and mineral supplementation, avoidance of alcohol and other harmful substances, and safe food handling. Pregnancy is a critical period during which maternal nutrition and lifestyle choices are major influences on mother and child health. Inadequate levels of key nutrients during crucial periods of fetal development may lead to reprogramming within fetal tissues, predisposing the infant to chronic conditions in later life. Improving the well-being of mothers, infants, and children is key to the health of the next generation.

Reproduced from Procter S, Campbell C. Position of the Academy of Nutrition and Dietetics: nutrition and lifestyle for a healthy pregnancy outcome. *J Am Diet Assoc*. 2014;114(7):1099–1103.

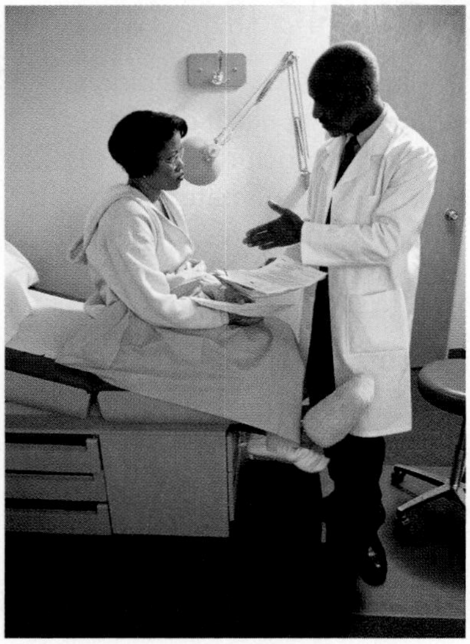

© Photodisc

FIGURE 16.1 Preconception care. Planning and care before pregnancy are recommended for all prospective mothers.

Although extending prenatal health care is a worthy goal, it is important to realize that about half the pregnancies in the United States are unplanned. Hence, good nutrition for all women of childbearing age is an important public health objective.

Preconception care can be defined as a set of interventions that identify and modify biomedical, behavioral, and social risks to a woman's health or pregnancy outcome through prevention and management.[1] The overall goals are to (1) screen for risks; (2) promote health and education; and (3) identify, prevent, and manage risks. Nutrition is an important aspect of all three goals. Risk screening includes an evaluation of a prospective mother's vitamin status and weight as well as her health habits—including use of alcohol, tobacco, and other substances—and her overall medical condition. Health promotion and education means providing information to the would-be mother about steps she can take to maximize her chances of a trouble-free pregnancy, an uneventful delivery, and a healthy, full-term baby. Intervention can be as simple as recommending a folic acid supplement or as complex as treating an eating disorder or a substance abuse problem. Before conception, the goal is to resolve the nutrition and health issues that could harm a mother or her baby. **TABLE 16.1** lists 10 recommendations for preconception health developed by the Centers for Disease Control and Prevention.

Weight

Although everyone should be concerned about maintaining a healthful weight, a woman contemplating pregnancy needs to pay special attention to weight. Maternal obesity can complicate pregnancy and delivery and compromise a baby's health. Being too thin likewise carries its own risks.

Body mass index (BMI) is an indicator of a prospective mother's weight status. Lean women with a BMI less than 20 kg/m^2 have increased risks of **preterm delivery**.[2] Inadequate weight gain and poor nutrition—marked by a low white blood cell count and high serum ferritin—during the first stages of pregnancy are also associated with preterm birth,[3] as are inadequate intakes of protein and energy, calcium, zinc, omega-3 fatty acids, and multiple micronutrients.[4] At the other end of the spectrum, nearly two-thirds of U.S. women of childbearing age are overweight or obese, and one-fifth are obese at the start of pregnancy.[5] Overweight and obese women have increased risks of several problems, including preterm delivery and stillbirth.[6] In addition, obese women are at higher risk for the following[7]:

▶ **preterm delivery** A delivery that occurs before the thirty-seventh week of gestation.

- High blood pressure
- Gestational diabetes—a form of diabetes associated with pregnancy that is often controlled through diet alone
- Preeclampsia—a condition marked by high blood pressure and protein in the urine
- Prolonged labor
- Unplanned cesarean section
- Difficulty initiating and continuing breastfeeding

Studies show that overweight and obesity during pregnancy are also linked to a variety of issues for the baby later in life, including higher BMI and waist circumference, increased subcutaneous adipose tissue, higher triglyceride levels and reduced high-density lipoprotein (HDL) cholesterol.[8]

TABLE 16.1
Recommendations for Preconception Health

Individual responsibility	Each woman, man, and couple should be encouraged to have a reproductive life plan.
Consumer awareness	Increase public awareness of appropriate preconception health behaviors.
Preventive visits	Provide risk assessment and health promotion counseling to all women of childbearing age during primary care visits.
Interventions for identified risks	Provide interventions to women following risk identification.
Interconception care	Use the interconception period for intensive interventions.
Prepregnancy checkups	Offer prepregnancy visits as a component of maternity care.
Health insurance coverage	Increase coverage to ensure access for low-income women.
Public health programs	Integrate preconception health into existing public health programs.
Research	Increase the evidence base for methods to improve preconception health.
Monitoring	Use public health surveillance mechanisms to monitor the effectiveness of preconception care.

Modified from Centers for Disease Control and Prevention. Recommendations to improve preconception health and health care—United States. *MMWR*. 2006;55(RR–06):1–23. http://www.cdc.gov/mmwr/preview/mmwrhtml/rr5506a1.htm. Accessed January 9, 2016.

THINK About It 2

Of course, the time to lose or gain weight is well before a pregnancy begins. It is not a good idea for pregnant women, even obese pregnant women, to try to lose weight or follow a restrictive diet during pregnancy. Even a thin woman who finds it hard to put on weight under normal circumstances is unlikely to find it any easier when she's pregnant, especially if she experiences **morning sickness**.

Women with eating disorders have special pregnancy-related risks. Ideally, anorexia nervosa or bulimia nervosa is diagnosed and treated well before conception, to give the prospective mother's body plenty of time to recover and prepare for the demands of pregnancy, birth, and breastfeeding. A woman who begins her pregnancy with an active eating disorder may not gain enough weight—or may vomit too much—to sustain a growing fetus. Risks can include premature delivery, a **low-birth-weight infant**, and even fetal death.

Vitamins

A good diet goes a long way toward meeting the demands of pregnancy, but even a diet that includes all the food groups can lack enough of certain nutrients. This is especially true for folic acid, a nutrient needed to prevent neural tube defects, which are birth defects that involve the spinal column.[9] One of the most common neural tube defects is spina bifida, a birth defect in which part of the spinal cord protrudes through the spinal column, causing varying degrees of paralysis and lack of bowel and bladder control (see **FIGURE 16.2**).

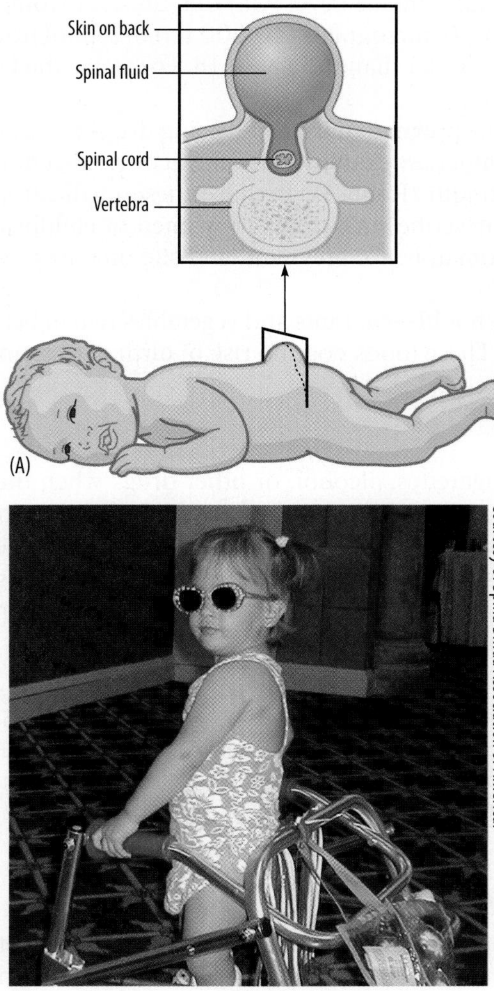

(B)

Courtesy of Spina Bifida Association of America.

FIGURE 16.2 Spina bifida: a neural tube defect. (a) Low folate status during the early stages of pregnancy can cause neural tube defects. (b) Spina bifida causes varying degrees of limb paralysis. Some children will be able to walk using leg braces or crutches whereas others will require a wheelchair.

Dietary Guidelines for Americans, 2015–2020

Key Recommendations

- Maintain appropriate calorie balance during each stage of life—childhood, adolescence, adulthood, pregnancy and breastfeeding, and older age.

Key Recommendations for Specific Population Groups
Women Capable of Becoming Pregnant

- Choose foods that supply heme iron, which is more readily absorbed by the body, additional iron sources, and enhancers of iron absorption such as vitamin C–rich foods.
- Consume 400 micrograms (mcg) per day of synthetic folic acid (from fortified foods and/or supplements) in addition to food forms of folate from a varied diet.

Women Who Are Pregnant or Breastfeeding

- Consume 8 to 12 ounces of seafood per week from a variety of seafood types.
- Due to their high methyl mercury content, limit white (albacore) tuna to 6 ounces per week and do not eat the following four types of fish: tailfish, shark, swordfish, and king mackerel.
- If pregnant, take an iron supplement, as recommended by an obstetrician or other healthcare provider.

Source: U.S. Department of Agriculture and U.S. Department of Health and Human Services. *Dietary Guidelines for Americans, 2015–2020*. 8th ed. Washington, DC: U.S. Government Printing Office; 2015.

▶ **morning sickness** A persistent or recurring nausea that often occurs in the morning during early pregnancy.

▶ **low-birth-weight infant** A newborn who weighs less than 2,500 grams (5.5 pounds) as a result of either premature birth or inadequate growth in utero.

TABLE 16.2
Folate in Grain Products

Foods	Folate (µg DFE)*
Ready-to-eat cereals (25% DV), 1 cup	170
Pasta, enriched, cooked, 1 cup	125–180
Rice, enriched, cooked, 1 cup	180
Tortilla, flour, enriched, 1 (10-inch diameter)	145
Bagel, enriched, 1 (3-inch diameter)	92
Bread, white, enriched, 1 slice	15–51

*DFE = Dietary Folate Equivalents

Data from U.S. Department of Agriculture, Agricultural Research Service. USDA National Nutrient Database for Standard Reference, Release 28. 2015. http://www.ars.usda.gov/ba/bhnrc/ndl. Accessed January 10, 2016.

The U.S. Preventive Services Task Force recommends that all women of childbearing age take a daily supplement of 400 to 800 micrograms of synthetic folic acid to reduce the risk of producing a fetal neural tube defect.[10] The CDC estimates that 50 to 70 percent of the birth defects spina bifida and anencephaly could be avoided if women consumed 400 micrograms of folic acid daily before and during pregnancy.[11]

This recommendation includes all women of childbearing age—not just pregnant women—because neural tube development occurs before the sixth week of fetal life. During this period, a woman may not know she is pregnant or may not have made appropriate dietary changes. This intake of folic acid is recommended in addition to folate (the natural form of the supplement) consumed from other foods. Folic acid is added to all enriched grain products and many ready-to-eat cereals. **TABLE 16.2** presents the folate content of selected grain products. The rate of neural tube defects has been declining in recent years, in part as a result of folic acid fortification.

Just as it is important to get enough folic acid, it is also crucial to avoid getting too much vitamin A (retinol) during pregnancy. Some vitamin A is good for you; too much can be teratogenic. A teratogen is a substance that causes birth defects—literally, the term means "monster-producing." The Institute of Medicine considered this link between excessive retinol intake and birth defects in setting the Tolerable Upper Intake Level (UL) of retinol for women of childbearing age. The UL is 3,000 micrograms (10,000 IU) of retinol from food and supplements for women older than the age of 18. For teens, the UL is 2,800 micrograms (9,300 IU).

Any woman who may become pregnant must avoid using drugs that contain vitamin A or vitamin A analogues; examples are the acne medications isotretinoin (Accutane) and tretinoin (Retin-A). Because these medications are potent teratogens, doctors prescribe such drugs to women of childbearing age only if tests show the woman is not pregnant, and she practices two forms of birth control.

Pregnant women can—and should—eat fruits and vegetables rich in beta-carotene and other carotenoids. These foods pose no risk of birth defects and offer many health benefits.

Substance Use

Many women plan to give up cigarettes, alcohol, or other drugs when they get pregnant. It is important to give up these substances well before becoming pregnant, which emphasizes the need for preconception guidance[12] (see **FIGURE 16.3**). A woman who uses or abuses tobacco, alcohol, or illicit drugs during pregnancy is likely to have higher pregnancy-related complications and more infant health problems.

THINK About It 3

Key Concepts Ideally, the time to prepare nutritionally for pregnancy is well before conceiving. A woman who has adequate nutrient stores, particularly of folic acid, and is at a healthy weight can reduce the risk for maternal and fetal complications during pregnancy. In addition to healthful diet selections, avoiding tobacco, alcohol, and other drugs is important when contemplating pregnancy.

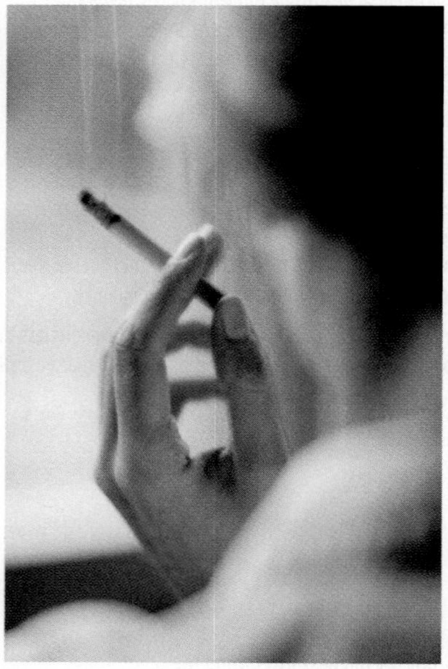

© Photodisc

FIGURE 16.3 Substance use. Using tobacco, alcohol, or illicit drugs before and during pregnancy puts the baby at risk. If you use these substances, stop before becoming pregnant.

Physiology of Pregnancy

Pregnancy is an awe-inspiring interactive process of growth and development for both mother and fetus. An understanding of the stages of growth and development of the fetus, along with the physiological changes that occur in the mother during pregnancy, helps to explain the nutrient needs of a pregnant woman.

Stages of Human Fetal Growth

How long does pregnancy last? Nine months, right? Well, it depends on when you start counting. When a health care provider gives an expectant mother a due date, it is typically calculated as 40 weeks from the date of the start of her last menstrual period, roughly 10 to 14 days before the actual date of conception. This 40-week period is often considered as three **trimesters** of 13 or 14 weeks each; however, these time divisions do not coincide with specific stages in fetal development.

FIGURE 16.4 illustrates the early stages of pregnancy. Fertilization of the egg (ovum) sets off the **blastogenic stage**—a period of rapid cell division. As these cells divide, they begin to differentiate. The inner cells in this growing mass will form the fetus; the outer layer of cells will become the **placenta**. During this stage, which lasts about two weeks, the fertilized ovum implants itself in the wall of the mother's uterus.

The next period of pregnancy, the **embryonic stage**, extends from the end of the second week through the eighth week after conception. The placenta, a vital organ that serves as filter and conduit between mother and child, forms on the uterine wall during this stage. Attached to the placenta by the umbilical cord, the embryo now receives its nourishment from its mother; nearly everything the mother eats, drinks, or smokes reaches the embryo.

The embryonic stage also is a period of **organogenesis**. By the time the embryo is eight weeks old, all its main internal organs have formed, along with the major external body structures (see **FIGURE 16.5**). Because nutrient deficiencies or excesses and intake of harmful substances during this time can result in congenital abnormalities (birth defects) or spontaneous abortion (miscarriage), this stage is a **critical period of development**.

The longest period of pregnancy is the **fetal stage**, the period from the end of the embryonic period until the baby is born. During this time, the fetus is growing rapidly, with dramatic changes in body proportions. From the end of the third month of pregnancy until delivery at full term, fetal weight increases nearly 500-fold. The typical newborn is about 20 inches (50 cm) long and weighs approximately 7 pounds 7 ounces (3.4 kg).

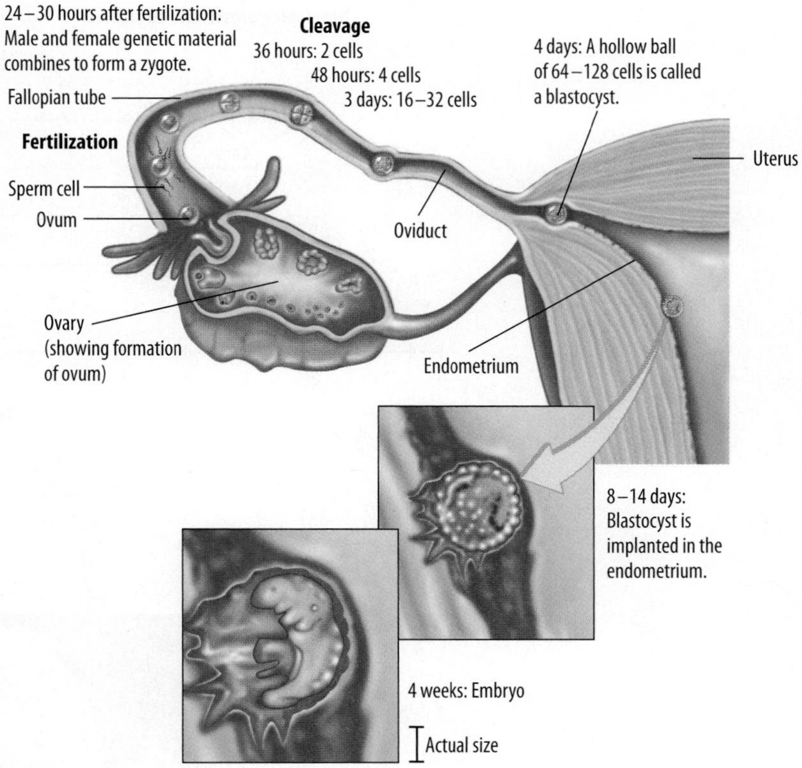

FIGURE 16.4 Early stages of pregnancy. The fertilized egg divides rapidly and begins to differentiate. The inner cells become the fetus, and the outer cells become the placenta.

- **trimesters** Three equal time periods of pregnancy, each lasting approximately 13 to 14 weeks, that do not coincide with specific stages in fetal development.
- **blastogenic stage** The first stage of gestation, during which tissue proliferation by rapid cell division begins.
- **placenta** The organ formed during pregnancy that produces hormones for the maintenance of pregnancy and across which oxygen and nutrients are transferred from mother to infant; it also allows waste materials to be transferred from infant to mother.
- **embryonic stage** The developmental stage between the time of implantation (about two weeks after fertilization) through the seventh or eighth week; the stage of major organ system differentiation and development of main external features.
- **organogenesis** The period when organ systems are developing in a growing fetus.
- **critical period of development** Time during which the environment has the greatest impact on the developing embryo.
- **fetal stage** The period of rapid growth from the end of the embryonic stage until birth.

Key Concepts From conception to full-term baby, the process of fetal development is typically described in three stages. The blastogenic stage involves rapid cell division of the fertilized ovum and its implantation in the uterine wall. During the embryonic stage, cells differentiate and organ systems and body structures are formed. The fetal stage, the longest stage of pregnancy, is marked by growth in size and change in body proportions.

Maternal Physiological Changes and Nutrition

While the fertilized ovum is developing from a mass of dividing cells into an embryo, and then into a fetus, changes are occurring in the mother's body as well (see **FIGURE 16.6**). These changes occur as the result of various hormones, secreted mainly by the placenta.

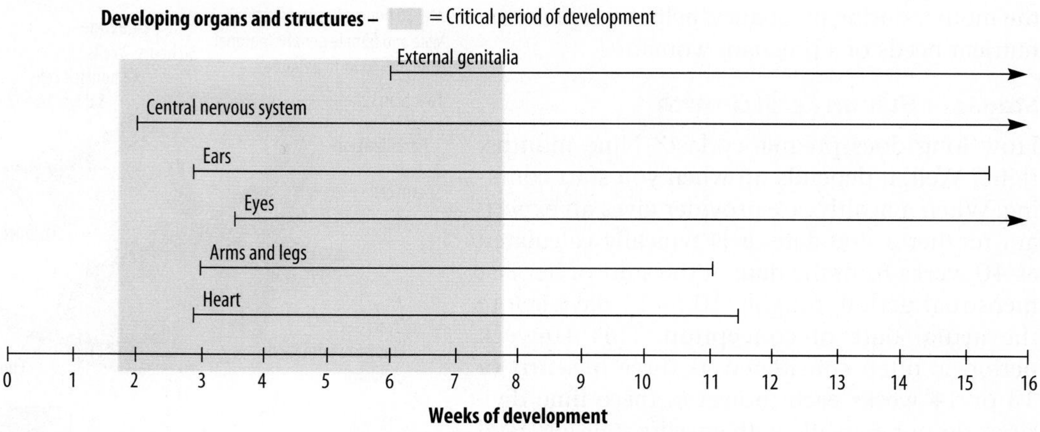

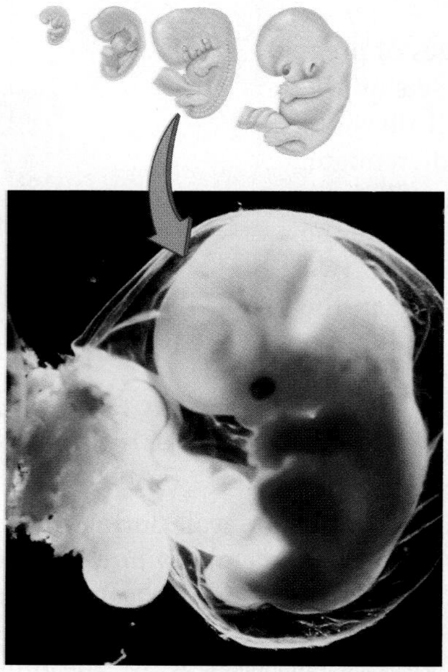

FIGURE 16.5 Embryonic development. During the embryonic stage—week 2 through week 8—all the major organ systems are forming. During this critical period of development, the embryo is highly vulnerable to nutrient deficiencies and toxicities as well as harmful substances, such as tobacco smoke.

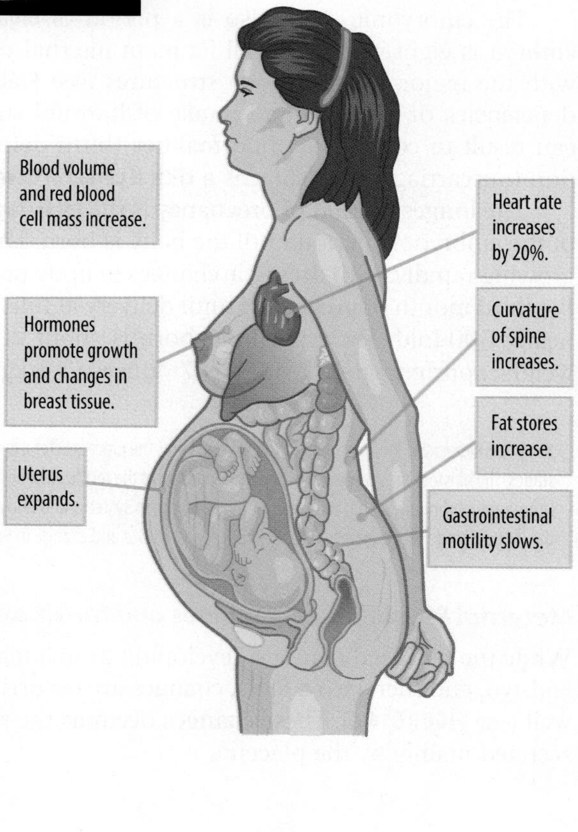

FIGURE 16.6 Maternal changes during pregnancy. Hormones released throughout pregnancy influence the growth of the baby and alter the way the mother's organs function.

Growth of Maternal Tissue Maternal tissues, including breasts, uterus, and adipose stores, enlarge during pregnancy. Hormones promote growth and changes in the breast tissue to prepare for **lactation**. Fat stores increase to provide energy for late pregnancy and for lactation and are a major component of maternal weight gain.

Maternal Blood Volume During the course of pregnancy, maternal blood volume expands by nearly 50 percent. Production of red blood cells also increases. Iron, folate, and vitamin B_{12} are all key nutrients in red blood cell production. Hemoglobin and hematocrit values during pregnancy are lower than when a woman is not pregnant, but this is more often the result of increased plasma volume diluting the blood cells than nutrient deficiency.

Gastrointestinal Changes During pregnancy, gastrointestinal motility slows, and food moves more slowly through the intestinal tract. Because nutrients spend more time in the small intestine, their slower transit permits greater nutrient absorption. On the other hand, slower motility can contribute to nausea, heartburn, constipation, and hemorrhoids.

Key Concept The mother's body changes during pregnancy, responding to changing levels of hormones. Uterine, breast, and adipose tissues grow; blood volume expands; and gastrointestinal motility slows. All these changes have nutritional and dietary implications for pregnant women.

▶ **lactation** The process of synthesizing and secreting breast milk.

Quick Bite

Would It Be Healthier to Menstruate *Less* Often?

Women in industrialized countries, who start menstruating at an average age of 12.5 years, will generate 350 to 400 menstrual cycles in their lifetimes. In populations that do not use birth control, however, women spend the majority of their fertile years either pregnant or lactating. Menarche in these populations occurs at an average age of 16. In addition, because menstrual cycles do not occur during pregnancy and may not occur during lactation, women in natural-fertility populations, such as the Dogon of West Africa, experience only about 110 menstrual cycles in a lifetime. Women who produce fewer menstrual cycles are exposed to less estrogen and other steroid hormones. Researchers hypothesize that this can partly explain why nonindustrialized societies have lower cancer rates than do industrialized societies.

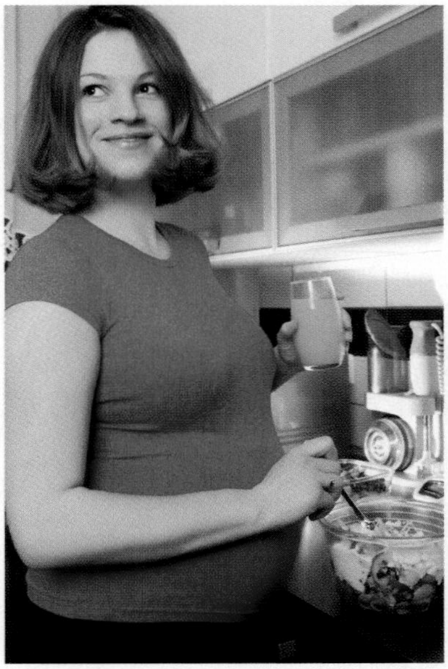

© Hemera/Thinkstock

Maternal Weight Gain

How much weight should a woman gain during pregnancy? Doctors' recommendations have varied over the years from minimal weight gain to unlimited weight gain to recommendations based on prepregnancy BMI, as shown in **TABLE 16.3**. The most recent pregnancy weight gain guidelines from the Institute of Medicine and the National Research Council consider that a woman's health and that of her infant are affected by the woman's weight at the start of pregnancy as well as how much she gains throughout the pregnancy.[13]

For underweight women with a BMI of less than 18.5 kg/m^2, the recommended weight gain is 28 to 40 pounds (12.5–18 kg). Normal-weight women with a starting BMI of 18.5 to 24.9 kg/m^2 should gain 25 to 35 pounds (11.5–16 kg). Women beginning pregnancy with an overweight BMI of 25.0 to 29.9 kg/m^2 are recommended to gain 15 to 25 pounds (7–11.5 kg). For the heaviest women—those with BMIs greater than 30.0 kg/m^2 at the start of pregnancy—a weight gain of 11 to 20 pounds (5–9 kg) is recommended.

TABLE 16.3
Guidelines for Weight Gain During Pregnancy

	Weight Gain[a]	
Prepregnancy BMI (kg/m^2)	Pounds	Kilograms
Underweight (< 18.5)	28–40	12.5–18
Normal (18.5–24.9)	25–35	11.5–16
Overweight (25.0–29.9)	15–25	7.0–11.5
Obese (> 30.0)	11–20	5–9

[a] Young pregnant adolescents should strive for gains at the upper end of the recommended range. Short pregnant women (< 157 cm or 62 in.) should strive for gains at the lower end of the range.

Reprinted with permission from *Weight Gain During Pregnancy: Reexamining the Guidelines*. © 2009 by the National Academy of Sciences, Courtesy of the National Academies Press, Washington, D.C.

When maternal weight gain is within these limits, infants are more likely to be born normal weight and at term. These guidelines reflect the greater number of overweight and obese women currently in the United States and advise women to choose a healthy diet and exercise to achieve a normal BMI prior to getting pregnant. Although weight gain varies widely among women who give birth to healthy, full-term infants, pregnancy weight gain guidelines aim to lower risks associated with pregnancy weight change.[14]

Twin births account for 1 of every 34 live births in the United States. Of course, women who carry two or more fetuses need to gain more weight than women who carry just one. For normal-weight women, the recommended weight gain for carrying twins is 37 to 54 pounds (17–25 kg). Overweight women are recommended to gain 31 to 50 pounds (14–23 kg), and obese women should gain 25 to 42 pounds (11–19 kg).[15] There is currently not enough information to establish weight gain guidelines for underweight women with multiple fetuses. However, a higher weight gain is often recommended for women who were underweight prior to pregnancy.

The pattern of weight gain also is important to a healthy pregnancy outcome. During the first trimester, average weight gain is low, less than 5 pounds for most women. Over the second and third trimesters, the suggested weight gain for normal-weight women is a little less than 1 pound per week (0.4 kg per week), with more gain suggested for underweight women and those carrying twins and a lower gain for women who are overweight or obese.[16] Monitoring the amount and rate of weight gain is an important component of prenatal care.

The weight gained during pregnancy is divided between (1) the fetus and associated tissues and fluids and (2) maternal tissue growth. In a typical final weight gain of 27.5 pounds (12.5 kg), the fetus, placenta, and **amniotic fluid** account for nearly 40 percent of that weight. Maternal tissues (i.e., adipose stores, breast and uterine growth, and expanded blood and extracellular fluid volumes) account for the remaining 60 percent (see **FIGURE 16.7**).

▶ **amniotic fluid** The fluid that surrounds the fetus; contained in the amniotic sac inside the uterus.

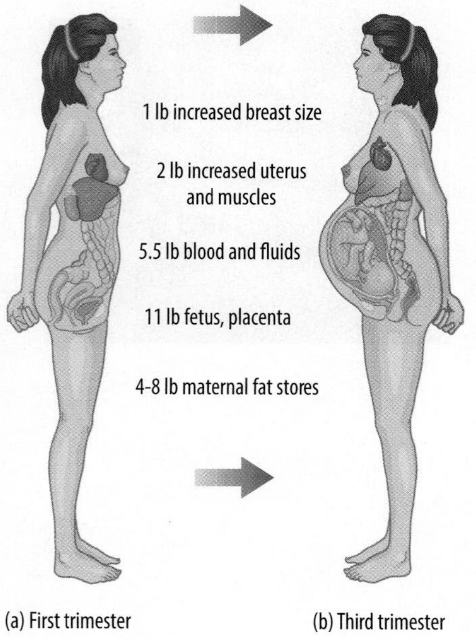

FIGURE 16.7 Components of maternal weight gain. During the first trimester, most women gain less than 5 pounds. Over the second and third trimesters, the suggested weight gain is a little less than 1 pound per week.

> **Key Concepts** Weight gained during pregnancy is a combination of increased weight in fetal and maternal tissues and fluids. Weight gain recommendations are based on BMI prior to pregnancy. Women of normal weight (BMI = 18.5–24.9 kg/m^2) should gain 25 to 35 pounds over the course of pregnancy. Most of this weight gain occurs during the second and third trimesters.

Energy and Nutrition During Pregnancy

A pregnant woman requires added calories to grow and maintain not just her developing fetus, but also its support system: placenta, increased breast tissue, and fat stores. Growth and development of the fetus also require protein, vitamins, and minerals.

Energy

Resting energy expenditure (REE) increases during pregnancy because of the energy requirements of the fetus and placenta and the increased workload on the heart and lungs.[17] Energy also is needed to support weight gain, primarily in the second and third trimesters. Using median energy expenditure as a guide, pregnant women need approximately 340 extra kilocalories per day during the second trimester and an extra 450 kilocalories per day during the third trimester.[18] Because actual energy expenditure varies widely, weight gain during pregnancy is probably the best indicator of adequate calorie intake.[19]

Nutrients to Support Pregnancy

Most healthy women who eat a well-balanced diet have no trouble meeting the majority of their nutrient requirements during pregnancy without vitamin and mineral supplements. However, despite even the best effort, many women have difficulty meeting increased recommendations during pregnancy for numerous nutrients, most often iron and folic acid. As a preventive measure, it is therefore recommended that all women planning to become pregnant take a multivitamin/mineral supplement containing folic acid.[20]

Essential nutrients can be divided into two broad categories: macronutrients (proteins, fats, and carbohydrates) and micronutrients (vitamins and minerals). **TABLE 16.4** shows the nutrient recommendations for pregnant women compared with nonpregnant women. The U.S. Department of Agriculture (USDA) Daily Food Plan for Moms is an interactive website that provides nutritional guidance to help pregnant and nursing mothers meet their individual nutritional requirements.[21]

TABLE 16.4
Nutritional Recommendations for Pregnancy

	Nonpregnant	Pregnant	% Increase
Energy (kcal)	2,400	2,740/2,852	14–18
Protein (g)	46	71	54
Vitamin A (μg RAE)	700	770	10
Vitamin D (μg)	5	5	0
Vitamin E (mg)	15	15	0
Vitamin K (μg)	90	90	0
Thiamin (mg)	1.1	1.4	27
Riboflavin (mg)	1.1	1.4	27
Niacin (mg)	14	18	29
Vitamin B_6 (mg)	1.3	1.9	46
Folate (μg)	400	600	50
Vitamin B_{12} (μg)	2.4	2.6	8
Pantothenic acid (mg)	5	6	20
Biotin (μg)	30	30	0
Choline (mg)	425	450	6
Vitamin C (mg)	75	85	13
Calcium (mg)	1,000	1,000	0
Phosphorus (mg)	700	700	0
Magnesium (mg)	310	350	13
Iron (mg)	18	27	50
Zinc (mg)	8	11	38
Selenium (μg)	55	60	9
Iodine (μg)	150	220	47
Fluoride (mg)	3	3	0
Copper (μg)	900	1,000	11
Chromium (μg)	25	30	20
Manganese (mg)	1.8	2	11
Molybdenum (μg)	45	50	11
Sodium (mg)	1,500	1,500	0
Chloride (mg)	2,300	2,300	0
Potassium (mg)	4,700	4,700	0
Water (mL)	2,700	3,000	11

Needs for most nutrients increase during pregnancy. Generally, vitamin and mineral needs increase more than energy needs, which means that food choices should be nutrient-dense. Values for energy are based on Estimated Energy Requirements (EER) for a reference 19-year-old active woman. The first number for pregnancy represents the second trimester; the other number is for the third trimester. Values for protein, vitamins, minerals, and water are RDAs or AIs for ages 19 to 30.

Macronutrients

Macronutrients supply energy and provide the building blocks for protein synthesis. The recommended balance of energy sources does not change during pregnancy. A low-fat, moderate-protein, high-carbohydrate diet is still appropriate.

Protein Extra protein is needed during pregnancy for synthesizing new maternal, placental, and fetal tissues. A pregnant woman's Recommended Dietary Allowance (RDA) for protein is 1.1 grams per kilogram per day (an additional 25 grams per day over nonpregnant needs). This amount of protein is easily supplied in typical American diets consumed by nonpregnant women. Thus, many women need not increase their protein intake to reach the levels recommended for pregnancy. Pregnant women who are vegetarians, including vegans, also should be able to meet their protein needs from food sources alone—as long as they select a variety of protein sources and consume enough total calories. (See the FYI feature "Vegetarianism and Pregnancy.")

Fats Dietary fats provide vital fuel for the mother and for the development of placental tissues. Needs for essential fatty acids during pregnancy are slightly higher than those of nonpregnant women.[22] The pregnant woman's body also stores fats to support breastfeeding after childbirth. Very-low-fat diets (in which less than 10 percent of daily calories comes from dietary fats) are not recommended for pregnancy. Such diets are unlikely to supply sufficient amounts of essential fatty acids, fat-soluble vitamins, or calories.

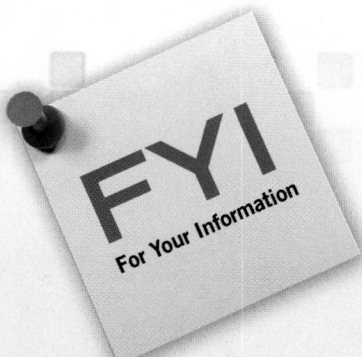

FYI
For Your Information

Vegetarianism and Pregnancy

Can pregnant women meet all their nutritional needs on a vegetarian diet? A fair question. Common vegetarian practices include the avoidance of meat, poultry, and fish (lacto-ovo-vegetarian and lactovegetarian) and the avoidance of all animal foods (vegan). These foods are important sources of iron, zinc, calcium, vitamin B_{12}, and other nutrients. Although vegetarian diets can provide reasonable quantities of trace elements, animal-derived foods frequently contribute larger amounts that the body absorbs more easily. To meet the demands of pregnancy, supplementation can be in order.

Supplemental iron is generally recommended for all pregnant women. Supplemental vitamin B_{12} (2.0 micrograms per day) is also recommended for vegan mothers. If their sun exposure is limited, they also may need daily supplementation of 10 micrograms of vitamin D.[a] Vegetarians with low calcium intake (< 600 milligrams per day) should consume a supplement that provides at least 500 milligrams per day. Some vegan foods, such as fortified soy milks, may contain these important nutrients. It is important to check the label to be sure.

The overall nutrient content of a vegetarian diet depends on both the energy content and the variety of the foods consumed. The sample meal plan in **TABLE A** provides an example of a vegan diet for pregnant women.

[a] Institute of Medicine, Food and Nutrition Board. *Dietary Reference Intakes for Calcium and Vitamin D.* Washington, DC: National Academies Press; 2011.

TABLE A
Sample Meal Plan for a Vegan Pregnancy

Breakfast	Medium apple
1/2 cup oatmeal with maple syrup	1 cup fortified soy milk
1 slice whole wheat toast with	**Afternoon Snack**
Fruit spread	3/4 cup ready-to-eat cereal with
1 cup fortified soy milk	1 cup blueberries
1/2 cup calcium-fortified orange juice	1 cup fortified soy milk
Morning Snack	**Dinner**
1/2 whole-wheat bagel with	3/4 cup tofu stir-fried with
Margarine	1 cup vegetables
1 banana	1 cup brown rice
Lunch	1 medium orange
Veggie burger on whole-wheat bun with	**Evening Snack**
Mustard	Whole-grain crackers with
Ketchup	2 tablespoons peanut butter
1 cup steamed collard greens	4 oz apple juice

Carbohydrate Carbohydrates provide the main source of extra calories during pregnancy. Food choices should emphasize complex carbohydrates such as whole-grain breads, fortified cereals, rice, and pasta. In addition to supplying vitamins and minerals, these foods can increase fiber intake substantially. A fiber-rich diet is recommended during pregnancy to help prevent constipation and hemorrhoids. The Adequate Intake (AI) for fiber increases from 25 to 28 grams per day during pregnancy.

Key Concepts Most healthy women with well-balanced diets meet the majority of their nutrient requirements during pregnancy. The actual increase in energy needs varies substantially among women. The adequacy of energy intake can be measured by the amount of weight gained. Weight loss is not advised during pregnancy, even for obese women. As long as energy intake is adequate and a variety of foods is eaten, protein intake should be more than adequate to support prenatal growth and development.

Micronutrients

A pregnant woman has an increased need for many vitamins and minerals that support fetal growth and development. In addition, her increased energy needs mean she requires higher amounts of nutrients such as the B vitamins thiamin, riboflavin, niacin, and pantothenic acid, which are essential for energy metabolism.

Needs for the other B vitamins (except biotin) also increase. Folate and vitamin B_{12} are used to synthesize DNA and red blood cells, and vitamin B_6 is crucial for metabolizing amino acids. Of these vitamins, folate needs increase the most, from 400 micrograms per day to 600 micrograms per day during pregnancy. Vitamin C needs increase slightly during pregnancy, from 75 to 85 milligrams per day for women aged 19 to 50 years. For the fat-soluble vitamins, the RDA for vitamin A increases slightly during pregnancy, whereas recommended intake levels for vitamins D, E, and K are unchanged.

For most minerals, recommended intakes are higher during pregnancy—most dramatically for iron. The RDA for iron increases from 18 milligrams per day to 27 milligrams per day. Iron is necessary to make red blood cells and is important for normal growth and energy metabolism. Iron deficiency and its associated anemia is the most common nutrient deficiency in pregnancy. **TABLE 16.5** lists the characteristics of women who are at particularly high risk for iron deficiency.

TABLE 16.5
Factors Associated with Increased Risk for Iron Deficiency During Pregnancy

- Young age (e.g., 15 to 19 years)
- Multiple sequential pregnancies
- Twin or triplet pregnancy
- Diet low in meat
- Diet high in coffee and tea
- Low socioeconomic status
- Low level of education
- Black or Hispanic ethnicity
- Previous diagnosis of iron deficiency or iron-deficiency anemia

Because getting 27 milligrams of iron in the daily diet is not easy, experts recommend iron supplementation for the general population of pregnant women.[23] A woman can maximize absorption of an iron supplement by eating it on an empty stomach (between meals or at bedtime) and washing it down with liquids other than milk, tea, or coffee, which inhibit absorption.

Key Concepts Needs for vitamins and minerals increase during pregnancy, some more than others. Extra vitamins and minerals are needed to support growth and development as well as increased energy use. Recommended intake levels increase most dramatically for folate and iron.

Food Choices for Pregnant Women

You may be surprised to learn that the recommended diet for a pregnant woman is not much different from that for adults in the general population. Variety is the key to a well-balanced diet. The extra calories needed for pregnancy are easy to obtain from an additional serving from each of the following food groups: grains, vegetables, fruits, and low-fat milk. Because the increased need for energy is proportionately less than the increased need for most nutrients, nutrient-dense foods are important. There is little room in the diet plan for high-calorie, high-fat, low-nutrient "extras."

Supplementation

Other than iron and folate, a pregnant woman can usually get all the nutrients she needs by making healthful choices, guided by the food intake patterns of MyPlate. Health care providers often evaluate the dietary intake of all prenatal patients and recommend dietary changes to improve nutrition where needed. However, to reduce preventable complications of nutrient deficiencies, pregnant women in the United States and Canada routinely receive prescriptions for prenatal vitamin/mineral supplements. The amount and balance of nutrients in prenatal formulations is appropriate for pregnancy. Because toxic levels can be reached quickly, especially for vitamins A and D, pregnant women should avoid high doses and multiple supplements. In addition, because most herbal preparations have not been evaluated for safety during pregnancy, they are not recommended.

Foods to Avoid

Alcohol is completely off-limits to pregnant women. And if a mother-to-be is experiencing problems with nausea and vomiting, she may want to abstain for a while from foods that aggravate these symptoms. Cultural traditions can dictate changes in diet during pregnancy, but these tend to reflect traditional beliefs and practices rather than health science.

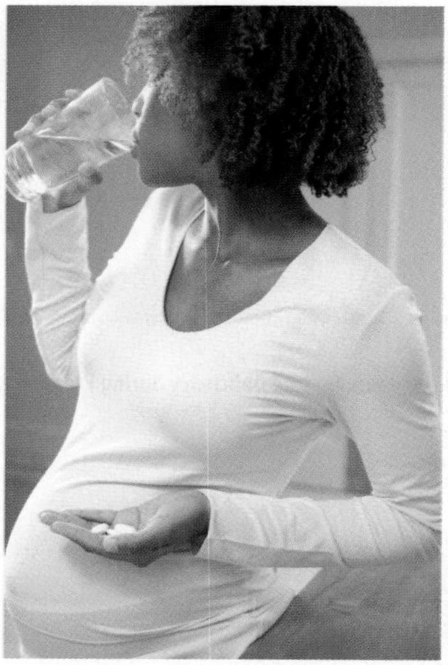

The *Dietary Guidelines for Americans, 2015–2020* advises that women who are pregnant or breastfeeding consume 8 to 12 ounces of a variety of seafood types weekly; however, because of a high mercury content, it limits albacore tuna to 6 ounces per week and suggests avoiding tilefish, shark, swordfish, and king mackerel.[24] In addition, the Food and Drug Administration (FDA) and the Environmental Protection Agency (EPA) advise that women who may become pregnant, pregnant women, lactating mothers, and young children check local advisories about the safety of fish caught by family and friends in local lakes, rivers, and coastal areas.[25]

The question of whether to reduce or eliminate caffeine intake during pregnancy continues to be debated. High caffeine intake has been linked to delayed conception, spontaneous miscarriage, and low birth weight.[26,27] However, caffeine intake during pregnancy does not appear to be associated with birth defects[28] or preterm birth.[29] The Academy of Nutrition and Dietetics recommends that pregnant women consume less than 300 milligrams of caffeine per day.[30] **TABLE 16.6** shows the caffeine content of common beverages and foods.

TABLE 16.6
Caffeine Content of Common Beverages and Foods

Food	Serving Size	Caffeine (mg)
Coffee, regular, brewed	8 fl. oz.	130
Coffee, Starbucks, brewed	8 fl. oz.	160
Espresso, regular	1 fl. oz.	40
Espresso, Starbucks	1 fl. oz.	75
Frappuccino beverage, Starbucks	9.5 fl. oz.	115
Tea, regular, brewed	8 fl. oz.	50
Tea, fruited, Snapple	8 fl. oz.	20
Tea, latte, Starbucks Tazo Chai	8 fl. oz.	50
Vault	12 fl. oz.	70
Mountain Dew	12 fl. oz.	55
Coca-Cola/Pepsi, regular, flavored, diet	12 fl. oz.	35–45
Sprite/7-Up	12 fl. oz.	0
Red Bull	8.3 fl. oz.	80
Ice cream, coffee	8 fl. oz.	50–80
Milk chocolate, Hershey's	1.55 oz.	10
Dark chocolate, Hershey's	1.45 oz.	20

Adapted from Center for Science in the Public Interest. Caffeine content of food and drugs. http://www.cspinet.org/new/cafchart.htm. Accessed January 10, 2016.

Key Concepts With the exception of iron and folate, a well-balanced, varied diet can often meet all of a pregnant woman's nutrient needs. Pregnant women should choose nutrient-dense and high-carbohydrate foods in the proportions found in MyPlate. Although vitamin/mineral supplementation is common during pregnancy, it probably is not needed other than for iron and folate. When supplements are used, they should be designed for pregnant women. Pregnant women should avoid alcohol and moderate their intake of caffeine.

Substance Use and Pregnancy Outcome

When a pregnant woman eats, she eats for two. When she smokes, drinks, or uses drugs, she does so for two as well. The consequences of these behaviors can be felt for generations.

Tobacco and Alcohol

Smoking during pregnancy increases the risks of miscarrying, delivering a stillborn infant, giving birth prematurely, and delivering a low-birth-weight baby.[31] Women in lower socioeconomic groups have the highest rates of cigarette use before, during, and after pregnancy. Women in the highest socioeconomic groups, meanwhile, are the most likely to quit smoking during pregnancy but are just as likely as other women to take up the habit again after giving birth.

All women of childbearing age should be aware of alcohol's effects on a developing fetus. Exposure to alcohol can lead to a range of physical, cognitive, and behavioral conditions collectively known as fetal alcohol syndrome (FAS).[32] Most importantly, alcohol exposure affects the development of the brain during critical periods of differentiation and growth. Children severely afflicted by the syndrome show marked growth deficiencies before and after birth; physical anomalies such as a small head, certain characteristic facial deformities (see **FIGURE 16.8**), heart defects, and joint and limb irregularities; mental retardation; and central nervous system disorders. The greater a mother's alcohol use during pregnancy, the more severe the symptoms of FAS tend to be in the child. There is no known safe threshold for alcohol use in pregnancy. The only way to avoid alcohol-related risks to a fetus is to avoid all alcohol during pregnancy.

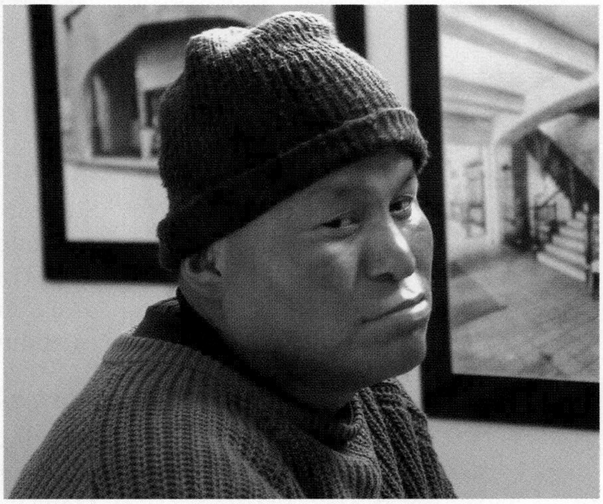

FIGURE 16.8 Fetal alcohol syndrome. The facial characteristics of a person with fetal alcohol syndrome include a short nose with a flattened bridge, eyelids with extra folds, and a thin upper lip with no groove below the nose.

Drugs

Approximately 5 percent of pregnant women take street drugs, including cocaine, ecstasy, heroin, marijuana, and prescription drugs that are abused.[33]

Marijuana use increases the risk for premature delivery and low birth weight. In addition, maternal marijuana use can result in some of the same physical abnormalities seen in infants with FAS. Effects on the fetus vary depending on the mother's diet, frequency of marijuana use, and the use of other drugs. Marijuana also reduces fertility in both women and men.

Cocaine use increases risks of stroke, prematurity, fetal growth retardation, miscarriage, and certain birth defects. Some of these problems could stem from nutritional deficiencies in the mother both before and during pregnancy, as well as from concurrent tobacco and alcohol use, which is common among cocaine users. **FIGURE 16.9** illustrates the possible effects of a woman's use of drugs, alcohol, or tobacco while she is pregnant.

Key Concepts Smoking, alcohol, and illicit drug use during pregnancy can all have devastating effects on fetal development. Low birth weight, preterm delivery, and birth defects are some of the consequences. Fetal alcohol syndrome is a specific set of physical, mental, and behavioral defects caused by maternal alcohol consumption during pregnancy. A pregnant woman should avoid all these substances.

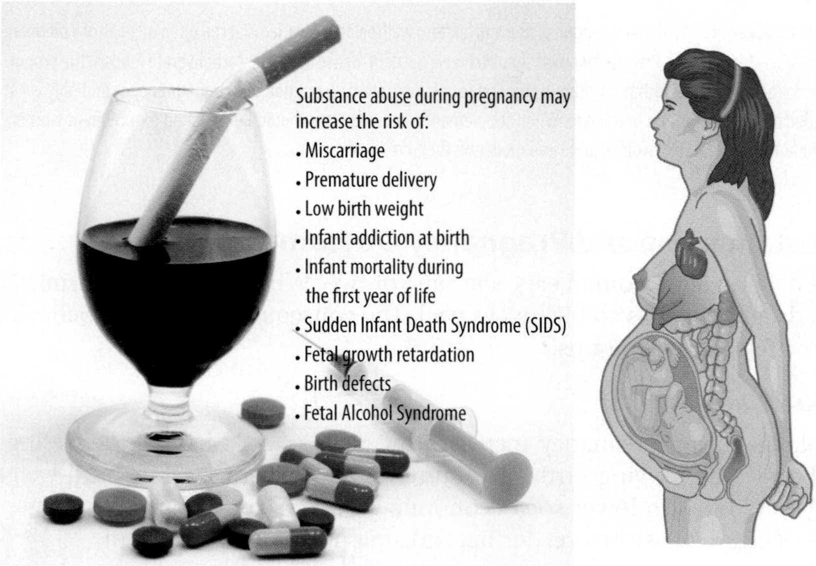
Substance abuse during pregnancy may increase the risk of:
• Miscarriage
• Premature delivery
• Low birth weight
• Infant addiction at birth
• Infant mortality during the first year of life
• Sudden Infant Death Syndrome (SIDS)
• Fetal growth retardation
• Birth defects
• Fetal Alcohol Syndrome

FIGURE 16.9 Substance use can lead to birth defects. When a pregnant woman smokes, drinks, or uses drugs, so does her growing baby. The consequences of these behaviors can be felt for generations.

Photo ©Stockphoto/Thinkstock.

Special Situations During Pregnancy

Some women progress through pregnancy with no more than a mild period of morning sickness or problems with constipation or heartburn. However, even these conditions, as well as complications such as abnormal glucose tolerance or elevated blood pressure, can affect dietary choices and nutritional status. In addition, some women have unique nutritional needs during pregnancy.

Gastrointestinal Distress

Morning sickness, or nausea associated with pregnancy, is most common early in pregnancy as the mother's body adjusts to changes in hormone levels. Many pregnant women find they experience less morning sickness if they eat dry cereal, toast, or crackers about half an hour before getting out of bed (see **FIGURE 16.10**). Keeping some food in the stomach throughout the day helps, too. This means eating smaller, more frequent meals, and drinking liquids between meals instead of with food. Avoiding food aromas that trigger nausea is another useful tactic.

Heartburn and constipation are the result of slowed gastrointestinal (GI) movement. Remaining upright for at least an hour after eating and having smaller, more frequent meals can prevent heartburn. Getting plenty of fiber and fluids in the diet and getting regular mild to moderate exercise can limit constipation. Of course, a pregnant woman should always consult her health care provider before using a prescription drug, over-the-counter medicine, herbal supplement, or home remedy for nausea, vomiting, heartburn, or constipation.

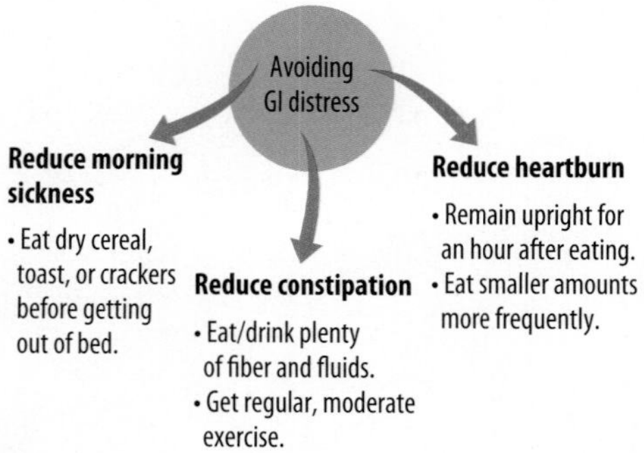
Avoiding GI distress
Reduce morning sickness
• Eat dry cereal, toast, or crackers before getting out of bed.
Reduce constipation
• Eat/drink plenty of fiber and fluids.
• Get regular, moderate exercise.
Reduce heartburn
• Remain upright for an hour after eating.
• Eat smaller amounts more frequently.

FIGURE 16.10 Strategies for avoiding GI distress. During pregnancy, most women experience GI distress as morning sickness, constipation, or heartburn.

Food Cravings and Aversions

Many pregnant women experience specific food cravings and/or aversions, and we often laugh at stories about unusual combinations such as pickles and ice cream. These changes in food preferences can be linked to taste and metabolic changes, but they rarely are based on a nutrient deficiency or other physiological conditions. Most cravings and aversions do not affect the quality of the diet unless food choices become very narrow.

Some pregnant women crave nonfood items such as starch or clay. The term *pica* describes routine consumption of nonfood items such as dirt, clay, laundry starch, ice, or burnt matches. Although this behavior may seem outlandish, in many cases it is a culturally accepted practice that affects significant numbers of pregnant women worldwide.[34] Pica can be harmful if nonfood items crowd nutritious foods out of the diet. In addition, nonfood items can contain toxins, bacteria, and parasites; and in the case of laundry starch, a significant number of calories can be consumed without providing any vitamins or minerals.

Hypertension

Measurement of maternal blood pressure is a routine part of prenatal care. When not accompanied by other symptoms, increased blood pressure during pregnancy is usually temporary and carries little risk. However, the combination of hypertension and proteinuria (protein in the urine) indicates a serious medical condition called **preeclampsia**. If preeclampsia progresses to **eclampsia**, it can threaten the lives of both mother and baby.

Preeclampsia is more common in first pregnancies, as well as adolescents, women older than 35 years, and women with preexisting diabetes or hypertension. In mild cases, bed rest and close monitoring are the treatments of choice. Sodium restriction and drug therapy are not recommended. Ensuring adequate intake of zinc may help early detection of gestational hypertension. Early identification of preeclampsia through routine prenatal care is important for good maternal and fetal outcomes.

▶ **preeclampsia** A condition of late pregnancy characterized by hypertension, edema, and proteinuria.

▶ **eclampsia** The occurrence of seizures in a pregnant woman that are unrelated to brain conditions.

Diabetes

A woman with diabetes faces special challenges in pregnancy. She has an increased risk of developing preeclampsia and a greater-than-average chance of problems that affect the fetus, including fetal death. However, with early prenatal intervention and careful control of blood glucose levels, these risks can be reduced to the same level as in nondiabetic pregnancies.[35]

Pregnancy can require frequent adjustments of both diet and insulin to keep blood glucose in check. Insulin requirements often decrease during the first half of pregnancy but increase during the second half. Women who did not need insulin before they became pregnant and were able to control their blood glucose through diet alone may begin to need insulin during their pregnancy.

Gestational Diabetes

Gestational diabetes is a condition in which abnormal glucose tolerance exists only during pregnancy and resolves after delivery. The hormones of pregnancy tend to counteract insulin, and in about 4 percent of pregnancies, this results in a rise in blood glucose. **TABLE 16.7** lists factors associated with an increased risk of gestational diabetes. Gestational diabetes often can be controlled through diet, although some cases require insulin therapy.

TABLE 16.7
Factors Associated with Risk for Gestational Diabetes

- Being older than 25 years
- Obesity, at any age
- Family history of diabetes mellitus
- Previous poor pregnancy outcome
- History of abnormal glucose tolerance
- Ethnicity associated with high incidence of diabetes

HIV/AIDS

Women with the human immunodeficiency virus (HIV) can potentially pass the virus to their children during pregnancy, delivery, or breastfeeding. Medical treatments used routinely in the United States and other developed countries reduce the risk of transmission during pregnancy and delivery in the approximately 6,000 HIV-infected women who give birth each year.[36] More than 90 percent of all cases of childhood HIV infection are attributable to mother-to-child transmission of HIV, especially in countries where effective HIV/AIDS drugs are not available.[37] In developing countries where treatments are not available, women with HIV or acquired immune deficiency syndrome (AIDS) are likely to have multiple nutrition problems, including protein-energy malnutrition, vitamin and mineral deficiencies, and inadequate weight gain, all of which pose risks to the fetus.

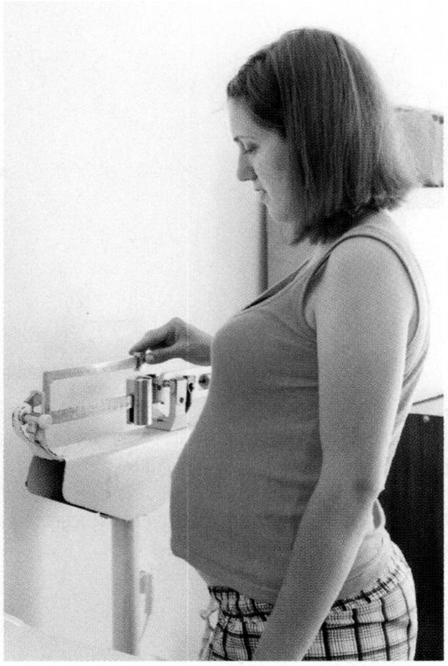

Adolescence

Despite prevention efforts, about 367,750 infants were born to teenagers in 2010; the majority of these pregnancies were unintended.[38] Pregnant adolescents are nutritionally at risk. Their own needs for growth and development are compromised by the extra demands posed by the growth and development of the fetus. Risks for preeclampsia, anemia, premature birth, low-birth-weight babies, infant mortality, and sexually transmitted diseases are all increased for pregnant adolescents under the age of 16.[39]

Even before becoming pregnant, many teenagers do not demonstrate healthful eating patterns. Their diets are likely to be inadequate in total calories, calcium, iron, zinc, riboflavin, folic acid, and vitamins A, D, and B_6. Poverty, smoking, and abuse of alcohol and other substances compound the negative effects of adolescent nutritional inadequacies.

Nutrition care for pregnant teens starts with determining daily energy needs. The Institute of Medicine recommends that pregnant adolescents be encouraged to strive for weight gains toward the upper end of the range recommended for adult mothers (see Table 16.3). The need for supplemental vitamins and minerals is also greater in this age group.

Key Concepts Numerous factors affect the dietary needs and choices of pregnant women. Routine prenatal care is important to identify unhealthful eating behaviors and potential complications such as preeclampsia and gestational diabetes. Pregnant women with diabetes or HIV/AIDS need special dietary intervention. Pregnant teens have especially high nutrient needs to support not only fetal growth, but also their own adolescent growth.

Lactation

During pregnancy, physiological changes in breast tissue and fat stores prepare the woman's body for the demands of lactation. Preparation for lactation also involves education. Although breastfeeding is a natural function of a woman's body, knowledge about lactation can make breastfeeding a success for both mother and infant.

Breastfeeding Trends

Public health goals since the late 1970s have sought to increase the percentage of infants who are breastfed. The goal of Healthy People 2020 is to increase the proportion of newborns who are initially breastfed to almost 82 percent.[40] Efforts to promote breastfeeding have been successful; 74 percent of infants are now breastfed initially.[41] However, only 44 percent of infants are still being breastfed at 6 months of age.[42] What are the reasons for this trend? Lack of knowledge about the benefits of breastfeeding for both mother and baby surely plays a role. Societal attitudes regarding the acceptability of breastfeeding also are influential and vary across cultural and demographic groups. Some states have actually had to pass laws stating that breastfeeding in public is not indecent exposure. In addition, the decline in breastfeeding through the 1950s and 1960s affected the attitudes and knowledge base of today's grandmothers.

Parents should make decisions about feeding their infants based on accurate information, so providing information about the mechanics of breastfeeding as well as the benefits for both mother and baby should be an integral part of prenatal care.

Physiology of Lactation

Virtually every woman who wants to breastfeed her newborn can do so. The size or shape of the breast has no impact on the lactation process. **FIGURE 16.11** shows the anatomy of a normal breast.

Position Statement: Academy of Nutrition and Dietetics

Promoting and Supporting Breastfeeding

It is the position of the Academy of Nutrition and Dietetics that exclusive breastfeeding provides optimal nutrition and health protection for the first 6 months of life, and breastfeeding with complementary foods for 6 months until at least 12 months is the ideal feeding pattern for infants. Breastfeeding is an important public health strategy for improving infant and child morbidity and mortality, and improving maternal morbidity, and helping to control health care costs.

Reproduced from James DC, Lessen R. Position of the American Dietetic Association: promoting and supporting breastfeeding. *J Am Diet Assoc.* 2009;109(11):1926–1942.

Changes During Adolescence and Pregnancy

Although mammary tissue is present in newborns, that tissue does not grow and develop until the onset of puberty. Throughout adolescence, the amount of breast tissue grows and the mammary glands and ducts develop. An adolescent who becomes pregnant shortly after her first period or who has had only irregular periods prior to becoming pregnant may have underdeveloped mammary glands and insufficient breast tissue to support lactation. However, most teen mothers have no difficulty breastfeeding their babies.

During pregnancy, breast tissue changes so milk production is possible. Not only does the breast change in size, but the structure of the glands and ducts also becomes more intricate, and secretory cells form. Mammary tissue is mature and capable of producing milk by the start of the third trimester.

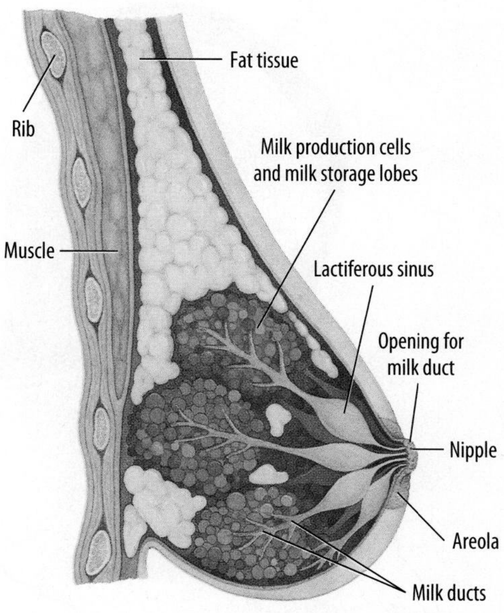

FIGURE 16.11 Anatomy of the breast. During pregnancy, breasts increase in size and undergo internal development. By the start of the third trimester, breasts are capable of producing milk.

After Delivery

Although birth triggers a rapid increase in a mother's milk production and secretion, full lactation does not begin as soon as the baby is born. An efficient way to establish lactation is to put the newborn to the breast as soon after delivery as possible. During the first two or three days after birth, a nursing infant receives **colostrum**, an immature milk that is quite high in protein and immunoglobulins (immunoprotective factors). If the newborn is fed regularly at the breast, lactation will be firmly established within two or three weeks after birth, and mature milk will be produced.

Hormonal Controls

Several hormones control the maturation of breast tissue and the production and release of breast milk (see **FIGURE 16.12**). During lactation, the pituitary gland produces two important hormones—**prolactin** and **oxytocin**. The infant suckling at the breast stimulates the release of prolactin from the mother's pituitary gland. In turn, prolactin stimulates the production of milk in the breast tissue. Giving water or infant formula to the baby reduces the time spent nursing at the breast, and milk production declines.

The second hormone, oxytocin, allows milk to be released from the mammary glands to the nipple and therefore to the hungry infant. It would be inconvenient and messy if milk were released from the breast as soon as it was produced! So, the infant suckling at the breast signals the pituitary gland to release oxytocin, which in turn stimulates the release of milk. This process, often called the **let-down reflex**, may be accompanied by a tingling or burning sensation in the breast that lets the mother know the infant is receiving milk. Let-down can be inhibited by anxiety, stress, and fatigue. It can also be stimulated by thoughts of the baby or hearing the baby cry.

- **colostrum** A thick, yellow fluid secreted by the breast during pregnancy and the first days after delivery.
- **prolactin** A pituitary hormone that stimulates the production of milk in breast tissue.
- **oxytocin** A pituitary hormone that stimulates the release of milk from the breast.
- **let-down reflex** The release of milk from the breast tissue in response to the stimulus of the hormone oxytocin. The major stimulus for oxytocin release is the infant suckling at the breast.

Key Concepts Increasing the proportion of infants who are breastfed is an important public health goal. Prenatal care should include information about the physiology of lactation and its benefits for mother and baby. Changes in breast tissue that allow lactation culminate at delivery. Breast milk composition changes in the two or three weeks following the infant's birth. The first milk, colostrum, is high in protein and immune factors. Key hormones that regulate milk production and release are prolactin and oxytocin.

Nutrition for Breastfeeding Women

To provide adequate nutrition for her baby while protecting her own nutritional status, a breastfeeding mother must choose a varied, healthful, nutrient-dense diet. Dietary inadequacies will lead to mobilization of stored maternal nutrients in an effort to produce nutritionally complete breast milk. Her needs for energy and most nutrients are higher or the same as for pregnancy.

Quick Bite

Breastfeeding and Birth Control

Does breastfeeding prevent pregnancy? No. But under certain conditions, breastfeeding can dramatically reduce the chances of becoming pregnant. During the first six months after giving birth, a woman who has not yet had a period and fully breastfeeds her baby (no other liquids or solids) has less than a 2 percent chance of pregnancy. Still, it's important to use a reliable method of birth control while breastfeeding.

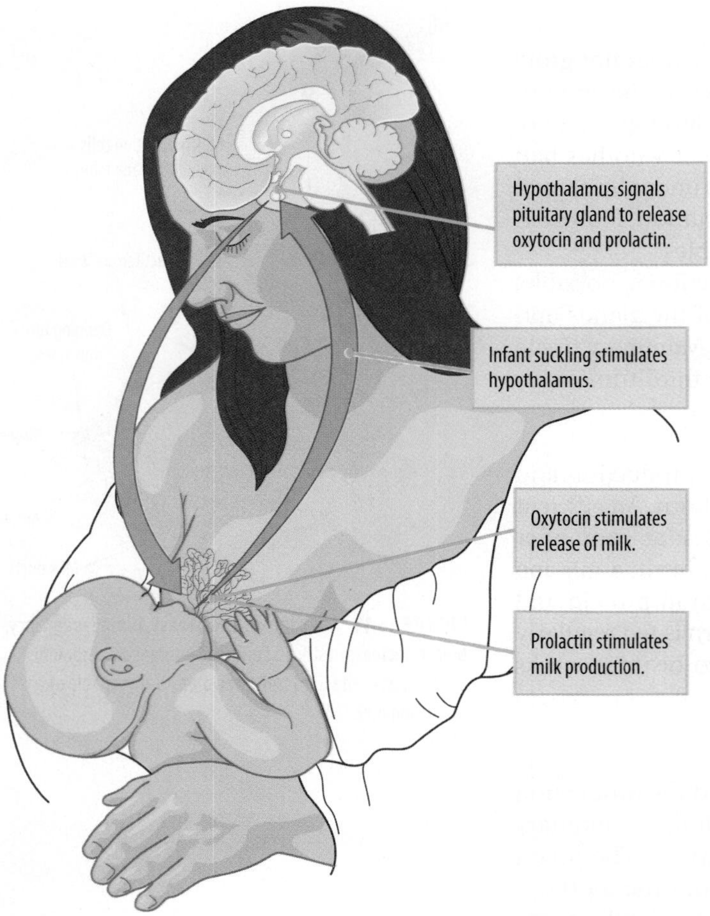
Hypothalamus signals pituitary gland to release oxytocin and prolactin.
Infant suckling stimulates hypothalamus.
Oxytocin stimulates release of milk.
Prolactin stimulates milk production.

FIGURE 16.12 Hormonal control of lactation. When an infant nurses, the infant's suckling stimulates the nipple, which sends nerve signals to the hypothalamus. In turn, the hypothalamus signals the pituitary gland to release hormones that stimulate milk production and release.

Energy

The energy needed to support milk production is obtained in part by mobilization of fat stores, with the remaining kilocalories provided by the diet. On average, well-nourished breastfeeding women lose weight slowly, about 0.8 kilograms (approximately 1¾ pounds) per month, with weight stabilizing after about six months. Based on this rate of weight loss, a breastfeeding woman needs an extra intake of 330 kilocalories per day during the first six months of lactation and 400 extra kilocalories daily during the second six months.[43] However, this may be an overestimation of actual needs for many women, especially those who are sedentary. To ensure adequate milk production and avoid nutrient deficiencies, a nursing mother should consume at least 1,800 kilocalories per day.

Protein

Adequate protein intake is very important while nursing. The RDA for protein is 1.3 grams per kilogram per day, or an additional 25 grams over the nonpregnant RDA. Unless calorie intake is very low, lack of dietary protein is uncommon among women in the United States and Canada.

Vitamins and Minerals

Breastfeeding women need higher amounts of most vitamins than they do during pregnancy. Exceptions include vitamins D and K, for which the recommended intake is the same during lactation and pregnancy, and niacin and folate, for which the RDA is lower during lactation than during pregnancy (although still higher than for women in the general population). When vitamin intake is inadequate, the vitamin content of breast milk can diminish, which puts the infant at risk for deficiency.

For minerals, current RDA and AI values suggest increased needs during lactation (as compared with pregnancy) for all minerals except sodium, chloride, calcium, phosphorus, magnesium, fluoride, and molybdenum. Iron needs decrease below nonpregnant values because iron losses from menstruation often do not occur during the early months of exclusive breastfeeding. Maternal intake of minerals has less influence on levels in breast milk than is true for vitamins.

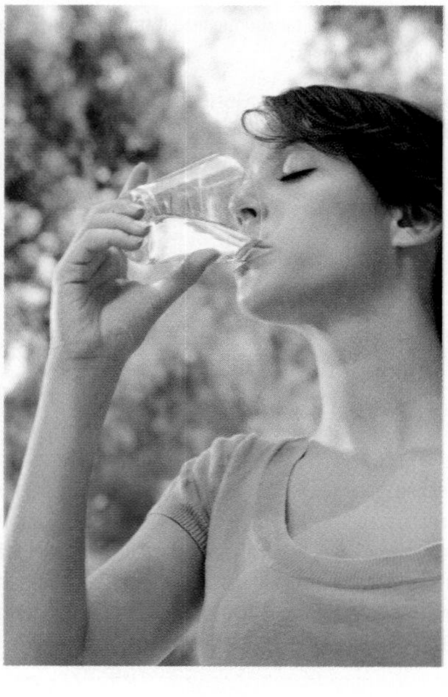

© iStockphoto/Thinkstock

Water

Breastfeeding women require plenty of fluids. A nursing mother should drink about 2 liters (about 8 cups) of water per day and at least 1 cup of water each time she breastfeeds her baby. The AI for total water (beverages plus foods) is 3.8 liters per day. Coffee and other caffeinated beverages are acceptable if limited to 1 or 2 cups per day—and if they do not replace other fluids. Because caffeine passes into the breast milk, caffeine can make some breastfed infants wakeful and jittery.

Key Concepts Energy and nutrient needs are usually even higher during lactation than during pregnancy. Intake recommendations suggest an additional 330 to 400 kilocalories and 25 extra grams of protein each day above nonpregnant needs. Low vitamin intake affects the nutritional quality of breast milk. Recommended intake levels for minerals are generally higher during lactation than during pregnancy. Fluids are also important for adequate milk production.

Food Choices

Choosing a variety of foods from MyPlate for Pregnancy and Breastfeeding is the best way to meet the nutritional demands of lactation. Following the food intake patterns of MyPlate for Pregnancy and Breastfeeding, diets of 2,000 to 2,800 kilocalories per day can easily meet most nutrient needs.

Nursing mothers should eat plenty of vegetables, the source of many essential micronutrients. Although vegetables in the cabbage family, including broccoli, cauliflower, kale, and Brussels sprouts, have long been considered causes of **colic** symptoms in breastfed infants, these vegetables may have an unwarranted bad reputation. Scientific evidence that these vegetables cause distress for infants remains weak. Removal of numerous foods from the diet should be done only under the supervision of a registered dietitian.

▶ **colic** Periodic inconsolable crying in an otherwise healthy infant that appears to result from abdominal cramping and discomfort.

Supplementation

Some breastfeeding women need routine vitamin/mineral supplementation.[44] This group would include, for example, those women who do not follow dietary guidelines and vegan women, who avoid all animal products. Vitamin B_{12} is likely to be too low in the milk of nursing vegans, and they should take a B_{12} supplement.[45] For breastfeeding women who do not get regular sun exposure and do not drink milk or other fortified products, a vitamin D supplement can be warranted.[46] For most nursing mothers, though, dietary counseling to improve food choices is the preferred way to address nutrient imbalances.

Practices to Avoid During Lactation

When a nursing mother smokes or uses alcohol or other drugs, these substances wind up in her breast milk. Women who smoke are encouraged to quit smoking. However, breast milk remains the ideal food for their infants.[47] It is a myth that drinking alcohol enhances the letdown reflex, making it easier to nurse. Rather, alcohol inhibits the milk-ejection reflex so that the baby gets less milk with a higher concentration of alcohol. An occasional drink may not be harmful, but breastfeeding should be avoided for two hours after alcohol consumption.[48] Illicit drugs also show up in breast milk and can be transferred to the infant. If a new mother cannot abstain from using these drugs, she should not breastfeed.

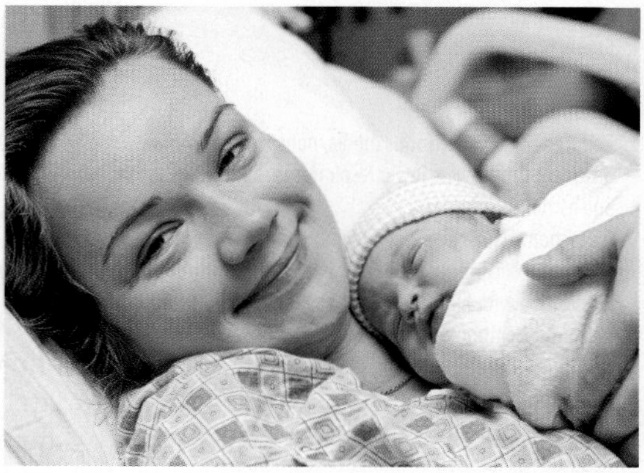

Key Concepts Food choices during lactation should follow MyPlate for Pregnancy and Breastfeeding and emphasize nutrient-dense foods. With good choices and adequate calories, a lactating woman may not need vitamin and mineral supplements.

Benefits of Breastfeeding

Breast milk is the optimal food for the health, growth, and development of infants. Both infants and mothers benefit from breastfeeding: breastfed infants have lower rates of childhood obesity and higher protection from infections and illnesses such as diarrhea; mothers have reduced risk of breast and ovarian cancers.[49] It is estimated that $13 billion in U.S. healthcare costs could be saved annually if 90 percent of babies were breastfed exclusively for six months.[50]

Benefits for Infants

Human milk provides optimal nutrition for babies, as you will see in the section "Energy and Nutrient Needs During Infancy." Breast milk provides more than nutrients, however, and the health-promoting factors in breast milk are difficult, if not impossible, to replicate in infant formula.

Breast milk has been shown to protect infants from infections and illnesses, including diarrhea, ear infections, pneumonia, and asthma,[51] leading to fewer healthcare visits, less prescription medication use, and fewer hospitalizations and resulting in decreased health care costs.[52] Breastfeeding also reduces an infant's risk of sudden infant death syndrome (SIDS).[53] In addition, a baby's risk of obesity declines with each month of breastfeeding.[54] Babies who are breastfed for at least six months are less likely to develop obesity, and breastfeeding for nine months reduces a baby's chance of being overweight by more than 30 percent.[55] Evidence suggests that these effects occur in a dose–response relationship, with the best outcomes for infants who are exclusively breastfed for at least six months.[56] Prolonged and exclusive breastfeeding also improves children's cognitive development.[57]

What makes human milk so important for infant health? Colostrum contains substantial amounts of antibodies, including immunoglobulin A (IgA), the first line of defense against most infectious agents.[58] Breastfeeding also appears to stimulate development of the infant's own immune system.[59]

Breastfeeding promotes a close bond between mother and infant that can be important to normal psychological development. It is important for mothers (and fathers) who bottle-feed to promote the same type of closeness while feeding.

As long as mother and baby are in relatively close proximity, breast milk is always ready when the baby is ready to eat. There's nothing to prepare, mix, or heat; and for a hungry infant who doesn't want to wait, that's an important advantage! Breast milk is always the perfect temperature and is sterile. In addition, links between breastfeeding and reduced risk of disorders such as type 1 diabetes, cardiovascular diseases, childhood obesity, and Crohn's disease have been suggested, although these need further study. **TABLE 16.8** lists some possible protective benefits of human milk.

TABLE 16.8
Potential Benefits of Breastfeeding for Infants and Mothers

Benefits for Infants
- Optimal nutrition for infant
- Strong bonding with mother
- Safe, fresh milk
- Enhanced immune system
- Reduced risk for acute otitis media, nonspecific gastroenteritis, severe lower respiratory tract infections, and asthma
- Protection against allergies and intolerances
- Promotion of correct development of jaw and teeth
- Association with higher intelligence quotient and school performance through adolescence
- Reduced risk for chronic disease such as obesity, types 1 and 2 diabetes, heart disease, hypertension, hypercholesterolemia, and childhood leukemia
- Reduced risk for sudden infant death syndrome
- Reduced risk for infant morbidity and mortality

Benefits for Mothers
- Strong bonding with infant
- Increased energy expenditure, which may lead to faster return to prepregnancy weight
- Faster shrinking of the uterus
- Reduced postpartum bleeding and delayed menstrual cycle
- Decreased risk for chronic diseases such as type 2 diabetes, and breast and ovarian cancer
- Improved bone density and decreased risk for hip fracture
- Decreased risk for postpartum depression
- Enhanced self-esteem in the maternal role
- Time saved from preparing and mixing formula
- Money saved from not buying formula and increased medical expenses

Reproduced with permission from Position of the American Dietetic Association: promoting and supporting breastfeeding. *J Am Diet Assoc.* 2009;109:1926–1942.

Benefits for Mother

Following childbirth, breastfeeding stimulates uterine contractions, which help the uterus return to its normal size. If the baby is put to the breast immediately after delivery, these same contractions (an effect of oxytocin) also can help control blood loss. Although not an effective method of birth control, exclusive breastfeeding suppresses ovulation in many women.

Breastfeeding is as convenient for mother as it is for baby and is certainly less expensive than formula feeding. Although more comprehensive studies are needed, there is some evidence that breastfeeding will reduce a woman's risk of ovarian cancer, breast cancer, and osteoporosis,[60] as well as postpartum depression. If, as expected, a breastfed baby has fewer episodes of infectious illness, this saves healthcare costs and reduces employee absence and lost income for working mothers.[61]

Contraindications to Breastfeeding

Nearly all women who want to breastfeed can do so successfully, and breastfeeding rates are steadily increasing. There are times, however, when breastfeeding is inappropriate because of infant or maternal disease or drug use.[62] Depending on the specifics of the operation, breast enlargement or reduction surgery may or may not preclude breastfeeding. The main concern is whether milk ducts and major nerves are cut or damaged.[63]

In the case of infectious or chronic diseases, individual situations should be discussed with the healthcare provider. For example, a woman with untreated tuberculosis should not breastfeed because the illness can be transmitted to her child. In the United States and Canada, where safe feeding alternatives exist, women infected with HIV are advised not to breastfeed because HIV can be transmitted to the baby through breast milk.

Some medications pass directly into human milk, and some prescribed medications preclude breastfeeding. If the mother is using an illegal drug such as cocaine, she should not breastfeed. Women taking prescription or over-the-counter medicines or herbal supplements should discuss the effects of these products on breast milk with their healthcare providers.

Key Concepts Health benefits and convenience are key advantages of breastfeeding. For the infant, breastfeeding has been linked to reduced incidence of many infectious diseases, as well as other conditions. For a mother, breastfeeding speeds recovery of normal uterine size and can reduce her disease risk. Although breastfeeding is the preferred method of infant feeding, there are times when breastfeeding is contraindicated. These situations should be identified and discussed as part of prenatal care.

Resources for Pregnant and Lactating Women and Their Children

Many agencies support research and education programs that promote the health of pregnant and breastfeeding women and their children. You may be familiar with the March of Dimes and its efforts to reduce birth defects and prematurity through optimal nutrition during pregnancy. La Leche League is a voluntary health and education organization that offers programs and educational materials to help breastfeeding mothers learn about the benefits and practice of breastfeeding.

The **Special Supplemental Nutrition Program for Women, Infants, and Children (WIC)** is a much-acclaimed program of the Food and Nutrition Service of the U.S. Department of Agriculture. WIC provides food assistance, nutrition education, and referrals to healthcare services for low-income pregnant, postpartum, and breastfeeding women, as well as infants and children up to age 5.

Although WIC services include breastfeeding education and support, WIC participants are less likely to breastfeed their infants.[64] Continued promotion of breastfeeding by WIC and other public health programs can have both health and economic benefits, including improved household food security and reduced hunger.[65] Periodically, WIC participants are required to bring their infants into the local WIC office. These visits give WIC staff an opportunity to evaluate the infant's growth and provide the caregiver with additional nutrition education.

▶ **Special Supplemental Nutrition Program for Women, Infants, and Children (WIC)** A USDA program that provides federal grants to states for supplemental foods, health care referrals, and nutrition education for low-income pregnant, breastfeeding, and nonbreastfeeding postpartum women, and to infants and children at nutritional risk.

Infancy

Infancy is the period of a child's life between birth and 1 year. Because of the rapid growth that occurs during this time, nutritional needs are higher per unit of body weight than at any other time in the life cycle. Despite the critical importance of nutrition at this stage, feeding an infant is a fairly simple process. Human milk provides all the nutrients an infant needs and is the model for infant formulas. By 4 to 6 months, the infant's physical development and physiological maturation signal readiness for the addition of "solid" foods to the diet.

Human infants need love as much as they need food. Without love and nurturing, a baby can fail to thrive even if she is offered all the right nutrients. If an infant is not nourished emotionally, nutrition recommendations and requirements become meaningless.

▶ **infancy** The period between birth and 12 months of age.

Quick Bite

Breastfeeding to Control Blood Pressure?

Oxytocin, the hormone produced while breastfeeding, can lower the blood pressure of nursing mothers. Research shows that breastfeeding mothers have lower blood pressures after nursing than do bottle-feeding mothers. When asked to discuss stressful events, nursing mothers show smaller increases in blood pressure than the bottle-feeders. Mothers often claim that they feel relaxed during breastfeeding, which can account for the difference in blood pressure.

Quick Bite

Flavored Breast Milk

When lactating mothers exercise vigorously, the amount of lactic acid in breast milk can increase. Some babies dislike the taste and tend to nurse less. Alcohol also can cause a taste that babies dislike. What flavors do babies like? When mothers consume vanilla, mint, or garlic, some babies nurse more.

Infant Growth and Development

Birth weight is the best predictor of a child's health in the first year of life; however, it is important to correlate weight with length of development. The risk profile of an infant who has a low birth weight because of **prematurity** differs from that of a **full-term baby** with a low birth weight.

Immediately after birth, an infant loses about 6 percent of his body weight. This is normal and expected. By 10 to 14 days, the infant should return to his birth weight. Over the next 12 months, the infant's growth will be phenomenal.

By the age of 4 to 6 months, a healthy infant will have doubled his birth weight. By his first birthday, the infant will have tripled his birth weight and increased his length by about 50 percent. The infant's body proportions change, too, so that by age 1 he is looking less like a baby and more like a **toddler** (see **FIGURE 16.13**).

Length (used instead of height because infants can't stand) and **head circumference** are more sensitive measures than weight for assessing a baby's growth and nutritional status. Weight alone reflects just recent nutritional intake. Head circumference measures brain growth and development. Chronic malnutrition can limit this growth and is reflected in inadequate gains in head size. Regular measurements of head circumference, therefore, can verify desirable growth. Head circumference measurements are useful in infants and children up to age 2.

Growth Charts

During routine checkups throughout infancy (and during childhood and adolescence), health care practitioners measure weight, length or height, and head circumference and plot these values on **growth charts** (see **FIGURE 16.14**).

Charts for weight-for-age, length- (or height-) for-age, head circumference-for-age, weight-for-length, and BMI-for-age are available for boys and girls and for two age ranges: birth to 36 months and 2 to 20 years. Healthcare practitioners use growth charts to show the growth of an individual child over time. These charts also allow comparison of one child's growth to that of children in the general population.

- **prematurity** Birth before 37 weeks of gestation.
- **full-term baby** A baby delivered during the normal period of human gestation, between 38 and 41 weeks.
- **toddler** A child between 12 and 36 months of age.
- **head circumference** Measurement of the largest part of the infant's head (just above the eyebrows and ears); used to determine brain growth.
- **growth charts** Charts that plot the weight, length, and head circumference of infants and children as they grow.

Key Concepts A typical infant doubles her birth weight by age 4 to 6 months and triples it by 12 months. Infant length increases about 50 percent during the first year. Healthcare practitioners use growth charts to follow and assess an infant's growth in weight, length, and head circumference.

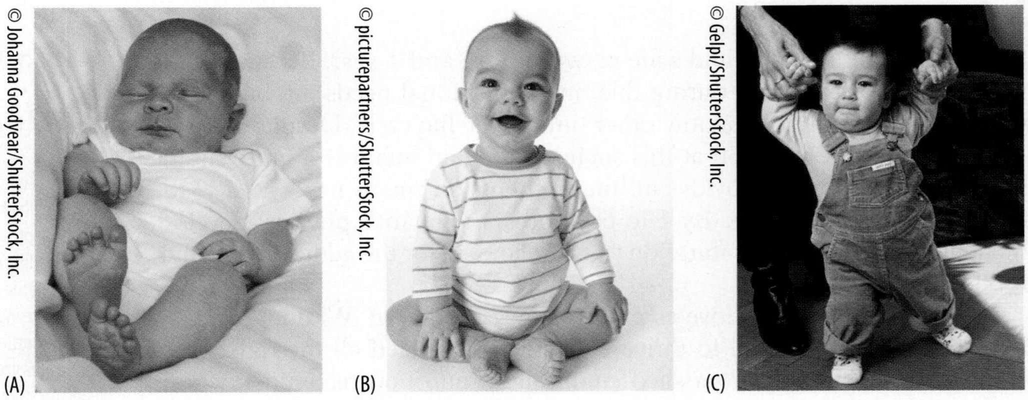

FIGURE 16.13 Different stages of infancy. (A) Newborn. (B) 4 to 6 months. (C) 12 months.

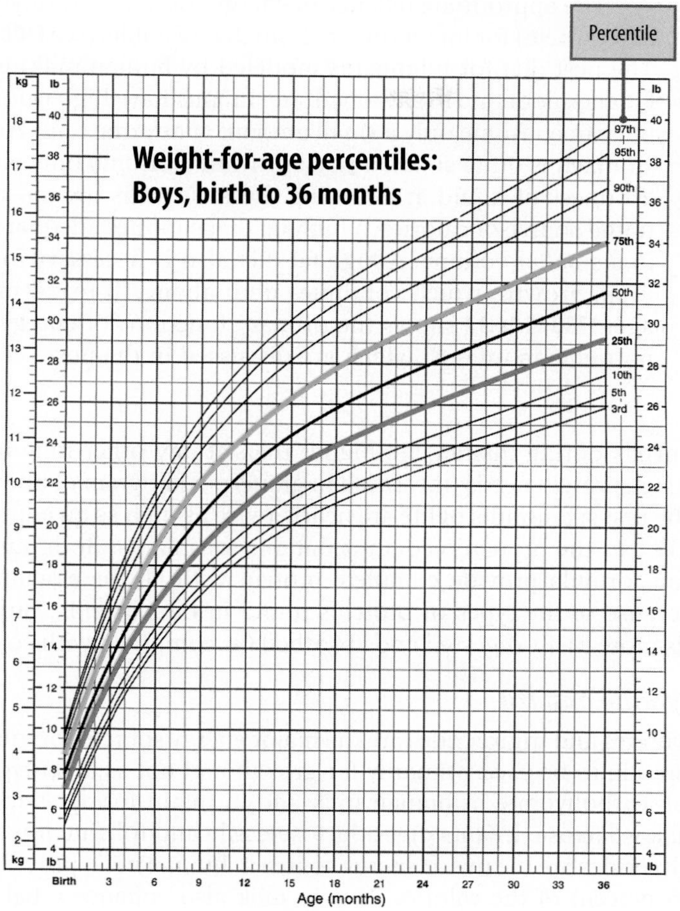

FIGURE 16.14 Growth chart. The Centers for Disease Control and Prevention (CDC) has complete sets of growth charts available on the Internet at www.cdc.gov/growthcharts.

Reproduced from the National Center for Health Statistics in collaboration with the National Center for Chronic Disease Prevention and Health Promotion (2000).

Energy and Nutrient Needs During Infancy

How do you suppose scientists determine the nutrient needs of newborns and young infants? Studies with babies as subjects are rare—the logistical and ethical questions are daunting! So, how else can we know what babies need? It's simple; we just look at human milk—the food designed especially for babies. The composition of human milk is the gold standard by which infant nutrient needs are determined. Babies who are not breastfed are given infant formula. In the United States, most infant formulas have a base of modified cow's milk or soy protein. To ensure that formula meets all of an infant's nutrient needs, federal regulations require that the formula's composition complies with nutritional standards.

Energy

An infant's energy need is the amount of energy he or she requires for basal functions, such as respiration and metabolism, in addition to growth and activity. An infant's basal energy needs, relative to his or her size, are about twice those of an adult. The amount of energy an infant needs for activity varies throughout the first year of life, increasing as the child becomes more mobile (see **FIGURE 16.15**). In general, a newborn requires about 100 kilocalories per kilogram of body weight.[66] **TABLE 16.9** lists the specific equations for calculating infants' Estimated Energy Requirements (EER).

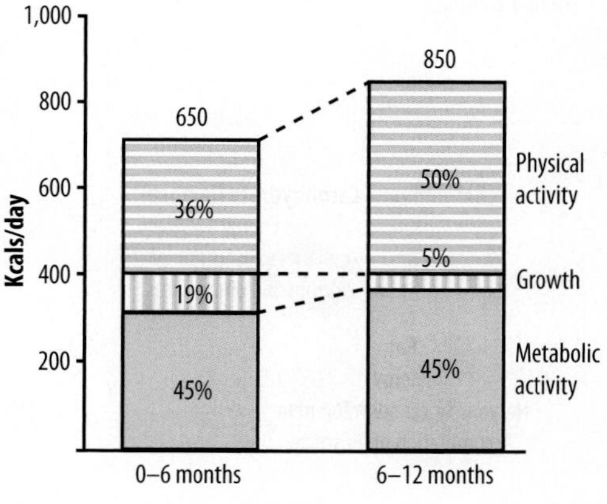

FIGURE 16.15 Allocation of energy expenditure. During the second six months, infants increase their energy expenditure for physical activity.

Adapted from Foman SJ, Bell EF. Energy. In: Foman SJ, ed. Nutrition of Normal Infants. St. Louis: Mosby; 1993.

TABLE 16.9
Estimated Energy Requirement RDA During Infancy

Age (mo)	EER Equation
0–3	(89 × wt [kg] – 100) + 175 kcal/day
4–6	(89 × wt [kg] – 100) + 56 kcal/day
7–12	(89 × wt [kg] – 100) + 22 kcal/day

Reproduced from Institute of Medicine, Food and Nutrition Board. *Dietary Reference Intakes for Energy, Carbohydrate, Fiber, Fat, Fatty Acids, Cholesterol, Protein, and Amino Acids (Macronutrients)*. Copyright © 2005 by the National Academy of Sciences, courtesy of the National Academies Press, Washington, DC.

The appropriate balance of energy sources (carbohydrate, fat, and protein) for infants differs from that of adults (see **FIGURE 16.16**). The best diet for infants (as modeled by human milk) is high in fat and moderate in carbohydrate. Infants have high calorie needs but can consume only a small amount at any one time. An infant's stomach is quite small; a newborn can consume only about 1 to 2 ounces of liquid at a feeding. Because fat is the most concentrated source of calories, a high-fat diet supplies adequate calories in a smaller volume. A high-fat diet also is necessary for normal brain growth, which continues until about 18 to 24 months of age. **FIGURE 16.17** shows the primary functions of energy-yielding nutrients in infants, which are discussed in the next sections.

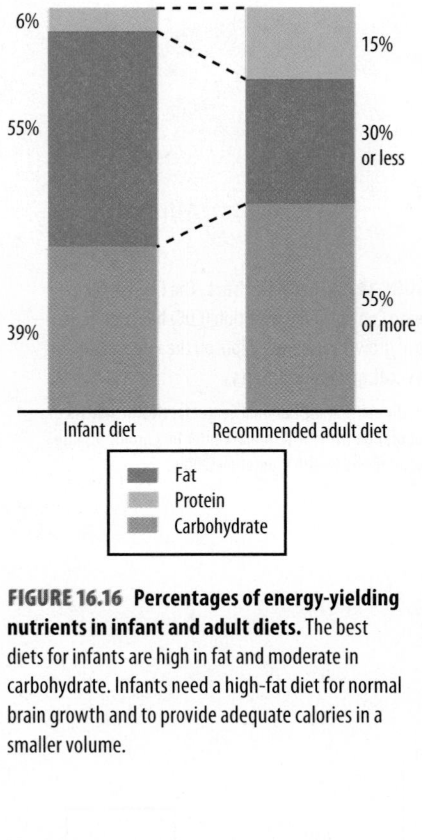

FIGURE 16.16 Percentages of energy-yielding nutrients in infant and adult diets. The best diets for infants are high in fat and moderate in carbohydrate. Infants need a high-fat diet for normal brain growth and to provide adequate calories in a smaller volume.

Protein

Protein needs during infancy are higher than at any other time in the life cycle. In fact, protein needs (measured in grams per kilogram of body weight) during the first six months of life are nearly twice as high as an adult's needs. **TABLE 16.10** lists the protein recommendations for infants. Both human milk and infant formula provide complete protein with all the essential amino acids. Because of the types of proteins found in human milk, human milk protein is more easily digested and absorbed (as compared with cow's milk).

Carbohydrate and Fat

Carbohydrates and triglycerides are the major energy sources for infants. This allows protein to be used primarily for growth and not as an energy source. Nearly all carbohydrate in human milk and in infant formulas made from cow's milk is lactose. Infants digest lactose easily and tolerate it well.

Triglycerides are the major energy source in human milk, providing about 50 to 55 percent of the calories. Fats in milk also enhance a baby's sense of fullness between feedings. Experts recommend that infants get at least 30 grams of fat per day.[67] Human milk is rich in essential fatty acids: the omega-6 fatty acid arachidonic acid and two long-chain omega-3 fatty acids, eicosapentaenoic acid and docosahexaenoic acid. These fatty acids have roles in neurological development. The Food and Nutrition Board has set an AI for newborns (0 to 6 months of age) of 4.4 grams per day of linoleic acid and 0.5 gram per day of alpha-linolenic acid.[68] Infants also need cholesterol for brain development. Human milk is rich in cholesterol, containing about 20 to 30 milligrams per 100 milliliters.[69]

Water

Because water as a percentage of body weight is higher in babies than in adults, infants need more fluids. The AI for water during infancy is 0.7 liter per day

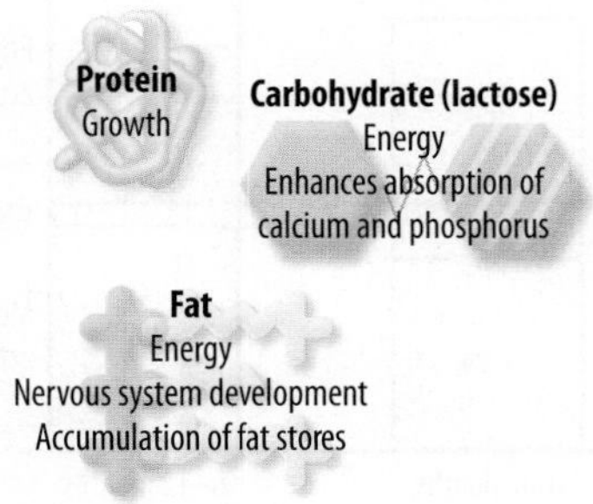

FIGURE 16.17 Primary functions of energy-yielding nutrients for infants. To support growth, protein needs (per kg body weight) are higher in infancy than in any other life stage.

TABLE 16.10
Protein AI or RDA for Infants

Age (mo)	g/kg	g/d[a]
0–6	1.52	
7–12	1.2	11

[a] The values for grams per day are based on reference weights of infants.

Data from Institute of Medicine, Food and Nutrition Board. *Dietary Reference Intakes for Energy, Carbohydrate, Fiber, Fat, Fatty Acids, Cholesterol, Protein, and Amino Acids (Macronutrients)*. Copyright © 2005 by the National Academy of Sciences, courtesy of the National Academies Press, Washington, DC.

in the first six months (assumed to be from human milk) and 0.8 liter per day from 7 months to 1 year of age. Human milk fulfills not only the nutrient needs of the **neonate**, but also the fluid requirements. Properly prepared formula accomplishes the same task. During the first four to six months, supplemental water is not necessary for healthy infants who are exclusively breastfed or who receive properly mixed formula. This is true even in hot, humid weather.[70] Once solid foods are introduced, a baby's water needs change, and additional water may be required.

▶ **neonate** An infant less than four weeks old.

Vitamins and Minerals

Human milk provides the amounts of vitamins and minerals that human babies need. Therefore, the micronutrient composition of human milk is the reference point for designing infant formula. As long as an infant is receiving adequate calories from breast milk or infant formula, nearly all vitamin and mineral needs also are being met. Human milk is lower in a few nutrients (e.g., iron, vitamin D), but infants absorb these nutrients more efficiently from breast milk than from formula. This section focuses on a few vitamins and minerals that are of concern for infants (see **FIGURE 16.18**).

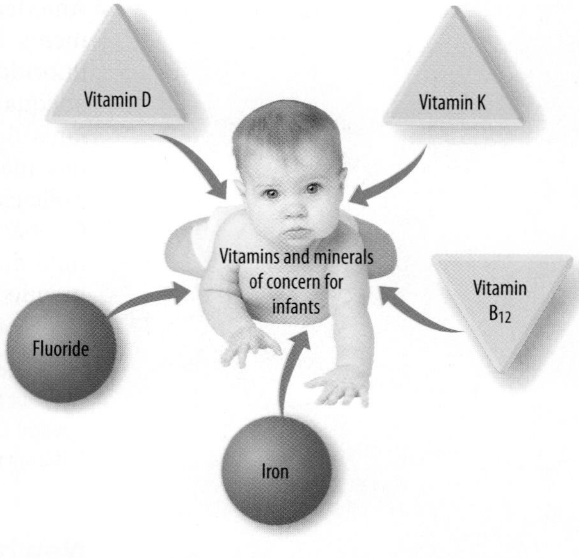

FIGURE 16.18 Micronutrients of concern during infancy. Infants who lack sun exposure can become deficient in vitamin D. A dose of vitamin K usually is given to babies at birth to ensure a sufficient supply. Because vegan mothers can have breast milk deficient in vitamin B_{12}, their babies may need a B_{12} supplement. By the age of 6 months, breastfed infants need additional iron. Formula-fed infants should consume iron-fortified formula. Human milk is low in fluoride.

Vitamin D Vitamin D is a key nutrient for absorbing calcium and mineralizing bone. Rickets is attributable to inadequate vitamin D intake and insufficient sunlight exposure in infants and children.[71] Recent evidence also suggests a role for vitamin D in maintaining innate immunity and preventing diseases such as cancer and diabetes.[72] Although human milk is low in vitamin D, infants absorb it well. Despite this, inadequate vitamin D levels are a concern for those infants who are exclusively breastfed, those not exposed to sunlight, and those with darkly pigmented skin who make less vitamin D from the same amount of sunlight exposure than do lighter-skinned infants. If a breastfed baby does not get adequate sunlight exposure and if the baby's mother is deficient in vitamin D, the infant's risk is especially high. In 2008 the American Academy of Pediatrics (AAP) increased its recommendation for daily vitamin D to 400 IU per day for all infants, children, and adolescents, beginning the first few days after birth.[69]

Vitamin K Vitamin K is necessary for the production of prothrombin, a substance needed for blood to clot. Although intestinal bacteria synthesize vitamin K, the gut is sterile at birth. Because babies are born with minimal stores of vitamin K, it is recommended that a single dose of vitamin K be given at birth. Both human milk and infant formula provide adequate vitamin K, and as feeding begins, helpful bacteria begin to flourish in the infant's intestinal tract.

Vitamin B_{12} Vitamin B_{12} is essential for cell division and normal folate metabolism. Mothers who include meat, fish, and dairy products in their diets produce milk that is adequate in vitamin B_{12}. This may not be true of strict vegetarians, whose diet—and therefore breast milk—can be deficient in vitamin B_{12}. Breastfed infants of vegan mothers may need a vitamin B_{12} supplement.

Iron Iron is essential for growth and development, and iron-deficiency anemia is the most common nutritional deficiency in the United States. Human milk is not a rich source of iron, but it does not need to be. Approximately 50 percent of the iron in breast milk is absorbed, compared with only 4 percent of the iron in infant formula. If the mother has consumed

Quick Bite

What's a Biberon?

Many people consider Dr. Nils Rosen von Rosenstein to be the father of pediatrics. In his 1764 textbook, he describes a "biberon," a leather nipple used for artificial infant feeding. He also describes 14 types of infant diarrhea.

an iron-rich diet during pregnancy, the fetus builds up large enough iron stores during gestation to meet most of its iron needs for the first few months of life. These stores begin to diminish during the fourth month of life. By the age of 6 months, a breastfed infant needs an additional iron source. Iron-fortified infant cereals can meet this need. For formula-fed babies, iron supplementation is needed from birth. The AAP therefore recommends iron-fortified formula for all formula-fed babies.[74]

Fluoride Human milk, although optimal in so many ways, is low in fluoride, a mineral important for dental health. Current research has led the American Dental Association and the AAP to recommend fluoride supplements for breastfed infants after the age of 6 months, depending on the fluoride content of the local water supply.[75] If the local water supply has adequate fluoride and the formula is mixed with tap water, formula-fed infants do not need fluoride supplements. If the water used to mix formula has inadequate fluoride, fluoride supplements are indicated. Fluoridation policies and the fluoride content of tap water vary among municipalities. Oversupplementation with fluoride in children has been associated with mild fluorosis in developing teeth; therefore, ingestion of higher than recommended levels is discouraged.[76]

Key Concepts Energy and nutrient needs for infants are estimated based on the composition of human milk. Because of their rapid growth and development, infants have high energy and nutrient needs per kilogram of body weight. Caregivers must give special attention to vitamin D, iron, and fluoride to ensure that the infant obtains enough. If breast milk or formula (properly mixed) is meeting energy needs, the fluid needs of the infant also are being met.

Newborn Breastfeeding

The AAP has identified breastfeeding as the ideal method of feeding to achieve optimal growth and development[77] and recommends that breastfeeding begin as soon after birth as possible and continue at least through the first 12 months of life.[78] Feedings should occur at least every two to three hours, for a total of 8 to 12 feedings per day. Duration of feedings is guided by the infant's behavior and can last from 10 to 15 minutes per breast. Hospitals should provide every opportunity for breastfeeding to begin before the baby goes home. Nurses or **lactation consultants** should be available to offer professional breastfeeding support to new mothers. The AAP recommends that no supplements of formula or water be given to breastfed neonates unless medically indicated.

▶ **lactation consultants** Health professionals trained to specialize in education about and promotion of breastfeeding; can be certified as an International Board Certified Lactation Consultant (IBCLC).

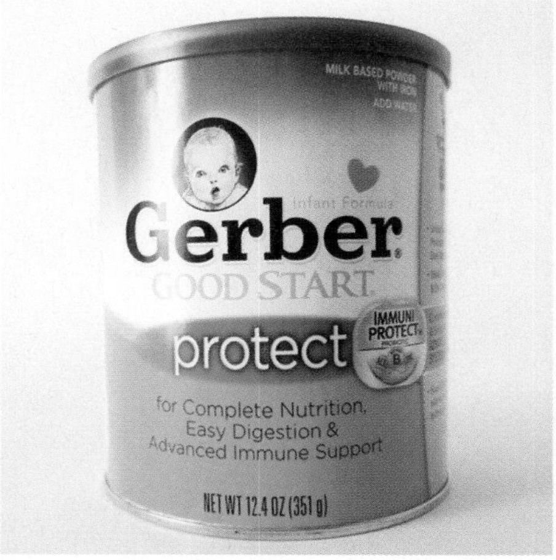

© Jones & Bartlett Learning. Photo by Amy Rathburn.

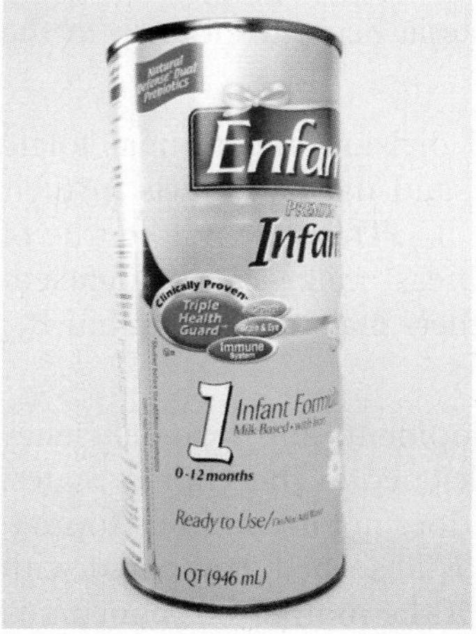

© Jones & Bartlett Learning. Photo by Amy Rathburn.

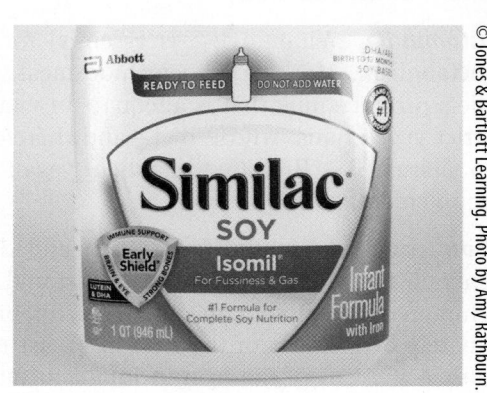

© Jones & Bartlett Learning. Photo by Amy Rathburn.

Alternative Feeding: Infant Formula

Women may decide not to breastfeed or to breastfeed only briefly. Their infants need infant formulas designed to provide adequate nutrition.

Standard Infant Formulas

Standard infant formulas have cow's milk as a base. In making infant formula, manufacturers first remove the milk fat and replace it with vegetable oils. Infant formula is fortified with all the essential vitamins and minerals according to guidelines established by the AAP and enforced by the Food and Drug Administration. Infant formulas are available with or without added iron, but because of the decreased bioavailability of iron in infant formulas and the infant's high needs, the AAP recommends using only iron-fortified formulas.

Although formula manufacturers try to mimic the composition of human milk, formula remains an imperfect copy. Several brands of infant formula contain three fatty acids that are prevalent in human milk: arachidonic acid (ARA), eicosapentaenoic acid (EPA), and docosahexaenoic acid (DHA). Some studies show that supplemental ARA and EPA benefit infants' visual function and cognitive development; however, a large review of studies found that most randomized controlled trials have not shown a beneficial effect of long-chain polyunsaturated fatty acid supplementation of formula milk on the neurodevelopmental, visual, and physical outcomes of full-term newborns.[79] Human milk also contains more cholesterol than infant formulas.

Soy-Based Formulas

Formula-fed infants who develop vomiting, diarrhea, constipation, abdominal pain, or colic are frequently switched to soy-based formulas. In these formulas, soy is the source of protein. To compensate for the inferior digestibility of soy protein, soy formulas contain more protein than formulas based on cow's milk. Soy formulas are lactose-free and iron-fortified. Corn syrup and sucrose are the carbohydrate sources.

Other Types of Formula

Formulas can be classified according to three basic criteria: caloric density, carbohydrate source, and protein composition.[80] Special formulas are available for infants who are allergic to both cow's milk and soy protein, those who are premature, and those who have rare defects in metabolic pathways. These special formulas often have their protein content modified in either its digestibility or its amino acid composition. Antireflux formulas are designed to decrease emesis and regurgitation. Many special formulas contain medium-chain triglycerides as the major fat source. This type of fat is very well digested and absorbed. These special formulas are expensive and often taste bad, but they are essential for many infants.

Formula Preparation

Formulas come in three forms: ready-to-feed, concentrate, and powdered. Although the ready-to-feed version is the most convenient, it is also the most expensive. As the name implies, the formula can be poured directly into a bottle and fed to the baby. Liquid concentrate formula is mixed with an equal amount of water before feeding. Powdered formula also is mixed with water and is the least expensive.

When using infant formulas, principles of food safety must be observed. Infants have immature immune systems and can develop infections from improperly prepared or stored formula. Prepared formula should be refrigerated

Going Green

How Safe Are Plastics?

Reduce, recycle, and reuse—even hard plastic water bottles? No, not those with the following symbol, They may actually leave a harmful substance behind in your body known as bisphenol A (BPA). Human exposure to BPA is widespread. According to scientists at the Centers for Disease Control and Prevention, 92 percent of Americans aged 6 and older have measurable levels of BPA in their bodies. Children had the highest levels, followed by teens, women, and then men.

Bisphenol A is a human-made industrial chemical used primarily in the production of plastics used in some food and drink packages, such as refillable water bottles, infant feeding bottles, reusable food storage containers, and some plastic eating utensils. BPA is also found in epoxy resins that coat water supply pipes as well as metal food cans and bottle tops.

BPA is classified as an endocrine disruptor. This means that it alters the function of the endocrine system by mimicking the role of hormones that occur naturally in the body. BPA can be most harmful in the early stages of development. In animals, it has been shown to have hormonelike effects on the developing reproductive system, but whether the adverse effects observed in animals could also occur in people exposed to low environmental levels of these chemicals is still not clear. The National Toxicology Program (NTP), which is part of the National Institutes of Health, has concerns about the possibility that BPA could cause prostate and breast problems in adults and brain problems in infants and children.

BPA from food and beverage packages leaches into foods and then gets into the body through the diet. How much BPA enters the foods depends on such factors as food temperature and the age of the container. The temperature of the liquid can have the most impact. Researchers at the Harvard School of Public Health found that after just one week of drinking cold liquids from water bottles, urinary BPA levels increased by 69 percent. Once hard water bottles are exposed to boiling water, BPA is released into the water at faster and much higher levels. Bisphenol A is released from polycarbonate drinking bottles and mimics the neurotoxic actions of estrogen in developing cerebellar neurons. This would be of significant concern for infants, who may be particularly susceptible to BPAs because formula often is warmed and served in the bottle.

In 2008, Canada banned the use of BPA in baby bottles, and the FDA followed in 2012 by banning the use of BPA in baby bottles and children's drinking cups. According to the NTP, parents and caregivers can further reduce exposures of their infants and children to BPA by opting for glass or porcelain containers for heating or serving hot foods and beverages and by reducing the use of canned foods.

immediately and kept in the refrigerator until needed. If formula is not used within 48 hours, it should be discarded. For at least the first few months, the AAP recommends sterilizing all equipment used for feeding.

Failure to follow instructions can result in an improperly mixed formula. Some caregivers on limited budgets may purposefully overdilute formula to make it last longer. This deprives the infant of necessary calories and protein and provides too much water. Other caregivers may overconcentrate the formula in the misguided belief that this may encourage faster growth. Overconcentrated formula provides too much protein and too little water and can cause problems with an infant's kidney function and hydration.

Breast Milk or Formula: How Much Is Enough?

It is fairly simple to use DRI values and breast milk or formula composition to estimate an infant's needs based on body weight. For example, a newborn who weighs 7 pounds, 11 ounces (3.5 kilograms) requires approximately 390 kilocalories and 5 grams of protein each day. This amount is provided by approximately 600 milliliters (approximately 20 fluid ounces) of breast milk or infant formula.

It's easy to keep track of how much formula an infant has consumed, but what about the breastfed baby? Although you can't see how much breast milk a nursing infant is consuming, there are other ways to tell that a baby is getting enough to eat. An adequately fed newborn will breastfeed daily 8 to 12 times, wet at least six diapers, and have at least three loose stools each day in the first week of life. The newborn will also regain his or her birth weight within the first two weeks. Normal growth, regular elimination patterns, and a satisfied demeanor are the best indicators that a baby is getting enough to eat.

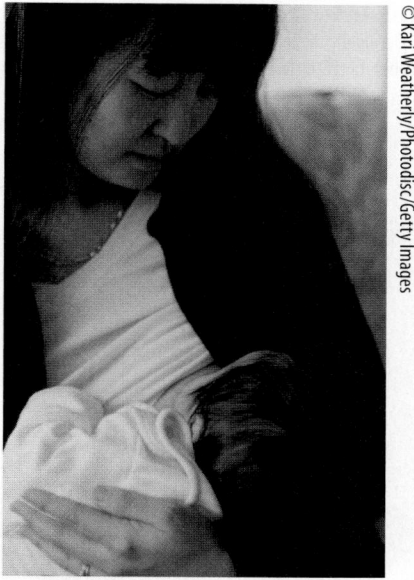

© Kari Weatherly/Photodisc/Getty Images

FIGURE 16.19 Breastfeeding. Breastfeeding nurtures an infant emotionally as well as physically. This intensely rewarding time helps to bond a mother and her child.

Feeding Technique

Feeding should take place in a loving and affectionate environment. A breastfeeding mother holds her baby close, at a distance that encourages mother–baby eye contact (see **FIGURE 16.19**). During bottle-feeding, the caregiver should also hold the baby close and make eye contact. Propping the bottle against a pillow or other object so that the baby can feed alone should be avoided.

Babies swallow air while feeding, whether at the breast or with a bottle, and they need to be burped. Babies generally need to be burped after 15 minutes or 2 to 3 ounces of formula.

Just as the infant sends signals of readiness for feeding, he also signals fullness. Fullness cues include fussiness, playfulness, sleep, or just turning away. Parents need to learn these cues and respond to them.

Key Concepts Human milk provides all the necessary nutrients for growth and development and enhances the immune system of the maturing infant. Infants who are not breastfed receive infant formula, which should be fortified with iron. Careful preparation and storage of the formula ensures proper nutrient composition and food safety. Formula feedings should nourish the baby emotionally as well as nutritionally.

Introduction of Solid Foods into the Infant's Diet

Based on an infant's physiological needs (e.g., depletion of iron stores) and physical development (e.g., the ability to sit up), solid foods, also called **complementary foods**, are introduced. To say that we are introducing solid foods is a bit of a misnomer: We are really referring to pureed and liquefied cereals, fruits, vegetables, and meats that are added to the infant's diet of breast milk or infant formula. According to the AAP, solid foods should be introduced when infants are developmentally ready, around 4 to 6 months of age, to ensure that they get adequate nutrition.[81]

▶ **complementary foods** Any foods or liquids other than breast milk or infant formula fed to an infant.

Physiological Indicators of Infant Readiness for Solid Foods

Before a baby reaches 6 months of age, solid food is not necessary for nutrition; in fact, early introduction of supplemental foods can be detrimental. By the age of 4 to 6 months, however, an infant is physiologically ready to expand his or her diet. For example, at this age a baby has increased levels of digestive enzymes so that foods other than human milk or formula can be digested with ease. In addition, the infant is better able to maintain adequate hydration by the age of 6 months. Before this age, adding cereals or other solid foods to the diet can negatively affect an infant's hydration. It is probably no coincidence that the iron stores acquired in the mother's womb become depleted at the same time the baby is physiologically ready to expand his or her diet. However, solid food is a supplement to, not a replacement for, human milk or formula at this time.

Quick Bite

Ancient Baby Bottle

The earliest infant feeding vessel ever discovered is Egyptian and dates from 2000 B.C.E. Art found in the ruins of the palace of King Sardanapalus of Nineveh, who died in 888 B.C.E., depicts a mother holding a modern-looking baby bottle.

▶ **extrusion reflex** A young infant's response when a spoon is put in its mouth; the tongue is thrust forward, indicating that the baby is not ready for spoon feeding.

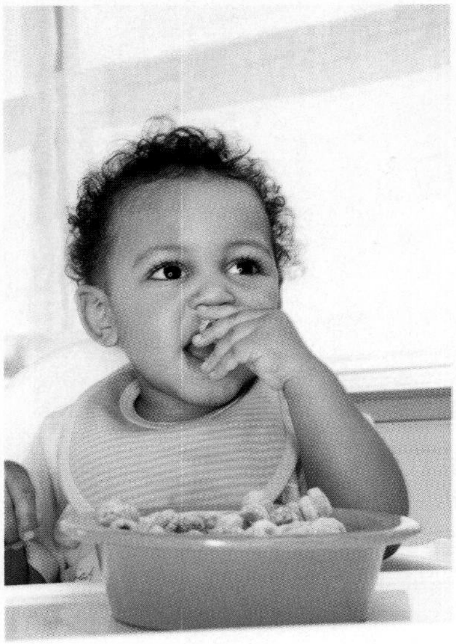

© James Woodson/Digital Vision/Thinkstock

Developmental Readiness for Solid Foods

If you attempt to spoon-feed a very young infant, for example, at 3 weeks of age, the infant's tongue will push the spoon and food right back out. This **extrusion reflex** is a sign that the infant is not ready for solid foods. By 4 to 6 months of age, the infant will no longer push the food out and is capable of transferring food from the front of the mouth to the back, an ability necessary for swallowing solid foods. Also, the infant can purposefully bring her hand to her mouth, an ability necessary for self-feeding. In addition, if the baby is able to control her head and neck while sitting with minimal support, she is ready to be fed solids.

Start Healthy Feeding Guidelines

The *Start Healthy Feeding Guidelines for Infants and Toddlers* are science-based, practical guidelines for feeding healthy babies for the first two years.[82] The *Start Healthy Feeding Guidelines* were designed to answer parents' and caregivers' questions, such as "When is my baby ready for complementary foods? What foods should I feed my baby? How do I feed these foods?"[83] The appropriate age for introduction of complementary foods balances physiological and developmental readiness with nutritional requirements for growth and development. **FIGURE 16.20** summarizes the *Start Healthy Feeding Guidelines*.

Signs of readiness for the introduction of infant cereals and thin, pureed foods include the ability to sit with support and the ability to take food from a spoon and move it forward and backward in the mouth with the tongue. As the infant's body control improves and he or she can sit independently, she will also develop the ability to pick up and hold objects in her hand. She will be able to take in thicker, pureed foods and soft, mashed foods without lumps.

Babies who can crawl also are likely to be ready to self-feed finger foods such as baby biscuits or crackers. Babies at this stage can hold small foods between the thumb and first finger and also hold a cup (preferably one with a cap and spout) independently. A baby is able to participate in the feeding process, and as his dexterity improves, he will be able to pick up small pieces of food. It is important that caregivers monitor the child's eating to make sure the youngster does not choke on food or on nonfood items.

At the end of the first year, when a baby is standing alone and beginning to walk, his diet can expand even further with bite-size pieces of table foods and a wider variety of textures. Self-feeding with his fingers is much easier, and he desires to self-feed with a spoon as well—a messy but developmentally appropriate thing to do. Most table foods are appropriate for the child at this stage.

There is no scientific evidence to support introduction of complementary foods in any particular order; cultural practices play a large role in determining which foods are introduced first. Introducing a source of iron, such as an iron-fortified infant cereal or pureed meats, is necessary because iron stores developed in pregnancy are declining. No matter what food is introduced first, new foods should be introduced one at a time, at intervals of about one week, to see how well the infant tolerates each food and to be on the lookout for allergic reactions. Throughout the first year, breast milk or infant formula still forms the major portion of the infant's diet. Ideally, however, the child will have been introduced to a variety of foods by his or her first birthday.

Parents and caregivers should take care that complementary foods are soft in texture to avoid the risk of choking. Delaying—until age 1—the introduction of common food allergens, particularly cow's milk, egg whites, and wheat, can prevent food allergies for many infants. In addition to its allergic potential, whole cow's milk provides too much protein and too little iron, is low in essential fatty acids, can impair kidney function and lead to dehydration, and has been linked to development of type 1 diabetes.[84] In families with

Development Stage	Newborn	Head Up	Supported Sitter	Independent Sitter	Crawler	Beginning to Walk	Independent Toddler
	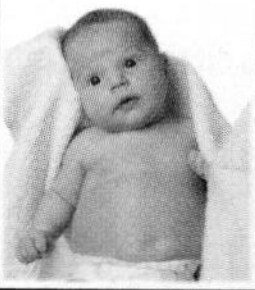	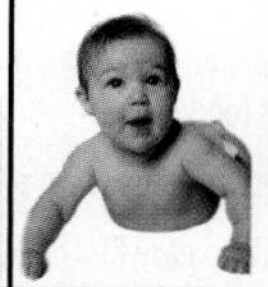	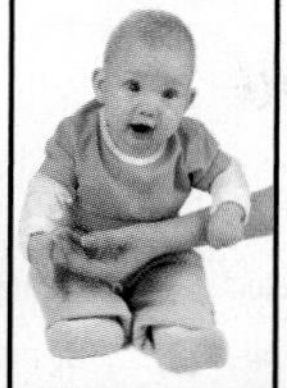	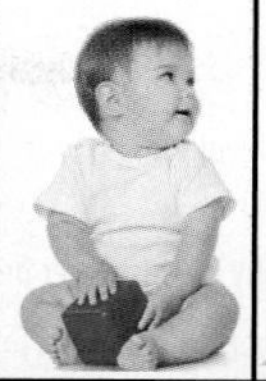	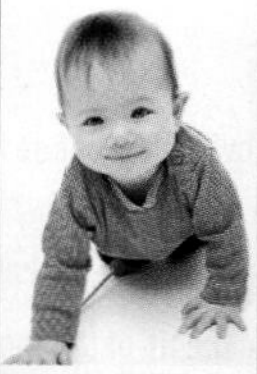	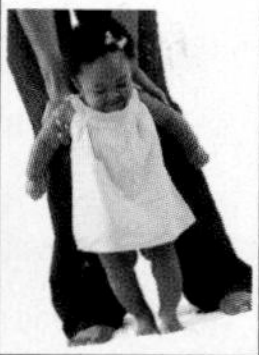	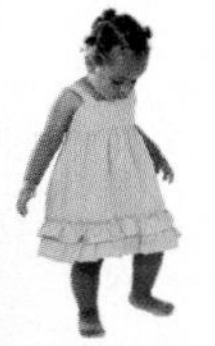
Physical Skills	• Needs head support	• More skillful head control with support emerging	• Sits with help or support • On tummy, pushes up on arms with straight elbows	• Sits independently • Can pick up and hold small object in hand • Leans toward food	• Learns to crawl • May pull self to stand	• Pulls self to stand • Stands alone • Takes early steps	• Walks well alone • Runs
Eating Skills	• Baby establishes a suck-swallow-breathe pattern during breast or bottle feeding	• Breastfeeds or bottle feeds • Tongue moves forward and back to suck	• May push food out of mouth with tongue, which gradually decreases with age • Moves pureed food forward and backward in mouth with tongue to swallow • Recognizes spoon and holds mouth open as spoon approaches	• Learns to keep thick purees in mouth • Pulls head downward and presses upper lip to draw food from spoon • Tries to rake foods toward self into fist • Can transfer food from one hand to the other • Can drink from a cup held by feeder	• Learns to move tongue from side to side to transfer food and push food to the side of the mouth so food can be mashed • Begins to use jaw to mash food • Plays with spoon at mealtime, may bring it to mouth, but does not use it for self-feeding yet • Can feed self finger foods • Holds cup independently	• Feeds self easily with fingers • Can drink from a straw • Can hold cup with two hands and take swallows • More skillful at chewing • Dips spoon in food rather than scooping • Demands to spoon-feed self • Bites through a variety of textures	• Chews and swallows firmer foods skillfully • Learns to use a fork for spearing • Uses spoon with less spilling • Can hold cup in one hand and set it down skillfully
Baby's Hunger and Fullness Cues	• Cries or fusses to show hunger • Gazes at caregiver, opens mouth during feeding indicating desire to continue • Spits out nipple when full • Stops sucking when full	• Cries or fusses to show hunger • Smiles, gazes, or coos during feeding to indicate desire to continue • Spits out nipple when full • Stops sucking when full	• Moves head forward to reach spoon when hungry • May swipe the food toward the mouth • Turns head away when full • May be distracted when full	• Reaches for or points spoon or food when hungry • Slows down in eating when full • Clenches mouth shut or pushes food away when full	• Reaches for food when hungry • Points to food and shows excitement when hungry • Pushes food away when full • Slows down in eating when full	• Expresses desire for specific foods with words or sounds • Shakes head to say "no more" when full	• Combines phrases with gestures, such as pointing • Can lead parent to refrigerator and point to a desired food or drink • Uses words like "all done" • Plays with food when full
Appropriate Foods and Textures	• Breast milk or infant formula	• Breast milk or infant formula	• Breast milk or infant formula • Infant cereals • Thin pureed foods	• Breast milk or infant formula • Infant cereals • Thin, pureed baby foods • Thicker pureed baby foods • Soft mashed foods without lumps • 100% juice	• Breast milk or infant formula • 100% juice • Pureed foods • Ground or soft mashed foods with noticeable lumps • Crunchy foods that dissolve (such as baby biscuits or crackers) • Increase variety of flavors offered	• Breast milk or infant formula or whole milk • 100% juice • Coarsely chopped foods, including foods with noticeable pieces • Foods with soft to moderate texture • Bite sized pieces of food	• Whole milk • 100% juice • Coarsely chopped foods • Bite-sized pieces of food • Becomes efficient at eating foods of varying textures and taking controlled bites by 2 years

FIGURE 16.20 The Start Healthy Feeding Guidelines. Summary of physical and eating skills, hunger and fullness cues, and appropriate food textures for children 0 to 24 months of age.

Reproduced from Butte N, Cobb K, Dwyer J, et al. The Start Healthy Feeding Guidelines for Infants and Toddlers. J Am Diet Assoc. 2004;104(3):442–454. Photos (left to right): © Barbara Penoyar/Stockbyte /Getty Images; © Barbara Penoyar/Stockbyte/Getty Images; © Olga Sapegina/ShutterStock, Inc.; © iStockphoto/Thinkstock; © iStockphoto/Thinkstock; © iStockphoto/Thinkstock; © Hemera/Thinkstock.

a history of allergies, introduction of eggs should be delayed until age 2, and peanuts, tree nuts, fish, and shellfish should not be introduced before age 3.

Along with observing the infant's developmental readiness for complementary foods, parents and caregivers need to be alert to an infant's hunger and satiety cues. Hunger cues include crying and fussing, reaching for spoonfuls of food, opening mouth and leaning toward bowl or spoon, and also staring at you while eating. Conversely, if full, the infant may turn away from food, push the bowl or food away, clench her mouth shut, and spit out food. The

TABLE 16.11
Suggestions for Establishing a Healthy Feeding Relationship with a Child

Do	Why
Wash the baby's hands before feeding.	To clean any dirt or germs off the hands to keep the baby's food clean.
Use a small spoon or let the baby use his or her fingers.	To help the baby learn proper eating habits.
Place food on the tip of the spoon and put food in the middle of the baby's tongue.	To make it easy for the baby to swallow.
Remove food from the jar before feeding. Do not feed the baby food from the jar.	To prevent the saliva from the baby's mouth from spoiling the remainder of the food in the jar.
Give only one new food at a time, and wait at least 1 week before giving another new food.	To give the baby time to get used to each new flavor and texture, and to see if the baby is allergic to the new food.

Reproduced from U.S. Department of Agriculture, Food and Nutrition Service. *A Guide for Use in the Child Nutrition Programs*. FNS-258. 2002. http://www.FNS.usda.gov/tn/resources/feeding_infants.html. Accessed January 11, 2016.

suggestions in **TABLE 16.11** can help new parents establish a healthy feeding relationship with their child.

Various caregivers may be involved in a child's nutrition. In today's society, it is inappropriate to assume that the caregiver is solely the mother, father, grandparent, or even a relative of the child. Many children spend the majority of their feeding time in a child-care setting. Child-care staff can develop and implement strategies to overcome challenges and support healthy eating behaviors of children.[85]

Quick Bite

Pumping Iron

The use of cow's milk for children younger than 1 year is a common cause of iron deficiency. Cow's milk is low in iron, and drinking it can cause intestinal bleeding in infants. Although the amount of iron in breast milk also is low, this iron is highly bioavailable. Breast milk also contains proteins that bind iron, thereby inhibiting the growth of diarrhea-causing bacteria that feed on iron. If formula is used, the AAP recommends that it be iron-fortified.

Key Concepts An infant's physiological needs and developmental readiness usually indicate the appropriate time to introduce solid foods. Semisolid and solid foods should be introduced slowly to check for infant food intolerances and allergic reactions. The caregiver should choose foods that meet the child's nutritional needs and suit his or her developmental capabilities.

Feeding Problems During Infancy

Colic

The term *colic* refers to continuous crying and distress in a healthy infant—apparently because of abdominal cramping and discomfort. Infants with colic usually cry for hours, despite efforts to comfort them. In some cases, a change in formula or a change in the breastfeeding mother's diet provides some relief. However, diet (of either mother or infant) is not considered a cause of colic.[86] Most often, colic goes away on its own, usually by the age of 3 to 4 months.

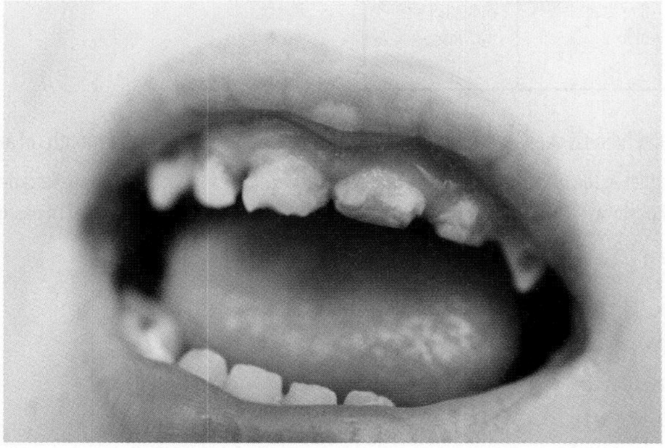

FIGURE 16.21 Early childhood caries. A baby routinely put to bed with a bottle can develop extensive tooth decay.

Early Childhood Caries

Decay in the primary teeth, known as early childhood caries and sometimes called "baby-bottle tooth decay" (see **FIGURE 16.21**), can result if baby teeth are bathed too long in milk, formula, or juice, which nourish decay-producing bacteria. Other factors, such as inadequate development of tooth enamel, can also contribute to tooth decay.[87] The problem is often associated with routinely putting a baby to bed with a bottle so the baby's teeth are awash in formula or juice for much or all of the night. Children with early childhood caries are more susceptible to caries in the permanent teeth and lifelong dental problems.[88]

Iron-Deficiency Anemia: Milk Anemia

Human milk and cow's milk both are low in iron. As discussed earlier, this is usually not a problem: The iron in breast milk is well absorbed, and regular cow's milk is not recommended for babies younger than 1 year; however, iron deficiency may develop in older infants who do not eat enough iron-rich foods.

Gastroesophageal Reflux

Gastroesophageal reflux is the regurgitation of the stomach contents into the esophagus after a feeding. This type of spitting up occurs in 3 percent of newborns, usually males, and typically disappears within 12 to 18 months. Concern is warranted if reflux makes a child difficult to feed or results in coughing, choking, or frequent vomiting. Adding cereal to bottle feedings is not recommended for a baby who has reflux.

Diarrhea

Stool patterns vary from infant to infant, as well as in the same infant over time. Healthy, thriving breastfed infants can have up to 12 stools per day—or only 1 per week. Formula-fed infants usually have one to seven bowel movements per day. Diarrhea—the frequent passage of loose, watery stools—can rapidly dehydrate an infant. Infants with diarrhea require increased fluids, and caregivers should consult the child's pediatrician for specific advice about how to meet this need.

Failure to Thrive

Full-term infants who experience poor growth in the absence of disease or physical defect suffer from **failure to thrive (FTT)** (see **FIGURE 16.22**). Although this can occur at any age, in infancy it usually occurs in the second half of the first year. Common causes include poverty and a resulting shortage of food, inappropriate foods in an infant's diet, improper formula preparation, or excessive consumption of fruit juice or fruit drinks. (See the FYI feature "Fruit Juices and Drinks.") In addition, well-meaning parents may introduce low-fat or nonfat milk in an attempt to prevent obesity. Babies need a high-fat diet to support normal growth and brain development. As stated, regular cow's milk should not be introduced before age 1. Low-fat milks are inappropriate for children younger than 2 years.

Untreated, FTT can delay cognitive, motor, and language development. Studies indicate, however, that intensive intervention can correct FTT and allow resumption of a normal growth pattern. Such intervention includes nutrition education for caregivers, maintenance of food records by the caregiver, frequent weight checks of the infant, and perhaps social service intervention for the family.

Although there is nothing complex about the nutrient needs and food choices appropriate for babies, it is important for caregivers to receive some education about proper feeding. Some practices that we learn from friends, parents, and other family members, or remember from our own childhood, are inappropriate for babies. Studies show that even people who receive nutrition education in the WIC program introduce solid foods much too early and feed infants sweetened tea, soft drinks, and other inappropriate foods.[89] Newborns don't come with instructions, but caregivers can always turn to a pediatrician or registered dietitian for answers to feeding questions.

Key Concepts Feeding-related problems of infancy include colic, baby-bottle tooth decay, iron-deficiency anemia, gastroesophageal reflux, diarrhea, and failure to thrive. Usually minor adjustments in food choices or feeding techniques solve these problems; however, caregivers may need the guidance of a pediatrician or registered dietitian.

Quick Bite

But the Breast Milk Looks Weak . . .

Mature breast milk looks similar to nonfat milk—thin, pale, and bluish. Not to worry! This appearance is normal, and breast milk always contains the right amount of nutrients for the baby. It is never too weak.

▶ **gastroesophageal reflux** A backflow of stomach contents into the esophagus, accompanied by a burning pain because of the acidity of the gastric juices.

▶ **failure to thrive (FTT)** Abnormally low gains in length (height) and weight during infancy and childhood; can result from physical problems or poor feeding, but many affected children have no apparent disease or defect.

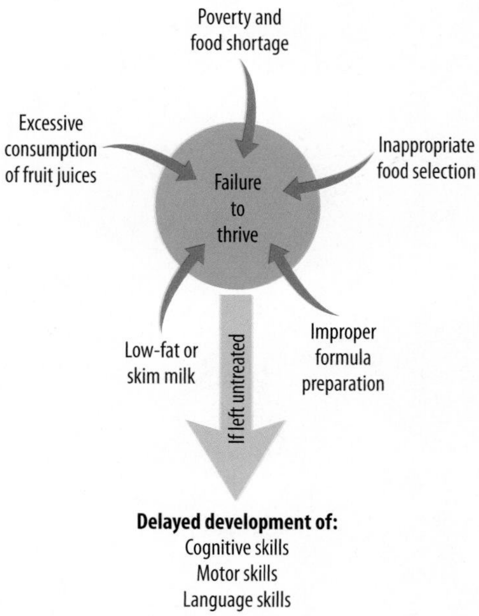

FIGURE 16.22 Failure to thrive. Failure to thrive can result from many different causes. If untreated, the effects are lifelong.

FYI For Your Information

Fruit Juices and Drinks

Fruit juices are popular beverages for children ages 6 months to 5 years. Apple, citrus, and other fruit juices, in addition to bananas and dried fruits, constitute a large amount of their total fruit intake, compared to youth ages 6 to 11 years.[a] A glass of 100-percent fruit juice counts as one fruit serving. If juice is being used as a source of vitamin C, drinking just 3 to 6 fluid ounces per day meets vitamin C intake recommendations.

Juices do provide benefits to the diet. They are refreshing and sweet; accessible and affordable; more healthful than soft drinks; and provide energy, water, and selected minerals and vitamins.

However, high fruit juice consumption among young children may also contribute to obesity and a failure to thrive. The link between excessive juice consumption and obesity has not been proven; however, studies suggest that it is more likely to be a factor in those children who are at risk for overweight and obesity.[b] Failure to thrive may result if fruit juices replace other food sources (particularly milk) or if sorbitol and fructose, found in higher amounts in apple and pear juice, cause diarrhea and malabsorption. If juice is substituted with fresh fruit, energy intake could be reduced and the adequacy of fiber intake improved. This would likely increase costs for schools, childcare providers, and families, but the nutritional gains would be achieved.[c]

To keep intake of fruit juices to a healthy level, the American Academy of Pediatrics (AAP) recommends the following practices[d]:

- Wait until at least 6 months of age before introducing juice.
- Avoid giving infants juice in bottles or other containers that allow easy consumption throughout the day. Avoid giving juice at bedtime.
- Limit consumption of fruit juice to 4 to 6 fluid ounces per day for children 1 to 6 years old.
- Encourage caregivers to offer fruit rather than fruit juice to children.
- Determine the amount of juice being consumed when evaluating children with malnutrition (overnutrition and undernutrition) and in children with dental caries.
- Educate parents about the differences between fruit juice and fruit drinks.
- Fruit juice should be pasteurized (e.g., children should not drink fresh-pressed apple cider).
- Make sure that juice does not replace breast milk, formula, or cow's milk.

[a] Herrick KA, Rossen LM, Nielsen SJ, et al. Fruit consumption by youth in the United States. *Pediatrics.* 2015;136(4):664–671.

[b] Monsivais P, Rehm C. Potential nutritional and economic effects of replacing juice with fruit in the diets of children in the United States. *Arch Pediatr Adolesc Med.* 2012;166(5):459–464.

[c] Ibid.

[d] American Academy of Pediatrics, Committee on Nutrition. In: Kleinman RE, Greer FR, eds., *Pediatric Nutrition.* 7th ed. Elk Grove Village, IL: American Academy of Pediatrics; 2014:123.

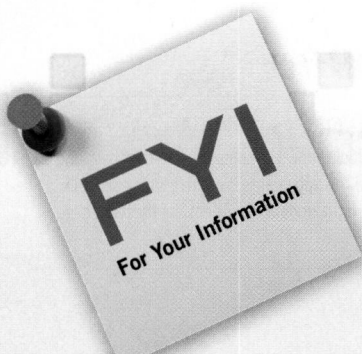

Label to Table

A pregnant woman requires more nutrients than usual. The RDA for both iron and folate increases by 50 percent during pregnancy. Iron, especially, is difficult to get in this quantity from the diet. Enriched grains and fortified foods, such as cereals, make it easier to obtain these essential nutrients. Let's take a look at the Nutrition Facts label from a popular breakfast cereal.

Take a look at how much folic acid a 1-cup serving of this breakfast cereal contains—50% DV (DV = 400 micrograms). The DV for folate is the same as the RDA for nonpregnant women; for pregnancy, the RDA increases to 600 micrograms. If orange juice accompanies the cereal, another 15% DV (60 mg) is added for a 1-cup serving. So, these two foods provide a substantial amount of the folate that a pregnant woman would need.

Iron also is extremely important for pregnancy because of its role in growth and its importance as blood volume increases during pregnancy. One serving of this breakfast cereal provides almost half of the DV of 18 milligrams (45 percent of 18 milligrams equals 8 milligrams). However, during pregnancy, the RDA for iron is 27 milligrams. So, one serving of this cereal provides nearly one-third of the iron needed each day—a good start. Having orange juice with the/cereal will enhance iron absorption.

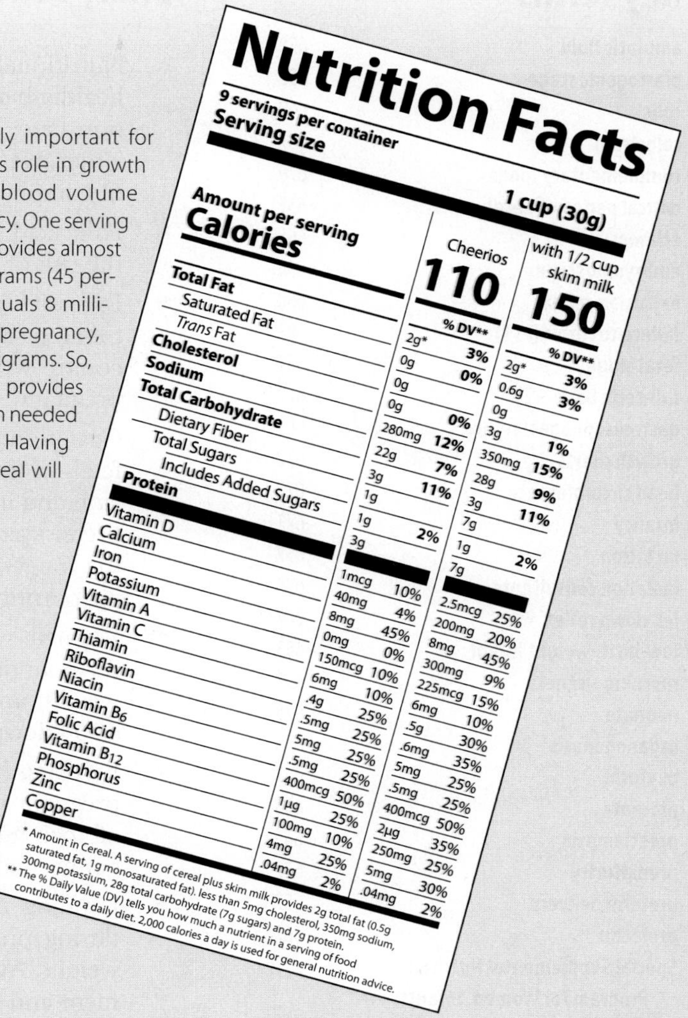
Nutrition Facts
9 servings per container
Serving size
1 cup (30g)
Amount per serving
Calories
Cheerios
110
with 1/2 cup skim milk
150
% DV**
Total Fat 2g* 3% 2g* 3%
Saturated Fat 0g 0% 0.6g 3%
Trans Fat 0g 0g
Cholesterol 0g 0% 3g 1%
Sodium 280mg 12% 350mg 15%
Total Carbohydrate 22g 7% 28g 9%
Dietary Fiber 3g 11% 3g 11%
Total Sugars 1g 7g
Includes Added Sugars 1g 2% 1g 2%
Protein 3g 7g
Vitamin D 1mcg 10% 2.5mcg 25%
Calcium 40mg 4% 200mg 20%
Iron 8mg 45% 8mg 45%
Potassium 0mg 0% 300mg 9%
Vitamin A 150mcg 10% 225mcg 15%
Vitamin C 6mg 10% 6mg 10%
Thiamin .4g 25% .5g 30%
Riboflavin .5mg 25% .6mg 35%
Niacin 5mg 25% 5mg 25%
Vitamin B6 .5mg 25% .5mg 25%
Folic Acid 400mcg 50% 400mcg 50%
Vitamin B12 1μg 25% 2μg 35%
Phosphorus 100mg 10% 250mg 25%
Zinc 4mg 25% 5mg 30%
Copper .04mg 2% .04mg 2%
* Amount in Cereal. A serving of cereal plus skim milk provides 2g total fat (0.5g saturated fat, 1g monosaturated fat). less than 5mg cholesterol, 350mg sodium, 300mg potassium, 28g total carbohydrate (7g sugars) and 7g protein.
** The % Daily Value (DV) tells you how much a nutrient in a serving of food contributes to a daily diet. 2,000 calories a day is used for general nutrition advice.

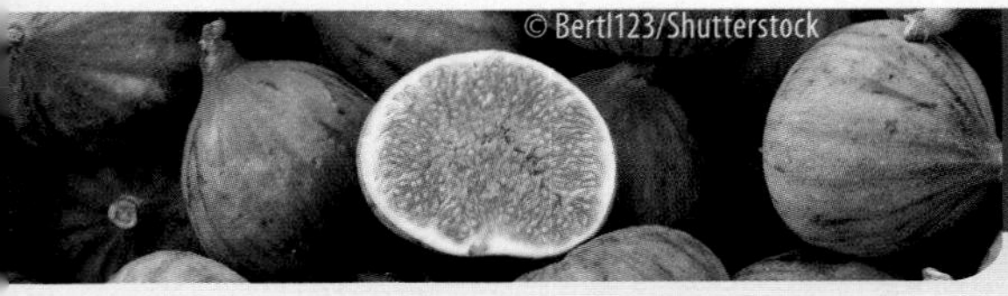

Learning Portfolio

Key Terms

Study Points

- Nutritional status before pregnancy is an important part of having a healthy baby. Moreover, it is an integral part of all aspects of preconception care: risk assessment, health promotion, and intervention. Being either overweight or underweight prior to pregnancy increases the risk of complications.
- Folic acid supplementation before pregnancy has been shown to reduce the risk of neural tube defects such as spina bifida.
- Excessive intake of some vitamins (vitamin A, in particular) and use of tobacco, alcohol, and drugs increase the risk of poor pregnancy outcomes; women should discontinue these practices before they become pregnant.
- Gestation can be divided into three stages: blastogenic, embryonic, and fetal. In the blastogenic stage, the fertilized ovum begins rapid cell division and implants itself in the uterine wall. During the embryonic stage, organ systems and other body structures form. During the fetal stage, the longest period of gestation, the fetus grows in size and changes in proportions.
- Women who enter pregnancy at a normal BMI should gain 25 to 35 pounds during pregnancy. Underweight women should gain more weight, and overweight women less. Energy needs increase by 340 to 450 kilocalories per day for the second and third trimesters.
- By using MyPlate for Pregnancy and Breastfeeding to plan food intake, pregnant women who consume enough energy should be able to meet all their nutrient needs with the exception of iron and folate. They should get needed extra calories mainly from grains, fruits, and vegetables.
- Limiting caffeine intake during pregnancy is recommended. Smoking during pregnancy increases the risk of preterm delivery and low birth weight. Alcohol and drug use can interfere with normal fetal development and should be avoided during pregnancy.
- Gastrointestinal distress such as morning sickness, heartburn, and constipation are common during pregnancy and result from the action of various hormones on the GI tract. Although most food cravings or aversions present no problems, excessive consumption of nonfood items, known as pica, interferes with adequate nutrition.
- During pregnancy, hormones control the development of breast tissue in preparation for milk production. Colostrum, the first milk, which is rich in protein and antibodies, is produced soon after delivery. By two to three weeks after delivery, lactation is well established, and mature milk is being produced.
- The pituitary hormone prolactin stimulates milk production. Oxytocin, another pituitary hormone, stimulates milk release, which is known as the let-down reflex.

- Unless they reduce their physical activity, breastfeeding women need 330 to 400 more kilocalories per day than they did when they were not pregnant. By obtaining adequate energy and using MyPlate for Pregnancy and Breastfeeding to balance choices, most lactating women can obtain all the nutrients they need from their diet. Cigarettes, alcohol, and illicit drugs should not be used while breastfeeding.
- Mothers benefit from breastfeeding through enhanced physiological recovery, convenience, and emotional bonding. Contraindications to breastfeeding include infection with HIV or active tuberculosis, and regular use of certain medications.
- Infants receive optimal nutrition from human milk. Breastfeeding can reduce the incidence of infectious diseases, allergies, and other problems during infancy.
- La Leche League, the March of Dimes, and the WIC program for low-income women are among the numerous resources for support and education of pregnant and breastfeeding women.
- Infancy is the fastest growth stage in the life cycle; infants double their birth weight in 4 to 6 months and triple it by 1 year of age. The nutritional status of infants is assessed primarily through measurements of growth.
- Infants' energy needs must be met through a high-fat diet, which provides the maximum calories in minimal volume. Infants' protein and fluid needs also are high.
- Human milk is low in vitamin D; breastfed babies need regular sun exposure or supplemental vitamin D. For breastfed infants, iron-fortified foods need to be introduced by 6 months of age. Formula-fed infants should be given iron-fortified formula.
- Infant formulas usually are based on either cow's milk or soy protein. Unmodified cow's milk is inappropriate for infants throughout the first year of life.
- The FDA regulates the vitamin and mineral composition of infant formulas to ensure adequate infant nutrition. Formula is available in ready-to-feed, liquid concentrate, and powdered forms.
- A nurturing environment is important to the feeding of infants, no matter what the milk source.
- Solid foods are introduced to the infant one at a time, usually beginning with iron-fortified infant cereal. Potential allergens, such as cow's milk, egg whites, and wheat, should be delayed until the baby is at least 12 months old. Developmental markers, such as head and body control and the absence of the extrusion reflex, show readiness for solid foods.
- Colic, although troublesome to infant and caregiver, is not caused by diet. Iron-deficiency anemia is common in infants who lack iron-rich foods. Infants are susceptible to dehydration, especially when diarrhea is prolonged. Failure to thrive describes an infant who is not growing well; intervention can be required to correct the feeding practices of caregivers.

Study Questions

1. Describe the three stages of fetal growth.
2. What are some physiological changes that occur in a woman during pregnancy?
3. How do the recommended intake values for calories, protein, folate, and iron change for pregnancy?
4. What contributes to morning sickness, and how can a woman minimize its effects?
5. What are some benefits of breastfeeding for the infant? For the mother?
6. Is it okay for an infant to experience weight loss immediately after birth? If an infant does lose weight, does it mean he or she is at nutritional risk?
7. How much water does a breastfed or formula-fed infant need each day?
8. Is it necessary to give breastfed infants supplements of vitamins and/or minerals? If so, which ones?
9. Describe the process for introducing solid foods into an infant's diet.
10. List the feeding problems that can occur during infancy.

Try This

For Just One Week, Can You Eat Like You're Expecting?

The purpose of this exercise is to see if you can follow the nutrition guidelines for pregnancy for just one week. Keep in mind that pregnant women attempt to do this for 38 to 40 weeks! Your goal is to reduce or eliminate caffeine,

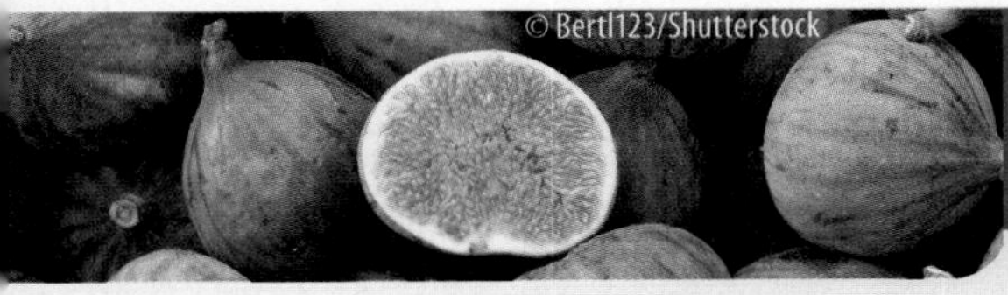

Learning Portfolio (continued)

alcohol, and over-the-counter medications. Make an effort to eat according to MyPlate each day, selecting the most nutrient-dense choices from each group. You should also take a basic multivitamin/mineral tablet (in place of a woman's prenatal supplement) daily. This will ensure that you consume the amounts of vitamins and minerals recommended for pregnancy.

Costs of Infant Formula

The purpose of this exercise is to find out how much it may cost to feed an infant. An average 3-month-old baby weighs about 13 pounds (6 kilograms) and would need about 650 kilocalories per day. Using standard infant formula, this baby would need about 32 ounces of formula each day. Now, go to a grocery store and find the infant formulas. If you were to purchase ready-to-feed formula, how much would it cost to feed this baby for one day? What if you were to use concentrated liquid formula? Powdered formula?

References

1. Farahi N, Zolotor A. Recommendations for preconception counseling and care. *Am Fam Physician*. 2013;88(8):499–506.
2. Salihu HM, Mbah AK, Alio AP, et al. Low pre-pregnancy body mass index and risk of medically indicated versus spontaneous preterm singleton birth. *Eur J Obstet Gynecol Reprod Biol*. 2009;144(2):119–123.
3. Hsu WY, Wu CH, Hsieh CT, et al. Low body weight gain, low white blood cell count and high serum ferritin as markers of poor nutrition and increased risk for preterm delivery. *Asia Pac J Clin Nutr*. 2013;22(1):90–99.
4. Ramakrishnan U, Imhoff-Kunsch B, Martorell R. Maternal nutrition interventions to improve maternal, newborn, and child health outcomes. *Nestle Nutrition Institute Workshop Series*. 2014;78:71–80.
5. Rasmussen KM, Yaktine AL, eds. *Weight Gain During Pregnancy: Reexamining the Guidelines*. Washington, DC: National Academies Press; 2009.
6. Ibid.
7. Ibid.
8. Kaar JL, Crume T, Brinton JT, et al. Maternal obesity, gestational weight gain, and offspring adiposity: the Exploring Perinatal Outcomes Among Children Study. *J Pediatr*. 2014;165(3):509–515.
9. Centers for Disease Control and Prevention. Folic acid. http://www.cdc.gov/ncbddd/folicacid/index.html. Accessed January 11, 2016.
10. U.S. Preventive Services Task Force. Folic acid to prevent neural tube defects: preventive medication. 2009. http://www.uspreventiveservicestaskforce.org/uspstf/uspsnrfol.htm. Accessed January 11, 2016.
11. Centers for Disease Control and Prevention. Folic acid. Op cit.
12. Lum KJ, Sundaram R, Buck Louis GM. Women's lifestyle behaviors while trying to become pregnant: evidence supporting preconception guidance. *Am J Obstet Gynecol*. 2011;205(3):203.e1–203.e7.
13. Rasmussen KM, Yaktine AL, eds. *Weight Gain During Pregnancy*. Op cit.
14. Ibid.
15. Ibid.
16. Ibid.
17. Institute of Medicine, Food and Nutrition Board. *Dietary Reference Intakes for Energy, Carbohydrate, Fiber, Fat, Fatty Acids, Cholesterol, Protein, and Amino Acids*. Washington, DC: National Academies Press; 2002.
18. Ibid.
19. Procter S, Campbell C. Position of the Academy of Nutrition and Dietetics: nutrition and lifestyle for a healthy pregnancy outcome. *J Acad Nutr Diet*. 2014;114(7):1099–1103.
20. U.S. Preventive Services Task Force. Folic acid for the prevention of neural tube defects: U.S. Preventive Services Task Force recommendation statement. *Ann Intern Med*. 2009;150(9):626–631.
21. U.S. Department of Agriculture. http://www.choosemyplate.gov/moms-pregnancy-breastfeeding Accessed July 8, 2015.
22. Institute of Medicine, Food and Nutrition Board. *Dietary Reference Intakes for Energy, Carbohydrate*. Op cit.
23. Academy of Nutrition and Dietetics. Op cit.
24. U.S. Department of Health and Human Services and U.S. Department of Agriculture. *Dietary Guidelines for Americans, 2015*. 8th ed. Washington, DC: U.S. Government Printing Office; December 2015.
25. U.S. Food and Drug Administration. What you need to know about mercury in fish and shellfish. March 2004. http://www.fda.gov/food/foodborneillnesscontaminants/metals/ucm351781.htm. Accessed January 11, 2016.
26. Higdon JV, Frei B. Coffee and health: a review of recent human research. *Crit Rev Food Sci Nutr*. 2006;46:101–123.
27. Greenwood DC, Alwan N, Boylan S, et al. Caffeine intake during pregnancy, late miscarriage and stillbirth. *Eur J Epidemiol*. 2010;25(4):275–280.
28. Browne ML, Hoyt AT, Feldkamp ML, et al. Maternal caffeine intake and risk of selected birth defects in the National Birth Defects Prevention Study. *Birth Defects Res A Clin Mol Teratol*. 2011;91(2):93–101.
29. Maslova E, Bhattacharya S, Lin SW, Michels KB. Caffeine consumption during pregnancy and risk of preterm birth: a meta-analysis. *Am J Clin Nutr*. 2010;92(5):1120–1132.
30. Academy of Nutrition and Dietetics. Op cit.
31. Phelan S. Smoking cessation in pregnancy. *Obstet Gynecol Clin North Am*. 2014;4(2):255–266.
32. Ungerer M, Knezovich J, Ramsay M. In utero alcohol exposure, epigenetic changes, and their consequences. *Alcohol Res*. 2013;35(1):37–46.
33. March of Dimes. Street drugs and pregnancy. http://www.marchofdimes.org/pregnancy/street-drugs-and-pregnancy.aspx. Accessed May 20, 2016.
34. Young SL. Pica in pregnancy: new ideas about an old condition. *Ann Rev Nutr*. 2010;21:30:403–422.
35. Tande DL, Ralph JL, Johnson LK, et al. First trimester dietary intake, biochemical measures, and subsequent gestational hypertension among nulliparous women. *J Midwifery Women Health*. 2013;58(4):423–430.
36. March of Dimes. HIV and AIDS in pregnancy. http://americanpregnancy.org/pregnancy-complications/hiv-aids-during-pregnancy/ Accessed July 8, 2015.
37. U.S. Department of Health and Human Services, National Institutes of Health, National Institute of Allergy and Infectious Disease. Family planning. http://www.aids.gov/hiv-aids-basics/staying-healthy-with-hiv-aids/friends-and-family/having-children/. Accessed January 11, 2016.
38. Centers for Disease Control and Prevention. Reproductive health: teen pregnancy. The importance of prevention. http://www.cdc.gov/TeenPregnancy/index.htm. Accessed January 11, 2016.
39. Ibid.
40. March of Dimes. Quick references fact sheet: Teenage pregnancy. http://www.marchofdimes.com/professionals/14332_1159.asp. Accessed July 8, 2015.
41. U.S. Department of Health and Human Services. Healthy People 2020. Maternal, infant, and child health. http://www.healthypeople.gov/2020/topics-objective Accessed July 8, 2015
42. Ibid.
43. Centers for Disease Control and Prevention. Breastfeeding report card—United States, 2014. http://www.cdc.gov/breastfeeding/pdf/2041BreastfeedingReportCard.pdf. Accessed January 11, 2016.
44. Institute of Medicine, Food and Nutrition Board. *Dietary Reference Intakes for Energy, Carbohydrate*. Op cit.
45. Statement from Surgeon General Dr. Regina M. Benjamin on World Breastfeeding Week, August 1–7, 2011. Press release. August 1, 2011.

46. National Institutes of Health, Office of Dietary Supplements. Vitamin B12: dietary supplement fact sheet. http://ods.od.nih.gov/factsheets/VitaminB12-HealthProfessional. Accessed January 11, 2016.
47. U.S. Department of Agriculture. Health & nutrition programs for pregnant & breastfeeding women. Op cit.
48. American Academy of Pediatrics policy statement. Breastfeeding and the use of human milk. *Pediatrics*. 2005;115:496–506.
49. Ibid.
50. Academy of Nutrition and Dietetics. Position of the American Dietetic Association: promoting and supporting breastfeeding. *J Am Diet Assoc*. 2014;114(7):1099–1103.
51. Bartick M, Reinhold A. The burden of suboptimal breastfeeding in the United States: a pediatric cost analysis. *Pediatrics*. 2010;125(5):e1048–e1056.
52. SurgeonGeneral.gov. The surgeon general's call to action to support breastfeeding. Fact sheet. January 20, 2011. http://www.surgeongeneral.gov/topics/breastfeeding/factsheet.html. Accessed January 1, 2016.
53. National Conference of State Legislatures. Breastfeeding state laws. http://www.ncsl.org/default.aspx?tabid=14389. Accessed January 11, 2016.
54. Academy of Nutrition and Dietetics. Position of the American Dietetic Association: promoting and supporting breastfeeding. Op cit.
55. SurgeonGeneral.gov. The surgeon general's call to action to support breastfeeding. Op cit.
56. Centers for Disease Control and Prevention. Vital signs. Hospital support for breastfeeding. Preventing obesity begins in hospitals. http://www.cdc.gov/vitalsigns/BreastFeeding/?s_cid=vitalsigns_081. Accessed January 11, 2016.
57. Ibid.
58. Hogue MM, Ahmed NU, Khan FH, et al. Breastfeeding and cognitive development of children: assessment at one year of age. *Mymensingh Med J*. 2012;21(2):316–321.
59. American Academy of Pediatrics policy statement. Breastfeeding and the use of human milk. Op cit.
60. Ibid.
61. Ballard O, Morrow AL. Human milk composition: nutrients and bioactive factors. *Pediatr Clin North Am*. 2013;60(1):49–74.
62. Walker A. Breast milk as the gold standard for protective nutrients. *J Pediatr*. 2010;156(2 suppl):S3–S7.
63. Hennet T, Weiss A, Borsig L. Decoding breast milk oligosaccharides. *Swiss Med Wkly*. 2014;144:w13927.
64. U.S. Department of Agriculture. Pregnancy and breastfeeding. Weight loss during breastfeeding. http://www.choosemyplate.gov. Accessed July 8, 2014.
65. American Academy of Pediatrics. Breastfeeding and the use of human milk. Op cit.
66. Academy of Nutrition and Dietetics. Position of the American Dietetic Association: promoting and supporting breastfeeding. Op cit.
67. National Conference of State Legislatures. Breastfeeding state laws. Op cit.
68. Ibid.
69. Centers for Disease Control and Prevention. 2011 pediatric nutrition surveillance: national summary of trends in breastfeeding children aged < 5 years. http://www.cdc.gov/pednss/pednss_tables/pdf/national_table13.pdf. Accessed January 11, 2016.
70. Riordan J, Wambach K. *Breastfeeding and Human Lactation*. 4th ed. Burlington, MA: Jones & Bartlett Learning; 2010.
71. Hadberg IC. Barriers to breastfeeding in the WIC population. *MCN Am J Matern Child Nurs*. 2013;38(4):244–249.
72. Metallinos-Katsaras E, Gorman KS, Wilde P, Kallio J. A longitudinal study of WIC participation on household food insecurity. *Matern Child Health J*. 2011;15(5):627–633.
73. Institute of Medicine, Food and Nutrition Board. *Dietary Reference Intakes for Energy, Carbohydrate*. Op cit.
74. Ibid.
75. Ibid.
76. Ibid.
77. Institute of Medicine, Food and Nutrition Board. *Dietary Reference Intakes for Water, Potassium, Sodium, Chloride, and Sulfate*. Washington, DC: National Academies Press; 2004.
78. Elder CJ, Bishop NJ. Rickets. *Lancet*. 2014;383(9929):1665–1676.
79. Institute of Medicine, Food and Nutrition Board. *Dietary Reference Intakes for Calcium and Vitamin D*. Washington, DC: National Academies Press; 2011.
80. Wagner CL, Greer FR. Op cit.
81. Kleinman RE, ed. *Pediatric Nutrition Handbook*. 6th ed. Elk Grove Village, IL: American Academy of Pediatrics; 2008.
82. http://www.ada.org/3088.aspx#dosschedule. Accessed 5-3-2016.
83. Vernacchio L, Kelly JP, Kaufman DW, Mitchell AA. Vitamin, fluoride, and iron use among US children younger than 12 years of age: results from the Slone survey, 1998–2007. *J Am Diet Assoc*. 2011;111:285–289.
84. Ibid.
85. National Treasury Employees Union. Why EPA's headquarters union of scientists opposes fluoridation. May 1, 1999. http://fluoridation.com/epa2.htm. Accessed January 11, 2016.
86. American Academy of Pediatrics policy statement. Breastfeeding and the use of human milk. Op cit.
87. Ibid.
88. Simmer K, Patole SK, Rao SC. Long-chain polyunsaturated fatty acid supplementation in infants born at term. *Cochrane Database Syst Rev*. 2011, December 7;12.
89. Kleinman RE, ed. Pediatric Nutrition Handbook. 6th ed. Elk Grove Village, IL: American Academy of Pediatrics; 2008.
90. American Academy of Pediatrics. Ages and stages. Starting solid foods. http://www.healthychildren.org/english/ages-stages/baby/feeding-nutrition/pages/Switching-To-Solid-Foods.aspx. Accessed January 11, 2016.
91. Pac S, McMahon K, Ripple M, et al. Development of the *Start Healthy Feeding Guidelines* for infants and toddlers. *J Am Diet Assoc*. 2004;104:455–467.
92. Gerber. Home page. https://www.gerber.com/Home. Accessed January 11, 2016.
93. Butte N, Cobb K, Dwyer J, et al. The *Start Healthy Feeding Guidelines* for infants and toddlers. *J Am Diet Assoc*. 2004;104:442–454.
94. Thorsdottir L, Thorisdottir AV. Whole cow's milk in early life. *Nestle Nutrition Workshop Series Pediatric Program*. 2011;67:29–40.
95. Academy of Nutrition and Dietetics. Position of the American Dietetic Association: benchmarks for nutrition in child care. *J Am Diet Assoc*. 2011;111:607–615.
96. U.S. Department of Agriculture, Food and Nutrition Service. Special Supplemental Nutrition Program for Women, Infants, and Children (WIC). Infant nutrition and feeding. http://www.nal.usda.gov/wicworks/Topics/FG/CompleteIFG.pdf. Accessed January 11, 2016.
97. Sheiham A, James WPT. A reappraisal of the quantitative relationship between sugar intake and dental caries: the need for new criteria for developing goals for sugar intake. *BMC Public Health*. 2014;14:863.
98. Ibid.
99. American Academy of Pediatric Dentistry. Policy on early childhood caries (ECC): unique challenges and treatment options. http://www.aapd.org/media/Policies_Guidelines/P_ECCUniqueChallenges.pdf. Accessed January 11, 2016.
100. National Maternal and Child Oral Health Resource Center. Promoting awareness, preventing pain: facts on early childhood caries (ECC). 2004. http://www.mchoralhealth.org/PDFs/ECCFactSheet. Accessed July 8, 2014.
101. Colak H, Dulgergil CT, Dalli M, Hamidi MM. Early childhood caries update: a review of causes, diagnoses, and treatments. *J Nat Sci Biol Med*. 2013;4(1):29–38.
102. Deming DM, Briefel RR, Reidy KC. Infant feeding practices and food consumption patterns of children participating in WIC. *J Nutr Educ Behav*. 2014;46(3 suppl):S29–S37.

Chapter 17

Life Cycle: From Childhood to Adulthood

Revised by Paul Insel

THINK About It

1. Were you a "picky" eater as a child? What about now?
2. What's your experience with acne and eating particular foods?
3. What behavior changes would you now consider making that would help you live longer?
4. Your grandfather lives by himself and relies on frozen foods for his nutritional needs. How do you feel about his diet?

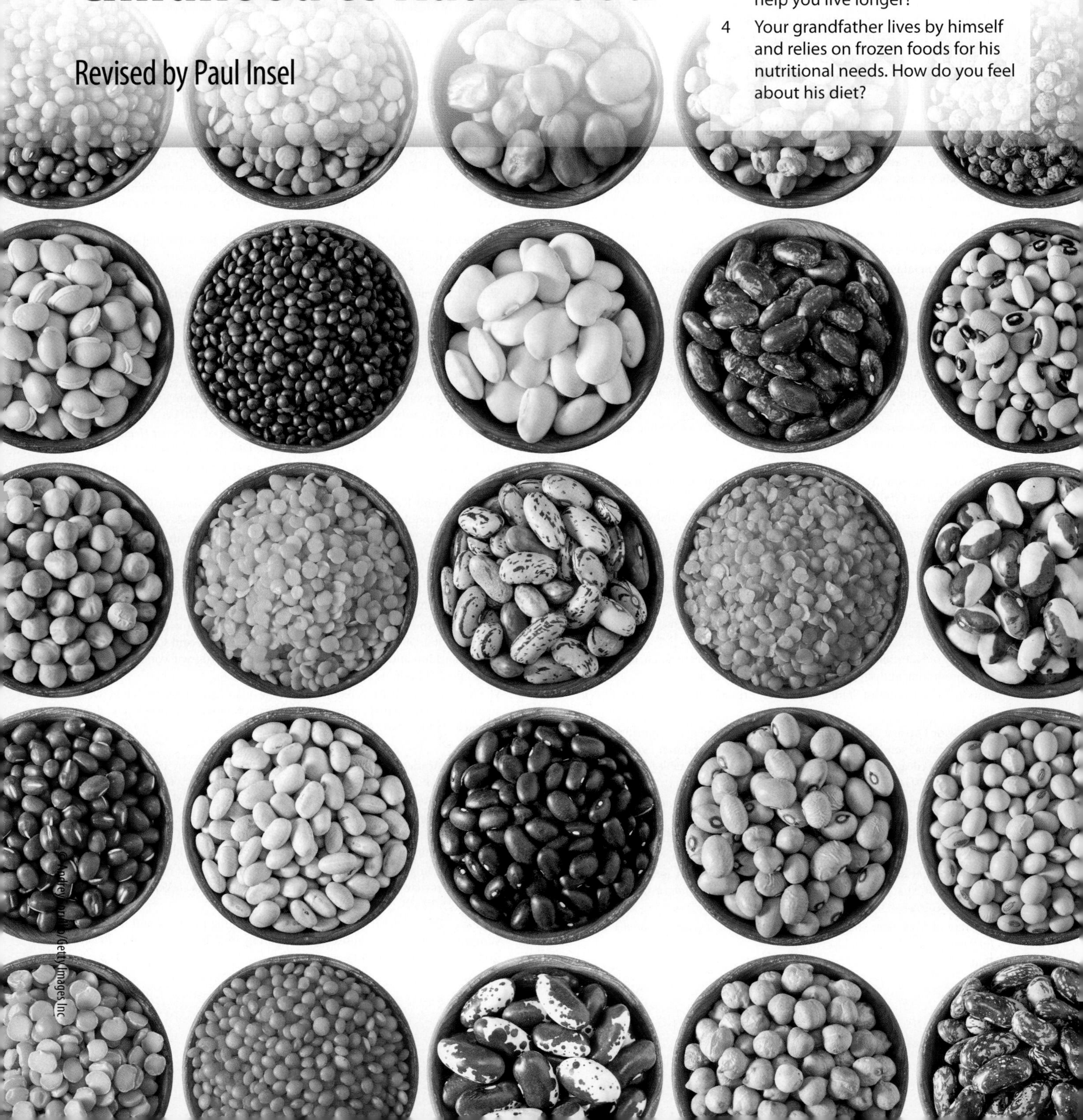

CHAPTER Menu

- Childhood
- Adolescence
- Staying Young While Growing Older
- Nutrient Needs of the Mature Adult
- Nutrition-Related Concerns of Mature Adults
- Meal Management for Mature Adults
- Key Terms
- Study Points
- Study Questions
- Try This
- References

LEARNING Objectives

- Discuss nutritional needs and concerns during childhood.
- Discuss nutritional needs and concerns during adolescence.
- Discuss age-related changes, nutritional needs, and concerns with aging.
- Analyze nutrition-related issues and concerns associated with older adults.
- Apply meal management strategies to older adults.

It's the year 2060. Who are you? Where do you live? What is your life like? How healthy are you? If projections made earlier in the century were accurate, you are part of the largest segment of the population—in 2060, between one-third and one-fourth of Americans are older than 65. Perhaps you have retired recently, or maybe you continue to work in your profession. Think about how technology has changed in your lifetime; new methods of communication have been developed that make email and the Internet seem old-fashioned, so late twentieth century!

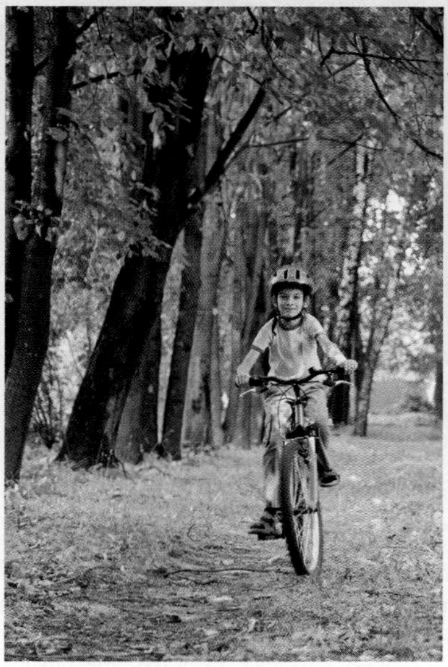

Consider how much you have changed over the years. Throughout childhood and adolescence you were growing, sometimes quite rapidly! Whether you fueled that growth with burgers and fries, black beans and rice, chips and soft drinks, or yogurt and salads will have determined a lot about your health status in 2060. Did you continue the eating habits you had in college, and did these allow you to control your weight, blood cholesterol, and blood pressure? Or perhaps, in the year 2060, these conditions are no longer of concern. Advances in genetics may have allowed gene therapy to replace diet therapy and medications for chronic diseases.

This chapter looks at how continued growth in childhood and adolescence affects nutritional needs. In addition, we'll see how nutritional needs change as we age, and we'll consider feeding practices, meal planning, and obstacles to healthful eating for each age group.

Childhood

Childhood is the term that refers to the years from age 1 through the beginning of **adolescence**. Growth in childhood, although continuous, occurs at a significantly slower rate than in infancy. During the childhood years, a typical child will gain about 5 pounds and grow 2 to 3 inches each year. Children can be divided into three groups based on their age and development: toddlers (ages 1–3), preschoolers (ages 4–5), and school-aged children (ages 6–10).

▶ **childhood** The period of life from age 1 to the onset of puberty.

▶ **adolescence** The period between onset of puberty and adulthood.

Energy and Nutrient Needs During Childhood

An average 1-year-old requires about 850 to 1,000 kilocalories per day.[1] This daily energy requirement gradually increases until it almost doubles by around age 10.

TABLE 17.1
Estimated Energy Requirement Equations for Children (Ages 3 Through 8)

Males
EER = 88.5 – 61.9 × age [y] + PA × (26.7 × weight [kg] + 903 × height [m]) + 20 kcal/day
Physical activity (PA): Sedentary = 1.00; Low active = 1.13; Active = 1.26; Very active = 1.42
Females
EER = 135.3 – 30.8 × age [y] + PA × (10.0 × weight [kg] + 934 × height [m]) + 20 kcal/day
Physical activity (PA): Sedentary = 1.00; Low active = 1.16; Active = 1.31; Very active = 1.56

TABLE 17.2
Protein RDAs for Childhood

Age (y)	Protein (g/kg)	Reference Weight[a] (kg)	Protein (g/d)
1–3	1.05	12	13
4–8	0.95	20	19
9–13	0.95	36	34

[a] Reference weights are based on median weights of children in that age group.

Energy and Protein

Estimated Energy Requirements (EERs) for children can be calculated based on sex, age, height, weight, and activity level (see **TABLE 17.1**). In contrast to the 175 kilocalories per day needed during early infancy, the added energy cost for growth during childhood is only 20 kilocalories per day.

Although total energy requirements increase, the kilocalories needed per kilogram of body weight slowly decrease as children move through childhood. The same is true for protein requirements (see **TABLE 17.2**).

Vitamins and Minerals

As long as a healthy child cooperates by eating a variety of healthful foods, a well-planned diet should provide most of the nutrients a child needs. One exception is iron. Children ages 4 to 8 years require 10 milligrams of iron per day but may not get that amount without careful meal planning.

Children should limit their consumption of sugar-sweetened beverages and calorie-dense snack foods, which are poor sources of iron. This allows room in the diet for high-iron food sources such as lean meats, legumes, fish, poultry, and iron-enriched breads and cereals (see **TABLE 17.3**). Iron deficiency not only affects growth, but also can impair the child's mood, attention span, focus, and ability to learn.[2]

TABLE 17.3
Iron-Rich Foods and Snacks

- Ground beef
- Poultry
- Fish
- Legumes
- Dark-green vegetables
- Protein
- Sloppy Joe
- Casseroles with meat

Iron-Rich Snacks

- Cream of wheat
- Cooked macaroni or pasta
- Enriched cereals, either dry or with milk
- Tortillas filled with refried beans
- Dried apricots
- Raisins (for older children)
- Bean dip
- Chili, mildly seasoned
- Peanut butter on enriched bread or graham crackers
- Enriched breads, cereals, rice, and pasta

Seventy percent of U.S. children do not get enough vitamin D. Among U.S. children ages 1 to 21, 7.6 million, or 9 percent, are vitamin D deficient, and another 50.8 million, or 61 percent, have insufficient levels of vitamin D.[3] Traditionally, rickets was the primary disease of concern with childhood vitamin D deficiency. New evidence links low levels of vitamin D to increased adverse cardiovascular risks, including high blood pressure and lower levels of high-density lipoprotein in children[4] and hypertension, hyperglycemia, and metabolic syndrome in adolescents regardless of body weight.[5] The American Academy of Pediatrics recommends that children and adolescents who do not obtain enough dietary vitamin D from fortified foods receive a supplement of 400 IU per day.[6]

A child's diet also may be low in other micronutrients, especially calcium, magnesium, potassium, and vitamin E[7] (see **FIGURE 17.1**). American children do not consistently meet the recommendations of MyPlate for the fruit, grain, and dairy groups, important sources of these nutrients.

Vitamin and Mineral Supplements

Many caregivers would rather give a child a vitamin/mineral pill than plan and prepare the meals necessary to ensure an adequate diet. However, the balanced diet a child needs is not much different from the diet an adult needs. In fact, MyPlate Kid's Place (see **FIGURE 17.2**) shows the same balance of food groups as is recommended for adults. Caregivers who understand this may be less tempted to rely on supplements and make the effort to achieve a balanced diet.

Some children should receive supplements. Among them are children whose diets are restricted for medical reasons, those with chronic diseases, those who are malnourished, and those with food allergies that require them to avoid multiple foods or food groups.[8] (For more on food allergies, see the FYI feature "Food Hypersensitivities and Allergies.") Caregivers need to be reminded that vitamin and mineral supplements for children are dangerous in large doses. Vitamin and mineral preparations must be treated like all medicines and kept safely out of children's reach. Supplements containing iron in doses of more than 30 milligrams are especially dangerous to children. Accidental consumption of vitamin and mineral or iron supplements should be treated as a poisoning emergency.

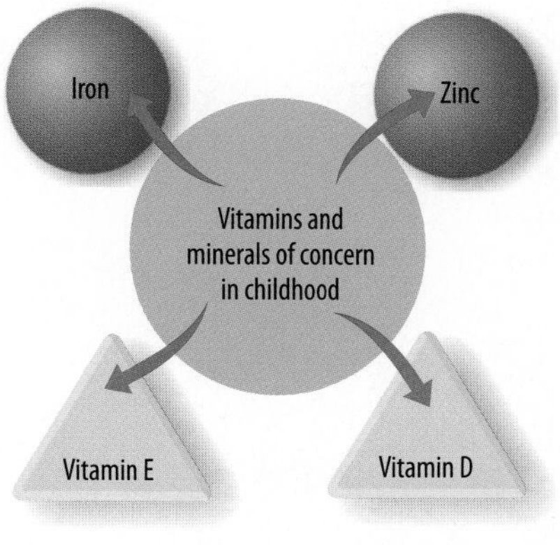

FIGURE 17.1 Micronutrients of concern in childhood. Milk is low in iron, and small children also might have low intakes of magnesium, potassium, calcium, and vitamin E.

Influences on Childhood Food Habits and Intake

Children develop food preferences at an early age. Toddlers start to exhibit unique feeding practices and styles. For some, this means that one food cannot touch another, or that foods cannot be green, or that all foods must be green. All of these "preferences" are merely the toddler's way of exhibiting control over his or her environment while experimenting and exploring. Although it may seem like an eternity to even the most patient caregiver, these food habits are

Position Statement: Academy of Nutrition and Dietetics

Dietary Guidance for Healthy Children Aged 2 to 11 Years

It is the position of the Academy of Nutrition and Dietetics that children ages 2 to 11 years should achieve optimal physical and cognitive development, attain a healthy weight, enjoy food, and reduce the risk of chronic disease through appropriate eating habits and participation in regular physical activity.

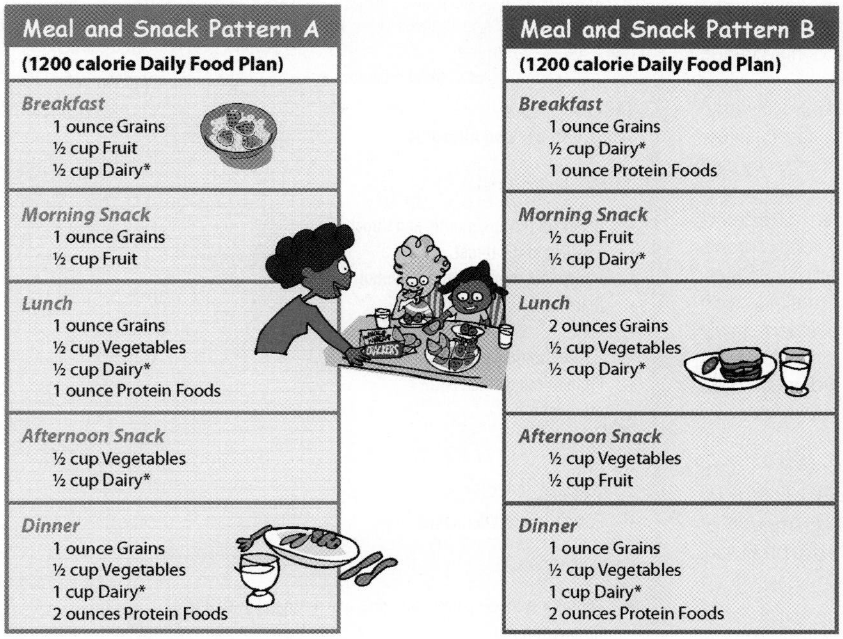

Meal and Snack Pattern A (1200 calorie Daily Food Plan)	Meal and Snack Pattern B (1200 calorie Daily Food Plan)
Breakfast 1 ounce Grains ½ cup Fruit ½ cup Dairy*	***Breakfast*** 1 ounce Grains ½ cup Dairy* 1 ounce Protein Foods
Morning Snack 1 ounce Grains ½ cup Fruit	***Morning Snack*** ½ cup Fruit ½ cup Dairy*
Lunch 1 ounce Grains ½ cup Vegetables ½ cup Dairy* 1 ounce Protein Foods	***Lunch*** 2 ounces Grains ½ cup Vegetables ½ cup Dairy*
Afternoon Snack ½ cup Vegetables ½ cup Dairy*	***Afternoon Snack*** ½ cup Vegetables ½ cup Fruit
Dinner 1 ounce Grains ½ cup Vegetables 1 cup Dairy* 2 ounces Protein Foods	***Dinner*** 1 ounce Grains ½ cup Vegetables 1 cup Dairy* 2 ounces Protein Foods

*Offer your child fat-free or low-fat milk, yogurt, and cheese.

FIGURE 17.2 MyPlate Meal and Snack Patterns for a 1,200-calorie daily food plan for preschoolers. Sample patterns also are available for 1,000, 1,400, and 1,600 calories at ChooseMyPlate.com.

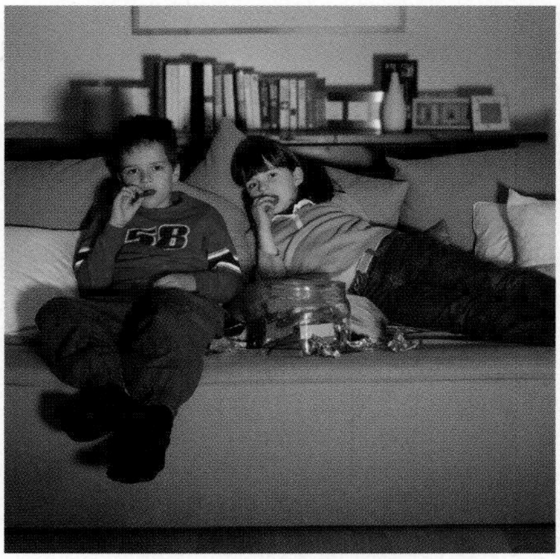

usually temporary. The wise caregiver allows this process to occur naturally, rather than wage food battles that ultimately are always won by the child. Nutrition professionals advocate child-feeding practices in which caregivers are responsible for positive structure, age-appropriate support, and healthful food and beverage choices, and children are responsible for whether and how much to eat. This division of responsibility promotes self-regulation of energy intake.[9] THINK About It 1

More and more children spend time in organized daycare settings. In these early years, child-care workers are playing an increasingly important role in the development of children's health and nutritional habits.[10]

FYI For Your Information

Food Hypersensitivities and Allergies

Food allergies, or food hypersensitivities, are allergic reactions to food proteins. Allergies are different from food intolerances (such as lactose intolerance) that can involve digestive problems rather than an immune response. Allergies are less likely than intolerances to be transient and tend to have more serious consequences. Proteins that trigger allergies are known as allergens. The most common food allergens are found in milk, eggs, tree nuts, peanuts, soy, wheat, fish, and shellfish.

Food allergies occur when the immune system mounts a specific reaction to a food protein. About 25 percent of people in the general population think they suffer from food allergies. In 2007, 3.9 percent of children younger than 18 years—that's 3 million, or 4 of every 100 children—were reported to have food or digestive allergies, a figure 18 percent higher than in 1997.[a]

In a true allergic reaction, the immune system responds to an allergen with a cascade of chemical reactions that can cause wheezing, difficulty breathing, and hives as well as a host of other symptoms (see **Table A**). Food allergy symptoms often affect more than one body system and may change in severity from one reaction to the next.

Anaphylaxis, the most severe allergic reaction, usually takes place within the first hour after eating the offending food. Shock and respiratory failure can rapidly ensue. Anaphylaxis can be fatal, so immediate emergency care is essential.

Allergy symptoms that occur immediately after a food is eaten make detective work easier. If symptoms are slow to evolve, a child may suffer chronic diarrhea and even experience failure to thrive before the problem is identified.

When identification of the food culprit isn't so obvious, an elimination diet can help. All suspected foods are eliminated from the diet and slowly reintroduced, one by one, on a specific schedule. Both intake and reactions are carefully recorded. Prolonged or improper use of such a diet can have severe nutritional consequences. A registered dietitian can help with diet planning to ensure nutritional adequacy.

The double-blind, placebo-controlled food challenge is the gold standard of food allergy testing. Although definitive, it can be dangerous for people prone to anaphylactic reactions. In this test, increasing amounts of a suspected food are given to the child under the supervision of a physician, who looks for allergy symptoms and signs. This test must be done by trained personnel with emergency equipment handy.

The treatment for food allergy is avoidance of the offending allergen. Each child with a food allergy needs a nutrition assessment that pays attention to the specific nutrients missing as a result of avoiding the offending foods. For example, if a toddler is avoiding milk and milk products because of a cow's milk allergy, the nutrients most at risk would be protein, vitamin D, and calcium. As a child's diet includes more and more foods, careful label reading is the key to identifying allergen-containing foods. Organizations such as the Food Allergy & Anaphylaxis Network (FAAN) provide materials for deciphering food labels.[b] FAAN also offers tips for successful traveling and dining with a child who has food allergies.

Many children naturally outgrow food allergies by the time they are 3 years old. Once outgrown, the food allergy will not return.

[a] Branum AM, Lukacs SL. Food allergy among U.S. children: trends in prevalence and hospitalizations. October 2008. NCHS Data Brief 10. http://www.cdc.gov/nchs/data/databriefs/db10.htm. Accessed January 11, 2016.

[b] Food Allergy & Anaphylaxis Network. http://www.foodallergy.org. Accessed January 11, 2016.

TABLE A
Symptoms of Food Allergies

Symptoms of Food Allergies
Gastrointestinal Tract
• Itching of the lips, mouth, and throat • Swelling of the throat • Abdominal cramping and distention • Diarrhea • Colic • Gastrointestinal bleeding • Protein-losing enteropathy
Skin
• Hives • Swelling • Eczema, contact dermatitis
Respiratory Tract
• Runny or stuffed-up nose, sneezing, and postnasal discharge • Recurrent croup • Chronic pneumonia • Middle-ear infections
Systemic
• Anaphylaxis • Heart rhythm irregularities • Low blood pressure

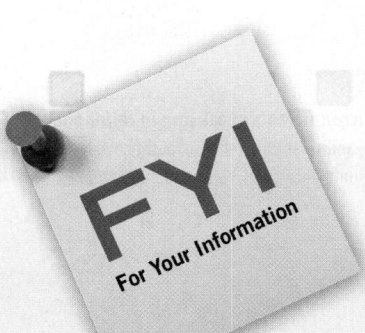

As a child's environment expands, an increasing number of external factors influence the child's diet. Sedentary behavior in children, such as long periods of television watching, is associated with unhealthy dietary habits.[11] It is estimated that children spend more time watching television than doing most other activities. Television advertising influences children's food preferences, purchasing requests, and consumption.[12] Recognizing the influence that children have on household purchases, advertisers target commercials specifically at children during prime children's viewing hours. Cartoons, for example, feature countless ads for sweetened cereals, fast foods, candy, and other foods high in sugar or fat, none of which are necessary or desirable. Ninety-one percent of food ads during Saturday morning television programming push foods of poor nutritional quality.[13] Children are more likely to eat an unhealthy diet if they watch a lot of television.[14] Studies show an association among young children watching morning television and poor diet, including higher intakes of sugar-sweetened beverages, fast food, and red and processed meat; total energy intake and percent energy intake from trans fat; and lower intakes of fruit and vegetables, calcium, and dietary fiber.[15]

Social events and parties often promote unhealthful eating habits. No matter what the occasion, the menu for children's parties rarely varies. Popular snacks and beverages also tend to be too high in sugar and fat. Serving more healthful but still child-friendly snacks, such as those in **TABLE 17.4**, breaks this tradition.

Who has the most important influence on the development of healthful eating habits? Parents![16] Parents not only are models for children's eating behaviors, but also can make it easier for children to accept new foods. Parents can offer a variety of healthy food choices that help ensure that their children get all the nutrients they need from each food group. Eating healthy meals together as a family has also been found to reduce the risk of obesity in children.[17]

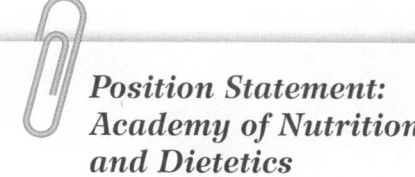

Position Statement: Academy of Nutrition and Dietetics

Benchmarks for Nutrition in Child Care

It is the position of the Academy of Nutrition and Dietetics that child-care programs should achieve recommended benchmarks for meeting children's nutrition needs in a safe, sanitary, and supportive environment that promotes optimal growth and development. Use of child care has become increasingly common and is now the norm for the majority of families in the United States.

Reproduced from Position of the American Dietetic Association: benchmarks for nutrition in child care. *J Am Diet Assoc.* 2011;111:607–615.

Key Concepts Children grow at a slower rate than they did as infants but still gain 2 to 3 inches and about 5 pounds per year. They should be able to obtain adequate energy and nutrients from their meals and snacks. Iron-deficiency anemia is the most common nutritional deficiency among American children. Many children in the United States also do not get enough calcium and vitamin D. Sugar-sweetened beverages and high-calorie snacks fail to provide needed nutrients and contribute to obesity. Outside influences, such as television viewing, affect children's preferences for foods with low nutrient density. Parents are the most important influence on the food habits of their children.

Nutritional Concerns of Childhood

The major challenges to promoting healthful childhood nutrition are combating malnutrition and hunger, chronic disease, overweight, lead toxicity, food and behavior and nutrition concerns regarding vegetarian practices.

Malnutrition and Hunger in Childhood

Of all issues facing children with respect to growth and nutrition, none is so devastating as hunger and malnutrition. Throughout the world, 60 percent of the deaths of young children can be attributed to undernutrition.[18] Deficiencies in vitamin A, zinc, iron, and protein also result in illness, stunted growth, limited development, and, in the case of vitamin A, possibly permanent blindness. In the United States, in 2013, 3.8 million households were unable to provide adequate, nutritious food for their children.[19] In many of these households, young children are protected from substantial reductions in food intake.

TABLE 17.4
Healthy Snacks

- Cereal and milk
- Yogurt shake: plain yogurt, fresh fruit
- Popcorn sprinkled with Parmesan cheese
- Fresh vegetables and a yogurt dip
- Pretzels
- Peanut butter on celery
- Bananas with peanut butter
- Graham crackers and peanut butter
- Sliced apples with cheese
- Bagel and melted cheese
- Bran muffins
- Pumpkin, banana, or zucchini bread
- Mini pizza on English muffin
- Homemade pita pocket sandwiches
- Yogurt with fresh fruit or granola
- Vegetable soup
- Fresh fruit
- Colored peppers and hummus
- Cucumbers with plain yogurt
- Cheese and whole-grain crackers

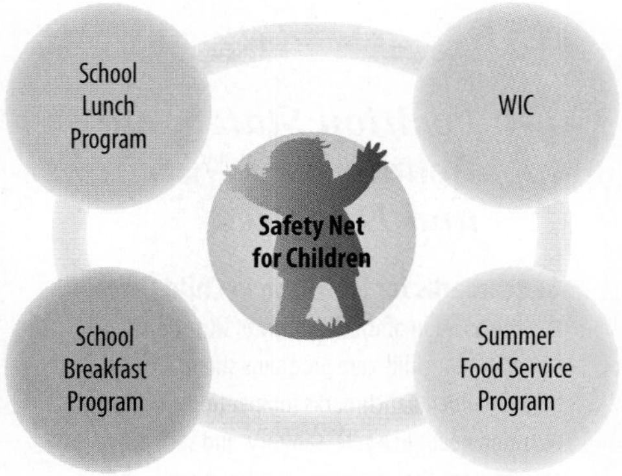

FIGURE 17.3 Federal safety net for children. Children are more vulnerable than adults to the effects of malnutrition. For many children, these federal programs provide the major—and, in some cases, the only—sources of calories and other nutrients.

▶ **hyperactivity** A maladaptive and abnormal increase in activity that is inconsistent with developmental levels. Includes frequent fidgeting, inappropriate running, excessive talking, and difficulty in engaging in quiet activities.

Federal programs help to create a safety net for these children. The U.S. Department of Agriculture (USDA) has 15 nutrition assistance programs that address hunger, including the Supplemental Nutrition Assistance Program (SNAP)—formerly the Food Stamp Program—the National School Breakfast and Lunch Programs, and the Special Supplemental Nutrition Program for Women, Infants, and Children (WIC). (See **FIGURE 17.3**.) For many children, the meals provided through the National School Lunch, Breakfast, and Summer Food Service Programs are the major—and, in some cases, the only—sources of calories and other nutrients. Those who plan and serve meals have the challenge of balancing popular foods that children will eat with foods that provide good nutrition. To ensure that the nutritional needs of the more than 31 million children receiving meals through school lunch programs are met, the Child Nutrition Reauthorization Healthy Hunger-Free Kids Act of 2010 represents a national effort to provide children with healthier and more nutritious food choices.[20] The main objectives of the Healthy Hunger-Free Kids Act focus on improving nutrition and reducing childhood obesity, increasing access to school meal programs, and increasing monitoring and the integrity of school meal programs.[21]

Food and Behavior

The term **hyperactivity** usually is defined as an abnormal increase in activity that is maladaptive and inconsistent with developmental level, but common usage has exaggerated its meaning. Parents often use this term to describe what they view as unruly behavior in children, particularly in classroom settings or structured home settings such as meal time. In social settings, children typically react to situations surrounding parties (where high-sugar foods are often served) in excitable ways. This is not proof of a cause-and-effect relationship between those foods and hyperactivity.

Attention-deficit hyperactivity disorder (ADHD) is characterized by inattentive, hyperactive, and impulsive behavior that is unrestrained and frenetic. ADHD is estimated to affect 5 percent of children worldwide.[22] Genetic and environmental factors are both involved in the etiology of ADHD. Sugar and certain food additives, including preservatives and colorings, have all been thought to cause or exacerbate behavioral disorders. Many parents and caregivers often blame sugar for "hyper" behavior in children. However, this association has not been clearly demonstrated.[23] Although the cause remains controversial, studies do suggest that certain food colorings and additives enhance hyperactive behaviors in some children. Further research is needed.[24,25] For some children, ADHD can be triggered by various foods, and a diet that eliminates these foods can produce a favorable response in sensitive children.[26]

Caffeine products can make children jittery and interfere with their sleep. Because children have small body sizes, the effects of a caffeinated beverage are intensified. Many soft drinks are high in caffeine; examples include Mountain Dew (55 milligrams per 12-oz can), Surge (51 milligrams per 12-oz can), and Coca-Cola (37 milligrams per 12-oz can). Popular energy drinks can also be substantial sources of caffeine.

Childhood Overweight

In the United States, overweight in childhood is increasing at an alarming rate. Approximately 32 percent of children aged 2 to 19 years are overweight (body mass index in the 85th to 94th percentile) or obese (body mass index at or above the 95th percentile).[27] An overweight child is likely to reach maturity earlier than a child of normal weight but perhaps at the expense of height. Some overweight children already deal with the cardiovascular consequences of obesity, such as lipid abnormalities and hypertension, and many overweight children develop type 2 diabetes prior to the teen years. Finally, overweight children are likely to have social and academic problems[28] and experience the psychological trauma associated with obesity in our culture. Factors involved in the development of overweight in childhood include genetics, environment, behavior, and activity levels (see **FIGURE 17.4**).

Programs designed to treat childhood obesity generally provide behavior modification, exercise counseling, psychological support or therapy, family counseling, and family meal-planning advice. In some cases, the goal is not weight loss, but rather to allow the child's height to catch up with his or her weight. Instead of restricting caloric intake or food choices, the first strategy is usually to increase physical activity and improve food choices. To meet the challenge of childhood obesity and direct children toward healthy, active lifestyles, the White House Task Force on Childhood Obesity launched a comprehensive campaign, called Let's Move![29] Let's Move! aims to end childhood obesity within a generation with strategies that include providing parents with helpful information, creating environments that support healthy choices, providing healthier foods in schools, ensuring that every family has access to healthy and affordable foods, and helping children become more physically active.[30]

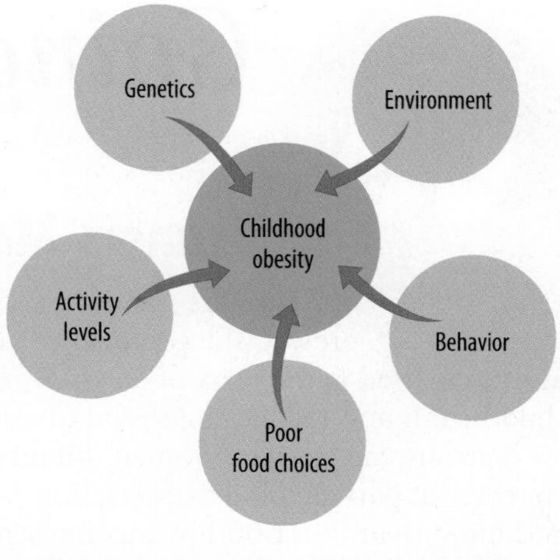

FIGURE 17.4 Factors that contribute to childhood obesity. Childhood obesity is on the rise and predisposes children to health problems when they become adults.

Nutrition and Chronic Disease in Childhood

When is it appropriate to adopt adult dietary guidelines for children? It is well documented that early signs of chronic disease can appear in childhood. Evidence of early plaque development has been seen in the coronary arteries of adolescents and is associated with adult cardiovascular diseases. However, the low-fat, high-fiber diet advocated for adults can jeopardize a very young child's growth. Infants and toddlers younger than 2 years old need fat in their diets for growth, organ protection, and central nervous system development. Dietary restrictions at this age are not appropriate.

For children older than 2 years, however, efforts to lower fat, saturated fat, and cholesterol intake can reduce risks of chronic disease. Dietary choices in line with the *Dietary Guidelines for Americans* are recommended. But it's important that parents and caregivers not misinterpret the recommendations and restrict children's energy intake. During the preschool and school years, gradual changes can bring food choices in line with the *Dietary Guidelines for Americans.* Caregivers should offer children healthful choices and, as they grow, educate them about proper nutrition.

Because of the rising rates of childhood obesity and incidence of chronic diseases related to weight, the American Academy of Pediatrics (AAP) now recommends screening children who have a positive family history of abnormal blood lipids or premature cardiovascular disease for blood lipid abnormalities.[31] For those children with high levels of low-density lipoprotein (LDL) cholesterol, lifestyle interventions such as changes in diet and physical activity are recommended. In some circumstances, medication may be warranted.

Lead Toxicity

Reducing elevated blood lead levels among children is one of the Healthy People 2020 objectives.[32] The Centers for Disease Control and Prevention (CDC) reports that the percentage of children with elevated levels (equal to or greater than 10 micrograms per deciliter) dropped significantly, from 7.61 percent in 1997 to 0.56 percent in 2013.[33] Lead toxicity can result in slow growth and iron-deficiency anemia and can damage the brain and central nervous system, leading to a host of learning disabilities and behavior

Quick Bite

Television Tubbies

The number of obese children in the United States has doubled in the past 20 years, and one in five U.S. children is now overweight. Today's kids spend more time watching television and playing video games than engaging in physical activity. Advertisers know it. When programs for children are broadcast, 80 percent of commercials advertise food, most of it high in sugar or fat.

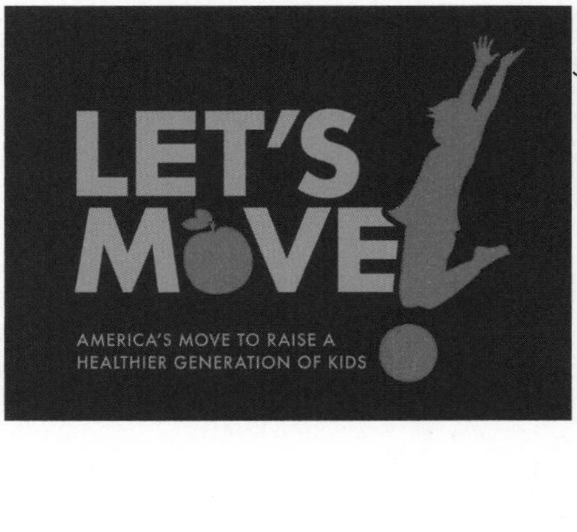

Courtesy of Let's Move!

Going Green

Farmers' Markets

Farmers' markets serve up a fresh harvest for those of us who don't have gardens. Direct from the grower, the produce of farmers' markets supports healthy lifestyles by offering unique varieties of fresh, nutritious food at the peak of flavor. By increasing children's access to fresh fruits and vegetables, these markets promote child health and reduce childhood obesity.

Patrons can redeem Women, Infants, and Children (WIC) and Senior Farmers Market Nutrition Program (SFMNP) vouchers at participating markets, thus providing fresh fruits and vegetables to more than 2.3 million low-income families and more than 835,000 low-income seniors.[a] Many farmers' markets also accept electronic benefit transfer (EBT) cards that accompany the Supplemental Nutrition Assistance Program (formerly known as food stamps). They also donate hundreds of thousands of pounds of unsold, fresh produce to food banks, shelters, and other social service agencies.

Farmers' markets support small family farms and preserve America's rural landscapes. They maintain opportunities for farmers, promote diversity, preserve agricultural land from overdevelopment, and keep farmers farming. Farmers' markets strengthen communities and stimulate local economies by creating jobs, strengthening local economies, reducing the distance food travels, and making local food affordable.

[a] U.S. Department of Agriculture, Food and Nutrition Service. Senior Farmers' Market Nutrition Program. http://www.fns.usda.gov/sfmnp/overview. Accessed January 11, 2016.

problems. Increased blood lead levels are associated with reduced IQ, even at levels less than the CDC's reference value of 5 micrograms per deciliter.[34]

Lead is present in the plumbing of old homes; old paint; house dust in homes with cracked or peeling lead-based paint; and, in some areas, the soil. Children can ingest lead by drinking contaminated water, eating paint chips, or sucking their fingers after playing in or around lead-contaminated house dust or soil. Lead toxicity occurs more frequently in areas of poverty, where lead contamination is more common and where iron-deficiency anemia is present.

Low intakes of iron, calcium, and zinc tend to result in increased lead absorption. Children with an adequate intake of these micronutrients show less incidence of lead toxicity. Therefore, many of the programs established to reduce the incidence of lead toxicity in children also promote good nutrition, with an emphasis on adequate iron, calcium, and zinc consumption.

Vegetarianism in Childhood

Well-planned lactovegetarian, lacto-ovo-vegetarian, and vegan diets can satisfy the nutrient needs of children.[35] Vegetarian children have lower intakes of total fat, saturated fat, and cholesterol, and higher intakes of fruits, vegetables, and fiber. Sources of calcium, iron, zinc, vitamin B_{12}, and vitamin D need to be emphasized, especially for children following vegan diets. For a vegan child, legumes and nuts should be substituted for meats, and calcium- and vitamin B_{12}–fortified soy milk should be substituted for cow's milk. Because of the risks associated with direct sunlight exposure, current AAP guidelines advocate decreasing sunlight exposure,[36] recommending daily intake of 400 IU of vitamin D per day for all infants beginning in the first few days of life. Children and adolescents who do not get regular sunlight exposure or drink at least 32 ounces of vitamin D–fortified milk each day should take supplemental vitamin D daily.[37]

Key Concepts Hunger and malnutrition affect a significant number of our nation's children. To combat the growing number of hungry children, programs such as WIC, SNAP, and the National School Breakfast and Lunch Programs are vital. Other concerns common to childhood include overweight, lead toxicity, and chronic disease prevention. Infants and toddlers should not be given low-fat, high-fiber diets; when children reach the age of 2, caregivers should begin to adjust children's diets to follow appropriate dietary guidelines. For vegetarian children, dietary sources of calcium, iron, zinc, vitamin D, and vitamin B_{12} require special attention.

Adolescence

Adolescents seem to add inches overnight. Many caregivers complain that they cannot keep enough food in the house to satisfy an adolescent's appetite. Adolescence commonly is defined as the time between the onset of **puberty** and adulthood. This maturation process involves both physical growth and emotional maturation.

Physical Growth and Development

Hormones drive growth, which varies from child to child. In general, growth spurts begin between ages 10 and 12 for girls and between ages 12 and 14 for boys.[38] This spurt, or period of maximal growth, lasts about two years.

Height

The first phase of adolescent growth is linear. On average, boys grow 8 inches and girls grow 6 inches during puberty. This growth is uneven. The hands and feet enlarge first. The calves and forearms lengthen next, followed by expansion of the hips, chest, shoulders, and trunk. As a result, adolescents often appear awkward or clumsy. After the main growth spurt, growth continues for two to three years, but at a much slower rate.

For girls, peak growth occurs about one year before **menarche**, the onset of menstruation. A typical girl has achieved about 95 percent of her adult height by menarche and grows only 2 to 4 inches during the remainder of adolescence. Growth rates are closely related to sexual maturation, reflected in breast development (girls), change of voice (boys), development of sexual organs, and growth of pubic hair. When the growth plates at the ends of the long bones (**epiphyses**) close, skeletal growth is complete. This is a critical point in development. An adolescent who is malnourished and of small stature at the point of epiphyseal closure may not achieve his or her full potential height.

Weight

The second growth phase of adolescence involves lateral growth. Here, the adolescent "fills out," or gains weight. External factors such as diet and exercise affect weight gain more than linear growth, so weight gain can vary widely among adolescents. However, a typical healthy girl will gain 35 pounds during adolescence; a typical boy will gain 45 pounds. In our weight-sensitive society, adolescents should be prepared for this normal, expected weight gain. Although the bulk of an adolescent's lateral growth occurs after the linear growth spurt, a significant portion of the two growth stages overlap. For girls, for example, peak weight gain usually occurs around the time of menarche.

Body Composition

Before puberty, the body composition of boys and girls does not differ greatly. This changes dramatically during adolescence. Boys experience greater increases in lean body mass, resulting in more obvious muscle definition. Girls accumulate greater stores of body fat, specifically around the hips and buttocks, upper arms, breasts, and upper back.

Overweight in Children

American Heart Association suggests **that** overweight children are more likely to be overweight adults. Successfully preventing or treating overweight in childhood may reduce the risk of adult overweight. This may help reduce the risk of heart disease and other diseases.

Reproduced from American Heart Association, Inc.

Quick Bite

Are Minority Children at High Risk for Cardiovascular Disease?

Early risk factors for cardiovascular disease are increasing in the United States. African American and Mexican American children are more likely to exhibit high blood pressure and high body mass index and to consume a higher percentage of calories from fat than are Caucasian children. The three ethnic groups have similar blood cholesterol levels, however, and Caucasian children are more likely to smoke.

▶ **puberty** The period of life during which the secondary sex characteristics develop and the ability to reproduce is attained.

▶ **menarche** First menstrual period.

▶ **epiphyses** The heads of the long bones that are separated from the shaft of the bone until the bone stops growing.

Dietary Guidelines for Americans, 2015–2020

Key Recommendations

Balancing Calories to Manage Weight

- Maintain appropriate calorie balance during each stage of life—childhood, adolescence, adulthood, pregnancy and breastfeeding, and older age.

Reproduced from U.S. Department of Agriculture and U.S. Department of Health and Human Services. *Dietary Guidelines for Americans, 2015–2020.* 8th ed. Washington, DC: US Government Printing Office; December 2015.

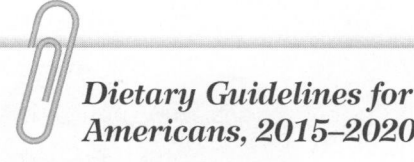

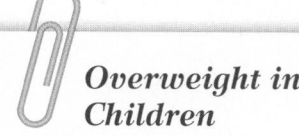

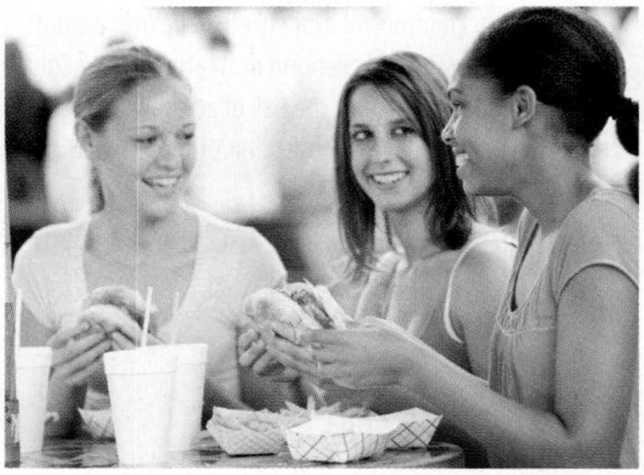

© iStockphoto/Thinkstock

TABLE 17.5
Estimated Energy Requirement Equations for Adolescence (Ages 9 Through 18)

Males
$EER = 88.5 - 61.9 \times age\ [y] + PA \times (26.7 \times weight\ [kg] + 903 \times height\ [m]) + 25$ kcal/day
Physical activity (PA): Sedentary = 1.00; Low active = 1.13; Active = 1.26; Very active = 1.42
Females
$EER = 135.3 - 30.8 \times age\ [y] + PA \times (10.0 \times weight\ [kg] + 934 \times height\ [m]) + 25$ kcal/day
Physical activity (PA): Sedentary = 1.00; Low active = 1.16; Active = 1.31; Very active = 1.56

Reproduced from Institute of Medicine, Food and Nutrition Board. *Dietary Reference Intakes for Energy, Carbohydrate, Fiber, Fat, Fatty Acids, Cholesterol, Protein, and Amino Acids (Macronutrients).* Copyright © 2005 by the National Academy of Sciences, courtesy of the National Academies Press, Washington, DC.

TABLE 17.6
Protein RDAs for Adolescence

Age (y)	Protein (g/kg)	Reference Weight[a] (kg)	Protein (g/d)
14–18, female	0.85	54	46
14–18, male	0.85	61	52

[a] Reference weights are based on median weights for that sex and age group.

Reproduced from Institute of Medicine, Food and Nutrition Board. *Dietary Reference Intakes for Energy, Carbohydrate, Fiber, Fat, Fatty Acids, Cholesterol, Protein, and Amino Acids (Macronutrients).* Copyright © 2005 by the National Academy of Sciences, courtesy of the National Academies Press, Washington, DC.

Emotional Maturity: Developmental Tasks

Adolescence is a time not only of great physical growth, but also of tremendous emotional growth. This psychological development affects food choices, eating habits, and body image. Many teens become more interested in the healthful aspects of nutrition. Others experiment with unhealthful food choices, as an exercise in independence or in an attempt to achieve an idealized body.

Nutrient Needs of Adolescents

Although growth, not age, should be the ultimate indicator of nutrient needs, Daily Reference Intakes (DRIs) are established based on age. Separate recommendations for males and females reflect the differences in growth rates and body composition during adolescence.

Energy and Protein

Energy needs, as total kilocalories per day, are greater during adolescence than at any other time of life, with the exception of pregnancy and lactation. Equations used to calculate Estimated Energy Requirements (EERs) are the same as for children, except for the added energy factor for growth, which is higher for adolescents (see **TABLE 17.5**). Recommended energy intakes are guidelines only; adjustments often are needed to meet individual requirements.

To support growth, an adolescent's protein needs per unit body weight are higher than an adult's but less than a rapidly growing infant's (see **TABLE 17.6**). By age 14 to 18, the protein RDA has declined nearly to adult levels (as g/kg body weight), reflecting the end of linear growth for most teens. American teens rarely have a problem with adequate protein intake, but teen girls risk a lack of protein if they cut calories too drastically in attempts to control weight.

Vitamins and Minerals

Along with increased needs for energy and protein, adolescents have higher vitamin and mineral needs compared with people at most other life stages. Nutrients of particular concern for adolescents are vitamin A, vitamin D, calcium, and iron, each of which plays an important role in growth and development (see **FIGURE 17.5**).

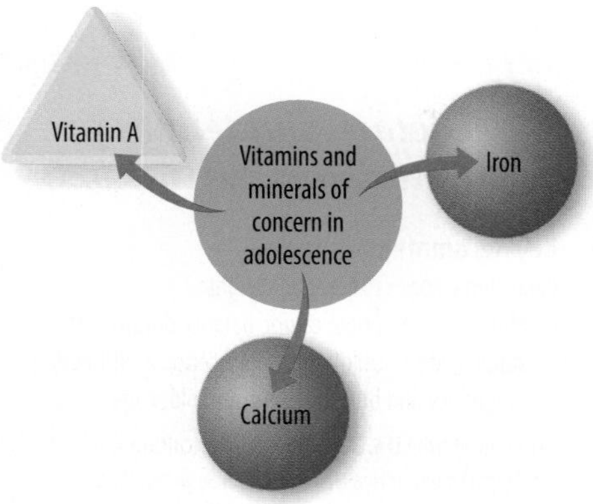

FIGURE 17.5 Micronutrients of concern in adolescence. Vitamin A is important for growth, and calcium and vitamin D are essential for building strong bones. Teen girls especially need adequate iron intake to replace iron lost during menstruation.

Teens can improve their vitamin A intake by including more fruits and vegetables in their diets. Adequate calcium and vitamin D are essential for bone formation, and maximal bone density can be hard to obtain if diets are deficient in these nutrients. Many teens, especially girls, actually reduce their calcium and vitamin D intake by replacing the milk in their diets with soft drinks. During puberty, adolescents gain 15 percent of their full adult height and accumulate half of their ultimate adult bone mass. Adolescents who do not achieve sufficient bone density have a greater risk of developing osteoporosis later in life. The RDA for calcium for adolescents aged 9 to 18 years is 1,300 milligrams per day, and the RDA for vitamin D is 600 IU every day.[39] Fortified milk and dairy products are rich in these nutrients and convenient to eat; without these or other fortified products, meeting the recommended intake is difficult.

Adolescent boys need added iron to support growth of muscle and lean body mass. Teenage girls need added iron to replace what is lost in blood during menstruation. The recommended iron intake for boys aged 14 to 18 years is 11 milligrams per day; for teen girls, it is 15 milligrams per day. As long as they take in enough calories, both groups should be able to obtain this iron from nutrient-dense foods. During adolescence, however, food selection often is less than optimal. Careful meal planning is required to maximize teenagers' iron consumption.

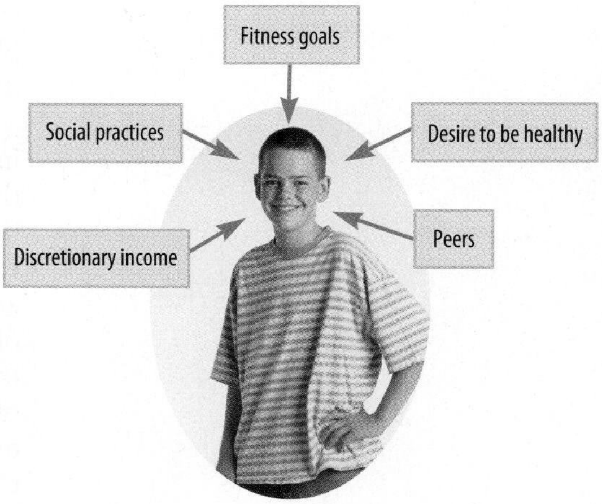

FIGURE 17.6 Factors that influence adolescent food choices. Social, cultural, and psychological factors, especially peer pressure, strongly influence adolescent food choices.

Photo © Patrick Foto/ShutterStock, Inc.

Influences on Adolescent Food Intake

Teenagers want and need to make their own food choices and purchases and may want to take over preparation of their own food. Although the parent can set a good example, parental influence is much weaker now. Factors that influence an adolescent's food selection and consumption include the desire to be healthy, fitness goals, amount of discretionary income, social practices, and peers (see **FIGURE 17.6**).

Teens have more access to foods than children. They also usually have their own money and may have access to independent transportation. Along with this increased freedom comes greater spending power. Teens enjoy spending money on food and making their own selections. The food industry responds accordingly by marketing directly to teens. The message is enjoyment and pleasure, and advertised products may not be nutritionally adequate.

Teens perceive benefits to eating healthful foods, such as enhanced physical and mental performance, increased energy, and psychological well-being. However, while at school, teens are faced with more food choices than ever before. In addition to the standard school lunch or breakfast program outlined earlier, most middle schools and high schools have vending machines, snack carts, school stores, or even private vendors supplying foods for cafeteria meals. Vending and other food sales can be a major source of revenue for many schools, supporting athletic programs and other after-school activities. Although healthier choices may be available, the strongest risk factor for eating unhealthy snacks and beverages is simply the proximity of vending machines in schools.[40] More than half of middle and high schools in the United States offer sugary drinks and less healthy foods for their students to purchase.[41-43] Sugar-sweetened beverages (SSBs) are the largest source of added sugars in the diets of children and adolescents in the United States. The increased caloric intake resulting from SSBs is a leading dietary contributor to the prevalence of obesity among adolescents.[44]

Health professionals and others have expressed concern about the presence of low-nutrient-density "competitive" foods (e.g., snacks and soft drinks sold side-by-side with school lunches), and many states have pursued legislation to either remove vending machines or change the products available during the school day. The Healthy Hunger-Free Kids Act of 2010 gives the USDA authority to establish national nutrition standards for all food and beverages sold and served in schools at any time during the school day.[44-46]

However, despite efforts to provide healthier options in schools, vending machines continue to offer foods and beverages that are high in fat, sugar, and

> ### *American Heart Association*
>
> **Fiber and Children's Diets**
>
> Children older than 2 years should gradually adopt American Heart Association dietary recommendations. That means saturated fat intake should be less than 7 percent of total calories, trans fat intake should be less than 1 percent of total calories, and dietary cholesterol should be limited to no more than 300 milligrams daily. Children also should get the majority of calories from complex carbohydrates high in fiber. Both children and adults should consume 14 grams of fiber per 1,000 calories consumed. Read the Nutrition Facts panel on the food label to determine how much fiber is in the food you are choosing.
>
> Based on www.heart.org, © 2013 American Heart Association, Inc.

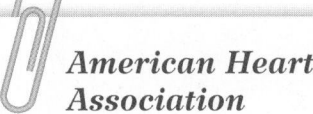

calories with minimal nutritional value.[47] The most frequently consumed competitive products are foods and beverages that are low in nutrients and energy dense, consumed by more than 40 percent of children daily while at school.[48]

Vending machines are widely available in U.S. schools, placing schools in a unique position to influence the diet of their students.[49] Consistent with the recommendation of the 2015 *Dietary Guidelines for Americans* to reduce the intake of calories from solid fats and added sugars, the American Academy of Pediatrics states that routine ingestion of sports drinks by children and adolescents should be avoided or restricted.[50] To reduce consumption of SSBs, the CDC is encouraging schools to improve access to free drinking water and to implement other strategies to reduce student consumption of SSBs through changes in school policies.[51] Also necessary is the involvement of families, media, and other institutions that interact with adolescents to discourage their consumption of SSBs and increase their awareness of the potential detrimental health effects of a poor diet.[52]

Key Concepts Humans need more calories and nutrients during adolescence than at any other stage of life, with the exception of pregnancy and lactation. During this stage, boys grow about 8 inches, gain about 45 pounds, and increase their lean body mass. Girls grow about 6 inches, gain about 35 pounds, and increase their body fat. As at earlier ages, calcium, vitamin D, iron, and vitamin A are often lacking in adolescent diets. Factors that determine food selection and consumption include the desire to be healthy, fitness goals, amount of discretionary income, social practices, and peers.

Nutrition-Related Concerns for Adolescents

Adolescents are often preoccupied with weight, appearance, and eating habits. They need to know whether and how their eating practices can affect body image and development, fitness, acne, and obesity.

Fitness and Sports

For many adolescents, an interest in fitness becomes the catalyst for learning about nutrition and improving dietary habits. Some teens, unfortunately, become obsessed with their athletic performance, food intake, and body appearance and go to extremes that can jeopardize not only their current athletic performance, but also their long-term health.

Acne

▶ **acne** An inflammatory skin eruption that usually occurs in or near the sebaceous glands of the face, neck, shoulders, and upper back.

Many teens blame certain foods for their **acne**. Myths surrounding acne and diet abound, but research has not found any correlation between acne and chocolate, greasy foods, soft drinks, nuts, or milk. Nevertheless, differences in acne incidence between Westernized and non-Westernized societies are striking, and researchers are investigating the connections between diets and acne.[53,54] Specifically, dietary components such as dairy products, high-glycemic-index foods, fat intake, and fatty acid composition have recently been investigated as contributors to acne.[55] Preliminary research suggests that a low-glycemic-load diet can be helpful, but further controlled testing is needed before specific recommendations can be made.[56] THINK About It 2

Effective treatments for acne include topical benzoyl peroxide, low-dose oral antibiotics, and two medications derived from vitamin A—Retin-A and Accutane. Although both of these medications are derivatives of vitamin A, there is no correlation between dietary vitamin A and acne.

Eating Disorders

Eating disorders frequently begin during adolescence. Adolescents often become preoccupied with their weight, appearance, and eating habits.

Although eating disorders are still found more often in girls than in boys, the prevalence in males is increasing. Thus, eating disorders shouldn't be ignored or dismissed as only a "girl's problem."

Adolescent Obesity

As in childhood, obesity rates in adolescence are climbing. One contributing factor is a decline in physical activity by many teens.[57] Obese adolescents have an increased risk of developing high blood pressure, abnormal glucose tolerance and type 2 diabetes, breathing problems, joint pain, and heartburn.[58] They also suffer psychologically with poor self-esteem from teasing, being ostracized by peers, and longing to be slimmer. In addition, adolescent obesity sets the stage for adult obesity, with all its attendant health consequences.[59] Finally, overweight adolescents who spend on average 7.5 hours daily watching television or using other forms of entertainment media could be otherwise spending some of this time being physically active.[60] Nutrition education can positively influence the knowledge, attitudes, and eating behaviors of high school students, leading to a healthier lifestyle and reducing their risk of becoming overweight.[61] See **TABLE 17.7** for factors that put an adolescent at risk for obesity.

TABLE 17.7
Risk Factors for Obesity in Adolescents

- Genetics
- Extent and duration of breastfeeding
- Early menarche
- Participation in high-risk behaviors such as smoking, alcohol use, and sexual experimentation
- Family and parental dynamics
- Food insecurity
- Socioeconomic status
- Lack of safe place for physical activity
- Inconsistent access to healthful food choices
- Low cognitive stimulation at home
- Parental food choices
- Parental food-related behaviors
- Lack of regular family meals
- Low level of physical activity—leisure time activities and activities of daily living, school physical activity programs
- Television, computer, and video games

Data from American Academy of Pediatrics. Prevention of pediatric overweight and obesity. *Pediatrics.* 2003;112(2):424–430.

Tobacco, Alcohol, and Recreational Drugs

Developmentally, adolescence is a period of experimentation, and many adolescents experiment with smoking and/or prescription or illegal drugs. Although survey results from 2010 show a continuing decline in alcohol use and binge drinking among teenagers, alcohol use remains widespread in this group.[62] Marijuana use, along with use of tobacco, illicit drugs, and the nonmedical use of prescription medications, continues to be high.[63] Nearly one-fourth of high school seniors graduate as users of tobacco products. An adolescent who smokes tobacco often has a lower energy intake and subsequently decreased nutrient intake. Although the use of cigarettes declined among middle and high school students between 2011 and 2014, there was no decline in overall tobacco use in this period, in part due to a rise in the use of electronic cigarettes. Between 2013 and 2014 alone, e-cigarette use more than tripled among middle and high school students, increasing from 4.5 percent to 13.4 percent. With 2 million American students now using e-cigarettes, 2014 marked the first year in which e-cigarette use surpassed the use of every other tobacco product, including conventional cigarettes.[64] Studies have not yet reported consistent results on the potential risks they carry.

Marijuana has the opposite effect on hunger. Many teens who smoke marijuana experience "the munchies," a desire to snack and munch—usually on snacks high in calories but with low nutrient density. Smoking marijuana carries the same risks as smoking tobacco. In addition, marijuana sometimes is laced with other drugs, including LSD and amphetamines.

Almost all the alcohol consumed by those younger than the age of 21 occurs during binge drinking—more than five drinks within two hours for men and four drinks within two hours for women. Through violence and accidental injury, adolescents who drink alcohol are at increased risk of harming themselves or others.[65] In addition, teens who drink are replacing needed nutrients with empty alcohol calories. Finally, alcohol can interfere with the absorption and metabolism of necessary nutrients. Growing adolescents cannot afford to have nutrients replaced or poorly absorbed during growth.

Other drugs, such as cocaine, pose further risks. In using illegal drugs, the adolescent becomes preoccupied with both the acquisition and use of the drug; these activities take priority over food intake or selection. Teens who use drugs are usually underweight and report poor appetites.

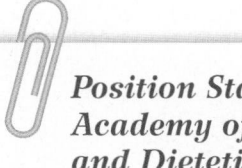

Position Statement: Academy of Nutrition and Dietetics

Child and Adolescent Nutrition Assistance Programs

It is the position of the Academy of Nutrition and Dietetics that children and adolescents should have access to an adequate supply of healthful and safe foods that promote optimal physical, cognitive, and social growth and development. Nutrition assistance programs, such as food assistance and meal service programs and nutrition education initiatives, play a vital role in meeting this critical need.

Reproduced from Stang J, Bayerl CT. Position of the American Dietetic Association: child and adolescent nutrition assistance programs. *J Am Diet Assoc.* 2010;110:791–799.

Quick Bite

The Dangers of Teenage Smoking

The CDC estimates that more than 3 million adolescents smoke regularly. Each day, more than 3,800 young people try a cigarette for the first time, and more than 2,000 become regular smokers. The CDC predicts that if smoking continues at the current rate among U.S. youth, 5.6 million of today's Americans younger than 18 years of age will die prematurely from a smoking-related illness. Research shows that the earlier a person begins to smoke, the greater the damage.

Quick Bite

Longevity Champions

In the United States, women live an average of five years longer than men.

Key Concepts Adolescence can be an uncomfortable time for the teen who is concerned with body image, body changes, or athletic activities. Although many teens blame certain foods for their acne, research has not found a definite correlation between acne and diet. Many adolescents are preoccupied with their weight, appearance, and eating habits. Adolescent obesity is on the rise, and eating disorders frequently begin during adolescence. Use of tobacco, alcohol, or recreational drugs can influence nutrient intake and interfere with good nutrition.

Staying Young While Growing Older

Just when does old age begin? The answer is increasingly elusive, as more people remain healthy and active well into their seventies, eighties, and even nineties. Today, older adults represent the fastest-growing segment of the U.S. population; in 2013, the percentage of the older population (Americans age 65 years and older) had more than tripled since 1900, from 4.1 percent to 14.1 percent of the U.S. population.[66] (See **FIGURE 17.7**.) The baby boomers started turning 65 in 2011, and experts estimate that by 2030 approximately 72.1 million Americans will be older than 65 years. During the current decade, the population aged 85 and older is projected to increase almost 20 percent, from 5.5 million in 2010 to 6.6 million by 2020.[67]

Age-related changes in body composition, sensory abilities, organ systems, and immune function are normal (see **FIGURE 17.8**). We age at different rates, and many age-related declines will have little impact on our day-to-day lives. Other changes affect our nutrient needs and nutrient status (see **TABLE 17.8**), so it becomes especially important to eat nutrient-dense food.

As we get older, many of us fear loss of mental function even more than loss of physical function. Yet, as the years advance, most people maintain cognitive function with only subtle changes. Staying physically and mentally active is a key factor in maintaining function and independence. In most cases, slight changes involving sensory acuity, secondary memory, and information-processing speed do not affect quality of life or lead to progressive or rapid declines in mental function. However, when depression or dementia is suspected, professional evaluation becomes necessary. Overmedication or drug interactions, rather than disease, could be responsible for the changes in behavior.

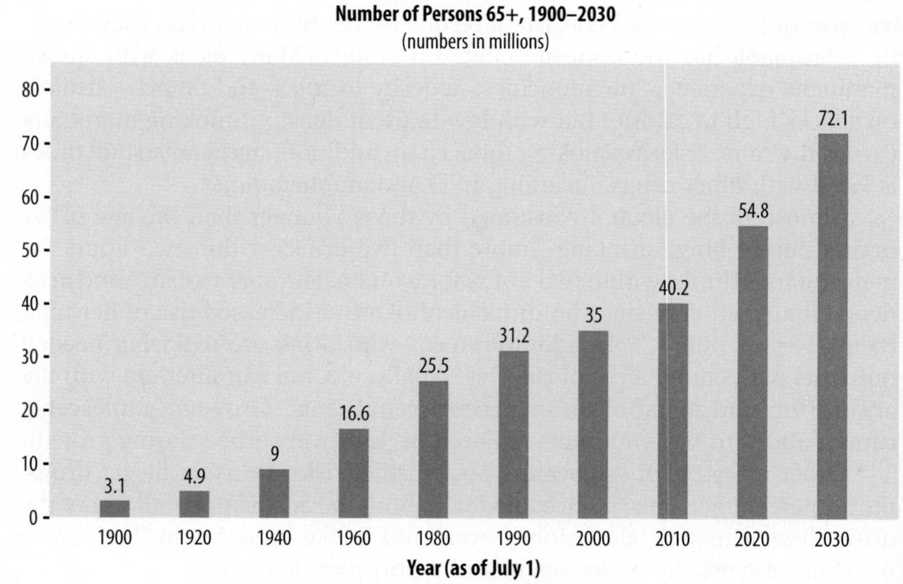

FIGURE 17.7 The aging U.S. population. The number of people older than age 65 is growing rapidly.

Reproduced from Administration on Aging. A Profile of Older Americans, 2010 future growth. http://www.aoa.gov/aoaroot/aging_statistics/Profile/2010/4.aspx. Accessed August 8, 2011.

Although it is not possible to stop the aging process, we can control aspects of our lifestyle that contribute to a healthier old age. Many of our choices—food, exercise, smoking, and alcohol—affect not only our risk for chronic disease, but also the rate at which we age. Nutrition is a key factor in promoting health and ability to function at advanced ages and plays a role in medical nutrition therapy for disease management.[68] Eating is not only a necessity of everyday life, but also an important pleasure and social component at every age.

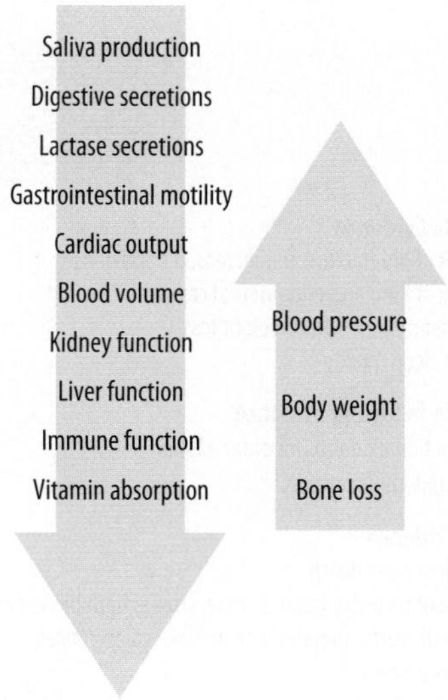

FIGURE 17.8 Age-related physiological changes. As we age, most physiological changes emerge gradually.

Weight and Body Composition

Poor food choices and too many calories combined with a sedentary lifestyle have resulted in a growing number of overweight and obese older adults.[69] Older people who are overweight or who gain weight with age have an increased risk of chronic diseases such as heart disease, diabetes, metabolic syndrome, and cancer.[70] In addition, many older adults who have an increase in body fat and loss of muscle mass decline physically and are unable to function independently in their normal activities of daily living.

In contrast, people who enter their mature years on the lean side—and who remain lean as a result of a healthy, active lifestyle—increase their chances of enjoying a healthy old age. But thinness alone is not always a health advantage. Obviously, older adults who lose weight because of illness enjoy no health benefits from losing these pounds. Weight loss puts them at increased risk for further illness, including cardiovascular disease and osteoporosis—especially if the original illness also limits activity. And, of course, leanness caused by tobacco use or alcoholism increases a person's vulnerability to a decline in health.

THINK About It 3

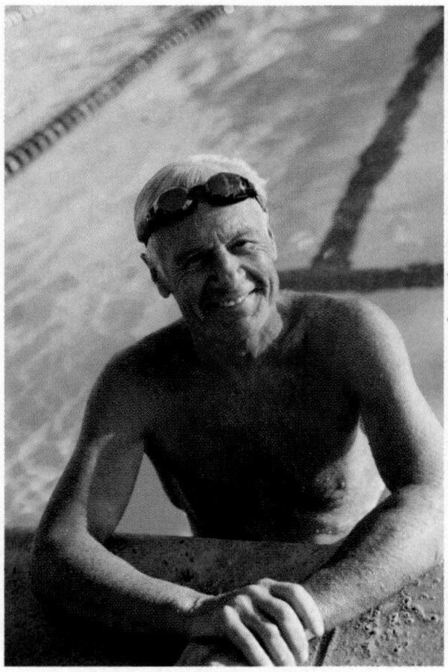

Physical Activity

Lean body mass (muscle mass) and strength are commonly observed to decline with age. However, this decline might not be a simple physiological consequence of aging. Decreases in physical activity that accompany age contribute to loss of lean mass and muscle strength, a condition called sarcopenia.[71] Sarcopenia contributes to functional disability and loss of independence.

TABLE 17.8
Age-Related Changes and Nutrient Needs

Change in Body Composition or Physiologic Function	Impact on Nutrient Requirement
Decreased muscle mass	Decreased need for energy Increased need for high-quality protein
Decreased bone density	Increased need for calcium and vitamin D
Decreased immune function	Increased need for vitamin B_6, antioxidants, vitamin E, zinc, and high-quality protein
Increased gastric pH	Increased need for vitamin B_{12}, folic acid, calcium, iron, and zinc
Decreased skin capacity for cholecalciferol synthesis	Increased need for vitamin D
Decreased kidney ability to concentrate urine, constipation, and reduced thirst sensation	Increased fluid needs
Increased oxidative stress, cognitive impairment, cataracts, and age-related macular degeneration	Increased need for antioxidants such as beta-carotene, vitamin C, and vitamin E
Slowed gastric motility	Increased need for fiber

Our posture begins deteriorating in our fifties—a result of bad habits, bone loss, and a decrease in muscle tone. Poor posture can affect lung and cardiovascular function, mobility, and balance. Diseases such as stroke, heart disease, arthritis, and diabetes become more common and can cause severe physical disability. These conditions, however, do not automatically preclude older adults from participating in physical activity with qualified supervision. In fact, they might instead provide additional justification for appropriate exercises for the older adult.[72] Medications and nutritional deficiencies can lead to impaired motor function; therefore, older adults should be evaluated by their physician prior to beginning a new exercise program.

Although physical activity cannot stop biological aging, regular exercise can help to minimize the physiological effects of a sedentary lifestyle and limit the progression of disabling conditions and chronic diseases.[73] The U.S. Department of Health and Human Services' 2008 *Physical Activity Guidelines for Americans* states that "regular physical activity is essential for healthy aging" and that all adults should avoid inactivity.[74] These recommendations for physical activity for older adults are included in the 2015 *Dietary Guidelines for Americans.* Canada also addresses this issue in its *Physical Activity Guide for Older Adults*. The benefits of an individualized exercise prescription designed to increase physical activity that includes aerobic activities, flexibility exercises, and progressive resistance strength training can be most profound for those who are aging. Increased self-confidence, better balance and mobility, fewer falls and fractures, enhanced mental acuity, and improved appetite and nutrient intake are but a few of the physical and psychological benefits of exercise during our older years. The bottom line is that all adults should avoid inactive lifestyles and regularly engage in various forms of physical activity.[75] (See **FIGURE 17.9** and **TABLE 17.9**.)

Moderate Evidence
Lower risk of hip fracture and increased bone density
Lower risk of lung and endometrial cancers
Weight maintenance after weight loss
Improved sleep quality

Moderate to Strong Evidence
Better functional health (for older adults)
Reduced abdominal obesity

Strong Evidence
Lower risk of early death
Lower risk of coronary heart disease, stroke, high blood pressure, type 2 diabetes, metabolic syndrome, colon cancer, and breast cancer
Prevention of weight gain
Weight loss, particularly when combined with reduced calorie intake
Improved cardiorespiratory and muscular fitness
Prevention of falls
Reduced depression
Better cognitive function (for older adults)

FIGURE 17.9 The health benefits associated with regular physical activity for adults and older adults.
Physical activity helps adults maintain their health and independence as they age.

Note: The Advisory Committee rated the evidence of health benefits of physical activity as strong, moderate, or weak. To do so, the committee considered the type, number, and quality of studies available, as well as consistency of findings across studies that addressed each outcome. The committee also considered evidence for causality and dose response in assigning the strength-of-evidence rating.

Modified from U.S. Department of Health and Human Services. 2008 Physical Activity Guidelines for Americans. ODPHP Publication No. U0036. Washington, DC: U.S. Department of Health and Human Services; 2008. http://www.health.gov/paguidelines/guidelines/chapter2.aspx. Accessed 8/8/11.

TABLE 17.9
2008 *Physical Activity Guidelines for Americans*: Key Guidelines for Adults and Older Adults

The following guidelines are the same for adults and older adults:

- All older adults should avoid inactivity. Some physical activity is better than none, and older adults who participate in any amount of physical activity gain some health benefits.
- For substantial health benefits, older adults should do at least 150 minutes (2 hours and 30 minutes) a week of moderate-intensity, or 75 minutes (1 hour and 15 minutes) a week of vigorous-intensity aerobic physical activity, or an equivalent combination of moderate- and vigorous-intensity aerobic activity. Aerobic activity should be performed in episodes of at least 10 minutes, and preferably, it should be spread throughout the week.
- For additional and more extensive health benefits, older adults should increase their aerobic physical activity to 300 minutes (5 hours) a week of moderate-intensity, or 150 minutes a week of vigorous-intensity aerobic physical activity, or an equivalent combination of moderate- and vigorous-intensity activity. Additional health benefits are gained by engaging in physical activity beyond this amount.
- Older adults should also do muscle-strengthening activities that are moderate or high intensity and involve all major muscle groups two or more days a week, as these activities provide additional health benefits.

The following guidelines are just for older adults:

- When older adults cannot do 150 minutes of moderate-intensity aerobic activity a week because of chronic conditions, they should be as physically active as their abilities and conditions allow.
- Older adults should do exercises that maintain or improve balance if they are at risk of falling.
- Older adults should determine their level of effort for physical activity relative to their level of fitness.
- Older adults with chronic conditions should understand whether and how their conditions affect their ability to do regular physical activity safely.

Reproduced from U.S. Department of Health and Human Services. *2008 Physical Activity Guidelines for Americans.* Chapter 5: active older adults. http://www.health.gov/paguidelines/guidelines/chapter5.aspx. Accessed January 11, 2016.

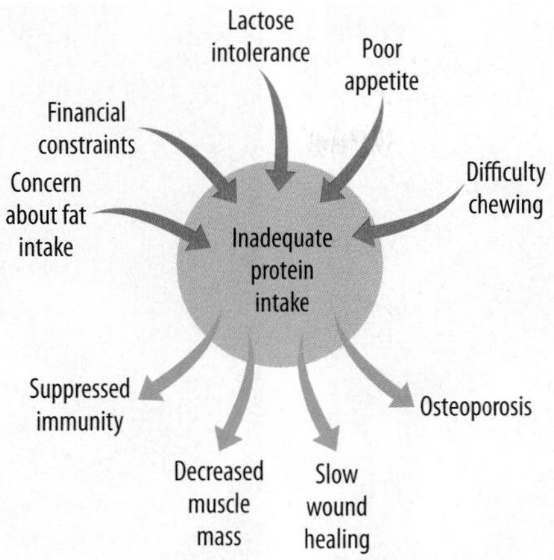

FIGURE 17.10 Protein malnutrition in older adults. A combination of several factors can lead to inadequate protein intake that compromises immunity and health.

Immunity

In the fifth decade of life, the body's defense mechanisms begin to weaken. The immune system loses some of its ability to fight viruses, bacteria, and other foreign bodies. Older adults are more vulnerable to upper respiratory tract infections such as influenza, pneumonia, **urinary tract infections (UTIs)**, pressure sores, and foodborne illnesses. Physical barriers to infectious agents, foreign bodies, and chemicals weaken as well. These barriers include the skin, the acid environment in the stomach, and the swallowing and coughing reflexes.

▶ **urinary tract infection (UTI)** An infection of one or more of the structures in the urinary tract; usually caused by bacteria.

Inadequate consumption of protein and some antioxidant nutrients can compromise immunity and health in older adults. Because of poor appetite, difficulty chewing, financial constraints, concerns about fat intake, or lactose intolerance, older adults might reduce their intake of meat, dairy products, and fresh fruits and vegetables, making it difficult for them to get all the calories, protein, and other essential nutrients they need (see **FIGURE 17.10**). Poor dietary intake can lead to suppressed immunity, decreased muscle mass, slowed wound healing, and osteoporosis.

Key Concepts Lifestyle choices, such as diet and exercise, affect how we age. Control of body weight can reduce our risk for many chronic diseases associated with aging. Adequate nutrient intake can protect our immune status. Regular physical activity not only helps us to maintain the ability to function in daily activities and enables our independence, but also reduces disease risk and overall well-being.

Taste and Smell

In older adults, the **taste threshold**—the minimum amount of a flavor that must be present to detect the taste—is more than double that of college-aged adults. Sensitivity to sweet and salty tastes goes first, so older adults often increase their intake of foods high in sugar and sodium—increasing health problems that stem from overconsumption of these nutrients. Along with taste, our sense of smell diminishes with age, especially in the seventh decade of life (60 to 70 years old) and beyond. Medication use also can alter taste and flavor perception. The idea that older adults should be served bland foods is misguided. Intensifying flavors and aromas of food and varying temperature and textures are strategies older adults can use to compensate for the diminished taste and smell of foods (see **FIGURE 17.11**).

▶ **taste threshold** The minimum amount of flavor that must be present for a taste to be detected.

Gastrointestinal Changes

Saliva production tends to decrease as we age, especially in people who take medications for conditions such as congestive heart failure. Lack of saliva

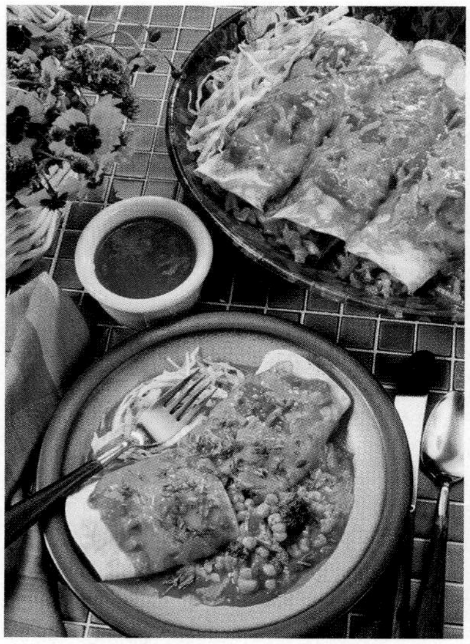
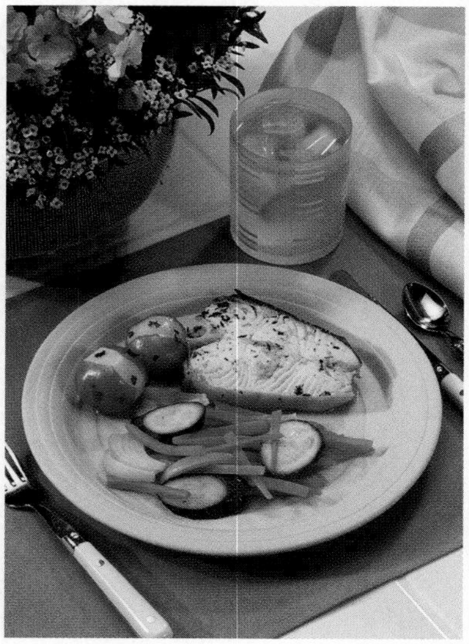

FIGURE 17.11 Older adults need stronger flavors. More highly spiced meals rather than bland ones can encourage an older adult to eat more.

© Photodisc

© Photodisc

affects the preparation of food for digestion and contributes to gum disease—a breach in one of the immune system's first lines of defense against infection.

With age, digestive secretions decline. Most significant are reductions in the stomach secretions of hydrochloric acid and pepsin. These reductions can allow the development of atrophic gastritis—a chronic inflammation of the stomach lining that is common among older adults. Atrophic gastritis can interfere with normal absorption of vitamin B_{12}, leading to a deficiency of this vitamin.[76] Although reduced lactase production also is associated with aging, a complete intolerance to milk and dairy products is less common than older adults often suspect. Most people with reduced lactase production can include some milk, cheese, and yogurt in their diets.

Constipation, gas, and bloating are common complaints of old age. These problems are caused by a slowing of gastrointestinal motility with age, along with decreased physical activity, a diet low in fiber, and low fluid intake. Feelings of fullness can cause older adults to eat less. Reduced digestive secretions lower the amount of nutrients older adults absorb from the foods they do eat. Myths and misinformation about the gastrointestinal (GI) effects of various foods, even among the medical community, can steer a person away from nutrient-dense foods such as dairy products, legumes, broccoli, cauliflower, tomatoes, and citrus products. Although many older adults mistakenly blame these foods for causing problems with gas, others may be sensitive to lactose in dairy products or may have had an adverse reaction to members of the cabbage family or "acid"-containing foods. GI distress also can be caused by factors totally unrelated to the food itself—inappropriate food preparation, lack of adequate fluid, and physical inactivity. Regardless of the cause, once people have an adverse reaction, they may associate it with a recently consumed food and become reluctant to try it again.

Key Concepts The perception of taste declines with age. To detect flavors, older adults often need food with stronger flavors and odors. This loss of taste can contribute to loss of appetite and poor food intake. Age-related changes in the GI tract reduce nutrient absorption. Decreased motility contributes to constipation.

Nutrient Needs of the Mature Adult

At any age, to live life to its fullest, you need good nutrition. A lifestyle that incorporates the *Dietary Guidelines for Americans* and MyPlate eating plan, together with regular physical activity, is essential to a long and productive

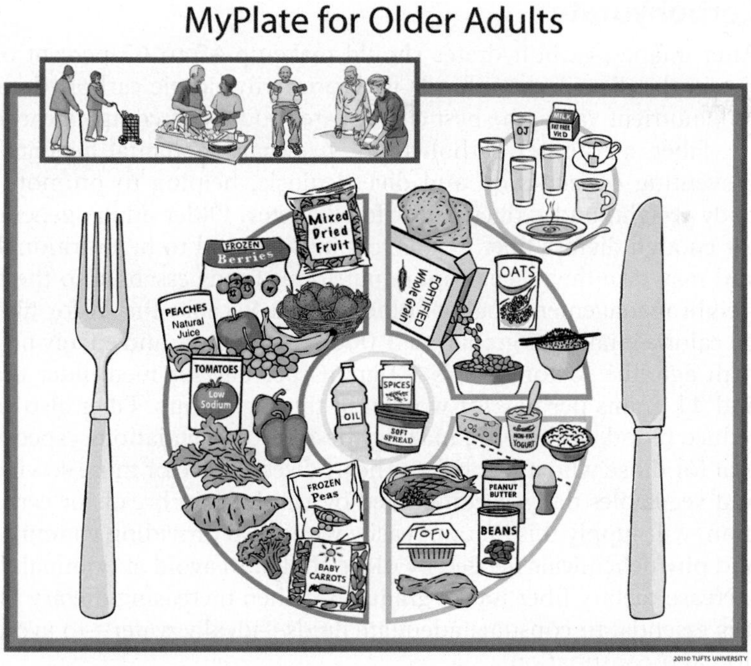

FIGURE 17.12 MyPlate for older adults.

© 2011 Tufts University. For details about the MyPlate for Older Adults, please see http://nutrition.tufts.edu/research/myplate-older-adults.

life. **FIGURE 17.12** shows how MyPlate has been adapted to illustrate the nutritional concerns of older adults.

Energy

Mainly because of reduced physical activity and loss of lean body mass, our energy requirements decline as we age. In other words, a 60-year-old man will need to increase his physical activity and/or decrease his caloric intake to maintain his weight as he ages. Physical activity increases energy requirements while also helping to delay some of the loss in lean mass, thus allowing us to eat more without gaining weight and increasing the likelihood that our diets will be adequate in essential nutrients.

The EER equations are the same for older adults as for younger adults. Individual energy needs depend on activity, lean body mass, and the presence of disease; a person who is bed- or chair-ridden, for example, usually requires fewer calories than a mobile person.

Quick Bite

Losing Water

At birth, 75 percent of the body is composed of water. By the time a person reaches old age, that number has dwindled to 50 percent as a result of changes in body composition.

Protein

Protein needs (as grams per kilogram of body weight) can be somewhat harder for us to meet as our overall energy needs decrease and our tastes change. As our caloric needs decrease and our protein needs remain constant, an adequate diet must contain relatively more protein. For healthy older adults, the RDA for protein is 0.8 gram per kilogram of body weight, or on average 46 grams per day for women and 56 grams for men. To meet their protein needs and maximize muscle protein synthesis, older adults should aim to include 25 to 30 grams of high-quality protein with each meal.[77] Eating enough protein can be challenging for older adults, so choosing foods with high-quality protein as recommended by MyPlate throughout the day is a helpful strategy. Chronically ill individuals might need more protein to maintain nitrogen balance. Trauma, stress, and infection also increase protein needs. However, there are risks associated with high protein intake, including dehydration, nitrogen overload, and adverse effects on the kidneys.

Carbohydrate

After infancy, carbohydrates should make up 45 to 65 percent of the calories in the diet. Because foods with primarily simple carbohydrates provide little nutrient value, the best choices are foods with complex carbohydrates.

Fiber, a complex carbohydrate, has many potential benefits, including preventing constipation and diverticulosis, helping to promote a healthy body weight, and reducing risk for diabetes. Older adults generally do not eat enough dietary fiber. Foods low in fiber tend to be nutritionally inferior and may take the place of more nutritious foods essential to the health and weight management goals of older adults. Because the AI for fiber is based on calorie intake (14 grams per 1,000 kcal per day), and energy needs decline with age, the AI for fiber is 30 grams per day for men older than age 50 and 21 grams per day for women in that age group. Fiber also can help to reduce blood cholesterol, making these recommendations especially important for those who are at risk for heart disease. Five or more servings of fruits and vegetables daily, accompanied by whole-grain breads or cereals high in bran, will supply this amount easily while also providing vitamins, minerals, and phytochemicals needed by older adults. To avoid abdominal discomfort, increase dietary fiber intake gradually. When increasing dietary fiber intake, it is essential to consume adequate fluids—ideally water—to avoid dehydration and constipation.

Fat

Excess dietary fat can lead to obesity, which in turn increases the risk for diabetes, heart disease, and some types of cancer. Younger people should limit their dietary cholesterol and fat, but severe restrictions in older adults may be counterproductive. Extreme fat phobia could contribute to nutritional deficiencies among older adults who are afraid to drink milk, eat red meat, or even eat poultry or fish. Too few animal products in the diet can contribute to a lack of dietary protein; deficiency of minerals such as calcium, iron, and zinc; and poor vitamin D and vitamin B_{12} intake.

Healthy people who are at low risk for heart disease should obtain 20 to 35 percent of their daily calories from fat, with no more than 8 to 10 percent of the calories from saturated fat. They should limit their cholesterol intake to 300 milligrams per day. People at increased risk for heart disease should limit saturated fat and cholesterol even more, according to their physicians' advice. Older adults in general should limit excess dietary fat to prevent eating too many calories, which could contribute to difficulty maintaining a healthy body weight.

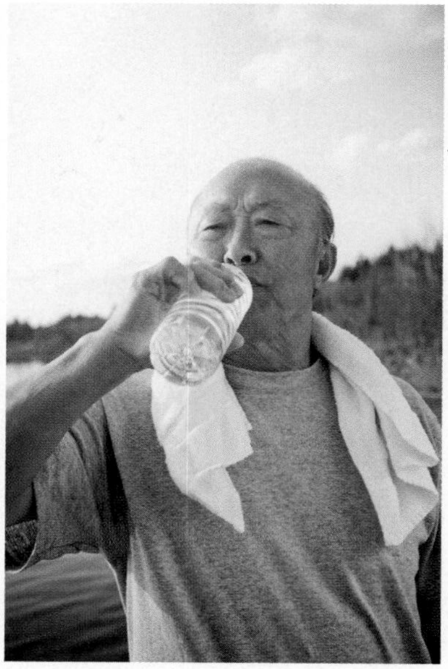

Water

Nutritionists often call water the forgotten nutrient. Water is essential to all body functions; if intake is inadequate, cellular metabolism becomes difficult, if not impossible. In older adults, a decreased thirst response and a reduction in kidney function can increase the risk of dehydration.[78] Diuretic medications, alcohol, and caffeine all increase fluid excretion and can contribute to dehydration. Fluid recommendations for older adults are the same as for younger adults: 3,700 milliliters per day for men, and 2,700 milliliters (91 fluid ounces) per day for women.[79] These fluids should be obtained from both beverages and foods.

Key Concepts Although caloric needs decline with loss of lean tissue and reduced physical activity, protein needs do not change for older adults. A high-carbohydrate, moderate-fat diet is still recommended. Water is important; because of their diminished thirst response, older adults may not drink enough.

Vitamins and Minerals

As we age, our micronutrient status changes, especially our needs for vitamin D, vitamin B_{12}, and calcium (see **FIGURE 17.13**). In many cases, our vitamin needs remain stable, while our energy needs decline. This often creates a challenge for older adults who become inactive with age, reducing their calorie needs. To maintain body weight or prevent gaining, this means that older adults must eat a more nutrient-dense diet to eat all the nutrients they need for good health without overeating calories. In other cases, age-related declines in absorption, use, or activation of nutrients lead to increased dietary vitamin and mineral needs. Therefore, it is especially important for older adults to eat nutrient-dense foods.

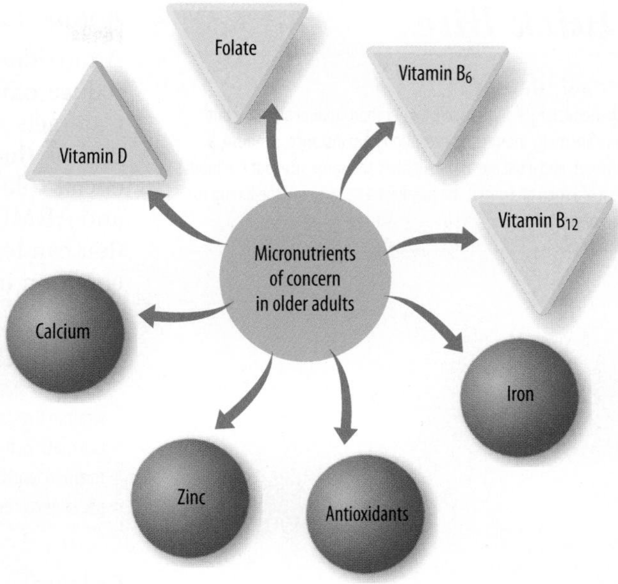

FIGURE 17.13 Micronutrients of particular concern for older adults. As we age, our energy needs decline, but our vitamin and mineral needs remain stable. This makes nutrient-dense foods especially important for older adults.

Vitamin D

Vitamin D promotes bone health; too little dietary vitamin D can lead to brittle and porous bones that are susceptible to fracture. Recently, vitamin D has been investigated for its role in the prevention and treatment of cancer, types 1 and 2 diabetes mellitus, hypertension, glucose metabolism, heart disease, arthritis, and multiple sclerosis.[80] Older adults often have low vitamin D status.[81] Not only are aging tissues less able to take up vitamin D from the blood, but also aging skin is less effective in synthesizing vitamin D when exposed to sunlight. In addition, many older adults spend more time indoors and have reduced exposure to sunlight. When they go outside, many avoid the sun and use sunscreens—a good strategy for skin cancer prevention, but one that reduces vitamin D synthesis. Older adults with lactose intolerance often avoid dairy products, reducing their vitamin D intake and further compromising vitamin D status. The RDA for vitamin D for adults aged 51 through 70 years is 600 IU per day. Younger adults also need 600 IU per day. For adults 70 years and older, the RDA is 800 IU per day.[82]

B Vitamins

The B vitamins deserve special consideration in adults and aging adults. Extensive research links inadequate folate, vitamin B_6, and vitamin B_{12} to elevated levels of plasma homocysteine, which is associated with an increased risk for cardiovascular disease and mortality.[83] High homocysteine levels also have been found to be an independent risk factor for cognitive impairment and dementia.[84] Since the 1998 fortification of the food supply with folic acid, ready-to-eat cereals and grain products now play a significant role in the dietary folic acid intake of older adults.[85]

The prevalence of vitamin B_{12} deficiency increases with age. Six percent of adults aged 60 years or older are vitamin B_{12} deficient, and close to 20 percent have marginal status.[86] Although most adults consume adequate amounts of dietary vitamin B_{12}, 10 to 30 percent of older adults lose their ability to absorb protein-bound vitamin B_{12} from foods. Folic acid intake in excess of recommended levels can mask a vitamin B_{12} deficiency and delay diagnosis.[87] Neurological symptoms such as changes in mental status require further investigation in older adults and should not simply be attributed to old age. An intake of 2.4 micrograms per day of vitamin B_{12} is recommended for all adults older than 51 years. Because it is easier to absorb synthetic B_{12} than food-bound B_{12}, scientists suggest that adults older than 50 years use fortified foods or B_{12}-containing supplements to meet their vitamin B_{12} requirements.

Quick Bite

Animal Lifetimes

In general, larger animals live longer than smaller animals, but there are many interesting exceptions. For instance, a mouse, a parakeet, and a bat are approximately the same size, but the mouse has a life span of 2 years, the parakeet 13 years, and the bat up to 50 years!

Antioxidants

Antioxidants such as those found in fruits and vegetables are important to reduce oxidative stress and degenerative diseases common in older adults. Cataracts and age-related macular degeneration (ARMD) are common conditions that affect the vision of older adults. Antioxidants can have a beneficial role in preventing, slowing the progression of, and treating cataracts and ARMD.[88] In addition, antioxidants protect against damage to the brain that can lead to Alzheimer's disease and other declines in cognition that are common in aging.[89]

Key Concepts Vitamin D, folate, vitamin B_6, vitamin B_{12}, and antioxidants are key nutrients for older adults. Vitamin D status can decline as a result of reduced intake, synthesis, and activation. Poor folate, vitamin B_6, and vitamin B_{12} status might result in high homocysteine levels, a risk factor for heart disease. Excessive folic acid intake can mask a vitamin B_{12} deficiency. Vitamin B_{12} absorption declines with age; vitamin B_{12} is more easily absorbed from fortified foods and supplements, so these become important sources for older adults. Antioxidants help to lower the prevalence and progression of degenerative diseases such as ARMD and Alzheimer's.

Calcium

Maintaining adequate calcium intake reduces the rate of age-related bone loss and the incidence of fractures, especially of the hip.[90] For women aged 51 to 70 years, the RDA for calcium is 1,200 milligrams per day, 200 milligrams per day higher than the RDA for men of the same age. For both men and women older than the age of 70, the RDA for calcium is 1,200 milligrams per day.[91]

As we age we are less able to absorb calcium, partly because of a loss of vitamin D receptors in the gut. Stomach inflammation also reduces calcium absorption, as does an increase in the consumption of fiber—a practice that doctors recommend for its laxative effects. Because of real or perceived lactose intolerance, many older adults have a low intake of dairy foods and therefore of calcium.

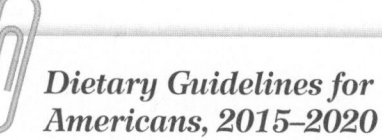

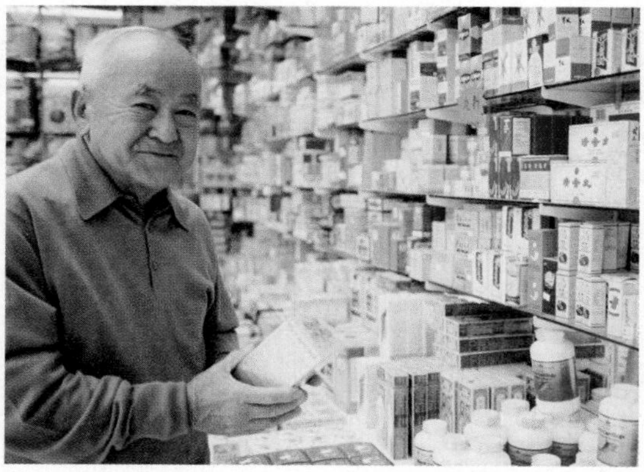

© Paul Edmondson/Corbis

Zinc

Although clinical zinc deficiencies are uncommon, older adults frequently have marginal zinc intakes. Stress, especially in hospitalized older adults, appears to increase the risk of zinc deficiency and suppress immune function. Studies show that zinc supplementation hastens wound healing, but only in those who are zinc deficient. Because excess zinc can interfere with immune function and the absorption of other minerals and may work to lower high-density lipoprotein (HDL) cholesterol, people of all ages should avoid excessive and continuous zinc supplementation.

Iron

Iron remains an important nutrient throughout the life cycle. Following menopause, the RDA for women drops to the same level as for men, 8 milligrams per day. Iron deficiency is a concern for older adults who have limited intake of iron from the best sources—red meats, fish, and poultry. Reduced meat consumption may result from taste changes, economics, poor dentition, or a combination of factors.

Dietary Guidelines for Americans, 2015–2020

Key Recommendations

Recommendations for Specific Population Groups: Individuals Aged 50 Years and Older

- Consume foods fortified with vitamin B_{12} such as fortified cereals, or dietary supplements.

Reproduced from U.S. Department of Agriculture and U.S. Department of Health and Human Services. *Dietary Guidelines for Americans, 2015–2020.* 8th ed. Washington, DC: U.S. Government Printing Office; December 2015.

To Supplement or Not to Supplement

Increased use of dietary supplements, including vitamins, minerals, and herbal and botanical products, is widespread.[92] Although food is "the best medicine," some older adults feel they need a supplement to meet their nutrient needs. Older adults take nutritional supplements for two main reasons: first, to delay age-related chronic diseases, and second, for the potential health-promoting effects of these nutrients.[93] Food is more than the sum of its known nutrients, however, and replacing food with supplements is a poor trade-off. In addition, some nutrients in large amounts can be toxic; they also can affect the absorption of other nutrients or interfere with the absorption and metabolism of prescription medications.

Excessive use of vitamin supplements by older adults might result in **hypervitaminosis**. The need for vitamin A decreases with age, increasing the chances that supplementation might lead to liver dysfunction, bone and joint pain, headaches, and other problems. Also, taking large amounts of vitamin C can increase the likelihood of kidney stones and gastric bleeding. Because we know that many older adults use vitamin supplements and that megadoses can have negative effects on health, it is important to inform older adults of the Tolerable Upper Intake Levels (ULs) for micronutrients. The UL represents a level of intake from a combination of food and dietary supplements that should not be exceeded on a routine basis (see **TABLE 17.10**).

▶ **hypervitaminosis** High levels of vitamins in the blood, usually a result of excess supplement intake.

Key Concepts Important minerals for older adults are calcium, zinc, and iron. Calcium is important to reduce the risk for osteoporosis. Marginal zinc deficiency has been suspected in many older adults and might be the result of reduced intake of red meats. Iron needs decline for women as they go through menopause. Excessive supplementation with certain vitamins or minerals can lead to health problems.

TABLE 17.10
The UL Values for Vitamins and Minerals for Adults

Vitamin/Mineral	Daily UL
Vitamin A (as retinol)	3,000 µg/d
Vitamin C	2,000 mg/d
Vitamin D	4,000 IU/d
Vitamin E [a]	1,000 mg/d
Niacin [a]	35 mg/d
Vitamin B_6	100 mg/d
Folic acid	1,000 µg/d
Choline	3,500 mg/d
Boron	20 mg/d
Calcium	2,500 mg/d (19–50 years)
	2,000 mg/d (51+ years)
Chloride	3,600 mg/d
Copper	10,000 µg/d
Fluoride	10 mg/d
Iodine	1,100 µg/d
Iron	45 mg/d
Magnesium	350 mg/d
Manganese	11 mg/d
Molybdenum	2,000 µg/d
Nickel	1 mg/d
Phosphorus	4,000 mg/d
	3,000 mg/d (70+ years)
Selenium	400 µg/d
Sodium	2,300 mg/d
Vanadium	1.8 mg/d
Zinc	40 mg/d

[a] From fortified foods and supplements only.

Nutrition-Related Concerns of Mature Adults

Many factors can interfere with intake or use of nutrients by older adults. Therefore, caretakers, healthcare practitioners, and seniors themselves must pay attention to nutritional status. To manage acute or chronic nutrition-related conditions, older adults may need to make specific dietary changes.

Drug–Drug and Drug–Nutrient Interactions

Drugs not only affect the way the body uses nutrients, but also can alter the activities of other drugs. In turn, foods and nutrients can enhance or interfere with the effects of drugs (see **TABLE 17.11**). Some drugs interfere with appetite; others cause a dry mouth. Because many older adults take several medications or are on long-term drug therapy, they can find themselves at increased nutritional risk.

Herbal supplements and vitamins or minerals in high doses should be viewed as drugs, particularly when taken in conjunction with prescription or over-the-counter medications. Although herbal products almost certainly interact with other medicines, many interactions are not well documented. In addition to the health and safety issues, supplement therapies can be costly. It is critical that older adults tell their healthcare providers all the drugs and supplements that they take on a regular basis so that possible interactions can be identified and avoided.

Depression

Many studies report high levels of well-being among older adults, especially those who remain independent. Although depression is one of the most common psychological effects of aging, it is most common among institutionalized and low-income people.

TABLE 17.11
Examples of Food–Drug Interactions

Drug	Food That Interacts	Effect of the Food	What to Do
Analgesic			
Acetaminophen (Tylenol)	Alcohol	Increases risk for liver toxicity	Avoid alcohol.
Antibiotic			
Tetracyclines	Dairy products; iron supplements	Decreases drug absorption	Do not take with milk. Take 1 hr before or 2 hr after food or milk.
Amoxicillin, penicillin	Food	Decreases drug absorption	Take 1 hr before or 2 hr after meals.
Azithromycin (Zithromax), erythromycin	Food	Decreases drug absorption	Take 1 hr before or 2 hr after meals.
Nitrofurantoin (Macrobid)	Food	Decreases GI distress, slows drug absorption	Take with food or milk.
Anticoagulant			
Warfarin (Coumadin)	Foods rich in vitamin K	Decreases drug effectiveness	Limit foods high in vitamin K: liver, broccoli, spinach, kale, cauliflower, and Brussels sprouts.
Antifungal			
Griseofulvin (Fulvicin)	High-fat meal	Increases absorption	Take with high-fat meal.
Antihistamine			
Diphenhydramine (Benadryl), chlorpheniramine (Chlor-Trimeton)	Alcohol	Increases drowsiness	Avoid alcohol.
Antihypertensive			
Felodipine (Plendil), nifedipine	Grapefruit juice	Increases drug absorption	Consult physician or pharmacist before changing diet.
Anti-inflammatory			
Naproxen (Aleve)	Food or milk	Decreases GI irritation	Take with food or milk.
Ibuprofen (Advil, Motrin)	Alcohol	Increases risk for liver damage or stomach bleeding	Avoid alcohol.
Diuretic			
Spironolactone (Aldactone)	Food	Decreases GI irritation	Take with food.
Psychotherapeutic (MAO inhibitors)			
Tranylcypromine (Parnate)	Foods high in tyramine: aged cheeses, Chianti wine, pickled herring, brewer's yeast, fava beans	Risk for hypertensive crisis	Avoid foods high in tyramine.

Note: This table includes major food–drug and drug–nutrient interactions. This is only a sample of the medications and interactions in each of these common medication categories. Not all categories of medications are included in the table. Check with your doctor or pharmacist for specific information about your medications.

Reproduced from Bobroff LB, Lentz A, Turner RE. *Food/Drug and Drug/Nutrient Interactions: What You Should Know About Your Medications.* Gainesville, FL: University of Florida; 2009. Publication FCS 8092 in a series of the Department of Family, Youth and Community Sciences, Florida Cooperative Extension Service, Institute of Food and Agricultural Sciences. http://edis.ifas.ufl.edu/pdffiles/HE/HE77600.pdf. Accessed January 11, 2016. Reprinted by permission.

In older adults, life transitions and stressful events can become frequent companions that increase the likelihood and severity of depression. Among these stressors are the loss of loved ones, including spouse and friends; physical disability; perceived loss of physical attractiveness; inability to psychologically defend oneself from unpleasant events; inability to care for oneself, which forces one to depend upon caregivers and long-term care; social isolation; and, inevitably, the approach of death. In later life, depression often leads to malnutrition and can manifest itself as either anorexia (loss of appetite) or obesity.

Alcoholism is prevalent among socially isolated or depressed older adults. People who consume excessive amounts of alcohol often have diets low in essential nutrients.

Anorexia of Aging

Poor food intake that accompanies age can result from **anorexia of aging**. Reductions in appetite and food intake contribute to undernutrition in older adults.[94] Malnutrition, in turn, can contribute to numerous problems, including immune deficiencies, anemia, falls, and cognitive decline.

It can be difficult to pinpoint treatment strategies for anorexia in older adults. However, treating even one aspect of the problem can provide at least temporary improvement. Unfortunately, lifelong inappropriate food habits, social factors, living conditions, and fear of injury can interfere with a person's ability and desire to stay or become healthy.

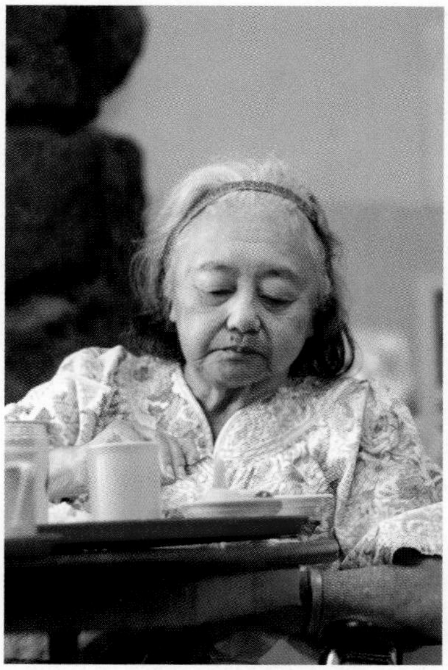

© Photos.com

▶ **anorexia of aging** Loss of appetite and wasting associated with old age.

Key Concepts Among the problems older adults face are lack of appetite and the side effects and interactions of medications they use. Medicines have the potential to interact with food and nutrients in the diet, and a lack of knowledge of these possibilities increases the risk for harmful effects. Although many older adults have high levels of well-being, depression is common among institutionalized and low-income seniors.

Arthritis

Arthritis is a general term that describes more than 100 diseases that cause pain and swelling of joints and connective tissue (see **FIGURE 17.14**). Arthritis is a chronic, lifelong affliction that, at its worst, can make movement difficult or even impossible. Unfortunately, there is no proven cure for arthritis. At best, appropriate treatment programs reduce symptoms. In terms of nutrition, arthritis pain can impair appetite or make it hard to prepare meals, and some arthritis medications interfere with nutrient absorption. These factors underscore the importance of a nutrient-dense diet for arthritis sufferers.

Weight management is important in treating arthritis. Excess weight puts undue pressure on the hips and knees. Weight loss by people who are overweight or obese can reduce the risk of developing osteoarthritis, particularly of the knee.[95]

People who have rheumatoid arthritis can benefit from adding foods that are high in unsaturated fatty acids, particularly the omega-3 fatty acids in flaxseed and cold-water fish. There is some evidence that the right ratio of these fatty acids has beneficial effects on chronic inflammatory diseases such as rheumatoid arthritis, thus helping to reduce discomfort.[96] Other factors found to be protective against arthritis include dietary antioxidants; however, high coffee consumption, alcohol intake (especially among smokers), and obesity tend to increase risk of rheumatoid arthritis.[97]

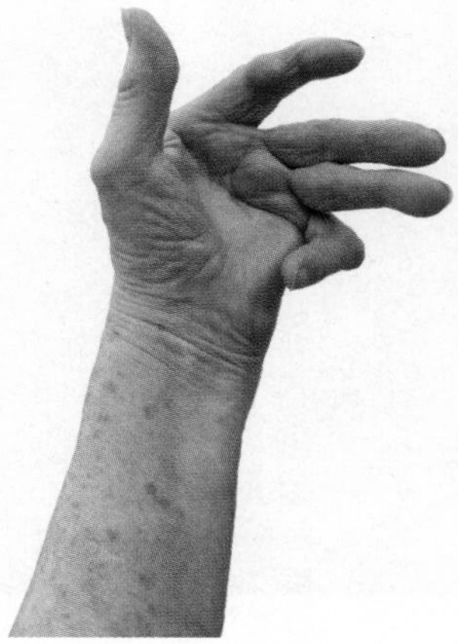

© Peterfactors/Dreamstime.com

FIGURE 17.14 Arthritis. Degeneration of the finger joints can cause a debilitating lack of function.

Bowel and Bladder Regulation

As a result of physiological and lifestyle changes, older adults are susceptible to problems with their bowels and bladder. Inadequate hydration not only affects the bladder, but also makes constipation more likely. Age-related decreases in intestinal motility and transit time, accompanied by poor food intake, can exacerbate the problem. In addition, lack of physical activity contributes to loss of muscle tone needed for regular elimination.

Chronic constipation is one of the most common health complaints among older adults. Excessive use of laxatives can cause nutritional deficiencies by decreasing transit time and preventing adequate absorption of nutrients. Decreased transit time also reduces water re-absorption by the GI tract and contributes to dehydration.

Increasing dietary fiber and fluid is one of the most effective treatments for bowel and bladder problems. Older adults should gradually switch to—and then maintain—a high-fiber diet. They also should be careful to maintain adequate fluid intake and exercise regularly. Supplementation with prebiotics, such as fructooligosaccharides, and probiotics, such as *Lactobacillus acidophilus*, can also improve their gastrointestinal health.[98]

Key Concepts Arthritis and changes in bowel and bladder habits are common problems in older adults. Weight management is an important component of arthritis treatment. Because of an increased risk of dehydration and constipation, older adults should be encouraged to follow a high-fiber diet and consume plenty of fluids.

Dental Health

The mouth is the gateway to the rest of the gastrointestinal system. Poor oral health can impair the ability to eat and obtain adequate nutrition. Missing teeth or poorly fitting dentures make some older adults self-conscious about eating, which leaves them unable to eat comfortably in public. Mouth pain and difficulty swallowing interfere with the process of eating, and tooth loss can alter choices and quality of food. Meats, fresh fruits, and fresh vegetables often are avoided. Oral infections affect the whole body and increase the risk of other chronic diseases, including heart disease.

Vision Problems

▶ **macular degeneration** Progressive deterioration of the macula, an area in the center of the retina, that eventually leads to loss of central vision.

Poor vision and blindness interfere with the ability to buy and prepare food; people with visual impairments cannot read food labels, cookbooks, or the settings on stoves or microwave ovens. **Macular degeneration** is a common disease of the eye that gradually leads to loss of vision. It affects about 6 percent of people between the ages of 65 and 74 years, and about 20 percent of those aged 75 to 85 years. Research has found that people with a higher intake of green leafy vegetables are less likely to develop this sight-robbing disorder. Foods that contain the carotenoids lutein and zeaxanthin are widely investigated for their ability to reduce risk.[99] By preventing free radical damage, antioxidants in these foods may protect the eye and the blood vessels that supply it. The National Eye Institute's Age-Related Eye Disease Study (AREDS) found that taking a specific high-dose formulation of antioxidants and zinc (beta-carotene; vitamins A, C, and E; copper; and zinc) significantly reduces the risk of advanced age-related macular degeneration and its associated vision loss.[100] Preventing or slowing progression of the disease will save the vision of many people.

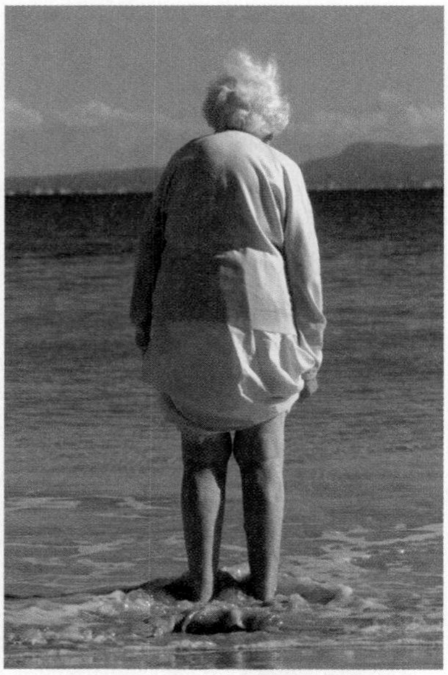

FIGURE 17.15 Osteoporosis. A hunched back (sometimes called a dowager's hump) caused by collapsed vertebrae is a visible symptom of osteoporosis.

Osteoporosis

Although osteoporosis affects older adults of both genders, it is most common in postmenopausal women. Osteoporosis is the deterioration of bone structure (see **FIGURE 17.15**) until, often without warning, the fragile bone breaks upon the slightest impact.

Nutritional factors, particularly early in life, are thought to play an important role in the development of osteoporosis. Whereas regular weight-bearing exercise helps prevent osteoporosis, inactivity increases osteoporosis risk. Long periods of inactivity, such as may be imposed by complete bed rest or illnesses that limit mobility, can promote the disease.

Although prevention is the best treatment for osteoporosis, many people enter later life with bad habits—poor nutrition and physical inactivity—that put them at risk. Adopting a diet that is rich in calcium and vitamin D and engaging in regular physical activity, particularly weight-bearing exercises, minimizes osteoporosis risks.

Alzheimer Disease

Among its other ravages, **Alzheimer disease (AD)** eventually destroys the ability to obtain, prepare, and consume an optimal diet. Although genetic factors can affect the risk for Alzheimer disease, other risk factors include age, head trauma, and possibly exposure to environmental toxins. Although much more research is needed to determine their effects, antioxidants offer some protection from the disease.[101] Antioxidant supplements, however, have not been shown conclusively to be beneficial and can lead to undesirable side effects. Therefore, antioxidants from food should be encouraged for older adults to reduce risk of Alzheimer disease.[102]

▶ **Alzheimer disease (AD)** A presenile dementia characterized by accumulation of plaques in certain regions of the brain and degeneration of a certain class of neurons.

Most cases of Alzheimer disease begin after age 70, but it can strike genetically predisposed people at a younger age. During the first stage of the disease, the afflicted person can have difficulty recalling names, frequently lose possessions, and easily become lost. Sensory sensitivity, such as loss of the sense of smell, is common, but because changes often occur gradually, they may not be readily noticed.

As the disease progresses, the person becomes unable to complete simple tasks that require learned motor movement, such as using a can opener. There is an increase in behavior problems and wandering that can affect the person's ability to maintain weight and nutritional status.

In late stages of the disease, about one-third of those with AD develop overactivity, which drains the nutritional reserve and increases calorie needs. At each stage the caregiver must carefully plan the person's diet to meet psychological and physical needs, paying particular attention to optimum nutrition without excess weight gain.

Overweight and Obesity

Maintaining a healthy body weight is critical at every life stage, the importance of which is underscored in older adults. Both underweight and overweight have significant consequences for the quality of life, health, and well-being of older adults. In addition to the health implications that accompany too much body weight, obesity in older adults can affect their ability to remain independent and accomplish their daily activities by interfering with normal physical functioning. Weight loss in this population is complicated by other health risks; however, additional weight gain is discouraged for overweight and obese older adults.[103] The presence of nutritional deficiencies in overweight and obese older adults can be a consequence of the long-term consumption of a high-calorie, poor-nutrient diet and a physically inactive lifestyle.[104]

Key Concepts Oral health, vision, and bone health all decline with aging. Tooth loss and oral pain can reduce food intake and nutrient quality. Loss of vision can make food shopping and preparation difficult. Osteoporosis, most common in postmenopausal women, can cause debilitating fractures. Alzheimer disease eventually destroys the ability to obtain, prepare, and consume an optimal diet. Overweight and obesity are increasingly common and significantly affect the quality of life and health of older adults. Management of these conditions depends first on their identification by healthcare professionals.

Meal Management for Mature Adults

Many older adults are at nutritional risk because of economics, social isolation, physical restrictions, inability to shop for or prepare food, and medical conditions. Fortunately, there are a number of ways that older adults can remain independent and have access to an adequate diet.

- **Meals on Wheels** A voluntary, not-for-profit organization established to provide nutritious meals to homebound people (regardless of age) so they can maintain their independence and quality of life.
- **Older Americans Act Nutrition Program** A federally funded program (formerly known as the Elderly Nutrition Program) that provides older persons with nutritionally sound meals through home-delivered nutrition services, congregate nutrition services, and the nutrition services' incentive.
- **Supplemental Nutrition Assistance Program (SNAP)** A USDA program that helps single people and families with little or no income to buy food. Formerly known as the Food Stamp Program.

Quick Bite

Why Elephants Don't Need Dentures

Elephants are the only mammals with a built-in tooth replacement system. As they age, elephants go through six sets of teeth, changing about every 10 years. When elephants are around 70 years old, about the maximum life span, the last set of molars wears out.

Quick Bite

Meno-What?

Most animal species do not go through menopause.

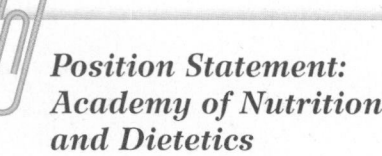

Position Statement: Academy of Nutrition and Dietetics

Food and Nutrition for Older Adults: Promoting Health and Wellness

It is the position of the Academy of Nutrition and Dietetics that all Americans aged 60 years and older receive appropriate nutrition care; have access to coordinated, comprehensive food and nutrition services; and receive the benefits of ongoing research to identify the most effective food and nutrition programs, interventions, and therapies.

Reproduced from Position of the Academy of Nutrition and Dietetics: food and nutrition for older adults: promoting health and wellness. *J Acad Nutr Diet*. 2012;112:1255–1277. Copyright © 2012. Reprinted with permission from Elsevier.

Managing Independently

Independent and assisted-living programs allow people to live relatively carefree yet independent lives. Senior citizen apartment buildings and retirement villages offer a variety of services, including balanced meals. Programs such as **Meals on Wheels** and the **Older Americans Act Nutrition Program** (formerly known as the Elderly Nutrition Program) provide meals to home-bound people as well as those in congregate (group) settings. Most programs provide meals at least five times per week. The Older Americans Act Nutrition Program is supported primarily with federal funds; volunteer time, in-kind donations, and participant contributions make up the remainder. The **Supplemental Nutrition Assistance Program (SNAP)**, formerly the Food Stamp Program, is another option that provides low-income older adults with the means to purchase food. Unfortunately, because SNAP carries a "welfare" stigma, some older adults are reluctant to participate. In addition, many people who need some help buying food do not meet the eligibility requirements.

An evaluation of the Older Americans Act Nutrition Program showed that program participants had higher nutrient intake levels than nonparticipants and had a higher number of regular social contacts—another important factor in eating well.[105] Participation in food assistance programs can reduce the incidence of depression and overweight associated with food insecurity.[106]

Wise Eating for One or Two

Preparing meals that are healthful and tasty is a challenge for those living alone or in small households. As discussed earlier in this chapter, our nutrition needs—with the exception of calories—do not decrease as we age, but our ability to meet them does. Reliance on convenience foods, fast foods, and eating out can adversely affect the nutritional status of older adults. Men who live alone are especially likely to eat out or skip meals rather than prepare food for themselves. For both men and women, physical disability or illness can diminish the desire to prepare and eat meals.

Some simple changes in appliances and food-preparation techniques can help older adults overcome common obstacles to food preparation. Those who can't or won't cook can use microwaves, toaster ovens, and small appliances to prepare simple meals. A meal based on a lower-sodium, low-fat convenience entrée can meet nutritional needs if accompanied by vegetables, whole-grain bread, milk, and fruit. THINK About It 4

Finding Community Resources

An older person's need for community support typically changes from decade to decade. Sometimes, identifying community resources can be challenging, and financial considerations might further limit access to resources that can assist older adults in their own homes. Within local communities, area agencies on aging, social and rehabilitation services, cooperative extension services, churches, and extended-care facilities might have lists of resources and educational programs for older adults. **TABLE 17.12** lists important resources for older adults.

Key Concepts Older adults who obtain adequate food and nutrient intake while living independently can require assistance from time to time. This assistance might take the form of help with food shopping or preparation or identification of community resources that can stretch the food dollar. Numerous resources exist to assist older adults in maintaining a productive, high-quality life.

TABLE 17.12
Important Resources for Older Adults

Resource Directory for Older People: www.aoa.gov (https://chs-nhlbi.org/node/5868) The Resource Directory for Older People is a cooperative effort of the National Institute on Aging and the Administration on Aging. This directory provides resources for elders, their caregivers and family members, and those in the legal and healthcare professions. Available on the Internet, it provides telephone numbers (some toll free), names, addresses, and fax numbers for organizations that work with older adults.
The Eldercare Locator: www.eldercare.gov and (800) 677-1116 (toll free) The National Association of Area Agencies on Aging and the National Association of State Units on Aging administer the Eldercare Locator, a public service of the Administration on Aging, U.S. Department of Health and Human Services. The Eldercare Locator is a nationwide directory-assistance service that helps older persons and their families identify resources for aging Americans.

Look Into the Future

You are 65 years old. Revisit your eating habits as a child, teenager, and college student, and assign the most appropriate descriptor to each item. Consider how your past nutritional behavior has helped determine your current health status.

0 = seldom or never true
1 = sometimes true
2 = frequently true

As a child,

1. I was a picky eater, rejecting the food usually offered.
2. I was not permitted to decide how much to eat.
3. I rarely drank milk.
4. I ate candy every day.

As an adolescent,

5. I let peer pressure influence my nutrition choices.
6. I ate in front of the TV.
7. I worried about my weight.

As a college student,

8. I didn't think about healthy food choices.
9. I resisted changing my eating habits.
10. I was influenced by food fads.

Add up your score. Scores over 12 should signal that your healthy nutrition behavior can be improved. Highlight the items you feel can be affected by behavior change.

Label to Table

What is it about fruit snacks that attracts kids? The sweet flavors, bright colors, different shapes, or logos of favorite movie or TV characters? Probably all of these. Parents may be attracted by claims for vitamins. So, are these nutritious snacks or little more than candy? Let's look at the label.

On the positive side, this is a fat-free snack and contains little sodium. However, most of the calories—56 of 80—come from sugar (14 g × 4 kcal/g), and the remainder from starch and protein. The ingredient list shows that the first three ingredients are sugars: corn syrup, sucrose, and fruit juice from concentrate.

The vitamins added to fruit snacks are the only redeeming feature of the product, providing 25 percent of the DV for vitamins A, C, and E. But is there a better way to get these nutrients? One-half cup of orange juice provides two-thirds of the DV for vitamin C and significant amounts of thiamin, folate, and potassium as well. Just a handful of baby carrots provides more than 100 percent DV for vitamin A, along with some fiber. Vitamin E is widespread in the food supply—a small amount of salad dressing as a dip for the carrots would add vitamin E.

So, the fruit snacks are not as devoid of nutrients as candy, but are not as nutrient dense as fruits and vegetables. The fruit snacks may have some nutrient value, but they are high in sugar and, like all sugary snacks, should be limited.

Nutrition Facts

10 servings per container
Serving size 1 pouch (26g/0.9 oz)

Amount per serving	
Calories	**80**
	% Daily Value*
Total Fat 0g	**0%**
Sodium 15mg	**1%**
Total Carbohydrate 19g	**6%**
Total Sugars 14g	
Includes 14g Added Sugars	**28%**
Protein 1g	
Vitamin D 0mcg	0%
Calcium 0mg	0%
Iron 0mg	0%
Potassium 2mg	0%
Vitamin A 375mcg	25%
Vitamin C 15mg	25%
Vitamin E 5mg	25%

Not a significant source of calories from fat, saturated fat, trans fat, cholesterol, dietary fiber, calcium, or iron.

*The % Daily Value (DV) tells you how much a nutrient in a serving of food contributes to a daily diet. 2,000 calories a day is used for general nutrition advice.

Learning Portfolio

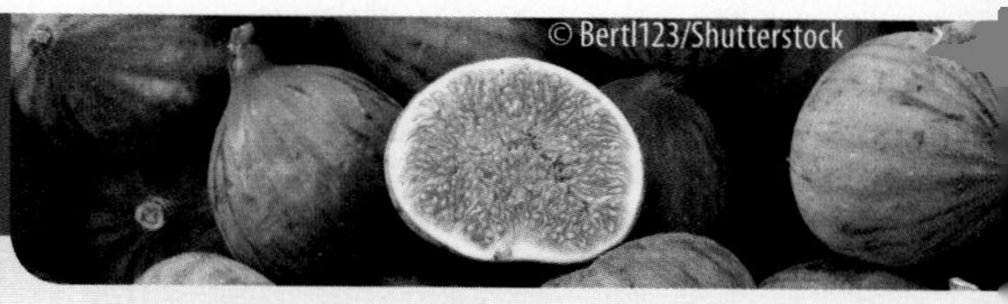

Key Terms

acne	702	Meals on Wheels	718
adolescence	691	menarche	699
Alzheimer disease (AD)	717	Older Americans Act Nutrition Program	718
anorexia of aging	715	puberty	699
childhood	691	Supplemental Nutrition Assistance Program (SNAP)	718
epiphyses	699	taste threshold	707
hyperactivity	696	urinary tract infections (UTIs)	707
hypervitaminosis	713		
macular degeneration	716		

Study Points

- For children and adolescents, growth is the key determinant of nutrient needs. If diets are planned carefully, children do not need vitamin/mineral supplementation.
- Federally funded nutrition and feeding programs reduce malnutrition and hunger among American children.
- Adoption of adult food plans to reduce risk of chronic disease should begin gradually after the age of 2.
- The prevalence of obesity and eating disorders is rising among American children and teens; treatment programs should address food choices and activity levels rather than impose strict calorie limits. Vegetarian diets for children need to be planned carefully to avoid nutrient deficiencies.
- The total energy and nutrient needs of adolescents are high to support growth and maturation. Girls need more iron than boys do to compensate for losses after the onset of menstruation. Active teens need more calories and nutrients than sedentary teens; fluid intake is also a priority.
- Nutrition and physical activity are two important, controllable components of a healthy life and healthful aging. Moreover, numerous physiological and psychological aspects of the aging process affect food intake and nutritional status.
- Energy needs decline with age, reflecting loss of lean body mass and reduced physical activity. The protein RDA and the recommended balance of carbohydrate and fat calories in the diet are similar for young and older adults. Fluid intake needs special attention because of the reduced thirst response that occurs with age.
- Because of reduced intake, synthesis, and activation, vitamin D status declines with age; recommended intake levels are therefore raised. Vitamin B_{12} status might be compromised by inadequate absorption. Antioxidants can help in the protection against degenerative diseases.
- Calcium and zinc intakes are likely to be marginal in the diets of older adults. Iron also remains important.
- Dietary supplements, both vitamin/mineral and herbal/botanical, should be used with caution, preferably with professional advice.
- Because many older adults take multiple medications, they are at risk for drug–nutrient, food–drug, and drug–drug interactions. Anorexia of aging is also a major public health problem.
- Arthritis is a prevalent chronic health problem in this age group. Weight management is a key element of arthritis treatment.
- Chronic constipation is a common complaint among older adults. Fluids, fiber, and regular exercise can reduce the likelihood of constipation.
- Both poor oral and visual health can compromise the ability of older adults to consume a nutritionally adequate diet.
- Osteoporosis is a major health problem that can be addressed through adequate calcium and vitamin D, regular weight-bearing exercise, and medication if needed.
- Adults can maintain independence while aging but may require special assistance to obtain and prepare food. Community resources can help respond to the needs of older adults and those of their caretakers and family.

Study Questions

1. Which vitamins and minerals are most likely to be deficient in a child's diet?
2. Identify several chronic nutrition problems that can affect children. How can these problems be avoided?
3. What are typical nutritional concerns for adolescents?

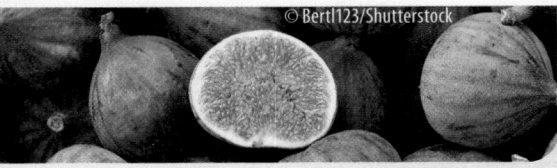

Learning Portfolio (continued)

4. What are some consequences of decreased immunity among older adults?
5. Compared with a younger adult, does a person older than 65 years need more, less, or about the same amount of protein?
6. Why are older adults at risk of vitamin D deficiency?
7. Discuss minerals that may need special attention in assessment of an older adult's nutrition status.
8. What problems might older adults encounter with dietary supplements?
9. What is the role of physical activity in osteoporosis prevention? What nutritional factors are important?

Try This

Eat Like a Kid

Children, especially toddlers, tend to be exploratory and take in the sensory nature of food—the textures, smells, and tastes. In fact, you were probably once this way. The purpose of this exercise is to eat a meal like a kid and gain an appreciation of food's textures and taste. Make some mashed potatoes, macaroni and cheese, buttered peas, or spaghetti (favorite "kid food") and eat it with your fingers. Explore your food and play with it. Try mixing foods. How does this experience make you feel?

Aging Simulation

The purpose of this exercise is to simulate what it can be like to age and experience age-related declines in health. Have you ever thought of how difficult it is to be an older person with health problems and do routine tasks? Invite a few friends over and do the following:

- Put gloves on to simulate the difficulty of losing sensitivity in your hands.
- Use cotton balls in your ears to decrease your hearing ability.
- Apply some petroleum jelly to a pair of glasses or sunglasses to give yourself poor vision.

Now try a simple activity. Make a salad, send a text message, or play a video. After completing the activity, switch disabilities with your friends so that everyone has experienced each of the limitations. What is it like to do these activities with your impairment?

References

1. Institute of Medicine, Food and Nutrition Board. *Dietary Reference Intakes for Energy, Carbohydrate, Fiber, Fat, Fatty Acids, Cholesterol, Protein, and Amino Acids*. Washington, DC: National Academies Press; 2002.
2. Kleinman RE, Greer FR. *Pediatric Nutrition Handbook*. 7th ed. Elk Grove Village, IL: American Academy of Pediatrics; 2013.
3. Nicklas T, Johnson R, American Dietetic Association. Position of the American Dietetic Association: nutrition guidance for healthy children ages 2 to 11 years. *J Am Diet Assoc*. 2008;108:1038–1047.
4. Kumar J, Muntner P, Kaskel FJ, et al. Prevalence and associations of 25-hydroxyvitamin D deficiency in U.S. children: NHANES 2001–2004. *Pediatrics*. 2009;124(3):e362–e370.
5. Reis JP, von Mühlen D, Miller ER III, et al. Vitamin D status and cardiometabolic risk factors in the United States adolescent population. *Pediatrics*. 2009;124(3):e371–e379.
6. Wagner CL, Greer FR, Section on Breastfeeding and Committee on Nutrition. Prevention of rickets and vitamin D deficiency in infants, children, and adolescents. *Pediatrics*. 2008;122(5):1143–1152.
7. Nicklas T, Johnson R, American Dietetic Association. Position of the American Dietetic Association: nutrition guidance for healthy children ages 2 to 11 years. Op cit.
8. Kleinman RE, Greer FR. *Pediatric Nutrition Handbook*. Op cit.
9. Nicklas T, Johnson R, American Dietetic Association. Position of the American Dietetic Association: nutrition guidance for healthy children ages 2 to 11 years. Op cit.
10. Neelon SE, Briley ME, American Dietetic Association. Position of the American Dietetic Association: benchmarks for nutrition in child care. *J Am Diet Assoc*. 2011;111:607–615.
11. Pearson N, Biddle SJ. Sedentary behavior and dietary intake in children, adolescents, and adults: a systematic review. *Am J Prev Med*. 2011;41(2):178–188.
12. Kelly B, Halford JCG, Boyland EJ, et al. Television food advertising to children: a global perspective. *Am J Pub Health*. 2011;100(9):1730–1736.
13. Batada A, Seitz M, Wootan M. Nine out of 10 food advertisements shown during Saturday morning children's television programming are for foods high in fat, sodium, or added sugars, or low in nutrients. *J Am Diet Assoc*. 2008;108(4):673–678.
14. Boyland EJ, Harrold JA, Kirkham TC, et al. Food commercials increase preference for energy-dense foods, particularly in children who watch more television. *Pediatrics*. 2011;128(1): e93–e100.
15. Miller SA, Taveras EM, Rifas-Shiman SL, Gillman MW. Association between television viewing and poor diet quality in young children. *Int J Pediatr Obes*. 2008;3(3):168–176.
16. U.S. Department of Agriculture. Choose MyPlate. Be a healthy role model for children. http://www.choosemyplate.gov/food-groups/downloads/TenTips/DGTipsheet12BeAHealthyRoleModel. Accessed May 21, 2016.
17. Lehto R, Ray C, Roos E. Longitudinal associations between family characteristics and measures of childhood obesity. *Int J Public Health*. 2012;57(3):495–503.
18. World Food Programme. Hunger statistics. http://www.wfp.org/hunger/stats. Accessed January 11, 2016.
19. Coleman-Jensen A, Gregory C, Singh A. Household food security in the United States in 2013. U.S. Department of Agriculture. http://www.ers.usda.gov/media/1565410/err173_summary.pdf. Accessed January 11, 2016.
20. Let's Move! Child Nutrition Reauthorization Healthy Hunger-Free Kids Act of 2010 fact sheet. www.heart.org/idc/groups/ahaecc-public/@wcm/@adv/documents/downloadable/ucm_463491.pdf.
21. Ibid.

22. American Psychiatric Association. *Diagnostic and Statistical Manual of Mental Disorders*. 5th ed. Arlington, VA: Author; 2013.
23. Kim Y, Chang H. Correlation between attention deficit hyperactivity disorder and sugar consumption, quality of diet, and dietary behavior in school children. *Nutr Res Pract*. 2011;5(3):236–245.
24. Stevens LJ, Kuczek T, Burgess JR, Hurt E, Arnold LE. Dietary sensitivities and ADHD symptoms: thirty-five years of research. *Clin Pediatr (Phila)*. 2011;50(4):279–293.
25. McCann D, Barrett A, Cooper A, et al. Food additives and hyperactive behaviour in 3-year-old and 8/9-year-old children in the community: a randomized, double-blinded, placebo-controlled trial. *Lancet*. 2007;370:1560–1567.
26. Pelsser LM, Frankena K, Toorman J, et al. Effects of a restricted elimination diet on the behaviour of children with attention-deficit hyperactivity disorder (INCA study): a randomised controlled trial. *Lancet*. 2011;377:494–503.
27. Ogden CL, Carroll MD, Curtin LR, Lamb MM, Flegal KM. Prevalence of high body mass index in US children and adolescents, 2007–2008. *JAMA*. 2010;303:242–249.
28. Let's Move! Health problems and childhood obesity. http://www.letsmove.gov/health-problems-and-childhood-obesity. Accessed January 12, 2016.
29. Let's Move! http://www.letsmove.gov. Accessed January 12, 2016.
30. Ibid.
31. National Heart, Lung, and Blood Institute. Integrated guidelines for cardiovascular health and risk reduction in children and adolescents. The Report of the Expert Panel. www.nhlbi.nih.gov/files/docs/peds_**guidelines**_sum.pdf. Accessed February 22, 2016.
32. Office of Disease Prevention and Health Promotion. Healthy People 2020: environmental health. http://www.healthypeople.gov/2020/topicsobjectives2020/overview.aspx?topicid=12. Accessed January 21, 2016.
33. Centers for Disease Control and Prevention. Lead: CDC's national surveillance data (1997–2014). 2015. http://www.cdc.gov/nceh/lead/data/national.htm. Accessed January 12, 2016.
34. Centers for Disease Control and Prevention. Lead. http://www.cdc.gov/lead.Accessed January 12, 2016.
35. Craig WJ, Mangels AR, American Dietetic Association. Position of the American Dietetic Association: vegetarian diets. *J Am Diet Assoc*. 2009; 109(7):1266–1282.
36. Wagner CL, Greer FR, Section on Breastfeeding and Committee on Nutrition. Prevention of rickets and vitamin D deficiency in infants, children, and adolescents. Op cit.
37. American Academy of Pediatrics. Vitamin D: on the double. http://www.healthychildren.org/English/healthy-living/nutrition/Pages/Vitamin-D-On-the-Double.aspx. Accessed January 12, 2016.
38. Kleinman RE, Greer FR. *Pediatric Nutrition Handbook*. Op cit.
39. Institute of Medicine. *Dietary Reference Intakes for Calcium and Vitamin D*. Washington, DC: National Academies Press; 2011.
40. Park S, Sappenfield WM, Huang Y, Sherry B, Bensyl DM. The impact of the availability of school vending machines on eating behavior during lunch: the Youth Physical Activity and Nutrition Survey. *J Am Diet Assoc*. 2010;110(10):1532–1536.
41. Minaker LM, Storey KE, Raine KD, et al. Associations between the perceived presence of vending machines and food and beverage logos in schools and adolescents' diet and weight status. *Public Health Nutr*. 2011;14(8):1350–1356.
42. Fox MK, Dodd AH, Wilson A, Gleason PM. Association between school food environment and practices and body mass index of US public school children. *J Am Diet Assoc*. 2009;109(2 suppl):S108–S117.
43. Centers for Disease Control and Prevention. Overweight and obesity: a growing problem. April 2012. www.cdc.gov/obesity/childhood/causes.html. Accessed February 22, 2016.
44. Reedy J, Krebs-Smith SM. Dietary sources of energy, solid fats, and added sugars among children and adolescents in the United States. *J Am Diet Assoc*. 2010;110:1477–1484.
45. Centers for Disease Control and Prevention. Beverage consumption among high school students—United States, 2010. *MMWR*. 2011;60(23):778–780.
46. Let's Move! Child Nutrition Reauthorization Healthy, Hunger-Free Kids Act of 2010.
47. Pasch KE, Lytle LA, Samuelson AC, et al. Are school vending machines loaded with calories and fat: an assessment of 106 middle and high schools. *J Sch Health*. 2011;81(4):212–218.
48. Fox MK, Gordon A, Nogales R, Wilson A. Availability and consumption of competitive foods in US public schools. *J Am Diet Assoc*. 2009;109 (2 suppl):S57–S66.
49. Rovner AJ, Nansel TR, Wang J, Iannotti RJ. Food sold in school vending machines is associated with overall student dietary intake. *J Adolesc Health*. 2011;48(1):13–19.
50. American Academy of Pediatrics Committee on Nutrition and the Council on Sports Medicine. Clinical report—sports drinks and energy drinks for children and adolescents: are they appropriate? *Pediatrics*. 2011;127:1182–1189.
51. Centers for Disease Control and Prevention. Beverage consumption among high school students—United States, 2010. *MMWR*. 2011;60(23):778–780.
52. Ibid.
53. Danby FW. Nutrition and acne. *Clin Dermatol*. 2010;28(6):598–604.
54. Spencer EH, Ferdowsian HR, Barnard ND. Diet and acne: a review of the evidence. *Int J Dermatol*. 2009;48:339–347.
55. Marcason W. Milk consumption and acne—is there a link? *J Am Diet Assoc*. 2010;110(1):152.
56. Berra B, Rizzo AM. Glycemic index, glycemic load: new evidence for a link with acne. *J Am Coll Nutr*. 2009;28(suppl):450S–454S.
57. Nader PR, Bradley RH, Houts RM, et al. Moderate-to-vigorous physical activity from ages 9 to 15 years. *JAMA*. 2008;300:295–305.
58. Centers for Disease Control and Prevention. Overweight and obesity. Basics about childhood obesity. April 2012 **www.cdc.gov/obesity/childhood/**causes.html Accessed February 22, 2016.
59. Ibid.
60. Centers for Disease Control and Prevention. Overweight and obesity. Basics about childhood obesity. www.cdc.gov/obesity/childhood/causes.html Op cit.
61. Watson LC, Kwon J, Nichols D, Rew M. Evaluation of the nutrition knowledge, attitudes, and food consumption behaviors of high school students before and after completion of a nutrition course. *Fam Consumer Sci Res J*. 2009;37(4):523–534.
62. Johnston LD, O'Malley PM, Bachman JG, Schulenberg JE. *Monitoring the Future: National Results on Adolescent Drug Use: Overview of Key Findings, 2010*. Ann Arbor, MI: Institute for Social Research, the University of Michigan; 2011. http://www.monitoringthefuture.org/pubs/monographs/mtf-overview2010.pdf. Accessed January 12, 2016.
63. Ibid.
64. Centers for Disease Control and Prevention. E-cigarette use triples among middle and high school students in just one year. http://www.cdc.gov/media/releases/2015/p0416-e-cigarette-use.html. Accessed January 12, 2016.
65. Centers for Disease Control and Prevention. Alcohol and public health: fact sheets—binge drinking. http://www.cdc.gov/alcohol/quickstats/binge_drinking.htm. Accessed January 12, 2016.
66. U.S. Department of Health and Human Services, Administration on Aging. A profile of older Americans: 2013. http://www.aoa.acl.gov/Aging_Statistics/index.aspx

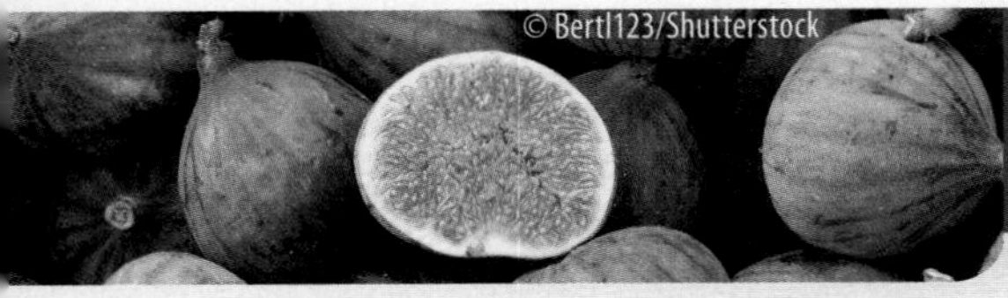
© Bertl123/Shutterstock

Learning Portfolio (continued)

67. U.S. Department of Health and Human Services, Administration on Aging. A profile of older Americans: 2011. Future growth. /Profile/2011/4. http://www.aoa.acl.gov/Aging_Statistics/index.aspx. Accessed July 10, 2012.
68. Position of the Academy of Nutrition and Dietetics: food and nutrition for older adults: promoting health and wellness. *J Acad Nutr Diet*. 2012;112:1255–1277.
69. Federal Interagency Forum on Aging Related Statistics. Older Americans 2010. Key indicators of well-being. 2010. http://www.aoa.acl.gov/Aging_Statistics/index.aspx. Accessed August 7, 2011.
70. Bernstein MA, Munoz NM, eds. *Nutrition for the Older Adult*. 2nd ed. Burlington, MA: Jones & Bartlett; 2016.
71. Sayer AA, Robinson SM, Patel HP, Shavlakadze T, Cooper C, Grounds MD. New horizons in the pathogenesis, diagnosis and management of sarcopenia. *Age Ageing*. 2013;42(2):145–150. doi: 10.1093/ageing/afs191.
72. Bernstein MA, Munoz NM. *Nutrition for the Older Adult*. Op cit.
73. Salem GJ, Skinner JS, Chodzko-Zajko WJ, et al. Exercise and physical activity for older adults. *Med Sci Sports Exer*. 2009;41(7):1510–1530.
74. U.S. Department of Health and Human Services. Active older adults. In: *2008 Physical Activity Guidelines for Americans*. Rockville, MD: Author; 2008.
75. Chodzko-Zajki W, Proctor D, Fiatarone-Singh M, et al. American College of Sports Medicine position stand. Exercise and physical activity for older adults. *Med Sci Sport Exerc*. 2009;41(7):1510–1530.
76. Moskovitz DN, Saltzman J, Kim YI. The aging gut. In: Chernoff R, ed. *Geriatric Nutrition: The Health Professional's Handbook*. 3rd ed. Sudbury, MA: Jones & Bartlett; 2006.
77. Paddon-Jones D, Rasmussen BB. Dietary protein recommendations and the prevention of sarcopenia. *Curr Opin Clin Nutr Metab Care*. 2009;12(1):86–90.
78. Institute of Medicine, Food and Nutrition Board. *Dietary Reference Intakes for Water, Potassium, Sodium, Chloride, and Sulfate*. Washington, DC: National Academies Press; 2004.
79. Ibid.
80. National Institutes of Health, Office of Dietary Supplements. Vitamin D: fact sheet for health professionals. http://ods.od.nih.gov/factsheets/vitamind/. Accessed January 12, 2016.
81. Ibid.
82. Institute of Medicine. *Dietary Reference Intakes for Calcium and Vitamin D*. Op cit.
83. Bernstein MA, Munoz NM. *Nutrition for the Older Adult*. Op cit.
84. Schalinske KL, Smazal AL. Homocysteine imbalance: A pathological metabolic marker. *Adv Nutr*. 2012;3(6):755–762. doi: 10.3945/an.112.002758.
85. Position of the Academy of Nutrition and Dietetics: food and nutrition for older adults. Op cit.
86. Allen LH. How common is vitamin B-12 deficiency? *Am J Clin Nutr*. 2009;89(2):693S–696S.
87. Position of the Academy of Nutrition and Dietetics: food and nutrition for older adults. Op cit.
88. Academy of Nutrition and Dietetics. Food and nutrition for older adults (FNOA) promoting health and wellness (2011-2012). Evidence Analysis Library. http://www.andevidenceanalysislibrary.com/topic.cfm?cat=3987. Accessed January 12, 2016.

89. Devore E, Kang J, Stampfer M, Grodstein F. Total antioxidant capacity of diet in relation to cognitive function. *Am J Clin Nutr*. 2010;92:1157–1164.

90. Institute of Medicine. *Dietary Reference Intakes for Calcium and Vitamin D*. Op cit.

91. Ibid.

92. Nahin R, Pecha M, Welmerink D, et al. Concomitant use of prescription drugs and dietary supplements in ambulatory elderly people. *J Am Geriatr Soc*. 2009;57(7):1197–1205.

93. Buhr G, Bales CW. Nutritional supplements for older adults: review and recommendations—part II. *J Nutr Elder*. 2010;29(1):42–71.

94. Bernstein MA, Munoz NM. *Nutrition for the Older Adult*. Op cit.

95. National Institute of Arthritis and Musculoskeletal and Skin Diseases. Handout on health: osteoarthritis. July 2010. http://www.niams.nih.gov/Health_Info/Osteoarthritis. Accessed January 12, 2016.

96. Patterson E, Wall R, Fitzgerald GF, Ross RP, Stanton C. Health implications of high dietary omega-6 polyunsaturated fatty acids. *J Nutr Metab*. 2012;2012:539426.

97. Lahiri M, Morgan C, Symmons DP, Bruce IN. Modifiable risk factors for RA: prevention, better than a cure? *Rheumatology (Oxford)*. 2012;51(3):499–512.

98. Sarubin Fragakis A, Thomson CA. *The Health Professional's Guide to Popular Dietary Supplements*. 3rd ed. Chicago: American Dietetic Association; 2006.

99. Position of the Academy of Nutrition and Dietetics: food and nutrition for older adults. Op cit.

100. National Eye Institute. The AREDS formulation and age-related macular degeneration. Are these high levels of antioxidants and zinc right for you? http://www.nei.nih.gov/amd/summary.asp. Accessed January 12, 2016.

101. Devore E, Kang J, Stampfer M, Grodstein F. Total antioxidant capacity of diet in relation to cognitive function. Op cit.

102. Position of the Academy of Nutrition and Dietetics: food and nutrition for older adults. Op cit.

103. U.S. Department of Agriculture and U.S. Department of Health and Human Services. *Dietary Guidelines for Americans, 2015*. http://www.cnpp.usda.gov/2015-2020-dietary-guidelines-americans.

104. Position of the Academy of Nutrition and Dietetics: food and nutrition for older adults. Op cit.

105. Academy of Nutrition and Dietetics. Nutrition across the spectrum of aging. Evidence Analysis project. Aging Programs. Evidence Analysis Library. http://www.eatrightpro.org/resources/research/applied-practice/evidence-analysis-library. Accessed July 12, 2012.

106. Kim K, Frongillo EA. Participation in food assistance programs modifies the relation of food insecurity with weight and depression in older adults. *J Nutr*. 2007;137:1005–1010.

Chapter 18

Food Safety and Technology: Microbial Threats and Genetic Engineering

Revised by Paul Insel

THINK About It

1 Do you worry about getting sick from the food you eat?
2 To what extent do you rely on organically grown food to avoid pesticides?
3 What food safety measures, such as thawing meat in the refrigerator, do you practice at home?
4 Would genetically engineered rice be welcome at your dinner table?

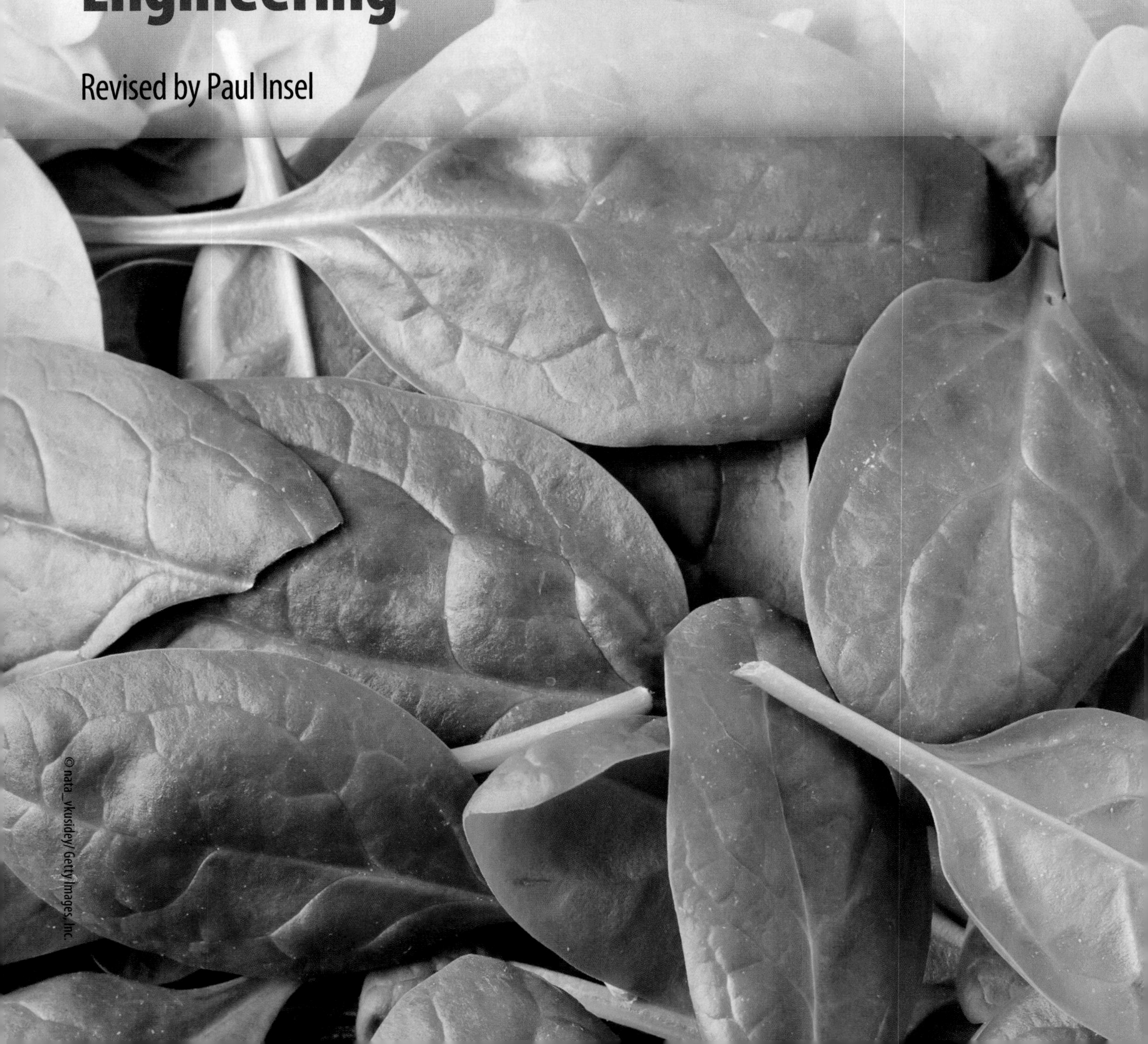

CHAPTER Menu

LEARNING Objectives

- Identify common food pathogens and related illnesses.
- Identify common food contaminants and related health concerns.
- Discuss governmental agencies and their strategies that help keep food safe in the United States.
- Compare food technology methods and their impact when used on the food supply in the United States.
- List the issues related to genetically engineered foods.

The newspaper headline screams, "Contaminated Peanut Butter Proves Fatal." You read further and discover that a child's death has been traced to bacteria thriving in improperly packaged peanut butter that has since been recalled. Additionally, several adults have become ill from the same source. This worries you; the peanut butter is your favorite brand, and several jars are in your pantry. The lot numbers on your jars don't match what was recalled. "I think I'll throw them away anyway," you decide, and wonder if you should change brands. Have you made the right choice? Or should you investigate this issue further?

Although once confined mainly to cookbooks and textbooks, today food safety advice shows up in many places—the popular press, the classroom, the Internet, even the *Dietary Guidelines for Americans*. What has prompted such enthusiasm? Recent headlines tell part of the story. Microbial contamination of such foods as hamburger, apple juice, eggs, raw sprouts, peanuts, pistachios, melon, and both fresh and frozen berries has seriously sickened thousands and killed many, especially those most susceptible: young children, people with compromised immune systems, and seniors.

Consumers are voicing concerns about other food safety issues as well—including fears about excessive pesticide residues in plant foods, antibiotics and hormones in animals used for food, and hidden food allergens (e.g., nuts, milk, eggs) in prepared foods. Increasingly, they are checking prepared foods for ingredients to which they are allergic (e.g., caseinates as milk protein) and questioning preparation methods to avoid an allergen that might be an unintentional food additive (e.g., peanut material found in a milk chocolate candy might be residue left on machinery from earlier processing of peanut butter cups). Other, less frequently discussed food hazards include physical contamination with glass fragments and other sharp objects, heavy metals, and naturally occurring toxins in seafood and some agricultural products (see **FIGURE 18.1**).

Quick Bite

A Morbid Marginal Note

Every day, more than 130,000 Americans get sick from something they ate. Eight of them die.

Food Safety

This chapter reviews major food safety hazards and examines controversial issues such as the merits of organic foods, the use of food irradiation, and the production of genetically engineered foods.

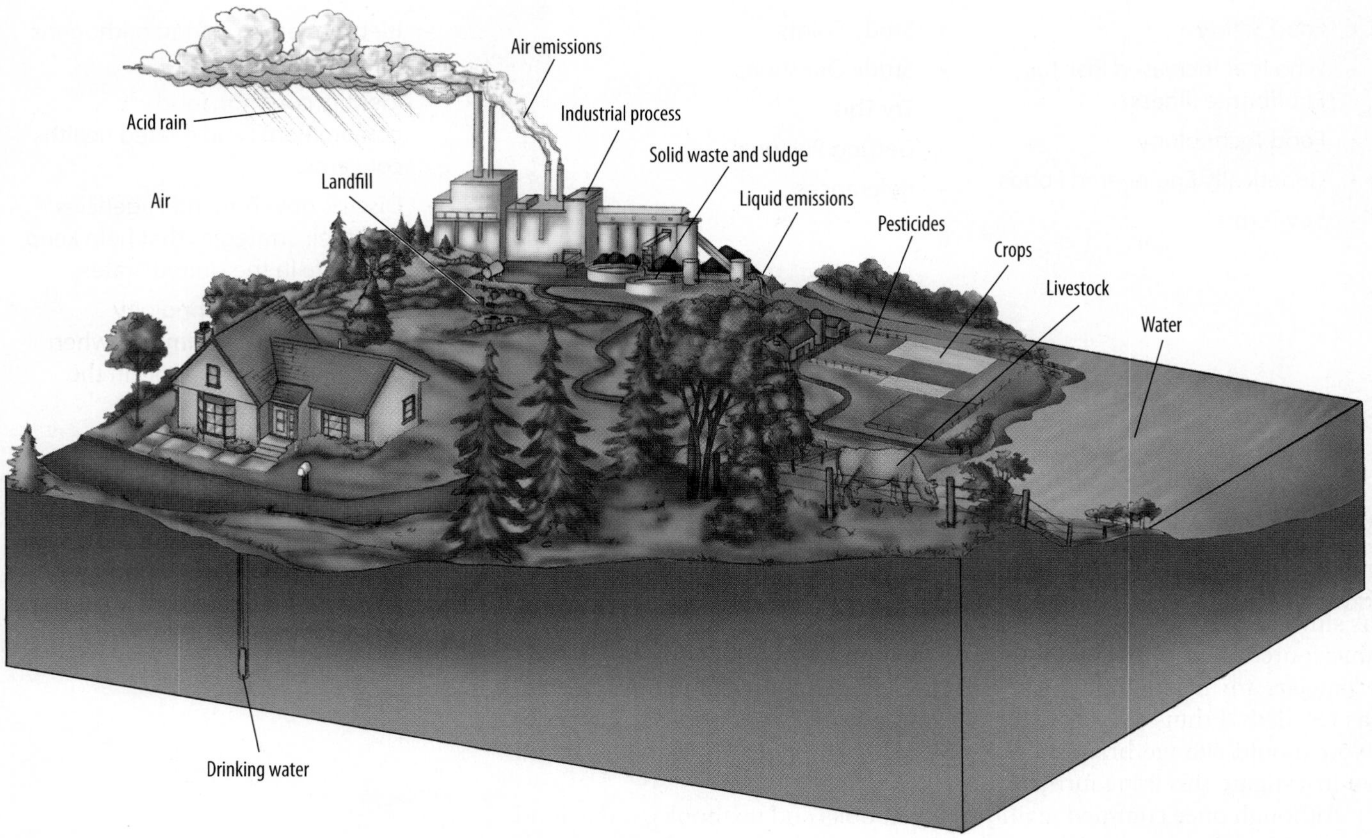

FIGURE 18.1 Heavy metals and other contaminants can be found in foods. Industrial plants and automobiles release heavy metals and other contaminants into the air. Rainfall carries these contaminants to the soil. Plants for food crops and animal feed absorb contaminants from the soil. Runoff can pick up contaminants from pesticides, fertilizers, and animal manure. This pollutes surface water (lakes and streams), groundwater, and coastal water. Polluted water contaminates seafood and other fish that people eat.

Harmful Substances in Foods

In the United States and Canada, most foodborne diseases are caused by microorganisms and can be prevented by cleaning hands and surfaces, cooking raw foods sufficiently, and refrigerating foods promptly.

Pathogens

▶ **foodborne illness** A sickness caused by food contaminated with microorganisms, chemicals, or other substances hazardous to human health.

In North America, most food safety experts agree that the chief cause of **foodborne illness** is pathogenic (disease-causing) microorganisms, including bacteria, viruses, and parasites. See **TABLE 18.1** for a list of common foodborne microbes and the serious illnesses they cause. Each year in the United States, approximately 48 million Americans (that's 1 in 6) become sick, 128,000 are hospitalized, and 3,000 die from foodborne illnesses, according to researchers at the Centers for Disease Control and Prevention (CDC).[1] Illness can range from relatively mild stomach upset to severe symptoms that can be fatal. Foodborne illnesses cost the United States about $15 billion annually.[2]

THINK About It 1

Development of foodborne illness results from the interaction of three factors: the pathogen, the host, and the environment in which they exist and

TABLE 18.1
Common Foodborne Pathogens and Illnesses

Organism	Sources	Diseases and Symptoms
Bacteria		
Campylobacter jejuni	Raw poultry and meat and unpasteurized milk 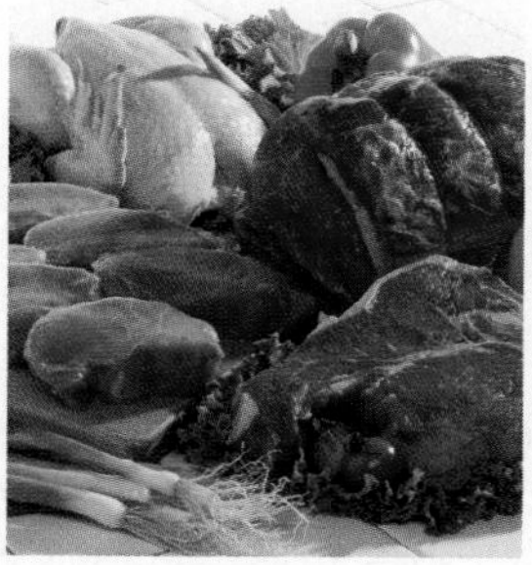 © Purestock/Getty Images	Campylobacteriosis **Onset:** usually 2 to 5 days after eating **Symptoms:** diarrhea, stomach cramps, fever, bloody stools; lasts 7 to 10 days
Clostridium botulinum—illness is caused by a toxin produced by this organism	Improperly canned foods, such as corn, green beans, soups, beets, asparagus, mushrooms, tuna, and liver pate; also, luncheon meats, ham, sausage, garlic in oil, lobster, and smoked and salted fish 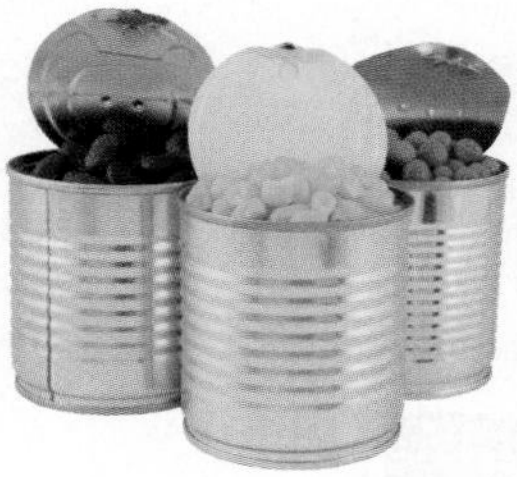 © Evlakhov Valeriy/Shutterstock	Botulism **Onset:** 18 to 36 hours after eating **Symptoms:** nerve dysfunction, such as double vision, inability to swallow, speech difficulty, and progressive paralysis of respiratory system; can lead to death
Escherichia coli 0157:H7	Raw or undercooked meat, raw vegetables, unpasteurized milk, minimally processed ciders and juices, contaminated water 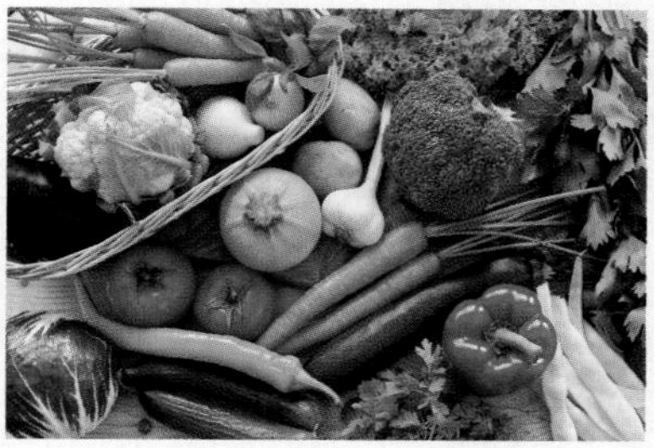 © Ana Blazic Pavlovic/Shutterstock	*E. coli* infection **Onset:** 2 to 5 days after eating **Symptoms:** watery and bloody diarrhea, severe stomach cramps, dehydration, colitis, neurological symptoms, stroke, and hemolytic uremic syndrome (HUS), a particularly serious disease in young children that can cause kidney failure and death
Listeria monocytogenes	Soft cheeses, unpasteurized milk, hot dogs, luncheon meats, cold cuts, other deli-style meat and poultry **Note:** resists salt, heat, nitrites, and acidity better than most microorganisms 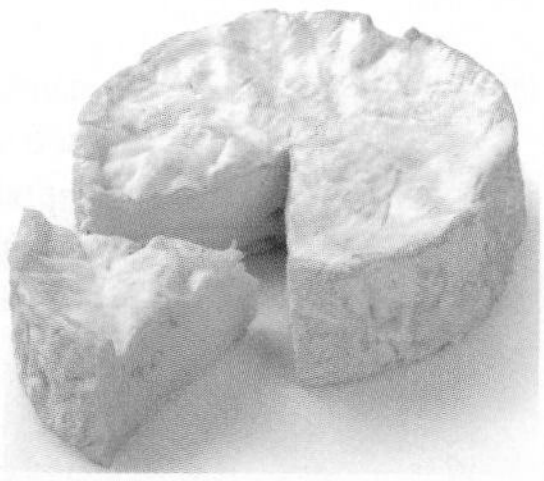 © kaband/Shutterstock	Listeriosis **Onset:** from 7 to 21 days after eating, but symptoms have been reported 9 to 48 hours after eating **Symptoms:** fever, headache, nausea, and vomiting; primarily affects pregnant women and their fetuses, newborns, older adults, and people with cancer and compromised immune systems; can cause death in fetuses and babies

(*continues*)

TABLE 18.1
Common Foodborne Pathogens and Illnesses (continued)

Organism	Sources	Diseases and Symptoms
Salmonella	Raw or undercooked meats, poultry, eggs; raw milk and other dairy products; seafood; fresh produce, including raw sprouts; coconut; pasta; chocolate; foods containing raw eggs 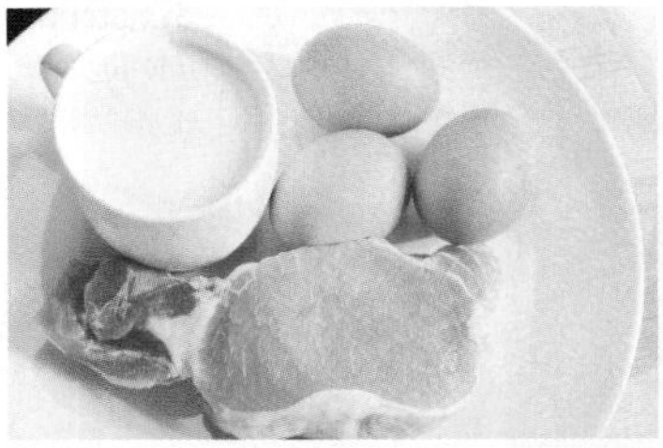 © Supattra Luasook/Shutterstock	Salmonellosis **Onset:** 1 to 3 days after eating **Symptoms:** nausea, abdominal cramps, diarrhea, fever, and headache
Shigella	Undercooked liquid or moist food that has been handled by an infected person 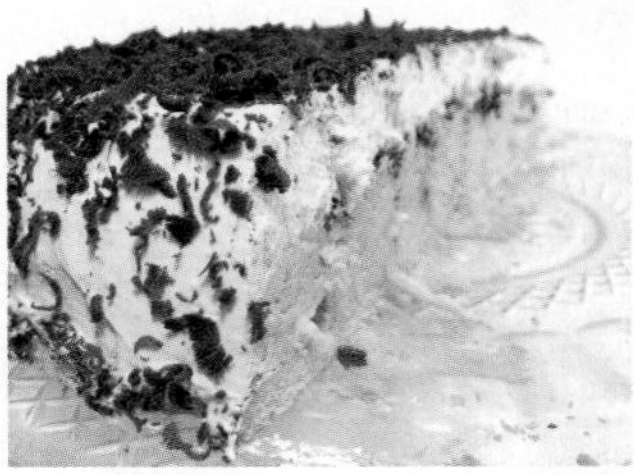 © Hirurg/Shutterstock	Shigellosis (bacillary dysentery) **Onset:** 12 to 50 hours after eating **Symptoms:** stomach cramps; diarrhea; fever; sometimes vomiting; and blood, pus, and mucus in stools
Staphylococcus aureus—illness is caused by a toxin produced by this organism	Meat and poultry; egg products; tuna, potato, and macaroni salads; cream-filled pastries and other foods left unrefrigerated for long periods **Note:** *S. aureus* is frequently found in cuts on skin and in nasal passages 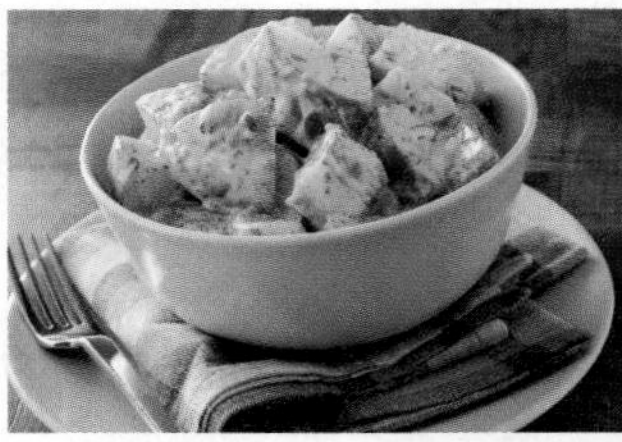 © Rohit Seth/Shutterstock	Staphylococcal food poisoning **Onset:** 1 to 6 hours after eating **Symptoms:** diarrhea, vomiting, nausea, stomach pain, and cramps; lasts 1 to 2 days
Vibrio vulnificus	Raw seafood, especially raw oysters 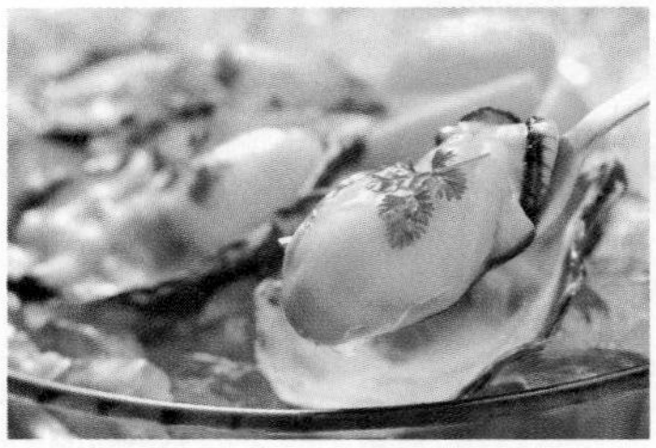 © gori910/Shutterstock	*Vibrio* infection **Onset:** 1 to 7 days **Symptoms:** chills, fever, nausea and vomiting, and possibly death, especially in people with underlying health problems
Viruses		
Hepatitis A	Raw shellfish from polluted water, food handled by an infected person 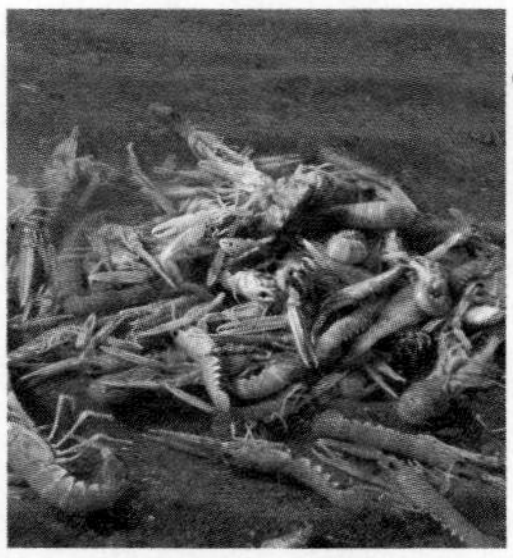 © Ewan Loughlin/iStock/Getty Images	Hepatitis A **Onset:** averages about 1 month after exposure **Symptoms:** at first, malaise, loss of appetite, nausea, vomiting, and fever; after 3 to 10 days, jaundice and darkened urine; severe cases can result in liver damage and death

TABLE 18.1
Common Foodborne Pathogens and Illnesses (continued)

Organism	Sources	Diseases and Symptoms
Noroviruses Norwalk-like virus	Raw shellfish from polluted water; salads, sandwiches, and other ready-to-eat foods handled by an infected person. Noroviruses are highly contagious and spread rapidly from person to person because of the ease of transmission by touch. 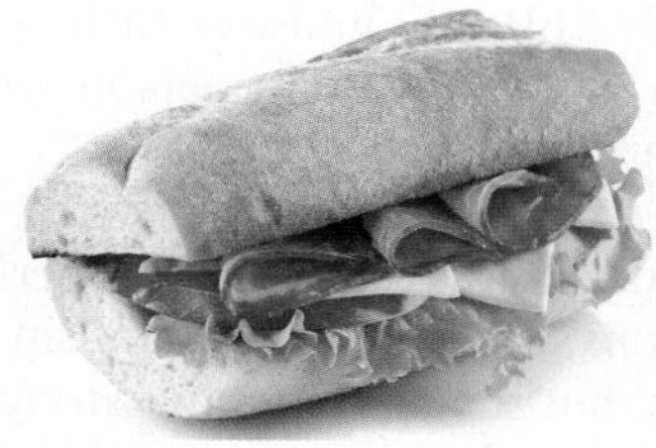 © MaraZe/Shutterstock	Gastroenteritis **Onset:** 1 to 3 days **Symptoms:** nausea, vomiting, diarrhea, stomach pain, headache, and low-grade fever
Protozoa		
Anisakis	Raw fish 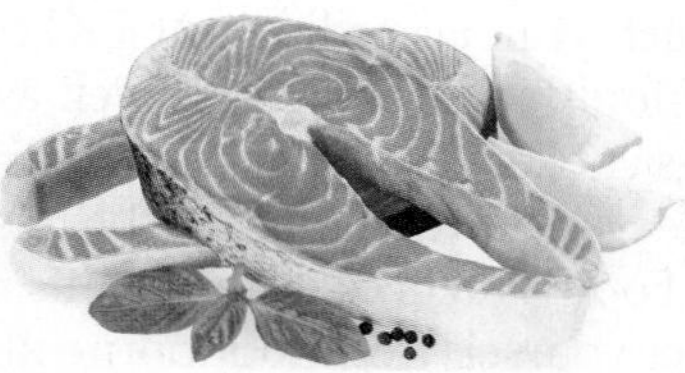 © Abramova Elena/Shutterstock	Anisakiasis **Onset:** 12 to 24 hours **Symptoms:** abdominal pain, can be severe
Cryptosporidium	Food that comes in contact with sewage-contaminated water; foods handled by a person who did not wash hands after using the toilet 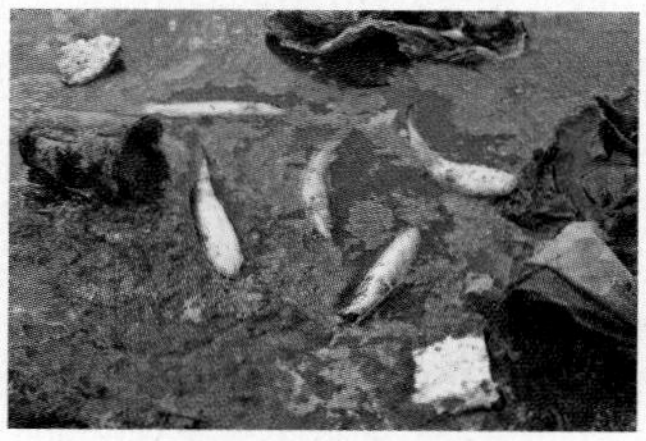 © wk1003mike/Shutterstock	Cryptosporidiosis **Onset:** 1 to 12 days **Symptoms:** profuse, watery stools, stomach pain, loss of appetite, vomiting, and low-grade fever
Giardia lamblia	Consumption of contaminated water, contamination of food by an infected person 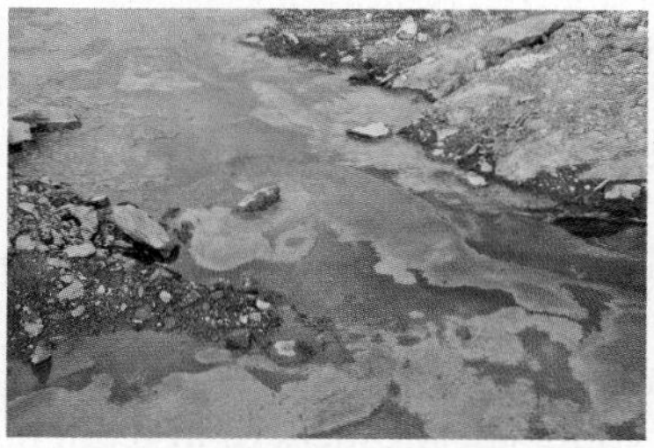 © dominique landau/Shutterstock	Giardiasis **Onset:** 1 to 3 days **Symptoms:** diarrhea, abdominal cramps, nausea
Toxoplasma gondii	Raw or undercooked meat and, under certain conditions, unwashed fruits and vegetables; also, cats shed cysts in their feces during acute infection—organism may be transmitted to humans, if feces are handled 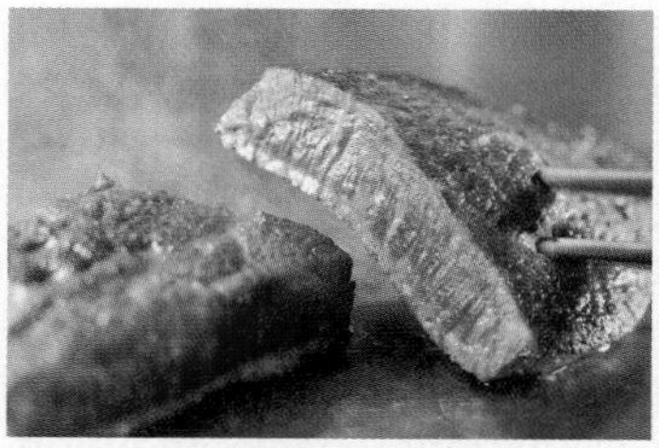 © TAGSTOCK1/Shutterstock	Toxoplasmosis **Onset:** 10 to 13 days **Symptoms:** fever, headache, rash, sore muscles, diarrhea; can kill a fetus or cause severe defects, such as mental retardation

interact.[3] Foodborne illnesses can result directly from infection with a pathogen or from toxins produced by a pathogenic microorganism. For example, the bacterium *Staphylococcus aureus*, a common bacterium found on the skin of many healthy people, creates havoc with the gastrointestinal tract by producing a toxin. When food containing *S. aureus* stands unrefrigerated, the bacteria begin multiplying. After several hours, the expanding bacterial population can produce enough of a nasty toxin to cause nausea, vomiting, and abdominal cramps. Staphylococcal food poisoning is common and causes approximately 250,000 illnesses each year.[4] Fortunately, the illness usually resolves after a day or so of a person vomiting and feeling miserable, with no further harmful effects.

▶ **botulism** An often-fatal type of food poisoning caused by a toxin released from *Clostridium botulinum*, a bacterium that can grow in improperly canned low-acid foods.

Another toxin-producing bacterium, *Clostridium botulinum*, causes the rare, but deadly, illness **botulism**. Improperly canned foods, as well as garlic-in-oil preparations, are sources of botulism. Honey can be contaminated with *C. botulinum*, but the acid in adult stomachs kills the bacteria. Infants produce insufficient amounts of stomach acid to kill botulinum, so even small amounts of contaminated honey can be fatal.

▶ ***Salmonella*** Rod-shaped bacteria responsible for many foodborne illnesses.

▶ ***Escherichia coli (E. coli)*** Bacteria that are the most common cause of urinary tract infections. Because they release toxins, some types of *E. coli* can rapidly cause shock and death.

Salmonella causes more than 1 million cases of foodborne illness and almost 400 deaths each year, according to CDC estimates.[5] *Salmonella* bacteria are prevalent on poultry and in eggs as well as in a wide variety of other foods. Choosing eggs cooked "over easy" is potentially disastrous because inadequate cooking can leave you vulnerable to the misery of salmonellosis. (See the FYI feature "Safe Food Practices" later in this chapter for more information on how to protect yourself from foodborne illness.)

Escherichia coli (E. coli) are a diverse group of bacteria. Although most varieties are harmless, others can make you sick. Some types cause diarrhea, whereas others cause more serious illnesses, even death. Many foods, including eggs, dairy products, meat and poultry, seafood, fresh produce, unpasteurized juices, and cereal grains, can harbor these disease-causing bacteria.

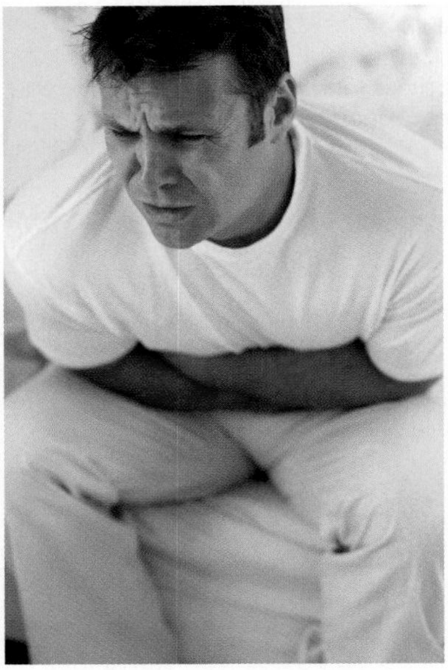
© Bananastock/Thinkstock

Because bacteria and other infectious organisms are pervasive in the environment, the contamination of food can occur anywhere from the farm to your plate. Many organisms capable of causing foodborne illness in humans are naturally present in food-producing animals and their environment. For example, *Salmonella enteritidis* bacteria enter eggs directly from the egg-laying hen, and *E. coli* are normally present in the intestines of cattle. Microorganisms natural to the marine environment, but toxic to humans, can contaminate seafood. (See the FYI feature "Seafood Safety.")

Exposure to animal manure or sewage runoff can contaminate crops. Sewage runoff into rivers and streams also can contaminate fish that live there. In the food-processing stage, contamination can occur from dirty equipment, rodent droppings, improper food storage, and infectious employees who fail to wash their hands adequately or take proper precautions when handling food. Poor food safety practices in retail facilities and at home also can contaminate food.

Patterns of foodborne illness have changed dramatically over the last several decades as our food production has become more centralized. When food animals and produce were grown, prepared, and eaten on the family farm, the consequences of errors in food handling were generally limited to a single family. Now, much of the food we eat is mass-produced at central locations and distributed widely to restaurant chains and supermarkets. Although most food poisoning cases arise from poor food handling in homes and restaurants, contamination at a processing plant can make hundreds or even thousands of people ill. This can have nationwide implications and therefore receives intense national media attention.

Quick Bite

Sticky *Salmonella*

One in six Americans suffers a foodborne illness each year. In 2013, 818 foodborne disease outbreaks resulted in 13,360 people reporting illness, 1,062 people going to the hospital, 16 people dying. What made all these people sick? The most common causes were norovirus in fruits and *Salmonella* in chicken and pork.

http://www.niaid.nih.gov/topics/foodborne/pages/default.aspx

FYI
For Your Information

Seafood Safety

Seafood can be a delicious and heart-healthy part of our diets. However, as with all food, contamination can have serious consequences. Seafood is one of the most rapidly perishable foods, so proper refrigeration and rapid processing and transport to the consumer are essential. Although certain types of microbial contaminants and toxins are unique to seafood, properly handled and cooked seafood is as safe to eat as most other foods. To kill seafood parasites, cook the fish or freeze it for at least 72 hours.

Eating raw seafood is risky business. Despite the popularity of such dishes as sashimi, sushi, and raw oysters, uncooked fish, no matter how carefully prepared, poses a risk for infection. People with liver disease, diabetes, cancer, or other diseases that impair immune function should be especially careful to stay away from raw seafood. Pregnant women also should avoid uncooked seafood; some physicians recommend that pregnant women avoid seafood altogether. The rest of us should think twice before enjoying those raw oysters and sashimi and, at the very least, should make sure they are fresh and from a reliable source before letting those slippery delicacies pass our lips.

Seafood-related illness falls into several categories (see **Table A**). Sources of infection include bacteria, viruses, and parasites. Toxins occur naturally in some fish, and human pollution can contaminate seafood. The following are several examples of seafood-caused illness:

- Raw or undercooked shellfish such as oysters, clams, and mussels can be contaminated with bacteria such as *Salmonella*, *Vibrio* species, and *Staphylococcus aureus*. Hepatitis A (caused by a virus) and gastroenteritis are other illnesses that can be contracted by eating uncooked shellfish from polluted waters.
- Fish such as mahi-mahi, tuna, and bluefish that have begun to spoil can cause scombroid poisoning. A toxin in these decomposing fish causes flushing, itching, and headache. Cooking does not destroy the toxin, so the best prevention is proper refrigeration and rapid use of fresh fish.
- Some tropical fish, such as red snapper and barracuda, might contain ciguatera toxin, which can cause gastrointestinal and neurological problems in humans. Larger warm-water fish are most often implicated in this illness. The toxin is actually produced by tiny plants that are eaten by small fish. When larger fish consume many small fish, the toxin can accumulate. The flesh of these large fish can contain enough of the toxin to make humans very ill. Heating or freezing does not destroy this toxin.
- *Anisakis* is a parasite found in raw fish. After a person eats an infected fish, the larvae of this roundworm can invade the human stomach, causing severe abdominal pain. Thoroughly cooking the fish, or freezing it for at least 72 hours, can kill this parasite.
- Red tide is a well-known phenomenon in which huge numbers of tiny, toxic organisms called dinoflagellates infest seawater. Shellfish in the area become poisonous as a result. Respiratory paralysis and death are possible effects of eating shellfish from red tide areas.
- Human pollution is a serious problem, especially near population centers where industrial wastes and human sewage flow into the water. Heavy metals such as mercury can accumulate in larger fish (e.g., sharks, swordfish) that have been exposed to mercury in their environment for long periods. The *Dietary Guidelines for Americans, 2015–2020* advises pregnant and breastfeeding women to limit white (albacore) tuna to 6 ounces per week and completely avoid eating tilefish, shark, swordfish, and king mackerel.[a]
- Dioxin and polychlorinated biphenols (PCBs) also can accumulate in fish living in polluted water. Commercial seafood companies tend to avoid contaminated areas, but local fishers who frequently catch and eat fish from these waters may be at some risk.

[a]http://health.gov/dietaryguidelines/2015/guidelines/

TABLE A
Understanding Seafood Safety

Condition	Explanation
Scombroid poisoning	Scombroid poisoning is a type of food intoxication caused by the consumption of scombroid and scombroid-like marine fish species that have begun to spoil with the growth of particular types of food bacteria. Fish most commonly involved are members of the *Scombridae* family (tunas and mackerels) and a few nonscombroid relatives (bluefish, mahi-mahi, and amberjacks). The suspect toxin is an elevated level of histamine generated by bacterial degradation of substances in the muscle protein.
Anisakis	*Anisakis simplex* (herring worm) and *Pseudoterranova* (*Phocanema*, *Terranova*) *decipiens* (cod or seal worm) are anisakid nematodes (roundworms) that have been implicated in human infections caused by the consumption of raw or undercooked seafood. *Anisakiasis* is the term generally used to refer to the acute disease in humans.
Red tide	When temperature, salinity, and nutrients reach certain levels, algae grow very fast or "bloom" and accumulate into dense, visible patches near the surface of the water. *Red tide* is a common name for such a phenomenon where certain species of phytoplankton contain reddish pigments and bloom such that the water appears to be colored red. The term *red tide* is a misnomer because the reddish color is not associated with tides. A small number of species produces potent neurotoxins that can cause illness and even death.
Polychlorinated biphenols (PCBs)	Polychlorinated biphenols are a group of toxic, persistent chemicals used as insulation for electrical transformers and capacitors and as lubricants in gas pipeline systems. PCBs are a serious health problem because of their persistence in the environment, accumulation in the body, and potential for a long-term negative effect on health. In the United States, their manufacture was stopped in 1976.

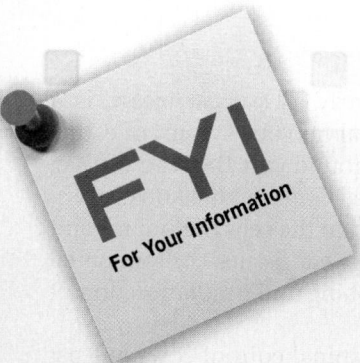

▶ **bovine spongiform encephalopathy (BSE)** A chronic degenerative disease, widely referred to as "mad cow disease," that affects the central nervous system of cattle.

▶ **mad cow disease** See *bovine spongiform encephalopathy (BSE).*

▶ **prions** Short for *proteinaceous infectious particle*. Self-reproducing protein particles that can cause disease.

Prions and Mad Cow Disease

Bovine spongiform encephalopathy (BSE), known popularly as **mad cow disease**, is a chronic degenerative disease that affects the central nervous system of cattle. Once thought to infect only cows, scientists have found that BSE can cause a rare, but fatal, brain-wasting disease in humans called Creutzfeldt-Jakob disease.

Researchers believe that **prions**—proteins found in the cells of humans and other mammals—are responsible. When mammals eat tissues contaminated with abnormal prions, they can develop BSE. Cooking and irradiation do not kill or deactivate abnormal prions.

The skull, brain, eyes, vertebral column, and spinal cord of cows at least 30 months of age are most likely to harbor abnormal prions. The tonsils and a portion of the small intestine of all cattle also can contain the agent. To protect the safety of meat, milk, and dairy products, Canadian and U.S. agencies prohibit these cow parts in the human food supply. Government agencies also regulate and provide guidance to manufacturers who produce cow-derived foods, such as gelatin and some dietary supplements.

Key Concepts Foodborne pathogens are a major cause of illness in the United States and Canada. Pathogenic (disease-causing) agents include bacteria, viruses, parasites, and prions. Contamination of food can occur at many points along the chain from farm to table.

▶ **organic foods** Foods that originate from farms or handling operations that meet the standards set by the USDA National Organic Program.

Chemical Contamination

To avoid foods exposed to chemicals, more and more people are turning to **organic foods**. (See the section "Organic Alternatives" later in this chapter.) Yet food safety experts consider contamination by pathogenic microorganisms to be a much greater risk to public health than contamination by chemicals. Chemical contaminants include pesticides, drugs, pollutants, and natural toxins.

▶ **pesticides** Chemicals used to control insects, diseases, weeds, fungi, and other pests on plants, vegetables, fruits, and animals.

Pesticides **Pesticides** play an important role in food production—controlling plant diseases, weeds, insects, and other pests. Pesticides protect crops and ensure a substantial yield, thus ensuring that consumers have a wide variety of foods at affordable prices. Without these chemicals, many argue that crop production would fall and prices for food would rise.

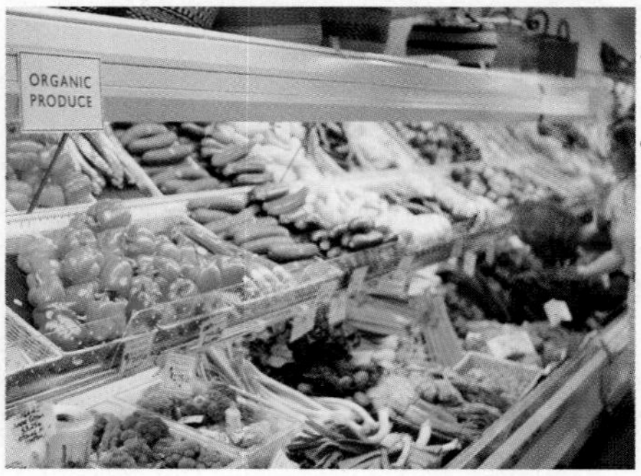

© Jupiterimages/Creatas/Thinkstock

Every year, the U.S. Food and Drug Administration (FDA) collects thousands of domestic and imported food samples and analyzes them for pesticide residues.[6] Nearly two-thirds of the produce samples tested by the U.S. Department of Agriculture (USDA) in 2013 contained pesticide residues; however, according to the USDA, the levels were not high enough to pose a safety concern.[7] The FDA also samples and analyzes domestic and imported animal feeds for pesticide residues. This monitoring focuses on feeds for livestock and poultry—animals that become or produce foods for human consumption. Processing methods can either reduce or concentrate pesticide residues in foods (see **FIGURE 18.2**). Despite these results that reassure consumers about low pesticide residues, concerns about pesticides in food persist. According to a 2014 survey by *Consumer Reports*' Food Safety and Sustainability Center, 85 percent of Americans worry about pesticide exposure in food.[8]

Infants and young children are particularly susceptible to the hazards of pesticides. Their small size and rapid growth make them especially vulnerable to pesticide residues, which can accumulate in their bodies over their lifetimes. Enacted in 1996, the Food Quality Protection Act includes landmark protections for the young. For the first time, manufacturers had to show that pesticide levels are safe for infants and children. In addition, when determining a safe level for a pesticide in a food, the U.S. Environmental Protection

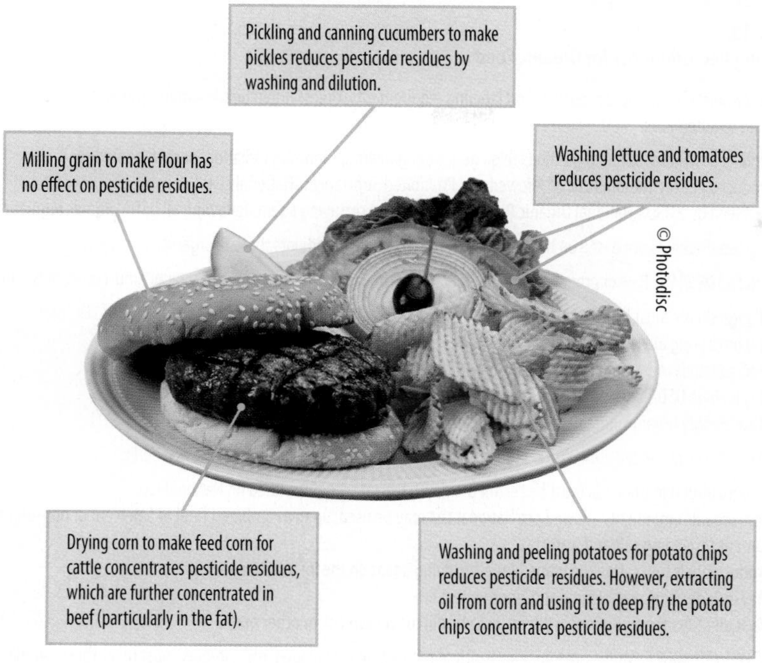

Pickling and canning cucumbers to make pickles reduces pesticide residues by washing and dilution.
Milling grain to make flour has no effect on pesticide residues.
Washing lettuce and tomatoes reduces pesticide residues.
© Photodisc
Drying corn to make feed corn for cattle concentrates pesticide residues, which are further concentrated in beef (particularly in the fat).
Washing and peeling potatoes for potato chips reduces pesticide residues. However, extracting oil from corn and using it to deep fry the potato chips concentrates pesticide residues.

FIGURE 18.2 Pesticide pathways to dinner. Food processing and preparation methods can either reduce or concentrate pesticide residues in foods.

Agency (EPA) must account for the cumulative effect of exposures to similar pesticides and toxic chemicals.[9]

Excessive use of synthetic pesticides, herbicides, and fertilizers contributes substantially to the pollution of soil and water. Overuse can be particularly hazardous to farm workers, whose exposure to these chemicals typically is much higher than that of consumers. Overuse also threatens wildlife. Today, many farmers use **integrated pest management (IPM)** to reduce pesticide use (see **FIGURE 18.3**). IPM methods include crop rotation, use of natural rather than synthetic pesticides, and planting nonfood crops nearby that lure pests away from food crops. Releasing sterile fruit flies into orchards also allows reductions in pesticide use. Because fruit flies produce no offspring when they mate with sterile partners, the overall fruit fly population drops.

Organic Alternatives Organic foods are grown or produced without most synthetic pesticides and without synthetic fertilizers. In the United States, growth of the organic food industry can be seen in the expanding number of retailers offering a variety of organic foods and the widespread introduction of new organic products.[10] In 2013, sales of organic foods exceeded $35 billion, and they continue to grow.[11] Growth of the industry reflects, in part, America's distrust of technology and a desire to return to a simpler, more "natural" way of food production.

The Organic Foods Production Act and the National Organic Program (NOP) are intended to assure U.S. consumers that the organic foods they purchase are produced, processed, and certified to consistent national standards. The labeling requirements of this program apply to raw meats, fresh produce, and processed foods that contain organic ingredients. Foods that are sold, labeled, or represented as organic must be produced and processed in accordance with the NOP standards.[12] **TABLE 18.2** outlines the requirements for labeling a food product as being organic.

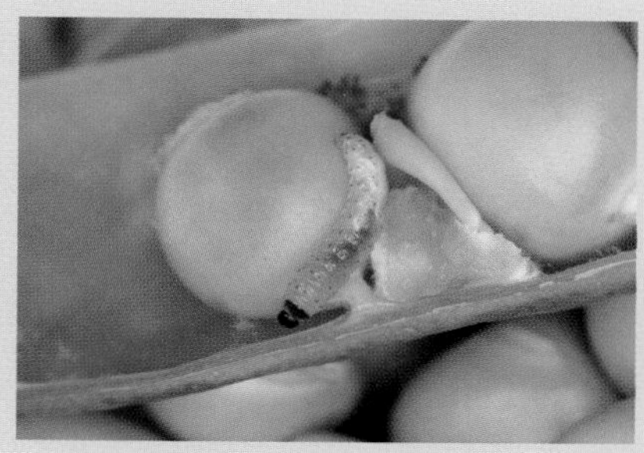

1. **Legal control**
   State and federal guidelines are designed to limit the spread of pests.
2. **Biological control**
   Beneficial organisms, such as predators, parasites, and viruses, are released into the environment to suppress pest organisms.
3. **Cultural control**
   Rotation, sanitation, and other good farming techniques are employed to help reduce pest populations.
4. **Physical control**
   Barriers, traps, and the location and timing of planting are all used to control pest infestations.
5. **Genetic control**
   Resistant plant strains are developed to reduce the impact of pests.
6. **Chemical control**
   Conventional pesticides, biopesticides, pheromones, and other chemicals are used to prevent or suppress pest outbreaks. The chemical controls are specific to a pest species and are ideally short-lived in the environment. In addition, the chemicals are used at their lowest effective rate and may be alternated to help prevent the development of pest resistance.

FIGURE 18.3 Integrated pest management. Integrated pest management is a sustainable approach that combines prevention, avoidance, monitoring, and suppression strategies in a way that minimizes economic, health, and environmental risks. It minimizes pesticide use and promotes economically sound practices.

▶ **integrated pest management (IPM)** Economically sound pest control techniques that minimize pesticide use, enhance environmental stewardship, and promote sustainable systems.

Quick Bite

How Many *Salmonella* Does It Take?

In 1994, 224,000 people in 41 states came down with *Salmonella* food poisoning from eating contaminated ice cream. The amazing part? The ice cream contained only about six *Salmonella* bacteria per serving.

TABLE 18.2
Labeling Requirements for Organic Food

Organic products have strict production and labeling requirements. Unless noted below, organic products must meet the following requirements:

- Produced without excluded methods (e.g., genetic engineering), ionizing radiation, or sewage sludge
- Produced per the National List of Allowed and Prohibited Substances (National List)
- Overseen by a USDA National Organic Program–authorized certifying agent, following all USDA organic regulations

Labeling requirements are based on the percentage of a product's ingredients that are organic.

100 PERCENT ORGANIC: Raw or processed agricultural products in the "100 percent organic" category must meet these criteria:

- All ingredients must be certified organic.
- Any processing aids must be organic.
- Product labels must state the name of the certifying agent on the information panel.
- May include USDA organic seal and/or 100 percent organic claim.
- Must identify organic ingredients (e.g., organic dill) or via asterisk or other mark.

ORGANIC: Raw or processed agricultural products in the "organic" category must meet these criteria:

- All agricultural ingredients must be certified organic, except where specified on National List.
- Non-organic ingredients allowed per National List may be used, up to a combined total of 5 percent of non-organic content (excluding salt and water).
- Product labels must state the name of the certifying agent on the information panel.
- May include USDA organic seal and/or organic claim.
- Must identify organic ingredients (e.g., organic dill) or via asterisk or other mark.

"MADE WITH" ORGANIC: Multi-ingredient agricultural products in the "made with" category must meet these criteria:

- At least 70 percent of the product must be certified organic ingredients (excluding salt and water).
  - Any remaining agricultural products are not required to be organically produced but must be produced without excluded methods.
  - Non-agricultural products must be specifically allowed on the National List.
- Product labels must state the name of the certifying agent on the information panel.
- May state "made with organic (insert up to three ingredients or ingredient categories)." Must not include USDA organic seal anywhere, represent finished product as organic, or state "made with organic ingredients."
- Must identify organic ingredients (e.g., organic dill) or via asterisk or other mark.

SPECIFIC ORGANIC INGREDIENTS: Multi-ingredient products with less than 70 percent certified organic content (excluding salt and water) don't need to be certified. Any non-certified product:

- Must not include USDA organic seal anywhere or the word "organic" on principal display panel.
- May only list certified organic ingredients as organic in the ingredient list and the percentage of organic ingredients. Remaining ingredients are not required to follow the USDA organic regulations.

USDA National Organic Program, Agricultural Marketing Service. Labeling organic products. October 2012. http://www.ams.usda.gov/AMSv1.0/getfile?dDocName=STELDEV3004446. Accessed June 2, 2014.

Quick Bite

A Not So Dirty Dozen

The Environmental Working Group (EWG), an environmental advocacy organization, publishes an annual list of the "Dirty Dozen"—fruits and vegetables suspected of having the greatest potential for contamination with pesticide residues. According to UC Davis researchers, however, "findings conclusively demonstrate that consumer exposures to the ten most frequently detected pesticides on EWG's 'Dirty Dozen' commodity list are at negligible levels and that the EWG methodology is insufficient to allow any meaningful rankings among commodities."

Quick Bite

Is It Stomach Flu or Food Poisoning?

Both can have similar symptoms—miserable vomiting, abdominal cramping, and diarrhea. Although we often do not know the exact cause, stomach flu tends to occur in the winter months and is preceded by other symptoms, such as sore throat. Food poisoning tends to occur in summer months, and symptoms usually appear suddenly without warning. Symptoms may not begin until 12 to 72 hours after eating tainted food. If many people who ate the same food get sick around the same time, it's probably food poisoning.

Under the NOP, farm and processing operations that grow and process organic foods must be certified by the USDA. The certification process includes an on-site inspection to verify that the applicant's operation complies with strict national organic standards. Certifying agents may collect and test soil, water, waste, plant and animal tissues, and processed products. A certified operation may label its products or ingredients as organic and may use the "USDA Organic" seal.[13]

Organic farming has its drawbacks. The use of manure as a natural fertilizer raises food safety concerns. The organic producer must manage animal and plant waste materials so they do not contribute to contamination of crops, soil, or water. Manure runoff can pollute nearby lakes and streams. Some critics charge that organic farming is "elitist" and that synthetic fertilizers and pesticides are necessary to meet the food needs of an expanding world population. They also point out that complete freedom from pesticides cannot be guaranteed, no matter how carefully a food is produced, because pesticide residues may still exist in soil, water, and air.

Organic foods are not pesticide-free foods. Organic farmers can use natural and approved synthetic pesticides to control weeds and insects.[14,15] A 2012 audit by the USDA's National Organic Program revealed that 43 percent of organic produce had some degree of prohibited pesticides.[16] Microbial contaminants that cause foodborne illness can be found in organic as well as conventional foods. Consumers must handle all food appropriately, whether organically or conventionally grown.

THINK About It 2

Courtesy of the USDA

Animal Drugs Current agricultural practice depends heavily on the use of drugs in food animals and food-producing animals raised specifically to provide meat, milk, and eggs. Producers use drugs to maintain animal health and well-being as well as to increase production. Keeping animals in good health reduces the chance that disease will spread from animals to humans, and healthy animals can use nutrients for growth and production rather than to fight infection. But there is a possibility that drugs used in animals could enter human food and possibly increase the risk of ill health in humans.

There are five major classes of drugs used in animals raised for food.[17]

1. Topical antiseptics, bactericides, and fungicides used to treat skin or hoof infections, cuts, and abrasions
2. Ionophores, which are feed additives that alter stomach microorganisms to more efficiently digest feeds and to help protect against some parasites
3. Hormone and hormone-like production enhancers (anabolic hormones for meat production and bovine somatotropin for increased milk production in dairy cows)
4. Antiparasitics
5. Antibiotics used to prevent infections, treat disease, and promote growth

Can drugs used to raise animals for food affect your health? The FDA is responsible for ensuring that drugs approved for use in animals are safe not only for the animals, but also for humans who eat food produced from the animals. Because antibiotics used in both humans and animals contribute to the development of antimicrobial resistance, in 2013 the FDA implemented a voluntary plan working with industry to phase out the use of certain antibiotics for enhanced food production in farm animals.[18] The FDA recommends that use of medically important antimicrobial drugs in food-producing animals be limited to situations where the use of these drugs is necessary for ensuring animal health, and their use includes veterinary oversight or consultation.

Pollutants **Pollutants** from animal manure and other wastes, factories, human sewage, and industrial runoff can contaminate food-production areas. For example, some scientists theorize that dioxin contamination of foods can cause human cancer. **Dioxins** are chemical compounds created in the manufacturing, combustion, and chlorine bleaching of pulp and paper and in other industrial processes.[19] Dioxins can accumulate in the food chain and are potent animal carcinogens.[20]

Mercury occurs both naturally in the environment and is produced by human activities. It is soluble in water, where bacteria can cause chemical changes that transform mercury to **methylmercury**, a more toxic form. Fish absorb methylmercury from water passing over their gills and by eating other contaminated aquatic species. Larger predatory fish can consume many contaminated smaller fish, thereby accumulating higher levels of methylmercury (see **FIGURE 18.4**). Although women seem to be making more informed seafood choices, shark, swordfish, king mackerel, and tilefish contain high levels of mercury, and therefore the FDA and EPA continue to recommend that women who may become pregnant, pregnant women, nursing mothers, and young children avoid eating these fish.[21] In addition, the *Dietary Guidelines for Americans, 2015–2020* recommends that women who are pregnant or breastfeeding also limit white (albacore) tuna to 6 ounces per week because it is higher in methylmercury.[22]

▶ **pollutants** Gaseous, chemical, or organic waste that contaminates air, soil, or water.

▶ **dioxins** Chemical compounds created in the manufacturing, combustion, and chlorine bleaching of pulp and paper and in other industrial processes.

▶ **methylmercury** A toxic compound that results from the chemical transformation of mercury by bacteria. Mercury is water-soluble in trace amounts and contaminates many bodies of water.

Quick Bite

Well-Traveled Dioxin

In Nunavut, a Canadian province, the breast milk of native Inuits has twice the average concentration of dioxin as does the milk of women in southern Quebec. Native Inuits primarily eat fatty animals high on the food chain. These animals accumulate dioxin, but where did the dioxin originate? Not Canada. Carried by the wind, most comes from industrial combustion in the eastern and midwestern United States, and some originates as far away as Mexico.

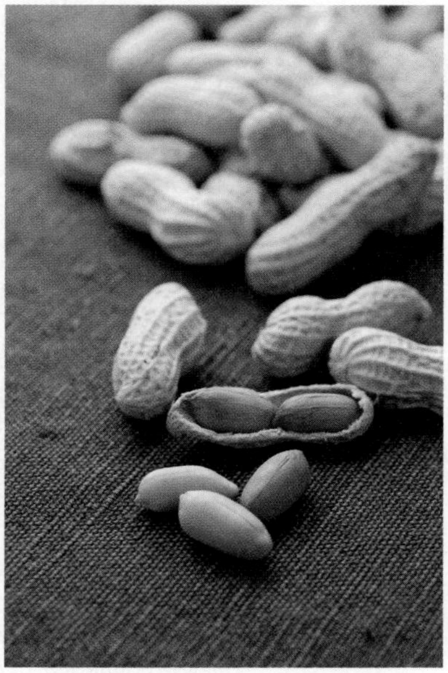

© matin/ShutterStock, Inc.

▶ **natural toxins** Poisons that are produced by or naturally occur in plants or microorganisms.

▶ **aflatoxins** A toxin produced by a mold that grows on crops, such as peanuts, tree nuts, corn, wheat, and oil seeds (like cottonseed).

▶ **ciguatera** A toxin found in more than 300 species of Caribbean and South Pacific fish. It is a nonbacterial source of food poisoning.

▶ **poisonous mushrooms** Mushrooms that contain toxins that can cause stomach upset, dizziness, hallucinations, and other neurological symptoms.

▶ **solanine** A potentially toxic alkaloid that is present with chlorophyll in the green areas on potato skins.

Natural Toxins Other chemical contamination of food can occur from **natural toxins**. Examples include the following:

- **Aflatoxins**, found in contaminated food or animal feed. Aflatoxins are produced by certain strains of *Aspergillus* fungi under certain conditions of temperature and humidity. The most pronounced contamination has been found in tree nuts, peanuts, and other oilseeds, such as corn and cottonseed.
- **Ciguatera** and other marine toxins. These toxins can accumulate in seafood (mainly in large tropical fish) and, when ingested, cause serious problems, including paralysis, amnesia, and nerve toxicity. Cooking does not destroy these toxins.
- **Poisonous mushrooms**. These plants produce toxic substances that can cause stomach upset, dizziness, hallucinations, and other neurological symptoms. The more lethal mushroom species can cause liver and kidney failure, coma, and death.
- **Solanine**, a toxic substance in raw potato skins. Solanine develops in the greenish layer of improperly stored potatoes. It can be removed by thoroughly peeling the potato.

A variety of compounds in herbs and spices also can be toxic. However, foodborne illness caused by these and other natural toxins is relatively rare compared with illness from pathogenic microorganisms.

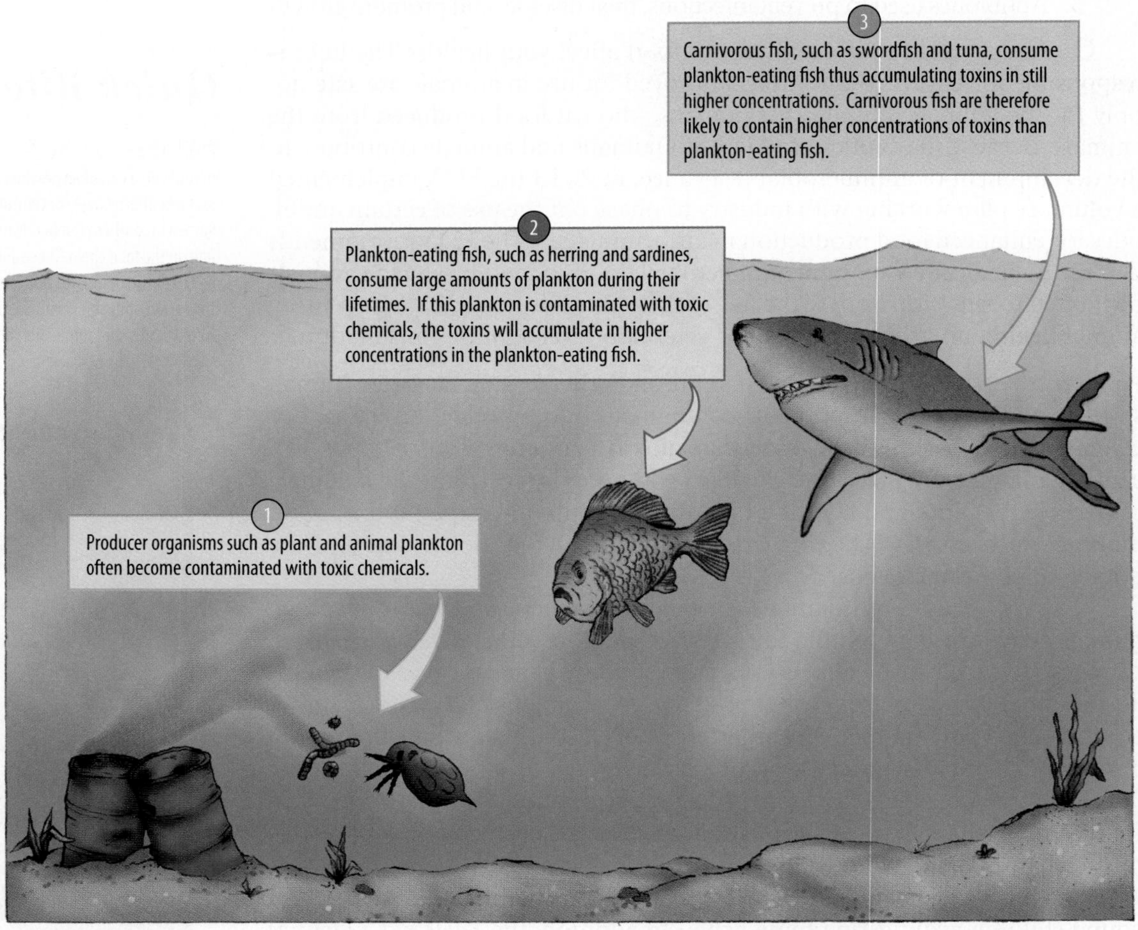

3
Carnivorous fish, such as swordfish and tuna, consume plankton-eating fish thus accumulating toxins in still higher concentrations. Carnivorous fish are therefore likely to contain higher concentrations of toxins than plankton-eating fish.
2
Plankton-eating fish, such as herring and sardines, consume large amounts of plankton during their lifetimes. If this plankton is contaminated with toxic chemicals, the toxins will accumulate in higher concentrations in the plankton-eating fish.
1
Producer organisms such as plant and animal plankton often become contaminated with toxic chemicals.

FIGURE 18.4 Toxins in the food chain. As toxins travel up the food chain, they become concentrated in larger fish. The longer a fish lives, the higher the level of toxins it will accumulate.

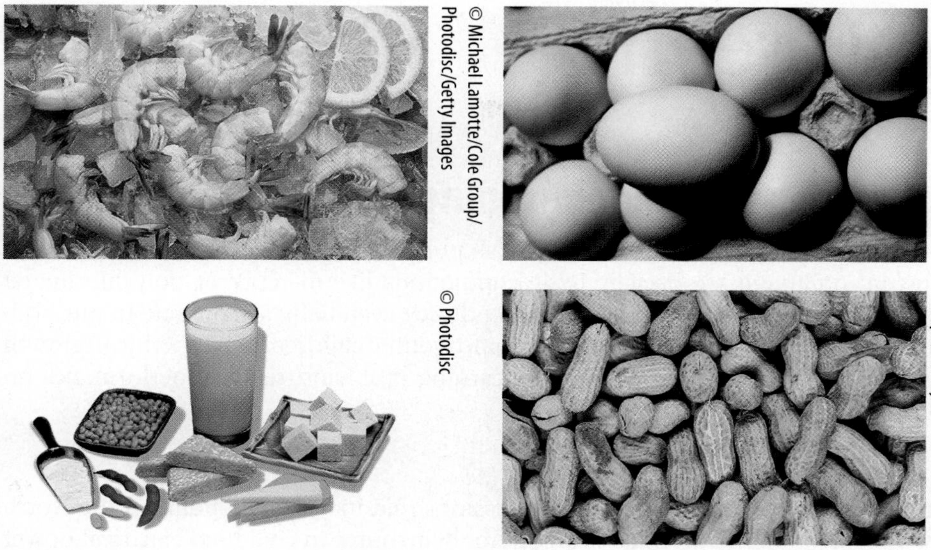

© Michael Lamotte/Cole Group/Photodisc/Getty Images

© Photodisc

© Photodisc

© LiquidLibrary

FIGURE 18.5 Foods that commonly cause allergic reactions. In sensitive people, an allergic reaction to food can be life threatening.

Other Food Contaminants In the United States, about 2 percent of adults and 5 percent of infants and young children (nearly 11 million people) have food allergies. Eight major foods or food groups—milk, eggs, fish, shellfish, tree nuts, peanuts, wheat, and soybeans—account for 90 percent of allergic reactions (see **FIGURE 18.5**). Whenever these foods (or ingredients derived from them) are present in a food product, food labels must identify them.[23] In an allergic person, these foods can cause a variety of reactions, including gastrointestinal problems, skin irritation, breathing difficulty, shock, and even death.

Contaminants, such as glass, metal, and other objects, can be introduced unintentionally during food production. Improper use of cleaning agents in food-contact areas can add these undesirable substances to food. Insects, dirt, and other undesirable items, although generally not a health hazard, also can find their way into food.

Key Concepts Chemical contaminants in foods include pesticides, natural toxins, and contamination related to pollution. Although organic foods are grown without synthetic pesticides or fertilizers, they still can contain chemical contaminants. Other potential food hazards are allergens and nonfood contaminants.

Keeping Food Safe

Having safe foods to eat requires the efforts of a great many people along the way from the farm to your plate. Imagine yourself enjoying a piece of broiled chicken. Consider that harmful contamination of that chicken could have occurred at the farm, in the processing plant, or during transportation to the supermarket. Once at the supermarket, the chicken might have been underrefrigerated or kept too long before being sold. After buying the chicken, you might have left it in a warm car or kept it in a refrigerator that was not cold enough. Your kitchen hygiene might not have been the best; finally, you could have undercooked the chicken. Considering the many opportunities for contamination, it is truly amazing that most of the time our food does not make us sick.

Keeping foods free from contamination is a job that falls to many parties. It is the responsibility not only of government officials at the national, state, and local levels, but also of everyone who comes in contact with food—the producer, the manufacturer, the retailer, and ultimately, the consumer.

Quick Bite

Chill Out!

In 1939, Fred McKinley Jones, a prolific African-American inventor, and Joe Numero received a patent for a vehicle refrigeration device for large trucks. Their invention eliminated the problem of food spoilage during long shipping times and permitted year-round delivery of fresh produce across the country. Refrigerated shipping launched international markets for food; helped create new industries such as frozen foods, fast foods, and container shipping; and forever altered consumers' eating habits.

Going Green

Ocean Pollution and Mercury Poisoning

Humans suffer, of course, when ocean pollution reduces fish populations or stains the pristine nature of beach recreation. Industrial pollutants—especially toxic compounds like mercury or polychlorinated biphenyls (PCBs)—that end up in water bodies are absorbed by fish we eat, and they eventually accumulate in our bodies. Mercury exposure is especially dangerous to fetuses, newborn infants, and young children during critical growth phases when the brain and other organs are rapidly developing. It leads to learning problems, reduced performance on intelligence tests, and other health problems later in life.

Source of Mercury Emissions

Studies in 2009 and then in 2013 identified escalating mercury-laden air emissions that increasingly polluted the North Pacific Ocean and contaminated tuna, swordfish, and other popular seafood, to their source in coal-fired electrical power plants in Asia.[a] The emissions transform into methylmercury, a potent neurotoxin, and enter long-range eastward transport by large ocean circulation currents. A 2013 treaty, the Minamata Convention on Mercury, calls for a substantial reduction in marine predator mercury levels just to keep levels where they are currently, which is higher than recommended for consumption. This sort of reduction is predicted to be unlikely, so the human health concern remains ongoing.[b]

EPA Declares "Major Health Threat"

The implications of the mercury cycle for human health are grave. According to the U.S. Geological Survey, more than 90 percent of human methylmercury exposure in the United States can be attributed to consumption of ocean fish and shellfish. Pacific tuna consumption accounts for 40 percent of Americans' exposure, and the EPA is suggesting new diplomatic efforts to persuade Asian nations "to significantly cut mercury pollution in the years ahead and protect the health of millions of people." There are still those who argue that the benefits of eating mercury-tainted seafood might outweigh the risks. In recent years, however, the EPA and the FDA have issued more-specific recommendations about population subgroups that should limit their fish consumption and which low-mercury fish people can eat in place of species that tend to have elevated mercury levels such as tuna and swordfish.

[a]McLendon R. Mercury will rise in Pacific fish, study finds. Mother Nature Network. August 2013. http://www.mnn.com/food/healthy-eating/blogs/mercury-will-rise-in-pacific-fish-study-finds. Accessed February 16, 2016.

[b]McKinney MA, Dean K, Hussey NE, et al. Global versus local causes and health implications of high mercury concentrations in sharks from the east coast of South Africa. *Sci Total Environ.* 2016;541:176–183.

Government Agencies

The basis of modern U.S. food law is the Federal Food, Drug, and Cosmetic (FD&C) Act of 1938, which gives the Food and Drug Administration authority over food and food ingredients and defines requirements for truthful labeling of ingredients.

To update and reform the food safety system in the United States, the FDA Food Safety Modernization Act (FSMA) was signed into law on January 4, 2011. The primary objective of FSMA is to ensure that the U.S. food supply is safe by enabling the FDA to increase its focus on prevention of food safety problems rather than primarily reacting after problems occur. Under the new law, the FDA has higher authority to enforce compliance with prevention- and risk-based food safety standards and to better respond to and contain problems when they do occur. The law also enables the FDA to better ensure the safety of imported foods and build an integrated national food safety system in partnership with state and local authorities.[24] In late 2011, the FDA launched the Coordinated Outbreak Response and Evaluation

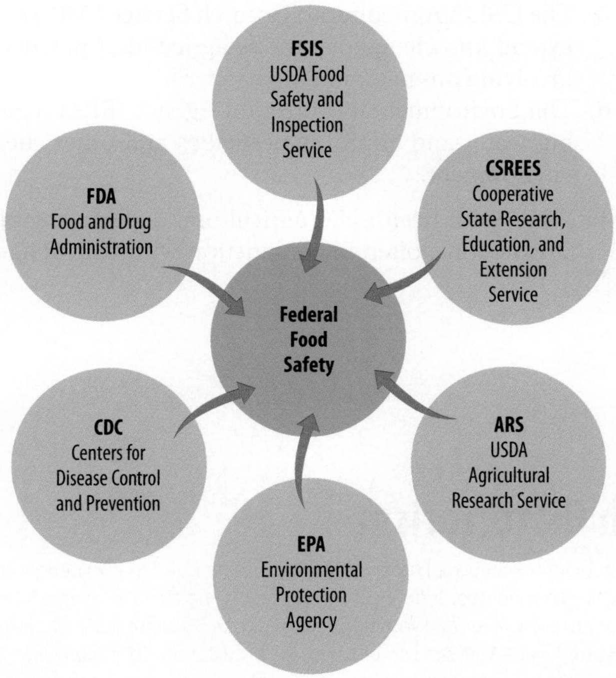

Other Agencies with Food Safety Responsibilities

Federal Trade Commission (FTC)

- Regulates the advertising and marketing of food products.
- Has the authority to take legal action against unwarranted advertising claims.

Department of Justice

- Seizes products when federal food safety laws are violated.
- Prosecutes suspected violators of food safety laws.

Bureau of Alcohol, Tobacco, and Firearms (BATF)

- Enforces laws that involve the production, distribution, and labeling of most alcoholic beverages.
- Sometimes shares responsibilities with FDA when alcoholic beverages are adulterated or contain food or color additives, pesticides, or contaminants.

National Marine Fisheries Service (NMFS)

- Responsible for seafood quality and identification, fisheries management and development, habitat conservation, and aquaculture production.

State and Local Governments

- Inspect restaurants, retail food outlets, dairies, grain mills, and other food establishments within their areas of jurisdiction.
- Embargo illegal food products in many situations.

FIGURE 18.6 Government agencies that help protect our food supply. Although the FDA has primary responsibility for the safety of much of our food supply, many government agencies provide oversight.

(CORE) Network to strengthen and streamline its efforts to prevent, investigate, and control outbreaks of foodborne illnesses.

At the federal level, six agencies (see **FIGURE 18.6**) share responsibility for food safety.

1. The Food and Drug Administration (FDA) enforces laws governing the safety of domestic and imported food, except meat and poultry.
2. The Centers for Disease Control and Prevention (CDC) monitors outbreaks of foodborne diseases, investigates their causes, and determines proper prevention.
3. The USDA Food Safety and Inspection Service (FSIS) enforces laws governing the safety of domestic and imported meat and poultry products.
4. The USDA Cooperative State Research, Education, and Extension Service (CSREES) develops research and education programs on food safety for farmers and consumers.

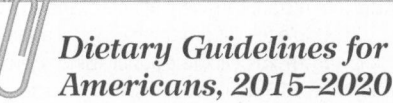

Dietary Guidelines for Americans, 2015–2020

Key Recommendations for Building Healthy Eating Patterns

- Follow food safety recommendations when preparing and eating foods to reduce the risk of foodborne illnesses.
- Four basic food safety principles work together to reduce the risk of foodborne illness:
  1. *Clean* hands, food contact surfaces, and vegetables and fruit.
  2. *Separate* raw, cooked, and ready-to-eat foods while shopping, storing, and preparing foods.
  3. *Cook* foods to a safe temperature to kill microorganisms.
  4. *Chill* (refrigerate) perishable food promptly.
- *Women who are pregnant or breastfeeding.* Due to their high methylmercury content, limit white (albacore) tuna to 6 ounces per week and do not eat the following four types of fish: tilefish, shark, swordfish, and king mackerel.

Reproduced from U.S. Department of Agriculture and U.S. Department of Health and Human Services. *Dietary Guidelines for Americans, 2015–2020.* 8th ed. Washington, DC: U.S. Government Printing Office; December 2015.

5. The USDA Agricultural Research Service (ARS) conducts research to extend knowledge of various agricultural practices, including those involving animal and crop safety.
6. The Environmental Protection Agency (EPA) regulates public drinking water and approves pesticides and other chemicals used in the environment.

State and local health and agricultural departments oversee food safety in their jurisdictions, often in conjunction with federal agencies.

FYI For Your Information

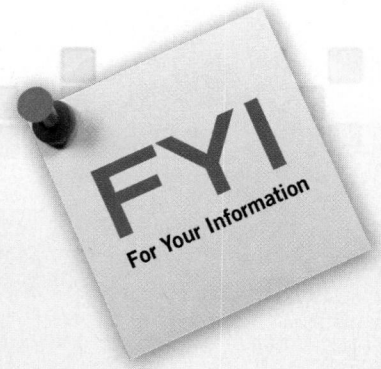

At War with Bioterrorism

Late one afternoon, restaurant owner Dave Lutgens first felt nauseated, and then experienced mild stomach cramps. By evening he was dizzy and disoriented. Suffering from diarrhea, he had to crawl to reach the toilet. Weak and dehydrated, he was wracked with chills, fever, and vomiting. Two days later his wife became ill with the same symptoms. By the end of the week, 13 employees were sick as well as dozens of customers. The culprit was *Salmonella typhimurium*, a rod-shaped bacterium responsible for many foodborne illnesses. But this was not a simple case of food poisoning. Occurring in 1984, this was a criminal assault on the small Oregon town of Dalles. The Rajaneesh religious cult attempted to sway local election results by poisoning people to keep them away from the polls. The cult deliberately perpetrated this terrifying food experience by contaminating a number of self-service salad bars and coffee creamers with home-grown *Salmonella*. Ten restaurants were affected, and more than 700 people fell ill from the biological attack.

Bioterrorism is a deliberate attack using agents typically found in nature, such as viruses, bacteria, or other germs, to cause illness or death.[a] Biological agents can be spread through food or water and could be used by terrorists because they can be difficult to detect and might not cause illness for hours or days.[b] Biocriminals have also struck in Canada. In 1970, four students in Montreal, Quebec, were admitted to the hospital after eating eggs inoculated with a parasitic nematode, *Ascaris suum*. They had signs of a parasitic infection and suffered from asthma and other lung problems. In 2000, 27 people suffered food poisoning after drinking coffee from a single vending machine at Lavalle University in Quebec City. The coffee had been laced with arsenic. In 2003, arsenic-laced coffee also poisoned more than a dozen people after a church service in New Sweden, Maine. One person died.

After September 11, 2001, food bioterrorism received a surge of attention, and efforts focused on protecting against a large-scale terrorist attack on the nation's food or water supply.[c]

Food and water poisonings can be divided into three categories[d]:

1. *Bioterrorism and biowarfare:* Terrorist acts by state-sponsored organizations or hate groups. Few such events have occurred to date.
2. *Biocrime:* Intent to harm for personal gain or revenge. A few dozen events have occurred during recent decades.
3. *Biomisfortune:* Naturally occurring foodborne disease. Virtually all foodborne disease falls into this category, which is a daily concern for public health agencies everywhere.

Americans enjoy one of the safest food supplies in the world; however, our food supply is an obvious route for the delivery of certain chemical and biological agents. Food production and distribution form a complex system not protected easily from the deliberate introduction of toxic agents. The attacks on the World Trade Center and Pentagon and the anthrax assaults increased the concern and vigilance of the U.S. and Canadian governments, which are acutely aware that public food and water supplies are among the most vulnerable avenues for terrorist attacks.

At ports of entry, food inspection facilities, and research labs and buildings, government personnel are at a heightened state of alert. To prevent the entry of animal or plant pests and diseases, product and cargo inspections of travelers and baggage are intensified. Food safety inspectors have been given a mandate to be alert to any irregularities at food-processing facilities. Within processing facilities, specific plans for security should be developed to reduce the risk of tampering and other malicious, criminal, or terrorist actions. Employees FIRST is an initiative from the FDA designed to educate food industry workers about the risk of intentional food contamination and identify actions to reduce risk (see **TABLE A**).[e]

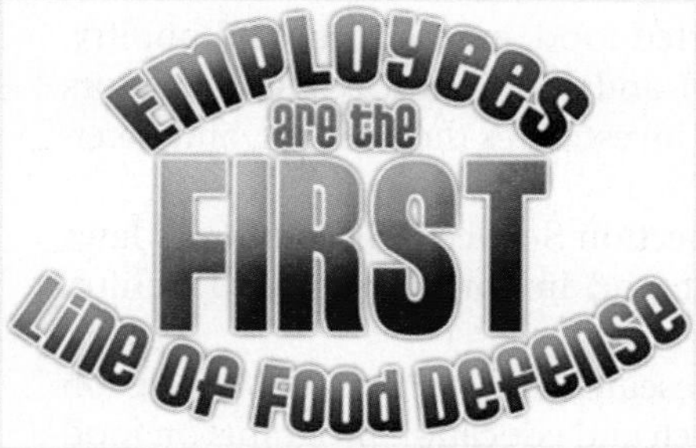

Courtesy of the U.S. Food and Drug Administration.

The Public Health Security and Bioterrorism Preparedness and Response Act of 2002 (called the Bioterrorism Act) mandated that the FDA take numerous steps to protect the safety and security of the food and drug supply. Since then, the FDA has developed additional food safety regulations, increased domestic and foreign surveillance, and continued to work toward reducing threats and vulnerabilities. To protect the nation's food supply from both unintentional contamination and deliberate attack, the Food Protection Plan (2007) was developed by the FDA to address changes in food sources, production, and consumption as a strategy.[f] The Food Protection Plan focuses on the three main areas of prevention using risk-based interventions and rapid responses to contaminated foods or animal feeds.

The FDA's ALERT tool is intended to raise food defense awareness of state and local government agencies and industry representatives in the farm-to-table supply chain. ALERT identifies five key points to decrease the risk of intentional food contamination (see **TABLE B**).[g]

What can consumers do to protect themselves from food contamination? We must be the final judges of the safety of the food we buy. At a minimum, we should:

1. Make sure the food package or can is intact before opening it. If it has been damaged or dented or opened prior to purchase, call it to the attention of the appropriate person.
2. Be alert to abnormal color, taste, and appearance of a food item. If you have any doubt, don't eat it.
3. If the food appears to be tampered with, report it immediately.
4. Follow safe food-handling practices. (See the FYI feature "Safe Food Practices.")

[a]Centers for Disease Control and Prevention. Bioterrorism overview. http://www.bt.cdc.gov/bioterrorism/overview.asp. Accessed February 16, 2016.

[b]Ibid.

[c]Position of the American Dietetic Association: food and water safety. *J Am Diet Assoc.* 2009;109:1449–1460.

[d]Sobel J. *Epidemiologic preparedness and response to terrorist events involving the nation's food supply.* Paper presented at: Centers for Disease Control and Prevention's Health Preparedness Conference; February 2005.

[e]U.S. Food and Drug Administration. Employees FIRST. Food defense awareness for front-line food industry workers. March 2012. http://www.fda.gov/EmergencyPreparedness/default.htm Accessed March, 2016.

[f]U.S. Food and Drug Administration. Food: food protection plan 2007. November 2011. http://www.fda.gov/Food/GuidanceRegulation/FoodProtectionPlan2007/. Accessed July 17, 2015.

[g]U.S. Food and Drug Administration. Food: ALERT. The basics. March 2012. http://www.fda.gov/EmergencyPreparedness/default.htm Accessed March, 7, 2016

TABLE A
Employees FIRST

F	FOLLOW company food defense plans and procedures.
I	INSPECT your work area and surrounding areas.
R	RECOGNIZE anything out of the ordinary.
S	SECURE all ingredients, supplies, and finished product.
T	TELL management if you notice anything unusual or suspicious.

Courtesy of the U.S. Food and Drug Administration.

TABLE B
ALERT

A	How do you ASSURE that the supplies and ingredients you use are from safe and secure sources?
L	How do you LOOK after the security of the products and ingredients in your facility?
E	What do you know about your EMPLOYEES and people coming in and out of your facility?
R	Could you provide REPORTS about the security of your products while under your control?
T	What do you do and who do you notify if you have a THREAT or issue at your facility, including suspicious behavior?

Courtesy of the U.S. Food and Drug Administration.

Hazard Analysis Critical Control Point

Hazard Analysis Critical Control Point (HACCP) is a food industry program that focuses on preventing contamination by identifying areas in food production and retail where contamination could occur. HACCP also is an important line of defense against intentional contamination by bioterrorists. (See the FYI feature "At War with Bioterrorism.")

Companies and retailers analyze their food-production processes and determine **critical control points (CCPs)**—points at which hazards could occur. They then determine measures that they can institute at these points to prevent, control, or eliminate the hazards.[25] (See **TABLE 18.3**.) Critical control points can occur anywhere in a food's production—from its raw state through processing and shipping to purchase by the consumer. Preventive measures can include proper cooking, chilling, and sanitizing, as well as preventing cross-contamination and improving employee hygiene.

The USDA requires HACCP for the food products it regulates—meat and poultry. The FDA, which regulates all other foods, requires HACCP in the seafood and low-acid canned-food industries and the juice industry.[26] Also, the FDA has incorporated HACCP principles in its ***Food Code***, a reference for restaurants, grocery stores, institutional food services, vending operations, and other retailers on how to store, prepare, and serve food to prevent foodborne illness.[27] The FDA updates and publishes the *Food Code* periodically as a model for states to adopt and use to regulate retail food establishments in their jurisdictions.

Key Concepts Food safety is the responsibility of many agencies at the federal and state levels. The use of the Hazard Analysis Critical Control Point system allows government and industry to identify possible sites of food contamination and correct problems before they occur.

Quick Bite

Wood vs. Plastic: The Cutting Controversy

Which type of cutting board is safer to use while cutting meat: wood or plastic? Both have drawbacks. A wood cutting board tends to absorb bacteria, sucking them down into the wood fibers. This may be safer than a plastic board, which keeps bacteria on the surface, in an easy position to rub off onto food and other objects. But with use, wooden cutting boards tend to keep more on the surface than new wooden boards, acting more like plastic boards. What's the solution? Keep cutting boards clean by heating wooden boards in the microwave or putting plastic boards in the dishwasher.

▶ **critical control points (CCPs)** Operational steps or procedures in a process, production method, or recipe at which control can be applied to prevent, reduce, or eliminate a food safety hazard.

▶ ***Food Code*** A reference published periodically by the Food and Drug Administration for restaurants, grocery stores, institutional food services, vending operations, and other retailers on how to store, prepare, and serve food to prevent foodborne illness.

Quick Bite

Link Between Food Satisfaction and General Happiness among College Students

Students satisfied with their food life were found to be correspondingly satisfied with their general life.[28]

TABLE 18.3
HACCP: Hazard Analysis and Critical Control Point

Step 1: Analyze hazards.	Identify the potential hazards associated with a food. The hazard could be biological (e.g., a microbe), chemical (e.g., mercury), or physical (e.g., ground glass, metal).
Step 2: Identify critical control points (CCPs).	Identify points in a food's production path—from its raw state through processing and shipping to consumption—where a potential hazard can be controlled or eliminated. Examples of CCPs are cooking, chilling, handling, cleaning, and storage.
Step 3: Establish preventive measures with critical limits for each control point.	An example is setting the minimum cooking temperature and time to ensure safety for a particular food. (The temperature and time are critical limits.)
Step 4: Establish procedures to monitor the control points.	Such procedures might include determining how and by whom cooking time and temperature should be monitored.
Step 5: Establish corrective actions to be taken when a critical limit has not been met.	For example, reprocessing or disposing of food if the minimum cooking temperature is not met.
Step 6: Establish effective record keeping to document the HACCP system.	For example, recording hazards and their control methods, the monitoring of safety requirements, and action taken to correct potential problems.
Step 7: Establish procedures to verify that the system is working consistently.	For example, test time-recording and temperature-recording devices to verify that a cooking unit is working properly.

Modified from U.S. Food and Drug Administration. Hazard Analysis and Critical Control Point principles and application guidelines. http://www.fda.gov/Food/GuidanceRegulation/HACCP/. Accessed July 19, 2012.

Position Statement: Academy of Nutrition and Dietetics

Food and Water Safety

It is the position of the Academy of Nutrition and Dietetics that the public has the right to a safe food and water supply. The Association supports collaboration among food and nutrition professionals, academics, representatives of the agriculture and food industries, and appropriate government agencies to ensure the safety of the food and water supply by providing education to the public and industry, promoting technological innovation and applications, and supporting further research.

Reproduced from Albrecht JA, Nagy-Nero D. Position of the American Dietetic Association: food and water safety. *J Am Diet Assoc*. 2009;109:1449–1460.

The Consumer's Role in Food Safety

Food safety advice to consumers used to consist of a simple message: "Keep hot foods hot and cold foods cold" (see **FIGURE 18.7**). Now food safety experts also urge consumers to adhere to the following four rules (see **FIGURE 18.8**)[29,30]:

1. *Clean.* Wash hands and surfaces often. Clean fruits and vegetables. Meat and poultry should not be washed or rinsed.
2. *Separate.* Don't cross-contaminate. When shopping, preparing, or storing food, separate raw, cooked, and ready-to-eat foods.

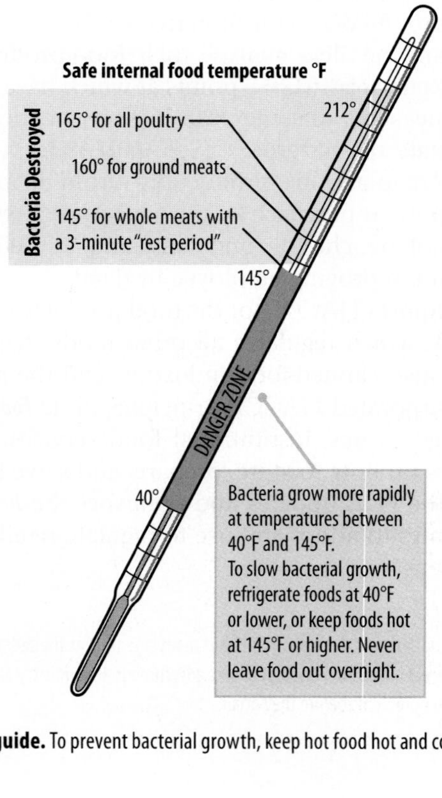
Safe internal food temperature °F
Bacteria Destroyed
165° for all poultry
160° for ground meats
145° for whole meats with a 3-minute "rest period"
212°
145°
DANGER ZONE
40°
Bacteria grow more rapidly at temperatures between 40°F and 145°F.
To slow bacterial growth, refrigerate foods at 40°F or lower, or keep foods hot at 145°F or higher. Never leave food out overnight.

FIGURE 18.7 Temperature guide. To prevent bacterial growth, keep hot food hot and cold food cold.

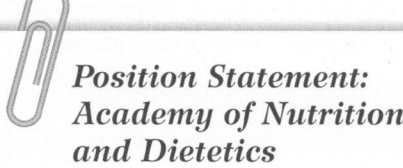

TABLE 18.4
Dangerous Food Safety Mistakes

Here are some common food safety mistakes that have been proven to cause serious illness:
Mistake #1: Tasting food to see if it's still good
Mistake #2: Putting cooked meat back on a plate that held raw meat
Mistake #3: Thawing food on the counter
Mistake #4: Washing meat or poultry
Mistake #5: Letting food cool before putting it in the fridge
Mistake #6: Eating raw cookie dough (or other foods with uncooked eggs)
Mistake #7: Marinating meat or seafood on the counter
Mistake #8: Using raw meat marinade on cooked food
Mistake #9: Undercooking meat, poultry, seafood, or eggs
Mistake #10: Not washing your hands

Modified from http://www.niaaa.nih.gov/alcohol-health/overview-alcohol-consumption/alcohol-facts-and-statistics.

3. *Cook.* Cook to proper temperatures. Avoid unpasteurized milk and juices, raw sprouts, raw or partially cooked eggs, and raw or undercooked meat and poultry.
4. *Chill.* Refrigerate promptly. Defrost foods properly and quickly refrigerate perishable foods.

THINK About It 3

Once a consumer takes possession of a food, food safety becomes his or her responsibility. Unfortunately, studies show that many consumers fail to follow safe food practices in the home (see **TABLE 18.4**). Current public health efforts focus on teaching consumers—from young children to older Americans—safe food practices in the home. (See the FYI feature "Safe Food Practices.")

Some food-handling practices are so important that the federal government requires specific instructions or warnings on labels of certain foods. Following outbreaks of illness from *E. coli* O157:H7 in contaminated hamburger in 1993, the USDA mandated instructions on labels of raw meat and poultry to encourage consumers to follow recommendations for safe handling and cooking of these products.

Labels of unpasteurized or otherwise untreated, packaged juice products carry a warning statement about the product's possible danger to children, older adults, and people with weakened immune systems. The warning states that the product has not been pasteurized and therefore might contain harmful bacteria that can cause serious illness in these high-risk groups. This requirement was made after a number of people became seriously ill from drinking unpasteurized apple juice that was contaminated with *E. coli*.

Fresh eggs must be handled carefully, and even eggs with clean, uncracked shells occasionally contain *Salmonella* that can cause an intestinal infection. The FDA requires the following safe handling statement on egg cartons[31]:

SAFE HANDLING INSTRUCTIONS: To prevent illness from bacteria: keep eggs refrigerated, cook eggs until yolks are firm, and cook foods containing eggs thoroughly.

Food manufacturers may voluntarily place other safe handling instructions on the label, such as those for proper cooking and storage of the item. Consumers should always follow these instructions.

Who Is at Increased Risk for Foodborne Illness?

Although everyone should follow safe food practices, infants and young children, pregnant women, older adults, and those who are immunocompromised or have certain chronic conditions must be especially careful. In particular,

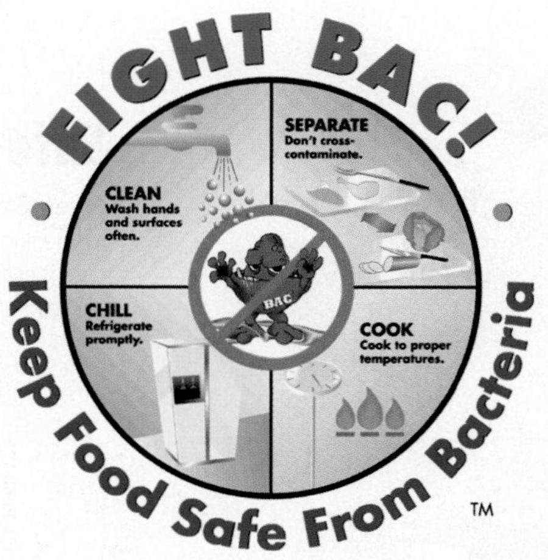

Clean: Wash hands and surfaces often
Separate: Don't cross-contaminate
Cook: Cook to proper temperatures
Chill: Refrigerate properly

FIGURE 18.8 Keeping harmful bacteria at bay. Although our food supply generally is safe, home food safety practices are the weakest link in the food chain from farm to kitchen table. Be sure to follow the four basic practices: clean, separate, cook, and chill.

Reprinted by permission from Partnership for Food Safety Education, www.fightbac.org.

FYI For Your Information

Safe Food Practices

Because bacteria grow rapidly between 40°F and 140°F (4–60°C), most food should be kept out of this temperature range, known as the Danger Zone. Cold temperatures keep bacteria from multiplying; the fewer bacteria, the less the risk of illness. Proper cooking (or other heat treatment, such as pasteurization) kills the bacteria. These principles serve as the basis for many of the following recommended food-handling practices.

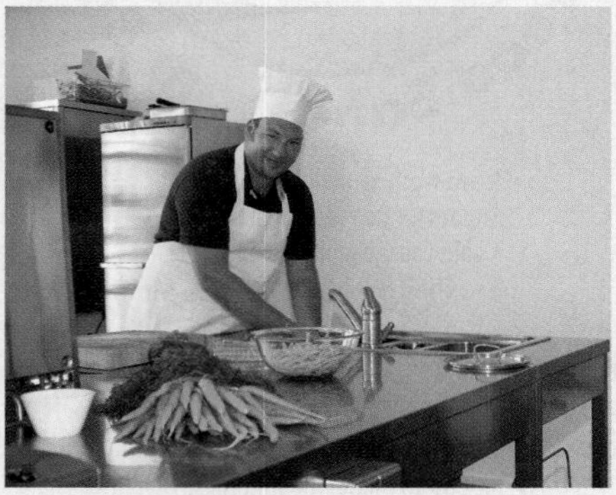

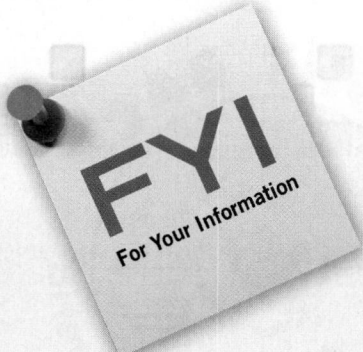

Buying Food

- Buy from reputable dealers and grocers who keep their selling areas and facilities clean and sanitary and maintain food at the appropriate temperature—for example, holding dairy foods, eggs, meats, seafood, and certain produce such as cut melons and raw sprouts at refrigerator temperatures.
- Don't buy canned goods with dents or bulges. Avoid torn, crushed, or open food packages. Also, avoid buying packages that are above the frost line in the store's freezer. If the package cover is transparent, look for frost or ice crystals, signs that the product has been stored for a long time or thawed and refrozen.

Storing Food

- Separate raw, cooked, and ready-to-eat foods while shopping, preparing, and storing.
- Refrigerate perishable items as quickly as possible after purchase. The refrigerator temperature should be 40°F or colder. Check it periodically with a thermometer to make sure the correct temperature is being maintained.
- Keep eggs in their original carton and store them in the refrigerator itself, not the door, where the temperature is warmer.
- If raw meat, poultry products, or fresh seafood will be used within two days, store them in the coldest part of the refrigerator, usually under the freezer compartment or in a special "meat keeper." Store the packages loosely to allow air to circulate freely around each package, and be sure to wrap them tightly so raw juices can't leak out and contaminate other foods.
- If raw meat, poultry, and seafood will not be used within two days, store them in the freezer, which should have a temperature of 0°F. Check this temperature periodically, too, and adjust as needed.
- Read label directions for storing other foods; for example, mayonnaise and ketchup need to be refrigerated after they have been opened.
- Store potatoes and onions in a cool dark place, but not under the sink because leakage from pipes can contaminate and damage them. Keep them away from household cleaning products and other chemicals as well.

Preparing Food

- Wash hands thoroughly with warm, soapy water for at least 20 seconds before beginning food preparation and every time you handle raw foods, including fresh produce.
- Defrost meat, poultry, and seafood products in the refrigerator, microwave oven, or a watertight plastic bag submerged in cold water (the water must be changed every 30 minutes). Never defrost at room temperature—an ideal temperature for bacteria to grow and multiply.
- Marinate foods in the refrigerator. Discard the marinade after use because it contains raw juices, which can harbor bacteria; make a separate batch for basting food while cooking.
- Always use a clean cutting board. Wash cutting boards with hot water, soap, and a scrub brush. Then sanitize them in an automatic dishwasher or by rinsing with a solution of 5 milliliters (1 teaspoon) chlorine bleach to about 1 liter (1 quart) of water. If possible, use one cutting board for fresh produce and a separate one for raw meat, poultry, and seafood. Once cutting boards become excessively worn or develop hard-to-clean grooves, you should replace them.
- Before opening canned foods, wash the top of the can to prevent dirt from coming in contact with the food.
- Wash fresh fruits and vegetables thoroughly with cold water. It is not necessary to wash or rinse meat or poultry.
- Avoid eating dough or batter containing raw eggs because of the risk of *Salmonella enteritidis*, a bacterium that can live in eggs.

Cooking Food

- Cook foods to the USDA Recommended Safe Minimum Internal Temperatures.[a]
  - 145°F for whole meats with a three-minute rest period
  - 160°F for ground meats
  - 165°F for all poultry
- The only safe way to know whether food is "done" is to use a food thermometer. According to the USDA, one of every four hamburgers turns brown before reaching a safe internal temperature.
- During the three-minute rest period after meat is removed from the heat source, the internal temperature remains constant or continues to rise, which destroys pathogens.
- Never place cooked food on a plate that previously held raw meat, poultry, or seafood.
- When microwaving foods, rotate the dish and stir its contents several times to ensure even cooking. Follow recommended standing times, then check meat, poultry, and seafood products with a thermometer to make sure they have reached the correct internal temperature.
- Cook eggs until the white is firm and the yolk is firm.

Serving Food

- Keep hot foods at 140°F (60°C) or higher and cold foods at 40°F (4°C) or lower.
- Refrigerate or freeze leftovers and perishables within two hours or sooner.
- Date leftovers so they can be used within a safe time—generally, three to five days in the refrigerator.

[a]U.S. Department of Agriculture, Food Safety and Inspection Service. USDA revises recommended cooking temperature for all whole cuts of meat, including pork, to 145°F. *Constituent Update.* 2011;13(21). http://www.fsis.usda.gov/PDF/Const_Update_052711.pdf. Accessed February 16, 2016.

they should not eat or drink raw (unpasteurized) milk or any products made from raw milk. They also should not eat raw or partially cooked eggs or foods containing raw eggs, raw or undercooked meat and poultry, raw or undercooked fish or shellfish, unpasteurized juices, and raw sprouts.

A Final Word on Food Safety

A totally risk-free system of food production is an unreasonable and unattainable goal. The United States and Canada enjoy a reputation as having food supplies that are among the safest in the world. We expect our food to be clean, fresh, and not contaminated with debris, chemicals, or organisms that cause sickness or discomfort. To make sure it stays that way, food safety experts are continually trying to ensure that every participant in the food production chain—from the farmer who produces the food to the manufacturer who processes it to the retailer who sells it and the consumer who buys it—undertakes measures to help reduce and perhaps even eliminate foodborne disease. That's one reason food safety advice today is turning up in so many places—to ensure that everyone gets the word on food safety.

Key Concepts Consumers play a huge role in food safety. They can avoid foodborne illness by following a few simple food-handling and preparation rules: Keep hands and food-preparation areas clean; avoid cross-contamination of foods; cook foods adequately; refrigerate foods promptly. People who have weak or less-developed immune systems are at higher risk for foodborne illnesses.

Quick Bite

How Good Are Your Food Safety Habits?

Do Americans practice food safety in their own kitchens? Apparently not. A study conducted by the FDA and the Centers for Disease Control and Prevention showed that one-half of people surveyed ate undercooked eggs in the past year. Twenty percent of people ate undercooked hamburger, and 25 percent of men and 14 percent of women failed to wash their hands with soap after handling raw meat.

Food Technology

Technology is having a larger and larger impact on the food we eat. Our use of preservatives, other preservation techniques, and genetic engineering has implications for our food supply in the years to come and has triggered debates about the risks and benefits of such practices.

Food Preservation

In our modern society, few people grow their own vegetables, fruits, and grains, or keep livestock as a source of meat and milk. Rather, we shop for our food, typically at a large, full-service supermarket. Because we don't often consume our food at the point of harvest or slaughter, we use food preservation methods to help maintain the quality of the foods we purchase. Among food preservation methods are the addition of chemical preservatives, canning or freezing, **pasteurization**, and irradiation.

▶ **pasteurization** A process for destroying pathogenic bacteria by heating liquid foods to a prescribed temperature for a specified time.

Preservatives

Preservatives are added to foods to prevent spoilage and increase shelf life. The most common antimicrobial agents are salt and sugar. Other preservatives, such as potassium sorbate and sodium propionate, extend the shelf life of baked goods and many other products. Antioxidants are a type of preservative that prevents the changes in color and flavor caused by exposure to air. Common antioxidants include vitamin C and vitamin E, sulfites, and BHA and BHT.

▶ **preservatives** Chemicals or other agents that slow the decomposition of a food.

Preparation for Preservation

Some preservation techniques, such as salting and fermenting, date to ancient times and are still practiced along with their modern counterparts—freezing, canning, pasteurization, and the like. Salting, drying, or fermenting foods creates an environment in which bacteria cannot multiply and therefore cannot cause food spoilage. Canned foods are heated quickly to a temperature that kills microbes and then are sealed airtight to prevent both contamination and oxidative damage. Freezing temperatures not only keep bacteria from multiplying, but also prevent normal enzymatic changes in food that would cause spoilage. Pasteurization of milk or other beverages uses a very high temperature for a very short time to kill bacteria but minimizes changes that would result from longer heating. The food industry and the North American public readily accept these food preservation methods. One of the most modern preservation techniques—irradiation—also is the most controversial, in part because of our fear of anything that has to do with radiation.

▶ **irradiation** A food preservation technique in which foods are exposed to measured doses of radiation to reduce or eliminate pathogens and kill insects, reduce spoilage, and, in certain fruits and vegetables, inhibit sprouting and delay ripening.

Irradiation

Before it received official approval, food **irradiation** underwent more than 40 years of scientific research and testing—more than any other food technology.[32] During irradiation, foods are exposed to a measured dose of radiation to reduce or eliminate pathogenic bacteria, including *E. coli* O157:H7, *Salmonella*, and *Campylobacter*, the chief causes of foodborne illness today. Irradiation also can destroy insects and parasites, reduce spoilage, and inhibit sprouting and delay ripening of certain fruits and vegetables. Irradiated strawberries, for example, stay unspoiled for up to three weeks versus three to five days for untreated berries. Irradiation also is effective in raw poultry and meat, where it can reduce levels of many pathogens significantly. Although some people fear irradiation will make the food radioactive, the energy used to irradiate foods passes through the food and leaves no residue—in the same way that microwaves pass through food. Despite its benefits, use of irradiation remains rare in North America.

Quick Bite

Where Do *E. coli* Hang Out?
Ground beef is the most common source of *E. coli* bacteria, but *E. coli* also have been found on apples, spinach, and lettuce.

Quick Bite

Bacteria at the Supermarket
Bacteria abound on the surface of supermarket meat. A piece of pork, on average, can harbor a few hundred bacteria per cubic centimeter, and a piece of chicken might have 10,000 in the same area.

Because food manufacturers fear consumer rejection, they have been reluctant to use irradiation on their products. Some consumers and advocacy groups protest its use because they are concerned that irradiation may compromise a food's nutritional value and change its texture, taste, or appearance. In fact, irradiation may cause less nutritive loss than conventional methods of food preservation.[33] At appropriate doses, irradiation of food does not significantly change its flavor, texture, or appearance.[34] Many organizations, including the Academy of Nutrition and Dietetics, the American Medical Association, and the World Health Organization, endorse irradiation as a means of providing the public with a safer food supply.

The FDA requires labels of irradiated foods to state that the product was "treated with irradiation" or "treated by irradiation" and display the international symbol for irradiation, the radura (see **FIGURE 18.9**).

▶ **bacteriophages** Viruses that infect bacteria.

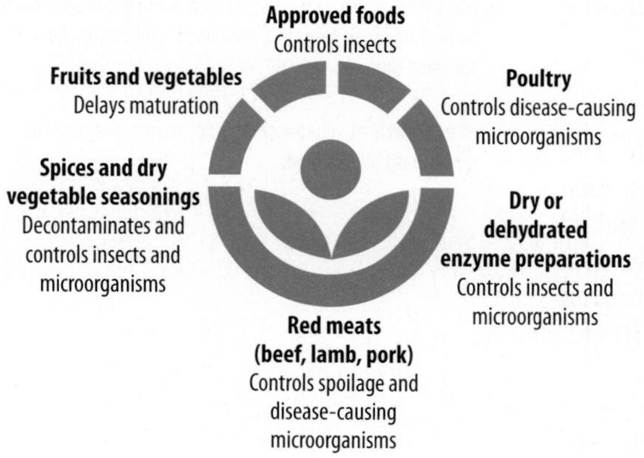

FIGURE 18.9 Irradiation. Irradiation can retard spoilage and reduce risk of foodborne illness.

Bacteriophages

The Food and Drug Administration has approved a mixture of viruses as a food additive to protect people from bacterial infections. The viruses used in the additive are called **bacteriophages** ("bacteria eaters"). A bacteriophage is any virus that infects bacteria.

Bacteriophages are common in soil, water, and our bodies. In the human gut and oral cavity, bacteriophages are normal and beneficial microbial inhabitants. Bacteriophages infect only bacteria and do not bother mammalian or plant cells. The increase in concern regarding antibiotic-resistant and virulent bacteria has renewed scientific interest in bacteriophages for use in clinical and medical settings and commercial food safety.[35,36]

Under the Federal Meat Inspection Act and the Poultry Products Inspection Act, both administered by the USDA, the use of the bacteriophage preparation must be declared on labeling as an ingredient. Consumers will see "bacteriophage preparation" on the label of meat or poultry products that have been treated with the additive.[37]

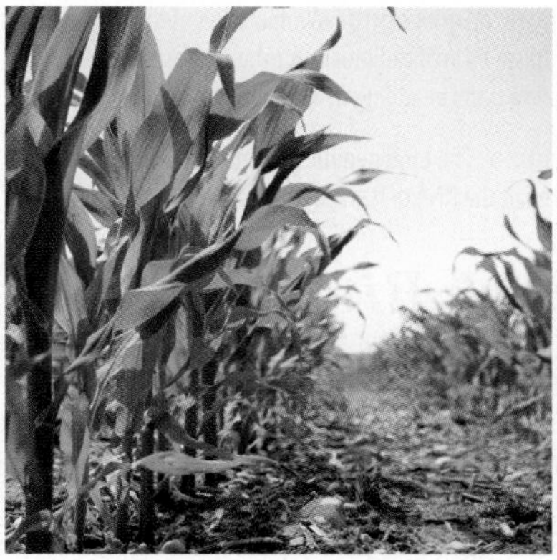

© ryasick photography/ShutterStock, Inc.

Key Concepts Various processing methods help protect us from contamination of food by pathogens. Drying, salting, canning, freezing, and pasteurizing are methods that consumers accept. Irradiation is a process in which foods are exposed to a measured dose of radiation to reduce or eliminate pathogenic bacteria. Although government and professional organizations deem irradiation a safe procedure, consumers are still wary. The FDA has also approved spraying ready-to-eat meats and poultry products with bacteriophages, viruses that infect bacteria.

Genetically Engineered Foods

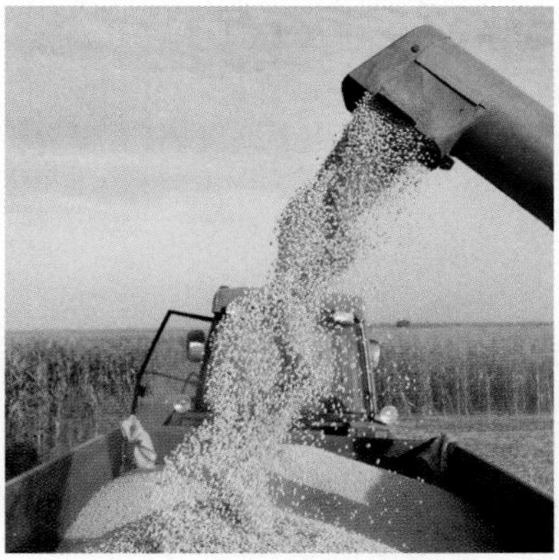

© sima/ShutterStock, Inc.

Genetically engineered (GE) foods have arrived, and most of us are already dining on them. When you prepare a dinner of broccoli and tofu, some of the soybeans used to make the tofu probably came from plants genetically engineered to resist herbicide sprays or insect pests or both. And although your broccoli is currently "natural," you can be sure that in a lab somewhere genetically engineered broccoli seeds are sprouting, perhaps with enhanced nutrient or other phytochemical levels. If you are eating tenderloin tonight, the steak probably came from a steer fed on genetically engineered corn that had its DNA altered by the addition of foreign genes to allow the plant to resist insect pests and herbicides.

Should you be indignant that these new foods are showing up on your table without any indication on the label, or should you be grateful that these high-tech methods are keeping crop yields high and food costs low? An informed answer to this question requires some understanding of how genetic engineering works, how new crops and foods are regulated, and how gene modification of crops and animals differs from the classical methods of agricultural breeding that have been practiced for thousands of years.

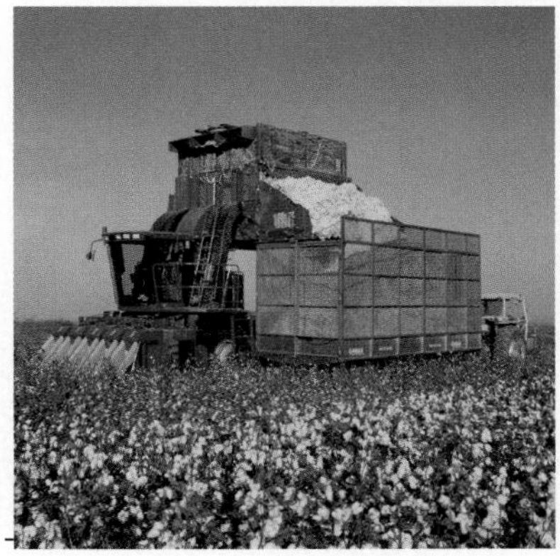

© Alaettin YILDIRIM/ShutterStock, Inc.

A Short Course in Plant Genetics

How do GE plants differ from those developed through traditional cross-pollination and hybridization? The answer, surprisingly, is that most crop modifications achieved by DNA manipulation and associated techniques of **biotechnology** also could be achieved with classical techniques, but the time scale and expense are very different (see **FIGURE 18.10**).

The classical techniques for breeding a plant with new characteristics have been practiced for hundreds of years. They involve crossing two plants with different characteristics, and then growing the resulting hybrid seeds and looking for plants with the desired combination of characteristics. Hybrid plants get half of their genes from one parent and half from the other. Though the hybrid might combine favorable qualities from both parents, a lot of undesirable genetic baggage must be sorted out after formation of such a hybrid. It usually takes dozens of additional crosses, and many years, to separate the desirable genes from the undesirable, and the process has a large element of chance. As a result of human intervention, today virtually every crop plant species differs greatly from its original, wild form.

▶ **genetically engineered (GE) foods** Foods produced using plant or animal ingredients that have been modified using gene technology.

▶ **biotechnology** The set of laboratory techniques and processes used to modify the genome of plants or animals and thus create desirable new characteristics. Genetic engineering in the broad sense.

▶ **genetic engineering** Manipulation of the genome of an organism by artificial means for the purpose of modifying existing traits or adding new genetic traits.

▶ **genome** The total genetic information of an organism, stored in the DNA of its chromosomes.

Quick Bite

Biotechnology in the 1930s

One of the first examples of genetic theory successfully applied to food production was hybrid corn. When first introduced, it seemed miraculous and convinced skeptical farmers of the potential benefits of this emerging agricultural science. To this day, tougher and healthier new hybrids continue to outyield their predecessors.

Genetic engineering, in contrast, allows scientists to transform a plant one gene at a time, using well-established methods for manipulating DNA sequences and integrating them into the plant **genome** (its set of genes). In some cases, a gene can be selected and introduced into plant cells, and new GE seeds can be prepared within a year or two. When we consider that it took centuries of selection and breeding to transform the weedy wild maize plant of pre-Columbian Mexico into our modern varieties of corn, the scale and speed of the gene revolution in agriculture are astounding.

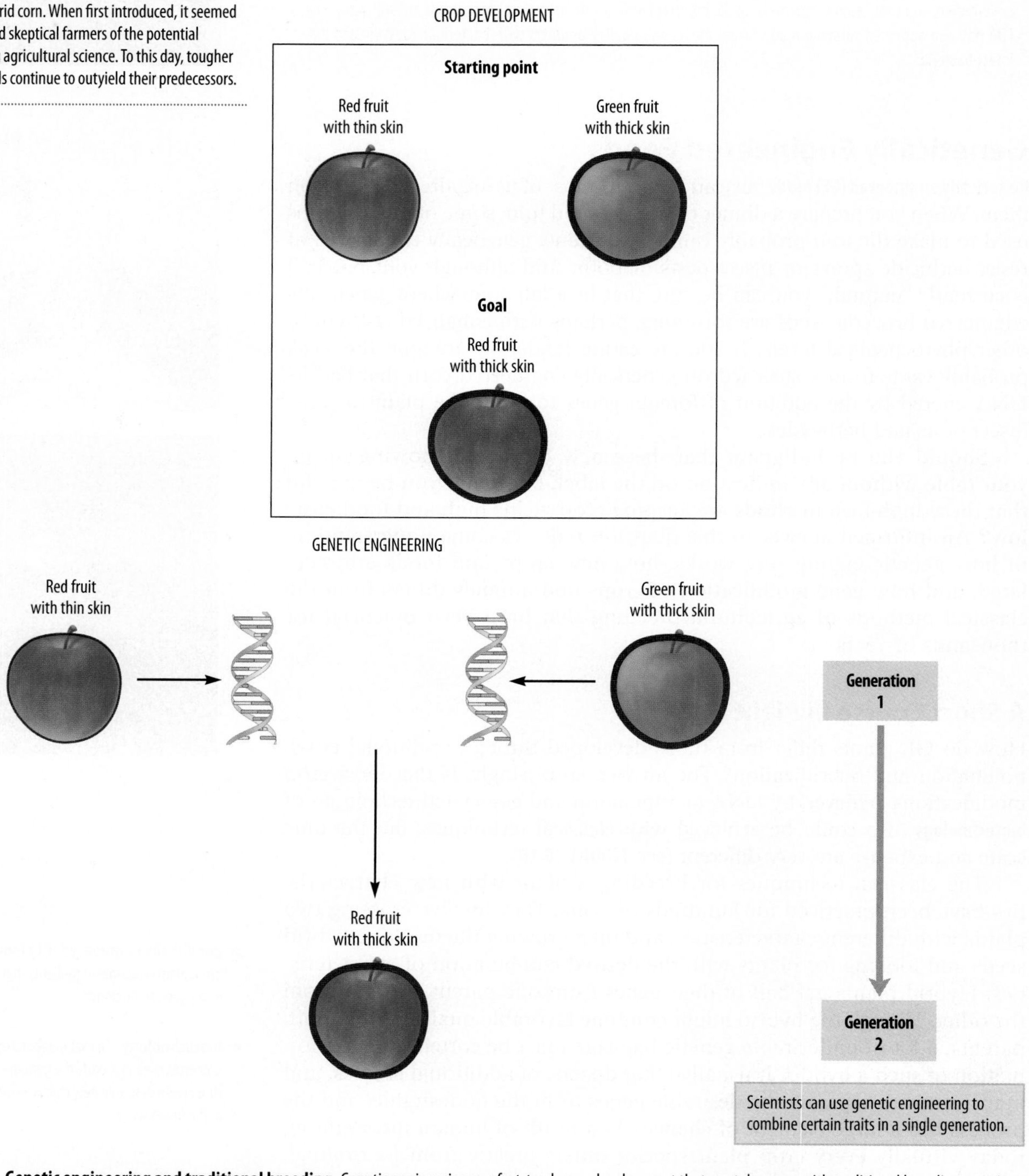

FIGURE 18.10 Genetic engineering and traditional breeding. Genetic engineering can fast-track crop development that can take years with traditional breeding practices.

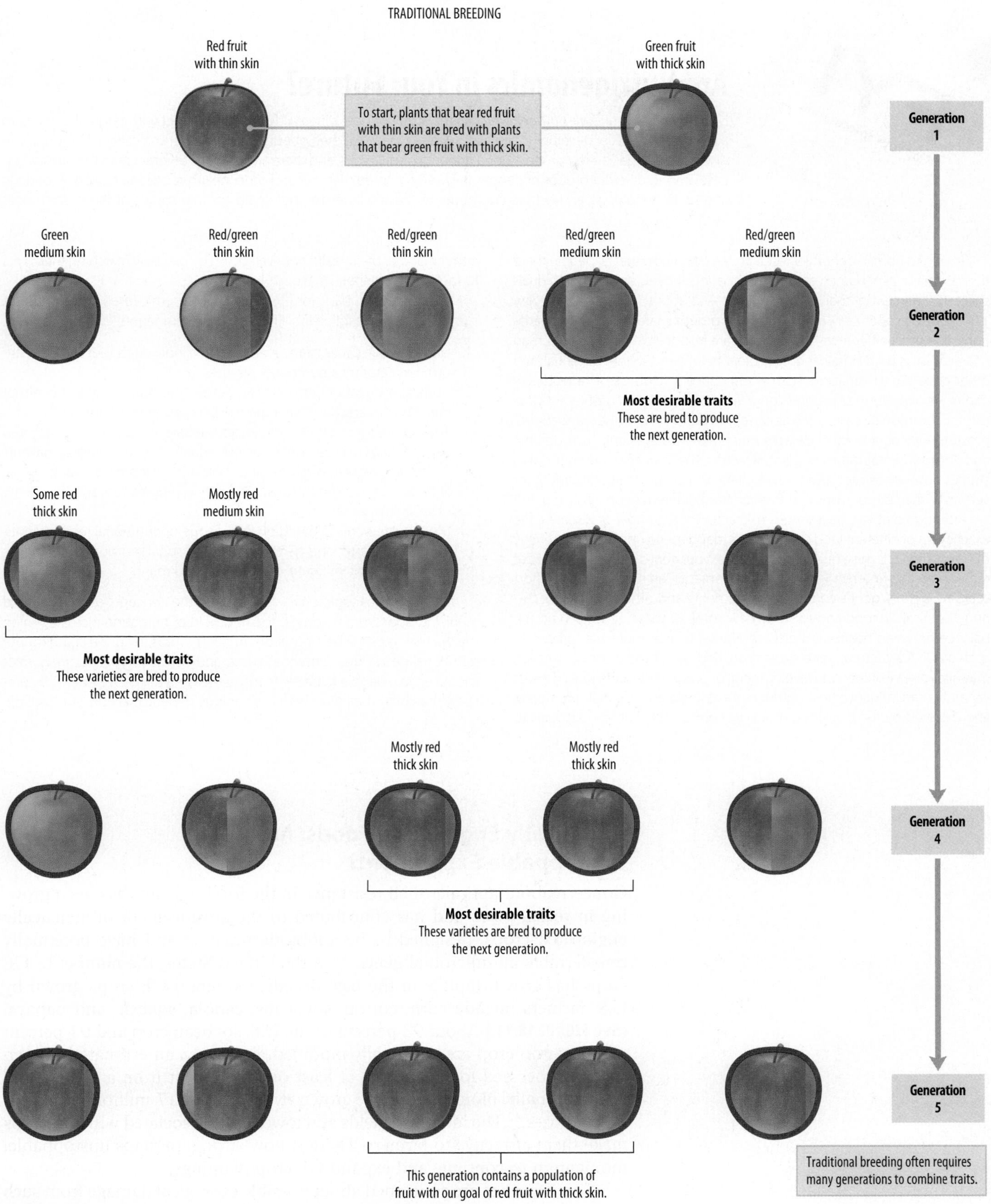
TRADITIONAL BREEDING
Red fruit with thin skin
Green fruit with thick skin
To start, plants that bear red fruit with thin skin are bred with plants that bear green fruit with thick skin.
Generation 1
Green medium skin
Red/green thin skin
Red/green thin skin
Red/green medium skin
Red/green medium skin
Generation 2
Most desirable traits
These are bred to produce the next generation.
Some red thick skin
Mostly red medium skin
Generation 3
Most desirable traits
These varieties are bred to produce the next generation.
Mostly red thick skin
Mostly red thick skin
Generation 4
Most desirable traits
These varieties are bred to produce the next generation.
Generation 5
This generation contains a population of fruit with our goal of red fruit with thick skin.
Traditional breeding often requires many generations to combine traits.

FIGURE 18.10 Genetic engineering and traditional breeding. *(continued)*

FYI For Your Information

Are Nutrigenomics in Your Future?

Nutritional genomics, or ***nutrigenomics***, is the study of how different foods can interact with particular genes to alter a person's risk of developing diseases such as type 2 diabetes, obesity, heart disease, and cancer. Many of these diseases are especially common among minority populations, and there are dramatic differences in the rates of disease among different groups of people. It is well accepted that diet and other health-related behaviors, economic and social conditions, and culture contribute to these differences, but could another source of these differences lie in our genes?

Thanks to human genomics research, we now know that all people share the vast majority of human genetic information. Indeed, any two individuals share 99.9 percent of their DNA sequence—or about 1 difference in every 1,000 base pairs. Similarly, racial and ethnic groups share most genetic variations. The small differences that do exist are responsible for diverse human characteristics such as hair and skin colors; height and weight potential; and other "gene-based" variations, such as susceptibility to disease. The incidence of disease or patterns of progression differ among different groups. Risk factors for common diseases such as obesity, coronary heart disease, diabetes, prostate cancer, and birth defects must take into account both genetic and environmental/behavioral/social factors. The science of nutrigenomics studies how genes, diet, and disease interact to create health disparities for certain human populations that evolved from different geographic regions.

Although diet can be a serious risk factor for a number of diseases, the exact effect of different food components may depend on a person's genetic makeup. Thus, it is not a question of whether your genes are good or bad but rather how they interact with your environment. The nutrigenomics effort seeks to identify genes controlled by nutrients and other naturally occurring chemicals in food and to study how some of these genes can tip the balance between health and disease. Nutrients alter molecular processes such as DNA structure, gene expression, and metabolism, which, in turn, may alter disease initiation, development, or progression. Individual genetic variations can influence how nutrients are assimilated, metabolized, stored, and excreted by the body. Nutritional genomics will enable individuals to better manage their health and well-being by precisely matching their diets to their unique genetic makeup.

The conceptual basis for this branch of genomic research can best be summarized by the following "Five Tenets of Nutrigenomics"[a]:

1. Under certain circumstances and in some individuals, diet can be a serious risk factor for a number of diseases.
2. Common dietary chemicals can act on the human genome, either directly or indirectly, to alter gene expression or structure.
3. The degree to which diet influences the balance between healthy and disease states may depend on an individual's particular genetic makeup.
4. Some diet-regulated genes (and their normal, common variants) are likely to play a role in the onset, incidence, progression, and/or severity of chronic diseases.
5. Dietary intervention based on knowledge of nutritional requirements, nutritional status, and genotype (i.e., "personalized nutrition") can be used to prevent, mitigate, or cure chronic disease.

Just as pharmacogenomics has inspired the concepts of "personalized medicine" and "designer drugs," the new field of nutrigenomics is opening the way for "personalized nutrition." In other words, by understanding our nutritional needs, our nutritional status, and our genotype, nutrigenomics should enable people to better manage their health and well-being by precisely matching their diets with their unique genetic makeup. Stay tuned!

Genetically Engineered Foods: An Unstoppable Experiment?

Concern about antimicrobial resistance in the food industry has been growing in recent years and has contributed to the advancement of genetically engineered crops, designed to be antibiotic resistant and have potentially transferrable antimicrobial genes.[38] In the United States, the number of GE crops has grown rapidly in the past decade. Common GE crops grown by U.S. farmers include corn, cotton, soybeans, canola, squash, and papaya. (See **FIGURE 18.11**.) About 93 percent of the U.S. soybean crop and 94 percent of the cotton crop are genetically modified.[39] Already, an estimated 70 percent of processed foods contain at least one ingredient from a GE plant.[40] Internationally, biotech crops are grown by more than 17 million farmers in 28 countries.[41] The increased yields and lower costs associated with GE crops make them attractive to farmers. There is now strong, perhaps unstoppable, momentum to continue and expand GE crop plantings.

Some farmers are concerned about possible ecological damage from such crops and fear potential unintended consequences of genetic "tampering" with the food supply. Although some U.S. consumer groups voice similar concerns,

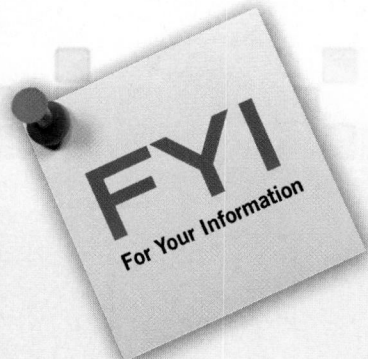

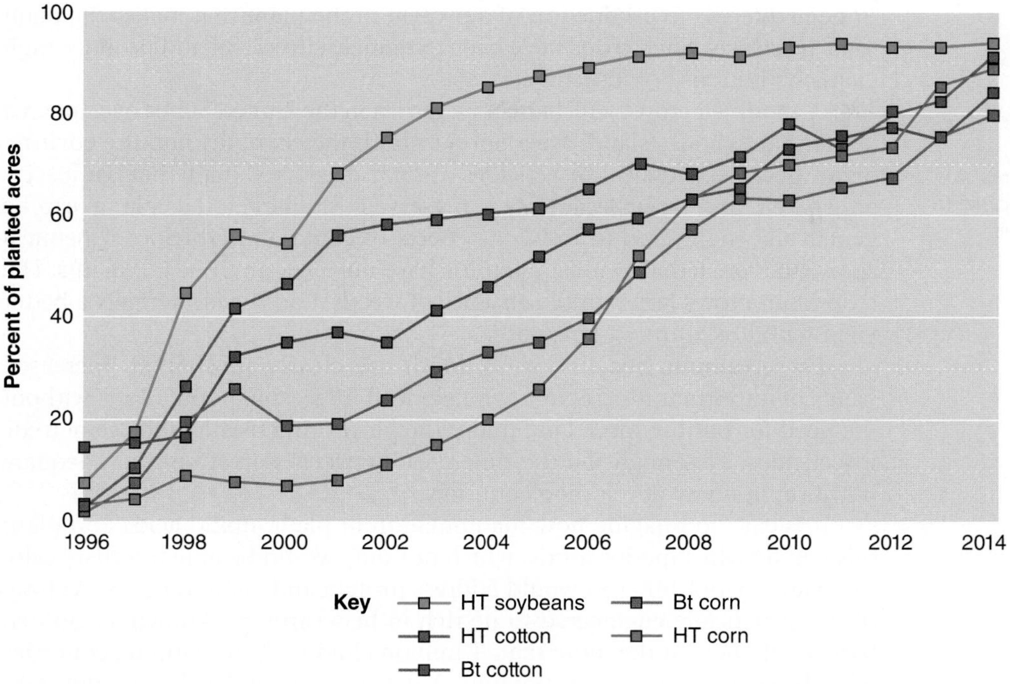

FIGURE 18.11 Adoption of genetically engineered crops in the United States, 1996–2013.

Reproduced from U.S. Department of Agriculture, Economic Research Service. Recent trends in GE adoption. http://ers.usda.gov/data-products/adoption-of-genetically-engineered-crops-in-the-us/recent-trends-in-ge-adoption.aspx#.VEpkOiLF-Sp. Accessed February 16, 2016.

agribusiness, the Academy of Nutrition and Dietetics, the American Medical Association, the National Academy of Sciences, and the Food and Agriculture Organization of the United Nations have been supportive of the trend toward GE foods.[42]

The GE crops mentioned earlier are just the tip of the genetic-modification iceberg; hundreds more are under development in university laboratories and in the labs of giant agribusinesses. Research in plant biotechnology has focused primarily on characteristics that improve resistance to pests, reduce the need for pesticides, and increase the ability of the plant to survive adverse growing conditions such as drought, soil salinity, and cold. Many of these goals would be achievable with classical selection techniques, but with genetic engineering, they move from laboratory to table in decades rather than centuries.

If only plant genes were involved in GE food production, there would be much less controversy. However, *any* gene, including genes from bacteria and animals, can be introduced into a plant genome. Some people find this frightening, and an imaginative term, *Frankenfoods*, has been coined to express the "unnatural" nature of some GE products. But how unnatural is the exchange of DNA between species? It may be reassuring to realize that organisms have been swapping DNA for eons, with no help from humans. Foreign DNA can be carried from one species to another by a variety of viruses, for example. Nature has already performed millions of "gene modifications" on its own, and exchange of DNA is an established part of the evolutionary process. Now that we can do our own experiments with DNA manipulation, we hope the benefits will be increased.

Benefits of Genetic Engineering

Whatever the risks, no one can argue with the success of these GE techniques. For instance, a bacterial gene was used to create insect-resistant varieties of corn, potatoes, and soybeans. This gene, the ***Bt* gene**, was taken from the soil bacterium *Bacillus thuringiensis*. When inserted into a plant genome, the

▶ ***Bt* gene** *Bacillus thuringiensis (Bt)* is a bacterium that produces a protein called the *Bt* toxin. One of the bacterium's genes, the *Bt* gene, carries the information for the *Bt* toxin. Inserting a copy of the *Bt* gene into plants enables them to produce *Bt* toxin protein and resist some insect pests. The *Bt* protein is not toxic to humans.

Bt gene directs the production of a protein in the plant that makes the plant toxic to insects. Such crops have been extremely successful and produce high yields without use of insecticides.

Bt-modified crops, which are now grown in the United States over an area larger than Rhode Island, are a boon to both the economy and the environment. Because chemical insecticides are not necessary, many benign insects are spared, and insect **biodiversity** is preserved. Similarly, other plants can be genetically engineered to resist the effects of common herbicides. Chemical sprays that are lethal to most plant life have no effect on these GE plants. The crop plant grows larger in the absence of weeds, and the farmer gets a better yield with less effort and expense.

▶ **biodiversity** The countless species of plants, animals, and insects that exist on the earth. An undisturbed tropical forest is an example of the biodiversity of a healthy ecosystem.

The economic benefits of GE foods are clearly substantial. Increased yields of important food plants can help feed increasing populations without the need for putting more land under the plow or increasing the use of toxic insecticides. This might be the difference between starvation and adequate nutrition in many developing countries.

It is easy to imagine how manipulation of plant amino acids and plant oils could yield superior foods, which not only would be able to satisfy calorie requirements, but also would address protein and vitamin needs. A strain of rice genetically engineered to be rich in beta-carotene, known as Golden Rice, could benefit the more than 1 million children in developing countries who die or are weakened by vitamin A deficiency.[43] In developed countries, where heart disease and cancer loom as greater risks than malnutrition, the ability to adjust the saturation level of plant lipids or to boost beneficial phytochemicals would be of great value to public health. But do these undoubted benefits outweigh the risks?

Risks

What are the specific risks of GE foods? Many consumers are concerned about whether these new foods are safe to eat. The answer to this concern is a fairly unequivocal "yes." When a new protein or other substance is introduced into a food, the FDA requires substantial testing to demonstrate its safety. With GE foods, the potential risk appears to be the possibility of introducing a new allergen into a GE food.[44] To be cautious, the FDA has focused on allergy issues. Under the law and the FDA's biotech food policy, companies must tell consumers on the food label when a product includes a gene from a food that commonly causes an allergic reaction.

Of greater concern, and more difficult to predict, are environmental effects, although no ecological disasters have occurred thus far. For example, what if the *Bt*-containing plants lead to the development of insects resistant to *Bt*-modified plants and to other insecticides? Another concern is the development of herbicide-resistant weeds, or "superweeds." When herbicide-resistant crops are planted in proximity to related wild plants, pollen can drift from food plant to weed, and the resistant genes might be passed to the weedy cousins of the GE plants. In the presence of herbicide, this might lead to the rapid selection of herbicide-resistant weeds.

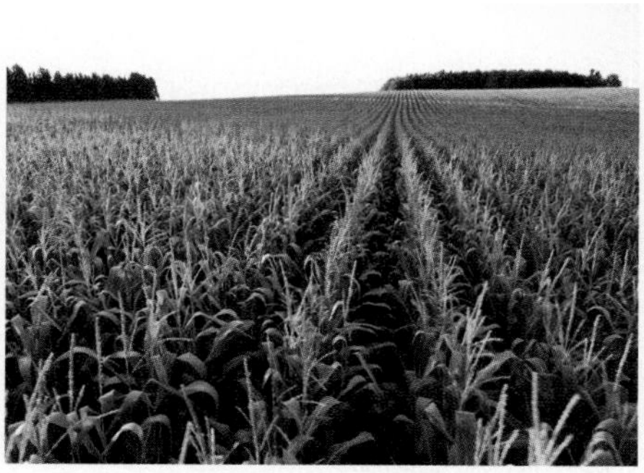

© Anderl/ShutterStock, Inc.

A final concern is that the herbicide-resistant food plants might become so successful that they are planted over a vast acreage. In the worst scenario, this could lead to a loss of many species of unmodified plants as well as the insect and animal communities that depend on them. Many scientists feel that the loss of biodiversity is one of the greatest threats to the planet today. Because of the complexity and interdependence of the biosphere, this is perhaps the greatest unknown and the greatest danger of unmonitored use of GE crops. **TABLE 18.5** summarizes benefits and current controversies.

TABLE 18.5
GE Products: Benefits and Controversies

Benefits
Crops
• Enhanced taste and quality
• Reduced maturation time
• Increased nutrients, yields, and stress tolerance
• Improved resistance to diseases, pests, and herbicides
• New products and growing techniques
Animals
• Increased resistance, productivity, hardiness, and feed efficiency
• Better yields of meat, eggs, and milk
• Improved animal health and diagnostic methods
Environment
• "Friendly" bioherbicides and bioinsecticides
• Conservation of soil, water, and energy
• Bioprocessing for forestry products
• Better natural waste management
• More efficient processing
Society
• Increased food security for growing populations
Controversies
Safety
• Potential human health impacts, including allergens, transfer of antibiotic resistance markers, and unknown effects
• Potential environmental impacts, including unintended transfer of transgenes through cross-pollination, unknown effects on other organisms (e.g., soil microbes), and loss of flora and fauna biodiversity
Access and Intellectual Property
• Domination of world food production by a few companies
• Increasing dependence on industrialized nations by developing countries
• Biopiracy, or foreign exploitation of natural resources
Ethics
• Violation of natural organisms' intrinsic values
• Tampering with nature by mixing genes among species
• Objections to consuming animal genes in plants and vice versa
• Stress for animals
Labeling
• Not mandatory in some countries (e.g., United States)
• Mixing GE crops with non-GE products confounds labeling attempts
Society
• New advances might be skewed to interests of rich countries

Reproduced from U.S. Department of Energy, Human Genome Project. Genetically modified foods and organisms. November 2008. fog.ccsf.edu/~cpogge/Bio41L/GMfoods.pdf. Accessed February 16, 2016.

Regulation

The FDA regulates foods and food safety, and it oversees genetically engineered foods and animals as well as conventional foods. For foods derived from new varieties of plants, the FDA takes the position that whether modified by traditional breeding or genetic engineering, testing for safe human consumption is the legal responsibility of the producer or manufacturer of the foods. Crops such as genetically engineered soybeans do not require special testing, labeling, or FDA approval. Except for some foreign DNA sequences, the beans are identical to unmodified soybeans. However, when a new substance is added to a food, FDA review and approval are necessary. Thus, if a new substance is produced or introduced into a food by genetic means, it must be tested as though it were a food additive.

Some consumer groups are pushing for mandatory labeling of GE foods. They believe consumers have the right to know whether a food is bioengineered. Other groups desire labeling so they can adhere to cultural or religious beliefs that might ban certain animal foods. Because the FDA believes the way a food is developed or produced is irrelevant information, current FDA policy does not require labeling of GE foods.

The FDA supports the voluntary labeling of products that contain genetically engineered ingredients and requires that food labels disclose any significant difference between the bioengineered food and its conventional counterpart.[45] Such differences would include changes in nutritional properties, the presence of an allergen that consumers would not expect in the food, or any property that would require special handling, storage, cooking, or preservation.

Similar to U.S. regulations, Health Canada requires special labeling for genetically engineered foods when there is a potential for allergic reactions or a difference in composition or nutritional value. Voluntary positive ("does contain") and voluntary negative ("does not contain") labeling is permitted, provided the statements are factual and not misleading or deceptive.[46]

Many groups (government agencies, such as the FDA; professional organizations, such as the ADA; and consumer advocacy groups) are monitoring developments in biotechnology. Websites for these organizations can be a source of policy statements and breaking news in this area. Regardless of our views on genetic manipulation of food plants, research and development will continue.

Position Statement: Academy of Nutrition and Dietetics

Agricultural and Food Biotechnology

It is the position of the Academy of Nutrition and Dietetics that agricultural and food biotechnology techniques can enhance the quality, safety, nutritional value, and variety of food available for human consumption and increase the efficiency of food production, food processing, food distribution, and environmental and waste management. The AND encourages the government, food manufacturers, food commodity groups, and qualified food and nutrition professionals to work together to inform consumers about this new technology and encourage availability of these products in the marketplace.

Reproduced from Bruhn C, Earl R. Position of the American Dietetic Association: agricultural and food biotechnology. *J Am Diet Assoc.* 2006;106(2):285–293.

Key Concepts Genetic engineering allows scientists to transform a plant one gene at a time, using well-established methods for manipulating DNA sequences. The goals of genetic modification of foods are higher yields, lower costs, increased amounts of critical nutrients, and a healthier mix of plant oils. Because of the complexity and interdependence of the biosphere, loss of genetic biodiversity is perhaps the greatest unknown and the greatest danger of unmonitored GE crops.

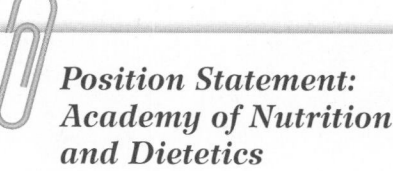

Learning Portfolio

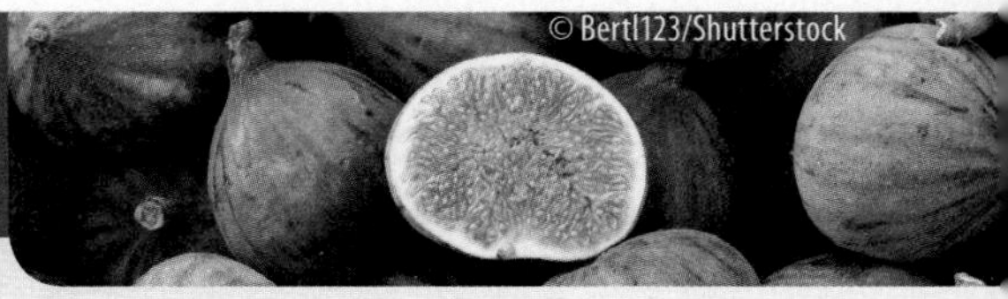

Key Terms

aflatoxins	738
bacteriophages	748
biodiversity	754
biotechnology	749
botulism	732
bovine spongiform encephalopathy (BSE)	734
***Bt* gene**	753
ciguatera	738
critical control points (CCPs)	743
dioxins	737
Escherichia coli (E. coli)	732
Food Code	743
foodborne illness	728
genetic engineering	750
genetically engineered (GE) foods	749
genome	750
integrated pest management (IPM)	735
irradiation	748
mad cow disease	734
methylmercury	737
natural toxins	738
organic foods	734
pasteurization	747
pesticides	734
poisonous mushrooms	738
pollutants	737
preservatives	747
prions	734
Salmonella	732
solanine	738

Study Points

- Foodborne illness is extremely common; it affects millions of Americans each year. Estimates of the frequency of foodborne illness are difficult because the vast majority of foodborne illnesses go unreported.
- The incidence of foodborne illness may be on the rise in the United States and Canada. Many factors are responsible, including the increased centralization of food preparation, food imports, an increasing population of especially susceptible individuals (such as older adults and those with weakened immune systems), and failure of consumers and retail establishments to follow appropriate food safety measures.
- Microorganisms cause most foodborne diseases in the United States and Canada. Most of these illnesses are preventable.
- *Staphylococcus aureus* is one of the most common causes of foodborne illness. Onset of illness is rapid, typically occurring between 30 minutes and a few hours after consuming the contaminated food.
- Common symptoms of foodborne illness are diarrhea, nausea, abdominal cramps, and sometimes fever. The severity of the illness depends on the type of organism and the amount of contaminant eaten.
- Ensuring a safe food supply is a farm-to-table continuum involving producers, manufacturers, retailers, and consumers.
- Pesticides, animal drugs, natural toxins, and pollutants are the major forms of chemical food contamination.
- The government monitors imported and domestic foods for pesticide residues by testing food samples for both amounts and types of pesticides. Efforts are under way to reduce the allowable amounts of certain pesticides to avoid harm to infants and children.
- The FDA evaluates drugs used in food-producing animals for safety in both animals and humans. Overuse of animal antibiotics could contribute to the emergence of antibiotic-resistant microorganisms that could threaten human health.
- The government and the food industry use the Hazard Analysis Critical Control Point system to prevent food contamination.
- Consumers must take responsibility for food safety in their homes. Cleaning hands and surfaces, avoiding cross-contamination, cooking adequately, and refrigerating foods promptly are important steps that prevent foodborne illness.
- Food preservation techniques inhibit growth of microorganisms. Canning, drying, freezing, fermentation, and pasteurization are common methods.
- Although the FDA has approved food irradiation for numerous uses, it is rarely used, mostly because of consumer fears. Food irradiation does not make foods radioactive. It can kill insects and most microorganisms. Appropriate doses of radiation extend the shelf life of many foods.
- Genetically engineered (GE) foods are most likely already on your table. Soybeans, corn, and potatoes are some of the GE foods being commercially produced. Concerns about GE foods include worries about decreasing biodiversity and the development of herbicide-resistant weeds.

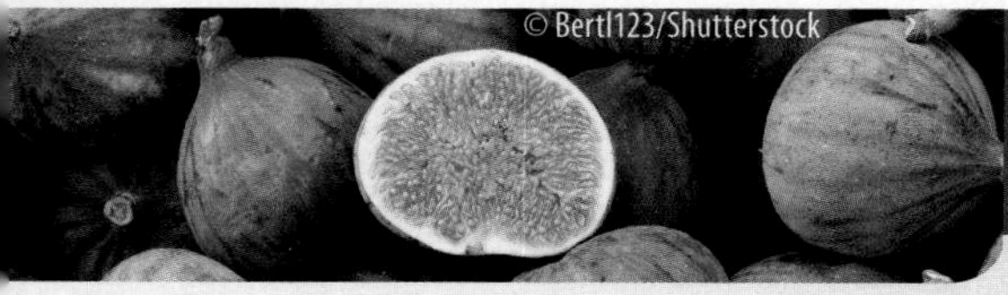

© Bertl123/Shutterstock

Learning Portfolio (continued)

Study Questions

1. What are the two main ways that pathogenic bacteria can cause foodborne illness?
2. Why shouldn't your 97-year-old great-grandmother drink homemade eggnog made from raw eggs?
3. List four naturally occurring toxins.
4. What does HACCP stand for, and what is its purpose?
5. What are some ways to keep food safe at home?
6. List the most common food preservation techniques.
7. What are scientists' two major concerns about genetically engineered crops?

Try This

Bacterial Detective

What sources of bacteria do you encounter in your everyday activities? Here's an experiment to find out. First, you'll need the following:

- Cotton swabs
- Six or more Petri dishes with agar

If you are unable to obtain a set of agar-filled Petri dishes from your school or local health department, you can make your own culture medium. Here's how:

- Add 2 teaspoons of unflavored gelatin (1 packet) and 2 teaspoons of sugar to one cup of water.
- Bring the solution to a boil and stir for 1 minute until everything is dissolved. Pour ¼ inch of the solution into each Petri dish or other suitable container.

Then, using separate Petri dishes,

1. Pluck a hair and lay it in one Petri dish, labeled "Hair."
2. Sneeze or cough into another Petri dish, labeled "Cough."
3. Run a cotton swab around a nostril and carefully zigzag it across the agar in another Petri dish, labeled "Nose."
4. Run a cotton swab across a dampened kitchen sink sponge and carefully zigzag it across the agar in another Petri dish, labeled "Sponge."
5. Run a cotton swab around a clean kitchen countertop and carefully zigzag it across the agar in another Petri dish, labeled "Countertop."
6. Use the same procedure to collect additional samples from any other area in which bacteria might be present.
7. Store the Petri dishes in a warm environment, at a constant temperature around 80°F. Check your specimens periodically. Within a week, you should see something growing! What do you observe? Which Petri dishes show the most growth? Which show the least?

Does this change your ideas about cleaning habits?

Organic Foods

Organic foods are increasing in popularity. Are organic foods widely available in your neighborhood? What types of organic produce can you find? Go to either a natural food store or the local grocery store and look at the array of organic produce. Compare the prices of organic produce and nonorganic produce. Do you think the cost differences outweigh possible benefits? Compare the look of the organic and nonorganic produce. Do you see any differences? What other organic products can you find?

Getting Personal

Using the numbers shown, please indicate how often you engage in the following food safety practices:

1. Rarely or never
2. Sometimes
3. Frequently
4. Always

___ Wash hands before handling food and after touching raw meat.

___ Reheat leftovers to 165 degrees Fahrenheit.

___ Refrigerate leftovers within two hours of preparation.

___ Avoid using food products whose use-buy date has expired.

___ Do not eat foods containing uncooked eggs.

___ Wash fresh produce including prepackaged greens.

___ Avoid eating fish high in mercury levels.

___ Defrost food in the refrigerator, the microwave, or cold water, not on the counter.

___ Use separate cutting boards for raw meat, poultry, and fish.

___ Wash cutting boards after use before putting them away.

Total the numbers you have selected. If your score is less than 20, you should revisit the items to which you assigned a number less than 2 and consider a plan to incorporate a food safety practice that will raise your total score.

References

1. Centers for Disease Control and Prevention. Foodborne germs and illnesses. http://www.cdc.gov/foodsafety/facts.html#howmanycases. Accessed February 16, 2016.
2. Institute of Food Technologists. Foodborne illness costs US 152 B annually. March 2010. http://www.ift.org/food-technology/daily-news/2010/march/10/foodborne-illness-costs-us-152-b-annually.aspx. Accessed February 16, 2016.
3. Institute of Food Technologists. *IFT Expert Report on Emerging Microbiological Food Safety Issues: Implications for Control in the 21st Century*. Chicago, IL: Institute of Food Technologies; April 2010. http://www.ift.org/knowledge-center/read-ift-publications/science-reports/expert-reports/~/media/Knowledge%20Center/Science%20Reports/Expert%20Reports/Emerging%20Microbiological/Emerging%20Micro.pdf. Accessed February 16, 2016.
4. Centers for Disease Control and Prevention. Foodborne germs and illnesses. Op cit.
5. Ibid.
6. U.S. Food and Drug Administration. Residue monitoring reports. FDA Pesticide Program residue monitoring: 1993–2008. 2010. http://www.fda.gov/Food/FoodborneIllnessContaminants/default.htm Accessed March 7, 2016
7. Ibid.
8. Zuraw L. Consumer Reports guides shoppers through produce pesticide residues. Food Safety News. March 19, 2015. http://www.foodsafetynews.com/2015/03/consumer-reports-guides-shoppers-through-produce-pesticide-residues/#.VnCUn79URMc. Accessed February 16, 2016.
9. http://www.epa.gov/pesticide-science-and-assessing-pesticide-risks/overview-risk-assessment-pesticide-program Accessed March 7, 2016
10. Dimitri C, Oberholtzer L. Marketing U.S. organic foods: recent trends from farms to consumers. September 2009. Economic Information Bulletin No. 58. http://www.ers.usda.gov/publications/eib58/eib58.pdf. Accessed February 16, 2016.
11. Organic Trade Association. American appetite for organic products breaks through $35 billion mark. May 2014. http://www.ota.com/news/press-releases/17165. Accessed February 16, 2016.
12. https://www.ams.usda.gov/about-ams/programs-offices/national-organic-program, Accessed, March 7, 2016
13. https://www.ams.usda.gov/about-ams/programs-offices/national-organic-program.
14. Ibid.
15. U.S. Department of Agriculture, Agricultural Marketing Service. NOSB meetings. http://www.ams.usda.gov/AMSv1.0/nosbmeetings. Accessed February 16, 2016.
16. Porterfield A. Fraud or drift? USDA finds 43 percent of organic foods contain 'prohibited' substances. Genetic Literacy Project. July 2015. http://www.geneticliteracyproject.org/2015/07/22/fraud-or-drift-usda-finds-43-percent-of-organic-foods-contain-prohibited-substances/. Accessed February 16, 2016.
17. National Research Council, Committee on Drug Use in Food Animals, Panel on Animal Health, Food Safety, and Public Health. *The Use of Drugs in Food Animals*. Washington, DC: National Academies Press; 1999.
18. U.S. Food and Drug Administration. Phasing out certain antibiotic use in farm animals. http://www.fda.gov/forconsumers/consumerupdates/ucm378100.htm. Accessed February 16, 2016.
19. Food and Agriculture Organization of the United Nations. Fact sheet: dioxins in the food chain: prevention and control of contamination. April 2008. http://www.fao.org/AG/AGAINFO/PROGRAMMES/documents/VPH_factsheets/FAO_Fact_Sheet_020408.pdf. Accessed February 16, 2016.
20. Food and Agriculture Organization of the United Nations. Dioxins: food safety – needs a solid food chain approach. http://www.fao.org/food/food-safety-quality/a-z-index/dioxins/en/. Accessed February 16, 2016.
21. http://www.fda.gov/food/resourcesforyou/consumers/ucm110591.htm
22. U.S. Department of Agriculture and U.S. Department of Health and Human Services. *Dietary Guidelines for Americans, 2015*. 8th ed. Washington, DC: U.S. Government Printing Office; December 2015.
23. U.S. Food and Drug Administration. Food allergies: what you need to know. May 2012. http://www.fda.gov/Food/ResourcesForYou/Consumers/ucm079311.htm. Accessed February 16, 2016.
24. U.S. Department of Health and Human Services. Food Safety Modernization Act (FSMA). http://www.fda.gov/Food/FoodSafety/FSMA/default.htm. Accessed February 19, 2016.
25. U.S. Food and Drug Administration. Hazard Analysis and Critical Control Point principles and application guidelines. November 2015. http://www.fda.gov/Food/GuidanceRegulation/HACCP/ucm2006801.htm. Accessed May 24, 2016.
26. http://www.fda.gov/Food/GuidanceRegulation/HACCP/ Accessed March 7, 2016
27. U.S. Food and Drug Administration. Food: FDA Food Code. February 2012. http://www.fda.gov/Food/GuidanceRegulation/RetailFoodProtection/ucm2006807.htm
28. Schnettler B, Orellana L, Lobos G, et al. Relationship between the domains of the Multidimensional Students' Life Satisfaction Scale, satisfaction with food-related life and happiness in university students. *Nutr Hosp*. 2015;31(6):2752–2763.
29. Partnership for Food Safety Education. Fight Bac! Four simple steps to food safety. http://www.fightbac.org. Accessed February 16, 2016.
30. U.S. Department of Agriculture and U.S. Department of Health and Human Services. *Dietary Guidelines for Americans, 2015*
31. Food labeling, safe handling statements, labeling of shell eggs; refrigeration of shell eggs held for retail distribution, final rule. *Federal Register*. 2000;65:76091–76114.
32. http://www.fda.gov/Food/ResourcesForYou/Consumers/ucm261680.htm accessed March 7, 2016
33. Iowa State University. Consumer questions about food irradiation. June 2010.
34. http://www.fda.gov/Food/ResourcesForYou/Consumers/ucm261680.htm Accessed March 7,2016
35. Maura D1, Debarbieux L. Bacteriophages as twenty-first century antibacterial tools for food and medicine. *Appl Microbiol Biotechnol*. 2011;90(3):851–859. doi: 10.1007/s00253-011-3227-1. Epub March 29, 2011.
36. Lu TK, Koeris MS. The next generation of bacteriophage therapy. *Curr Opin Microbiol*. 2011;14(5):524–531. doi: 10.1016/j.mib.2011.07.028. Epub August 23, 2011.
37. Bren L. Bacteria-eating virus approved as food additive. *FDA Consumer*. January–February 2007.
38. Capita R, Alonso-Calleja C. Antibiotic-resistant bacteria: a challenge for the food industry. *Crit Rev Food Sci Nutr*. 2013;53(1):11–48. doi: 10.1080/10408398.2010.519837.
39. U.S. Department of Agriculture. Biotechnology: frequently asked questions about biotechnology. http://www.usda.gov/wps/portal/usda/usdahome?navid=AGRICULTURE&contentid=BiotechnologyFAQs.xml Accessed March 7, 2016
40. ibid
41. U.S. Department of Agriculture. Biotechnology. Frequently asked questions about biotechnology. Op cit.
42. Position of the American Dietetic Association: agricultural and food biotechnology. *J Am Diet Assoc*. 2006;106(2):285–293.
43. Tang G, Qin J, Dolnikowski GG, et al. Golden Rice is an effective source of vitamin A. *Am J Clin Nutr*. 2009;89(6):1776–1783.
44. Selgrade MK, Bowman CC, Ladics GS, et al. Safety assessment of biotechnology products for potential risk of food allergy: implications of new research. *Toxicol Sci*. 2009;110(1):31–39.
45. U.S. Food and Drug Administration. FDA's role in regulating safety of GE foods. https://njfb.org/wp-content/uploads/2013/07/FDA-GE- Accessed March 7,
46. Health Canada. The regulation of genetically modified food. November 2005. http://www.hc-sc.gc.ca/sr-sr/pubs/biotech/reg_gen_mod-eng.php. Accessed February 16, 2016.

Chapter **19**

World View of Nutrition: The Faces of Global Malnutrition

Revised by Cynthia Blanton

THINK About It

1 Have you ever experienced hunger without being able to satisfy it within a day?
2 Have you seen evidence of hunger or malnutrition in your community?
3 What can you do to help eliminate hunger in North America?
4 How do you feel about the United States sending food to impoverished nations?

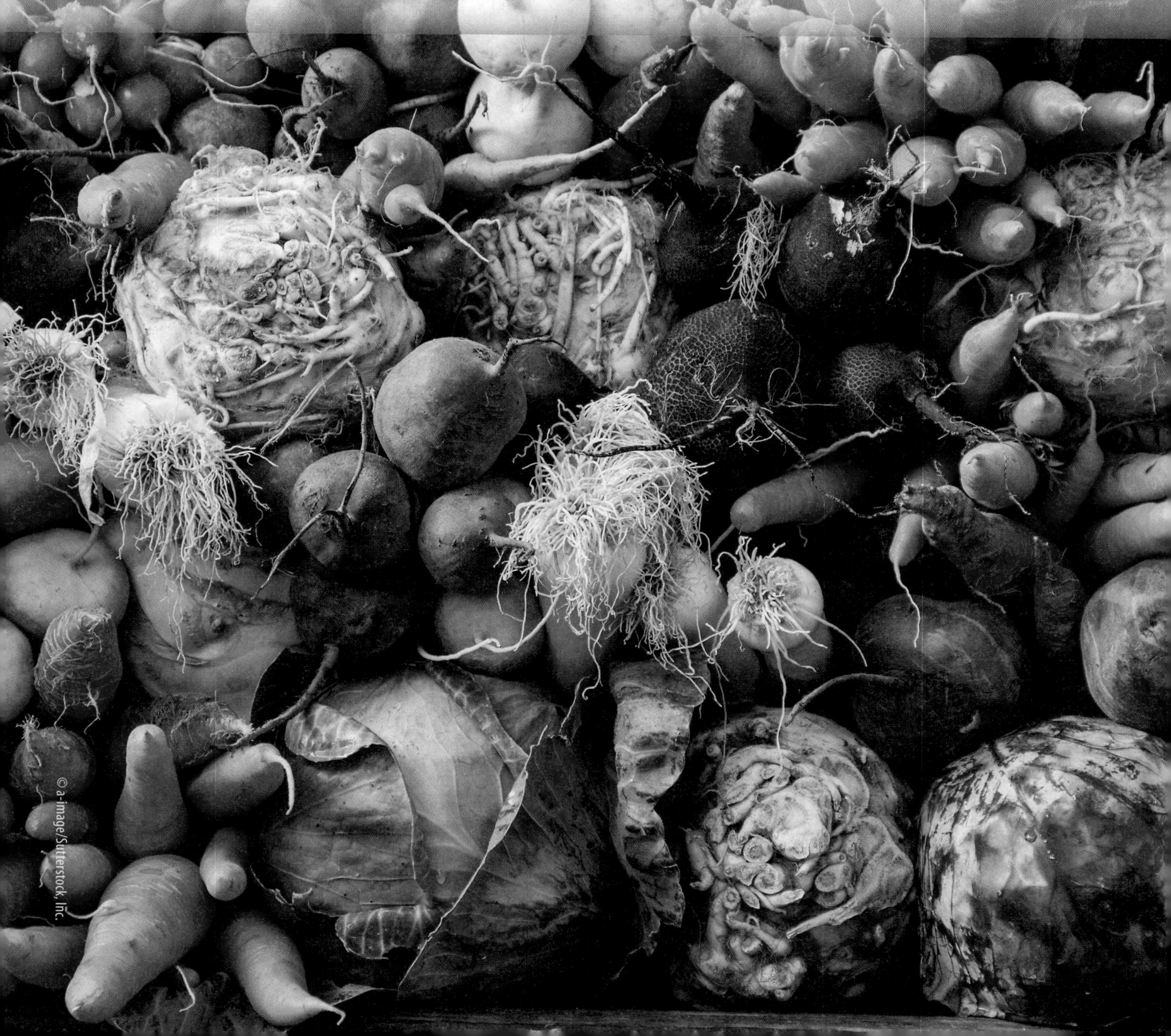

CHAPTER Menu

- Malnutrition in the United States
- Malnutrition in the Developing World
- Key Terms
- Study Points
- Study Questions
- Try This
- Getting Personal
- References

LEARNING Objectives

- Define food insecurity.
- List populations at risk for malnutrition.
- Discuss domestic food programs that combat hunger.
- Explain the causes of world hunger.
- Describe the key features of protein-energy malnutrition.
- Identify and discuss the major nutritional deficiencies worldwide.

Whether it be a family in rural Iowa struggling to stretch groceries through to the end of the month or a single parent in New York working 60 hours a week, yet still unable to buy enough food for the children, hunger due to inadequate access to food is a common experience across America. If **hunger** exists in our rich country, what about people living in poor countries?

Worldwide, 795 million people do not have enough to eat.[1] Although this figure includes 14 million in developed countries, most of the world's hungry live in developing countries.[2] The most undernourished region is Asia (525 million people), and the region with the highest proportion of undernutrition is sub-Saharan Africa (20 percent, 226 million people).[3] Worldwide, 45 percent of the deaths of children younger than 5 years (more than 3 million children per year) are caused directly or indirectly by **malnutrition**.[4]

In this chapter, we look at hunger and malnutrition. By *hunger* we don't mean that mildly empty feeling one gets before mealtime. We mean the inability, day after day, to satisfy basic nutrition needs, the gnawing emptiness that creates a constant focus on eating and how to obtain food. In contrast to the hunger dieters feel from cutting calories, this deprivation is involuntary and unwanted.

Technically speaking, malnutrition can be any kind of unhealthy nutritional status, including the result of imbalance and excess—obesity or toxicity from oversupplementation, for example. And although we touch on obesity as an emerging issue, even in developing countries, by and large in this chapter, *malnutrition* means undernutrition resulting from hunger.

Along the spectrum of malnutrition and hunger is the less extreme condition of **food insecurity**, the ongoing worry about having enough to eat. At the opposite end of the spectrum is **food security**, access to nutritionally adequate and safe food. Most people in the industrialized world are food-secure. Overabundance and obesity are the primary problems in these populations, but malnutrition is a serious problem among certain groups such as the homeless and urban poor.

▶ **hunger** The internal, physiological drive to find and consume food. Unlike appetite, hunger is often experienced as a negative sensation, often manifesting as an uneasy or painful sensation; the recurrent and involuntary lack of access to food that can produce malnutrition over time.

▶ **malnutrition** Failure to achieve nutrient requirements, which can impair physical and/or mental health. It can result from consuming too little food or a shortage or imbalance of key nutrients.

▶ **food insecurity** (1) Limited or uncertain availability of nutritionally adequate and safe foods, or (2) limited or uncertain ability to acquire acceptable foods in socially acceptable ways.

▶ **food security** Access to enough food for an active, healthy life, including (1) the ready availability of nutritionally adequate and safe foods and (2) an assured ability to acquire acceptable foods in socially acceptable ways.

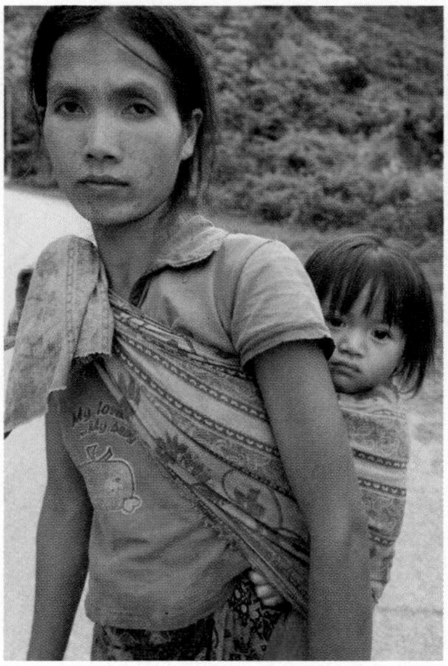

© iStockphoto/Thinkstock

Malnutrition in the United States

Malnutrition and hunger are serious problems not only in developing countries, but also in the United States and other industrialized countries. Among those who suffer the worst malnutrition are the homeless, children, older adults, the working poor, and the rural poor.

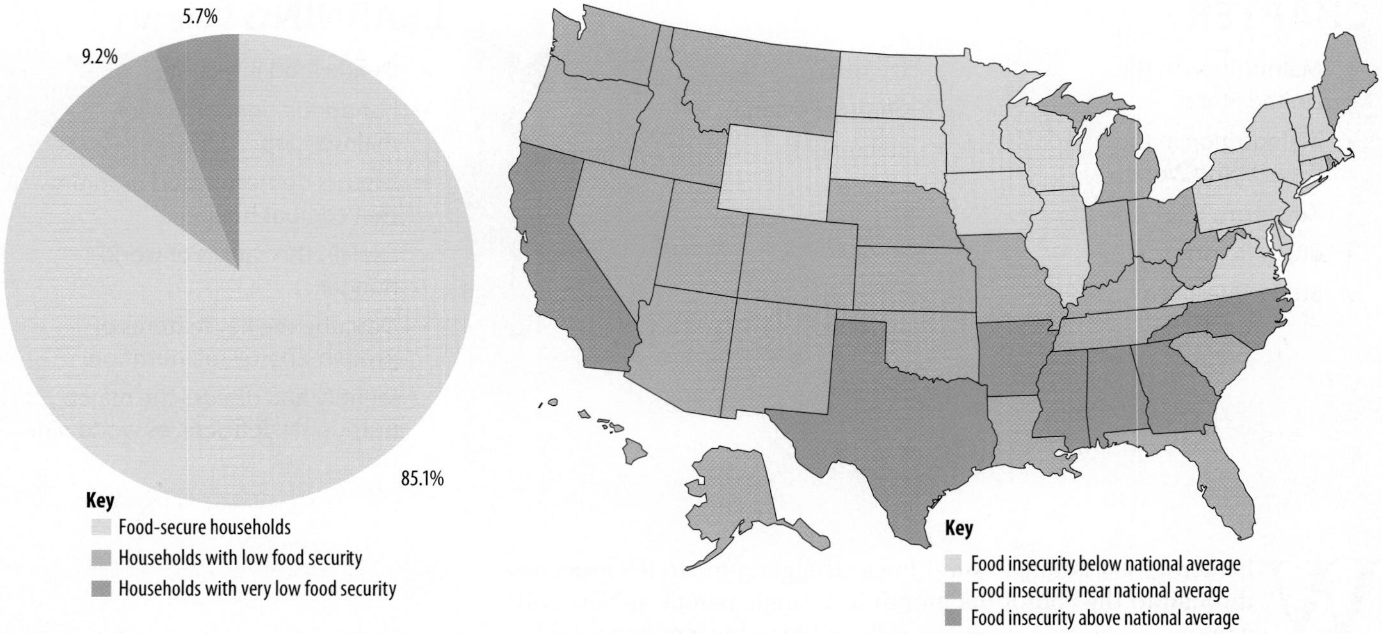

FIGURE 19.1 Prevalence of food insecurity. State-to-state differences in food insecurity reflect both differences in the makeup of state populations, such as the income, employment, age, education, and family structure of their residents, and differences in state characteristics, such as economic conditions, the accessibility and use of food assistance programs, and tax policies.

Reproduced from ERS using data from the Current Population Survey Food Security Supplement.

The Face of American Malnutrition

In the food-rich United States, food insecurity remains a problem[5] (see **FIGURE 19.1**). It is characterized by anxiety about having enough to eat and about running out of food and having no money to purchase more. Some people actually go hungry in the United States: During 2014, 17.4 million households, including 3.7 million households with children, experienced food insecurity.[6]

Households that are struggling to meet basic food needs tend to follow a typical pattern as their plight worsens. First, adults worry about having enough food. Then, they stretch resources and juggle other necessities, with more of the budget going for fixed expenses than for food. The quality and variety of the diet decline. Next, the adults eat less and less often. And, finally, as food becomes more limited, the children also eat less. Families cope with food insecurity in various ways. When there is not enough food, common strategies include eating less varied diets and participating in local and federal emergency relief and food assistance programs.[7]

THINK About It 1

Surprisingly, obesity is more prevalent among low-income, food-insecure groups than among those with higher incomes. Households with little money often rely on cheaper, high-calorie foods to stave off hunger. Families try to maximize caloric intake for each dollar spent, which can lead to overconsumption of calories and a less healthful diet. Historically, obesity has hit low-income Americans the hardest. Their limited financial resources and worsening food insecurity shift food purchases to cheaper, easier, high-energy, and affordable options, which can contribute to obesity.[8]

Those who live in a state of food insecurity consume significantly fewer healthful foods and micronutrients. Although such suboptimal diets usually do not lead to overt deficiency diseases, more subtle effects are serious and costly, showing up years later as chronic illness or more immediately as reduced immune function. More illness, more medicines, more doctor visits and hospital stays, more missed days and poorer performance at school and work,

TABLE 19.1
2015 Poverty Guidelines: Income Levels Defined as Poverty for a Given Household Size

Persons in Family	48 Contiguous States and DC	Alaska	Hawaii
1	$11,770	$14,720	$13,550
2	15,930	19,920	18,330
3	20,090	25,120	23,110
4	24,250	30,320	27,890
5	28,410	35,520	32,670
6	32,570	40,720	37,450
7	36,730	45,920	42,230
8	40,890	51,120	47,010
For each additional person, add	4,160	5,200	4,780

Reproduced from U.S. Department of Health and Human Services, Office of the Secretary. Annual update of the HHS poverty guidelines. *Federal Register.* 2015;80(14):3236–3237.

poor pregnancy outcome, delayed growth and development—suboptimal nutrition contributes to them all.

Prevalence and Distribution

How much hunger and food insecurity exists in the United States? Until recently, it was difficult to measure. Estimates were based on the percentage of the population living in poverty, with the assumption that they were at risk of undernutrition. Such estimates are somewhat flawed because being at risk does not necessarily mean that people are poorly nourished. Many people with limited financial resources manage to eat well. However, under certain circumstances, such as loss of a job, people who live well above the poverty line (see **TABLE 19.1**) may be food-insecure.

The U.S. Department of Agriculture (USDA) tracks hunger with an annual **Food Security Supplement Survey**, which asks about food availability and hunger in the household (see **TABLE 19.2**). Food insecurity is strongly associated with

TABLE 19.2
Sample Questions from the Food Security Questionnaire

Light Food Insecurity
"We worried whether our food would run out before we got money to buy more." Was that often, sometimes, or never true for you in the last 12 months? "The food that we bought just didn't last and we didn't have money to get more." Was that often, sometimes, or never true for you in the last 12 months?
Moderate Food Insecurity
In the last 12 months, did you or other adults in the household ever cut the size of your meals or skip meals because there wasn't enough money for food? In the last 12 months, were you ever hungry but didn't eat because you couldn't afford enough food?
Severe Food Insecurity
In the last 12 months, did you or other adults in the household ever not eat for a whole day because there wasn't enough money for food? (For households with children) In the last 12 months, did any of the children ever not eat for a whole day because there wasn't enough money for food?

Modified from Nord M, Coleman-Jensen A, Gregory C. *Prevalence of U.S. Food Insecurity Is Related to Changes in Unemployment, Inflation, and the Price of Food.* ERR-167. Washington, DC: U.S. Department of Agriculture, Economic Research Service; June 2014.

Quick Bite

Food Recovery and Gleaning

Each year, 40 percent of the food produced in this country is wasted.[9,10] Programs throughout the country are rescuing much of this wholesome food and distributing it to people in need. *Gleaning* is harvesting excess food from farms, orchards, and packing houses. Perishable items are also salvaged from wholesale and retail markets; fresh foods that are wholesome but will spoil before they can be sold are given to local food pantries and meal providers. Canned goods and other staples are collected from groceries, distributors, food processors, and individual homes. Even surplus food from restaurants, caterers, and other food services is collected by some charities for local food programs.

▶ **Food Security Supplement Survey** A federally funded survey that measures the prevalence and severity of food insecurity and hunger.

poverty and is interlinked with economic and social factors. Food insecurity and hunger were highest in households headed by single women with children and in Hispanic and African American households.[11] Geographically, food insecurity is more common in large cities and rural areas and, regionally, more prevalent in the South. To combat food insecurity and hunger effectively, nutrition programs must be accompanied by social and economic efforts.

The Working Poor

Employment does not guarantee that families always have enough to eat. Often the pay is too little to lift households out of poverty, and work-related expenses, such as transportation or child care, further deplete family budgets. Food insecurity can be as common among the working poor as it is among the unemployed. Low-paid workers may be unaware that they still qualify for food-assistance programs. However, their work hours can preclude program participation.

Migrant farm workers may have access to plenty of fresh produce but are poorly paid and may not have the money to buy other foods. Farm workers and undocumented workers (illegal aliens) do not qualify for government programs to help the poor or may not sign up for fear of deportation.

Food Deserts

People in remote rural areas often live far from food resources and lack access to transportation. Areas that lack access to affordable healthful foods such as low-fat milk products, whole grains, fruits, and vegetables are termed **food deserts.**[12] Do food deserts exist in wealthy nations? The answer is yes. Researchers have counted 6,501 food deserts in the United States, and the poor access to healthful food can negatively affect the health of residents in the region[13] (see **FIGURE 19.2**). Even in populated cities, some people can become isolated despite living in a crowded neighborhood or apartment building. Usually, they live alone and are physically or mentally unable to obtain adequate food.

▶ **food deserts** Geographic area where affordable and nutritious food is hard to obtain, particularly for those without access to an automobile.

Older Adults

The infirmities of age, along with feelings of vulnerability, keep some older people homebound and lonely, conditions hardly conducive to a healthy appetite. Physical ailments can make cooking and eating difficult while actually

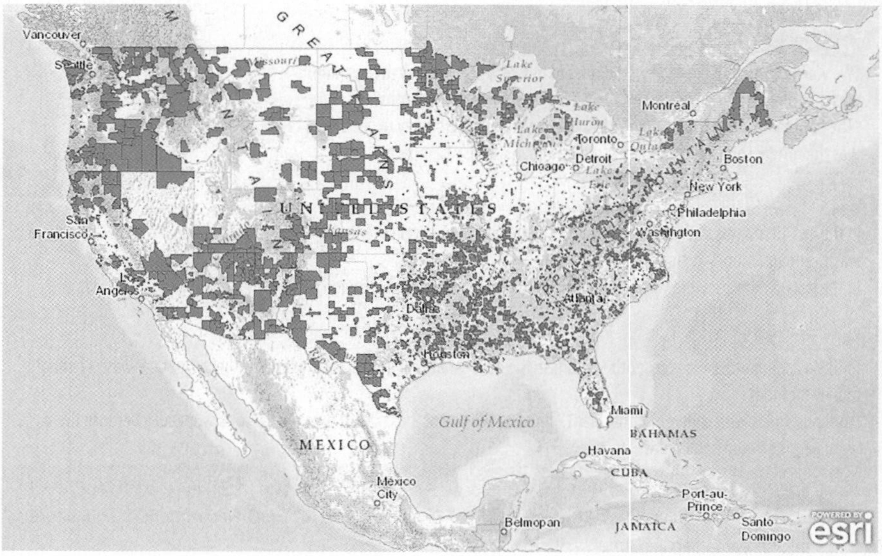

FIGURE 19.2 Food deserts in the United States.

Courtesy of US Department of Agriculture (USDA), Economic Research Service (ERS). Food Access Research Atlas. www.ers.usda.gov/data-products/food-access-research-atlas/.

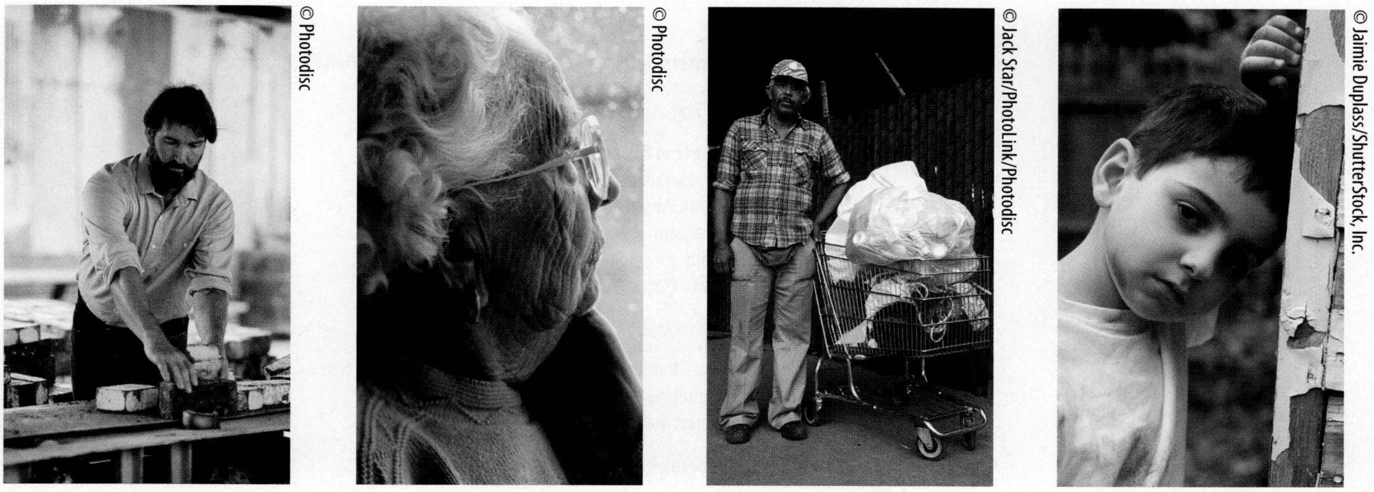

© Photodisc © Photodisc © Jack Star/PhotoLink/Photodisc © Jaimie Duplass/ShutterStock, Inc.

FIGURE 19.3 Americans at risk. Americans most at risk for hunger include working poor, older adults, homeless people, and children.

increasing nutrient needs. Older adults often have small incomes, with little prospect for improvement. Like others with limited resources, they cut food purchases to pay for other necessities. Although food assistance may be available, pride, shame, health conditions, or physical limitations can keep an older person from participating in such programs.

The Homeless or Inadequately Housed

People experiencing homelessness rely on soup kitchens and other public programs for much of their food. Some resort to handouts and even forage through garbage. Many are mentally ill or substance abusers. Those who suffer from addiction often have little interest in eating and may sell available food to buy more drugs. Many other people live in welfare hotels, single-room-occupancy facilities, or rooming houses without storage or cooking facilities. Budget-stretching strategies such as buying food in bulk and carefully using leftovers are out of the question for these people, like some others at risk (see **FIGURE 19.3**); as the monthly budget dwindles, they often rely on fast-food meals and then soup kitchens.

Children

Perhaps no group is more vulnerable to hunger than the young. Growth and development are delayed in poorly nourished children. They get sick more often. It is harder for them to concentrate in school. Children are captives of their family circumstances; poverty and lack of nutritious food in the household are beyond a child's control. In the United States, 9.4 percent of adults and children in households with children experienced times of low food security during 2014, and 1.1 percent experienced instances of very low food security.[14] Note that low food security describes having reduced quality, variety, or desirability of the diet, but with little or no reduction in food intake, while very low food security is when eating patterns are disrupted and food intake is reduced.[15]

Attacking Hunger in America

Government efforts to fight hunger began during the Great Depression of the 1930s. From that modest beginning, the USDA has grown to include numerous food and nutrition assistance programs and services that address hunger, including the Supplemental Nutrition Assistance Program (SNAP,

Quick Bite

Urban Food Production

Local food production is gaining support across U.S. urban areas. City governments have passed legislation that encourages urban agriculture, such as legalizing the sale of food produced from local gardens in San Francisco in 2011[16] and allowing commercial urban farmers to lease government farmland from the City of Seattle in 2014.[17] Local community gardens and farms are increasingly recognized as effective strategies for improving food security and access to fresh produce in urban areas.[18]

TABLE 19.3
USDA Food and Nutrition Service Food Assistance and Distribution Programs

Child Nutrition Programs
• Child and Adult Care Food Program • Fresh Fruit & Vegetable Program • National School Lunch Program • School Breakfast Program • Special Milk Program • Summer Food Service Program
Supplemental Nutrition Assistance Programs
• Special Supplemental Nutrition Program for Women, Infants, and Children • Farmers' Market Nutrition Programs • Senior Farmers' Market Nutrition Programs
Food Distribution Programs
• Commodity Supplemental Food Program • Food Distribution Program on Indian Reservations • Emergency Food Assistance Program

Data from U.S. Department of Agriculture, Food and Nutrition Service. Programs and services. http://www.fns.usda.gov/programs-and-services. Accessed January 14, 2016.

formerly the Food Stamp Program), the School Meals Programs, and the Special Supplemental Nutrition Program for Women, Infants, and Children (WIC) (see **TABLE 19.3**). The School Lunch Program was created in 1946 after many young men had failed the physical requirements for military service in World War II because of poor nutrition.

The Supplemental Nutrition Assistance Program (Food Stamp Program) was greatly expanded in the early 1970s following an exposé of hunger in Appalachia and the Mississippi Delta and the television documentary "Hunger in America." The federal government initiated WIC in the 1970s as a response to concerns about maternal and child health. Other government programs have since been added to meet the special needs of the young, the elderly, the disadvantaged, and the disabled.

▶ **Food Research and Action Center (FRAC)** Founded in 1970 as a public interest law firm, FRAC is a nonprofit child advocacy group that works to improve public policies to eradicate hunger and undernutrition in the United States.

▶ **Electronic Benefits Transfer (EBT)** Electronic delivery of government benefits by a single plastic card that allows access to food benefits at point-of-sale locations.

The **Food Research and Action Center (FRAC)** is a national nonprofit advocacy group that fights hunger and undernutrition at the national, state, and local levels. Nonprofit community agencies, charities, religious organizations, and similar groups create a large network of food pantries, soup kitchens, and services for home-delivered meals. Most of the federal government's programs for direct distribution of food or meals operate at the local level through these networks. Both laypeople and professionals, such as dietitians, work in these programs, either as volunteers or as staff, to fight hunger and malnutrition. THINK About It 2

Food assistance programs have greatly reduced the prevalence of hunger, but not of food insecurity, which requires social and economic change. The following are among the federal government's most far-reaching programs against hunger.

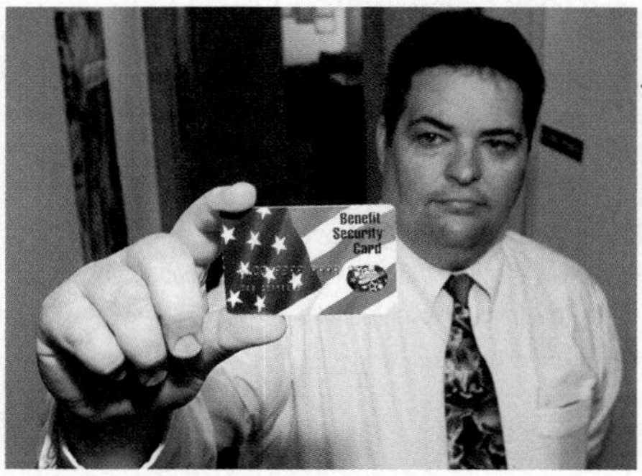

© Danny Johnston/AP Photos

FIGURE 19.4 Electronic Benefits Transfer card. Electronic Benefits Transfer (EBT) is an electronic system that allows recipients to authorize transfer of their government benefits from a federal account to a retailer account to pay for products received.

The Supplemental Nutrition Assistance Program

On October 1, 2008, the Food Stamp Program was renamed the Supplemental Nutrition Assistance Program (SNAP). SNAP is our main food security program. Recipients can use benefits to purchase food, but not nonfood items such as paper goods, pet food, cigarettes, or alcohol. The benefit amount varies according to household size and income level.

Actually, the term *food stamp* is becoming a misnomer. Most people who receive benefits use **Electronic Benefits Transfer (EBT)** cards (see **FIGURE 19.4**). The card

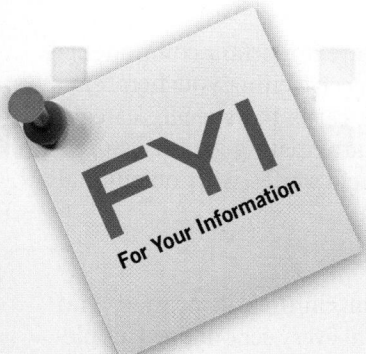

FYI
For Your Information

Hungry and Homeless

A shabbily dressed man slowly pushes a shopping cart along the sidewalk. It is laden with bottles and cans that he can redeem for cash. In front of a supermarket, a woman and child clutch a sign scrawled with the words "Hungry. Please help." On a street corner, a man confronts every passing car with a sign that says "Will work for food." When faced with a homeless person, do you feel uncomfortable? Do you turn away? Or do you try to help?

The U.S. Conference of Mayors' Task Force on Hunger and Homelessness reports that between 2013 and 2014, among the people who requested emergency food assistance, 56 percent were persons in families, 38 percent were employed, 20.5 percent were elderly, and 7 percent were homeless.[a]

Who are the people who experience homelessness? Roughly, 28 percent of homeless adults are severely mentally ill, 22 percent are physically disabled, 18 percent are employed, 15 percent are victims of domestic violence, 13 percent are veterans, and 3 percent are HIV positive.[b]

Hunger in people without housing is caused by a number of interrelated factors, including low-paying jobs, unemployment and related problems, high housing costs, substance abuse, poverty or lack of income, and food assistance cuts. Family members—children and their parents—most frequently request emergency food assistance. Among households with children, lack of affordable housing is the primary cause of homelessness, followed by unemployment, poverty, and low-paying jobs. Lack of affordable housing is the leading cause of homelessness for unaccompanied individuals, followed by unemployment, poverty, mental illness and the lack of needed services, and substance abuse and the lack of needed services.[c]

Complex challenges face those who are homeless, who may sleep in the streets or in emergency shelters. They get food from many sources—shelters, drop-in centers, fast food restaurants, and garbage bins. Approximately 46.5 million Americans (including 12 million children and 7 million seniors) obtained food from pantries at least once in 2013.[d] Soup kitchens are a primary source of meals, yet navigating this system to obtain adequate food can be a formidable and time-consuming task. Almost 70 percent of food-insecure households did not use a food pantry despite knowing that they were available in their community.[e] Also, although people who are homeless in America often are eligible for SNAP, they are extremely limited in their ability to store and prepare food, and few restaurants are authorized to accept SNAP benefits.

A major public health concern for people without housing is not only whether they are getting enough to eat, but also the nutritional quality of their diet. This concern is complicated by the special needs of infants, children, and women, especially pregnant women. The diet of food-insecure people is often nutritionally inadequate for numerous key nutrients including lower intake of fruits and vegetables, especially in children.[f] Poor diets put individuals who are homeless at an increased risk for illness and chronic conditions. Pregnant women, children, and people with compromised health status are particularly vulnerable.

Families and individuals experiencing homelessness rely on emergency food assistance facilities not only during emergencies, but also for extended periods. Unfortunately, these facilities are strained beyond their capacities. Because of limited space, emergency shelters must turn away families with children experiencing homelessness and unaccompanied individuals. During 2009–2010, an average of 27 percent of homeless persons in need of food assistance did not receive it.[g]

Some shelters have resorted to rationing to extend their food resources to a greater number of people. Because of a lack of resources, more than half can be forced to turn people away. Addressing hunger is a top priority. Once access to food is secure, obtaining a nutritionally adequate diet and dealing with health issues become reasonable goals.

[a] U.S. Conference of Mayors. *A Status Report on Hunger and Homelessness in America's Cities: A 25-City Survey.* December 2014. Accessed May 20, 2015.

[b] Ibid.

[c] Ibid.

[d] Feeding America. *Hunger in America 2014: A Report on Charitable Food Distribution in the United States in 2013, Executive Summary.* August 2014. http://www.feedingamerica.org/hunger-in-america/our-research/hunger-in-america/. Accessed January 14, 2016.

[e] Position of the Academy of Nutrition and Dietetics: food insecurity in the United States. *J Am Diet Assoc.* 2010;110:1368–1377.

[f] Ibid.

[g] Ibid.

resembles and functions like a debit card. Each month the household's benefit amount is credited to the card, which is then used at participating retailers and farmers' markets.

Special Supplemental Nutrition Program for Women, Infants, and Children

The WIC program provides food to pregnant and breastfeeding women, infants, and preschoolers. More than 8 million women and children receive WIC benefits each month.[19] To be eligible for WIC services, the participant must be at nutritional risk, and household income must meet federal poverty guidelines. For a family of four in fiscal year 2015–2016, the eligibility cutoff point was an annual income of no more than $44,863.[20]

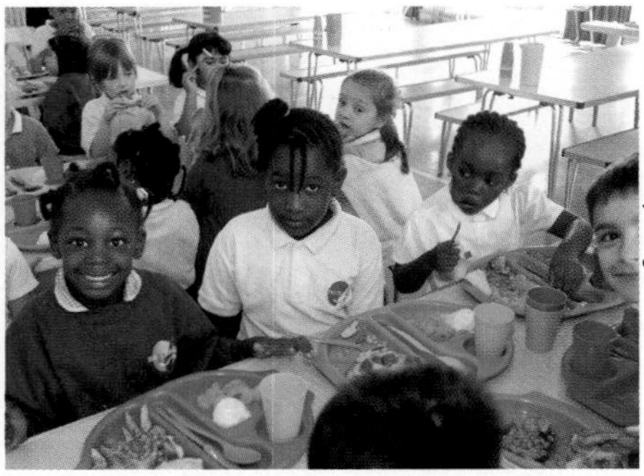
© Mike Booth/Alamy Images

FIGURE 19.5 National School Lunch Program.

Nutrition assessment and nutrition education are important components of the WIC program. In most states, participants receive either vouchers, also known as checks, or Electronic Benefits Transfer cards for specific categories of healthful foods, and they "cash" them at participating grocery stores. Unlike food stamps, the amount of the WIC benefit varies with nutritional need, not income.

National School Lunch Program

The National School Lunch Program ensures that children in primary and secondary schools receive at least one healthful meal every school day (supplemented in many areas by the School Breakfast Program). For a family of four in the year 2015–2016, the child's meals were free if the household income was less than $31,525; the meals were reduced in price if household income was less than $44,863.[21] School lunches must be in compliance with applicable *Dietary Guidelines for Americans* and the lunch must provide one-third or more of dietary requirements for key nutrients. The program operates in more than 100,000 public and nonprofit private schools and residential child-care institutions. It provided nutritionally balanced low-cost or free lunches to more than 31 million children each school day in 2012[22] (see **FIGURE 19.5**).

▶ **Child and Adult Care Food Program** A federally funded program that reimburses approved family child-care providers for USDA-approved foods served to preschool children; it also provides funds for meals and snacks served at after-school programs for school-age children and to adult day care centers serving chronically impaired adults or people older than age 60.

Child and Adult Care Food Program

The **Child and Adult Care Food Program** provides funds for children's meals and snacks at nonprofit licensed child-care centers, day care homes, after-school programs, and similar settings. Nutritious meals for the elderly or people with disabilities are also funded at nonprofit facilities such as adult day care centers and recreation centers.

▶ **Feeding America** The largest charitable hunger-relief organization in the United States. Its mission is to feed America's hungry through a nationwide network of member food banks and to engage the country in the fight to end hunger.

Feeding America

Feeding America, formerly known as America's Second Harvest, is the largest charitable hunger-relief organization in the United States. This network of more than 200 member food banks and food-rescue organizations secures and distributes more than 3.3 billion meals throughout the United States. Each year, Feeding America provides food assistance to more than 46 million hungry people, including 12 million children and 7 million seniors.[23]

Feeding America focuses on nutritious products such as fresh produce, seafood, meat, cereal, rice, and pasta. The organization also works to effect changes in public attitudes and laws that assist Americans who are hungry or at risk of being hungry. Feeding America also works to educate the general public and keep them informed about hunger in America.

Quick Bite

Tackling Food Insecurity

The National Commission on Hunger was established as part the Consolidated Appropriations Act of 2014 to develop a report on new strategies to solve the problem of hunger and food insecurity in America. The 9-member commission is charged with finding innovative ways to strengthen domestic anti-hunger policies and develop public–private partnerships. The commission conducted public hearings in cities across the United States in 2015 and will release its final recommendations in November 2015 and released its recommendations in January 2016. Twenty specific reommendations were provided to USDA and Congress, including enhancing nutrition assistance programs and offering incentives to increase corporate and non-profit support of hunger relief.[24]

Key Concepts Although overt malnutrition in the United States is uncommon, more than 17 million American households experience food insecurity at some time during the year. Food insecurity and hunger are interlinked with poverty. Groups at risk include the working poor, the isolated, those who are homeless, children, and elders. A large network of individual volunteers, nonprofit agencies, and charities, together with major government programs such as SNAP, WIC, and the School Lunch Program, have done much to reduce hunger. However, food insecurity, which continues among an unacceptably large number of people, must be overcome by social and economic improvements. Feeding America is the largest charitable hunger-relief organization in the United States.

▶ **World Health Organization (WHO)** A global organization that directs and coordinates international health work. Its goal is the attainment by all peoples of the highest possible level of health, defined as a state of complete physical, mental, and social well-being and not merely the absence of disease or infirmity.

Malnutrition in the Developing World

"Proper nutrition and health are fundamental human rights," according to the **World Health Organization (WHO)**. "Nutrition is a key element in any strategy to reduce the global burden of disease. Hunger, malnutrition, obesity and unsafe food all cause disease, and better nutrition will translate into large improvements in health among all of us, irrespective of our wealth and home country."[25]

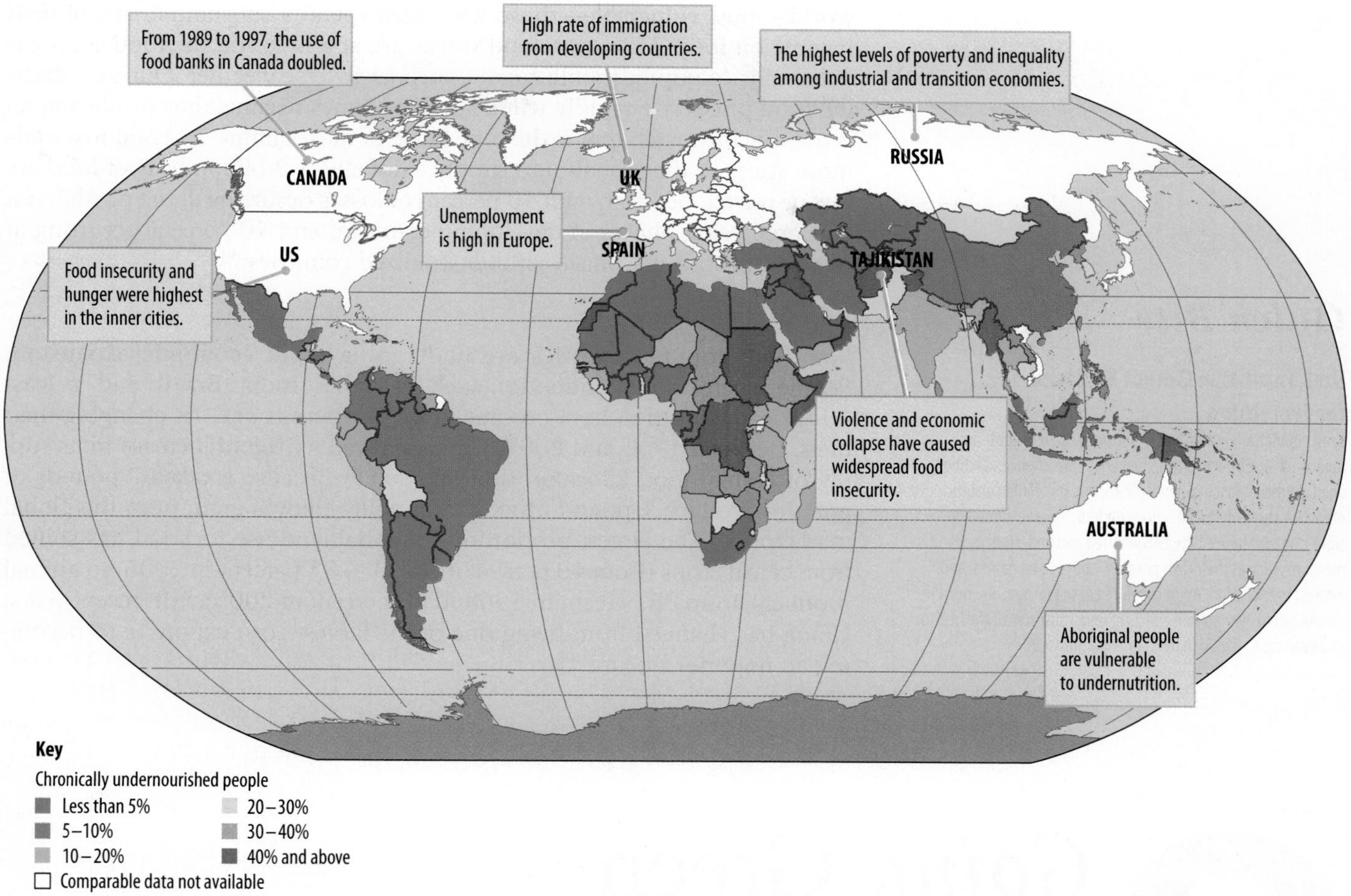
From 1989 to 1997, the use of food banks in Canada doubled.
High rate of immigration from developing countries.
The highest levels of poverty and inequality among industrial and transition economies.
RUSSIA
CANADA
UK
Unemployment is high in Europe.
SPAIN
US
TAJIKISTAN
Food insecurity and hunger were highest in the inner cities.
Violence and economic collapse have caused widespread food insecurity.
AUSTRALIA
Aboriginal people are vulnerable to undernutrition.
Key
Chronically undernourished people
Less than 5%
5–10%
10–20%
20–30%
30–40%
40% and above
Comparable data not available

FIGURE 19.6 Global hunger. Although the proportion of the world's population that is chronically undernourished has been decreasing over the last few decades, undernutrition is still widespread, particularly in certain regions. Furthermore, projections suggest that there will be little change in the absolute number of chronically undernourished people.

Reproduced from Food and Agriculture Organization of the United Nations, 2015. Hunger: Interactive world hunger map. www.fao.org/hunger/en. Accessed December 17, 2015.

Hunger is a global problem (see **FIGURE 19.6**). "Sustained political commitment at the highest level is a prerequisite for hunger eradication. It entails placing food security and nutrition at the top of the political agenda and creating an enabling environment for improving food security and nutrition," says the **Food and Agriculture Organization (FAO)** of the United Nations.[26] Although undernutrition persists, its prevalence declined by nearly 50 percent between 1990 and 2014 in developing regions. This reduction in undernutrition marked success in reaching one of the 2015 United Nations Millennium Development Goals.[27]

► **Food and Agriculture Organization (FAO)** The largest autonomous United Nations agency; the FAO works to alleviate poverty and hunger by promoting agricultural development, improved nutrition, and the pursuit of food security.

THINK About It 3

"We face a double imperative: we must end hunger and malnutrition, and we must do so sustainably. Our progress in improving global food security is fragile and in many ways environmentally unsustainable. Meeting both imperatives is doable, but it will demand more strategic use of resources, stronger responsibility and accountability, and more creativity from all of us," states the *2014–2015 Global Food Policy Report* of the International Food Policy Research Institute.[28]

The World Food Equation

Income growth, climate change, high energy prices, globalization, and urbanization are transforming food consumption. Soaring food prices are hitting the world's most vulnerable—those who must spend a substantial part of their income on food. Moreover, food stocks are at a low, and the food supply is vulnerable to unpredictable factors, such as adverse weather. During a disaster, food prices rise rapidly while family incomes decline, thus producing an economic mismatch that is the root cause of most famines.[29] Food loss adds more stress to the global food supply. Globally, 1.3 billion tons of food are lost or wasted per year, with 40 percent of losses occurring at the postharvest and processing phases in developing countries and 40 percent occurring at retail and consumer phases in industrialized countries.[30]

Quick Bite

Undernutrition Cannot Be Blamed for Everything

In all populations in the developing world, low weight- and height-for-age affect 10 to 15 percent of preschool and school-aged children. Most experts attribute this shortfall to insufficiency of food. A study of African schoolchildren, however, found no significant difference between well-fed and underfed pupils on measures such as their class position, aptitude for games, and interest in education. Among children of school age, one must be careful not to overrate the effects of undernutrition or the health disadvantages of mild to moderate malnutrition.

Global Economic Boom

Some developing countries are undergoing rapid economic expansion. People in emerging economies, such as China, India, Brazil, and at least 10 African countries, have become more prosperous and are changing their diets. Between 1961 and 2007, China showed a fivefold increase in its supply of animal food kilocalories per person.[31] Because it takes 7 pounds of grain to produce 1 pound of meat, this shift removes grain from the global marketplace. The largest proportion of global land use for food has shifted from cereal crops (from 40 percent in 1963 to 31 percent in 2005) to animal products (from 35 percent in 1963 to 38 percent in 2005).[32] In recent years, China has changed from being one of the largest corn exporters to becoming an importer of corn.[33]

Going Green

Can Chocolate Help the Planet?

Cacao trees, the source of chocolate, used to be a thriving industry in the Mata Atlantica, a rainforest area of eastern Brazil. But now the shrinking price of chocolate in the world market and several decades of plant disease are working against chocolate production. The precious rainforest trees that produce cacao beans have been marked for destruction by logging interests. The short-sighted logging interests see more profit in cutting down these trees for wood, or burning them to make room for pasture land, than in cultivating the cacao. Thus, there is little incentive for farmers to cultivate cacao beans for chocolate.

But how does that affect the environment? Dario Anhert, a researcher at the University of Santa Cruz in eastern Brazil, suggests that the chocolate industry can help reduce global climate change. These rainforest trees store massive amounts of carbon and thus prevent the carbon from getting into the air as carbon dioxide. When a tree is burned, it releases the stored carbon, thereby affecting climate change and contributing to a warmer planet.

One alternative to destroying the trees is cabruca farming. This method entails planting cacao trees among other trees, cutting down just a few of the tall rainforest trees, and planting the midheight cacao trees underneath. Inside a cabruca forest, the ground is covered in a thick layer of composting leaves. It's moist, shady, and cool in the cabruca.

Planting inside the forest means fewer cacao trees to the acre, and in turn less production. But farming in the forest avoids drawbacks other farmers struggle with when they grow cacao trees on more open land, including disease and more insects.

There's also an expanding market for environmentally friendly chocolate. Some forest farmers have been able to get a premium for their crop. Anhert hopes that cabruca can become part of the carbon credit market. Farmers would then get money for preserving forest trees, as well as for their chocolate. Anhert hopes to persuade farmers to preserve rainforest ecosystems and provide a viable, long-term economic opportunity with the chocolate option. A complicated process—but, yes, producing chocolate in the rainforest can contribute to a better planet.

Oil Prices and Biofuels

Oil prices affect costs along the entire food production chain—from fertilizer to diesel for tilling, planting, and harvesting to storage and shipping. High oil prices reduce global food availability by diverting food stocks and cropland toward the manufacture of biofuels.[34] Research models estimate that 25–50 percent of net kilocalories in corn or wheat diverted to ethanol biofuel manufacture are not replaced, resulting in less food energy for human consumption.[35] Production of biodiesel and other biofuels is pressuring the global markets for wheat, corn, sugar, oil-containing seeds, cassava, palm oil, and other crops.

Global Climate Change and Severe Weather Events

As a consequence of climate change, farmers will face growing unpredictability and variability in water supplies and increasing frequency of droughts and floods. However, these impacts will vary tremendously from place to place. According to experts with the FAO, "The livelihoods of rural communities and the food security of a predominantly urban population are at risk from water-related impacts linked primarily to climate variability. The rural poor, who are the most vulnerable, are likely to be disproportionately affected."[36]

Water is fundamental to the stability of global food production. Reliable access to water increases agricultural yields, and a lack of sustainable water management places global food security at risk. In developing countries, drought is the single most common natural cause of severe food shortages. Floods are another major cause of food emergencies. To the extent that climate change increases rainfall variability and the frequency of extreme weather events, it will threaten food security.

The Fight Against Global Hunger

International relief agencies and government programs help combat food shortages and hunger. Some U.S. agencies involved in the fight against global hunger are the USDA; the U.S. State Department, through its Agency for International Development; and the Centers for Disease Control and Prevention (CDC), through the Center for Communicable Diseases. These agencies offer both short-term emergency efforts and long-term programs for repair and rebuilding.

Long-term solutions to hunger are tremendously complex; they require economic, political, and social change, as well as improvements in nutrition, food production, and environmental safeguards. As you study the critical nutrient deficiencies in the developing world, you will see that poverty, infection, poor sanitation, and social upheaval interact with nutrient shortages to bring about these deficiencies.

Social and Economic Factors

Poverty, overpopulation, and migration to overcrowded cities are closely interrelated causes of hunger (see **FIGURE 19.7**). Each situation worsens the effects of the others as they steadily drive a population toward malnutrition.

Poverty

Poverty, hunger, and malnutrition stalk one another in a vicious circle, compromising health and wreaking havoc on the development of entire countries and regions. A large

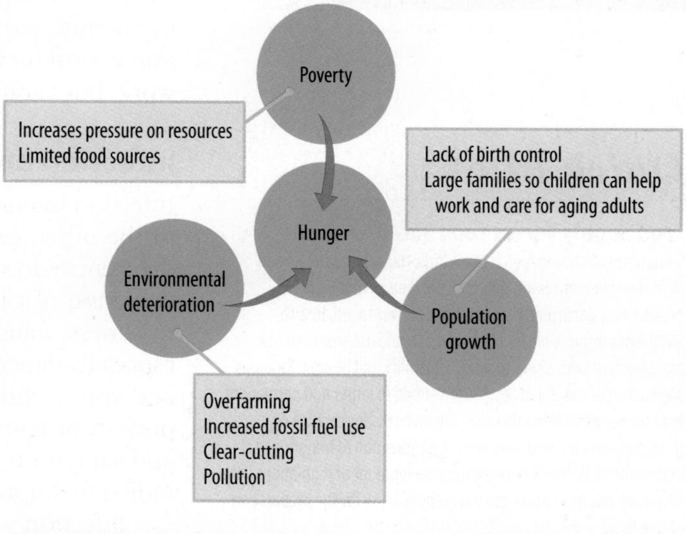

FIGURE 19.7 Major problems causing hunger. Poverty, population growth, and environmental degradation interact to make hunger worse.

Position Statement: Academy of Nutrition and Dietetics

Addressing World Hunger, Malnutrition, and Food Insecurity

It is the position of the Academy of Nutrition and Dietetics that all people should have consistent access to an appropriately nutritious diet of food and water, coupled with a sanitary environment, adequate health services, and care that ensures a healthy and active life for all household members. The Academy supports policies, systems, programs, and practices that work with developing nations to achieve nutrition security and self-sufficiency while being environmentally and economically sustainable.

Reproduced from Struble MB, Aomari LL. Position of the American Dietetic Association: addressing world hunger, malnutrition, and food insecurity. *J Am Diet Assoc.* 2003;103(8):1046–1057.

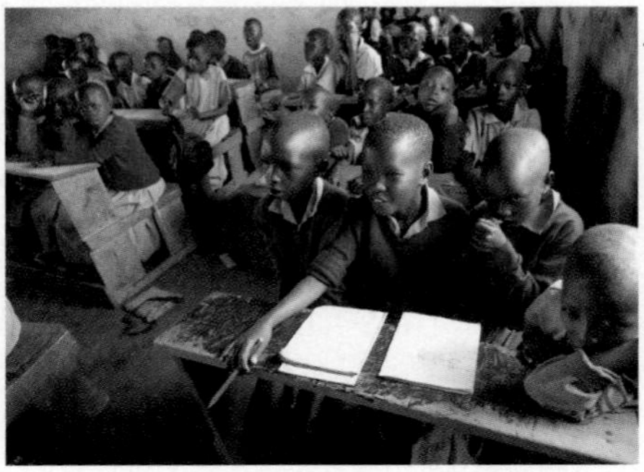
© spirit of america/ShutterStock, Inc.

Quick Bite

Food Supply Versus Food Safety

Sometimes obtaining food is more important than safety. Food from street vendors is important in the diets of many urban populations, particularly the socially disadvantaged. Health authorities responsible for food safety should balance their risk management with issues of food availability and hunger. Rigorous application of codes and regulations suited to larger and permanent food service establishments may cause the disappearance of the street vendors, with consequent aggravation of hunger and malnutrition. WHO encourages the development of regulations that empower vendors to take greater responsibility for the preparation of safe food.

percentage of the global population—especially those in developing countries—bear this triple burden.

Poverty is the most important underlying reason for chronic hunger.[37] Obviously, it limits access to food. It limits purchase of farming supplies to grow food, boats and equipment to fish, and storage equipment to prevent spoilage. It limits access to medical care. It compromises sanitation efforts. It discourages education and the chance for personal advancement.

For nations, poverty means paralyzed economic development and too few jobs; inadequate investments in infrastructure and basic housing; and too few resources to train doctors, nutritionists, nurses, and other healthcare workers.

Population Growth

Population growth in many regions is outstripping gains in food production, education, employment, health care, and economic progress. The burgeoning numbers stress limited environmental resources, contributing to environmental degradation and pollution. In rural areas where farmland is limited, each small parcel of family land is subdivided with each generation, until there is too little land to support each family.

You may think that poverty would pressure parents to limit family size, but ironically, poverty and sickness do just the reverse. Where child mortality rates are high, having many babies is a guarantee some children will survive. In countries that have no economic safeguards for disability, unemployment, or old age, parents consider their children a source of security and support in times of need. Many other factors contribute to large families, from ignorance of birth control methods to the attitude that big families reflect the father's masculinity. Some political groups also encourage high birth rates and fast population growth as a way to achieve political or military dominance.

To slow population growth, socioeconomic and cultural changes that make smaller family size acceptable, even desirable, must accompany access to birth control.

Urbanization

Urbanization is a worldwide trend. As rural lands become too crowded or exhausted farmland no longer supports good crops, rural people migrate to the city in hopes of jobs and a better life. Unfortunately, in fast-growing cities, social disorder, sanitary conditions, and living standards can be much worse. Hunting, fishing, foraging, and gardening—sources of accessible food in the rural setting—are seldom an option in the city. Breastfeeding becomes impractical for many mothers who could nurse their babies while doing farm work, but cannot do so with jobs in the city.

Infection and Disease

Infection interacts with malnutrition, each making its victim more vulnerable to the other, each making the other worse, in a downward spiral. Nutrient deficiencies lower resistance to infections. In turn, the fever of infection speeds depletion of calories and nutrients. Other symptoms (e.g., loss of appetite, weakness, nausea, mouth lesions) limit ability to eat. Infectious diarrhea is especially dangerous, quickly wasting what few nutrients are consumed; infants and young children can die quickly from loss of electrolytes. Programs that prevent or control infection (e.g., immunizations, improvements in hygiene and sanitation, safe water supplies, access to medicine and medical care) all indirectly improve nutrition status.

Infection with the human immunodeficiency virus (HIV) provides a dramatic demonstration of the interaction between malnutrition and infection.

Among those who are afflicted, the infection progresses fastest in people who are poorly nourished. Severe loss of weight and muscle is a hallmark of the advanced disease, acquired immune deficiency syndrome (AIDS).

Globally, 1.5 million people died from AIDS-related causes in 2014. More than 35 million people are living with HIV because infected people are living longer than before, and AIDS-related deaths have declined in recent years.[38] Ninety-seven percent of people living with HIV/AIDS live in low- and middle-income countries, and an estimated 70 percent of new HIV cases worldwide occur in sub-Saharan Africa, where it is the leading cause of death. Other areas experiencing severe epidemics include eastern Europe, Latin America, and Central Asia. In 2013, approximately 240,000 children were newly infected with HIV, bringing the total number of children living with HIV to 3.2 million.[39]

Quick Bite

Where Were You Born?

Your survival was greatly influenced by the location of your birth. In 2013, infant mortality rates (the probability of dying between birth and age 1 per 1,000 live births) ranged from 53 in low-income countries to 5 in high-income countries.[40] Across continents, the highest infant mortality rate was seen in Africa (6%) and the lowest in Europe (1.1%) and the Americas (1.2%).[41]

Political Disruptions

Social upheavals and natural disasters such as floods and drought can leave famine in their wake. The resulting displacement of populations and inequitable food distribution usually lead to hunger and malnutrition.

War

Whereas poverty is the underlying cause of chronic mild to moderate malnutrition, war and its aftermath cause severe malnutrition and famine. War diverts limited financial resources from development efforts to expenditures for fighting and destruction. Men and women no longer farm, fish, or bring home a paycheck—they are in the army. Households become fatherless and sometimes motherless, often permanently. Crops and croplands are destroyed, along with irrigation systems, food-processing facilities, and transportation infrastructure, which may have taken decades to develop.

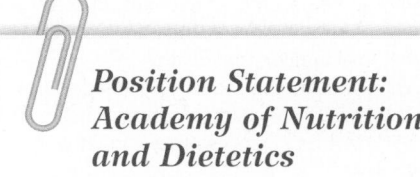

Position Statement: Academy of Nutrition and Dietetics

Nutrition Intervention and Human Immunodeficiency Virus Infection

It is the position of the Academy of Nutrition and Dietetics that efforts to optimize nutritional status through individualized medical nutrition therapy, assurance of food and nutrition security, and nutrition education are essential to the total system of health care available to people with human immunodeficiency virus (HIV) infection throughout the continuum of care.

Reproduced from Position of the American Dietetic Association: nutrition intervention and human immunodeficiency virus infection. *J Am Diet Assoc.* 2010;110:1105–1119.

Refugees

Masses of refugees—many very young, old, infirm, and already weakened by chronic hunger—find themselves without the basic elements of sustenance. The resulting famine has become an all-too-common sight on the evening news.

International relief agencies have learned to respond to these emergencies quickly and with great determination, but logistic difficulties (e.g., mobilizing manpower, obtaining foods, transporting supplies, setting up feeding stations) can slow relief until it is too late for the sickest or weakest. Some refugee groups are inaccessible, hidden, or intentionally kept hungry as part of a political plan; emergency food may never reach many of them.

Sanctions

International sanctions and embargoes create food shortages, both directly and indirectly, by limiting access to agricultural supplies, fuel, and food-processing supplies. Some people argue that shortages created by embargoes hurt powerless people rather than government officials; others say that such actions are preferable to war.

Quick Bite

Rehydration Therapy for Diarrhea

Simple and inexpensive packets of carbohydrate and salts diluted with sterile water replace lost fluids and electrolytes. These packets are saving thousands of people each year.

Floods, Droughts, Mudslides, and Hurricanes

Many countries are not equipped to deal with food shortages, water and food sanitation concerns, and hunger caused by disruptions in food supply and distribution resulting from natural disasters. International relief agencies and other governments step in to help when possible. Emergency relief efforts in the United States that include food distribution have taken more of a prominent role in disaster preparedness. In the wake of terrorist attacks such as those on September 11, 2001, and natural disasters such as Hurricane Katrina, the U.S.

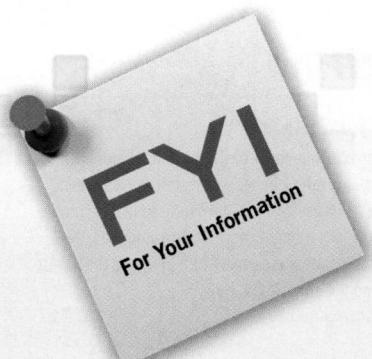

FYI For Your Information

AIDS and Malnutrition

Like other infections, HIV interacts with malnutrition in a vicious, devastating cycle. Left untreated, HIV infection progresses to acquired immune deficiency syndrome (AIDS). The virus attacks by destroying its victim's immune system. When a person is unable to fight infections and malignancies, disease quickly depletes marginal nutrient stores, speeding the way to severe malnutrition and death. But, malnutrition and HIV interact on several other levels as well, such as[a]:

- Poor nutrition contributes to declining immune function, HIV progression, and further health deterioration.
- HIV can be transmitted to infants in breast milk; but in impoverished regions, substitutions for breast milk can lead to increased infantile diarrhea, malnutrition, and death.
- AIDS leaves mothers too weak to feed and care for their children. Eventually, AIDS turns children into orphans.
- AIDS disables parents so they cannot work to support and feed their families.
- Among those who are afflicted, the infection progresses faster in people who are poorly nourished.
- Weight loss and muscle wasting in an infected person are associated with faster progression of HIV disease and AIDS.
- Infections that accompany AIDS cause fever and diarrhea, making malnutrition worse. Nausea and loss of appetite also contribute to malnutrition.
- Severe protein-energy malnutrition (PEM) is characteristic of untreated AIDS and frequently the ultimate cause of death.
- Adequate dietary intake and nutrient absorption are essential to achieving the maximum benefit of antiretroviral treatment for HIV/AIDS.

More than 35 million people are living with HIV. Sub-Saharan Africa, Southeast Asia, Latin America, eastern Europe, and central Asia continue to be areas with a high prevalence of HIV.[b] Although fewer people are dying from AIDS-related causes, only about 34 percent of HIV-infected people in low- and middle-income countries received antiretroviral therapy in 2013.[c] The untreated people are doomed to death, usually within 10 years of the initial infection. The fate of severe PEM in millions of people appears unavoidable. If we do not arrest the continued transmission of HIV, the number of PEM victims will climb even higher.

[a]World Food Programme, World Health Organization, and UNAIDS. Policy brief. HIV, food security and nutrition. May 2008. http://www.unaids.org/en/media/unaids/contentassets/dataimport/pub/manual/2008/jc1515_policy_brief_nutrition_en.pdf. Accessed January 14, 2016.

[b]UNAIDS. Global Report: UNAIDS report on the global AIDS epidemic 2013. http://www.unaids.org/sites/default/files/en/media/unaids/contentassets/documents/epidemiology/2013/gr2013/UNAIDS_Global_Report_2013_en.pdf. Accessed January 16, 2016.

[c]Ibid.

Quick Bite

Emergency Management

Imagine a civil war in a developing country that displaces tens of thousands of people. What are the most important measures for preventing sickness and death among these refugees? Protection from violence heads the list, closely followed by adequate food rations, clean water and sanitation, diarrheal disease control, measles immunization, and maternal and child health care.

military and both domestic and international relief agencies reevaluated their level of preparedness to respond to these types of emergencies. Some U.S. agencies involved are the U.S. military, the USDA, the U.S. State Department through its Agency for International Development (USAID), the Federal Emergency Management Agency (FEMA), and the CDC. These agencies offer both short-term emergency efforts and long-term programs for repair and rebuilding.

Agriculture and Environment: A Tricky Balance

Advances in agriculture increase food supplies and reduce food costs. Because the economies of most developing countries are based on agriculture, improvements boost rural incomes and buying power, increase demand for agricultural labor, stimulate commerce among small vendors and food processors, and ultimately help a nation's economy.

Dramatic gains in agricultural productivity took place in the 1960s and 1970s with the development of new seed varieties, especially rice and corn. The seeds greatly increased crop yields. Expectations were so strong that these seeds would finally solve the world's food shortage that their development and use was dubbed the "Green Revolution." Despite its successes, the Green Revolution had limitations. The seeds required irrigation and heavy use of pesticides and fertilizers, which poor farmers could not afford. The farming techniques were sometimes hard on the environment. Proponents of agricultural biotechnology see it as another step along the continuum of plant-breeding techniques and a promising tool to increase crop production.

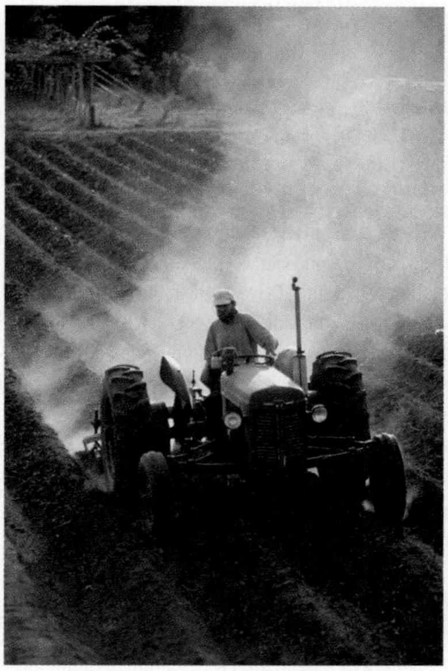

Some uses of biotechnology are well accepted—for example, diagnostic kits that identify plants and insects by DNA and tissue culture for plant reproduction, a technique already in widespread commercial use. More controversial is the modification of plant genetic material. The technology has the potential to improve plants' resistance to disease, tolerance to adverse conditions, yield, and nutritional quality.

At the other end of the technology spectrum is a renewed appreciation and conservation of traditional seed varieties, those selected over the generations by local farmers because they do well in local conditions. In developing countries, farmers typically save some of these seeds at each harvest to use in the next planting season. The seeds grow well in the regions where they've evolved, whereas imported seeds, no matter how carefully bred, often fail.

In addition to seed selection, strategies to optimize agriculture include irrigation, soil preparation, improved planting and harvest methods, erosion prevention, fertilization, pest control, and flood control. The methods should be affordable, suitable for the level of local development, and protective of the environment. For example, where there is an abundant supply of willing farm laborers and gasoline is expensive, using heavy-duty farm machinery makes little sense. Other examples include mulching to conserve water and control weeds, and using manure (after composting to kill pathogens) to reduce the need for fertilizer.

Environmental Degradation

Environmental degradation is a growing concern in both the developing and the industrialized world. In developing countries, there is pressure for more land to support rapidly expanding populations. In industrialized countries, there is pressure from the affluent for more land, more houses, larger properties, more recreation areas, and so on. Residents of the industrialized world consume vast amounts of resources (e.g., water, fuel, wood, paper, textiles, food), often without a thought or making a small effort to conserve or recycle. Residents of the developing world consume much less per person, but the impact of their numbers is greater.

Environmental degradation has nutritional consequences because it threatens food production. Urbanization and the expansion of cities reduce acreage available for farming. The pressure to supply food to growing populations leads to clear-cutting marginal land, eventually eroding hilly terrain or quickly exhausting fragile rainforest soils. Overdependence on irrigation can drain water, eventually creating deserts. The destruction of vast areas of natural ground cover can lead to global climate changes. Overuse of pesticides and fertilizers pollutes waterways, destroying fish and seafood.

Key Concepts Despite gains in eradicating malnutrition, almost all of the undernourished people in the world live in developing countries. Factors that allow hunger to continue include rising food prices, poverty, poor sanitation, urbanization, and inefficient food distribution. Infection, especially AIDS; rapid population growth; wars; and environmental degradation threaten to reverse hard-won gains.

Malnutrition: Its Nature, Its Victims, and Its Eradication

Previous chapters discussed the diseases of nutritional deficiency. Most of these diseases exist throughout the developing world, but seldom in isolation. Typically, the malnourished person has two or more coexisting deficiencies, each increasing the severity of the other. Additionally, the increasing prevalence of obesity worldwide has presented a new nutritional paradox. The growing number of overweight, overfat individuals who are malnourished with worsening health status, increased disability, and higher risk of chronic degenerative conditions presents a new global health problem. Keep the potential for this deadly synergy in mind as we discuss some of the major categories of malnutrition.

Quick Bite

Who Produces the World's Soybeans?

Before 1900, the soybean was rarely grown in the United States. Today, the U.S. is the world's largest producer and exporter of soybeans. Ninety percent of U.S. oilseed production is composed of soybeans. Soybeans provide 75 percent of the dietary fats and oils in the United States and are an important ingredient in high-protein feed for livestock poultry, swine, beef, and dairy. Over half a metric ton of soybean meal per year is used to produce food for America's pets.[43,44]

Protein-Energy Malnutrition

Lack of protein and also energy can have devastating consequences, especially on the young. In kwashiorkor, the body and face swell with excess fluid, the hair turns wispy and red, and a terrible rash develops; without treatment, the person dies. Marasmus paints an even more dramatic picture of sunken eyes, shriveled limbs, and a clearly visible outline of the skeleton; it is as deadly as kwashiorkor.

Protein-energy malnutrition (PEM) is by far the most lethal form of malnutrition, and children are its most visible victims.[42] Their rapid growth creates high nutrient demands, leaving them especially vulnerable to inappropriate food distribution in the family, inappropriate infant and child feeding practices, and interactions of infection with malnutrition. PEM typically develops after a child is weaned from the breast. Men in the household may have priority for nutritious food. In big families, the young child must also compete for food with many siblings.

In the developing world, breastfeeding is almost always essential to an infant's survival. Inappropriate bottle-feeding puts a baby at grave risk. Relative to income, formula is usually very expensive and is often diluted to make it "stretch." Contaminated water and lack of other hygienic requirements for bottle preparation cause diarrhea. The combination of diarrhea and nutritional deficiency from watered-down formula often is fatal.

A tremendous educational effort, including promotion of breastfeeding, has reduced the global prevalence and severity of infant and childhood PEM. Still, globally, acute malnutrition, defined as wasting or low body weight for height, affects 52 million children under the age of 5 years. Of these children, over 17 million suffer severe acute malnutrition. Worldwide, wasting accounts for 4.7 percent of child deaths, and children who are wasted and

FYI
For Your Information

Tough Choices

Imagine you live in a poor village of a developing country. How would you make these choices?

- You've learned you must boil your drinking water to prevent diarrhea. But that means cutting young trees for firewood. You recently planted those trees to stop erosion. What do you do?
- You've recently given birth to your fourth child. Your husband was injured in an accident and is unable to work. But you can work at a nearby factory and use your pay to buy food and clothes for the older children. How would you feed the new baby?
- Your small herd of goats provides milk for your young children. You like the goats because they can survive in the rough, hilly countryside. But the goats are overgrazing the grasses on the hillside. What can you do?
- Insects have destroyed your crop. In the past, you burned fields after harvest to control insects, but you've learned that "slash and burn" is bad for the land. You've thought about using a chemical pesticide, but it is too expensive. You could clear the jungle for another growing field. Do you have other choices? What should you do?
- You can grow either vegetables to feed your family or a "cash crop" to sell for export. The cash crop would help pay for medicine and other necessities. Which should you grow?

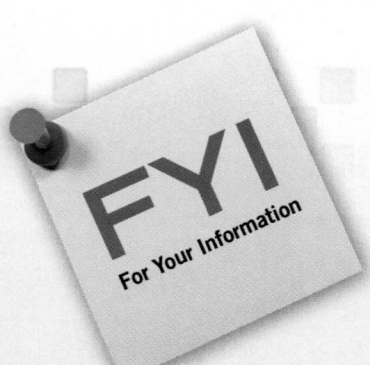

stunted (low height-for-age) experience the highest rates of mortality. Wasting increases the risk of death from infectious disease such as measles, pneumonia, and diarrhea.[45]

Iodine Deficiency Disorders

Iodine deficiency is the world's most common cause of preventable brain damage and one of the main causes of impaired cognitive development in children.[46] Its impairment of intellectual ability and work performance is potentially so widespread that **iodine deficiency disorders (IDDs)** can actually slow a nation's social and economic development.

Iodine deficiency is most devastating during pregnancy, causing spontaneous abortions, stillbirths, and birth defects, including cretinism, a disease of mental retardation that is often severe. Deafness and spastic paralysis are likely to accompany the retardation. Dietary goitrogens, which interfere with iodine uptake or metabolism by the thyroid gland, can worsen the effects of an iodine-deficient diet. People consuming diets centered around food staples that contain high levels of goitrogens (cruciferous vegetables, soy, cassava, and sweet potatoes) and whose iodine intake is minimal are at particular risk for iodine deficiency disorders. Moreover, iodine deficiency is damaging at all ages, limiting mental development in infants and children and producing apathy and marginal mental function in adults.[47]

Iodine deficiency disorders are endemic throughout much of the developing world where the soil is low in iodine. These areas typically are mountainous or far from the oceans. They often are isolated and impoverished. Although imported food is a potential source of iodine, it often is not consumed; according to WHO reports, 54 countries are still iodine-deficient.[48] Globally, 35 million newborns are at risk of iodine deficiency disorders (see **FIGURE 19.8**).[49]

Disturbing though these figures are, great strides have been made in IDD prevention, mainly through iodizing salt over the past 30 years. Currently, 75 percent of households now use iodized salt, and East Asia and the Pacific are close to reaching the target of 90 percent of households.[50] Iodized salt is manufactured using simple technology and costs only $0.04 per year per person.[51]

▶ **iodine deficiency disorders (IDDs)** A wide range of disorders caused by iodine deficiency that affect growth and development.

Vitamin A Deficiency

Vitamin A deficiency is the leading cause of preventable blindness in children. It also increases the risk of disease and death from severe infections. Vitamin A deficiency causes night blindness, and in pregnant women can increase the risk of maternal mortality.[52]

Vitamin A deficiency is a public health problem in more than half of all countries, especially those in Africa and Southeast Asia, hitting young children and pregnant women in low-income countries hardest. The nutrient is crucial for maternal and child survival, and supplying adequate vitamin A in high-risk areas can significantly reduce mortality. Conversely, its absence causes a needlessly high risk of disease and death. An estimated 250 million preschool children are vitamin A–deficient, 250,000 to 500,000 children become blind every year, and one-half of them die within 12 months of losing their sight.[53]

Vitamin A deficiency often coexists with marginal PEM. The vitamin deficiency predisposes infants and children to diarrheal diseases, which, in turn, worsen the child's nutritional status, leading to severe PEM. Common childhood infections, most notably measles, are much more serious in vitamin A–deficient children, with a much greater risk of death or permanent damage from complications.

In communities where vitamin A deficiency exists, pregnant and breastfeeding women often experience night blindness, an early symptom of

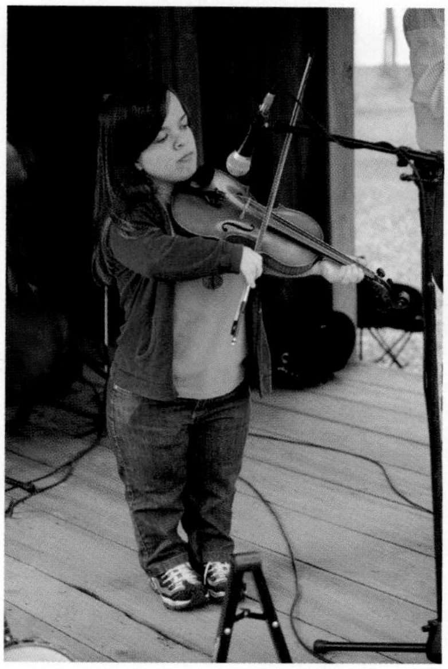

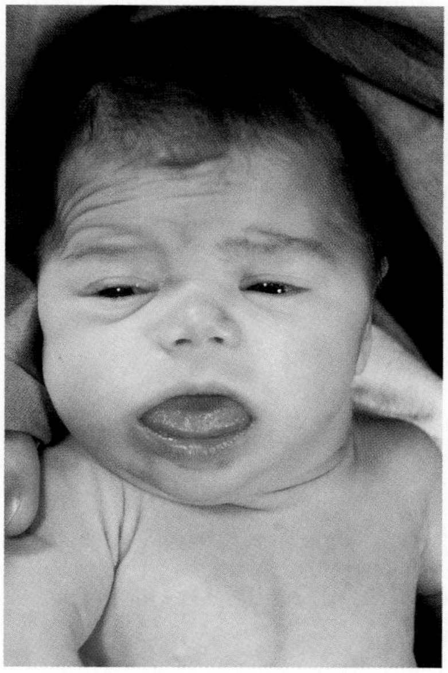

FIGURE 19.8 The toll of iodine deficiency. Iodine deficiency remains the single greatest cause of preventable brain damage and mental retardation worldwide.

deficiency. Maternal death, poor pregnancy outcome, and failure to lactate are all increased with vitamin A deficiency. Vitamin A levels in the breast milk of these women are likely to be low as well, putting their infants at risk of deficiency.

Many countries are taking a multipronged approach to vitamin A deficiency that includes promotion of breastfeeding, fortification of foods, supplementation, and nutrition education. Foods such as eggs, dairy foods, and liver are promoted as important for women and children; educational programs also encourage growing and eating fruits and vegetables high in beta-carotene. However, dietary change can be difficult and slow. The best sources of vitamin A are often the most expensive or inaccessible. For absorption and conversion to vitamin A, beta-carotene requires dietary fat—another expensive item in many areas. Meanwhile, periodic single, large-dose vitamin A supplements, often given in tandem with maternal–child immunizations, are proving an effective short-term measure.

Biotechnology can have a significant impact on vitamin A deficiency. Through genetic engineering, scientists have developed a strain of rice that is rich in beta-carotene. When these rice plants are crossed with locally grown strains of rice, they become suited to a particular region's climate and growing conditions. If local farmers and consumers accept such crops, bioengineered rice may play a critical role in feeding the world's burgeoning population and alleviating widespread vitamin A deficiency.[54,55] Considerable public controversy surrounds the development of genetically modified (GM) food, however. Concerns about inadequate safety testing of GM food and the contamination of non-GM cropland with GM seeds from nearby farms have resulted in activist protests and the vandalism of GM crop fields. Government regulation of GM organisms (plant and animal) is an active area of public policy debate at the local, state, and federal levels.[56-58]

Iron-Deficiency Anemia

Iron deficiency is the most common nutritional disorder in the world. The numbers are astounding: 2 billion people—more than 30 percent of the world's population—are anemic, mainly because of iron deficiency. In resource-poor areas, the condition frequently is worsened by infectious diseases, including malaria, HIV/AIDS, and hookworm infestation.[59] Although iron deficiency occurs in all age groups, fast growth in young children and reproductive blood loss in women make them especially vulnerable to low-iron diets. Anemia impairs childhood development, work capacity, learning capacity, and resistance to disease.[60] Anemia during pregnancy increases illness and death rates for mother and baby. For all groups of people, anemia can cause profound fatigue, and severe anemia causes death.

The anemias of the developing world demonstrate the interaction of multiple nutrient deficiencies, which in turn interact with infection, sanitation, and poverty. Supplying iron alone is seldom enough to correct the problem.

Iron-deficient diets are typically high in starch and cereal grains. During digestion, cereals can bind with the very limited iron the diet provides, preventing its absorption. Other blood-building nutrients, such as vitamins B_6 and B_{12} and folate, are often in short supply as well.

Anemia-producing parasites are common in areas of iron deficiency, aggravating the effects of poor diet. Blood cells are destroyed by malarial infections. Intestinal malabsorption and intestinal bleeding are caused by hookworm, prevalent where human waste contaminates the fields where people walk barefoot, and by other parasites, acquired when human waste contaminates the water that people drink or in which people bathe.

Quick Bite

Is Breastfeeding Always Best?

An HIV-positive mother can transmit the virus to her baby through breast milk. HIV-positive women whose infants were spared HIV transmission during pregnancy face the dilemma of how to feed those babies. In developing countries, the WHO is working to prevent HIV transmission through breastfeeding while continuing to protect, promote, and support breastfeeding as the best way to feed babies of women who are HIV negative and women who do not know their status. Unfortunately, alternatives such as formula feeding are expensive, carry the risk of food poisoning from contaminated water, and often carry a social stigma.

Quick Bite

A Dire Doubling in Less Than Three Decades

In less than three decades (from 1998 to 2025), the number of people with obesity-related diabetes is expected to double. Three-quarters of this growth is projected to occur in developing countries.

People debilitated by anemia can be too weak to build outhouses, too poor to buy shoes or fuel to boil water, or too apathetic to clear standing water where malaria-carrying mosquitoes breed. Moreover, they often do not understand the connection between sanitation, infection, and malnutrition. Added to this mix are excessive blood loss from repeated pregnancies, inherited blood disorders such as sickle cell disease, and chronic bacterial or viral infections such as HIV.

Timely treatment can restore personal health and raise national productivity levels by as much as 20 percent.[61] The WHO has developed a comprehensive package of public health measures based on a three-pronged approach[62]:

1. *Increase iron intake:* Dietary diversification, including iron-rich foods and enhancement of iron absorption, food fortification, and iron supplementation
2. *Control infection:* Immunization and control programs for malaria and parasitic worm diseases
3. *Improve nutritional status:* Prevention and control of other nutritional deficiencies, such as vitamin B_{12}, folate, and vitamin A

Deficiencies of Other Micronutrients

Deficiencies of zinc and calcium often coexist with other deficiencies, contributing to illness and death during periods of growth and threatening immune function and skeletal health in people who survive to old age.

Selenium deficiency, although limited to only a few countries, has serious consequences. It occurs where the soil is selenium-poor, in distinct regional patterns in China and Russia. In China, where the deficiency is most severe, it predisposes individuals to the fatal Keshan disease, in which heart muscle is destroyed. Keshan disease affects mainly women and children. The condition can be prevented by selenium supplementation or by fortification, as in programs undertaken in New Zealand, where soil is also low in selenium.

The classical deficiency diseases beriberi, pellagra, and scurvy still occur among the world's poorest and most underprivileged people. Most often, however, these diseases strike the victims of war and political strife—the refugees. Diets based on milled cereals and starchy roots, all poor thiamin sources, predispose refugee populations to beriberi. People who rely on corn-based diets low in niacin and tryptophan are susceptible to pellagra. The disruption of refugee life can easily tip the balance from marginal deficiency to overt deficiency disease.

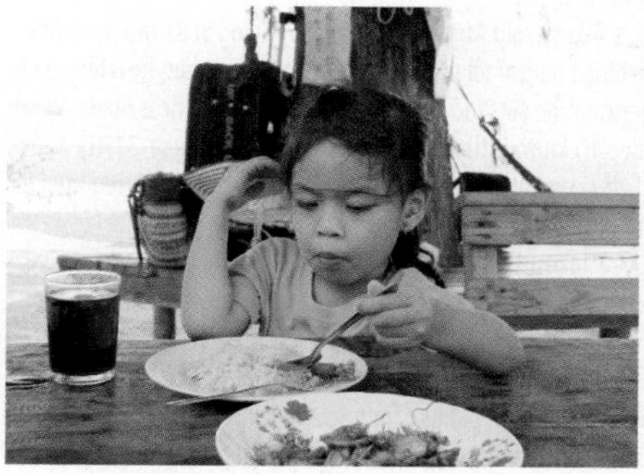
© netsuthep summat/123RF

Overweight and Obesity

Obesity is a growing health problem worldwide and is increasingly being recognized as a form of malnutrition. Overweight and obesity have reached epidemic proportions globally, with 39 percent of adults overweight and more than half a billion obese. An estimated 42 million children under age 5 years are overweight,[63] and obesity is a major contributor to the global burden of chronic disease and disability.[64] In developed countries, obesity often exists right alongside undernutrition. Obesity is more likely in areas of economic advancement and in urban areas. Its prevalence is rising rapidly in Latin America and the Caribbean, but obesity still is relatively uncommon in Asia and Africa.

Societal changes and the worldwide nutrition transition are driving the obesity epidemic (see **FIGURE 19.9**). Economic growth, modernization, urbanization, and globalization of food markets are just some of the forces thought to underlie the epidemic.

Quick Bite

The Importance of Rice

Rice is the principal food crop for one-half of the world's population, serving as the predominant staple food for 17 countries in Asia and the Pacific, nine countries in the Americas, and eight countries in Africa. It provides 20 percent of the world's dietary energy supply.

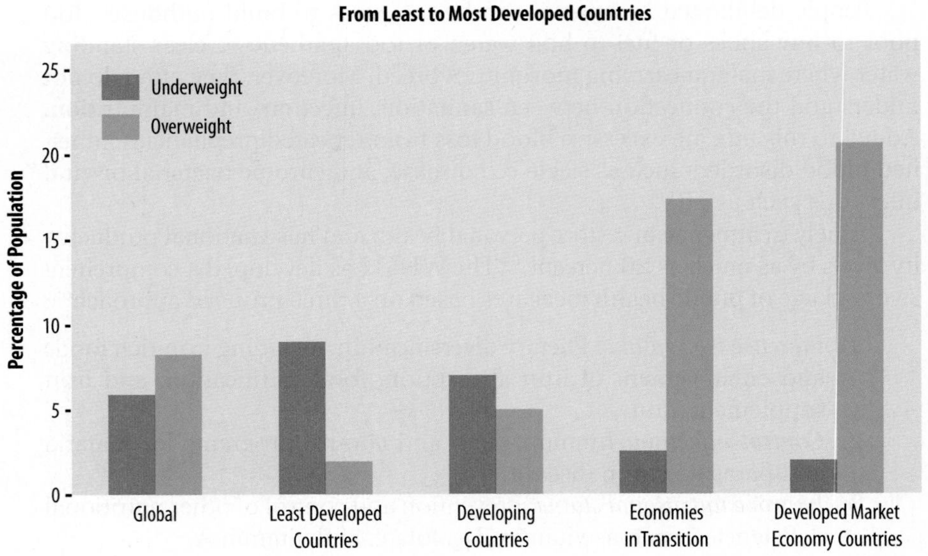

FIGURE 19.9 Global nutrition transition and obesity. As poor countries become more prosperous, they acquire some of the problems, including obesity, along with the benefits of becoming a more developed nation. In the developing world, a number of changes in diet, physical activity, health, and nutrition, collectively known as the "nutrition transition," lead to increased rates of obesity.

Reproduced from Food and Agriculture Organization of the United Nations using data from the World Health Organization. The nutrition transition and obesity. http://www.fao.org/FOCUS/E/obesity/obes2.htm.

Quick Bite

Overweight and Malnourished—It Knows No Boundaries

Take a 14-year-old African American boy living in Baltimore. While watching hours of television or playing video games, he is like many Americans: he eats too much junk food. He knows he is obese. What he doesn't know is that his body is starving for omega-3 fatty acids and other essential nutrients like vitamins and minerals required for good development and health.

Now take a 14-year-old boy from Nigeria. He has poor, uneducated parents and has to share a small bowl of rice and legumes with his three siblings every day. He walks several miles to school daily, often in intense heat. He is emaciated and frequently endures pangs of hunger. For Nigerian children like this, malnutrition usually starts before they are born due to poor prenatal care.

They are an ocean apart, yet both boys suffer from malnutrition, ranging from undernutrition with resulting short stature and below normal weight for the Nigerian to overconsumption of high-fat foods with little or no exercise leading to obesity for the American. Research tells us that both these forms of malnutrition weaken a person's defenses against various infections and make one more prone to diseases, including measles, malaria, tuberculosis, respiratory and diarrheal diseases, HIV/AIDS, and some cancers.

Source: Courtesy of Dr. Cyril O. Enwonwu, Professor of Biochemistry, University of Maryland. First published in *The Baltimore Sun*.

As incomes rise and populations become more urban, diets high in complex carbohydrates give way to more varied diets with a higher proportion of fats, saturated fats, and sugars. Calorie-dense foods that have few other nutrients are often cheap, satisfying, convenient, and heavily promoted; some are foreign brands that have become affordable status symbols. In poor communities, cultural attitudes toward overweight may be more accepting and even admiring.

Large shifts toward less physically demanding work have been observed worldwide. Moves toward less physical activity are also found in the increasing use of automated transport, technology in the home, and more passive leisure pursuits. The reductions in energy expenditure can be dramatic. If an individual is overweight, can we assume that the person is well nourished? Not necessarily. A new trend in developed countries is the presence of malnutrition with obesity. With too little physical activity, obese individuals can be eating too many calories of poor-nutrient foods and not enough nutritious foods including vegetables and fruit. The availability of an overabundance of inexpensive poor food choices in combination with lack of accessible opportunities for physical activity are just some of the factors contributing to the obesogenic environment in which many people are currently living.[65]

Key Concepts The most critical nutritional deficiencies in today's developing world are deficiencies of protein, calories, iodine, vitamin A, and iron. There have been gains in reducing the severity and prevalence of protein-energy malnutrition through breastfeeding promotion, nutrition education, and improvements in food supplies. Fortification and supplementation programs are effectively attacking iodine and vitamin A deficiencies but have had less success overcoming iron deficiency. All of the underlying causes of malnutrition must be addressed to reduce and eliminate these and other deficiencies.

Learning Portfolio

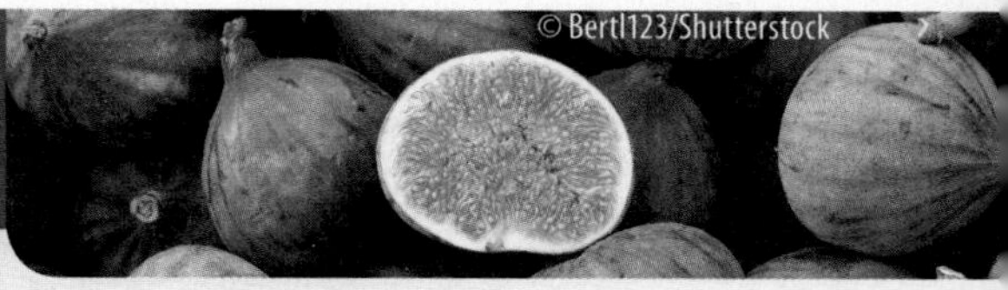
© Bertl123/Shutterstock

Key Terms

Study Points

- Hunger and malnutrition continue to be problems in both industrialized and developing countries.
- Although most people in the United States are food-secure, malnutrition is a serious problem among the working poor, the rural poor, the homeless, elders, and children.
- The Supplemental Nutrition Assistance Program (SNAP), the Special Supplemental Nutrition Program for Women, Infants, and Children (WIC), the National School Lunch and Breakfast Programs, and the Child and Adult Care Food Program are among the many federal programs that address hunger in the United States. Feeding America is the largest charitable hunger-relief organization in the United States.
- Progress against global hunger and malnutrition is slow and uneven. It is estimated that more than 795 million people in the developing world do not have enough to eat.
- Social and economic factors, infection, disease, political disruptions, natural disasters, and inequitable food distribution all contribute to hunger in the developing world.
- Advances in agricultural practices have increased food supplies and reduced food costs in the developing world; however, the increase in production has led to environmental degradation as a result of urbanization, clear-cutting, overirrigation, and soil erosion.
- Protein-energy malnutrition (PEM) refers to conditions, such as kwashiorkor and marasmus, that result from not having enough to eat.
- Infants and children are most likely to suffer from PEM. However, nutrition education efforts, including promotion of breastfeeding, have reduced the severity and prevalence of PEM.
- Iodine deficiency is the largest cause of preventable brain damage and impaired cognitive development in the developing world. It can cause damage to people of all ages.
- Great strides have been made in preventing iodine deficiency disorders (IDDs) through salt iodization programs. More than two-thirds of households in IDD-affected countries now use iodized salt.
- Vitamin A deficiency is the leading cause of preventable childhood blindness. It also makes its victims more vulnerable to infection, diarrheal diseases, and PEM.
- Pregnant and breastfeeding women with vitamin A deficiency are at increased risk of death, poor pregnancy outcomes, and lactation failure.
- Many countries are taking a multipronged approach to vitamin A deficiency that includes promotion of breastfeeding, fortification of foods, supplementation, and nutrition education.
- The best sources of vitamin A often are expensive and inaccessible to people in developing countries. Scientists have developed bioengineered strains of rice that are rich in beta-carotene and that may play a critical role in alleviating widespread vitamin A deficiency.

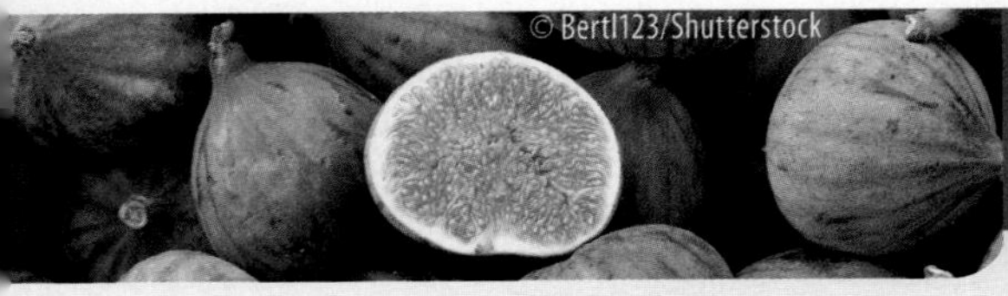
© Bertl123/Shutterstock

Learning Portfolio (continued)

- The anemias of the developing world demonstrate the interaction of multiple nutrient deficiencies, which in turn interact with infection, poor sanitation, and poverty.
- Food fortification and iron supplementation for women and children are the mainstays of anemia prevention and treatment, along with efforts to overcome poverty and improve sanitation.
- The classical deficiency diseases beriberi and pellagra still occur among the world's poorest and most underprivileged people.
- In some developed countries, obesity exists right alongside undernutrition.

Study Questions

1. What is the difference between food insecurity and hunger?
2. What is food security?
3. Which groups are most at risk for food insecurity in the United States?
4. List some of the organizations and programs fighting hunger and food insecurity in the United States.
5. List four causes of malnutrition worldwide.
6. List four common nutritional deficiencies worldwide and what is being done to combat the problem.
7. What populations are at increased risk of nutritional deficiencies, and why?

Try This

Try Giving Up Your Stove and Refrigerator

A person experiencing homelessness has no kitchen facilities to store or prepare food. For one day, eat a balanced diet without resorting to cooking or using your refrigerator. Some of the foods you could eat include the following:

- Breads, bagels, tortillas, rolls
- Cereals
- Crackers
- Milk—canned, evaporated, or aseptically packaged
- Cheese—hard cheeses keep well
- Pudding cups (single-serve, nonrefrigerated type)
- Tuna, chicken—canned
- Sardines, salmon—canned
- Nuts, peanut butter
- Beans—canned
- Fruits and vegetables—fresh, canned, dried fruits

How satisfying did you find this eating pattern? What did you miss most? What would it be like to eat this way for an extended time?

Community Food Programs

The purpose of this exercise is to see how you can contribute to decreasing or eliminating food insecurity in your community. Look in the phone book or search the Web (under "Food Programs" and "Human Services") to see what programs are available. Consider volunteering at your local food bank or another community program to help feed people who do not have the means to feed themselves.

References

1. Food and Agriculture Organization of the United Nations, International Fund for Agricultural Development, and World Food Programme. *The State of Food Insecurity in the World 2014. Strengthening the Enabling Environment for Food Security and Nutrition*. Rome, Author; 2014. This is the citation to use for 1-3: FAO, IFAD and WFP. 2015. The State of Food Insecurity in the World 2015. Meeting the 2015 international hunger targets: taking stock of uneven progress. Rome, FAO Web site: http://www.fao.org/3/a-i4646e.pdf
2. Ibid.
3. Ibid.
4. Black R, Victoria CG, Walker SP, et al. Maternal and child undernutrition and overweight in low-income and middle-income countries. *Lancet*. 2013;382:427–451.
5. Position of the Academy of Nutrition and Dietetics: food insecurity and hunger in the United States. *J Am Diet Assoc*. 2010;110(9):1368–1377.
6. Coleman-Jensen A, Rabbit M, Gregory C. Household food security in the United States in 2014. ERR-194. U.S. Department of Agriculture, Economic Research Service. September 2015. Accessed September 10, 2015.
7. Position of the Academy of Nutrition and Dietetics: food insecurity and hunger in the United States. Op cit.
8. Finkelstein EA, Strombotne KL. The economics of obesity. *Am J Clin Nutr*. 2010;91(5):1520S–1524S.
9. Gunders D. Wasted: How America is losing up to 40 percent of its food from farm to fork to landfill. Natural Resources Defense Council (NRDC) Issue Paper 12-06-B. August 2012.
10. Food and Agriculture Organization of the United Nations. *Global Food Losses and Food Waste—Extent, Causes and Prevention*. Rome: Author; 2011.
11. Coleman-Jensen A, Gregory C, Singh A. Household food security in the United States in 2013. ERR-173. U.S. Department of Agriculture, Economic Research Service. September 2014.
12. Centers for Disease Control and Prevention. A look inside food deserts. http://www.cdc.gov/features/FoodDeserts/index.html. Accessed January 14, 2016.
13. U.S. Department of Agriculture. Food access research atlas. http://www.ers.usda.gov/data-products/food-access-research-atlas.aspx#. Accessed January 14, 2016.
14. Coleman-Jensen A, Rabbit M, Gregory C. Household food security in the United States in 2014. Op cit.
15. U.S. Department of Agriculture, Economic Research Service. Definitions of food security. http://www.ers.usda.gov/topics/food-nutrition-assistance/food-security-in-the-us/definitions-of-food-security.aspx. Accessed January 14, 2016.

16. San Francisco Urban Agriculture Alliance. SF urban agriculture zoning proposal. http://www.sfuaa.org/urban-ag-zoning-proposal.html. Accessed January 14, 2016.
17. Seattle.gov. Food. http://www.seattle.gov/environment/food. Accessed January 14, 2016.
18. Kremer P. Quantifying urban agriculture impacts, one tomato at a time. http://www.triplepundit.com/2012/05/quantifying-urban-agriculture-impacts-one-tomato-time/. Accessed January 14, 2016.
19. U.S. Department of Agriculture, Special Supplemental Nutrition Program for Women, Infants, and Children (WIC). WIC program participation and costs. Data as of May 8, 2015. http://www.fns.usda.gov/sites/default/files//pd/wisummary.pdf. Accessed May 20, 2015.
20. U.S. Department of Agriculture, Food and Nutrition Service. WIC eligibility requirements. http://www.fns.usda.gov/wic/wic-eligibility-requirements. Accessed January 14, 2016.
21. U.S. Department of Agriculture, Food and Nutrition Service. Child nutrition programs—income eligibility guidelines. *Federal Register*. 2015;80(61). http://www.gpo.gov/fdsys/pkg/FR-2015-03-31/pdf/2015-07358.pdf. Accessed January 14, 2016.
22. U.S. Department of Agriculture, Food and Nutrition Service. National School Lunch Program. September 2013. http://www.fns.usda.gov/nslp/national-school-lunch-program-nslp. Accessed January 14, 2016.
23. Feeding America. About us http://www.feedingamerica.org/about-us/?_ga=1.244128261.1038510502.1454017935. Accessed May 20, 2015.
24. National Commission on Hunger. http://cybercemetery.unt.edu/archive/hungercommission/20151216222336/ https://hungercommission.rti.org/Activities/FinalReport. Accessed January 28, 2016.
25. Brundtland GH. *Nutrition, Health, and Human Rights*. Geneva, Switzerland: World Health Organization; 2003. http://apps.who.int/iris/bitstream/10665/66505/1/WHO_NHD_00.7.pdf. Accessed June 17, 2012.
26. Food and Agriculture Organization of the United Nations. *The State of Food Insecurity in the World 2014*. http://www.fao.org/publications/sofi/2014/en/. Accessed January 16, 2016.
27. United Nations. The millennium development goals report 2015. http://www.un.org/millenniumgoals/2015_MDG_Report/pdf/MDG%202015%20rev%20(July%201).pdf. Accessed January 14, 2016.
28. International Food Policy Research Institute. *2014–2015 Global Food Policy Report*. Washington, DC: International Food Policy Research Institute; 2015. http://ebrary.ifpri.org/cdm/singleitem/collection/p15738coll2/id/129072/rec/2. Accessed January 14, 2016.
29. World Food Programme. What causes hunger? http://www.wfp.org/hunger/causes. Accessed January 14, 2016.
30. Food and Agriculture Organization of the United Nations. Global food losses and food waste. http://www.fao.org/docrep/014/mb060e/mb060e.pdf. Accessed January 14, 2016.
31. Kastner T, Rivas M, Koch W, Nonhebel S. Global changes in diets and the consequences for land requirements for food. PNAS 2012;109(18) 6868-6872.
32. Ibid.
33. Sheeran J. *The new face of hunger*. Keynote address presented at Center for Strategic and International Studies, Washington DC. April 18, 2008.
34. Timilsina G, Mevel S, Shrestha A. World oil price and biofuels : a general equilibrium analysis. Research working paper 5673. The World Bank Development Research Group Environment and Energy Team. June 2011.
35. Searchinger T, Edwards R, Mulligan D, Heimlich R, Plevin R. Do biofuel policies seek to cut emissions by cutting food? *Science*. 2015;347(6229):1420–1422.
36. Turral H, Burke J, Faurès J-M. *Climate Change, Water and Food Security*. Rome: Food and Agriculture Organization of the United Nations; 2011.
37. Hunger Notes. 2015 world hunger and poverty facts and statistics. http://www.worldhunger.org/articles/Learn/world%20hunger%20facts%202002.htm#What_are_the_causes_of_hunger. Accessed January 14, 2016.
38. UNAIDS. Global report: UNAIDS report on the global AIDS epidemic 2013. http://www.unaids.org/sites/default/files/en/media/unaids/contentassets/documents/epidemiology/2013/gr2013/UNAIDS_Global_Report_2013_en.pdf. Accessed January 14, 2016.
39. World Health Organization. HIV/AIDS: data and statistics. http://www.who.int/hiv/data/en/. Accessed January 14, 2016.
40. World Health Organization. Global Health Observatory data repository. http://apps.who.int/gho/data/view.main.200?lang=en. Accessed January 14, 2016.
41. Ibid.
42. Hunger in America: 2015 United States Hunger and Poverty Facts http://www.worldhunger.org/articles/Learn/us_hunger_facts.htm accessed January 28, 2016.
43. U.S. Department of Agriculture, Economic Research Service. Soybeans and oil crops. http://ers.usda.gov/topics/crops/soybeans-oil-crops.aspx. Accessed January 14, 2016.
44. American Soybean Association. SoyStats. http://soystats.com/. Accessed September 8, 2015.
45. World Health Organization, UNICEF, and World Food Programme. *Global Nutrition Targets 2025: Wasting Policy Brief*. Geneva, Switzerland: World Health Organization; 2014.
46. World Health Organization. Micronutrient deficiencies: iodine deficiency disorders. http://www.who.int/nutrition/topics/idd/en/. Accessed January 14, 2016.
47. Eastman CJ, Zimmermann M. The iodine deficiency disorders. In: De Groot LJ, Beck-Peccoz P, Chrousos G, et al., eds. Endotext [Internet]. http://www.ncbi.nlm.nih.gov/books/NBK285556/. Accessed January 14, 2016.
48. World Health Organization. Micronutrient deficiencies: iodine deficiency disorders. Op cit.
49. UNICEF. Adequately iodized salt can protect children from brain damage, but only three quarters of the world's households are using it. http://data.unicef.org/nutrition/iodine.html#sthash.GpIczvv6.dpuf http://data.unicef.org/nutrition/iodine.html. Accessed January 28, 2016.
50. Ibid.
51. Iodine Global Network. Protecting children. http://www.ign.org/p142000273.html. Accessed January 14, 2016.
52. World Health Organization. Micronutrient deficiencies: vitamin A deficiency. 2009. http://www.who.int/nutrition/topics/vad/en/index.html. Accessed January 14, 2016.
53. Ibid.
54. De Moura FF, Palmer AC, Finkelstein JL, et al. Are biofortified staple food crops improving vitamin A and iron status in women and children? New evidence from efficacy trials. *Adv Nutr*. 2014;5:568–570.
55. Hefferon KL. Nutritionally enhanced food crops; progress and perspectives. *Int J Mol Sci*. 2015;16:3895–3914.
56. McClurg CF. Making hunger yield. *Science*. 2014. http://www.sciencemag.org/content/344/6185/699.full.pdf?sid=e13f1a6c-dc52-4b06-a0b3-fde222793f79. Accessed January 14, 2016.
57. Around the world. *Science*. http://www.sciencemag.org/content/341/6147/698.2.full.pdf?sid=71908d79-340a-461c-8c76-f75041d73250. Accessed January 14, 2016.
58. European Commission. Genetically modified organisms. http://ec.europa.eu/food/plant/gmo/new/index_en.htm. Accessed January 14, 2016.
59. World Health Organization. Micronutrient deficiencies: iron deficiency anaemia. http://www.who.int/nutrition/topics/ida/en/. Accessed January 14, 2016.
60. Ibid.
61. Ibid.
62. World Health Organization. *Global Nutrition Targets 2025: Anaemia Policy Brief*. Geneva, Switzerland: Author; 2014.
63. World Health Organization. Obesity and overweight fact sheet. http://www.who.int/mediacentre/factsheets/fs311/en//. Accessed May 28, 2015.
64. Ibid.
65. World Health Organization. Global status report on noncommunicable diseases 2014. http://apps.who.int/iris/bitstream/10665/148114/1/9789241564854_eng.pdf?ua=1. Accessed January 14, 2016.

Appendix A Dietary Reference Intakes

The Food and Nutrition Board of the National Academy of Sciences determines recommended nutrient intakes that apply to healthy individuals. Beginning in 1997, the Food and Nutrition Board (with the involvement of Health Canada) began releasing updated recommendations under a new framework called the Dietary Reference Intakes (DRIs). In these revisions,

Dietary Reference Intakes (DRIs)

Life stage group	Vitamin A (µg/d)[1]	Vitamin D (IU/d)[2]	Vitamin E (mg/d)[3]	Vitamin K (µg/d)	Thiamin (mg/d)	Riboflavin (mg/d)	Niacin (mg/d)[4]	Pantothenic Acid (mg/d)	Biotin (µg/d)	Vitamin B_6 (mg/d)	Folate (µg/d)[5]	Vitamin B_{12} (µg/d)	Vitamin C (mg/d)	Choline (mg/d)	Sodium (g/d)
Infants															
0-6 mo	400*	400*	4*	2.0*	0.2*	0.3*	2*	1.7*	5*	0.1*	65*	0.4*	40*	125*	0.12*
6-12 mo	500*	400*	5*	2.5*	0.3*	0.4*	4*	1.8*	6*	0.3*	80*	0.5*	50*	150*	0.37*
Children															
1-3 y	300	600	6	30*	0.5	0.5	6	2*	8*	0.5	150	0.9	15	200*	1.0*
4-8 y	400	600	7	55*	0.6	0.6	8	3*	12*	0.6	200	1.2	25	250*	1.2*
Males															
9-13 y	600	600	11	60*	0.9	0.9	12	4*	20*	1.0	300	1.8	45	375*	1.5*
14-18 y	900	600	15	75*	1.2	1.3	16	5*	25*	1.3	400	2.4	75	550*	1.5*
19-30 y	900	600	15	120*	1.2	1.3	16	5*	30*	1.3	400	2.4	90	550*	1.5*
31-50 y	900	600	15	120*	1.2	1.3	16	5*	30*	1.3	400	2.4	90	550*	1.5*
51-70 y	900	600	15	120*	1.2	1.3	16	5*	30*	1.7	400	2.4[7]	90	550*	1.3*
>70 y	900	800	15	120*	1.2	1.3	16	5*	30*	1.7	400	2.4[7]	90	550*	1.2*
Females															
9-13 y	600	600	11	60*	0.9	0.9	12	4*	20*	1.0	300	1.8	45	375*	1.5*
14-18 y	700	600	15	75*	1.0	1.0	14	5*	25*	1.2	400[6]	2.4	65	400*	1.5*
19-30 y	700	600	15	90*	1.1	1.1	14	5*	30*	1.3	400[6]	2.4	75	425*	1.5*
31-50 y	700	600	15	90*	1.1	1.1	14	5*	30*	1.3	400[6]	2.4	75	425*	1.5*
51-70 y	700	600	15	90*	1.1	1.1	14	5*	30*	1.5	400	2.4[7]	75	425*	1.3*
>70 y	700	800	15	90*	1.1	1.1	14	5*	30*	1.5	400	2.4[7]	75	425*	1.2*
Pregnancy															
≤18 y	750	600	15	75*	1.4	1.4	18	6*	30*	1.9	600	2.6	80	450*	1.5*
19-30 y	770	600	15	90*	1.4	1.4	18	6*	30*	1.9	600	2.6	85	450*	1.5*
31-50 y	770	600	15	90*	1.4	1.4	18	6*	30*	1.9	600	2.6	85	450*	1.5*
Lactation															
≤18 y	1,200	600	19	75*	1.4	1.6	17	7*	35*	2.0	500	2.8	115	550*	1.5*
19-30 y	1,300	600	19	90*	1.4	1.6	17	7*	35*	2.0	500	2.8	120	550*	1.5*
31-50 y	1,300	600	19	90*	1.4	1.6	17	7*	35*	2.0	500	2.8	120	550*	1.5*

This table presents Recommended Dietary Allowances (RDAs) and Adequate Intakes (AIs). An asterisk (*) indicates AI. RDAs and AIs may both be used as goals for individual intake.

[1] As retinol activity equivalents (RAE).

[2] As cholecalciferol.

[3] As α-tocopherol.

[4] As niacin equivalents (NE).

[5] As dietary folate equivalents (DFE).

[6] In view of evidence linking folate intake with neural-tube defects in the fetus, it is recommended that all women capable of becoming pregnant consume 400 µg of folic acid from supplements or fortified foods in addition to intake of food folate from a varied diet.

[7] Because 10 to 30% of older people may malabsorb food-bound vitamin B_{12}, it is advisable for those older than 50 years to meet their RDA mainly by consuming foods fortified with vitamin B_{12} or a supplement containing vitamin B_{12}.

[8] The AI for water represents total water from drinking water, beverages, and moisture from food.

target intake levels for healthy individuals in the U.S. and Canada are listed as either Adequate Intake (AI) levels or Recommended Dietary Allowances (RDAs). Also, the DRI values include a set of Tolerable Upper Intake Levels (ULs), which are levels of nutrient intake that should not be exceeded due to the potential for adverse effects from excessive consumption.

Life stage group	Potassium (g/d)	Chloride (g/d)	Calcium (mg/d)	Phosphorus (mg/d)	Magnesium (mg/d)	Iron (mg/d)	Zinc (mg/d)	Selenium (μg/d)	Iodine (μg/d)	Copper (μg/d)	Manganese (mg/d)	Fluoride (mg/d)	Chromium (μg/d)	Molybdenum (μg/d)	Water (L/d)[8]
Infants															
0-6 mo	0.4*	0.18*	200*	100*	30*	0.27*	2*	15*	110*	200*	0.003*	0.01*	0.2*	2*	0.7*
6-12 mo	0.7*	0.57*	260*	275*	75*	11	3*	20*	130*	220*	0.6*	0.5*	5.5*	3*	0.8*
Children															
1-3 y	3.0*	1.5*	700	460	80	7	3	20	90	340	1.2*	0.7*	11*	17	1.3*
4-8 y	3.8*	1.9*	1,000	500	130	10	5	30	90	440	1.5*	1*	15*	22	1.7*
Males															
9-13 y	4.5*	2.3*	1,300	1,250	240	8	8	40	120	700	1.9*	2*	25*	34	2.4*
14-18 y	4.7*	2.3*	1,300	1,250	410	11	11	55	150	890	2.2*	3*	35*	43	3.3*
19-30 y	4.7*	2.3*	1,000	700	400	8	11	55	150	900	2.3*	4*	35*	45	3.7*
31-50 y	4.7*	2.3*	1,000	700	420	8	11	55	150	900	2.3*	4*	35*	45	3.7*
51-70 y	4.7*	2.0*	1,000	700	420	8	11	55	150	900	2.3*	4*	30*	45	3.7*
>70 y	4.7*	1.8*	1,200	700	420	8	11	55	150	900	2.3*	4*	30*	45	3.7*
Females															
9-13 y	4.5*	2.3*	1,300	1,250	240	8	8	40	120	700	1.6*	2*	21*	34	2.1*
14-18 y	4.7*	2.3*	1,300	1,250	360	15	9	55	150	890	1.6*	3*	24*	43	2.3*
19-30 y	4.7*	2.3*	1,000	700	310	18	8	55	150	900	1.8*	3*	25*	45	2.7*
31-50 y	4.7*	2.3*	1,000	700	320	18	8	55	150	900	1.8*	3*	25*	45	2.7*
51-70 y	4.7*	2.0*	1,200	700	320	8	8	55	150	900	1.8*	3*	20*	45	2.7*
>70 y	4.7*	1.8*	1,200	700	320	8	8	55	150	900	1.8*	3*	20*	45	2.7*
Pregnancy															
≤18 y	4.7*	2.3*	1,300	1,250	400	27	12	60	220	1,000	2.0*	3*	29*	50	3.0*
19-30 y	4.7*	2.3*	1,000	700	350	27	11	60	220	1,000	2.0*	3*	30*	50	3.0*
31-50 y	4.7*	2.3*	1,000	700	360	27	11	60	220	1,000	2.0*	3*	30*	50	3.0*
Lactation															
≤18 y	5.1*	2.3	1,300	1,250	360	10	13	70	290	1,300	2.6*	3*	44*	50	3.8*
19-30 y	5.1*	2.3	1,000	700	310	9	12	70	290	1,300	2.6*	3*	45*	50	3.8*
31-50 y	5.1*	2.3	1,000	700	320	9	12	70	290	1,300	2.6*	3*	45*	50	3.8*

Tolerable Upper Intake Levels (ULs[1])

Life stage group	Vitamin A[2] (µg/d)	Vitamin D (µg/d)	Vitamin E[3,4] (mg/d)	Niacin[4] (mg/d)	Vitamin B_6 (mg/d)	Folate[4] (µg/d)	Vitamin C (mg/d)	Choline (g/d)	Calcium (g/d)	Phosphorus (g/d)	Magnesium[5] (mg/d)	Sodium (g/d)
Infants												
0-6 mo	600	25	ND[7]	ND	ND	ND	ND	ND	ND	ND	ND	ND
7-12 mo	600	25	ND	ND	ND	ND	ND	ND	ND	ND	ND	ND
Children												
1-3 y	600	50	200	10	30	300	400	1.0	2.5	3	65	1.5
4-8 y	900	50	300	15	40	400	650	1.0	2.5	3	110	1.9
Males, females												
9-13 y	1,700	50	600	20	60	600	1,200	2.0	2.5	4	350	2.2
14-18 y	2,800	50	800	30	80	800	1,800	3.0	2.5	4	350	2.3
19-70 y	3,000	50	1,000	35	100	1,000	2,000	3.5	2.5	4	350	2.3
>70 y	3,000	50	1,000	35	100	1,000	2,000	3.5	2.5	3	350	2.3
Pregnancy												
≤18 y	2,800	50	800	30	80	800	1,800	3.0	2.5	3.5	350	2.3
19-50 y	3,000	50	1,000	35	100	1,000	2,000	3.5	2.5	3.5	350	2.3
Lactation												
≤18 y	2,800	50	800	30	80	800	1,800	3.0	2.5	4	350	2.3
19-50 y	3,000	50	1,000	35	100	1,000	2,000	3.5	2.5	4	350	2.3

Life stage group	Iron (mg/d)	Zinc (mg/d)	Selenium (µg/d)	Iodine (µg/d)	Copper (µg/d)	Manganese (mg/d)	Fluoride (mg/d)	Molybdenum (µg/d)	Boron (mg/d)	Nickel (mg/d)	Vanadium[6] (mg/d)	Chloride (g/d)
Infants												
0-6 mo	40	4	45	ND	ND	ND	0.7	ND	ND	ND	ND	ND
7-12 mo	40	5	60	ND	ND	ND	0.9	ND	ND	ND	ND	ND
Children												
1-3 y	40	7	90	200	1,000	2	1.3	300	3	0.2	ND	2.3
4-8 y	40	12	150	300	3,000	3	2.2	600	6	0.3	ND	2.9
Males, females												
9-13 y	40	23	280	600	5,000	6	10	1,100	11	0.6	ND	3.4
14-18 y	45	34	400	900	8,000	9	10	1,700	17	1.0	ND	3.6
19-70 y	45	40	400	1,100	10,000	11	10	2,000	20	1.0	1.8	3.6
>70 y	45	40	400	1,100	10,000	11	10	2,000	20	1.0	1.8	3.6
Pregnancy												
≤18 y	45	34	400	900	8,000	9	10	1,700	17	1.0	ND	3.6
19-50 y	45	40	400	1,100	10,000	11	10	2,000	20	1.0	ND	3.6
Lactation												
≤18 y	45	34	400	900	8,000	9	10	1,700	17	1.0	ND	3.6
19-50 y	45	40	400	1,100	10,000	11	10	2,000	20	1.0	ND	3.6

[1] UL = The maximum level of daily nutrient intake that is likely to pose no risk of adverse effects. Unless otherwise specified, the UL represents total intake from food, water, and supplements. Due to lack of suitable data, ULs could not be established for vitamin K, thiamin, riboflavin, vitamin B_{12}, pantothenic acid, biotin, or carotenoids. In the absence of ULs, extra caution may be warranted in consuming levels above recommended intakes.

[2] As preformed vitamin A (retinol) only.

[3] As α-tocopherol; applies to any form of supplemental α-tocopherol.

[4] The ULs for vitamin E, niacin, and folate apply to synthetic forms obtained from supplements, fortified foods, or a combination of the two.

[5] The ULs for magnesium represent intake from a pharmacological agent only and do not include intake from food and water.

[6] Although vanadium in food has not been shown to cause adverse effects in humans, there is no justification for adding vanadium to food and vanadium supplements should be used with caution. The UL is based on adverse effects in laboratory animals and these data could be used to set a UL for adults but not children or adolescents.

[7] ND = Not determinable due to lack of data on adverse effects in this age group and concern with regard to lack of ability to handle excess amounts. Source of intake should be from food only to prevent high levels of intake.

Daily Values for Food Labels

The Daily Values are standard values developed by the Food and Drug Administration (FDA) for use on food labels.

Nutrient	Amount
Protein[1]	50 g
Thiamin	1.5 mg
Riboflavin	1.7 mg
Niacin	20 mg
Pantothenic Acid	10 mg
Biotin	300 µg
Vitamin B_6	2 mg
Folate	400 µg
Vitamin B_{12}	6 µg
Vitamin C	60 mg
Vitamin A[2]	5,000 IU
Vitamin D[2]	400 IU
Vitamin E[2]	30 IU
Vitamin K	80 µg
Chloride	3,400 mg
Calcium	1,000 mg
Phosphorus	1,000 mg
Magnesium	400 mg
Iron	18 mg
Zinc	15 mg
Selenium	70 µg
Iodine	150 µg
Copper	2 mg
Manganese	2 mg
Chromium	120 µg
Molybdenum	75 µg

[1] The Daily Values for protein vary for different groups of people: pregnant women, 60 g; nursing mothers, 65 g; infants under 1 year, 14 g; children 1 to 4 years, 16 g.

[2] The Daily Values for fat-soluble vitamins are expressed in International Units (IU), an old system of measurement.

Food Component	Amount	Calculation Factors
Fat	65 g	30% of kcalories
Saturated fat	20 g	10% of kcalories
Cholesterol	300 mg	Same regardless of kcalories
Carbohydrate (total)	300 g	60% of kcalories
Fiber	25 g	11.5 g per 1,000 kcalories
Protein	50 g	10% of kcalories
Sodium	2,400 mg	Same regardless of kcalories
Potassium	3,500 mg	Same regardless of kcalories

Note: Daily Values were established for adults and children over 4 years old. The values for energy-yielding nutrients are based on 2,000 kcalories a day.

Dietary Reference Intakes (DRIs) for Carbohydrates, Fiber, Fat, Fatty Acids, and Protein

Life stage group	Carbohydrate (g/d)	Fiber (g/d)	Fat (g/d)	Linoleic Acid (g/d)	α-Linolenic Acid (g/d)	Protein[1] (g/d)
Infants						
0-6 mo	60*	ND[2]	31*	4.4*	0.5*	9.1*
7-12 mo	95*	ND	30*	4.6*	0.5*	11
Children						
1-3 y	130	19*	ND	7*	0.7*	13
4-8 y	130	25*	ND	10*	0.9*	19
Males						
9-13 y	130	31*	ND	12*	1.2*	34
14-18 y	130	38*	ND	16*	1.6*	52
19-30 y	130	38*	ND	17*	1.6*	56
31-50 y	130	38*	ND	17*	1.6*	56
51-70 y	130	30*	ND	14*	1.6*	56
> 70 y	130	30*	ND	14*	1.6*	56
Females						
9-13 y	130	26*	ND	10*	1.0*	34
14-18 y	130	26*	ND	11*	1.1*	46
19-30 y	130	25*	ND	12*	1.1*	46
31-50 y	130	25*	ND	12*	1.1*	46
51-70 y	130	21*	ND	11*	1.1*	46
> 70 y	130	21*	ND	11*	1.1*	46
Pregnancy						
≤ 18 y	175	28*	ND	13*	1.4*	71
19-30 y	175	28*	ND	13*	1.4*	71
31-50 y	175	28*	ND	13*	1.4*	71
Lactation						
≤ 18 y	210	29*	ND	13*	1.3*	71
19-30 y	210	29*	ND	13*	1.3*	71
31-50 y	210	29*	ND	13*	1.3*	71

This table presents Recommended Dietary Allowances (RDAs) and Adequate Intakes (AIs).

An asterisk (*) indicates AI. RDAs and AIs may both be used as goals for individual intake.

[1] Based on 1.52 g/kg/day for infants 0-6 mo, 1.2 g/kg/day for infants 7-12 mo, 1.05 g/kg/day for 1-3 y, 0.95 g/kg/day for 4-13 y, 0.85 g/kg/day for 14-18 y, 0.8 g/kg/day for adults, and 1.3 g/kg/day for pregnant women (using pre-pregnancy weight) and lactating women.

[2] ND = Not determinable due to lack of data on adverse effects in this age group and concern with regard to lack of ability to handle excess amounts. Source of intake should be from food only to prevent high levels of intake.

Data compiled from Dietary Reference Intakes for Calcium, Phosphorus, Magnesium, Vitamin D, and Fluoride. Washington, DC: National Academies Press; 1997. Dietary Reference Intakes for Thiamin, Riboflavin, Niacin, Vitamin B_6, Folate, Vitamin B_{12}, Pantothenic Acid, Biotin, and Choline. Washington, DC: National Academies Press; 1998. Dietary Reference Intakes for Vitamin C, Vitamin E, Selenium, and Carotenoids. Washington, DC: National Academies Press; 2000. Dietary Reference Intakes for Vitamin A, Vitamin K, Arsenic, Boron, Chromium, Copper, Iron, Manganese, Molybdenum, Nickel, Silicon, Vanadium, and Zinc. Washington, DC: National Academies Press; 2000. Dietary Reference Intakes for Water, Potassium, Sodium, Chloride, and Sulfate. Food and Nutrition Board. Washington, DC: National Academies Press; 2005. Dietary Reference Intakes for Calcium and Vitamin D. Washington, DC: National Academies Press; 2011.

These reports may be accessed via http://nap.edu.

Appendix B Food Composition Tables

Baking/Cooking, first page; Bars, first page; Beverages, p. 790; Condiments and Sauces, p. 796; Dairy Products and Substitutes, p. 802; Desserts, p. 806; Eggs and Substitutes, p. 818; Fats, p. 820; Fruits, p. 822; Grain Products, p. 826; Grains and Flours, p. 840; Infant Foods, p. 840; Meats and Substitutes, p. 840; Nuts and Seeds, p. 852; Prepared Foods, p. 854; Restaurants, p. 870; Vegetables, p. 880

ESHA CODE	FOOD DESCRIPTION	AMT	UNIT	WT (g)	CAL (kcal)	KILO (kJ)	WTR (g)	PROT (g)	CARB (g)	FIBR (g)	FAT (g)	SATF (g)	MONO (g)	POLY (g)
BAKING/COOKING														
Baking/Cooking Ingredients														
23012	Baking Chips, chocolate, semi sweet	1	Tbs	10.5	50	209	<1	<1	7	1	3	1.9	1	0.1
23010	Baking Chocolate, unswtnd, square	1	ea	29	145	607	<1	4	9	5	15	9.4	4.7	0.5
28003	Baking Soda	0.25	tsp	1.15	0	0	<1	0	0	0	0	0	0	0
28200	Cocoa, unswntd, pwd	1	Tbs	5.375	12	50	<1	1	3	2	1	0.4	0.2	<0.1
30000	Cornstarch	1	Tbs	8	30	126	1	<1	7	<1	<1	<0.1	<0.1	<0.1
53002	Sauce, soy, f/soy and wheat	1	Tbs	16	8	33	11	1	1	<1	<1	<0.1	<0.1	<0.1
53099	Sauce, worcestershire	1	Tbs	17	13	54	13	0	3	0	0	0	0	0
27205	Vinegar, malt, ale	1	Tbs	16	0	0		0	0	0	0	0	0	0
28000	Yeast, baker's, dry active	1	tsp	4	13	54	<1	2	2	1	<1	<0.1	0.2	<0.1
Sweeteners														
63655	Agave, nectar	1	Tbs	21	60	251		0	16	0	0	0	0	0
25001	Honey, extracted	1	Tbs	21	64	268	4	<1	17	<1	0	0	0	0
31183	Molasses, blackstrap	1	Tbs	21	55	230	5	1	14	1	<1	<0.1	<0.1	<0.1
25005	Sugar, brown, packed	1	tsp	4.6	17	71	<1	<1	5	0	0	0	0	0
25009	Sugar, powdered, unsftd	1	tsp	2.5	10	42	<1	0	2	0	0	0	0	0
63348	Sugar, raw, turbinado, natural, bulk	1	tsp	4	15	63	0	0	4	0	0	0	0	0
25006	Sugar, white, granulated	1	tsp	4.2	16	67	<1	0	4	0	0	0	0	0
25010	Syrup, corn, dark	2	Tbs	40	114	477	9	0	31	0	0	0	0	0
25000	Syrup, corn, light	2	Tbs	44	125	523	10	0	34	0	<1	0	0	0
25002	Syrup, maple	0.25	cup	80	208	870	26	<1	54	0	<1	<0.1	<0.1	<0.1
23042	Syrup, pancake	0.25	cup	80	187	782	30	0	49	0	0	0	0	0
23172	Syrup, pancake, rducd cal	0.25	cup	60	99	414	33	0	27	0	0	0	0	0
23090	Syrup, pancake, with butter	0.25	cup	80	237	992	19	<1	59	0	1	0.8	0.4	<0.1
BARS														
53227	Bar, cereal, mixed berry	1	ea	37	137	573	5	2	27	1	3	0.6	1.8	0.4
62640	Bar, diet, breakfast and lunch, Dutch chocolate	1	ea	34	140	586		5	20	2	5	3		
62641	Bar, diet, snack, crispy peanut caramel	1	ea	28	120	502		1	20	1	4	3		
62643	Bar, diet, snack, rich chewy caramel	1	ea	28	120	502		2	18	1	4	3		
62205	Bar, energy, peanut butter	1	ea	35	140	586		6	18	1	5	1		
23100	Bar, granola, almond, hard	1	ea	24	119	498	1	2	15	1	6	3	1.9	0.9
23105	Bar, granola, chocolate chip, uncoated, soft, 1.5 oz	1	ea	42.5	178	745	3	2	30	2	7	2.6	3	0.7

< = Trace amount present   Blank = Not available

ESHA, EatRight Analysis; **AMT**, amount; **WT**, weight; **CAL**, calories; **KILO**, KiloJoule; **WTR**, water; **PROT**, protein; **CARB**, carbohydrate; **FIBR**, fiber; **FAT**, fat; **SATF**, saturated fat; **MONO**, monounsaturated fat; **POLY**, polyunsaturated fat; **CHOL**, cholesterol; **V**, vitamin; **THI**, thiamin; **RIB**, riboflavin; **NIA**, niacin; **FOL**, folate; **CALC**, calcium; **PHOS**, phosphorus; **SOD**, sodium; **POT**, potassium; **MAG**, magnesium

CHOL (mg)	V-A (IU)	THI (mg)	RIB (mg)	NIA (mg)	$V\text{-}B_6$ (mg)	FOL (µg)	$V\text{-}B_{12}$ (µg)	V-C (mg)	V-E (mg)	CALC (mg)	PHOS (mg)	SOD (mg)	POT (mg)	MAG (mg)	IRON (mg)	ZINC (mg)
0	0	<0.1	<0.1	<0.1	<0.1	1	0	0	<0.1	3	14	1	38	12	0.3	0.2
0	0	<0.1	<0.1	0.4	<0.1	8	0	0	0.1	29	116	7	241	95	5	2.8
0	0	0	0	0	0	0	0	0	0	0	0	315	0	0	0	0
0	0	<0.1	<0.1	0.1	<0.1	2	0	0	<0.1	7	39	1	82	27	0.7	0.4
0	0	0	0	0	0	0	0	0	0	<1	1	1	<1	<1	<0.1	<0.1
0	0	<0.1	<0.1	0.4	<0.1	2	0	0	0	5	27	879	70	12	0.2	0.1
0	13	<0.1	<0.1	0.1	0	1	0	2.2	<0.1	18	10	167	136	2	0.9	<0.1
0	0							0		0		0	5		0	
0	0	0.4	0.2	1.6	0.1	94	<0.1	<1	0	1	25	2	38	2	0.1	0.3
0	0							0		0		0			0	
0	0	0	<0.1	<0.1	<0.1	<1	0	0.1	0	1	1	1	11	<1	0.1	<0.1
<1	2	<0.1	<0.1	0.6				0.4		218		72	441		3.2	
0	0	0	0	<0.1	<0.1	<1	0	0	0	4	<1	1	6	<1	<0.1	<0.1
0	0	0	<0.1	0	0	0	0	0	0	<1	0	<1	<1	0	<0.1	<0.1
0	0							0		0		0			0	
0	0	0	<0.1	0	0	0	0	0	0	<1	0	<1	<1	0	<0.1	<0.1
0	0	<0.1	<0.1	<0.1	<0.1	0	0	0	0	7	4	62	18	3	0.1	<0.1
0	0	<0.1	0	0	0	0	0	0	0	6	0	27	<1	<1	0	0.2
0	0	0.1	1	0.1	<0.1	0	0	0	0	82	2	10	170	17	0.1	1.2
0	0	<0.1	<0.1	0	0	0	0	0	0	2	7	66	12	2	<0.1	0.1
0	0	<0.1	<0.1	<0.1	<0.1	0	0	0	0	6	26	107	2	1	<0.1	0.1
3	49	<0.1	<0.1	<0.1	0	0	0	0		2	8	78	2	2	0.1	<0.1
0	750	0.4	0.4	5	0.5	40	0	0		14	36	105	70	10	1.8	1.5
5	1250	0.4	0.4	5	0.4	40	1.5	15	3.4	100	100	85	150	16	4.5	3.8
5	750	0.2	0.3	3	0.3	60	0.9	9	2	250	100	120			2.7	
5	750	0.2	0.3	3	0.3	60	0.9	9	2	250	100	50			2.7	
0	750	1.3	0.6	3	0.6		1.5	6		300	100	75		100	2.7	
0	9	0.1	<0.1	0.1	<0.1	3	0	0		8	55	61	66	19	0.6	0.4
0	0	0.1	<0.1	0.3	<0.1	7	0	0	0.1	17	75	76	101	27	0.9	0.6

ESHA, EatRight Analysis; **AMT**, amount; **WT**, weight; **CAL**, calories; **KILO**, KiloJoule; **WTR**, water; **PROT**, protein; **CARB**, carbohydrate; **FIBR**, fiber; **FAT**, fat; **SATF**, saturated fat; **MONO**, monounsaturated fat; **POLY**, polyunsaturated fat; **CHOL**, cholesterol;

ESHA CODE	FOOD DESCRIPTION	AMT	UNIT	WT (g)	CAL (kcal)	KILO (kJ)	WTR (g)	PROT (g)	CARB (g)	FIBR (g)	FAT (g)	SATF (g)	MONO (g)	POLY (g)
BARS (CONTINUED)														
23108	Bar, granola, peanut butter, uncoated, soft	1	ea	28	119	498	2	3	18	1	4	1	1.8	1.2
23059	Bar, granola, plain, hard	1	ea	25	118	494	1	3	16	1	5	0.6	1.1	3
23104	Bar, granola, plain, uncoated, soft	1	ea	28	124	519	2	2	19	1	5	2	1.1	1.5
23097	Bar, granola, raisin, uncoated, soft	1	ea	43	193	808	3	3	29	2	8	4.1	1.2	1.4
44221	Bar, snack, Kudos, chocolate chip, whole grain	1	ea	28	118	494	1	1	20	1	4	1.3	1.3	0.8
BEVERAGES														
Alcoholic Beverages														
22543	Alcohol, gin, 100 proof	1	fl-oz	27.8	82	343	16	0	0	0	0	0	0	0
22514	Alcohol, gin, 80 proof	1	fl-oz	27.8	64	268	19	0	0	0	0	0	0	0
22516	Alcohol, gin, 86 proof	1	fl-oz	27.8	70	293	18	0	<1	0	0	0	0	0
22542	Alcohol, gin, 94 proof	1	fl-oz	27.8	76	318	17	0	0	0	0	0	0	0
22500	Beer, can/btl, 12 fl oz	12	fl-oz	356	153	640	327	2	13	0	0	0	0	0
22512	Beer, light, can/btl, 12 fl oz	12	fl-oz	354	103	431	336	1	6	0	0	0	0	0
20276	Beer, non alcoholic, Sharp's	12	fl-oz	340.5	56	234		<1	12		0	0	0	0
22519	Liqueur, coffee, 53 proof	1	fl-oz	34.8	113	473	11	<1	16	0	<1	<0.1	<0.1	<0.1
22521	Liqueur, Creme De Menthe, 72 proof	1	fl-oz	33.6	125	523	10	0	14	0	<1	<0.1	<0.1	0.1
22601	Mixed Drink, Sangria	6	fl-oz	177	118	494	153	<1	16	<1	<1	<0.1	<0.1	<0.1
22518	Wine, dessert, dry	1	fl-oz	29.5	45	188	21	<1	3	0	0	0	0	0
22507	Wine, dessert, sweet	1	fl-oz	29.5	47	197	21	<1	4	0	0	0	0	0
20076	Wine, non alcoholic	4	fl-oz	116	7	29	114	1	1	0	0	0	0	0
20077	Wine, non alcoholic, light	5	fl-oz	122.5	7	29	120	1	1	0	0	0	0	0
22501	Wine, red	5	fl-oz	147	125	523	127	<1	4	0	0	0	0	0
22638	Wine, sherry, spray dried	1	oz	28.35	100	418	1	0	25	0	0	0	0	0
22504	Wine, white, med, 5 fl oz svg	5	fl-oz	147	121	506	128	<1	4	0	0	0	0	0
22862	Wine, white, riesling, 5 fl oz svg	5	fl-oz	148	118	494	128	<1	6		0	0	0	0
Carbonated Drinks														
20006	Soda, club	8	fl-oz	236.67	0	0	236	0	0	0	0	0	0	0
90615	Soda, cola	12	fl-oz	368.4	136	569	333	<1	35	0	<1	0	0	0
20054	Soda, cola, caff free	1	cup	240	107	448	765	0	27	0	0	0	0	0
90617	Soda, cola, diet, with asp	12	fl-oz	355.2	7	29	354	<1	1	0	<1	0	0	0
20007	Soda, cola, diet, with sacc	12	fl-oz	355	0	0	354	0	<1	0	0	0	0	0
20056	Soda, cola, diet, with sacc and asp, caff free	1	cup	240	0	0		0	0	0	0	0	0	0
20028	Soda, cream	1	cup	247.2	126	527	214	0	33	0	0	0	0	0
20189	Soda, cream, diet, with sacc and asp	1	cup	240	0	0		0	0	0	0	0	0	0
20008	Soda, ginger ale	1	cup	244	83	347	223	0	21	0	0	0	0	0
20031	Soda, grape	1	cup	248	107	448	220	0	28	0	0	0	0	0
20029	Soda, orange	1	cup	248	119	498	217	0	31	0	0	0	0	0
20027	Soda, pepper type, with caff	1	cup	245.6	101	423	220	0	26	0	<1	0.2	0	0

< = Trace amount present   Blank = Not available

V, vitamin; **THI**, thiamin; **RIB**, riboflavin; **NIA**, niacin; **FOL**, folate; **CALC**, calcium; **PHOS**, phosphorus; **SOD**, sodium; **POT**, potassium; **MAG**, magnesium

CHOL (mg)	V-A (IU)	THI (mg)	RIB (mg)	NIA (mg)	V-B_6 (mg)	FOL (µg)	V-B_{12} (µg)	V-C (mg)	V-E (mg)	CALC (mg)	PHOS (mg)	SOD (mg)	POT (mg)	MAG (mg)	IRON (mg)	ZINC (mg)
<1	4	0.1	<0.1	0.9	<0.1	9	0.1	0		25	70	115	81	24	0.6	0.5
0	8	0.1	<0.1	0.4	<0.1	6	0	0.2	0.5	15	69	74	84	24	0.7	0.5
<1	0	0.1	<0.1	0.1	<0.1	7	0.1	0		29	64	78	91	21	0.7	0.4
<1	0	0.1	0.1	0.5	<0.1	9	0.1	0		43	95	121	156	31	1	0.6
38	16	<0.1	0.1	0.4	<0.1	4	<0.1	<1	3	304	58	69	78	20	0.4	0.4
0	0	<0.1	<0.1	<0.1	<0.1	0	0	0		0	1	<1	1	0	<0.1	<0.1
0	0	<0.1	<0.1	<0.1	<0.1	0	0	0	0	0	1	<1	1	0	<0.1	<0.1
0	0	<0.1	<0.1	<0.1	<0.1	0	0	0	0	0	1	<1	1	0	<0.1	<0.1
0	0	<0.1	<0.1	<0.1	<0.1	0	0	0		0	1	<1	1	0	<0.1	<0.1
0	0	<0.1	0.1	1.8	0.2	21	0.1	0	0	14	50	14	96	21	0.1	<0.1
0	0	<0.1	0.1	1.4	0.1	21	0.1	0	0	14	42	14	74	18	0.1	<0.1
0												3				
0	0	<0.1	<0.1	0.1	0	0	0	0	0	<1	2	3	10	1	<0.1	<0.1
0	0	0	0	<0.1	0	0	0	0	0	0	0	2	0	0	<0.1	<0.1
0	26	<0.1	<0.1	0.1	<0.1	5	<0.1	8.1	<0.1	8	8	12	63	6	0.2	0.1
0	0	<0.1	<0.1	0.1	0	0	0	0	0	2	3	3	27	3	0.1	<0.1
0	0	<0.1	<0.1	0.1	0	0	0	0	0	2	3	3	27	3	0.1	<0.1
0	0	0	<0.1	0.1	<0.1	1	0	0	0	10	17	8	102	12	0.5	0.1
0	0	0	<0.1	0.1	<0.1	1	0	0	0	11	18	9	108	12	0.5	0.1
0	3	<0.1	<0.1	0.3	0.1	1	0	0	0	12	34	6	187	18	0.7	0.2
0	0						0	0		4		14			0.3	
0	0	<0.1	<0.1	0.2	0.1	1	0	0	0	13	26	7	104	15	0.4	0.2
0	0	0	0	0	0	0	0	0	0	12	0	50	5	2	<0.1	0.2
0	0	0	0	0	0	0	0	0	0	7	37	15	7	0	0.4	0.1
0							0				33	30	0			
0	0	<0.1	0.1	0	0	0	0	0	0	11	32	28	28	4	0.4	<0.1
0	0	0	0	0	0	0	0	0	0	14	39	57	14	4	0.1	0.1
0							0				33	37	36			
0	0	0	0	0	0	0	0	0	0	12	0	30	2	2	0.1	0.2
0							0				0	37	0			
0	0	0	0	0	0	0	0	0	0	7	0	17	2	2	0.4	0.1
0	0	0	0	0	0	0	0	0		7	0	37	2	2	0.2	0.2
0	0	0	0	0	0	0	0	0		12	2	30	5	2	0.1	0.2
0	0	0	0	0	0	0	0	0		7	27	25	2	0	0.1	0.1

ESHA, EatRight Analysis; **AMT**, amount; **WT**, weight; **CAL**, calories; **KILO**, KiloJoule; **WTR**, water; **PROT**, protein; **CARB**, carbohydrate; **FIBR**, fiber; **FAT**, fat; **SATF**, saturated fat; **MONO**, monounsaturated fat; **POLY**, polyunsaturated fat; **CHOL**, cholesterol;

ESHA CODE	FOOD DESCRIPTION	AMT	UNIT	WT (g)	CAL (kcal)	KILO (kJ)	WTR (g)	PROT (g)	CARB (g)	FIBR (g)	FAT (g)	SATF (g)	MONO (g)	POLY (g)
BEVERAGES (CONTINUED)														
20009	Soda, root beer	1	cup	246.4	101	423	220	0	26	0	0	0	0	0
20032	Soda, Sprite	8	fl-oz	264.4	106	444	237	<1	27	0	<1	0	0	0
20010	Water, tonic	1	fl-oz	30.5	10	42	28	0	3	0	0	0	0	0
4793	Water, tonic, diet	1	cup	244	0	0	595	0	0	0	0	0	0	0
Coffees														
20048	Coffee Substitute, cereal grain, prep f/pwd with water	1	cup	240.8	14	59	237	<1	3	1	<1	<0.1	<0.1	<0.1
20012	Coffee, brewed with tap water	1	cup	236.8	2	8	235	<1	0	0	<1	<0.1	<0.1	<0.1
20686	Coffee, decaf, brewed with tap water	1	cup	236.8	0	0	235	<1	0	0	<1	<0.1	0	<0.1
20091	Coffee, decaf, inst, prep with water	1	cup	239.2	5	21	237	<1	1	0	<1	<0.1	0	<0.1
20931	Coffee, French vanilla cappuccino, inst, pkt	1	indv pkt	28	120	502		2	22		3	1		
20023	Coffee, reg, inst, prep with water	1	cup	238.4	5	21	236	<1	1	0	<1	<0.1	0	<0.1
20093	Coffee, with chicory, inst, prep with water	1	cup	239.2	7	29	237	<1	2	0	<1	<0.1	0	<0.1
20972	Espresso, decaf, restaurant prep	8	fl-oz	240	22	92	235	<1	4	0	<1	0.2	0	0.2
20439	Espresso, restaurant prep	8	fl-oz	240	22	92	235	<1	4	0	<1	0.2	0	0.2
Dairy Mixed Drinks and Substitutes														
101	Drink, Instant Breakfast, prep with 1% milk	1	cup	281	233	975	626	15	36	<1	3	1.8		
25	Drink, Instant Breakfast, prep with 2% milk	1	cup	281	253	1059	619	15	36	<1	5	3.1		
27	Drink, Instant Breakfast, prep with nonfat milk	1	cup	282	216	904	635	16	36		1	0.7		
26	Drink, Instant Breakfast, prep with whole milk	1	cup	281	280	1172	611	15	36	<1	9	5.3		
41	Drink, strawberry, prep f/dry mix with whole milk	1	cup	266	234	979	215	8	33	0	8	5.1	2.4	0.3
20925	Eggnog Substitute, low fat	0.5	cup	127	90	377		3	15	0	2	0		
48	Hot Cocoa, prep f/dry mix with water	8	fl-oz	274.4	151	632	237	3	32	1	2	0.9	0.5	<0.1
21	Hot Cocoa, prep f/recipe with milk	8	fl-oz	249.6	192	803	206	9	27	2	6	3.6	1.7	0.2
46	Hot Cocoa, sugar free, prep f/dry with water	8	fl-oz	256.8	74	310	237	3	14	2	1	0.4	0.2	<0.1
38	Malted Milk, choc, with add nutrients, prep f/pwd with whole milk	1	cup	265	231	967	215	9	30	1	9	5	2.2	0.5
Fruit Flavored Drinks														
20004	Drink, breakfast, orange, prep f/pwd	1	cup	271.2	133	556	236	0	34	<1	0	0	0	0
20035	Drink, fruit punch, prep f/fzn conc with water	8	fl-oz	247.2	114	477	218	<1	29	<1	<1	<0.1	<0.1	<0.1
20131	Drink, fruit punch, prep f/pwd with water	8	fl-oz	261.6	97	406	236	0	25	0	<1	<0.1	<0.1	<0.1
20024	Drink, fruit punch, with add nutrients, cnd	8	fl-oz	248	117	490	218	0	30	<1	<1	0	<0.1	<0.1
20967	Drink, fruit, low cal, with high vitamin C, pwd	1	tsp	2	5	21	<1	<1	2	<1	<1	<0.1	<0.1	<0.1
20101	Drink, grape, cnd	8	fl-oz	250.4	153	640	211	0	39	0	0	0	0	0

< = Trace amount present   Blank = Not available

V, vitamin; **THI**, thiamin; **RIB**, riboflavin; **NIA**, niacin; **FOL**, folate; **CALC**, calcium; **PHOS**, phosphorus; **SOD**, sodium; **POT**, potassium; **MAG**, magnesium

CHOL (mg)	V-A (IU)	THI (mg)	RIB (mg)	NIA (mg)	V-B_6 (mg)	FOL (µg)	V-B_{12} (µg)	V-C (mg)	V-E (mg)	CALC (mg)	PHOS (mg)	SOD (mg)	POT (mg)	MAG (mg)	IRON (mg)	ZINC (mg)
0	0	0	0	0	0	0	0	0	0	12	0	32	2	2	0.1	0.2
0	0	0	0	<0.1	0	0	0	0	0	5	0	24	3	3	0.3	0.1
0	0	0	0	0	0	0	0	0	0	<1	0	4	0	0	<0.1	<0.1
	0							0				35				
0	0	<0.1	<0.1	0.7	<0.1	2	0	0	<0.1	10	24	12	99	12	0.2	<0.1
0	0	<0.1	0.2	0.5	<0.1	5	0	0	<0.1	5	7	5	116	7	<0.1	<0.1
0	0	0	0	0.5	0	0	0	0	0	5	2	5	128	12	0.1	<0.1
0	0	0	<0.1	0.7	0	0	0	0	0	10	7	10	86	10	0.1	<0.1
0	0							0		40		70			0	
0	0	0	<0.1	0.6	0	0	0	0	0	10	7	10	72	10	0.1	<0.1
0	0	0	<0.1	0.5	0	0	0	0	0	10	7	17	84	7	0.1	<0.1
0	0	<0.1	0.4	12.5	<0.1	2	0	0.5	0	5	17	34	276	192	0.3	0.1
0	0	<0.1	0.4	12.5	<0.1	2	0	0.5	<0.1	5	17	34	276	192	0.3	0.1
14	2345	0.4	0.5	5.5	0.5	118	1.5	30.9	5.4	406	392	267	731	119	4.9	4.1
24	2345	0.4	0.5	5.5	0.5	118	1.5	30.9	5.5	403	390	264	726	119	4.9	4.1
9	2343	0.4	0.4	5.5	0.5	118	1.6	30.8	5.3	407	406	268	755	112	4.8	4.1
38	2152	0.4	0.5	5.5	0.5	118	1.5	30.7	5.5	396	386	262	721	117	4.9	4.1
32	309	0.1	0.4	0.2	0.1	13	0.9	2.4		293	229	128	370	32	0.2	0.9
0	0							0		20		75			0.7	
0	3	<0.1	0.2	0.2	<0.1	3	0.1	0	0.1	58	118	200	272	33	0.5	0.6
20	439	0.1	0.5	0.3	0.1	12	1.2	0.5	0.1	285	262	110	492	57	1	1.6
0	3	0.1	0.3	0.2	0.1	3	0.2	0	0	123	180	185	542	44	1	0.7
26	3177	0.8	1.3	11	1	13	1.1	31.8	0.2	368	289	231	575	45	3.8	1.1
0	694	0	0.2	2.8	0.3	0	0	80	0	141	52	14	68	3	0	<0.1
0	27	<0.1	<0.1	0.1	<0.1	2	0	108.3	0	10	2	12	32	5	0.2	<0.1
0	0	0	<0.1	<0.1	0	0	0	30.9	0	44	0	18	3	3	0.1	0.1
0	69	<0.1	0.1	0.1	<0.1	2	0	73.4	<0.1	20	7	94	77	7	0.2	<0.1
0	400	<0.1	0.1	1.6	0.2	<1	0	48	<0.1	16	10	<1	50	5	<0.1	<0.1
0	0	<0.1	<0.1	<0.1	<0.1	0	0	78.6	0	130	0	40	30	3	0.2	0.3

ESHA, EatRight Analysis; **AMT**, amount; **WT**, weight; **CAL**, calories; **KILO**, KiloJoule; **WTR**, water; **PROT**, protein; **CARB**, carbohydrate; **FIBR**, fiber; **FAT**, fat; **SATF**, saturated fat; **MONO**, monounsaturated fat; **POLY**, polyunsaturated fat; **CHOL**, cholesterol;

ESHA CODE	FOOD DESCRIPTION	AMT	UNIT	WT (g)	CAL (kcal)	KILO (kJ)	WTR (g)	PROT (g)	CARB (g)	FIBR (g)	FAT (g)	SATF (g)	MONO (g)	POLY (g)
BEVERAGES (CONTINUED)														
20047	Drink, lemonade, low cal, prep f/pwd with water	8	fl-oz	239	7	29	237	<1	2	0	<1	0	0	<0.1
20045	Drink, lemonade, prep f/pwd	8	fl-oz	255	69	289	237	0	18	0	<1	0	0	0
20070	Drink, orange, with add Vit C, cnd	8	fl-oz	248	122	510	217	0	31	0	<1	<0.1	<0.1	<0.1
20052	Juice Drink, citrus fruit, prep f/fzn conc with water	8	fl-oz	248	114	477	218	1	28	<1	<1	<0.1	<0.1	<0.1
3276	Juice Drink, cran cocktail, low cal, with calc sacc and swtnr btl	1	cup	236.8	45	188	225	<1	11	0	<1	0	0	0
3042	Juice Drink, cranberry cocktail, btl	1	cup	252.8	137	573	218	0	34	0	<1	<0.1	<0.1	0.1
20158	Juice Drink, flashin' fruit punch, box	1	box	197.78	90	377		0	25	0	0	0	0	0
3064	Juice Drink, grape, swtnd, with add vit C, prep f/fzn conc	8	fl-oz	249.6	127	531	217	<1	32	<1	<1	0.1	<0.1	0.1
20117	Juice Drink, lemonade, pink, prep f/fzn conc with water	8	fl-oz	247.2	106	444	220	<1	27	<1	<1	<0.1	<0.1	<0.1
20000	Juice Drink, lemonade, white, prep f/fzn conc with water	8	fl-oz	247.2	99	414	221	<1	26	0	<1	<0.1	<0.1	<0.1
20002	Juice Drink, limeade, prep f/fzn conc with water	8	fl-oz	247.2	129	540	213	0	34	0	0	0	0	0
20025	Juice Drink, pineapple orange, cnd	1	cup	250.4	125	523	218	3	30	<1	0	0	0	0
45437	Juice Drink, sparkling, cranberry	10.5	fl-oz can	327.25	120	502		0	29	0	0	0	0	0
Juices														
3015	Juice Drink, apricot nectar, w/o add vit C, cnd	1	cup	251	141	590	213	1	36	2	<1	<0.1	0.1	<0.1
3304	Juice Drink, guava nectar	1	cup	250	149	623	211	<1	38	2	<1	0.1	<0.1	0.1
4949	Juice Drink, mango nectar	8	fl-oz	250	120	502		0	29	0	0	0	0	0
3095	Juice Drink, papaya nectar, cnd	1	cup	250	142	594	213	<1	36	2	<1	0.1	0.1	0.1
3008	Juice, apple, unswtnd, btl	1	cup	248	114	477	219	<1	28	<1	<1	0.1	<0.1	0.1
3010	Juice, apple, unswtnd, prep f/fzn conc with water	1	cup	239	112	469	210	<1	28	<1	<1	<0.1	<0.1	0.1
5226	Juice, carrot, cnd	1	cup	236	94	393	210	2	22	2	<1	0.1	<0.1	0.2
41498	Juice, grape, unswtnd, btl	1	cup	253	152	636	214	1	37	1	<1	0.1	<0.1	0.1
3052	Juice, grapefruit, unswtnd, cnd	1	cup	247	94	393	223	1	22	<1	<1	<0.1	<0.1	0.1
3053	Juice, grapefruit, unswtnd, prep f/fzn conc with water	1	cup	247	101	423	221	1	24	<1	<1	<0.1	<0.1	0.1
3069	Juice, lemon, btl	1	Tbs	15.25	3	13	14	<1	1	<1	<1	<0.1	<0.1	<0.1
3073	Juice, lime, unswtnd, btl	1	Tbs	15.375	3	13	14	<1	1	<1	<1	<0.1	<0.1	<0.1
3988	Juice, orange strawberry banana	1	cup	247.2	120	502	538	1	28	0	0	0	0	0
14460	Juice, orange tangerine, no pulp	8	fl-oz	245	110	460		2	25	0	0	0	0	0
3092	Juice, orange, chilled	1	cup	249	122	510	217	2	29	1	<1	<0.1	0.1	0.1
21113	Juice, orange, chilled, with add calcium and vitamin D	1	cup	249	117	490	217	2	28	1	<1	<0.1	0.1	0.1
3090	Juice, orange, fresh	1	cup	248	112	469	219	2	26	<1	<1	0.1	0.1	0.1
3091	Juice, orange, unswtnd, prep f/fzn conc with water	1	cup	249	112	469	219	2	27	<1	<1	<0.1	<0.1	<0.1

< = Trace amount present Blank = Not available

V, vitamin; **THI**, thiamin; **RIB**, riboflavin; **NIA**, niacin; **FOL**, folate; **CALC**, calcium; **PHOS**, phosphorus; **SOD**, sodium; **POT**, potassium; **MAG**, magnesium

CHOL (mg)	V-A (IU)	THI (mg)	RIB (mg)	NIA (mg)	V-B_6 (mg)	FOL (µg)	V-B_{12} (µg)	V-C (mg)	V-E (mg)	CALC (mg)	PHOS (mg)	SOD (mg)	POT (mg)	MAG (mg)	IRON (mg)	ZINC (mg)
0	0	0	0	0	0	0	0	7.6	0	67	31	10	2	2	0.1	<0.1
0	0	0	<0.1	0	0	0	0	7.4	0	10	18	33	8	33	<0.1	<0.1
0	20	0	0	<0.1	0	5	0	142.1	<0.1	12	2	7	45	5	0.1	<0.1
0	92	<0.1	<0.1	0.2	<0.1	17	0	67.2	0.1	22	25	10	278	15	2.8	0.1
0	5	0	<0.1	<0.1	<0.1	0	0	76.2	0.1	21	2	7	59	5	0.1	<0.1
0	20	0	0	0.1	0	0	0	106.9	0.6	8	3	5	35	3	0.3	0.1
0	0							60		0		15			0	
0	20	<0.1	0.1	0.3	0.1	2	0	59.7	0	10	10	5	52	10	0.2	0.1
0	0	<0.1	0	0.1	<0.1	5	0	7.7	<0.1	10	5	10	42	5	<0.1	<0.1
0	2	<0.1	0.1	<0.1	<0.1	2	0	9.6	<0.1	10	5	10	37	5	0.4	<0.1
0	0	<0.1	<0.1	<0.1	<0.1	2	0	7.7	0	5	2	7	25	5	0	<0.1
0	48	0.1	<0.1	0.5	0.1	23	0	56.3	0.1	13	10	8	115	15	0.7	0.2
0	0							0		0		25	105		0.4	
0	3303	<0.1	<0.1	0.7	0.1	3	0	1.5	0.8	18	23	8	286	13	1	0.2
0	215	<0.1	<0.1	0.4	<0.1	3	0	46.5	0.4	11	10	7	93	5	0.2	0.1
0	500							12		40		10	105		0.7	
0	902	<0.1	<0.1	0.4	<0.1	5	0	7.5	0.6	25	0	12	78	8	0.8	0.4
0	2	0.1	<0.1	0.2	<0.1	0	0	2.2	<0.1	20	17	10	250	12	0.3	<0.1
0	0	<0.1	<0.1	0.1	0.1	0	0	1.4	<0.1	14	17	17	301	12	0.6	0.1
0	45133	0.2	0.1	0.9	0.5	9	0	20.1	2.7	57	99	156	689	33	1.1	0.4
0	20	<0.1	<0.1	0.3	0.1	0	0	0.3	0	28	35	13	263	25	0.6	0.2
0	17	0.1	<0.1	0.6	<0.1	25	0	72.1	0.1	17	27	2	378	25	0.5	0.2
0	22	0.1	0.1	0.5	0.1	10	0	83.2	0.1	20	35	2	336	27	0.3	0.1
0	2	<0.1	<0.1	<0.1	<0.1	2	0	3.8	<0.1	2	1	3	16	1	<0.1	<0.1
0	2	<0.1	<0.1	<0.1	<0.1	1	0	1	<0.1	2	2	2	12	1	<0.1	<0.1
0	0	0		0	0	0		60	0	0		30	290		0	
0	0	0.2	0.1	0.4	0.2	60		72		20		0	450	24	0	
0	105	0.1	0.1	0.7	0.2	47	0	83.7	0.5	27	42	5	443	27	0.3	0.2
0	105	0.1	0.1	0.7	0.2	47	0	83.7	0.5	349	117	5	443	27	0.3	0.2
0	496	0.2	0.1	1	0.1	74	0	124	0.1	27	42	2	496	27	0.5	0.1
0	266	0.2	<0.1	0.5	0.1	110	0	96.9	0.5	22	40	2	473	25	0.2	0.1

ESHA, EatRight Analysis; **AMT**, amount; **WT**, weight; **CAL**, calories; **KILO**, KiloJoule; **WTR**, water; **PROT**, protein; **CARB**, carbohydrate; **FIBR**, fiber; **FAT**, fat; **SATF**, saturated fat; **MONO**, monounsaturated fat; **POLY**, polyunsaturated fat; **CHOL**, cholesterol;

ESHA CODE	FOOD DESCRIPTION	AMT	UNIT	WT (g)	CAL (kcal)	KILO (kJ)	WTR (g)	PROT (g)	CARB (g)	FIBR (g)	FAT (g)	SATF (g)	MONO (g)	POLY (g)
BEVERAGES (CONTINUED)														
3120	Juice, pineapple, unswtnd, w/o add vit C, cnd	1	cup	250	132	552	216	1	32	<1	<1	<0.1	<0.1	0.1
3128	Juice, prune, cnd	1	cup	256	182	761	208	2	45	3	<1	<0.1	0.1	<0.1
5397	Juice, tomato, unsalted, cnd	1	cup	243	41	172	228	2	10	1	<1	<0.1	<0.1	0.1
5188	Juice, tomato, with salt, cnd	1	cup	243	41	172	228	2	10	1	<1	<0.1	<0.1	0.1
20080	Juice, vegetable cocktail, cnd	1	cup	242	46	192	226	2	11	2	<1	<0.1	<0.1	0.1
Other Beverages														
20421	Drink, sports, Body Quencher, fruit punch, rtd	8	fl-oz	244	60	251		0	16	0	0	0	0	0
63629	Drink, sports, Gatorade, orange, dry scoop	2	Tbs	25.875	100	418	1	0	24	0	<1			
20042	Juice Drink, clam and tomato, 5.5oz can	5.5	fl-oz	166	80	335	145	1	18	1	<1	0	0	0
62652	Shake, diet, milk chocolate, dry mix, scoop	0.33	cup	26	100	418		2	18	4	3	0.5	2	0.5
62599	Shake, diet, strawberry supreme, dry mix, scoop	0.33	cup	26	110	460		2	18	4	4	0.5	3	0
20050	Water, bottled, Perrier	1	cup	237	0	0	237	0	0	0	0	0	0	0
20051	Water, bottled, Poland Spring	1	cup	237	0	0	237	0	0	0	0	0	0	0
20041	Water, tap, municipal	1	cup	237	0	0	237	0	0	0	0	0	0	0
Teas														
20014	Tea, black, brewed with tap water	1	cup	237	2	8	236	0	1	0	<1	<0.1	<0.1	<0.1
20079	Tea, brewed, black, decaf, with asp	1	cup	245	6	25	243	<1	2	0	<1	<0.1	<0.1	<0.1
20924	Tea, chai, soy milk, rtd	1	cup	248	140	586		6	19	0	4	0		
20118	Tea, herbal, chamomile, brewed	1	cup	237	2	8	236	0	<1	0	<1	<0.1	<0.1	<0.1
20036	Tea, herbal, not chamomile, brewed	1	cup	237	2	8	236	0	<1	0	<1	<0.1	<0.1	<0.1
20040	Tea, lemon flvr, low calorie, prep f/inst pwd	1	cup	238	5	21	237	<1	1	0	0	0	0	0
20022	Tea, lemon flvr, swtnd, prep f/inst pwd	1	cup	259	91	381	236	<1	22	<1	<1	<0.1	<0.1	<0.1
20020	Tea, unswtnd, prep f/inst pwd	1	cup	238	2	8	237	<1	<1	0	0	0	0	0
CONDIMENTS AND SAUCES														
Condiments														
9149	Catsup	1	Tbs	17	19	79	12	<1	4	<1	<1	<0.1	<0.1	<0.1
8046	Dressing, mayonnaise	1	Tbs	13.8	94	393	3	<1	<1	0	10	1.6	2.3	6.2
8021	Dressing, mayonnaise type	1	Tbs	14.7	57	238	6	<1	4	0	5	0.7	1.3	2.6
8122	Dressing, mayonnaise type, low cal	1	Tbs	14.5	38	159	8	<1	3	0	3	0.4	0.7	1.5
8032	Dressing, mayonnaise type, soybean	1	Tbs	15	35	146	9	<1	2	0	3	0.5	0.7	1.6
8069	Dressing, mayonnaise, fat free	1	Tbs	16	11	46	13	<1	2	<1	<1	0.1		
44462	Dressing, mayonnaise, low sod, low cal	1	Tbs	14	32	134	9	<1	2	0	3	0.5	0.6	1.5
27000	Ketchup	1	Tbs	17	19	79	12	<1	4	<1	<1	<0.1	<0.1	<0.1
435	Mustard, yellow, prep	1	tsp	5	3	13	4	<1	<1	<1	<1	<0.1	0.1	<0.1
27004	Spice, horseradish, prep	1	tsp	5	2	8	4	<1	1	<1	<1	<0.1	<0.1	<0.1
Gravies														
53023	Gravy, beef, cnd	0.25	cup	58.25	31	130	51	2	3	<1	1	0.7	0.6	<0.1
53006	Gravy, beef, prep f/recipe	0.25	cup	67.5	53	222	58	1	4	<1	4	1	1.7	1
53005	Gravy, chicken giblet, prep f/recipe	0.5	cup	130	97	406	110	6	6		5	1.4	2.2	1.3

< = Trace amount present   Blank = Not available

V, vitamin; **THI**, thiamin; **RIB**, riboflavin; **NIA**, niacin; **FOL**, folate; **CALC**, calcium; **PHOS**, phosphorus; **SOD**, sodium; **POT**, potassium; **MAG**, magnesium

CHOL (mg)	V-A (IU)	THI (mg)	RIB (mg)	NIA (mg)	V-B_6 (mg)	FOL (µg)	V-B_{12} (µg)	V-C (mg)	V-E (mg)	CALC (mg)	PHOS (mg)	SOD (mg)	POT (mg)	MAG (mg)	IRON (mg)	ZINC (mg)
0	12	0.1	0.1	0.5	0.2	45	0	25	<0.1	32	20	5	325	30	0.8	0.3
0	8	<0.1	0.2	2	0.6	0	0	10.5	0.3	31	64	10	707	36	3	0.5
0	1094	0.1	0.1	1.6	0.3	49	0	44.5	0.8	24	44	24	556	27	1	0.4
0	1094	0.1	0.1	1.6	0.3	49	0	44.5	0.8	24	44	654	556	27	1	0.4
0	3770	0.1	0.1	1.8	0.3	51	0	67	0.8	27	41	479	467	27	1	0.5
0	0							24		0		55	60		0	
0		<0.1	0.2	0.1	<0.1			0.1		10	31	16	8	<1	0.1	<0.1
0	247	<0.1	<0.1	0.4	0.1	13	<0.1	8.3	0.2	13	18	601	148	8	0.2	0.1
0	750	0.4	0.2	10	0.6	100	2.1	27	13.6	200	100	120	260	100	5.4	4.5
0	750	0.4	0.2	10	0.6	100	2.1	27	13.6	200	100	130	160	100	6.3	4.5
0	0	0	0	0	0	0	0	0		33	0	2	0	0	0	0
0	0	0	0	0	0	0	0	0		2	0	2	0	2	<0.1	0
0	0	0	0	0	0	0	0	0	0	7	0	7	2	2	0	0
0	0	0	<0.1	0	0	12	0	0	0	0	2	7	88	7	<0.1	<0.1
0	0	0	<0.1	0	0	13	0	0	0	<1	2	7	90	7	<0.1	<0.1
0	300		0.3				0.9	0		300		50			1.1	0.9
0	47	<0.1	<0.1	0	0	2	0	0	0	5	0	2	21	2	0.2	0.1
0	0	<0.1	<0.1	0	0	2	0	0	0	5	0	2	21	2	0.2	0.1
0	0	0	<0.1	<0.1	<0.1	0	0	0	0	7	2	14	33	5	0.1	<0.1
0	0	<0.1	0	<0.1	<0.1	0	0	0	0	5	0	5	39	3	0.1	<0.1
0	0	0	<0.1	0.1	<0.1	0	0	0	0	7	2	10	43	5	<0.1	<0.1
0	87	<0.1	<0.1	0.2	<0.1	2	0	0.7	0.2	3	5	154	54	3	0.1	<0.1
6	9	<0.1	<0.1	0	<0.1	1	<0.1	0	0.5	1	3	88	3	<1	<0.1	<0.1
4	32	<0.1	<0.1	<0.1	<0.1	1	<0.1	0	0.3	2	4	105	1	<1	<0.1	<0.1
4	32	<0.1	<0.1	0	<0.1	1	<0.1	0	0.4	2	4	121	3	<1	<0.1	<0.1
4	0	0	0	0	0	0	0	0	0.3	0	0	75	2	0	0	<0.1
2	16							0		1	4	120	8		<0.1	
3	0	0	<0.1	0	0	0	<0.1	0	0.9	0	0	15	1	0	0	<0.1
0	87	<0.1	<0.1	0.2	<0.1	2	0	0.7	0.2	3	5	154	54	3	0.1	<0.1
0	4	<0.1	<0.1	<0.1	<0.1	<1	0	0.1	<0.1	3	5	57	7	2	0.1	<0.1
0	<1	<0.1	<0.1	<0.1	<0.1	3	0	1.2	<0.1	3	2	21	12	1	<0.1	<0.1
2	2	<0.1	<0.1	0.4	<0.1	1	0.1	0	<0.1	3	17	326	47	1	0.4	0.6
1	249	<0.1	<0.1	0.3	<0.1	1	0.1	0	0.1	14	20	389	74	1	0.3	0.5
55	1091	<0.1	0.2	1.6	0.1	49	2.3	0.6	0.3	16	62	683	151	5	1.5	1.5

ESHA, EatRight Analysis; **AMT**, amount; **WT**, weight; **CAL**, calories; **KILO**, KiloJoule; **WTR**, water; **PROT**, protein; **CARB**, carbohydrate; **FIBR**, fiber; **FAT**, fat; **SATF**, saturated fat; **MONO**, monounsaturated fat; **POLY**, polyunsaturated fat; **CHOL**, cholesterol;

ESHA CODE	FOOD DESCRIPTION	AMT	UNIT	WT (g)	CAL (kcal)	KILO (kJ)	WTR (g)	PROT (g)	CARB (g)	FIBR (g)	FAT (g)	SATF (g)	MONO (g)	POLY (g)
CONDIMENTS AND SAUCES (CONTINUED)														
53022	Gravy, chicken, cnd	0.25	cup	59.5	47	197	51	1	3	<1	3	0.8	1.5	0.9
53026	Gravy, mushroom, cnd	0.25	cup	59.5	30	126	53	1	3	<1	2	0.2	0.7	0.6
53033	Gravy, turkey, cnd	1	Tbs	14.9	8	33	13	<1	1	<1	<1	0.1	0.1	0.1
Jams														
23000	Fruit butter, apple	1	Tbs	17	29	121	10	<1	7	<1	<1	<0.1	<0.1	<0.1
23054	Jam	1	Tbs	20	56	234	6	<1	14	<1	<1	<0.1	<0.1	0
23003	Jelly	1	Tbs	21	56	234	6	<1	15	<1	<1	<0.1	<0.1	<0.1
23165	Jelly, rducd sug, prep f/recipe	1	Tbs	19	34	142	10	<1	9	<1	<1	<0.1	<0.1	<0.1
23005	Marmalade, orange	1	Tbs	20	49	205	7	<1	13	<1	0	0	0	0
23278	Preserves, strawberry, low sugar	1	Tbs	17	25	105		0	6	0	0	0	0	0
Salad Dressings														
27135	Dip, French onion	2	Tbs	31	60	251		1	3	0	4	3		
8530	Dip, honey mustard	2	Tbs	30	140	586		0	6	0	13	2		
8013	Salad Dressing, blue cheese	1	Tbs	15	71	297	6	<1	1	<1	8	1.2	2	4.1
44705	Salad Dressing, Caesar	1	Tbs	14.7	80	335	5	<1	<1	<1	9	1.3	2	4.8
8498	Salad Dressing, Catalina, fat free, Free	2	Tbs	33	35	146		0	8	1	0	0	0	0
8015	Salad Dressing, French	1	Tbs	16	73	305	6	<1	2	0	7	0.9	1.3	3.4
44467	Salad Dressing, French, fat free	1	Tbs	16	21	88	10	<1	5	<1	<1	<0.1	<0.1	<0.1
8014	Salad Dressing, French, rducd fat	1	Tbs	16	36	151	9	<1	5	<1	2	0.1	0.7	0.6
8504	Salad Dressing, honey dijon, fat free, Free	2	Tbs	34	50	209		1	10	1	0	0	0	0
8020	Salad Dressing, Italian	1	Tbs	14.7	35	146	9	<1	2	0	3	0.4	0.8	1.6
8491	Salad Dressing, Italian, fat free, Free	2	Tbs	28	20	84		0	4	0	0	0	0	0
8016	Salad Dressing, Italian, reduced fat	1	Tbs	15	15	63	12	<1	1	0	1	0.1	0.3	0.5
44718	Salad Dressing, peppercorn	1	Tbs	13.4	76	318	4	<1	<1	0	8	1.4	2	4.4
8555	Salad Dressing, ranch	1	Tbs	15	60	251		0	2	0	6	1		
8493	Salad Dressing, ranch, fat free, Free	2	Tbs	34	50	209		0	11	0	0	0	0	0
8022	Salad Dressing, Russian	1	Tbs	15	53	222	6	<1	5	<1	4	0.4	0.9	2.2
8024	Salad Dressing, thousand island	1	Tbs	16	59	247	7	<1	2	<1	6	0.8	1.3	2.9
8023	Salad Dressing, thousand island, rducd fat	1	Tbs	15	29	121	9	<1	4	<1	2	0.1	1	0.4
8035	Salad Dressing, vinegar and oil, prep f/recipe	1	Tbs	16	72	301	8	0	<1	0	8	1.5	2.4	3.9
Sauces														
7081	Hummus, prep f/recipe	1	Tbs	15	27	113	10	1	3	1	1	0.2	0.7	0.3
53466	Salsa, rts	2	Tbs	32	9	38	29	<1	2	1	<1	<0.1	<0.1	<0.1
53388	Sauce, alfredo, microwv	0.25	cntr	62	180	753		3	3	0	18	7		
53000	Sauce, barbecue	2	Tbs	34	58	243	19	<1	14	<1	<1	<0.1	<0.1	<0.1
53016	Sauce, curry, prep f/recipe	0.5	cup	115	74	310	182	3	3	<1	6	1		
9054	Sauce, enchilada	0.25	cup	61	20	84		0	3	1	1	0		
53233	Sauce, enchilada, green chile, mild	0.25	cup	61	20	84		0	3	0	1	0		
53406	Sauce, horseradish	1	tsp	5	20	84		0	1	0	2	0		

< = Trace amount present Blank = Not available

V, vitamin; **THI**, thiamin; **RIB**, riboflavin; **NIA**, niacin; **FOL**, folate; **CALC**, calcium; **PHOS**, phosphorus; **SOD**, sodium; **POT**, potassium; **MAG**, magnesium

CHOL (mg)	V-A (IU)	THI (mg)	RIB (mg)	NIA (mg)	$V-B_6$ (mg)	FOL (µg)	$V-B_{12}$ (µg)	V-C (mg)	V-E (mg)	CALC (mg)	PHOS (mg)	SOD (mg)	POT (mg)	MAG (mg)	IRON (mg)	ZINC (mg)
1	2	<0.1	<0.1	0.3	<0.1	1	0.1	0	0.1	12	17	252	65	1	0.3	0.5
0	0	<0.1	<0.1	0.4	<0.1	7	0	0		4	9	339	63	1	0.4	0.4
<1	0	<0.1	<0.1	0.2	<0.1	<1	<0.1	0	<0.1	1	4	86	16	<1	0.1	0.1
0	4	<0.1	<0.1	<0.1	<0.1	<1	0	0.1	<0.1	2	1	3	15	1	0.1	<0.1
0	0	<0.1	<0.1	<0.1	<0.1	2	0	1.8	<0.1	4	4	6	15	1	0.1	<0.1
0	1	<0.1	<0.1	<0.1	<0.1	<1	0	0.2	0	1	1	6	11	1	<0.1	<0.1
0	1	<0.1	<0.1	<0.1	<0.1	<1	0	0	0	1	1	<1	13	1	<0.1	<0.1
0	12	<0.1	<0.1	<0.1	<0.1	2	0	1	<0.1	8	1	11	7	<1	<0.1	<0.1
0	0							0		0		0			0	
0	0							0		0		210			0	
10	0	<0.1	<0.1	<0.1	<0.1	2	<0.1	0	1	0	9	220	31	2	0	0.1
5	11	<0.1	<0.1	<0.1	<0.1	1	<0.1	0.1	0.6	6	11	156	13	1	<0.1	<0.1
6	5	<0.1	<0.1	<0.1	<0.1	<1	<0.1	<1	0.7	7	3	178	4	<1	0.2	<0.1
0	0							0		0		320			0	
0	74	<0.1	<0.1	<0.1	0	0	<0.1	0.6	0.8	4	3	134	11	1	0.1	<0.1
0	12	<0.1	<0.1	<0.1	0	2	0	0	<0.1	1	0	136	13	<1	0.1	<0.1
0	87	<0.1	<0.1	0.1	<0.1	<1	0	0.8	0.2	2	3	134	17	1	0.1	<0.1
0	0							0		0		340			0	
0	5	<0.1	0	<0.1	<0.1	0	0	0.1	0.3	2	2	146	12	1	<0.1	<0.1
0	0							0		0		380			0	
0	2	<0.1	<0.1	<0.1	<0.1	<1	0	0	0.6	2	2	150	14	1	<0.1	<0.1
7	5	0	0	0	<0.1	1	<0.1	0.1	0.6	3	3	148	24	<1	<0.1	<0.1
0	0							0		0		185			0	
0	0							0		0		330			0	
0	87	<0.1	<0.1	0.1	<0.1	1	0	0.9	0.5	2	3	170	26	2	0.1	<0.1
4	34	0.2	<0.1	0.1	0	0	0	0	0.6	3	4	138	17	1	0.2	<0.1
2	47	<0.1	<0.1	0.1	0	0	0	0.2	0.2	4	2	143	30	1	0.1	<0.1
0	0	0	0	0	0	0	0	0	0.7	0	0	<1	1	0	0	0
0	1	<0.1	<0.1	0.1	0.1	9	0	1.2	0.1	7	16	36	26	4	0.2	0.2
0	154	<0.1	<0.1	0.4	0.1	1	0	0.6	0.4	10	11	226	91	5	0.1	0.1
25	0							0		0		600			0	
0	76	<0.1	<0.1	0.2	<0.1	1	0	0.2	0.3	11	7	349	79	4	0.2	0.1
0	221	<0.1	<0.1	1.6	<0.1	5	0.1	0.1	0.8	9	38	392	103	3	0.5	0.1
0												370				
0	0							1.2		0		340			0	
5	0							0		0		35			0	

ESHA, EatRight Analysis; **AMT**, amount; **WT**, weight; **CAL**, calories; **KILO**, KiloJoule; **WTR**, water; **PROT**, protein; **CARB**, carbohydrate; **FIBR**, fiber; **FAT**, fat; **SATF**, saturated fat; **MONO**, monounsaturated fat; **POLY**, polyunsaturated fat; **CHOL**, cholesterol;

ESHA CODE	FOOD DESCRIPTION	AMT	UNIT	WT (g)	CAL (kcal)	KILO (kJ)	WTR (g)	PROT (g)	CARB (g)	FIBR (g)	FAT (g)	SATF (g)	MONO (g)	POLY (g)
CONDIMENTS AND SAUCES (CONTINUED)														
7563	Sauce, miso	2	Tbs	31	49	205	18	2	9	1	1	0.1	0.2	0.5
9570	Sauce, pasta, alfredo, creamy garlic, jar	0.25	cup	61	100	418		2	3	0	10	4		
92544	Sauce, pasta, mini meatball	0.5	cup	130	100	418	107	4	13	3	3	1		
91140	Sauce, pasta, pesto, traditional basil	0.25	cup	57	230	962		3	6	1	21	3		
53471	Sauce, pepper, Tabasco, rts	1	tsp	4.7	1	4	4	<1	<1	<1	<1	<0.1	<0.1	<0.1
53267	Sauce, soy, lite	1	Tbs	16	15	63		1	2	0	0	0	0	0
53524	Sauce, spaghetti, rts	0.5	cup	132	65	272	115	2	10	2	2	0.2	0.5	0.7
53718	Sauce, spaghetti, with meat, cnd	0.5	cup	125	60	251		3	14	3	1	0		
51018	Sauce, spaghetti, with mushrooms, cnd	0.5	cup	125	60	251	132	2	14	2	1	0		
53415	Sauce, tartar, fat free, Free	2	Tbs	32	25	105		0	5	0	0	0	0	0
53004	Sauce, teriyaki, rts	1	Tbs	18	16	67	12	1	3	<1	<1	0	0	0
53468	Sauce, white, med, prep f/recipe	0.25	cup	62.5	92	385	47	2	6	<1	7	1.8	2.8	1.8
Spices and Seasonings														
26001	Herb, basil, dried, ground	1	tsp	1.4	3	13	<1	<1	1	1	<1	<0.1	<0.1	<0.1
26038	Herb, coriander, leaf, fresh	1	Tbs	1	<1		1	<1	<1	<1	<1	<0.1	<0.1	<0.1
26021	Herb, dill weed, dried	1	tsp	1	3	13	<1	<1	1	<1	<1	<0.1		
26009	Herb, oregano, ground	1	tsp	1.8	5	21	<1	<1	1	1	<1	<0.1	<0.1	<0.1
26012	Herb, parsley, fresh, chpd	1	Tbs	3.8	1	4	3	<1	<1	<1	<1	<0.1	<0.1	<0.1
26031	Herb, sage, ground	1	tsp	0.7	2	8	<1	<1	<1	<1	<1	<0.1	<0.1	<0.1
7503	Miso	0.5	cup	137.5	274	1146	59	16	36	7	8	1.6	1.7	4.4
26091	Salt Substitute, seasoned	0.25	tsp	1.1	1	4	<1	<1	<1	0	<1			
26048	Salt, lite, mixture	0.25	tsp	1.4	<1		<1	0	<1		<1			
26014	Salt, table	0.25	tsp	1.5	0	0	<1	0	0	0	0	0	0	0
26004	Spice Blend, curry, pwd	1	tsp	2	6	25	<1	<1	1	1	<1	<0.1	0.1	0.1
26040	Spice, celery seeds	1	tsp	2	8	33	<1	<1	1	<1	1	<0.1	0.3	0.1
26002	Spice, chili pepper, pwd	1	tsp	2.7	8	33	<1	<1	1	1	<1	0.1	0.1	0.2
26003	Spice, cinnamon, ground	1	tsp	2.6	6	25	<1	<1	2	1	<1	<0.1	<0.1	<0.1
26007	Spice, garlic, pwd	1	tsp	3.1	10	42	<1	1	2	<1	<1	<0.1	<0.1	<0.1
26023	Spice, ginger, ground	1	tsp	1.8	6	25	<1	<1	1	<1	<1	<0.1	<0.1	<0.1
26008	Spice, onion, pwd	1	tsp	2.4	8	33	<1	<1	2	<1	<1	<0.1	<0.1	<0.1
26010	Spice, paprika	1	tsp	2.3	6	25	<1	<1	1	1	<1	<0.1	<0.1	0.2
26016	Spice, pepper, black, ground	1	tsp	2.3	6	25	<1	<1	1	1	<1	<0.1	<0.1	<0.1
26037	Spice, pepper, white	1	tsp	2.4	7	29	<1	<1	2	1	<1	<0.1	<0.1	<0.1
DAIRY PRODUCTS AND SUBSTITUTES														
Cheese														
1001	Cheese Product, American, cold pack	1	oz	28.35	94	393	12	6	2	0	7	4.4	2	0.2
1287	Cheese Product, American, past, proc, nonfat, slice	1	slice	21	31	130	12	5	2	<1	<1	0.1		
1071	Cheese Product, Swiss, past, proc, 8oz pkg	1	oz	28.35	92	385	12	6	1	0	7	4.4	1.9	0.2
1002	Cheese Spread, American, past, proc	2	Tbs	32	93	389	15	5	3	0	7	4.3	2	0.2

< = Trace amount present   Blank = Not available

V, vitamin; **THI**, thiamin; **RIB**, riboflavin; **NIA**, niacin; **FOL**, folate; **CALC**, calcium; **PHOS**, phosphorus; **SOD**, sodium; **POT**, potassium; **MAG**, magnesium

CHOL (mg)	V-A (IU)	THI (mg)	RIB (mg)	NIA (mg)	V-B_6 (mg)	FOL (µg)	V-B_{12} (µg)	V-C (mg)	V-E (mg)	CALC (mg)	PHOS (mg)	SOD (mg)	POT (mg)	MAG (mg)	IRON (mg)	ZINC (mg)
0	12	<0.1	<0.1	0.1	<0.1	5	0	0	<0.1	10	22	508	26	7	0.4	0.5
30	200							0		40		360			0	
5	500							2.3		20		480	360		1.1	
0	0							0		60		720			0.7	
0	77	<0.1	<0.1	<0.1	<0.1	<1	0	0.2	<0.1	1	1	30	6	1	0.1	<0.1
0	0							0		0		550			0	
3	858	<0.1	0.1	5.2	0.2	17	0	2.6	3.2	36	45	553	421	24	1	0.3
0	750							9		40		720			1.4	
0	750							9		40		630			1.4	
0	0							0		0		200			0	
0	0	<0.1	<0.1	0.2	<0.1	1	0	0	0	4	28	690	40	11	0.3	<0.1
4	236	<0.1	0.1	0.3	<0.1	5	0.2	0.5	0.2	74	61	221	98	9	0.2	0.3
0	10	<0.1	<0.1	0.1	<0.1	4	0	<1	0.1	31	4	1	37	10	1.3	0.1
0	67	<0.1	<0.1	<0.1	<0.1	1	0	0.3	<0.1	1	<1	<1	5	<1	<0.1	<0.1
0	58	<0.1	<0.1	<0.1	<0.1		0	0.5		18	5	2	33	5	0.5	<0.1
0	31	<0.1	<0.1	0.1	<0.1	4	0	<1	0.3	29	3	<1	23	5	0.7	<0.1
0	320	<0.1	<0.1	<0.1	<0.1	6	0	5.1	<0.1	5	2	2	21	2	0.2	<0.1
0	41	<0.1	<0.1	<0.1	<0.1	2	0	0.2	0.1	12	1	<1	7	3	0.2	<0.1
0	120	0.1	0.3	1.2	0.3	26	0.1	0	<0.1	78	219	5126	289	66	3.4	3.5
0							0					<1	476			
							0			1		276	354	1		
0	0	0	0	0	0	0	0	0	0	<1	0	581	<1	<1	<0.1	<0.1
0	20	<0.1	<0.1	0.1	<0.1	3	0	0.2	0.4	10	7	1	31	5	0.6	0.1
0	1	<0.1	<0.1	0.1	<0.1	<1	0	0.3	<0.1	35	11	3	28	9	0.9	0.1
0	801	<0.1	<0.1	0.3	0.1	1	0	<1	1	9	8	44	53	4	0.5	0.1
0	8	<0.1	<0.1	<0.1	<0.1	<1	0	0.1	0.1	26	2	<1	11	2	0.2	<0.1
0	0	<0.1	<0.1	<0.1	0.1	1	0	<1	<0.1	2	13	2	37	2	0.2	0.1
0	1	<0.1	<0.1	0.2	<0.1	<1	0	<1	0	2	3	<1	24	4	0.4	0.1
0	0	<0.1	<0.1	<0.1	<0.1	2	0	0.6	<0.1	9	8	2	24	3	0.1	0.1
0	1133	<0.1	<0.1	0.2	<0.1	1	0	<1	0.7	5	7	2	52	4	0.5	0.1
0	13	<0.1	<0.1	<0.1	<0.1	<1	0	0	<0.1	10	4	<1	31	4	0.2	<0.1
0	0	<0.1	<0.1	<0.1	<0.1	<1	0	0.5		6	4	<1	2	2	0.3	<0.1
18	200	<0.1	0.1	<0.1	<0.1	1	0.4	0		141	113	274	103	9	0.2	0.9
3	455		0.1					<1		150	194	273	50		<0.1	0.5
23	243	<0.1	0.1	<0.1	<0.1	2	0.7	0		205	149	440	81	8	0.2	1
18	209	<0.1	0.1	<0.1	<0.1	2	0.1	0	0.1	180	280	520	77	9	0.1	0.8

ESHA, EatRight Analysis; **AMT**, amount; **WT**, weight; **CAL**, calories; **KILO**, KiloJoule; **WTR**, water; **PROT**, protein; **CARB**, carbohydrate; **FIBR**, fiber; **FAT**, fat; **SATF**, saturated fat; **MONO**, monounsaturated fat; **POLY**, polyunsaturated fat; **CHOL**, cholesterol;

ESHA CODE	FOOD DESCRIPTION	AMT	UNIT	WT (g)	CAL (kcal)	KILO (kJ)	WTR (g)	PROT (g)	CARB (g)	FIBR (g)	FAT (g)	SATF (g)	MONO (g)	POLY (g)
DAIRY PRODUCTS AND SUBSTITUTES (CONTINUED)														
48313	Cheese Spread, cream cheese base	1	Tbs	30	88	368	18	2	1	0	9	5.4	2.4	0.3
1272	Cheese Spread, Velveeta, past, proc	1	svg	30	91	381	14	5	3	0	7	4.3		
1000	Cheese, American, past, proc, with add vit D	1	slice	28	102	427	11	5	1	0	9	5.1	2.3	0.4
1003	Cheese, blue, crumbled	0.25	cup	33.75	119	498	14	7	1	0	10	6.3	2.6	0.3
1037	Cheese, brick, shredded	0.25	cup	28.25	105	439	12	7	1	0	8	5.3	2.4	0.2
1004	Cheese, brie, sliced	0.25	cup	36	120	502	17	7	<1	0	10	6.3	2.9	0.3
1006	Cheese, camembert	0.25	cup	61.5	184	770	32	12	<1	0	15	9.4	4.3	0.4
1448	Cheese, cheddar, low fat, shredded	0.25	cup	28.25	49	205	18	7	1	0	2	1.2	0.6	0.1
1451	Cheese, cheddar, low sod, shredded	0.25	cup	28.25	112	469	11	7	1	0	9	5.9	2.6	0.3
1423	Cheese, cheddar, rducd fat, 1" cube	1	cube	28	90	377		7	0	0	7	4.5		
1008	Cheese, cheddar, shredded	0.25	cup	28.25	114	477	10	7	<1	0	9	6	2.7	0.3
1010	Cheese, colby, shredded	0.25	cup	28.25	111	464	11	7	1	0	9	5.7	2.6	0.3
1050	Cheese, edam	1	oz	28.35	101	423	12	7	<1	0	8	5	2.3	0.2
1016	Cheese, feta, crumbled	0.25	cup	37.5	99	414	21	5	2	0	8	5.6	1.7	0.2
1052	Cheese, fontina, shredded	0.25	cup	27	105	439	10	7	<1	0	8	5.2	2.3	0.4
1078	Cheese, goat, hard	1	oz	28.35	128	536	8	9	1	0	10	7	2.3	0.2
1080	Cheese, goat, soft	1	oz	28.35	75	314	17	5	<1	0	6	4.1	1.4	0.1
1054	Cheese, gouda	1	oz	28.35	101	423	12	7	1	0	8	5	2.2	0.2
1074	Cheese, gruyere, shredded	0.25	cup	27	112	469	9	8	<1	0	9	5.1	2.7	0.5
1017	Cheese, Monterey jack, shredded	0.25	cup	28.25	105	439	12	7	<1	0	9	5.4	2.5	0.3
15403	Cheese, mozzarella, low sod	1	slice	28	78	326	14	8	1	0	5	3	1.4	0.1
1058	Cheese, mozzarella, part skim	1	oz	28.35	72	301	15	7	1	0	5	2.9	1.3	0.1
48252	Cheese, mozzarella, string, low moist, part skim	1	stick	28	80	335	3	8	1	0	6	3.5		
1056	Cheese, mozzarella, whole milk, shredded	0.25	cup	28	84	351	14	6	1	0	6	3.7	1.8	0.2
1021	Cheese, muenster, shredded	0.25	cup	28.25	104	435	12	7	<1	0	8	5.4	2.5	0.2
1075	Cheese, parmesan, grated	1	Tbs	5	22	92	1	2	<1	0	1	0.9	0.4	0.1
1112	Cheese, parmesan, shredded	1	Tbs	5	21	88	1	2	<1	0	1	0.9	0.4	<0.1
1069	Cheese, pimento, past, proc, shredded	0.25	cup	28.25	106	444	11	6	<1	<1	9	5.6	2.5	0.3
1062	Cheese, port de salut, shredded	0.25	cup	28.25	99	414	13	7	<1	0	8	4.7	2.6	0.2
1023	Cheese, provolone, diced	0.25	cup	33	116	485	14	8	1	0	9	5.6	2.4	0.3
1024	Cheese, ricotta, part skim	0.25	cup	62	86	360	46	7	3	0	5	3.1	1.4	0.2
1064	Cheese, ricotta, whole milk	0.25	cup	62	108	452	44	7	2	0	8	5.1	2.2	0.2
1428	Cheese, Swiss, rducd fat, 1" cube	1	cube	28	90	377		8	1	0	6	3.5		
1027	Cheese, Swiss, shredded	0.25	cup	27	103	431	10	7	1	0	8	4.8	2	0.3
1047	Cottage Cheese, 1% fat	0.5	cup	113	81	339	93	14	3	0	1	0.7	0.3	<0.1
1014	Cottage Cheese, 2% fat	0.5	cup	113	97	406	91	13	4	0	3	1.1	0.5	0.1
1013	Cottage Cheese, creamed, lrg curd, not packed	0.5	cup	105	103	431	84	12	4	0	5	1.8	0.8	0.1
1012	Cottage Cheese, creamed, sml curd, not packed	0.5	cup	112.5	110	460	90	13	4	0	5	1.9	0.9	0.1

< = Trace amount present Blank = Not available

V, vitamin; **THI**, thiamin; **RIB**, riboflavin; **NIA**, niacin; **FOL**, folate; **CALC**, calcium; **PHOS**, phosphorus; **SOD**, sodium; **POT**, potassium; **MAG**, magnesium

CHOL (mg)	V-A (IU)	THI (mg)	RIB (mg)	NIA (mg)	V-B$_6$ (mg)	FOL (μg)	V-B$_{12}$ (μg)	V-C (mg)	V-E (mg)	CALC (mg)	PHOS (mg)	SOD (mg)	POT (mg)	MAG (mg)	IRON (mg)	ZINC (mg)
27	309	<0.1	0.1	0.3	<0.1	4	0.1	0	0.2	21	27	152	34	2	0.3	0.2
24	332		0.1					0.1		140	259	450	100		0.1	0.6
28	317	<0.1	0.1	<0.1	<0.1	2	0.4	0	0.2	293	179	468	37	7	0.2	0.7
25	258	<0.1	0.1	0.3	0.1	12	0.4	0	0.1	178	131	471	86	8	0.1	0.9
27	305	<0.1	0.1	<0.1	<0.1	6	0.4	0	0.1	190	127	158	38	7	0.1	0.7
36	213	<0.1	0.2	0.1	0.1	23	0.6	0	0.1	66	68	226	55	7	0.2	0.9
44	504	<0.1	0.3	0.4	0.1	38	0.8	0	0.1	239	213	518	115	12	0.2	1.5
6	58	<0.1	0.1	<0.1	<0.1	3	0.1	0	<0.1	117	137	173	19	5	0.1	0.5
28	281	<0.1	0.1	<0.1	<0.1	5	0.2	0	0.1	199	137	6	32	8	0.2	0.9
20	300							0		200		170			0.4	
30	283	<0.1	0.1	<0.1	<0.1	5	0.2	0	0.1	204	145	175	28	8	0.2	0.9
27	281	<0.1	0.1	<0.1	<0.1	5	0.2	0	0.1	194	129	171	36	7	0.2	0.9
25	234	<0.1	0.1	<0.1	<0.1	5	0.4	0	0.1	207	152	274	53	9	0.1	1.1
33	158	0.1	0.3	0.4	0.2	12	0.6	0	0.1	185	126	418	23	7	0.2	1.1
31	247	<0.1	0.1	<0.1	<0.1	2	0.5	0	0.1	148	93	216	17	4	0.1	0.9
30	495	<0.1	0.3	0.7	<0.1	1	<0.1	0	0.1	254	207	98	14	15	0.5	0.5
13	293	<0.1	0.1	0.1	0.1	3	0.1	0	0.1	40	73	104	7	5	0.5	0.3
32	160	<0.1	0.1	<0.1	<0.1	6	0.4	0	0.1	198	155	232	34	8	0.1	1.1
30	256	<0.1	0.1	<0.1	<0.1	3	0.4	0	0.1	273	163	91	22	10	<0.1	1.1
25	217	<0.1	0.1	<0.1	<0.1	5	0.2	0	0.1	211	125	151	23	8	0.2	0.8
15	145	<0.1	0.1	<0.1	<0.1	3	0.3	0	<0.1	205	147	4	27	7	0.1	0.9
18	136	<0.1	0.1	<0.1	<0.1	3	0.2	0	<0.1	222	131	175	24	7	0.1	0.8
15	200							0		200		240			0	
22	189	<0.1	0.1	<0.1	<0.1	2	0.6	0	0.1	141	99	176	21	6	0.1	0.8
27	286	<0.1	0.1	<0.1	<0.1	3	0.4	0	0.1	203	132	177	38	8	0.1	0.8
4	43	<0.1	<0.1	<0.1	<0.1	<1	0.1	0	<0.1	55	36	76	6	2	<0.1	0.2
4	43	<0.1	<0.1	<0.1	<0.1	<1	0.1	0	<0.1	63	37	85	5	3	<0.1	0.2
27	291	<0.1	0.1	<0.1	<0.1	2	0.2	0.6	0.1	173	210	403	46	6	0.1	0.8
35	308	<0.1	0.1	<0.1	<0.1	5	0.4	0	0.1	184	102	151	38	7	0.1	0.7
23	290	<0.1	0.1	0.1	<0.1	3	0.5	0	0.1	249	164	289	46	9	0.2	1.1
19	238	<0.1	0.1	<0.1	<0.1	8	0.2	0	<0.1	169	113	78	78	9	0.3	0.8
32	276	<0.1	0.1	0.1	<0.1	7	0.2	0	0.1	128	98	52	65	7	0.2	0.7
20	200							0		250		115			0	
25	224	<0.1	0.1	<0.1	<0.1	2	0.9	0	0.1	214	153	52	21	10	0.1	1.2
5	46	<0.1	0.2	0.1	0.1	14	0.7	0	<0.1	69	151	459	97	6	0.2	0.4
11	84	<0.1	0.2	0.1	<0.1	11	0.5	0	<0.1	103	184	373	95	8	0.2	0.5
18	147	<0.1	0.2	0.1	<0.1	13	0.5	0	0.1	87	167	382	109	8	0.1	0.4
19	158	<0.1	0.2	0.1	0.1	14	0.5	0	0.1	93	179	410	117	9	0.1	0.4

ESHA, EatRight Analysis; **AMT**, amount; **WT**, weight; **CAL**, calories; **KILO**, KiloJoule; **WTR**, water; **PROT**, protein; **CARB**, carbohydrate; **FIBR**, fiber; **FAT**, fat; **SATF**, saturated fat; **MONO**, monounsaturated fat; **POLY**, polyunsaturated fat; **CHOL**, cholesterol;

ESHA CODE	FOOD DESCRIPTION	AMT	UNIT	WT (g)	CAL (kcal)	KILO (kJ)	WTR (g)	PROT (g)	CARB (g)	FIBR (g)	FAT (g)	SATF (g)	MONO (g)	POLY (g)
DAIRY PRODUCTS AND SUBSTITUTES (CONTINUED)														
1015	Cream Cheese	1	Tbs	14.5	50	209	8	1	1	0	5	2.8	1.2	0.2
1115	Cream Cheese, fat free, svg	1	svg	33	30	126	9	5	1	0	0	0	0	0
1098	Cream Cheese, low fat	1	Tbs	15	30	126	10	1	1	0	2	1.4	0.6	0.1
1060	Cream Cheese, neufchatel	1	oz	28.35	72	301	18	3	1	0	6	3.6	1.6	0.3
1083	Cream Cheese, regular, svg	1	svg	31	90	377	5	2	2	0	9	5		
Creams and Substitutes														
54237	Cream Substitute, Irish creme	1	Tbs	17	40	167		0	7	0	2	0		
540	Cream Substitute, original, dry	1	tsp	2	10	42	0	0	1	0	1	1	0	0
54316	Cream Substitute, soy milk, French vanilla	1	Tbs	16	21	88	12	0	3	0	1	0		
54317	Cream Substitute, soy milk, hazelnut	1	Tbs	16	21	88	12	0	3	0	1	0		
54315	Cream Substitute, soy milk, plain	1	Tbs	15.38	15	63	13	0	1	0	1	0		
500	Cream, half and half	1	indv pkt	15	20	84	12	<1	1	0	2	1.1	0.5	0.1
501	Cream, light	1	Tbs	15	29	121	11	<1	1	0	3	1.8	0.8	0.1
502	Cream, whipping, heavy	1	Tbs	15	52	218	9	<1	<1	0	6	3.5	1.6	0.2
503	Cream, whipping, heavy, whipped	1	Tbs	7.5	26	109	4	<1	<1	0	3	1.7	0.8	0.1
511	Cream, whipping, light	1	Tbs	15	44	184	10	<1	<1	0	5	2.9	1.4	0.1
504	Sour Cream, cultured	2	Tbs	24	46	192	18	<1	1	0	5	2.8	1.2	0.2
505	Sour Cream, imitation, cultured	2	Tbs	28.75	60	251	20	1	2	0	6	5.1	0.2	<0.1
515	Sour Cream, rducd fat, cultured	2	Tbs	30	40	167	24	1	1	0	4	2.2	1	0.1
Milks and Substitutes														
28100	Almond Milk, Almond Breeze, original	8	fl-oz	227	60	251		1	8	1	2	0		
7	Buttermilk, low fat, cultured	1	cup	245	98	410	221	8	12	0	2	1.3	0.6	0.1
17	Eggnog	1	cup	254	224	937	210	12	20	0	11	6.6	3.3	0.5
72	Eggnog, prep f/dry mix with whole milk	1	cup	272	258	1079	215	8	39	0	8	4.6	2.1	0.5
130	Milk Substitute, fluid, with lauric acid oil	1	cup	244	149	623	215	4	15	0	8	7.4	0.4	<0.1
54	Milk, 1%, low lactose	1	cup	246	103	431	222	8	12	0	3	1.6	0.8	0.1
4	Milk, 1%, with add vit A and D	1	cup	244	102	427	219	8	12	0	2	1.5	0.7	0.1
2	Milk, 2%, with add vit A and D	1	cup	244	122	510	218	8	12	0	5	3.1	1.4	0.2
18	Milk, chocolate, 2%, with add vit A and D	1	cup	250	190	795	205	7	30	2	5	2.9	1.1	0.2
21109	Milk, chocolate, rducd fat, with add calc	1	cup	250	195	816	205	7	30	2	5	2.9	1.1	0.2
20	Milk, chocolate, with add vit A and D	1	cup	250	208	870	206	8	26	2	8	5.3	2.5	0.3
11	Milk, cond, swtnd, cnd	1	fl-oz	38.2	123	515	10	3	21	0	3	2.1	0.9	0.1
164	Milk, evaporated, 2%, Carnation, with add vit A and D	2	Tbs	32.12	25	105	8	2	3	0	<1	0		
10	Milk, evaporated, nonfat/skim, with add vit A and D, cnd	1	fl-oz	31.9	25	105	25	2	4	0	<1	<0.1	<0.1	<0.1
23	Milk, goat, with add vit D	1	cup	244	168	703	212	9	11	0	10	6.5	2.7	0.4
19	Milk, low fat, chocolate, with add vit A and D	1	cup	250	178	745	206	8	32	1	2	1.5	0.8	0.1
6	Milk, nonfat/skim, with add vit A and D	1	cup	245	83	347	223	8	12	0	<1	0.1	0.1	<0.1
35299	Milk, nonfat/skim, with omega 3 and vit E, lactose free	1	cup	245	110	460		10	14	0	2	0	0.5	0

< = Trace amount present   Blank = Not available

V, vitamin; **THI**, thiamin; **RIB**, riboflavin; **NIA**, niacin; **FOL**, folate; **CALC**, calcium; **PHOS**, phosphorus; **SOD**, sodium; **POT**, potassium; **MAG**, magnesium

CHOL (mg)	V-A (IU)	THI (mg)	RIB (mg)	NIA (mg)	V-B_6 (mg)	FOL (µg)	V-B_{12} (µg)	V-C (mg)	V-E (mg)	CALC (mg)	PHOS (mg)	SOD (mg)	POT (mg)	MAG (mg)	IRON (mg)	ZINC (mg)
16	195	<0.1	<0.1	<0.1	<0.1	2	<0.1	0	<0.1	14	15	47	20	1	0.1	0.1
5	500							0		150		200			0	
8	83	<0.1	<0.1	<0.1	<0.1	3	0.1	0	<0.1	22	23	70	37	1	<0.1	0.1
21	238	<0.1	<0.1	0.1	<0.1	4	0.1	0	0.1	33	39	95	43	3	<0.1	0.2
35	300							0		20		130			0	
0	0	0	<0.1	0	0	0	0	0		0	<1	5	<1	<1	0	<0.1
0	0	0	<0.1	0	0	0	0	0		0	<1	10	15	<1	0	<0.1
0	0							0		0		11			0	
0	0							32		0		11			0	
0	0							0		0		10			0	
6	53	<0.1	<0.1	<0.1	<0.1	<1	<0.1	0.1	<0.1	16	14	6	20	2	<0.1	0.1
10	98	<0.1	<0.1	<0.1	<0.1	<1	<0.1	0.1	0.1	14	12	6	18	1	<0.1	<0.1
21	220	<0.1	<0.1	<0.1	<0.1	1	<0.1	0.1	0.2	10	9	6	11	1	<0.1	<0.1
10	110	<0.1	<0.1	<0.1	<0.1	<1	<0.1	<1	0.1	5	5	3	6	1	<0.1	<0.1
17	152	<0.1	<0.1	<0.1	<0.1	1	<0.1	0.1	0.1	10	9	5	15	1	<0.1	<0.1
12	150	<0.1	<0.1	<0.1	<0.1	2	0.1	0.2	0.1	26	28	19	34	2	<0.1	0.1
0	0	0	0	0	0	0	0	0	0.2	1	13	29	46	2	0.1	0.3
12	112	<0.1	<0.1	<0.1	<0.1	3	0.1	0.3	0.1	31	28	27	39	3	<0.1	0.2
0	500							0	10.1	200	100	150	180	16	0.4	
10	115	0.1	0.4	0.1	0.1	12	0.5	2.4	0.1	284	218	257	370	27	0.1	1
150	523	0.1	0.5	0.3	0.1	3	1.1	3.8	0.5	330	277	137	419	48	0.5	1.2
30	256	0.1	0.5	0.3	0.1	14	1.1	0	0.2	250	209	150	329	27	0.3	1
0	0	<0.1	0.2	0	0	0	0	0		81	181	190	278	15	1	2.9
10	504	0.1	0.4	0.2	0.1	13	0.9	2.4	0.1	303	237	124	384	34	0.1	1
12	478	<0.1	0.5	0.2	0.1	12	1.1	0	<0.1	305	232	107	366	27	0.1	1
20	464	0.1	0.5	0.2	0.1	12	1.3	0.5	0.1	293	224	115	342	27	<0.1	1.2
20	568	0.1	0.5	0.4	0.1	5	0.8	0	0.1	272	255	165	422	35	0.6	1
20	568	0.1	1.4	0.4	0.1	5	0.8	0	0.1	485	190	165	308	35	0.6	1
30	245	0.1	0.4	0.3	0.1	12	0.8	2.2	0.2	280	252	150	418	32	0.6	1
13	102	<0.1	0.2	0.1	<0.1	4	0.2	1	0.1	108	97	49	142	10	0.1	0.4
5	100		0.1					0		80	60	35	100		0	
1	126	<0.1	0.1	0.1	<0.1	3	0.1	0.4	0	93	62	37	106	9	0.1	0.3
27	483	0.1	0.3	0.7	0.1	2	0.2	3.2	0.2	327	271	122	498	34	0.1	0.7
8	490	0.1	0.4	0.3	0.1	12	0.8	2.2	<0.1	290	258	152	425	32	0.7	1
5	500	0.1	0.4	0.2	0.1	12	1.2	0	<0.1	299	247	103	382	27	0.1	1
5	500							0	23.2	350		160			0	

ESHA, EatRight Analysis; **AMT**, amount; **WT**, weight; **CAL**, calories; **KILO**, KiloJoule; **WTR**, water; **PROT**, protein; **CARB**, carbohydrate; **FIBR**, fiber; **FAT**, fat; **SATF**, saturated fat; **MONO**, monounsaturated fat; **POLY**, polyunsaturated fat; **CHOL**, cholesterol;

ESHA CODE	FOOD DESCRIPTION	AMT	UNIT	WT (g)	CAL (kcal)	KILO (kJ)	WTR (g)	PROT (g)	CARB (g)	FIBR (g)	FAT (g)	SATF (g)	MONO (g)	POLY (g)
DAIRY PRODUCTS AND SUBSTITUTES (CONTINUED)														
1	Milk, whole, 3.25%, with add vit D	1	cup	244	149	623	215	8	12	0	8	4.6	2	0.5
20033	Soy Milk	1	cup	243	131	548	214	8	15	1	4	0.5	1	2.3
7801	Soy Milk, carob	8	fl-oz	244	170	711		7	27	0	4	0.5	1	2
20920	Soy Milk, chocolate	1	cup	250	145	607	216	5	24	2	4	0.5		
20916	Soy Milk, plain	1	cup	245	100	418	224	7	8	1	4	0.5		
20144	Soy Milk, So Good, INTL	1	cup	255	158	661	222	8	13	2	8	0.8	2	4.6
20145	Soy Milk, So Good, light, INTL	1	cup	260	114	477	229	9	17	2	2	0.3	0.5	1
20918	Soy Milk, vanilla	1	cup	246	101	423	225	6	10	1	4	0.5		
7775	Soy Milk, vanilla delight	8	fl-oz	244	120	502	532	7	13	1	4	0.5		
Yogurts and Substitutes														
2001	Yogurt, fruit, low fat, 10g prot, 8oz cntr	1	cup	245	250	1046	182	11	47	0	3	1.7	0.7	0.1
2428	Yogurt, Grande, creamy strawberry, low fat	1	cup	245	237	992	422	9	45	0	3	1.6		
39884	Yogurt, Greek, blueberry, nonfat	1	cntr	170	140	586		14	20	1	0	0	0	0
39871	Yogurt, Greek, honey, nonfat	1	cntr	170	150	628		16	20	0	0	0	0	0
2000	Yogurt, plain, low fat, 12g prot, 8oz cntr	1	cup	245	154	644	208	13	17	0	4	2.4	1	0.1
2012	Yogurt, plain, skim, 13g prot, 8oz cntr	1	cup	245	137	573	209	14	19	0	<1	0.3	0.1	<0.1
2013	Yogurt, plain, whole milk, 8g prot, 8oz cntr	1	cup	245	149	623	215	9	11	0	8	5.1	2.2	0.2
11994	Yogurt, soy, strawberry, cultured, svg	1	cntr	170.1	140	586		5	22	3	4	0		
7546	Yogurt, tofu	1	cup	262	246	1029	203	9	42	1	5	0.7	1	2.7
11982	Yogurt, vanilla, nonfat	1	cup	226	220	920		12	40	0	0	0	0	0
72086	Yogurt, vanilla, nonfat, with low cal swtnr	1	cntr	170	73	305	149	7	13	0	<1	0.2	0.1	<0.1
DESSERTS														
Cakes														
46004	Cake, angel food, 1/12 of 9"	1	slice	28	72	301	9	2	16	<1	<1	<0.1	<0.1	0.1
46098	Cake, applesauce, w/o icing	1	pce	87	313	1310	20	3	52	2	12	2.4	5	3.5
46275	Cake, chocolate fudge, three layer, fzn, 1/8 pce	1	slice	69	250	1046		3	31	1	11	3		
16392	Cake, chocolate, with chocolate icing, f/in-store bakery	1	pce	64	249	1042	14	2	34	1	13	3.8	4.7	3
46118	Cake, chocolate, with vanilla icing, 1/12 piece	1	pce	103	367	1536	48	3	53	1	17	4.3		
46093	Cake, coffee, cinnamon, with crumb topping, enrich, 20oz	1	pce	63	263	1100	14	4	29	1	15	3.7	8.2	2
46097	Cake, coffee, fruit, 14oz	1	pce	50	156	653	16	3	26	1	5	1.2	2.8	0.7
51192	Cake, funnel, sticks	1	order	60	210	879		2	31	1	8	1.5		
46000	Cake, gingerbread, prep f/rec, 1/9 of 8" square	1	pce	74	263	1100	21	3	36		12	3.1	5.3	3.1
71650	Cake, lemon, layer, 9"	1	slice	88	290	1213		2	43	0	12	3.5		
46070	Cake, pineapple upside down, prep f/rec, 1/9 of 8" square	1	pce	115	367	1536	37	4	58	1	14	3.4	6	3.8
46016	Cake, pound, with butter, 12oz	1	pce	28	109	456	7	2	14	<1	6	3.2	1.7	0.3

< = Trace amount present Blank = Not available

V, vitamin; **THI**, thiamin; **RIB**, riboflavin; **NIA**, niacin; **FOL**, folate; **CALC**, calcium; **PHOS**, phosphorus; **SOD**, sodium; **POT**, potassium; **MAG**, magnesium

CHOL (mg)	V-A (IU)	THI (mg)	RIB (mg)	NIA (mg)	V-B$_6$ (mg)	FOL (µg)	V-B$_{12}$ (µg)	V-C (mg)	V-E (mg)	CALC (mg)	PHOS (mg)	SOD (mg)	POT (mg)	MAG (mg)	IRON (mg)	ZINC (mg)
24	395	0.1	0.4	0.2	0.1	12	1.1	0	0.2	276	205	105	322	24	0.1	0.9
0	7	0.1	0.2	1.2	0.2	44	0	0	0.3	61	126	124	287	61	1.6	0.3
0	0	0.3	0.1	2	0.2	80		0		75	125	95	350	58	1.3	0.8
0	515		0.5			25	3.1	0		308		102	360	40	1.5	0.6
0	505		0.5			24	3	0		301		120	301	39	1.1	0.6
0	994	0.2	0.5		0.2	26	0.8	5.1		252		92	316		2	0.5
0	1014	0.2	0.5		0.2	26	0.8	5.2		257		94	322		2.1	0.5
0	507		0.5			25	3	0		303		96	303	39	1.1	0.6
0	0							0		40		115	320		0.7	
10	88	0.1	0.4	0.2	0.1	22	1.2	1.7	<0.1	372	292	142	478	37	0.2	1.8
16	1079	0.1	0.2					0		270	216	140	421		0	
0	0							0		200	240	65	250		0	
0	0							0		200	240	75	250		0	
15	125	0.1	0.5	0.3	0.1	27	1.4	2	0.1	448	353	172	573	42	0.2	2.2
5	17	0.1	0.6	0.3	0.1	29	1.5	2.2	0	488	385	189	625	47	0.2	2.4
32	243	0.1	0.3	0.2	0.1	17	0.9	1.2	0.1	296	233	113	380	29	0.1	1.4
0	0							96	23.2	150		20			1.1	
0	86	0.2	0.1	0.6	0.1	16	0	6.6	0.8	309	100	92	123	105	2.8	0.8
5	500							3.6		450		180			0	
3	10	0.1	0.3	0.1	0.1	14	0.7	1.9	0	243	185	100	301	22	0.2	1.1
0	0	<0.1	0.1	0.2	<0.1	10	<0.1	0		39	91	210	26	3	0.1	<0.1
22	38	0.1	0.1	1.1	0.1	6	<0.1	0.9	1.6	17	45	141	145	11	1.4	0.2
30	0							0		0		160			1.1	
14	1	0	<0.1	0.5	0	11	0	0.1	2.8	19	88	223	173	20	1.9	0.4
23	258	0.1	0.1	1	<0.1	33	0.1	0.2	0.9	23	47	232	61	11	1	0.3
20	70	0.1	0.1	1.1	<0.1	38	0.1	0.2		34	68	221	77	14	1.2	0.5
4	70	<0.1	0.1	1.3	<0.1	24	<0.1	0.4		22	59	192	45	8	1.2	0.3
6												200				
24	36	0.1	0.1	1.3	0.1	24	<0.1	0.1		53	40	242	325	52	2.1	0.3
35												250				
25	291	0.2	0.2	1.4	<0.1	30	0.1	1.4		138	94	367	129	15	1.7	0.4
62	170	<0.1	0.1	0.4	<0.1	11	0.1	0		10	38	111	33	3	0.4	0.1

ESHA, EatRight Analysis; **AMT**, amount; **WT**, weight; **CAL**, calories; **KILO**, KiloJoule; **WTR**, water; **PROT**, protein; **CARB**, carbohydrate; **FIBR**, fiber; **FAT**, fat; **SATF**, saturated fat; **MONO**, monounsaturated fat; **POLY**, polyunsaturated fat; **CHOL**, cholesterol;

ESHA CODE	FOOD DESCRIPTION	AMT	UNIT	WT (g)	CAL (kcal)	KILO (kJ)	WTR (g)	PROT (g)	CARB (g)	FIBR (g)	FAT (g)	SATF (g)	MONO (g)	POLY (g)
DESSERTS (CONTINUED)														
46077	Cake, shortcake, biscuit type, prep f/recipe	1	svg	55	190	795	16	3	27	1	8	2.1	3.3	2
46008	Cake, snack, sponge, with cream filling	1	ea	42	157	657	8	1	27	<1	5	1.7	2.1	0.8
46116	Cake, spice, with icing	1	pce	109	368	1540	29	5	62	1	12	3.2	5.9	1.9
46078	Cake, sponge, prep f/recipe, 1/12 of 10"	1	slice	63	187	782	19	5	36	1	3	0.8	1	0.4
46007	Cake, white, with chocolate icing, prep f/recipe, 1/12 piece	1	pce	100	428	1791	6	2	75	1	14	7.2		
16393	Cake, yellow, with chocolate icing, f/in-store bakery	1	pce	64	243	1017	14	2	35	1	11	3.7	4.6	3
49004	Cheesecake, 17oz	1	pce	80	257	1075	36	4	20	<1	18	7.9	6.9	1.3
71626	Cheesecake, chocolate ganache	1	pce	153	580	2427		9	52		39	20		
49001	Cheesecake, no bake, prep f/dry mix, 1/12 of 9"	1	pce	99	271	1134	44	5	35	2	13	6.6	4.5	0.8
46011	Cupcake, snack, chocolate, with frosting and cream filling	1	ea	50	200	837	9	2	30	2	8	2.4	4.3	0.9
Candies														
23136	Candy Bar, 100 Grand, 1.5 oz bar	1	ea	43	201	841	3	1	31	<1	8	5.1	2.6	0.6
23075	Candy Bar, 3 Musketeers, 2.13oz bar	1	ea	60	262	1096	3	2	47	1	8	5.2	1.4	0.2
23076	Candy Bar, 3 Musketeers, fun size	2	ea	28	122	510	2	1	22	<1	4	2.4	0.7	0.1
23125	Candy Bar, 5th Avenue, 2oz	1	ea	56	270	1130	1	5	35	2	13	3.7	5.9	1.9
23129	Candy Bar, almond chocolate, Pot of Gold, 2.8oz pkg	1	pkg	78	450	1883		10	36	3	30	13		
23049	Candy Bar, Almond Joy, 1.7oz	1	ea	49	235	983	4	2	29	2	13	8.6	2.6	0.6
23110	Candy Bar, Baby Ruth, 2.1oz bar	1	ea	60	275	1151	4	3	39	1	13	7.3	3.3	1.6
23066	Candy Bar, Butterfinger, 2.16oz bar	1	ea	60	275	1151	1	3	44	1	11	5.7	3.1	1.9
23116	Candy Bar, Caramello, 1.6oz	1	ea	45	208	870	3	3	29	1	10	5.7	2.4	0.3
23060	Candy Bar, Kit Kat, 1.5oz bar	1	ea	42	218	912	1	3	27	<1	11	7.5	2.5	0.4
23061	Candy Bar, Krackel, 1.45oz	1	ea	41	210	879	<1	3	26	1	11	6.5	2.6	0.2
23037	Candy Bar, Mars almond, 1.76oz bar	1	ea	50	234	979	2	4	31	1	12	3.6	5.3	2
92671	Candy Bar, milk chocolate, roast almond	7	pce	39	210	879	<1	4	21	1	13	6		
23058	Candy Bar, milk chocolate, with crisped rice, 1.4oz bar	1	ea	40	204	854	1	3	24	1	12	6.4	3.5	0.3
23038	Candy Bar, Milky Way, 2.05oz bar	1	ea	58	264	1105	4	2	41	1	10	7	1.3	0.2
23035	Candy Bar, Mounds, 1.9oz	1	ea	53	258	1079	5	2	31	2	14	10.9	0.2	0.1
23062	Candy Bar, Mr. Goodbar, 1.75oz	1	ea	49	264	1105	<1	5	27	2	16	6.9	4	2.1
23135	Candy Bar, Oh Henry!, 2oz bar	1	ea	57	263	1100	1	4	37	1	13	5.5	3.2	1.5
23036	Candy Bar, Skor, toffee bar, 1.4oz	1	ea	39	209	874	1	1	24	1	13	7.3	3.6	0.5
23040	Candy Bar, Snickers, 2oz bar	1	ea	57	280	1172	3	4	35	1	14	5.2	4.5	1.7
23151	Candy Bar, Whatchamacallit, 1.7oz	1	ea	48	237	992	1	4	30	1	11	8.2	1.8	0.4
23130	Candy, almond solitaires, choc cvrd, Golden Collection	13	ea	41	234	979		5	19	2	15	6.2		
91520	Candy, almonds, sugar coated	1	ea	3.5	17	71	<1	<1	2	<1	1	0.1	0.4	0.1
23115	Candy, butterscotch	3	ea	16	63	264	1	<1	14	0	1	0.3	0.1	<0.1

< = Trace amount present   Blank = Not available

V, vitamin; **THI**, thiamin; **RIB**, riboflavin; **NIA**, niacin; **FOL**, folate; **CALC**, calcium; **PHOS**, phosphorus; **SOD**, sodium; **POT**, potassium; **MAG**, magnesium

CHOL (mg)	V-A (IU)	THI (mg)	RIB (mg)	NIA (mg)	$V\text{-}B_6$ (mg)	FOL (μg)	$V\text{-}B_{12}$ (μg)	V-C (mg)	V-E (mg)	CALC (mg)	PHOS (mg)	SOD (mg)	POT (mg)	MAG (mg)	IRON (mg)	ZINC (mg)
2	40	0.2	0.1	1.4	<0.1	29	<0.1	0.1		113	79	278	58	9	1.4	0.3
17	7	0.1	0.1	0.7	0	16	0.1	<1	0.3	10	78	197	30	3	0.6	0.3
50	145	0.1	0.2	1.1	<0.1	9	0.1	0.1	2.2	76	209	281	136	13	1.5	0.4
107	163	0.1	0.2	0.8	<0.1	25	0.2	0		26	63	144	89	6	1	0.4
21	278	0.1	0.1	1.1	<0.1	30	<0.1	<1	0.5	43	148	356	80	19	0.9	0.3
10		<0.1	0.1	0.5	0		0		2.9	20	88	198	120	13	1.3	0.3
44	438	<0.1	0.2	0.2	<0.1	14	0.1	0.3	0.4	41	74	350	72	9	0.5	0.4
135	150							0		60		330			0.4	
29	362	0.1	0.3	0.5	0.1	30	0.3	0.5		170	232	376	209	19	0.5	0.5
0	1	<0.1	<0.1	0.5	0.1	13	<0.1	1	0.5	58	44	166	88	18	1.8	0.5
5	55	<0.1	0.1	0.1	<0.1	2	0.1	0.3	0.2	33	37	87	70	11	0.1	0.4
3	40	<0.1	<0.1	0.1	<0.1	2	0.1	0.1	0.6	32	41	116	80	17	0.4	0.3
1	19	<0.1	<0.1	0.1	<0.1	1	<0.1	0.1	0.3	15	19	54	37	8	0.2	0.2
3	29	0.1	0.1	2.2	0.1	20	0.1	0.2	1.5	41	79	126	194	35	0.7	0.6
10								0		150		50			1.4	
2	21							0.3		31	55	70	124		0.6	
0	0	<0.1	0.1	0.8	<0.1	7	<0.1	0	0.6	28	56	138	149	26	0.4	0.4
0	0	0.1	<0.1	1.6	<0.1	17	<0.1	0	1	22	58	138	132	29	0.5	0.6
12	136							0.8		96	68	55	153		0.5	
5	34	<0.1	0.1	0.2	<0.1	6	0.2	0	0.1	52	57	23	97	16	0.4	<0.1
5	42	<0.1	0.1	0.1	<0.1	2		0.3		65	50	80	133	5	0.4	0.2
8	26	<0.1	0.2	0.5	<0.1	4	0.2	0.4	3.9	84	117	85	162	36	0.6	0.6
10	67	<0.1	0.1	0.3	<0.1	6	0.3	0	1.4	80	93	35	159	34	0.4	0.9
9	87	0.1	0.1	0.3	<0.1	7	0.3	0.2	0.2	75	83	34	148	25	1.1	0.9
5	64	<0.1	0.1	0.1	<0.1	2	0.1	0.4	0.5	67	39	97	72	12	0.3	0.4
1	0	<0.1	<0.1	0.1	<0.1	3	0	0.2	0.1	11	48	77	170	29	1.1	0.6
5	61	0.1	0.1	1.7	<0.1	19	0.2	0.4	1.6	54	80	20	193	23	0.7	0.5
4	0	0.1	0.1	1.5	<0.1	25	0.1	0	1.3	39	80	110	148	29	0.3	0.7
21	280	<0.1	<0.1	0.1		1		0.2			24	124	60	4	0.2	0.1
7	92	<0.1	0.1	2.1	0.1	15	0.1	0.3	0.9	53	108	136	184	41	0.4	1.4
6	64	0.1	0.1	1.2	<0.1	9	0.2	0.4	0.6	57	66	144	145	13	0.5	0.2
5	0							0		83		21			1	
0	<1	<0.1	<0.1	<0.1	<0.1	1	0	0	0.4	4	6	<1	9	5	0.1	0.1
1	16	<0.1	<0.1	<0.1	0	0	0	0	<0.1	1	<1	63	<1	0	<0.1	<0.1

ESHA, EatRight Analysis; **AMT**, amount; **WT**, weight; **CAL**, calories; **KILO**, KiloJoule; **WTR**, water; **PROT**, protein; **CARB**, carbohydrate; **FIBR**, fiber; **FAT**, fat; **SATF**, saturated fat; **MONO**, monounsaturated fat; **POLY**, polyunsaturated fat; **CHOL**, cholesterol;

ESHA CODE	FOOD DESCRIPTION	AMT	UNIT	WT (g)	CAL (kcal)	KILO (kJ)	WTR (g)	PROT (g)	CARB (g)	FIBR (g)	FAT (g)	SATF (g)	MONO (g)	POLY (g)
DESSERTS (CONTINUED)														
23507	Candy, California Gold, raisins, yogurt cvrd, natural	35	pce	40	160	669	2	1	28	1	5	1		
23117	Candy, caramel, chocolate flvr roll	6	ea	39.6	153	640	3	1	35	<1	1	0.4	0.8	0.1
23015	Candy, caramels	1	ea	10.1	39	163	1	<1	8	0	1	0.3	0.2	0.4
92197	Candy, chocolate cvrd, low cal	1	oz	28.35	168	703	1	3	11	1	12	6.2	3.1	1.2
93360	Candy, divinity, prep f/recipe	1	pce	11	40	167	1	<1	10	0	<1	0	0	0
23024	Candy, fondant, prep f/recipe	1	oz	28.35	106	444	2	0	26	0	<1	0	0	0
23023	Candy, fondants, chocolate cvrd	1	sml	11	40	167	1	<1	9	<1	1	0.6	0.3	<0.1
23025	Candy, fudge, chocolate, prep f/recipe	1	pce	17	70	293	2	<1	13	<1	2	1.1	0.5	0.1
23026	Candy, fudge, chocolate, with nuts, prep f/recipe	1	oz	28.35	131	548	2	1	19	1	5	1.8	1.1	2.1
23132	Candy, Goobers, peanuts, chocolate cvrd	0.25	cup	41	210	879	1	4	22	4	14	5		
23029	Candy, gumdrops	0.25	cup	45.5	180	753	<1	0	45	<1	0	0	0	0
23030	Candy, gummy bears	10	ea	22	87	364	<1	0	22	<1	0	0	0	0
23031	Candy, hard, all flvrs	1	ea	6	24	100	<1	0	6	0	<1	0	0	0
23074	Candy, hard, low cal	1	ea	3	12	50	<1	0	3	0	0	0	0	0
4148	Candy, honey, chews, Bit-O-Honey	6	ea	40	150	628	3	1	32	<1	3	2.2	0.4	0.1
23033	Candy, jellybeans	10	sml	11	41	172	1	0	10	<1	<1	0	0	0
92647	Candy, licorice, Good and Plenty	33	ea	40	140	586	1	1	35	<1	0	0	0	0
23047	Candy, milk chocolate peanut, M&Ms	0.25	cup	42.5	219	916	1	4	26	2	11	4.3	3.4	1.5
23063	Candy, milk chocolate, Kisses	9	ea	41	200	837		3	25	1	12	7		
23045	Candy, milk chocolate, M&Ms	0.25	cup	52	256	1071	1	2	37	1	11	6.8	2.7	0.5
23018	Candy, milk chocolate, with almonds, 1.45oz bar	1	ea	41	216	904	1	4	22	3	14	7.3	4.9	1.2
23226	Candy, mints, spearmint	1	ea	1.8	5	21		0	2		0	0	0	0
23081	Candy, peanut brittle, prep f/recipe	1	oz	28.35	138	577	<1	2	20	1	5	1.2	2.3	1.3
23043	Candy, peanut butter cups, Reese's, 1.6oz pkg	1	pkg	45	232	971	1	5	25	2	14	4.8	5.9	2.5
23021	Candy, peanuts, milk chocolate cvrd	10	ea	40	208	870	1	5	20	2	13	5.8	5.2	1.7
90803	Candy, pralines, prep f/recipe	1	pce	39.94	174	728	3	1	22	1	10	2.7		
23022	Candy, raisins, milk chocolate cvrd	0.25	cup	45	176	736	5	2	31	1	7	4.6	1.4	0.3
23140	Candy, Reese's Pieces	0.25	cup	47	234	979	<1	6	28	1	12	7.7	2.1	0.9
23141	Candy, Rolo, caramels in milk chocolate	7	ea	42	199	833	2	2	29	<1	9	6.1	0.9	0.1
23142	Candy, sesame crunch	20	ea	35	181	757	1	4	18	3	12	1.6	4.4	5.1
23431	Candy, Skittles, original, bite size	0.25	cup	51.25	208	870	2	<1	47	0	2	2.1	0	0
23144	Candy, Starburst, fruit chews, original	8	ea	40	163	682	3	<1	33	0	3	3.1	0	0
93430	Candy, taffy, prep f/recipe	1	pce	15	60	251	1	<1	14	0	<1	0.3	0.1	<0.1
23486	Candy, Turtles, milk choc pecan caramels, grain swtnd	2	pce	40	160	669		2	16	1	11	3		
23154	Candy, Twizzlers, strawberry twists, 5 oz pkg	4	pce	38	133	556		1	30	0	1	0		
23152	Candy, York peppermint patty, 1.5 oz	1	ea	43	165	690	4	1	35	1	3	1.9	0.2	<0.1

< = Trace amount present Blank = Not available

V, vitamin; **THI**, thiamin; **RIB**, riboflavin; **NIA**, niacin; **FOL**, folate; **CALC**, calcium; **PHOS**, phosphorus; **SOD**, sodium; **POT**, potassium; **MAG**, magnesium

CHOL (mg)	V-A (IU)	THI (mg)	RIB (mg)	NIA (mg)	V-B_6 (mg)	FOL (µg)	V-B_{12} (µg)	V-C (mg)	V-E (mg)	CALC (mg)	PHOS (mg)	SOD (mg)	POT (mg)	MAG (mg)	IRON (mg)	ZINC (mg)
0	4							1		30		10			0	
1	0	<0.1	<0.1	0.1	<0.1	4	0	0	0.3	14	23	17	46	9	0.3	0.2
1	4	<0.1	<0.1	<0.1	<0.1	<1	<0.1	<1	<0.1	14	12	25	22	2	<0.1	<0.1
6	57	<0.1	0.1	0.4	<0.1	7	0.2	0.5	0.8	81	93	32	172	28	0.8	0.8
0	0	<0.1	<0.1	<0.1	<0.1	0	<0.1	0	0	1	<1	4	3	<1	<0.1	<0.1
0	0	<0.1	<0.1	0	0	0	0	0	0	1	0	3	1	0	<0.1	<0.1
0	0	<0.1	<0.1	0.1	<0.1	<1	0	0	<0.1	2	10	3	18	7	0.2	<0.1
2	27	<0.1	<0.1	<0.1	<0.1	1	<0.1	0	<0.1	8	12	8	23	6	0.3	0.2
3	40	<0.1	<0.1	0.1	<0.1	5	<0.1	0.1	0.1	16	32	11	52	16	0.6	0.4
5	28							0.1		36		15	206		0.5	
0	0	<0.1	<0.1	<0.1	<0.1	0	0	0	0	1	<1	20	2	<1	0.2	0
0	0	<0.1	<0.1	<0.1	<0.1	0	0	0	0	1	<1	10	1	<1	0.1	0
0	0	<0.1	<0.1	<0.1	<0.1	0	0	0	0	<1	<1	2	<1	<1	<0.1	<0.1
0	0	0	0	0	0	0	0	0	0	0	0	0	0	0	0	0
0	0	<0.1	<0.1	<0.1	<0.1	1	<0.1	0.3	0.1	14	11	118	18	3	0.1	0.2
0	0	<0.1	<0.1	<0.1	<0.1	0	0	0	0	<1	<1	6	4	<1	<0.1	<0.1
0	0	0.1	<0.1	0.5	<0.1	17	0	0	<0.1	0	10	120	15	3	0.4	0.1
3	31	<0.1	<0.1	1.4	<0.1	23	0.1	0	1.2	43	81	21	147	29	0.5	0.7
10								0		80		35			0.4	
7	97	<0.1	0.1	0.1	<0.1	4	0.3	0.3	0.2	55	76	32	136	23	0.6	0.8
8	72	<0.1	0.2	0.3	<0.1	6	0.3	0.1	1.3	92	108	30	182	37	0.7	0.5
								0		0					0	
3	40	<0.1	<0.1	0.8	<0.1	13	<0.1	0	0.7	8	30	126	48	12	0.3	0.2
3	25	0.1	<0.1	2	<0.1	22	0.1	0.1	0.1	35	72	161	154	28	0.5	0.6
4	52	<0.1	0.1	1.7	<0.1	20	0.2	0	1	42	85	16	201	38	0.5	1
10	148	0.1	<0.1	0.1	<0.1	2	<0.1	0.2	0.4	20	33	40	67	13	0.3	0.4
1	41	<0.1	0.1	0.2	<0.1	4	0.2	0.1	0.1	39	64	16	231	20	0.8	0.6
0	0	0.1	0.1	2.8	0.1	26	0.1	0	0.5	32	97	91	169	41	0.2	0.5
5	51	<0.1	0.1	<0.1	0	0	0.1	0.4	0.5	61	30	79	79	0	0.2	0
0	2	0.2	0.1	1.3	0.2	18	0	0	0.1	224	144	58	107	88	1.5	1.3
0	0	0	<0.1	<0.1	<0.1	0	0	34.2	0.1	0	1	8	6	1	0	<0.1
0	<1	<0.1	<0.1	<0.1	0	<1	0	23.5	0.1	0	2	1	1	<1	<0.1	0
1	15	<0.1	<0.1	<0.1	0	0	<0.1	0	<0.1	1	<1	8	<1	0	<0.1	<0.1
7	98							0		43		29			0	
0	0							0		0		109			0.2	
<1	3							0		5	0	12	48		0.4	

ESHA, EatRight Analysis; **AMT**, amount; **WT**, weight; **CAL**, calories; **KILO**, KiloJoule; **WTR**, water; **PROT**, protein; **CARB**, carbohydrate; **FIBR**, fiber; **FAT**, fat; **SATF**, saturated fat; **MONO**, monounsaturated fat; **POLY**, polyunsaturated fat; **CHOL**, cholesterol;

ESHA CODE	FOOD DESCRIPTION	AMT	UNIT	WT (g)	CAL (kcal)	KILO (kJ)	WTR (g)	PROT (g)	CARB (g)	FIBR (g)	FAT (g)	SATF (g)	MONO (g)	POLY (g)
DESSERTS (CONTINUED)														
23082	Chewing Gum, stick	1	stick	3	11	46	<1	0	3	<1	<1	<0.1	<0.1	<0.1
92196	Chewing Gum, sugarless	1	pce	2	5	21	<1	0	2	<1	<1	<0.1	<0.1	<0.1
23016	Chocolate Bar, milk, 1.55oz bar	1	ea	44	235	983	1	3	26	1	13	8.1	3.2	0.6
23146	Chocolate Bar, milk, 1.5oz bar	1	ea	42	223	933	<1	4	24	1	13	7.7	3.3	0.3
23057	Chocolate Bar, Special Dark, 1.45oz	1	ea	41	228	954	<1	2	25	3	13		2.1	0.2
23007	Marshmallows	1	ea	7.2	23	96	1	<1	6	<1	<1	<0.1	<0.1	<0.1
Cookies														
44219	Bar, dessert, crisp rice, square	1	ea	37	153	640	2	1	30	<1	3	0.5	0.9	1.9
32651	Bar, dessert, lemon	1	indv	128	370	1548		6	58	1	14	6		
24431	Brownie, butterscotch blondie	1	ea	76	350	1464		3	52	0	14	9		
47019	Brownie, prep f/recipe, 2" square	1	ea	24	112	469	3	1	12		7	1.8	2.6	2.3
47000	Brownie, twin wrap, pkg	1	pkg	61	247	1033	8	3	39	1	10	2.6	5.5	1.4
91664	Cookie, almond	2	ea	29	170	711		2	19	0	10	3		
32666	Cookie, biscotti, chocolate	1	ea	34	160	669		3	22	2	7	3		
47005	Cookie, butter, enrich	6	ea	30	140	586	1	2	21	<1	6	3.3	1.7	0.3
47032	Cookie, chocolate chip, lower fat	3	ea	30	136	569	1	2	22	1	5	1.1	1.8	1.4
47002	Cookie, chocolate chip, prep f/recipe with marg, med, 2¼"	2	ea	32	156	653	2	2	19	1	9	2.6	3.3	2.7
43728	Cookie, chocolate mint cake, SnackWell's	1	ea	16	50	209		1	12	0	<1	0		
47041	Cookie, chocolate wafer	5	ea	30	130	544	1	2	22	1	4	1.3	1.5	1.2
47042	Cookie, coconut macaroon, prep f/recipe, 2"	1	ea	24	97	406	3	1	17	<1	3	2.7	0.1	<0.1
47153	Cookie, devil's food, Snackwell's, fat free, svg	1	svg	16	49	205	3	1	12	<1	<1	0.1	<0.1	<0.1
47012	Cookie, fig bar	1	ea	16	56	234	3	1	11	1	1	0.2	0.5	0.4
47043	Cookie, fortune	1	ea	8	30	126	1	<1	7	<1	<1	0.1	0.1	<0.1
47376	Cookie, fruit bar, fat free	1	ea	28	90	377		2	21	0	0	0	0	0
47324	Cookie, fudge brownie, SnackWell's, sugar free	1	ea	24	90	377		1	17	0	4	1	1	0
47009	Cookie, ladyfinger, with lemon juice and rind	3	ea	33	120	502	6	3	20	<1	3	1	1.2	0.5
47046	Cookie, marshmallow, chocolate coated, sml, .75" × 1.5"	3	ea	39	164	686	4	2	26	1	7	1.8	3.6	0.8
47496	Cookie, oatmeal raisin, home style, svg	1	svg	26	106	444	3	1	18	1	3	0.7	1.3	0.3
47054	Cookie, oatmeal, prep f/recipe, 2⅝"	2	ea	30	134	561	2	2	20		5	1.1	2.3	1.7
47010	Cookie, peanut butter, prep f/recipe, 3"	1	ea	20	95	397	1	2	12		5	0.9	2.2	1.4
47006	Cookie, sandwich, chocolate, with creme	2	ea	23	108	452	1	1	16	1	5	1.5	2	0.8
47038	Cookie, sandwich, chocolate, with creme, chocolate coated	1	ea	17	82	343	<1	1	11	1	4	1.3	2.5	0.5
47180	Cookie, sandwich, Oreo, chocolate	3	ea	34	160	669	<1	1	24	1	7	1.5		
47059	Cookie, sandwich, peanut butter	1	ea	14	67	280	<1	1	9	<1	3	0.7	1.6	0.5
47160	Cookie, sandwich, SnackWell's, creme, rducd fat	2	ea	26	110	460		1	20	0	3	0.5		

< = Trace amount present   Blank = Not available

V, vitamin; **THI**, thiamin; **RIB**, riboflavin; **NIA**, niacin; **FOL**, folate; **CALC**, calcium; **PHOS**, phosphorus; **SOD**, sodium; **POT**, potassium; **MAG**, magnesium

CHOL (mg)	V-A (IU)	THI (mg)	RIB (mg)	NIA (mg)	V-B_6 (mg)	FOL (μg)	V-B_{12} (μg)	V-C (mg)	V-E (mg)	CALC (mg)	PHOS (mg)	SOD (mg)	POT (mg)	MAG (mg)	IRON (mg)	ZINC (mg)
0	0	0	0	0	0	0	0	0	0	0	0	<1	<1	0	0	0
0	0	0	0	0	0	0	0	0	0	<1	0	<1	0	0	0	0
10	86	<0.1	0.1	0.2	<0.1	5	0.3	0	0.2	83	92	35	164	28	1	1
10	96							0.9		105	87	42	184		0.4	
2		0	<0.1	0	0	0		0		12	21	2	206	13	0.9	<0.1
0	0	<0.1	<0.1	<0.1	<0.1	<1	0	0	0	<1	1	6	<1	<1	<0.1	<0.1
0	400	0.5	0.5	6	0.3	40	0	0		1	16	130	14	5	0.5	0.2
140	500							12		40		220			1.1	
70	500							2.4		0		25			1.1	
18	198	<0.1	<0.1	0.2	<0.1	7	<0.1	0.1		14	32	82	42	13	0.4	0.2
10	42	0.2	0.1	1	<0.1	29	<0.1	0	0.1	18	62	174	91	19	1.4	0.4
0	0							0		0		75			0	
5	0							0		0		15			1.4	
35	202	0.1	0.1	1	<0.1	23	0.1	0	0.2	9	31	85	33	4	0.7	0.1
0	1	0.1	0.1	0.8	0.1	21	0	0		6	25	113	37	8	0.9	0.2
10	219	0.1	0.1	0.4	<0.1	11	<0.1	0.1		12	32	116	72	18	0.8	0.3
0	0							0		0		40			0.4	
1	4	0.1	0.1	0.9	<0.1	18	<0.1	0	0.2	9	40	207	63	16	1.2	0.3
0	0	<0.1	<0.1	<0.1	<0.1	1	<0.1	0	<0.1	2	10	59	37	5	0.2	0.2
0	<1	<0.1	<0.1	0.2	<0.1	3	<0.1	<1		5	11	28	18	4	0.4	0.1
0	5	<0.1	<0.1	0.3	<0.1	6	<0.1	<1	0.1	10	10	56	33	4	0.5	0.1
<1	<1	<0.1	<0.1	0.1	<0.1	5	<0.1	0	<0.1	1	3	2	3	1	0.1	<0.1
0	0							0	<0.1	0		95			0.4	
0	0							0		0		130			1.1	
73	16	0.1	0.1	0.7	<0.1	20	0.2	1.2	0.2	16	57	49	37	4	1.2	0.4
0	2	<0.1	0.1	0.3	<0.1	9	0.1	<1	0.1	18	38	73	71	14	1	0.3
2	4	0.1	<0.1	0.4		12		0		10		88	74		0.6	
11	227	0.1	0.1	0.4	<0.1	10	<0.1	0.1		32	50	179	55	13	0.8	0.3
6	129	<0.1	<0.1	0.7	<0.1	11	<0.1	<1		8	23	104	46	8	0.4	0.2
0	<1	<0.1	<0.1	0.5	0	16	0	0	0.6	5	23	106	49	11	2	0.2
0	1	<0.1	<0.1	0.2	<0.1	3	<0.1	0	<0.1	6	15	55	41	7	0.5	0.1
0	0							0		0		180			1.4	
0	1	<0.1	<0.1	0.5	<0.1	9	<0.1	<1	0.3	7	26	52	27	7	0.4	0.1
0	0							0		0		130			0.4	

ESHA, EatRight Analysis; **AMT**, amount; **WT**, weight; **CAL**, calories; **KILO**, KiloJoule; **WTR**, water; **PROT**, protein; **CARB**, carbohydrate; **FIBR**, fiber; **FAT**, fat; **SATF**, saturated fat; **MONO**, monounsaturated fat; **POLY**, polyunsaturated fat; **CHOL**, cholesterol;

ESHA CODE	FOOD DESCRIPTION	AMT	UNIT	WT (g)	CAL (kcal)	KILO (kJ)	WTR (g)	PROT (g)	CARB (g)	FIBR (g)	FAT (g)	SATF (g)	MONO (g)	POLY (g)
DESSERTS (CONTINUED)														
47071	Cookie, sandwich, vanilla, with creme, 1¾"	3	ea	30	145	607	1	1	22	<1	6	0.9	2.5	2.3
47062	Cookie, shortbread, pecan, 2"	1	ea	14	76	318	<1	1	8	<1	5	1.1	2.6	0.6
47007	Cookie, shortbread, plain, 1 ⅝" square	3	ea	24	120	502	1	1	15	<1	6	1.5	3.2	0.8
47045	Cookie, snap, ginger	4	ea	28	116	485	1	2	22	1	3	0.7	1.5	0.4
47011	Cookie, snickerdoodle, prep f/recipe	1	ea	20	80	335	1	1	12	<1	3	2.1		
47064	Cookie, sugar	1	ea	15	72	301	1	1	10	<1	3	0.8	1.8	0.4
47069	Cookie, sugar wafer, creme filled	3	ea	30.3	152	636	1	1	21	<1	7	3.6	2.3	0.8
47068	Cookie, sugar, prep f/recipe with margarine, 3"	2	ea	28	132	552	2	2	17	<1	7	1.3	2.9	2
47065	Cookie, sugar, sugar and sodium free, med, 1 ⅝"	4	ea	28	121	506	2	1	22	<1	4	0.5	1.5	1.3
47171	Cookie, vanilla wafers, Nilla	8	ea	30	140	586	<1	1	21	1	6	1	1.5	0
Doughnuts and Pastries														
49018	Blintz, fruit filled	1	ea	70	124	519	44	4	17	<1	4	1.3	1.8	0.9
42094	Bread, sweet, mex-pan dulce with crumb topping	1	ea	79	291	1218	17	5	48	1	9	1.8	4	2.5
45523	Croissant, cheese	1	med	57	236	987	12	5	27	1	12	6.1	3.7	1.4
45505	Doughnut, cake, med, 3¼"	1	ea	54	226	946	12	3	25	1	13	3.8	6.9	1.4
45524	Doughnut, cake, with chocolate icing, med, 3"	1	ea	43	194	812	7	2	22	1	11	5.8	3.7	0.8
45563	Doughnut, creme filled, 3½" oval	1	ea	85	307	1284	32	5	26	1	21	4.6	10.3	2.6
45507	Doughnut, filled, jelly, 3½" oval	1	ea	85	289	1209	30	5	33	1	16	4.1	8.7	2
45527	Doughnut, French crullers, glazed, 3"	1	ea	41	169	707	7	1	24	<1	8	1.9	4.3	0.9
45506	Doughnut, glazed, enrich, med, 3 ¾"	1	ea	64	269	1125	14	4	31	1	15	6	4.6	2.3
45560	Doughnut, okinawan	1	ea	18	76	318	3	1	10	<1	4	0.9	2	0.5
14118	Doughnut, raised, French cruller	1	ea	49	150	628		2	17	1	8	2		
34535	Pastry, baklava	1	ea	69	375	1569		6	50	2	16	2		
45557	Pastry, Chinese	1	svg	55	132	552	25	1	25	1	3	0.4	0.9	1.7
45509	Pastry, cream puff, custard filled, prep f/recipe	1	ea	130	335	1402	70	9	30	1	20	4.8	8.5	5.4
45508	Pastry, eclair, chocolate, custard filled, prep f/rec, 5×2	1	ea	100	262	1096	52	6	24	1	16	4.1	6.5	3.9
45504	Pastry, toaster, apple	1	ea	54	211	883	8	3	37	1	6	1.4	3.5	0.6
45604	Pastry, toaster, raspberry, frosted	1	ea	52	205	858	6	2	37	1	6	1	3.2	1.3
42164	Sweet Roll, cheese	1	ea	66	238	996	19	5	29	1	12	4	6	1.3
42166	Sweet Roll, cinnamon, frosted, prep f/refrig dough	1	ea	30	109	456	7	2	17		4	1	2.2	0.5
42266	Turnover, apple, with icing, kit, refrig	1	ea	57	180	753		2	24	0	8	2		
45555	Turnover, guava	1	ea	78	234	979	34	2	28	3	13	2.5	5.5	3.9
Frozen Desserts														
72682	Cake, ice cream, Chocolate Chipper, 6" round	1	slice	132	430	1799		5	49	3	24	12		
23174	Frozen Dessert Bar, fruit juice, 2.5 fl oz	1	ea	77	67	280	60	1	16	1	<1	0	0	<0.1

< = Trace amount present   Blank = Not available

V, vitamin; **THI**, thiamin; **RIB**, riboflavin; **NIA**, niacin; **FOL**, folate; **CALC**, calcium; **PHOS**, phosphorus; **SOD**, sodium; **POT**, potassium; **MAG**, magnesium

CHOL (mg)	V-A (IU)	THI (mg)	RIB (mg)	NIA (mg)	V-B$_6$ (mg)	FOL (µg)	V-B$_{12}$ (µg)	V-C (mg)	V-E (mg)	CALC (mg)	PHOS (mg)	SOD (mg)	POT (mg)	MAG (mg)	IRON (mg)	ZINC (mg)
0	0	0.1	0.1	0.8	<0.1	15	0	0	0.5	8	22	105	27	4	0.7	0.1
5	<1	<0.1	<0.1	0.3	<0.1	9	<0.1	0		4	12	39	10	3	0.3	0.1
5	21	0.1	0.1	0.8	<0.1	17	<0.1	0	0.1	8	26	126	24	4	0.7	0.1
0	1	0.1	0.1	0.9	<0.1	24	0	0	0.3	22	23	140	97	14	1.8	0.2
9	127	0.1	<0.1	0.4	<0.1	14	<0.1	0.1	0.1	8	10	75	23	2	0.5	0.1
8	14	<0.1	<0.1	0.4	<0.1	8	<0.1	<1	<0.1	3	12	45	9	2	0.3	0.1
0	<1	<0.1	<0.1	0.7	<0.1	23	0	0	0.8	8	22	31	35	5	1.1	0.1
7	288	0.1	0.1	0.7	<0.1	17	<0.1	<1	0.7	20	25	137	22	3	0.7	0.1
0	0	0.1	0.1	1	<0.1	20	0	0	0.3	7	20	32	29	3	1.1	0.1
5										20		115	30		0.7	
53	376	0.1	0.1	0.4	<0.1	8	0.2	0.5	0.5	35	59	93	78	7	0.8	0.3
26	287	0.2	0.2	2	<0.1	19	0.1	0.1	1.2	13	56	75	57	9	1.8	0.4
32	459	0.3	0.2	1.2	<0.1	42	0.2	0.1	0.8	30	74	206	75	14	1.2	0.5
5	6	0.1	0.1	1.1	<0.1	43	<0.1	0.7	1	14	141	243	61	9	1.6	0.4
8	7	0.1	0.1	0.7	<0.1	28	<0.1	0.6	0.9	10	90	140	86	13	1.7	0.4
20	34	0.3	0.1	1.9	0.1	60	0.1	0	0.2	21	65	263	68	17	1.6	0.7
22	60	0.3	0.1	1.8	0.1	58	0.2	0	0.4	21	72	387	67	17	1.5	0.6
5	3	0.1	0.1	0.9	<0.1	17	<0.1	0	0.1	11	50	141	32	5	1	0.1
19	15	0.2	0.1	1.7	<0.1	69	0.1	0.8	0.9	65	75	202	65	11	1.5	0.4
13	23	<0.1	0.1	0.4	<0.1	2	<0.1	<1	0.5	24	22	38	15	2	0.4	0.1
20	0	<0.1	<0.1	<0.1	<0.1	3	0.1	0	0.7	0	23	105	18	2	0	0.1
0	0							0		20		181			2	
0	1	<0.1	<0.1	0.5	0.1	2	0	0	0.5	12	30	5	49	14	0.3	0.3
174	768	0.2	0.4	1.1	0.1	48	0.5	0.4	1.9	86	142	443	150	16	1.5	0.8
127	828	0.1	0.3	0.8	0.1	43	0.3	0.3	2	63	107	337	117	15	1.2	0.6
0	555	0.2	0.3	2.8	0.2	28	0	0	0.4	6	38	180	40	6	2.1	0.2
0	500	0.2	0.2	2	0.2	52	0	0		11	46	166	44	8	1.8	0.6
50	168	0.1	0.1	0.5	<0.1	28	0.2	0.1		78	65	236	90	13	0.5	0.4
0	1	0.1	0.1	1.1	<0.1	16	<0.1	0.1		10	104	250	19	4	0.8	0.1
0	0							0		0		260			0.7	
<1	264	0.1	0.1	1.5	0.1	6	<0.1	48	2	13	33	13	120	9	1.1	0.2
35	300							1.2		100		230			0.7	
0	14	<0.1	<0.1	0.1	<0.1	5	0	7.3	0	4	5	3	41	3	0.1	<0.1

ESHA, EatRight Analysis; **AMT**, amount; **WT**, weight; **CAL**, calories; **KILO**, KiloJoule; **WTR**, water; **PROT**, protein; **CARB**, carbohydrate; **FIBR**, fiber; **FAT**, fat; **SATF**, saturated fat; **MONO**, monounsaturated fat; **POLY**, polyunsaturated fat; **CHOL**, cholesterol;

ESHA CODE	FOOD DESCRIPTION	AMT	UNIT	WT (g)	CAL (kcal)	KILO (kJ)	WTR (g)	PROT (g)	CARB (g)	FIBR (g)	FAT (g)	SATF (g)	MONO (g)	POLY (g)
DESSERTS (CONTINUED)														
90723	Frozen Dessert Pop, 2 fl oz bar	1	ea	59.43	47	197	48	0	11	0	<1	<0.1	<0.1	<0.1
72190	Frozen Dessert Pop, orange, no sug add	1	ea	44	25	105	36	1	6	<1	<1	0.2		
2070	Frozen Dessert, banana split, with whipped cream	1	ea	425	1089	4556	217	15	124	1	65	37.5	18.7	5.3
71949	Frozen Dessert, French Vanilla	0.5	cup	70	140	586		1	17	1	7	0.5		
23051	Frozen Dessert, slushy	1	cup	193	247	1033	129	1	63	0	0	0	0	0
2043	Frozen Yogurt Bar, chocolate coated	1	ea	41	109	456	21	1	12	<1	7	5.3	0.8	0.2
72124	Frozen Yogurt, all flavors, not chocolate	0.5	cup	87	110	460	62	3	19	0	3	2	0.9	0.1
71819	Frozen Yogurt, chocolate, nonfat, with art swtnr	0.5	cup	93	100	418	68	4	18	2	1	0.5	0.2	<0.1
2035	Frozen Yogurt, soft serve, chocolate	0.5	cup	72	115	481	46	3	18	2	4	2.6	1.3	0.2
2064	Frozen Yogurt, soft serve, vanilla	0.5	cup	72	114	477	47	3	17	0	4	2.5	1.1	0.2
2592	Frozen Yogurt, vanilla raspberry swirl, low fat	0.5	cup	108	170	711		4	32	0	2	1.5		
72207	Ice Cream Bar, caramel crunch	1	ea	93	270	1130		3	26	0	17	13		
72208	Ice Cream Bar, chocolate, chocolate covered	1	ea	91	280	1172		3	23	1	19	14		
72330	Ice Cream Bar, Cookie and cream, cookie coated	1	ea	60	190	795		2	21	1	12	6		
72191	Ice Cream Bar, Creamsicle, orange	1	ea	65	100	418		1	18	0	2	1.5		
72255	Ice Cream Bar, Creamsicle, raspberry	1	ea	65	100	418		1	18	0	2	1.5		
72188	Ice Cream Bar, Fudgsicle	1	ea	61	90	377	24	3	16	1	2	1		
2050	Ice Cream, chocolate	0.5	cup	66	143	598	37	3	19	1	7	4.5	2.1	0.3
2216	Ice Cream, chocolate chip cookie dough	0.5	cup	104	270	1130		4	32	0	15	10		
18397	Ice Cream, Cookie 'n cream, light	0.5	cup	62	120	502		3	18	0	4	2		
2008	Ice Cream, soft serve, French vanilla	0.5	cup	86	191	799	51	4	19	1	11	6.4	3	0.4
2063	Ice Cream, strawberry, indv pkg	1	indv cup	58	111	464	35	2	16	1	5	3		
2004	Ice Cream, vanilla	0.5	cup	66	137	573	40	2	16	<1	7	4.5	2	0.3
2009	Ice Cream, vanilla, light	0.5	cup	76	137	573	45	4	22	<1	4	2.2	1	0.2
2006	Ice Cream, vanilla, rich	0.5	cup	107	266	1113	61	4	24	0	17	11.1	4.8	0.7
2011	Sherbet, orange	0.5	cup	74	107	448	49	1	22	1	1	0.9	0.4	0.1
19298	Sherbet, orange	1	reg	113	160	669		2	34	0	2	1.5		
49198	Sorbet, lemon	0.5	cup	70	90	377		0	22	0	0	0	0	0
49197	Sorbet, strawberry	0.5	cup	70	80	335		0	19	0	0	0	0	0
Pies														
49071	Bar, tart, blueberry, low fat	1	ea	40	130	544	3	2	28	1	2	0		
49063	Cobbler, peach, fzn	1	svg	113	330	1381		3	38	1	19	4		
48022	Pie, apple, prep f/recipe, ⅛ of 9"	1	slice	155	411	1720	73	4	58		19	4.7	8.4	5.2
70536	Pie, apple, rtb, 10"	1	slice	130	300	1255	95	2	39	2	15	3		
70557	Pie, Boston cream, 10"	1	slice	78	220	920		2	32	0	9	2.5		
70538	Pie, cherry, rtb, 10"	1	slice	130	330	1381	82	3	48	1	15	3		
70554	Pie, chocolate cream, 10"	1	slice	130	370	1548	79	3	44	1	21	13		
70562	Pie, lemon meringue, 10"	1	slice	120	250	1046		2	46	0	6	1.5		

< = Trace amount present Blank = Not available

V, vitamin; **THI**, thiamin; **RIB**, riboflavin; **NIA**, niacin; **FOL**, folate; **CALC**, calcium; **PHOS**, phosphorus; **SOD**, sodium; **POT**, potassium; **MAG**, magnesium

CHOL (mg)	V-A (IU)	THI (mg)	RIB (mg)	NIA (mg)	V-B_6 (mg)	FOL (µg)	V-B_{12} (µg)	V-C (mg)	V-E (mg)	CALC (mg)	PHOS (mg)	SOD (mg)	POT (mg)	MAG (mg)	IRON (mg)	ZINC (mg)
0	0	0	0	0	0	0	0	0.4	0	0	0	4	9	1	0.3	0.1
1	10							0.2		60		18			0.1	
204	1946	0.1	0.9	0.5	0.2	19	1.4	2.4	0.5	466	485	360	783	92	1.6	2.7
0	0	<0.1	<0.1	0.2	<0.1	5	0	0		0	26	70	49	11	0	0.1
0	0	<0.1	0	<0.1	<0.1	0	0	1.9	0	4	2	42	6	2	0.3	<0.1
1	68	<0.1	0.1	0.1	<0.1	2	0.1	0.3	<0.1	46	43	28	74	6	0.1	0.2
11	153	<0.1	0.2	0.1	<0.1	3	0.1	0.6	0.1	87	77	55	136	9	0.4	0.2
4	7	<0.1	0.2	0.2	<0.1	11	0.5	0.7	0.1	148	120	75	315	37	<0.1	0.5
4	115	<0.1	0.2	0.2	0.1	8	0.2	0.2		106	100	71	188	19	0.9	0.4
1	153	<0.1	0.2	0.2	0.1	4	0.2	0.6	0.1	103	93	63	152	10	0.2	0.3
25	0							1.2		100		35			0	
25	200							0		100		80			0	
20	200							0		80		55			1.1	
10	100							0		60		120			0.4	
5	0							0		40		30			0	
5	0							0		40		30			0	
5	0							0		80		65			0.4	
22	275	<0.1	0.1	0.1	<0.1	11	0.2	0.5	0.2	72	71	50	164	19	0.6	0.4
65	500							0		150		90			0.7	
20										60		60				
78	507	<0.1	0.2	0.1	<0.1	8	0.4	0.7	0.5	113	100	52	152	10	0.2	0.4
17	186	<0.1	0.1	0.1	<0.1	7	0.2	4.5		70	58	35	109	8	0.1	0.2
29	278	<0.1	0.2	0.1	<0.1	3	0.3	0.4	0.2	84	69	53	131	9	0.1	0.5
21	340	<0.1	0.2	0.1	<0.1	5	0.4	0.9	0.1	122	78	56	158	11	0.1	0.6
98	699	<0.1	0.2	0.1	<0.1	9	0.4	0	0.5	125	112	65	168	12	0.4	0.5
1	34	<0.1	0.1	<0.1	<0.1	3	0.1	1.7	<0.1	40	30	34	71	6	0.1	0.4
10	100							2.4		60		35			0	
0												33	3			
0												1	34			
0	100	0.2	0.2	2	0.2	40	0.6	1.2		250		80			0.7	
0	0							36		0		160			1.1	
0	90	0.2	0.2	1.9	<0.1	37	0	2.6		11	43	327	122	11	1.7	0.3
0	0	<0.1	<0.1	0.4	0.1			0		0		390	96		0.4	
30	0	<0.1	0.1	0.2	<0.1			0		20		170	77		0.4	
0	400	<0.1	<0.1	0.2	0.1			0		80		360	112		0.4	
20	99	<0.1	0.1	1.4	<0.1			0		35		359	176		0.9	
0	0							0		0		290	23		0	

ESHA, EatRight Analysis; **AMT**, amount; **WT**, weight; **CAL**, calories; **KILO**, KiloJoule; **WTR**, water; **PROT**, protein; **CARB**, carbohydrate; **FIBR**, fiber; **FAT**, fat; **SATF**, saturated fat; **MONO**, monounsaturated fat; **POLY**, polyunsaturated fat; **CHOL**, cholesterol;

ESHA CODE	FOOD DESCRIPTION	AMT	UNIT	WT (g)	CAL (kcal)	KILO (kJ)	WTR (g)	PROT (g)	CARB (g)	FIBR (g)	FAT (g)	SATF (g)	MONO (g)	POLY (g)
DESSERTS (CONTINUED)														
70559	Pie, pecan, 10"	1	slice	128	550	2301	24	7	75	2	26	6		
70561	Pie, pumpkin, 10"	1	slice	125	310	1297		5	47	2	12	3		
49015	Strudel, apple	1	pce	71	195	816	31	2	29	2	8	1.5	2.3	3.8
Puddings														
2613	Custard, egg, prep f/dry mix with whole milk	0.5	cup	141	172	720	104	6	25	0	6	2.9	1.6	0.4
2625	Custard, flan, prep f/dry mix with whole milk	0.5	cup	140	158	661	104	4	26	0	4	2.5	1.1	0.2
23052	Gelatin, prep f/dry mix with water	0.5	cup	135	84	351	114	2	19	0	0	0	0	0
23093	Gelatin, rducd cal, with asp, prep with water	0.5	cup	117	23	96	111	1	5	0	0	0	0	0
48044	Pie Filling, pumpkin, cnd	0.5	cup	135	140	586	97	1	36	11	<1	0.1	<0.1	<0.1
58203	Pudding, all flvrs, not choc, low cal, inst	1	dry svg	8	28	117	1	<1	7	<1	<1	<0.1	<0.1	<0.1
2628	Pudding, banana, inst, prep with 2% milk	0.5	cup	147	154	644	110	4	29	0	2	1.4	0.7	0.2
57915	Pudding, bread, prep f/recipe, svg	1	svg	270.91	475	1987	459	15	66	2	17	8		
2636	Pudding, chocolate, prep f/dry mix with 2% milk	0.5	cup	128	142	594	95	4	25	1	3	1.6	0.8	0.1
2604	Pudding, chocolate, prep f/dry mix with whole milk	0.5	cup	142	170	711	104	4	28	1	4	2.6	1.2	0.3
45888	Pudding, tapioca, old fashioned	1	indv cup	113	140	586		3	24	0	4	3		
2653	Pudding, tapioca, prep f/dry mix with 2% milk	0.5	cup	128	134	561	96	4	25	0	2	1.3	0.6	0.1
Toppings														
39909	Spread, dark chocolate peanut	2	Tbs	32	180	753	<1	5	12	1	13	2		
23013	Syrup, chocolate	2	Tbs	39	109	456	12	1	25	1	<1	0.2	0.1	<0.1
23069	Topping, butterscotch	2	Tbs	41	103	431	13	1	27	<1	<1	<0.1	<0.1	0
23070	Topping, caramel	2	Tbs	41	103	431	13	1	27	<1	<1	<0.1	<0.1	0
23014	Topping, chocolate fudge	2	Tbs	38	133	556	8	2	24	1	3	1.5	1.5	0.1
23071	Topping, marshmallow cream	2	Tbs	12	39	163	2	<1	9	<1	<1	<0.1	<0.1	<0.1
23064	Topping, marshmallow creme	2	Tbs	12	40	167	<1	0	10	0	0	0	0	0
23162	Topping, syrup, with nuts	2	Tbs	41	184	770	6	2	24	1	9	0.8	2	5.6
510	Topping, whipped cream, pressurized	2	Tbs	7	18	75	4	<1	1	0	2	1	0.4	0.1
569	Topping, whipped, dry mix, svg, Dream Whip	1	dry svg	2	10	42	0	0	2		0	0	0	0
509	Topping, whipped, prep with .5 cup milk f/1.5oz dry mix	2	Tbs	8	16	67	5	<1	1	0	1	0.9	0.1	<0.1
508	Topping, whipped, semi-solid, fzn	2	Tbs	8	25	105	4	<1	2	0	2	1.7	0.1	<0.1
EGGS AND SUBSTITUTES														
19522	Egg White, ckd	1	ea	33.4	17	71	29	4	<1	0	0	0	0	0
19507	Egg White, raw	0.25	cup	60.75	32	134	53	7	<1	0	<1	0	0	0
19506	Egg White, raw, lrg	1	ea	33	17	71	29	4	<1	0	<1	0	0	0
19523	Egg Yolk, ckd	1	ea	16.6	59	247	8	3	<1	0	5	1.6	1.9	0.7

< = Trace amount present   Blank = Not available

V, vitamin; **THI**, thiamin; **RIB**, riboflavin; **NIA**, niacin; **FOL**, folate; **CALC**, calcium; **PHOS**, phosphorus; **SOD**, sodium; **POT**, potassium; **MAG**, magnesium

CHOL (mg)	V-A (IU)	THI (mg)	RIB (mg)	NIA (mg)	$V\text{-}B_6$ (mg)	FOL (µg)	$V\text{-}B_{12}$ (µg)	V-C (mg)	V-E (mg)	CALC (mg)	PHOS (mg)	SOD (mg)	POT (mg)	MAG (mg)	IRON (mg)	ZINC (mg)
85	200							0		0		510	90		0.7	
45	3500	<0.1	0.2	0.5				0		80		390	193		1.4	
4	21	<0.1	<0.1	0.2	<0.1	20	0.2	1.2	1	11	23	96	106	6	0.3	0.1
72	257	0.1	0.3	0.2	0.1	13	0.7	0.1	0.1	196	183	118	292	23	0.5	0.7
17	158	<0.1	0.2	0.1	<0.1	6	0.4	1		155	118	157	224	17	0.1	0.5
0	0	0	<0.1	<0.1	0	1	0	0	0	4	30	101	1	1	<0.1	<0.1
0	0	0	0	0	0	0	0	0	0	4	80	56	1	1	<0.1	0
0	11202	<0.1	0.2	0.5	0.2	47	0	4.7		50	61	281	186	22	1.4	0.4
0	0	<0.1	<0.1	<0.1	<0.1	<1	<0.1	0	<0.1	11	189	340	2	<1	<0.1	<0.1
9	250	<0.1	0.2	0.1	0.1	6	0.4	1.2		150	318	435	193	18	0.1	0.5
243	855	0.3	0.6	2.2	0.2	78	1	1.7	1	241	267	666	406	39	2.7	1.4
9	209	<0.1	0.2	0.2	<0.1	5	0.5	0.1	<0.1	143	120	131	200	27	0.4	0.7
13	197	0.1	0.2	0.2	<0.1	6	0.4	0	0.1	151	124	139	213	28	0.5	0.7
0	0							0		100		180			0	
8	205	<0.1	0.2	0.1	<0.1	5	0.3	0.9		134	105	155	170	15	0.1	0.4
0	0	0.1	0.1	1.6	0.1	31	0.1	0	1.8	40	90	30	170	36	0.7	0.7
0	0	<0.1	<0.1	0.1	<0.1	1	0	0.1	<0.1	5	50	28	87	25	0.8	0.3
<1	37	<0.1	<0.1	<0.1	<0.1	1	<0.1	0.1		22	19	143	34	3	0.1	0.1
<1	37	<0.1	<0.1	<0.1	<0.1	1	<0.1	0.1		22	19	143	34	3	0.1	0.1
<1	1	<0.1	<0.1	0.1	<0.1	2	<0.1	0.1	1	19	37	131	108	18	0.5	0.3
0	<1	<0.1	<0.1	<0.1	<0.1	<1	0	0	0	<1	1	10	1	<1	<0.1	<0.1
0	0							0		0		10			0	
0	3	0.1	<0.1	0.2	0.1	11	0	0.1	0.1	14	48	17	62	22	0.4	0.4
5	48	<0.1	<0.1	<0.1	<0.1	<1	<0.1	0	<0.1	7	6	1	10	1	<0.1	<0.1
0	0							0		0		0			0	
1	10	<0.1	<0.1	<0.1	<0.1	<1	<0.1	0.1	<0.1	7	7	5	12	1	<0.1	<0.1
0	11	0	0	0	0	0	0	0	0.1	<1	1	2	1	<1	<0.1	<0.1
0	0	<0.1	0.1	<0.1	<0.1	1	0.1	0	0	2	4	55	48	4	<0.1	<0.1
0	0	<0.1	0.3	0.1	<0.1	2	0.1	0	0	4	9	101	99	7	<0.1	<0.1
0	0	<0.1	0.1	<0.1	<0.1	1	<0.1	0	0	2	5	55	54	4	<0.1	<0.1
213	323	<0.1	0.1	<0.1	0.1	18	0.4	0	0.5	23	81	7	16	1	0.6	0.5

ESHA, EatRight Analysis; **AMT**, amount; **WT**, weight; **CAL**, calories; **KILO**, KiloJoule; **WTR**, water; **PROT**, protein; **CARB**, carbohydrate; **FIBR**, fiber; **FAT**, fat; **SATF**, saturated fat; **MONO**, monounsaturated fat; **POLY**, polyunsaturated fat; **CHOL**, cholesterol;

ESHA CODE	FOOD DESCRIPTION	AMT	UNIT	WT (g)	CAL (kcal)	KILO (kJ)	WTR (g)	PROT (g)	CARB (g)	FIBR (g)	FAT (g)	SATF (g)	MONO (g)	POLY (g)
EGGS AND SUBSTITUTES (CONTINUED)														
19508	Egg Yolk, raw, lrg	1	ea	17	55	230	9	3	1	0	5	1.6	2	0.7
19511	Egg, hard bld, chpd	0.25	cup	34	53	222	25	4	<1	0	4	1.1	1.4	0.5
19510	Egg, hard bld, lrg	1	ea	50	78	326	37	6	1	0	5	1.6	2	0.7
19585	Egg, original, liquid	0.25	cup	61	30	126		6	1	0	0	0	0	0
19517	Egg, poached, lrg	1	ea	50	72	301	38	6	<1	0	5	1.6	1.8	1
19509	Egg, whole, lrg, fried	1	ea	46	90	377	32	6	<1	0	7	2	2.8	1.5
19500	Egg, whole, raw	0.25	cup	60.75	87	364	46	8	<1	0	6	1.9	2.2	1.2
FATS														
44466	Butter Substitute, low fat, pwd	1	Tbs	5	19	79	<1	<1	4	0	<1	<0.1	<0.1	<0.1
44469	Butter, light, salted	1	Tbs	14	71	297	6	<1	0	0	8	4.8	2.2	0.3
8000	Butter, salted	1	Tbs	14.2	102	427	2	<1	<1	0	12	7.3	3	0.4
8142	Butter, salted, whipped	1	Tbs	9.4	67	280	1	<1	<1	0	8	4.7	2.2	0.3
8025	Butter, unsalted	1	Tbs	14.2	102	427	3	<1	<1	0	12	7.3	3	0.4
8002	Cooking Spray, butter flavor	0.25	sec spray	0.27	0	0		0	0	0	0	0	0	0
8004	Fat, beef, tallow	1	Tbs	12.8	115	481	0	0	0	0	13	6.4	5.4	0.5
8005	Fat, chicken	1	Tbs	12.8	115	481	<1	0	0	0	13	3.8	5.7	2.7
90219	Margarine, hard, hydrog soybean oil, stick	1	Tbs	14.1	101	423	2	<1	<1	0	11	2.4	5.5	2.9
8485	Margarine, hard, soybean and safflower oil, unsalted	1	Tbs	14	100	418	<1	0	0	0	11	1.2	6.5	1.2
44784	Margarine, industrial, cttnsd and part hydrog soy, non dairy	1	Tbs	14	100	418	2	<1	0	0	11	2.9	6.5	1.3
8790	Margarine, soft, part hydrog and reg soybean oil	1	Tbs	14	100	418	<1	0	0	0	11	2	3	5
8031	Oil, butter, anhydrous	1	Tbs	12.8	112	469	<1	<1	0	0	13	7.9	3.7	0.5
8084	Oil, canola	1	Tbs	14	124	519	0	0	0	0	14	1	8.9	3.9
8037	Oil, coconut	1	Tbs	13.6	117	490	0	0	0	0	14	11.8	0.8	0.2
8009	Oil, corn, salad or cooking	1	Tbs	13.6	122	510	0	0	0	0	14	1.8	3.8	7.4
8081	Oil, cottonseed, salad or cooking	1	Tbs	13.6	120	502	0	0	0	0	14	3.5	2.4	7.1
8067	Oil, fish, cod liver	1	Tbs	13.6	123	515	0	0	0	0	14	3.1	6.4	3.1
8008	Oil, olive, salad or cooking	1	Tbs	13.5	119	498	0	0	0	0	14	1.9	9.8	1.4
8082	Oil, palm	1	Tbs	13.6	120	502	0	0	0	0	14	6.7	5	1.3
8083	Oil, palm kernel	1	Tbs	13.6	117	490	0	0	0	0	14	11.1	1.6	0.2
8026	Oil, peanut, salad or cooking	1	Tbs	13.5	119	498	0	0	0	0	14	2.3	6.2	4.3
8010	Oil, safflower, salad or cooking, greater than 70% linoleic	1	Tbs	13.6	120	502	0	0	0	0	14	0.8	2	10.1
8027	Oil, sesame, salad or cooking	1	Tbs	13.6	120	502	0	0	0	0	14	1.9	5.4	5.7
8012	Oil, soybean, salad or cooking	1	Tbs	13.6	120	502	0	0	0	0	14	2.1	3.1	7.9
8028	Oil, soybean, salad or cooking, part hydrog, with cttnsd oil	1	Tbs	13.6	120	502	0	0	0	0	14	2.4	4	6.5
8011	Oil, sunflower, 65% linoleic	1	Tbs	13.6	120	502	0	0	0	0	14	1.4	2.7	8.9
8085	Oil, walnut	1	Tbs	13.6	120	502	0	0	0	0	14	1.2	3.1	8.6

< = Trace amount present   Blank = Not available

V, vitamin; **THI**, thiamin; **RIB**, riboflavin; **NIA**, niacin; **FOL**, folate; **CALC**, calcium; **PHOS**, phosphorus; **SOD**, sodium; **POT**, potassium; **MAG**, magnesium

CHOL (mg)	V-A (IU)	THI (mg)	RIB (mg)	NIA (mg)	V-B_6 (mg)	FOL (µg)	V-B_{12} (µg)	V-C (mg)	V-E (mg)	CALC (mg)	PHOS (mg)	SOD (mg)	POT (mg)	MAG (mg)	IRON (mg)	ZINC (mg)
184	245	<0.1	0.1	<0.1	0.1	25	0.3	0	0.4	22	66	8	19	1	0.5	0.4
127	177	<0.1	0.2	<0.1	<0.1	15	0.4	0	0.4	17	58	42	43	3	0.4	0.4
186	260	<0.1	0.3	<0.1	0.1	22	0.6	0	0.5	25	86	62	63	5	0.6	0.5
0	750	0.2	0.8	0.1	0.1	60	1.2	0		20	9	115	95	7	1.1	0.6
185	269	<0.1	0.2	<0.1	0.1	18	0.4	0	0.5	28	98	148	69	6	0.9	0.6
184	362	<0.1	0.2	<0.1	0.1	23	0.4	0	0.6	29	99	95	70	6	0.9	0.6
226	328	<0.1	0.3	<0.1	0.1	29	0.5	0	0.6	34	120	86	84	7	1.1	0.8
<1	0	0	0	0	0	0	0	0	0	1	<1	60	<1	0	0.1	0
15	238	<0.1	<0.1	<0.1	<0.1	<1	<0.1	0	0.2	7	5	63	10	1	0.2	<0.1
31	355	<0.1	<0.1	<0.1	<0.1	<1	<0.1	0	0.3	3	3	101	3	<1	<0.1	<0.1
21	235	<0.1	<0.1	<0.1	<0.1	<1	<0.1	0	0.2	2	2	78	2	<1	<0.1	<0.1
31	355	<0.1	<0.1	<0.1	<0.1	<1	<0.1	0	0.3	3	3	2	3	<1	<0.1	<0.1
0	0							0		0		0			0	
14	0	0	0	0	0	0	0	0	0.3	0	0	0	0	0	0	0
11	0	0	0	0	0	0	0	0	0.3	0	0	0	0	0	0	0
0	504	<0.1	<0.1	<0.1	<0.1	<1	<0.1	<1	0.4	4	3	133	6	<1	0	0
0	500							0	3	0		0			0	
0	600	<0.1	<0.1	<0.1	<0.1	<1	<0.1	0.1	0.6	9	7	123	13	1	0	0
0	500							0		0		95			0	
33	393	<0.1	<0.1	<0.1	<0.1	0	<0.1	0	0.4	1	<1	<1	1	0	0	<0.1
0	0	0	0	0	0	0	0	0	2.4	0	0	0	0	0	0	0
0	0	0	0	0	0	0	0	0	<0.1	0	0	0	0	0	<0.1	0
0	0	0	0	0	0	0	0	0	1.9	0	0	0	0	0	0	0
0	0	0	0	0	0	0	0	0	4.8	0	0	0	0	0	0	0
78	13600		0	0	0	0	0	0		0	0	0	0	0	0	0
0	0	0	0	0	0	0	0	0	1.9	<1	0	<1	<1	0	0.1	0
0	0	0	0	0	0	0	0	0	2.2	0	0	0	0	0	<0.1	0
0	0	0	0	0	0	0	0	0	0.5	0	0	0	0	0	0	0
0	0	0	0	0	0	0	0	0	2.1	0	0	0	0	0	<0.1	<0.1
0	0	0	0	0	0	0	0	0	4.6	0	0	0	0	0	0	0
0	0	0	0	0	0	0	0	0	0.2	0	0	0	0	0	0	0
0	0	0	0	0	0	0	0	0	1.1	0	0	0	0	0	<0.1	<0.1
0	0	0	0	0	0	0	0	0	1.6	0	0	0	0	0	0	0
0	0	0	0	0	0	0	0	0	5.6	0	0	0	0	0	0	0
0	0	0	0	0	0	0	0	0	0.1	0	0	0	0	0	0	0

ESHA, EatRight Analysis; **AMT**, amount; **WT**, weight; **CAL**, calories; **KILO**, KiloJoule; **WTR**, water; **PROT**, protein; **CARB**, carbohydrate; **FIBR**, fiber; **FAT**, fat; **SATF**, saturated fat; **MONO**, monounsaturated fat; **POLY**, polyunsaturated fat; **CHOL**, cholesterol;

ESHA CODE	FOOD DESCRIPTION	AMT	UNIT	WT (g)	CAL (kcal)	KILO (kJ)	WTR (g)	PROT (g)	CARB (g)	FIBR (g)	FAT (g)	SATF (g)	MONO (g)	POLY (g)
FATS (CONTINUED)														
8038	Oil, wheat germ	1	Tbs	13.6	120	502	0	0	0	0	14	2.6	2.1	8.4
8007	Shortening, household, part hydrog, soybean and cttnsd oil	1	Tbs	12.8	113	473	0	0	0	0	13	3.2	5.7	3.3
250	Spread, Benecol	1	Tbs	14	70	293	1	0	0	0	8	1	4.5	2
8825	Spread, light, Benecol	1	Tbs	14	50	209	8	0	1		5	0.7	2.7	1.7
8176	Spread, tub	1	Tbs	14	60	251	1	0	0	0	7	1.5		
8698	Spread, tub	1	Tbs	14	90	377	1	0	0	0	10	2		
FRUITS														
3000	Apple, fresh, sml 2 ¾", USDA	1	ea	149	77	322	127	<1	21	4	<1	<0.1	<0.1	0.1
3003	Apple, peeled, fresh, sml 2 ¾"	1	ea	132	63	264	114	<1	17	2	<1	<0.1	<0.1	<0.1
3005	Apple, rings, sulfured, dried	0.25	cup	21.5	52	218	7	<1	14	2	<1	<0.1	<0.1	<0.1
3388	Apple, slices, peeled, ckd f/fresh	0.5	cup	85.5	45	188	73	<1	12	2	<1	<0.1	<0.1	0.1
3147	Applesauce, swtnd, cnd	1	cup	246	167	699	202	<1	43	3	<1	0.1	<0.1	0.1
3006	Applesauce, unswtnd, cnd	0.5	cup	122	51	213	108	<1	14	1	<1	<0.1	<0.1	<0.1
3013	Apricot, halves, sulfured, dried	0.25	cup	32.5	78	326	10	1	20	2	<1	<0.1	<0.1	<0.1
3152	Apricot, halves, with skin and juice, cnd	0.5	cup	122	59	247	106	1	15	2	<1	<0.1	<0.1	<0.1
3157	Apricot, whole, fresh, USDA	1	ea	35	17	71	30	<1	4	1	<1	<0.1	0.1	<0.1
3016	Avocado, avg, fresh	0.25	ea	50.25	80	335	37	1	4	3	7	1.1	4.9	0.9
3307	Banana, chips	1	oz	28.35	147	615	1	1	17	2	10	8.2	0.6	0.2
3020	Banana, fresh, med, 7" to 7 ⅞" long	1	ea	118	105	439	88	1	27	3	<1	0.1	<0.1	0.1
3024	Blackberries, fresh	0.5	cup	72	31	130	63	1	7	4	<1	<0.1	<0.1	0.2
3028	Blackberries, unswtnd, fzn	0.5	cup	75.5	48	201	62	1	12	4	<1	<0.1	<0.1	0.2
3029	Blueberries, fresh	0.5	cup	74	42	176	62	1	11	2	<1	<0.1	<0.1	0.1
3232	Blueberries, swtnd, fzn, 10oz pkg	1	pkg	284	241	1008	220	1	62	6	<1	<0.1	0.1	0.2
3031	Blueberries, unswtnd, fzn, 20oz pkg	0.5	cup	77.5	40	167	67	<1	9	2	<1	<0.1	0.1	0.2
3663	Breadfruit, fresh	0.5	cup	110	113	473	78	1	30	5	<1	0.1	<0.1	0.1
3036	Cherries, sweet, fresh	0.5	cup	77	49	205	63	1	12	2	<1	<0.1	<0.1	<0.1
3158	Cherries, sweet, swtnd, fzn, thawed	0.5	cup	129.5	115	481	98	1	29	3	<1	<0.1	<0.1	0.1
3039	Cranberries, fresh, whole	0.5	cup	50	23	96	44	<1	6	2	<1	<0.1	<0.1	<0.1
3040	Cranberry Sauce, swtnd, cnd, ½" slice	1	slice	57	86	360	35	<1	22	1	<1	<0.1	<0.1	<0.1
3043	Date, Deglet Noor, pitted, chopped	0.25	cup	36.75	104	435	8	1	28	3	<1	<0.1	<0.1	<0.1
3044	Date, Deglet Noor, whole	1	ea	7.1	20	84	1	<1	5	1	<1	<0.1	<0.1	<0.1
3271	Feijoa, fresh	1	ea	42	23	96	36	<1	5	2	<1	0.1	<0.1	0.1
3162	Fig, dried	1	ea	8.4	21	88	3	<1	5	1	<1	<0.1	<0.1	<0.1
3160	Fig, fresh, med, 2¼"	1	ea	50	37	155	40	<1	10	1	<1	<0.1	<0.1	0.1
3045	Fruit Cocktail, cnd, with heavy syrup	0.5	cup	124	91	381	100	<1	23	1	<1	<0.1	<0.1	<0.1
3164	Fruit Cocktail, cnd, with juice	0.5	cup	118.5	55	230	104	1	14	1	<1	<0.1	<0.1	<0.1
3163	Fruit Cocktail, cnd, with light syrup	0.5	cup	121	69	289	102	<1	18	1	<1	<0.1	<0.1	<0.1
3313	Fruit Cocktail, cnd, with water	0.5	cup	118.5	38	159	108	<1	10	1	<1	<0.1	<0.1	<0.1
61363	Fruit Leather, summer strawberry	1	ea	14	45	188	<1	0	12	1	0	0	0	0

< = Trace amount present   Blank = Not available

V, vitamin; **THI**, thiamin; **RIB**, riboflavin; **NIA**, niacin; **FOL**, folate; **CALC**, calcium; **PHOS**, phosphorus; **SOD**, sodium; **POT**, potassium; **MAG**, magnesium

CHOL (mg)	V-A (IU)	THI (mg)	RIB (mg)	NIA (mg)	V-B_6 (mg)	FOL (µg)	V-B_{12} (µg)	V-C (mg)	V-E (mg)	CALC (mg)	PHOS (mg)	SOD (mg)	POT (mg)	MAG (mg)	IRON (mg)	ZINC (mg)
0	0	0	0	0	0	0	0	0	20.3	0	0	0	0	0	0	0
0	0	0	0	0	0	0	0	0	0.8	0	0	0	0	0	0	0
0	500							0	2.7	0		110			0	
	639	<0.1	0	0	0				5.2	1	1	94	1	<1	0	0
0	500							0				110			0	
0	500							0		0		90			0	
0	80	<0.1	<0.1	0.1	0.1	4	0	6.9	0.3	9	16	1	159	7	0.2	0.1
0	50	<0.1	<0.1	0.1	<0.1	0	0	5.3	0.1	7	15	0	119	5	0.1	0.1
0	0	0	<0.1	0.2	<0.1	0	0	0.8	0.1	3	8	19	97	3	0.3	<0.1
0	38	<0.1	<0.1	0.1	<0.1	1	0	0.2	<0.1	4	7	1	75	3	0.2	<0.1
0	15	<0.1	0.1	0.2	0.1	2	0	4.2	0.4	7	15	5	184	7	0.3	0.1
0	35	<0.1	<0.1	0.1	<0.1	4	0	1.2	0.2	5	6	2	90	4	0.3	<0.1
0	1171	<0.1	<0.1	0.8	<0.1	3	0	0.3	1.4	18	23	3	378	10	0.9	0.1
0	2063	<0.1	<0.1	0.4	0.1	2	0	6	0.7	15	24	5	201	12	0.4	0.1
0	674	<0.1	<0.1	0.2	<0.1	3	0	3.5	0.3	5	8	<1	91	4	0.1	0.1
0	73	<0.1	0.1	0.9	0.1	41	0	5	1	6	26	4	244	15	0.3	0.3
0	24	<0.1	<0.1	0.2	0.1	4	0	1.8	0.1	5	16	2	152	22	0.4	0.2
0	76	<0.1	0.1	0.8	0.4	24	0	10.3	0.1	6	26	1	422	32	0.3	0.2
0	154	<0.1	<0.1	0.5	<0.1	18	0	15.1	0.8	21	16	1	117	14	0.4	0.4
0	86	<0.1	<0.1	0.9	<0.1	26	0	2.3	0.9	22	23	1	106	17	0.6	0.2
0	40	<0.1	<0.1	0.3	<0.1	4	0	7.2	0.4	4	9	1	57	4	0.2	0.1
0	139	0.1	0.1	0.7	0.2	20	0	2.8	1.5	17	20	3	170	6	1.1	0.2
0	36	<0.1	<0.1	0.4	<0.1	5	0	1.9	0.4	6	9	1	42	4	0.1	0.1
0	0	0.1	<0.1	1	0.1	15	0	31.9	0.1	19	33	2	539	28	0.6	0.1
0	49	<0.1	<0.1	0.1	<0.1	3	0	5.4	0.1	10	16	0	171	8	0.3	0.1
0	245	<0.1	0.1	0.2	<0.1	5	0	1.3	0.1	16	21	1	258	13	0.5	0.1
0	30	<0.1	<0.1	0.1	<0.1	<1	0	6.6	0.6	4	6	1	42	3	0.1	<0.1
0	24	<0.1	<0.1	0.1	<0.1	1	0	1.1	0.5	2	3	17	15	2	0.1	<0.1
0	4	<0.1	<0.1	0.5	0.1	7	0	0.1	<0.1	14	23	1	241	16	0.4	0.1
0	1	<0.1	<0.1	0.1	<0.1	1	0	<1	<0.1	3	4	<1	47	3	0.1	<0.1
0	3	<0.1	<0.1	0.1	<0.1	10	0	13.8	0.1	7	8	1	72	4	0.1	<0.1
0	1	<0.1	<0.1	0.1	<0.1	1	0	0.1	<0.1	14	6	1	57	6	0.2	<0.1
0	71	<0.1	<0.1	0.2	0.1	3	0	1	0.1	18	7	<1	116	8	0.2	0.1
0	254	<0.1	<0.1	0.5	0.1	4	0	2.4	0.5	7	14	7	109	6	0.4	0.1
0	361	<0.1	<0.1	0.5	0.1	4	0	3.2	0.5	9	17	5	113	8	0.2	0.1
0	252	<0.1	<0.1	0.5	0.1	4	0	2.3	0.6	7	13	7	108	6	0.4	0.1
0	296	<0.1	<0.1	0.4	0.1	4	0	2.5	0.5	6	13	5	111	8	0.3	0.1
0	0							2.4		0		0	95		0	

ESHA, EatRight Analysis; **AMT**, amount; **WT**, weight; **CAL**, calories; **KILO**, KiloJoule; **WTR**, water; **PROT**, protein; **CARB**, carbohydrate; **FIBR**, fiber; **FAT**, fat; **SATF**, saturated fat; **MONO**, monounsaturated fat; **POLY**, polyunsaturated fat; **CHOL**, cholesterol;

ESHA CODE	FOOD DESCRIPTION	AMT	UNIT	WT (g)	CAL (kcal)	KILO (kJ)	WTR (g)	PROT (g)	CARB (g)	FIBR (g)	FAT (g)	SATF (g)	MONO (g)	POLY (g)
FRUITS (CONTINUED)														
3048	Grapefruit, pink, fresh, sections	0.5	cup	115	37	155	105	1	9	1	<1	<0.1	<0.1	<0.1
3047	Grapefruit, white, fresh, 3 ¾"	0.5	ea	118	39	163	107	1	10	1	<1	<0.1	<0.1	<0.1
71089	Grapes, concord, fresh	0.5	cup	46	31	130	37	<1	8	<1	<1	0.1	<0.1	<0.1
3056	Grapes, red European type varieties, fresh	0.5	cup	75.5	52	218	61	1	14	1	<1	<0.1	<0.1	<0.1
3055	Grapes, Thompson seedless, fresh	0.5	cup	75.5	52	218	61	1	14	1	<1	<0.1	<0.1	<0.1
3207	Guava, fresh, whole	1	ea	55	37	155	44	1	8	3	1	0.1	<0.1	0.2
3065	Kiwi, fresh, 2"	1	ea	69	42	176	57	1	10	2	<1	<0.1	<0.1	0.2
3066	Lemon, peeled, fresh, 2 ⅛"	1	ea	58	17	71	52	1	5	2	<1	<0.1	<0.1	0.1
3071	Limes, peeled, fresh, 2"	1	ea	67	20	84	59	<1	7	2	<1	<0.1	<0.1	<0.1
3257	Lychees, fresh	0.5	cup	95	63	264	78	1	16	1	<1	0.1	0.1	0.1
3221	Mango, fresh, whole	1	ea	336	202	845	280	3	50	5	1	0.3	0.5	0.2
3075	Melon, cantaloupe, fresh, cubes	0.5	cup	80	27	113	72	1	7	1	<1	<0.1	<0.1	0.1
3076	Melon, cantaloupe, fresh, med, 5"	0.25	ea	138	47	197	124	1	11	1	<1	0.1	<0.1	0.1
3079	Melon, casaba, fresh	1	ea	1640	459	1920	1506	18	108	15	2	0.4	<0.1	0.6
3078	Melon, casaba, fresh, cubes	0.5	cup	85	24	100	78	1	6	1	<1	<0.1	<0.1	<0.1
3080	Melon, honeydew, fresh, diced	0.5	cup	85	31	130	76	<1	8	1	<1	<0.1	<0.1	0.1
3081	Melon, honeydew, fresh, wedge, ⅛ of 6-7"	1	pce	160	58	243	144	1	15	1	<1	0.1	<0.1	0.1
3215	Nectarines, fresh, medium 2 ½"	1	ea	142	62	259	124	2	15	2	<1	<0.1	0.1	0.2
27010	Olives, black, cnd	1	Tbs	8.4	10	42	7	<1	1	<1	1	0.1	0.7	0.1
3082	Oranges, all types, fresh, med, 2 ⅝"	1	ea	131	62	259	114	1	15	3	<1	<0.1	<0.1	<0.1
3083	Oranges, all types, fresh, sections	0.5	cup	90	42	176	78	1	11	2	<1	<0.1	<0.1	<0.1
3720	Papaya, fresh	0.25	lrg	195.25	84	351	172	1	21	3	1	0.2	0.1	0.1
3098	Peaches, cnd, with heavy syrup	0.5	cup	131	97	406	104	1	26	2	<1	<0.1	<0.1	0.1
3174	Peaches, cnd, with light syrup, halves	0.5	cup	125.5	68	285	106	1	18	2	<1	<0.1	<0.1	<0.1
3096	Peaches, fresh, med, 2 ⅔"	1	ea	150	58	243	133	1	14	2	<1	<0.1	0.1	0.1
3107	Pears, cnd, with heavy syrup	0.5	cup	133	98	410	107	<1	25	2	<1	<0.1	<0.1	<0.1
3179	Pears, cnd, with juice, halves	0.5	cup	124	62	259	107	<1	16	2	<1	<0.1	<0.1	<0.1
3177	Pears, cnd, with light syrup, halves	0.5	cup	125.5	72	301	106	<1	19	2	<1	<0.1	<0.1	<0.1
3103	Pears, fresh	1	med	178	101	423	149	1	27	6	<1	<0.1	0.1	0.1
3183	Pineapple, crushed, cnd, with juice	0.5	cup	124.5	75	314	104	1	20	1	<1	<0.1	<0.1	<0.1
3181	Pineapple, crushed, cnd, with light syrup	0.5	cup	126	66	276	108	<1	17	1	<1	<0.1	<0.1	0.1
3113	Pineapple, fresh, slices, 3 ½" × ¾"	1	pce	84	42	176	72	<1	11	1	<1	<0.1	<0.1	<0.1
3115	Pineapple, slices, cnd, with heavy syrup	1	slice	49	38	159	39	<1	10	<1	<1	<0.1	<0.1	<0.1
3195	Plantain, fresh, slices	0.5	cup	74	90	377	48	1	24	2	<1	0.1	<0.1	0.1
24122	Plantain, yellow, fried, ¼" slices	0.5	cup	84.5	199	833	41	1	34	3	6	1.5	2	1.9
3121	Plums, fresh, 2 ⅛"	1	ea	66	30	126	58	<1	8	1	<1	<0.1	0.1	<0.1
3126	Prunes, dried	1	ea	9.5	23	96	3	<1	6	1	<1	<0.1	<0.1	<0.1
3129	Raisins, seedless, packed cup	0.25	cup	41.25	123	515	6	1	33	2	<1	<0.1	<0.1	<0.1
3130	Raisins, seedless, unpacked cup	0.25	cup	36.25	108	452	6	1	29	1	<1	<0.1	<0.1	<0.1
3648	Raspberries, fresh	0.5	cup	61.5	32	134	53	1	7	4	<1	<0.1	<0.1	0.2

< = Trace amount present   Blank = Not available

V, vitamin; **THI**, thiamin; **RIB**, riboflavin; **NIA**, niacin; **FOL**, folate; **CALC**, calcium; **PHOS**, phosphorus; **SOD**, sodium; **POT**, potassium; **MAG**, magnesium

CHOL (mg)	V-A (IU)	THI (mg)	RIB (mg)	NIA (mg)	V-B$_6$ (mg)	FOL (µg)	V-B$_{12}$ (µg)	V-C (mg)	V-E (mg)	CALC (mg)	PHOS (mg)	SOD (mg)	POT (mg)	MAG (mg)	IRON (mg)	ZINC (mg)
0	1066	<0.1	<0.1	0.3	<0.1	12	0	39.6	0.1	14	9	0	160	9	0.1	0.1
0	39	<0.1	<0.1	0.3	0.1	12	0	39.3	0.2	14	9	0	175	11	0.1	0.1
0	46	<0.1	<0.1	0.1	0.1	2	0	1.8	0.1	6	5	1	88	2	0.1	<0.1
0	50	0.1	0.1	0.1	0.1	2	0	2.4	0.1	8	15	2	144	5	0.3	0.1
0	50	0.1	0.1	0.1	0.1	2	0	2.4	0.1	8	15	2	144	5	0.3	0.1
0	343	<0.1	<0.1	0.6	0.1	27	0	125.6	0.4	10	22	1	229	12	0.1	0.1
0	60	<0.1	<0.1	0.2	<0.1	17	0	64	1	23	23	2	215	12	0.2	0.1
0	13	<0.1	<0.1	0.1	<0.1	6	0	30.7	0.1	15	9	1	80	5	0.3	<0.1
0	34	<0.1	<0.1	0.1	<0.1	5	0	19.5	0.1	22	12	1	68	4	0.4	0.1
0	0	<0.1	0.1	0.6	0.1	13	0	67.9	0.1	5	29	1	162	10	0.3	0.1
0	3636	0.1	0.1	2.2	0.4	144	0	122.3	3	37	47	3	564	34	0.5	0.3
0	2706	<0.1	<0.1	0.6	0.1	17	0	29.4	<0.1	7	12	13	214	10	0.2	0.1
0	4667	0.1	<0.1	1	0.1	29	0	50.6	0.1	12	21	22	368	17	0.3	0.2
0	0	0.2	0.5	3.8	2.7	131	0	357.5	0.8	180	82	148	2985	180	5.6	1.1
0	0	<0.1	<0.1	0.2	0.1	7	0	18.5	<0.1	9	4	8	155	9	0.3	0.1
0	42	<0.1	<0.1	0.4	0.1	16	0	15.3	<0.1	5	9	15	194	8	0.1	0.1
0	80	0.1	<0.1	0.7	0.1	30	0	28.8	<0.1	10	18	29	365	16	0.3	0.1
0	471	<0.1	<0.1	1.6	<0.1	7	0	7.7	1.1	9	37	0	285	13	0.4	0.2
0	34	<0.1	0	<0.1	<0.1	0	0	0.1	0.1	7	<1	62	1	<1	0.3	<0.1
0	295	0.1	0.1	0.4	0.1	39	0	69.7	0.2	52	18	0	237	13	0.1	0.1
0	202	0.1	<0.1	0.3	0.1	27	0	47.9	0.2	36	13	0	163	9	0.1	0.1
0	1855	<0.1	0.1	0.7	0.1	72	0	118.9	0.6	39	20	16	355	41	0.5	0.2
0	435	<0.1	<0.1	0.8	<0.1	4	0	3.7	0.6	4	14	8	121	7	0.4	0.1
0	444	<0.1	<0.1	0.7	<0.1	4	0	3	0.6	4	14	6	122	6	0.5	0.1
0	489	<0.1	<0.1	1.2	<0.1	6	0	9.9	1.1	9	30	0	285	14	0.4	0.3
0	0	<0.1	<0.1	0.3	<0.1	1	0	1.5	0.1	7	9	7	86	5	0.3	0.1
0	7	<0.1	<0.1	0.2	<0.1	1	0	2	0.1	11	15	5	119	9	0.4	0.1
0	0	<0.1	<0.1	0.2	<0.1	1	0	0.9	0.1	6	9	6	83	5	0.4	0.1
0	44	<0.1	<0.1	0.3	0.1	12	0	7.7	0.2	16	21	2	206	12	0.3	0.2
0	47	0.1	<0.1	0.4	0.1	6	0	11.8	<0.1	17	7	1	152	17	0.3	0.1
0	48	0.1	<0.1	0.4	0.1	6	0	9.4	<0.1	18	9	1	132	20	0.5	0.2
0	49	0.1	<0.1	0.4	0.1	15	0	40.2	<0.1	11	7	1	92	10	0.2	0.1
0	7	<0.1	<0.1	0.1	<0.1	2	0	3.6	<0.1	7	3	<1	51	8	0.2	0.1
0	834	<0.1	<0.1	0.5	0.2	16	0	13.6	0.1	2	25	3	369	27	0.4	0.1
	1114	0.1	<0.1	0.7	0.2				0.9	5	36	5	428	38	0.5	0.2
0	228	<0.1	<0.1	0.3	<0.1	3	0	6.3	0.2	4	11	0	104	5	0.1	0.1
0	74	<0.1	<0.1	0.2	<0.1	<1	0	0.1	<0.1	4	7	<1	70	4	0.1	<0.1
0	0	<0.1	0.1	0.3	0.1	2	0	0.9	<0.1	21	42	5	309	13	0.8	0.1
0	0	<0.1	<0.1	0.3	0.1	2	0	0.8	<0.1	18	37	4	272	12	0.7	0.1
0	20	<0.1	<0.1	0.4	<0.1	13	0	16.1	0.5	15	18	1	93	14	0.4	0.3

ESHA, EatRight Analysis; **AMT**, amount; **WT**, weight; **CAL**, calories; **KILO**, KiloJoule; **WTR**, water; **PROT**, protein; **CARB**, carbohydrate; **FIBR**, fiber; **FAT**, fat; **SATF**, saturated fat; **MONO**, monounsaturated fat; **POLY**, polyunsaturated fat; **CHOL**, cholesterol;

ESHA CODE	FOOD DESCRIPTION	AMT	UNIT	WT (g)	CAL (kcal)	KILO (kJ)	WTR (g)	PROT (g)	CARB (g)	FIBR (g)	FAT (g)	SATF (g)	MONO (g)	POLY (g)
FRUITS (CONTINUED)														
71120	Raspberries, red, swtnd, fzn, 10oz pkg	0.5	cup	125	129	540	91	1	33	6	<1	<0.1	<0.1	0.1
3133	Rhubarb, ckd f/fzn with sugar	0.5	cup	120	139	582	81	<1	37	2	<1	<0.1	<0.1	<0.1
3209	Rhubarb, fresh, diced	0.5	cup	61	13	54	57	1	3	1	<1	<0.1	<0.1	0.1
3664	Star Fruit, fresh, cubes	0.5	cup	66	20	84	60	1	4	2	<1	<0.1	<0.1	0.1
3240	Star Fruit, fresh, lrg, 4 ½" long	1	ea	124	38	159	113	1	8	3	<1	<0.1	<0.1	0.2
3136	Strawberries, fresh, med, 1 ¼"	1	ea	12	4	17	11	<1	1	<1	<1	<0.1	<0.1	<0.1
3135	Strawberries, fresh, sliced	0.5	cup	83	27	113	75	1	6	2	<1	<0.1	<0.1	0.1
3236	Strawberries, swtnd, fzn, thawed, slices	0.5	cup	127.5	122	510	93	1	33	2	<1	<0.1	<0.1	0.1
3089	Tangerines, cnd, with juice	0.5	cup	124.5	46	192	111	1	12	1	<1	<0.1	<0.1	<0.1
3138	Tangerines, fresh, med, 2 ½"	1	ea	88	47	197	75	1	12	2	<1	<0.1	0.1	0.1
3142	Watermelon, fresh, diced	0.5	cup	76	23	96	70	<1	6	<1	<1	<0.1	<0.1	<0.1
GRAIN PRODUCTS														
Bagels														
42100	Bagel, cinnamon raisin, 3 ½"	1	ea	105	288	1205	34	10	58	2	2	0.3	0.2	0.7
42041	Bagel, egg, 3 ½"	1	ea	105	292	1222	34	11	56	2	2	0.4	0.4	0.7
42103	Bagel, oat bran, 3 ½"	1	ea	105	268	1121	35	11	56	4	1	0.2	0.3	0.5
42000	Bagel, plain, enrich, with calc proprionate, 3 ½"	1	ea	105	270	1130	38	11	53	2	2	0.4	0.5	0.7
72307	Bagel, whole wheat, 100%	1	ea	95	260	1088	27	11	52	9	2	0.5		
Biscuits														
42110	Biscuit, buttermilk, low fat, prep f/refrig dough, 2 ¼"	1	ea	21	63	264	6	2	12	<1	1	0.3	0.6	0.2
42002	Biscuit, buttermilk, prep f/dry mix	1	ea	55	184	770	16	4	27	1	7	1.5	2.3	2.4
42001	Biscuit, buttermilk, prep f/recipe, 2 ½"	1	ea	60	212	887	17	4	27	1	10	2.6	4.2	2.5
26739	Biscuit, cheddar	1	ea	57	180	753		3	20	1	9	6		
42325	Biscuit, crumpet, whole wheat, INTL	1	ea	43	74	310	22	2	15	1	<1			
42111	Biscuit, mixed grain, refrig dough, 2 ½"	1	ea	44	116	485	17	3	21		2	0.6	1.3	0.4
Bread Crumbs and Stuffing														
42004	Bread Crumbs, plain, grated, dry	0.25	cup	27	107	448	2	4	19	1	1	0.3	0.3	0.6
42144	Bread Crumbs, seasoned, grated, dry	0.25	cup	30	115	481	2	4	21	1	2	0.4	0.4	0.7
42016	Croutons, plain, dry	0.25	cup	7.5	31	130	<1	1	6	<1	<1	0.1	0.2	0.1
42148	Croutons, seasoned, cubes	0.25	cup	10	46	192	<1	1	6	<1	2	0.5	0.9	0.2
42037	Stuffing, bread, prep f/dry mix	0.5	cup	100	177	741	65	3	22	3	9	1.7	3.8	2.6
42147	Stuffing, cornbread, prep f/dry mix, 6oz pkg	0.5	cup	100	179	749	65	3	22	3	9	1.8	3.9	2.7
Breads and Tortillas														
52431	Bread, banana	1	slice	55	200	837		3	27	1	10	3		
42039	Bread, banana, prep f/recipe with margarine, slice	1	slice	60	196	820	18	3	33	1	6	1.3	2.7	1.9
42052	Bread, Boston brown, cnd, slice	1	slice	45	88	368	21	2	19	2	1	0.1	0.1	0.3
42042	Bread, cracked wheat	1	slice	25	65	272	9	2	12	1	1	0.2	0.5	0.2
42090	Bread, egg, slice	1	slice	40	115	481	14	4	19	1	2	0.6	0.9	0.4

< = Trace amount present Blank = Not available

V, vitamin; **THI**, thiamin; **RIB**, riboflavin; **NIA**, niacin; **FOL**, folate; **CALC**, calcium; **PHOS**, phosphorus; **SOD**, sodium; **POT**, potassium; **MAG**, magnesium

CHOL (mg)	V-A (IU)	THI (mg)	RIB (mg)	NIA (mg)	$V\text{-}B_6$ (mg)	FOL (µg)	$V\text{-}B_{12}$ (µg)	V-C (mg)	V-E (mg)	CALC (mg)	PHOS (mg)	SOD (mg)	POT (mg)	MAG (mg)	IRON (mg)	ZINC (mg)
0	75	<0.1	0.1	0.3	<0.1	32	0	20.6	0.9	19	21	1	142	16	0.8	0.2
0	88	<0.1	<0.1	0.2	<0.1	6	0	4	0.2	174	10	1	115	14	0.3	0.1
0	62	<0.1	<0.1	0.2	<0.1	4	0	4.9	0.2	52	9	2	176	7	0.1	0.1
0	40	<0.1	<0.1	0.2	<0.1	8	0	22.7	0.1	2	8	1	88	7	0.1	0.1
0	76	<0.1	<0.1	0.5	<0.1	15	0	42.7	0.2	4	15	2	165	12	0.1	0.1
0	1	<0.1	<0.1	<0.1	<0.1	3	0	7.1	<0.1	2	3	<1	18	2	<0.1	<0.1
0	10	<0.1	<0.1	0.3	<0.1	20	0	48.8	0.2	13	20	1	127	11	0.3	0.1
0	31	<0.1	0.1	0.5	<0.1	19	0	52.8	0.3	14	17	4	125	9	0.8	0.1
0	1061	0.1	<0.1	0.6	0.1	6	0	42.6	0.1	14	12	6	166	14	0.3	0.6
0	599	0.1	<0.1	0.3	0.1	14	0	23.5	0.2	33	18	2	146	11	0.1	0.1
0	432	<0.1	<0.1	0.1	<0.1	2	0	6.2	<0.1	5	8	1	85	8	0.2	0.1
0	77	0.4	0.3	3.2	0.1	117	0	0.7	0.3	20	105	361	155	29	4	1.2
25	114	0.6	0.2	3.6	0.1	92	0.2	0.6		14	88	530	71	26	4.2	0.8
0	4	0.3	0.4	3.1	<0.1	103	0	0.2	0.3	13	116	620	121	33	3.2	0.9
0	0	0.6	0.3	4.2	0.1	152	0	1	0.1	93	91	501	79	23	6.4	2
0	0	0.2	0.1	4	0.3	32	<0.1	0		100	225	450	238	81	2.7	1.8
0	0	0.1	<0.1	0.7	<0.1	17	0	0	<0.1	4	98	214	39	4	0.6	0.1
2	52	0.2	0.2	1.7	<0.1	29	0.1	0.2		102	258	525	103	14	1.1	0.3
2	49	0.2	0.2	1.8	<0.1	37	<0.1	0.1		141	98	348	73	11	1.7	0.3
40												370				
	0	<0.1	0	0.6				0		31		372	49	12	0.7	0.2
0	0	0.2	0.1	1.5	<0.1	37	0	0		7	104	295	201	13	1.2	0.3
0	0	0.3	0.1	1.8	<0.1	29	0.1	0	<0.1	49	45	198	53	12	1.3	0.4
<1	58	0.3	0.1	1.8	0.1	36	0.1	0.8	0.1	55	53	401	69	14	1.5	0.4
0	0	<0.1	<0.1	0.4	<0.1	10	0	0		6	9	52	9	2	0.3	0.1
1	3	0.1	<0.1	0.5	<0.1	10	<0.1	0	<0.1	10	14	109	18	4	0.3	0.1
0	313	0.1	0.1	1.5	<0.1	39	<0.1	0	1.4	32	42	479	74	12	1.1	0.3
0	340	0.1	0.1	1.2	<0.1	97	<0.1	0.8	0.8	26	34	455	62	13	0.9	0.2
15	63	0.1	0.1	0.7	0.1	23	0.1	1.2		40	37	190	69	6	0.7	0.2
26	296	0.1	0.1	0.9	0.1	20	0.1	1		13	35	181	80	8	0.8	0.2
<1	39	<0.1	0.1	0.5	<0.1	5	<0.1	0	0.1	32	50	284	143	28	0.9	0.2
0	0	0.1	0.1	0.9	0.1	15	<0.1	0		11	38	134	44	13	0.7	0.3
20	84	0.2	0.2	1.9	<0.1	42	<0.1	0	0.1	37	42	152	46	8	1.2	0.3

ESHA, EatRight Analysis; **AMT**, amount; **WT**, weight; **CAL**, calories; **KILO**, KiloJoule; **WTR**, water; **PROT**, protein; **CARB**, carbohydrate; **FIBR**, fiber; **FAT**, fat; **SATF**, saturated fat; **MONO**, monounsaturated fat; **POLY**, polyunsaturated fat; **CHOL**, cholesterol;

ESHA CODE	FOOD DESCRIPTION	AMT	UNIT	WT (g)	CAL (kcal)	KILO (kJ)	WTR (g)	PROT (g)	CARB (g)	FIBR (g)	FAT (g)	SATF (g)	MONO (g)	POLY (g)
GRAIN PRODUCTS (CONTINUED)														
42091	Bread, egg, tstd, slice	1	slice	37	117	490	10	4	19	1	2	0.6	1.1	0.4
42043	Bread, French	1	slice	64	185	774	18	8	36	2	1	0.3	0.2	0.5
72411	Bread, Indian fry, made with lard, Navajo	1	ea	152	502	2100	48	10	73		19	7	6.7	1.6
71219	Bread, Italian	1	slice	20	54	226	7	2	10	1	1	0.2	0.2	0.3
42047	Bread, multigrain	1	slice	26	69	289	10	3	11	2	1	0.2	0.2	0.5
62746	Bread, multigrain, stay trim, low fat	1	slice	31	60	251		3	14	5	1	0		
42007	Bread, pita, white, enrich, lrg, 6 ½"	1	lrg	60	165	690	19	5	33	1	1	0.1	0.1	0.3
71227	Bread, pita, white, enrich, sml, 4"	1	sml	28	77	322	9	3	16	1	<1	<0.1	<0.1	0.1
42080	Bread, pita, whole wheat, lrg, 6 ½"	1	lrg	64	170	711	20	6	35	5	2	0.3	0.2	0.7
42006	Bread, pumpernickel	1	slice	26	65	272	10	2	12	2	1	0.1	0.2	0.3
42051	Bread, raisin, enrich	1	slice	26	71	297	9	2	14	1	1	0.3	0.6	0.2
42005	Bread, rye	1	slice	32	83	347	12	3	15	2	1	0.2	0.4	0.3
42045	Bread, sourdough	1	slice	64	185	774	18	8	36	2	1	0.3	0.2	0.5
42173	Bread, Spanish	1	pce	20	55	230	7	2	10	1	1	0.1	0.2	0.1
12485	Bread, sprouted, multigrain	1	slice	56	128	536	13	6	26	4	0	0	0	0
42190	Bread, sweet, pannetone, Italian style	1	pce	27	87	364	8	2	15	1	2	1.2	0.7	0.2
42136	Bread, wheat bran, slice	1	slice	36	89	372	14	3	17	1	1	0.3	0.6	0.2
42599	Bread, wheat germ, slice	1	slice	28	73	305	10	3	14	1	1	0.2	0.4	0.2
42095	Bread, wheat, rducd calorie, slice	1	slice	21	46	192	8	3	9	2	1	0.2	0.1	0.3
42012	Bread, wheat, slice	1	slice	29	78	326	10	3	14	1	1	0.2	0.2	0.5
42084	Bread, white, rducd calorie, slice	1	slice	23	48	201	10	2	10	2	1	0.1	0.2	0.1
71242	Bread, white, soft	1	slice	25	66	276	9	2	12	1	1	0.2	0.1	0.4
42014	Bread, whole wheat, slice	1	slice	28	69	289	11	4	12	2	1	0.2	0.4	0.2
42020	Bun, hamburger	1	ea	42	117	490	14	4	21	1	2	0.4	0.4	0.7
42021	Bun, hot dog, plain	1	ea	42	117	490	14	4	21	1	2	0.4	0.4	0.7
42717	Cornbread, deluxe, dry mix	1	dry svg	19.4	74	310	2	1	14	<1	2	0.4		
49012	Cornbread, hush puppies, prep f/recipe	1	ea	22	74	310	6	2	10	1	3	0.5	0.7	1.6
42115	Cornbread, prep f/dry mix	1	pce	60	198	828	16	4	33	1	6	2.2	2.1	1.2
42116	Cornbread, prep f/recipe with 2% milk	1	pce	65	173	724	25	4	28	2	5	1	1.2	2.1
42015	Croissant, butter	1	med	57	231	967	13	5	26	1	12	6.6	3.1	0.6
42070	Roll, dinner, oat bran	1	ea	33	78	326	15	3	13	1	2	0.2	0.5	0.5
42157	Roll, dinner, sml, 2" × 2"	1	ea	25	78	326	7	3	13	<1	2	0.3	0.5	0.6
42160	Roll, dinner, wheat	1	ea	28	76	318	10	2	13	1	2	0.4	0.9	0.3
42057	Roll, dinner, whole wheat	1	ea	28	74	310	9	2	14	2	1	0.2	0.3	0.6
16617	Roll, garlic, fzn dough	1	ea	38	140	586		3	17	1	6	1.5		
42022	Roll, hard, 3 ½"	1	ea	57	167	699	18	6	30	1	2	0.3	0.6	1
42381	Roll, hoagie, soft	1	ea	69	200	837		7	33	2	5	1.5		
42185	Roll, Mexican, bolillo	1	ea	117	307	1284	43	10	61	2	2	0.5	0.2	0.6
42168	Taco Shells, bkd, med, 5"	1	ea	13.3	63	264	1	1	9	1	3	0.8	0.8	0.9
42023	Tortilla, corn, rtb	1	ea	24	52	218	11	1	11	2	1	0.1	0.2	0.3

< = Trace amount present   Blank = Not available

V, vitamin; **THI**, thiamin; **RIB**, riboflavin; **NIA**, niacin; **FOL**, folate; **CALC**, calcium; **PHOS**, phosphorus; **SOD**, sodium; **POT**, potassium; **MAG**, magnesium

CHOL (mg)	V-A (IU)	THI (mg)	RIB (mg)	NIA (mg)	V-B_6 (mg)	FOL (µg)	V-B_{12} (µg)	V-C (mg)	V-E (mg)	CALC (mg)	PHOS (mg)	SOD (mg)	POT (mg)	MAG (mg)	IRON (mg)	ZINC (mg)
21	85	0.1	0.2	1.8	<0.1	36	<0.1	0	0.1	38	43	154	47	8	1.2	0.3
0	0	0.3	0.2	3	0.1	95	0	0.1	0.1	28	73	328	82	18	2.3	0.6
11		0.7	0.3	7	0.1	185	0		0	87	187	500	117	27	6.1	0.5
0	0	0.1	0.1	0.9	<0.1	38	0	0	0.1	16	21	123	22	5	0.6	0.2
0	0	0.1	<0.1	1.1	0.1	20	0	<1	0.1	27	59	99	60	20	0.6	0.4
0	0	0.2	0.2	2	0.2	40	0.9	0		60		90		40	1.1	2.2
0	0	0.4	0.2	2.8	<0.1	64	0	0	0.2	52	58	322	72	16	1.6	0.5
0	0	0.2	0.1	1.3	<0.1	30	0	0	0.1	24	27	150	34	7	0.7	0.2
0	0	0.2	0.1	1.8	0.2	22	0	0	0.4	10	115	284	109	44	2	1
0	0	0.1	0.1	0.8	<0.1	24	0	0	0.1	18	46	155	54	14	0.7	0.4
0	0	0.1	0.1	0.9	<0.1	28	0	<1	0.1	17	28	90	59	7	0.8	0.2
0	2	0.1	0.1	1.2	<0.1	35	0	0.1	0.1	23	40	193	53	13	0.9	0.4
0	0	0.3	0.2	3	0.1	95	0	0.1	0.1	28	73	328	82	18	2.3	0.6
0	0	0.1	0.1	0.9	<0.1	6	0	0	<0.1	9	21	122	23	5	0.5	0.2
0	0							0		20		3			1.8	
19	88	0.1	0.1	1	<0.1	19	0.1	0.3	0.1	16	40	28	54	5	0.8	0.2
0	0	0.1	0.1	1.6	0.1	38	0	0	0.1	27	67	175	82	29	1.1	0.5
0	1	0.1	0.1	1.3	<0.1	33	<0.1	0.1	0.1	25	34	155	71	8	1	0.3
0	<1	0.1	<0.1	0.8	<0.1	19	0	<1	0.1	34	31	70	32	9	0.6	0.3
0	1	0.1	0.1	1.7	<0.1	25	0	0.1	0.1	40	44	151	53	13	1	0.3
0	1	0.1	0.1	0.8	<0.1	22	0.1	0.1	<0.1	22	28	110	17	5	0.7	0.3
0	<1	0.1	0.1	1.2	<0.1	28	0	0	0.1	65	26	123	29	6	0.9	0.2
0	1	0.1	0.1	1.3	0.1	14	0	0	0.2	30	57	112	69	23	0.7	0.5
0	<1	0.3	0.1	2	<0.1	47	0.1	0.5	<0.1	73	45	210	53	10	1.4	0.4
0	<1	0.3	0.1	2	<0.1	47	0.1	0.5	<0.1	73	45	210	53	10	1.4	0.4
2	2					16		<1		48		296			0.7	
10	41	0.1	0.1	0.6	<0.1	20	<0.1	<1	0.3	61	42	147	32	5	0.7	0.1
34	100	0.1	0.1	1.2	0.1	33	0.1		0.3	80	234	359	80	10	1.1	0.4
26	180	0.2	0.2	1.5	0.1	50	0.1	0.2		162	110	428	96	16	1.6	0.4
38	424	0.2	0.1	1.2	<0.1	50	0.1	0.1	0.5	21	60	266	67	9	1.2	0.4
0	0	0.1	0.1	1.6	<0.1	31	0	0	0.2	28	38	136	40	11	1.4	0.3
1	1	0.1	0.1	1.3	<0.1	25	<0.1	<1	0.1	44	30	117	35	6	0.9	0.2
0	0	0.1	0.1	1.1	<0.1	17	0	0	0.1	49	29	147	32	10	1	0.3
0	0	0.1	<0.1	1	0.1	8	0	0	0.3	30	63	146	76	24	0.7	0.6
0	0							0		0		220			1.1	
0	0	0.3	0.2	2.4	<0.1	54	0	0	0.2	54	57	310	62	15	1.9	0.5
0	0	0.2	0.1	2		40		0		80		320			1.4	
1	15	0.7	0.5	6.6	<0.1	41	<0.1	<1	0.1	14	90	7	98	22	3.8	0.8
0	2	<0.1	<0.1	0.2	<0.1	9	0	0	0.1	13	31	32	31	11	0.2	0.2
0	<1	<0.1	<0.1	0.4	0.1	1	0	0	0.1	19	75	11	45	17	0.3	0.3

ESHA, EatRight Analysis; **AMT**, amount; **WT**, weight; **CAL**, calories; **KILO**, KiloJoule; **WTR**, water; **PROT**, protein; **CARB**, carbohydrate; **FIBR**, fiber; **FAT**, fat; **SATF**, saturated fat; **MONO**, monounsaturated fat; **POLY**, polyunsaturated fat; **CHOL**, cholesterol;

ESHA CODE	FOOD DESCRIPTION	AMT	UNIT	WT (g)	CAL (kcal)	KILO (kJ)	WTR (g)	PROT (g)	CARB (g)	FIBR (g)	FAT (g)	SATF (g)	MONO (g)	POLY (g)
GRAIN PRODUCTS (CONTINUED)														
42025	Tortilla, flour, rtb, 10"	1	ea	72	217	908	23	6	37	2	5	1.2	2.5	1
71938	Tortilla, whole wheat	1	ea	47	140	586		4	22	2	3	0		
Cereals - Hot														
40006	Cereal, hot, farina, enrich, ckd with water w/o salt	1	cup	233	123	515	202	4	25	2	1	0.2	0.1	0.3
40016	Cereal, hot, multigrain, plain, ckd with water w/o salt	1	cup	241	147	615	199	7	33	8	1	0.1		
40083	Cereal, hot, multigrain, plain, dry	0.33	cup	31	100	418	3	4	22	6	1	0.1	0.1	0.3
40431	Cereal, hot, oat bran, dry	0.5	cup	40	146	611	4	7	25	6	3	0.6	1	1.2
40167	Cereal, hot, oatmeal, maple and brown sugar, inst	1	indv pkt	43	157	657	3	4	32	3	2	0.4	0.8	0.7
40239	Cereal, hot, oatmeal, maple, ckd with water and salt	1	cup	240	170	711	198	6	32	5	2	0.4	0.6	0.5
40015	Cereal, hot, oatmeal, maple, ckd with water w/o salt	1	cup	240	170	711	198	6	32	6	2	0.4	0.7	0.9
40072	Cereal, hot, oatmeal, plain, fort, inst, prep with water	1	cup	234	159	665	197	6	27	4	3	0.5	0.9	1
38008	Cereal, hot, oatmeal, quick, unenrich, dry	0.5	cup	40.5	153	640	4	5	27	4	3	0.4	0.8	0.9
40000	Cereal, hot, oatmeal, quick, unenrich, prep with water w/o salt	1	cup	234	166	695	196	6	28	4	4	0.7	1	1.3
40078	Cereal, hot, rice, ckd with water w/o salt	1	cup	244	127	531	214	2	28	<1	<1	0.1	0.1	0.1
40088	Cereal, hot, wheat, ckd with water w/o salt	1	cup	253	134	561	218	6	28	6	1	0.1	0.1	0.4
40080	Cereal, hot, wheat, tstd, ckd with water	1	cup	243	136	569	208	5	29	7	1	0.2	0.2	0.6
40191	Cereal, hot, wheat, tstd, ckd with water and salt	1	cup	243	143	598	208	5	29	5	1	0.2	0.2	0.6
40002	Cereal, hot, whole wheat, natural, ckd with water w/o salt	1	cup	242	150	628	202	5	33	4	1	0.1	0.1	0.5
40093	Grits, corn, white, quick, enrich, ckd with water w/o salt	0.5	cup	128.5	91	381	107	2	19	1	1	0.1	0.1	0.2
40094	Grits, corn, white, reg, unenrich, ckd with water w/o salt	0.5	cup	121	71	297	103	2	16	<1	<1	<0.1	0.1	0.1
40178	Grits, corn, yellow, reg, unenrich, ckd with water and salt	0.5	cup	121	71	297	103	2	16	<1	<1	<0.1	0.1	0.1
Cereals — Ready to Eat														
61644	Cereal, 7 whole grain flakes	1	cup	50	175	732	2	6	41	6	1	0.2	0.2	0.6
60959	Cereal, 7 whole grain, puffed	1	cup	19	64	268	1	2	15	2	<1	0.1	0.1	0.2
12430	Cereal, 8 Grain Synergy, flakes	0.75	cup	30	100	418		3	24	5	1	0		
40029	Cereal, All-Bran Buds	0.33	cup	30	75	314	1	2	24	13	1	0.1	0.2	0.4
61198	Cereal, Alpha-Bits	1	cup	28	108	452	<1	2	23	2	1	0.3	0.3	0.4
61702	Cereal, Apple Zings	1	cup	33	130	544	1	2	29	1	1	0.1	0.4	0.3
61388	Cereal, Autumn Wheat	1	cup	54	183	766	3	6	43	6	1	0.2	0.1	0.5
14903	Cereal, bran flakes, enriched, USDA	0.75	cup	29	90	377	1	3	23	5	1	0.1	0.1	0.4

< = Trace amount present   Blank = Not available

V, vitamin; **THI**, thiamin; **RIB**, riboflavin; **NIA**, niacin; **FOL**, folate; **CALC**, calcium; **PHOS**, phosphorus; **SOD**, sodium; **POT**, potassium; **MAG**, magnesium

CHOL (mg)	V-A (IU)	THI (mg)	RIB (mg)	NIA (mg)	V-B_6 (mg)	FOL (µg)	V-B_{12} (µg)	V-C (mg)	V-E (mg)	CALC (mg)	PHOS (mg)	SOD (mg)	POT (mg)	MAG (mg)	IRON (mg)	ZINC (mg)
0	0	0.4	0.1	2.6	<0.1	89	0	0	0.1	76	137	494	110	14	2.4	0.4
0	0							0		0		170			1.1	
0	0	0.3	0.2	3.5	0.2	179	0	0	0.1	226	86	42	54	16	12.4	0.5
0	0	0.2	0.1	3.1	0.1	24	0	0		29	214	2	301	108	2.1	1.8
0	0	0.2	0.1	2.1	0.1	22	0	0		20	146	2	205	73	1.4	1.2
0	40	0.4	0.1	0.3	<0.1	15	0	0		32	278	2	232	96	3.2	1.7
0	1000	0	<0.1	0.3	<0.1	6	0	0	0.2	106	148	258	123	44	3.9	0.8
0	2335	0.7	0.8	9.4	0.9	12	2.8	28.3	0.2	130	247	259	211	53	8.4	1.5
0	2338	0.7	0.7	9.4	1	10	2.9	28.8	0.2	125	247	10	211	50	8.4	1.5
0	1013	0.6	0.5	7.1	0.7	103	0	0	0.2	187	180	115	143	61	13.9	1.5
0	0	0.2	0.1	0.5	<0.1	13	0	0	0.2	21	166	2	147	56	1.7	1.5
0	0	0.2	<0.1	0.5	<0.1	14	0	0	0.2	21	180	9	164	63	2.1	2.3
0	0	0	0	1	0.1	7	0	0	<0.1	7	41	2	49	7	0.5	0.4
0	0	0.2	0.2	2	0.1	18	0.1	0		13	147	5	154	58	1.6	1.4
0	0	<0.1	<0.1	1.3	<0.1	17	0	0		194	146	5	187	49	1.4	1.7
0	7	<0.1	0.1	1.3	<0.1	22	0	0	1.3	194	146	578	187	51	1.4	1.7
0	0	0.2	0.1	2.2	0.2	34	0	0	0.6	17	167	0	172	53	1.5	1.2
0	0	0.1	0.1	1	0.1	36	0	0	<0.1	1	26	3	35	9	0.7	0.2
0	1	<0.1	<0.1	0.2	<0.1	1	0	0	<0.1	4	13	2	25	6	0.2	0.1
0	38	<0.1	<0.1	0.2	<0.1	1	0	0	<0.1	4	13	270	25	6	0.2	0.1
0	0							0		15	142	152	160	50	1.5	1.2
0	1	<0.1	<0.1	0.6	0.1	5	0	0	0.2	7	46	2	53	29	0.6	0.6
0	0							0		20		0			2.7	
0	510	0.4	0.4	5.1	2	404	6	6	0.2	19	150	203	300	62	4.5	1.5
0	751	0.4	0.4	5	0.5	100	1.5	5.9	0.1	8	70	178	61	22	1.8	1.5
<1	921	0.4	0.7	6.6	0.9	116	2.1	19.7	0.1	142	41	150	46	12	5.6	4.8
0	0	0.2	0.1	2.8	0.2	19	0	0	0.5	0	122	2	185	44	1.7	0.8
	514	1.4	2.1	26.3	2			69.5	23.3	13	155	236	183	55	19.6	18.7

ESHA, EatRight Analysis; **AMT**, amount; **WT**, weight; **CAL**, calories; **KILO**, KiloJoule; **WTR**, water; **PROT**, protein; **CARB**, carbohydrate; **FIBR**, fiber; **FAT**, fat; **SATF**, saturated fat; **MONO**, monounsaturated fat; **POLY**, polyunsaturated fat; **CHOL**, cholesterol;

ESHA CODE	FOOD DESCRIPTION	AMT	UNIT	WT (g)	CAL (kcal)	KILO (kJ)	WTR (g)	PROT (g)	CARB (g)	FIBR (g)	FAT (g)	SATF (g)	MONO (g)	POLY (g)
GRAIN PRODUCTS (CONTINUED)														
40032	Cereal, Cap'n Crunch	0.75	cup	27	107	448	1	1	23	1	1	0.9	0.2	0.2
40033	Cereal, Cap'n Crunch, crunchberries	0.75	cup	26	103	431	1	1	22	1	1	0.8	0.2	0.2
40034	Cereal, Cap'n Crunch, peanut butter	0.75	cup	27	113	473	1	2	21	1	2	1.1	0.7	0.6
40297	Cereal, Cheerios	1	cup	28	104	435	1	3	21	3	2	0.4	0.7	0.7
40051	Cereal, Cheerios, honey nut	0.75	cup	28	105	439	1	2	22	2	1	0.3	0.5	0.5
40333	Cereal, Chex, rice	1	cup	27	101	423	1	2	23	1	<1	0.1	0.1	0.1
40335	Cereal, Chex, wheat	0.75	cup	47	162	678	1	5	39	6	1	0.2	0.1	0.5
60927	Cereal, Cinnamon Oat Crunch	1	cup	60	228	954	2	6	48	5	3	0.5	0.9	0.8
60929	Cereal, Cocoa Bumpers	1	cup	33	124	519	1	2	29	1	1	0.1	0.1	0.2
12440	Cereal, corn flakes, Honey'd	0.75	cup	30	120	502	<1	2	26	2	<1	0		
40205	Cereal, Cracklin' Oat Bran	0.75	cup	49	197	824	1	4	35	6	7	3	2.3	1.5
40017	Cereal, crispy rice	1	cup	28	102	427	1	2	24	<1	<1	0.1	0.1	0.1
40217	Cereal, Frosted Flakes	0.75	cup	31.5	116	485	1	1	28	1	1	0.1	0.1	0.2
40043	Cereal, Frosted Mini Wheats, Big Bite	5	ea	51	176	736	2	5	43	6	1	0.2	0.1	0.5
61261	Cereal, frosted oat, with marshmallows	0.75	cup	30	116	485	1	2	25	1	1	0.2	0.3	0.4
61546	Cereal, Fruit and Bran, dates raisins and walnuts	1	cup	55	200	837	3	4	42	6	3	0		
61204	Cereal, Fruity Pebbles	0.75	cup	30	120	502	1	1	26	<1	1	1.1	<0.1	<0.1
61213	Cereal, Golden Crisp	0.75	cup	27	105	439	<1	2	24	1	<1	0.1	0.1	0.1
61688	Cereal, Golden Puffs	0.75	cup	27	107	448	1	2	24	1	<1	<0.1	0.1	0.1
60961	Cereal, Good Friends	1	cup	53	158	661	2	5	42	12	2	0.3	0.3	0.6
61310	Cereal, granola, oat bran, crunchy with almond and raisin	0.5	cup	50	210	879		6	31	5	8	1		
40063	Cereal, granola, oats and honey	0.5	cup	51	215	900	1	5	38	5	6	0.6	3.5	1.4
38361	Cereal, granola, w/o raisins, low fat	0.5	cup	49	191	799	2	4	40	3	3	0.7	1.2	0.8
40197	Cereal, granola, with raisins, low fat	0.66	cup	60	226	946	2	5	48	4	3	0.8	1.1	0.9
61208	Cereal, Grape-Nuts, flakes	0.75	cup	29	107	448	1	3	24	3	1	0.1	0.4	0.4
60928	Cereal, Groovy Graham Bumpers	0.75	cup	28	104	435	1	2	24	1	<1	0.1	0.1	0.2
61526	Cereal, Honey Nut O's	1	cup	30	120	502	<1	3	24	2	2	0	0.5	0.5
60960	Cereal, Honey Puffs, 7 whole grain	1	cup	30	105	439	1	3	24	2	1	0.1	0.2	0.3
40068	Cereal, Honey Smacks	0.75	cup	27	103	431	1	2	24	1	1	0.1	0.1	0.1
40055	Cereal, hot, pilaf, 7 whole grain, ckd	0.5	cup	140	170	711		6	30	6	3	0		
61340	Cereal, Just Flakes, oats	0.75	cup	28	100	418		4	19	3	2	0		
40054	Cereal, King Vitamin	1.5	cup	31	118	494	1	2	26	1	1	0.5	0.2	0.3
40010	Cereal, Kix	1.25	cup	30	107	448	1	2	25	3	1	0.2	0.3	0.4
40011	Cereal, Life, plain	0.75	cup	32	120	502	1	3	25	2	1	0.3	0.5	0.5
40300	Cereal, Lucky Charms	0.75	cup	27	103	431	1	2	22	1	1	0.2	0.4	0.4
40451	Cereal, maple buckwheat flakes	1	cup	43	170	711		4	35	1	1	0	0.5	0.5
40418	Cereal, Mueslix, with raisins dates and almonds	0.67	cup	55	196	820	5	5	40	5	3	0.3	1.4	0.7
12432	Cereal, multigrain flakes, with oat bran	0.75	cup	30	110	460	<1	4	24	5	1	0		

< = Trace amount present Blank = Not available

V, vitamin; **THI**, thiamin; **RIB**, riboflavin; **NIA**, niacin; **FOL**, folate; **CALC**, calcium; **PHOS**, phosphorus; **SOD**, sodium; **POT**, potassium; **MAG**, magnesium

CHOL (mg)	V-A (IU)	THI (mg)	RIB (mg)	NIA (mg)	V-B_6 (mg)	FOL (µg)	V-B_{12} (µg)	V-C (mg)	V-E (mg)	CALC (mg)	PHOS (mg)	SOD (mg)	POT (mg)	MAG (mg)	IRON (mg)	ZINC (mg)
0	40	0.4	0.5	5.8	0.6	420	0	0	0.2	3	45	204	50	15	5.2	4.4
0	39	0.4	0.5	5.7	0.6	400	0	<1	0.2	3	44	188	49	14	5.2	4.3
0	40	0.4	0.5	5.5	0.6	420	0	0	0.2	2	52	200	64	19	5	4.1
0	924	0.4	0.4	5.9	0.7	200	1.9	6	0.2	112	135	161	179	36	9.3	4.7
0	500	0.4	0.4	5	0.5	200	1.5	6	0.1	100	80	152	114	24	4.5	3.8
0	500	0.4	0.4	5	0.5	200	1.5	6	0.3	100	40	242	44	8	9	3.8
0	500	0.4	0.4	5	0.5	400	1.5	6	0.3	100	150	268	173	40	14.4	5.3
0	5	0.2	0.2	1.4	0.1	22	0	0.1		44	215	251	322	64	2.2	1.5
0	54	<0.1	0.2	0.4	<0.1	4	0	0		46	55	156	260	20	1.7	0.4
0	100							0		0		170			0.4	
0	750	0.4	0.4	5	0.5	100	1.5	15.2	0.3	29	195	151	220	76	1.8	1.5
0	657	0.6	0.8	8.1	0.5	170	1.5	18.1	<0.1	1	27	214	31	6	9.2	0.4
0	509	0.6	0.5	8.7	1.1	120	2.6	7.6	<0.1	1	15	147	24	3	8.4	<0.1
0	0	0.3	0.4	4.4	0.4	88	1.3	0	0.3	17	188	1	185	44	14.3	1.4
0	1323	0.4	0.4	5.3	0.5	106	1.6	15.9	0.2	21	42	160	62	8	4.8	2.4
0	750							0		20		260			5.4	
0	750	0.4	0.4	5	0.5	100	1.5	6	<0.1	5	20	189	20	4	1.8	1.5
0	750	0.4	0.4	5	0.5	100	1.5	0	<0.1	4	47	25	48	22	1.8	1.5
0	1086	0.5	0.6	6.8	0.6	200	1.8	7.5	0.1	3	38	65	42	12	2.1	2
0	67	0.1	0.1	2.1	0.1	23	0	0	0.4	14	125	108	194	10	2.2	1.4
0	100							1.2		20		0			1.4	
1	4	0.2	0.1	1.2	0.1	19	0.1	0.1	0.7	56	200	26	246	62	1.4	1.2
0	750	0.4	0.4	5	2	400	6	2.9	1.2	16	112	126	105	33	1.8	3.8
0	653	0.5	0.5	5.4	2	433	5.9	1.2	1.4	19	132	144	118	38	2.5	5.2
0	750	0.4	0.4	5	0.5	200	1.5	0	0.2	12	81	125	99	30	8.1	2.3
0	41	<0.1	0.2	0.4	<0.1	4	0	0		39	45	230	211	16	1.4	0.3
0	500	0.4		5	0.5	100		6		100	80	250	70	24	4.5	3.8
0	0	<0.1	<0.1	0.8	0.1	8	0	0	0.3	13	79	2	67	34	0.8	0.8
0	500	0.4	0.4	5	0.5	100	1.5	5.9	0.1	6	58	38	49	16	0.4	0.5
0	0							0		20		15			1.4	
0	0							0		20		190	80		1.1	
0	1039	0.4	0.4	5.2	0.5	414	1.6	12.4	1.4	3	78	256	83	25	9	3.9
0	923	0.6	0.6	7.3	0.7	236	1.7	7.6	0.1	171	57	179	67	15	9.6	5.2
0	13	0.5	0.7	5	0.5	268	0	0	0.2	112	135	160	91	31	9.4	3.7
0	762	0.5	0.5	6.8	0.8	200	1.8	7.2	0.1	117	78	175	60	20	6	5
0	0	0.2	<0.1	1.6				6		20		190	100		0.7	
0	300	0.4	0.4	5.5	2	406	6	0.2	4	32	100	139	171	49	4.5	3.7
0	0							0		20		115			0.9	

ESHA, EatRight Analysis; **AMT**, amount; **WT**, weight; **CAL**, calories; **KILO**, KiloJoule; **WTR**, water; **PROT**, protein; **CARB**, carbohydrate; **FIBR**, fiber; **FAT**, fat; **SATF**, saturated fat; **MONO**, monounsaturated fat; **POLY**, polyunsaturated fat; **CHOL**, cholesterol;

ESHA CODE	FOOD DESCRIPTION	AMT	UNIT	WT (g)	CAL (kcal)	KILO (kJ)	WTR (g)	PROT (g)	CARB (g)	FIBR (g)	FAT (g)	SATF (g)	MONO (g)	POLY (g)
GRAIN PRODUCTS (CONTINUED)														
61168	Cereal, oat bran flakes	1	cup	50	190	795	2	5	39	4	2	0.5	0.4	0.4
61645	Cereal, Organic Promise, Cinnamon Harvest	28	ea	55	185	774	3	6	43	6	1	0.1	0.1	0.6
40066	Cereal, Quisp	1	cup	27	110	460	1	1	23	1	2	1.2	0.2	0.2
61212	Cereal, Raisin Bran	1	cup	59	189	791	5	5	46	8	1	0.2	0.2	0.5
61530	Cereal, raisin bran	1	cup	55	180	753	2	5	43	6	2			
61689	Cereal, raisin bran	1	cup	59	213	891	5	5	45	8	1	0.3	0.2	0.6
40393	Cereal, Raisin Nut Bran	0.75	cup	49	180	753	2	3	39	5	3	0.5	1.2	0.9
61681	Cereal, rice crisps, USDA	1	cup	28	107	448	1	2	24	<1	<1	0.1	0.1	0.1
40018	Cereal, rice, puffed	0.75	cup	14	54	226	1	1	12	<1	<1	<0.1	<0.1	<0.1
61558	Cereal, Shredded Wheat, biscuits	2	ea	47	160	669	2	5	37	6	1	0		
61218	Cereal, Shredded Wheat, spoon size	1	cup	49	172	720	1	6	40	6	1	0.2	0.1	0.6
40062	Cereal, shredded wheat, w/o sug and salt, rectangle biscuits	2	ea	46	155	649	3	5	36	6	1	0.2	0.2	0.6
40070	Cereal, Tasteeos	1	cup	30	119	498	1	4	22	3	2	0.3	0.5	0.6
60926	Cereal, Toasted Oat Bran	0.75	cup	32	119	498	1	4	24	3	2	0.3	0.5	0.6
17712	Cereal, Total, cranberry crunch	1.25	cup	58	190	795	2	4	45	4	1	0.2	0.2	0.5
40021	Cereal, Total, wheat	0.75	cup	30	96	402	1	3	22	3	1	0.2	0.1	0.2
40128	Cereal, Uncle Sam, original	0.75	cup	55	190	795	2	9	36	11	6	0.7	1.1	4.6
38026	Cereal, wheat germ, tstd	0.25	cup	28.25	108	452	2	8	14	4	3	0.5	0.4	1.9
40023	Cereal, wheat, puffed	1	cup	15	55	230	1	2	11	1	<1	0.1	<0.1	0.2
40242	Cereal, wheat, puffed, fort	1	cup	12	44	184	<1	2	10	1	<1	<0.1		
Crackers														
71273	Cracker, cheese, 1" square	15	ea	15	73	305	1	2	9	<1	3	0.8	0.9	1.5
43771	Cracker, cheese, Better Cheddars	22	ea	30	150	628	<1	3	18	1	8	2		
11759	Cracker, cheese, hot and spicy	25	ea	30	150	628	<1	2	18	1	8	2		
43527	Cracker, graham, chocolate coated, 2½" square	1	ea	14	68	285	<1	1	9	<1	3	1.8	1.1	0.1
43502	Cracker, graham, plain, 2½" square	1	ea	14	59	247	1	1	11	<1	1	0.2	0.6	0.5
43534	Cracker, matzoh, plain	1	ea	28	111	464	1	3	23	1	<1	0.1	<0.1	0.2
43509	Cracker, melba toast, plain, pce, 3¾" × 1¾" × ⅛"	3	ea	15	58	243	1	2	11	1	<1	0.1	0.1	0.2
43507	Cracker, oyster	15	ea	15	63	264	1	1	11	<1	1	0.3	0.3	0.6
43505	Cracker, oyster, crushed	0.25	cup	17.5	74	310	1	2	13	1	2	0.4	0.4	0.7
43532	Cracker, rye, crispbread	2	ea	20	73	305	1	2	16	3	<1	<0.1	<0.1	0.1
43506	Cracker, saltine	5	ea	15	63	264	1	1	11	<1	1	0.3	0.3	0.6
43586	Cracker, saltine, Premium, unsalted tops	5	ea	15	70	293	<1	1	11	0	2	0		
43818	Cracker, saltine, whole wheat, Zesta	5	ea	15	60	251		1	11	<1	2	0.5	0.5	0
43501	Cracker, sandwich, cheese, with peanut butter fill	2	ea	13	64	268	<1	2	7	<1	3	0.6	1.7	0.7
43541	Cracker, sandwich, rye, with cheese fill	2	ea	14	67	280	1	1	9	1	3	0.8	1.7	0.4
43548	Cracker, sandwich, wheat, with cheese fill	2	ea	14	70	293	<1	1	8	<1	4	0.6	1.4	1.3

< = Trace amount present Blank = Not available

V, vitamin; **THI**, thiamin; **RIB**, riboflavin; **NIA**, niacin; **FOL**, folate; **CALC**, calcium; **PHOS**, phosphorus; **SOD**, sodium; **POT**, potassium; **MAG**, magnesium

CHOL (mg)	V-A (IU)	THI (mg)	RIB (mg)	NIA (mg)	V-B_6 (mg)	FOL (µg)	V-B_{12} (µg)	V-C (mg)	V-E (mg)	CALC (mg)	PHOS (mg)	SOD (mg)	POT (mg)	MAG (mg)	IRON (mg)	ZINC (mg)
0	0	0.4	0.4	5	0.5	100	1.5	60	0.3	40	172	190	170	72	1.4	1.1
0	0							0		0		2	174		1.5	
0	40	0.4	0.5	5.5	0.5	420	0	0	0.2	2	45	200	50	15	5	4.1
0	750	0.4	0.4	5	0.5	200	1.5	0.5	0.3	31	234	250	318	97	10.8	2.2
0	500	0.4	0.1	5	0.5	100		0		20		340	270		4.5	3.8
1	743	0.6	0.8	13.9	0.9	200	1.9	7.7	0.4	27	239	340	341	84	5.8	6.5
0	0	0.4	0.4	5	0.5	100	1.5	0	0.8	20	100	226	172	40	4.5	3.8
	568	0.6	0.7	7.3	0.8			12.9	<0.1	1	27	238	30	7	2.9	0.3
0	0	0.1	<0.1	0.5	0	22	0	0	<0.1	1	17	1	16	4	0.4	0.2
0	0							0		20		0			1.1	
0	0	0.1	<0.1	2.8	0.1	20	0	0	0.3	28	188	1	190	65	1.2	1.5
0	0	0.1	0.1	2.4	0.5	20	0	4.6	0	23	170	3	173	61	1.4	1.4
0	513	0.5	0.6	7.2	0.7	200	1.6	4.5	0.1	107	157	204	92	37	9	4.3
	23	0.1	0.1	0.6	<0.1	13	0	0		21	147	202	157	46	1.3	1
0	500	1.5	1.7	20	2	400	6	0	13.5	1000	100	190	140	32	18	15
0	500	1.5	1.7	20	2	400	6	60	13.5	1000	80	141	92	24	18	15
0	0	0.4	0.1	2.6	0.5	29	0	1.3	0.5	52	206	113	245	113	2.2	2.1
0	29	0.5	0.2	1.6	0.3	99	0	1.7	4.5	13	324	1	268	90	2.6	4.7
0	2	0.1	0.1	0.8	<0.1	23	0.1	0	0	4	50	1	55	20	0.7	0.5
0	0	0.3	0.2	4.2	<0.1	4	0	0		3	43	<1	42	17	3.8	0.3
<1	23	0.1	0.1	0.9	<0.1	23	0.1	0	0.3	20	30	146	23	4	0.7	0.2
3	0							0		20		360			1.1	
0	100							0		0		280			1.4	
0	2	<0.1	<0.1	0.3	<0.1	3	0	0	<0.1	8	19	42	29	8	0.5	0.1
0	<1	<0.1	<0.1	0.6	<0.1	6	0	0	<0.1	3	15	67	19	4	0.5	0.1
0	0	0.1	0.1	1.1	<0.1	5	0	0	<0.1	4	25	0	31	7	0.9	0.2
0	0	0.1	<0.1	0.6	<0.1	19	0	0	0.1	14	29	90	30	9	0.6	0.3
0	<1	0.1	<0.1	0.8	<0.1	21	<0.1	0	0.2	3	17	153	24	4	0.8	0.1
0	<1	0.1	0.1	0.9	<0.1	24	<0.1	0	0.2	4	19	179	28	4	0.9	0.1
0	0	<0.1	<0.1	0.2	<0.1	9	0	0	0.2	6	54	82	64	16	0.5	0.5
0	<1	0.1	<0.1	0.8	<0.1	21	<0.1	0	0.2	3	17	153	24	4	0.8	0.1
0	0							0		0		115			0.7	
0	0							0		0		230			0.4	
0	<1	0.1	<0.1	0.8	<0.1	12	<0.1	0	0.3	6	35	108	28	7	0.4	0.1
1	47	0.1	0.1	0.5	<0.1	11	<0.1	0.1		31	47	146	48	5	0.3	0.1
1	10	0.1	0.1	0.4	<0.1	9	<0.1	0.2		29	53	117	43	8	0.4	0.1

ESHA, EatRight Analysis; **AMT**, amount; **WT**, weight; **CAL**, calories; **KILO**, KiloJoule; **WTR**, water; **PROT**, protein; **CARB**, carbohydrate; **FIBR**, fiber; **FAT**, fat; **SATF**, saturated fat; **MONO**, monounsaturated fat; **POLY**, polyunsaturated fat; **CHOL**, cholesterol;

ESHA CODE	FOOD DESCRIPTION	AMT	UNIT	WT (g)	CAL (kcal)	KILO (kJ)	WTR (g)	PROT (g)	CARB (g)	FIBR (g)	FAT (g)	SATF (g)	MONO (g)	POLY (g)
GRAIN PRODUCTS (CONTINUED)														
43549	Cracker, sandwich, wheat, with peanut butter fill	1	ea	7	35	146	<1	1	4	<1	2	0.3	0.8	0.6
139	Cracker, standard, snack, rectangle	4	ea	16	81	339	1	1	10	<1	4	0.9	1.1	2
43543	Cracker, standard, snack, round	5	ea	16	81	339	1	1	10	<1	4	0.9	1.1	2
72335	Cracker, stoned wheat, low fat	5	ea	14	60	251	<1	2	10	1	1	0		
43547	Cracker, wheat, reg	5	ea	10	46	192	<1	1	7	<1	2	0.3	0.4	0.9
12683	Cracker, wheat, Town House	5	ea	16	80	335	<1	1	10	<1	4	1	2	1
43747	Cracker, wheat, Wheat Thins, low sodium	16	ea	31	150	628	<1	3	21	1	6	1		
43508	Cracker, whole wheat	6	ea	27.6	118	494	1	3	19	3	4	0.6	0.9	1.9
Muffins														
42214	English Muffin, cheese	1	ea	63	153	640	26	5	28	2	2	0.8	0.5	0.6
42059	English Muffin, plain, with calc proprionate	1	ea	57	129	540	25	5	25	2	1	0.4	0.2	0.3
42060	English Muffin, sourdough, with calc proprionate	1	ea	57	129	540	25	5	25	2	1	0.4	0.2	0.3
42082	English Muffin, whole wheat	1	ea	66	134	561	30	6	27	4	1	0.2	0.3	0.6
44520	Muffin, blueberry, prep f/recipe with 2% milk	1	ea	57	162	678	23	4	23	1	6	1.2	1.5	3.1
44518	Muffin, blueberry, toaster	1	ea	33	103	431	10	2	18	1	3	0.5	0.7	1.8
11785	Muffin, chocolate chocolate chip, dry mix	0.25	cup	33	150	628		2	23	2	5	2		
44524	Muffin, corn, prep f/recipe with 2% milk, 2" × 2¾"	1	ea	57	180	753	19	4	25	2	7	1.3	1.7	3.5
44522	Muffin, cornmeal, toaster	1	ea	33	114	477	8	2	19	1	4	0.6	0.9	2.1
15486	Muffin, oat bran	1	sml	66	178	745	23	5	32	3	5	0.7	1.1	2.7
44515	Muffin, plain, prep f/recipe with 2% milk	1	ea	57	169	707	21	4	24	2	6	1.2	1.6	3.3
18098	Muffin, whole grain, Fiber One, mixed fruit nuts and honey	1	ea	65	170	711		3	34	7	4	1		
Pancakes and Cones														
49013	Cone, ice cream, cake type	1	ea	4	17	71	<1	<1	3	<1	<1	<0.1	0.1	0.1
49014	Cone, ice cream, sugar, rolled type	1	ea	10	40	167	<1	1	8	<1	<1	0.1	0.1	0.1
45194	Crepe	1	ea	12.8	30	126		1	5	0	<1	0		
42156	French Toast, prep f/recipe with 2% milk	1	pce	65	149	623	36	5	16		7	1.8	2.9	1.7
45023	Pancakes, blueberry, prep f/recipe, 4"	1	ea	38	84	351	20	2	11	<1	3	0.8	0.9	1.6
45025	Pancakes, buttermilk, prep f/recipe, 4"	1	ea	38	86	360	20	3	11	<1	4	0.7	0.9	1.7
45044	Pancakes, flour and water patty, also Chinese style	5	ea	112	232	971	56	5	51	1	<1	0.1	0.1	0.1
45002	Pancakes, plain, prep f/complete dry mix, 4"	1	ea	38	74	310	20	2	14	<1	1	0.2	0.3	0.3
45001	Pancakes, plain, prep f/recipe, 4"	1	ea	38	86	360	20	2	11	<1	4	0.8	0.9	1.7
45067	Pancakes, plain, rth, fzn, 6"	1	ea	73	170	711	35	4	28	1	5	0.8	1.1	2.8
45036	Pancakes, rye	5	ea	105	316	1322	36	7	48	3	11	2.4	4.6	3.2
45035	Pancakes, sourdough	5	ea	105	231	967	55	6	36	1	7	1.3	2	2.9
45008	Pancakes, whole wheat, prep f/incomplete dry mix, 4"	1	ea	44	92	385	23	4	13	1	3	0.8	0.8	1.1

< = Trace amount present   Blank = Not available

V, vitamin; **THI**, thiamin; **RIB**, riboflavin; **NIA**, niacin; **FOL**, folate; **CALC**, calcium; **PHOS**, phosphorus; **SOD**, sodium; **POT**, potassium; **MAG**, magnesium

CHOL (mg)	V-A (IU)	THI (mg)	RIB (mg)	NIA (mg)	V-B_6 (mg)	FOL (µg)	V-B_{12} (µg)	V-C (mg)	V-E (mg)	CALC (mg)	PHOS (mg)	SOD (mg)	POT (mg)	MAG (mg)	IRON (mg)	ZINC (mg)
0	0	<0.1	<0.1	0.4	<0.1	5	0	0		12	24	56	21	3	0.2	0.1
0	0	0.1	<0.1	0.7	<0.1	19	0	0	0.6	15	41	120	18	3	0.6	0.1
0	0	0.1	<0.1	0.7	<0.1	19	0	0	0.6	15	41	120	18	3	0.6	0.1
0	0							0		20		140			0.4	
0	0	0.1	<0.1	0.5	<0.1	12	<0.1	0	0.1	8	26	79	21	5	0.5	0.2
0	0							0		0		140			0.4	
0	0							0		0		80			1.1	
0	0	0.1	<0.1	1.3	0.1	8	0	0	0.4	10	91	194	95	30	0.9	0.7
3	33	0.3	0.2	2.3	<0.1	23	<0.1	0.1	0.1	127	96	297	82	13	1.5	0.5
0	0	0.3	0.1	2.3	<0.1	54	<0.1	1	0.2	93	52	206	62	14	2.3	0.6
0	0	0.3	0.1	2.3	<0.1	54	<0.1	1	0.2	93	52	206	62	14	2.3	0.6
0	3	0.2	0.1	2.3	0.1	32	0	0	0.3	175	186	240	139	47	1.6	1.1
21	80	0.2	0.2	1.3	<0.1	27	0.1	0.9		108	83	251	70	9	1.3	0.3
2	105	0.1	0.1	0.7	<0.1	21	<0.1	0	0.3	4	19	138	27	4	0.2	0.1
0	0							0		20		200			1.4	
24	137	0.2	0.2	1.4	0.1	43	0.1	0.2		148	101	333	83	13	1.5	0.3
4	32	0.1	0.1	0.8	<0.1	19	<0.1	0		6	50	142	30	5	0.5	0.1
0	0	0.2	0.1	0.3	0.1	59	<0.1	0	0.4	42	248	259	335	104	2.8	1.2
22	80	0.2	0.2	1.3	<0.1	29	0.1	0.2		114	87	266	69	10	1.4	0.3
30	0							1.2		20		190			1.1	
0	0	<0.1	<0.1	0.2	<0.1	7	0	0	<0.1	1	4	10	4	1	0.1	<0.1
0	0	0.1	<0.1	0.5	<0.1	14	0	0	<0.1	4	10	30	14	3	0.4	0.1
5	0							0		0		50			0	
75	327	0.1	0.2	1.1	<0.1	28	0.2	0.2		65	76	311	87	11	1.1	0.4
21	76	0.1	0.1	0.6	<0.1	14	0.1	0.8		78	57	157	52	6	0.7	0.2
22	40	0.1	0.1	0.6	<0.1	14	0.1	0.2		60	53	198	55	6	0.6	0.2
0	0	<0.1	<0.1	1	0.1	5	0	0	0.1	19	73	5	73	16	0.5	0.7
5	12	0.1	0.1	0.7	<0.1	14	0.1	0.1		48	127	239	66	8	0.6	0.1
22	74	0.1	0.1	0.6	<0.1	14	0.1	0.1		83	60	167	50	6	0.7	0.2
13	1103	0.5	0.3	4.6	0.4	52	2	0.2	0.5	57	157	337	66	10	4.1	0.3
39	71	0.2	0.2	1.7	0.2	11	0.2	0.4	1.6	108	123	291	484	77	2.6	0.9
42	62	0.3	0.3	2.8	<0.1	34	0.1	<1	1.6	14	81	263	85	13	2.4	0.5
27	99	0.1	0.2	1	<0.1	13	0.1	0.2		110	164	252	123	20	1.4	0.5

ESHA, EatRight Analysis; **AMT**, amount; **WT**, weight; **CAL**, calories; **KILO**, KiloJoule; **WTR**, water; **PROT**, protein; **CARB**, carbohydrate; **FIBR**, fiber; **FAT**, fat; **SATF**, saturated fat; **MONO**, monounsaturated fat; **POLY**, polyunsaturated fat; **CHOL**, cholesterol;

ESHA CODE	FOOD DESCRIPTION	AMT	UNIT	WT (g)	CAL (kcal)	KILO (kJ)	WTR (g)	PROT (g)	CARB (g)	FIBR (g)	FAT (g)	SATF (g)	MONO (g)	POLY (g)
GRAIN PRODUCTS (CONTINUED)														
45094	Waffles, blueberry, fzn	2	ea	70	190	795	20	4	30	1	6	1.5		
45093	Waffles, buttermilk, fzn	1	ea	35	90	377	11	2	13	<1	3	0.8		
45003	Waffles, plain, prep f/recipe, round, 7"	1	ea	75	218	912	32	6	25	1	11	2.1	2.6	5.1
45005	Waffles, plain, tstd f/fzn, 4"	2	ea	66	206	862	20	5	33	2	6	1.1	3.2	1.5
45083	Waffles, whole grain, fzn	2	ea	71	154	644	21	6	29	3	3	0.9	1.1	0.6
Pastas														
38048	Chow Mein Noodles, dry	0.5	cup	28	129	540	<1	3	19	1	5	0.5	1.5	3
38076	Couscous, ckd	1	cup	157	176	736	114	6	36	2	<1	<0.1	<0.1	0.1
38092	Pasta, ckd f/fresh	3	oz	85.5	112	469	59	4	21	1	1	0.1	0.1	0.4
38047	Pasta, egg, enrich, ckd	1	cup	160	221	925	108	7	40	2	3	0.7	0.9	0.9
38260	Pasta, egg, unenrich, ckd	1	cup	160	221	925	108	7	40	2	3	0.7	0.9	0.9
38102	Pasta, macaroni, enrich, ckd	1	cup	140	221	925	87	8	43	3	1	0.2	0.2	0.4
38551	Pasta, rice, ckd	1	cup	176	192	803	130	2	44	2	<1	<0.1	<0.1	<0.1
38105	Pasta, shells, sml, enrich, ckd	1	cup	115	182	761	71	7	35	2	1	0.2	0.2	0.4
38118	Pasta, spaghetti, enrich, ckd	1	cup	140	221	925	87	8	43	3	1	0.2	0.2	0.4
38121	Pasta, spaghetti, enrich, ckd with salt	1	cup	140	220	920	87	8	43	3	1	0.2	0.2	0.4
38066	Pasta, spaghetti, spinach, ckd	1	cup	140	182	761	95	6	37	6	1	0.1	0.1	0.4
38060	Pasta, spaghetti, whole wheat, ckd	1	cup	140	174	728	94	7	37	6	1	0.1	0.1	0.3
38163	Rice and Pasta, mix, ckd	0.5	cup	101	123	515	72	3	22	3	3	0.5	1.1	1
38067	Soup, ramen noodles, ckd	1	cup	227	154	644	195	3	20	1	7	1.7	1.2	3.3
Snack Foods														
44029	Chips, corn cones, plain, extruded	1	oz	28.35	145	607	1	2	18	<1	8	6.4	0.5	0.2
44006	Chips, potato, plain, 8oz bag	1	oz	28.35	154	644	1	2	14	1	10	1.1	4.5	4.5
44043	Chips, potato, rducd fat, 6 oz bag	1	oz	28.35	134	561	<1	2	19	2	6	1.2	1.4	3.1
61056	Chips, sweet potato, spiced	1	oz	28.35	140	586		1	16	3	7	1		
61250	Chips, tortilla, low fat, bkd	1	svg	28	116	485	<1	3	22	1	2	0.2	0.5	0.8
44054	Chips, tortilla, nacho flvr, rducd fat, 6oz bag	1	oz	28.35	126	527	<1	2	20	1	4	0.8	2.5	0.6
44266	Chips, tortilla, original, bite size, bkd	20	ea	28	110	460		3	24	2	1	0		
44031	Corn Nuts, original	0.33	cup	28.33	126	527	<1	2	20	2	4	0.7	2.7	0.9
44012	Popcorn, air popped	1	cup	8	31	130	<1	1	6	1	<1	<0.1	0.1	0.2
44014	Popcorn, caramel coated, with opeanuts	1	oz	28.35	122	510	1	1	22	1	4	1	0.8	1.3
44037	Popcorn, caramel coated, with peanuts	1	cup	42.5	170	711	1	3	34	2	3	0.4	1.2	1.4
44038	Popcorn, cheese flvrd	1	cup	11	58	243	<1	1	6	1	4	0.7	1.1	1.7
44013	Popcorn, oil popped, microwaved	1	cup	11	64	268	<1	1	5	1	5	0.8	1.1	2.6
44039	Pork Skins, bbq flvr	1	oz	28.35	153	640	1	16	<1		9	3.3	4.3	1
44015	Pretzels, hard	5	ea	30	114	477	1	3	24	1	1	0.1	0.3	0.3
44312	Rice Cake, caramel corn, mini, Quakers	7	ea	15	60	251		1	13	0	0	0	0	0
44016	Rice Cake, plain	1	ea	9	35	146	<1	1	7	<1	<1	0.1	0.1	0.1
44028	Rice Cake, plain, salt free	1	ea	9	35	146		1	7	0	0	0	0	0
44032	Snack, mix, Chex	1	cup	47	199	833	1	4	35	2	5	0.7	1.4	2.1

< = Trace amount present Blank = Not available

V, vitamin; **THI**, thiamin; **RIB**, riboflavin; **NIA**, niacin; **FOL**, folate; **CALC**, calcium; **PHOS**, phosphorus; **SOD**, sodium; **POT**, potassium; **MAG**, magnesium

CHOL (mg)	V-A (IU)	THI (mg)	RIB (mg)	NIA (mg)	V-B$_6$ (mg)	FOL (µg)	V-B$_{12}$ (µg)	V-C (mg)	V-E (mg)	CALC (mg)	PHOS (mg)	SOD (mg)	POT (mg)	MAG (mg)	IRON (mg)	ZINC (mg)
15	1000	0.3	0.3	4	0.4	40	1.2	0		100	200	370	55		3.6	
8	500	0.2	0.2	2	0.2	20	0.6	0		50	100	210	30		1.8	
52	171	0.2	0.3	1.6	<0.1	34	0.2	0.3		191	142	383	119	14	1.7	0.5
10	878	0.3	0.5	5.9	0.7	50	1.9	0	0.6	203	283	482	95	16	4.6	0.3
5	0							0		221	406	676	176	34	5.8	0.6
0	0	0.2	0.1	1.7	<0.1	31	0	0	0.7	6	45	237	34	15	1.3	0.4
0	0	0.1	<0.1	1.5	0.1	24	0	0	0.2	13	35	8	91	13	0.6	0.4
28	17	0.2	0.1	0.8	<0.1	55	0.1	0		5	54	5	21	15	1	0.5
46	34	0.5	0.2	3.3	0.1	134	0.1	0	0.3	19	122	8	61	34	2.4	1
46	34	<0.1	<0.1	0.6	0.1	11	0.1	0	0.3	19	122	8	61	34	1	1
0	0	0.4	0.2	2.4	0.1	102	0	0	0.1	10	81	1	62	25	1.8	0.7
0	0	<0.1	<0.1	0.1	<0.1	5	0	0		7	35	33	7	5	0.2	0.4
0	0	0.3	0.2	1.9	0.1	84	0	0	0.1	8	67	1	51	21	1.5	0.6
0	0	0.4	0.2	2.4	0.1	102	0	0	0.1	10	81	1	62	25	1.8	0.7
0	0	0.4	0.2	2.4	0.1	102	0	0	0.1	10	81	183	62	25	1.8	0.7
0	213	0.1	0.1	2.1	0.1	17	0	0		42	151	20	81	87	1.5	1.5
0	4	0.2	0.1	1	0.1	7	0	0	0.4	21	125	4	62	42	1.5	1.1
1	0	0.1	0.1	1.8	0.1	44	0.1	0.2		8	37	574	42	12	0.9	0.3
<1	8	<0.1	<0.1	0.3	<0.1	3	<0.1	<1	2.3	13	24	802	49	10	0.4	0.2
0	90	0.1	0.1	0.4	<0.1	1	0	0		1	12	290	23	3	0.7	0.1
0	0	<0.1	0.1	1.2	0.2	21	0	5.3	1.9	7	44	136	466	20	0.5	0.7
0	0	0.1	0.1	2	0.2	8	0	7.3	1.6	6	55	139	494	25	0.4	<0.1
0	4000							4.8		60		105			1.1	
0	29	0.1	0.1	0.1	0.1	4	0	0.1	0.2	45	89	117	76	27	0.4	0.3
1	108	0.1	0.1	0.1	0.1	7	0	0.1		45	90	284	77	27	0.5	
0	0	0.1			0.1			0		40	60	200			0.4	
0	0	<0.1	<0.1	0.5	0.1	0	0	0	0.6	3	78	160	79	32	0.5	0.5
0	16	<0.1	<0.1	0.2	<0.1	2	0	0	<0.1	1	29	1	26	12	0.3	0.2
1	2	<0.1	<0.1	0.6	<0.1	1	<0.1	0	0.3	12	24	58	31	10	0.5	0.2
0	33	<0.1	0.1	0.8	0.1	7	0	0	0.4	28	54	125	151	34	1.7	0.5
1	27	<0.1	<0.1	0.2	<0.1	1	0.1	0.1		12	40	98	29	10	0.2	0.2
0	17	<0.1	<0.1	0.1	<0.1	3	0	<1	0.3	<1	22	116	20	9	0.2	0.3
33	189	<0.1	0.1	1	<0.1	9	<0.1	0.4		12	62	756	51	0	0.3	0.2
0	0	0.2	0.1	1.5	<0.1	56	0	0	0.1	5	34	380	41	9	1.6	0.4
0	0							0		0		150			0	
0	0	<0.1	<0.1	0.6	<0.1	2	0	0	<0.1	1	33	14	25	14	0.1	2
0	0							0		0		0			0	
	0	0.2	0.1	2	<0.1	24				16	72	348	92	19	1.4	0.5

ESHA, EatRight Analysis; **AMT**, amount; **WT**, weight; **CAL**, calories; **KILO**, KiloJoule; **WTR**, water; **PROT**, protein; **CARB**, carbohydrate; **FIBR**, fiber; **FAT**, fat; **SATF**, saturated fat; **MONO**, monounsaturated fat; **POLY**, polyunsaturated fat; **CHOL**, cholesterol;

ESHA CODE	FOOD DESCRIPTION	AMT	UNIT	WT (g)	CAL (kcal)	KILO (kJ)	WTR (g)	PROT (g)	CARB (g)	FIBR (g)	FAT (g)	SATF (g)	MONO (g)	POLY (g)
GRAIN PRODUCTS (CONTINUED)														
44033	Snack, pretzel, Combos, with cheddar cheese	0.33	cup	28.35	131	548	<1	3	19		5	2.8		
44058	Trail Mix, regular	0.25	cup	37.5	173	724	3	5	17		11	2.1	4.7	3.6
44085	Trail Mix, regular, unsalted	0.25	cup	37.5	173	724	3	5	17		11	2.1	4.7	3.6
44060	Trail Mix, tropical	0.25	cup	35	155	649	3	2	23		6	3	0.9	1.8
GRAINS AND FLOURS														
40123	Amaranth, flakes	1	cup	38	134	561	1	6	27	4	3	0.5	0.8	1
38003	Barley, pearled, ckd	0.5	cup	78.5	97	406	54	2	22	3	<1	0.1	<0.1	0.2
38078	Bran, oat, ckd	0.5	cup	109.5	44	184	92	4	13	3	1	0.2	0.3	0.4
38064	Bran, oat, dry	1	Tbs	5.88	14	59	<1	1	4	1	<1	0.1	0.1	0.2
38024	Bran, wheat, crude	1	Tbs	3.63	8	33	<1	1	2	2	<1	<0.1	<0.1	0.1
38004	Cornmeal, yellow, degerminated, enrich	0.25	cup	39.25	145	607	4	3	31	2	1	0.1	0.1	0.2
38030	Flour, all purpose, white, bleached, enrich	0.25	cup	31.25	114	477	4	3	24	1	<1	<0.1	<0.1	0.1
38548	Flour, barley	0.25	cup	37	128	536	4	4	28	4	1	0.1	0.1	0.3
38277	Flour, bread, white, enrich	0.25	cup	34.25	124	519	5	4	25	1	1	0.1	<0.1	0.2
38053	Flour, buckwheat, whole groat	0.25	cup	30	100	418	3	4	21	3	1	0.2	0.3	0.3
46086	Flour, cake, white, enrich, unsifted	0.25	cup	34.25	124	519	4	3	27	1	<1	<0.1	<0.1	0.1
38023	Flour, rye, light	0.25	cup	25.5	91	381	3	3	20	2	<1	<0.1	<0.1	0.1
38438	Flour, white, unbleached, enriched	0.25	cup	34	120	502	1	5	26	1	<1	0		
38032	Flour, whole wheat	0.25	cup	30	102	427	3	4	22	3	1	0.1	0.1	0.4
38052	Millet, ckd	0.5	cup	87	104	435	62	3	21	1	1	0.1	0.2	0.4
38080	Oats, unprocessed whole grain	0.25	cup	39	152	636	3	7	26	4	3	0.5	0.8	1
38010	Rice, brown, long grain, ckd	0.5	cup	97.5	108	452	71	3	22	2	1	0.2	0.3	0.3
38082	Rice, brown, med grain, ckd	0.5	cup	97.5	109	456	71	2	23	2	1	0.2	0.3	0.3
38083	Rice, white, glutinous, ckd	0.5	cup	87	84	351	67	2	18	1	<1	<0.1	0.1	0.1
38013	Rice, white, long grain, ckd	0.5	cup	79	103	431	54	2	22	<1	<1	0.1	0.1	0.1
38019	Rice, white, long grain, enrich, prep f/inst	0.5	cup	82.5	97	406	59	2	21	<1	<1	<0.1	0.1	<0.1
38097	Rice, white, med grain, ckd	0.5	cup	93	121	506	64	2	27	<1	<1	0.1	0.1	0.1
38021	Rice, wild, ckd	0.5	cup	82	83	347	61	3	17	1	<1	<0.1	<0.1	0.2
38028	Wheat, bulgur, ckd	0.5	cup	91	76	318	71	3	17	4	<1	<0.1	<0.1	0.1
38055	Wheat, germ, honey crunch, Kretschmer	2	Tbs	16.8	62	259	1	4	10	2	1	0.2	0.2	0.8
INFANT FOODS														
60616	Infant Cereal, rice, with mixed fruit, jr	6	oz jar	170	139	582	137	2	31	1	<1	0.1	0.1	0.1
60491	Infant Dinner, beef stew, toddler	6	oz jar	170	87	364	148	9	9	2	2	1	0.7	0.2
62893	Infant Dinner, vegetable beef, jr	6	oz jar	170	131	548	144	4	15	2	6	2.3	2.2	0.5
60638	Infant Meat, turkey, sticks, jr	2.5	oz jar	71	133	556	50	10	1	<1	10	2.9	3.3	2.6
60500	Infant Vegetable, carrot, jr	6	oz jar	170	54	226	155	1	12	3	<1	0.1	<0.1	0.2
60632	Infant Vegetable, sweet potato, jr	6	oz jar	170	102	427	143	2	24	3	<1	<0.1	<0.1	0.1
MEATS AND SUBSTITUTES														
Beef and Veal														
10268	Beef, average of all cuts, lean, ckd, 0" trim	3	oz	85.05	179	749	50	25	0	0	8	3	3.3	0.3

< = Trace amount present   Blank = Not available

V, vitamin; **THI**, thiamin; **RIB**, riboflavin; **NIA**, niacin; **FOL**, folate; **CALC**, calcium; **PHOS**, phosphorus; **SOD**, sodium; **POT**, potassium; **MAG**, magnesium

CHOL (mg)	V-A (IU)	THI (mg)	RIB (mg)	NIA (mg)	V-B_6 (mg)	FOL (µg)	V-B_{12} (µg)	V-C (mg)	V-E (mg)	CALC (mg)	PHOS (mg)	SOD (mg)	POT (mg)	MAG (mg)	IRON (mg)	ZINC (mg)
<1	19	0.1	0.2	0.9	<0.1	2	<0.1	0.1		51	41	440	37	6	0.3	0.2
0	7	0.2	0.1	1.8	0.1	27	0	0.5		29	129	86	257	59	1.1	1.2
0	7	0.2	0.1	1.8	0.1	27	0	0.5		29	129	4	257	59	1.1	1.2
0	17	0.2	<0.1	0.5	0.1	15	0	2.7		20	65	33	248	34	0.9	0.4
0	0	<0.1	<0.1	1	<0.1	4	0	1	0.5	6	126	13	134	10	0.7	0.1
0	5	0.1	<0.1	1.6	0.1	13	0	0	<0.1	9	42	2	73	17	1	0.6
0	0	0.2	<0.1	0.2	<0.1	7	0	0		11	130	1	101	44	1	0.6
0	0	0.1	<0.1	0.1	<0.1	3	0	0	0.1	3	43	<1	33	14	0.3	0.2
0	<1	<0.1	<0.1	0.5	<0.1	3	0	0	0.1	3	37	<1	43	22	0.4	0.3
0	84	0.2	0.1	1.9	0.1	82	0	0	<0.1	1	39	3	56	13	1.7	0.3
0	0	0.2	0.2	1.8	<0.1	57	0	0	<0.1	5	34	1	33	7	1.4	0.2
0	0	0.1	<0.1	2.3	0.1	3	0	0	0.2	12	110	1	114	36	1	0.7
0	1	0.3	0.2	2.6	<0.1	63	0	0	0.1	5	33	1	34	9	1.5	0.3
0	0	0.1	0.1	1.8	0.2	16	0	0	0.1	12	101	3	173	75	1.2	0.9
0	0	0.3	0.1	2.3	<0.1	64	0	0	<0.1	5	29	1	36	5	2.5	0.2
0	0	0.1	<0.1	0.2	0.1	6	0	0	0.2	3	33	1	57	8	0.2	0.3
0	0	0.1	0.1	1.2				0		0		0	35		1.1	
0	3	0.2	<0.1	1.5	0.1	13	0	0	0.2	10	107	1	109	41	1.1	0.8
0	3	0.1	0.1	1.2	0.1	17	0	0	<0.1	3	87	2	54	38	0.5	0.8
0	0	0.3	0.1	0.4	<0.1	22	0	0		21	204	1	167	69	1.8	1.5
0	0	0.1	<0.1	1.5	0.1	4	0	0	<0.1	10	81	5	42	42	0.4	0.6
0	0	0.1	<0.1	1.3	0.1	4	0	0		10	75	1	77	43	0.5	0.6
0	0	<0.1	<0.1	0.3	<0.1	1	0	0	<0.1	2	7	4	9	4	0.1	0.4
0	0	0.1	<0.1	1.2	0.1	46	0	0	<0.1	8	34	1	28	9	0.9	0.4
0	0	0.1	<0.1	1.4	<0.1	58	0	0	<0.1	7	31	3	7	4	1.5	0.4
0	0	0.2	<0.1	1.7	<0.1	54	0	0		3	34	0	27	12	1.4	0.4
0	2	<0.1	0.1	1.1	0.1	21	0	0	0.2	2	67	2	83	26	0.5	1.1
0	2	0.1	<0.1	0.9	0.1	16	0	0	<0.1	9	36	5	62	29	0.9	0.5
0	0	0.2	0.1	0.8	0.1	102	0	0	3.4	8	170	2	162	46	1.4	2.3
0	26	0.2	0.3	3.6	0.2	2	<0.1	15.8	0.1	27	36	17	85	8	4.4	0.2
22	2803	<0.1	0.1	2.2	0.1	10	0.9	5.1	0.8	15	75	180	241	19	1.2	1.5
12	8374	<0.1	0.1	1.3	0.1	10	0.6	0.3	0.8	29	56	53	246	17	0.6	0.6
46	13	<0.1	0.1	1.4	<0.1	8	0.9	1.1	0.1	59	85	312	85	7	0.7	1.7
0	20077	<0.1	0.1	0.8	0.1	29	0	9.4	0.9	39	34	83	343	19	0.7	0.3
0	11281	<0.1	0.1	0.7	0.2	17	0	16.3	0.9	27	41	31	413	20	0.7	0.2
73	0	0.1	0.2	3.4	0.3	7	2.2	0	0.1	7	196	56	302	22	2.5	5.8

ESHA, EatRight Analysis; **AMT**, amount; **WT**, weight; **CAL**, calories; **KILO**, KiloJoule; **WTR**, water; **PROT**, protein; **CARB**, carbohydrate; **FIBR**, fiber; **FAT**, fat; **SATF**, saturated fat; **MONO**, monounsaturated fat; **POLY**, polyunsaturated fat; **CHOL**, cholesterol;

ESHA CODE	FOOD DESCRIPTION	AMT	UNIT	WT (g)	CAL (kcal)	KILO (kJ)	WTR (g)	PROT (g)	CARB (g)	FIBR (g)	FAT (g)	SATF (g)	MONO (g)	POLY (g)
MEATS AND SUBSTITUTES (CONTINUED)														
11237	Beef, bottom round steak, brsd, 0" trim	3	oz	85.05	190	795	49	29	0	0	8	2.7	3.2	0.3
10035	Beef, breakfast strips, cured, ckd	3	ea	34	153	640	9	11	<1	0	12	4.9	5.7	0.5
10008	Beef, corned, cured, cnd, slices	3	oz	85.05	213	891	49	23	0	0	13	5.3	5.1	0.5
10020	Beef, flank steak, lean, brld, choice, 0" trim	3	oz	85.05	165	690	54	24	0	0	7	2.9	2.8	0.3
58117	Beef, ground, hamburger patty, brld, 15% fat	3	oz	85.05	213	891	49	22	0	0	13	5	5.7	0.4
58122	Beef, ground, hamburger patty, brld, 20% fat	3	oz	85.05	230	962	48	22	0	0	15	5.7	6.7	0.4
58107	Beef, ground, hamburger patty, brld, 5% fat	1	ea	82	140	586	54	22	0	0	5	2.4	2.2	0.3
10015	Beef, heart, ckd	3	oz	85.05	140	586	56	24	<1	0	4	1.2	0.9	0.8
10051	Beef, jerky, lrg pce	1	pce	20	82	343	5	7	2	<1	5	2.2	2.3	0.2
10010	Beef, liver, fried	3	oz	85.05	149	623	53	23	4	0	4	1.3	0.6	0.5
10920	Beef, porterhouse steak, brld, choice, ⅛" trim	3	oz	85.05	254	1063	45	20	0	0	19	7.2	8.3	0.7
10706	Beef, rib eye steak, lean, brld, choice, 0" trim	3	oz	85.05	174	728	52	25	0	0	8	2.9	3.1	0.3
10624	Beef, short ribs, brsd, choice	3	oz	85.05	401	1678	30	18	0	0	36	15.1	16.1	1.3
10922	Beef, T-bone steak, brld, choice, ⅛" trim	3	oz	85.05	243	1017	46	20	0	0	17	6.7	7.6	0.6
11280	Beef, tenderloin, steak, lean, brld, 0" trim	3	oz	85.05	164	686	54	24	0	0	7	2.5	2.7	0.2
11286	Beef, top loin, strip steak, lean, brld, 0" trim	3	oz	85.05	155	649	55	25	0	0	5	2.1	2.2	0.2
15383	Beef, top round steak, lean, pan fried, choice, ⅛" trim	3	oz	85.05	194	812	46	29	2	0	7	2	2.6	1.3
10913	Beef, top round steak, pan fried, choice, ⅛" trim	3	oz	85.05	226	946	45	28	0	0	12	3.9	4.4	1.5
58327	Beef, top sirloin steak, lean, brld, choice, ⅛" trim	3	oz	85.05	159	665	54	25	0	0	6	2.2	2.3	0.2
10089	Beef, tripe, ckd	3	oz	85.05	80	335	69	10	2	0	3	1.2	1.4	0.2
11530	Veal, ground, brld, 8% fat	3	oz	85.05	146	611	57	21	0	0	6	2.6	2.4	0.5
11517	Veal, loin cutlet, brsd	3	oz	85.05	242	1013	44	26	0	0	15	5.7	5.7	1
11519	Veal, short ribs, rstd	3	oz	85.05	194	812	51	20	0	0	12	4.6	4.6	0.8
11527	Veal, sirloin steak, rstd	3	oz	85.05	172	720	53	21	0	0	9	3.8	3.5	0.6
Chicken														
15004	Chicken, breast, w/o skin, rstd	1	ea	86	142	594	56	27	0	0	3	0.9	1.1	0.7
15001	Chicken, breast, with skin, rstd	1	ea	98	193	808	61	29	0	0	8	2.1	3	1.6
15027	Chicken, dark meat, w/o skin, rstd	3	oz	85.05	174	728	54	23	0	0	8	2.3	3	1.9
15035	Chicken, drumstick, w/o skin, rstd	1	ea	97	145	607	69	23	0	0	5	1.4	2	1.1
15008	Chicken, drumstick, with skin, rstd	3	oz	85.05	158	661	57	19	0	0	8	2.3	3.4	1.7
15025	Chicken, gizzard, avg, chpd, simmered	1	oz	28.35	44	184	19	9	0	0	1	0.2	0.1	0.1
15032	Chicken, light meat, w/o skin, rstd	3	oz	85.05	147	615	55	26	0	0	4	1.1	1.3	0.8
15012	Chicken, thigh, w/o skin, rstd	3	oz	85.05	151	632	57	20	0	0	7	1.9	2.9	1.4
15010	Chicken, thigh, with skin, rstd	3	oz	85.05	195	816	53	19	0	0	13	3.5	5.3	2.5
15016	Chicken, w/o skin, with broth, can	3	oz	85.05	140	586	58	19	0	0	7	1.9	2.7	1.5

< = Trace amount present   Blank = Not available

V, vitamin; **THI**, thiamin; **RIB**, riboflavin; **NIA**, niacin; **FOL**, folate; **CALC**, calcium; **PHOS**, phosphorus; **SOD**, sodium; **POT**, potassium; **MAG**, magnesium

CHOL (mg)	V-A (IU)	THI (mg)	RIB (mg)	NIA (mg)	V-B_6 (mg)	FOL (µg)	V-B_{12} (µg)	V-C (mg)	V-E (mg)	CALC (mg)	PHOS (mg)	SOD (mg)	POT (mg)	MAG (mg)	IRON (mg)	ZINC (mg)
81	0	0.1	0.2	5	0.4	9	1.6	0	0.4	7	177	37	230	19	2.3	4.8
40	0	<0.1	0.1	2.2	0.1	3	1.2	0	0.1	3	80	766	140	9	1.1	2.2
73	0	<0.1	0.1	2.1	0.1	8	1.4	0	0.1	10	94	763	116	12	1.8	3
68	0	0.1	0.1	7	0.5	8	1.5	0	0.3	13	179	48	287	20	1.6	4.3
77	0	<0.1	0.1	4.6	0.3	8	2.2	0	0.4	15	168	61	270	18	2.2	5.4
77	0	<0.1	0.2	4.3	0.3	9	2.3	0	0.4	20	165	64	259	17	2.1	5.3
62	0	<0.1	0.1	4.9	0.3	6	2	0	0.3	6	169	53	285	18	2.3	5.3
180	0	0.1	1	5.7	0.2	4	9.2	0	0.2	4	216	50	186	18	5.4	2.4
10	0	<0.1	<0.1	0.3	<0.1	27	0.2	0	0.1	4	81	416	119	10	1.1	1.6
324	22188	0.2	2.9	14.9	0.9	221	70.7	0.6	0.4	5	412	65	299	19	5.2	4.4
63	0	0.1	0.2	3.5	0.3	6	1.8	0		7	159	54	274	20	2.3	3.9
77	0	0.1	0.1	7.2	0.5	9	1.5	0	0.3	14	193	51	309	21	1.7	4.7
80	0	<0.1	0.1	2.1	0.2	4	2.2	0	0.2	10	138	43	191	13	2	4.2
55	0	0.1	0.2	3.5	0.3	6	1.8	0		7	162	56	284	20	2.4	3.9
69	0	0.1	0.1	6.9	0.5	9	1.4	0	0.3	15	191	50	308	20	1.5	4.5
67	0	0.1	0.1	7.1	0.5	9	1.4	0	0.3	16	195	51	315	21	1.6	4.6
87	0	0.1	0.3	4.6	0.5	12	3.3	0	0.1	5	243	55	412	30	2.9	3.9
82	0	0.1	0.2	4.4	0.5	10	2.8	0	0.2	5	233	58	408	28	2.5	3.7
69	0	0.1	0.1	6.6	0.5	8	1.4	0	0.3	14	196	52	314	21	1.7	4.7
134	0	0	<0.1	0.4	0	3	0.6	0	0.1	69	56	58	36	13	0.6	1.5
88	0	0.1	0.2	6.8	0.3	9	1.1	0	0.1	14	185	71	287	20	0.8	3.3
100	0	<0.1	0.3	7.7	0.2	12	1	0	0.3	24	187	68	238	20	0.9	3.1
94	0	<0.1	0.2	5.9	0.2	11	1.2	0	0.3	9	168	78	251	19	0.8	3.5
87	0	0.1	0.3	7.5	0.3	13	1.2	0	0.4	11	190	71	299	22	0.8	2.8
73	18	0.1	0.1	11.8	0.5	3	0.3	0	0.2	13	196	64	220	25	0.9	0.9
82	91	0.1	0.1	12.5	0.5	4	0.3	0	0.3	14	210	70	240	26	1	1
79	61	0.1	0.2	5.6	0.3	7	0.3	0	0.2	13	152	79	204	20	1.1	2.4
126	20	0.1	0.2	5.4	0.4	4	0.4	0	0.2	12	194	114	257	23	1	2.3
111	34	0.1	0.1	4.6	0.3	3	0.3	0	0.2	10	165	97	218	20	0.8	1.9
105	0	<0.1	0.1	0.9	<0.1	1	0.3	0	0.1	5	54	16	51	1	0.9	1.3
72	25	0.1	0.1	10.6	0.5	3	0.3	0	0.2	13	184	65	210	23	0.9	1
115	23	0.1	0.2	5.3	0.4	4	0.3	0	0.2	9	185	74	236	20	0.9	1.5
115	47	0.1	0.1	4.9	0.3	3	0.4	0	0.2	9	174	73	221	19	0.9	1.4
53	100	<0.1	0.1	5.4	0.3	3	0.2	1.7	0.2	12	94	428	117	10	1.3	1.2

ESHA, EatRight Analysis; **AMT**, amount; **WT**, weight; **CAL**, calories; **KILO**, KiloJoule; **WTR**, water; **PROT**, protein; **CARB**, carbohydrate; **FIBR**, fiber; **FAT**, fat; **SATF**, saturated fat; **MONO**, monounsaturated fat; **POLY**, polyunsaturated fat; **CHOL**, cholesterol;

ESHA CODE	FOOD DESCRIPTION	AMT	UNIT	WT (g)	CAL (kcal)	KILO (kJ)	WTR (g)	PROT (g)	CARB (g)	FIBR (g)	FAT (g)	SATF (g)	MONO (g)	POLY (g)
MEATS AND SUBSTITUTES (CONTINUED)														
15000	Chicken, whole, w/o skin, rstd	3	oz	85.05	162	678	54	25	0	0	6	1.7	2.3	1.4
15006	Chicken, whole, w/o skin, stwd	3	oz	85.05	151	632	57	23	0	0	6	1.6	2	1.3
15002	Chicken, wing, with skin, rstd	1	ea	34	99	414	19	9	0	0	7	1.9	2.6	1.4
15050	Chicken, fried, back, w/o skin	1	ea	116	334	1397	56	35	7	0	18	4.8	6.6	4.2
15057	Chicken, fried, breast, w/o skin	3	oz	85.05	159	665	51	28	<1	0	4	1.1	1.5	0.9
15042	Chicken, fried, drumstick, w/o skin	1	ea	42	82	343	26	12	0	0	3	0.9	1.2	0.8
15011	Chicken, fried, thigh, w/o skin	1	ea	52	113	473	31	15	1	0	5	1.4	2	1.3
15028	Chicken, fried, whole, w/o skin, chpd	3	oz	85.05	186	778	49	26	1	<1	8	2.1	2.8	1.8
Fish and Shellfish														
17034	Caviar, black, granular	1	Tbs	16	42	176	8	4	1	0	3	0.6	0.7	1.2
19036	Crab, Alaska king, leg, stmd	1	ea	134	130	544	104	26	0	0	2	0.2	0.2	0.7
19004	Crab, dungeoness, stmd	3	oz	85.05	94	393	62	19	1	0	1	0.1	0.2	0.3
19022	Crayfish, wild, mixed species, raw	8	ea	27	21	88	22	4	0	0	<1	<0.1	<0.1	0.1
19038	Crayfish, wild, mixed species, stmd	3	oz	85.05	70	293	68	14	0	0	1	0.2	0.2	0.3
17124	Fish, anchovies, European, cnd, with oil, drnd	5	ea	20	42	176	10	6	0	0	2	0.4	0.8	0.5
17086	Fish, bass, sea, mixed species, fillet, bkd	3	oz	85.05	105	439	61	20	0	0	2	0.6	0.5	0.8
17104	Fish, bass, striped, fillet, bkd	3	oz	85.05	105	439	62	19	0	0	3	0.6	0.7	0.9
17106	Fish, butterfish, fillet, bkd	3	oz	85.05	159	665	57	19	0	0	9			
17179	Fish, catfish, channel, farmed, fillet, bkd	3	oz	85.05	122	510	63	16	0	0	6	1.3	2.6	1.2
17107	Fish, cod, Pacific, fillet, bkd	3	oz	85.05	72	301	68	16	0	0	<1	0.1	0.1	0.2
17071	Fish, grouper, mixed species, fillet, bkd	3	oz	85.05	100	418	62	21	0	0	1	0.3	0.2	0.3
17090	Fish, haddock, fillet, bkd	3	oz	85.05	77	322	68	17	0	0	<1	0.1	0.1	0.2
17047	Fish, herring, Atlantic, fillet, bkd	3	oz	85.05	173	724	55	20	0	0	10	2.2	4.1	2.3
17013	Fish, herring, Atlantic, pickled	0.25	cup	35	92	385	19	5	3	0	6	0.8	4.2	0.6
17072	Fish, mullet, striped, fillet, bkd	3	oz	85.05	128	536	60	21	0	0	4	1.2	1.2	0.8
17121	Fish, orange roughy, fillet, bkd	3	oz	85.05	89	372	57	19	0	0	1	<0.1	0.4	0.2
17123	Fish, salmon, Atlantic, fillet, bkd, wild	3	oz	85.05	155	649	51	22	0	0	7	1.1	2.3	2.8
17060	Fish, sardines, Atlantic, with bones, cnd, with oil, drnd	2	oz	56.7	118	494	34	14	0	0	6	0.9	2.2	2.9
17022	Fish, snapper, mixed species, fillet, bkd	3	oz	85.05	109	456	60	22	0	0	1	0.3	0.3	0.5
17068	Fish, sole, fillet, bkd	3	oz	85.05	73	305	69	13	0	0	2	0.5	0.6	0.4
17080	Fish, surimi	3	oz	85.05	84	351	65	13	6	0	1	0.2	0.1	0.4
17066	Fish, swordfish, fillet, bkd	3	oz	85.05	146	611	58	20	0	0	7	1.6	3	1.2
17101	Fish, tuna, bluefin, fillet, bkd	3	oz	85.05	156	653	50	25	0	0	5	1.4	1.7	1.6
17024	Fish, tuna, light, with oil, drnd, can	2	oz	56.7	112	469	34	17	0	0	5	0.9	1.7	1.6
17026	Fish, tuna, light, with water, drnd, 12.5 oz can	2	oz	56.7	49	205	44	11	0	0	1	0.1	0.1	0.2
19006	Lobster, northern, stmd	3	oz	85.05	76	318	66	16	0	0	1	0.2	0.2	0.3
19086	Mollusks, abalone, stmd	3	oz	85.05	179	749	42	29	10	0	1	0.3	0.2	0.2
19002	Mollusks, clam, mixed species, cnd, drnd	2	oz	56.7	81	339	37	14	3	0	1	0.2	0.1	0.2
19000	Mollusks, clam, mixed species, stmd	3	oz	85.05	126	527	54	22	4	0	2	0.2	0.1	0.5

< = Trace amount present   Blank = Not available

V, vitamin; **THI**, thiamin; **RIB**, riboflavin; **NIA**, niacin; **FOL**, folate; **CALC**, calcium; **PHOS**, phosphorus; **SOD**, sodium; **POT**, potassium; **MAG**, magnesium

CHOL (mg)	V-A (IU)	THI (mg)	RIB (mg)	NIA (mg)	V-B$_6$ (mg)	FOL (µg)	V-B$_{12}$ (µg)	V-C (mg)	V-E (mg)	CALC (mg)	PHOS (mg)	SOD (mg)	POT (mg)	MAG (mg)	IRON (mg)	ZINC (mg)
76	45	0.1	0.2	7.8	0.4	5	0.3	0	0.2	13	166	73	207	21	1	1.8
71	43	<0.1	0.1	5.2	0.2	5	0.2	0	0.2	12	128	60	153	18	1	1.7
29	54	<0.1	<0.1	2.3	0.1	1	0.1	0	0.1	5	51	28	63	6	0.4	0.6
108	114	0.1	0.3	8.9	0.4	10	0.4	0		30	204	115	291	29	1.9	3.2
77	20	0.1	0.1	12.6	0.5	3	0.3	0	0.4	14	209	67	235	26	1	0.9
39	26	<0.1	0.1	2.6	0.2	4	0.1	0		5	78	40	105	10	0.6	1.4
53	36	<0.1	0.1	3.7	0.2	5	0.2	0		7	103	49	135	14	0.8	1.5
80	50	0.1	0.2	8.2	0.4	6	0.3	0	0.4	14	174	77	219	23	1.1	1.9
94	145	<0.1	0.1	<0.1	0.1	8	3.2	0	0.3	44	57	240	29	48	1.9	0.2
71	39	0.1	0.1	1.8	0.2	68	15.4	10.2		79	375	1436	351	84	1	10.2
65	88	<0.1	0.2	3.1	0.1	36	8.8	3.1		50	149	321	347	49	0.4	4.7
31	14	<0.1	<0.1	0.6	<0.1	10	0.5	0.3	0.8	7	69	16	82	7	0.2	0.4
113	43	<0.1	0.1	1.9	0.1	37	1.8	0.8	1.3	51	230	80	252	28	0.7	1.5
17	8	<0.1	0.1	4	<0.1	3	0.2	0	0.7	46	50	734	109	14	0.9	0.5
45	181	0.1	0.1	1.6	0.4	5	0.3	0		11	211	74	279	45	0.3	0.4
88	88	0.1	<0.1	2.2	0.3	9	3.8	0		16	216	75	279	43	0.9	0.4
71	93	0.1	0.2	4.9	0.3	14	1.6	0		24	262	97	409	27	0.5	0.8
56	2	<0.1	0.1	2.2	0.2	10	2.4	0	0.8	8	210	101	311	20	0.2	0.5
48	6	<0.1	<0.1	1.1	0.1	7	2	0	0.6	9	293	316	246	20	0.2	0.3
40	140	0.1	<0.1	0.3	0.3	9	0.6	0		18	122	45	404	31	1	0.4
56	53	<0.1	0.1	3.5	0.3	11	1.8	0	0.5	12	236	222	299	22	0.2	0.3
65	102	0.1	0.3	3.5	0.3	10	11.2	0.6	1.2	63	258	98	356	35	1.2	1.1
5	301	<0.1	<0.1	1.2	0.1	1	1.5	0	0.6	27	31	304	24	3	0.4	0.2
54	120	0.1	0.1	5.4	0.4	9	0.2	1		26	208	60	390	28	1.2	0.7
68	68	<0.1	0.1	1.5	0.1	4	0.4	0	1.6	9	87	59	154	15	1	0.3
60	37	0.2	0.4	8.6	0.8	25	2.6	0		13	218	48	534	31	0.9	0.7
81	61	<0.1	0.1	3	0.1	6	5.1	0	1.2	217	278	286	225	22	1.7	0.7
40	98	<0.1	<0.1	0.3	0.4	5	3	1.4		34	171	48	444	31	0.2	0.4
48	31	<0.1	<0.1	1.1	0.1	5	1.1	0	0.7	21	263	309	168	19	0.2	0.3
26	57	<0.1	<0.1	0.2	<0.1	2	1.4	0	0.5	8	240	122	95	37	0.2	0.3
66	110	0.1	0.1	7.9	0.5	2	1.4	0	2	5	259	82	424	30	0.4	0.7
42	2143	0.2	0.3	9	0.4	2	9.3	0		9	277	43	275	54	1.1	0.7
10	44	<0.1	0.1	7	0.1	3	1.2	0	0.5	7	176	201	117	18	0.8	0.5
20	32	<0.1	<0.1	5.7	0.2	2	1.4	0	0.2	10	79	140	101	13	0.9	0.4
124	3	<0.1	<0.1	1.6	0.1	9	1.2	0	0.9	82	157	413	196	37	0.2	3.4
145	8	0.3	0.1	1.9	0.2	6	0.7	2.6	6.8	50	226	435	298	69	4.9	1.4
28	281	<0.1	<0.1	0.3	<0.1	4	10.6	0	0.6	37	185	64	356	18	1.5	0.5
57	485	0.1	0.4	2.9	0.1	25	84.1	18.8		78	287	1022	534	15	23.8	2.3

ESHA, EatRight Analysis; **AMT**, amount; **WT**, weight; **CAL**, calories; **KILO**, KiloJoule; **WTR**, water; **PROT**, protein; **CARB**, carbohydrate; **FIBR**, fiber; **FAT**, fat; **SATF**, saturated fat; **MONO**, monounsaturated fat; **POLY**, polyunsaturated fat; **CHOL**, cholesterol;

ESHA CODE	FOOD DESCRIPTION	AMT	UNIT	WT (g)	CAL (kcal)	KILO (kJ)	WTR (g)	PROT (g)	CARB (g)	FIBR (g)	FAT (g)	SATF (g)	MONO (g)	POLY (g)
MEATS AND SUBSTITUTES (CONTINUED)														
19044	Mollusks, mussel, blue, stmd	3	oz	85.05	146	611	52	20	6	0	4	0.7	0.9	1
19025	Mollusks, octopus, raw	4	oz	113.4	93	389	91	17	2	0	1	0.3	0.2	0.3
19048	Mollusks, octopus, stmd	3	oz	85.05	139	582	51	25	4	0	2	0.4	0.3	0.4
19026	Mollusks, oyster, eastern, wild, raw	4	oz	113.4	58	243	101	6	3	0	2	0.5	0.3	0.6
19027	Mollusks, oyster, eastern, wild, stmd, med	12	ea	84	86	360	66	10	5	0	3	0.8	0.4	0.9
19011	Mollusks, scallop, stmd	2	oz	56.7	63	264	40	12	3	0	<1	0.1	<0.1	0.1
19068	Mollusks, squid, bkd	0.5	cup	70	97	406	50	13	3	0	3	0.7	1.1	1
19040	Mollusks, whelk, stmd	3	oz	85.05	234	979	27	41	13	0	1	0.1	<0.1	<0.1
19012	Shrimp, mixed species, stmd, lrg	4	ea	22	26	109	16	5	<1	0	<1	0.1	0.1	0.1
Game Meat														
14008	Beefalo, rstd	3	oz	85.05	160	669	52	26	0	0	5	2.3	2.3	0.2
14009	Bison, rstd	3	oz	85.05	122	510	57	24	0	0	2	0.8	0.8	0.2
40551	Deer, rstd	3	oz	85.05	134	561	55	26	0	0	3	1.1	0.7	0.5
40570	Deer, top round steak, lean, 1" thick, brld	3	oz	85.05	129	540	56	27	0	0	2	0.9	0.4	0.1
14014	Elk, rstd	3	oz	85.05	124	519	56	26	0	0	2	0.6	0.4	0.3
14029	Frog, leg, stmd	2	ea	100	106	444	74	24	0	0	<1	0.1	0.1	0.1
14004	Rabbit, domestic, rstd	3	oz	85.05	168	703	52	25	0	0	7	2	1.8	1.3
14013	Venison, rstd	3	oz	85.05	134	561	55	26	0	0	3	1.1	0.7	0.5
Goat and Lamb														
13623	Goat, rstd	3	oz	85.05	122	510	58	23	0	0	3	0.8	1.2	0.2
13524	Lamb, ground, brld, 20% fat	3	oz	85.05	241	1008	47	21	0	0	17	6.9	7.1	1.2
13522	Lamb, kabob meat, lean, brld, ¼" trim	3	oz	85.05	158	661	54	24	0	0	6	2.2	2.5	0.6
13501	Lamb, leg, whole, lean, rstd, choice, ¼" trim	3	oz	85.05	162	678	54	24	0	0	7	2.3	2.9	0.4
13513	Lamb, loin chop, lean, brld, choice, ¼" trim	1	ea	46	99	414	28	14	0	0	4	1.6	2	0.3
13523	Lamb, stew meat, lean, brsd, choice, ¼" trim	3	oz	85.05	190	795	48	29	0	0	7	2.7	3	0.7
Lunchmeat														
57877	Frankfurter, beef	1	ea	50	156	653	27	6	2	0	14	5.5	6	0.4
13010	Frankfurter, beef and pork	1	ea	45	137	573	25	5	1	0	12	4.8	6.2	1.2
13012	Frankfurter, turkey	1	ea	45	100	418	28	6	2	0	8	1.8	2.6	1.8
57966	Hot Dog, beef, 97% fat free	1	ea	45	40	167		6	3	0	1	0		
13051	Lunchmeat Loaf, pickle pimiento, with pork, slice	1	slice	38	86	360	23	4	3	<1	6	2	2.7	1.1
13095	Lunchmeat Spread, chicken, cnd	1	oz	28.35	45	188	16	5	1	<1	5	0.9	1.4	0.7
13034	Lunchmeat Spread, ham salad	1	Tbs	15	32	134	9	1	2	0	2	0.8	1.1	0.4
56007	Lunchmeat Spread, tuna salad	1	Tbs	12.8	24	100	8	2	1	0	1	0.2	0.4	0.5
13000	Lunchmeat, beef, thin slice, oval	1	thin slc	9.3	11	46	7	2	<1	0	<1	0.1	0.1	<0.1
13006	Lunchmeat, bologna, beef and pork, 4½" × ⅛" slice	2	oz	56.7	175	732	29	9	3	0	14	5.3	6	0.6

< = Trace amount present   Blank = Not available

V, vitamin; **THI**, thiamin; **RIB**, riboflavin; **NIA**, niacin; **FOL**, folate; **CALC**, calcium; **PHOS**, phosphorus; **SOD**, sodium; **POT**, potassium; **MAG**, magnesium

CHOL (mg)	V-A (IU)	THI (mg)	RIB (mg)	NIA (mg)	V-B_6 (mg)	FOL (µg)	V-B_{12} (µg)	V-C (mg)	V-E (mg)	CALC (mg)	PHOS (mg)	SOD (mg)	POT (mg)	MAG (mg)	IRON (mg)	ZINC (mg)
48	259	0.3	0.4	2.6	0.1	65	20.4	11.6		28	242	314	228	31	5.7	2.3
54	170	<0.1	<0.1	2.4	0.4	18	22.7	5.7	1.4	60	211	261	397	34	6	1.9
82	255	<0.1	0.1	3.2	0.6	20	30.6	6.8	1	90	237	391	536	51	8.1	2.9
45	50	<0.1	0.1	1	<0.1	8	9.9	0	1	67	110	96	177	20	5.2	44.6
66	74	<0.1	0.2	1.6	0.1	12	14.7	0	1.4	97	163	139	117	29	7.7	66
23	3	<0.1	<0.1	0.6	0.1	11	1.2	0	0	6	242	378	178	21	0.3	0.9
198	118	<0.1	0.3	1.8	<0.1	4	1	3.8	1.3	28	188	62	210	28	0.6	1.3
111	138	<0.1	0.2	1.7	0.6	9	15.4	5.8		96	240	350	590	146	8.6	2.8
46	66	<0.1	<0.1	0.6	0.1	5	0.4	0	0.5	20	67	208	37	8	0.1	0.4
49	0	<0.1	0.1	4.2		15	2.2	7.7		20	213	70	390		2.6	5.4
70	0	0.1	0.2	3.2	0.3	7	2.4	0	0.3	7	178	48	307	22	2.9	3.1
95	0	0.2	0.5	5.7				0		6	192	46	285	20	3.8	2.3
72	0	0.2	0.4	7.1	0.6	9	1.9	0	0.5	3	231	38	321	26	3.6	3.1
62	0					8		0		4	153	52	279	20	3.1	2.7
72	65	0.2	0.3	1.6	0.2	16	0.5	0	1.4	26	160	84	372	29	2	1.4
70	0	0.1	0.2	7.2	0.4	9	7.1	0		16	224	40	326	18	1.9	1.9
95	0	0.2	0.5	5.7				0		6	192	46	285	20	3.8	2.3
64	0	0.1	0.5	3.4	0	4	1	0	0.3	14	171	73	344	0	3.2	4.5
82	0	0.1	0.2	5.7	0.1	16	2.2	0	0.1	19	171	69	288	20	1.5	4
77	0	0.1	0.3	5.6	0.1	20	2.6	0	0.2	11	191	65	285	26	2	4.9
76	0	0.1	0.2	5.4	0.1	20	2.2	0	0.2	7	175	58	287	22	1.8	4.2
44	0	0.1	0.1	3.2	0.1	11	1.2	0	0.1	9	104	39	173	13	0.9	1.9
92	0	0.1	0.2	5.1	0.1	18	2.3	0	0.2	13	174	60	221	24	2.4	5.6
28	0	<0.1	<0.1	1	0.1	5	0.7	0	0.1	6	78	518	145	6	0.6	1
22	26	0.1	0.1	1.2	0.1	2	0.6	0	0.1	5	39	369	75	4	0.5	0.8
35	0	<0.1	0.1	1.7	0.1	4	0.4	0	0.3	67	77	410	176	6	0.7	0.8
10	0							0		0		520	140		0.7	
22	99	0.1	<0.1	0.9	0.2	14	0.2	3	0.2	41	58	395	141	13	0.5	0.6
16	28	<0.1	<0.1	0.8	<0.1	1	<0.1	0		5	25	205	30	3	0.2	0.3
6	0	0.1	<0.1	0.3	<0.1	<1	0.1	0	0.3	1	18	161	22	2	0.1	0.2
2	12	<0.1	<0.1	0.9	<0.1	1	0.2	0.3		2	23	51	23	2	0.1	0.1
4	0	<0.1	<0.1	0.4	<0.1	<1	0.2	0	<0.1	1	24	82	29	2	0.2	0.3
34	48	0.1	0.1	1.4	0.2	3	1	0.5	0	48	92	544	179	10	0.7	1.3

ESHA, EatRight Analysis; **AMT**, amount; **WT**, weight; **CAL**, calories; **KILO**, KiloJoule; **WTR**, water; **PROT**, protein; **CARB**, carbohydrate; **FIBR**, fiber; **FAT**, fat; **SATF**, saturated fat; **MONO**, monounsaturated fat; **POLY**, polyunsaturated fat; **CHOL**, cholesterol;

ESHA CODE	FOOD DESCRIPTION	AMT	UNIT	WT (g)	CAL (kcal)	KILO (kJ)	WTR (g)	PROT (g)	CARB (g)	FIBR (g)	FAT (g)	SATF (g)	MONO (g)	POLY (g)
MEATS AND SUBSTITUTES (CONTINUED)														
13007	Lunchmeat, bologna, turkey	1	slice	28.35	59	247	18	3	1	<1	5	1.2	1.9	1.1
11913	Lunchmeat, pork and ham, Spam, cnd, svg	1	svg	56.7	176	736	30	8	2	0	15	5.6	7.8	1.7
13112	Lunchmeat, turkey breast, Louis Rich, hickory, 98% fat free	1	svg	28	30	126	6	5	1		<1	0		
13114	Lunchmeat, turkey breast, oven rstd, fat free	1	oz	28.35	24	100	22	4	1	0	<1	0.1	0.1	<0.1
45862	Meat Stick, super, slim	1	ea	18	90	377		4	1	0	8	3		
13020	Pastrami, turkey, slices	1	pce	28.5	38	159	20	5	1	<1	2	0.5	0.6	0.5
13026	Salami, beef and pork, hard, slice	3	slice	27	101	423	11	5	<1	0	9	3.1	3.9	1.2
13023	Salami, beef, ckd, slice	1	slice	26	68	285	16	3	<1	0	6	2.6	2.8	0.3
13079	Sausage, bratwurst, pork, ckd	1	ea	85	283	1184	44	12	2	0	25	8.5	12.5	2.2
13066	Sausage, braunschweiger, liver, pork 2 ½" × ¼"slice	1	slice	18	59	247	9	3	1	0	5	1.7	2.3	0.6
13070	Sausage, chorizo, pork and beef, 4" link, smkd	1	ea	60	273	1142	19	14	1	0	23	8.6	11	2.1
13015	Sausage, Italian, pork, link, ckd, ⅕ lb	1	ea	67	230	962	32	13	3	<1	18	6.5	8.6	2.3
13043	Sausage, kielbasa, beef pork and nonfat dry milk, link	1	ea	75	232	971	41	9	2	0	20	6.9	8.8	2.9
13019	Sausage, liverwurst, pork, 2 ½" × ¼" slice	1	slice	18	59	247	9	3	<1	0	5	1.9	2.4	0.5
13021	Sausage, pepperoni, beef and pork, slice	1	slice	2	10	42	1	<1	0	0	1	0.3	0.3	0.1
13022	Sausage, Polish, pork, 10" × 1 ¼"	1	ea	227	740	3096	121	32	4	0	65	23.4	30.7	7
13267	Sausage, pork, ckd	1	oz	28.35	96	402	14	6	0	0	8	2.6	3.5	1.1
58007	Sausage, turkey, breakfast link, mild	2	ea	56.7	133	556	36	9	1	0	10	2.2	2.9	2.6
Meat Substitutes														
7564	Tempeh	0.5	cup	83	160	669	50	15	8		9	1.8	2.5	3.2
7518	Tofu, firm, prep with nigari and calc sulfate, ¼ block pce	0.5	cup	126	88	368	107	10	2	1	5	1.1	1.5	2.3
7520	Tofu, fried, pce	3	oz	85.05	230	962	43	15	9	3	17	2.5	3.8	9.7
7500	Tofu, soft, with calc sulfate and nigari, ½" cubes	0.5	cup	124	76	318	108	8	2	<1	5	0.7	1	2.6
7752	Vegetarian Meat, bacon, Stripples, breakfast strips, fzn	2	ea	16	55	230	7	2	2	1	4	0.7	1	2.6
7732	Vegetarian Meat, beef, burger	0.25	cup	55	68	285	39	10	3	1	2	0.3	0.3	0.9
7610	Vegetarian Meat, beef, Choplets, cnd	2	pce	92	95	397	68	18	4	3	1	0.1	0.1	0.5
7642	Vegetarian Meat, beef, fillet, fzn	2	ea	85	180	753		16	8	4	9	1	3.5	4.5
91501	Vegetarian Meat, beef, ground	0.5	cup	57	60	251		13	6	3	<1			
7552	Vegetarian Meat, beef, meatballs	0.5	cup	72	142	594	42	15	6	3	6	1	1.6	3.4
7561	Vegetarian Meat, beef, patty	1	ea	56	110	460	32	12	4	3	5	0.8	1.2	2.6
8178	Vegetarian Meat, bologna, Smart Deli	4	slice	57	70	293		14	4	1	0	0	0	0
7726	Vegetarian Meat, burger, black bean, spicy, fzn	1	ea	67	115	481	38	11	13	5	4	0.5	1	2.2
7722	Vegetarian Meat, burger, Garden Veggie Patties, fzn	1	ea	67	118	494	40	12	9	3	4	0.5	1	2.1

< = Trace amount present   Blank = Not available

V, vitamin; **THI**, thiamin; **RIB**, riboflavin; **NIA**, niacin; **FOL**, folate; **CALC**, calcium; **PHOS**, phosphorus; **SOD**, sodium; **POT**, potassium; **MAG**, magnesium

CHOL (mg)	V-A (IU)	THI (mg)	RIB (mg)	NIA (mg)	V-B_6 (mg)	FOL (µg)	V-B_{12} (µg)	V-C (mg)	V-E (mg)	CALC (mg)	PHOS (mg)	SOD (mg)	POT (mg)	MAG (mg)	IRON (mg)	ZINC (mg)
21	9	<0.1	<0.1	0.7	0.1	3	0.1	3.8	0.1	35	32	304	38	5	0.9	0.4
40	0					2		0.5		8		776	130	8	0.5	1
10	0							0		0		260			0	
9	0							0		3	66	338	58	8	0.3	0.2
10	0							0		0		280			0.7	
19	7	<0.1	0.1	1	0.1	1	0.1	2.3	0.1	3	57	320	98	4	1.2	0.6
29	10	0.1	0.1	1.6	0.1	0	0.3	0	0.2	8	49	447	90	5	0.4	0.7
18	0	<0.1	<0.1	0.8	<0.1	1	0.8	0	<0.1	2	53	296	49	3	0.6	0.5
63	5	0.4	0.3	4.1	0.3	3	0.6	0	0.2	24	177	719	296	18	0.5	2.8
32	2529	<0.1	0.3	1.5	0.1	8	3.6	0	0.1	2	30	176	36	2	2	0.5
53	0	0.4	0.2	3.1	0.3	1	1.2	0	0.1	5	90	741	239	11	1	2
38	11	0.4	0.2	2.8	0.2	3	0.9	0.1	0.2	14	114	809	204	12	1	1.6
50	0	0.2	0.2	2.5	0.1	1	0.5	0	0.2	13	128	500	225	10	0.6	1.2
28	4980	<0.1	0.2	0.8	<0.1	5	2.4	0		5	41	155	31	2	1.2	0.4
2	0	<0.1	<0.1	0.1	<0.1	<1	<0.1	<1	0	<1	4	35	6	<1	<0.1	<0.1
159	0	1.1	0.3	7.8	0.4	5	2.2	2.3		27	309	1989	538	32	3.3	4.4
24	12	0.1	0.1	1.8	0.1	1	0.3	0.2	0.2	4	46	254	83	5	0.4	0.6
91	0	<0.1	0.1	2.1	0.1	2	0.4	0.3	0.1	18	88	362	130	9	0.6	1.7
0	0	0.1	0.3	2.2	0.2	20	0.1	0		92	221	7	342	67	2.2	0.9
0	0	0.1	0.1	0.1	0.1	24	0	0.3	<0.1	253	152	15	186	47	2	1
0	23	0.1	<0.1	0.1	0.1	23	0	0	<0.1	316	244	14	124	51	4.1	1.7
0	9	0.1	<0.1	0.7	0.1	55	0	0.2	<0.1	138	114	10	149	33	1.4	0.8
<1	0	1.6	0.1	1.4	0.1		0.5	0		7	46	234	16		0.6	0.1
0	0	0.1	0.1	1.6	0.2		2.4	0		4	54	248	24		1.4	0.7
0	0	0	0					0		7	69	420	35		1.4	0.9
0	0	0.4	0.1	0.8	0.4		2.7	0		20		650	130		1.8	
0	0							0		60		270			1.8	
0	0	0.7	0.2	1.8	0.1	56	1.1	0	1.2	18	248	396	130	13	1.6	1.3
0	0	0.5	0.3	5.6	0.7	44	1.3	0	1	16	193	308	101	10	1.2	1
0	0							0		250		490	50		1.8	
1		9.1	0.2	1.2	0.1	33	0			69	127	348	255	34	1.5	0.7
1	250	7.5	0.2	0.9	0.6					40	110	352	141		1.5	0.7

ESHA, EatRight Analysis; **AMT**, amount; **WT**, weight; **CAL**, calories; **KILO**, KiloJoule; **WTR**, water; **PROT**, protein; **CARB**, carbohydrate; **FIBR**, fiber; **FAT**, fat; **SATF**, saturated fat; **MONO**, monounsaturated fat; **POLY**, polyunsaturated fat; **CHOL**, cholesterol;

ESHA CODE	FOOD DESCRIPTION	AMT	UNIT	WT (g)	CAL (kcal)	KILO (kJ)	WTR (g)	PROT (g)	CARB (g)	FIBR (g)	FAT (g)	SATF (g)	MONO (g)	POLY (g)
MEATS AND SUBSTITUTES (CONTINUED)														
7746	Vegetarian Meat, burger, Grillers, fzn	1	ea	64	136	569	36	15	5	3	6	1.1	1.7	3.2
7674	Vegetarian Meat, burger, Harvest Burger, original, fzn	1	ea	90	138	577	58	18	7	6	4	1	2.1	0.3
91060	Vegetarian Meat, burger, mushroom and pepper, fzn	1	ea	67	120	502		12	9	3	4	0.5	1	2.5
91489	Vegetarian Meat, burger, original vegan	1	ea	71	70	293	35	13	6	4	1			
91059	Vegetarian Meat, burger, tomato and basil pizza, fzn	1	ea	67	121	506	42	10	7	2	6	1.5	1.4	2.6
7718	Vegetarian Meat, burger, veggie, black bean and salsa	1	ea	142	200	837		19	20	3	4	1.5		
7548	Vegetarian Meat, chicken, brd, fried	1	pce	36	84	351	20	8	3	2	5	0.4	1.2	1.6
7636	Vegetarian Meat, chicken, chicken style roll, sliced	1	slice	55	85	356	37	9	2	1	4	0.7	1	2.5
7727	Vegetarian Meat, chicken, Chik Nuggets, fzn	5	ea	85	250	1046		13	14	2	15	2	4.5	8
42772	Vegetarian Meat, cutlet, Smart Cutlets, original	1	ea	85	110	460		17	8	3	<1			
7549	Vegetarian Meat, fish sticks	1	ea	28	81	339	13	6	3	2	5	0.8	1.2	2.6
7624	Vegetarian Meat, fish, tuno, fzn	0.5	cup	55	90	377		7	3	2	6	1	2	3
7665	Vegetarian Meat, Grillers, Chik'n, patty, fzn	1	ea	67	132	552	36	8	15	2	5	0.5	0.9	3.1
92148	Vegetarian Meat, hot dog	1	ea	70	163	682	41	14	5	3	10	1.4	2.7	5.5
7744	Vegetarian Meat, hot dog, Big Franks, cnd	1	ea	51	111	464	30	11	3	2	6	0.8	1.6	3.8
7734	Vegetarian Meat, hot dog, Leanies, fzn	1	ea	40	100	418	22	8	2	2	7	1.1	2.5	2.9
8127	Vegetarian Meat, hot dog, Smart Dogs, jumbo	1	ea	76	80	335		15	3	2	1	0		
8835	Vegetarian Meat, hot dog, Tofu Dogs	1	ea	38	45	188		9	2	0	<1	0		
7551	Vegetarian Meat, lunchmeat, slices	1	pce	14	26	109	9	2	1	0	2	0.2	0.3	0.6
8173	Vegetarian Meat, lunchmeat, Smart Deli, baked ham	4	slice	52	70	293		12	3	0	1	0		
7618	Vegetarian Meat, salami, slices, fzn	3	slice	57	120	502		12	3	2	7	1	1	5
7555	Vegetarian Meat, sandwich spread	1	Tbs	15	22	92	11	1	1	<1	1	0.2	0.3	0.7
7511	Vegetarian Meat, sausage, links	1	ea	25	64	268	13	5	2	1	5	0.7	1.1	2.3
7512	Vegetarian Meat, sausage, patty	1	ea	38	98	410	19	7	4	1	7	1.1	1.7	3.5
8166	Vegetarian Meat, sausage, Smart Sausages, breakfast, link	2	ea	56	100	418		10	8	3	3	0	1	1.5
8159	Vegetarian Meat, sausage, Smart Sausages, italian, link	1	ea	85	140	586		13	7	1	7	1		
Other Poultry														
15240	Cornish Game Hen, whole, with skin, rstd	3	oz	85.05	220	920	50	19	0	0	15	4.3	6.8	3.1
14000	Duck, domesticated, whole, w/o skin, rstd	3	oz	85.05	171	715	55	20	0	0	10	3.4	3.3	1.3
16295	Duck, domesticated, whole, with skin, rstd	3	oz	85.05	287	1201	44	16	0	0	24	8.2	11	3.1
81166	Emu, top loin, brld	3	oz	85.05	129	540	57	25	0	0	3	0.7	1.1	0.4

< = Trace amount present Blank = Not available

V, vitamin; **THI**, thiamin; **RIB**, riboflavin; **NIA**, niacin; **FOL**, folate; **CALC**, calcium; **PHOS**, phosphorus; **SOD**, sodium; **POT**, potassium; **MAG**, magnesium

CHOL (mg)	V-A (IU)	THI (mg)	RIB (mg)	NIA (mg)	$V\text{-}B_6$ (mg)	FOL (μg)	$V\text{-}B_{12}$ (μg)	V-C (mg)	V-E (mg)	CALC (mg)	PHOS (mg)	SOD (mg)	POT (mg)	MAG (mg)	IRON (mg)	ZINC (mg)
2	0	1.8	0.2	4.1	0.4		2.9	0		39	118	270	116		2.7	0.8
0	0	0.3	0.2	6.3	0.4	22	0	0		102	225	411	432	70	3.9	8.1
0	0							0		20		470	250		1.4	
0	0							0		60		330			1.8	
7	285	0.1	0.2					14.7		32	93	261	159		1.2	
0												660				
0	0	0.5	0.1	4.6	0.3	20	1.8	0	0.7	15	88	144	108	4	1.4	0.2
1	0	0.4	0.1	4.1	0.3		2	0		150	134	249	227		2.1	0.4
0	0	0.4	0.2	6	0.8		3	0		20		490	210		1.4	
0	0							0		40		360	530		1.4	
0	0	0.3	0.3	3.4	0.4	29	1.2	0	1.1	27	126	137	168	6	0.6	0.4
0	0	0.2	<0.1	4	0.3		2.1	0		20		300	45		1.8	
0	17	0.2	0.1	2.8	0.1	8	1.1	0		27	84	559	263		1.7	0.3
0	0	0.3	0.6	2.2	0.1	55	1.6	0	1.3	23	241	330	69	13	1	0.8
0	0	0.3	0.5	7.5	0.7		6.7	0		9	72	217	59		1.3	1.2
1	0	0.2	0.1	0.8	0.2		0.9	0		29	82	431	41		0.7	0.3
0	0							0		20		560	490		1.8	
0	0	0.2					0.6	0		20		240	90	8	2.2	0.6
0	0	0.6	<0.1	1.6	0.1	14	0.6	0	0.4	6	62	100	28	3	0.3	0.2
0	0							0		0		390	20		1.4	
0	0	0.8	0.2	4	0.2		0.6	0		0		800	95		1.1	
0	2	0.1	0.1	2	0.2	15	0.5	0	0.3	7	33	94	51	19	0.2	0.2
0	0	0.6	0.1	2.8	0.2	6	0	0	0.5	16	56	222	58	9	0.9	0.4
0	0	0.9	0.2	4.3	0.3	10	0	0	0.8	24	86	337	88	14	1.4	0.6
0	0							0		40		500	570		1.4	
0	0							0		0		500	330		0.4	
111	90	0.1	0.2	5	0.3	2	0.2	0.4	0.3	11	124	54	208	15	0.8	1.3
76	65	0.2	0.4	4.3	0.2	9	0.3	0	0.6	10	173	55	214	17	2.3	2.2
71	179	0.1	0.2	4.1	0.2	5	0.3	0	0.6	9	133	50	174	14	2.3	1.6
75	0	0.3	0.5	7.8	0.7	8	7.4	0	0.2	8	233	49	318	26	4.3	2.9

ESHA, EatRight Analysis; **AMT**, amount; **WT**, weight; **CAL**, calories; **KILO**, KiloJoule; **WTR**, water; **PROT**, protein; **CARB**, carbohydrate; **FIBR**, fiber; **FAT**, fat; **SATF**, saturated fat; **MONO**, monounsaturated fat; **POLY**, polyunsaturated fat; **CHOL**, cholesterol;

ESHA CODE	FOOD DESCRIPTION	AMT	UNIT	WT (g)	CAL (kcal)	KILO (kJ)	WTR (g)	PROT (g)	CARB (g)	FIBR (g)	FAT (g)	SATF (g)	MONO (g)	POLY (g)
MEATS AND SUBSTITUTES (CONTINUED)														
14002	Goose, whole, w/o skin, rstd	3	oz	85.05	202	845	49	25	0	0	11	3.9	3.7	1.3
14003	Goose, whole, with skin, rstd	3	oz	85.05	259	1084	44	21	0	0	19	5.8	8.7	2.1
81180	Ostrich, tenderloin, raw	4	oz	113.4	139	582	84	25	0	0	4	1.3	1.4	0.9
16048	Pate, goose liver, smkd, pate de foie gras, cnd	1	Tbs	13	60	251	5	1	1	0	6	1.9	3.3	0.1
Pork														
12000	Bacon, brld, med slice	1	slice	8	43	180	1	3	<1	0	3	1.1	1.5	0.4
12002	Canadian Bacon, cured, grilled	2	slice	47	87	364	29	11	1	0	4	1.3	1.9	0.4
12035	Pork, chop, whole loin, lean, brld	1	ea	79	166	695	48	23	0	0	8	2.9	3.5	0.6
12031	Pork, chop, whole, loin, rstd	3	oz	85.05	211	883	49	23	0	0	12	4.6	5.5	1
12225	Pork, cured ham, lean, 7% fat, cnd	3	oz	85.05	122	510	60	15	0	0	6	2.1	3	0.6
12006	Pork, cured ham, whole, lean, rstd	3	oz	85.05	134	561	56	21	0	0	5	1.6	2.2	0.5
12175	Pork, cured shoulder, arm, lean, rstd	3	oz	85.05	145	607	54	21	0	0	6	2	2.7	0.7
12098	Pork, ribs, country style, lean, brsd	1	ea	80	198	828	45	22	0	0	11	4.1	5	1.3
12236	Pork, ribs, country style, lean, rstd	1	svg	85.05	193	808	50	25	0	0	10	3.2	3.7	1.2
Turkey														
51101	Turkey, dark meat, w/o skin, rstd	3	oz	85.05	147	615	55	24	0	0	5	1.5	1.8	1.4
16003	Turkey, ground, patty, ckd, 4oz raw	1	ea	82	166	695	51	22	0	0	9	2.2	2.8	2.4
16158	Turkey, light meat, w/o skin, rstd	3	oz	85.05	125	523	58	26	0	0	2	0.5	0.5	0.4
51152	Turkey, light, chunk, premium, with water, cnd	2	oz	56.7	80	335		16	0	0	2	0.5		
16000	Turkey, w/o skin, rstd	3	oz	85.05	135	565	57	25	0	0	3	1	1.1	0.9
NUTS AND SEEDS														
4649	Coconut, cream, cnd	1	Tbs	19	68	285	6	<1	10	<1	3	2.9	0.1	<0.1
4511	Coconut, dried, shredded, swtnd, 7oz pkg	2	Tbs	11.625	58	243	1	<1	6	1	4	3.7	0.2	<0.1
4510	Coconut, dried, unswtnd	3	Tbs	15	99	414	<1	1	4	2	10	8.6	0.4	0.1
4508	Coconut, fresh, 2" × 2" × ½" pce	1	pce	45	159	665	21	1	7	4	15	13.4	0.6	0.2
4528	Coconut, milk, fresh	2	Tbs	30	69	289	20	1	2	1	7	6.3	0.3	0.1
4572	Nut Butter, almond	2	Tbs	32	196	820	1	7	6	3	18	2.1	10.4	4.4
4534	Nut Butter, almond, unsalted	2	Tbs	32	196	820	1	7	6	3	18	1.3	10.4	4.4
4626	Nut Butter, peanut, chunky	2	Tbs	32	188	787	<1	8	7	3	16	2.4	7.4	4.5
4576	Nut Butter, peanut, chunky, unsalted	2	Tbs	32	188	787	<1	8	7	3	16	2.4	7.4	4.5
39907	Nut Butter, sunflower seed, hint of sea salt, rstd	2	Tbs	32	180	753		9	8	4	12	1.5		
4503	Nuts, almonds, slivered	0.25	cup	27	155	649	1	6	6	3	13	1	8.3	3.3
4519	Nuts, cashews, dry rstd, salted, whole	0.25	cup	34.25	197	824	1	5	11	1	16	3.1	9.4	2.7
4621	Nuts, cashews, dry rstd, unsalted	0.25	cup	34.25	197	824	1	5	11	1	16	3.1	9.4	2.7
4596	Nuts, cashews, oil rstd, salted, whole	0.25	cup	32.25	187	782	1	5	10	1	15	2.7	8.4	2.8
4622	Nuts, cashews, oil rstd, unsalted, whole	0.25	cup	32.25	187	782	1	5	10	1	15	2.7	8.4	2.8
4538	Nuts, chestnuts, European, rstd	0.25	cup	35.75	88	368	14	1	19	2	1	0.1	0.3	0.3
4514	Nuts, hazelnuts, chpd	0.25	cup	28.75	181	757	2	4	5	3	17	1.3	13.1	2.3

< = Trace amount present   Blank = Not available

V, vitamin; **THI**, thiamin; **RIB**, riboflavin; **NIA**, niacin; **FOL**, folate; **CALC**, calcium; **PHOS**, phosphorus; **SOD**, sodium; **POT**, potassium; **MAG**, magnesium

CHOL (mg)	V-A (IU)	THI (mg)	RIB (mg)	NIA (mg)	$V\text{-}B_6$ (mg)	FOL (µg)	$V\text{-}B_{12}$ (µg)	V-C (mg)	V-E (mg)	CALC (mg)	PHOS (mg)	SOD (mg)	POT (mg)	MAG (mg)	IRON (mg)	ZINC (mg)
82	34	0.1	0.3	3.5	0.4	10	0.4	0		12	263	65	330	21	2.4	2.7
77	60	0.1	0.3	3.5	0.3	2	0.3	0	1.5	11	230	60	280	19	2.4	2.2
91	0	0.2	0.3	5.4	0.6	9	5.7	0	0.2	7	249	98	363	25	5.5	4.4
20	433	<0.1	<0.1	0.3	<0.1	8	1.2	0.3		9	26	91	18	2	0.7	0.1
9	3	<0.1	<0.1	0.9	<0.1	<1	0.1	0	<0.1	1	43	137	45	3	0.1	0.3
27	0	0.4	0.1	3.3	0.2	2	0.4	0	0.2	5	139	727	183	10	0.4	0.8
62	6	0.7	0.3	4.1	0.4	5	0.6	0.6	0.2	13	200	51	346	23	0.7	2
70	8	0.8	0.3	4.7	0.4	5	0.6	0.5	0.2	16	206	50	347	22	0.8	2
32	0	0.7	0.2	3.9	0.4	5	0.7	0	0.2	5	176	1085	284	14	0.8	1.6
47	0	0.6	0.2	4.3	0.4	3	0.6	0	0.2	6	193	1129	269	19	0.8	2.2
41	0	0.6	0.2	4.1	0.3	3	0.9	0	0.2	9	207	1047	248	14	0.9	2.5
84	0	0.4	0.2	4.6	0.4	0	0.8	0	0.1	26	166	48	238	18	1.1	3.6
84	4	0.5	0.4	6.7	0.4	0	0.8	0	0.2	26	200	77	332	19	0.8	3.4
109	15	0.1	0.3	5.7	0.4	8	1.4	0	0.1	14	180	88	193	23	1.2	3
76	65	0.1	0.2	7.2	0.5	6	1.1	0	0.1	23	208	64	241	25	1.2	2.6
68	9	<0.1	0.2	10	0.7	9	0.3	0	0.1	8	196	84	212	27	0.6	1.5
55	0							0		0		150			0	
86	12	<0.1	0.2	8.1	0.5	8	0.8	0	0.1	11	189	86	203	25	0.9	2.1
0	0	<0.1	<0.1	<0.1	<0.1	3	0	0	<0.1	1	4	7	19	3	<0.1	0.1
0	0	<0.1	<0.1	0.1	<0.1	1	0	0.1	<0.1	2	12	30	39	6	0.2	0.2
0	0	<0.1	<0.1	0.1	<0.1	1	0	0.2	0.1	4	31	6	81	14	0.5	0.3
0	0	<0.1	<0.1	0.2	<0.1	12	0	1.5	0.1	6	51	9	160	14	1.1	0.5
0	0	<0.1	0	0.2	<0.1	5	0	0.8	<0.1	5	30	4	79	11	0.5	0.2
0	<1	<0.1	0.3	1	<0.1	17	0	0	7.7	111	163	73	239	89	1.1	1.1
0	<1	<0.1	0.3	1	<0.1	17	0	0	7.7	111	163	2	239	89	1.1	1.1
0	0	<0.1	<0.1	4.4	0.1	29	0	0	2	14	102	156	238	51	0.6	0.9
0	0	<0.1	<0.1	4.4	0.1	29	0	0	2	14	102	5	238	51	0.6	0.9
0	0							0	4	0		65		100	1.4	
0	<1	0.1	0.3	0.9	<0.1	14	0	0	7.1	71	131	<1	190	72	1	0.8
0	0	0.1	0.1	0.5	0.1	24	0	0	0.3	15	168	219	194	89	2.1	1.9
0	0	0.1	0.1	0.5	0.1	24	0	0	0.3	15	168	5	194	89	2.1	1.9
0	0	0.1	0.1	0.6	0.1	8	0	0.1	0.3	14	171	99	204	88	2	1.7
0	0	0.1	0.1	0.6	0.1	8	0	0.1	0.3	14	171	4	204	88	2	1.7
0	9	0.1	0.1	0.5	0.2	25	0	9.3	0.2	10	38	1	212	12	0.3	0.2
0	6	0.2	<0.1	0.5	0.2	32	0	1.8	4.3	33	83	0	196	47	1.4	0.7

ESHA, EatRight Analysis; **AMT**, amount; **WT**, weight; **CAL**, calories; **KILO**, KiloJoule; **WTR**, water; **PROT**, protein; **CARB**, carbohydrate; **FIBR**, fiber; **FAT**, fat; **SATF**, saturated fat; **MONO**, monounsaturated fat; **POLY**, polyunsaturated fat; **CHOL**, cholesterol;

ESHA CODE	FOOD DESCRIPTION	AMT	UNIT	WT (g)	CAL (kcal)	KILO (kJ)	WTR (g)	PROT (g)	CARB (g)	FIBR (g)	FAT (g)	SATF (g)	MONO (g)	POLY (g)
NUTS AND SEEDS (CONTINUED)														
4513	Nuts, hazelnuts, whole	10	ea	14	88	368	1	2	2	1	9	0.6	6.4	1.1
4594	Nuts, mixed, w/o peanuts, oil rstd, unsalted	0.25	cup	36	221	925	1	6	8	2	20	3.3	11.9	4.1
4533	Nuts, mixed, with peanuts, oil rstd, unsalted	0.25	cup	33.5	203	849	1	7	7	2	18	2.9	9.5	4.9
4542	Nuts, peanuts, oil rstd, unsalted, chpd	0.25	cup	36	216	904	1	10	5	3	19	3.1	9.4	5.5
4577	Nuts, pecans, chpd	0.25	cup	27.25	188	787	1	2	4	3	20	1.7	11.1	5.9
4578	Nuts, pecans, halves	0.25	cup	24.75	171	715	1	2	3	2	18	1.5	10.1	5.3
4554	Nuts, pine, dried	1	oz	28.35	178	745	2	3	5	3	17	2.7	6.5	7.3
4521	Nuts, pistachio, raw	0.25	cup	30.75	173	724	1	6	8	3	14	1.7	7.3	4.2
4525	Nuts, walnuts, black, dried, chpd	0.25	cup	31.25	193	808	1	8	3	2	18	1.1	4.7	11
4556	Nuts, walnuts, English, dried, chpd	0.25	cup	29.25	191	799	1	4	4	2	19	1.8	2.6	13.8
4557	Nuts, walnuts, English, dried, halves	0.25	cup	25	164	686	1	4	3	2	16	1.5	2.2	11.8
4564	Seeds, pumpkin and squash, whole, rstd, salted	0.25	cup	16	71	297	1	3	9	3	3	0.6	1	1.4
4523	Seeds, sesame, whole, dried	0.25	cup	36	206	862	2	6	8	4	18	2.5	6.8	7.8
4545	Seeds, sunflower, kernels, dried	0.25	cup	35	204	854	2	7	7	3	18	1.6	6.5	8.1
4552	Seeds, sunflower, oil rstd, salted	0.25	cup	33.75	200	837	1	7	8	4	17	2.4	2.7	11.6
4532	Tahini, f/unrstd kernels	2	Tbs	28	170	711	1	5	5	3	16	2.2	6	6.9
PREPARED FOODS														
Canned Soups and Dishes														
7038	Baked Beans, vegetarian, cnd	0.5	cup	127	119	498	91	6	27	5	<1	0.1	0.1	0.2
7040	Baked Beans, with pork, cnd	0.5	cup	126.5	134	561	90	7	25	7	2	0.8	0.9	0.3
40704	Broth, beef, clear, rducd sodium, cnd, rts	1	cup	198	15	63	382	2	1	0	0	0	0	0
20057	Broth, beef, with tomato juice, 5.5 fl oz can	1	cup	244	90	377	219	1	21	<1	<1	0.1	0.1	0.1
50004	Broth, chicken, prep f/cnd with water	1	cup	244	39	163	234	5	1	0	1	0.4	0.6	0.3
50007	Chili, beef, prep f/cnd with water	1	cup	261	149	623	224	6	24	3	3	1.6	1.3	0.1
56001	Chili, with beans, cnd	1	cup	256	287	1201	193	15	30	11	14	6	6	0.9
17406	Chili, vegetarian, cnd	1	cup	230	290	1213	167	24	25	8	10	1.6	2.1	6.7
70688	Chow Mein, beef, bi-pack, cnd	1	cup	246	80	335		7	11	3	1	0		
70699	Chow Mein, chicken, bi-pack, cnd	1	cup	250	100	418		5	11	3	4	1		
50093	Chowder, clam, Manhattan style, chunky, cnd, rts	1	cup	240	134	561	206	7	19	3	3	2.1	1	0.1
50008	Chowder, clam, New England, prep f/cnd with milk	1	cup	252	154	644	215	8	19	1	5	2.8	0.7	1.3
50098	Consomme, beef, prep with water, 10.5oz can	1	cup	241	29	121	232	5	2	0	0	0	0	0
70696	Dish, beef, pepper oriental, bi-pack, cnd	1	cup	252	80	335		7	11	1	1	0		
5068	Dish, creamed corn, yellow, sweet, cnd	0.5	cup	128	92	385	101	2	23	2	1	0.1	0.2	0.3
5552	Dish, sweet potatoes, with syrup, 4oz can	1	cup	228	203	849	176	2	48	6	<1	0.1	<0.1	0.2
7023	Pork and Beans, with sweet sauce, cnd	0.5	cup	124.5	138	577	88	6	26	5	2	0.4	0.4	0.7
7004	Pork and Beans, with tomato sauce, cnd	0.5	cup	123	116	485	90	6	23	5	1	0.4	0.3	0.2

< = Trace amount present   Blank = Not available

V, vitamin; **THI**, thiamin; **RIB**, riboflavin; **NIA**, niacin; **FOL**, folate; **CALC**, calcium; **PHOS**, phosphorus; **SOD**, sodium; **POT**, potassium; **MAG**, magnesium

CHOL (mg)	V-A (IU)	THI (mg)	RIB (mg)	NIA (mg)	V-B_6 (mg)	FOL (μg)	V-B_{12} (μg)	V-C (mg)	V-E (mg)	CALC (mg)	PHOS (mg)	SOD (mg)	POT (mg)	MAG (mg)	IRON (mg)	ZINC (mg)
0	3	0.1	<0.1	0.3	0.1	16	0	0.9	2.1	16	41	0	95	23	0.7	0.3
0	7	0.2	0.2	0.7	0.1	20	0	0.2		38	162	4	196	90	0.9	1.7
0	1	0.1	0.1	2.6	0.1	28	0	0.2	2.6	39	153	2	212	77	0.9	1.1
0	0	<0.1	<0.1	5	0.2	43	0	0.3	2.5	22	143	2	261	63	0.5	1.2
0	15	0.2	<0.1	0.3	0.1	6	0	0.3	0.4	19	75	0	112	33	0.7	1.2
0	14	0.2	<0.1	0.3	0.1	5	0	0.3	0.3	17	69	0	101	30	0.6	1.1
0	8	0.4	0.1	1.2	<0.1	16	0	0.6		2	10	20	178	66	0.9	1.2
0	128	0.3	<0.1	0.4	0.5	16	0	1.7	0.7	32	151	<1	315	37	1.2	0.7
0	12	<0.1	<0.1	0.1	0.2	10	0	0.5	0.6	19	160	1	163	63	1	1.1
0	6	0.1	<0.1	0.3	0.2	29	0	0.4	0.2	29	101	1	129	46	0.9	0.9
0	5	0.1	<0.1	0.3	0.1	24	0	0.3	0.2	24	86	<1	110	40	0.7	0.8
0	10	<0.1	<0.1	<0.1	<0.1	1	0	<1		9	15	407	147	42	0.5	1.6
0	3	0.3	0.1	1.6	0.3	35	0	0	0.1	351	226	4	168	126	5.2	2.8
0	18	0.5	0.1	2.9	0.5	79	0	0.5	12.3	27	231	3	226	114	1.8	1.8
0	3	0.1	0.1	1.4	0.3	79	0	0.4	12.3	29	384	247	163	43	1.4	1.8
0	19	0.4	<0.1	1.6	<0.1	27	0	0		39	221	<1	129	99	1.8	2.9
0	137	0.1	<0.1	0.5	0.1	15	0	0	0.2	43	94	436	284	34	1.5	2.9
9	0	0.1	<0.1	0.6	0.1	46	0	2.5		67	137	524	391	43	2.2	1.8
5	0							0		0		440			0	
0	312	<0.1	0.1	0.4	0.1	10	0.1	2.2		27	32	320	234	7	1.4	<0.1
0	0	<0.1	0.1	3.3	<0.1	5	0.2	0	<0.1	10	73	747	210	2	0.5	0.2
13	1469	0.1	0.1	1	0.2	10	0.4	3.9	1.4	47	144	1013	512	26	2.1	2
44	863	0.1	0.3	0.9	0.3	59	0	4.4	1.3	120	394	1336	934	115	8.8	5.1
0	0	0.2	0.2	2.1	0.7		1.6	0		41	177	1042	370		3.7	1.8
10	1250							12		20		920			1.1	
15	1500							12		20		1520			0.7	
14	3216	0.1	0.1	1.8	0.3	10	7.9	12.2	1.6	67	84	1001	384	19	2.6	1.7
18	320	0.2	0.4	2	0.2	23	12.2	5.3	0.6	176	436	688	451	30	3	1.1
0	0	<0.1	<0.1	0.7	<0.1	2	0	1		10	31	636	154	0	0.5	0.4
15	750							4.8		20		1240			1.8	
0	95	<0.1	0.1	1.2	0.1	58	0	5.9	0.1	4	65	365	172	22	0.5	0.7
0	17168	0.1	0.1	1	0.1	16	0	23.9	2.1	34	62	100	422	30	1.8	0.4
1	20	0.1	0.1	0.4	0.1	10	0	3.4	0.1	71	126	420	317	40	2.1	1
9	103	0.1	0.1	0.6	0.1	18	0	3.7	0.1	69	143	538	363	42	4	6.7

ESHA, EatRight Analysis; **AMT**, amount; **WT**, weight; **CAL**, calories; **KILO**, KiloJoule; **WTR**, water; **PROT**, protein; **CARB**, carbohydrate; **FIBR**, fiber; **FAT**, fat; **SATF**, saturated fat; **MONO**, monounsaturated fat; **POLY**, polyunsaturated fat; **CHOL**, cholesterol;

ESHA CODE	FOOD DESCRIPTION	AMT	UNIT	WT (g)	CAL (kcal)	KILO (kJ)	WTR (g)	PROT (g)	CARB (g)	FIBR (g)	FAT (g)	SATF (g)	MONO (g)	POLY (g)
PREPARED FOODS (CONTINUED)														
38948	Ravioli, meat, with tomato/meat sauce, cnd	1	cup	262	259	1084	205	9	36	4	9	3.7	4.2	0.6
7024	Refried Beans, cnd	0.5	cup	119	108	452	91	6	18	6	1	0.5	0.5	0.4
50000	Soup, bean and bacon, prep f/cnd with water	1	cup	266	168	703	227	8	22	8	6	1.5	2.1	1.8
90356	Soup, beef mushroom, prep with water, 10.75oz can	1	cup	244	73	305	226	6	6	<1	3	1.5	1.2	0.1
90299	Soup, beef noodle, prep with water, 10.75oz can	1	cup	244	83	347	225	5	9	1	3	1.1	1.2	0.5
50066	Soup, beef, chunky, rts, 19oz can	1	cup	245	162	678	204	10	25	1	3	1.4	1.1	0.1
50060	Soup, black bean, prep with water, 11oz can	1	cup	247	114	477	216	6	19	8	2	0.4	0.6	0.5
50071	Soup, cheese, prep with milk, 11oz can	1	cup	251	231	967	207	9	16	1	15	9.1	4.1	0.5
90302	Soup, chicken dumplings, prep with water, 10.5oz can	1	cup	241	96	402	221	6	6	<1	6	1.3	2.5	1.3
50005	Soup, chicken noodle, prep f/cnd with water	1	cup	248	62	259	233	3	7	<1	2	0.6	1	0.7
50020	Soup, chicken rice, prep f/cnd with water	1	cup	243	58	243	228	4	7	1	2	0.4	0.9	0.4
50921	Soup, chicken veg, chunky, rducd fat and sod, rts, cnd	1	cup	240	96	402	215	6	15		1	0.3	0.4	0.3
50091	Soup, chicken vegetable, prep f/cnd with water	1	cup	248	77	322	230	4	9	1	3	0.9	1.3	0.6
40675	Soup, cream of broccoli, At Hand, rts, microwv	1	svg	305	143	598	275	3	17	7	7	2		
90284	Soup, cream of chicken, prep with milk, 10.75oz can	1	cup	248	191	799	210	7	15	<1	11	4.6	4.5	1.6
90305	Soup, cream of chicken, prep with water, 10.75oz can	1	cup	244	117	490	221	3	9	<1	7	2.1	3.3	1.5
50011	Soup, cream of mushroom, prep f/cnd with milk	1	cup	252	161	674	219	6	15	1	9	2.8	2.2	3.6
50049	Soup, cream of mushroom, prep f/cnd with water	1	cup	248	97	406	229	2	8	1	6	1.2	1.5	3.5
90290	Soup, cream of potato, prep with milk, 10.75oz can	1	cup	248	149	623	215	6	17	<1	6	3.8	1.7	0.6
50103	Soup, gazpacho, rts, 13oz can	1	cup	244	46	192	229	7	4	<1	<1	<0.1	<0.1	0.1
50999	Soup, gumbo, zesty, chicken and sausage, rts, cnd	1	can	244	100	418		5	15	2	2	0.5		
39764	Soup, lentil, traditional, rts, microwv	1	cup	250	150	628		7	27	5	2	0.5		
50105	Soup, lentil, with ham, rts, 20oz can	1	cup	248	139	582	213	9	20		3	1.1	1.3	0.3
28181	Soup, lobster bisque, with white wine, semi-cond	0.67	cup	152.5	160	669		4	12	1	11	5		
50009	Soup, minestrone, prep f/cnd with water	1	cup	241	82	343	220	4	11	1	3	0.6	0.7	1.1
50025	Soup, split pea, with ham, prep f/cnd with water	1	cup	253	190	795	207	10	28	2	4	1.8	1.8	0.6
50135	Soup, tomato bisque, prep f/cnd with water	1	cup	247	124	519	215	2	24	<1	3	0.5	0.7	1.1
50012	Soup, tomato, prep f/cnd with milk	1	cup	252	139	582	217	6	23	2	3	1.8	0.8	0.3

< = Trace amount present   Blank = Not available

V, vitamin; **THI**, thiamin; **RIB**, riboflavin; **NIA**, niacin; **FOL**, folate; **CALC**, calcium; **PHOS**, phosphorus; **SOD**, sodium; **POT**, potassium; **MAG**, magnesium

CHOL (mg)	V-A (IU)	THI (mg)	RIB (mg)	NIA (mg)	V-B_6 (mg)	FOL (μg)	V-B_{12} (μg)	V-C (mg)	V-E (mg)	CALC (mg)	PHOS (mg)	SOD (mg)	POT (mg)	MAG (mg)	IRON (mg)	ZINC (mg)
13	582	0.1	0.2	3.4	0.2	55	0.4	0	1.4	34	113	927	443	34	2.8	1.2
0	0	<0.1	<0.1	0.5	0.1	13	0	7.1	0.1	39	132	534	400	45	2	0.8
3	862	0.1	<0.1	0.5	<0.1	32	<0.1	1.6	1.1	82	128	928	391	45	2	1
7	0	<0.1	0.1	1	<0.1	10	0.2	4.6		5	34	942	154	10	0.9	1.5
5	246	0.1	0.1	1	<0.1	20	0.2	0.5	1.2	20	46	793	98	7	1.1	1.5
15	2666	0.1	0.2	2.8	0.1	15	0.6	7.1	0.7	32	122	828	343	5	2.4	2.7
0	548	0.1	<0.1	0.5	0.1	82	0	0.2	0.4	47	94	1203	309	42	1.9	1.4
48	1242	0.1	0.3	0.5	0.1	10	0.4	1.3		289	251	1019	341	20	0.8	0.7
34	525	<0.1	0.1	1.8	<0.1	2	0.2	0	0.6	14	60	735	116	5	0.6	0.4
12	498	0.1	0.1	1.3	<0.1	20	<0.1	0	0.1	15	42	866	55	10	1.6	0.4
7	413	<0.1	<0.1	1.1	<0.1	0	0.2	0.2	0.1	22	22	578	100	0	0.8	0.3
10	3079											461				
10	1905	<0.1	0.1	1.3	<0.1	5	0.1	1	0.4	17	42	972	159	7	0.9	0.4
6	101							0		21		891			0.7	
27	714	0.1	0.3	0.9	0.1	7	0.5	1.2		181	151	898	273	17	0.7	0.7
10	561	<0.1	0.1	0.8	<0.1	2	0.1	0.2		34	37	847	88	2	0.6	0.6
10	257	0.1	0.3	0.5	0.1	8	0.7	0.3	0.7	171	149	900	260	18	0.3	0.8
0	10	<0.1	<0.1	0.4	<0.1	2	0	0	0.6	17	30	843	77	5	0.2	0.1
22	444	0.1	0.2	0.6	0.1	10	0.5	1.2		166	161	570	322	17	0.5	0.7
0	298	<0.1	<0.1	0.9	0.1	20	0	7.1	0.4	24	37	739	224	7	1	0.2
10	100							0		60		460			0.7	
5	750							0		80		440			2.7	
7	360	0.2	0.1	1.4	0.2	50	0.3	4.2		42	184	1319	357	22	2.7	0.7
40	200							0		40		1090			0.7	
2	2338	0.1	<0.1	0.9	0.1	36	0	1.2		34	55	612	313	7	0.9	0.7
8	445	0.1	0.1	1.5	0.1	3	0.3	1.5		23	213	1007	400	48	2.3	1.3
5	721	0.1	0.1	1.1	0.1	15	0	5.9		40	59	1047	417	10	0.8	0.6
10	723	0.1	0.3	1.4	0.2	5	0.7	15.9	0.5	174	156	529	461	30	1.4	0.9

ESHA, EatRight Analysis; **AMT**, amount; **WT**, weight; **CAL**, calories; **KILO**, KiloJoule; **WTR**, water; **PROT**, protein; **CARB**, carbohydrate; **FIBR**, fiber; **FAT**, fat; **SATF**, saturated fat; **MONO**, monounsaturated fat; **POLY**, polyunsaturated fat; **CHOL**, cholesterol;

ESHA CODE	FOOD DESCRIPTION	AMT	UNIT	WT (g)	CAL (kcal)	KILO (kJ)	WTR (g)	PROT (g)	CARB (g)	FIBR (g)	FAT (g)	SATF (g)	MONO (g)	POLY (g)
PREPARED FOODS (CONTINUED)														
50028	Soup, tomato, prep f/cnd with water	1	cup	248	74	310	227	2	16	1	1	0.2	0.2	0.2
50145	Soup, vegetable, chunky, rts, 19oz can	1	can	539	275	1151	472	8	43	3	8	1.2	3.6	3.1
50013	Soup, vegetable, vegetarian, prep f/cnd with water	1	cup	244	68	285	225	2	12	1	2	0.3	0.8	0.7
90291	Soup, vichyssoise, prep with milk, 10.75oz can	1	cup	248	149	623	215	6	17	<1	6	3.8	1.7	0.6
50181	Soup, won ton	1	cup	241	182	761	203	14	14	1	7	2.3	3	1
57659	Stew, beef, cnd, svg	1	svg	196	194	812	158	9	15	2	11	4.3	5	0.5
50024	Stew, oyster, prep with milk, 10.5oz can	1	cup	245	135	565	218	6	10	0	8	5	2.1	0.3
Dried Soups and Dishes														
15764	Broth, beef, prep f/dry cube with water	1	cup	240	7	29	237	1	1	0	<1	0.1	0.1	<0.1
50193	Broth, chicken, dehyd, cube	1	cube	4.8	10	42	<1	1	1	0	<1	0.1	0.1	0.1
50035	Broth, chicken, prep f/dehyd cube with water	1	cup	243	12	50	237	1	2		<1	0.1	0.1	0.1
5276	Casserole, potato au gratin, prep f/dry with water milk butter	1	svg	137	127	531	108	3	18	1	6	3.5	1.6	0.2
5271	Casserole, scalloped potatoes, prep f/dry with whl milk btr, svg	1	svg	137	127	531	108	3	17	2	6	3.6	1.7	0.3
52166	Fried Rice, Country Inn, Oriental, dry	1	dry svg	57	200	837		6	42	1	1	0		
5464	Mashed Potatoes, flakes, prep f/dry with milk and butter	0.5	cup	105	102	427	85	2	11	1	5	3.4	1.4	0.2
57711	Pasta Dish, Hamburger Helper, cheeseburger macaroni, dry mix	0.33	cup	32	110	460		3	23	1	<1	0		
57323	Pasta Dish, with creamy garlic sauce, dry	0.67	cup	69	270	1130		8	47	1	5	3.5		
57331	Pilaf, rice, dry	0.5	cup	61	220	920	4	6	46	1	1	0		
38613	Pilaf, rice, herb and butter, dry	0.33	cup	70	240	1004		5	52	1	2	0.5		
38619	Pilaf, rice, with red beans, dry	0.33	cup	70	240	1004		8	51	5	2	0		
57333	Rice Dish, Spanish, dry	0.5	cup	67	240	1004		6	51	2	1	0		
50037	Soup, chicken noodle, prep f/dehyd with water	1	cup	245	56	234	231	2	9	<1	1	0.3	0.5	0.4
15770	Soup, onion, prep f/dehyd with water	1	cup	230	28	117	220	1	6	1	<1	<0.1	<0.1	<0.1
57534	Stroganoff, Hamburger Helper, dry svg	0.5	cup	36	130	544		4	26	1	1	0		
Frozen Meals														
11118	Meal, beef, pot roast, with red potatoes, carrots, dessert, fzn	1	meal	312	280	1172		17	41	6	4	1.5	1	2
70127	Meal, cabbage, stuffed with meat and tomato sauce, low cal, fzn	1	ea	305	247	1033	253	16	22	3	11	3.9	4.5	0.9
16194	Meal, chicken enchilada suiza, with Mexican style rice, fzn	1	meal	255.15	280	1172		10	48	3	5	2	1	1
17888	Meal, chicken fajita, supreme, with veg rice and beans, fzn	1	pkg	262	260	1088		17	32	4	7	3	2	1.5
16263	Meal, chicken, country herb, with red potato, veg, dessert, fzn	1	meal	322	270	1130		17	37	7	5	1.5	1.5	2

< = Trace amount present   Blank = Not available

V, vitamin; **THI**, thiamin; **RIB**, riboflavin; **NIA**, niacin; **FOL**, folate; **CALC**, calcium; **PHOS**, phosphorus; **SOD**, sodium; **POT**, potassium; **MAG**, magnesium

CHOL (mg)	V-A (IU)	THI (mg)	RIB (mg)	NIA (mg)	$V\text{-}B_6$ (mg)	FOL (µg)	$V\text{-}B_{12}$ (µg)	V-C (mg)	V-E (mg)	CALC (mg)	PHOS (mg)	SOD (mg)	POT (mg)	MAG (mg)	IRON (mg)	ZINC (mg)
0	476	<0.1	0.1	1.3	0.1	0	0	15.6	0.4	20	35	471	278	17	1.3	0.3
0	13200	0.2	0.1	2.7	0.4	38	0	13.5	2.9	124	162	1935	889	16	3.7	7
0	3467	0.1	<0.1	0.9	0.1	10	0	1.5	1.4	24	34	825	210	7	1.1	0.5
22	444	0.1	0.2	0.6	0.1	10	0.5	1.2		166	161	570	322	17	0.5	0.7
53	896	0.4	0.3	4.6	0.2	19	0.4	3.4	0.4	31	153	543	316	21	1.8	1.1
25	437	0.1	0.1	2.1	0.2	27	1	1.4	0.5	24	82	760	319	16	4.9	2
32	225	0.1	0.2	0.3	0.1	10	2.6	4.4		167	162	1041	235	20	1.1	10.3
0	0	<0.1	<0.1	0.1	<0.1	0	<0.1	0	<0.1	10	7	624	14	5	<0.1	<0.1
1	<1	<0.1	<0.1	0.2	<0.1	2	<0.1	<1	<0.1	9	9	1152	18	3	0.1	<0.1
0	17	<0.1	<0.1	0.3	0	2	<0.1	0		12	12	792	24	2	0.1	<0.1
21	292	<0.1	0.1	1.3	0.1	10	0	4.2		114	130	601	300	21	0.4	0.3
15	203	<0.1	0.1	1.4	0.1	14	0	4.5		49	77	467	278	19	0.5	0.3
0	1000	0.4		3		120		2.4		20		580			3.6	
15	181	0.1	0.1	0.8	0.1	7	0.1	10.2	0.1	34	41	172	172	12	0.2	0.2
0	0	0.2	0.1	1.6		40		0		0		810	60		0.7	
10	0	0.5	0.2	4		120		0		40		740	0		1.8	
0	0	0.4	0.1	4		100		0		20		880	0		1.8	
0	100	0.3	0.1	2		100		1.2		20		1070			1.8	
0	200	0.2	0.1	1.6		140		15		60		1110			1.8	
0	200	0.4	0.1	4		100		4.8		20		880	0		2.7	
10	27	0.2	0.1	1.1	<0.1	17	<0.1	0	0.1	5	29	561	32	7	0.5	0.2
0	2	<0.1	<0.1	0.1	0.1	0	0	0.2	<0.1	21	21	796	71	9	0.1	0.1
0	0	0.2	0.1	1.6		40		0		20		780	120		0.7	
40	2500		0.2	3	0.2	100	1.5	30		40	200	500	800		1.8	3
49	3269	0.2	0.2	4.1	0.4	31	1.3	26.2	1	49	163	691	553	39	2.1	3.2
20												600	380			
40	1000							15		100		600			1.1	
40	750	0.2	0.2	5	0.2	100	0.6	12		60	200	430	760	40	0.7	

ESHA, EatRight Analysis; **AMT**, amount; **WT**, weight; **CAL**, calories; **KILO**, KiloJoule; **WTR**, water; **PROT**, protein; **CARB**, carbohydrate; **FIBR**, fiber; **FAT**, fat; **SATF**, saturated fat; **MONO**, monounsaturated fat; **POLY**, polyunsaturated fat; **CHOL**, cholesterol;

ESHA CODE	FOOD DESCRIPTION	AMT	UNIT	WT (g)	CAL (kcal)	KILO (kJ)	WTR (g)	PROT (g)	CARB (g)	FIBR (g)	FAT (g)	SATF (g)	MONO (g)	POLY (g)
PREPARED FOODS (CONTINUED)														
15967	Meal, chicken, parmesan, with spaghetti and cheese, fzn	1	cntr	308.31	310	1297	729	21	39	5	8	2	2	3
16260	Meal, chicken, pesto alfredo, with pasta, veg, dessert, fzn	1	meal	326	300	1255		20	39	7	7	2.5	1.5	2.5
70379	Meal, fish and chips, fried battered portions	1	cntr	284	490	2050		19	59	5	20	4		
18260	Meal, fish, breaded, lemon pepper, with rice and vegetables, fzn	1	cntr	255.15	330	1381		15	50	2	8	2.5	2	3.5
18825	Meal, fish, lemon pepper, with rice, broccoli, dessert, fzn	1	meal	303	300	1255		14	49	5	5	1	1.5	2
81080	Meal, manicotti, marinara formaggio, with broccoli, dessert, frozen	1	meal	333	350	1464		13	61	8	6	3	1	2
11093	Meal, meatloaf, with whipped potatoes and gravy, fzn	1	cntr	265.78	260	1088		21	25	3	8	3	2.5	2.5
70767	Meal, Mexican style	1	meal	567	690	2887	2382	26	87	13	27	9		
11063	Meal, steak, salisbury	1	cntr	312	340	1423		16	35	6	15	6		
Frozen Dishes														
56737	Cannelloni, four cheese, fzn	1	cntr	258.69	240	1004		17	30	3	6	3	1.5	1
18820	Casserole, tuna noodle, fzn	1	cntr	340.2	450	1883	835	22	45	3	20	6		
18139	Chicken and Dumplings, skillet, Easy Express, fzn	1	svg	340.2	370	1548	884	23	41	5	13	3.5		
49343	Chile Relleno, fire rstd, with salsa, fzn	1	pkg	284	350	1464		22	27	4	18	11		
15964	Chow Mein, chicken, with stir fry vegetables and rice, fzn	1	cntr	255.15	260	1088		14	41	3	4	1	1.5	1.5
4104	Dish, chicken and noodles, escalloped, fzn, family	1	svg	226.8	330	1381	372	14	28	2	18	4		
81223	Dish, chicken breast, patty, brd, ckd f/fzn	1	ea	90	210	879		13	10	0	13	3		
16252	Dish, chicken, alfredo florentine, with penne, fzn	1	entree	241	220	920		16	28	4	4	2	1	1.5
17880	Dish, chicken, Oriental, with veg and rice, fzn	1	pkg	255	230	962		12	39	2	2	0.5	0.5	1
16200	Dish, chicken, parmigiana, with spaghetti, fzn	1	cntr	340.2	410	1715	858	23	47	4	14	3.5		
39707	Dish, chicken, rosemary and sweet potato, fzn	1	entree	255	170	711		12	23	5	2	1	0.5	1
17927	Dish, chicken, Thai style, with peanut sauce and noodles, fzn	1	pkg	255	260	1088		14	43	2	4	0.5	1.5	1
18229	Dish, chicken, Tuscan, with linguine and vegetables, fzn	1	svg	340.2	280	1172		22	34	5	6	2	2	1.5
83170	Dish, chicken, Voila, teriyaki, with veg, rducd carb, fzn	1	svg	212	150	628		17	15	4	2	0.5		
70259	Dish, fish fillet, battered, fzn	1	svg	75	180	753	31	8	12	0	11			
4110	Dish, green peppers, stuffed, with beef and rice, fzn, family	1	cntr	226.8	210	879		11	20	3	9	3		
7758	Dish, loaf, vegetarian, lentil rice, fzn, 1" slice	1	in slc	90	160	669		8	16	4	7	1	1.5	4.5

< = Trace amount present Blank = Not available

V, vitamin; **THI**, thiamin; **RIB**, riboflavin; **NIA**, niacin; **FOL**, folate; **CALC**, calcium; **PHOS**, phosphorus; **SOD**, sodium; **POT**, potassium; **MAG**, magnesium

CHOL (mg)	V-A (IU)	THI (mg)	RIB (mg)	NIA (mg)	V-B_6 (mg)	FOL (µg)	V-B_{12} (µg)	V-C (mg)	V-E (mg)	CALC (mg)	PHOS (mg)	SOD (mg)	POT (mg)	MAG (mg)	IRON (mg)	ZINC (mg)
35	500							18		150		660	820			
45	1000	0.2	0.2	4		60	0.6	6		100	250	580	670	60	1.4	
45	100							2.4		60		1030			1.4	
40	500	1	0.9	8.3	1.1	131	1.9	30	1.2	60	231	590	370	58	2.9	1.1
25	400	0.2	0.2		0.2	140	1.2	24		40	150	360	480	40	0.7	
30	500	0.2	0.3			140	0.9	21		350	350	570	670	60	1.8	1.5
35	0							0		80		610	880			
35	1500							36		300		2170			3.6	
30	5000							6		80		920			2.7	
20	400	0.2	0.4	2.5	0.2	54	0.7	2.4	2.3	250	291	690	480	47	2.9	1.7
70	200							1.2		200		990			1.1	
60	4500							2.4		80		1120			1.4	
50	2500							264		450		1160			3.6	
25	2250	0.2	0.2	5.1	0.3	73	0.7	3.6	0.8	60	177	550	380	35	2.3	0.8
35	400							0		100		910			0.7	
45	0							0		0		400			0.7	
30	1250	0.2	0.1	1.6	0.1	140	0.6	4.8		100	200	560	280	60	1.1	1.5
35	1000							1.2		40		640			0.4	
40	500							0		150		900			1.8	
30	5000			3		60	0.5	2.4		40	150	500	690	40	0.7	
25	2500							1.2		40		570			0.7	
40	750							4.8		60		780	640			
25	1750							12		20		990			0.4	
20											200		190			
20	100							6		60		1180			1.4	
0	500							0		20		350	150		1.1	

ESHA, EatRight Analysis; **AMT**, amount; **WT**, weight; **CAL**, calories; **KILO**, KiloJoule; **WTR**, water; **PROT**, protein; **CARB**, carbohydrate; **FIBR**, fiber; **FAT**, fat; **SATF**, saturated fat; **MONO**, monounsaturated fat; **POLY**, polyunsaturated fat; **CHOL**, cholesterol;

ESHA CODE	FOOD DESCRIPTION	AMT	UNIT	WT (g)	CAL (kcal)	KILO (kJ)	WTR (g)	PROT (g)	CARB (g)	FIBR (g)	FAT (g)	SATF (g)	MONO (g)	POLY (g)
PREPARED FOODS (CONTINUED)														
7669	Dish, loaf, vegetarian, nine bean, fzn, 1" slice	1	in slc	91	150	628		8	15	4	7	1.5	2	3.5
5265	Dish, potato puffs, ckd f/fzn	1	cup	128	243	1017	76	3	36	3	11	2.3	7.7	0.6
977	Dish, skillet, Easy Express, steak teriyaki, with rice veg, fzn	1	cntr	333.11	310	1297		17	49	6	5	2		
36301	Egg Roll, chicken, w/o sauce, fzn	1	ea	70	120	502		5	12	2	6	1		
31465	Flauta, chipotle chicken and cheese	2	ea	142	310	1297		20	38	2	9	2		
31466	Flauta, shredded steak, with cheese and green chilies	2	ea	142	330	1381		21	39	2	10	3		
5791	French Fries, cottage cut, fzn	10	ea	65	99	414	43	2	16	2	4	1.8	1.5	0.3
5139	French Fries, extruded, ckd f/fzn w/o salt	10	ea	50	166	695	18	2	20	2	9	3	5.7	0.7
42368	Garlic Bread, hot and crusty, fzn, 2" slice	2	in slc	50	170	711		5	21	1	8	2		
56740	Lasagna, with meat sauce, fzn	1	cntr	297.68	320	1339		20	43	4	7	3.5	2	1
56702	Macaroni and Cheese, fzn	1	cntr	283.5	290	1213		15	41	1	7	4	1.5	1
14072	Meatloaf, with beef and pork	1	pce	108	214	895	69	19	7	<1	12	4.2	5.2	0.7
5190	Onion Rings, breaded, par fried, ckd f/fzn, lrg, 3-4" ea	10	ea	71	289	1209	20	4	27	1	19	6.1	7.7	3.6
39699	Pasta Dish, portabella spinach parmesan, fzn	1	entree	266	270	1130		12	38	5	7	2.5	1	3.5
56997	Pizza, bagel, cheese sausage pepperoni, fzn	4	ea	88	210	879	36	8	30	2	7	3		
92888	Pizza, chicken tomato and spinach, thin crispy crust, fzn	1	slice	133	260	1088		16	33	2	8	3.5		
56733	Pizza, French bread, cheese, fzn	1	cntr	170.1	340	1423		17	53	5	7	3	1.5	1
56735	Pizza, French bread, pepperoni, fzn	1	cntr	148.84	330	1381		17	46	4	9	2.5	2.5	3
56736	Pizza, French bread, with pepperoni sausage mushroom, fzn	1	cntr	173.64	340	1423		16	46	4	10	3.5	2.5	1.5
70734	Pot Pie, beef	1	ea	198	415	1736	239	11	41	2	23	9		
16234	Pot Pie, beef, fzn	1	ea	198	390	1632		12	36	3	22	9		
70893	Pot Pie, beef, prep f/fzn	1	ea	268	590	2469	156	19	59	2	31	11.1	14.2	3.9
18493	Pot Pie, chicken, white meat, fzn, large	1	svg	226.8	580	2427		21	50	0	33	13		
16928	Pot Pie, turkey, fzn	1	ea	198	380	1590		10	35	3	21	8		
5269	Potatoes O'Brien, prep f/fzn	0.5	cup	97	198	828	60	2	21	2	13	3.2	5.6	3.4
56868	Ravioli, cheese, with tomato sauce, fzn	1	cntr	340.2	380	1590		19	47	5	13	8		
56901	Ravioli, cheese, with tomato sauce, fzn	1	cntr	240.98	240	1004		11	38	3	6	3.5	1	0.5
39697	Ravioli, lobster, cheese, with zucchini, fzn	1	entree	255	260	1088		11	40	4	6	2.5	1	2
39700	Ravioli, pumpkin squash, with asparagus, fzn	1	entree	261	300	1255		9	52	5	6	2.5	1	2.5
57544	Sandwich, pocket, bbq beef, fzn	1	ea	127	310	1297		11	42	1	10	3.3	3.3	3.3
56076	Souffle, spinach	1	cup	136	230	962	96	11	8	1	18	10.1	5	1
56732	Spaghetti, with meatballs and sauce, fzn	1	svg	269	270	1130		16	38	3	6	2	2	1
17002	Sticks, fish, ckd f/fzn, 4" × 1" × ½"	1	ea	28	70	293	15	3	6	<1	4	0.8	1.2	1.6

< = Trace amount present   Blank = Not available

V, vitamin; **THI**, thiamin; **RIB**, riboflavin; **NIA**, niacin; **FOL**, folate; **CALC**, calcium; **PHOS**, phosphorus; **SOD**, sodium; **POT**, potassium; **MAG**, magnesium

CHOL (mg)	V-A (IU)	THI (mg)	RIB (mg)	NIA (mg)	$V\text{-}B_6$ (mg)	FOL (µg)	$V\text{-}B_{12}$ (µg)	V-C (mg)	V-E (mg)	CALC (mg)	PHOS (mg)	SOD (mg)	POT (mg)	MAG (mg)	IRON (mg)	ZINC (mg)
5	500							1.2		40		320	200		0.7	
0	6	0.2	<0.1	1.9	0.2	18	0	8.1	0.3	18	132	591	399	22	0.8	0.4
25	3000							2.4		40		1390			1.4	
15	1750	0.1	0.1	1.4	0.1	34	<0.1	6		20	64	330	138	14	1.1	0.5
35	100							3.6		60		670			2.7	
35	100							15		60		730			3.6	
0	0	0.1	<0.1	1.2	0.1	10	0	5.5		5	30	21	220	10	0.7	0.2
0	0	<0.1	<0.1	1.3	0.1	11	0	3.1		6	48	306	270	12	0.8	0.2
6	200							3.6		40		310			1.1	
30	500	0.4	0.5	3.4	0.5	75	0.7	3.6	0.9	200	313	590	710	50	3.8	2.2
20	0	0.9	1	5.1	0.7	101	1.1	0	0.1	300	264	630	560	40	1.7	1.5
87	70	0.2	0.3	4.1	0.2	11	1.4	0.7	0.2	44	176	129	317	23	1.8	3.2
0	160	0.2	0.1	2.6	0.1	47	0	1		22	58	266	92	13	1.2	0.3
10	750	0.1		0.4	0.2	24	0.5	2.4		150	200	580	290	60	1.1	1.5
14	200							0		80		410	280		0.7	
25	500							1.2		200		550			1.4	
15	400							4.8		350		680	310			
15	300							6		200		690	290			
20	400	0.5	0.4	4.1	0.2	101	0.3	12	1.3	150	191	760	330	30	3.2	1.2
25	750							0		20		740			1.8	
30	40	0.1	0.1	1.6		24	0.5	0		0	100	1010	190	16	1.1	
56		0.5	0.2	4.4	0.4	48	0.9	0.8	0.7	38	180	978	308	35	3.4	2.9
60	1250							0		100		890			2.7	
30	1000	0.1	0.1	1.2		32	0.5	0		40	150	1030	210		0.7	1.5
0	182	0.1	0.1	1.4	0.4	12	0	10.1		19	90	42	459	33	0.9	0.5
80	1000							9		300		1000			1.8	
40	400							1.2		150		600	540			
15	300		0.2		0.2	60	1.2	6		200	150	600	590	40	1.1	
10	2000	0.4	0.2	0.8		140	0.5	6		80	150	600	410	40	1.1	1.2
25	100	0.3	0.2	3		60	0.6			100	100	800			2.7	
160	3932	0.1	0.4	0.7	0.1	99	0.5	9.9	1.3	224	189	770	314	41	1.6	1.2
25					0.2	26	0.7		0.5		88	579	509	19		1.2
8	24	<0.1	<0.1	0.4	<0.1	9	0.4	0	0.3	7	51	118	60	8	0.3	0.1

ESHA, EatRight Analysis; **AMT**, amount; **WT**, weight; **CAL**, calories; **KILO**, KiloJoule; **WTR**, water; **PROT**, protein; **CARB**, carbohydrate; **FIBR**, fiber; **FAT**, fat; **SATF**, saturated fat; **MONO**, monounsaturated fat; **POLY**, polyunsaturated fat; **CHOL**, cholesterol;

ESHA CODE	FOOD DESCRIPTION	AMT	UNIT	WT (g)	CAL (kcal)	KILO (kJ)	WTR (g)	PROT (g)	CARB (g)	FIBR (g)	FAT (g)	SATF (g)	MONO (g)	POLY (g)
PREPARED FOODS (CONTINUED)														
11050	Stroganoff, beef, fzn	1	cntr	276.41	380	1590		22	34	2	17	5		
16811	Tamales, beef, fzn	1	ea	112	210	879		10	21	3	10	1.5		
57140	Tortellini, three cheese, fzn	0.33	pkg	81	250	1046	20	11	37	2	7	3.5		
41284	Twice Baked Potato, gourmet, with sour cream cheese bacon, fzn	1	ea	147	230	962		8	23	2	12	7		
5154	Vegetables, succotash, ckd f/fzn, drnd	0.5	cup	85	79	331	63	4	17	3	1	0.1	0.1	0.4
Prepared Soups and Dishes														
7037	Baked Beans, prep f/recipe	0.5	cup	126.5	196	820	82	7	27	7	7	2.5	2.7	0.9
7084	Bean Cake, Japanese style	1	ea	32	130	544	7	2	16	1	7	1	2.9	2.6
57428	Cannelloni, beef, 3oz	2	ea	170.1	391	1636		20	28	1	22	7.8		
5270	Casserole, scalloped potatoes, prep f/recipe with margarine	1	cup	245	216	904	198	7	26	5	9	3.4	3.3	1.8
56234	Chop Suey, pork, with noodles	1	cup	220	448	1874	136	22	31	4	27	4.8	7.7	12.8
57618	Chow Mein, pork, with noodles	1	cup	220	448	1874	136	22	31	4	27	4.8	7.7	12.8
42854	Chowder, shrimp and corn, bowl	1	bowl	492	360	1506		9	31	2	23	12		
19420	Crab Cake, made with blue crab	1	ea	60	93	389	43	12	<1	0	5	0.9	1.7	1.4
18807	Croquette, salmon	1	ea	120	261	1092	72	16	14	1	16	3.6	6.5	4.5
24640	Deviled Eggs	1	ea	31	70	293	7	3	1	0	5	1		
10081	Dish, beef cube steak, lean, brd/flour fried	1	ea	165	460	1925	79	44	18	1	22	6.2	8.2	5.8
15915	Dish, chicken breast, teriyaki	3	oz	85.05	118	494	57	18	4	<1	2	0.6	0.7	0.6
15916	Dish, chicken drumstick, teriyaki	1	ea	68	94	393	45	14	4	<1	2	0.5	0.6	0.5
15907	Dish, chicken, almond	1	cup	242	280	1172	186	22	16	3	15	1.9	6.1	5.6
38857	Dish, chicken, sweet and sour	3	pce	55	138	577	29	6	13	1	7	1.1	1.5	3.5
19080	Dish, clams, mixed species, brd, fried, sml	20	ea	188	380	1590	116	27	19		21	5	8.5	5.4
19009	Dish, eastern oysters, brd, fried, med	6	ea	88	175	732	57	8	10		11	2.8	4.1	2.9
18805	Dish, fish ball, cod	1	ea	63	125	523	39	9	8	1	7	1.4	2.8	1.9
17103	Dish, gefilte fish, sweet	1	pce	42	35	146	34	4	3	0	1	0.2	0.3	0.1
56236	Dish, grape leaves, stuffed with lamb and rice	6	ea	126	333	1393	73	11	15	4	26	6.7	15.2	2.8
13900	Dish, lamb curry	1	cup	236	256	1071	189	28	3	1	14	3.9	4.9	3.4
7086	Dish, loaf, lentil	1	pce	47	83	347	29	4	10	3	4	0.4	0.9	2.1
18800	Dish, lobster newberg	1	cup	244	611	2556	150	30	11	<1	50	29.6	14.7	2.3
56250	Dish, moo goo gai pan	1	cup	216	272	1138	168	15	12	3	19	3.8	6.7	7
56080	Dish, moussaka, lamb and eggplant, prep f/recipe	1	svg	250	238	996	937	17	13	4	13	4.6		
5514	Dish, mushrooms, battered, fried	5	ea	70	156	653	44	2	11	1	12	1.5	3.6	6
5644	Dish, okra, battered, fried	0.5	cup	46	88	368	31	1	7	1	6	0.8	1.6	3.5
27042	Dish, olives, green, stuffed	10	ea	40	41	172	32	1	1	<1	4	0.6	3.2	0.4
19403	Dish, oyster, rockefeller	1	cup	224	301	1259	165	16	21	3	17	7.7	5.7	2.4
12082	Dish, pork chop, breaded, lean, bkd	1	ea	80	184	770	44	21	5	<1	8	2.9	3.7	0.9
56292	Dish, pork dumpling, fried	1	ea	100	341	1427	41	13	25	1	21	4.8	9.1	5.7

< = Trace amount present Blank = Not available

V, vitamin; **THI**, thiamin; **RIB**, riboflavin; **NIA**, niacin; **FOL**, folate; **CALC**, calcium; **PHOS**, phosphorus; **SOD**, sodium; **POT**, potassium; **MAG**, magnesium

CHOL (mg)	V-A (IU)	THI (mg)	RIB (mg)	NIA (mg)	V-B_6 (mg)	FOL (µg)	V-B_{12} (µg)	V-C (mg)	V-E (mg)	CALC (mg)	PHOS (mg)	SOD (mg)	POT (mg)	MAG (mg)	IRON (mg)	ZINC (mg)
70	200							0		80		990			2.7	
15	300							2.4		40		630			2.7	
35	0							0		0		300			0	
30	400							12		150		310			4.5	
0	165	0.1	0.1	1.1	0.1	28	0	5	0.2	13	60	38	225	20	0.8	0.4
6	0	0.2	0.1	0.5	0.1	61	0	1.4		77	138	534	453	54	2.5	0.9
0	0	0.1	<0.1	0.5	<0.1	9	0	0	1.2	3	21	1	58	6	0.7	0.2
137										149		672			2.1	
15	368	0.2	0.2	2.6	0.4	27	0	26		140	154	821	926	47	1.4	1
48	183	0.8	0.4	6.2	0.4	42	0.4	20.2	2.7	45	249	848	489	53	3.3	2.6
48	183	0.8	0.4	6.2	0.4	42	0.4	20.2	2.7	45	249	848	489	53	3.3	2.6
												890				
90	151	0.1	<0.1	1.7	0.1	32	3.6	1.7		63	128	198	194	20	0.6	2.5
57	90	0.1	0.2	5.4	0.4	20	2.2	4	2.5	181	276	506	387	32	0.9	0.9
110	200							0		20		70			0.4	
125	16	0.3	0.5	7	0.7	17	4.7	0.1	1.7	80	380	316	653	54	6.4	8.4
55	43	0.1	0.1	5.8	0.3	8	0.2	2.1	0.2	18	132	1118	205	23	1.1	1.3
44	34	<0.1	0.1	4.7	0.2	6	0.2	1.7	0.2	14	105	894	164	19	0.9	1
40	351	0.1	0.2	9.5	0.4	26	0.3	6.9	3.8	69	252	526	549	60	2	1.6
15	174	<0.1	<0.1	2	0.1		<0.1	1.3	0.5	25	74	135	87	8	1.2	0.2
115	568	0.2	0.5	3.9	0.1	68	75.7	18.8		118	353	684	613	26	26.2	2.7
62	266	0.1	0.2	1.5	0.1	27	13.8	3.3		55	140	367	215	51	6.1	76.7
35	44	0.1	0.1	1.3	0.2	7	0.3	2.4	0.9	18	108	175	275	20	0.4	0.3
13	37	<0.1	<0.1	0.4	<0.1	1	0.4	0.3		10	31	220	38	4	1	0.3
32	8702	0.1	0.2	3.5	0.2	33	0.8	9	2.8	133	113	84	246	48	2.4	2
89	18	0.1	0.3	8.1	0.2	28	2.9	1.3	1.2	36	284	323	496	40	3	6.6
0	4	0.1	<0.1	0.7	0.1	61	<0.1	0.8	2.2	18	88	44	156	27	1.5	0.6
369	1886	0.1	0.4	1.6	0.2	32	4	0.8	2	241	398	647	607	55	1.2	4.1
35	1386	0.2	0.3	4.4	0.3	42	0.3	34.3	3.7	131	199	304	488	34	1.7	1.6
97	543	0.2	0.3	4.1	0.2	46	1.5	5.9	1	75	185	460	565	40	1.7	2.6
2	22	0.1	0.3	2.3	<0.1	8	<0.1	1.2	2.3	15	119	112	154	7	1.2	0.4
1	172	0.1	0.1	0.7	0.1	19	<0.1	5.2	1.5	30	61	61	95	18	0.6	0.2
0	252	<0.1	<0.1	<0.1	<0.1	1	0	4.8	1.1	21	7	826	28	8	0.6	0.1
87	7430	0.4	0.4	4	0.3	122	21	26.8	2.2	195	254	708	583	115	10.3	97.9
57	5	0.7	0.3	3.9	0.4	5	0.5	0.5	0.4	17	197	333	331	22	0.8	1.8
27	106	0.5	0.3	3.6	0.2	9	0.3	0.3	2.3	33	131	86	198	18	1.8	1.1

ESHA, EatRight Analysis; **AMT**, amount; **WT**, weight; **CAL**, calories; **KILO**, KiloJoule; **WTR**, water; **PROT**, protein; **CARB**, carbohydrate; **FIBR**, fiber; **FAT**, fat; **SATF**, saturated fat; **MONO**, monounsaturated fat; **POLY**, polyunsaturated fat; **CHOL**, cholesterol;

ESHA CODE	FOOD DESCRIPTION	AMT	UNIT	WT (g)	CAL (kcal)	KILO (kJ)	WTR (g)	PROT (g)	CARB (g)	FIBR (g)	FAT (g)	SATF (g)	MONO (g)	POLY (g)
PREPARED FOODS (CONTINUED)														
56244	Dish, sukiyaki	1	cup	162	172	720	126	19	7	1	8	2.9	3.1	0.7
5166	Dish, sweet potatoes, candied, prep f/recipe	1	pce	105	172	720	66	1	34	2	4	2.3	0.9	0.2
11583	Dish, veal leg, top round steak, brd, fried	3	oz	85.05	202	845	44	23	8	<1	8	2.6	2.9	1.3
11902	Dish, veal, scallopini	1	pce	96	238	996	57	18	1	<1	17	4.8	7.4	3.2
56132	Egg Foo Yung, patty	1	ea	86	113	473	67	6	3	1	8	2	3.4	2.1
56288	Egg Foo Yung, pork	1	ea	86	124	519	65	8	4	1	8	2.1	3	2.3
26825	Egg Roll, pork and shrimp	1	ea	85	146	611		8	21	1	3	1		
14971	Egg Roll, pork, ckd	1	ea	85	189	791	44	8	25	2	6	1.3	2	2.1
19516	Egg, scrambled	1	ea	61	91	381	47	6	1	0	7	2	2.7	1.5
18806	Fish Cake, cod	1	ea	120	237	992	75	16	15	1	13	2.7	5.3	3.7
17039	Fish Cake, fried	1	ea	69	149	623	42	13	6	<1	8	1.6	3.2	2.4
15003	Fried Chicken, breast, with skin, flour fried	1	ea	98	218	912	55	31	2	<1	9	2.4	3.4	1.9
15009	Fried Chicken, thigh, with skin, flour fried	1	ea	62	162	678	34	17	2	<1	9	2.5	3.6	2.1
15029	Fried Chicken, wing, with skin, flour fried	1	ea	32	103	431	16	8	1	<1	7	1.9	2.8	1.6
56150	Hash, beef	1	cup	190	312	1305	131	21	21	2	16	4.9	5.7	3.3
24685	Jambalaya, with shrimp	0.5	cup	120	140	586		15	4	1	7	2.5		
56296	Knish, meat	1	ea	50	175	732	19	7	13	1	11	2.6	4.9	2.3
56294	Knish, potato	1	ea	61	215	900	22	5	21	1	12	2.6	5.8	3.3
52430	Lasagna, beef and three cheese	1	cup	215	350	1464		25	28	4	15	6		
5569	Mashed Potatoes, prep f/recipe with whole milk and butter	0.5	cup	105	119	498	79	2	18	2	4	2.7	1.1	0.2
52434	Meal, seafood bouillabaisse, for two, with roll	1	svg	543.3	470	1966		49	46	7	8	1.5		
19534	Omelette, plain	1	ea	61	94	393	46	6	<1	0	7	2	3	1.7
19543	Omelette, with mushrooms, one egg	1	ea	69	88	368	54	6	2	<1	6	1.8	2.4	1
25603	Quiche, Lorraine, with bacon and swiss cheese, indiv	1	indv	307	710	2971		26	47	4	46	17		
57400	Ravioli, beef, brd	1	cup	120	270	1130		11	43	2	6	2		
57416	Ravioli, beef, round, jumbo, preckd	1	cup	214	450	1883		22	48	3	19	9		
57411	Ravioli, beef, square, preckd	9	pce	146.3	300	1255		14	40	1	8	3.8		
8954	Ravioli, chicken and jalapeno filled, brd	6	pce	137.45	316	1322		15	49	2	7	2.7		
57420	Ravioli, chicken, round, jumbo, preckd	1	cup	214	450	1883		21	52	2	17	10		
40067	Salisbury Steak, beef, flame brld, fzn, 3820	1	ea	72.3	162	678		16	2		10	3.9		
56075	Souffle, cheese, prep f/recipe	1	svg	112	192	803	93	11	6	<1	14	5.1		
17396	Soup, egg drop	1	cup	241	65	272	224	3	10	1	1	0.4	0.5	0.3
18912	Soup, gumbo, chicken and sausage, with rice	1	bowl	306	190	795	796	11	24	2	6	2		
17397	Soup, hot and sour	1	cup	233	91	381	211	6	10	1	3	0.5	0.7	0.7
50207	Soup, pork, with rice and veg	1	cup	244	124	519	219	12	8	1	4	1.5	2.1	0.4
50209	Soup, sweet and sour	1	cup	244	72	301	222	3	14	2	1	0.3	0.3	0.1
50186	Soup, vegetable, low sod, prep with water	1	cup	253	83	347	231	3	15	3	1	0.2	0.3	0.5

< = Trace amount present   Blank = Not available

V, vitamin; **THI**, thiamin; **RIB**, riboflavin; **NIA**, niacin; **FOL**, folate; **CALC**, calcium; **PHOS**, phosphorus; **SOD**, sodium; **POT**, potassium; **MAG**, magnesium

CHOL (mg)	V-A (IU)	THI (mg)	RIB (mg)	NIA (mg)	V-B$_6$ (mg)	FOL (μg)	V-B$_{12}$ (μg)	V-C (mg)	V-E (mg)	CALC (mg)	PHOS (mg)	SOD (mg)	POT (mg)	MAG (mg)	IRON (mg)	ZINC (mg)
148	2220	0.1	0.4	3.1	0.4	61	1.5	4.5	0.7	62	204	675	463	47	3.2	3.6
9	6850	<0.1	<0.1	0.4	0.1	6	<0.1	9.4	0.9	27	26	125	187	14	0.8	0.2
95	29	0.1	0.3	8.8	0.3	23	1.1	0	0.5	33	213	386	316	26	1.4	2.3
65	451	<0.1	0.2	5.1	0.2	12	0.9	0.7	1.7	54	172	278	253	19	1	2.8
185	307	<0.1	0.3	0.4	0.1	30	0.4	4.8	1.2	31	93	317	117	12	1	0.7
167	299	0.1	0.2	0.8	0.1	22	0.4	3.2	1.1	27	105	131	157	12	0.8	0.9
26	700							10.2		40		399			1.6	
12	6633	0.2	0.1	1.9	0.1	68	0.1	24.9	0.2	29	77	346	180	17	1.3	0.8
169	353	<0.1	0.2	<0.1	0.1	22	0.5	0	0.7	40	101	88	81	7	0.8	0.6
67	84	0.1	0.1	2.5	0.3	13	0.6	4.5	1.6	34	206	334	523	38	0.8	0.7
54	63	0.1	0.1	1.7	0.1	6	1.3	0.3	1.3	30	207	127	257	32	0.7	0.5
87	49	0.1	0.1	13.5	0.6	6	0.3	0		16	228	74	254	29	1.2	1.1
60	61	0.1	0.2	4.3	0.2	7	0.2	0		9	116	55	147	16	0.9	1.6
26	40	<0.1	<0.1	2.1	0.1	2	0.1	0		5	48	25	57	6	0.4	0.6
57	<1	0.2	0.2	3.7	0.5	16	1.8	7.1	1.2	19	204	470	587	36	2.5	5
100	750							30		40		570			1.1	
52	379	0.1	0.2	1.5	<0.1	8	0.3	0.4	1.2	12	61	107	88	8	1.2	1
59	548	0.2	0.2	1.5	0.1	10	0.1	0.9	1.7	16	60	140	96	10	1.3	0.4
50	1250	0.3	0.3	4.2	0.2	87	1.1	9		500	356	870	356	40	3.6	3.7
12	145	0.1	<0.1	1.1	0.2	8	0.1	6.3	0.1	25	47	333	298	19	0.3	0.3
110	1000	0.4	0.3	9.1	0.8	80	16.6	27		150	765	1380	1008	150	10.8	3.6
191	376	<0.1	0.2	<0.1	0.1	24	0.5	0	0.8	29	102	95	71	7	0.9	0.7
177	361	<0.1	0.2	0.3	0.1	17	0.4	0.1	0.7	43	100	147	97	9	0.7	0.6
262	700							3		460		2564			2.9	
25	0							1.2		60		660			2.7	
135	100							0		100		930			3.6	
77										119		400			2.1	
49										83		841			3	
115	300							0		200		420			2.7	
	91							1.5		29		503			2	
195	590	0.1	0.4	0.3	0.1	27	0.8	0.5	1.3	191	191	274	146	16	0.8	1
55	214	<0.1	<0.1	0.4	<0.1	17	0.1	15.7	0.3	17	36	892	53	5	0.6	0.2
25	500							15		40		1410			1.8	
49	79	0.1	0.1	1.2	0.1	19	0.2	0	0.9	44	75	876	128	21	1.5	0.5
41	2946	0.3	0.1	2.5	0.2	6	0.3	1.1	0.2	16	96	55	206	15	1.1	2
5	315	0.1	0.1	0.9	0.1	16	<0.1	16.7	0.5	27	43	1292	227	15	0.6	0.3
0	2176	0.1	0.1	1.9	0.2	15	0	1	1.8	30	58	491	549	33	0.8	0.5

ESHA, EatRight Analysis; **AMT**, amount; **WT**, weight; **CAL**, calories; **KILO**, KiloJoule; **WTR**, water; **PROT**, protein; **CARB**, carbohydrate; **FIBR**, fiber; **FAT**, fat; **SATF**, saturated fat; **MONO**, monounsaturated fat; **POLY**, polyunsaturated fat; **CHOL**, cholesterol;

ESHA CODE	FOOD DESCRIPTION	AMT	UNIT	WT (g)	CAL (kcal)	KILO (kJ)	WTR (g)	PROT (g)	CARB (g)	FIBR (g)	FAT (g)	SATF (g)	MONO (g)	POLY (g)
PREPARED FOODS (CONTINUED)														
2995	Spring Roll, fresh, vegetable, Thai, prep f/recipe	1	svg	63.22	158	661	40	4	20	1	7	0.9		
7559	Stew, vegetarian	1	cup	247	304	1272	173	42	17	3	7	1.2	1.8	3.8
91818	Sushi, California roll	1	ea	198	292	1222		8	49	3	3	1		
91912	Sushi, crab salad roll	1	ea	198	306	1280		8	49	3	5	1		
91814	Sushi, Maki, roll, cucumber	6	pce	85	120	502		3	25	2	1	0		
92384	Sushi, Maki, roll, vegetarian	4.5	pce	110	140	586		4	27	1	2	0		
91816	Sushi, roll, tuna	6	pce	105	150	628		8	30	1	0	0	0	0
56061	Taco, chicken, prep f/recipe	1	ea	77.3	175	732	34	15	9	1	9	2.8		
57407	Tortellini, beef filled, preckd	1	cup	128	250	1046		11	38	2	6	3.5		
57408	Tortellini, spinach, cheese filled, preckd	1	cup	128	280	1172		13	40	2	8	5		
56062	Tostada, bean and chicken, prep f/recipe	1	ea	156.2	242	1013	168	19	16	3	11	4.5		
Prepared Salads														
52035	Salad, cucumber, Alliant	0.5	cup	100	50	209		1	13		0	0	0	0
52066	Salad, egg	0.5	cup	100	230	962		9	8	0	18	4		
56005	Salad, potato, prep f/recipe	0.5	cup	125	179	749	95	3	14	2	10	1.8	3.1	4.7
52065	Salad, seafood	0.5	cup	100	230	962		6	14	8	17	2.5		
52064	Salad, shrimp	0.5	cup	100	170	711		7	5	3	14	2		
5537	Salad, spinach, w/o dressing	1	cup	74	108	452	51	5	11	2	5	1.4	2.2	0.7
56917	Salad, tabbouleh	1	cup	160	589	2464	15	17	122	13	4	0.8	0.6	2.1
52060	Salad, tuna	0.5	cup	100	260	1088		12	9	2	19	3		
56006	Salad, waldorf, prep f/recipe	1	svg	137	411	1720	113	4	12	3	41	4.3		
Prepared Sandwiches														
56038	Sandwich, beef, patty melt, with rye	1	ea	181.9	561	2347	143	37	22	6	37	12.7		
56009	Sandwich, BLT, with white	1	ea	123.8	318	1331	86	10	29	2	18	4.1		
56281	Sandwich, bologna	1	ea	83	256	1071	34	7	26	1	13	4.1	6.3	2.1
56020	Sandwich, corned beef swiss, with rye	1	ea	156	427	1787	111	28	22	6	26	9.5		
56013	Sandwich, grilled cheese, with white	1	ea	119	399	1669	54	17	30	1	23	11.9		
56066	Sandwich, ham salad, with part wheat	1	ea	130.6	357	1494	75	11	33	2	20	4.7		
56033	Sandwich, ham swiss, with rye	1	ea	149.5	385	1611	118	22	30	4	19	6.5		
56031	Sandwich, ham, with part wheat	1	ea	156.3	356	1490	125	25	26	2	17	3.6		
13093	Sandwich, hot dog, chicken, plain	1	ea	85	235	983	38	9	24	1	11	3	5	2.2
56040	Sandwich, peanut butter and jam, with white	1	ea	101	348	1456	29	11	47	3	14	2.7		
56046	Sandwich, roast beef, with part wheat	1	ea	155.8	397	1661	109	30	30	2	17	3.2		
32854	Sandwich, sub, pastrami, hot, with white, 12"	1	ea	413	880	3682		59	83	3	32	14		
56048	Sandwich, tuna salad, with white	1	ea	121.8	326	1364	68	13	35	1	14	1.9		
56059	Sandwich, turkey ham cheese, with part whole wheat	1	ea	156.3	396	1657	122	23	28		22	8.2		
56103	Sandwich, turkey ham, with rye	1	ea	149.5	279	1167	131	21	20	6	13	2.5		
56053	Sandwich, turkey, with whole wheat	1	ea	168.8	360	1506	142	27	29	4	16	2.3		

< = Trace amount present   Blank = Not available

V, vitamin; **THI**, thiamin; **RIB**, riboflavin; **NIA**, niacin; **FOL**, folate; **CALC**, calcium; **PHOS**, phosphorus; **SOD**, sodium; **POT**, potassium; **MAG**, magnesium

CHOL (mg)	V-A (IU)	THI (mg)	RIB (mg)	NIA (mg)	V-B_6 (mg)	FOL (µg)	V-B_{12} (µg)	V-C (mg)	V-E (mg)	CALC (mg)	PHOS (mg)	SOD (mg)	POT (mg)	MAG (mg)	IRON (mg)	ZINC (mg)
3	698	0.2	0.1	1.9	<0.1	32	<0.1	0.9	1.3	58	42	263	75	12	1.8	0.4
0	2317	1.7	1.5	29.6	2.7	254	5.4	0	1.2	77	543	988	296	314	3.2	2.7
3	450							4.8		20		952			1.1	
6	450							4.8		20		968			1.1	
0	250							0		0		90			0.4	
0	1000							2.4		0		105			0.7	
3	500							1.2		0		120			0.7	
45	192	0.1	0.1	4.1	0.3	13	0.2	0.6	0.6	82	156	132	157	28	1	1.3
40	100							1.2		60		490			1.8	
30	600							0		150		320			1.8	
55	316	0.1	0.1	4.3	0.3	25	0.3	5.1	0.7	146	220	387	263	41	1.6	1.9
0												580				
240	0							0		40		570			1.4	
85	196	0.1	0.1	1.1	0.2	9	0	12.5		24	65	661	318	19	0.8	0.4
20	0							0		20		770			0.4	
85	0							0		4		620			0.7	
77	1551	0.1	0.3	1.7	0.1	60	0.2	6.7	0.9	46	83	227	242	27	1.5	0.6
	1267							6.2		105		54			4.9	
30	100							0		20		580			0.4	
21	182	0.1	0.1	0.5	0.4	34	0.1	5.4	8.6	44	89	235	258	37	1	0.7
113	477	0.2	0.5	6.1	0.4	37	2.4	0.2	3.5	221	324	714	391	39	4.2	7
20	247	0.4	0.3	3.7	0.2	66	0.3	6	2.3	68	123	631	239	22	2.2	1
16	164	0.3	0.2	2.7	0.1	19	0.4	<1	0.8	60	74	598	112	15	2	0.9
83	290	0.2	0.3	2.8	0.2	32	1.7	0.2	2.6	267	269	1470	232	28	3	3.6
53	837	0.3	0.4	2.4	0.1	60	0.4	<1	1	407	470	1155	162	26	2	2
30	28	0.5	0.2	3.6	0.2	44	0.5	0	3.7	65	164	947	212	32	2.3	1.3
56	256	0.6	0.4	5	0.3	55	1	0.4	2.5	240	345	1392	369	42	2.7	3
56	34	0.9	0.4	6.9	0.4	44	0.6	0.2	2.7	68	307	1254	439	43	3.1	2.9
45	58	0.2	0.1	2.7	0.2	17	0.1	0	0.1	83	82	819	76	13	2	0.8
1	2	0.3	0.2	5.4	0.1	79	<0.1	1.7	2.6	76	143	429	240	52	2.3	1.1
45	40	0.3	0.3	6.9	0.4	51	2.3	0	3.6	67	232	1640	492	41	4.2	4.1
130	500							0		400		2780			7.2	
13	76	0.3	0.2	5.9	0.1	63	0.7	1.1	2.8	76	152	588	168	25	2.4	0.7
64	369	0.3	0.4	4.4	0.3	30	0.4	0	3.2	246	411	1389	354	44	3.7	3.2
55	35	0.2	0.3	4.3	0.3	29	0.3	0.3	2.9	51	211	1175	342	26	4	2.9
47	42	0.3	0.2	10.1	0.5	35	1.9	0	3.9	53	356	1734	417	71	2.5	2.2

ESHA, EatRight Analysis; **AMT**, amount; **WT**, weight; **CAL**, calories; **KILO**, KiloJoule; **WTR**, water; **PROT**, protein; **CARB**, carbohydrate; **FIBR**, fiber; **FAT**, fat; **SATF**, saturated fat; **MONO**, monounsaturated fat; **POLY**, polyunsaturated fat; **CHOL**, cholesterol;

ESHA CODE	FOOD DESCRIPTION	AMT	UNIT	WT (g)	CAL (kcal)	KILO (kJ)	WTR (g)	PROT (g)	CARB (g)	FIBR (g)	FAT (g)	SATF (g)	MONO (g)	POLY (g)
RESTAURANTS														
Arby's														
8987	French Fries, curly	1	sml	128	408	1707		5	48	4	22	3.2		
81476	Sandwich, Arby's melt, roast beef	1	ea	146	320	1339		18	38	2	11	3.5		
69056	Sandwich, beef'n cheddar	1	reg	195	430	1799		23	42	2	19	6		
56341	Sandwich, chicken, rstd	1	ea	189	400	1674		24	40	3	16	2.5		
81477	Sandwich, Market Fresh, roast beef gyro, with flatbread	1	ea	220	420	1757		20	32	2	23	6		
56336	Sandwich, roast beef	1	reg	154	350	1464		23	37	2	13	4.5		
56337	Sandwich, roast beef, jr	1	ea	125	300	1255		18	37	2	9	3.5		
69049	Sandwich, roast beef, patty melt, tstd, with sourdough	1	ea	200	460	1925		26	43	3	21	6		
69048	Sandwich, sub, classic Italian, tstd, with ciabatta	1	ea	291	590	2469		24	57	3	30	8		
69055	Sandwich, sub, Philly beef, tstd, with ciabatta	1	ea	254	570	2385		29	55	3	27	8		
69044	Sandwich, sub, turkey bacon club, tstd, with ciabatta	1	ea	292	570	2385		33	56	3	24	6		
48162	Turnover, cherry, w/o icing	1	ea	89	270	1130		4	31	1	15	7		
Auntie Anne's														
71911	Blended Drink, Dutch Ice, strawberry, lrg	1	lrg	539	230	962		0	58	0	0	0	0	0
71907	Frozen Dessert, Dutch Ice, pina colada, lrg	1	med	430	241	1008		0	59	0	0	0	0	0
71884	Pretzels, soft, cinnamon sugar	1	ea	136	380	1590		8	84	2	1	0		
42454	Pretzels, soft, original	1	ea	119	310	1297		8	65	2	1	0		
Burger King														
57001	Cheeseburger, double	1	ea	171	450	1883		26	29	1	26	12		
56355	Cheeseburger, Whopper	1	ea	316	790	3305	174	35	53	3	48	18.3	16	12
57000	Cheeseburger, Whopper Jr	1	ea	159	380	1590		16	29	2	23	8		
56354	Hamburger, Whopper	1	ea	291	678	2837	164	31	54	5	37	12.4	13.6	9.9
56999	Hamburger, Whopper Jr	1	ea	147	340	1423		14	28	2	19	5		
9040	Onion Rings	1	sml	91	320	1339		3	41	3	16	2.9		
40809	Sandwich, chicken, American original	1	ea	271	730	3054		29	49	3	47	12		
56360	Sandwich, chicken, original	1	ea	218	630	2636		24	46	3	39	7		
56362	Sandwich, fish, BK Big	1	ea	228	590	2469		21	57	3	31	5		
Carl's Junior														
91402	Hamburger, Famous Star	1	ea	269	620	2594		25	56	3	34	10		
48698	Salad, grilled chicken, original	1	ea	411	270	1130		25	23	4	9	3		
91408	Sandwich, chicken club, charbroiled	1	ea	264	580	2427		36	45	2	29	8		
91413	Sandwich, fish, Carl's Catch	1	ea	298	700	2929		21	73	5	37	6		
Dairy Queen														
56371	Cheeseburger, homestyle	1	ea	156	400	1674		19	34	1	18	9		
69027	Cheeseburger, Ultimate, double, homestyle	1	ea	259	780	3264		41	33	1	48	22		

< = Trace amount present   Blank = Not available

V, vitamin; **THI**, thiamin; **RIB**, riboflavin; **NIA**, niacin; **FOL**, folate; **CALC**, calcium; **PHOS**, phosphorus; **SOD**, sodium; **POT**, potassium; **MAG**, magnesium

CHOL (mg)	V-A (IU)	THI (mg)	RIB (mg)	NIA (mg)	V-B_6 (mg)	FOL (µg)	V-B_{12} (µg)	V-C (mg)	V-E (mg)	CALC (mg)	PHOS (mg)	SOD (mg)	POT (mg)	MAG (mg)	IRON (mg)	ZINC (mg)
0	0							2.3		25		930			1.7	
30	0							0		80		900			3.6	
45	100							1.2		100		1220			4.5	
50	100							1.2		80		950			1.8	
50	500							9		80		1040			3.6	
45	0							0		60		960			3.6	
30	0							0		60		750			2.7	
55	200							2.4		200		1790			4.5	
55	500							12		150		1870			2.7	
65	300							24		150		1490			3.6	
65	500							9		150		1700			2.7	
0	750							0		0		300			1.1	
0	0							3.6		20		50			0	
0	0							10.3		23		34			0	
0	0							0		20		400			0.7	
0	0							0		20		990			0.7	
95												960				
114		0.7	0.6	8.1	0.2	161		0.6	0.3	259	357	1431	534	57	6.3	5.1
55												730				
87		0.6	0.5	8.4	0.3	137		0.6	0.4	113	262	911	492	52	12.7	8.2
40												510				
0												840				
85												1830				
65												1390				
45												1480				
65	200							6		100		940			4.5	
70	4500							27		200		800			2.7	
95	300							6		150		1280			3.6	
40	200							6		100		1300			3.6	
65	500							0		100		920			2.7	
155	1000							12		200		1390			8.1	

ESHA, EatRight Analysis; **AMT**, amount; **WT**, weight; **CAL**, calories; **KILO**, KiloJoule; **WTR**, water; **PROT**, protein; **CARB**, carbohydrate; **FIBR**, fiber; **FAT**, fat; **SATF**, saturated fat; **MONO**, monounsaturated fat; **POLY**, polyunsaturated fat; **CHOL**, cholesterol;

ESHA CODE	FOOD DESCRIPTION	AMT	UNIT	WT (g)	CAL (kcal)	KILO (kJ)	WTR (g)	PROT (g)	CARB (g)	FIBR (g)	FAT (g)	SATF (g)	MONO (g)	POLY (g)
RESTAURANTS (CONTINUED)														
2133	Frozen Dessert Bar, Buster	1	ea	148	480	2008		11	45	2	31	15		
2135	Frozen Dessert Bar, Dilly, chocolate	1	ea	87	240	1004		4	24	1	15	9		
2131	Frozen Dessert, banana split	1	ea	374	520	2176		9	94	3	13	10		
72141	Frozen Dessert, Blizzard, banana split, med	1	med	382	570	2385		13	93	1	16	10		
2368	Frozen Dessert, Blizzard, Oreo Cookie, med	1	med	334	680	2845		14	100	1	25	12		
2154	Frozen Dessert, sundae, chocolate, med	1	med	234	400	1674		8	70	0	10	6		
56368	Hamburger, homestyle	1	ea	142	350	1464		17	33	1	14	7		
2222	Ice Cream Cone, chocolate, med	1	med	199	340	1423		9	54	0	10	7		
2136	Ice Cream Cone, soft serve, vanilla, choc dipped, med	1	med	220	480	2008		9	59	0	23	15		
2134	Ice Cream Sandwich, DQ	1	ea	85	190	795		4	31	1	5	3		
2348	Ice Cream, soft serve, chocolate	1	sml	135	215	900		6	32	0	7	5		
2224	Milk Shake, chocolate, med	1	med	550	790	3305		18	130	0	21	13		
2151	Parfait, Peanut Buster	1	ea	304	700	2929		16	94	2	30	16		
56374	Sandwich, hot dog, beef	1	ea	110	290	1213		11	22	1	17	7		
13236	Sandwich, hot dog, beef, foot long	1	ea	199	560	2343		20	39	2	35	14		
69069	Sandwich, hot dog, beef, with chili and cheese, foot long	1	ea	233	670	2803		28	41	2	43	19		
Denny's														
25240	Dish, steak, t-bone, with eggs, w/o sides	1	entree	481.95	790	3305		110	4	0	36	19		
12756	Meal, tilapia, lemon pepper, grilled, with bread, w/o sides	1	meal	425.25	800	3347		58	59	3	35	15		
51342	Meal, western omelette, with hash browns, w/o sides	1	meal	453.6	700	2929		38	32	2	46	13		
12766	Milk Shake, Oreo Blender Blaster	1	reg	218.9	890	3724		15	113	3	44	20		
56612	Omelette, veggie cheese, w/o sides	1	ea	368.55	460	1925		28	9	2	33	12		
Hardee's														
69061	Cheeseburger, Thickburger, Frisco, ⅓ lb	1	ea	311	930	3891		42	44	2	64	20		
56411	Dish, biscuit, with gravy	1	order	227	410	1715		9	50	2	23	6		
48946	Ice Cream Cone, vanilla, single scoop	1	ea	126	285	1192		6	37	0	13	8		
56420	Sandwich, ham and cheese, Big Hot	1	ea	236	450	1883		35	46	3	18	7		
56418	Sandwich, roast beef	1	ea	128	300	1255		18	28	2	14	5		
Jack in the Box														
56430	Breakfast Sandwich, Breakfast Jack	1	ea	125	280	1172		16	30	1	11	4.5		
69040	Breakfast Sandwich, with sourdough	1	ea	152	410	1715		20	35	2	21	8		
56437	Cheeseburger, Jumbo Jack	1	ea	253	580	2427		23	45	2	34	15		
69033	Cheeseburger, Sourdough Jack	1	ea	227	660	2761		28	40	3	44	16		
62547	Cheeseburger, Ultimate, with bacon	1	ea	301	920	3849		44	45	2	63	27		
56436	Hamburger, Jumbo Jack	1	ea	230	500	2092		19	45	2	27	10		
69035	Sandwich, chicken	1	ea	147	410	1715		15	42	2	21	3.5		
51213	Sandwich, pocket, chicken fajita, with whl grain pita	1	ea	192	320	1339		24	33	4	11	5		

< = Trace amount present Blank = Not available

V, vitamin; **THI**, thiamin; **RIB**, riboflavin; **NIA**, niacin; **FOL**, folate; **CALC**, calcium; **PHOS**, phosphorus; **SOD**, sodium; **POT**, potassium; **MAG**, magnesium

CHOL (mg)	V-A (IU)	THI (mg)	RIB (mg)	NIA (mg)	$V\text{-}B_6$ (mg)	FOL (µg)	$V\text{-}B_{12}$ (µg)	V-C (mg)	V-E (mg)	CALC (mg)	PHOS (mg)	SOD (mg)	POT (mg)	MAG (mg)	IRON (mg)	ZINC (mg)
20	400							0		200		220			1.1	
15	300							0		100		70			0	
30	750							18		250		160			2.7	
55	1250							9		450		230			3.6	
50	1000							0		400		530			3.6	
30	750							0		250		170			2.7	
50	300							0		40		680			2.7	
30	1000							0		200		160			1.8	
30	750							0		300		160			1.8	
10	200							0		100		135			1.1	
22	750							0		150		110			0.9	
70	1250							0		600		350			4.5	
35	750							0		400		360			3.6	
35	200							0		60		900			1.8	
65	200							0		100		1600			3.6	
95	500							0		250		1720			4.5	
555												2070				
155												1740				
770												2180				
105												590				
740												680				
125												2010				
10												1370				
45												140				
90												2140				
40												850				
240												780	190			
250												1010	220			
60												1190	360			
75												1210	430			
125												1840	510			
40												780	330			
30												880	250			
65												870	380			

ESHA, EatRight Analysis; **AMT**, amount; **WT**, weight; **CAL**, calories; **KILO**, KiloJoule; **WTR**, water; **PROT**, protein; **CARB**, carbohydrate; **FIBR**, fiber; **FAT**, fat; **SATF**, saturated fat; **MONO**, monounsaturated fat; **POLY**, polyunsaturated fat; **CHOL**, cholesterol;

ESHA CODE	FOOD DESCRIPTION	AMT	UNIT	WT (g)	CAL (kcal)	KILO (kJ)	WTR (g)	PROT (g)	CARB (g)	FIBR (g)	FAT (g)	SATF (g)	MONO (g)	POLY (g)
RESTAURANTS (CONTINUED)														
56441	Sandwich, pocket, chicken fajita, with whl grain pita, with salsa	1	ea	215	330	1381		24	35	4	11	5		
Kentucky Fried Chicken														
15169	Fried Chicken, breast, extra crispy	1	ea	212	568	2377	109	45	18		35	7.5	11.5	13.3
15163	Fried Chicken, breast, original rec	1	ea	201	444	1858	115	45	11		24	5.5	8.6	7.6
81291	Fried Chicken, drumstick, extra crispy	1	ea	81	222	929	42	17	6		14	3.1	4.9	5.1
81293	Fried Chicken, drumstick, original rec	1	ea	75	179	749	42	17	4		11	2.4	3.8	3.2
45236	Fried Chicken, drumstick, spicy crispy	1	ea	55	160	669		11	5	0	10	2		
45234	Fried Chicken, wing, spicy crispy	1	ea	51	170	711		11	6	0	12	2.5		
15177	Hot Wings	1	ea	22	70	293		4	4	0	4	0.5		
Long John Silver's														
56461	Dish, pollock, Alaskan, batter fried	1	ea	92	260	1088		12	17	0	16	4		
69030	Sandwich, pollock, Alaskan	1	ea	176	470	1966		18	49	3	23	5		
91388	Sticks, mozzarella, brd, fried	3	ea	50	150	628		5	13	1	9	3.5		
56457	Strips, chicken, brd, fried	1	ea	52	140	586		8	9	0	8	2		
91383	Strips, clam, brd, fried	1	order	85	320	1339		9	29	2	19	4.5		
McDonald's														
34752	Biscuit, with spread	1	ea	76	260	1088		5	33	2	12	7		
56675	Breakfast Burrito, sausage	1	ea	113	296	1238	56	13	24	1	17	6.1	6.5	2.4
69005	Breakfast Sandwich, McMuffin, egg cheese	1	ea	126	287	1201	66	17	27	1	12	4.5	3.4	2.2
69006	Breakfast Sandwich, McMuffin, sausage cheese	1	ea	115	383	1602	45	15	28	2	24	8.3	8.9	3.7
69009	Cheeseburger	1	ea	119	313	1310	54	15	33	1	14	5.3	4.3	0.4
69010	Cheeseburger, Big Mac	1	ea	219	563	2356	112	26	44	4	33	8.3	7.6	0.7
69012	Cheeseburger, Quarter Pounder	1	ea	199	513	2146	97	29	40	3	28	11.2	9.2	0.9
47147	Cookie, McDonaldland, pkg	1	indv pkg	57	255	1067	2	4	41	1	9	1.8	4.6	1.2
19579	Egg, scrambled, svg	1	svg	102.06	197	824	68	15	2		15	4.1	5.3	2.2
69008	Hamburger	1	ea	95	251	1050	42	12	29	1	10	3.3	3.6	1.3
69011	Hamburger, Quarter Pounder	1	ea	171	417	1745	86	24	38	3	20	6.9	7.2	0.5
6155	Hash Browns	1	svg	56	147	615	30	1	15	2	9	1.3	4.8	2.8
2166	Ice Cream Cone, vanilla, low fat	1	ea	90	146	611	57	4	24	<1	4	2.2	1.1	0.3
72911	Milk Shake, chocolate, triple thick	1	kids'	267	435	1820	168	10	74	1	12	6.1	3	0.6
72914	Milk Shake, strawberry, triple thick, 12 fl oz	1	kids'	265	419	1753	171	9	71	0	12	6	2.9	0.6
72890	Milk Shake, vanilla, triple thick	1	kids'	266	415	1736	172	9	71	0	12	6	2.9	0.6
49153	Nuggets, chicken, McNuggets	10	pce	159	480	2008	75	25	24		31	5.2	12.9	8.9
81453	Pancakes, Hotcake, with 2 pats marg and syrup	1	entree	221	601	2515	90	9	102	2	18	1.8	1.9	4.6
34699	Sandwich, chicken club, premium grld	1	ea	250	530	2218		39	52	4	17	6		
69013	Sandwich, Filet O Fish	1	ea	134	378	1582	61	15	35	2	20	3.8	5.4	8
42747	Sweet Roll, cinnamon	1	ea	105	418	1749	21	8	56	2	19	4.7	9.5	3

< = Trace amount present Blank = Not available

V, vitamin; **THI**, thiamin; **RIB**, riboflavin; **NIA**, niacin; **FOL**, folate; **CALC**, calcium; **PHOS**, phosphorus; **SOD**, sodium; **POT**, potassium; **MAG**, magnesium

CHOL (mg)	V-A (IU)	THI (mg)	RIB (mg)	NIA (mg)	V-B_6 (mg)	FOL (µg)	V-B_{12} (µg)	V-C (mg)	V-E (mg)	CALC (mg)	PHOS (mg)	SOD (mg)	POT (mg)	MAG (mg)	IRON (mg)	ZINC (mg)
65												990	390			
161		0.1	0.2	17.3	0.7		0.7			57	456	1287	547	51	1.2	1.7
165		0.1	0.2	17.8	0.7		0.6			62	458	1184	547	52	1.2	1.6
88		<0.1	0.2	3.7	0.2		0.4			20	160	512	192	17	0.7	1.5
88		<0.1	0.2	3.7	0.2		0.4			22	158	469	188	17	0.7	1.5
50												440				
45												470				
20												140				
35	0							0		0		790			0	
40	100							1.2		60		1180			1.8	
10	200							0		100		350			0.7	
20	0							2.4		0		480			0.7	
35	0							0		20		1190			1.4	
0	0							0		60		740			1.8	
173	382	0.2	0.3	1.9	0.4	70	0.6	0.9	0.2	203	247	763	155	19	1.8	1.3
208		0.3	0.5	3.9	0.2	100		1.5	0.7	242	252	777	218	25	2.9	1.6
45	299	0.4	0.3	4.8	0.2	79	0.5	0	0.3	258	187	797	216	24	2.3	1.5
42	289	0.3	0.3	4.8		70	1	0.7		199	167	745	238	24	2.8	2.3
79	412	0.4	0.5	7.4		101	1.9	0.9		254	267	1007	396	44	4.4	4.2
94	557	0.3	0.7	7.7		101	2.5	1.6		287	320	1152	436	44	4.2	5.2
	0	0.2	0.2	2.1	0.1	58			1.1	10	63	275	56	10	1.9	0.3
436	618	0.1	0.6	0.1	0.2	71	1.1		1.5	67	266	196	142	12	2.1	1.5
26	52	0.2	0.2	4.3		61	0.8	0.6		121	102	469	182	20	2.7	1.9
67	96	0.3	0.6	7.6		96	2.2	1.5		144	212	730	388	38	4.1	4.6
0	0	0.1	<0.1	1.3	0.1	21		1		8	60	307	219	12	0.3	0.2
14	289	<0.1	0.2	0.4	<0.1	8	0.5		<0.1	116	100	60	174	12	0.3	0.4
37	806	0.1	0.6	0.4	0.1	3	1.4		0	326	280	190	603	43	1.4	1.3
37	806	0.1	0.6	0.3	0.1	8	1.5	1.1	0	323	265	130	488	32	0.2	1.1
37	809	0.1	0.6	0.3	0.1	0	1.5		0	322	266	141	468	32	0.2	1.1
70		0.3	0.2	11.8	0.6		0.5	1.9		17	432	900	401	38	1.4	0.9
20	533	0.4	0.4	3.2	0.1	144	<0.1	0		126	391	625	276	29	2.8	0.6
95	400							6		200		1410			3.6	
43		0.3	0.2	3		28	1.4	0.4	1.6	161	184	582	295	36	2.1	0.8
61	441	0.3	0.3	2.5	0.1	108		0	1.9	60	109	397	147	20	1.8	0.9

ESHA, EatRight Analysis; **AMT**, amount; **WT**, weight; **CAL**, calories; **KILO**, KiloJoule; **WTR**, water; **PROT**, protein; **CARB**, carbohydrate; **FIBR**, fiber; **FAT**, fat; **SATF**, saturated fat; **MONO**, monounsaturated fat; **POLY**, polyunsaturated fat; **CHOL**, cholesterol;

ESHA CODE	FOOD DESCRIPTION	AMT	UNIT	WT (g)	CAL (kcal)	KILO (kJ)	WTR (g)	PROT (g)	CARB (g)	FIBR (g)	FAT (g)	SATF (g)	MONO (g)	POLY (g)
RESTAURANTS (CONTINUED)														
Pizza Hut														
56490	Pizza, hand tossed, pepperoni, 12" med	1	slice	96	269	1125	40	12	30	2	11	5	3.9	2
56481	Pizza, pan, cheese, 12" med	1	slice	100	280	1172	43	12	30	2	13	5.2	3.2	2.8
56482	Pizza, pan, pepperoni, 12" med	1	slice	96	286	1197	39	11	29	2	14	5.1	4.2	3.3
56483	Pizza, pan, supreme, 12" med	1	slice	112	290	1213		12	27	2	14	5		
56493	Pizza, personal pan, pepperoni	1	indv	201	610	2552		26	67	3	26	10		
56486	Pizza, thin 'n crispy, pepperoni, 12" med	1	slice	63	200	837		9	21	1	9	4		
56487	Pizza, thin 'n crispy, supreme, 12" med	1	slice	88	240	1004		10	23	1	12	5		
Starbucks														
20592	Coffee, cappuccino, with 2% milk, tall	1	sml	169	90	377		6	9	0	4	2		
20639	Coffee, cappuccino, with whole milk, tall	1	sml	169	110	460		6	9	0	6	3		
20659	Coffee, iced, latte, Caffe, with 2% milk, tall	1	sml	289	100	418		6	10	0	4	2.5		
20662	Coffee, iced, latte, Caffe, with whole milk, tall	1	sml	289	110	460		6	9	0	6	3.5		
20668	Coffee, latte, Caffe, with 2% milk, tall	1	sml	352	150	628		10	14	0	6	3.5		
20671	Coffee, latte, Caffe, with whole milk, tall	1	sml	352	180	753		10	14	0	9	5		
20677	Coffee, mocha, Caffe, with 2% milk, tall	1	sml	327	200	837		10	31	1	6	3.5		
20680	Coffee, mocha, Caffe, with whole milk, tall	1	sml	327	230	962		10	31	1	9	4.5		
27563	Muffin, zucchini walnut	1	ea	123	490	2050		7	52	2	28	2.5		
27571	Scone, vanilla bean, petite	1	ea	33	140	586		0	21	0	5	2.5		
Subway														
52125	Salad, turkey breast and ham, w/o dressing and croutons	1	ea	328	110	460		12	11	4	2	0.5		
52113	Salad, Veggie Delite, w/o dressing and croutons	1	ea	271	50	209		3	9	4	1	0		
69117	Sandwich, club, Subway, with wheat	6	in	240	310	1297		23	46	5	4	1.5		
69129	Sandwich, meatball marinara, with wheat	6	in	301	480	2008		21	59	8	18	7		
69143	Sandwich, tuna salad, with wheat	6	in	233	470	1966		20	44	5	24	4		
69109	Sandwich, Veggie Delite, with wheat	6	in	162	230	962		8	44	5	2	0.5		
Taco Bell														
56522	Burrito, beef, supreme	1	ea	248	469	1962	150	20	52	8	20	7.6	8.1	2
56688	Burrito, chicken, supreme	1	ea	248	444	1858	151	24	51	6	16	5.8	6.3	2
56691	Burrito, seven layer	1	ea	283	510	2134		16	69	11	19	7		
45585	Dessert, cinnamon twists	1	order	35	170	711		1	26	1	7	0		
56536	Dish, pintos 'n cheese	1	ea	128	180	753		9	20	7	7	3		
56534	Nachos, BellGrande	1	order	305	780	3264		18	79	12	43	7		
56684	Nachos, supreme, svg	1	svg	195	480	2008	105	15	45	8	27	7.8	13.7	2.8
56531	Pizza, Mexican	1	ea	213	540	2259		20	47	7	31	8		
56524	Taco, beef	1	ea	69	158	661	39	6	14	3	9	3	3	2.1
56692	Taco, crunchy, beef, supreme	1	ea	113	200	837		9	15	3	12	4.5		
56525	Taco, soft, beef	1	ea	102	210	879	60	9	21	3	10	4.2	3.3	1.6
56526	Taco, soft, beef, supreme	1	ea	131	230	962		10	22	3	11	5		

< = Trace amount present Blank = Not available

V, vitamin; **THI**, thiamin; **RIB**, riboflavin; **NIA**, niacin; **FOL**, folate; **CALC**, calcium; **PHOS**, phosphorus; **SOD**, sodium; **POT**, potassium; **MAG**, magnesium

CHOL (mg)	V-A (IU)	THI (mg)	RIB (mg)	NIA (mg)	V-B_6 (mg)	FOL (µg)	V-B_{12} (µg)	V-C (mg)	V-E (mg)	CALC (mg)	PHOS (mg)	SOD (mg)	POT (mg)	MAG (mg)	IRON (mg)	ZINC (mg)
25	196	0.3	0.3	3.9	0.1		0.7	0	0.7	149	209	769	199	22	2.1	1.6
21	260	0.2	0.3	3.9	0.1		0.6	0	1.1	208	241	624	168	21	1.9	1.6
24	164	0.3	0.2	3.7	0.1		0.6	0	0.7	140	197	664	191	21	2.1	1.5
30												650				
55												1410				
25												610				
30												670				
15	300							0		200		70			0	
15	200							0		200		70			0	
15	300							0		200		80			0	
20	200							0		200		75			0	
25	500							0		350		115			0	
30	300							0		300		115			0	
20	500							0		300		100			2.7	
25	0							0		300		100			2.7	
65	100							4.8		60		480			3.6	
15	100							0		20		90			0.7	
20	1250							27		60		580			1.4	
0	1250							27		40		65			1.1	
40	400							12		300		880			3.6	
30	1250							21		350		950			4.5	
35	400							12		300		620			3.6	
0	400							12		300		310			2.7	
40	203	0.4	0.4	4.3	0.3	112	1.2		1.1	231	337	1424	608	62	5.6	2.6
52	203	0.4	0.4	9.7	0.3	119	0.8		1	233	404	1399	655	69	3.9	1.6
20												1070				
0												200				
10												560				
30												1000				
37	136	0.2	0.3	1.9	0.3	57	0.8		1.4	142	384	838	472	90	4.2	2.7
40												860				
19	53	<0.1	<0.1	1.1	0.1	13	0.6	0.3	0.4	61	123	274	144	22	0.8	1.2
35												320				
26	81	0.2	0.1	2.9	0.1	53	0.9	0.1	0.4	125	170	571	164	19	1.7	1.4
35												530				

ESHA, EatRight Analysis; **AMT**, amount; **WT**, weight; **CAL**, calories; **KILO**, KiloJoule; **WTR**, water; **PROT**, protein; **CARB**, carbohydrate; **FIBR**, fiber; **FAT**, fat; **SATF**, saturated fat; **MONO**, monounsaturated fat; **POLY**, polyunsaturated fat; **CHOL**, cholesterol;

ESHA CODE	FOOD DESCRIPTION	AMT	UNIT	WT (g)	CAL (kcal)	KILO (kJ)	WTR (g)	PROT (g)	CARB (g)	FIBR (g)	FAT (g)	SATF (g)	MONO (g)	POLY (g)
RESTAURANTS (CONTINUED)														
56689	Taco, soft, chicken	1	ea	98	185	774	57	13	19	1	6	2.5	1.6	1.6
56693	Taco, soft, steak	1	ea	127	286	1197	72	15	22	2	15	4.3	5	4.4
20980	Tea, lemon, can	8	fl-oz	245	86	360	223	0	22	0	0	0	0	0
Taco Time														
56540	Burrito, bean, crisp	1	ea	134.66	360	1506		13	47	5	14	3.5		
56544	Burrito, beef bean and cheese	1	ea	248.06	490	2050		26	55	11	17	7		
56541	Burrito, beef, crisp	1	ea	134.66	430	1799		22	36	4	21	6		
12417	Hash Browns, cheddar fries	1	sml	134.66	350	1464		8	26	2	24	8		
12414	Hash Browns, Mexi Fries	1	sml	113.4	265	1109		2	26	2	18	3		
50979	Quesadilla, cheddar melt	1	ea	77.96	250	1046		11	25	4	12	7		
7273	Salad, taco, chicken	1	ea	269.33	310	1297		25	22	2	13	4		
Wendy's														
56574	Cheeseburger, deluxe, with bacon	1	ea	275	640	2678		37	46	2	35	14		
69058	Cheeseburger, jr, deluxe	1	ea	152	300	1255		15	28	2	14	6		
56571	Cheeseburger, jr, with bacon	1	ea	137	310	1297		17	25	1	16	6		
2176	Frozen Dessert, Frosty	1	sml	227	300	1255	157	8	54	7	6	3.7	1.6	0.3
56566	Hamburger, classic single	1	ea	218	464	1941	127	28	37	3	23	8	8.9	3.4
69057	Hamburger, jr	1	ea	117	284	1188	56	15	33	2	10	4.1	4.1	1.3
71596	Salad, spring mix, with cheese and bacon	1	ea	241	240	1004		15	9	3	16	8		
81443	Sandwich, chicken, Ultimate Grill	1	ea	225	403	1686	134	33	42	2	11	2.3	3.3	4.1
31401	Sauce, barbecue	1	indv pkt	28	45	188		1	11	0	0	0	0	0
Generic Fast Foods														
56629	Burrito, bean and cheese, fast food	1	ea	185	379	1586	98	14	58	8	11	4.3	2.3	4.1
66025	Burrito, bean, fast food	1	ea	108.5	224	937	57	7	36		7	3.4	2.4	0.6
66024	Burrito, beef, fast food	1	ea	110	262	1096	55	13	29		10	5.2	3.7	0.4
56634	Chimichanga, beef, fast food	1	ea	174	425	1778	88	20	43		20	8.5	8.1	1.1
47109	Cookie, molasses	1	med	15	64	268	1	1	11	<1	2	0.5	1.1	0.3
56668	Corn Dog, fast food	1	ea	175	460	1925	82	17	56		19	5.2	9.1	3.5
28439	Dish, chicken, kung pao	1	order	604	779	3259	452	59	41	9	42	8.2	13.1	18.2
66020	Dish, Enchirito, beef bean and cheese, fast food	1	ea	193	344	1439	121	18	34		16	7.9	6.5	0.3
17187	Dish, fish fillet, batter fried	3	oz	85.05	197	824	46	12	14	<1	10	2.4	2.2	5.3
56638	Dish, frijoles beans, with cheese, fast food	0.5	cup	83.5	113	473	58	6	14		4	2	1.3	0.3
19114	Dish, scallops, brd, fried, fast food	6	pce	144	386	1615	69	16	38		19	4.9	12.6	0.6
66021	Enchilada, cheese, fast food	1	ea	163	319	1335	103	10	29		19	10.6	6.3	0.8
42064	English Muffin, with butter, fast food	1	ea	63	189	791	21	5	30	2	6	2.4	1.5	1.3
90736	French Fries, fried in veg oil, fast food	1	med	117	365	1527	45	4	48	4	17	2.7	7	6.3
23938	Fried Rice	0.5	cup	70	114	477	43	3	22	1	2	0.3	0.4	0.7
2032	Frozen Dessert, sundae, hot fudge, fast food	1	ea	158	284	1188	94	6	48	0	9	5	2.3	0.8

< = Trace amount present   Blank = Not available

V, vitamin; **THI**, thiamin; **RIB**, riboflavin; **NIA**, niacin; **FOL**, folate; **CALC**, calcium; **PHOS**, phosphorus; **SOD**, sodium; **POT**, potassium; **MAG**, magnesium

CHOL (mg)	V-A (IU)	THI (mg)	RIB (mg)	NIA (mg)	V-B_6 (mg)	FOL (µg)	V-B_{12} (µg)	V-C (mg)	V-E (mg)	CALC (mg)	PHOS (mg)	SOD (mg)	POT (mg)	MAG (mg)	IRON (mg)	ZINC (mg)
28	24	0.2	0.1	5.1	0.1	47	0.1	0.2	0.3	120	239	601	213	24	1.6	0.7
39	29	0.4	0.2	3.8	0.1	47	1.2		0.5	149	197	700	232	27	2.8	2.7
0										2	64	51	47	0	0	<0.1
10	750							2.4		200		1910			3.6	
45	750							3.6		300		2310			7.2	
45	200							1.2		150		830			3.6	
22	250							12		150		790			0.9	
0	0							12		0		650			0.9	
30	300							0		250		470			1.8	
50	400							6		150		680			1.4	
125	750							12		200		1620			5.4	
45	500							3.6		100		740			2.7	
50	500							3.6		100		670			2.7	
36		0.1	1.6	0.8	0		1.3	0		291	254	222	420	45	2.4	1
76		0.6	0.4	7	0.2		3.2	1.1		74	225	861	425	39	6	5.4
32		0.5	0.3	4.5	0.1		1.5	0.6		53	125	631	205	25	3.9	2.5
45	3500							27		250		490			1.1	
90		0.9	0.6	9.4	0.3		0.7	2.5		56	378	961	497	54	3.5	1.3
0	0							2.4		0		160			0	
9	215	0.4	0.2	3.7	0.2	192	0.3	0.7	1	229	302	1042	483	63	4.4	1.6
2	166	0.3	0.3	2	0.2	43	0.5	1		56	49	493	327	43	2.3	0.8
32	139	0.1	0.5	3.2	0.2	65	1	0.6		42	87	746	370	41	3	2.4
9	146	0.5	0.6	5.8	0.3	84	1.5	4.7		63	124	910	586	63	4.5	5
0	0	0.1	<0.1	0.5	<0.1	13	0	0	<0.1	11	14	69	52	8	1	0.1
79	206	0.3	0.7	4.2	0.1	103	0.4	0		102	166	973	262	18	6.2	1.3
157	7846	0.2	0.3	16.7	1.5		0.7	42.9	6.2	121	568	2428	1317	145	4.6	4.5
50	1015	0.2	0.7	3	0.2	95	1.6	4.6		218	224	1251	560	71	2.4	2.8
29	32	0.1	0.1	1.8	0.1	14	0.9	0		15	145	452	272	20	1.8	0.4
18	228	0.1	0.2	0.7	0.1	56	0.3	0.8		94	88	441	302	43	1.1	0.9
108	138	0.2	0.8	0	0.1	53	0.4	0		19	292	919	294	32	2	1.1
44	1161	0.1	0.4	1.9	0.4	65	0.7	1		324	134	784	240	51	1.3	2.5
13	136	0.3	0.3	2.6	<0.1	57	<0.1	0.8	0.1	103	85	386	69	13	1.6	0.4
0	0	0.2	<0.1	3.5	0.4	35	0	5.5	2	21	146	246	677	41	0.9	0.6
16	24	<0.1	<0.1	0.4	<0.1	4	0	0	0.1	10	38	277	62	7	0.5	0.5
21	221	0.1	0.3	1.1	0.1	9	0.6	2.4	0.7	207	228	182	395	33	0.6	0.9

ESHA, EatRight Analysis; **AMT**, amount; **WT**, weight; **CAL**, calories; **KILO**, KiloJoule; **WTR**, water; **PROT**, protein; **CARB**, carbohydrate; **FIBR**, fiber; **FAT**, fat; **SATF**, saturated fat; **MONO**, monounsaturated fat; **POLY**, polyunsaturated fat; **CHOL**, cholesterol;

ESHA CODE	FOOD DESCRIPTION	AMT	UNIT	WT (g)	CAL (kcal)	KILO (kJ)	WTR (g)	PROT (g)	CARB (g)	FIBR (g)	FAT (g)	SATF (g)	MONO (g)	POLY (g)
RESTAURANTS (CONTINUED)														
2033	Frozen Dessert, sundae, strawberry, fast food	1	ea	153	268	1121	93	6	45	0	8	3.7	2.7	1
5463	Hash Browns, fast food	0.5	cup	72	235	983	30	2	23	2	16	3.6	8.3	2.7
2020	Milk Shake, chocolate, fast food	8	fl-oz	188	239	1000	134	6	39	4	7	4.3	2	0.3
2022	Milk Shake, strawberry, fast food	8	fl-oz	188	212	887	139	6	36	1	5	3.3		
56639	Nachos, with cheese, fast food	7	pce	113	346	1448	46	9	36		19	7.8	8	2.2
6176	Onion Rings, breaded, fried, svg, fast food	18	ea	117	481	2013	29	5	51	3	30	4.9	8.1	14.2
23949	Rice Pudding	0.5	cup	126.5	185	774	85	4	32	1	5	2.4	1.3	0.6
56628	Salad, chef, with turkey ham and cheese, w/o dressing, fast food	1.5	cup	326	267	1117	269	26	5		16	8.2	5.2	1.4
56643	Salad, taco, fast food	1.5	cup	198	279	1167	143	13	24		15	6.8	5.2	1.7
56623	Salad, tossed, veg, w/o dressing, fast food	1.5	cup	207	33	138	198	3	7		<1	<0.1	<0.1	0.1
56656	Sandwich, chicken, fillet, with cheese, fast food	1	ea	228	632	2644	105	29	42		39	12.4	13.7	9.9
56606	Sandwich, croissant, with egg and cheese, fast food	1	ea	127	368	1540	58	13	24		25	14.1	7.5	1.4
66011	Sandwich, fish, with cheese and tartar sauce, fast food	1	ea	134	374	1565	61	15	35		20	3.8	5.4	8
66004	Sandwich, hot dog, plain, fast food	1	ea	98	242	1013	53	10	18		15	5.1	6.9	1.7
56667	Sandwich, hot dog, with chili and bun, fast food	1	ea	114	296	1238	54	14	31		13	4.9	6.6	1.2
56670	Sandwich, steak, fast food	1	ea	204	459	1920	104	30	52		14	3.8	5.3	3.3
56671	Sandwich, sub, with cold cuts, fast food	1	ea	228	456	1908	132	22	51		19	6.8	8.2	2.3
56672	Sandwich, sub, with roast beef, fast food	1	ea	216	410	1715	127	29	44		13	7.1	1.8	2.6
56645	Tostada, beef and cheese, fast food	1	ea	163	315	1318	101	19	23		16	10.4	3.3	1
VEGETABLES														
5000	Artichoke, globe, ckd, drnd, med	1	med	120	64	268	101	3	14	10	<1	0.1	<0.1	0.2
5191	Artichokes, hearts, marinated	2	ea	28	25	105		1	3	1	2	0		
5007	Asparagus, cnd, drnd, 5" long	4	ea	72	14	59	68	2	2	1	<1	0.1	<0.1	0.2
5004	Asparagus, spears, ckd, drnd, ½" base	4	ea	60	13	54	56	1	2	1	<1	<0.1	0	0.1
5842	Asparagus, unsalted, with liquid, 300 can	0.5	cup	122	18	75	115	2	3	1	<1	0.1	<0.1	0.1
5249	Bamboo Shoots, slices, ckd, drnd	0.5	cup	60	7	29	58	1	1	1	<1	<0.1	<0.1	0.1
5401	Bamboo shoots, slices, cnd, drnd	0.5	cup	65.5	12	50	62	1	2	1	<1	0.1	<0.1	0.1
5250	Bamboo Shoots, whole, ckd, drnd	1	ea	144	17	71	138	2	3	1	<1	0.1	<0.1	0.1
7012	Beans, black, mature, ckd	0.5	cup	86	114	477	57	8	20	7	<1	0.1	<0.1	0.2
7027	Beans, broad, mature, ckd	0.5	cup	85	94	393	61	6	17	5	<1	0.1	0.1	0.1
7055	Beans, fava, mature, cnd	0.5	cup	128	91	381	103	7	16	5	<1	<0.1	0.1	0.1
7021	Beans, great northern, mature, ckd	0.5	cup	88.5	104	435	61	7	19	6	<1	0.1	<0.1	0.2
7087	Beans, kidney, all types, mature, cnd	0.5	cup	128	105	439	100	7	19	7	1	0.1	0.5	0.2
7047	Beans, kidney, red, mature, ckd	0.5	cup	88.5	112	469	59	8	20	7	<1	0.1	<0.1	0.2
7292	Beans, kidney, red, mature, cnd	0.5	cup	128	104	435	100	7	19	7	<1	0.1	0.1	0.3
7006	Beans, lentils, mature, ckd	0.5	cup	99	115	481	69	9	20	8	<1	0.1	0.1	0.2

< = Trace amount present　　Blank = Not available

V, vitamin; **THI**, thiamin; **RIB**, riboflavin; **NIA**, niacin; **FOL**, folate; **CALC**, calcium; **PHOS**, phosphorus; **SOD**, sodium; **POT**, potassium; **MAG**, magnesium

CHOL (mg)	V-A (IU)	THI (mg)	RIB (mg)	NIA (mg)	V-B$_6$ (mg)	FOL (μg)	V-B$_{12}$ (μg)	V-C (mg)	V-E (mg)	CALC (mg)	PHOS (mg)	SOD (mg)	POT (mg)	MAG (mg)	IRON (mg)	ZINC (mg)
21	222	0.1	0.3	0.9	0.1	18	0.6	2	0.8	161	155	92	271	24	0.3	0.7
0	0	0.1	0.1	1.2	0.2	14	0	2.1	0.7	12	79	373	256	14	0.5	0.2
24	175	0.1	0.5	0.3	0.1	9	0.6	0.8	0.2	212	192	182	376	32	0.6	0.8
21	226	0.1	0.4	0.3	0.1	6	0.6	1.5		212	188	156	342	24	0.2	0.7
18	559	0.2	0.4	1.5	0.2	10	0.8	1.2		272	276	816	172	55	1.3	1.8
	7	0.1	0.1	0.8	0.2			1.6	5.8	135	185	908	195	22	0.9	0.6
10		<0.1	0.1	0.4	<0.1		0.1		0.3	114	105	134	180	14	0.3	0.6
140	1053	0.4	0.4	6	0.4	101	0.8	16.3		235	401	743	401	49	2	3.1
44	588	0.1	0.4	2.5	0.2	83	0.6	3.6		192	143	762	416	51	2.3	2.7
0	2352	0.1	0.1	1.1	0.2	77	0	48		27	81	54	356	23	1.3	0.4
78	620	0.4	0.5	9.1	0.4	109	0.5	3		258	406	1238	333	43	3.6	2.9
216	1001	0.2	0.4	1.5	0.1	47	0.8	0.1		244	348	551	174	22	2.2	1.8
50		0.3	0.3	3.1	0.1		0.8	2		161	184	582	295	36	2.1	0.8
44	0	0.2	0.3	3.6	<0.1	48	0.5	0.1		24	97	670	143	13	2.3	2
51	58	0.2	0.4	3.7	<0.1	73	0.3	2.7		19	192	480	166	10	3.3	0.8
73	367	0.4	0.4	7.3	0.4	90	1.6	5.5		92	298	798	524	49	5.2	4.5
36	424	1	0.8	5.5	0.1	87	1.1	12.3		189	287	1651	394	68	2.5	2.6
73	413	0.4	0.4	6	0.3	71	1.8	5.6		41	192	845	330	67	2.8	4.4
41	712	0.1	0.6	3.1	0.2	75	1.2	2.6		217	179	896	572	64	2.9	3.7
0	16	0.1	0.1	1.3	0.1	107	0	8.9	0.2	25	88	72	343	50	0.7	0.5
0	0	<0.1	<0.1	0.2	<0.1	17	0	6		0	14	105	54	8	0	0.1
0	592	<0.1	0.1	0.7	0.1	69	0	13.2	0.9	12	31	207	124	7	1.3	0.3
0	604	0.1	0.1	0.7	<0.1	89	0	4.6	0.9	14	32	8	134	8	0.5	0.4
0	947	0.1	0.1	1	0.1	104	0	20.1	0.4	18	46	32	210	11	0.7	0.6
0	0	<0.1	<0.1	0.2	0.1	1	0	0		7	12	2	320	2	0.1	0.3
0	9	<0.1	<0.1	0.1	0.1	2	0	0.7	0.4	5	16	5	52	3	0.2	0.4
0	0	<0.1	0.1	0.4	0.1	3	0	0		17	29	6	768	4	0.3	0.7
0	5	0.2	0.1	0.4	0.1	128	0	0		23	120	1	305	60	1.8	1
0	13	0.1	0.1	0.6	0.1	88	0	0.3	<0.1	31	106	4	228	37	1.3	0.9
0	13	<0.1	0.1	1.2	0.1	42	0	2.3		33	101	580	310	41	1.3	0.8
0	1	0.1	0.1	0.6	0.1	90	0	1.2		60	146	2	346	44	1.9	0.8
0	0	0.1	0.1	0.5	0.1	46	0	1.5	<0.1	44	115	379	303	35	1.5	0.6
0	0	0.1	0.1	0.5	0.1	115	0	1.1	<0.1	25	126	2	357	40	2.6	0.9
0	0	0.1	0.1	0.6	0.1	33	0	1	<0.1	37	136	328	333	38	1.6	0.8
0	8	0.2	0.1	1	0.2	179	0	1.5	0.1	19	178	2	365	36	3.3	1.3

ESHA, EatRight Analysis; **AMT**, amount; **WT**, weight; **CAL**, calories; **KILO**, KiloJoule; **WTR**, water; **PROT**, protein; **CARB**, carbohydrate; **FIBR**, fiber; **FAT**, fat; **SATF**, saturated fat; **MONO**, monounsaturated fat; **POLY**, polyunsaturated fat; **CHOL**, cholesterol;

ESHA CODE	FOOD DESCRIPTION	AMT	UNIT	WT (g)	CAL (kcal)	KILO (kJ)	WTR (g)	PROT (g)	CARB (g)	FIBR (g)	FAT (g)	SATF (g)	MONO (g)	POLY (g)
VEGETABLES (CONTINUED)														
7058	Beans, lima, baby, mature, ckd	0.5	cup	91	115	481	61	7	21	7	<1	0.1	<0.1	0.2
5319	Beans, lima, immature, ckd, drnd	0.5	cup	85	105	439	57	6	20	5	<1	0.1	<0.1	0.1
7022	Beans, navy, mature, ckd	0.5	cup	91	127	531	58	7	24	10	1	0.1	0.1	0.4
7013	Beans, pinto, mature, ckd	0.5	cup	85.5	122	510	54	8	22	8	1	0.1	0.1	0.2
7051	Beans, pinto, mature, cnd	0.5	cup	120	98	410	94	6	18	6	1	0.1	0.1	0.2
7053	Beans, white, mature, ckd	0.5	cup	89.5	124	519	56	9	22	6	<1	0.1	<0.1	0.1
5022	Beet, ckd, drnd, sliced	0.5	cup	85	37	155	74	1	8	2	<1	<0.1	<0.1	0.1
5310	Beet, pickled, cnd, with liquid, slices	0.5	cup	113.5	74	310	93	1	18	3	<1	<0.1	<0.1	<0.1
9542	Broccoli rabe, bunch, ckd	1	svg	85	28	117	78	3	3	2	<1	<0.1	<0.1	0.1
9799	Broccoli rabe, fresh, chpd	0.5	cup	20	4	17	19	1	1	<1	<1	<0.1	<0.1	<0.1
5030	Broccoli, chpd, ckd f/fzn, drnd	0.5	cup	92	26	109	83	3	5	3	<1	<0.1	<0.1	0.1
5028	Broccoli, chpd, ckd, drnd	0.5	cup	78	27	113	70	2	6	3	<1	0.1	<0.1	0.1
6091	Broccoli, ckd with salt, drnd, chpd	0.5	cup	78	27	113	70	2	6	3	<1	0.1	<0.1	0.1
5029	Broccoli, stalk, med, 7½" - 8" long, ckd, drnd	1	ea	180	63	264	161	4	13	6	1	0.1	0.1	0.3
5035	Brussels Sprout, ckd f/fzn, drnd	0.5	cup	77.5	33	138	67	3	6	3	<1	0.1	<0.1	0.2
5033	Brussels Sprout, ckd, drnd	0.5	cup	78	28	117	69	2	6	2	<1	0.1	<0.1	0.2
5237	Cabbage, bok choy, ckd, drnd	0.5	cup	85	10	42	81	1	2	1	<1	<0.1	<0.1	0.1
15847	Cabbage, Chinese chard, ckd, drnd	0.5	cup	85	10	42	81	1	2	1	<1	<0.1	<0.1	0.1
5041	Cabbage, Chinese chard, shredded, fresh	1	cup	70	9	38	67	1	2	1	<1	<0.1	<0.1	0.1
5038	Cabbage, ckd, drnd, shredded	0.5	cup	75	17	71	69	1	4	1	<1	0	<0.1	<0.1
5036	Cabbage, fresh, shredded	1	cup	70	18	75	65	1	4	2	<1	<0.1	<0.1	<0.1
5075	Cabbage, kale, ckd, drnd	0.5	cup	65	18	75	59	1	4	1	<1	<0.1	<0.1	0.1
5235	Cabbage, pe-tsai, ckd, drnd, shredded	0.5	cup	59.5	8	33	57	1	1	1	<1	<0.1	<0.1	<0.1
5040	Cabbage, pe-tsai, fresh, chpd	1	cup	76	12	50	72	1	2	1	<1	<0.1	<0.1	0.1
5238	Cabbage, red, ckd, drnd, shredded	0.5	cup	75	22	92	68	1	5	2	<1	<0.1	<0.1	<0.1
5042	Cabbage, red, fresh, shredded	1	cup	70	22	92	63	1	5	1	<1	<0.1	<0.1	0.1
5358	Carrot, ckd f/fzn, drnd, slices	0.5	cup	73	27	113	66	<1	6	2	<1	0.1	<0.1	0.2
5047	Carrot, ckd, drnd, slices	0.5	cup	78	27	113	70	1	6	2	<1	<0.1	<0.1	0.1
5439	Carrot, fresh, baby	1	med	10	4	17	9	<1	1	<1	<1	<0.1	<0.1	<0.1
5046	Carrot, fresh, grated	0.5	cup	55	23	96	49	1	5	2	<1	<0.1	<0.1	0.1
90423	Carrot, fresh, lrg, 7¼" – 8½" long	1	ea	72	30	126	64	1	7	2	<1	<0.1	<0.1	0.1
5625	Cassava, yuca blanca, pieces, ckd	0.5	cup	68.5	111	464	41	1	26	1	<1	0.1	0.1	<0.1
5053	Cauliflower, ckd f/fzn, drnd, 1" pces	0.5	cup	90	17	71	85	1	3	2	<1	<0.1	<0.1	0.1
5052	Cauliflower, florets, ckd, drnd	3	ea	54	12	50	50	1	2	1	<1	<0.1	<0.1	0.1
5049	Cauliflower, fresh	0.5	cup	53.5	13	54	49	1	3	1	<1	<0.1	<0.1	<0.1
5054	Celery, fresh, diced	0.5	cup	50.5	8	33	48	<1	1	1	<1	<0.1	<0.1	<0.1
5055	Celery, stalk, med, 7.5" - 8" long, fresh	1	ea	40	6	25	38	<1	1	1	<1	<0.1	<0.1	<0.1
5399	Chili Pepper, green, hot, fresh, chpd	0.25	cup	37.5	15	63	33	1	4	1	<1	<0.1	<0.1	<0.1
5293	Chili Pepper, jalapeno, cnd, with liquid, chpd	0.25	cup	34	9	38	30	<1	2	1	<1	<0.1	<0.1	0.2
5288	Chili Pepper, red, hot, fresh, chpd	0.25	cup	37.5	15	63	33	1	3	1	<1	<0.1	<0.1	0.1

< = Trace amount present   Blank = Not available

V, vitamin; **THI**, thiamin; **RIB**, riboflavin; **NIA**, niacin; **FOL**, folate; **CALC**, calcium; **PHOS**, phosphorus; **SOD**, sodium; **POT**, potassium; **MAG**, magnesium

CHOL (mg)	V-A (IU)	THI (mg)	RIB (mg)	NIA (mg)	V-B_6 (mg)	FOL (µg)	V-B_{12} (µg)	V-C (mg)	V-E (mg)	CALC (mg)	PHOS (mg)	SOD (mg)	POT (mg)	MAG (mg)	IRON (mg)	ZINC (mg)
0	0	0.1	0.1	0.6	0.1	136	0	0		26	116	3	365	48	2.2	0.9
0	258	0.1	0.1	0.9	0.2	22	0	8.6	0.1	27	110	14	484	63	2.1	0.7
	0	0.2	0.1	0.6	0.1	127	0	0.8	<0.1	63	131	0	354	48	2.1	0.9
0	0	0.2	0.1	0.3	0.2	147	0	0.7	0.8	39	126	1	373	43	1.8	0.8
0	0	0.1	<0.1	0.3	0.1	29	0	0.8	0.7	56	110	322	331	40	1.8	0.7
0	0	0.1	<0.1	0.1	0.1	72	0	0	0.8	81	101	5	502	56	3.3	1.2
0	30	<0.1	<0.1	0.3	0.1	68	0	3.1	<0.1	14	32	65	259	20	0.7	0.3
0	56	<0.1	0.1	0.3	0.1	31	0	2.6	0.1	12	19	300	168	17	0.5	0.3
0	3853	0.1	0.1	1.7	0.2	60	0	31.4	2.2	100	70	48	292	23	1.1	0.5
0	524	<0.1	<0.1	0.2	<0.1	17	0	4	0.3	22	15	7	39	4	0.4	0.2
0	930	0.1	0.1	0.4	0.1	52	0	36.9	1.2	30	45	10	131	12	0.6	0.3
0	1207	<0.1	0.1	0.4	0.2	84	0	50.6	1.1	31	52	32	229	16	0.5	0.4
0	1207	<0.1	0.1	0.4	0.2	84	0	50.6	1.1	31	52	204	229	16	0.5	0.4
0	2786	0.1	0.2	1	0.4	194	0	116.8	2.6	72	121	74	527	38	1.2	0.8
0	718	0.1	0.1	0.4	0.2	78	0	35.4	0.4	20	43	12	225	14	0.4	0.2
0	604	0.1	0.1	0.5	0.1	47	0	48.4	0.3	28	44	16	247	16	0.9	0.3
0	3612	<0.1	0.1	0.4	0.1	35	0	22.1	0.1	79	25	29	315	9	0.9	0.1
0	3612	<0.1	0.1	0.4	0.1	35	0	22.1	0.1	79	25	29	315	9	0.9	0.1
0	3128	<0.1	<0.1	0.4	0.1	46	0	31.5	0.1	74	26	46	176	13	0.6	0.1
0	60	<0.1	<0.1	0.2	0.1	22	0	28.1	0.1	36	25	6	147	11	0.1	0.2
0	69	<0.1	<0.1	0.2	0.1	30	0	25.6	0.1	28	18	13	119	8	0.3	0.1
0	8854	<0.1	<0.1	0.3	0.1	8	0	26.6	0.6	47	18	15	148	12	0.6	0.2
0	575	<0.1	<0.1	0.3	0.1	32	0	9.4		19	23	5	134	6	0.2	0.1
0	242	<0.1	<0.1	0.3	0.2	60	0	20.5	0.1	59	22	7	181	10	0.2	0.2
0	25	0.1	<0.1	0.3	0.2	18	0	25.8	0.1	32	25	21	196	13	0.5	0.2
0	781	<0.1	<0.1	0.3	0.1	13	0	39.9	0.1	32	21	19	170	11	0.6	0.2
0	12357	<0.1	<0.1	0.3	0.1	8	0	1.7	0.7	26	23	43	140	8	0.4	0.3
0	13286	0.1	<0.1	0.5	0.1	11	0	2.8	0.8	23	23	45	183	8	0.3	0.2
0	1379	<0.1	<0.1	0.1	<0.1	3	0	0.3		3	3	8	24	1	0.1	<0.1
0	9188	<0.1	<0.1	0.5	0.1	10	0	3.2	0.4	18	19	38	176	7	0.2	0.1
0	12028	<0.1	<0.1	0.7	0.1	14	0	4.2	0.5	24	25	50	230	9	0.2	0.2
0	16	<0.1	<0.1	0.5	0.1	12	0	9.3	0.1	11	17	9	169	14	0.2	0.2
0	9	<0.1	<0.1	0.3	0.1	37	0	28.2	0.1	15	22	16	125	8	0.4	0.1
0	6	<0.1	<0.1	0.2	0.1	24	0	23.9	<0.1	9	17	8	77	5	0.2	0.1
0	0	<0.1	<0.1	0.3	0.1	30	0	25.8	<0.1	12	24	16	160	8	0.2	0.1
0	227	<0.1	<0.1	0.2	<0.1	18	0	1.6	0.1	20	12	40	131	6	0.1	0.1
0	180	<0.1	<0.1	0.1	<0.1	14	0	1.2	0.1	16	10	32	104	4	0.1	0.1
0	442	<0.1	<0.1	0.4	0.1	9	0	90.9	0.3	7	17	3	128	9	0.4	0.1
0	578	<0.1	<0.1	0.1	0.1	5	0	3.4	0.2	8	6	568	66	5	0.6	0.1
0	357	<0.1	<0.1	0.5	0.2	9	0	53.9	0.3	5	16	3	121	9	0.4	0.1

ESHA, EatRight Analysis; **AMT**, amount; **WT**, weight; **CAL**, calories; **KILO**, KiloJoule; **WTR**, water; **PROT**, protein; **CARB**, carbohydrate; **FIBR**, fiber; **FAT**, fat; **SATF**, saturated fat; **MONO**, monounsaturated fat; **POLY**, polyunsaturated fat; **CHOL**, cholesterol;

ESHA CODE	FOOD DESCRIPTION	AMT	UNIT	WT (g)	CAL (kcal)	KILO (kJ)	WTR (g)	PROT (g)	CARB (g)	FIBR (g)	FAT (g)	SATF (g)	MONO (g)	POLY (g)
VEGETABLES (CONTINUED)														
5515	Corn, with red and green peppers, cnd, with liquid	0.5	cup	113.5	85	356	88	3	21	2	1	0.1	0.2	0.3
5563	Corn, white, sweet, cnd, drnd	0.5	cup	82	66	276	63	2	15	2	1	0.1	0.2	0.4
5560	Corn, white, sweet, kernels f/one ear, ckd, drnd	0.5	cup	78.5	76	318	57	3	17	2	1	0.2	0.3	0.5
5393	Corn, white, sweet, kernels, ckd f/fzn, drnd	0.5	cup	82.5	66	276	63	2	16	2	<1	0.1	0.1	0.2
5562	Corn, white, sweet, kernels, unsalted, cnd, with liquid	0.5	cup	128	82	343	104	2	20	1	1	0.1	0.2	0.3
5364	Corn, yellow, sweet, cob, ckd f/fzn, drnd	1	ea	63	59	247	46	2	14	2	<1	0.1	0.1	0.2
5380	Corn, yellow, sweet, cob, ckd, drnd	1	ea	77	74	310	57	3	16	2	1	0.2	0.3	0.5
5065	Corn, yellow, sweet, kernels, ckd f/fzn, drnd	0.5	cup	82.5	67	280	64	2	16	2	1	0.1	0.2	0.3
5379	Corn, yellow, sweet, kernels, ckd, drnd	0.5	cup	74.5	72	301	55	3	16	2	1	0.1	0.3	0.4
5201	Corn, yellow, sweet, kernels, cnd, with brine	0.5	cup	128	78	326	106	2	18	2	1	0.1	0.2	0.3
5066	Corn, yellow, sweet, kernels, drnd, 12oz can	0.5	cup	82	65	272	64	2	15	2	1	0.1	0.2	0.3
5070	Cucumber, with skin, fresh, 8¼" long	1	ea	301	45	188	287	2	11	2	<1	0.1	<0.1	0.1
5071	Cucumber, with skin, fresh, slices	0.5	cup	52	8	33	50	<1	2	<1	<1	<0.1	<0.1	<0.1
5619	Dish, pickled radishes, Hawaiian	0.5	cup	75	21	88	69	1	4	2	<1	0.1	<0.1	0.1
5072	Eggplant, ckd, drnd, 1" cubes	0.5	cup	49.5	17	71	44	<1	4	1	<1	<0.1	<0.1	<0.1
9337	Eggplant, Japanese, ckd	0.66	cup	85	20	84	67	1	5	2	0	0	0	0
26005	Garlic, cloves, fresh	1	ea	3	4	17	2	<1	1	<1	<1	<0.1	<0.1	<0.1
6033	Greens, arugula, chpd, fresh	1	cup	20	5	21	18	1	1	<1	<1	<0.1	<0.1	0.1
48559	Greens, baby spring, mix, fresh	2	cup	85	15	63		2	4	2	0	0	0	0
5062	Greens, collard, chpd, ckd f/fzn, drnd	0.5	cup	85	31	130	75	3	6	2	<1	0.1	<0.1	0.2
5061	Greens, collard, chpd, ckd, drnd	0.5	cup	95	31	130	86	3	5	4	1	<0.1	<0.1	0.2
6811	Greens, corn salad, fresh	0.5	cup	28	6	25	26	1	1		<1			
5202	Greens, endive, fresh, chpd	1	cup	50	8	33	47	1	2	2	<1	<0.1	<0.1	<0.1
5096	Greens, mustard, ckd, drnd	0.5	cup	70	18	75	64	2	3	1	<1	<0.1	0.1	<0.1
5451	Greens, radicchio, fresh, shredded	1	cup	40	9	38	37	1	2	<1	<1	<0.1	<0.1	<0.1
24128	Greens, Swiss chard, bld, drnd, chpd	0.5	cup	87.5	18	75	81	2	4	2	<1	<0.1	<0.1	<0.1
5185	Greens, turnip, chpd, ckd, drnd	0.5	cup	72	14	59	67	1	3	3	<1	<0.1	<0.1	0.1
5186	Greens, turnip, ckd f/fzn, drnd	0.5	cup	82	24	100	74	3	4	3	<1	0.1	<0.1	0.1
5222	Greens, watercress, fresh, chpd	1	cup	34	4	17	32	1	<1	<1	<1	<0.1	<0.1	<0.1
5223	Greens, watercress, fresh, sprig	34	ea	85	9	38	81	2	1	<1	<1	<0.1	<0.1	<0.1
5140	Hash Browns, plain, prep f/fzn, 12 oz pkg	0.5	cup	39	85	356	22	1	11	1	4	1.8	2	0.5
5141	Hash Browns, plain, prep f/fzn, patty 3" × 1½" oval	1	ea	29	63	264	16	1	8	1	3	1.3	1.5	0.4
38077	Hominy, white, cnd	0.5	cup	82.5	59	247	68	1	12	2	1	0.1	0.2	0.3
5470	Hominy, yellow, cnd	0.5	cup	80	58	243	66	1	11	2	1	0.1	0.2	0.3
9181	Jicama, fresh, chpd	0.5	cup	65	25	105	59	<1	6	3	<1	<0.1	<0.1	<0.1
6832	Ladies Fingers, ckd f/fzn, drnd, slices	0.5	cup	92	27	113	84	1	6	2	<1	0.1	<0.1	0.1

< = Trace amount present   Blank = Not available

V, vitamin; **THI**, thiamin; **RIB**, riboflavin; **NIA**, niacin; **FOL**, folate; **CALC**, calcium; **PHOS**, phosphorus; **SOD**, sodium; **POT**, potassium; **MAG**, magnesium

CHOL (mg)	V-A (IU)	THI (mg)	RIB (mg)	NIA (mg)	V-B_6 (mg)	FOL (µg)	V-B_{12} (µg)	V-C (mg)	V-E (mg)	CALC (mg)	PHOS (mg)	SOD (mg)	POT (mg)	MAG (mg)	IRON (mg)	ZINC (mg)
0	263	<0.1	0.1	1.1	0.1	39	0	10		6	70	394	174	28	0.9	0.4
0	1	<0.1	0.1	1	<0.1	40	0	7	0.1	4	53	265	160	16	0.7	0.3
0	2	0.1	<0.1	1.3	0.1	16	0	4.9	0.1	2	72	2	198	24	0.4	0.4
0	2	0.1	0.1	1.1	0.1	26	0	2.6	0.1	3	47	4	121	16	0.3	0.3
0	1	<0.1	0.1	1.2	<0.1	49	0	7		5	65	15	210	20	0.5	0.5
0	146	0.1	<0.1	1	0.1	20	0	3	0.1	2	47	3	158	18	0.4	0.4
0	203	0.1	<0.1	1.3	0.1	18	0	4.2	0.1	2	59	1	168	20	0.3	0.5
0	164	<0.1	0.1	1.1	0.1	29	0	2.9	0.1	2	65	1	192	23	0.4	0.5
0	196	0.1	<0.1	1.3	0.1	17	0	4.1	0.1	2	57	1	162	19	0.3	0.5
0	44	<0.1	<0.1	1.1	<0.1	49	0	3.3	<0.1	5	59	250	174	19	0.5	0.5
0	37	<0.1	<0.1	0.6	0.1	29	0	1.3	0.1	3	39	153	113	11	0.5	0.3
0	316	0.1	0.1	0.3	0.1	21	0	8.4	0.1	48	72	6	442	39	0.8	0.6
0	55	<0.1	<0.1	0.1	<0.1	4	0	1.5	<0.1	8	12	1	76	7	0.1	0.1
0	0	<0.1	<0.1	0.2	0.1	7	0	0	0	21	23	592	250	6	0.2	0.2
0	18	<0.1	<0.1	0.3	<0.1	7	0	0.6	0.2	3	7	<1	61	5	0.1	0.1
0	0							1.2		0		0			0	
0	<1	<0.1	<0.1	<0.1	<0.1	<1	0	0.9	<0.1	5	5	1	12	1	0.1	<0.1
0	475	<0.1	<0.1	0.1	<0.1	19	0	3	0.1	32	10	5	74	9	0.3	0.1
0	5500							30		60		70			3.6	
0	9769	<0.1	0.1	0.5	0.1	65	0	22.4	1.1	178	23	42	213	26	1	0.2
0	7220	<0.1	0.1	0.5	0.1	15	0	17.3	0.8	134	30	14	111	20	1.1	0.2
0	1986	<0.1	<0.1	0.1	0.1	4	0	10.7		11	15	1	129	4	0.6	0.2
0	1084	<0.1	<0.1	0.2	<0.1	71	0	3.2	0.2	26	14	11	157	8	0.4	0.4
0	8659	<0.1	<0.1	0.3	0.1	6	0	17.7	1.2	83	29	6	113	9	0.6	0.2
0	11	<0.1	<0.1	0.1	<0.1	24	0	3.2	0.9	8	16	9	121	5	0.2	0.2
0	5358	<0.1	0.1	0.3	0.1	8	0	15.8	1.7	51	29	157	480	75	2	0.3
0	5490	<0.1	0.1	0.3	0.1	85	0	19.7	1.4	99	21	21	146	16	0.6	0.1
0	8827	<0.1	0.1	0.4	0.1	32	0	17.9	2.2	125	28	12	184	21	1.6	0.3
0	1085	<0.1	<0.1	0.1	<0.1	3	0	14.6	0.3	41	20	14	112	7	0.1	<0.1
0	2712	0.1	0.1	0.2	0.1	8	0	36.6	0.8	102	51	35	280	18	0.2	0.1
0	0	<0.1	<0.1	0.9	<0.1	3	0	2.5	0.1	6	28	13	170	7	0.6	0.1
0	0	<0.1	<0.1	0.7	<0.1	2	0	1.8	0.1	4	21	10	126	5	0.4	0.1
0	1	<0.1	<0.1	<0.1	<0.1	1	0	0	<0.1	8	29	285	7	13	0.5	0.9
0	88	<0.1	<0.1	<0.1	<0.1	1	0	0		8	28	276	7	13	0.5	0.8
0	14	<0.1	<0.1	0.1	<0.1	8	0	13.1	0.3	8	12	3	98	8	0.4	0.1
0	281	0.1	0.1	0.6	<0.1	92	0	8.8	0.3	68	34	3	169	37	0.5	0.5

ESHA, EatRight Analysis; **AMT**, amount; **WT**, weight; **CAL**, calories; **KILO**, KiloJoule; **WTR**, water; **PROT**, protein; **CARB**, carbohydrate; **FIBR**, fiber; **FAT**, fat; **SATF**, saturated fat; **MONO**, monounsaturated fat; **POLY**, polyunsaturated fat; **CHOL**, cholesterol;

ESHA CODE	FOOD DESCRIPTION	AMT	UNIT	WT (g)	CAL (kcal)	KILO (kJ)	WTR (g)	PROT (g)	CARB (g)	FIBR (g)	FAT (g)	SATF (g)	MONO (g)	POLY (g)
VEGETABLES (CONTINUED)														
5206	Leeks, bulb and lower leaf, fresh	1	ea	89	54	226	74	1	13	2	<1	<0.1	<0.1	0.1
5080	Lettuce, butterhead, fresh, chpd	1	cup	55	7	29	53	1	1	1	<1	<0.1	<0.1	0.1
5087	Lettuce, green leaf, fresh, outer leaf	1	cup	36	5	21	34	<1	1	<1	<1	<0.1	<0.1	<0.1
5086	Lettuce, green leaf, fresh, shredded	1	cup	36	5	21	34	<1	1	<1	<1	<0.1	<0.1	<0.1
90447	Lettuce, iceberg, fresh, leaf	1	med	8	1	4	8	<1	<1	<1	<1	<0.1	<0.1	<0.1
5083	Lettuce, iceberg, fresh, shred	1	cup	72	10	42	69	1	2	1	<1	<0.1	<0.1	0.1
5088	Lettuce, romaine, fresh, shred	1	cup	47	8	33	44	1	2	1	<1	<0.1	<0.1	0.1
5092	Mushrooms, ckd, drnd	0.5	cup	78	22	92	71	2	4	2	<1	<0.1	<0.1	0.1
5094	Mushrooms, cnd, drnd, slices	0.5	cup	78	20	84	71	1	4	2	<1	<0.1	<0.1	0.1
5090	Mushrooms, fresh, slices	0.5	cup	35	8	33	32	1	1	<1	<1	<0.1	0	0.1
6494	Mushrooms, fresh, whole	0.5	cup	48	11	46	44	1	2	<1	<1	<0.1	0	0.1
5385	Mushrooms, shiitake, ckd, pieces	0.5	cup	72.5	41	172	61	1	10	2	<1	<0.1	0.1	<0.1
7508	Natto, fermented soybeans	0.5	cup	87.5	186	778	48	16	13	5	10	1.4	2.1	5.4
5098	Okra, ckd, drnd, pods	8	ea	85	19	79	79	2	4	2	<1	<0.1	<0.1	<0.1
5099	Okra, ckd, drnd, slices	0.5	cup	80	18	75	74	1	4	2	<1	<0.1	<0.1	<0.1
5114	Onion, spring, tops and bulb, fresh, chpd	0.5	cup	50	16	67	45	1	4	1	<1	<0.1	<0.1	<0.1
5108	Onion, white, ckd, drnd, chpd	0.5	cup	105	46	192	92	1	11	1	<1	<0.1	<0.1	0.1
5101	Onion, white, fresh, chpd	0.5	cup	80	32	134	71	1	7	1	<1	<0.1	<0.1	<0.1
5106	Onion, white, fresh, lrg slice, ¼"	1	slice	38	15	63	34	<1	4	1	<1	<0.1	<0.1	<0.1
5104	Onion, white, fresh, med, whole, 2½"	1	ea	110	44	184	98	1	10	2	<1	<0.1	<0.1	<0.1
5212	Parsnips, ckd, drnd	0.5	cup	78	55	230	63	1	13	3	<1	<0.1	0.1	<0.1
5296	Pea Pods, ckd f/fzn, drnd	0.5	cup	80	42	176	69	3	7	2	<1	0.1	<0.1	0.1
5122	Pea Pods, ckd, drnd	0.5	cup	80	34	142	71	3	6	2	<1	<0.1	<0.1	0.1
7016	Peas, black eyed, mature, plain, cnd	0.5	cup	120	92	385	96	6	16	4	1	0.2	0.1	0.3
7018	Peas, cowpeas, mature, ckd	0.5	cup	85.5	99	414	60	7	18	6	<1	0.1	<0.1	0.2
7001	Peas, garbanzo, mature, ckd	0.5	cup	82	134	561	49	7	22	6	2	0.2	0.5	0.9
7088	Peas, garbanzo, mature, cnd	0.5	cup	120	106	444	94	6	16	5	2	0.2	0.5	1.1
5118	Peas, green, ckd f/fzn, drnd	0.5	cup	80	62	259	64	4	11	4	<1	<0.1	<0.1	0.1
5117	Peas, green, ckd, drnd	0.5	cup	80	67	280	62	4	13	4	<1	<0.1	<0.1	0.1
5214	Peas, green, cnd, with liquid	0.5	cup	124	72	301	106	4	13	4	1	0.1	0.1	0.3
7020	Peas, green, split, ckd	0.5	cup	98	116	485	68	8	21	8	<1	0.1	0.1	0.2
5267	Peas, green, unsalted, cnd, with liquid	0.5	cup	124	66	276	107	4	12	4	<1	0.1	<0.1	0.2
5126	Peppers, sweet, bell, green, ckd, drnd, chpd	0.5	cup	67.5	19	79	62	1	5	1	<1	<0.1	<0.1	0.1
5124	Peppers, sweet, bell, green, fresh, chpd	0.5	cup	74.5	15	63	70	1	3	1	<1	<0.1	<0.1	<0.1
5125	Peppers, sweet, bell, green, fresh, sml	1	ea	74	15	63	69	1	3	1	<1	<0.1	<0.1	<0.1
5128	Peppers, sweet, bell, red, fresh, chpd	0.5	cup	74.5	23	96	69	1	4	1	<1	<0.1	<0.1	0.1
5441	Peppers, sweet, bell, yellow, fresh, lrg, 3¾" long	1	ea	186	50	209	171	2	12	2	<1	0.1		
90580	Pickles, dill, lrg, 4" long	1	ea	135	16	67	127	1	3	1	<1	<0.1	<0.1	0.1
27013	Pickles, dill, slices	1	ea	7	1	4	7	<1	<1	<1	<1	<0.1	<0.1	<0.1

< = Trace amount present Blank = Not available

V, vitamin; **THI**, thiamin; **RIB**, riboflavin; **NIA**, niacin; **FOL**, folate; **CALC**, calcium; **PHOS**, phosphorus; **SOD**, sodium; **POT**, potassium; **MAG**, magnesium

CHOL (mg)	V-A (IU)	THI (mg)	RIB (mg)	NIA (mg)	V-B_6 (mg)	FOL (μg)	V-B_{12} (μg)	V-C (mg)	V-E (mg)	CALC (mg)	PHOS (mg)	SOD (mg)	POT (mg)	MAG (mg)	IRON (mg)	ZINC (mg)
0	1484	0.1	<0.1	0.4	0.2	57	0	10.7	0.8	53	31	18	160	25	1.9	0.1
0	1822	<0.1	<0.1	0.2	<0.1	40	0	2	0.1	19	18	3	131	7	0.7	0.1
0	2666	<0.1	<0.1	0.1	<0.1	14	0	3.3	0.1	13	10	10	70	5	0.3	0.1
0	2666	<0.1	<0.1	0.1	<0.1	14	0	3.3	0.1	13	10	10	70	5	0.3	0.1
0	40	<0.1	<0.1	<0.1	<0.1	2	0	0.2	<0.1	1	2	1	11	1	<0.1	<0.1
0	361	<0.1	<0.1	0.1	<0.1	21	0	2	0.1	13	14	7	102	5	0.3	0.1
0	4094	<0.1	<0.1	0.1	<0.1	64	0	1.9	0.1	16	14	4	116	7	0.5	0.1
0	0	0.1	0.2	3.5	0.1	14	0	3.1	<0.1	5	68	2	278	9	1.4	0.7
0	0	0.1	<0.1	1.2	<0.1	9	0	0	<0.1	9	51	332	101	12	0.6	0.6
0	0	<0.1	0.1	1.3	<0.1	6	<0.1	0.7	<0.1	1	30	2	111	3	0.2	0.2
0	0	<0.1	0.2	1.7	<0.1	8	<0.1	1	<0.1	1	41	2	153	4	0.2	0.2
0	0	<0.1	0.1	1.1	0.1	15	0	0.2	0	2	21	3	85	10	0.3	1
0	0	0.1	0.2	0	0.1	7	0	11.4	<0.1	190	152	6	638	101	7.5	2.7
0	241	0.1	<0.1	0.7	0.2	39	0	13.9	0.2	65	27	5	115	31	0.2	0.4
0	226	0.1	<0.1	0.7	0.1	37	0	13	0.2	62	26	5	108	29	0.2	0.3
0	498	<0.1	<0.1	0.3	<0.1	32	0	9.4	0.3	36	18	8	138	10	0.7	0.2
0	2	<0.1	<0.1	0.2	0.1	16	0	5.5	<0.1	23	37	3	174	12	0.3	0.2
0	2	<0.1	<0.1	0.1	0.1	15	0	5.9	<0.1	18	23	3	117	8	0.2	0.1
0	1	<0.1	<0.1	<0.1	<0.1	7	0	2.8	<0.1	9	11	2	55	4	0.1	0.1
0	2	0.1	<0.1	0.1	0.1	21	0	8.1	<0.1	25	32	4	161	11	0.2	0.2
0	0	0.1	<0.1	0.6	0.1	45	0	10.1	0.8	29	54	8	286	23	0.5	0.2
0	1049	0.1	0.1	0.5	0.1	28	0	17.6	0.4	47	46	4	174	22	1.9	0.4
0	824	0.1	0.1	0.4	0.1	23	0	38.3	0.3	34	44	3	192	21	1.6	0.3
0	16	0.1	0.1	0.4	0.1	61	0	3.2		24	84	359	206	34	1.2	0.8
0	13	0.2	<0.1	0.4	0.1	178	0	0.3	0.2	21	133	3	238	45	2.1	1.1
0	22	0.1	0.1	0.4	0.1	141	0	1.1	0.3	40	138	6	239	39	2.4	1.3
0	18	<0.1	<0.1	0.2	0.6	30	0	0.1		42	96	334	173	32	1.5	0.8
0	1680	0.2	0.1	1.2	0.1	47	0	7.9	<0.1	19	62	58	88	18	1.2	0.5
0	641	0.2	0.1	1.6	0.2	50	0	11.4	0.1	22	94	2	217	31	1.2	1
0	1896	0.1	<0.1	1.2	0.1	30	0	9.7	<0.1	25	78	229	131	24	1.6	0.9
0	7	0.2	0.1	0.9	<0.1	64	0	0.4	<0.1	14	97	2	355	35	1.3	1
0	1791	0.1	0.1	1	0.1	36	0	12.2	<0.1	22	66	11	124	21	1.3	0.9
0	316	<0.1	<0.1	0.3	0.2	11	0	50.2	0.3	6	12	1	112	7	0.3	0.1
0	276	<0.1	<0.1	0.4	0.2	7	0	59.9	0.3	7	15	2	130	7	0.3	0.1
0	274	<0.1	<0.1	0.4	0.2	7	0	59.5	0.3	7	15	2	130	7	0.3	0.1
0	2333	<0.1	0.1	0.7	0.2	34	0	95.1	1.2	5	19	3	157	9	0.3	0.2
0	372	0.1	<0.1	1.7	0.3	48	0	341.3		20	45	4	394	22	0.9	0.3
0	247	<0.1	<0.1	0.1	<0.1	1	0	1.1	0.1	57	16	1181	124	9	0.5	0.1
0	13	<0.1	<0.1	<0.1	<0.1	<1	0	0.1	<0.1	3	1	61	6	<1	<0.1	<0.1

ESHA, EatRight Analysis; **AMT**, amount; **WT**, weight; **CAL**, calories; **KILO**, KiloJoule; **WTR**, water; **PROT**, protein; **CARB**, carbohydrate; **FIBR**, fiber; **FAT**, fat; **SATF**, saturated fat; **MONO**, monounsaturated fat; **POLY**, polyunsaturated fat; **CHOL**, cholesterol;

ESHA CODE	FOOD DESCRIPTION	AMT	UNIT	WT (g)	CAL (kcal)	KILO (kJ)	WTR (g)	PROT (g)	CARB (g)	FIBR (g)	FAT (g)	SATF (g)	MONO (g)	POLY (g)
VEGETABLES (CONTINUED)														
27016	Pickles, sweet, lrg, 3" long	1	ea	35	32	134	27	<1	7	<1	<1	<0.1	<0.1	<0.1
5227	Pimentos, cnd	1	Tbs	12	3	13	11	<1	1	<1	<1	<0.1	<0.1	<0.1
5228	Pimentos, cnd, slices	20	pce	20	5	21	19	<1	1	<1	<1	<0.1	<0.1	<0.1
5130	Potatoes, baked, peeled	0.5	cup	61	57	238	46	1	13	1	<1	<0.1	<0.1	<0.1
5947	Potatoes, baked, with salt, med, 2¼" x 3¼"	1	ea	173	161	674	130	4	37	4	<1	0.1	<0.1	0.1
5352	Potatoes, cnd, drnd	0.5	cup	90	54	226	76	1	12	2	<1	<0.1	<0.1	0.1
5136	Potatoes, peeled, ckd, diced	0.5	cup	78	67	280	60	1	16	1	<1	<0.1	<0.1	<0.1
5339	Potatoes, skin, bkd	1	ea	58	115	481	27	2	27	5	<1	<0.1	<0.1	<0.1
5143	Radishes, fresh, med, ¾" to 1"	1	ea	4.5	1	4	4	<1	<1	<1	<1	<0.1	<0.1	<0.1
5144	Radishes, fresh, slices	0.5	cup	58	9	38	55	<1	2	1	<1	<0.1	<0.1	<0.1
7490	Radishes, Oriental, ckd, drnd, slices	0.5	cup	73.5	12	50	70	<1	3	1	<1	0.1	<0.1	0.1
5969	Rutabaga, ckd with salt, drnd, mashed	0.5	cup	120	36	151	110	1	8	2	<1	<0.1	<0.1	0.1
6255	Salad, bean, three, cnd	0.5	cup	121	80	335		3	18	3	0	0	0	0
5145	Sauerkraut, cnd, with liquid	0.5	cup	118	22	92	109	1	5	3	<1	<0.1	<0.1	0.1
5531	Sauerkraut, low sod, cnd	0.5	cup	71	16	67	66	1	3	2	<1	<0.1	<0.1	<0.1
5427	Shallots, chpd, fresh	1	Tbs	10	7	29	8	<1	2	<1	<1	<0.1	<0.1	<0.1
5013	Snap Beans, green, ckd f/fzn, drnd	0.5	cup	67.5	19	79	62	1	4	2	<1	<0.1	<0.1	0.1
5011	Snap Beans, green, ckd, drnd	0.5	cup	62.5	22	92	56	1	5	2	<1	<0.1	<0.1	0.1
6750	Snap Beans, green, cnd, drnd	0.5	cup	76.5	19	79	71	1	3	2	<1	0.1	<0.1	0.1
5231	Snap Beans, green, unsalted, cnd, with liquid	0.5	cup	120	18	75	114	1	4	2	<1	<0.1	<0.1	0.1
7015	Soybeans, mature, ckd	0.5	cup	86	149	623	54	14	9	5	8	1.1	1.7	4.4
48590	Spinach, baby, fresh, org	3	cup	85	30	126		2	5	2	0	0	0	0
5147	Spinach, ckd, drnd	0.5	cup	90	21	88	82	3	3	2	<1	<0.1	<0.1	0.1
5146	Spinach, fresh, chpd	1	cup	30	7	29	27	1	1	1	<1	<0.1	<0.1	<0.1
5010	Sprouts, alfalfa, fresh	1	cup	33	8	33	31	1	1	1	<1	<0.1	<0.1	0.1
5021	Sprouts, mung bean, mature, ckd, drnd	0.5	cup	62	13	54	58	1	3	<1	<1	<0.1	<0.1	<0.1
5197	Sprouts, mung bean, mature, cnd, drnd	0.5	cup	62.5	8	33	60	1	1	<1	<1	<0.1	<0.1	<0.1
5314	Squash, acorn, bkd, cubes	0.5	cup	102.5	57	238	85	1	15	5	<1	<0.1	<0.1	0.1
5317	Squash, butternut, bkd, cubes	0.5	cup	102.5	41	172	90	1	11	3	<1	<0.1	<0.1	<0.1
5453	Squash, hubbard, bkd, cubes	0.5	cup	102.5	51	213	87	3	11	5	1	0.1	<0.1	0.3
5455	Squash, spaghetti, ckd, drnd	0.5	cup	77.5	21	88	72	1	5	1	<1	<0.1	<0.1	0.1
5152	Squash, summer, all types, ckd, drnd, slices	0.5	cup	90	18	75	84	1	4	1	<1	0.1	<0.1	0.1
5303	Squash, winter, all types, bkd, cubes	0.5	cup	102.5	38	159	91	1	9	3	<1	0.1	<0.1	0.2
5667	Squash, zucchini, slices, stmd	0.5	cup	90	13	54	86	1	3	1	<1	<0.1	<0.1	0.1
5327	Squash, zucchini, with skin, ckd, drnd, slices	0.5	cup	90	14	59	86	1	2	1	<1	0.1	<0.1	0.1
5326	Squash, zucchini, with skin, fresh, chpd	0.5	cup	62	11	46	59	1	2	1	<1	0.1	<0.1	0.1
5158	Sweet Potatoes, dark orange, bkd in skin, peeled	0.5	cup	100	90	377	76	2	21	3	<1	<0.1	<0.1	0.1

< = Trace amount present   Blank = Not available

V, vitamin; **THI**, thiamin; **RIB**, riboflavin; **NIA**, niacin; **FOL**, folate; **CALC**, calcium; **PHOS**, phosphorus; **SOD**, sodium; **POT**, potassium; **MAG**, magnesium

CHOL (mg)	V-A (IU)	THI (mg)	RIB (mg)	NIA (mg)	V-B_6 (mg)	FOL (μg)	V-B_{12} (μg)	V-C (mg)	V-E (mg)	CALC (mg)	PHOS (mg)	SOD (mg)	POT (mg)	MAG (mg)	IRON (mg)	ZINC (mg)
0	267	<0.1	<0.1	<0.1	<0.1	<1	0	0.2	0.1	21	6	160	35	2	0.1	<0.1
0	319	<0.1	<0.1	0.1	<0.1	1	0	10.2	0.1	1	2	2	19	1	0.2	<0.1
0	531	<0.1	<0.1	0.1	<0.1	1	0	17	0.1	1	3	3	32	1	0.3	<0.1
0	0	0.1	<0.1	0.9	0.2	5	0	7.8	<0.1	3	30	3	239	15	0.2	0.2
0	17	0.1	0.1	2.4	0.5	48	0	16.6	0.1	26	121	17	926	48	1.9	0.6
0	0	0.1	<0.1	0.8	0.2	5	0	4.6		4	25	197	206	13	1.1	0.3
0	2	0.1	<0.1	1	0.2	7	0	5.8	<0.1	6	31	4	256	16	0.2	0.2
0	6	0.1	0.1	1.8	0.4	13	0	7.8	<0.1	20	59	12	332	25	4.1	0.3
0	<1	<0.1	<0.1	<0.1	<0.1	1	0	0.7	0	1	1	2	10	<1	<0.1	<0.1
0	4	<0.1	<0.1	0.1	<0.1	14	0	8.6	0	14	12	23	135	6	0.2	0.2
0	0	0	<0.1	0.1	<0.1	12	0	11.1	0	12	18	10	209	7	0.1	0.1
0	2	0.1	<0.1	0.9	0.1	18	0	22.6	0.3	22	49	6	259	12	0.2	0.1
0	200							0		20		470			1.1	
0	21	<0.1	<0.1	0.2	0.2	28	0	17.3	0.2	35	24	780	201	15	1.7	0.2
0	13	<0.1	<0.1	0.1	0.1	17	0	10.4	0.1	21	14	219	121	9	1	0.1
0	<1	<0.1	<0.1	<0.1	<0.1	3	0	0.8	<0.1	4	6	1	33	2	0.1	<0.1
0	376	<0.1	0.1	0.3	<0.1	16	0	2.8	<0.1	28	20	1	107	13	0.4	0.2
0	438	<0.1	0.1	0.4	<0.1	21	0	6.1	0.3	28	18	1	91	11	0.4	0.2
0	270	<0.1	<0.1	0.2	<0.1	21	0	2.1	<0.1	29	16	188	81	10	0.7	0.2
0	385	<0.1	0.1	0.2	<0.1	22	0	4.1	0.2	29	23	17	110	16	1.1	0.2
0	8	0.1	0.2	0.3	0.2	46	0	1.5	0.3	88	211	1	443	74	4.4	1
0	4500							24		80		90			2.7	
0	9433	0.1	0.2	0.4	0.2	131	0	8.8	1.9	122	50	63	419	78	3.2	0.7
0	2813	<0.1	0.1	0.2	0.1	58	0	8.4	0.6	30	15	24	167	24	0.8	0.2
0	51	<0.1	<0.1	0.2	<0.1	12	0	2.7	<0.1	11	23	2	26	9	0.3	0.3
0	8	<0.1	0.1	0.5	<0.1	18	0	7.1	<0.1	7	17	6	63	9	0.4	0.3
0	5	<0.1	<0.1	0.1	<0.1	6	0	0.2	<0.1	9	20	88	17	6	0.3	0.2
0	439	0.2	<0.1	0.9	0.2	19	0	11.1		45	46	4	448	44	1	0.2
0	11434	0.1	<0.1	1	0.1	19	0	15.5	1.3	42	28	4	291	30	0.6	0.1
0	6873	0.1	<0.1	0.6	0.2	16	0	9.7	0.2	17	24	8	367	23	0.5	0.2
0	85	<0.1	<0.1	0.6	0.1	6	0	2.7	0.1	16	11	14	91	9	0.3	0.2
0	191	<0.1	<0.1	0.5	0.1	18	0	5	0.1	24	35	1	173	22	0.3	0.4
0	5354	<0.1	0.1	0.5	0.2	20	0	9.8	0.1	23	19	1	247	13	0.5	0.2
0	292	0.1	<0.1	0.3	0.1	17	0	6.9	0.1	14	29	3	223	20	0.4	0.2
0	1005	<0.1	<0.1	0.5	0.1	25	0	11.6	0.1	16	33	3	238	17	0.3	0.3
0	124	<0.1	0.1	0.3	0.1	15	0	11.1	0.1	10	24	5	162	11	0.2	0.2
0	19218	0.1	0.1	1.5	0.3	6	0	19.6	0.7	38	54	36	475	27	0.7	0.3

ESHA, EatRight Analysis; **AMT**, amount; **WT**, weight; **CAL**, calories; **KILO**, KiloJoule; **WTR**, water; **PROT**, protein; **CARB**, carbohydrate; **FIBR**, fiber; **FAT**, fat; **SATF**, saturated fat; **MONO**, monounsaturated fat; **POLY**, polyunsaturated fat; **CHOL**, cholesterol;

ESHA CODE	FOOD DESCRIPTION	AMT	UNIT	WT (g)	CAL (kcal)	KILO (kJ)	WTR (g)	PROT (g)	CARB (g)	FIBR (g)	FAT (g)	SATF (g)	MONO (g)	POLY (g)
VEGETABLES (CONTINUED)														
5302	Taro, ckd, slices	0.5	cup	66	94	393	42	<1	23	3	<1	<0.1	<0.1	<0.1
5536	Tomatoes, green, ckd, fried	1	ea	144	284	1188	97	5	19	1	22	4.6	9.4	6.4
5172	Tomatoes, plum, fresh, year round avg	1	ea	62	11	46	59	1	2	1	<1	<0.1	<0.1	0.1
5476	Tomatoes, puree, cnd	0.5	cup	125	48	201	110	2	11	2	<1	<0.1	<0.1	0.1
90530	Tomatoes, red, cherry, fresh, year round avg	1	ea	17	3	13	16	<1	1	<1	<1	<0.1	<0.1	<0.1
5178	Tomatoes, red, ckd f/fresh	0.5	cup	120	22	92	113	1	5	1	<1	<0.1	<0.1	0.1
5179	Tomatoes, red, cnd, with tomato juice, whole	0.5	cup	120	20	84	113	1	5	1	<1	<0.1	<0.1	0.1
5169	Tomatoes, red, fresh, year round avg, med, 2 ⅗"	1	ea	123	22	92	116	1	5	1	<1	<0.1	<0.1	0.1
5170	Tomatoes, red, fresh, year round avg, sliced	0.5	cup	90	16	67	85	1	4	1	<1	<0.1	<0.1	0.1
5174	Tomatoes, red, fresh, year round avg, wedge, ¼ med	1	pce	31	6	25	29	<1	1	<1	<1	<0.1	<0.1	<0.1
5474	Tomatoes, red, stwd, cnd	0.5	cup	127.5	33	138	117	1	8	1	<1	<0.1	<0.1	0.1
5446	Tomatoes, sun dried	0.5	cup	27	70	293	4	4	15	3	1	0.1	0.1	0.3
5183	Turnips, ckd, drnd, cubes	0.5	cup	78	17	71	73	1	4	2	<1	<0.1	<0.1	<0.1
9667	Vegetables, Chinese stirfry, fzn	1	cup	85	25	105		2	6	2	0	0	0	0
42830	Vegetables, chop suey, cnd	0.5	cup	120	15	63		1	3	1	0	0	0	0
5187	Vegetables, ckd f/fzn, drnd, 10oz pkg	0.5	cup	91	59	247	76	3	12	4	<1	<0.1	<0.1	0.1
5305	Vegetables, cnd, drnd	0.5	cup	81.5	40	167	71	2	8	2	<1	<0.1	<0.1	0.1
9522	Vegetables, cnd, unsalted	0.5	cup	91	34	142	82	1	7	3	<1	<0.1	<0.1	0.1
5123	Vegetables, peas and carrots, ckd f/fzn, drnd	0.5	cup	80	38	159	69	2	8	2	<1	0.1	<0.1	0.2
5281	Vegetables, peas and carrots, cnd, with liquid	0.5	cup	127.5	48	201	112	3	11	3	<1	0.1	<0.1	0.2
5251	Vegetables, succotash, ckd, drnd	0.5	cup	96	110	460	66	5	23	4	1	0.1	0.1	0.4
5601	Vegetables, succotash, with whl kernel corn, cnd, with liquid	0.5	cup	127.5	80	335	104	3	18	3	1	0.1	0.1	0.3
5387	Water chestnuts, Chinese, cnd, with liquid, slices	0.5	cup	70	35	146	60	1	9	2	<1	<0.1	<0.1	<0.1
5160	Yams, domestic, ckd without skin, mashed	0.5	cup	164	125	523	131	2	29	4	<1	0.1	0	0.1

< = Trace amount present Blank = Not available

V, vitamin; **THI**, thiamin; **RIB**, riboflavin; **NIA**, niacin; **FOL**, folate; **CALC**, calcium; **PHOS**, phosphorus; **SOD**, sodium; **POT**, potassium; **MAG**, magnesium

CHOL (mg)	V-A (IU)	THI (mg)	RIB (mg)	NIA (mg)	V-B_6 (mg)	FOL (µg)	V-B_{12} (µg)	V-C (mg)	V-E (mg)	CALC (mg)	PHOS (mg)	SOD (mg)	POT (mg)	MAG (mg)	IRON (mg)	ZINC (mg)
0	55	0.1	<0.1	0.3	0.2	13	0	3.3	1.9	12	50	10	319	20	0.5	0.2
41	635	0.2	0.2	1.4	0.1	13	0.1	20.9	3	101	102	134	254	17	1.5	0.4
0	516	<0.1	<0.1	0.4	<0.1	9	0	8.5	0.3	6	15	3	147	7	0.2	0.1
0	638	<0.1	0.1	1.8	0.2	14	0	13.2	2.5	22	50	499	549	29	2.2	0.4
0	142	<0.1	<0.1	0.1	<0.1	3	0	2.3	0.1	2	4	1	40	2	<0.1	<0.1
0	587	<0.1	<0.1	0.6	0.1	16	0	27.4	0.7	13	34	13	262	11	0.8	0.2
0	140	0.1	0.1	0.9	0.1	10	0	11.2	0.8	37	23	172	226	13	1.2	0.2
0	1025	<0.1	<0.1	0.7	0.1	18	0	16.9	0.7	12	30	6	292	14	0.3	0.2
0	750	<0.1	<0.1	0.5	0.1	14	0	12.3	0.5	9	22	4	213	10	0.2	0.2
0	258	<0.1	<0.1	0.2	<0.1	5	0	4.2	0.2	3	7	2	73	3	0.1	0.1
0	219	0.1	<0.1	0.9	<0.1	6	0	10.1	1.1	43	26	282	264	15	1.7	0.2
0	236	0.1	0.1	2.4	0.1	18	0	10.6	<0.1	30	96	67	925	52	2.5	0.5
0	0	<0.1	<0.1	0.2	0.1	7	0	9	<0.1	26	20	12	138	7	0.1	0.1
0	3500							18		20		15	160		0.4	
0	400							15		0		640			0.4	
0	3892	0.1	0.1	0.8	0.1	17	0	2.9	0.3	23	46	32	154	20	0.7	0.4
0	9496	<0.1	<0.1	0.5	0.1	20	0	4.1	0.2	22	34	121	237	13	0.9	0.3
0	10602	<0.1	<0.1	0.4	0.1	16	0	3.5	0.3	19	34	24	126	14	0.6	0.5
0	7611	0.2	0.1	0.9	0.1	21	0	6.5	0.4	18	39	54	126	13	0.8	0.4
0	7357	0.1	0.1	0.7	0.1	23	0	8.4		29	59	332	128	18	1	0.7
0	282	0.2	0.1	1.3	0.1	32	0	7.9		16	112	16	394	51	1.5	0.6
0	186	<0.1	0.1	0.8	0.1	41	0	5.9		14	70	282	208	24	0.7	0.6
0	0	<0.1	<0.1	0.3	0.1	4	0	0.9	0.4	3	13	6	83	4	0.6	0.3
0	25814	0.1	0.1	0.9	0.3	10	0	21	1.5	44	52	44	377	30	1.2	0.3

Appendix C Exchange Lists for Diabetes

The following chart shows the amount of nutrients in one serving from each list.

Food List	Carbohydrate (g)	Protein (g)	Fat (g)	Calories
Carbohydrates				
Starch: breads, cereals and grains, starchy vegetables, crackers, snacks, and beans, peas, and lentils	15	0–3	0–1	80
Fruits	15	—	—	60
Milk				
Fat-free, low-fat, 1%	12	8	0–3	90
Reduced-fat, 2%	12	8	5	120
Whole	12	8	8	150
Sweets, Desserts, and Other Carbohydrates	15	Varies	Varies	Varies
Nonstarchy Vegetables	5	2	—	25
Meat and Meat Substitutes				
Very lean	—	7	1	35
Lean	—	7	3	5
Medium-fat	—	7	5	75
High-fat	—	7	8	100
Plant-based proteins	Varies	7	Varies	Varies
Fats	—	—	5	45
Alcohol	Varies	—	—	100

Starch List

Cereals, grains, pasta, breads, crackers, snacks, starchy vegetables, and cooked beans, peas, and lentils are starches. In general, one st arch choice is:

- ½ cup of cooked cereal, grain, or starchy vegetable
- ⅓ cup of cooked rice or pasta
- 1 ounce of a bread product, such as 1 slice of bread
- ¾ to 1 ounce of most snack foods (some snack foods may also have extra fat)

Bread

	Food	Serving Size
	Bagel, large	¼ (1 oz)
!	Biscuit, 2½ in. across	1
☺	Bread, reduced-calorie	2 slices (1½ oz)
	Bread, white, whole-grain, pumpernickel, rye, unfrosted raisin	1 slice (1 oz)
	Chapati, small, 6 in. across	1
!	Cornbread, 1¾ in. cube	1 (1½ oz)
	English muffin	½
	Hot dog or hamburger bun	½ (1 oz)
	Naan, 8 in. × 2 in.	¼
	Pancake, 4 in. across, ¼ in. thick	1
	Pita, 6 in. across	½
	Roll, plain, small	1 (1 oz)
!	Stuffing, bread	⅓ cup
!	Taco shell, 5 in. across	2
	Tortilla, corn, 6 in. across	1
	Tortilla, flour, 6 in. across	1
	Tortilla, flour, 10 in. across	⅓
!	Waffle, 4 in. square or 4 in. across	1

Cereals and Grains

	Food	Serving Size
	Barley, cooked	⅓ cup
	Bran, dry	
	☺ oat	¼ cup
	☺ wheat	½ cup
☺	Bulgur	½ cup
	Cereals	
	☺ bran	½ cup
	cooked (oats, oatmeal)	½ cup
	puffed	1½ cups
	shredded wheat, plain	½ cup
	sugar-coated	½ cup
	unsweetened, ready-to-eat	¾ cup
	Couscous	⅓ cup

< = Trace amount present   Blank = Not available

Granola	
low-fat	¼ cup
! regular	¼ cup
Grits, cooked	½ cup
Kasha	½ cup
Millet, cooked	⅓ cup
Muesli	¼ cup
Pasta, cooked	⅓ cup
Polenta, cooked	⅓ cup
Quinoa, cooked	⅓ cup
Rice, white or brown, cooked	⅓ cup
Tabbouleh (tabouli), prepared	½ cup
Wheat germ, dry	3 Tbsp
Wild rice, cooked	½ cup

Starchy Vegetables

Food	Serving Size
Cassava	⅓ cup
Corn	½ cup
on cob, large	½ cob (5 oz)
☺ Hominy, canned	¾ cup
☺ Mixed vegetables with corn, peas, or pasta	1 cup
☺ Parsnips	½ cup
☺ Peas, green	½ cup
Plantain, ripe	⅓ cup
Potato	
baked with skin	¼ large (3 oz)
boiled, all kinds	½ cup or ½ medium (3 oz)
! mashed, with milk and fat	½ cup
French fried (oven-baked)	1 cup (2 oz)
☺ Pumpkin, canned, no sugar added	1 cup
Spaghetti/pasta sauce	½ cup
☺ Squash, winter (acorn, butternut)	1 cup
☺ Succotash	½ cup
Yam, sweet potato, plain	½ cup

Crackers and Snacks

Food	Serving Size
Animal crackers	8
Crackers	
! round-butter type	6
saltine-type	6
! sandwich-style, cheese or peanut butter filling	3
! whole-wheat regular	2–5 (¾ oz)
☺ whole-wheat lower fat or crispbreads	2–5 (¾ oz)
Graham cracker, 2½ in. square	3
Matzoh	¾ oz
Melba toast, about 2 in. × 4 in. piece	4 pieces
Oyster crackers	20
Popcorn	3 cups
! ☺ with butter	3 cups
☺ no fat added	3 cups
☺ lower fat	3 cups
Pretzels	¾ oz
Rice cakes, 4 in. across	2
Snack chips	
fat-free or baked (tortilla, potato)	15–20 (¾ oz)
! regular (tortilla, potato)	9–13 (¾ oz)

Beans, Peas, and Lentils

(Count as 1 starch plus 1 lean meat.)

Food	Serving Size
☺ Baked beans	⅓ cup
☺ Beans, cooked (black, garbanzo, kidney, lima, navy, pinto, white)	½ cup
☺ Lentils, cooked (brown, green, yellow)	½ cup
☺ Peas, cooked (black-eyed, split)	½ cup
Δ☺ Refried beans, canned	½ cup

Fruits List

Fresh, frozen, canned, and dried fruits and fruit juices are on this list. In general, one fruit choice is:

- 1 small fresh fruit (4 oz)
- ½ cup of canned or fresh fruit or unsweetened fruit juice
- ¼ cup of dried fruit

Fruit

The weight listed includes skin, core, seeds, and rind.

Food	Serving Size
Apple, unpeeled, small	1 (4 oz)
Apples, dried	4 rings
Applesauce, unsweetened	½ cup
Apricots	
canned	½ cup
dried	8 halves
☺ fresh	4 whole (5½ oz)
Banana, extra small	1 (4 oz)
☺ Blackberries	¾ cup
Blueberries	¾ cup
Cantaloupe, small	⅓ melon or 1 cup cubed (11 oz)
Cherries, sweet	
canned	½ cup
fresh	12 (3 oz)

Dates	3
Dried fruits (blueberries, cherries, cranberries, mixed fruit, raisins)	2 Tbsp
Figs	
dried	1½
☺ fresh	1½ large or 2 medium (3½ oz)
Fruit cocktail	½ cup
Grapefruit	
large	½ (11 oz)
sections, canned	¾ cup
Grapes, small	17 (3 oz)
Honeydew melon	1 slice or 1 cup cubed (10 oz)
☺ Kiwi	1 (3½ oz)
Mandarin oranges, canned	¾ cup
Mango, small	½ fruit (5½ oz) or ½ cup
Nectarine, small	1 (5 oz)
☺ Orange, small	1 (6½ oz)
Papaya	½ fruit or 1 cup cubed (8 oz)
Peaches	
canned	½ cup
fresh, medium	1 (6 oz)
Pears	
canned	½ cup
fresh, large	½ (4 oz)
Pineapple	
canned	½ cup
fresh	¾ cup
Plums	
canned	½ cup
dried (prunes)	3
small	2 (5 oz)
☺ Raspberries	1 cup
☺ Strawberries	1¼ cup whole berries
☺ Tangerines, small	2 (8 oz)
Watermelon	1 slice or 1¼ cups cubed (13½ oz)

Fruit Juice

Food	Serving Size
Apple juice/cider	½ cup
Fruit juice blends, 100% juice	⅓ cup
Grape juice	⅓ cup
Grapefruit juice	½ cup
Orange juice	½ cup
Pineapple juice	½ cup
Prune juice	⅓ cup

Milk List

Different types of milk and milk products are on this list. However, two types of milk products are found on other lists:

- Cheeses are on the Meat and Meat Substitutes list (because they are rich in protein).
- Cream and other dairy fats are on the Fats list.

Milks and yogurts are grouped in three categories (fat-free/low-fat, reduced-fat, or whole) based on the amount of fat they have.

Fat-Free and Low-Fat Milk (1%; count as 1 fat-free milk)

Food	Serving Size
Milk, buttermilk, acidophilus milk, Lactaid	1 cup
Evaporated milk	½ cup
Yogurt, plain or flavored with an artificial sweetener (6 oz)	⅔ cup

Reduced-Fat Milk (2%; count as 1 reduced-fat milk)

Milk, acidophilus milk, kefir, Lactaid	1 cup
Yogurt, plain ⅔ cup (6 oz)	

Whole Milk (count as 1 whole milk)

Milk, buttermilk, goat's milk	1 cup
Evaporated milk	½ cup
Yogurt, plain	8 oz

Dairy-Like Foods

Food	Serving Size	Count as
Chocolate milk		
fat-free	1 cup	1 fat-free milk + 1 carbohydrate
whole	1 cup	1 whole milk + 1 carbohydrate
Eggnog, whole milk	½ cup	1 carbohydrate + 2 fats
Rice drink		
flavored, low-fat	1 cup	2 carbohydrates
plain, fat-free	1 cup	1 carbohydrate
Smoothies, flavored, regular	10 oz	1 fat-free milk + 2½ carbohydrates
Soy milk		
light	1 cup	1 carbohydrate + ½ fat
regular, plain	1 cup	1 carbohydrate + 1 fat
Yogurt		
and juice blends	1 cup	1 fat-free milk + 1 carbohydrate
low carbohydrate	⅔ cup (6 oz)	½ fat-free milk
with fruit, low-fat	⅔ cup (6 oz)	1 fat-free milk + 1 carbohydrate

< = Trace amount present   Blank = Not available

Sweets, Desserts, and Other Carbohydrates

Substitute food choices from this list for other carbohydrate-containing foods (such as those found on the Starch, Fruit or Milk lists) in your meal plan, even though these foods have added sugars and fat.

Beverages, Soda, and Energy/Sports Drinks

Food	Serving Size	Count as
Cranberry juice cocktail	½ cup	1 carbohydrate
Energy drink	1 can (8.3 oz)	2 carbohydrates
Fruit drink or lemonade	1 cup (8 oz)	2 carbohydrates
Hot chocolate		
regular	1 envelope added to 8 oz water	1 carbohydrate + 1 fat
sugar-free or light	1 envelope added to 8 oz water	1 carbohydrate
Soft drink (soda), regular	1 can (12 oz)	2½ carbohydrates
Sports drink	1 cup (8 oz)	1 carbohydrate

Brownies, Cake, Cookies, Gelatin, Pie, and Pudding

Food	Serving Size	Count as
Brownie, small, unfrosted	1¼ in. square (about 1 oz)	1 carbohydrate + 1 fat
Cake		
angel food, unfrosted	1/12 of cake (about 2 oz)	2 carbohydrates
frosted	2 in. square (about 2 oz)	2 carbohydrates + 1 fat
unfrosted	2 in. square (about 2 oz)	1 carbohydrate + 1 fat
Cookies		
chocolate chip	2 cookies (2¼ in. across)	1 carbohydrate + 2 fats
gingersnap	3 cookies	1 carbohydrate
sandwich, with crème filling	2 small (about ⅔ oz)	1 carbohydrate + 1 fat
sugar-free	3 small or 1 large (¾–1 oz)	1 carbohydrate + 1–2 fats
vanilla wafer	5 cookies	1 carbohydrate + 1 fat
Cupcake, frosted	1 small (about 1¾ oz)	2 carbohydrates + 1–1½ fats
Fruit cobbler	½ cup (3½ oz)	3 carbohydrates + 1 fat
Gelatin, regular	½ cup	1 carbohydrate
Pie		
commercially prepared fruit, 2 crusts	⅙ of 8-in. pie	3 carbohydrates + 2 fats
pumpkin or custard	⅛ of 8 in. pie	1½ carbohydrates + 1½ fats
Pudding		
regular (made with reduced-fat milk)	½ cup	2 carbohydrates
sugar-free or sugar- and fat-free (made with fat-free milk)	½ cup	1 carbohydrate

Candy, Spreads, Sweets, Sweeteners, Syrups, and Toppings

Food	Serving Size	Count as
Candy bar, chocolate/peanut	2 "fun size" bars (1 oz)	1½ carbohydrates + 1½ fats
Candy, hard	3 pieces	1 carbohydrate
Chocolate "kisses"	5 pieces	1 carbohydrate + 1 fat
Coffee creamer		
dry, flavored	4 tsp	½ carbohydrate + ½ fat
liquid, flavored	2 Tbsp	1 carbohydrate

Fruit snacks, chewy (pureed fruit concentrate)	1 roll (¾ oz)	1 carbohydrate
Fruit spreads, 100% fruit	1½ Tbsp	1 carbohydrate
Honey	1 Tbsp	1 carbohydrate
Jam or jelly, regular	1 Tbsp	1 carbohydrate
Sugar	1 Tbsp	1 carbohydrate
Syrup		
chocolate	2 Tbsp	2 carbohydrates
light (pancake type)	2 Tbsp	1 carbohydrate
regular (pancake type)	1 Tbsp	1 carbohydrate

Condiments and Sauces

Food	Serving Size	Count as
Barbeque sauce	3 Tbsp	1 carbohydrate
Cranberry sauce, jellied	¼ cup	1½ carbohydrates
Δ Gravy, canned or bottled	½ cup	½ carbohydrate + ½ fat
Salad dressing, fat-free, low-fat, cream-based	3 Tbsp	1 carbohydrate
Sweet and sour sauce	3 Tbsp	1 carbohydrate

Doughnuts, Muffins, Pastries, and Sweet Breads

Food	Serving Size	Count as
Banana nut bread	1-in. slice (1 oz)	2 carbohydrates + 1 fat
Doughnut		
cake, plain	1 medium (1½ oz)	1½ carbohydrates + 2 fats
yeast type, glazed	3¾ in. across	2 carbohydrates + 2 fats
Muffin (4 oz)	¼ muffin (1 oz)	1 carbohydrate + ½ fat
Sweet roll or Danish	1 (2½ oz)	2½ carbohydrates + 2 fats

Frozen Bars, Frozen Desserts, Frozen Yogurt, and Ice Cream

Food	Serving Size	Count as
Frozen pops	1	½ carbohydrate
Fruit juice bars, frozen, 100% juice	1 bar (3 oz)	1 carbohydrate
Ice cream		
fat-free	⅓ cup	1½ carbohydrates
light	½ cup	1 carbohydrate + 1 fat
no sugar added	½ cup	1 carbohydrate + 1 fat
regular	½ cup	1 carbohydrate + 2 fats
Sherbet, sorbet	½ cup	2 carbohydrates
Yogurt, frozen		
fat-free	⅓ cup	1 carbohydrate
regular	½ cup	1 carbohydrate + 0–1 fat

Granola Bars, Meal Replacement Bars/Shakes, and Trail Mix

Food	Serving Size	Count as
Granola or snack bar, regular or low-fat	1 bar (1 oz)	1½ carbohydrates
Meal replacement bar	1 bar (1⅓ oz)	1½ carbohydrates + 0–1 fat
Meal replacement bar	1 bar (2 oz)	2 carbohydrates + 1 fat

< = Trace amount present   Blank = Not available

Meal replacement shake, reduced calorie	1 can (10–11 oz)	1½ carbohydrates + 0–1 fat
Trail mix		
candy/nut-based	1 oz	1 carbohydrate + 2 fats
dried fruit-based	1 oz	1 carbohydrate + 1 fat

Nonstarchy Vegetable List

Vegetables that contain small amounts of carbohydrates and calories are on this list. In general, one nonstarchy vegetable choice is:

- ½ cup of cooked vegetables or vegetable juice
- 1 cup of raw vegetables

If you eat 3 cups or more of raw vegetables or 1½ cups of cooked vegetables at one meal, count them as 1 carbohydrate choice.

Amaranth or Chinese spinach
Artichoke
Artichoke hearts
Asparagus
Baby corn
Bamboo shoots
Beans (green, wax, Italian)
Bean sprouts
Beets
Δ Borscht
Broccoli
☺ Brussels sprouts
Cabbage (green, bok choy, Chinese)
☺ Carrots
Cauliflower
Celery
☺ Chayote
Coleslaw, packaged, no dressing
Cucumber
Eggplant
Gourds (bitter, bottle, luffa, bitter melon)
Green onions or scallions
Greens (collard, kale, mustard, turnip)
Hearts of palm
Jicama
Kohlrabi
Leeks
Mixed vegetables (without corn, peas, or pasta)
Mung bean sprouts
Mushrooms, all kinds, fresh
Okra
Onions
Oriental radish or daikon
Pea pods
☺ Peppers (all varieties)
Radishes
Rutabaga
Δ Sauerkraut
Soybean spouts
Spinach
Squash (summer, crookneck, zucchini)
Sugar pea snaps
☺ Swiss chard
Tomato
Tomatoes, canned
Δ Tomato sauce
Δ Tomato/vegetable juice
Turnips
Water chestnuts
Yard-long beans

Meat and Meat Substitutes

Meat and meat substitutes are rich in protein. Foods from this list are divided into 4 groups based on the amount of fat they contain.

Lean Meats and Meat Substitutes

Food	Amount
Beef: Select or Choice grades trimmed of fat: ground round, roast (chuck, rib, rump), round, sirloin, steak (cubed, flank, porterhouse, T-bone), tenderloin	1 oz
Δ Beef jerky	1 oz
Cheeses with 3 grams of fat or less per oz	1 oz
Cottage cheese	¼ cup
Egg substitutes, plain	¼ cup
Egg whites	2
Fish, fresh or frozen, plain: catfish, cod, flounder, haddock, halibut, orange roughy, salmon, tilapia, trout, tuna	1 oz
Δ Fish, smoked: herring or salmon (lox)	1 oz
Game: buffalo, ostrich, rabbit, venison	1 oz
Δ Hot dog with 3 grams of fat or less per oz. (8 hot dogs per 14 oz package) *Note: may be high in carbohydrate.*	1
Lamb: chop, leg, or roast	1 oz
Organ meats: heart, kidney, liver *Note: may be high in cholesterol.*	
Oysters, fresh or frozen	6 medium
Pork	
Δ Canadian bacon	1 oz
rib or loin chop/roast, ham, tenderloin	1 oz
Poultry, without skin: Cornish hen, chicken, domestic duck or goose (well drained of fat), turkey	1 oz

Processed sandwich meats with 3 grams or less fat per oz: chipped beef, deli thin-sliced meats, turkey ham, turkey kielbasa, turkey pastrami	1 oz
Salmon, canned	1 oz
Sardines, canned	2 medium
Δ Sausage with 3 grams of fat or less per oz	1 oz
Shellfish: clams, crab, imitation shellfish, lobster, scallops, shrimp	1 oz
Tuna, canned in water or oil, drained	1 oz
Veal: lean chop, roast	1 oz

Medium-Fat Meat and Meat Substitutes

Food	Amount
Beef: corned beef, ground beef, meatloaf, Prime grades trimmed of fat (prime rib), short ribs, tongue	1 oz
Cheeses with 4–7 grams of fat per oz: feta, mozzarella, pasteurized processed cheese spread, reduced-fat cheeses, string	1 oz
Egg	1
Note: high in cholesterol, limit to 3 per week.	
Fish: any fried product	1 oz
Lamb: ground, rib roast	1 oz
Pork: cutlet, shoulder roast	1 oz
Poultry: chicken with skin, dove, pheasant, wild duck or goose, fried chicken, ground turkey	1 oz
Ricotta cheese	2 oz or ¼ cup
Δ Sausage with 4–7 grams of fat per oz	1 oz
Veal, cutlet (no breading)	1 oz

High-Fat Meat and Meat Substitutes

These foods are high in saturated fat, cholesterol, and calories and may raise blood cholesterol levels if eaten on a regular basis. Try to eat 3 or fewer servings from this group per week.

Food	Amount
Bacon	
Δ pork	2 slices (16 slices/lb or 1 oz each before cooking)
Δ turkey	3 slices (½ oz each before cooking)
Cheese, regular: American, bleu, brie, cheddar, hard goat, Monterey Jack, queso, and Swiss	1 oz
Δ !Hot dog: beef, pork, or combination (10/lb)	1
Δ Hot dog: turkey or chicken (10/lb)	1
Pork: ground, sausage, spareribs	1 oz
Processed sandwich meats with 8 grams of fat or more per oz: bologna, pastrami, hard salami	1 oz
Δ Sausage with 8 grams of fat or more per oz: bratwurst, chorizo, Italian, knockwurst, Polish, smoked, summer	1 oz

Plant-Based Proteins

Because carbohydrate content varies among plant-based proteins, you should read the food label.

Food	Amount	Count as
"Bacon" strips, soy-based	3 strips	1 medium-fat meat
☺ Baked beans	⅓ cup	1 starch + 1 lean meat
☺ Beans, cooked: black, garbanzo, kidney, lima, navy, pinto, white	½ cup	1 starch + 1 lean meat
☺ "Beef" or "sausage" crumbles, soy-based	2 oz	½ carbohydrate + 1 lean meat
"Chicken" nuggets, soy-based	2 nuggets (1½ oz)	½ carbohydrate + 1medium-fat meat
☺ Edamame	½ cup	½ carbohydrate + 1 lean meat
Falafel (spiced chickpea and wheat patties)	3 patties (about 2 in. across)	1 carbohydrate + 1 high-fat meat
Hot dog, soy-based	1 (1½ oz)	½ carbohydrate + 1 lean meat
☺ Hummus	⅓ cup	1 carbohydrate + 1 high-fat meat
☺ Lentils, brown, green, or yellow	½ cup	1 carbohydrate + 1 lean meat
☺ Meatless burger, soy-based	3 oz	½ carbohydrate + 2 lean meats
☺ Meatless burger, vegetable- and starch-based	1 patty (about 2½ oz)	1 carbohydrate + 2 lean meats
Nut spread: almond butter, cashew butter, peanut butter, soy nut butter	1 Tbsp	1 high-fat meat
☺ Peas, cooked: black-eyed and split peas	½ cup	1 starch + 1 lean meat
Δ☺ Refried beans, canned	½ cup	1 starch + 1 lean meat
"Sausage" patties, soy-based	1 (1½ oz)	1 medium-fat meat
Soy nuts, unsalted	¾ oz	½ carbohydrate + 1 medium-fat meat
Tempeh	¼ cup	1 medium-fat meat
Tofu	4 oz (½ cup)	1 medium-fat meat
Tofu, light	4 oz (½ cup)	1 lean meat

< = Trace amount present   Blank = Not available

Fats

Fats are divided into three groups, based on the main type of fat they contain: unsaturated fats (omega-3, monounsaturated, and polyunsaturated) are primarily vegetable and are liquid at room temperature. These fats have good health benefits. Saturated fats have been linked with heart disease. Saturated fats are solid at room temperature. Trans fats are made in a process that changes vegetable oils into semi-solid fats. These fats can raise blood cholesterol and should be eaten in small amounts. Trans fats are found in the following types of food: solid vegetable shortening, stick margarines, and some tub margarines; crackers, candies, cookies, snack foods, fried foods, baked goods, and other food items made with partially hydrogenated vegetable oils.

Unsaturated Fats/Monounsaturated Fats

Food	Serving Size
Avocado, medium	2 Tbsp (1 oz)
Nut butters (trans fat-free): almond butter, cashew butter, peanut butter (smooth or crunchy)	1½ tsp
Nuts	
almonds	6
Brazil	2
cashews	6
filberts	5
macadamia	3
mixed (50 percent peanuts)	6
peanuts	10
pecans	4 halves
pistachios	16
Oil: canola, olive, peanut	1 tsp
Olives:	
black (ripe)	8 large
green, stuffed	10 large

Polyunsaturated Fats

Food	Serving Size
Margarine: lower-fat spread (30 to 50 percent vegetable oil, trans fat-free)	1 Tbsp
Margarine: stick, tub (trans fat-free), or squeeze (trans fat-free)	1 tsp
Mayonnaise	
reduced-fat	1 Tbsp
regular	1 tsp
Mayonnaise-type salad dressing	
reduced-fat	1 Tbsp
regular	2 tsp
Nuts	
pignolia (pine)	1 Tbsp
walnuts, English	4 halves
Oil: corn, cottonseed, flaxseed, grape seed, safflower, soybean, sunflower	1 tsp
Oil: made from soybean and canola oil—Enova	1 tsp
Plant stanol esters	
light	1 Tbsp
regular	2 tsp
Salad dressing	
Δ reduced-fat	2 Tbsp
Note: may be high in carbohydrate.	
Δ regular	1 Tbsp
Seeds	
flaxseed, whole	1 Tbsp
pumpkin, sunflower	1 Tbsp
sesame seeds	1 Tbsp
Tahini or sesame paste	2 tsp

Saturated Fats

Food	Serving Size
Bacon, cooked, regular or turkey	1 slice
Butter	
reduced-fat	1 Tbsp
stick	1 tsp
Butter blends made with oil	
reduced-fat or light	1 Tbsp
regular	1½ tsp
Chitterlings, boiled	2 Tbsp (½ oz)
Coconut, sweetened, shredded	2 Tbsp
Coconut milk	
light	⅓ cup
regular	1½ Tbsp
Cream	
half and half	2 Tbsp
heavy	1 Tbsp
light	1½ Tbsp
whipped	2 Tbsp
whipped, pressurized	¼ cup
Cream cheese	
reduced-fat	1½ Tbsp (¾ oz)
regular	1 Tbsp (½ oz)
Lard	1 tsp
Oil: coconut, palm, palm kernel	1 tsp
Salt pork	¼ oz
Shortening, solid	1 tsp

Sour cream	
reduced-fat	3 Tbsp
regular	2 Tbsp

Free Foods

A "free" food is any food or drink choice that contains less than 20 calories and 5 or fewer grams of carbohydrate per serving. Most foods on this list should be limited to three servings per day. Foods listed without a serving size can be eaten as often as you like.

Low Carbohydrate Foods

Food	Serving Size
Cabbage, raw	½ cup
Candy, hard (regular or sugar-free)	1 piece
Carrots, cauliflower, or green beans, cooked	¼ cup
Cranberries, sweetened with sugar substitute	½ cup
Cucumber, sliced	½ cup
Gelatin	
dessert, sugar-free	
unflavored	
Gum	
Jam or jelly, light or no sugar added	2 tsp
Rhubarb, sweetened with sugar substitute	½ cup
Salad greens	
Sugar substitutes (artificial sweeteners)†	
Syrup, sugar-free	2 Tbsp

†Sugar substitutes, alternatives, or replacements that are approved by the Food and Drug Administration (FDA) are safe to use. Common brand names include:

- Equal and Nutrasweet (aspartame)
- Splenda (sucralose)
- Sugar Twin, Sweet'N Low, and Sprinkle Sweet® (saccharin)
- Sweet One (acesulfame K)
- Sweet-10® (saccharin)

Although each sweetener is tested for safety before it can be marketed and sold, use a variety of sweeteners and in moderate amounts.

Modified Fat Foods with Carbohydrate

Food	
Cream cheese, fat-free	1 Tbsp (½ oz)
Creamers	
nondairy, liquid	1 Tbsp
nondairy, powdered	2 tsp
Margarine spread	
fat-free	1 Tbsp
reduced-fat	1 tsp
Mayonnaise	
fat-free	1 Tbsp
reduced-fat	1 tsp
Mayonnaise-style salad dressing	
fat-free	1 Tbsp
reduced-fat	1 tsp
Salad dressing	
fat-free or low-fat	1 Tbsp
fat-free, Italian	2 Tbsp
Sour cream, fat-free or reduced-fat	1 Tbsp
Whipped topping, light or fat-free	2 Tbsp
regular	1 Tbsp

Condiments

Food	Serving Size
Barbeque sauce	2 tsp
Catsup (ketchup)	1 Tbsp
Honey mustard	1 Tbsp
Horseradish	
Lemon juice	
Miso	1½ tsp
Mustard	
Parmesan cheese, freshly grated	1 Tbsp
Pickle relish	1 Tbsp
Pickles	
Δ dill	1½ medium
sweet, bread and butter	2 slices
sweet, gherkin	¾ oz
Salsa	¼ cup
Δ Soy sauce, light or regular	1 Tbsp
Sweet and sour sauce	2 tsp
Sweet chili sauce	2 tsp
Taco sauce	1 Tbsp
Vinegar	
Yogurt, any type	2 Tbsp

Drinks/Mixes

Any food on this list—without a serving size listed—can be consumed in any moderate amount

- Δ Bouillon, broth, consommé
- Δ Bouillon or broth, low-sodium
- Carbonated or mineral water
- Club soda
- Cocoa powder, unsweetened (1 Tbsp)
- Coffee, unsweetened or with sugar substitute
- Diet soft drinks, sugar-free
- Drink mixes, sugar-free
- Tea, unsweetened or with sugar substitute
- Tonic water, diet
- Water
- Water, flavored, carbohydrate-free

< = Trace amount present   Blank = Not available

Seasonings

Any food on this list can be consumed in any moderate amount.

Flavoring extracts (for example, vanilla, almond, peppermint)
Garlic
Herbs, fresh or dried
Hot pepper sauce
Nonstick cooking spray
Pimento
Spices
Wine, used in cooking
Worcestershire sauce

Δ *Be careful with seasonings that contain sodium or are salts, such as garlic or celery salt, and lemon pepper.*

Combination Foods

Many of the foods we eat are mixed together in various combinations, such as casseroles. These "combination" foods do not fit into any one choice list. This is a list of choices for some typical combination foods.

Entrees

Food	Serving Size	Count as
Δ Casserole-type (tuna noodle, lasagna, spaghetti with meatballs, chili with beans, macaroni and cheese)	1 cup (8 oz)	2 carbohydrates + 2 medium-fat meats
Δ Stews (beef/other meats and vegetables)	1 cup (8 oz)	1 carbohydrate + 1 medium-fat meats + 0–3 fats
Tuna salad or chicken salad	½ cup (3½ oz)	½ carbohydrate + 2 lean meats + 1 fat

Frozen Entrées and Meals

Food	Serving Size	Count as
Δ˜☺ Burrito (beef and bean)	1 (5 oz)	3 carbohydrates + 1 lean meat + 2 fats
Δ Dinner-type meal	generally 14–17 oz	3 carbohydrates + 3 medium-fat meats + 3 fats
Δ Entrée or meal with fewer than 340 calories	about 8–11 oz	2–3 carbohydrates + 1–2 lean meats
Pizza		
Δ cheese/vegetarian, thin crust	¼ of 12 in. (4½–5 oz)	2 carbohydrates + 2 medium-fat meats
Δ meat topping, thin crust	¼ of 12 in. (5 oz)	2 carbohydrates + 2 medium-fat meats + 1½ fats
Δ Pocket sandwich	1 (4½ oz)	3 carbohydrates + 1 lean meat + 1–2 fats
Δ Pot pie	1 (7 oz)	2½ carbohydrates + 1 medium-fat meat + 3 fats

Salads (Deli-Style)

Food	Serving Size	Count as
Coleslaw	½ cup	1 carbohydrate + 1½ fats
Macaroni/pasta salad	½ cup	2 carbohydrates + 3 fats
Δ Potato salad	½ cup	1½–2 carbohydrates + 1–2 fats

Soups

Food	Serving Size	Count as
Δ Bean, lentil or split pea	1 cup	1 carbohydrate + 1 lean meat
Δ Chowder (made with milk)	1 cup (8 oz)	1 carbohydrate + 1 lean meat + 1½ fats
Δ Cream (made with water)	1 cup (8 oz)	1 carbohydrate + 1 fat
Δ Instant	6 oz prepared	1 carbohydrate
Δ with beans/lentils	8 oz prepared	2½ carbohydrates + 1 lean meat
Δ Miso soup	1 cup	½ carbohydrate + 1 fat

Δ Oriental noodle	1 cup	2 carbohydrates + 2 fats
Rice (congee)	1 cup	1 carbohydrate
Δ Tomato (made with water)	1 cup (8 oz)	1 carbohydrate
Δ Vegetable beef, chicken noodle, or other broth-type	1 cup (8 oz)	1 carbohydrate

Fast Foods

The choices in the Fast Foods list are not specific fast food meals or items but are estimates based on popular foods. Ask at the restaurant or check its website for nutrition information about your favorite fast foods.

Breakfast Sandwiches

Food	Serving Size	Count as
Δ Egg, cheese, meat, English muffin	1 sandwich	2 carbohydrates + 2 medium-fat meats
Δ Sausage biscuit sandwich	1 sandwich	2 carbohydrates + 2 high-fat meats + 3½ fats

Main Dishes/Entrées

Food	Serving Size	Count as
Δ ☺ Burrito (beef and beans)	1 (about 8 oz)	3 carbohydrates + 3 medium-fat meats + 3 fats
Δ Chicken breast, breaded and fried	1 (about 5 oz)	1 carbohydrate + 4 medium-fat meats
Chicken drumstick, breaded and fried	1 (about 2 oz)	2 medium-fat meats
Δ Chicken nuggets	6 (about 3½ oz)	1 carbohydrate + 2 medium-fat meats + 1 fat
Δ Chicken thigh, breaded and fried	1 (about 4 oz)	½ carbohydrate + 3 medium-fat meats + 1½ fats
Δ Chicken wings, hot	6 (5 oz)	5 medium-fat meats + 1½ fats

Oriental

Food	Serving Size	Count as
Δ Beef/chicken/shrimp with vegetables in sauce	1 cup (about 5 oz)	1 carbohydrate + 1 lean meat + 1 fat
Δ Egg roll, meat	1 (about 3 oz)	1 carbohydrate + 1 lean meat + 1 fat
Fried rice, meatless	½ cup	1½ carbohydrates + 1½ fats
Δ Meat and sweet sauce (orange chicken)	1 cup	3 carbohydrates + 3 medium-fat meats + 2 fats
Δ ⊠ Noodles and vegetables in sauce (chow mein, lo mein)	1 cup	2 carbohydrates + 1 fat

Pizza

Food	Serving Size	Count as
Pizza		
Δ cheese, pepperoni, regular crust	⅛ of 14 in. (about 4 oz)	2½ carbohydrates + 1 medium-fat meat + 1½ fats
Δ cheese/vegetarian, thin crust	¼ of 12 in. (about 6 oz)	2½ carbohydrates + 2 medium-fat meats + 1½ fats

Sandwiches

Food	Serving Size	Count as
Δ Chicken sandwich, grilled	1	3 carbohydrates + 4 lean meats
Δ Chicken sandwich, crispy	1	3½ carbohydrates + 3 medium-fat meats + 1 fat
Fish sandwich with tartar sauce	1	2½ carbohydrates + 2 medium-fat meat + 2 fats
Hamburger		
Δ large with cheese	1	2½ carbohydrates + 4 medium-fat meats + 1 fat
regular	1	2 carbohydrates + 1 medium-fat meat + 1 fat

< = Trace amount present Blank = Not available

Δ Hot dog with bun	1	1 carbohydrate + 1 high-fat meat + 1 fat
Submarine sandwich		
Δ fewer than 6 grams fat	6-in. sub	3 carbohydrates + 2 lean meats
Δ regular	6-in. sub	3½ carbohydrates + 2 medium-fat meats + 1 fat
Taco, hard or soft shell (meat and cheese)	1 small	1 carbohydrate + 1 medium-fat meat + 1½ fats

Salads

Food	Serving Size	Count as
Δ☺ Salad, main dish (grilled chicken type, no dressing or croutons)	salad	1 carbohydrate + 4 lean meats
Salad, side, no dressing or cheese	small (about 5 oz)	1 vegetable

Sides/Appetizers

Food	Serving Size	Count as
! French fries, restaurant style	small	3 carbohydrates + 3 fats
	medium	4 carbohydrates + 4 fats
	large	5 carbohydrates + 6 fats
Δ Nachos with cheese	small (about 4½ oz)	2½ carbohydrates + 4 fats
Δ Onion rings	1 serving (about 3 oz)	2½ carbohydrates + 3 fats

Desserts

Food	Serving Size	Count as
Milkshake, any flavor	12 oz	6 carbohydrates + 2 fats
Soft-serve ice cream cone	1 small	2½ carbohydrates + 1 fat

Alcohol

In general, 1 alcohol choice (½ oz absolute alcohol) has about 100 calories.

Alcoholic Beverages	Serving Size	Count as
Beer		
light (4.2 percent)	12 fl oz	1 alcohol equivalent + ½ carbohydrate
regular (4.9 percent)	12 fl oz	1 alcohol equivalent + 1 carbohydrate
Distilled spirits: vodka, rum, gin, whiskey (80 or 86 proof)	1½ fl oz	1 alcohol equivalent
Liqueur, coffee (53 proof)	1 fl oz	1 alcohol equivalent + 1 carbohydrate
Sake	1 fl oz	½ alcohol equivalent
Wine		
dessert (sherry)	3½ fl oz	1 alcohol equivalent + 1 carbohydrate
dry, red, or white (10 percent)	5 fl oz	1 alcohol equivalent

☺ = More than 3 g of dietary fiber per serving ! = Extra fat or prepared with added fat Δ = ≥ 480 mg of sodium per serving; ≥ 600 mg of sodium per serving (for combination or fast food main dishes/meals)

Appendix D USDA Food Intake Patterns

The table below shows suggested amounts of food to consume from the basic food groups, subgroups, and oils to meet recommended nutrient intakes at 12 different calorie levels. Nutrient and energy contributions from each group are calculated according to the nutrient-dense forms of foods in each group (e.g., lean meats and fat-free milk). The table also shows the empty calories that can be accommodated within each calorie level, in addition to the suggested amounts of nutrient-dense forms of foods in each group.

Recommended Amounts of Food From Each Food Group at 12 Calorie Levels

Calorie Level of Pattern[a]	1,000	1,200	1,400	1,600	1,800	2,000	2,200	2,400	2,600	2,800	3,000	3,200
Food Group[b]	**Daily Amount[c] of Food from Each Group (vegetable and protein foods subgroup amounts are per week)**											
Vegetables	1 c-eq	1½ c-eq	1½ c-eq	2 c-eq	2½ c-eq	2½ c-eq	3 c-eq	3 c-eq	3½ c-eq	3½ c-eq	4 c-eq	4 c-eq
Dark-green vegetables (c-eq/wk)	½	1	1	1½	1½	1½	2	2	2½	2½	2½	2½
Red and orange vegetables (c-eq/wk)	2½	3	3	4	5½	5½	6	6	7	7	7½	7½
Legumes (beans and peas) (c-eq/wk)	½	½	½	1	1½	1½	2	2	2½	2½	3	3
Starchy vegetables (c-eq/wk)	2	3½	3½	4	5	5	6	6	7	7	8	8
Other vegetables (c-eq/wk)	1½	2½	2½	3½	4	4	5	5	5½	5½	7	7
Fruits	1 c-eq	1 c-eq	1½ c-eq	1½ c-eq	1½ c-eq	2 c-eq	2 c-eq	2 c-eq	2 c-eq	2½ c-eq	2½ c-eq	2½ c-eq
Grains	3 oz-eq	4 oz-eq	5 oz-eq	5 oz-eq	6 oz-eq	6 oz-eq	7 oz-eq	8 oz-eq	9 oz-eq	10 oz-eq	10 oz-eq	10 oz-eq
Whole grains[d] (oz-eq/day)	1½	2	2½	3	3	3	3½	4	4½	5	5	5
Refined grains (oz-eq/day)	1½	2	2½	2	3	3	3½	4	4½	5	5	5
Dairy	2 c-eq	2½ c-eq	2½ c-eq	3 c-eq	3 c-eq	3 c-eq	3 c-eq	3 c-eq	3 c-eq	3 c-eq	3 c-eq	3 c-eq
Protein Foods	2 oz-eq	3 oz-eq	4 oz-eq	5 oz-eq	5 oz-eq	5½ oz-eq	6 oz-eq	6½ oz-eq	6½ oz-eq	7 oz-eq	7 oz-eq	7 oz-eq
Seafood (oz-eq/wk)	3	4	6	8	8	8	9	10	10	10	10	10
Meats, poultry, eggs (oz-eq/wk)	10	14	19	23	23	26	28	31	31	33	33	33
Nuts seeds, soy products (oz-eq/wk)	2	2	3	4	4	5	5	5	5	6	6	6
Oils	15 g	17 g	17 g	22 g	24 g	27 g	29 g	31 g	34 g	36 g	44 g	51 g
Limit on Calories for Other Uses, calories (% of calories)[e,f]	150 (15%)	100 (8%)	110 (8%)	130 (8%)	170 (9%)	270 (14%)	280 (13%)	350 (15%)	380 (15%)	400 (14%)	470 (16%)	610 (19%)

[a] Food intake patterns at 1,000, 1,200, and 1,400 calories are designed to meet the nutritional needs of 2- to 8-year-old children. Patterns from 1,600 to 3,200 calories are designed to meet the nutritional needs of children 9 years and older and adults. If a child 4 to 8 years of age needs more calories and, therefore, is following a pattern at 1,600 calories or more, his/her recommended amount from the dairy group should be 2.5 cups per day. Children 9 years and older and adults should not use the 1,000-, 1,200-, or 1,400-calorie patterns.

[b] Foods in each group and subgroup are:

- **Vegetables**
  - Dark-green vegetables: All fresh, frozen, and canned dark-green leafy vegetables and broccoli, cooked or raw: for example, broccoli; spinach; romaine; kale; collard, turnip, and mustard greens.
  - Red and orange vegetables: All fresh, frozen, and canned red and orange vegetables or juice, cooked or raw: for example, tomatoes, tomato juice, red peppers, carrots, sweet potatoes, winter squash, and pumpkin.
  - Legumes (beans and peas): All cooked from dry or canned beans and peas: for example, kidney beans, white beans, black beans, lentils, chickpeas, pinto beans, split peas, and edamame (green soybeans). Does not include green beans or green peas.
  - Starchy vegetables: All fresh, frozen, and canned starchy vegetables: for example, white potatoes, corn, green peas, green lima beans, plantains, and cassava.
  - Other vegetables: All other fresh, frozen, and canned vegetables, cooked or raw: for example, iceberg lettuce, green beans, onions, cucumbers, cabbage, celery, zucchini, mushrooms, and green peppers.

< = Trace amount present   Blank = Not available

- **Fruits**
  - All fresh, frozen, canned, and dried fruits and fruit juices: for example, oranges and orange juice, apples and apple juice, bananas, grapes, melons, berries, and raisins.
- **Grains**
  - Whole grains: All whole-grain products and whole grains used as ingredients: for example, whole-wheat bread, whole-grain cereals and crackers, oatmeal, quinoa, popcorn, and brown rice.
  - Refined grains: All refined-grain products and refined grains used as ingredients: for example, white breads, refined grain cereals and crackers, pasta, and white rice. Refined grain choices should be enriched.
- **Dairy**
  - All milk, including lactose-free and lactose-reduced products and fortified soy beverages (soymilk), yogurt, frozen yogurt, dairy desserts, and cheeses. Most choices should be fat-free or low-fat. Cream, sour cream, and cream cheese are not included due to their low calcium content.
- **Protein Foods**
  - All seafood, meats, poultry, eggs, soy products, nuts, and seeds. Meats and poultry should be lean or low-fat and nuts should be unsalted. Legumes (beans and peas) can be considered part of this group as well as the vegetable group, but should be counted in one group only.

[c] Food group amounts shown in cup-(c) or ounce-equivalents (oz-eq). Oils are shown in grams (g). Quantity equivalents for each food group are:

- Vegetables and fruits, 1 cup-equivalent is: 1 cup raw or cooked vegetable or fruit, 1 cup vegetable or fruit juice, 2 cups leafy salad greens, ½ cup dried fruit or vegetable.
- Grains, 1 ounce-equivalent is: ½ cup cooked rice, pasta, or cereal; 1 ounce dry pasta or rice; 1 medium (1 ounce) slice bread; 1 ounce of ready-to-eat cereal (about 1 cup of flaked cereal).
- Dairy, 1 cup-equivalent is: 1 cup milk, yogurt, or fortified soymilk; 1½ ounces natural cheese such as cheddar cheese or 2 ounces of processed cheese.
- Protein Foods, 1 ounce-equivalent is: 1 ounce lean meat, poultry, or seafood; 1 egg; ¼ cup cooked beans or tofu; 1 Tbsp peanut butter; ½ ounce nuts or seeds.

[d] Amounts of whole grains in the Patterns for children are less than the minimum of 3 oz-eq in all Patterns recommended for adults.

[e] All foods are assumed to be in nutrient-dense forms, lean or low-fat and prepared without added fats, sugars, refined starches, or salt. If all food choices to meet food group recommendations are in nutrient-dense forms, a small number of calories remain within the overall calorie limit of the Pattern (i.e., limit on calories for other uses). The number of these calories depends on the overall calorie limit in the Pattern and the amounts of food from each food group required to meet nutritional goals. Nutritional goals are higher for the 1,200- to 1,600-calorie Patterns than for the 1,000-calorie Pattern, so the limit on calories for other uses is lower in the 1,200- to 1,600-calorie Patterns. Calories up to the specified limit can be used for added sugars, added refined starches, solid fats, alcohol, or to eat more than the recommended amount of food in a food group. The overall eating Pattern also should not exceed the limits of less than 10 percent of calories from added sugars and less than 10 percent of calories from saturated fats. At most calorie levels, amounts that can be accommodated are less than these limits. For adults of legal drinking age who choose to drink alcohol, a limit of up to 1 drink per day for women and up to 2 drinks per day for men within limits on calories for other uses applies; and calories from protein, carbohydrate, and total fats should be within the Acceptable Macronutrient Distribution Ranges (AMDRs).

[f] Values are rounded.

Reproduced from U.S. Department of Health and Human Services and U.S. Department of Agriculture. 2015 – 2020 Dietary Guidelines for Americans. 8th Edition. December 2015. Available at http://health.gov/dietaryguidelines/2015/guidelines/.

USDA Food Intake Pattern Calorie Levels

USDA food patterns assign individuals to a calorie level based on their sex, age, and activity level. The chart below identifies the calorie levels for males and females by age and activity level. Calorie levels are provided for each year of childhood, from 2-18 years, and for adults in five-year increments. The estimates are rounded to the nearest 200 calories. An individual's calorie needs may be higher or lower than these average estimates.

	Male				Female[d]		
Activity Level	**Sedentary[a]**	**Moderately Active[b]**	**Active[c]**	**Activity Level**	**Sedentary[a]**	**Moderately Active[b]**	**Active[c]**
Age				**Age**			
2	1,000	1,000	1,000	2	1,000	1,000	1,000
3	1,200	1,400	1,400	3	1,000	1,200	1,400
4	1,200	1,400	1,600	4	1,200	1,400	1,400

(continues)

	Male				Female[d]		
Activity Level	**Sedentary[a]**	**Moderately Active[b]**	**Active[c]**	**Activity Level**	**Sedentary[a]**	**Moderately Active[b]**	**Active[c]**
Age				**Age**			
5	1,200	1,400	1,600	5	1,200	1,400	1,600
6	1,400	1,600	1,800	6	1,200	1,400	1,600
7	1,400	1,600	1,800	7	1,200	1,600	1,800
8	1,400	1,600	2,000	8	1,400	1,600	1,800
9	1,600	1,800	2,000	9	1,400	1,600	1,800
10	1,600	1,800	2,200	10	1,400	1,800	2,000
11	1,800	2,000	2,200	11	1,600	1,800	2,000
12	1,800	2,200	2,400	12	1,600	2,000	2,200
13	2,000	2,200	2,600	13	1,600	2,000	2,200
14	2,000	2,400	2,800	14	1,800	2,000	2,400
15	2,200	2,600	3,000	15	1,800	2,000	2,400
16	2,400	2,800	3,200	16	1,800	2,000	2,400
17	2,400	2,800	3,200	17	1,800	2,000	2,400
18	2,400	2,800	3,200	18	1,800	2,000	2,400
19-20	2,600	2,800	3,000	19-20	2,000	2,200	2,400
21-25	2,400	2,800	3,000	21-25	2,000	2,200	2,400
26-30	2,400	2,600	3,000	26-30	1,800	2,000	2,400
31-35	2,400	2,600	3,000	31-35	1,800	2,000	2,200
36-40	2,400	2,600	2,800	36-40	1,800	2,000	2,200
41-45	2,200	2,600	2,800	41-45	1,800	2,000	2,200
46-50	2,200	2,400	2,800	46-50	1,800	2,000	2,200
51-55	2,200	2,400	2,800	51-55	1,600	1,800	2,200
56-60	2,200	2,400	2,600	56-60	1,600	1,800	2,200
61-65	2,000	2,400	2,600	61-65	1,600	1,800	2,000
66-70	2,000	2,200	2,600	66-70	1,600	1,800	2,000
71-75	2,000	2,200	2,600	71-75	1,600	1,800	2,000
76 and up	2,000	2,200	2,400	76 and up	1,600	1,800	2,000

[a] Sedentary means a lifestyle that includes only the physical activity of independent living.

[b] Moderately Active means a lifestyle that includes physical activity equivalent to walking about 1.5 to 3 miles per day at 3 to 4 miles per hour, in addition to the activities of independent living.

[c] Active means a lifestyle that includes physical activity equivalent to walking more than 3 miles per day at 3 to 4 miles per hour, in addition to the activities of independent living.

[d] Estimates for females do not include women who are pregnant or breastfeeding.

Reproduced from U.S. Department of Health and Human Services and U.S. Department of Agriculture. 2015 – 2020 Dietary Guidelines for Americans. 8th Edition. December 2015. Available at http://health.gov/dietaryguidelines/2015/guidelines/.

Appendix E Nutrition and Health for Canadians

- Canadian Guidelines for Nutrition
- Nutrient Intake Recommendations for Canadians
- *Canada's Food Guide to Healthy Eating*
- *Canada's Food Guide*
- *Canadian Physical Activity Guidelines*
- Nutrition Labeling for Canadians
- Canadian Diabetes Association's Meal Planning Guide

Canadian Guidelines for Nutrition

For more than 60 years, the Canadian government has worked to promote healthy and nutritious eating habits. In 1987, Health and Welfare Canada began a major review of the system for guiding Canadians on their food choices. To perform the review, the government appointed two advisory committees—the Scientific Review Committee and the Communications and Implementation Committee.

After examining research evidence available on nutrition and public health, the Scientific Review Committee issued a report in 1990 called *Nutrition Recommendations.* The report included both updated Recommended Nutrient Intakes (RNI) and a scientific description of a healthy dietary pattern that would deliver adequate nutrients for health and reduce the risk of nutrition-related chronic diseases.

Meanwhile, the Communications and Implementation Committee translated these scientific findings into understandable guidelines and outlined implementation strategies in a report called *Action Towards Healthy Eating: Technical Report* (1990). This report suggested that Canada develop a "total diet approach" toward healthy eating. A total diet approach would give consumers a better idea of eating patterns associated with reducing the risk of developing chronic diseases.

In 1990, the government issued *Nutrition Recommendations: A Call for Action*, a summary report produced jointly by the Scientific Review Committee and the Communications and Implementation Committee.

A Revised Food Guide

In accordance with the recommendations of its two advisory groups, the Health Department undertook to revise *Canada's Food Guide.* In 1992, the agency launched *Canada's Food Guide to Healthy Eating* and an explanatory document called *Using the Food Guide.* It promoted dietary diversity, a reduction in total fat intake, and an active lifestyle and offered consumers a pattern for establishing healthy eating habits in their daily selection of foods.

Moreover, the guide introduced a number of new concepts. A range of servings from the four food groups accommodated the wide range of energy needs for different ages, body sizes, activity levels, genders, and conditions such as pregnancy and nursing. The wide range of servings in grain products, vegetables, and fruits was designed to give consumers a better idea of the type of diet that would help reduce the risk of developing nutrition-related chronic diseases.

The guide also introduced a category of "other" foods such as sweets, fats such as butter, and drinks like coffee, that, though part of the diets of many Canadians, traditionally would not have been mentioned in a food guide. The guide recommended moderation in the consumption of these foods and acknowledged their role, along with the wide range of servings in grains, vegetables, and fruits, as a "total diet approach" to healthy eating.

A Work in Progress

Some groups and organizations challenged specific aspects of the government's *Nutrition Recommendations.* In a typically Canadian twist, the government responded to challengers by including them in the development process. When the Canadian Pediatric Society, for example, queried the dietary recommendations on fat consumption in children, the Society was invited to join Health Canada in researching the issue. The result was *Nutrition Recommendations Update: Dietary Fat and Children* (1993), which adjusted the recommendation of appropriate levels of dietary fat for growing children. In 1995, Health Canada issued *Canada's Food Guide to Healthy Eating: Focus on Preschoolers* as a background paper for educators and communicators.

A thorough review of the 1992 *Food Guide* began in 2002. Many strengths as well as some challenges in understanding and using the information from the 1992 *Food Guide* were identified. An assessment of the nutritional adequacy of the 1992 *Food Guide* using Dietary Reference Intakes was undertaken. The assessment also sought to address changes in the food supply and patterns of food use. Extensive stakeholder consultation was also carried out. Health Canada worked with three advisory groups, an external *Food Guide* Advisory Committee, an Interdepartmental Working Group, and the Expert Advisory Committee on Dietary Reference Intakes throughout the revision process. In 2007, Health Canada released *Eating Well with Canada's Food Guide*, which is available in 10 languages. In addition, *A Food Guide for First Nations, Inuit, and Métis,* which recognizes the cultural, spiritual, and physical importance of traditional aboriginal foods, was also released in 2007.

Health Canada has positioned nutrition in a broader health context, which includes physical activity and a positive outlook on life. One result of this comprehensive approach was the Vitality Leaders Kit (1994), intended to help community leaders promote healthy eating, active living, and positive self-image and body image in an integrated way. *Canada's Physical Activity Guide* was released in 1998, followed by the *Guide for Older Adults* and the *Guides for Children and Youth*. In 2011, the Public Health Agency of Canada released new physical activity guidelines. Canadians are now encouraged to refer to Get Active Tip Sheets for the latest information on physical activity.

Looking Ahead

The job of keeping Canada's nutrition policy and consumer guidelines up-to-date is an ongoing task. New scientific research on nutrition and health continually uncovers new relationships and connections between them. Consumer tastes in foods vary in response to prevailing fashions and shifting demographics. Global trade also influences the food choices that appear on the Canadian dinner table.

The science underlying nutrition recommendations knows no borders. An increasingly complex knowledge base on nutrients, food and health, global trade, and international agreements requires international efforts. Scientists from Canada and the United States worked with the National Academy of Sciences to develop the Dietary Reference Intakes (DRIs), recommended nutrient intake levels for healthy people in the United States and Canada.

To keep abreast of the latest developments in Canada's nutrition policies, visit the Food and Nutrition area of the Health Canada website at: http://www.hc-sc.gc.ca/fn-an/index-eng.php.

Nutrient Intake Recommendations for Canadians

Health Canada has reviewed and made recommendations on nutrient requirements on a periodic basis since 1938. Known as the Recommended Nutrient Intakes, or RNI, these values were last published in 1990 as part of *Nutrition Recommendations: The Report of the Scientific Review Committee*. Since that time, there have been advances in science, and by 1994, it was clear that it was time to initiate another review of the scientific data.

At the same time, the Food and Nutrition Board of the National Academy of Sciences was beginning a consultation process on the review of the Recommended Dietary Allowances, the nutrient recommendations used in the United States. Health Canada considered that participating in the U.S. review would offer several advantages to Canada. These were as follows:

- The science underlying nutrient requirements knows no borders, and scientists everywhere are utilizing the same knowledge produced from studies conducted all over the world.
- The knowledge base on nutrients, foods, and health is increasing rapidly in scope and complexity. This increases the need for specialized expertise. Participating in the U.S. review permits Canada to expand the base of scientific expertise that could be utilized.
- International trade considerations, including NAFTA, suggest that the harmonization of the science base underlying nutrition policy will facilitate harmonization of such trade-related matters as nutrition labeling and food composition.

Canadian and American scientists establish Dietary Reference Intakes (DRIs) through a review process overseen by the Food and Nutrition Board of the Institute of Medicine, National Academy of Sciences. DRIs have replaced the RNIs and are found printed inside the covers of this text.

The National Academy of Sciences is an American private, nonprofit society of distinguished scholars engaged in scientific and engineering research, dedicated to the advancement of science and technology and to their use for the general welfare. The Academy has a mandate that requires it to advise the U.S. federal government on scientific and technical matters.

The Food and Nutrition Board (FNB) is a unit of the Institute of Medicine, part of the National Academy of Sciences. The Board is a multidisciplinary group of biomedical scientists with expertise in various aspects of nutrition, food sciences, biochemistry, medicine, public health, epidemiology, food toxicology, and food safety. The major focus of the FNB is to evaluate emerging knowledge of nutrient requirements and relationships between diet and the reduction of risk of common chronic diseases and to relate this knowledge to strategies for promoting health and preventing disease.

Canada's Food Guide

Scientists have known for some time that adequate nutrition is essential for proper growth and development. More recently, healthy eating has been accepted as a significant factor in reducing the risk of developing nutrition-related problems, including heart disease, cancer, obesity, hypertension (high blood pressure), osteoporosis, anemia, dental decay, and some bowel disorders.

What "Reducing Risk" Means

Reducing risk means lowering the chances of developing a disease. It does not guarantee the prevention of a disease. Because the development of disease involves several factors, risk reduction usually involves several different strategies or approaches. Healthy eating is just one positive action that may help to avoid a potential problem.

Healthy Eating with *Canada's Food Guide*

The revised *Food Guide* was designed to meet the body's needs for vitamins, minerals, and other nutrients; to reduce the risk of obesity, type 2 diabetes, heart disease, and certain types of cancer and osteoporosis; and to enhance the overall health and vitality of Canadians over the age of 2. The *Food Guide* outlines the recommended number of servings from the different food groups based on age and gender. **FIGURE E.1** shows the current *Food Guide*.

Canadian Physical Activity Guidelines

High levels of physical inactivity are a serious threat to public health in Canada. Nearly two-thirds of Canadians are not active enough to achieve optimal health benefits. These Canadians are at risk for heart disease, obesity, high blood pressure, adult-onset diabetes, osteoporosis, stroke, depression, and colon cancer. Although physical activity levels increased during the 1980s and early 1990s, the progress has stalled. Health Canada estimates that physical inactivity results in at least 21,000 premature deaths annually.

The *Canadian Physical Activity Guidelines*, produced by the Canadian Society for Exercise Physiology, provides a standard set of Canadian guidelines for physical activity. It provides information to help Canadians understand how to achieve health benefits by being physically active. The guide complements the popular *Canada's Food Guide to Healthy Eating* and provides concrete examples of how to incorporate physical activity into daily life.

The guide recommends an adult 18–64 years should accumulate 105 minutes of physical activity each week to stay healthy or improve your health. Moderate to vigorous physical activity should occur in bouts of 10 minutes or more. **FIGURE E.2** shows the complete Physical Activity Guide, which provides physical activity recommendations for all ages.

Federal, provincial, and territorial governments are working to reduce the number of inactive Canadians. Canada's *Physical Activity Guidelines* are a major step toward building the knowledge and awareness necessary for all Canadians to become more active. These guidelines now include physical activity recommendations for children 5–11 years; youths 12–17 years; adults 18–64 years; and adults 65 years and older.

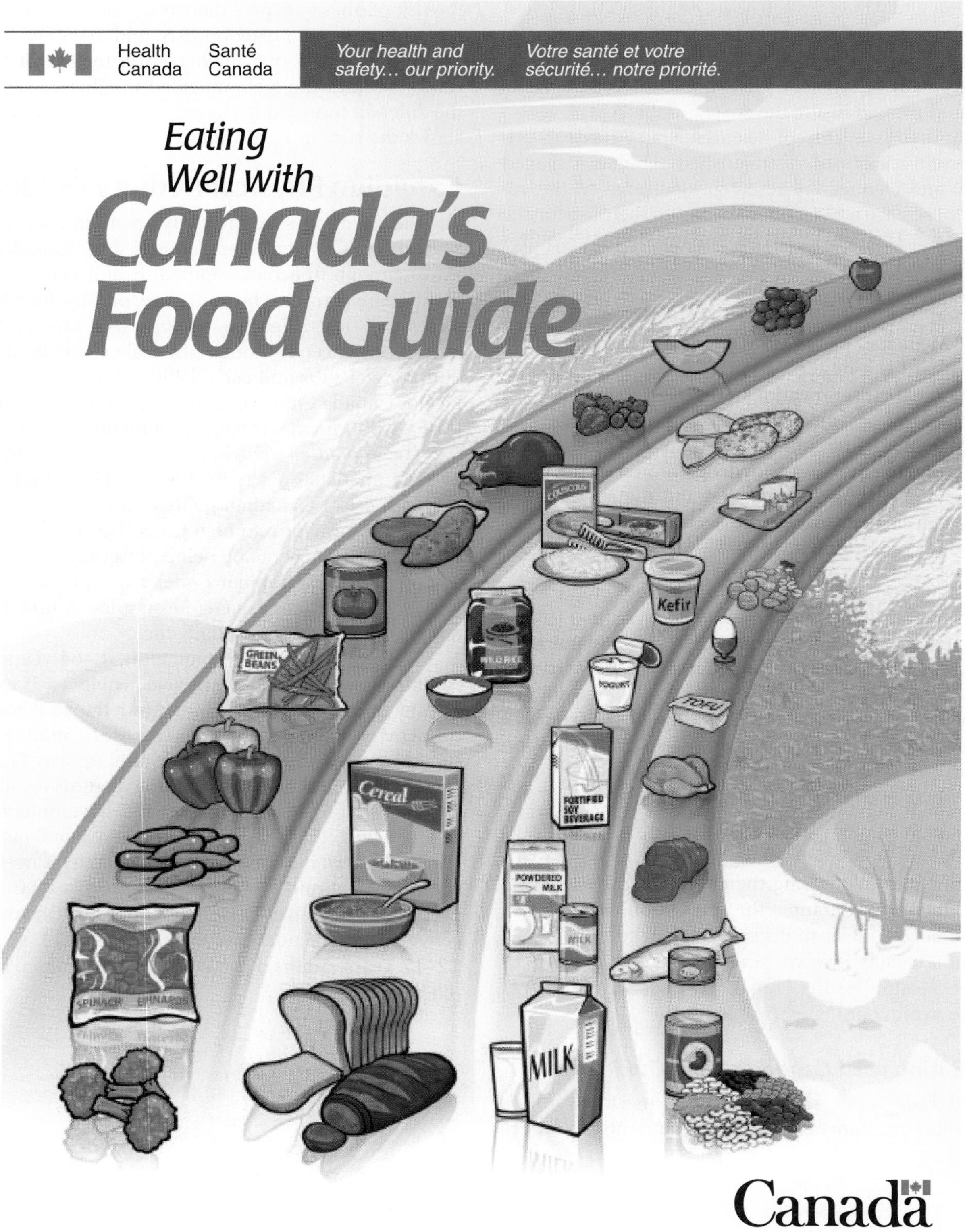

FIGURE E.1 Eating Well with Canada's Food Guide.

Recommended Number of Food Guide Servings per Day

	Children			Teens		Adults			
Age in Years	2-3	4-8	9-13	14-18		19-50		51+	
Sex	Girls and Boys			Females	Males	Females	Males	Females	Males
Vegetables and Fruit	4	5	6	7	8	7-8	8-10	7	7
Grain Products	3	4	6	6	7	6-7	8	6	7
Milk and Alternatives	2	2	3-4	3-4	3-4	2	2	3	3
Meat and Alternatives	1	1	1-2	2	3	2	3	2	3

The chart above shows how many Food Guide Servings you need from each of the four food groups every day.

Having the amount and type of food recommended and following the tips in *Canada's Food Guide* will help:

- Meet your needs for vitamins, minerals and other nutrients.
- Reduce your risk of obesity, type 2 diabetes, heart disease, certain types of cancer and osteoporosis.
- Contribute to your overall health and vitality.

What is One Food Guide Serving?
Look at the examples below.

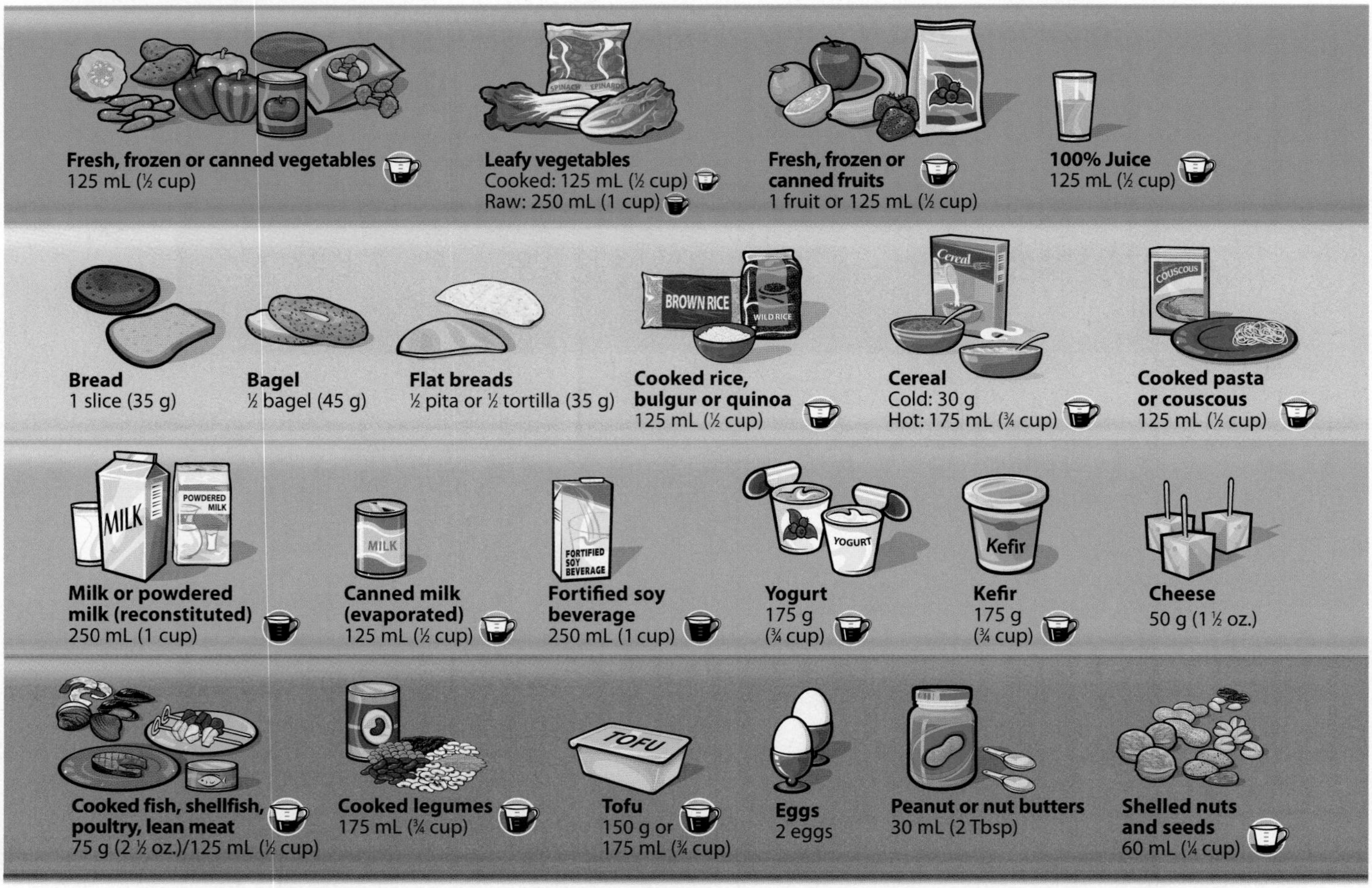
Fresh, frozen or canned vegetables
125 mL (½ cup)
Leafy vegetables
Cooked: 125 mL (½ cup)
Raw: 250 mL (1 cup)
Fresh, frozen or canned fruits
1 fruit or 125 mL (½ cup)
100% Juice
125 mL (½ cup)
Bread
1 slice (35 g)
Bagel
½ bagel (45 g)
Flat breads
½ pita or ½ tortilla (35 g)
Cooked rice, bulgur or quinoa
125 mL (½ cup)
Cereal
Cold: 30 g
Hot: 175 mL (¾ cup)
Cooked pasta or couscous
125 mL (½ cup)
Milk or powdered milk (reconstituted)
250 mL (1 cup)
Canned milk (evaporated)
125 mL (½ cup)
Fortified soy beverage
250 mL (1 cup)
Yogurt
175 g (¾ cup)
Kefir
175 g (¾ cup)
Cheese
50 g (1 ½ oz.)
Cooked fish, shellfish, poultry, lean meat
75 g (2 ½ oz.)/125 mL (½ cup)
Cooked legumes
175 mL (¾ cup)
Tofu
150 g or 175 mL (¾ cup)
Eggs
2 eggs
Peanut or nut butters
30 mL (2 Tbsp)
Shelled nuts and seeds
60 mL (¼ cup)

Oils and Fats

- Include a small amount – 30 to 45 mL (2 to 3 Tbsp) – of unsaturated fat each day. This includes oil used for cooking, salad dressings, margarine and mayonnaise.
- Use vegetable oils such as canola, olive and soybean.
- Choose soft margarines that are low in saturated and trans fats.
- Limit butter, hard margarine, lard and shortening.

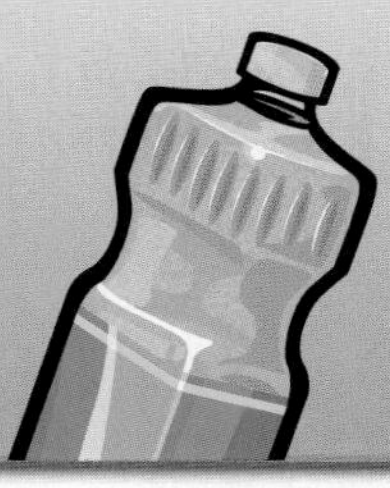

Make each Food Guide Serving count…
wherever you are – at home, at school, at work or when eating out!

▸ Eat at least one dark green and one orange vegetable each day.
- Go for dark green vegetables such as broccoli, romaine lettuce and spinach.
- Go for orange vegetables such as carrots, sweet potatoes and winter squash.

▸ Choose vegetables and fruit prepared with little or no added fat, sugar or salt.
- Enjoy vegetables steamed, baked or stir-fried instead of deep-fried.

▸ Have vegetables and fruit more often than juice.

▸ Make at least half of your grain products whole grain each day.
- Eat a variety of whole grains such as barley, brown rice, oats, quinoa and wild rice.
- Enjoy whole grain breads, oatmeal or whole wheat pasta.

▸ Choose grain products that are lower in fat, sugar or salt.
- Compare the Nutrition Facts table on labels to make wise choices.
- Enjoy the true taste of grain products. When adding sauces or spreads, use small amounts.

▸ Drink skim, 1%, or 2% milk each day.
- Have 500 mL (2 cups) of milk every day for adequate vitamin D.
- Drink fortified soy beverages if you do not drink milk.

▸ Select lower fat milk alternatives.
- Compare the Nutrition Facts table on yogurts or cheeses to make wise choices.

▸ Have meat alternatives such as beans, lentils and tofu often.

▸ Eat at least two Food Guide Servings of fish each week.*
- Choose fish such as char, herring, mackerel, salmon, sardines and trout.

▸ Select lean meat and alternatives prepared with little or no added fat or salt.
- Trim the visible fat from meats. Remove the skin on poultry.
- Use cooking methods such as roasting, baking or poaching that require little or no added fat.
- If you eat luncheon meats, sausages or prepackaged meats, choose those lower in salt (sodium) and fat.

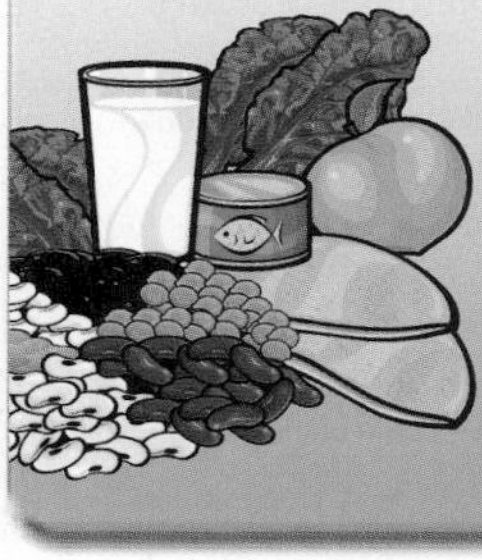

Enjoy a variety of foods from the four food groups.

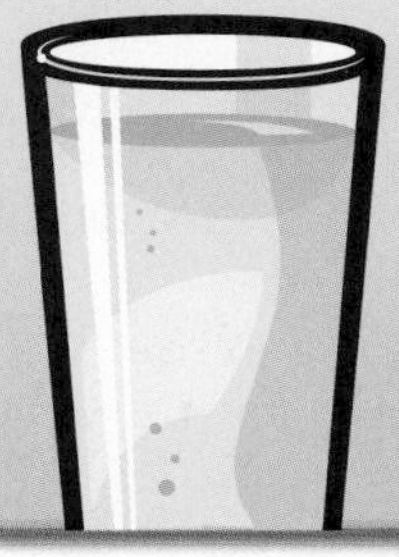

Satisfy your thirst with water!

Drink water regularly. It's a calorie-free way to quench your thirst. Drink more water in hot weather or when you are very active.

* Health Canada provides advice for limiting exposure to mercury from certain types of fish. Refer to www.healthcanada.gc.ca for the latest information.

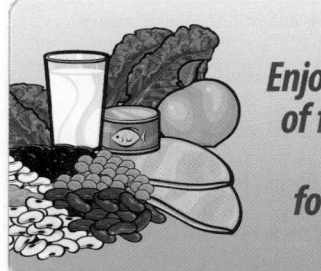

Advice for different ages and stages...

Children

Following *Canada's Food Guide* helps children grow and thrive.

Young children have small appetites and need calories for growth and development.

- Serve small nutritious meals and snacks each day.
- Do not restrict nutritious foods because of their fat content. Offer a variety of foods from the four food groups.
- Most of all... be a good role model.

Women of childbearing age

All women who could become pregnant and those who are pregnant or breastfeeding need a multivitamin containing **folic acid** every day. Pregnant women need to ensure that their multivitamin also contains **iron**. A health care professional can help you find the multivitamin that's right for you.

Pregnant and breastfeeding women need more calories. Include an extra 2 to 3 Food Guide Servings each day.

Here are two examples:

- Have fruit and yogurt for a snack, or
- Have an extra slice of toast at breakfast and an extra glass of milk at supper.

Men and women over 50

The need for **vitamin D** increases after the age of 50.

In addition to following *Canada's Food Guide*, everyone over the age of 50 should take a daily vitamin D supplement of 10 μg (400 IU).

How do I count Food Guide Servings in a meal?

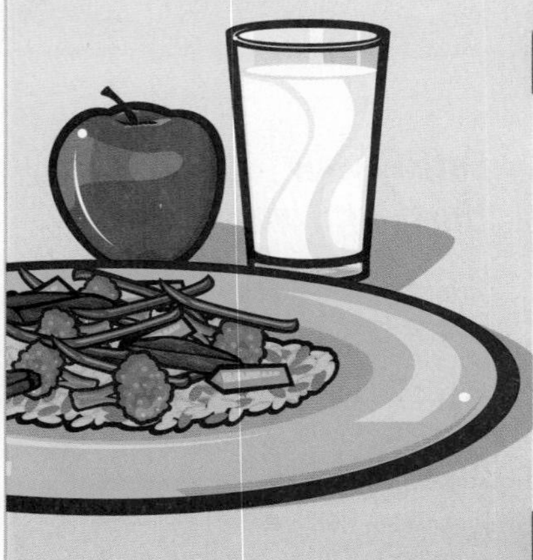

Here is an example:

Vegetable and beef stir-fry with rice, a glass of milk and an apple for dessert		
250 mL (1 cup) mixed broccoli, carrot and sweet red pepper	=	2 **Vegetables and Fruit** Food Guide Servings
75 g (2 ½ oz.) lean beef	=	1 **Meat and Alternatives** Food Guide Serving
250 mL (1 cup) brown rice	=	2 **Grain Products** Food Guide Servings
5 mL (1 tsp) canola oil	=	part of your **Oils and Fats** intake for the day
250 mL (1 cup) 1% milk	=	1 **Milk and Alternatives** Food Guide Serving
1 apple	=	1 **Vegetables and Fruit** Food Guide Serving

Eat well and be active today and every day!

The benefits of eating well and being active include:

- Better overall health.
- Lower risk of disease.
- A healthy body weight.
- Feeling and looking better.
- More energy.
- Stronger muscles and bones.

Be active

To be active every day is a step towards better health and a healthy body weight.

Canada's Physical Activity Guide recommends building 30 to 60 minutes of moderate physical activity into daily life for adults and at least 90 minutes a day for children and youth. You don't have to do it all at once. Add it up in periods of at least 10 minutes at a time for adults and five minutes at a time for children and youth.

Start slowly and build up.

Eat well

Another important step towards better health and a healthy body weight is to follow *Canada's Food Guide* by:

- Eating the recommended amount and type of food each day.
- Limiting foods and beverages high in calories, fat, sugar or salt (sodium) such as cakes and pastries, chocolate and candies, cookies and granola bars, doughnuts and muffins, ice cream and frozen desserts, french fries, potato chips, nachos and other salty snacks, alcohol, fruit flavoured drinks, soft drinks, sports and energy drinks, and sweetened hot or cold drinks.

Read the label

- Compare the Nutrition Facts table on food labels to choose products that contain less fat, saturated fat, trans fat, sugar and sodium.
- Keep in mind that the calories and nutrients listed are for the amount of food found at the top of the Nutrition Facts table.

Nutrition Facts
Per 0 mL (0 g)

Amount	% Daily Value
Calories 0	
Fat 0 g	0 %
Saturates 0 g + Trans 0 g	0 %
Cholesterol 0 mg	
Sodium 0 mg	0 %
Carbohydrate 0 g	0 %
Fibre 0 g	0 %
Sugars 0 g	
Protein 0 g	
Vitamin A 0 %	Vitamin C 0 %
Calcium 0 %	Iron 0 %

Limit trans fat

When a Nutrition Facts table is not available, ask for nutrition information to choose foods lower in trans and saturated fats.

Take a step today...

✓ Have breakfast every day. It may help control your hunger later in the day.

✓ Walk wherever you can – get off the bus early, use the stairs.

✓ Benefit from eating vegetables and fruit at all meals and as snacks.

✓ Spend less time being inactive such as watching TV or playing computer games.

✓ Request nutrition information about menu items when eating out to help you make healthier choices.

✓ Enjoy eating with family and friends!

✓ Take time to eat and savour every bite!

For more information, interactive tools, or additional copies visit Canada's Food Guide on-line at:
www.healthcanada.gc.ca/foodguide

or contact:

Publications
Health Canada
Ottawa, Ontario K1A 0K9
E-Mail: publications@hc-sc.gc.ca
Tel.: 1-866-225-0709
Fax: (613) 941-5366
TTY: 1-800-267-1245

Également disponible en français sous le titre :
Bien manger avec le Guide alimentaire canadien

This publication can be made available on request on diskette, large print, audio-cassette and braille.

Canadian Physical Activity Guidelines

FOR CHILDREN - 5 – 11 YEARS

Guidelines

For health benefits, children aged 5-11 years should accumulate at least 60 minutes of moderate- to vigorous-intensity physical activity daily. This should include:

Vigorous-intensity activities at least 3 days per week.

Activities that strengthen muscle and bone at least 3 days per week.

More daily physical activity provides greater health benefits.

Let's Talk Intensity!

Moderate-intensity physical activities will cause children to sweat a little and to breathe harder. Activities like:

- Bike riding
- Playground activities

Vigorous-intensity physical activities will cause children to sweat and be 'out of breath'. Activities like:

- Running
- Swimming

Being active for at least **60 minutes** daily can help children:

- Improve their health
- Do better in school
- Improve their fitness
- Grow stronger
- Have fun playing with friends
- Feel happier
- Maintain a healthy body weight
- Improve their self-confidence
- Learn new skills

Parents and caregivers can help to plan their child's daily activity. Kids can:

☑ Play tag – or freeze-tag!
☑ Go to the playground after school.
☑ Walk, bike, rollerblade or skateboard to school.
☑ Play an active game at recess.
☑ Go sledding in the park on the weekend.
☑ Go "puddle hopping" on a rainy day.

60 minutes a day. You can help your child get there!

PARTICIPACTION

CSEP | SCPE
THE GOLD STANDARD IN EXERCISE SCIENCE AND PERSONAL TRAINING
www.csep.ca/guidelines

FIGURE E.2A Canadian Physical Activity Guidelines for Children: 5–11 Years.

Canadian Physical Activity Guidelines

FOR YOUTH - 12 – 17 YEARS

Guidelines

For health benefits, youth aged 12-17 years should accumulate at least 60 minutes of moderate- to vigorous-intensity physical activity daily. This should include:

Vigorous-intensity activities at least 3 days per week.

Activities that strengthen muscle and bone at least 3 days per week.

More daily physical activity provides greater health benefits.

Let's Talk Intensity!

Moderate-intensity physical activities will cause teens to sweat a little and to breathe harder. Activities like:

- Skating
- Bike riding

Vigorous-intensity physical activities will cause teens to sweat and be 'out of breath'. Activities like:

- Running
- Rollerblading

Being active for at least **60 minutes** daily can help teens:

- Improve their health
- Do better in school
- Improve their fitness
- Grow stronger
- Have fun playing with friends
- Feel happier
- Maintain a healthy body weight
- Improve their self-confidence
- Learn new skills

Parents and caregivers can help to plan their teen's daily activity. Teens can:

☑ Walk, bike, rollerblade or skateboard to school.
☑ Go to a gym on the weekend.
☑ Do a fitness class after school.
☑ Get the neighbours together for a game of pick-up basketball, or hockey after dinner.
☑ Play a sport such as basketball, hockey, soccer, martial arts, swimming, tennis, golf, skiing, snowboarding...

Now is the time. 60 minutes a day can make a difference.

PARTICIPACTION

CSEP | SCPE
THE GOLD STANDARD IN EXERCISE SCIENCE AND PERSONAL TRAINING
www.csep.ca/guidelines

FIGURE E.2B Canadian Physical Activity Guidelines for Youth: 12–17 Years.

Canadian Physical Activity Guidelines

FOR ADULTS - 18 – 64 YEARS

Guidelines

To achieve health benefits, adults aged 18-64 years should accumulate at least 150 minutes of moderate- to vigorous-intensity aerobic physical activity per week, in bouts of 10 minutes or more.

It is also beneficial to add muscle and bone strengthening activities using major muscle groups, at least 2 days per week.

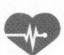

More physical activity provides greater health benefits.

Let's Talk Intensity!

Moderate-intensity physical activities will cause adults to sweat a little and to breathe harder. Activities like:

- Brisk walking
- Bike riding

Vigorous-intensity physical activities will cause adults to sweat and be 'out of breath'. Activities like:

- Jogging
- Cross-country skiing

Being active for at least **150 minutes** per week can help reduce the risk of:

- Premature death
- Heart disease
- Stroke
- High blood pressure
- Certain types of cancer
- Type 2 diabetes
- Osteoporosis
- Overweight and obesity

And can lead to improved:

- Fitness
- Strength
- Mental health (morale and self–esteem)

Pick a time. Pick a place. Make a plan and move more!

- ☑ Join a weekday community running or walking group.
- ☑ Go for a brisk walk around the block after dinner.
- ☑ Take a dance class after work.
- ☑ Bike or walk to work every day.
- ☑ Rake the lawn, and then offer to do the same for a neighbour.
- ☑ Train for and participate in a run or walk for charity!
- ☑ Take up a favourite sport again or try a new sport.
- ☑ Be active with the family on the weekend!

Now is the time. Walk, run, or wheel, and embrace life.

PARTICIPACTION

CSEP | SCPE
THE GOLD STANDARD IN EXERCISE SCIENCE AND PERSONAL TRAINING
www.csep.ca/guidelines

FIGURE E.2C Canadian Physical Activity Guidelines for Adults: 18–64 Years.

Canadian Physical Activity Guidelines

FOR OLDER ADULTS - 65 YEARS & OLDER

Guidelines

To achieve health benefits, and improve functional abilities, adults aged 65 years and older should accumulate at least 150 minutes of moderate- to vigorous-intensity aerobic physical activity per week, in bouts of 10 minutes or more.

It is also beneficial to add muscle and bone strengthening activities using major muscle groups, at least 2 days per week.

Those with poor mobility should perform physical activities to enhance balance and prevent falls.

More physical activity provides greater health benefits.

Let's Talk Intensity!

Moderate-intensity physical activities will cause older adults to sweat a little and to breathe harder. Activities like:

- Brisk walking
- Bicycling

Vigorous-intensity physical activities will cause older adults to sweat and be 'out of breath'. Activities like:

- Cross-country skiing
- Swimming

Being active for at least **150 minutes** per week can help reduce the risk of:

- Chronic disease (such as high blood pressure and heart disease) and,
- Premature death

And also help to:

- Maintain functional independence
- Maintain mobility
- Improve fitness
- Improve or maintain body weight
- Maintain bone health and,
- Maintain mental health and feel better

Pick a time. Pick a place. Make a plan and move more!

☑ Join a community urban poling or mall walking group.
☑ Go for a brisk walk around the block after lunch.
☑ Take a dance class in the afternoon.
☑ Train for and participate in a run or walk for charity!
☑ Take up a favourite sport again.
☑ Be active with the family! Plan to have "active reunions".
☑ Go for a nature hike on the weekend.
☑ Take the dog for a walk after dinner.

Now is the time. Walk, run, or wheel, and embrace life.

PARTICIPACTION

CSEP | SCPE THE GOLD STANDARD IN EXERCISE SCIENCE AND PERSONAL TRAINING

www.csep.ca/guidelines

FIGURE E.2D Canadian Physical Activity Guidelines for Older Adults: 65 Years and Older.

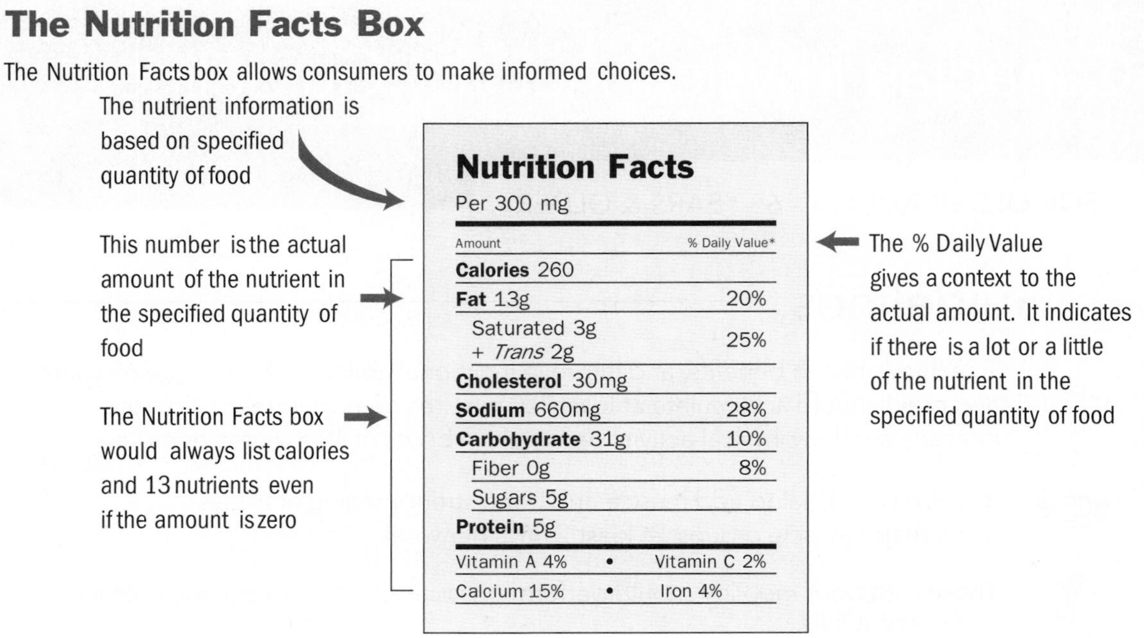
The Nutrition Facts Box
The Nutrition Facts box allows consumers to make informed choices.
The nutrient information is based on specified quantity of food
This number is the actual amount of the nutrient in the specified quantity of food
The Nutrition Facts box would always list calories and 13 nutrients even if the amount is zero
The % Daily Value gives a context to the actual amount. It indicates if there is a lot or a little of the nutrient in the specified quantity of food
Nutrition Facts
Per 300 mg
Amount
% Daily Value*
Calories 260
Fat 13g 20%
Saturated 3g
+ Trans 2g 25%
Cholesterol 30mg
Sodium 660mg 28%
Carbohydrate 31g 10%
Fiber 0g 8%
Sugars 5g
Protein 5g
Vitamin A 4% • Vitamin C 2%
Calcium 15% • Iron 4%

FIGURE E.3 How to read a food label.

Nutrition Labeling for Canadians

The nutrition label is one of the most useful tools in selecting foods for healthy eating (**FIGURE E.3**). The *Food Guide* outlines a pattern of healthy eating; the nutrition label supports the *Food Guide* by helping consumers to choose foods according to healthy eating messages.

Consumers can use labels to compare products and make choices on the basis of nutrient content. For example, consumers can choose a lower-fat product based on the fat content given on the labels.

Consumers also can use label information to evaluate products in relation to healthy eating. For instance, the *Nutrition Recommendations* advise Canadians to get 30 percent or less of their day's energy (kilocalories/kilojoules) from fat. This translates into a range of fat, in grams, that can be used as a benchmark against which individual foods and meals can be evaluated. The *Food Guide* covers a range of energy needs from 1,800 to 3,200 kilocalories (7,500 to 13,400 kilojoules) per day. A fat intake of 30 percent or less of a day's calories means a fat intake between 60 and 105 grams of fat.

Label Claims

A claim on a food label highlights a nutritional feature of a product. It is known to influence consumers' buying habits. Manufacturers often position label claims in a bold, banner-format on the front panel of a package or on the side panel along with the nutrition label. Because a label claim must be backed up by detailed facts relating to the claim, the consumer should look for the nutrition label for more information.

Nutrient Content Claims

A nutrient content claim describes the amount of a nutrient in a food. A food whose label carries the claim *high fibre* must contain 4 grams or more of fiber per reference amount and serving of stated size. A "sodium-free" food must contain less than 5 milligrams of sodium per reference amount and serving of stated size.

Diet-Related Health Claims

Optional health claims highlight the characteristics of a diet that reduces the chance of developing a disease such as cancer or heart disease. They also tell how the food fits into the diet.

Characteristic of the Diet:	Reduced Risk of:
Low in sodium and high in potassium	High blood pressure
Adequate in calcium and vitamin D	Osteoporosis
Low in saturated and trans fats	Heart disease
Rich in fruits and vegetables	Some types of cancer

For the latest information, visit the Nutrition Labeling area of the Health Canada website at http://www.inspection.gc.ca/english/fssa/lebeti/nutrition-pagee.shtml.

Canadian Diabetes Association's Meal Planning Guide

The Canadian Diabetes Association (CDA) works to promote the health of Canadians through diabetes research, education, service, and advocacy. In response to the introduction of new medications and new methods for the management of diabetes, the CDA has revised its meal planning guide. Like the Exchange Lists, the CDA meal planning guide was designed to make it easier for people with diabetes to eat the right amount of food for their insulin supply. The system is based on two concepts: Most foods are eaten by people with diabetes in measured amounts, and foods within each of the system's eight food groups can be interchanged.

The new guide, *Beyond the Basics: Meal Planning for Diabetes Prevention and Management,* has several features. First, food items have been modified to reflect current thinking on heart health, glycemic index, and carbohydrate counting. A wider range of multicultural foods have also been added. Portion sizes have been adjusted to be more similar to *Canada's Food Guide,* and to the Quebec and U.S. meal planning systems. The guide also used color coding to help consumers: green for "choose more often" or "everyday" foods and amber for "choose less often" or "special occasion foods." The listed portions of all carbohydrate-rich foods now contain 15 grams of available carbohydrate (total carbohydrate minus fiber and half of any sugar alcohols).

Beyond the Basics classifies foods into eight food groups:

- Grains & Starches
- Fruits
- Milk & Alternatives
- Other Choices
- Vegetables
- Meat & Alternatives
- Fats
- Extras

Within each group, food items are listed along with portions to show how much of one food is interchangeable with another food in the same group. In the past, symbols for the meal planning guide food groups were used on food labels, but this has been phased out with the new food labeling regulations. However, the CDA partnered with Dietitians of Canada to develop *Healthy Eating Is In Store for You*™, an educational program to help Canadians interpret the nutrition label. For more information visit the CDA site: http://www.diabetes.ca/diabetes-and-you/nutrition/healthy-eating.

Appendix F The Gastrointestinal Tract

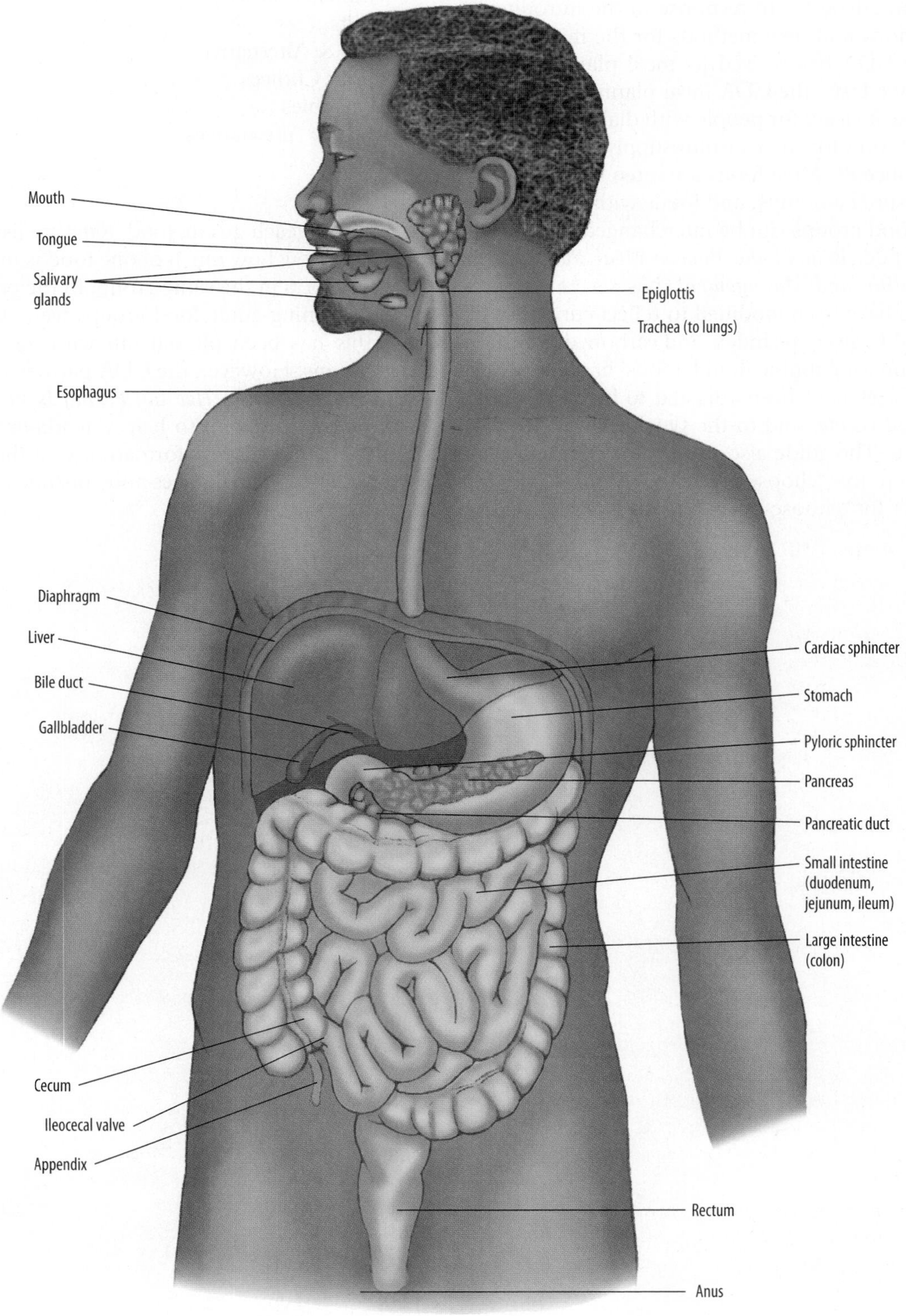

Mouth

- In the mouth, food is broken up by chewing with the teeth and tongue. Saliva lubricates food and makes swallowing easier. Salivary amylase begins the digestion of starch. The mouth warms or cools the food so that it is closer to body temperature. When the food bolus (a fairly liquid ball of food) is ready, swallowing is consciously initiated.

Tongue

- The tongue is a mobile mass of muscle that helps teeth tear food into pieces by forcing it against the bony palate. The tongue contains receptors for sweet, salty, sour, and bitter tastes. Umami, a fifth taste elicited by monosodium glutamate, is a meaty, savory sensation. Flavor is a complex combination of taste, smells (the nose has about 6 million olfactory receptor cells), physical sensations (e.g., spicy foods), and food texture.

Salivary Glands

- The three pairs of salivary glands produce saliva. The water in saliva helps dissolve food particles, facilitating taste sensations. The mucus in saliva lubricates food for swallowing and transport. Digestive enzymes begin breaking down foodstuffs. Salivary amylase begins the chemical breakdown of starches into simple sugars. Lingual lipase initiates the breakdown of fat. The mineral sodium and the enzyme lysozyme in the saliva act as disinfectants, destroying bacteria and other microorganisms in food.

Epiglottis

- The epiglottis is a flap of tissue that acts as a valve during swallowing. It closes the entrance to the larynx and prevents food from entering the respiratory passages.

Trachea

- These tubes allow air to pass to and from the lungs.

Esophagus

- The esophagus is the tube that connects the mouth to the stomach. Wavelike muscle action (peristalsis) moves food through the esophagus to the stomach. The upper one-third of the muscles of the esophagus are under voluntary control, the middle third are a mixture of voluntarily controlled muscle and automatically controlled smooth muscle, and the lower third is smooth muscle alone.

Cardiac Sphincter

- The cardiac sphincter is a muscular valve at the lower end of the esophagus. This control valve relaxes to allow food to pass into the stomach. When contracted, it prevents backflow (reflux) of stomach contents into the esophagus. Named for its proximity to the heart, a malfunction can cause painful esophageal reflux (heartburn), which can be so severe that it is mistaken for a heart attack.

Stomach

- The upper bag-like portion of the stomach acts as a hopper to receive and hold the food prior to delivery to the lower two-thirds. Three layers of smooth muscle surround this lower portion of the stomach. Muscular contractions churn the food, so the solids can ferment and mix with acids, fluid, and protein-splitting enzymes. The result is a sticky semiliquid, called chyme, that is gradually released into the duodenum (the first part of the small intestine). Stomach acid halts the digestion of starch, but the stomach also produces gastric lipase, an enzyme that acts on fat.

Pyloric Sphincter

- The pyloric sphincter is a muscular valve that controls passage of chyme from the stomach to the small intestine. When contracted, it prevents backflow from the small intestine into the stomach.

Liver

- The liver is the body's chemical factory and detoxification center. It has many functions in controlling metabolism and deactivating hormones, drugs, and toxins. It also produces bile—a mixture of bile salts, phospholipids, cholesterol, pigments, proteins, and inorganic ions such as sodium. The detergent-like action of bile emulsifies fat, facilitating fat digestion.

Gallbladder

- The gallbladder stores and concentrates bile. The arrival of fatty food in the duodenum stimulates the release of the duodenal hormone CCK, which signals the gallbladder to contract. The bile is then released into the duodenum, where it aids fat digestion.

Bile Duct

- The bile duct carries bile from the gallbladder to the duodenum.

Pancreas

- The pancreas is a complex gland that produces a pancreatic juice rich in bicarbonate and enzymes. The pancreatic juice is released into the duodenum, where it does its work. Pancreatic amylase breaks down starch into maltose. Lipase splits fats into monoglycerides, fatty acids, and glycerol. The pancreatic proenzyme trypsinogen is converted to the enzyme trypsin. Trypsin splits polypeptides and proteins into amino acids. Bicarbonate produced by the pancreas neutralizes the acid chyme that enters the small intestine. In addition, the pancreas produces insulin and glucagon—hormones that have important roles in regulating carbohydrate metabolism and blood sugar.

Pancreatic Duct

- The pancreatic duct carries pancreatic juice from the pancreas to the duodenum.

Small Intestine

- The small intestine is a tube approximately 10 feet long that is divided into three parts: the duodenum (the first 10 to 12 inches), the jejunum (about 4 feet), and the ileum (about 5 feet). Whereas the duodenum is mainly responsible for breaking down food, the jejunum and ileum primarily deal with the absorption of food. The duodenum secretes mucus, enzymes, and hormones to aid digestion. Most digestion and absorption occur in the small intestine. Intestinal cells secrete disaccharidases and peptidases to help complete carbohydrate and protein digestion. The intestinal lining is highly folded to increase its surface area and is richly supplied with circulatory vessels, which carry away absorbed nutrients in the blood and lymph. Undigested material is passed on to the large intestine.

Ileocecal Valve (sphincter)

- The ileocecal valve is the sphincter at the lower end of the small intestine. When open, it permits food residue to move from the small intestine to the large intestine. When closed, it prevents backflow from the large intestine.

Large Intestine

- The large intestine is made up of the appendix, cecum, colon, rectum, and anus. The colon is about 2.5 inches in diameter and about 4 feet long. In the large intestine, bacteria break down dietary fiber and other undigested carbohydrates, releasing acids and gas. The large intestine absorbs water and minerals while dehydrating and processing the remaining undigested material into solid feces. The colon walls secrete a viscous mucus to help lubricate and mold the feces. This mucus also helps protect the colon wall from mechanical damage.

Appendix

- The appendix is a fingerlike appendage attached to the cecum, the first part of the colon. The appendix has no known function.

Cecum

- The cecum is the pouchlike beginning of the large intestine. The small intestine's ileum empties into the cecum.

Rectum

- The rectum stores waste prior to elimination.

Anus

- The anal sphincter holds the rectum closed. Either voluntary or involuntary control may open it to allow elimination.

Appendix G Biochemical Structures

- Nomenclature
- ATP and Derivatives
- Carbohydrates
- Amino Acids
- Fatty Acids
- Fat-Soluble Vitamins
- Water-Soluble Vitamins and Coenzymes
- B Vitamins in Major Metabolic Pathways

Nomenclature

Prefixes

mono-	Means one subunit. For instance, *mono*saccharide means a one-unit saccharide.
bi-, di-, and tri-	Mean two and three subunits bonded together to form a larger molecule.
poly-	Means many or a lot. A *poly*saccharide has many linked monosaccharide subunits.
oligo-	Means a structure with typically 3 to 10 subunits, but smaller than a polymer.

Suffixes

-ose	Sugars are named with *-ose* as a suffix. They are subclassified with regard to the number of carbons, i.e., 3 = triose, 4 = tetrose, 5 = pentose, 6 = hexose, 7 = heptose. The suffix *-ose* refers to monosaccharides and disaccharides: sugars like gluc*ose*, fruct*ose*, sucr*ose*, etc.
-ase	Many enzymes are named by attaching the suffix *-ase* to the substrate of the enzyme (the compound altered by enzymatic action). For instance, a lipase cleaves a lipid substrate, a disaccharidase cleaves a disaccharide, and a peptidase breaks the peptide bond between two amino acids.
-ol	Suffix for naming alcohols and phenols (e.g., ethan*ol*, glycer*ol*).
-ic, -ate, -oic, -oate	Suffixes for naming acids and acid salts.

Although the terms *lactic acid* and *lactate* often are used interchangeably, they are not identical chemical compounds. Lactic acid ($C_3H_6O_3$), as its name implies, is an acid. Lactate is any salt of lactic acid, for instance, sodium lactate. When anaerobic glycolysis forms lactic acid, the acid quickly dissociates, releasing hydrogen (H^+) into the solution. The lactate ion then immediately associates with sodium (Na^+) or potassium (K^+) to form a salt–sodium or potassium lactate. In substances such as pyruvate and lactate, the carboxyl group is COO^- (one oxygen has an available bond). In acids such as pyruvic acid and lactic acid, the carboxyl group is COOH (the available bond is filled with hydrogen). The suffixes -ic and -ate are used for the acid and salt forms of most carboxyl groups. For reasons of pronunciation, some carboxyl groups require the *-oic* or *-oate* suffixes, for instance, butanoic acid, and its salt form butan*oate*.

-peptide	The suffix *peptide* refers to a molecule composed of 2 or more amino acids joined by peptide bonds. A di*peptide* is composed of 2 amino acids, a tri*peptide* of three, etc. A short string of amino acids is called a poly*peptide* and a long string is a protein.
-saccharide	The suffix *saccharide* refers to sugar. A poly*saccharide*, for example, is a large molecule composed of many sugar subunits. A polysaccharide may be composed of only one type of sugar (starch is made up of many glucose units) or of many different sugars. A lipopoly*saccharide*, for instance, is made up of a variety of sugars bonded to a lipid.
hydrogen ion	Also known as a proton, this lone hydrogen has a positive charge (H^+). It has lost its electron and associates readily with negatively charged ions, like the hydroxyl ion (OH^-).
atomic hydrogen	A hydrogen atom with a single electron. This proton-electron combination is unstable and is a short-lived intermediate in some enzymatically catalyzed reactions. During oxidation-reduction reactions it is atomic hydrogen (hydrogen 1 electron), not hydrogen ions (H^+), that is transferred.

Acids are substances that form hydrogen ions in solution. An acid dissociates to form a cation (H^+) and an anion (e.g., SO_4^-).

When the anion ends with the suffix *-ate*, its acid name is simply the anion with suffix *-ic*, followed by the word *acid*. Here are some examples:

- H_2SO_4 - hydrogen sulf*ate* becomes sulfur*ic acid*
- H_3PO_4 - hydrogen phosph*ate* becomes phosphor*ic acid*
- $HClO_3$ - hydrogen chlor*ate* becomes hydrochlor*ic acid*

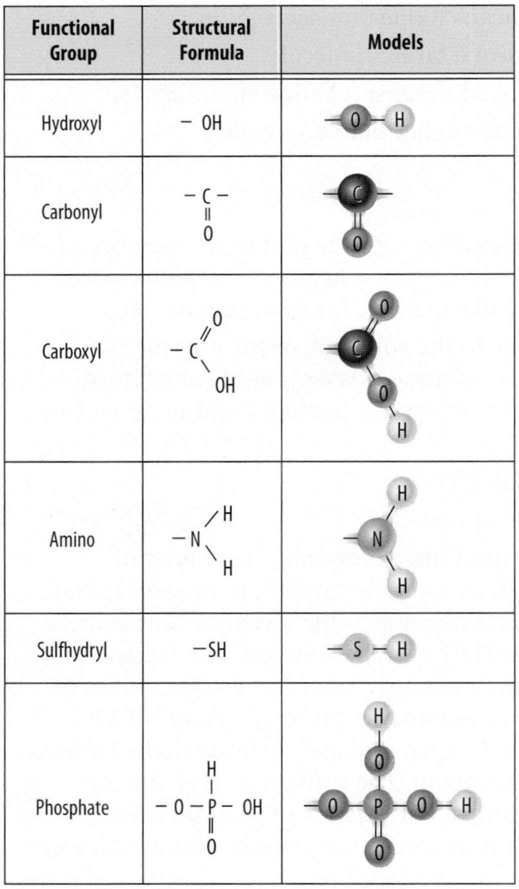
Functional Group
Structural Formula
Models
Hydroxyl
– OH
Carbonyl
Carboxyl
Amino
Sulfhydryl
–SH
Phosphate

Functional groups: These six functional groups are commonly involved in covalent and non-covalent bonding to form molecules such as proteins and DNA.

ATP and Derivatives

ATP, ADP, and AMP

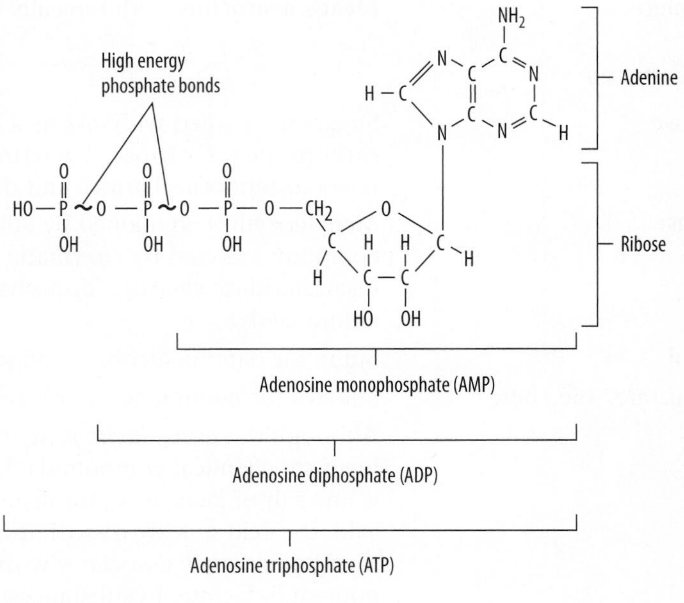

< = Trace amount present Blank = Not available

Carbohydrates

Monosaccharides

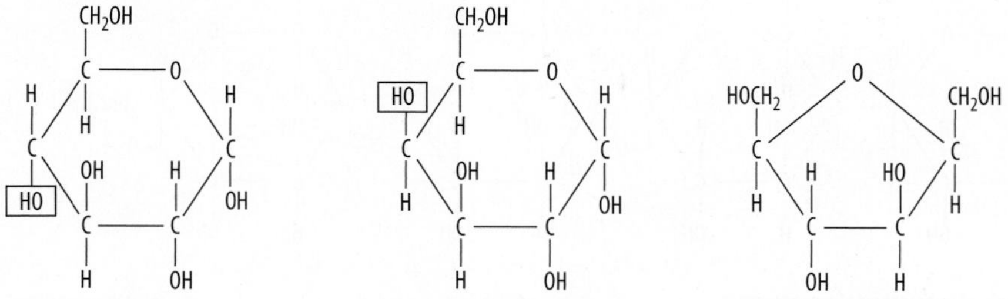

Glucose **Galactose** **Fructose**

The structures of glucose and galactose differ only by the location of the OH on carbon number 4.

Disaccharides

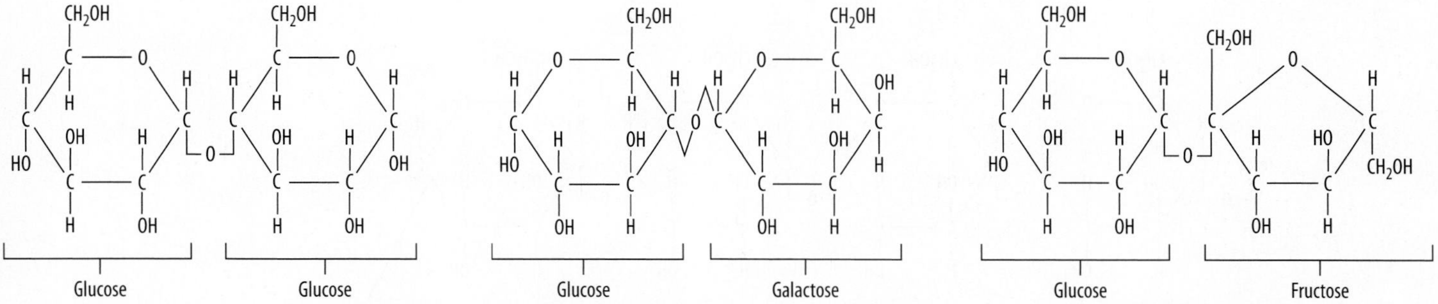

Maltose **Lactose** **Sucrose**

In maltose and sucrose, the monosaccharides are linked by alpha bonds. In lactose, a beta bond links galactose and glucose. The human digestive enzyme lactase can hydrolyze the beta bond in lactose.

Polysaccharides

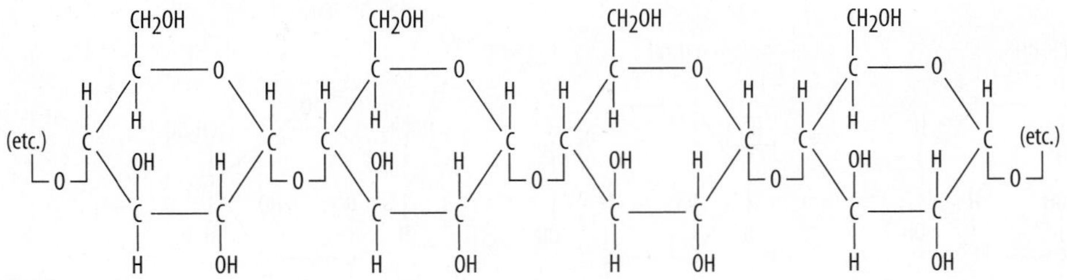

Amylose
Starch molecule made of unbranched glucose chains.

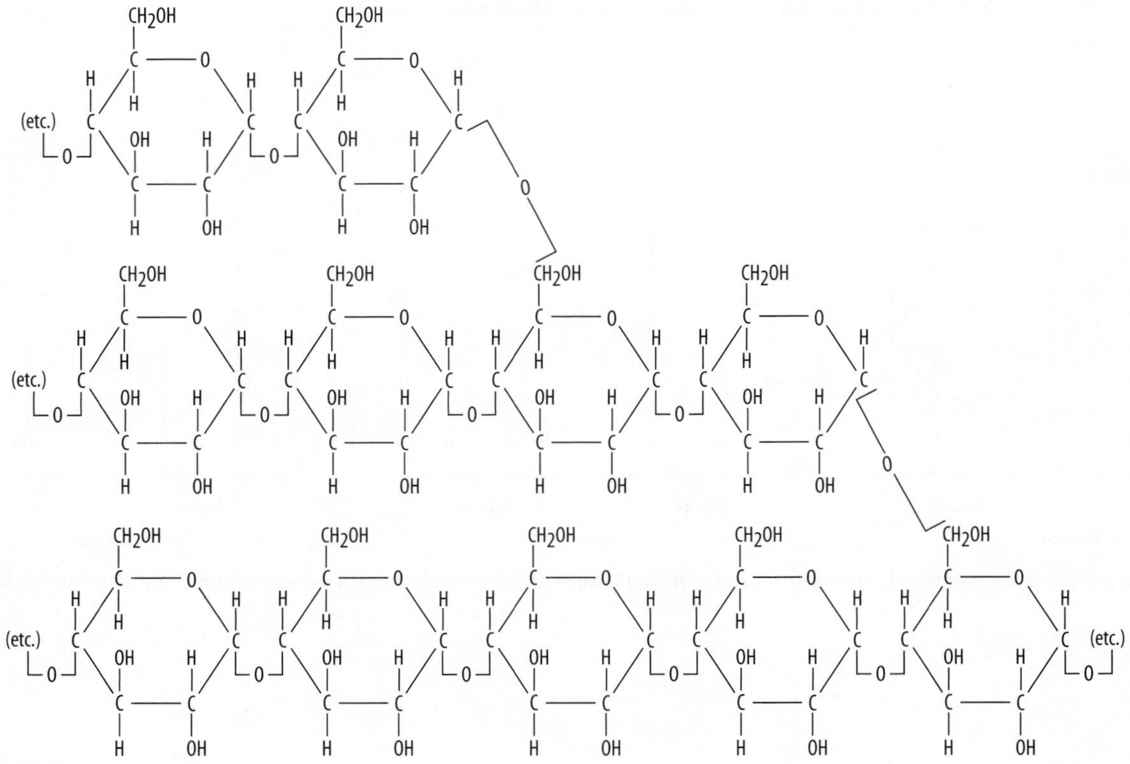

Amylopectin
Starch molecule made of branched glucose chains. In amylopectin, the chain branches every thirty glucose units. Glycogen is similar, but more highly branched (every ten glucose units).

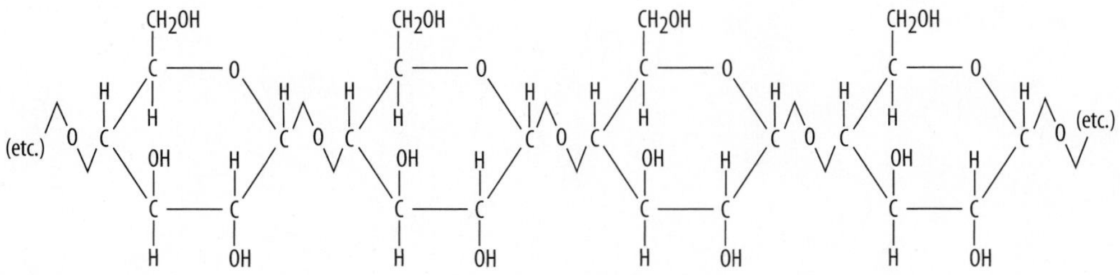

Cellulose
Cellulose is a nearly straight chain of glucose units where the glucose molecules are linked by beta bonds. Humans do not have the enzymes necessary to break the beta linkages in cellulose.

Amino Acids

Essential Amino Acids

Amino acids consist of a central carbon atom bonded to a carboxyl group, an amino group, a hydrogen, and a side group. The shaded areas show the structure common to all amino acids.

Valine (Val)

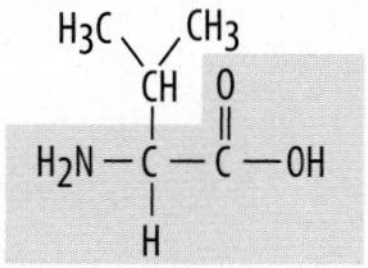

Leucine (Leu)

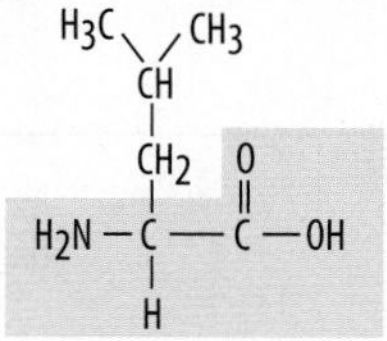

Isoleucine (Ile)

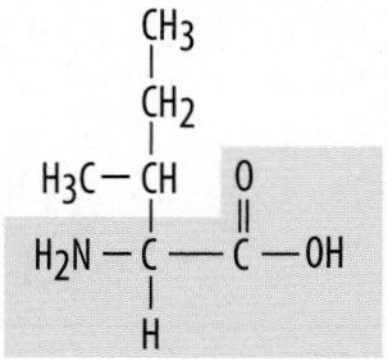

Threonine (Thr)

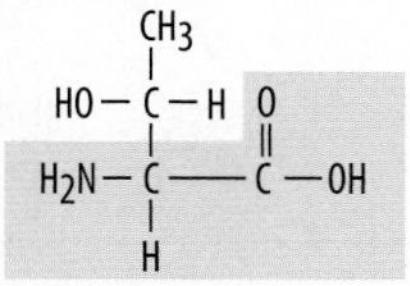

Lysine (Lys)

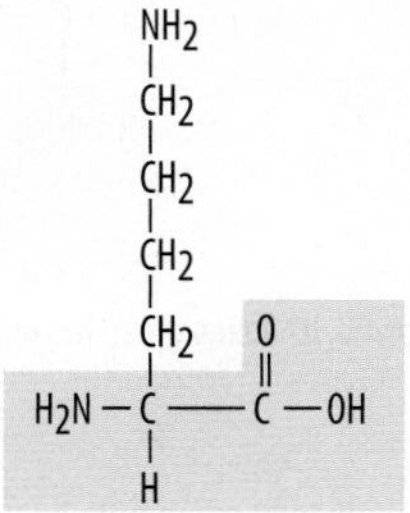

Histidine (His)

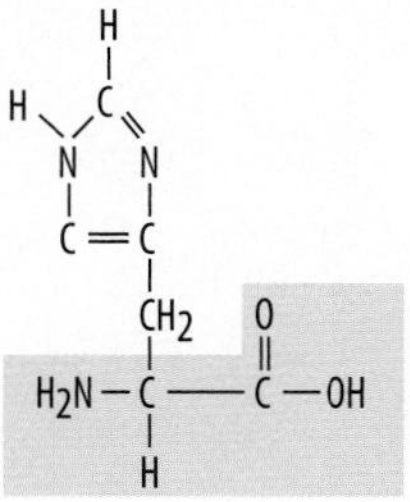

Phenylalanine (Phe)

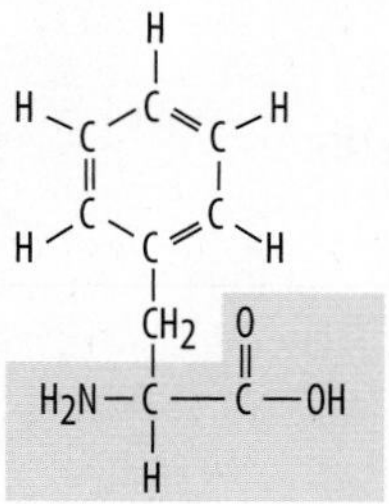

Tryptophan (Trp)

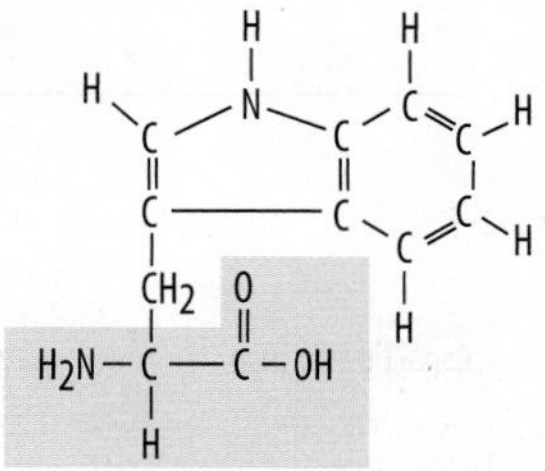

Methionine (Met)

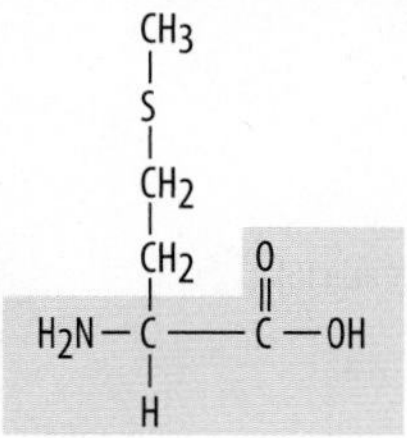

Nonessential Amino Acids

Glycine (Gly)

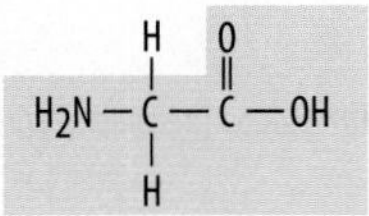

Alanine (Ala)

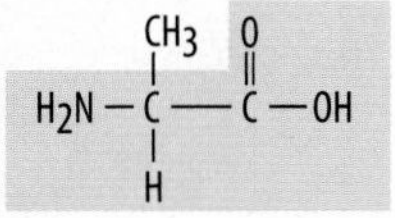

Serine (Ser)

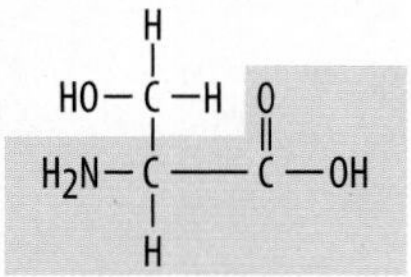

Aspartic acid (Asp)

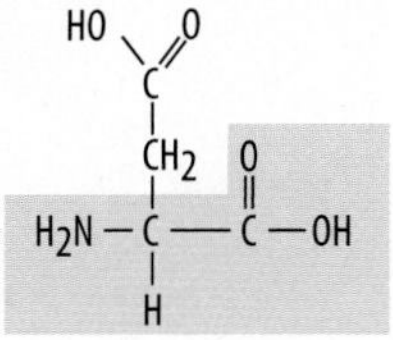

Glutamic acid (Glu)

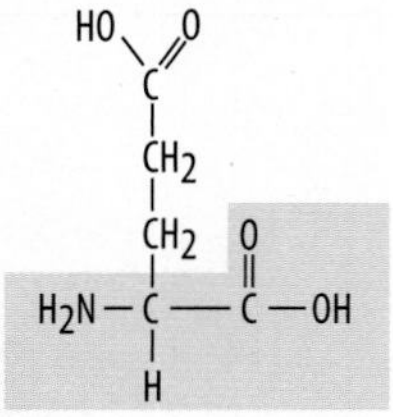

Asparagine (Asn)

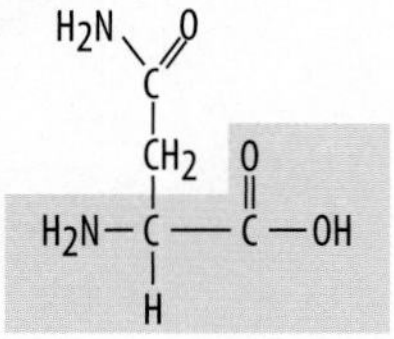

Glutamine (Gln)

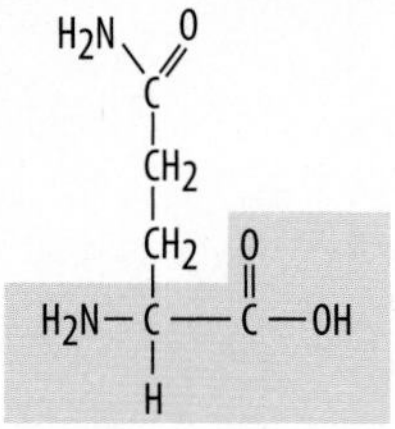

Arginine (Arg)

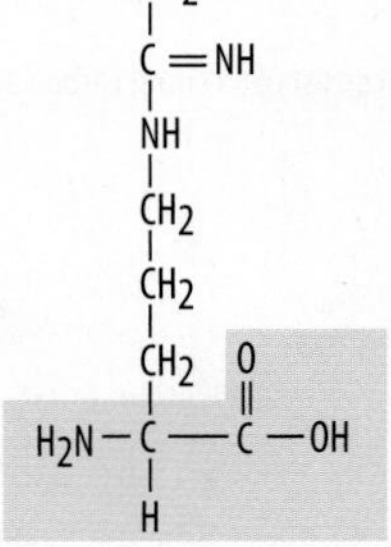

Tyrosine (Tyr)

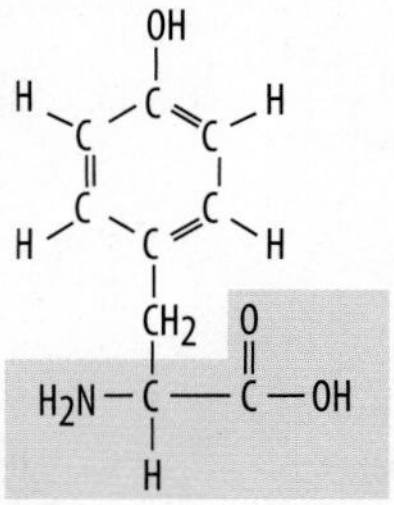

Cysteine (Cys)

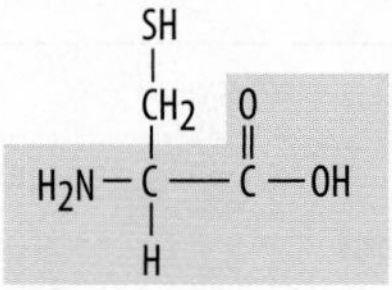

Proline (Pro)

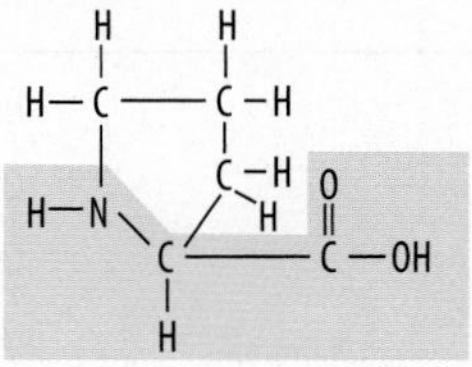

Proline is an amino acid. Its amino group has only one hydrogen and forms a ring.

< = Trace amount present   Blank = Not available

Fatty Acids

TABLE G.1
Saturated Fatty Acids Found in Food

Saturated Fatty Acid	Chemical Formula	Number of Carbons	Major Food Sources
Butyric	$CH_3(CH_2)_2COOH$	4	Small amounts in butterfat
Caproic	$CH_3(CH_2)_4COOH$	6	Small amounts in butterfat
Caprylic	$CH_3(CH_2)_6COOH$	8	Small amounts in many fats, including butterfat. Especially found in oils of plant origin.
Capric	$CH_3(CH_2)_8COOH$	10	Small amounts in many fats, including butterfat. Especially found in oils of plant origin.
Lauric	$CH_3(CH_2)_{10}COOH$	12	Cinnamon, palm kernel, coconut oil, butter
Myristic	$CH_3(CH_2)_{12}COOH$	14	Nutmeg, palm kernel, coconut oil, butter
Palmitic	$CH_3(CH_2)_{14}COOH$	16	Common in all animal and plant fats
Stearic	$CH_3(CH_2)_{16}COOH$	18	Common in all animal and plant fats
Arachidic	$CH_3(CH_2)_{18}COOH$	20	Peanut oil
Behenic	$CH_3(CH_2)_{20}COOH$	22	Seeds
Lignoceric	$CH_3(CH_2)_{22}COOH$	24	Peanut oil

TABLE G.2
Unsaturated Fatty Acids Found in Food

Unsaturated Fatty Acid	Chemical Formula	Number of Carbons	Number of Double Bonds	Omega Notation*	Major Food Sources
Palmitoleic	$CH_3(CH_2)_5CH = CH(CH_2)_7COOH$	16	1	16:1ω7	Nearly all fats
Oleic	$CH_3(CH_2)_7CH = CH(CH_2)_7COOH$	18	1	18:1ω9	Perhaps the most common fatty acid in food
Linoleic	$CH_3(CH_2)_4(CH = CHCH_2)_2(CH_2)_6COOH$	18	2	18:2ω6	Corn, peanut, cottonseed, soybean, and several oils from other plants
Linolenic	$CH_3CH_2(CH = CHCH_2)_3(CH_2)_6COOH$	18	3	18:3ω3	Often in foods with linoleic acid, but particularly found in linseed oil
Arachidonic	$CH_3(CH_2)_4(CH = CHCH_2)_4(CH_2)_2COOH$	20	4	20:4ω6	Animal fats and peanut oil
Eicosapentanoic	$CH_3(CH_2)_3(CH = CHCH_2)_4(CH_2)_3COOH$	20	5	20:5ω3	Fish oils such as cod liver, mackerel, and salmon
Docosahexanoic	$CH_3(CH_2)_2(CH = CHCH_2)_6COOH$	22	6	22:6ω3	Fish oils such as cod liver, mackerel, and salmon

*Omega Notation = number of carbons: number of double bonds, the number following the omega symbol (ω) represents the location of the first double bond counting from the methyl (CH_3) end.

Fat-Soluble Vitamins

Vitamin A and Beta-carotene

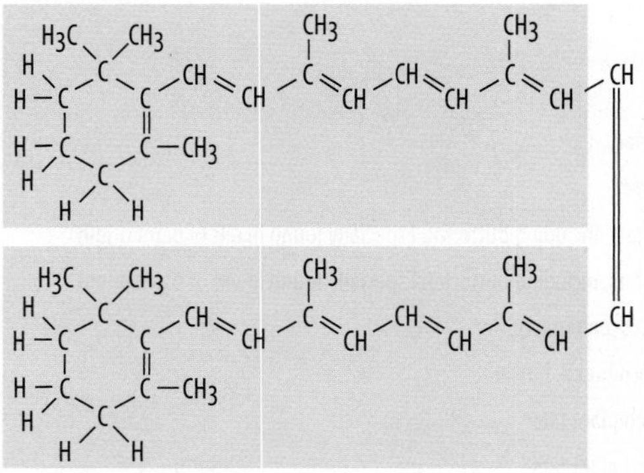

Vitamin A precursor: beta-carotene

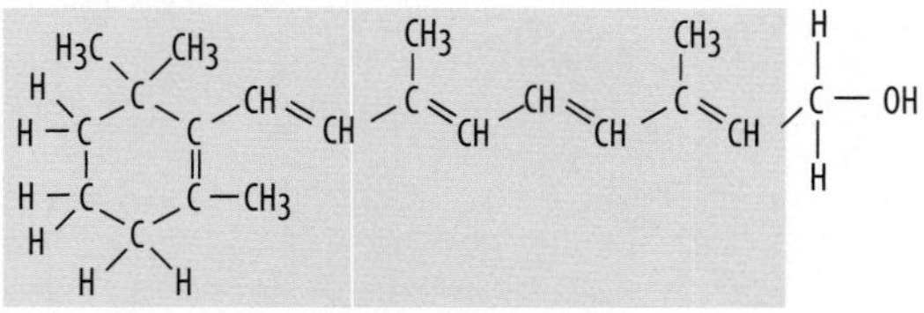

Vitamin A: retinol

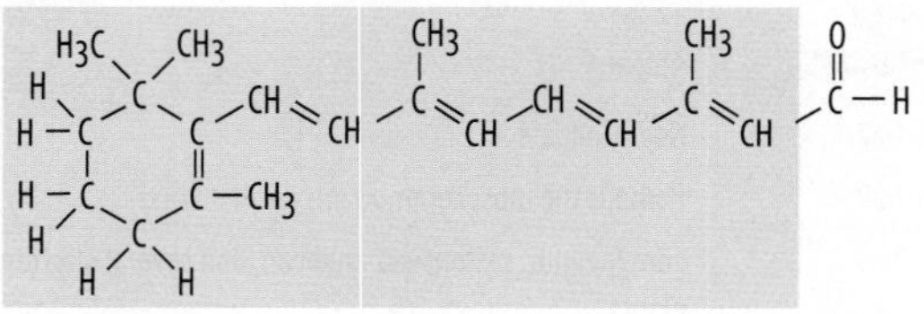

Vitamin A: retinal

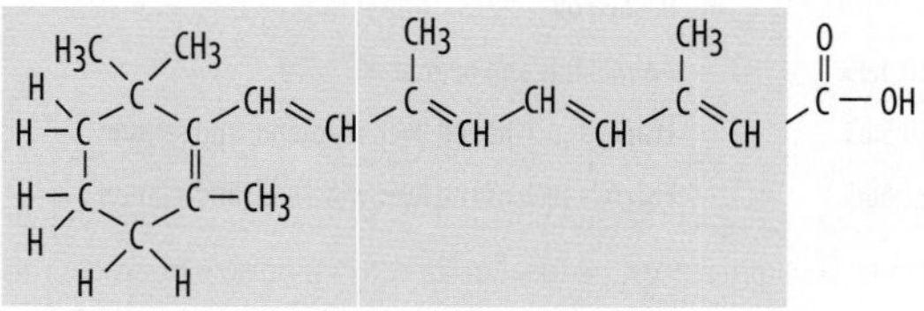

Vitamin A: retinoic acid

The shaded areas highlight the structure common to all four molecules.

Vitamin D

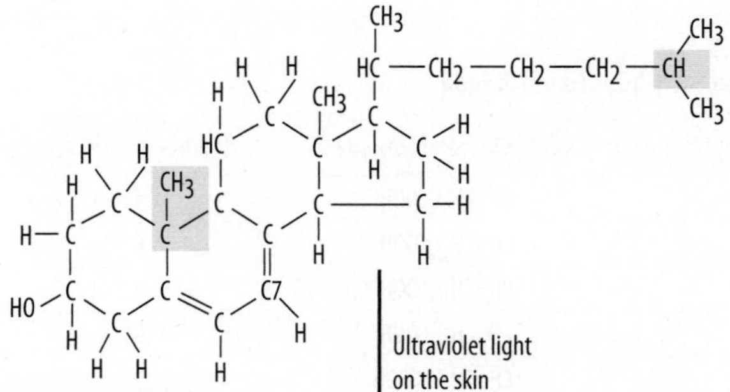

7–Dehydrocholesterol

Ultraviolet light on the skin

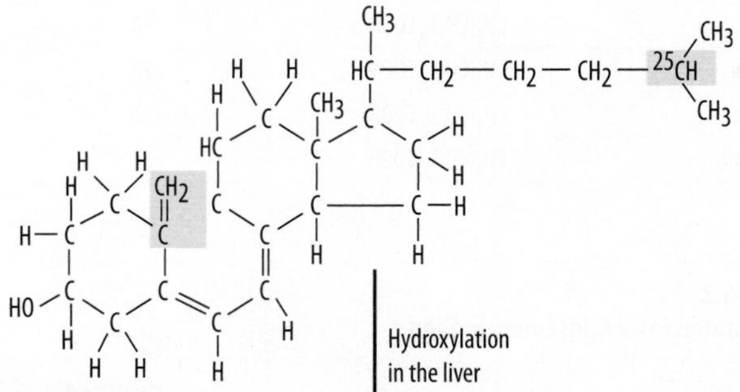

Cholecalciferol
(vitamin D_3)

Hydroxylation in the liver

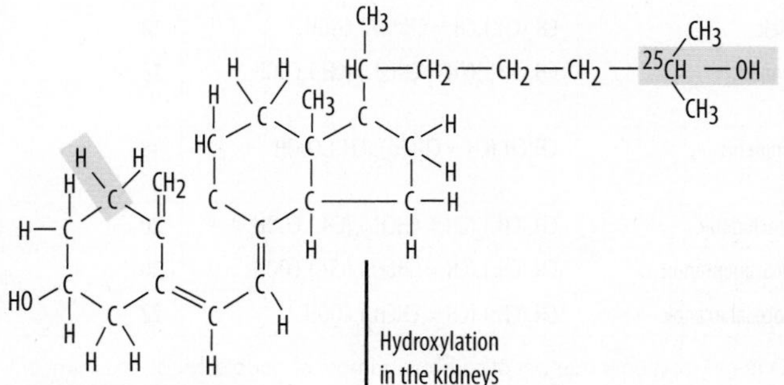

25–Hydroxycholecalciferol
(25–hydroxyvitamin D_3)

Hydroxylation in the kidneys

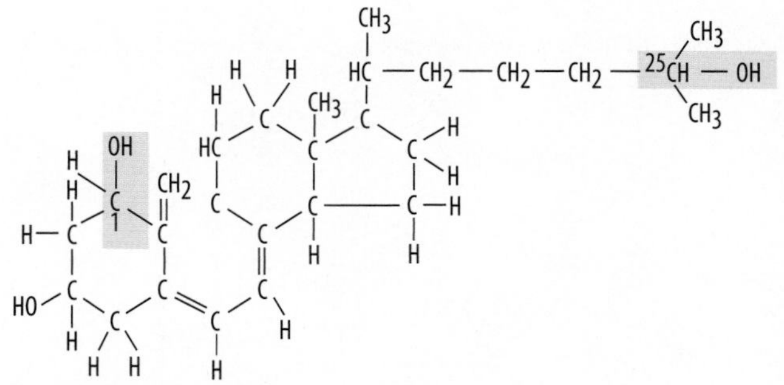

1, 25–Dihydroxycholecalciferol
(1, 25–dihydroxyvitamin D_3)
(calcitriol)

The shaded areas highlight the portion of the molecule that changes from stage to stage.

< = Trace amount present   Blank = Not available

Vitamin E

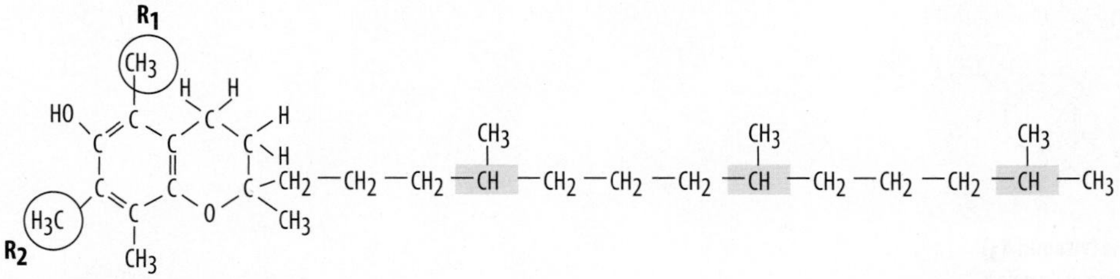

Vitamin E (alpha-tocopherol)
4 isomers α, β, γ, δ

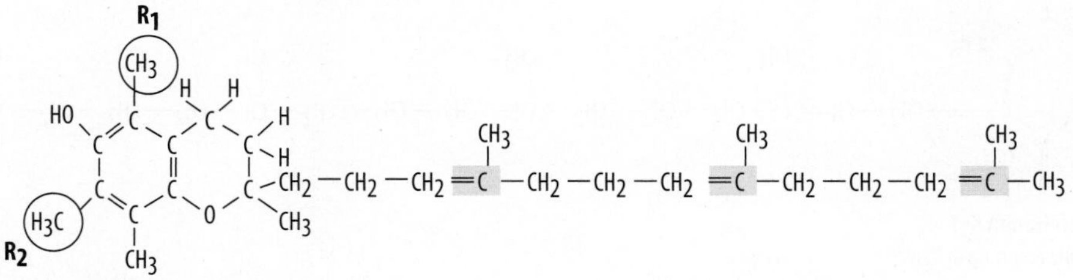

Vitamin E (alpha-tocotrienol)
4 isomers α, β, γ, δ

Isomers for tocopherols and tocotrienols

For α,	$R_1 = CH_3$	$R_2 = CH_3$
For β,	$R_1 = CH_3$	$R_2 = H$
For γ,	$R_1 = H$	$R_2 = CH_3$
For δ,	$R_1 = H$	$R_2 = H$

Vitamin E occurs in 8 forms but vitamin E activity is based on alpha-tocopherol. Humans do not convert β-, γ-, δ-tocopherols or the tocotrienols to alpha-tocopherol, so these forms do not contribute toward meeting the vitamin E requirement. The shading highlights the differences between tocopherols and tocotrienols.

Vitamin K

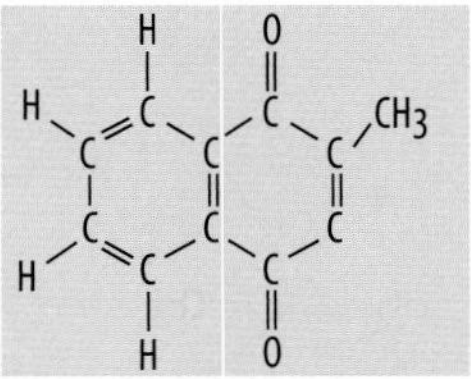

Menadione (vitamin K$_3$)
Synthetic form of Vitamin K

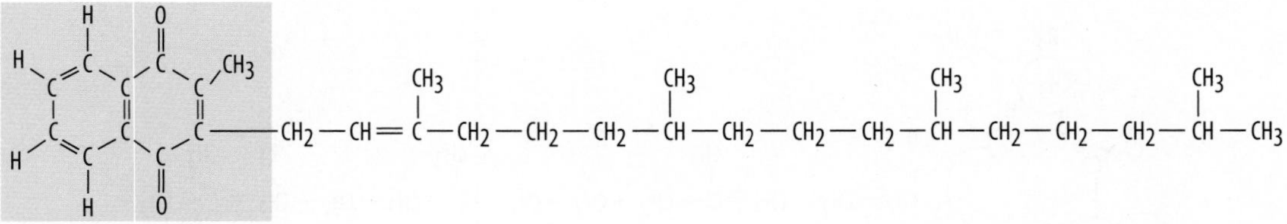

Phylloquinone (vitamin K$_1$)
Vitamin K naturally occurring in food

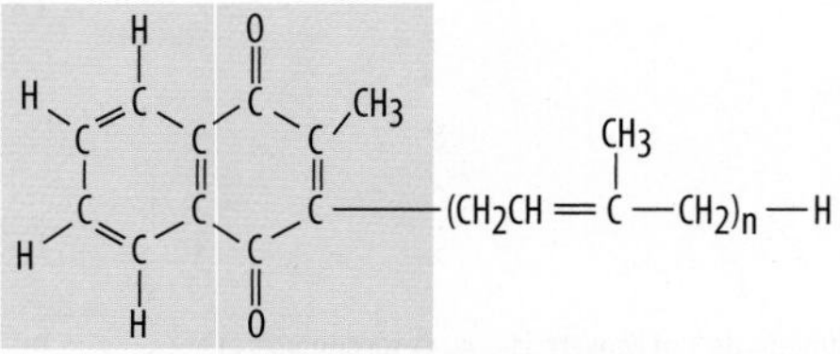

Menaquinone-n (vitamin K$_2$; n = 6, 7, or 9)
Vitamin K formed by bacteria in the large intestine

The shaded areas highlight the structure common to all three forms.

Water-Soluble Vitamins and Coenzymes

Thiamin and Coenzyme

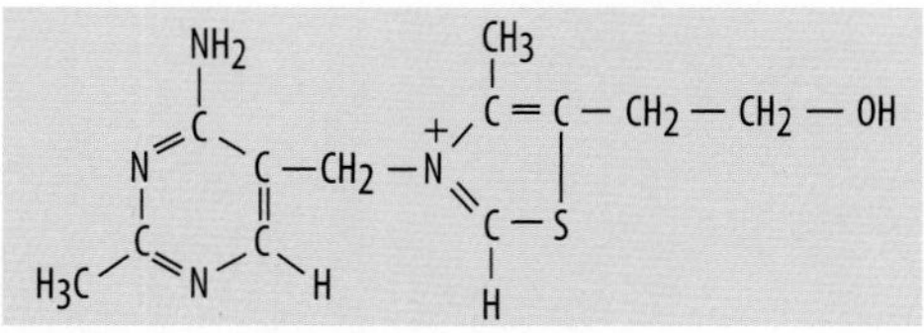

Thiamin

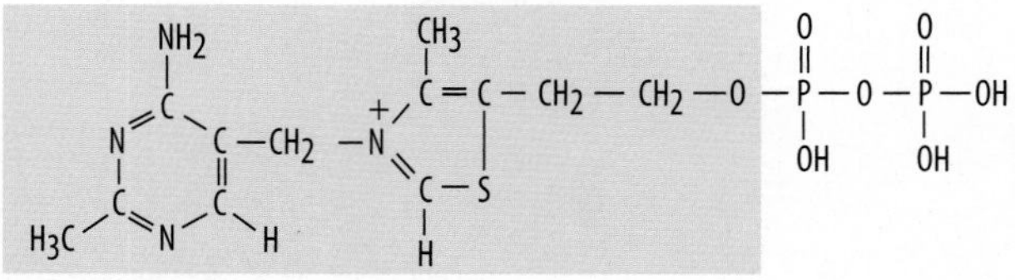

Thiamin pyrophosphate (TPP)

Thiamin is part of the active coenzyme TPP. The shaded areas highlight the structure common to both molecules.

< = Trace amount present   Blank = Not available

Riboflavin and Coenzymes

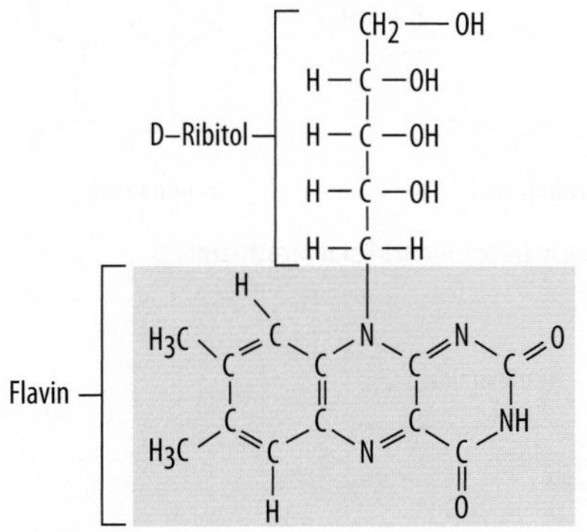

Riboflavin

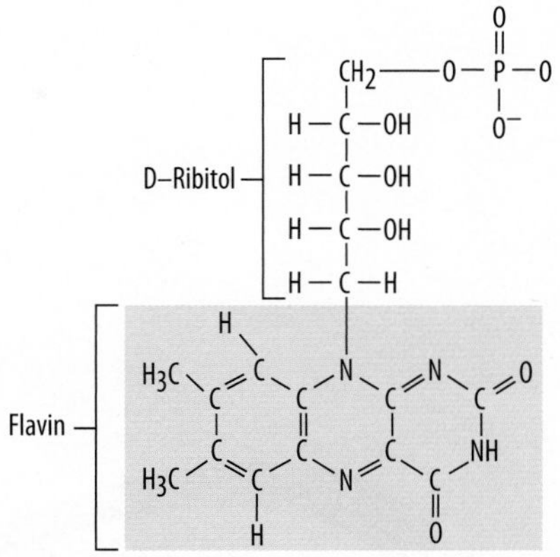

Flavin mononucleotide (FMN)

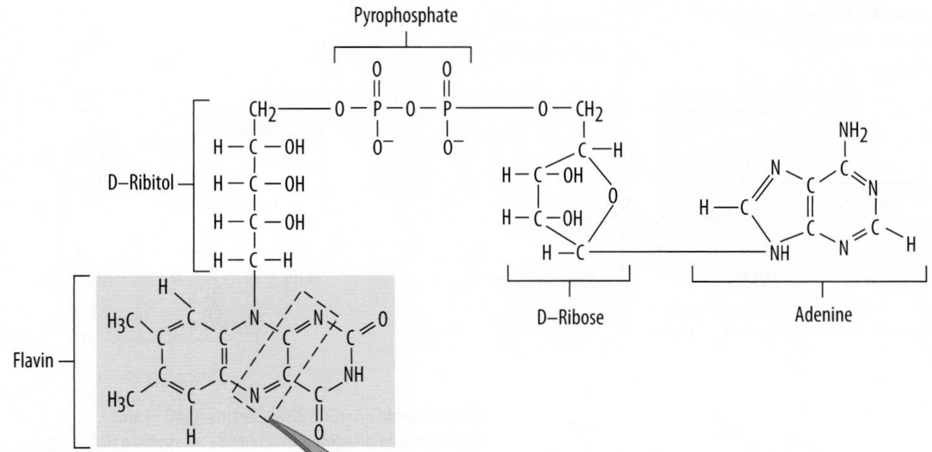

Flavin dinucleotide (FAD)

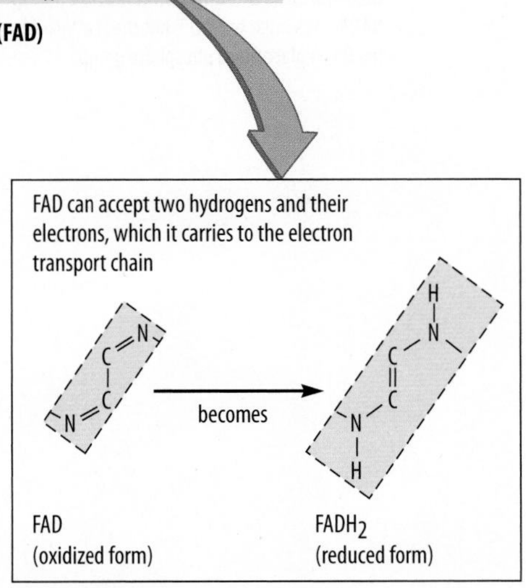
FAD can accept two hydrogens and their electrons, which it carries to the electron transport chain
becomes
FAD
(oxidized form)
FADH2
(reduced form)

FAD and $FADH_2$

The flavin portion of these molecules is highlighted.

Niacin and Coenzymes

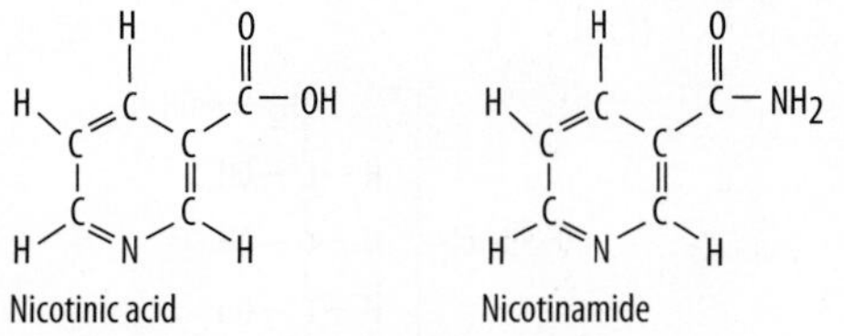

Niacin (nicotinic acid and nicotinamide)

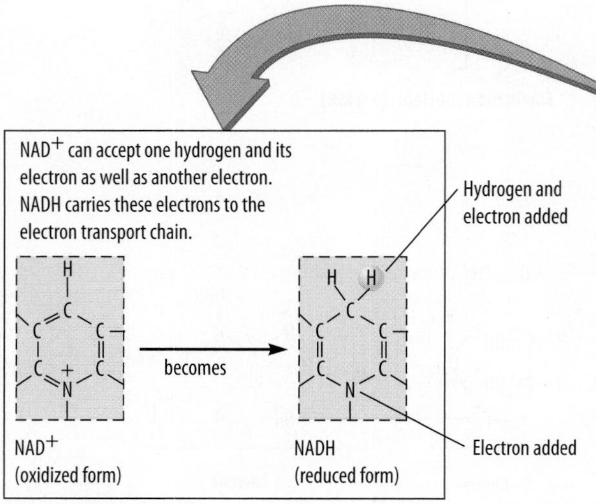

NAD^+ and NADH

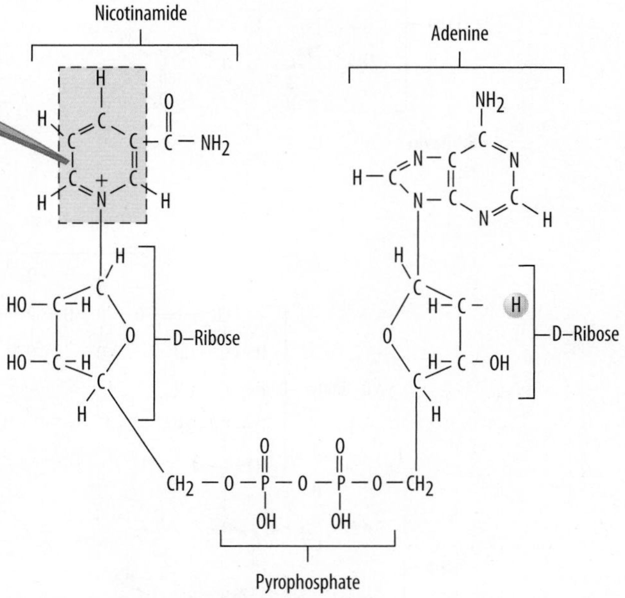

Nicotinamide adenine dinucleotide (NAD^+) and nicotinamide adenine dinucleotide phosphate ($NADP^+$)
$NADP^+$ is similar to NAD^+ but the H attached to the O is replaced by a phosphate group.

Pantothenic Acid and Coenzyme A

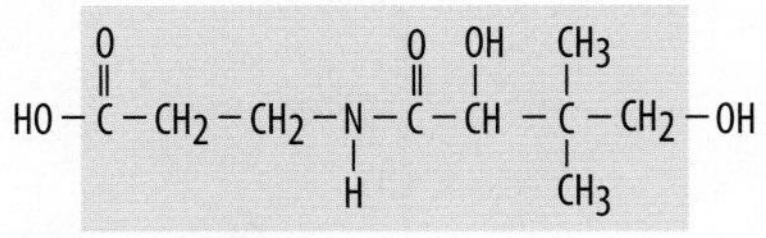

Pantothenic acid

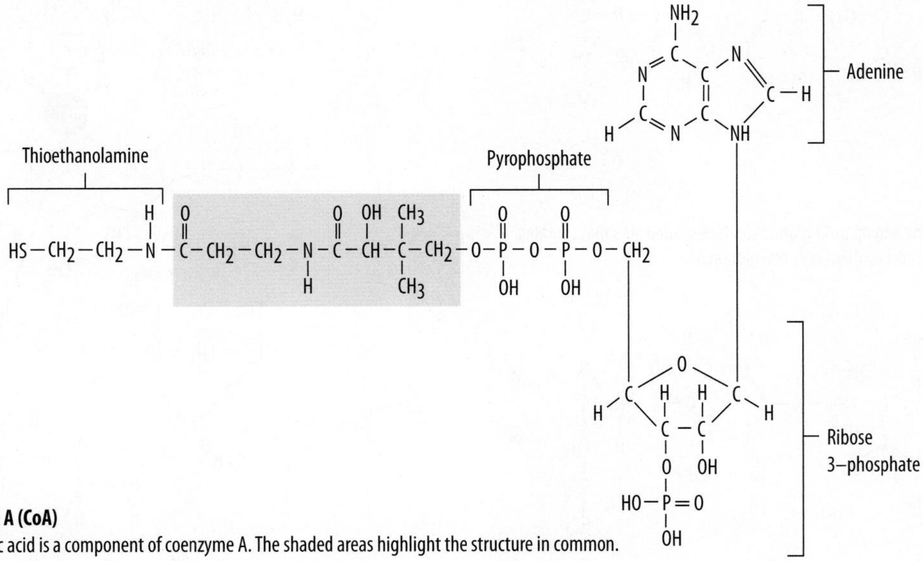

Coenzyme A (CoA)
Pantothenic acid is a component of coenzyme A. The shaded areas highlight the structure in common.

Biotin

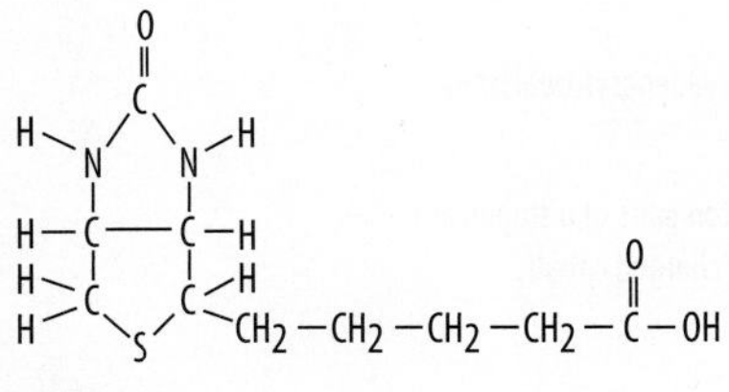

Biotin

Vitamin B_6 and Coenzymes

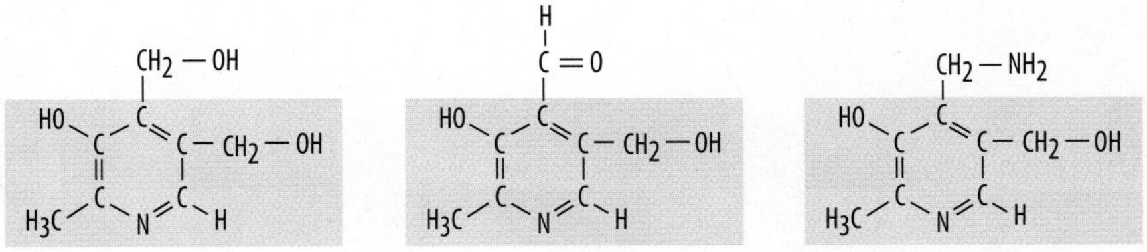

Pyridoxine Pyridoxal Pyridoxamine

Vitamin B_6 (pyridoxine, pyridoxal, and pyridoxamine)

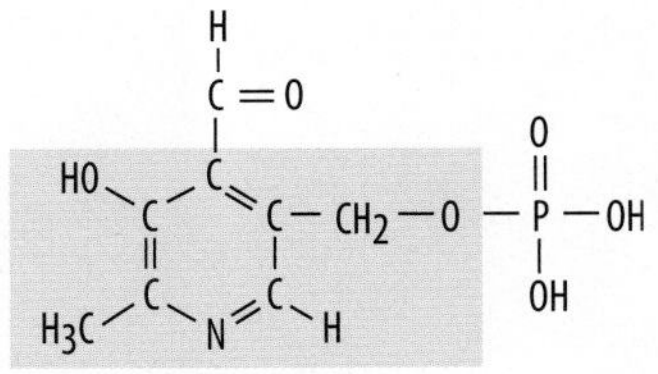

Pyridoxal phosphate (PLP)

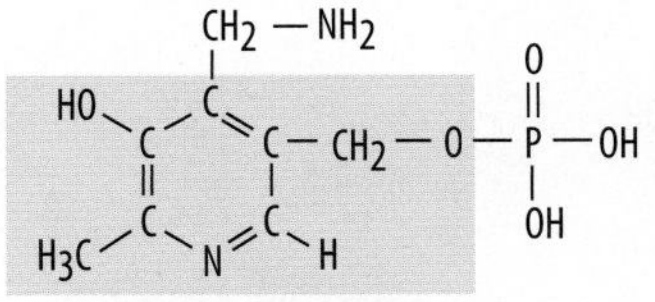

Pyridoxamine phosphate (PMP)

Pyridoxal phosphate (PLP) and pyridoxamine phosphate (PMP) are the two active coenzyme forms of vitamin B_6. The shaded areas highlight the structures in common.

Folate and Coenzyme

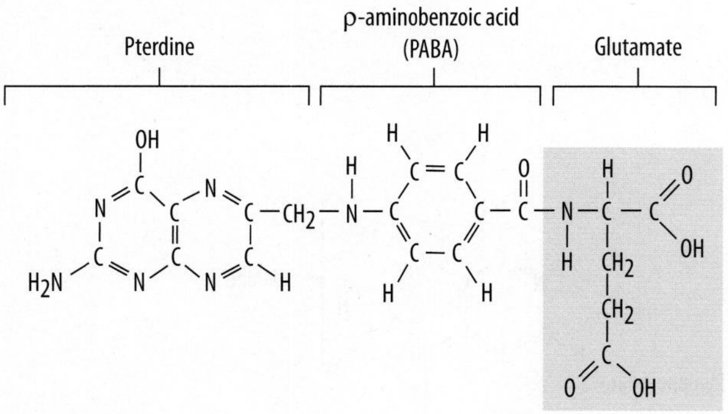

Folate
Folate contains at least one and up to 11 glutamates (see shaded area that contains a single glutamate). Folic acid contains only one glutamate.

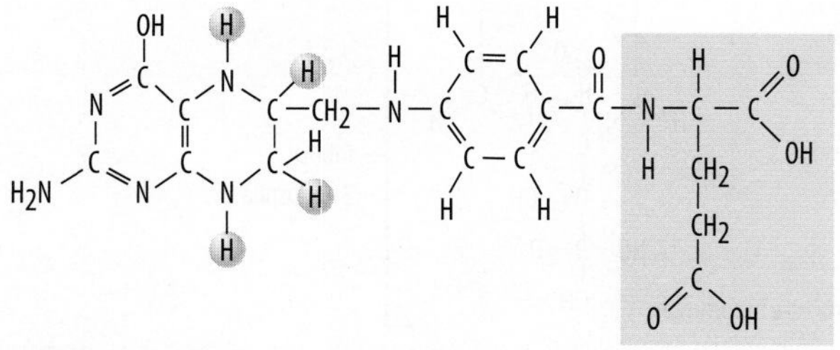

Tetrahydrofolic acid (THFA)
Adding 4 hydrogens to folate produces THFA, the active coenzyme form.

Vitamin C

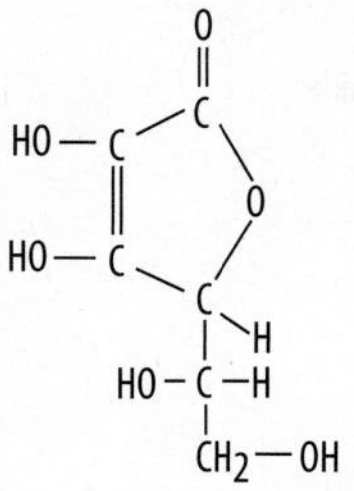

Vitamin C
(Ascorbic acid)

Vitamin B_{12}

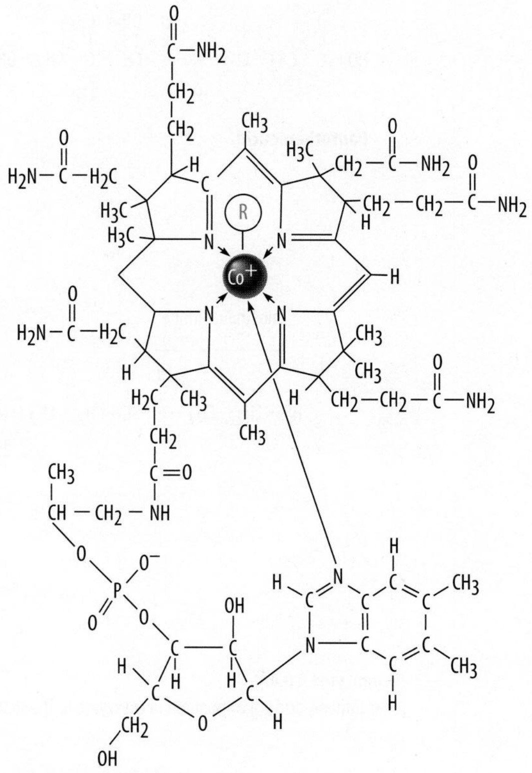

Vitamin B_{12} (cobalamin)

R = CN in cyanocobalamin
R = OH in hydroxocobalamin
R = 5′–deoxyadenosyl in 5′–deoxyadenosylcobalamin
R = CH_3 in methylcobalamin
Arrows indicate that the free electron pairs of nitrogen are in close proximity to the positively charged cobalt.

B Vitamins in Major Metabolic Pathways

Thiamin	Pyruvate to acetyl CoA (TPP) Citric acid cycle (TPP)
Riboflavin	Pyruvate to acetyl CoA (FAD) Citric acid cycle (FAD) Electron transport chain (FAD, FMN) Beta-oxidation (fatty acids to acetyl CoA) (FAD) Amino acid breakdown (FAD)
Niacin	Glycolysis (NAD^+) Pyruvate to acetyl CoA (NAD^+) Citric acid cycle (NAD^+) Electron transport chain (NAD^+) Beta-oxidation (fatty acids to acetyl CoA) (NAD^+) Fatty acid synthesis (acetyl CoA to fatty acids) (NADPH) Amino acid breakdown (NAD^+) Amino acid synthesis (NAD^+, NADPH) Gluconeogenesis (NAD^+)
Pantothenic acid	Pyruvate to acetyl CoA (coenzyme A) Citric acid cycle (coenzyme A) Beta-oxidation (fatty acids to acetyl CoA) (coenzyme A) Fatty acid synthesis (acetyl CoA to fatty acids) (coenzyme A)
Biotin	Fatty acid synthesis (acetyl CoA to fatty acids) (biotin-enzyme) Gluconeogenesis (biotin-enzyme)
Vitamin B6	Glycogen to glucose (PLP) Amino acid breakdown (PLP) Amino acid synthesis (PLP)
Folate	Amino acid synthesis (THFA) Synthesis of some components of DNA and RNA (THFA)
Vitamin B12	Amino acid breakdown (B_{12}) Synthesis of some components of DNA and RNA (B_{12})

Appendix H Major Metabolic Pathways

- Glycolysis
- Citric Acid Cycle
- Electron Transport Chain
- Urea Cycle

< = Trace amount present   Blank = Not available

Glycolysis

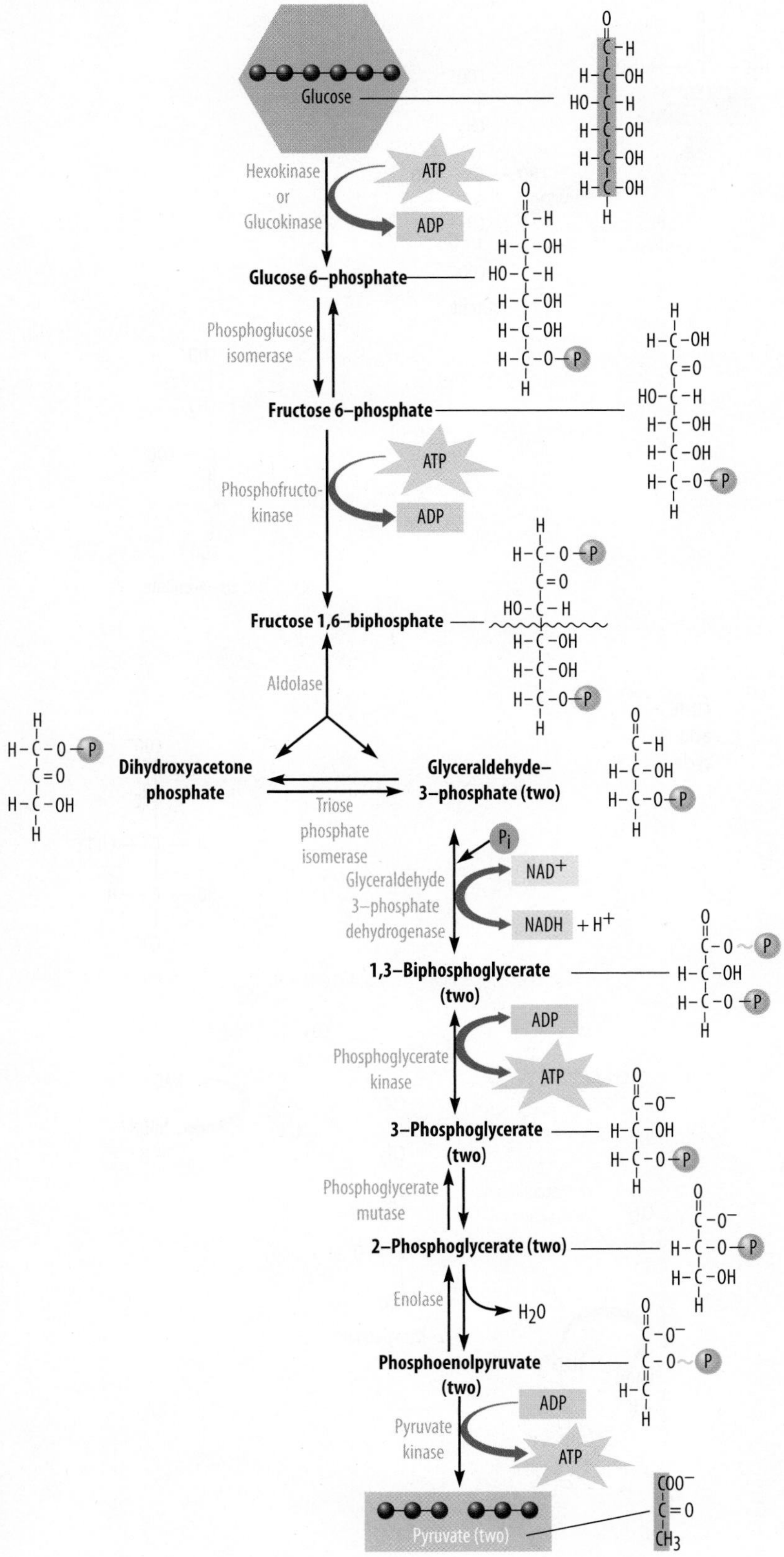

Glycolysis is the first step in metabolizing glucose and other monosaccharides for energy. Unlike the reaction that converts blood glucose to glucose 6-phosphate, the reaction that converts glucose from glycogen to glucose 6-phosphate does not require ATP. Thus the glycolysis of glucose from glycogen directly yields 3 ATP as compared to the 2 ATP from blood glucose. Additional ATP is produced from glycolytic NADH in the electron transport chain.

The reactions that convert fructose to fructose 6-phosphate require ATP so fructose produces the same amount of ATP as blood glucose. The same is true for galactose, which enters at glucose 6-phosphate.

Citric Acid Cycle

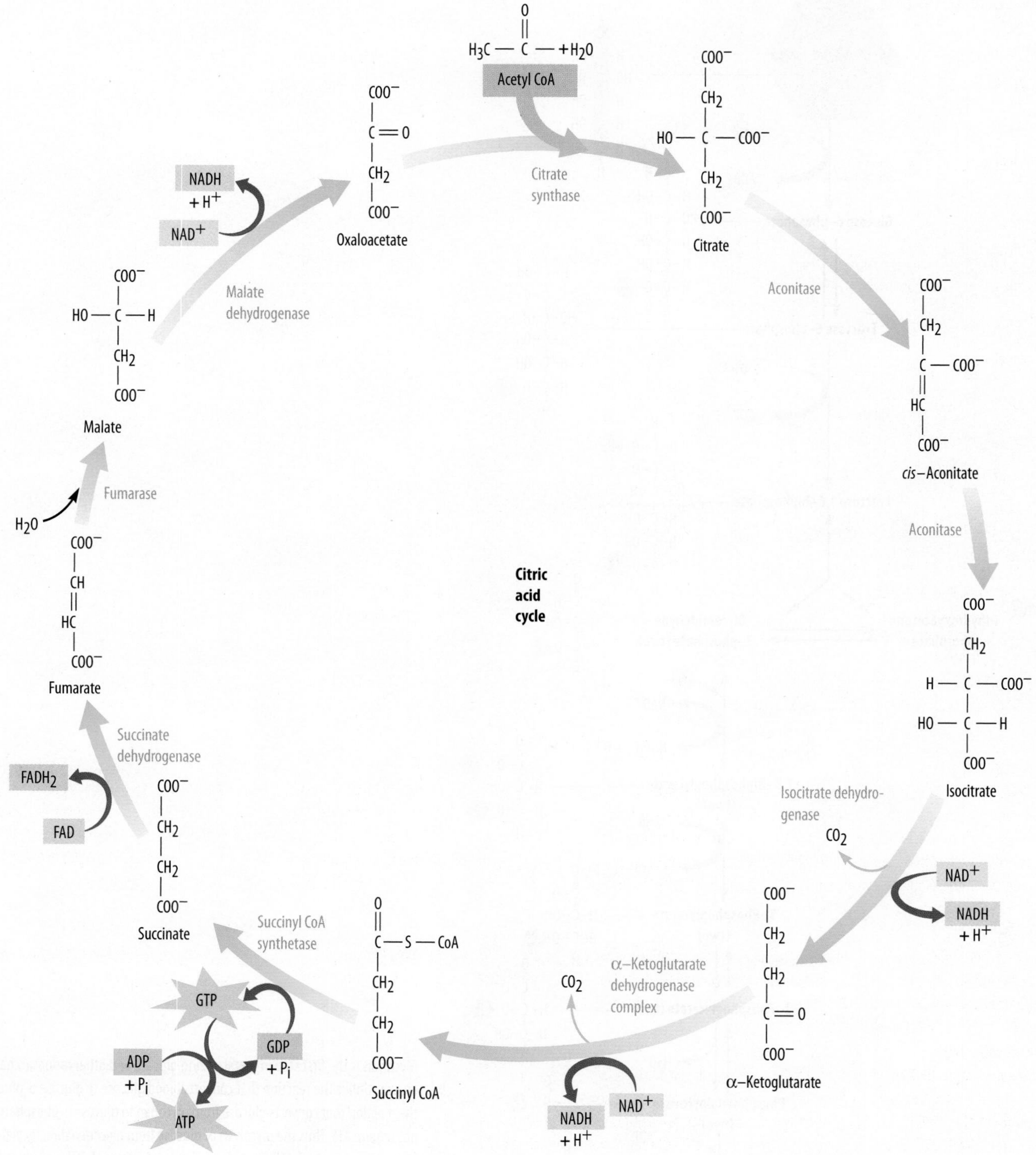

< = Trace amount present   Blank = Not available

Electron Transport Chain

(site of oxidative phosphorylation)

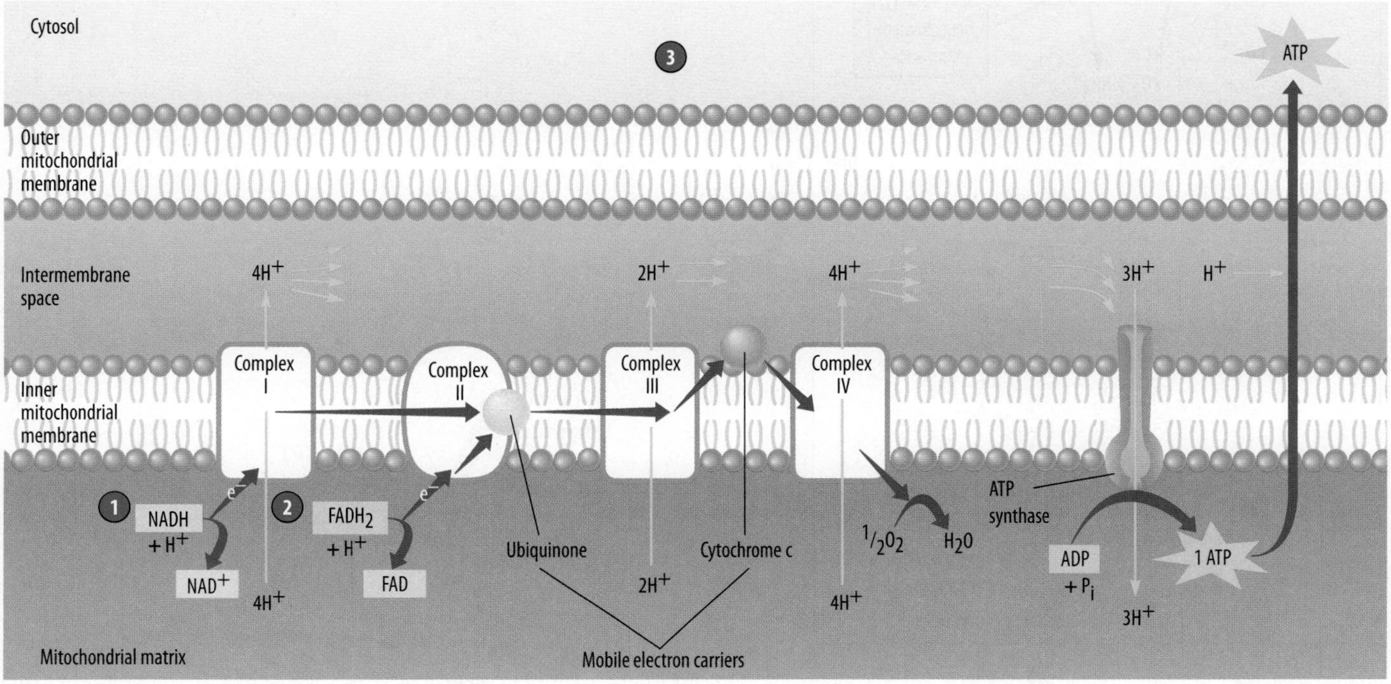

Complex I NADH–Q reductase
Complex II Succinate–Q reductase
Complex III Cytochrome reductase
Complex IV Cytochrome oxidase

Complexes I, III, and IV are proton (H^+) pumps. Complex II does not pump protons. The three proton pumps are linked by the mobile electron carriers ubiquinone and cytochrome c.

NADH

1 A pair of electrons from NADH enters the chain at complex I (NADH-Q reductase). The flow of electrons from NADH to ubiquinone leads to the pumping of 4 H^+ from the matrix to the intermembrane space. The flow of electrons from ubiquinone to cytochrome c through complex III (cytochrome reductase) pumps another 2 H^+ into the intermembrane space. As complex IV (cytochrome oxidase) catalyzes the transfer of electrons from cytochrome c to O_2, it pumps another 4 H^+. (Complex IV actually uses 4 electrons to produce 2 H_2O from a single O_2.) The transit of the NADH electron pair through the electron transport chain pumps a total of 10 H^+ into the intermembrane space. Each 3 H^+ returning to the matrix through the ATP synthase produces 1 ATP. Another H^+ is consumed in transporting ATP from the matrix to the cytosol. Thus the two electrons from NADH produce about 2.5 ATP (10 pumped $\div$ 4 = 2.5).

$FADH_2$

2 A pair of electrons from $FADH_2$ enter the chain at complex II (succinate-Q), which is the non-pumping complex. The flow of electrons from $FADH_2$ to ubiquinone does not pump any protons to the intermembrane space. The flow of electrons through complexes III and IV is the same as for NADH. Thus the transit of the two $FADH_2$ electrons through the electron transport chain pumps a total of 6 H^+ into the intermembrane space and produces about 1.5 ATP (6 $\div$ 4 = 1.5).

Cytosolic NADH

3 Glycolysis forms NADH in the cytosol, but the outer mitochondrial membrane is impervious to NADH. How can NADH deliver its electrons to the electron transport chain? NADH transfers its pair of electrons to special carriers that can cross the mitochondrial membrane. One carrier, glycerol 3-phosphate, shuttles the electrons to the matrix and delivers them to FAD, thereby forming $FADH_2$. This $FADH_2$ delivers the electrons to the chain where they form 1.5 ATP. In the heart and liver, malate shuttles the electrons from cytosolic NADH to the matrix. Malate crosses the mitochondrial membrane and delivers the electrons to NAD^+, thereby forming NADH inside the mitochondrion. This NADH delivers the electron pair to the chain where they form 2.5 ATP. Depending on the carrier, cytosolic NADH may produce 1.5 or 2.5 ATP.

Urea Cycle

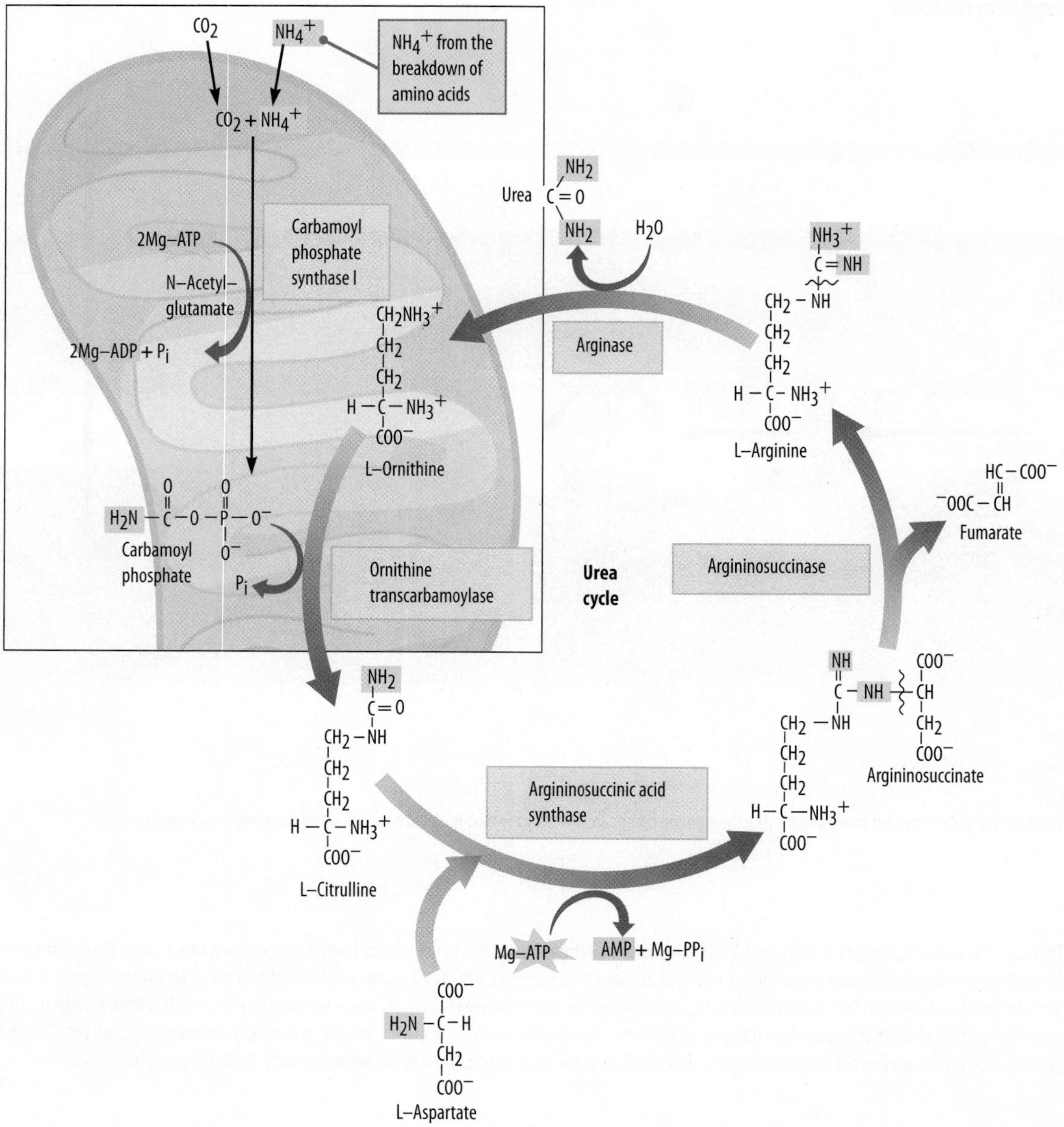

Some NH_4^+ from the breakdown of amino acids is used for biosynthesis of nitrogen compounds. Excess NH_4^+ is converted to urea and excreted.

< = Trace amount present Blank = Not available

Appendix I Calculations and Conversions

- Energy from Food
- Recommended Protein Intake for Adults
- Niacin Equivalents (NE)
- Dietary Folate Equivalents (DFE)
- Retinol Activity Equivalents (RAE)
- Vitamin D
- Vitamin E
- Estimating Energy Expenditure
- Body Mass Index (BMI)
- Metric Prefixes
- Length: Metric and U.S. Equivalents
- Capacities or Volumes
- Food Measurement Equivalents
- Food Measurement Conversions: U.S. to Metric
- Food Measurement Conversions: Metric to U.S.
- Conversion Factors
- Fahrenheit and Celsius (Centigrade) Scales
- Do You Speak Metric?

Energy from Food

grams carbohydrate × 4 kcal/g
grams protein × 4 kcal/g
grams fat × 9 kcal/g
grams alcohol × 7 kcal/g

total = energy from food

Example:

Carbohydrate	275 g × 4 kcal/g = 1,100 kcal
Protein	64 g × 4 kcal/g = 256 kcal
Fat	60 g × 9 kcal/g = 540 kcal
Alcohol	15 g × 7 kcal/g = 105 kcal
TOTAL ENERGY	2,001 kcal

Calculating the percentage of calories for each:

Carbohydrate	(1,100 kcal ÷ 2,001 kcal) × 100 = 54.97% (55%)
Protein	(256 kcal ÷ 2,001 kcal) × 100 = 12.79% (13%)
Fat	(540 kcal ÷ 2,001 kcal) × 100 = 26.99% (27%)
Alcohol	(105 kcal ÷ 2,001 kcal) × 100 = 5.25% (5%)

1 kilocalorie = 4.184 kilojoules
1 kilojoule = 0.239 kilocalories

Recommended Protein Intake for Adults

grams of recommended protein = weight in kilograms × 0.8 g/kg

Example:

A 70-kg (154-lb) person
grams of recommended protein = 70 kg × 0.8 g/kg = 56 grams protein, or
grams of recommended protein = (154 lb ÷ 2.2) × 0.8 g/kg = 56 grams protein

Note: Endurance athletes involved in heavy training may require 1.2 to 1.4 grams of protein per kilogram of body weight per day.

Niacin Equivalents (NE)

Determining the amount of niacin from tryptophan:

NE = milligrams niacin
NE from tryptophan = grams excess protein ÷ 6
NE from tryptophan = (grams dietary protein − protein RDA) ÷ 6

Example:

Assume dietary protein = 86 g and protein RDA = 56 g
NE from tryptophan = (86 g − 56 g) ÷ 6
NE from tryptophan = 5

Dietary Folate Equivalents (DFE)

Dietary folate equivalents account for differences in the absorption of food folate, synthetic folic acid in dietary supplements, and folic acid added to fortified foods. Food in the stomach also affects bioavailability. Folic acid taken as a supplement when fasting is two times more bioavailable than food folate. Folic acid taken with food and folic acid in fortified foods are 1.7 times more bioavailable than food folate.

1 μg DFE = 1 microgram of food folate
= 0.5 μg of folic acid supplement taken on an empty stomach
= 0.6 μg of folic acid supplement consumed with meals
= 0.6 μg of folic acid in fortified foods
1 μg folic acid as a fortificant = 1.7 μg DFE
1 μg folic acid as a supplement, fasting = 2.0 μg DFE

Example:

Food folate in cooked spinach	**100 μg = 100 μg DFE**
Ready-to-eat cereal fortified with folic acid	**100 μg = 170 μg DFE**
Supplemental folic acid taken without food	**100 μg = 200 μg DFE**

Estimating DFE from Daily Value:

DFE = %DV × DV × bioavailability factor

Example:

Assume that a serving of fortified breakfast cereal contains 10% of the Daily Value for folate

Daily Value = 400 μg folic acid

DFE = %DV × DV × bioavailability factor

DFE = 0.10 × 400 μg × 1.7
DFE = 68 μg, which can be rounded to 70 μg DFE

Retinol Activity Equivalents (RAE)

Retinol activity equivalents are a standardized measure of vitamin A activity that account for differences in the bioavailability of different sources of vitamin A. Of the provitamin A carotenoids, beta-carotene produces the most vitamin A.

1 μg RAE = 1 μg retinol
= 12 μg beta-carotene
= 24 μg of other vitamin A precursors

Many vitamin supplements still report vitamin A content as International Units (IU).

1 μg RAE = 3.33 IU from retinol
= 10 IU from beta-carotene in supplements
= 20 IU from beta-carotene in foods

Vitamin D

Many vitamin supplements still report vitamin D content as International Units (IU).

1 IU = 0.025 μg cholecalciferol

μg cholecalciferol = IU ÷ 40

Example:

A vitamin supplement contains 100 IU vitamin D
μg cholecalciferol = 100 ÷ 40 = 2.5

Vitamin E

Although outdated, many vitamin supplements still report vitamin E content as International Units (IU) rather than as milligrams of α-tocopherol. Two conversion factors are used to convert IU to milligrams of α-tocopherol. If the form of the supplement is "natural" or RRR-α-tocopherol (historically labeled as *d*-alpha-tocopherol), the conversion factor is 0.67 mg/IU. If the form of the supplement is *all rac*-α-tocopherol (historically labeled *dl*-α-tocopherol), the conversion factor is 0.45 mg/IU.

Examples:

A multivitamin supplement contains 30 IU of *d*-α-tocopherol
30 IU × 0.67 = 20 mg α-tocopherol
A multivitamin supplement contains 30 IU of *dl*-α-tocopherol
30 IU × 0.45 = 13.5 mg α-tocopherol

Estimating Energy Expenditure

The Estimated Energy Requirement (EER) is defined as the dietary energy intake (in kilocalories per day) that is predicted to maintain energy balance in a healthy adult of a defined age, gender, weight, height, and level of physical activity consistent with good health.* The EER equations predict Total Energy Expenditure (TEE).

Adult men (age 19 and older):

$$\mathbf{EER = 662 - 9.53 \times Age\,[yr] + PA \times (15.91 \times Weight\,[kg] + 539.6 \times Height\,[m])}$$

PA is the Physical Activity coefficient that represents physical activity level

Sedentary	**PA = 1.0**
Low active	**PA = 1.11**
Active	**PA = 1.25**
Very active	**PA = 1.48**

Adult women (age 19 and older):

$$\mathbf{EER = 354 - 6.91 \times Age\,[yr] + PA \times (9.36 \times Weight\,[kg] + 726 \times Height\,[m])}$$

PA is the Physical Activity coefficient that represents physical activity level

Sedentary	**PA = 1.0**
Low active	**PA = 1.12**
Active	**PA = 1.27**
Very active	**PA = 1.45**

Example:

A 21-year-old woman, 5'4" (1.6 m) tall, who weighs 120 pounds (54.5 kilograms) and is active.

$$\begin{aligned}
&= 354 - 6.91 \times 21\text{ yr} + 1.27 \\
&\times \quad (9.36 \times 54.5\text{ kg} + 726 \times 1.6\text{ m}) \\
&= 354 - 145.11 + 1.27 \times (510.12 + 1{,}161.6) \\
&= 354 - 145.11 + 1.27 \times 1{,}671.72 \\
&= 354 - 145.11 + 2{,}123.08 \\
&= 2{,}331.97 \\
&= 2{,}332\text{ kcal/day}
\end{aligned}$$

***Source:** Institute of Medicine, Food and Nutrition Board. *Dietary Reference Intakes for Energy, Carbohydrate, Fiber, Fat, Fatty Acids, Cholesterol, Protein, and Amino Acids*. Washington, DC: National Academy Press; 2005.

Total energy expenditure can also be estimated by first estimating resting energy expenditure (REE) and then adding additional energy to account for physical activity and the thermic effect of food.

Resting Energy Expenditure (REE)

Harris-Benedict Equations

Adult men	$\mathbf{REE = 66 + 13.7\mathit{W} + 5.0\mathit{H} - 6.8\mathit{A}}$
Adult women	$\mathbf{REE = 655 + 9.6\mathit{W} + 1.8\mathit{H} - 4.7\mathit{A}}$

(W = weight in kilograms, H = height in centimeters, A = age)

Note: Harris-Benedict equations may overestimate resting energy expenditure, especially for obese people.

Quick Estimate

Adult men	**REE – weight (kg) × 1.0 kcal/kg × 24 hours**
	REE = weight (kg) × 1.0 × 24
Adult women	**REE = weight (kg) × 0.9 kcal/kg × 24 hours**
	REE = weight (kg) × 0.9 × 24

Physical Activity (PA)

Physical activity can be estimated as a percentage of the resting energy expenditure (REE) based on the frequency and intensity of physical activity.

Percentage of REE	Activity Level	Descriptor
20–30%	Sedentary	Mostly resting, with little or no activity
30–45%	Light	Occasional unplanned activity (e.g., going for a stroll)
45–65%	Moderate	Daily planned activity, such as brisk walks
65–90%	Heavy	Daily workout routine requiring several hours of continuous exercise
90–120%	Exceptional	Daily vigorous workouts for extended hours; training for competition

Thermic Effect of Food (TEF)

The thermic effect of food can be estimated as 10% of the sum of REE + physical activity

Total energy expenditure (TEE) = REE + PA + TEF

Example using quick estimate of REE:

A 175-pound (79.5 kg), 30-year-old man engages in moderate activity (60% of REE).

$$\begin{aligned}
\textbf{REE} \quad &= 79.5\text{ kg} \times 1.0\text{ kcal/kg/hr} \times 24\text{ hr/day} \\
&= 1{,}908\text{ kcal/day} \\
\textbf{PA} \quad &= 60\%\text{ of REE} \\
&= 0.60 \times 1908\text{ kcal/day} \\
&= 1144.8\text{ kcal/day} \\
\textbf{TEF} \quad &= 10\%\text{ of REE} + \text{PA} \\
&= 0.10 \times (1908 + 1144.8\text{ kcal/day}) \\
&= 0.10 \times 3052.8\text{ kcal/day} \\
&= 305.3\text{ kcal/day} \\
\textbf{TEE} \quad &= \text{REE} + \text{PA} + \text{TEF} \\
&= 1908 + 1144.8 + 305.3\text{ kcal/day} \\
&= 3358\text{ kcal/day}
\end{aligned}$$

Body Mass Index (BMI)

U.S. Formula

BMI = [weight in pounds ÷ (height in inches)^2] × 703

Example:

A 154-pound man is 5 ft 8 inches (68 inches) tall
BMI = [154 ÷ (68 in × 68 in)] × 703
BMI = (154 ÷ 4,624) × 703
BMI = 23.41

Metric Formula

BMI = weight in kilograms ÷ [height in meters]^2
or
BMI = [weight in kilograms ÷ (height in cm)^2] × 10,000

Example:

A 70-kg man is 1.75 meters tall
BMI = 70 kg ÷ (1.75 m × 1.75 m)
BMI = 70 ÷ 3.0625
BMI = 22.86

Metric Prefixes

giga-	G	1,000,000,000
mega-	M	1,000,000
kilo-	k	1,000
hecto-	h	100
deka-	da	10
deci-	d	0.1
centi-	c	0.01
milli-	m	0.001
micro-	μ	0.000001
nano-	n	0.000000001

Length: Metric and U.S. Equivalents

1 centimeter	0.3937 inch
1 decimeter	3.937 inches
1 foot	0.3048 meter
1 inch	2.54 centimeters
1 meter	39.37 inches
	1.094 yards
1 micron	0.001 millimeter
	0.00003937 inch
1 millimeter	0.03937 inch
1 yard	0.9144 meter

Capacities or Volumes

1 cup, measuring	8 fluid ounces
	1/2 liquid pint
1 gallon (U.S.)	231 cubic inches
	3.785 liters
	0.833 British gallon
	128 U.S. fluid ounces
1 gallon (British Imperial)	277.42 cubic inches
	1.201 U.S. gallons
	4.546 liters
	160 British fluid ounces
1 liter	1.057 liquid quarts
	0.908 dry quart
	61.024 cubic inches
1 milliliter	0.061 cubic inches
1 ounce, fluid or liquid (U.S.)	1.805 cubic inches
	29.574 milliliters
	1.041 British fluid ounces
1 pint, dry	33.600 cubic inches
	0.551 liter
1 pint, liquid	28.875 cubic inches
	0.473 liter
1 quart, dry (U.S.)	67.201 cubic inches
	1.101 liters
	0.969 British quart
1 quart, liquid (U.S.)	57.75 cubic inches
	0.946 liter
	0.833 British quart
1 quart (British)	69.354 cubic inches
	1.032 U.S. dry quarts
	1.201 U.S. liquid quarts
1 tablespoon, measuring	3 teaspoons
	1/2 fluid ounce
1 teaspoon, measuring	1/3 tablespoon
	1/6 fluid ounce
1 kilogram	2.205 pounds
1 microgram (μg)	0.000001 gram

Food Measurement Equivalents

16 tablespoons = 1 cup
12 tablespoons = 3/4 cup
10 tablespoons + 2 teaspoons = 2/3 cup
8 tablespoons = 1/2 cup
6 tablespoons = 3/8 cup
5 tablespoons + 1 teaspoon = 1/3 cup
4 tablespoons = 1/4 cup

2 tablespoons = 1/8 cup
2 tablespoons + 2 teaspoons = 1/6 cup
1 tablespoon = 1/16 cup
2 cups = 1 pint
2 pints = 1 quart
3 teaspoons = 1 tablespoon
48 teaspoons = 1 cup

Food Measurement Conversions: U.S. to Metric

Capacity

1/5 teaspoon	1 milliliter
1 teaspoon	5 milliliters
1 tablespoon	15 milliliters
1 fluid ounce	30 milliliters
1/5 cup	47 milliliters
1 cup	237 milliliters
2 cups (1 pint)	473 milliliters
4 cups (1 quart)	0.95 liter
4 quarts (1 gal.)	3.8 liters

Weight

1 ounce	28 grams
1 pound	454 grams

Food Measurement Conversions: Metric to U.S.

Capacity

1 milliliter	1/5 teaspoon
5 milliliters	1 teaspoon
15 milliliters	1 tablespoon
100 milliliters	3.4 fluid oz
240 milliliters	1 cup
1 liter	34 fluid oz
	4.2 cups
	2.1 pints
	1.06 quarts
	0.26 gallon

Weight

1 gram	0.035 ounce
100 grams	3.5 ounces
500 grams	1.10 pounds
1 kilogram	2.205 pounds
	35 ounces

Conversion Factors

To change	To	Multiply by
centimeters	inches	0.3937
centimeters	feet	0.03281
cubic feet	cubic meters	0.0283
cubic meters	cubic feet	35.3145
cubic meters	cubic yards	1.3079
cubic yards	cubic meters	0.7646
feet	meters	0.3048
gallons (U.S.)	liters	3.7853
grams	ounces avdp	0.0353
grams	pounds	0.002205
inches	millimeters	25.4000
inches	centimeters	2.5400
inches	meters	0.0254
kilograms	pounds	2.2046
liters	gallons (U.S.)	0.2642
liters	pints (dry)	1.8162
liters	pints (liquid)	2.1134
liters	quarts (dry)	0.9081
liters	quarts (liquid)	1.0567
meters	feet	3.2808
meters	yards	1.0936
millimeters	inches	0.0394
ounces avdp	grams	28.3495
ounces	pounds	0.0625
pints (dry)	liters	0.5506
pints (liquid)	liters	0.4732
pounds	kilograms	0.4536
pounds	ounces	16
quarts (dry)	liters	1.1012
quarts (liquid)	liters	0.9463

Fahrenheit and Celsius (Centigrade) Scales

°Celsius	°Fahrenheit
–273.15	–459.67
–250	–418
–200	–328
–150	–238
–100	–148
–50	–58
–40	–40
–30	–22
–20	–4
–10	14
0	32
5	41
10	50
15	59
20	68
25	77
30	86
35	95

°Celsius	°Fahrenheit
40	104
45	113
50	122
55	131
60	140
65	149
70	158
75	167
80	176
85	185
90	194
95	203
100	212

Zero on the Fahrenheit scale represents the temperature produced by the mixing of equal weights of snow and common salt.

	°Fahrenheit	°Celsius
Boiling point of water	212°	100°
Freezing point of water	32°	0°
Normal body temperature	98.6°	37°
Comfortable room temperature	68–77°	20–25°
Absolute zero	−459.6°	−273.1°

Absolute zero is theoretically the lowest possible temperature, the point at which all molecular motion would cease.

To Convert Temperature Scales

To convert Fahrenheit to Celsius (Centigrade), subtract 32 and multiply by $^5/_9$.

$$°C = {}^5/_9(°F - 32)$$

To convert Celsius (Centigrade) to Fahrenheit, multiply by $^9/_5$ and add 32.

$$°F = ({}^9/_5 \times °C) + 32$$

Do You Speak Metric?

Although the metric system isn't really a language like English or Spanish, in some sense it is the language of science. Nutritionists must be fluent in metrics. Pick up any nutrition journal and you will find units of measurement expressed in terms like kilograms and liters.

The metric system is a decimal-based system of measurement units. Like our monetary system, units are related by factors of 10. There are 10 pennies in a dime, and 10 dimes equal 1 dollar. Calculations involve the simple process of moving the decimal point to the right or to the left.

There are only seven basic units in the metric system. The most common units are the meter (m) to measure length, the gram (g) for mass, the liter (L) for volume, and degree Celsius (°C) for temperature. The metric system avoids the confusing dual use of terms, such as the current use of ounces to measure both weight and volume.

One strategy for learning metric is to find common or familiar associations. For example, when using degrees Celsius you should equate 22 degrees Celsius (22°C) with room temperature, 37 degrees Celsius (37°C) with body temperature, and 0 and 100 degrees Celsius with the freezing and boiling points of water, respectively. A millimeter (1 mm) is about the thickness of a dime, and 2 centimeters (2 cm) is about the diameter of a nickel. When you pick up a 2-pound box of sugar, you are holding about 900 grams.

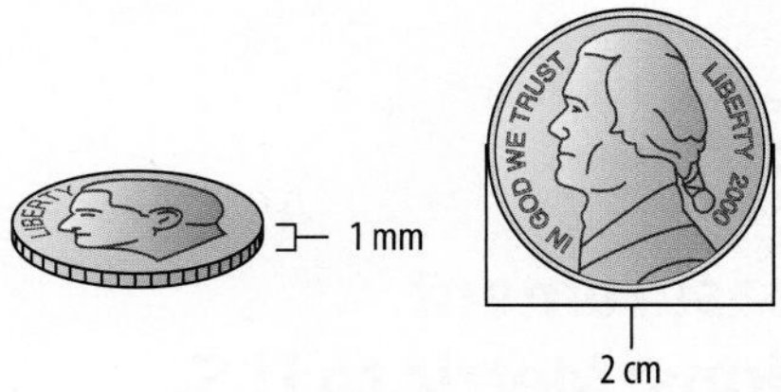

A fluid ounce can be tricky because it's a measure of liquid volume, not weight. Most people already recognize 1-liter and 2-liter soft-drink bottles. A 1-liter bottle equals 33.8 fluid ounces.

The United States is the only industrialized country in the world not officially using the metric system. Because of its many advantages (e.g., easy conversion between units of the same quantity), the metric system has become the internationally accepted system of measurement.

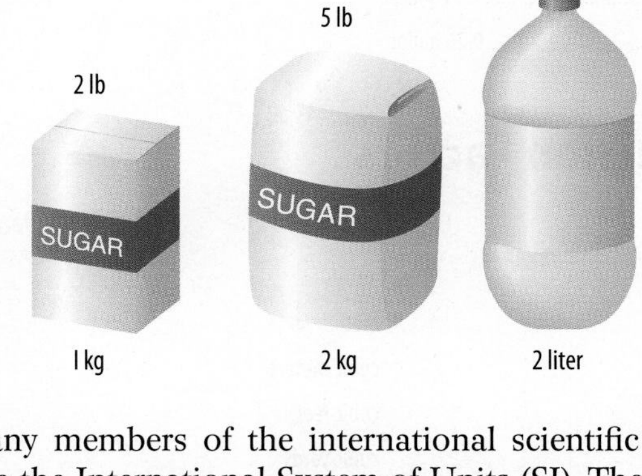

Many members of the international scientific community use the International System of Units (SI). The SI is the modern metric system and has adopted the joule rather than the calorie to measure food energy. Although we think of the calorie as a measure of energy, it is more accurately a measure of heat. Joules are a measure of work, not heat, and the amount of energy potential in foods is expressed best in kilojoules (kjoules). Each kilocalorie is equivalent to approximately 4.2 (4.184) kilojoules. For example, a 100-kilocalorie glass of juice provides about 420 kilojoules.

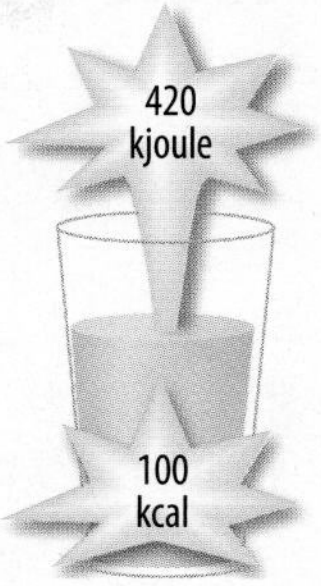

The Celsius (C) temperature scale should be used instead of the Fahrenheit (F) scale. The following are familiar points:

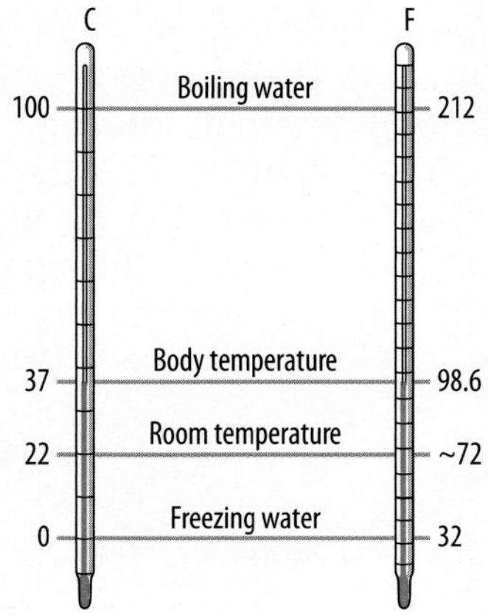

TABLE I.1
Measures Commonly Used in Nutrition

	Metric	English
Length	1 meter (m) 1 centimeter (cm) 2.54 centimeters (cm)	39.4 inches (in) 0.394 inch (in) 1 inch (in)
Weight (mass)	1 kilogram (kg) 454 grams (g) 5 grams (g) of salt	2.2 pounds (lb) 1 pound (lb) about 1 teaspoon (tsp)
Volume	1 liter (L) 236 milliliters (mL) 15 milliliters (mL) 5 milliliters (mL)	1.057 quarts (about 4 cups) about 1 cup (c) about 1 tablespoon (Tbsp) about 1 teaspoon (tsp)

Note:
1 gram = 1,000 milligrams
1 milligram = 1,000 micrograms (µg or mcg)

Appendix J Growth Charts

A complete set of growth charts is available on the Internet at www.cdc.gov/growthcharts. There are three sets, each with a different set of percentiles. Each set includes the -following charts for girls and boys:

Weight-for-age percentiles: birth to 36 months

Length-for-age percentiles: birth to 36 months

Weight-for-length percentiles: birth to 36 months

Head circumference-for-age percentiles: birth to 36 months

Weight-for-age percentiles: 2 to 20 years

Stature-for-age percentiles: 2 to 20 years

Weight-for-stature percentiles

Body mass index-for-age percentiles: 2 to 20 years

< = Trace amount present Blank = Not available

2 to 20 years: Girls
Stature-for-Age and Weight-for-Age Percentiles

NAME ____________________

RECORD # ____________

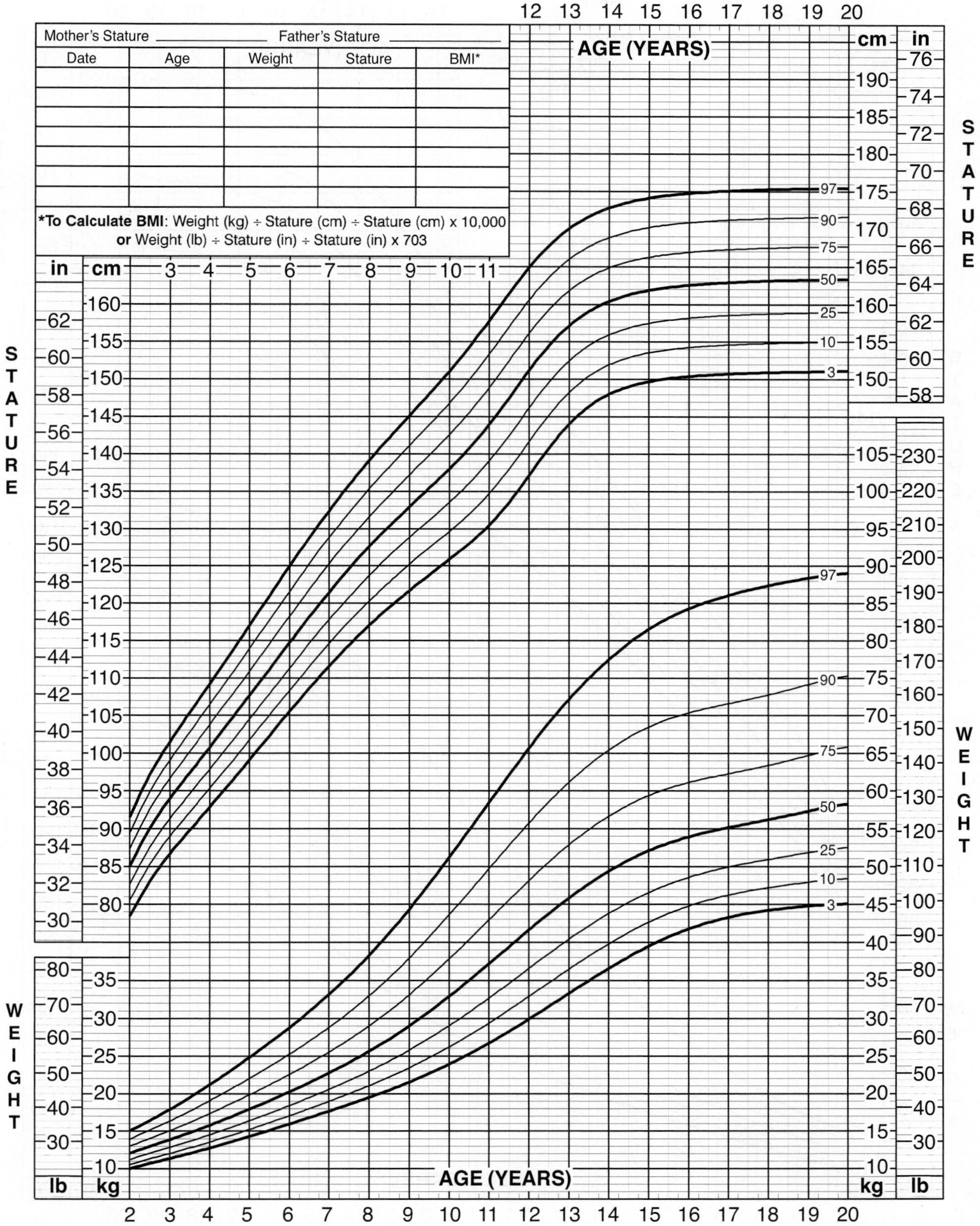

Developed by the National Center for Health Statistics in collaboration with
the National Center for Chronic Disease Prevention and Health Promotion (2000).
http://www.cdc.gov/growthcharts

CDC

2 to 20 years: Boys
Stature-for-Age and Weight-for-Age Percentiles

NAME ______________________

RECORD # ______________

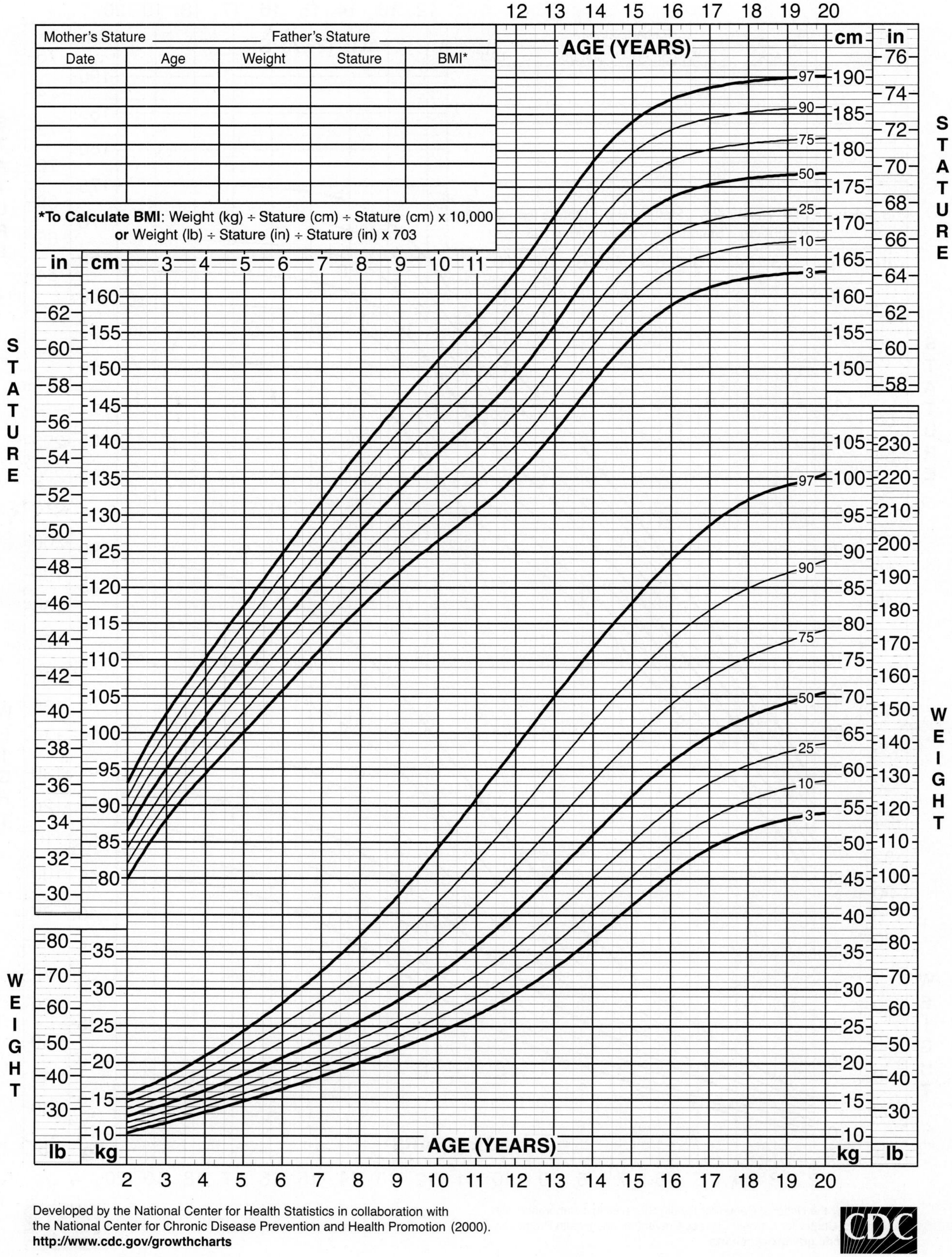

Developed by the National Center for Health Statistics in collaboration with
the National Center for Chronic Disease Prevention and Health Promotion (2000).
http://www.cdc.gov/growthcharts

< = Trace amount present Blank = Not available

Glossary

1,25-dihydroxyvitamin D_3 [$1,25(OH)_2D_3$] The active form of vitamin D. It is an important regulator of blood calcium levels.

24-hour dietary recall A form of dietary intake data collection. The interviewer takes the client through a recent 24-hour period (usually midnight to midnight) to determine what foods and beverages the client consumed.

ABC model of behavior A behavioral model that includes the external and internal events that precede and follow the behavior. The A stands for antecedents, the events that precede the behavior (B), which is followed by consequences (C) that positively or negatively reinforce the behavior.

ABCDs of nutrition assessment Nutrition assessment components: anthropometric measurements, biochemical tests, clinical observations, and dietary intake.

absorption The movement of substances into or across tissues; in particular, the passage of nutrients and other substances into the walls of the gastrointestinal tract and then into the bloodstream.

Acceptable Macronutrient Distribution Ranges (AMDRs) Range of intakes for a particular energy source that are associated with reduced risk of chronic disease while providing adequate intakes of essential nutrients.

acesulfame K [ay-SUL-fame kay] An artificial sweetener that is 200 times sweeter than common table sugar (sucrose). Because it is not digested and absorbed by the body, acesulfame contributes no calories to the diet and yields no energy when consumed.

acetaldehyde A toxic intermediate compound formed by the action of the alcohol dehydrogenase enzyme during the metabolism of alcohol.

acetyl CoA A key intermediate in the metabolic breakdown of carbohydrates, fatty acids, and amino acids. It consists of a two-carbon acetate group linked to coenzyme A, which is derived from pantothenic acid.

acidosis An abnormally low blood pH (below about 7.35) resulting from increased acidity.

acne An inflammatory skin eruption that usually occurs in or near the sebaceous glands of the face, neck, shoulders, and upper back.

acrolein A pungent decomposition product of fats, generated from dehydrating the glycerol components of fats; responsible for the coughing attacks caused by the fumes released by burning fat. This toxic water-soluble liquid vaporizes easily and is highly flammable.

active transport The movement of substances into or out of cells against a concentration gradient. Active transport requires energy (ATP) and involves carrier (transport) proteins in the cell membrane.

adenosine diphosphate (ADP) The compound produced upon hydrolysis of ATP and used to synthesize ATP. Composed of adenosine and two phosphate groups.

adenosine monophosphate (AMP) Hydrolysis product of ADP and of nucleic acids. Composed of adenosine and one phosphate group.

adenosine triphosphate (ATP) [ah-DEN-oh-seen try-FOS-fate] A high-energy compound that is the main direct fuel that cells use to synthesize molecules, contract muscles, transport substances, and perform other tasks.

Adequate Intake (AI) The nutrient intake that appears to sustain a defined nutritional state or some other indicator of health (e.g., growth rate or normal circulating nutrient values) in a specific population or subgroup. AI is used when there is insufficient scientific evidence to establish an EAR.

adipocytes Fat cells.

adipose tissue Body fat tissue.

adolescence The period between onset of puberty and adulthood.

aerobic [air-ROW-bic] Referring to the presence of or need for oxygen. The complete breakdown of glucose, fatty acids, and amino acids to carbon dioxide and water occurs only through aerobic metabolism. The citric acid cycle and electron transport chain are aerobic pathways.

aerobic endurance The ability of skeletal muscle to obtain a sufficient supply of oxygen from the heart and lungs to maintain muscular activity for a prolonged time.

aflatoxins A toxin produced by a mold that grows on crops, such as peanuts, tree nuts, corn, wheat, and oil seeds (like cottonseed).

albumin A protein that circulates in the blood and functions in the transport of many minerals and some drugs.

alcohol Common name for ethanol or ethyl alcohol. As a general term, it refers to any organic compound with one or more hydroxyl (–OH) groups.

alcohol dehydrogenase (ADH) The enzyme that catalyzes the oxidation of ethanol and other alcohols.

alcohol poisoning An overdose of alcohol. The body is overwhelmed by the amount of alcohol in the system and cannot break it down fast enough.

aldehyde dehydrogenase (ALDH) The enzyme that catalyzes the conversion of acetaldehyde to acetate, which forms acetyl CoA.

aldosterone [al-DOS-ter-own] A steroid hormone secreted from the adrenal glands that acts on the kidneys to regulate electrolyte and water balance. It raises blood pressure by promoting retention of sodium (and thus water) and excretion of potassium.

alkalosis An abnormally high blood pH (above about 7.45) resulting from increased alkalinity.

alpha (α) bonds Chemical bonds linking two monosaccharides (glycosidic bonds) that can be broken by human intestinal enzymes, releasing the individual monosaccharides. Maltose and sucrose contain alpha bonds.

alpha-linolenic acid [al-fah lin-oh-LEN-ik ah-sid] An essential omega-3 fatty acid that contains 18 carbon atoms and 3 carbon—carbon double bonds (18:3).

Alzheimer disease (AD) A presenile dementia characterized by accumulation of plaques in certain regions of the brain and degeneration of a certain class of neurons.

amenorrhea [A-men-or-EE-a] Absence or abnormal stoppage of menses in a female; commonly indicated by the absence of three to six consecutive menstrual cycles.

amino acid pool The amino acids in body tissues and fluids that are available for new protein synthesis.

amino acid scoring A method to determine the protein quality of a food by comparing its amino acid composition with that of a reference protein. Also called *chemical scoring*.

amino acids Organic compounds that function as the building blocks of protein.

amniotic fluid The fluid that surrounds the fetus; contained in the amniotic sac inside the uterus.

amylase [AM-ih-lace] A salivary enzyme that catalyzes the hydrolysis of amylose, a starch. Also called *ptyalin*.

amylopectin [am-ih-low-PEK-tin] A branched-chain polysaccharide composed of glucose units.

amylose [AM-ih-los] A straight-chain polysaccharide composed of glucose units.

anabolism [an-AH-bol-iz-um] Any metabolic process whereby cells convert simple substances into more complex ones.

anaerobic [AN-ah-ROW-bic] Referring to the absence of oxygen or the ability of a process to occur in the absence of oxygen.

android obesity [AN-droyd oh-BEE-sih-ty] Excess storage of fat located primarily in the abdominal area.

anemia Abnormally low concentration of hemoglobin in the bloodstream; can be caused by impaired synthesis of red blood cells, increased destruction of red cells, or significant loss of blood.

anencephaly A type of neural tube birth defect in which part or all of the brain is missing.

angiotensin I [an-jee-oh-TEN-sin one] A 10-amino-acid peptide that is a precursor of angiotensin II.

angiotensin II In the lungs, the eight-amino-acid peptide angiotensin II is formed from angiotensin I. Angiotensin II is a powerful vasoconstrictor that rapidly raises blood pressure.

angiotensinogen A circulating protein produced by the liver from which angiotensin I is cleaved by the action of renin.

angular stomatitis Inflammation and cracking of the skin at the corners of the mouth; a symptom of riboflavin deficiency.

anions Ions that carry a negative charge.

anorexia athletica Eating disorder associated with competitive participation in athletic activity.

anorexia nervosa [an-or-EX-ee-uh ner-VOH-sah] An eating disorder marked by prolonged decrease of appetite and refusal to eat, leading to self-starvation and excessive weight loss. It results in part from a distorted body image and intense fear of becoming fat, often linked to social pressures.

anorexia of aging Loss of appetite and wasting associated with old age.

anthropometric measurements Measurements of the physical characteristics of the body, such as height, weight, head circumference, girth, and skinfold measurements. Anthropometric measurements are particularly useful in evaluating the growth of infants, children, and adolescents and in determining body composition.

antibodies [AN-tih-bod-ees] Large blood proteins produced by B lymphocytes in response to exposure to particular antigens (e.g., a protein on the surface of a virus or bacterium). Each type of antibody specifically binds to and helps eliminate its matching antigen from the body. Once formed, antibodies circulate in the blood and help protect the body against subsequent infection.

antidiuretic hormone (ADH) A peptide hormone secreted by the pituitary gland. It increases blood pressure and prevents fluid excretion by the kidneys. Also called *vasopressin*.

antioxidant A substance that combines with or otherwise neutralizes a free radical, thus preventing oxidative damage to cells and tissues.

antirachitic Pertaining to activities of an agent used to treat rickets.

appetite A psychological desire to eat that is related to the pleasant sensations often associated with food.

ariboflavinosis Riboflavin deficiency.

aspartame [AH-spar-tame] An artificial sweetener composed of two amino acids and methanol. It is 200 times sweeter than sucrose. Its trade name is NutraSweet.

atherosclerosis A type of "hardening of the arteries" in which cholesterol and other substances in the blood build up in the walls of arteries. As the process continues, the arteries to the heart can narrow, cutting down the flow of oxygen-rich blood and nutrients to the heart.

ATP—CP energy system A simple and immediate anaerobic energy system that maintains ATP levels. Creatine phosphate is broken down, releasing energy and a phosphate group, which is used to form ATP.

atrophic gastritis An age-related condition in which the stomach loses its ability to secrete acid. In severe cases, ability to make intrinsic factor is also impaired.

autonomic nervous system The part of the central nervous system that regulates the automatic responses of the body; consists of the sympathetic and parasympathetic systems.

avidin A protein in raw egg whites that binds biotin, preventing its absorption. Avidin is destroyed by heat.

bacteriophages Viruses that infect bacteria.

basal energy expenditure (BEE) The basal metabolic rate (BMR) extrapolated to 24 hours. Often used interchangeably with REE.

basal metabolic rate (BMR) A clinical measure of resting energy expenditure performed upon awakening, 10 to 12 hours after eating, and 12 to 18 hours after significant physical activity. Often used interchangeably with RMR.

base pair Two nitrogenous bases (adenine and thymine or guanine and cytosine), held together by weak bonds, that form a "rung" of the "DNA ladder." The bonds between base pairs hold the DNA molecule together in the shape of a double helix.

benign [beh-NINE] Not cancerous; does not invade nearby tissue or spread to other parts of the body.

beriberi Thiamin-deficiency disease. Symptoms include muscle weakness, loss of appetite, nerve degeneration, and in some cases, edema.

beta (β) bonds Chemical bonds linking two monosaccharides (glycosidic bonds) that cannot be broken by human intestinal enzymes. Cellulose contains beta bonds.

β-glucans Functional fiber, consisting of branched polysaccharide chains of glucose, that helps lower blood cholesterol levels. Found in barley and oats.

beta-oxidation The breakdown of a fatty acid into numerous molecules of the two-carbon compound acetyl coenzyme A (acetyl CoA).

bile An alkaline, yellow-green fluid that is produced in the liver and stored in the gallbladder. The primary constituents of bile are bile salts, bile acids, phospholipids, cholesterol, and bicarbonate. Bile emulsifies dietary fats, aiding fat digestion and absorption.

binge drinking Consuming excessive amounts of alcohol in short periods of time.

binge eaters Individuals who routinely consume a very large amount of food in a brief period of time (e.g., two hours) and lose control over how much and what is eaten.

binge-eating disorder An eating disorder marked by repeated episodes of binge eating and a feeling of loss of control. The diagnosis is based on a person's having an average of at least two binge-eating episodes per week for six months.

binges Episodes of consuming a very large amount of food in a brief time (e.g., two hours) accompanied by a loss of control over how much and what is eaten.

bioavailability A measure of the extent to which a nutrient becomes available to the body after ingestion and thus is available to the tissues.

biochemical assessment Assessment by measuring a nutrient or its metabolite in one or more body fluids, such as blood and urine, or in feces. Also called laboratory assessment.

biocytin A biotin–lysine complex released from digested protein.

biodiversity The countless species of plants, animals, and insects that exist on the earth. An undisturbed tropical forest is an example of the biodiversity of a healthy ecosystem.

bioelectrical impedance analysis (BIA) Technique to estimate amounts of total body water, lean tissue mass, and total body fat. It uses the resistance of tissue to the flow of an alternating electric current.

bioflavonoids Naturally occurring plant chemicals, especially from citrus fruits, that reduce the permeability and fragility of capillaries.

biological value (BV) The extent to which protein in a food can be incorporated into body proteins. BV is expressed as the percentage of the absorbed dietary nitrogen retained by the body.

biosynthesis Chemical reactions that form simple molecules into complex biomolecules, especially carbohydrate, lipids, protein, nucleotides, and nucleic acids.

biotechnology The set of laboratory techniques and processes used to modify the genome of plants or animals and thus create desirable new characteristics. Genetic engineering in the broad sense.

biotinidase An enzyme in the small intestine that releases biotin from biocytin.

blastogenic stage The first stage of gestation, during which tissue proliferation by rapid cell division begins.

bleaching process A complex light-stimulated reaction in which rod cells lose color as rhodopsin is split into retinal and opsin.

blood glucose levels The amount of glucose in the blood at any given time. Also known as blood sugar levels.

blood pressure The pressure of blood against the walls of a blood vessel or heart chamber. Unless there is reference to another location, such as the pulmonary artery or one of the heart chambers, this term refers to the pressure in the systemic arteries, as measured, for example, in the forearm.

BOD POD A device used to measure the density of the body based on the volume of air displaced as a person sits in a sealed chamber of known volume.

body composition The chemical or anatomical composition of the body. Commonly defined as the proportions of fat, muscle, bone, and other tissues in the body.

body dysmorphic disorder (BDD) An eating disorder in which a distressing and impairing preoccupation with an imagined or slight defect in appearance is the primary symptom.

body fat distribution The pattern of fat distribution on the body.

body image A person's mental concept of his or her physical appearance, constructed from many different influences.

body mass index (BMI) Body weight (in kilograms) divided by the square of height (in meters), expressed in units of kg/m^2. Also called Quetelet index.

bolus [BOH-lus] A chewed, moistened lump of food that is ready to be swallowed.

bomb calorimeter A device that uses the heat of combustion to measure the energy content of a food.

botulism An often-fatal type of food poisoning caused by a toxin released from *Clostridium botulinum*, a bacterium that can grow in improperly canned low-acid foods.

bovine spongiform encephalopathy (BSE) A chronic degenerative disease, widely referred to as "mad cow disease," that affects the central nervous system of cattle.

bran The layers of protective coating around the grain kernel that are rich in dietary fiber and nutrients.

***Bt* gene** *Bacillus thuringiensis (Bt)* is a bacterium that produces a protein called the *Bt* toxin. One of the bacterium's genes, the *Bt* gene, carries the information for the *Bt* toxin. Inserting a copy of the *Bt* gene into plants enables them to produce *Bt* toxin protein and resist some insect pests. The *Bt* protein is not toxic to humans.

buffers Compounds or mixtures of compounds that can take up and release hydrogen ions to keep the pH of a solution constant. The buffering action of proteins and bicarbonate in the bloodstream plays a major role in maintaining the blood pH at 7.35 to 7.45.

built environment Any human-formed, developed, or structured areas, including the urban environment that consists of buildings, roads, fixtures, parks, and all other human developments that form the area's physical character.

bulimia nervosa [bull-EEM-ee-uh ner-VOH-sah] An eating disorder marked by consumption of large amounts of food at one time (binge eating) followed by a behavior such as self-induced vomiting, use of laxatives, excessive exercise, fasting, or other practices to avoid weight gain.

calcitonin A hormone secreted by the thyroid gland in response to elevated blood calcium. It stimulates calcium deposition in bone and calcium excretion by the kidneys, thus reducing blood calcium.

calcitriol See *1,25-dihydroxyvitamin* D_3 *[1,25(OH)*$_2$*D*$_3$*]*.

calmodulin A calcium-binding protein that regulates a variety of cellular activities, such as cell division and proliferation.

calorie The general term for energy in food; used synonymously with the term *energy*. Often used instead of *kilocalorie* on food labels, in diet books, and in other sources of nutrition information.

calorimeter [kal-oh-RIM-eh-ter] A device used to measure quantities of heat generated by various processes.

calorimetry [kal-oh-RIM-eh-tree] The measurement of the amount of heat given off by an organism. It is used to determine total energy expenditure.

Canada's Guidelines for Healthy Eating Key messages that are based on the 1990 *Nutrition Recommendations for Canadians* and that provide positive, action-oriented, scientifically accurate eating advice to Canadians.

cancer A term for diseases in which abnormal cells divide without control. Cancer cells can invade nearby tissues and can spread through the bloodstream and lymphatic system to other parts of the body.

carbohydrate loading Changes in dietary carbohydrate intake and exercise regimen before competition to maximize glycogen stores in the muscles. It is appropriate for endurance events lasting 60 to 90 consecutive minutes or longer. Also known as *glycogen loading.*

carbohydrates Compounds, including sugars, starches, and dietary fibers, that usually have the general chemical formula $(CH_2O)n$, where *n* represents the number of CH_2O units in the molecule. Carbohydrates are a major source of energy for body functions.

carboxylation A reaction that adds a carboxyl group (–COOH) to a substrate, replacing a hydrogen atom.

carcinogens [kar-SIN-o-jins] Any substances that cause cancer.

cardiac output The amount of blood expelled by the heart.

cardiovascular disease (CVD) Any abnormal condition characterized by dysfunction of the heart and blood vessels. CVD includes atherosclerosis (especially coronary heart disease, which can lead to heart attacks), cerebrovascular disease (e.g., stroke), and hypertension (high blood pressure).

carnitine [CAR-nih-teen] A compound that transports fatty acids from the cytosol into the mitochondria, where they undergo beta-oxidation.

carotenodermia A harmless yellow-orange cast to the skin caused by high levels of carotenoids in the bloodstream resulting from consumption of extremely large amounts of carotenoid-rich foods, such as carrot juice.

carotenoids A group of yellow, orange, and red pigments in plants, including foods. Many of these compounds are precursors of vitamin A.

case control studies Investigations that use a group of people with a particular condition rather than a randomly selected population. These cases are compared with a control group of people who do not have the condition.

catabolism [ca-TA-bol-iz-um] Any metabolic process whereby cells break down complex substances into simpler, smaller ones.

catalyze To speed up a chemical reaction.

cations Ions that carry a positive charge.

cecum The blind pouch at the beginning of the large intestine into which the ileum opens from one side and which is continuous with the colon.

celiac disease [SEA-lee-ak] A disease that involves an inability to digest gluten, a protein found in wheat, barley, rye, and oats. If untreated, it causes fattening of the villi in the intestine, leading to severe malabsorption of nutrients. Symptoms include diarrhea, fatty stools, swollen belly, and extreme fatigue.

cell differentiation The process by which an immature cell develops into a specific type of mature cell.

cells The basic structural units of all living tissues, which have two major parts: the nucleus and the cytoplasm.

cellulose [SELL-you-los] A straight-chain polysaccharide composed of hundreds of glucose units linked by beta bonds. It is nondigestible by humans and a component of dietary fiber.

central nervous system (CNS) The brain and the spinal cord. The central nervous system transmits signals that control muscular actions and glandular secretions along the entire GI tract.

cephalic phase responses The responses of the parasympathetic nervous system to the sight, smell, thought, and sound of food. Also called preabsorptive phase responses.

ceruloplasmin A copper-dependent enzyme responsible for the oxidation of ferrous iron (Fe^{2+}) to ferric iron (Fe^{3+}), enabling iron to bind to transferrin. Also known as ferroxidase I.

chain length The number of carbons that a fatty acid contains. Foods contain fatty acids with chain lengths of 4 to 24 carbons, and most have an even number of carbons.

cheilosis Inflammation and cracking of the lips; a symptom of riboflavin deficiency.

chelation therapy Use of a chelator (e.g., EDTA) to bind metal ions to remove them from the body.

chemical energy Energy contained in the bonds between atoms of a molecule.

chemical scoring A method to determine the protein quality of a food by comparing its amino acid composition with that of a reference protein. Also called *amino acid scoring*.

Child and Adult Care Food Program A federally funded program that reimburses approved family child-care providers for USDA-approved foods served to preschool children; it also provides funds for meals and snacks served at after-school programs for school-age children and to adult day care centers serving chronically impaired adults or people older than age 60.

childhood The period of life from age 1 to the onset of puberty.

chitin A long-chain structural polysaccharide of slightly modified glucose. Found in the hard exterior skeletons of insects, crustaceans, and other invertebrates; also occurs in the cell walls of fungi.

chitosan Polysaccharide derived from chitin.

chloride shift The movement of chloride ions into and out of red blood cells to maintain a lower level of chloride in red blood cells in the arteries than in the veins.

cholecystokinin (CCK) [ko-la-sis-toe-KY-nin] A hormone produced by cells in the small intestine that stimulates the release of digestive enzymes from the pancreas and bile from the gallbladder.

cholesterol [ko-LES-te-rol] A waxy lipid (sterol) whose chemical structure contains multiple hydrocarbon rings.

choline A nitrogen-containing compound that is part of phosphatidylcholine, a phospholipid. Choline is also part of the neurotransmitter acetylcholine. The body synthesizes choline from the amino acid methionine.

chylomicron [kye-lo-MY-kron] A large lipoprotein particle formed in intestinal cells following the absorption of dietary fats. A chylomicron has a central core of triglycerides and cholesterol surrounded by phospholipids and proteins.

chyme [KIME] A mass of partially digested food and digestive juices moving from the stomach into the duodenum.

chymotrypsinogen/chymotrypsin A protease produced by the pancreas that is converted from the inactive proenzyme form (chymotrypsinogen) to the active form (chymotrypsin) in the small intestine.

ciguatera A toxin found in more than 300 species of Caribbean and South Pacific fish. It is a nonbacterial source of food poisoning.

ciliary action Wavelike motion of small hairlike projections on some cells.

circular muscle Layers of smooth muscle that surround organs, including the stomach and the small intestine.

circulation Movement of substances through the vessels of the cardiovascular or lymphatic system.

cis fatty acid Unsaturated fatty acid in which the hydrogens surrounding a double bond are both on the same side of the carbon chain, causing a bend in the chain. Most naturally occurring unsaturated fatty acids are cis fatty acids.

citric acid cycle The metabolic pathway occurring in mitochondria in which the acetyl portion (CH_3COO–) of acetyl CoA is oxidized to yield two molecules of carbon dioxide and one molecule each of NADH, $FADH_2$, and GTP. Also known as the *Krebs cycle* and the *tricarboxylic acid (TCA) cycle*.

clinical observations Assessment by evaluating the characteristics of well-being that can be seen in a physical exam. Nonspecific, clinical observations can provide clues to nutrient deficiency or excess that can be confirmed or ruled out by biochemical testing.

clinical trials Studies that collect large amounts of data to evaluate the effectiveness of a treatment.

coenzyme A Coenzyme A is a cofactor derived from the vitamin pantothenic acid.

coenzymes Organic compounds, often B-vitamin derivatives, that combine with an inactive enzyme to form an active enzyme. Coenzymes associate closely with these enzymes, allowing them to catalyze certain metabolic reactions in a cell.

cofactors Compounds required for an enzyme to be active. Cofactors include coenzymes and metal ions such as iron (Fe^{2+}), copper (Cu^{2+}), and magnesium (Mg^{2+}).

colic Periodic inconsolable crying in an otherwise healthy infant that appears to result from abdominal cramping and discomfort.

collagen The most abundant fibrous protein in the body. Collagen is the major constituent of connective tissue, forms the foundation for bones and teeth, and helps maintain the structure of blood vessels and other tissues.

colon The portion of the large intestine extending from the cecum to the rectum. It is made up of four parts—the ascending, transverse, descending, and sigmoid colons. Although often used interchangeably with the term *large intestine*, these terms are not synonymous.

colostrum A thick yellow fluid secreted by the breast during pregnancy and the first days after delivery.

complementary foods Any foods or liquids other than breast milk or infant formula fed to an infant.

complementary protein An incomplete food protein whose assortment of amino acids makes up for, or complements, another food protein's lack of specific essential amino acids so that the combination of the two proteins provides sufficient amounts of all the essential amino acids.

complementary sequence Nucleic acid base sequence that can form a double-stranded structure with another DNA fragment by following base-pairing rules (A pairs with T, and C pairs with G). The complementary sequence to GTAC, for example, is CATG.

complete (high-quality) proteins Proteins that supply all the essential amino acids in the proportions the body needs.

complex carbohydrates Chains of more than two monosaccharides. May be oligosaccharides or polysaccharides.

compulsive overeating See *binge-eating disorder.*

condensation In chemistry, a reaction in which a covalent bond is formed between two molecules by removal of a water molecule.

conditionally essential amino acids Amino acids that are normally made in the body (nonessential) but become essential under certain circumstances, such as during critical illness.

cones Light-sensitive cells in the retina that are sensitive to bright light and translate it into color images.

congeners Biologically active compounds in alcoholic beverages that include nonalcoholic ingredients as well as other alcohols such as methanol. Congeners contribute to the distinctive taste and smell of the beverage and can increase intoxicating effects and subsequent hangover.

conjugated linoleic acid (CLA) A polyunsaturated fatty acid in which the position of the double bonds has moved so that a single bond alternates with two double bonds.

connective tissues Tissues composed primarily of fibrous proteins such as collagen, and which contain few cells. Their primary function is to bind together and support various body structures.

constipation Infrequent and difficult bowel movements, followed by a sensation of incomplete evacuation.

control group A set of people used as a standard of comparison to the experimental group. The people in the control group have characteristics similar to those in the experimental group and are selected at random.

Cori cycle The circular path that regenerates NAD^+ and glucose when oxygen is low and lactate and NADH build up in excess in muscle tissue.

cornea The transparent outer surface of the eye.

coronary heart disease (CHD) A type of heart disease caused by narrowing of the coronary arteries that feed the heart, which needs a constant supply of oxygen and nutrients carried by the blood in the coronary arteries. When the coronary arteries become narrowed or clogged by fat and cholesterol deposits and cannot supply enough blood to the heart, CHD results.

correlations Connections co-occurring more frequently than can be explained by chance or coincidence but without a proven cause.

C-reactive protein (CRP) A protein released by the body in response to acute injury, infection, or other inflammatory stimuli. CRP is associated with future cardiovascular events.

creatine An important nitrogenous compound found in meats and fish and synthesized in the body from amino acids (glycine, arginine, and methionine).

creatine phosphate An energy-rich compound that supplies energy and a phosphate group for the formation of ATP. Also called *phosphocreatine.*

cretinism A congenital condition often caused by severe iodine deficiency during gestation, which is characterized by arrested physical and mental development.

critical control points (CCPs) Operational steps or procedures in a process, production method, or recipe at which control can be applied to prevent, reduce, or eliminate a food safety hazard.

critical period of development Time during which the environment has the greatest impact on the developing embryo.

Crohn's disease A disease that causes inflammation and ulceration along sections of the intestinal tract.

cystic fibrosis An inherited disorder that causes widespread dysfunction of the exocrine glands, resulting in chronic lung disease, abnormally high levels of electrolytes (e.g., sodium, potassium, chloride) in sweat, and deficiency of pancreatic enzymes needed for digestion.

cytochromes Heme proteins that transfer electrons in the electron transport chain through the alternate oxidation and reduction of iron.

cytoplasm The material of the cell, excluding the cell nucleus and cell membranes. The cytoplasm includes the semifluid cytosol, the organelles, and other particles.

cytosol The semifluid inside the cell membrane, excluding organelles. The cytosol is the site of glycolysis and fatty acid synthesis.

Daily Values (DVs) A single set of nutrient intake standards developed by the Food and Drug Administration to represent the needs of the "typical" consumer; used as standards for expressing nutrient content on food labels.

dark adaptation The process that increases the rhodopsin concentration in your eyes, allowing them to detect images in the dark better.

DASH (Dietary Approaches to Stop Hypertension) An eating plan low in total fat, saturated fat, and cholesterol and rich in fruits, vegetables, and low-fat dairy products that has been shown to reduce elevated blood pressure.

deamination The removal of the amino group ($-NH_2$) from an amino acid.

decarboxylation Removal of a carboxyl group (–COOH) from a molecule. The carboxyl group is then released as carbon dioxide (CO_2).

denaturation An alteration in the three-dimensional structure of a protein resulting in an unfolded polypeptide chain that usually lacks biological activity.

densitometry A method for estimating body composition from measurement of total body density.

dental caries [KARE-ees] Destruction of the enamel surface of teeth caused by acids resulting from bacterial breakdown of sugars in the mouth.

desaturation Insertion of double bonds into fatty acids to change them into new fatty acids.

diabetes mellitus A chronic disease in which uptake of blood glucose by body cells is impaired, resulting in high glucose levels in the blood and urine. Type 1 is caused by decreased pancreatic release of insulin. In type 2, target cells (e.g., fat and muscle cells) lose the ability to respond normally to insulin.

diarrhea Loose, watery stools that occur more than three times in one day; it is caused by digestive products moving through the large intestine too rapidly for sufficient water to be reabsorbed.

diastolic Pertaining to the time between heart contractions, a period known as diastole. Diastolic blood pressure is measured at the point of maximum cardiac relaxation.

diet history Record of food intake and eating behaviors that includes recent and long-term habits of food consumption. Conducted by a skilled interviewer, the diet history is the most comprehensive form of dietary intake data collection.

dietary fiber Carbohydrates and lignins that are naturally in plants and are nondigestible; that is, they are not digested and absorbed in the human small intestine.

dietary folate equivalents (DFEs) A measure of folate intake used to account for the high bioavailability of folic acid taken as a supplement compared with the lower bioavailability of the folate found in foods.

Dietary Guidelines for Americans, 2015–2020 The *Dietary Guidelines for Americans* are the foundation of federal nutrition policy and are developed by the U.S. Department of Agriculture (USDA) and the U.S. Department of Health and Human Services (DHHS). These science-based guidelines are intended to reduce the number of Americans who develop chronic diseases such as hypertension, diabetes, cardiovascular disease, obesity, and alcoholism.

Dietary Reference Intakes (DRIs) A framework of dietary standards that includes Estimated Average Requirement (EAR), Recommended Dietary Allowance (RDA), Adequate Intake (AI), and Tolerable Upper Intake Level (UL).

dietary standards A set of values for the recommended intake of nutrients.

Dietary Supplement Health and Education Act (DSHEA) [da-SHAY] Legislation that regulates dietary supplements.

dietary supplements Products taken by mouth in tablet, capsule, powder, gelcap, or other nonfood form that contain one or more of the following: vitamins, minerals, amino acids, herbs, enzymes, metabolites, or concentrates.

digestion The process of transforming the foods we eat into units for absorption.

digestive secretions Substances released at different places in the GI tract to speed the breakdown of ingested carbohydrates, fats, and proteins into smaller compounds that can be absorbed by the body.

diglycerides Molecules composed of glycerol combined with two fatty acids.

dioxins Chemical compounds created in the manufacturing, combustion, and chlorine bleaching of pulp and paper and in other industrial processes.

dipeptide Two amino acids joined by a peptide bond.

direct calorimetry Determination of energy use by the body by measuring the heat released from an organism enclosed in a small insulated chamber surrounded by water. The rise in the temperature of the water is directly related to the energy used by the organism.

disaccharides [dye-SACK-uh-rides] Carbohydrates composed of two monosaccharide units linked by a glycosidic bond. They include sucrose (common table sugar), lactose (milk sugar), and maltose.

disordered eating An abnormal change in eating pattern related to an illness, a stressful event, or a desire to improve one's health or appearance. If it persists it can lead to an eating disorder.

disulfide bridge A bond between the sulfur components of two sulfur-containing amino acids that helps stabilize the structure of protein.

diuresis The formation and secretion of urine.

diuretics [dye-u-RET-iks] Drugs or other substances that promote the formation and release of urine. Diuretics are given to reduce body fluid volume in treating such disorders as high blood pressure, congestive heart disease, and edema. Both alcohol and caffeine act as diuretics.

DNA (deoxyribonucleic acid) The carrier of genetic information. Specific regions of each DNA molecule, called genes, act as blueprints for the synthesis of proteins.

double-blind study A research study set up so that neither the subjects nor the investigators know which study group is receiving the placebo and which is receiving the active substance.

doubly labeled water A method for measuring daily energy expenditure over extended time periods, typically 7 to 14 days, while subjects are living in their usual environments. Small amounts of water that is isotopically labeled with deuterium and oxygen-18 (^2H_2O and $H_2{}^{18}O$) are ingested. Energy expenditure can be calculated from the difference between the rates at which the body loses each isotope.

d-tagatose An artificial sweetener derived from lactose that has the same sweetness as sucrose with only half the calories.

dual-energy x-ray absorptiometry (DEXA) A body composition measurement technique originally developed to measure bone density.

duodenum [doo-oh-DEE-num or doo-AH-den-um] The portion of the small intestine closest to the stomach. The duodenum is 10 to 12 inches long and wider than the remainder of the small intestine.

dyspepsia A condition also known as upset stomach or indigestion; refers to difficulty with digestion.

eating disorders A spectrum of abnormal eating patterns that eventually can endanger a person's health or increase the risk for other diseases. Generally, psychological factors play a key role.

Eating Well with Canada's Food Guide Recommendations to help Canadians select foods to meet energy and nutrient needs while reducing the risk of chronic disease. The *Food Guide* is based on the *Nutrition Recommendations for Canadians* and *Canada's Guidelines for Healthy Eating* and is a key nutrition education tool for Canadians aged 4 years and older.

eclampsia The occurrence of seizures in a pregnant woman that are unrelated to brain conditions.

edema Swelling caused by the buildup of fluid between cells.

eicosanoids A class of hormonelike substances formed in the body from long-chain fatty acids.

electrolytes [ih-LEK-tro-lites] Substances that dissociate into charged particles (ions) when dissolved in water or other solvents and thus become capable of conducting an electrical current. The terms *electrolyte* and *ion* often are used interchangeably.

electron transport chain An organized series of carrier molecules—including flavin mononucleotide (FMN), coenzyme Q, and several cytochromes—that are located in mitochondrial membranes and shuttle electrons from NADH and $FADH_2$ to oxygen, yielding water and ATP.

Electronic Benefits Transfer (EBT) Electronic delivery of government benefits by a single plastic card that allows access to food benefits at point-of-sale locations.

elongation Addition of carbon atoms to fatty acids to lengthen them into new fatty acids.

embryonic stage The developmental stage between the time of implantation (about two weeks after fertilization) through the seventh or eighth week; the stage of major organ system differentiation and development of main external features.

emetics Agents that induce vomiting.

emulsifiers Agents that blend fatty and watery liquids by promoting the breakup of fat into small particles and stabilizing their suspension in aqueous solution.

endocytosis The uptake of material by a cell by the indentation and pinching off of its membrane to form a vesicle that carries material into the cell.

endosperm The largest, middle portion of a grain kernel. The endosperm is high in starch to provide food for the growing plant embryo.

endothelial cells Thin, flattened cells that line internal body cavities in a single layer.

endothelium See *endothelial cells.*

enemas Infusions of fluid into the rectum, usually for cleansing or other therapeutic purposes.

energy balance The balance in the body between amounts of energy consumed and expended.

energy equilibrium A balance of energy intake and output that results in little or no change in weight over time.

energy intake The caloric or energy content of food provided by the sources of dietary energy: carbohydrate (4 kcal/g), protein (4 kcal/g), fat (9 kcal/g), and alcohol (7 kcal/g).

energy The capacity to do work. The energy in food is chemical energy, which the body converts to mechanical, electrical, or heat energy.

energy output The use of calories or energy for basic body functions, physical activity, and processing of consumed foods.

enrich To add vitamins and minerals lost or diminished during food processing, particularly the addition of thiamin, riboflavin, niacin, folic acid, and iron to grain products.

enteric nervous system A network of nerves located in the gastrointestinal wall.

enterohepatic circulation [EN-ter-oh-heh-PAT-ik] Recycling of certain compounds between the small intestine and the liver. For example, bile acids move from the liver to the gallbladder, and then into the small intestine, where they are absorbed into the portal vein and transported back to the liver.

enzymes [EN-zimes] Large proteins in the body that accelerate the rate of chemical reactions but are not altered in the process.

epinephrine A hormone released in response to stress or sudden danger, epinephrine raises blood glucose levels to ready the body for "fight or flight." Also called adrenaline.

epiphyses The heads of the long bones that are separated from the shaft of the bone until the bone stops growing.

epithelial cells The millions of cells that line and protect the external and internal surfaces of the body. Epithelial cells form epithelial tissues such as skin and mucous membranes.

epithelial tissues Closely packed layers of epithelial cells that cover the body and line its cavities.

ergogenic aids Substances that can enhance athletic performance.

Escherichia coli (E. coli) Bacteria that are the most common cause of urinary tract infections. Because they release toxins, some types of *E. coli* can rapidly cause shock and death.

esophageal sphincter The opening between the esophagus and the stomach that relaxes and opens to allow the bolus to travel into the stomach, and then closes behind it. Also acts as a barrier to prevent the reflux of gastric contents. Commonly called the cardiac sphincter.

esophagitis Inflammation of the esophagus.

esophagus [ee-SOFF-uh-gus] The food pipe that extends from the pharynx to the stomach, about 25 centimeters long.

essential fatty acids The fatty acids that the body needs but cannot synthesize, and which must be obtained from diet.

essential hypertension Hypertension for which no specific cause can be identified. Ninety to 95 percent of people with hypertension have essential hypertension.

essential (indispensable) amino acids Amino acids that the body cannot make at all or cannot make enough of to meet physiological needs. Essential amino acids must be supplied in the diet.

essential nutrients Substances that must be obtained in the diet because the body either cannot make them or cannot make adequate amounts of them.

ester A chemical combination of an organic acid (e.g., fatty acid) and an alcohol. When hydrogen from the alcohol combines with the acid's hydrogen and oxygen, water is released and an ester linkage is formed. A triglyceride is an ester of three fatty acids and glycerol.

esterification [e-ster-ih-fih-KAY-shun] A condensation reaction in which an organic acid (e.g., fatty acid) combines with an alcohol with the loss of water, creating an ester.

Estimated Average Requirement (EAR) The intake value that meets the estimated nutrient needs of 50 percent of individuals in a specific life-stage and gender group.

Estimated Energy Requirement (EER) Dietary energy intake that is predicted to maintain energy balance in a healthy adult of a defined age, gender, weight, height, and level of physical activity consistent with good health.

ethanol Chemical name for alcohol that is consumed. Also known as ethyl alcohol.

ethyl alcohol See *ethanol.*

Exchange Lists Lists of foods that in specified portions provide equivalent amounts of carbohydrate, fat, protein, and energy. Any food in an Exchange List can be substituted for any other without markedly affecting macronutrient intake.

experimental group A set of people being studied to evaluate the effect of an event, substance, or technique.

extracellular fluid The fluid located outside of cells. It is composed largely of the liquid portion of the blood (plasma) and the fluid between cells in tissues (interstitial fluid), with fluid in the GI tract, eyes, joints, and spinal cord contributing a small amount. It constitutes about one-third of body water.

extreme obesity Obesity characterized by body weight exceeding 100 percent of normal; a condition so severe it often requires surgery.

extrusion reflex A young infant's response when a spoon is put in its mouth; the tongue is thrust forward, indicating that the baby is not ready for spoon feeding.

facilitated diffusion A process by which carrier (transport) proteins in the cell membrane transport substances into or out of cells down a concentration gradient.

$FADH_2$ The reduced form of flavin adenine dinucleotide (FAD). This coenzyme, which is derived from the B vitamin riboflavin, acts as an electron carrier in cells and undergoes reversible oxidation and reduction.

failure to thrive (FTT) Abnormally low gains in length (height) and weight during infancy and childhood; can result from physical problems or poor feeding, but many affected children have no apparent disease or defect.

fasting hypoglycemia A type of hypoglycemia that occurs because the body produces too much insulin even when no food is eaten.

fast-twitch (FT) fibers Muscle fibers that can develop high tension rapidly. These fibers can fatigue quickly but are well suited to explosive movements in sprinting, jumping, and weight lifting.

fat replacers Compounds that imitate the functional and sensory properties of fats, but contain less available energy than fats.

fatty acids Compounds containing a long hydrocarbon chain with a carboxyl group (—COOH) at one end and a methyl group (—CH_3) at the other end.

fatty liver Accumulation of fat in the liver, a sign of increased fatty acid synthesis.

Feeding America The largest charitable hunger-relief organization in the United States. Its mission is to feed America's hungry through a nationwide network of member food banks and to engage the country in the fight to end hunger.

female athlete triad A syndrome in young female athletes that involves disordered eating, amenorrhea, and lowered bone density.

fermentation The anaerobic conversion of various carbohydrates to carbon dioxide and an alcohol or organic acid.

ferric iron (Fe^{3+}) The oxidized form of iron able to be bound to transferrin for transport.

ferritin A complex of iron and apoferritin that is a major storage form of iron.

ferrous iron (Fe^{2+}) The reduced form of iron most commonly found in food.

fetal alcohol syndrome A set of physical and mental abnormalities observed in infants born to women who abuse alcohol during pregnancy. Affected infants exhibit poor growth, characteristic abnormal facial features, limited hand—eye coordination, and mental retardation.

fetal stage The period of rapid growth from the end of the embryonic stage until birth.

fibrin A stringy, insoluble protein that is the final product of the blood-clotting process.

flatus Lower intestinal gas that is expelled through the rectum.

flavin adenine dinucleotide (FAD) A coenzyme synthesized in the body from riboflavin. It undergoes reversible oxidation and reduction and thus acts as an electron carrier in cells. FAD is the oxidized form; $FADH_2$ is the reduced form.

flavor The collective experience that describes both taste and smell.

fluorosis Mottled discoloration and pitting of tooth enamel caused by prolonged ingestion of excessive fluoride.

Food and Agriculture Organization (FAO) The largest autonomous United Nations agency; the FAO works to alleviate poverty and hunger by promoting agricultural development, improved nutrition, and the pursuit of food security.

Food and Drug Administration (FDA) The federal agency responsible for ensuring that foods sold in the United States (except for eggs, poultry, and meat, which are monitored by the USDA) are safe, wholesome, and labeled properly. The FDA sets standards for the composition of some foods, inspects food plants, and monitors imported foods. The FDA is an agency of the U.S. Department of Health and Human Services (DHHS).

Food and Nutrition Board A board within the Institute of Medicine of the National Academy of Sciences. It is responsible for assembling the group of nutrition scientists who review available scientific data to determine appropriate intake levels of the known essential nutrients.

Food Code A reference published periodically by the Food and Drug Administration for restaurants, grocery stores, institutional food services, vending operations, and other retailers on how to store, prepare, and serve food to prevent foodborne illness.

food deserts Geographic area where affordable and nutritious food is alleged to be hard to obtain, particularly for those without access to an automobile.

food frequency questionnaire (FFQ) A questionnaire for nutrition assessment that asks how often the subject consumes specific foods or groups of foods, rather than what specific foods the subject consumes daily. Also called food frequency checklist.

food groups Categories of similar foods, such as fruits or vegetables.

food insecurity (1) Limited or uncertain availability of nutritionally adequate and safe foods, or (2) limited or uncertain ability to acquire acceptable foods in socially acceptable ways.

food label Labels required by law on virtually all packaged foods and having five requirements: (1) a statement of identity; (2) the net contents (by weight, volume, or measure) of the package; (3) the name and address of the manufacturer, packer, or distributor; (4) a list of ingredients; and (5) nutrition information.

food records Detailed information about day-to-day eating habits; typically includes all foods and beverages consumed for a defined period, usually three to seven consecutive days.

Food Research and Action Center (FRAC) Founded in 1970 as a public interest law firm, FRAC is a nonprofit child advocacy group that works to improve public policies to eradicate hunger and undernutrition in the United States.

food security Access to enough food for an active, healthy life, including (1) the ready availability of nutritionally adequate and safe foods and (2) an assured ability to acquire acceptable foods in socially acceptable ways.

Food Security Supplement Survey A federally funded survey that measures the prevalence and severity of food insecurity and hunger.

foodborne illness A sickness caused by food contaminated with microorganisms, chemicals, or other substances hazardous to human health.

fortify Refers to the addition of vitamins or minerals that were not originally present in a food.

free radicals Short-lived, highly reactive chemicals often derived from oxygen-containing compounds, which can have detrimental effects on cells, especially DNA and cell membranes.

French paradox A phenomenon observed in the French, who have a lower incidence of heart disease than people whose diets contain comparable amounts of fat. Part of the difference has been attributed to the regular and moderate drinking of red wine.

fructose [FROOK-tose] A common monosaccharide containing six carbons that is naturally present in honey and many fruits; often added to foods in the form of high-fructose corn syrup. Also called levulose or fruit sugar.

full-term baby A baby delivered during the normal period of human gestation, between 38 and 41 weeks.

functional fiber Isolated nondigestible carbohydrates, including some manufactured carbohydrates, that have beneficial effects in humans.

functional food A food that may provide a health benefit beyond basic nutrition.

galactose [gah-LAK-tose] A monosaccharide containing six carbons that can be converted into glucose in the body. In foods and living systems, galactose usually is joined with other monosaccharides.

gallbladder A pear-shaped sac that stores and concentrates bile from the liver.

galvanized Iron or steel with a thin layer of zinc plated onto it to protect against corrosion.

gastric inhibitory peptide (GIP) [GAS-trik in-HIB-ih-tor-ee PEP-tide] A hormone released from the walls of the duodenum that slows the release of the stomach contents into the small intestine and stimulates release of insulin from the pancreas.

gastric lipase An enzyme in the stomach that hydrolyzes certain triglycerides into fatty acids and glycerol.

gastrin [GAS-trin] A polypeptide hormone released from the walls of the stomach mucosa and duodenum that stimulates gastric secretions and motility.

gastritis Inflammation of the stomach.

gastroesophageal reflux A backflow of stomach contents into the esophagus, accompanied by a burning pain because of the acidity of the gastric juices.

gastroesophageal reflux disease (GERD) A condition in which gastric contents move backward (reflux) into the esophagus, causing pain and tissue damage.

gastrointestinal (GI) tract [GAS-troh-in-TES-tin-al] The connected series of organs and structures used for digestion of food and absorption of nutrients; also called the alimentary canal or the digestive tract. The GI tract contains the mouth, esophagus, stomach, small intestine, large intestine (colon), rectum, and anus.

gene expression The process by which proteins are made from the instructions encoded in DNA.

genes Sections of DNA that contain hereditary information. Most genes contain information for making proteins.

genetic code The instructions in a gene that tell the cell how to make a specific protein. A, T, G, and C are the "letters" of the DNA code; they stand for the chemicals adenine, thymine, guanine, and cytosine, respectively, which make up the nucleotide bases of DNA. Each gene's code combines the four chemicals in various ways to spell out three-letter "words" that specify which amino acid is needed at every step in making a protein.

genetic engineering Manipulation of the genome of an organism by artificial means for the purpose of modifying existing traits or adding new genetic traits.

genetically engineered (GE) foods Foods produced using plant or animal ingredients that have been modified using gene technology.

genome The total genetic information of an organism, stored in the DNA of its chromosomes.

geophagia Ingestion of clay or dirt.

germ The innermost part of a grain, located at the base of the kernel, that can grow into a new plant. The germ is rich in protein, oils, vitamins, and minerals.

gestational diabetes A condition that results in high blood glucose levels during pregnancy.

ghrelin A peptide hormone produced by the stomach that stimulates feeding; sometimes called the "hunger hormone."

glossitis Inflammation of the tongue; a symptom of riboflavin deficiency.

glucagon [GLOO-kuh-gon] Produced by alpha cells in the pancreas, this polypeptide hormone promotes the breakdown of liver glycogen to glucose, thereby increasing blood glucose. Glucagon secretion is stimulated by low blood glucose levels and by growth hormone.

glucogenic In the metabolism of amino acids, a term describing an amino acid broken down into pyruvate or an intermediate of the citric acid cycle; that is, any compound that can be used in gluconeogenesis to form glucose.

gluconeogenesis [gloo-ko-nee-oh-JEN-uh-sis] Synthesis of glucose within the body from noncarbohydrate precursors such as amino acids, lactate, and glycerol. Fatty acids cannot be converted to glucose.

glucose [GLOO-kose] A common monosaccharide containing six carbons that is present in the blood; also known as dextrose or blood sugar. It is a component of the disaccharides sucrose, lactose, and maltose and various complex carbohydrates.

glutathione A tripeptide of glycine, cysteine, and glutamic acid that is involved in protection of cells from oxidative damage.

glutathione peroxidase A selenium-containing enzyme that promotes the breakdown of fatty acids that have undergone peroxidation.

glycemic index A measure of the effect of food on blood glucose levels. It is the ratio of the blood glucose value after eating a particular food to the value after eating the same amount of white bread or glucose.

glycemic load The glycemic index of a food adjusted for the amount of carbohydrate in one serving: (glycemic index × g carbohydrate per serving)/100.

glycerol [GLISS-er-ol] An alcohol that contains three carbon atoms, each of which has an attached hydroxyl group (—OH). It forms the backbone of mono-, di-, and triglycerides.

glycogen [GLY-ko-jen] A very large, highly branched polysaccharide composed of multiple glucose units. Sometimes called animal starch, glycogen is the primary storage form of glucose in animals.

glycogen loading See *carbohydrate loading.*

glycogenesis The formation of glycogen from glucose.

glycogenolysis The breakdown of glycogen to glucose.

glycolysis [gligh-COLL-ih-sis] The anaerobic metabolic pathway that breaks a glucose molecule into two molecules of pyruvate and yields two molecules of ATP and two molecules of NADH. Glycolysis occurs in the cytosol of a cell.

goblet cells One of the many types of specialized cells that produce and secrete mucus. These cells are found in the stomach, intestines, and portions of the respiratory tract.

goiter A chronic enlargement of the thyroid gland, visible as a swelling at the front of the neck; usually associated with iodine deficiency.

goitrogens Compounds that can induce goiter.

gout An intensely painful form of inflammatory arthritis that results from deposits of needlelike crystals of uric acid in connective tissue and/or the joint space between bones.

growth charts Charts that plot the weight, length, and head circumference of infants and children as they grow.

guanosine triphosphate (GTP) A high-energy compound, similar to ATP but with three phosphate groups linked to guanosine.

gums Dietary fibers, which contain galactose and other monosaccharides, found between plant cell walls.

hangover The collection of symptoms experienced by someone who has consumed a large quantity of alcohol. Symptoms can include pounding headache, fatigue, muscle aches, nausea, stomach pain, heightened sensitivity to light and sound, dizziness, and possibly depression, anxiety, and irritability.

head circumference Measurement of the largest part of the infant's head (just above the eyebrows and ears); used to determine brain growth.

health claim Any statement that associates a food or a substance in a food with a disease or health-related condition. The FDA authorizes health claims.

health disparities Differences in health outcomes and their determinants between segments of the population, as defined by social, demographic, environmental, and geographic attributes.

heat capacity The amount of energy required to raise the temperature of a substance 1 degree Celsius.

hematocrit Percentage volume occupied by packed red blood cells in a centrifuged sample of whole blood.

heme A chemical complex with a central iron atom (ferric iron Fe^{3+}) that forms the oxygen-binding part of hemoglobin and myoglobin.

heme iron The iron found in the hemoglobin and myoglobin of animal foods.

hemicelluloses [hem-ih-SELL-you-los-es] A group of large polysaccharides in dietary fiber that are fermented more easily than cellulose.

hemochromatosis A metabolic disorder that results in excess iron deposits in the body.

hemoglobin [HEEM-oh-glow-bin] The oxygen-carrying protein in red blood cells that consists of four heme groups and four globin polypeptide chains. The presence of hemoglobin gives blood its red color.

hemolysis The breakdown of red blood cells that usually occurs at the end of a red blood cell's normal life span. This process releases hemoglobin.

hemosiderin An insoluble form of storage iron.

herbal therapy (phytotherapy) The therapeutic use of herbs and other plants to promote health and treat disease.

high-density lipoproteins (HDLs) The blood lipoproteins that contain high levels of protein and low levels of triglycerides. Synthesized primarily in the liver and small intestine, HDL picks up cholesterol released from dying cells and other sources and transfers it to other lipoproteins.

homocysteine An amino acid precursor of cysteine and a risk factor for heart disease.

hormones Chemical messengers that are secreted into the blood by one tissue and act on cells in another part of the body.

Human Genome Project An effort coordinated by the Department of Energy and the National Institutes of Health to map the genes in human DNA.

hunger The internal, physiological drive to find and consume food. Unlike appetite, hunger is often experienced as a negative sensation, often manifesting as an uneasy or painful sensation; the recurrent and involuntary lack of access to food that can produce malnutrition over time.

husk The inedible covering of a grain kernel. Also known as the chaff.

hydrochloric acid An acid of chloride and hydrogen atoms made by the gastric glands and secreted into the stomach. Also called gastric acid.

hydrogen bonds Noncovalent bonds between hydrogen and an atom, usually oxygen, in another molecule.

hydrogen ions Also called a proton. This lone hydrogen has a positive charge (H^+). It does not have its own electron, but it can share one with another atom.

hydrogenation [high-dro-jen-AY-shun] A chemical reaction in which hydrogen atoms are added to carbon—carbon double bonds, converting them to single bonds. Hydrogenation of monounsaturated and polyunsaturated fatty acids reduces the number of double bonds they contain, thereby making them more saturated.

hydrolysis A reaction that breaks apart a compound through the addition of water.

hydrophilic [high-dro-FILL-ik] Can mix with or dissolve in water ("water-loving"). Hydrophilic compounds are polar and soluble in water.

hydrophilic amino acids Amino acids that are attracted to water (water-loving).

hydrophobic Insoluble in water.

hydrophobic amino acids Amino acids that are repelled by water (water-fearing).

hydrostatic weighing See *underwater weighing.*

hydroxyapatite A crystalline mineral compound of calcium and phosphorus that makes up bone.

hyperactivity A maladaptive and abnormal increase in activity that is inconsistent with developmental levels. Includes frequent fidgeting, inappropriate running, excessive talking, and difficulty in engaging in quiet activities.

hypercalcemia Abnormally high concentrations of calcium in the blood.

hypercholesterolemia The presence of greater than normal amounts of cholesterol in the blood.

hyperglycemia [HIGH-per-gly-SEE-me-uh] Abnormally high concentration of glucose in the blood.

hyperkalemia Abnormally high potassium concentrations in the blood.

hyperkeratosis Excessive accumulation of the protein keratin that produces rough and bumpy skin, most commonly affecting the palms and soles, as well as flexure areas (elbows, knees, wrists, ankles). It can affect moist epithelial tissues and impair their ability to secrete mucus. Also called hyperkeratinization.

hypermagnesemia An abnormally high concentration of magnesium in the blood.

hypernatremia Abnormally high sodium concentrations in the blood resulting from increased kidney retention of sodium or rapid ingestion of large amounts of salt.

hyperparathyroidism Excessive secretion of parathyroid hormone, which alters calcium metabolism.

hyperphosphatemia Abnormally high phosphate concentration in the blood.

hypertension When resting blood pressure persistently exceeds 140 mm Hg systolic or 90 mm Hg diastolic.

hyperthermia A much higher than normal body temperature.

hypervitaminosis High levels of vitamins in the blood, usually a result of excess supplement intake.

hypervolemia An abnormal increase in the circulating blood volume.

hypocalcemia A deficiency of calcium in the blood.

hypoglycemia [HIGH-po-gly-SEE-mee-uh] Abnormally low concentration of glucose in the blood; any blood glucose value below 40 to 50 mg/dL of blood.

hypogonadism Decreased functional activity of the gonads (ovaries or testes) with retardation of growth and sexual development.

hypokalemia Inadequate levels of potassium in the blood.

hypomagnesemia An abnormally low concentration of magnesium in the blood.

hyponatremia Abnormally low sodium concentrations in the blood resulting from excessive excretion of sodium (by the kidneys), prolonged vomiting, or diarrhea.

hypophosphatemia Abnormally low phosphate concentration in the blood.

hypothalamus [high-po-THAL-ah-mus] A region of the brain involved in regulating hunger and satiety, respiration, body temperature, water balance, and other body functions.

hypotheses Scientists' educated guesses to explain phenomena.

hypothyroidism The result of a lowered level of circulating thyroid hormone, with slowing of mental and physical functions.

ileocecal valve The sphincter at the junction of the small and large intestines.

ileum [ILL-ee-um] The terminal segment (about 5 feet) of the small intestine, which opens into the large intestine.

immune response A coordinated set of steps, including production of antibodies, that the immune system takes in response to an antigen.

incomplete (low-quality) proteins Proteins that lack one or more amino acids.

indirect calorimetry Determination of energy use by the body without directly measuring the production of heat. Methods include gas exchange, the measurement of oxygen uptake and/or carbon dioxide output, and the doubly labeled water method.

infancy The period between birth and 12 months of age.

infantile anorexia Severe feeding difficulties that begin with the introduction of solid foods to infants. Symptoms include persistent food refusal for more than one month, malnutrition, parental concern about the child's poor food intake, and significant caregiver—infant conflict during feeding.

inorganic Any substance that does not contain carbon, excepting certain simple carbon compounds such as carbon dioxide and carbon monoxide. Common examples include table salt (sodium chloride) and baking soda (sodium bicarbonate).

insensible water loss The continual loss of body water by evaporation from the respiratory tract and diffusion through the skin.

insoluble fiber Nondigestible carbohydrates that do not dissolve in water.

insulin [IN-suh-lin] Produced by beta cells in the pancreas, this polypeptide hormone stimulates the uptake of blood glucose into muscle and adipose cells, the synthesis of glycogen in the liver, and various other processes.

integrated pest management (IPM) Economically sound pest control techniques that minimize pesticide use, enhance environmental stewardship, and promote sustainable systems.

integrative health care A comprehensive, often interdisciplinary approach to treatment, prevention, and health promotion that brings together complementary and conventional therapies.

intermediate-density lipoproteins (IDLs) The lipoproteins formed when lipoprotein lipase strips some of the triglycerides from VLDL. Containing about 40 percent triglycerides, this type of lipoprotein is more dense than VLDL and less dense than LDL. Also called a VLDL remnant.

interstitial fluid [in-ter-STISH-ul] The fluid between cells in tissues. Also called intercellular fluid.

intervention studies See *clinical trials*.

intracellular fluid The fluid in the body's cells. It usually is high in potassium and phosphate and low in sodium and chloride. It constitutes about two-thirds of total body water.

intravascular fluid The fluid portion of the blood (plasma) contained in arteries, veins, and capillaries. It accounts for about 15 percent of the extracellular fluid.

intrinsic factor A glycoprotein released from parietal cells in the stomach wall that binds to and aids in absorption of vitamin B_{12}.

iodine deficiency disorders (IDDs) A wide range of disorders caused by iodine deficiency that affect growth and development.

iodopsin Color-sensitive pigment molecules in cone cells that consist of opsin-like proteins combined with retinal.

ions Atoms or groups of atoms with an electrical charge resulting from the loss or gain of one or more electrons.

iron overload Toxicity from excess iron.

irradiation A food preservation technique in which foods are exposed to measured doses of radiation to reduce or eliminate pathogens and kill insects, reduce spoilage, and, in certain fruits and vegetables, inhibit sprouting and delay ripening.

irritable bowel syndrome (IBS) A disruptive state of intestinal motility with no known cause. Symptoms include constipation, abdominal pain, and episodic diarrhea.

isoflavones Plant chemicals that include genistein and daidzein and may have positive effects against cancer and heart disease. Also called *phytoestrogens*.

isotopes [EYE-so-towps] Forms of an element in which the atoms have the same number of protons but different numbers of neutrons.

jejunum [je-JOON-um] The middle section (about 4 feet) of the small intestine, lying between the duodenum and ileum.

keratin A water-insoluble fibrous protein that is the primary constituent of hair, nails, and the outer layer of the skin.

Keshan disease Selenium-deficiency disease that impairs the structure and function of the heart.

ketoacidosis Acidification of the blood caused by a buildup of ketone bodies. It is primarily a consequence of uncontrolled type 1 diabetes mellitus and can be life threatening.

ketogenesis The process in which excess acetyl CoA from fatty acid oxidation is converted into the ketone bodies acetoacetate, beta-hydroxybutyrate, and acetone.

ketogenic In the metabolism of amino acids, a term describing an amino acid broken down into acetyl CoA (which can be converted into ketone bodies).

ketone bodies Molecules formed when insufficient carbohydrate is available to completely metabolize fat. Formation of ketone bodies is promoted by a low glucose level and high acetyl CoA level within cells. Acetone, acetoacetate, and beta-hydroxybutyrate are ketone bodies.

ketones [KEE-tones] Organic compounds that contain a chemical group consisting of C=O (a carbon—oxygen double bond) bound to two hydrocarbons.

ketosis [kee-TOE-sis] Abnormally high concentration of ketone bodies in body tissues and fluids.

kilocalories (kcal) [KILL-oh-kal-oh-rees] Units used to measure food energy (1,000 calories = 1 kilocalorie).

Krebs cycle See *citric acid cycle*.

kwashiorkor A type of malnutrition that occurs primarily in young children who have an infectious disease and whose diets supply marginal amounts of energy and very little protein. Common symptoms include poor growth, edema, apathy, weakness, and susceptibility to infections.

lactate The ionized form of lactic acid, a three-carbon acid. It is produced when insufficient oxygen is present in cells to oxidize pyruvate.

lactation The process of synthesizing and secreting breast milk.

lactation consultants Health professionals trained to specialize in education about and promotion of breastfeeding; can be certified as an International Board Certified Lactation Consultant (IBCLC).

lacteal A small lymphatic vessel in the interior of each intestinal villus that picks up chylomicrons and fat-soluble vitamins from intestinal cells.

lactic acid energy system Anaerobic energy system; using glycolysis, it rapidly produces energy (ATP) and lactate. Also called anaerobic glycolysis.

lactose [LAK-tose] A disaccharide composed of glucose and galactose; also called milk sugar because it is the major sugar in milk and dairy products.

lanugo [lah-NEW-go] Soft, downy hair that covers a normal fetus from the fifth month but is shed almost entirely by the time of birth. It also appears on semistarved individuals who have lost much of their body fat, serving as insulation normally provided by body fat.

large intestine The tube (about 5 feet long) extending from the ileum of the small intestine to the anus. The large intestine includes the appendix, cecum, colon, rectum, and anal canal.

laxatives Substances that promote evacuation of the bowel by increasing the bulk of the feces, lubricating the intestinal wall, or softening the stool.

lean body mass The portion of the body exclusive of stored fat, including muscle, bone, connective tissue, organs, and water.

lecithin In the body, a phospholipid with the nitrogenous component choline. In foods, lecithin is a blend of phospholipids with different nitrogenous components.

legumes A family of plants with edible seed pods, such as peas, beans, lentils, and soybeans; also called *pulses*.

leptin A hormone produced by adipose cells that signals the amount of body fat content and influences food intake; sometimes called the "satiety hormone."

let-down reflex The release of milk from the breast tissue in response to the stimulus of the hormone oxytocin. The major stimulus for oxytocin release is the infant suckling at the breast.

leukemia [loo-KEE-mee-a] Cancer of blood-forming tissue.

lignins [LIG-nins] Insoluble fibers composed of multi-ring alcohol units that constitute the only noncarbohydrate component of dietary fiber.

limiting amino acid The amino acid in shortest supply during protein synthesis. Also the amino acid in the lowest quantity when evaluating protein quality.

linear growth Increase in body length/height.

lingual lipase A fat-splitting enzyme secreted by cells at the base of the tongue.

linoleic acid [lin-oh-LAY-ik ah-sid] An essential omega-6 fatty acid that contains 18 carbon atoms and 2 carbon—carbon double bonds (18:2).

lipid peroxidation Production of unstable, highly reactive lipid molecules that contain excess amounts of oxygen.

lipids A group of fat-soluble compounds that includes triglycerides, sterols, and phospholipids.

lipogenesis [lye-poh-JEN-eh-sis] Synthesis of fatty acids, primarily in liver cells, from acetyl CoA derived from the metabolism of alcohol and some amino acids.

lipophilic Attracted to fat and fat solvents; fat-soluble.

lipophobic Adverse to fat solvents; insoluble in fat and fat solvents.

lipoprotein Complexes that transport lipids in the lymph and blood. They consist of a central core of triglycerides and cholesterol surrounded by a shell composed of proteins and phospholipids. The various types of lipoproteins differ in size, composition, and density.

lipoprotein a [Lp(a)] A substance that consists of an LDL "bad cholesterol" part plus a protein (apoprotein a), whose exact function is currently unknown.

lipoprotein lipase The major enzyme responsible for the hydrolysis of plasma triglycerides.

liver The largest glandular organ in the body, it produces and secretes bile, detoxifies harmful substances, and helps metabolize carbohydrates, lipids, proteins, and micronutrients.

longitudinal muscle Muscle fibers aligned lengthwise.

low-birth-weight infant A newborn who weighs less than 2,500 grams (5.5 pounds) as a result of either premature birth or inadequate growth in utero.

low-density lipoproteins (LDLs) The cholesterol-rich lipoproteins that result from the breakdown and removal of triglycerides from intermediate-density lipoprotein in the blood.

lumen Cavity or hollow channel in any organ or structure of the body.

lycopene One of a family of plant chemicals, the carotenoids. Others in this big family include alpha-carotene and beta-carotene.

lymph Fluid that travels through the lymphatic system, made up of fluid drained from between cells and large fat particles.

lymph nodes [limf nodes] Rounded masses of lymphatic tissue that are surrounded by a capsule of connective tissue. Lymph nodes filter lymph (lymphatic fluid) and store lymphocytes (white blood cells). They are located along lymphatic vessels. Also called lymph glands.

lymphatic system A system of small vessels, ducts, valves, and organized tissue (e.g., lymph nodes) through which lymph moves from its origin in the tissues toward the heart.

lymphoma [lim-FO-ma] Cancer that arises in cells of the lymphatic system.

macrocytes Abnormally large red blood cells with short life spans.

macrominerals Major minerals required in the diet and present in the body in large amounts compared with trace minerals.

macronutrients Nutrients, such as carbohydrate, fat, or protein, that are needed in relatively large amounts in the diet.

macular degeneration Progressive deterioration of the macula, an area in the center of the retina, that eventually leads to loss of central vision.

mad cow disease See *bovine spongiform encephalopathy (BSE)*.

major mineral A mineral required in the diet and present in the body in large amounts compared with trace minerals.

malabsorption syndromes Conditions that result in imperfect, inadequate, or otherwise disordered gastrointestinal absorption.

malignant [ma-LIG-nant] Cancerous; a growth with a tendency to invade and destroy nearby tissue and spread to other parts of the body.

malnutrition Failure to achieve nutrient requirements, which can impair physical and/or mental health. It can result from consuming too little food or a shortage or imbalance of key nutrients.

maltose [MALL-tose] A disaccharide composed of two glucose molecules; sometimes called malt sugar. Maltose seldom occurs naturally in foods but is formed whenever long molecules of starch break down.

marasmus A type of malnutrition resulting from chronic inadequate consumption of protein and energy that is characterized by wasting of muscle, fat, and other body tissue.

Meals on Wheels A voluntary, not-for-profit organization established to provide nutritious meals to homebound people (regardless of age) so they can maintain their independence and quality of life.

megadoses Doses of a nutrient that are 10 or more times the recommended amount.

megaloblastic anemia Excess amounts of megaloblasts in the blood caused by deficiency of folate or vitamin B_{12}.

megaloblasts Large, immature red blood cells produced when precursor cells fail to divide normally because of impaired DNA synthesis.

melanocytes [mel-AN-o-sites] Cells in the skin that produce and contain the pigment called melanin.

melanoma A form of skin cancer that arises in melanocytes, the cells that produce pigment. Melanoma usually begins in a mole.

menadione A medicinal form of vitamin K that can be toxic to infants. Also known as vitamin K_3.

menaquinones Forms of vitamin K that come from animal sources. Also produced by intestinal bacteria, they are collectively known as vitamin K_2.

menarche First menstrual period.

Menkes syndrome A genetic disorder that results in copper deficiency.

messenger RNA (mRNA) Long, linear, single-stranded molecules of ribonucleic acids formed from DNA templates that carry the amino acid sequence of one or more proteins from the cell nucleus to the cytoplasm, where the ribosomes translate mRNA into proteins.

metabolic alkalosis An abnormal pH of body fluids, usually caused by significant loss of acid from the body or increased levels of bicarbonate.

metabolic pathway A series of chemical reactions that either break down a large compound into smaller units (catabolism) or synthesize more complex molecules from smaller ones (anabolism).

metabolic syndrome A cluster of at least three of the following risk factors for heart disease: hypertriglyceridemia (high blood triglycerides), low HDL cholesterol, hyperglycemia (high blood glucose), hypertension (high blood pressure), and excess abdominal fat.

metabolically healthy obesity Obesity accompanied by normal metabolic features such as lipid profile, glucose tolerance, blood pressure, and waist circumference.

metabolism All chemical reactions within organisms that enable them to maintain life. The two main categories of metabolism are catabolism and anabolism.

metabolites Any substances produced during metabolism.

metalloproteins Proteins with a mineral element as an essential part of their structure.

metallothionein An abundant, nonenzymatic, zinc-containing protein.

metastasis [meh-TAS-ta-sis] The spread of cancer from one part of the body to another. Tumors formed from cells that have spread are called *secondary tumors* and contain cells that are like those in the original (primary) tumor. The plural is metastases.

methanol The simplest alcohol. Also known as methyl alcohol and wood alcohol.

methyl alcohol See *methanol.*

methylmercury A toxic compound that results from the chemical transformation of mercury by bacteria. Mercury is water-soluble in trace amounts and contaminates many bodies of water.

micelles Tiny emulsified fat packets that can enter enterocytes. The complexes are composed of emulsifier molecules oriented with their hydrophobic part facing inward and their hydrophilic part facing outward toward the surrounding aqueous environment.

microbiota Community of beneficial and pathogenic microorganisms that inhabit the body.

microcytic hypochromic anemia Anemia characterized by small, pale red blood cells that lack adequate hemoglobin to carry oxygen; can be caused by deficiency of iron or vitamin B_6.

microminerals See *trace minerals.*

micronutrients Nutrients, such as vitamins and minerals, that are needed in relatively small amounts in the diet.

microsomal ethanol-oxidizing system (MEOS) An energy-requiring enzyme system in the liver that normally metabolizes drugs and other foreign substances. When the blood alcohol level is high, alcohol dehydrogenase cannot metabolize it fast enough, and the excess alcohol is metabolized by MEOS.

microvilli Minute, hairlike projections that extend from the surface of absorptive cells facing the intestinal lumen. Singular is microvillus.

mineralization The addition of minerals, such as calcium and phosphorus, to bones and teeth.

minerals Inorganic compounds needed for growth and for regulation of body processes.

mitochondria (mitochondrion) The sites of aerobic production of ATP, where most of the energy from carbohydrate, protein, and fat is captured. Called the "power plants" of the cell, the mitochondria contain two highly specialized membranes, an outer membrane and a highly folded inner membrane, that separate two compartments, the internal matrix space and the narrow intermembrane space. A human cell contains about 2,000 mitochondria.

mitochondrial membrane The mitochondria are enclosed by a double shell separated by an intermembrane space. The outer membrane acts as a barrier and gatekeeper, selectively allowing some molecules to pass through while blocking others. The inner membrane is where the electron transport chains are located.

monoglycerides Molecules composed of glycerol combined with one fatty acid.

monosaccharides Any sugars that are not broken down further during digestion and have the general formula CnH_2nOn, where n = 3 to 7. The common monosaccharides glucose, fructose, and galactose all have six carbon atoms (n = 6).

monounsaturated fatty acid (MUFA) A fatty acid in which the carbon chain contains one double bond.

morbid obesity See *extreme obesity.*

morning sickness A persistent or recurring nausea that often occurs in the morning during early pregnancy.

motor proteins Proteins that use energy and convert it into some form of mechanical work. Motor proteins are active in processes such as dividing cells, contracting muscle, and swimming sperm.

mucilages Gelatinous soluble fibers containing galactose, mannose, and other monosaccharides; found in seaweed.

mucosa [myu-KO-sa] The innermost layer of a cavity. The inner layer of the gastrointestinal tract, also called the intestinal wall. It is composed of epithelial cells and glands.

mucus A slippery substance secreted in the GI tract (and other body linings) that protects cells from irritants such as digestive juices.

muscle fibers Individual muscle cells.

mutation A permanent structural alteration in DNA. In most cases, DNA changes either have no effect or cause harm. Occasionally, a mutation can improve an organism's chance of surviving and passing the beneficial change on to its descendants. Certain mutations can lead to cancer or other diseases.

myelin sheath The protective coating that surrounds nerve fibers.

myelinization Development of the myelin sheath, a substance that surrounds nerve fibers.

myoglobin The oxygen-transporting protein of muscle that resembles blood hemoglobin in function.

NADH The reduced form of nicotinamide adenine dinucleotide (NAD^+). This coenzyme, derived from the B vitamin niacin, acts as an electron carrier in cells and undergoes reversible oxidation and reduction.

NADPH The reduced form of nicotinamide adenine dinucleotide phosphate. This coenzyme, which is derived from the B vitamin niacin, acts as an electron carrier in cells, undergoing reversible oxidation and reduction. The oxidized form is $NADP^+$.

National Center for Complementary and Integrative Health (NCCIH) A National Institutes of Health organization established to stimulate, develop, and support objective scientific research on complementary and alternative medicine for the benefit of the public.

National Institutes of Health (NIH) A U.S. Department of Health and Human Services agency composed of 27 separate institutes and centers with a mission to advance knowledge and improve human health.

natural toxins Poisons that are produced by or naturally occur in plants or microorganisms.

negative energy balance Energy intake is lower than energy expenditure, resulting in a depletion of body energy stores and weight loss.

negative nitrogen balance Nitrogen intake is less than the sum of all sources of nitrogen excretion.

negative self-talk Mental or verbal statements made to one's self that reinforce negative or destructive self-perceptions.

neophobia A dislike for anything new or unfamiliar.

neotame An artificial sweetener similar to aspartame, but that is sweeter and does not require a warning label for phenylketonurics.

net protein utilization (NPU) Percentage of ingested protein nitrogen retained by the body. It measures the amount of dietary protein the body uses.

neural tube defect (NTD) A birth defect resulting from failure of the neural tube to develop properly during early fetal development.

neuropeptide Y (NPY) A neurotransmitter widely distributed throughout the brain and peripheral nervous tissue. NPY activity has been linked to eating behavior, depression, anxiety, and cardiovascular function.

neurotransmitters Substances released at the end of a stimulated nerve cell that diffuse across a small gap and bind to another nerve cell or muscle cell, stimulating or inhibiting it.

niacin equivalents (NEs) A measure that includes preformed dietary niacin as well as niacin derived from tryptophan; 60 milligrams of tryptophan yield about 1 milligram of niacin.

nicotinamide adenine dinucleotide (NAD^+) The oxidized form of nicotinamide adenine dinucleotide. This coenzyme, which is derived from the B vitamin niacin, acts as an electron carrier in cells, undergoing reversible oxidation and reduction. The reduced form is NADH. When a phosphate is present, the energy-carrying molecule is NADPH.

night blindness The inability of the eyes to adjust to dim light or to regain vision quickly after exposure to a flash of bright light.

night-eating syndrome (NES) An eating disorder in which a habitual pattern of interrupting sleep to eat is the primary symptom.

nitrogen balance Nitrogen intake minus the sum of all sources of nitrogen excretion.

nitrogen equilibrium Nitrogen intake equals the sum of all sources of nitrogen excretion; nitrogen balance equals zero.

nonessential (dispensable) amino acids Amino acids that the body can make if supplied with adequate nitrogen. Nonessential amino acids do not need to be supplied in the diet.

nonessential fatty acids The fatty acids that your body can make when they are needed. It is not necessary to consume them in the diet.

nonexercise activity thermogenesis (NEAT) The output of energy associated with fidgeting, maintenance of posture, and other minimal physical exertions.

nonheme iron The iron in plants and the iron in animal foods that is not part of hemoglobin or myoglobin.

nonnutritive sweeteners Substances that impart sweetness to foods but supply little or no energy to the body; also called artificial sweeteners or alternative sweeteners. They include acesulfame, aspartame, saccharin, and sucralose.

nucleic acids A family of more than 25,000 molecules found in chromosomes, nucleoli, mitochondria, and the cytoplasm of cells.

nucleotides Subunits of DNA or RNA consisting of a nitrogenous base (adenine, guanine, thymine, or cytosine in DNA; adenine, guanine, uracil, or cytosine in RNA), a phosphate molecule, and a sugar molecule (deoxyribose in DNA and ribose in RNA). Thousands of nucleotides are linked to form a DNA or RNA molecule.

nucleus The primary site of genetic information in the cell, enclosed in a double-layered membrane. The nucleus contains the chromosomes and is the site of messenger RNA (mRNA) and ribosomal RNA (rRNA) synthesis, the "machinery" for protein synthesis in the cytosol.

nutrient content claims These claims describe the level of a nutrient or dietary substance in the product, using terms such as *good source*, *high*, or *free*.

nutrient density A description of the healthfulness of foods. Foods high in nutrient density are those that provide substantial amounts of vitamins and minerals and relatively few calories; foods low in nutrient density are those that supply calories but relatively small amounts of vitamins and minerals (or none at all).

nutrients Any substances in food that the body can use to obtain energy, synthesize tissues, or regulate functions.

nutrigenomics The study of how nutrition interacts with specific genes to influence a person's health.

nutrition The science of foods and their components (nutrients and other substances), including the relationships to health and disease (actions, interactions, and balances); processes within the body (ingestion, digestion, absorption, transport, functions, and disposal of end products); and the social, economic, cultural, and psychological implications of eating.

nutrition assessment Measurement of the nutritional health of the body. It can include anthropometric measurements, biochemical tests, clinical observations, and dietary intake, as well as medical histories and socioeconomic factors.

Nutrition Facts Panel A portion of the food label that states the content of selected nutrients in a food in a standard way prescribed by the Food and Drug Administration. By law, Nutrition Facts must appear on nearly all processed food products in the United States and the new Nutrition Fact Label is intended to make it easier for consumers to make informed decisions about the foods that they are eating. For example, the new Label includes the addition of nutrients which better reflect people's adequate, over- or under-consumption of nutrients and vitamins such as added sugar, Vitamin D and potassium.

nutrition informatics According to the Academy of Nutrition and Dietetics, this is "the effective retrieval, organization, storage and optimum use of information, data and knowledge for food- and nutrition-related problem solving and decision-making. Informatics is supported by the use of information standards, processes and technology."

Nutrition Recommendations for Canadians A set of scientific statements that provide guidance to Canadians for a dietary pattern that will supply recommended amounts of all essential nutrients while reducing the risk of chronic disease.

nutritive sweeteners Substances that impart sweetness to foods and that can be absorbed and yield energy in the body. Simple sugars, sugar alcohols, and high-fructose corn syrup are the most common nutritive sweeteners used in food products.

obesity BMI at or above 30 kg/m^2.

obesogenic environment Circumstances in which a person lives, works, and plays that promote the overconsumption of calories and discourage physical activity and calorie expenditure.

obsessive-compulsive disorder A disorder in which a person attempts to relieve anxiety by ritualistic behavior and continuous repetition of certain acts.

Older Americans Act Nutrition Program A federally funded program (formerly known as the Elderly Nutrition Program) that provides older persons with nutritionally sound meals through home-delivered nutrition services, congregate nutrition services, and the nutrition services' incentive.

oligopeptide Four to 10 amino acids joined by peptide bonds.

oligosaccharides Short carbohydrate chains composed of 3 to 10 sugar molecules.

omega-3 fatty acids Any polyunsaturated fatty acid in which the first double bond starting from the methyl (—CH_3) end of the molecule lies between the third and fourth carbon atoms.

omega-6 fatty acid Any polyunsaturated fatty acid in which the first double bond starting from the methyl (—CH_3) end of the molecule lies between the sixth and seventh carbon atoms.

omega-9 fatty acid Any polyunsaturated fatty acid in which the first double bond starting from the methyl (—CH_3) end of the molecule lies between the ninth and tenth carbon atoms.

opsin A protein that combines with retinal to form rhodopsin in rod cells.

orexin A class of hormones in the brain that may affect human food consumption.

organelles Various membrane-bound structures that form part of the cytoplasm. Organelles, including mitochondria and lysosomes, perform specialized metabolic functions.

organic In chemistry, any compound that contains carbon, except carbon oxides (e.g., carbon dioxide) and sulfides and metal carbonates (e.g., potassium carbonate). The term *organic* also is used to denote crops that are grown without synthetic fertilizers or chemicals.

organic foods Foods that originate from farms or handling operations that meet the standards set by the USDA National Organic Program.

organogenesis The period when organ systems are developing in a growing fetus.

orthomolecular medicine The preventive or therapeutic use of high-dose vitamins to treat disease.

osmolarity The concentration of dissolved particles (e.g., electrolytes) in a solution expressed per unit of volume.

osmoreceptors Neurons in the hypothalamus that detect changes in the fluid concentration in blood and regulate the release of antidiuretic hormone.

osmosis The movement of a solvent, such as water, through a semipermeable membrane from the low-solute to the high-solute solution until the concentrations on both sides of the membrane are equal.

osmotic pressure The pressure exerted on a semipermeable membrane by a solvent, usually water, moving from the side of low-solute to the side of high-solute concentration.

osteoblasts Bone cells that promote bone deposition and growth.

osteoclasts Bone cells that promote bone resorption and calcium mobilization.

osteomalacia A disease in adults that results from vitamin D deficiency; it is marked by softening of the bones, leading to bending of the spine, bowing of the legs, and increased risk for fractures.

osteoporosis A bone disease characterized by a decrease in bone mineral density and the appearance of small holes in bones resulting from loss of minerals.

overnutrition The long-term consumption of an excess of nutrients. The most common type of overnutrition in the United States results from the regular consumption of excess calories, fats, saturated fats, and cholesterol.

overweight BMI at or above 25 kg/m^2 and less than 30 kg/m^2.

oxalate (oxalic acid) An organic acid in some leafy green vegetables, such as spinach, that binds to calcium to form calcium oxalate, an insoluble compound the body cannot absorb.

oxaloacetate A four-carbon intermediate compound in the citric acid cycle. Acetyl CoA combines with free oxaloacetate in the mitochondria, forming citrate and beginning the cycle.

oxidation Oxygen attaches to the double bonds of unsaturated fatty acids. Rancid fats are oxidized fats.

oxidative phosphorylation Formation of ATP from ADP and P_i coupled to the flow of electrons along the electron transport chain.

oxygen energy system A complex energy system that requires oxygen. To release ATP, it completes the breakdown of carbohydrate and fatty acids through the citric acid cycle and electron transport chain.

oxytocin A pituitary hormone that stimulates the release of milk from the breast.

palatable Pleasant tasting.

pancreas An organ that secretes enzymes that affect the digestion and absorption of nutrients and that releases hormones, such as insulin, that regulate metabolism as well as the disposition of the end products of food in the body.

pancreatic amylase Starch-digesting enzyme secreted by the pancreas.

parathyroid hormone A hormone secreted by the parathyroid glands in response to low blood calcium. It stimulates calcium release from bone and calcium absorption by the intestines, while decreasing calcium excretion by the kidneys. It acts in conjunction with $1,25(OH)_2D_3$ to raise blood calcium. Also called parathormone.

passive diffusion The movement of substances into or out of cells without the expenditure of energy or the involvement of transport proteins in the cell membrane. Also called simple diffusion.

pasteurization A process for destroying pathogenic bacteria by heating liquid foods to a prescribed temperature for a specified time.

pathogenic Capable of causing disease.

pectins A type of dietary fiber found in fruits.

peer review An appraisal of research against accepted standards by professionals in the field.

pentoses Sugar molecules containing five carbon atoms.

pepsin A protein-digesting enzyme produced by the stomach.

pepsinogen The inactive form of the enzyme pepsin.

peptidases Enzymes that act on small peptide units by breaking peptide bonds.

peptide bond The bond between two amino acids formed when a carboxyl (—COOH) group of one amino acid joins an amino (—NH_2) group of another amino acid, releasing water in the process.

perceived exertion The subjective experience of how difficult an effort is.

peristalsis [per-ih-STAHL-sis] The wavelike, rhythmic muscular contractions of the GI tract that propel its contents down the tract.

pernicious anemia A form of anemia that results from an autoimmune disorder that damages cells lining the stomach and inhibits vitamin B_{12} absorption, leading to vitamin B_{12} deficiency.

pesticides Chemicals used to control insects, diseases, weeds, fungi, and other pests on plants, vegetables, fruits, and animals.

pH A measurement of the hydrogen ion concentration, or acidity, of a solution. It is equal to the negative logarithm of the hydrogen ion (H^+) concentration expressed in moles per liter.

phagocytosis The process by which cells engulf large particles and small microorganisms. Receptors on the surface of cells bind these particles and organisms to bring them into large vesicles in the cytoplasm. From *phago*, "eating," and *cyto*, "cell."

phenylketonuria (PKU) An inherited disorder caused by a lack or deficiency of the enzyme that converts phenylalanine to tyrosine.

phosphate group A chemical group ($—PO_4$) on a larger molecule, where the phosphorus is single-bonded to each of the four oxygens and the other bond of one of the oxygens is attached to the rest of the molecule. Often hydrogen atoms are attached to the oxygens. Sometimes there are double bonds between the phosphorus and an oxygen.

phosphocreatine See *creatine phosphate.*

phospholipids Compounds that consist of a glycerol molecule bonded to two fatty acid molecules and to a phosphate group with a nitrogen-containing component. Phospholipids have both hydrophilic and hydrophobic regions that make them good emulsifiers.

phosphorylation The addition of phosphate to an organic (carbon-containing) compound. Oxidative phosphorylation is the formation of high-energy phosphate bonds ($ADP + P_i = ATP$) from the energy released by oxidation of energy-yielding nutrients.

photosynthesis The process by which green plants use radiant energy from the sun to produce carbohydrates (hexoses) from carbon dioxide and water.

phylloquinone The form of vitamin K that comes from plant sources. Also known as vitamin K_1.

phytate (phytic acid) A phosphorus-containing compound in the outer husks of cereal grains that binds with minerals and inhibits their absorption.

phytochemicals Substances in plants that may possess health-protective effects, even though they are not essential for life.

phytoestrogens Compounds that have weak estrogen activity in the body.

phytosterols Sterols found in plants. Phytosterols are poorly absorbed by humans and reduce intestinal absorption of cholesterol. They have been used as a cholesterol-lowering food ingredient.

pinocytosis The process by which cells internalize fluids and macromolecules. To do so, the cell membrane invaginates and forms a pocket around the substance. From *pino*, "drinking," and *cyto*, "cell."

placebo An inactive substance that is outwardly indistinguishable from the active substance whose effects are being studied.

placebo effect A physical or emotional change that is not caused by properties of an administered substance. The change reflects participants' expectations.

placenta The organ formed during pregnancy that produces hormones for the maintenance of pregnancy and across which oxygen and nutrients are transferred from mother to infant; it also allows waste materials to be transferred from infant to mother.

plaque A buildup of substances that circulate in the blood (e.g., calcium, fat, cholesterol, cellular waste, fibrin) on a blood vessel wall, making it vulnerable to blockage from blood clots.

plasma The fluid portion of the blood that contains blood cells and other components.

platelets Tiny disk-shaped components of blood that are essential for blood clotting.

poisonous mushrooms Mushrooms that contain toxins that can cause stomach upset, dizziness, hallucinations, and other neurological symptoms.

pollutants Gaseous, chemical, or organic waste that contaminates air, soil, or water.

polyols See *sugar alcohols.*

polypeptide More than 10 amino acids joined by peptide bonds.

polyphenols Organic compounds that include an unsaturated ring containing more than one OH group as part of their chemical structures; they produce bitterness in coffee and tea.

polysaccharides Long carbohydrate chains composed of more than 10 sugar molecules. Polysaccharides can be straight or branched.

polyunsaturated fatty acid (PUFA) A fatty acid in which the carbon chain contains two or more double bonds.

positive energy balance Energy intake exceeds energy expenditure, resulting in an increase in body energy stores and weight gain.

positive nitrogen balance Nitrogen intake exceeds the sum of all sources of nitrogen excretion.

positive self-talk Constructive mental or verbal statements made to one's self to change a belief or behavior.

post-traumatic stress disorder (PTSD) An anxiety disorder characterized by an emotional response to a traumatic event or situation involving severe external stress.

prebiotics Group of compounds that promote growth and activity of bacteria that impart benefits on the host organism.

precursor A substance that is converted into another active substance. Enzyme precursors also are called *proenzymes*.

pre-diabetes Blood glucose levels higher than normal but not high enough to warrant a diagnosis of diabetes.

preeclampsia A condition of late pregnancy characterized by hypertension, edema, and proteinuria.

preformed vitamin A Retinyl esters, the main storage form of vitamin A. About 90 percent of dietary retinol is in the form of esters, mostly found in foods from animal sources.

pregorexia A term used to describe pregnant women who reduce calories and exercise in excess in an effort to control pregnancy weight gain.

prematurity Birth before 37 weeks of gestation.

preservatives Chemicals or other agents that slow the decomposition of a food.

preterm delivery A delivery that occurs before the thirty-seventh week of gestation.

prions Short for *proteinaceous infectious particle*. Self-reproducing protein particles that can cause disease.

proenzymes Inactive precursors of enzymes.

prolactin A pituitary hormone that stimulates the production of milk in breast tissue.

proteases [PRO-tea-ace-ez] Enzymes that break down protein into peptides and amino acids.

protein digestibility corrected amino acid score (PDCAAS) A measure of protein quality that takes into account the amino acid composition of the food and the digestibility of the protein. It is calculated by multiplying the amino acid score by the percentage of the digestible food protein.

protein efficiency ratio (PER) Protein quality calculated by comparing the weight gain of growing animals fed a test protein with growing animals fed a high-quality reference protein. It depends on both the digestibility and the amino acid composition of a protein.

protein-energy malnutrition (PEM) A condition resulting from long-term inadequate intakes of energy and protein that can lead to wasting of body tissues and increased susceptibility to infection.

protein hydrolysates Proteins that have been treated with acid or enzymes to break them down into amino acids and polypeptides.

protein turnover The constant synthesis and breakdown of proteins in the body.

proteins Large, complex compounds consisting of many amino acids connected in varying sequences and forming unique shapes.

protoporphyrin A chemical complex that combines with iron to form heme.

provitamin A Carotenoid precursors of vitamin A in foods of plant origin, primarily deeply colored fruits and vegetables.

provitamins Inactive forms of vitamins that the body can convert into active usable forms. Also referred to as *vitamin precursors.*

psyllium The dried husk of the psyllium seed.

puberty The period of life during which the secondary sex characteristics develop and the ability to reproduce is attained.

purges Episodes of emptying the gastrointestinal (GI) tract by self-induced vomiting and/or misuse of laxatives, diuretics, or enemas.

pyloric sphincter [pie-LORE-ic SFINGK-ter] A circular muscle that forms the opening between the stomach and the duodenum. It regulates the passage of food into the small intestine.

pyrophosphate (P_i) Inorganic phosphate. This high-energy phosphate group is an important component of ATP, ADP, and AMP.

pyruvate The three-carbon compound that results from glycolytic breakdown of glucose. Pyruvate, the salt form of pyruvic acid, also can be derived from glycerol and some amino acids.

reactive hypoglycemia A type of hypoglycemia that occurs about one hour after eating carbohydrate-rich food.

Recommended Dietary Allowances (RDAs) The nutrient intake levels that meet the nutrient needs of almost all (97 to 98 percent) individuals in a life-stage and gender group.

Recommended Nutrient Intakes (RNIs) Canadian dietary standards that have been replaced by Dietary Reference Intakes.

rectum The muscular final segment of the intestine, extending from the sigmoid colon to the anus.

reducing agent A compound that donates electrons or hydrogen atoms to another compound.

refined sweeteners Composed of monosaccharides and disaccharides that have been extracted and processed from other foods.

renin An enzyme, produced by the kidney, that affects blood pressure by catalyzing the conversion of angiotensinogen to angiotensin I.

requirement The lowest continuing intake level of a nutrient that prevents deficiency in an individual.

resistant starch A starch that is not digested.

resting energy expenditure (REE) The minimum energy needed to maintain basic physiological functions (e.g., heartbeat, muscle function, respiration). The resting metabolic rate (RMR) extrapolated to 24 hours. Often used interchangeably with BEE.

resting metabolic rate (RMR) A clinical measure of resting energy expenditure performed three to four hours after eating or performing significant physical activity. Often used interchangeably with BMR.

restrained eaters Individuals who routinely avoid food as long as possible, and then gorge on food.

retina A paper-thin tissue that lines the back of the eye and contains cells called rods and cones.

retinal The aldehyde form of vitamin A. One of the retinoids, it is the active form of vitamin A in the photoreceptors of the retina. It is interconvertible with retinol.

retinoic acid The acid form of vitamin A. One of the retinoids, it is formed from retinal but not interconvertible. It helps growth, cell differentiation, and the immune system, but does not have a role in vision or reproduction.

retinoids Compounds in foods that have chemical structures similar to vitamin A. Retinoids include the active forms of vitamin A (retinol, retinal, and retinoic acid) and the main storage forms of retinol (retinyl esters).

retinol The alcohol form of vitamin A. It is one of the retinoids, and thought to be the main physiologically active form of vitamin A. It is interconvertible with retinal.

retinol activity equivalents (RAEs) A unit of measurement of the vitamin A content of a food. One RAE equals 1 microgram (µg) of retinol.

retinol-binding protein (RBP) A carrier protein that binds to retinol and transports it in the bloodstream from the liver to destination cells.

retinyl esters The main storage form of vitamin A. It is one of the retinoids. Retinyl esters are retinol combined with fatty acids, usually palmitic acid. Also known as preformed vitamin A.

rhodopsin Found in rod cells, a light-sensitive pigment molecule that consists of a protein called opsin combined with retinal.

ribosomal RNA (rRNA) A type of ribonucleic acid that is a major component of ribosomes. It provides a structural framework for protein synthesis and orchestrates the process.

ribosomes Cell components composed of protein located in the cytoplasm that translate messenger RNA into protein sequences.

rickets A bone disease in children that results from vitamin D deficiency.

risk factors Anything that increases a person's chance of developing a disease, including substances, agents, genetic alterations, traits, habits, or conditions.

rods Light-sensitive cells in the retina that react to dim light and transmit black-and-white images.

R-protein A protein produced by the salivary glands that might protect vitamin B_{12} as it travels through the stomach and into the small intestine.

saccharin [SAK-ah-ren] An artificial sweetener that tastes about 300 to 700 times sweeter than sucrose.

salivary glands Glands in the mouth that release saliva.

Salmonella Rod-shaped bacteria responsible for many foodborne illnesses.

salts Compounds that result from the replacement of the hydrogen of an acid with a metal or a group that acts like a metal.

satiation Feeling of satisfaction and fullness that terminates a meal.

satiety The effects of a food or meal that delay subsequent intake. A feeling of satisfaction and fullness following eating that quells the desire for food.

saturated fatty acid A fatty acid completely filled by hydrogen with all carbons in the chain linked by single bonds.

seborrheic dermatitis Disease of the oil-producing glands of the skin; a symptom of riboflavin deficiency.

secondary hypertension Hypertension caused by an underlying condition such as a kidney disorder. Once the underlying condition is treated, the blood pressure usually returns to normal.

secretin [see-CREET-in] An intestinal hormone released during digestion that stimulates the pancreas to release water and bicarbonate.

segmentation Periodic muscle contractions at intervals along the GI tract that alternate forward and backward movement of the contents, thereby breaking apart chunks of the food mass and mixing in digestive juices.

selenocysteine A selenium-containing amino acid that is the biologically active form of selenium.

selenomethionine A selenium-containing amino acid derived from methionine that is the storage form of selenium.

semipermeable membrane Membrane that allows passage of some substances but blocks others.

serosa A smooth membrane composed of a mesothelial layer and connective tissue. The intestines are covered in serosa.

silicosis A disease that results from excess silicon exposure.

simple carbohydrates Sugars composed of a single sugar molecule (a monosaccharide) or two joined sugar molecules (a disaccharide).

skeletal muscles Muscles composed of bundles of parallel, striated muscle fibers under voluntary control. Also called voluntary muscle or striated muscle.

skinfold measurements A method to estimate body fat by measuring with calipers the thickness of a fold of skin and subcutaneous fat.

sleep apnea Periods of absence of breathing during sleep.

slow-twitch (ST) fibers Muscle fibers that develop tension more slowly and to a lesser extent than fast-twitch muscle fibers. ST fibers have high oxidative capacities and are slower to fatigue than fast-twitch fibers.

small intestine The tube (approximately 10 feet long) where the digestion of protein, fat, and carbohydrate is completed, and where the majority of nutrients are absorbed. The small intestine is divided into three parts: the duodenum, the jejunum, and the ileum.

soda loading Consumption of bicarbonate (baking soda) to raise blood pH. The intent is to increase the capacity to buffer acids, thus delaying fatigue. Also known as bicarbonate loading.

sodium—potassium pumps Mechanisms that pump sodium ions out of a cell, allowing potassium ions to enter the cell.

solanine A potentially toxic alkaloid that is present with chlorophyll in the green areas on potato skins.

soluble fiber Nondigestible carbohydrates that dissolve in water.

solutes Substances that are dissolved in a solvent.

Special Supplemental Nutrition Program for Women, Infants, and Children (WIC) A USDA program that provides federal grants to states for supplemental foods, health care referrals, and nutrition education for low-income pregnant, breastfeeding, and nonbreastfeeding postpartum women, and to infants and children at nutritional risk.

sphincters [SFINGK-ters] Circular bands of muscle fibers that surround the entrance or exit of a hollow body structure (e.g., the stomach) and act as valves to control the flow of material.

sphygmomanometer [sfig-mo-ma-NOM-eh-ter] An instrument for measuring blood pressure and especially arterial blood pressure.

spina bifida A type of neural tube birth defect.

sports anemia A lowered concentration of hemoglobin in the blood resulting from dilution. The increased plasma volume that dilutes the hemoglobin is a normal consequence of aerobic training.

squalene A cholesterol precursor found in whale liver and plants.

standard drink One serving of alcohol (about 15 grams), defined as 12 ounces of beer, 4 to 5 ounces of wine, or 1.5 ounces of liquor.

starch The major storage form of carbohydrate in plants; starch is composed of long chains of glucose molecules in a straight (amylose) or branching (amylopectin) arrangement.

statement of identity A mandate that commercial food products prominently display the common or usual name of the product or identify the food with an "appropriately descriptive term."

stem cells A formative cell whose daughter cells can differentiate into other cell types.

sterols A category of lipids that includes cholesterol. Sterols are hydrocarbons with several rings in their structures.

stevioside A dietary supplement, not approved for use as a sweetener, that is extracted and refined from *Stevia rebaudiana* leaves.

stomach The enlarged, muscular, saclike portion of the digestive tract between the esophagus and the small intestine, with a capacity of about 1 quart.

structure/function claims These statements may claim a benefit related to a nutrient-deficiency disease (e.g., *vitamin C prevents scurvy*) or describe the role of a nutrient or dietary ingredient intended to affect a structure or function in humans (e.g., *calcium helps build strong bones*).

subcutaneous fat Fat stores under the skin.

submucosa The layer of loose, fibrous connective tissue under the mucous membrane.

sucralose An artificial sweetener made from sucrose; it was approved for use in the United States in 1998 and has been used in Canada since 1992. Sucralose is nonnutritive and about 600 times sweeter than sugar.

sucrose [SOO-crose] A disaccharide composed of one molecule of glucose and one molecule of fructose joined together. Also known as table sugar.

sugar alcohols Compounds formed from monosaccharides by replacing a hydrogen atom with a hydroxyl group (—OH); commonly used as nutritive sweeteners. Also called polyols.

Supplement Facts panel Content label that must appear on all dietary supplements.

Supplemental Nutrition Assistance Program (SNAP) A USDA program that helps single people and families with little or no income to buy food. Formerly known as the Food Stamp Program.

systolic Pertaining to a heart contraction. Systolic blood pressure is measured during a heart contraction, a time period known as systole.

taste threshold The minimum amount of flavor that must be present for a taste to be detected.

teratogen Any substance that causes birth defects.

thermic effect of food (TEF) The energy used to digest, absorb, and metabolize energy-yielding foodstuffs. It constitutes about 10 percent of total energy expenditure but is influenced by various factors.

thiamin pyrophosphate (TPP) A coenzyme of which the vitamin thiamin is a part. It plays a key role in decarboxylation and helps drive the reaction that forms acetyl CoA from pyruvate during metabolism.

thyroglobulin The storage form of thyroid hormone in the thyroid gland.

thyroid-stimulating hormone (TSH) Secreted from the pituitary gland at the base of the brain, a hormone that regulates synthesis of thyroid hormones.

thyroxine (T4) An iodine-containing hormone secreted by the thyroid gland to regulate the rate of cell metabolism; known chemically as tetraiodothyronine.

tissue A group or layer of cells that are alike and that work together to perform a specific function.

tocopherol The chemical name for vitamin E. There are four tocopherols (alpha, beta, gamma, and delta), but only alpha-tocopherol is active in the body.

tocotrienols Four compounds (alpha, beta, gamma, and delta) chemically related to tocopherols. The tocotrienols and tocopherols are collectively known as vitamin E.

toddler A child between 12 and 36 months of age.

Tolerable Upper Intake Levels (ULs) The maximum levels of daily nutrient intakes that are unlikely to pose health risks to almost all of the individuals in the group for whom they are designed.

total body water All of the water in the body, including intracellular and extracellular water, and water in the urinary and GI tracts.

total energy expenditure (TEE) The total of the resting energy expenditure (REE), energy used in physical activity, and energy used in processing food (TEF); usually expressed in kilocalories per day.

total fiber The sum of dietary fiber and functional fiber.

total parenteral nutrition (TPN) Feeding a person by giving all essential nutrients intravenously.

trace minerals Minerals present in the body and required in the diet in relatively small amounts compared with major minerals; also known as *microminerals*.

trans fatty acids Unsaturated fatty acids in which the hydrogens surrounding a double bond are on opposite sides of the carbon chain. This straightens the chain, and the fatty acid becomes more solid.

transamination [TRANS-am-ih-NAY-shun] The transfer of an amino group from an amino acid to a carbon skeleton to form a different amino acid.

transfer RNA (tRNA) A type of ribonucleic acid that is composed of a complementary RNA sequence and an amino acid specific to that sequence. It inserts the appropriate amino acid when the messenger RNA sequence and the ribosome call for it.

transferrin A protein synthesized in the liver that transports iron in the blood to the erythroblasts for use in heme synthesis.

transferrin receptors Specialized receptors on the cell membrane that bind transferrin.

transferrin saturation The extent to which transferrin has vacant iron-binding sites (e.g., low transferrin saturation indicates a high proportion of vacant iron-binding sites).

trehalose A disaccharide of two glucose molecules, but with a linkage different from maltose. Used as a food additive and sweetener.

tricarboxylic acid (TCA) cycle See *citric acid cycle.*

triglycerides The major form of lipids in food and in the body. They are composed of three fatty acids attached to a glyceride backbone. Triglycerides are the body's main storage form of energy and source of fuel for the body cells, with the exception of nervous system and red blood cells, which prefer glucose.

triiodothyronine (T3) An iodine-containing thyroid hormone with several times the biologic activity of thyroxine (T4).

trimesters Three equal time periods of pregnancy, each lasting approximately 13 to 14 weeks, that do not coincide with specific stages in fetal development.

tripeptide Three amino acids joined by peptide bonds.

trypsinogen/trypsin A protease produced by the pancreas that is converted from the inactive proenzyme form (trypsinogen) to the active form (trypsin) in the small intestine.

tryptophan An amino acid that serves as a niacin precursor in the body. In the body, 60 milligrams of tryptophan yield about 1 milligram of niacin, or 1 niacin equivalent (NE).

tumor An abnormal mass of tissue that results from excessive cell division. Tumors perform no useful body function. They can be benign (not cancerous) or malignant (cancerous).

type 1 diabetes Diabetes that occurs when the body's immune system attacks beta cells in the pancreas, causing them to lose their ability to make insulin.

type 2 diabetes Diabetes that occurs when target cells (e.g., fat and muscle cells) lose the ability to respond normally to insulin.

ulcer A craterlike lesion that occurs in the lining of the stomach or duodenum; also called a peptic ulcer to distinguish it from a skin ulcer.

umami [ooh-MA-mee] A Japanese term that describes a delicious meaty or savory sensation. Chemically, this taste detects the presence of glutamate.

undernutrition Poor health resulting from depletion of nutrients caused by inadequate nutrient intake over time. It is now most often associated with poverty, alcoholism, and some types of eating disorders.

underwater weighing Determining body density by measuring the volume of water displaced when the body is fully submerged in a specialized water tank. Also called hydrostatic weighing.

underweight BMI less than 18.5 kg/m^2.

unsaturated fatty acid A fatty acid in which the carbon chain contains one or more double bonds.

urea The main nitrogen-containing waste product in mammals. Formed in liver cells from ammonia and carbon dioxide, urea is carried by the bloodstream to the kidneys, where it is excreted in the urine.

urinary tract infection (UTI) An infection of one or more of the structures in the urinary tract; usually caused by bacteria.

U.S. Department of Agriculture (USDA) The government agency that monitors the production of eggs, poultry, and meat for adherence to standards of quality and wholesomeness. The USDA also provides public nutrition education, performs nutrition research, and administers the WIC program.

U.S. Department of Health and Human Services (DHHS) The principal federal agency responsible for protecting the health of all Americans and providing essential human services. The agency is especially concerned with those Americans who are least able to help themselves.

U.S. Pharmacopeia (USP) Established in 1820, the USP is a nonprofit health care organization that sets quality standards for a range of health care products.

vascular system A network of veins and arteries through which the blood carries nutrients. Also called the circulatory system.

vasoconstrictor A substance that causes blood vessels to constrict.

vasopressin See *antidiuretic hormone.*

very-low-calorie diets (VLCDs) Diets supplying 400 to 800 kilocalories per day, which include adequate high-quality protein, little or no fat, and little carbohydrate.

very-low-density lipoproteins (VLDLs) The triglyceride-rich lipoproteins formed in the liver. VLDL enters the bloodstream and is gradually acted upon by lipoprotein lipase, releasing triglyceride to body cells.

villi Small, finger-like projections that blanket the folds in the lining of the small intestine. Singular is villus.

visceral fat Fat stores that cushion body organs.

vitamin precursors See *provitamins.*

vitamins Organic compounds necessary for reproduction, growth, and maintenance of the body. Vitamins are required in miniscule amounts.

waist circumference The waist measurement, as a marker of abdominal fat content; can be used to indicate health risks.

wasting The breakdown of body tissue such as muscle and organs for use as a protein source when the diet lacks protein.

weighed food records Detailed food records obtained by weighing foods before eating and then weighing leftovers to determine the exact amount consumed.

weight cycling Repeated periods of gaining and losing weight. Also called *yo-yo dieting*.

weight management The adoption of healthful and sustainable eating and exercise behaviors that reduce disease risk and improve well-being.

Wilson disease Genetic disorder of increased copper absorption, which leads to toxic levels in the liver and heart.

wood alcohol Common name for methanol.

World Health Organization (WHO) A global organization that directs and coordinates international health work. Its goal is the attainment by all peoples of the highest possible level of health, defined as a state of complete physical, mental, and social well-being and not merely the absence of disease or infirmity.

xerophthalmia A condition caused by vitamin A deficiency that dries the cornea and mucous membranes of the eye.

zoochemicals The animal equivalent of phytochemicals in plants that are believed to provide health benefits beyond the traditional nutrients that foods contain.

Index

Note: Page numbers followed by *f* or *t* indicate materials in figures or tables respectively.

B

E

F

N

O

P

T

W